Atlas of
Small Parts Ultrasound
with Color Flow Imaging

Atlas of Small Parts Ultrasound with Color Flow Imaging

Fourth Edition

PK Srivastava
MBBS MD (Radiol) FICR FICMU
Professor
Department of Radiodiagnosis
King George's Medical University
Director
Yashdeep Ultrasound Centres
Lucknow, Uttar Pradesh, India
yashdeep.pks@gmail.com, pks_yash@yahoo.co.in

Foreword

Ravi Kant

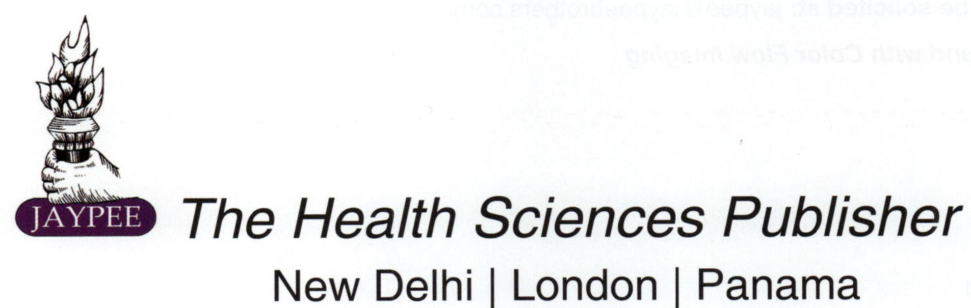

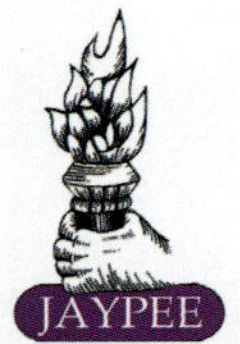

Jaypee Brothers Medical Publishers (P) Ltd

Headquarters
Jaypee Brothers Medical Publishers (P) Ltd
4838/24, Ansari Road, Daryaganj
New Delhi 110 002, India
Phone: +91-11-43574357
Fax: +91-11-43574314
Email: jaypee@jaypeebrothers.com

Overseas Offices

J.P. Medical Ltd
83 Victoria Street, London
SW1H 0HW (UK)
Phone: +44 20 3170 8910
Fax: +44 (0)20 3008 6180
Email: info@jpmedpub.com

Jaypee-Highlights Medical Publishers Inc
City of Knowledge, Bld. 235, 2nd Floor, Clayton
Panama City, Panama
Phone: +1 507-301-0496
Fax: +1 507-301-0499
Email: cservice@jphmedical.com

Jaypee Brothers Medical Publishers (P) Ltd
17/1-B Babar Road, Block-B, Shaymali
Mohammadpur, Dhaka-1207
Bangladesh
Mobile: +08801912003485
Email: jaypeedhaka@gmail.com

Jaypee Brothers Medical Publishers (P) Ltd
Bhotahity, Kathmandu
Nepal
Phone: +977-9741283608
Email: kathmandu@jaypeebrothers.com

Website: www.jaypeebrothers.com
Website: www.jaypeedigital.com

© 2017, Jaypee Brothers Medical Publishers

The views and opinions expressed in this book are solely those of the original contributor(s)/author(s) and do not necessarily represent those of editor(s) of the book.

All rights reserved. No part of this publication may be reproduced, stored or transmitted in any form or by any means, electronic, mechanical, photocopying, recording or otherwise, without the prior permission in writing of the publishers.

All brand names and product names used in this book are trade names, service marks, trademarks or registered trademarks of their respective owners. The publisher is not associated with any product or vendor mentioned in this book.

Medical knowledge and practice change constantly. This book is designed to provide accurate, authoritative information about the subject matter in question. However, readers are advised to check the most current information available on procedures included and check information from the manufacturer of each product to be administered, to verify the recommended dose, formula, method and duration of administration, adverse effects and contraindications. It is the responsibility of the practitioner to take all appropriate safety precautions. Neither the publisher nor the author(s)/editor(s) assume any liability for any injury and/or damage to persons or property arising from or related to use of material in this book.

This book is sold on the understanding that the publisher is not engaged in providing professional medical services. If such advice or services are required, the services of a competent medical professional should be sought.

Every effort has been made where necessary to contact holders of copyright to obtain permission to reproduce copyright material. If any have been inadvertently overlooked, the publisher will be pleased to make the necessary arrangements at the first opportunity.

Inquiries for bulk sales may be solicited at: jaypee@jaypeebrothers.com

Atlas of Small Parts Ultrasound with Color Flow Imaging

First Edition: 1997

Second Edition: 2002

Third Edition: 2006

Fourth Edition: **2017**

ISBN 978-93-86261-99-1

Printed at Replika Press Pvt. Ltd.

Dedicated to

All my patients who were generous enough to give permission to include the images of their pathologies in the book

Foreword

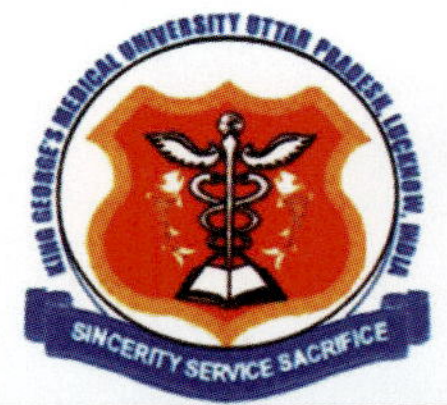

King George's Medical University
Uttar Pradesh, Lucknow – 226003, India

Prof. Ravi Kant,
FRCS (Engl) FRCS (Edin) FRCS (Glasg) FRCS (Irel)
FAMS MS DNB FACS FICS FAIS
Vice-Chancellor

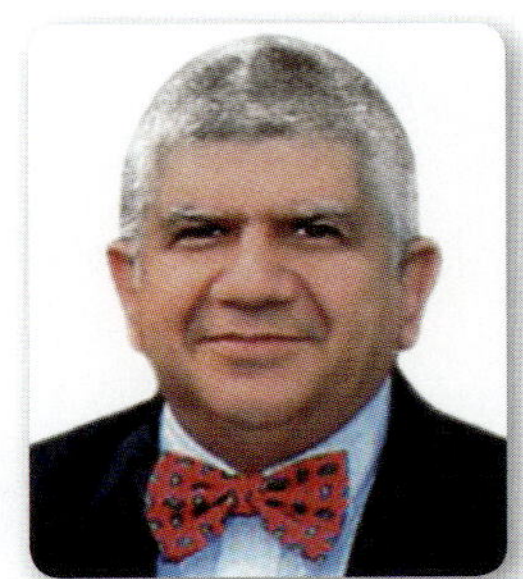

It is my pleasure to write Foreword to Dr PK Srivastava's book *Atlas of Small Parts Ultrasound with Color Flow Imaging*. In the present scenario of explosive advancement in the field of imaging with increasing pressure to contain the cost of investigation, high-resolution ultrasound with 3D imaging is an excellent modality for evaluation of small parts. Since it is a radiation-free modality, it very well suits the motto of keeping the radiation "As Low as Reasonably Achievable" (ALARA).

High-resolution ultrasound opens an entire new field for investigation of various body parts. In the last decade, there was tremendous advancement in the field of imaging as CT scan and MRI. However, these have developed as expensive procedures with fixed locations. Whereas high-resolution ultrasound provides cost effective, noninvasive imaging of tissue which can be performed in critical care areas and also at bedside critically ill patients, it is highly useful in the field of small parts imaging like infant brain, eye and orbit, breast, thyroid and neck, peripheral chest, pediatric abdomen and GIT. It is the first-line investigation in scrotal pathologies and also anterior abdominal wall. Dr PK Srivastava is one of the pioneers in the field of small parts ultrasound and brought the concept of 3D ultrasound in radiology. His vast experience of more than 30 years in the field of ultrasound has gone a long way in shaping this Atlas. The book is valuable in depicting multiple small parts pathologies in a pictorial essay. The 3D application of ultrasound increases diagnostic value of the Atlas.

I compliment Dr PK Srivastava for an excellent job and a fine accomplishment.

Ravi Kant

(Professor Ravi Kant)

Preface to the Fourth Edition

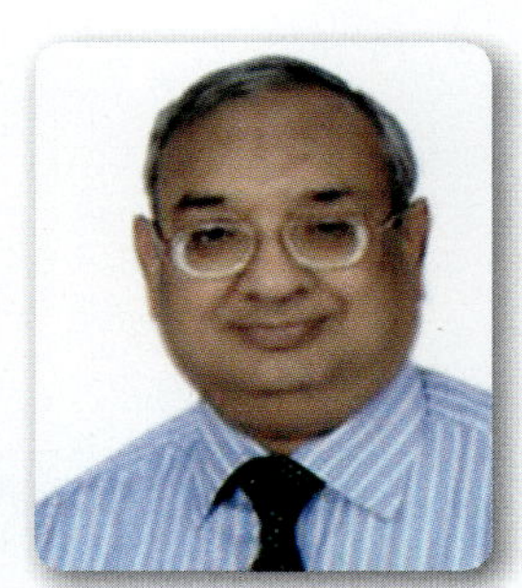

Since the publication of 2nd and 3rd editions of the book *Atlas of Small Parts Ultrasound with Color Flow Imaging*, which was a big success, tremendous advancement has taken place in diagnostic ultrasound in the form of high frequency broadband transducers. The tissue resolution has become improved tremendously and it is better than MRI and CT scan in many small parts imaging. With the application of 3D ultrasound in radiology, better assessment with global view of the large pathology is easily made. The fourth edition of the book has new chapters on face, sperm transport system, ambiguous genitalia and intersex. The book has been totally rewritten and more than 70% images are replaced with new images with 3D multiplanar tomographic ultrasound imaging. The 3D and TUI images provide excellent tissue details. The size of the Atlas has been completely changed. The Atlas has become a comprehensive book having more than 4,500 images which are self-explanatory and covering most common and also uncommon pathologies of small parts. I have tried to incorporate clinical images at most of the places with CT and MRI for better understanding of the subject. My main objective is to provide most illustrative and comprehensive Atlas on small parts ultrasound. I wish and hope this Atlas will serve the purpose of ready-reference book for all doctors in various specialties practising ultrasound.

PK Srivastava

Preface to the First Edition

The development of ultrasonographic imaging has been one of the most important breakthroughs in the field of diagnostic imaging in the last two decades. The ultrasonographic imaging has crossed its infancy and attained adulthood after improvement in technology and invention of high-resolution transducers. The application of high-resolution sonography in small parts imaging has opened a new horizon in the diagnosis, treatment and management of small parts pathology. It was a long-felt need to have a book on small parts imaging. This book has been written to give a detailed account of ultrasonographic applications in small parts, and the main focus of the book is on the commonly encountered problems involving small parts. This book is intended for practising sonologists, physicians and medical students. The book contains ten chapters covering almost all the small parts of body which are superficially placed and need high-resolution sonography for their imaging.

The authors who have contributed chapters in the book are recognized experts in their fields. They have provided most up-to-date information available in the literature to make this book comprehensive.

I hope this book will become a reference work for all who use ultrasonographic imaging in their clinical practice and further gain expertise in small parts imaging.

PK Srivastava

Acknowledgments

I am extremely thankful to Professor Mukund Joshi MD FICRI FAMS Chairman, National Academy of Medical Sciences for his encouragement and valuable guidance in completing the book. He is generous enough to contribute a chapter in the book.

I express my sincere thanks to my clinic staff without their help this would not have been possible.

I extend my sincere thanks to Mr Vivek Tripathi, Mr Sunil Kumar Gupta, and Mr Prem Chand Joshi, who have done an excellent job in typing the manuscript and formatting the Atlas and made the work simple and easy. I am also thankful to Mr Rizwan Ahmad and Mr Ashutosh Mishra, the staff members of Yashdeep Ultrasound Centres for their contribution and support in writing the book.

Lastly, I am extremely thankful to Shri Jitendar P Vij (Group Chairman), Mr Ankit Vij (Group President), Ms Sunita Katla (Publishing Manager), and Production team of M/s Jaypee Brothers Medical Publishers (P) Ltd, New Delhi, India, for constant support in giving the final shape to this Atlas and publishing it.

Contents

Chapter 1. **Eye and Orbit** 1
PK Srivastava

Chapter 2. **Face** 185
PK Srivastava

Chapter 3. **Thyroid** 233
PK Srivastava

Chapter 4. **Neck** 287
PK Srivastava

Chapter 5. **Salivary Glands** 351
PK Srivastava

Chapter 6. **Neurosonography of Neonatal Brain** 409
PK Srivastava

Chapter 7. **Peripheral Chest** 461
PK Srivastava

Chapter 8. **Breast** 515
PK Srivastava

Chapter 9. **Gastrointestinal Tract** 597
PK Srivastava

Chapter 10. **Prostate** 653
Mukund Joshi, PK Srivastava

Chapter 11. **Sperm Transprort System** 711
PK Srivastava

Chapter 12. **Testes** 741
PK Srivastava

Chapter 13. **Ambigous Genitalia and Intersex** 839
PK Srivastava

Chapter 14. **Penis** 857
PK Srivastava

Chapter 15. **Anterior Abdominal Wall** 891
PK Srivastava

Index *943*

CHAPTER 1

Eye and Orbit

PK Srivastava

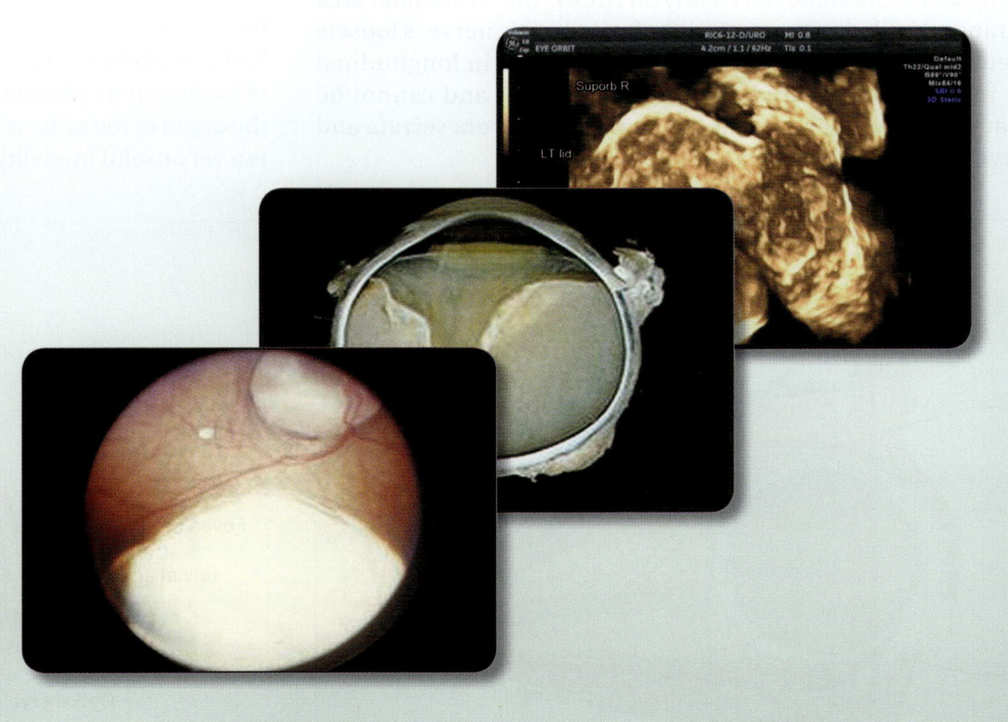

INTRODUCTION

Ultrasonic appearance of eye and orbit closely resemble the normal anatomical structures. Eye is the easiest structure to visualize within the orbit as its fluid content and superficial position makes it ideal for USG examination. Ultrasound is only practical method of obtaining images of the posterior segment of eye when the light conducting media are opaque and is the most useful investigation prior to vitrectomy. Ultrasound contributes more to tissue diagnosis than computed tomography. The characteristics of motion and topography of pathological intraocular structures enables to differentiation between retinal detachment and vitreous membrane or tumor and hemorrhage. The 2D ultrasound image displays ocular and orbital structures much more than a CT scan.

NORMAL ANATOMY

Eye is fluid-filled structure. It is situated in the anterior part of the orbit and embedded in the fat. The Tenon's capsule separates it from the orbital wall. The anterior segment forms 1/6th of eyeball and posterior segment forms 5/6th of eyeball. Normal axial length of eye is 22 mm

REFRACTIVE MEDIA

Cornea, lens, aqueous humor and vitreous gel form the refractive media. Aqueous humor is a saline solution which fills the anterior segment. Lens is a transparent biconvex body which rests over the vitreous gel. It is 3–4 mm in thickness. The vitreous is transparent gel which fills the posterior segment. All of these are very good sound conducting media and stand out clearly on HRSG. The retrobulbar area is predominantly filled with retrobulbar fat and optic nerve is loosely embedded in it. It comes out as an echo-poor strap in longitudinal axis. The retina is closely applied to the ocular coat and cannot be seen separately in normal eye. It is firmly adherent to ora serrata and optic nerve head.

EXAMINATION TECHNIQUE

2D Imaging

Short focus 7.5 MHz and 12 MHz real-time small part sector transducers are prerequisite for eye and orbital imaging. The quality of images produced by general purpose ultrasound with these probes, are good and made eye scanning a practical proposition. Sector imaging is done with patient lying supine. The main method of examination is direct contact method. The probe is directly placed on closed eyelid with intervening coupling gel.

Complete visualization of the ocular structures is achieved with careful movement and orientation of transducers with eye fixed in primary position and in all directions of gaze (Straight head position).

Color Flow Imaging and Doppler Study

Color Doppler study is highly useful in assessing vascular pathologies of eye and orbit. Ophthalmic artery and central artery of retina like short ciliary and posterior ciliary arteries supplying the choroids can be easily documented on color flow imaging. It is the useful method to examine intra ocular tumors like melanomas, retinoblastoma and metastasis. It is an important investigation in retinopathies. Neovascularisation of tumor and infiltration in adjoining tissues can be better evaluated on color flow imaging.

3D Imaging

3D ultrasound imaging increases the diagnostic accuracy particularly in localizing foreign bodies in dense intragel hemorrhage. It is also very useful in the proper assessment of intraocular tumors particularly to determine choroidal excavation. In difficult situation, it is a very handy technique to get the global view of eye and orbit. The capability of tomographic ultrasound imaging (TUI) to cut the slices of the eye or the organ in the same way as done in CT and MR making 3D ultrasound is a very useful modality.

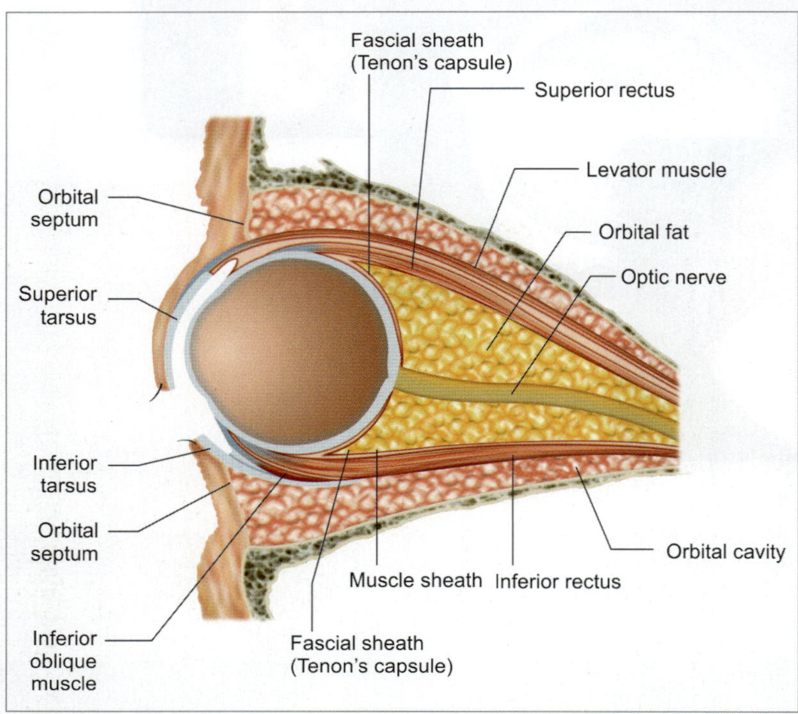

FIGURE 1.1: Sagittal section of orbit. Sagittal section of the orbit shows eyeball, retrobulbar fat, optic nerve and ocular muscles.

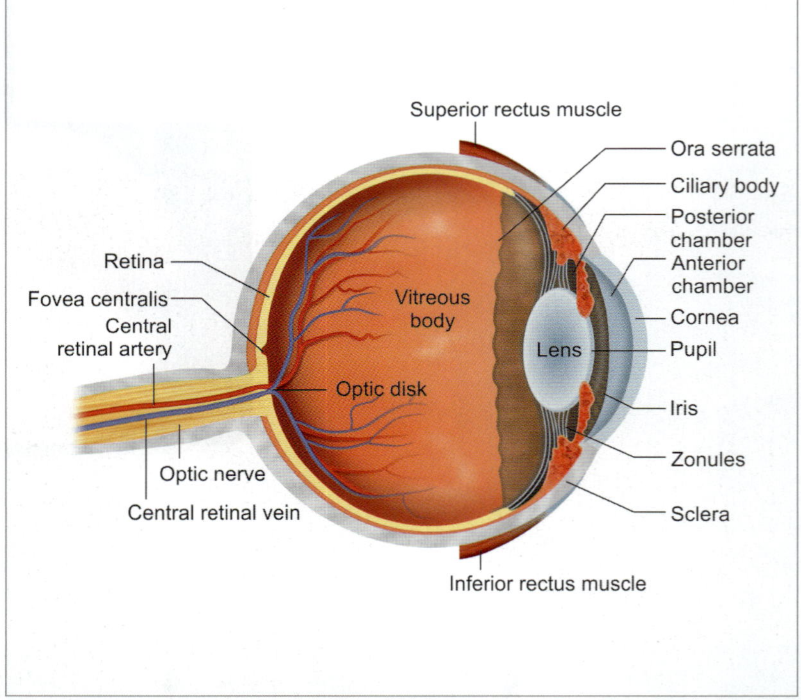

FIGURE 1.2: Cross section of eye. Cross section of the eye shows lens, anterior chamber, refractive media and posterior segment.

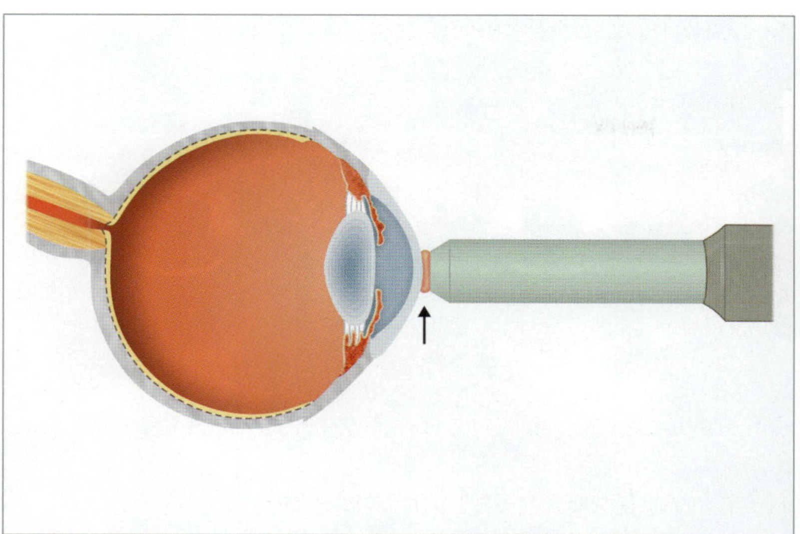

FIGURE 1.3: Diagrammatic presentation of keeping the probe over the eyelid to do ocular ultrasound.

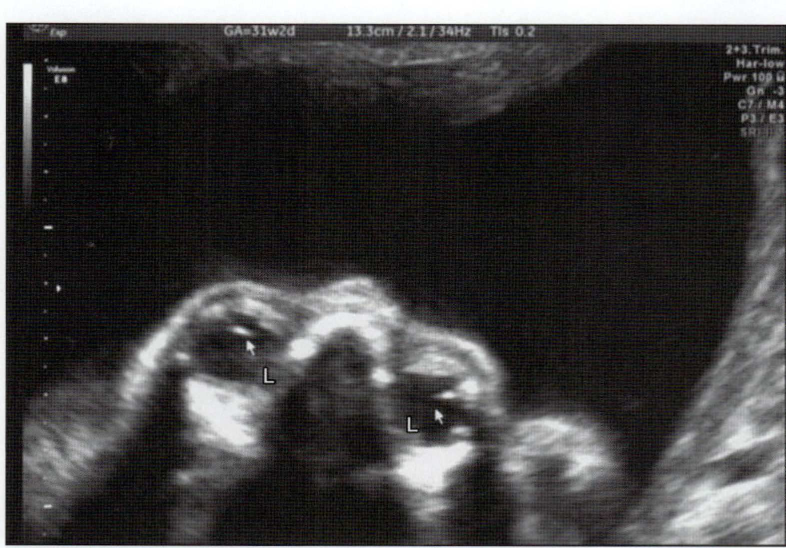

FIGURE 1.4: High-resolution sonography (HRSG) shows normal lens of fetal eyes. Both lens are seen as echogenic shadows.

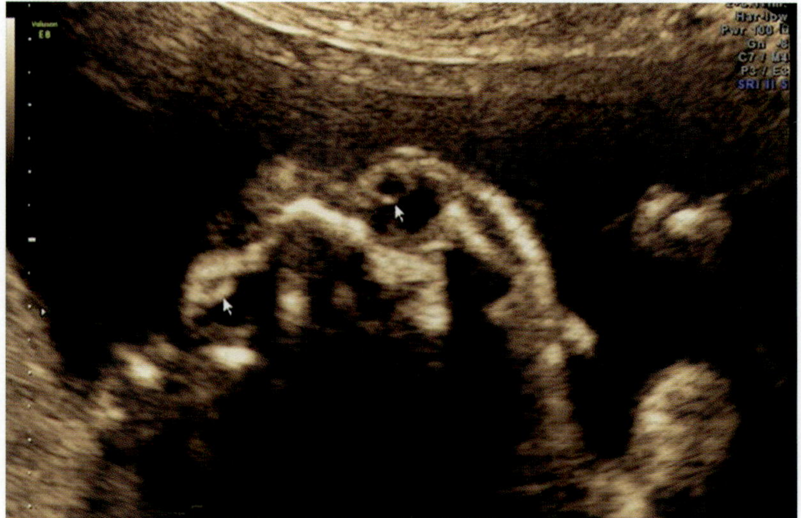

FIGURE 1.5: Fetal cataract. The ultrasound of fetus shows thickened opaque lens in left eye. Right eye shows normal lens.

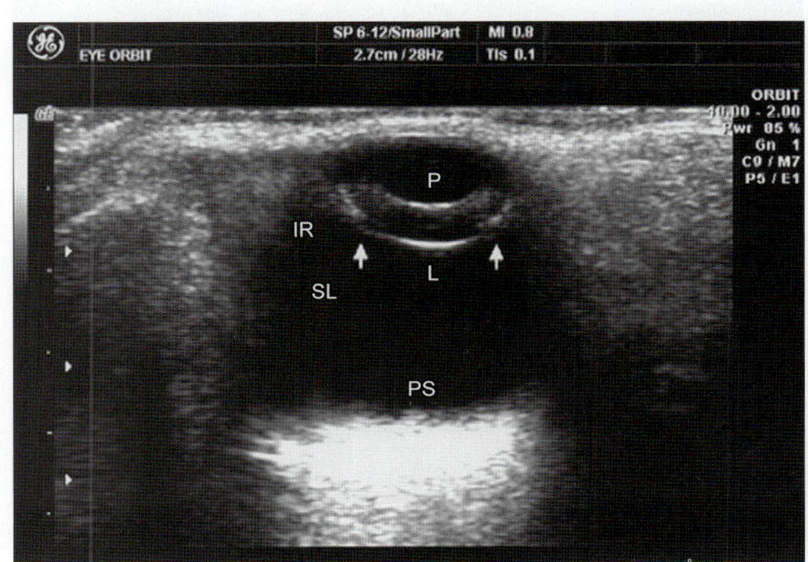

FIGURE 1.6

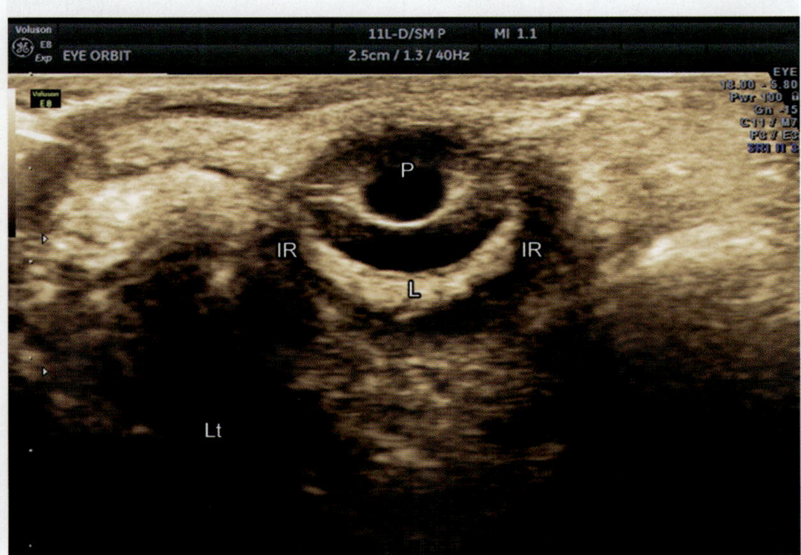

FIGURE 1.7

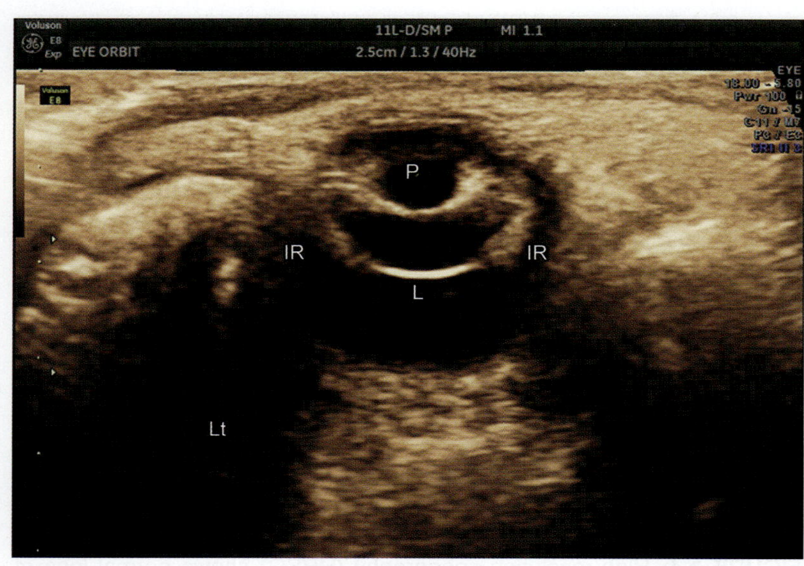

FIGURE 1.8

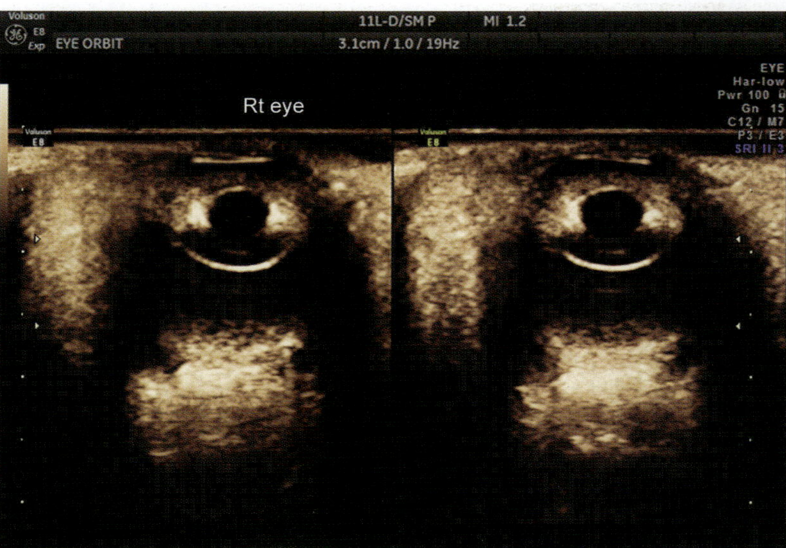

FIGURE 1.9

FIGURES 1.6 to 1.9: Normal lens. An anterior segment study – HRSG shows cornea, pupil, RIS and lens. Ir, Iris; P, pupil; L, lens.

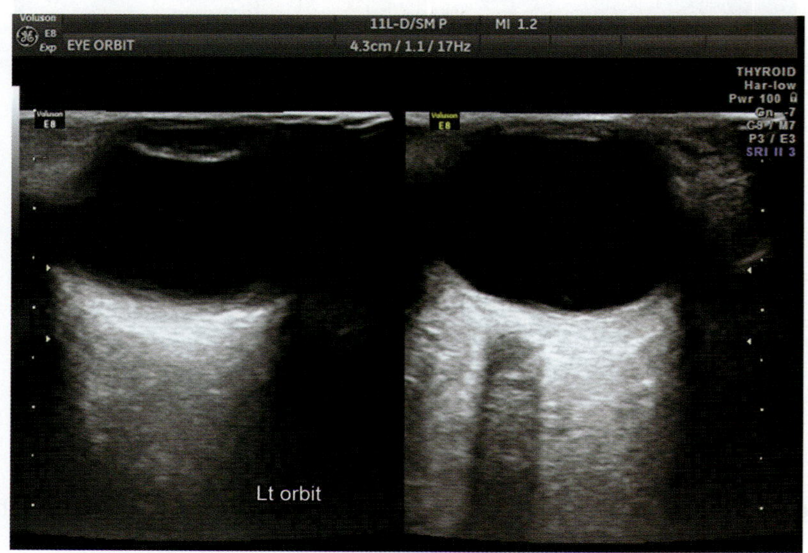

FIGURE 1.10

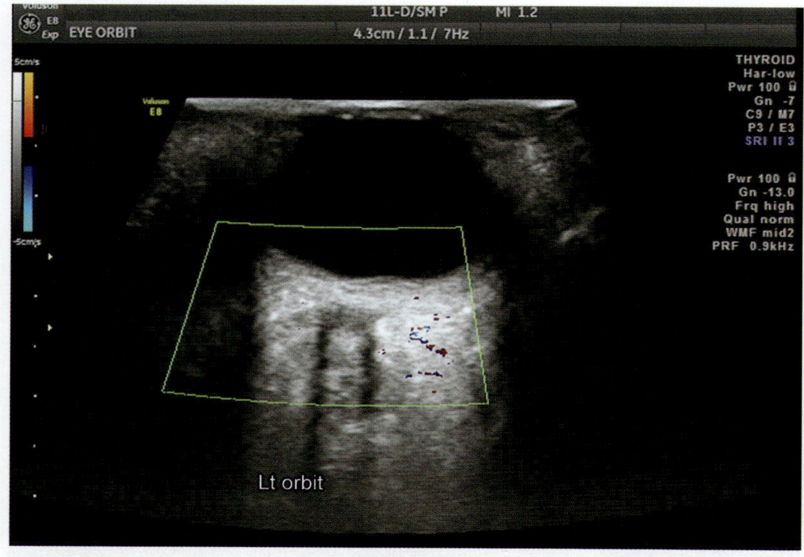

FIGURE 1.11

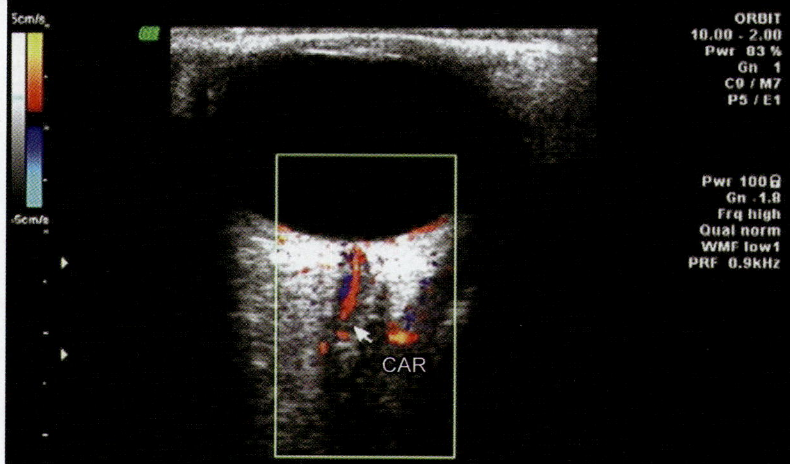

FIGURE 1.12

FIGURES 1.10 to 1.12: Normal image of posterior segment of eye. The vitreous gel is seen as anechoic body. The retinochoroid layer is seen as echogenic layer fused together. The optic nerve is seen as a hypoechoic band in long axis traversing through the retrobulbar fat.

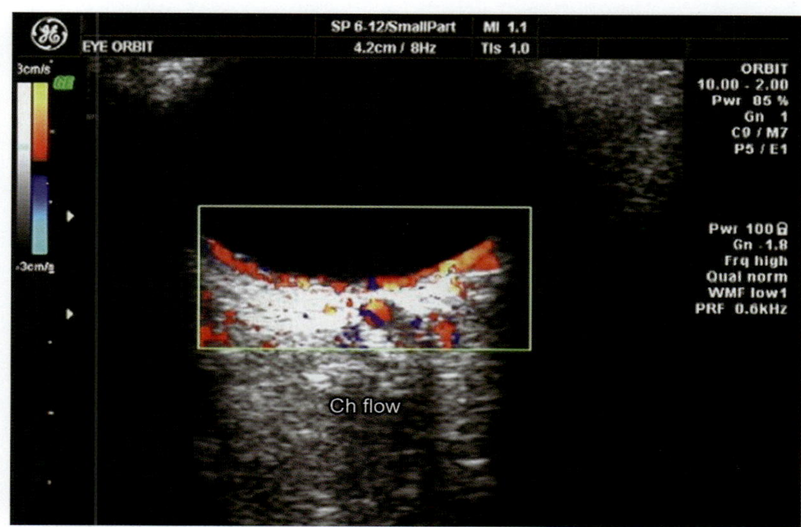

FIGURE 1.13

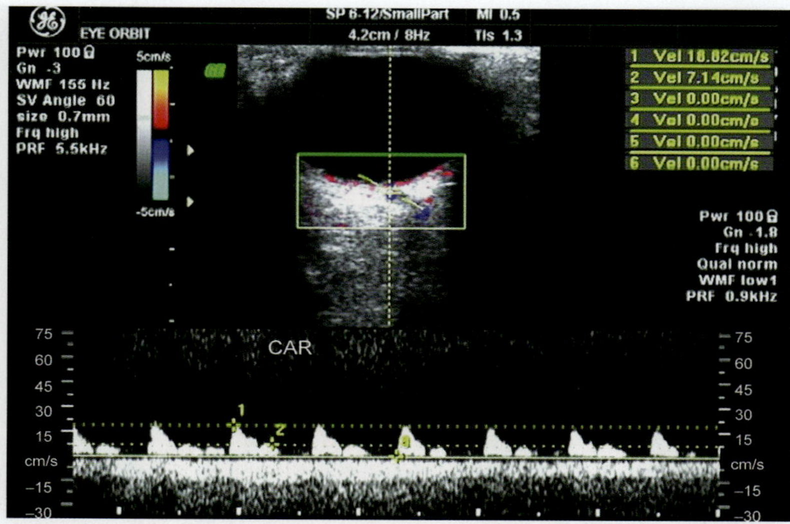

FIGURE 1.14

FIGURES 1.13 and 1.14: Choroidal flow. Color Doppler study shows central artery of retina and vein traversing through optic nerve. The posterior ciliary artery of central artery of retina (CAR) is seen supplying the choroid layer. It is seen as choroidal bluge on direct ophthalmoscopy. On spectral Doppler tracing, low arterial flow is seen in the central artery of retina.

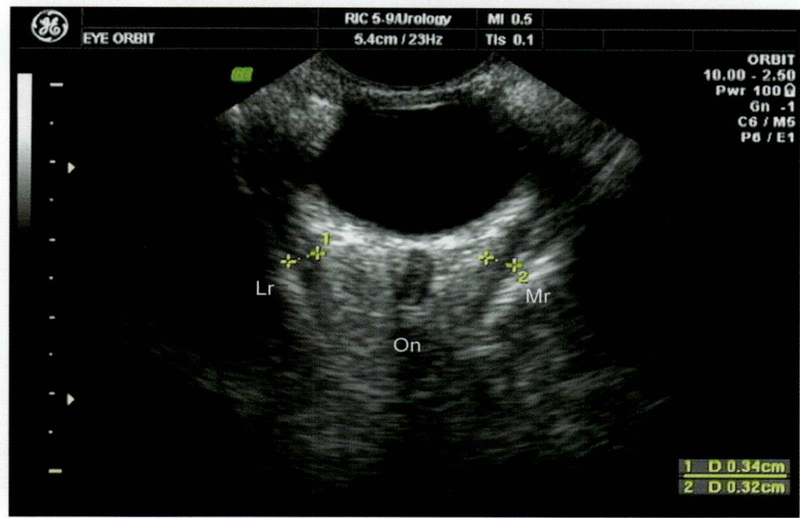

FIGURE 1.15: Extraocular muscle. HRSG shows normal extraocular muscles as a hypoechoic bands. The medial and the lateral rectus muscles are seen on nasal and temporal side. Maximum normal thickness of the muscles is 3 mm.

INDICATIONS FOR OCULAR ULTRASOUND

All the pathological conditions where direct ophthalmoscopy is not possible are the indication for high-resolution sonography (HRSG) of the globe. They are grouped as under:

Congenital Anomalies

High-resolution sonography is an excellent tool for evaluation of congenital developmental anomalies of eye and orbit. The following conditions can be very well evaluated on HRSG:

1. Anophthalmia.
2. Agenesis of eye.
3. Cryptophthalmos
4. Persistent hyperplastic primary vitreous.
5. Retrolental hyperplasia.
6. Congenital cataract.
7. Microophthalmos.
8. Macrophthalmos
9. Retinopathy of prematurity.
10. Congenital orbital cyst.
11. Congenital ocular tumors.
12. Congenital exophthalmoses.
13. Anterior staphyloma.

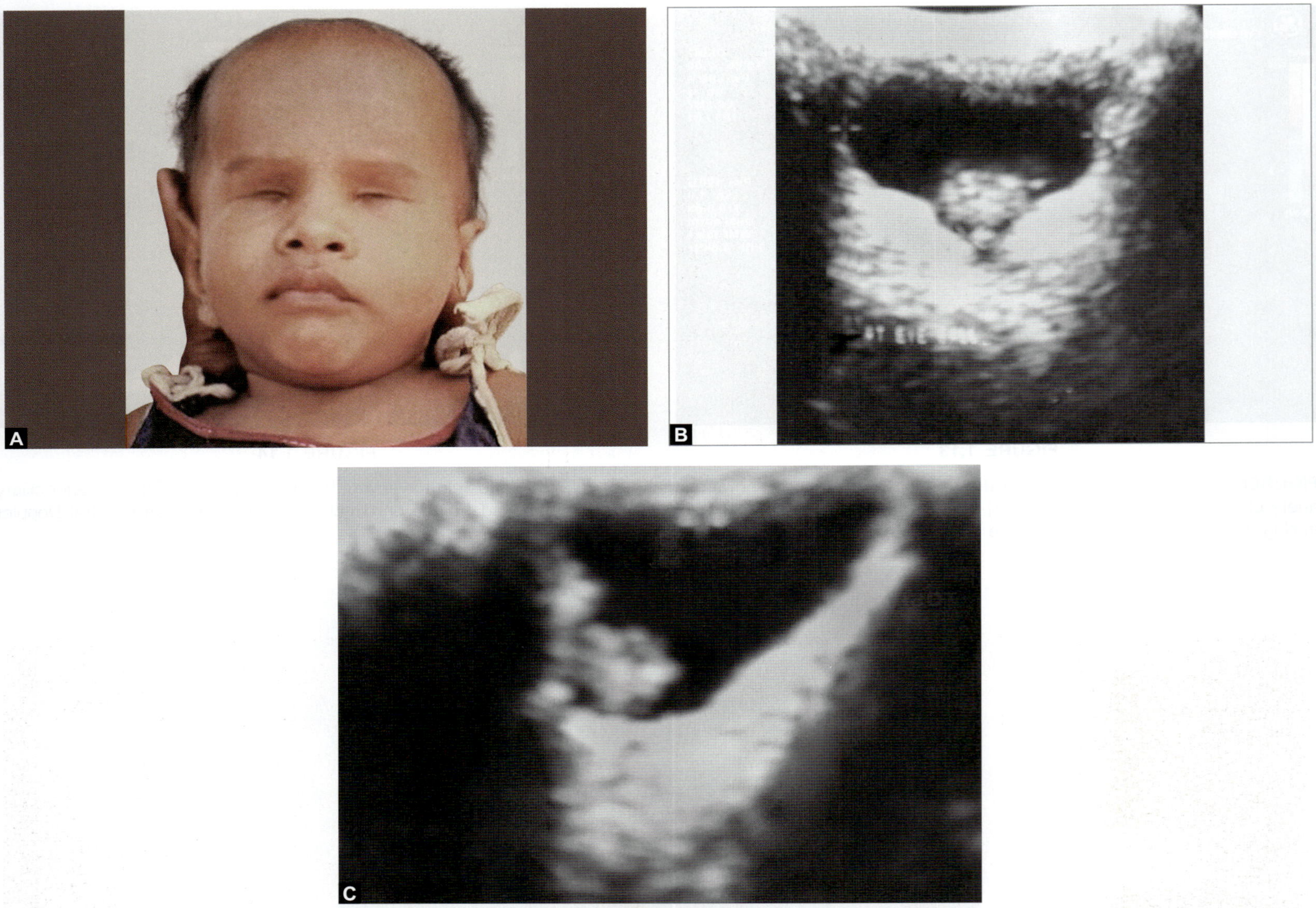

FIGURES 1.16A to C: A young child was born with small orbital sockets and thin palpebral fissure. Bilateral agenisis of eye—shows bilateral agenesis of eyeballs with small palpebral fissure in the orbital socket. Irregular cystic spaces are seen in both the orbits with small echogenic retrobulbar fat.

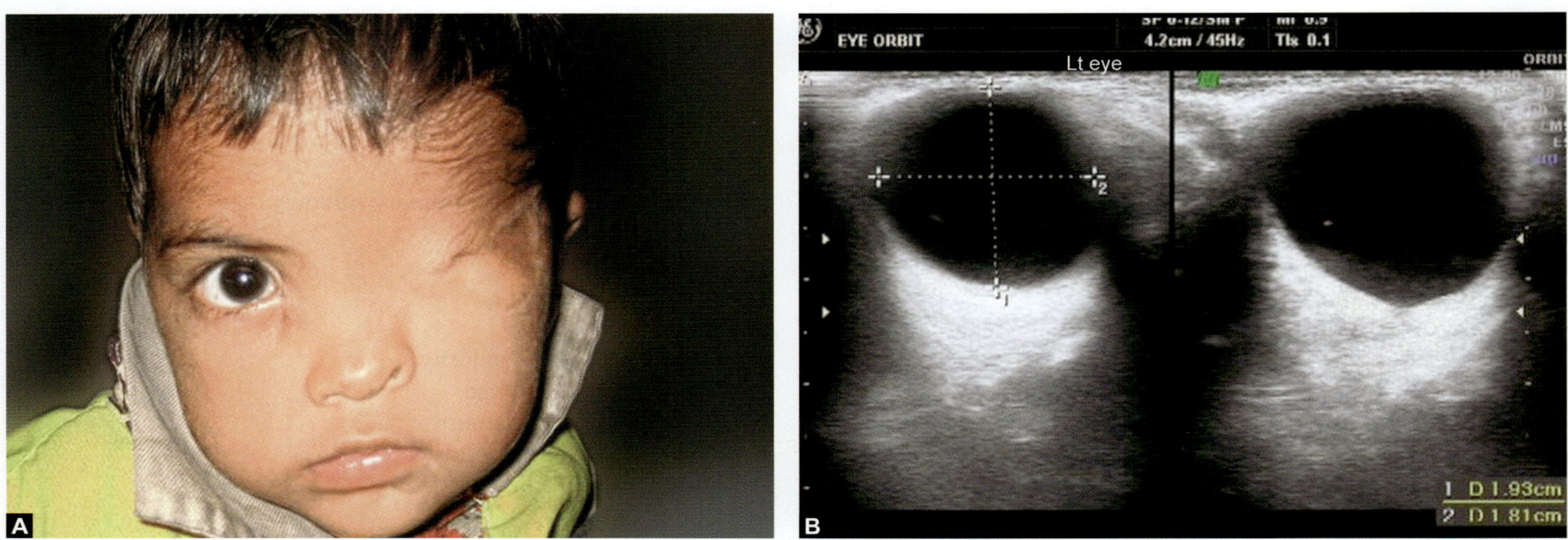

FIGURES 1.17A and B

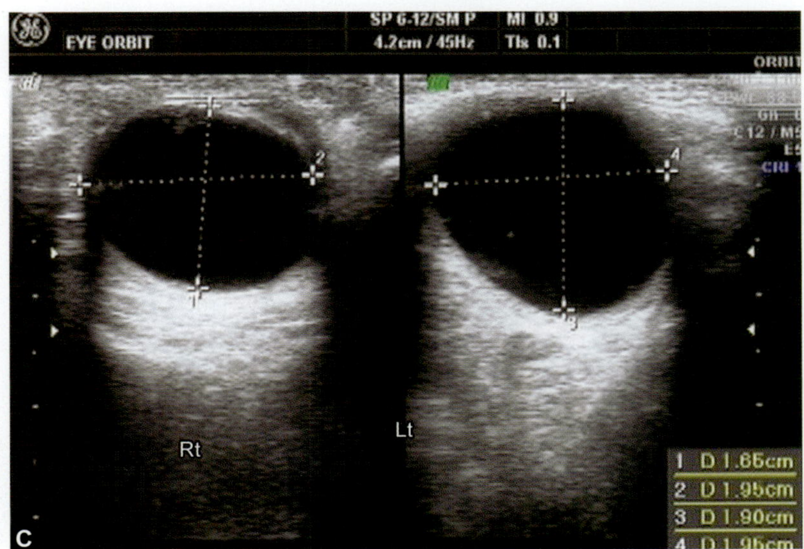

FIGURE 1.17C

FIGURES 1.17A to C: Cryptoophthalmos. Left eye covered with a skin fold in a infant child. HRSG reveals a small cystic mass with absent lens and iris in left orbit. The right eye was normal.

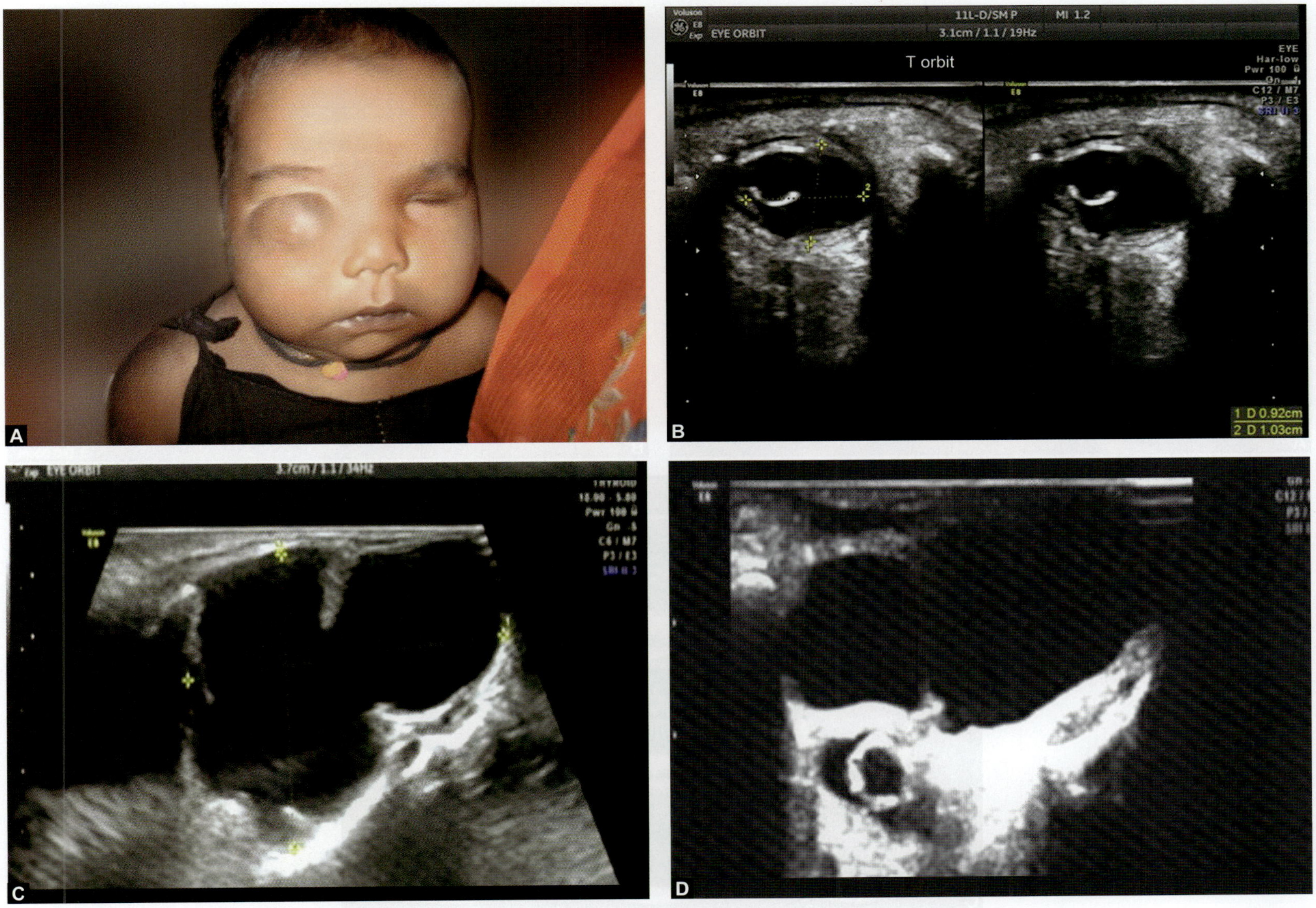

FIGURES 1.18A to D

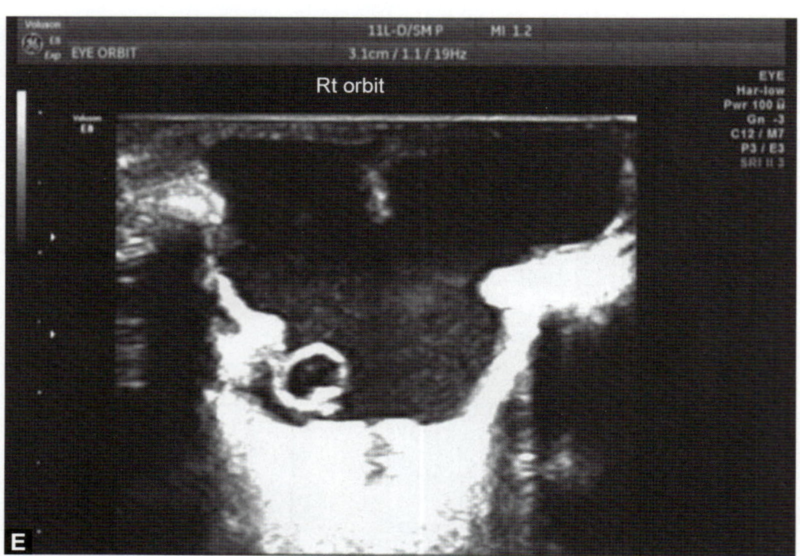

FIGURE 1.18E

FIGURES 1.18A to E: Bilateral anophthalmia. A young baby was born with right orbit covered with skin and left orbit shows small palpebral fissure. The left eye is small and 10 mm in axial length. Lens is displaced. The right eye shows an irregular cystic mass. A small eye is seen engulfed in the cystic mass. Normal anatomy of the orbit is distorted.

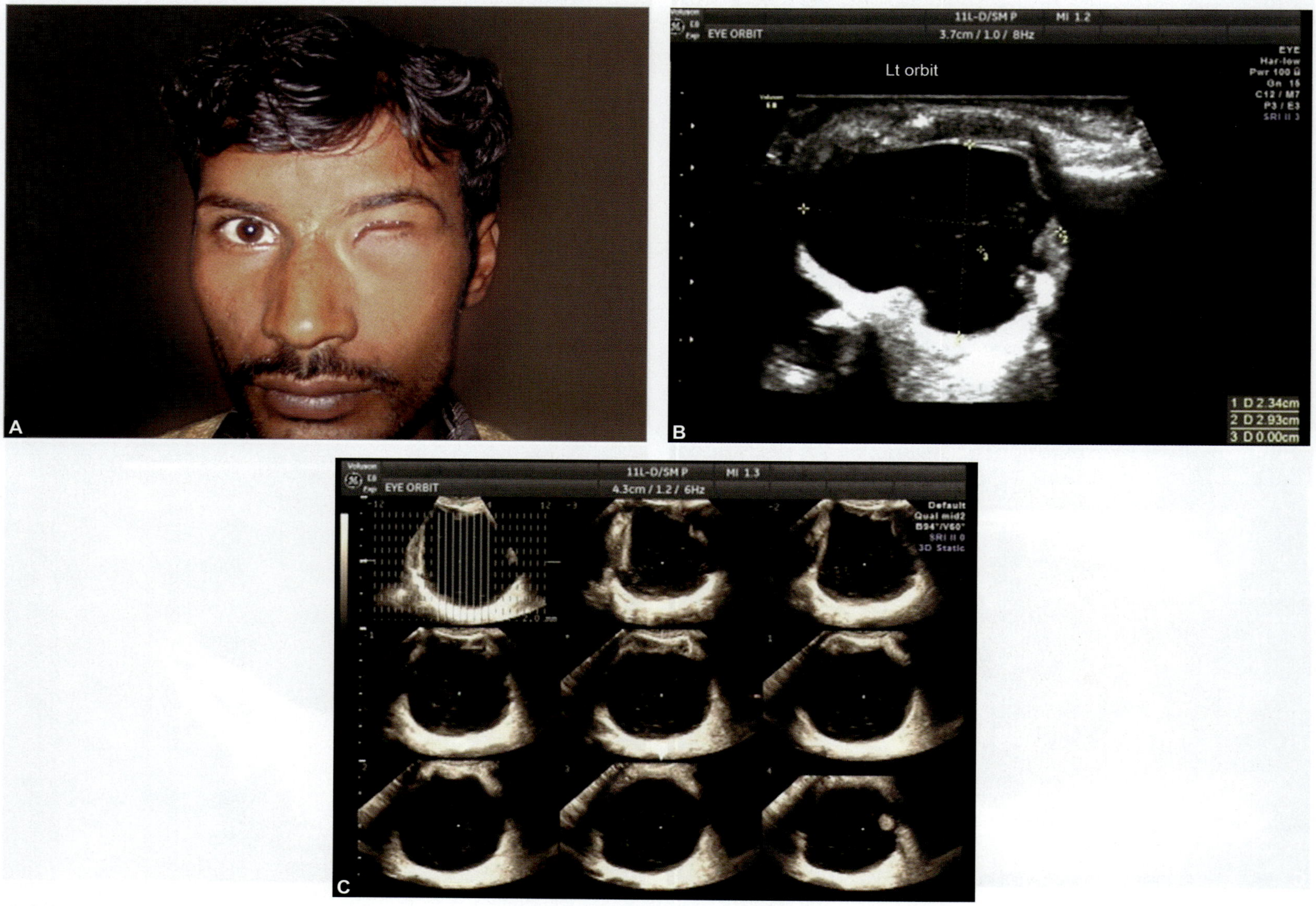

FIGURES 1.19A to C: Congenital cystic eye. A young man presented with soft tissue cystic mass in the left orbit. It is covered by a skin fold. HRSG shows an irregular cystic mass in the left orbit. Normal eye anatomy is distorted. Right eye is normal in appearance.

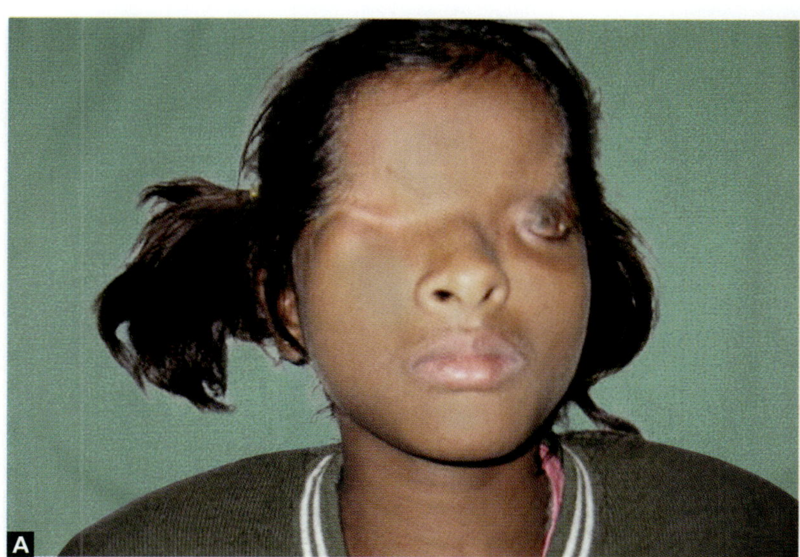

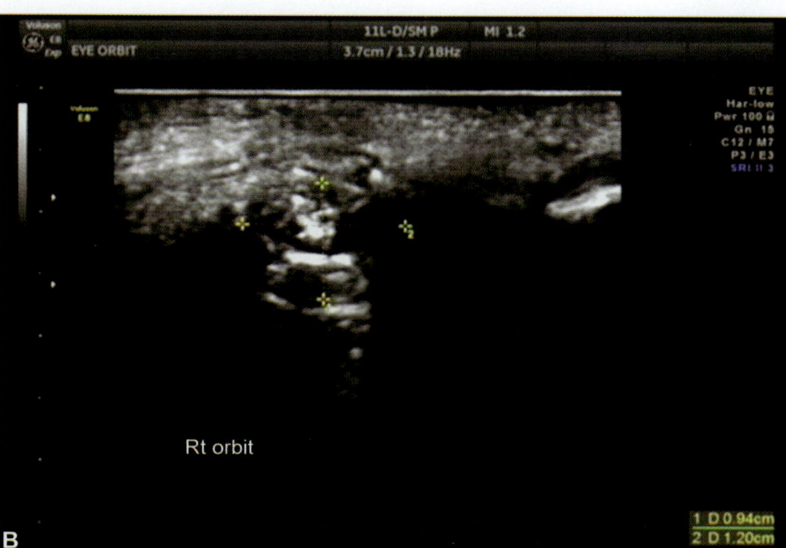

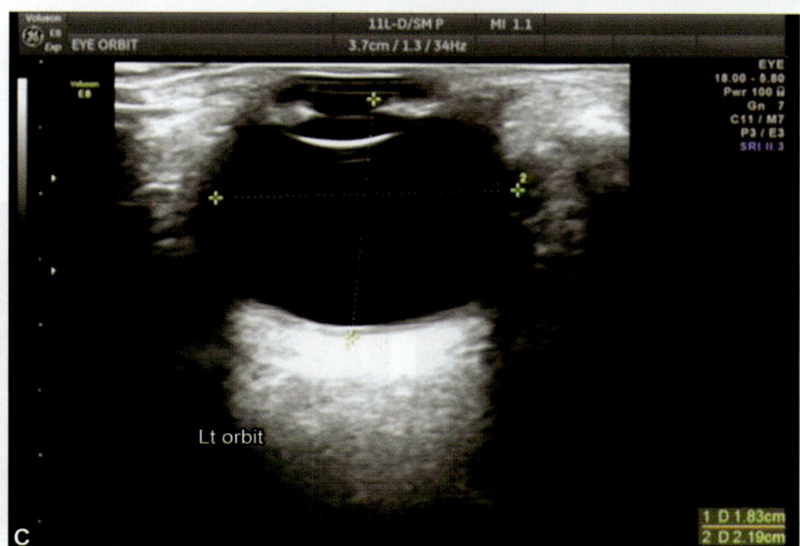

FIGURES 1.20A to C: A young girl presented with both orbit covered with skin. The right orbit shows small deformed right eye with multiple echogenic shadows filling it. The left orbit shows normal left eye. Lens and IRIS are well seen. The posterior segment of the eye is normal.

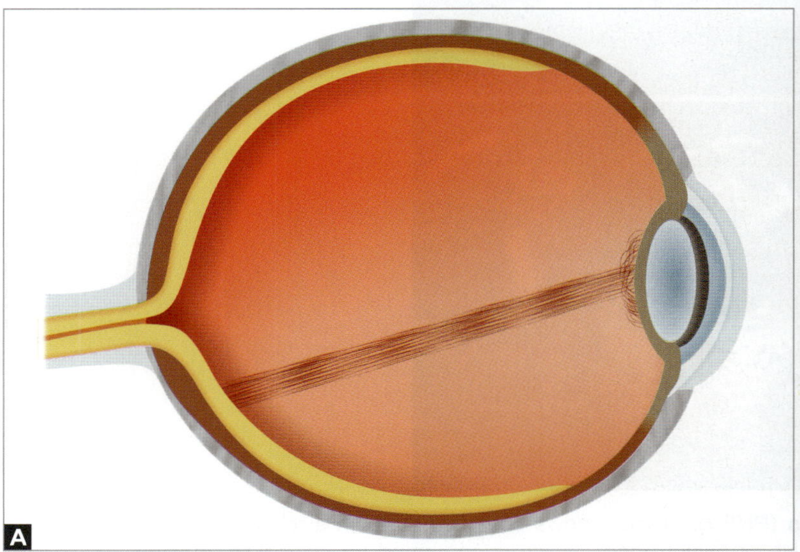

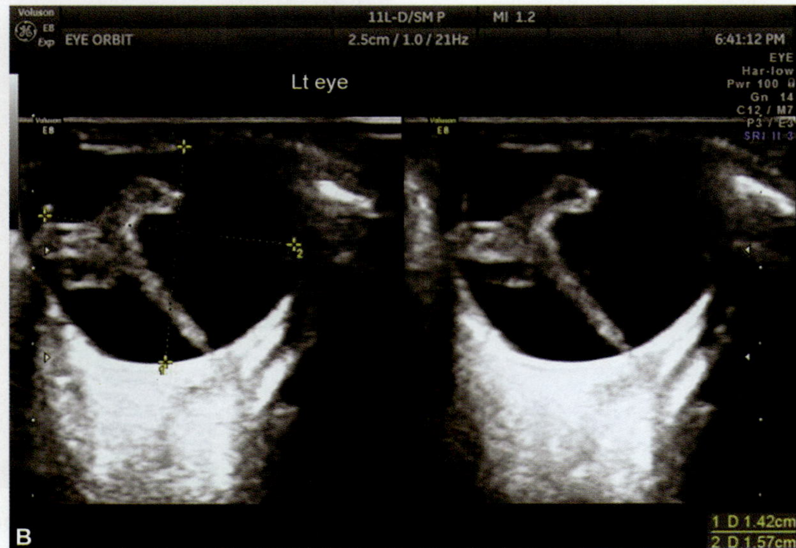

FIGURES 1.21A and B

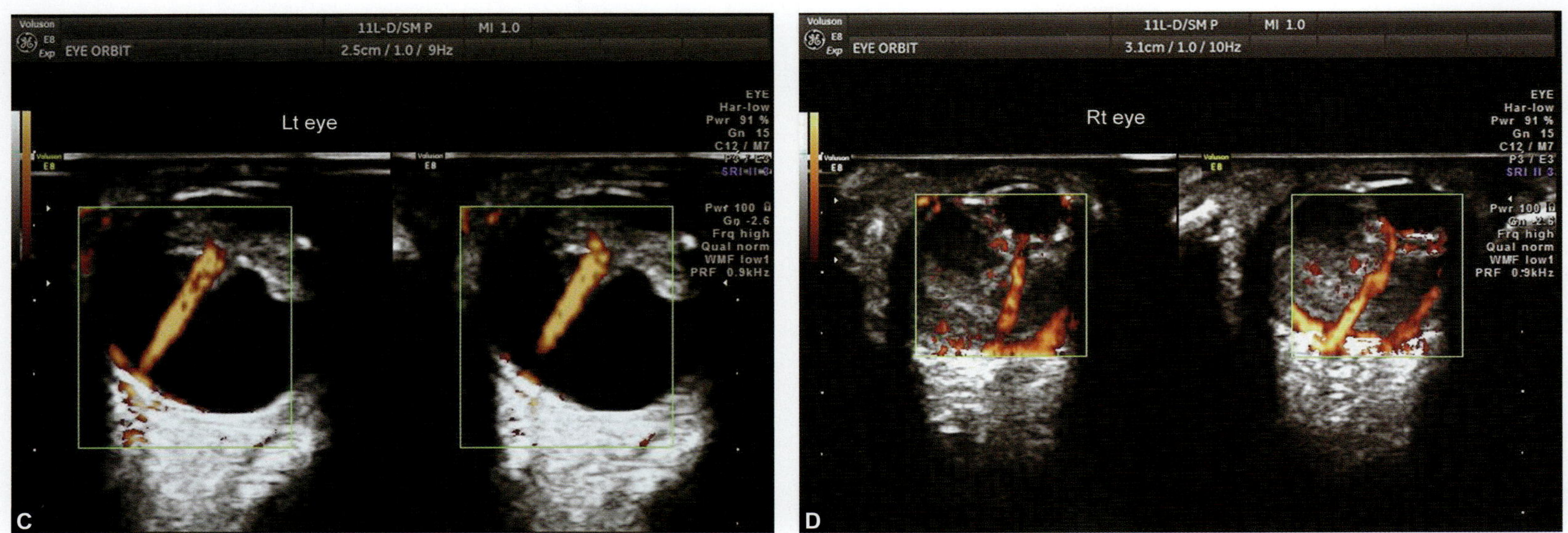

FIGURES 1.21C and D

FIGURES 1.21A to D: Proliferate hypertrophic primary vitreous (PHPV). HRSG shows small left eye. Lens is thickened. Thick band is seen going to the posterior pole from the lens. On color flow imaging, a vessel is seen feeding it suggestive of hyloid artery. The vitreous is also membranous. Findings are consistent with PHPV.

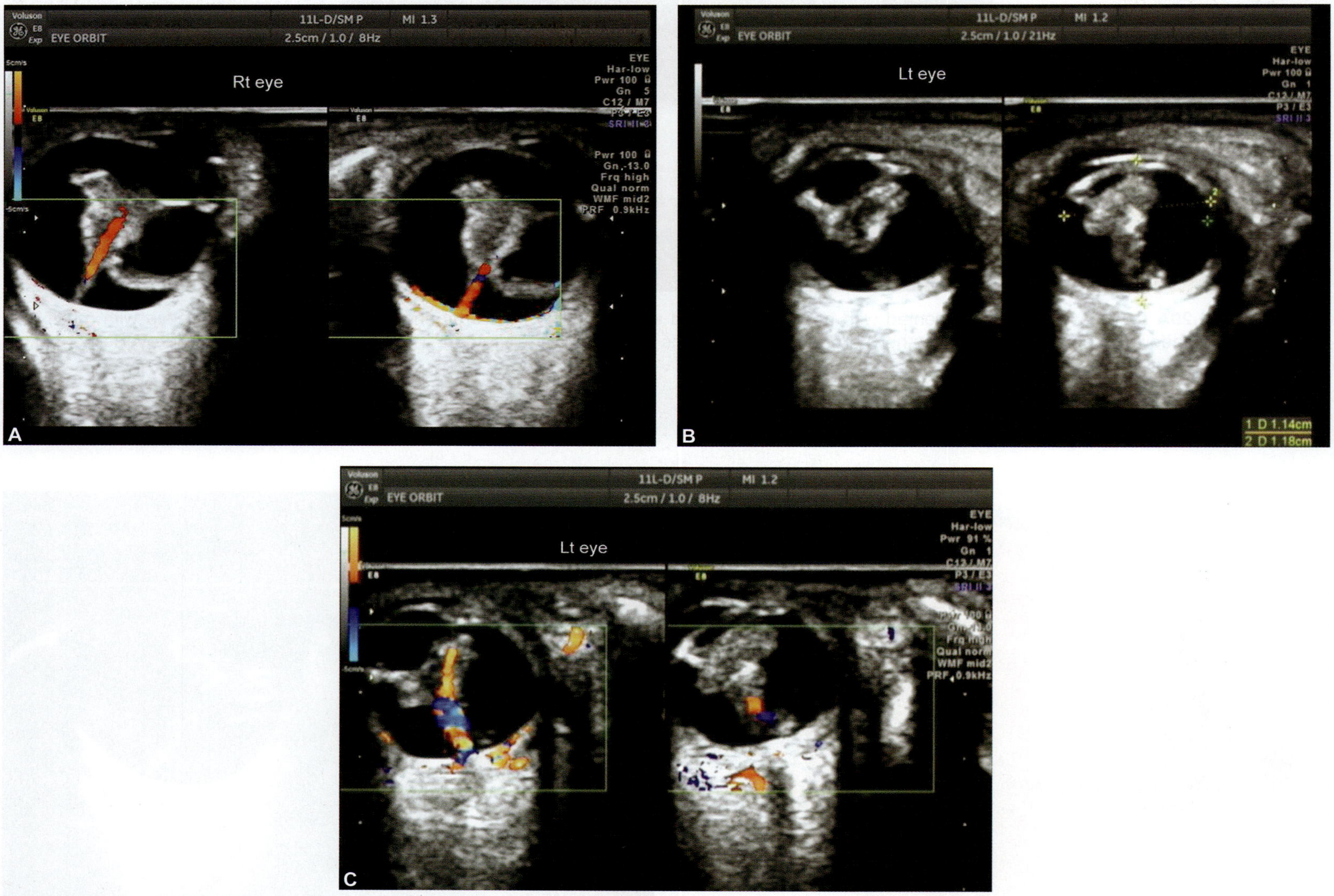

FIGURES 1.22A to C: Bilateral proliferate hypertrophic primary vitreous (PHPV). HRSG shows both eye small in size. Vitreous is membranous. An echogenic band is seen going to the posterior pole suggestive of hyloid artery, which is confirmed on color flow imaging.

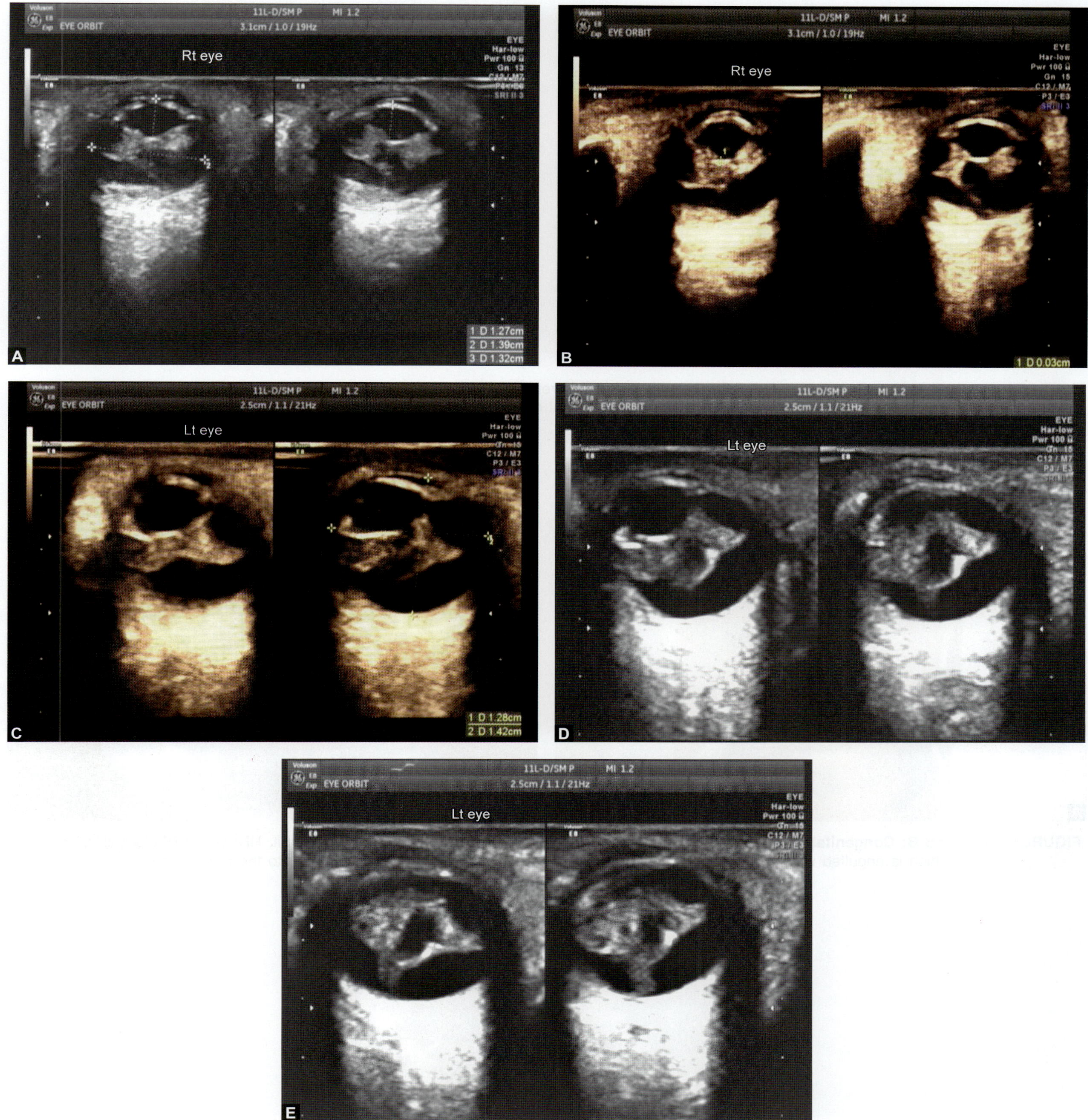

FIGURES 1.23A to E: Retinopathy of prematurity. A baby was born with white eye reflex in both eyes. HRSG shows echogenic membranous shadows filling the posterior segment. The eye is small. Multiple cysts are also seen in the posterior segment suggestive of retinopathy of prematurity.

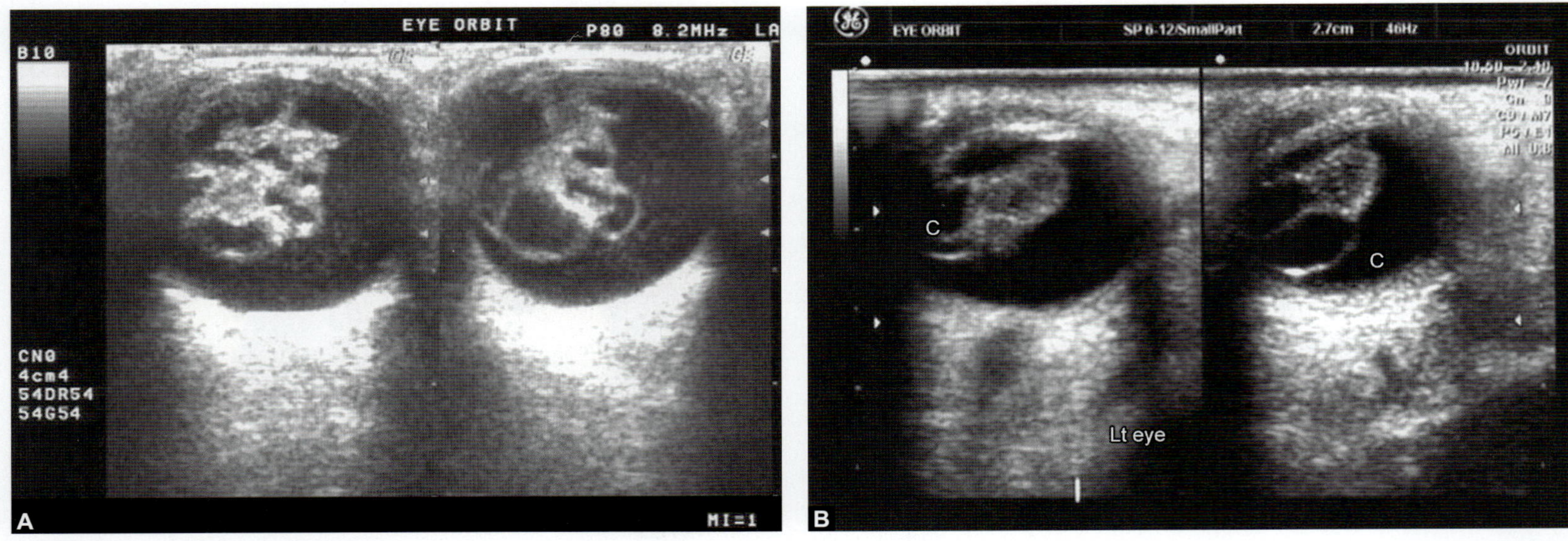

FIGURES 1.24A and B: Retinopathy of prematurity. Another case of retinopathy of prematurity. HRSG shows bilateral small eyes. Membranous shadows are seen in the posterior segment with retinal cyst formation suggestive of retinopathy of prematurity.

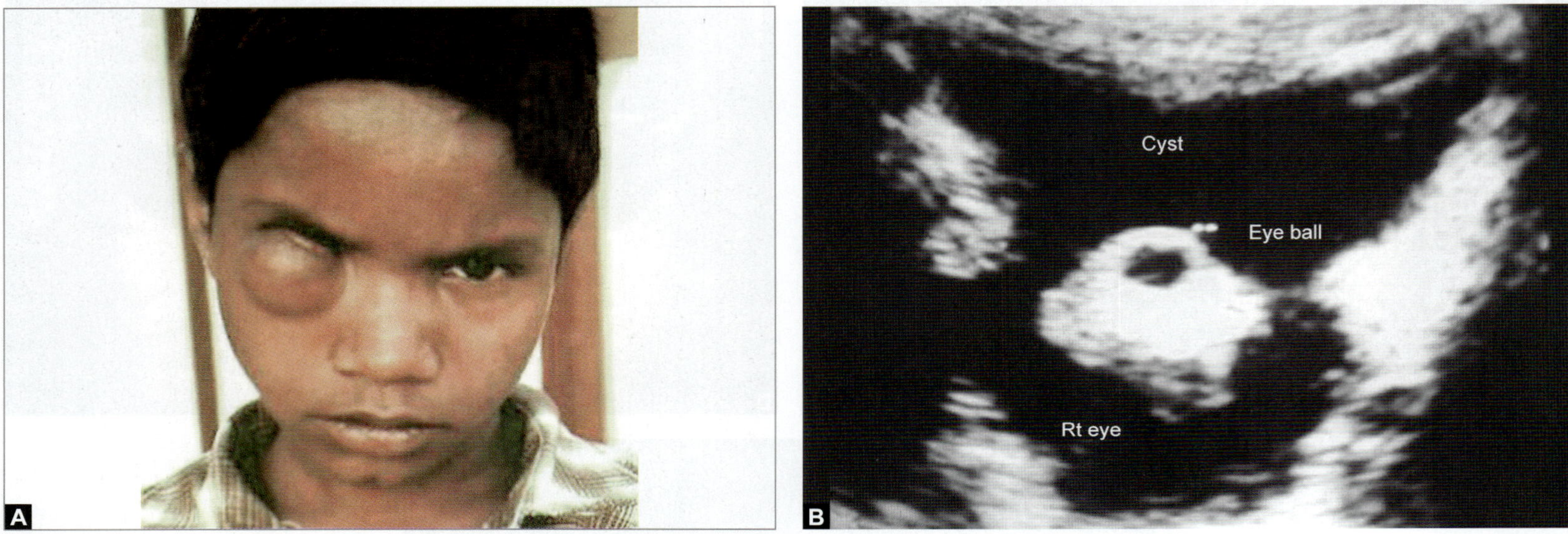

FIGURES 1.25A and B: Congenital cystic eye. A young boy presented with cystic mass over the right orbit. HRSG shows a small rudimentary eye which is engulfed with a big orbital cyst. Small amount of retrobulbar fat is seen posterior to the rudimentary eye.

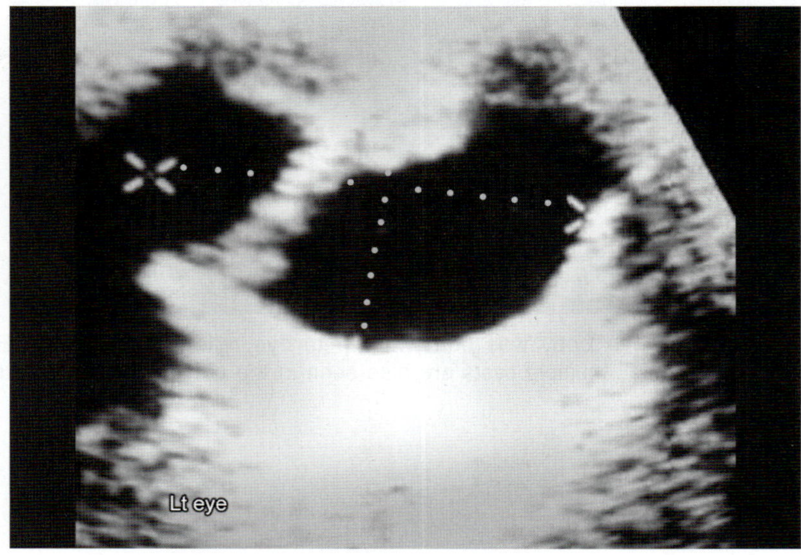

FIGURE 1.26: Retrolental fibroplasia. HRSG shows a thick opaque lens with posterior membrane and an echogenic band going from the membrane to the posterior pole in a newborn child.

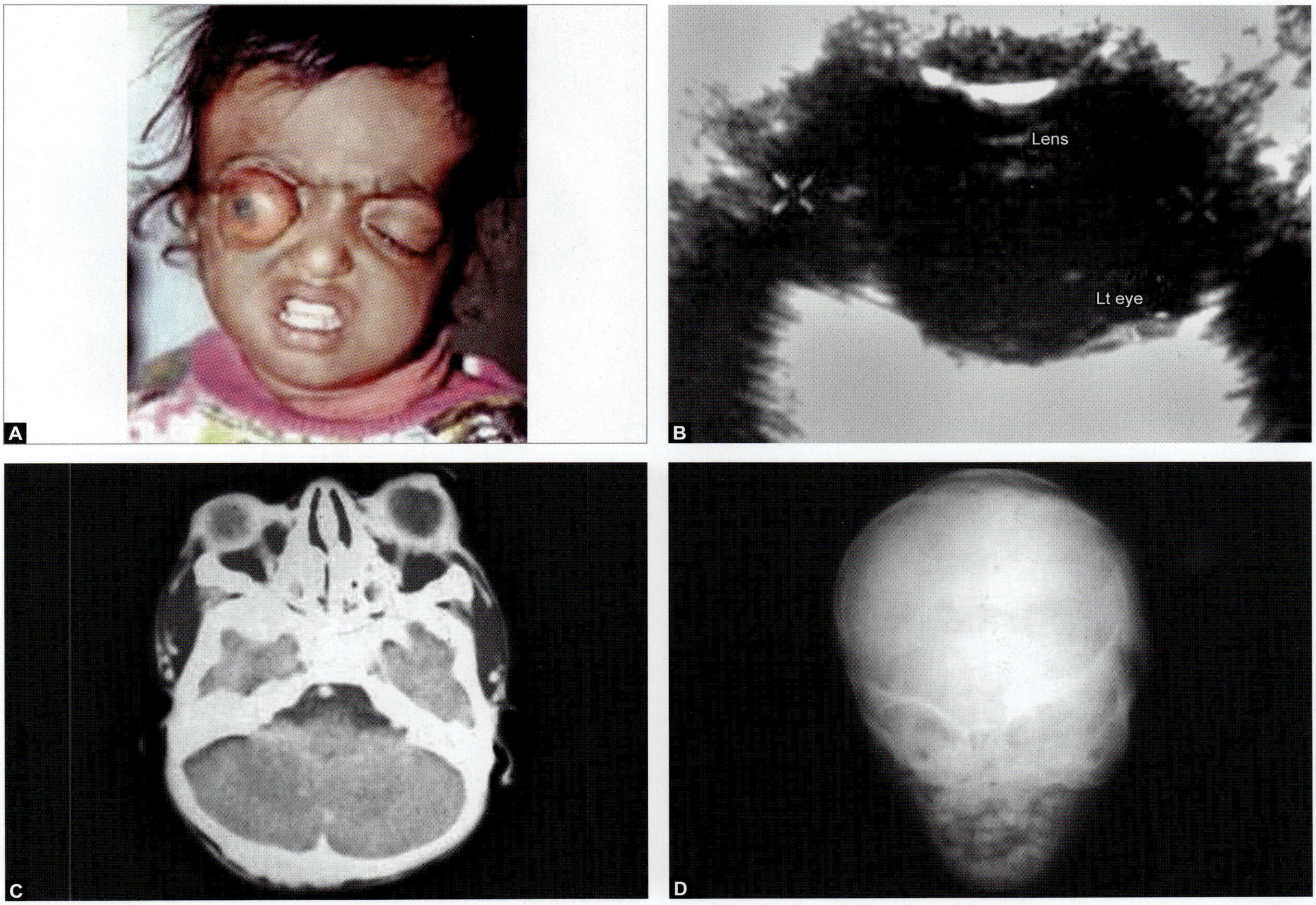

FIGURES 1.27A to D: Congenital exophthalmos. Patient shows bilateral exophthalmos with exposure keratitis of right eye in a case of craniostenosis – Crouzon's disease. Plain X-ray skull of same patient shows "tower skull" of Crouzon's disease. CT scan of the same patient shows bilateral proptosis of eyes more marked of right side with normal retrobulbar fat. HRSG shows normal appearance of the eye in the same patient.

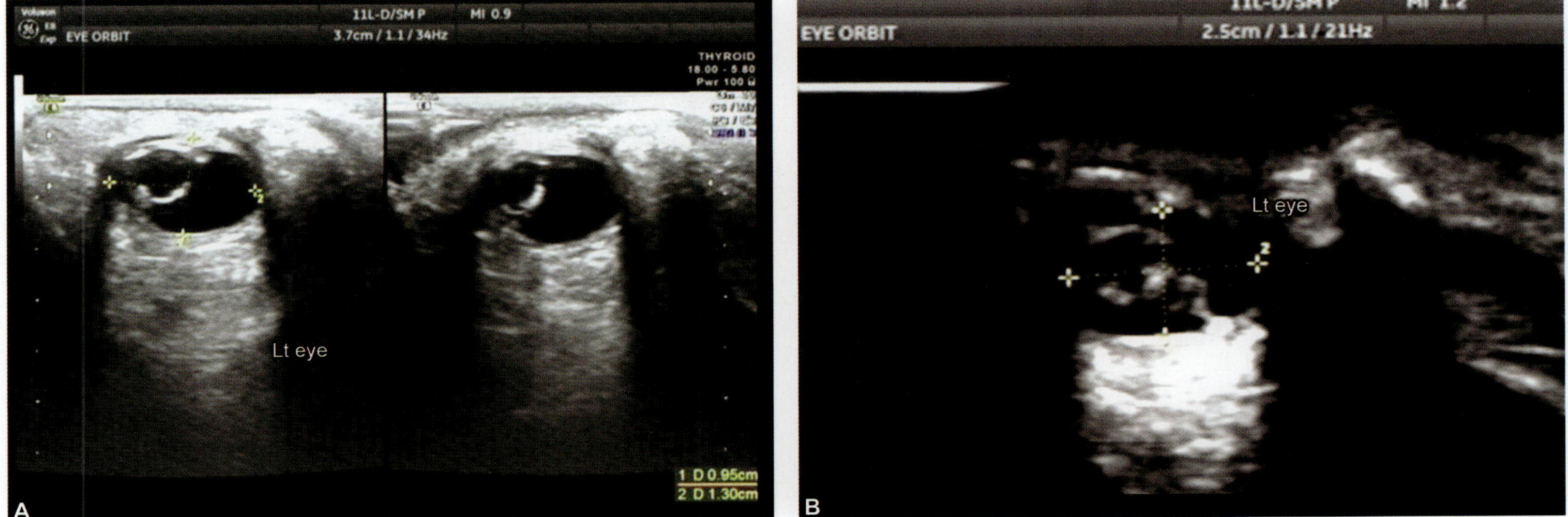

FIGURES 1.28A and B : Microphthalmos. HRSG shows bilateral small eyes. The left eye measures 10 × 13 mm. The right eye measures 10 × 8 mm in size suggestive of bilateral microphthalmos.

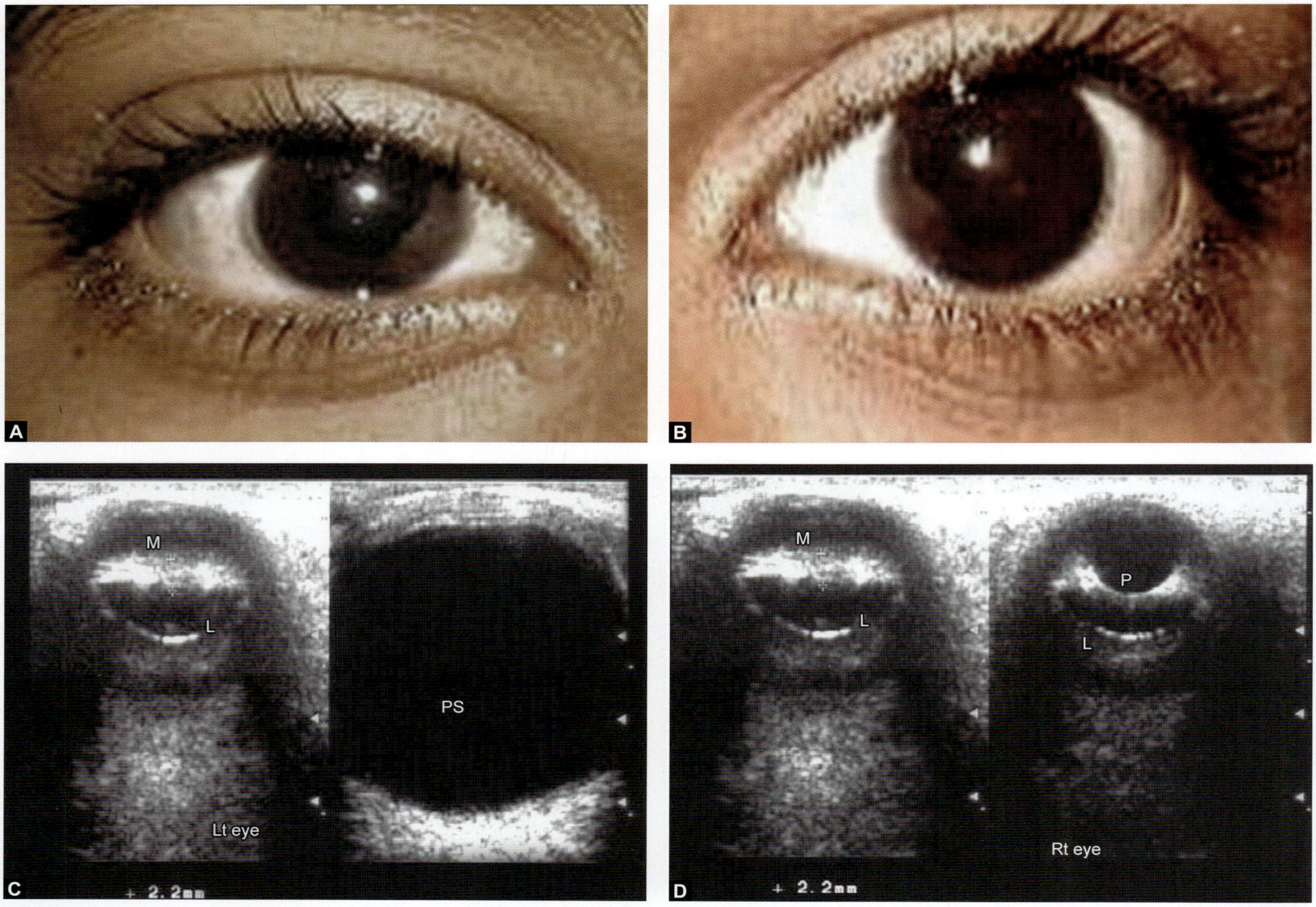

FIGURES 1.29A to D: Opaque corneal membrane. Young girl presented with opaque membrane covering the cornia. HRSG shows thick echogenic membrane covering the cornia. However, posterior segment of the eye is free. No intragel pathology is seen. HRSG shows normal pupil and cornia in the right eye and thickened echogenic membrane seen in the left eye covering the cornea.

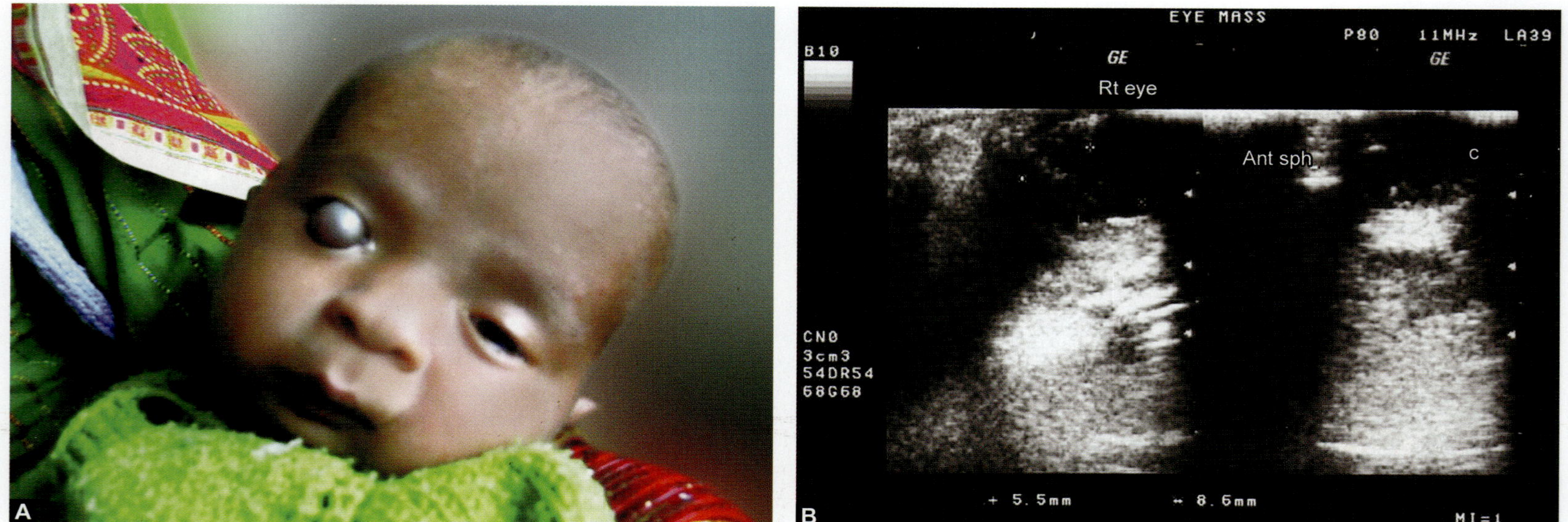

FIGURES 1.30A and B: Anterior staphyloma. An infant baby is seen born with right eye covered with membrane. HRSG shows a cystic mass seen coming out from the Iris and covering the cornea suggestive of anterior staphyloma.

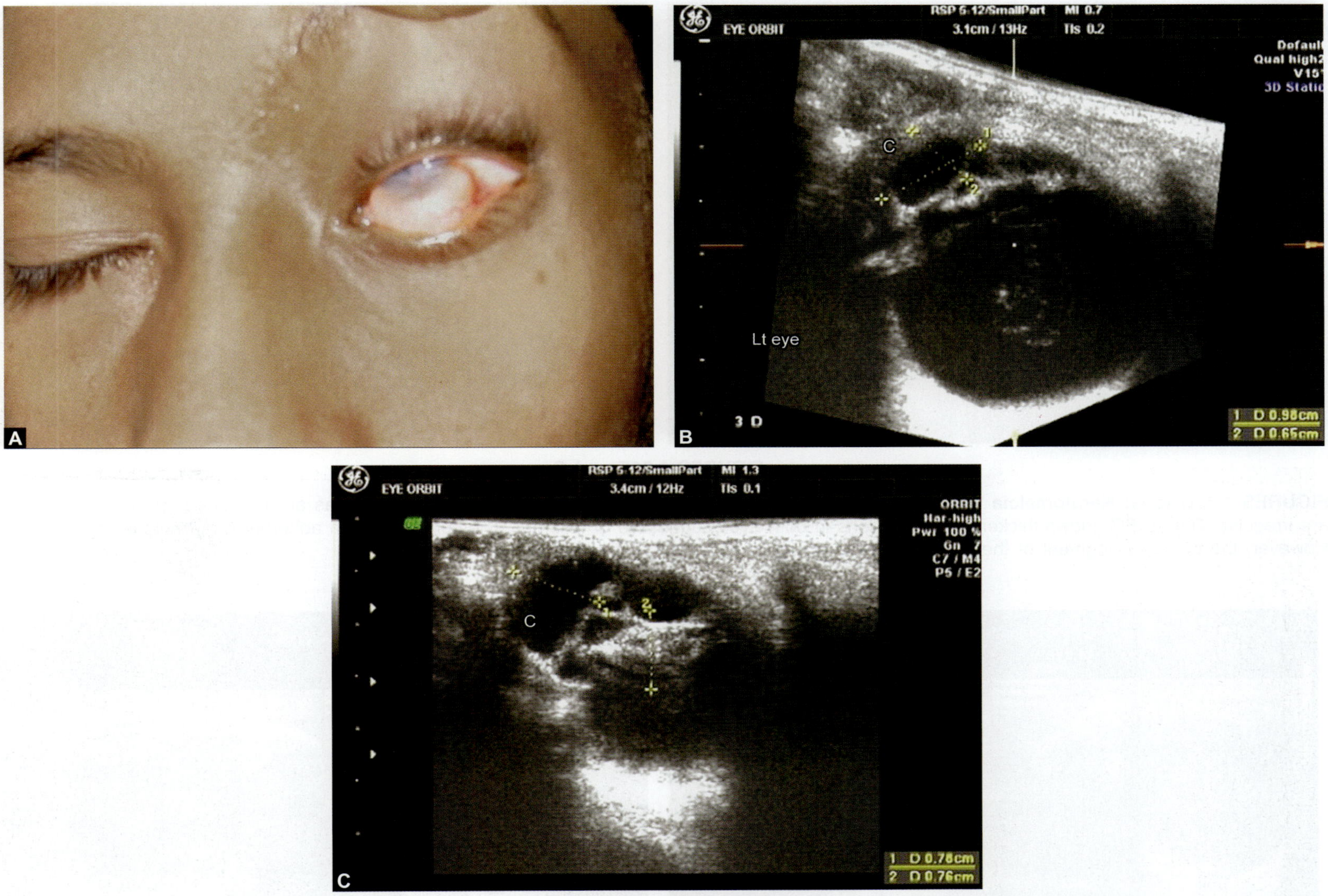

FIGURES 1.31A to C: Complicated traumatic anterior staphyloma. Patient presented with bulging shining membranous shadow in the left eye. HRSG shows a thick walled cystic mass coming out from the anterior chamber. Multiple internal echoes are also seen in it. 3D imaging of the same patient shows details of the complicated staphyloma. Multiple echogenic bands are seen going from the lens to the cyst. The cyst is adhered with the lens. Lens is thickened and opaque with calcification of the nucleus.

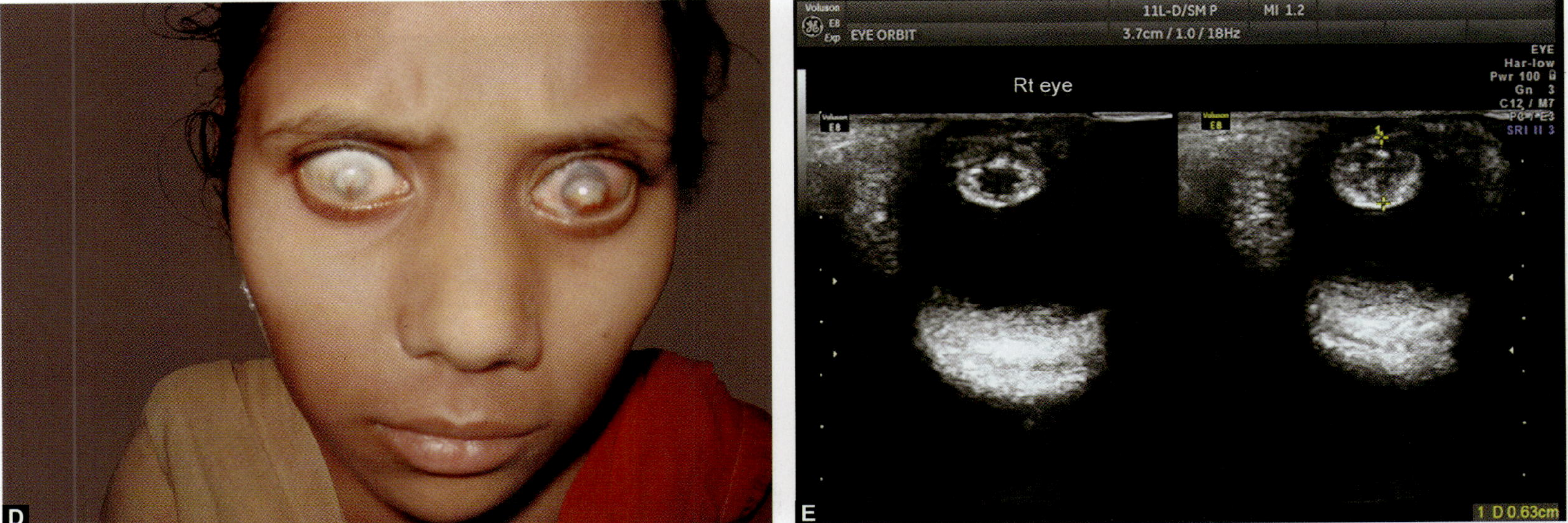

FIGURES 1.31D and E

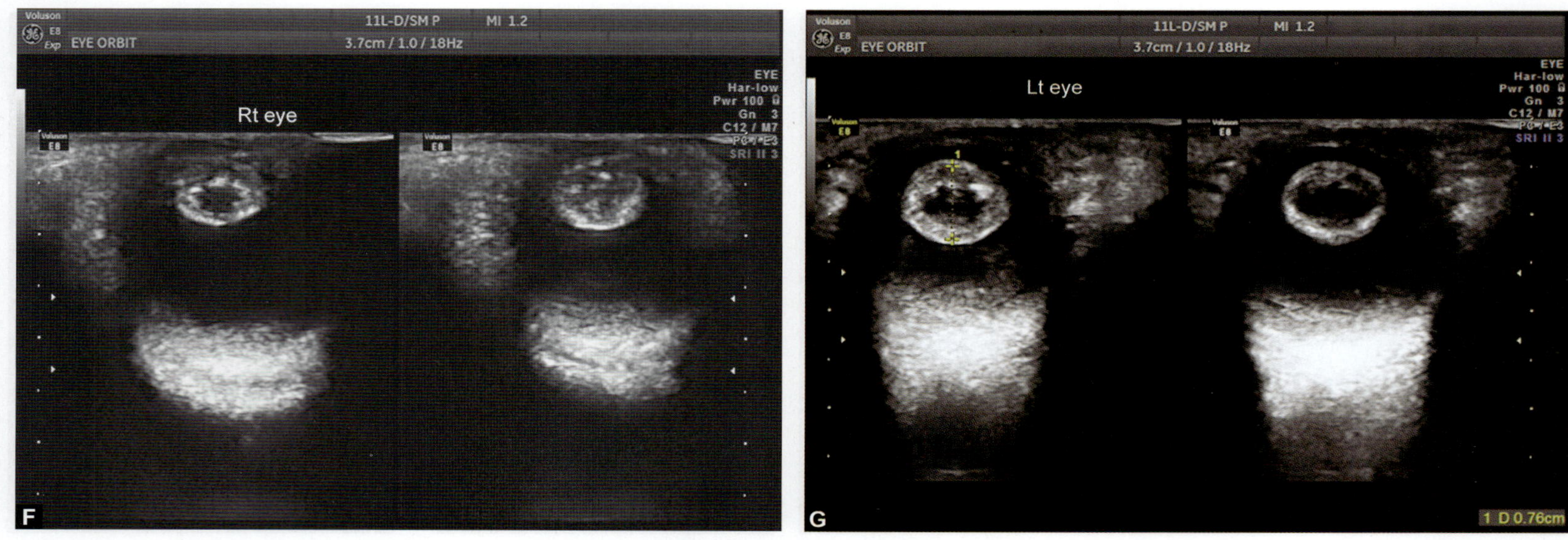

FIGURES 1.31F and G

FIGURES 1.31D to G: Keratomalcia with cataract. A young girl presented with white eye reflex. Both corneas are thickened and echogenic. They are irregular. The HRSG shows thickened opaque lens in both eyes suggestive of cataract. The cornea is seen adherent with the lens on both sides. However, the posterior segment of the eye is free. No intragel pathology is seen.

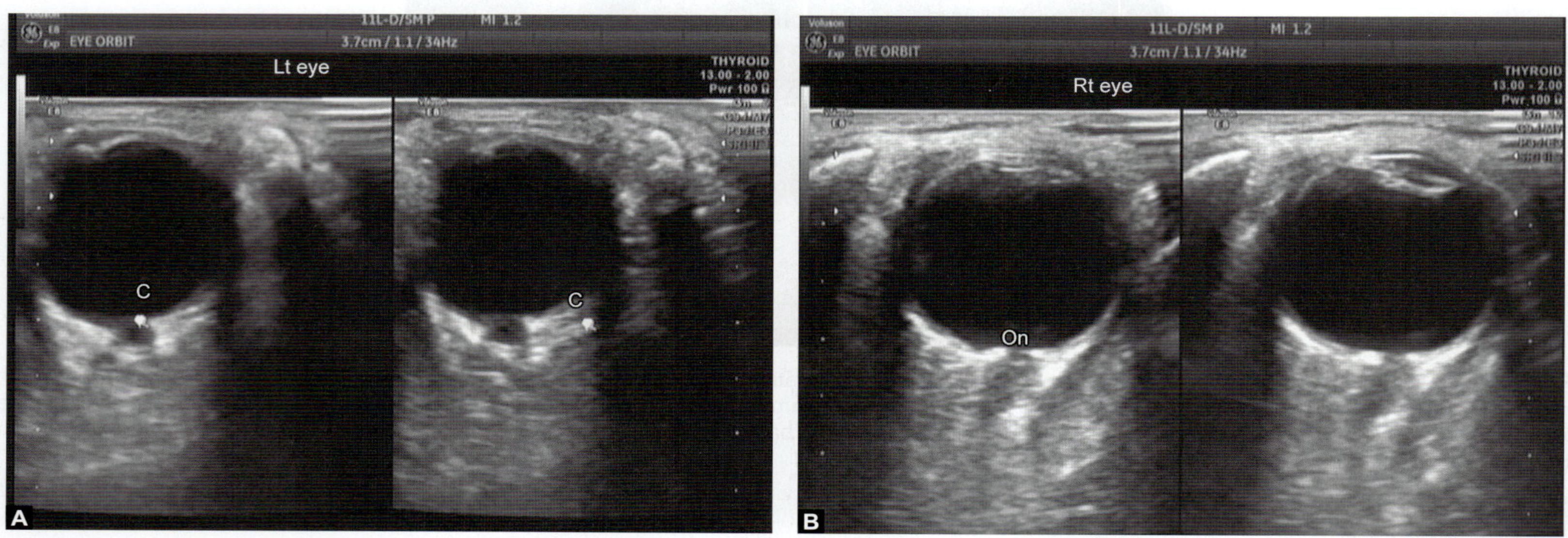

FIGURES 1.32A and B: Coloboma eye. A newborn baby presented with white eye reflex. HRSG shows a defect in the posterior pole of the eye suggestive of coloboma. The right eye is normal.

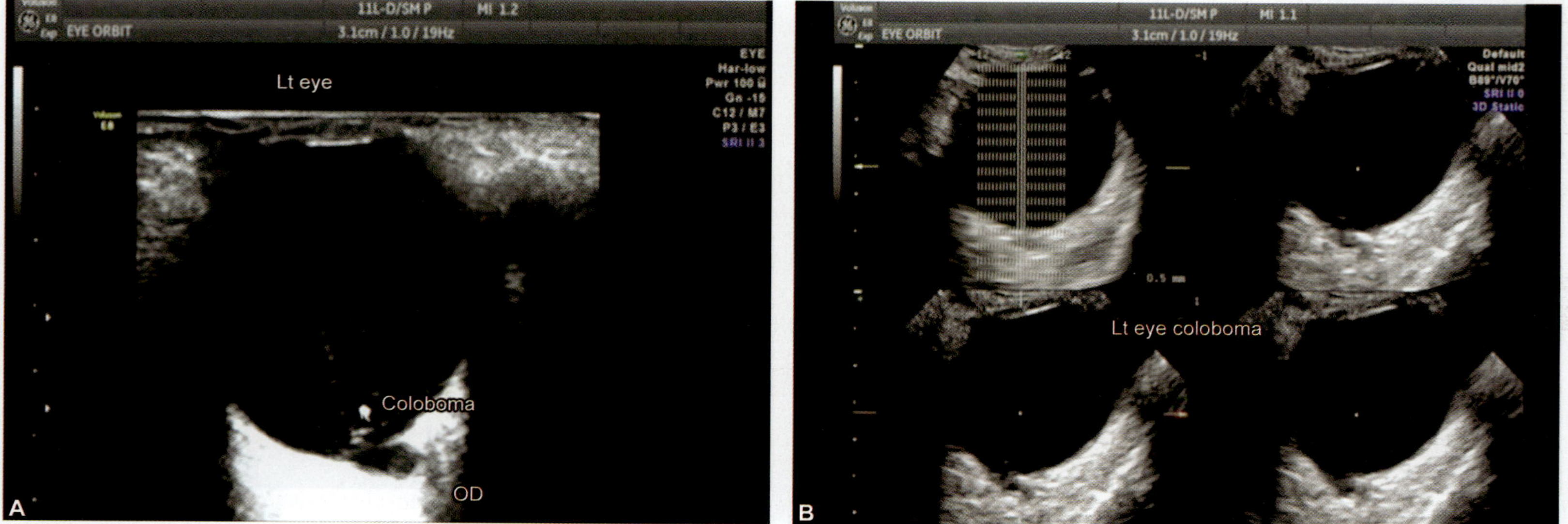

FIGURES 1.33A and B

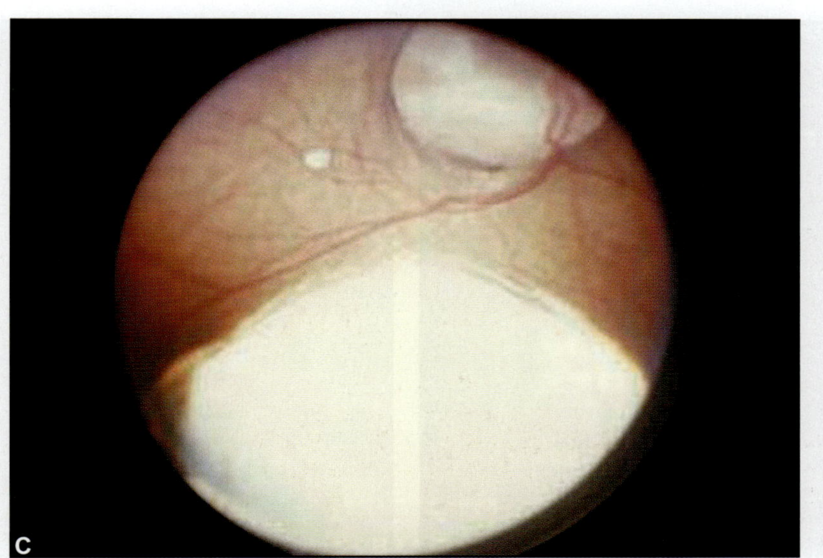

FIGURE 1.33C

FIGURES 1.33A to C: Coloboma eye. A patient presented with white eye reflex. (A and B) HRSG shows defect in the eye coat suggestive of coloboma. (C) Shows defect on direct ophthalmoscopy.

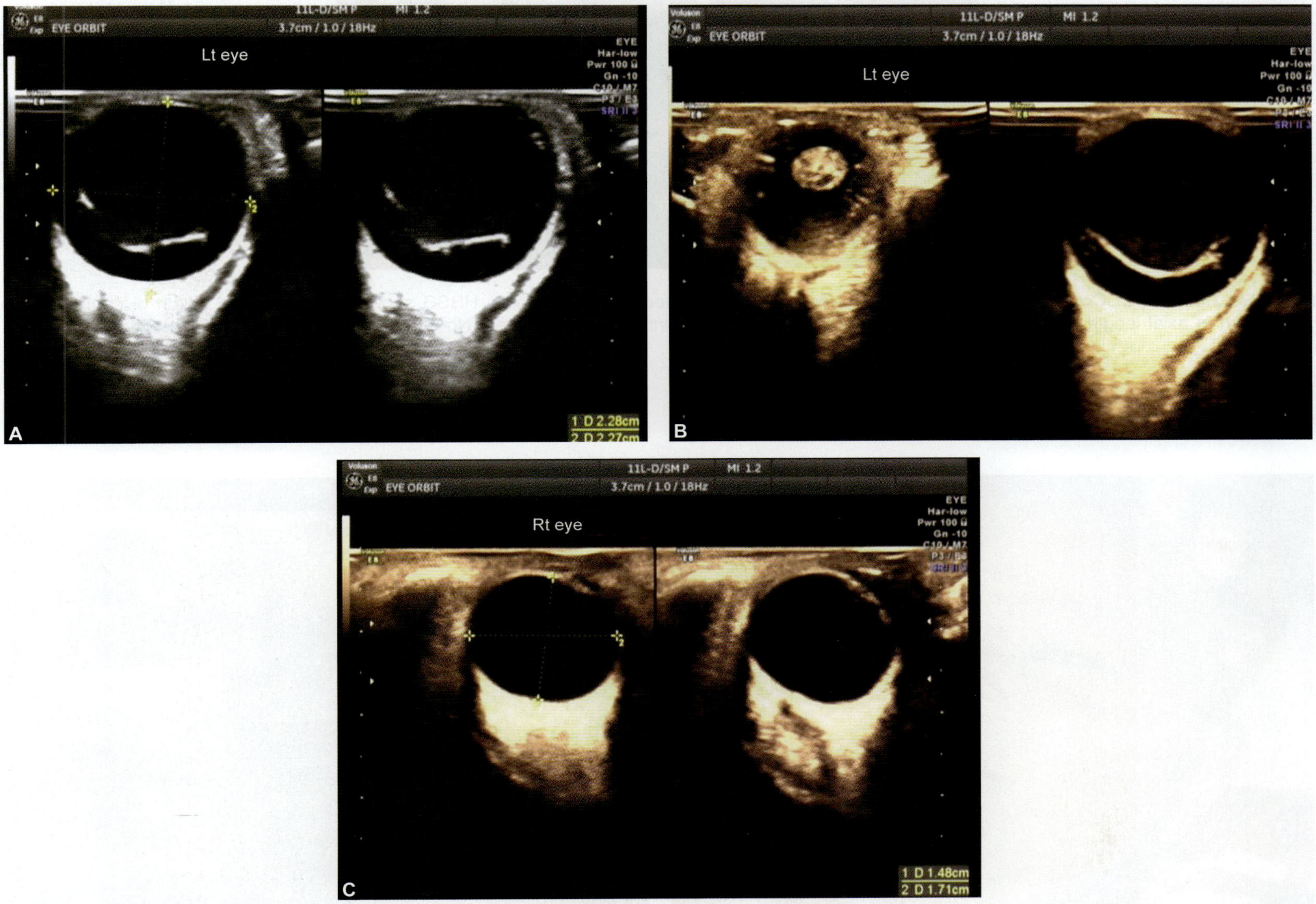

FIGURES 1.34A to C: Congenital glaucoma. A 4-month-baby presented with pseudo-proptosis in left eye. The axial length of the eye is increased. It is 22.8 mm. The lens is also thickened and opaque. An echogenic membrane is detached from its surface suggestive of associated retinal detachment. The right eye is normal on ultrasound.

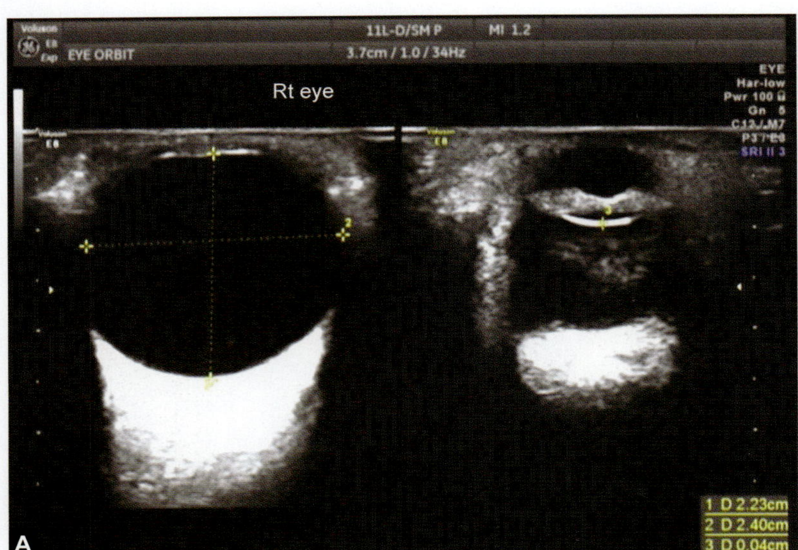

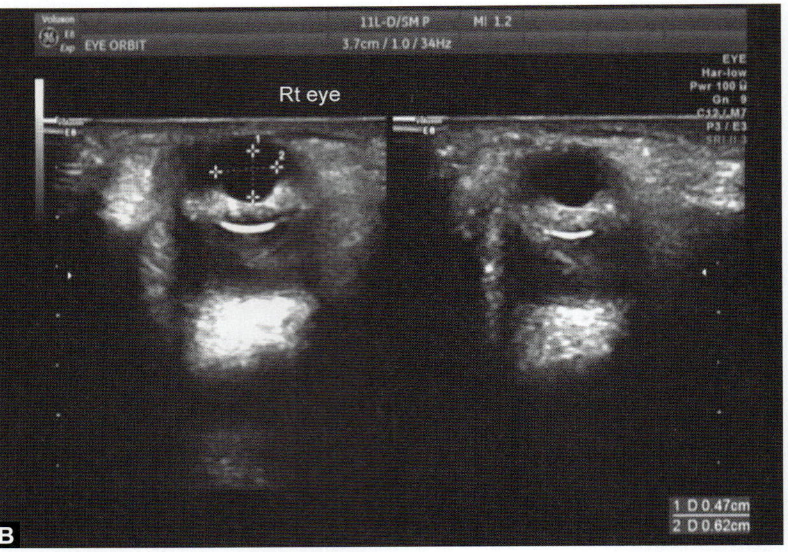

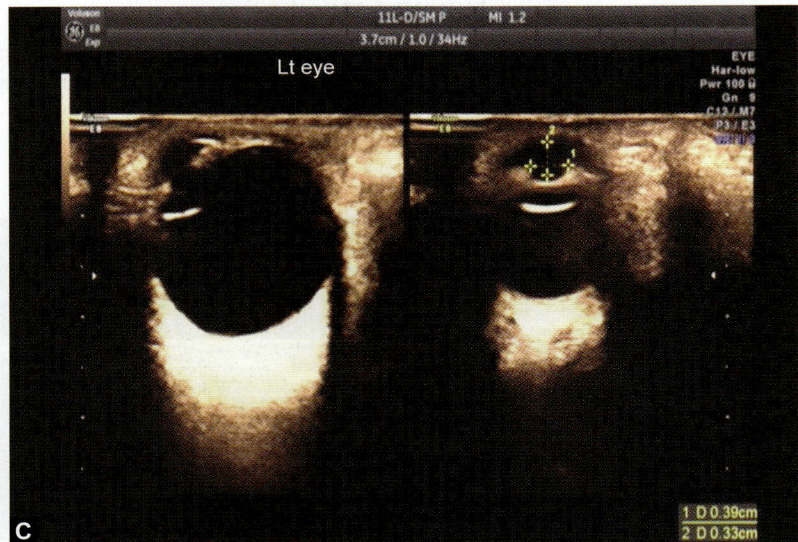

FIGURES 1.35A to C: Congenital Buphthalmos. A young child presented pseudoproptosis. HRSG shows increased axial length of right eye. It is 24 mm in axial length. Lens shows early thickening. Posterior segment of the eye is free. No intragel pathology is seen. left eye is normal.

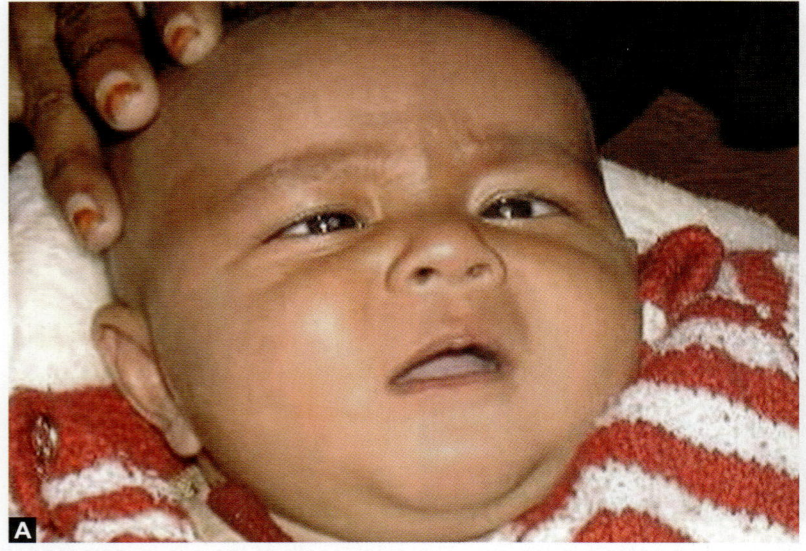

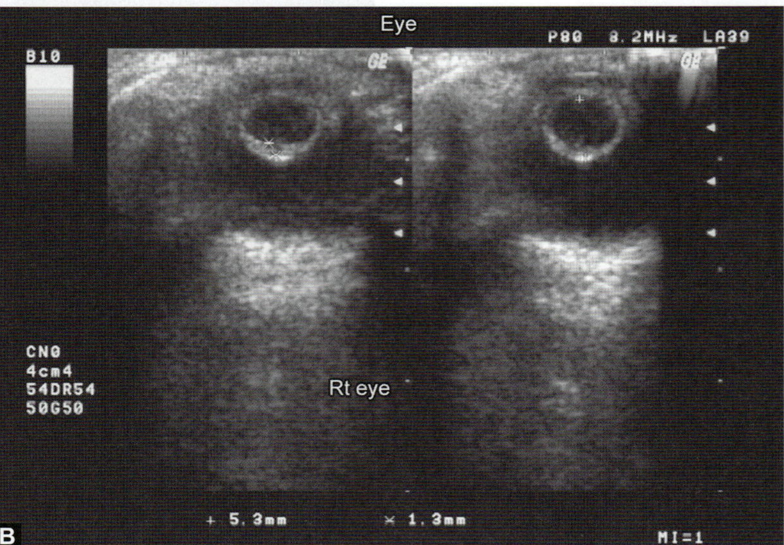

FIGURES 1.36A and B: Bilateral congenital cataract. An infant was born with white eye reflex in both eyes. HRSG shows echogenic thickened opaque lens in both eyes. Posterior segment of the eye is free.

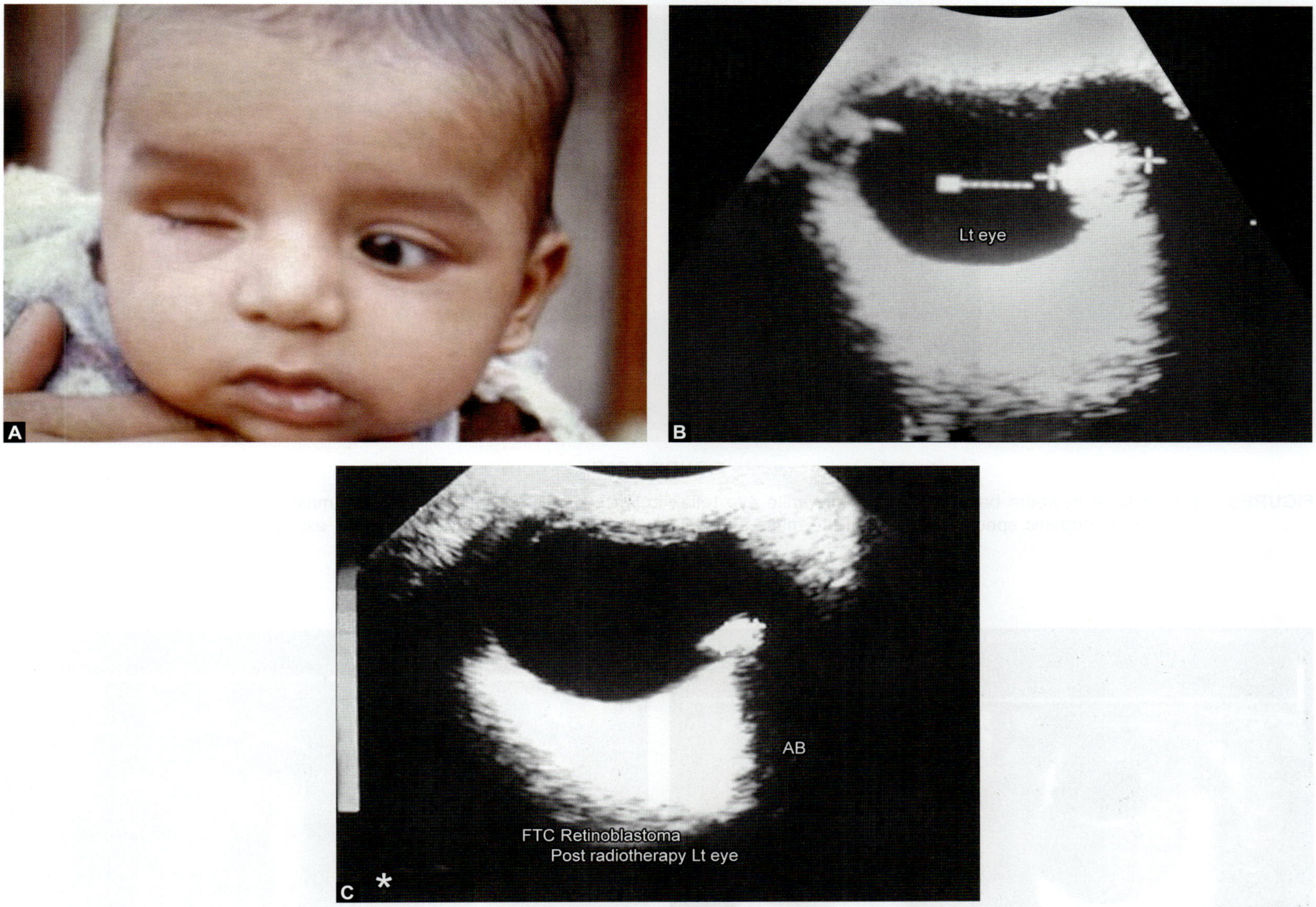

FIGURES 1.37A to C: An infant presented with congenital retinoblastoma in right eye, and it was operated. His father also had retinoblastoma in one eye. Another eye also showed white reflex after 3 month of his birth. HRSG shows an echogenic mass on temporal side with wide base typical of retinoblastoma. Post-teleradiotherapy—The mass has regressed in size. Echogenic calcification is seen at the base of the mass. HRSG is an excellent modality to evaluate treatment response. It is noninvasive, cost effective and does not require any sedation.

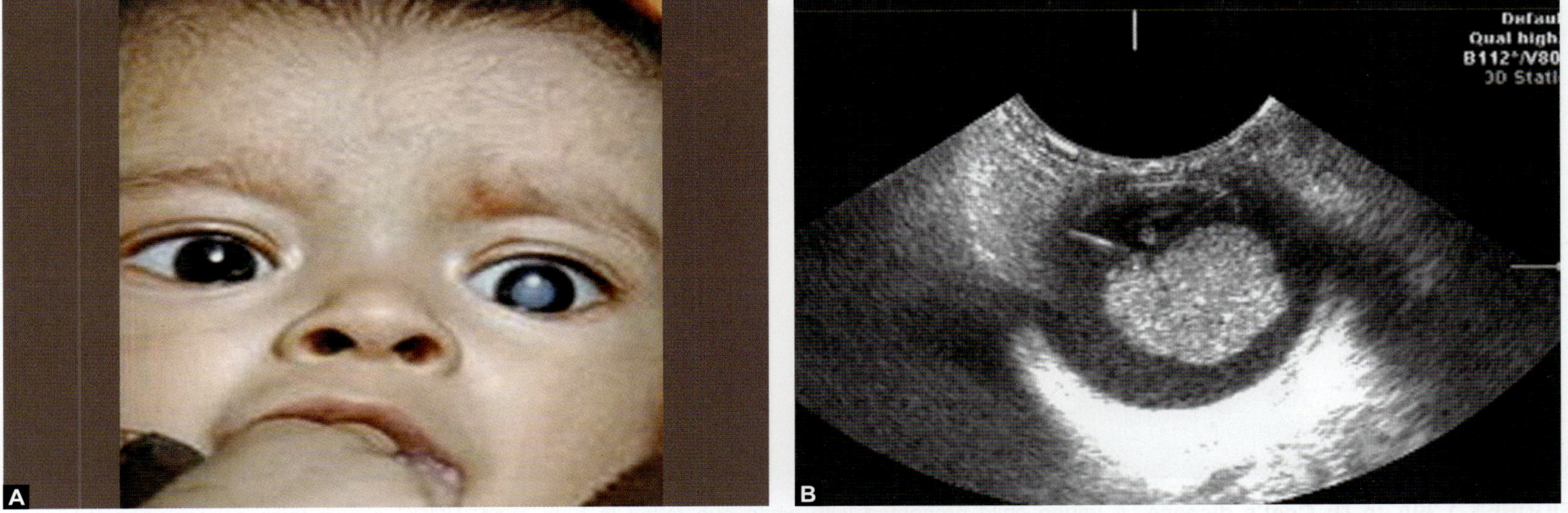

FIGURES 1.38A and B

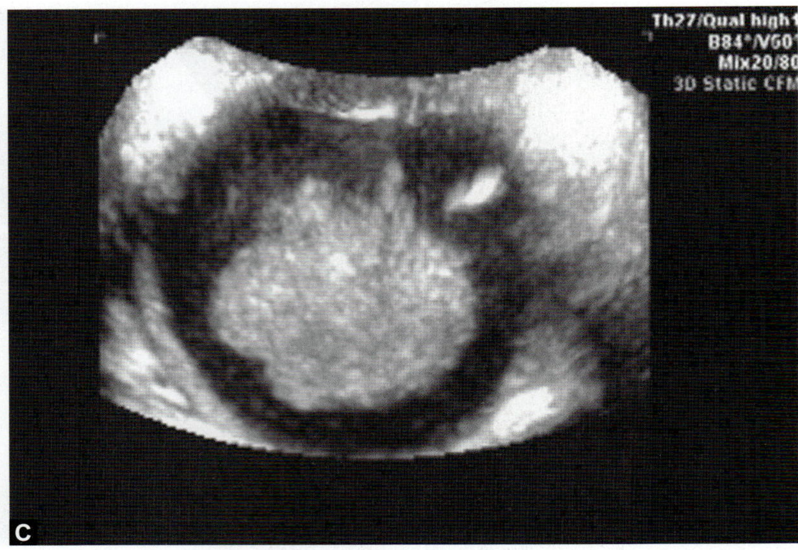

FIGURE 1.38C

FIGURES 1.38A to C: A newborn baby presented with white eye reflex in left eye. HRSG shows soft tissue mass in the posterior segment of the eye. Echogenic specks are seen in the mass suggestive of retinoblastoma. But no choroidal excavation is seen.

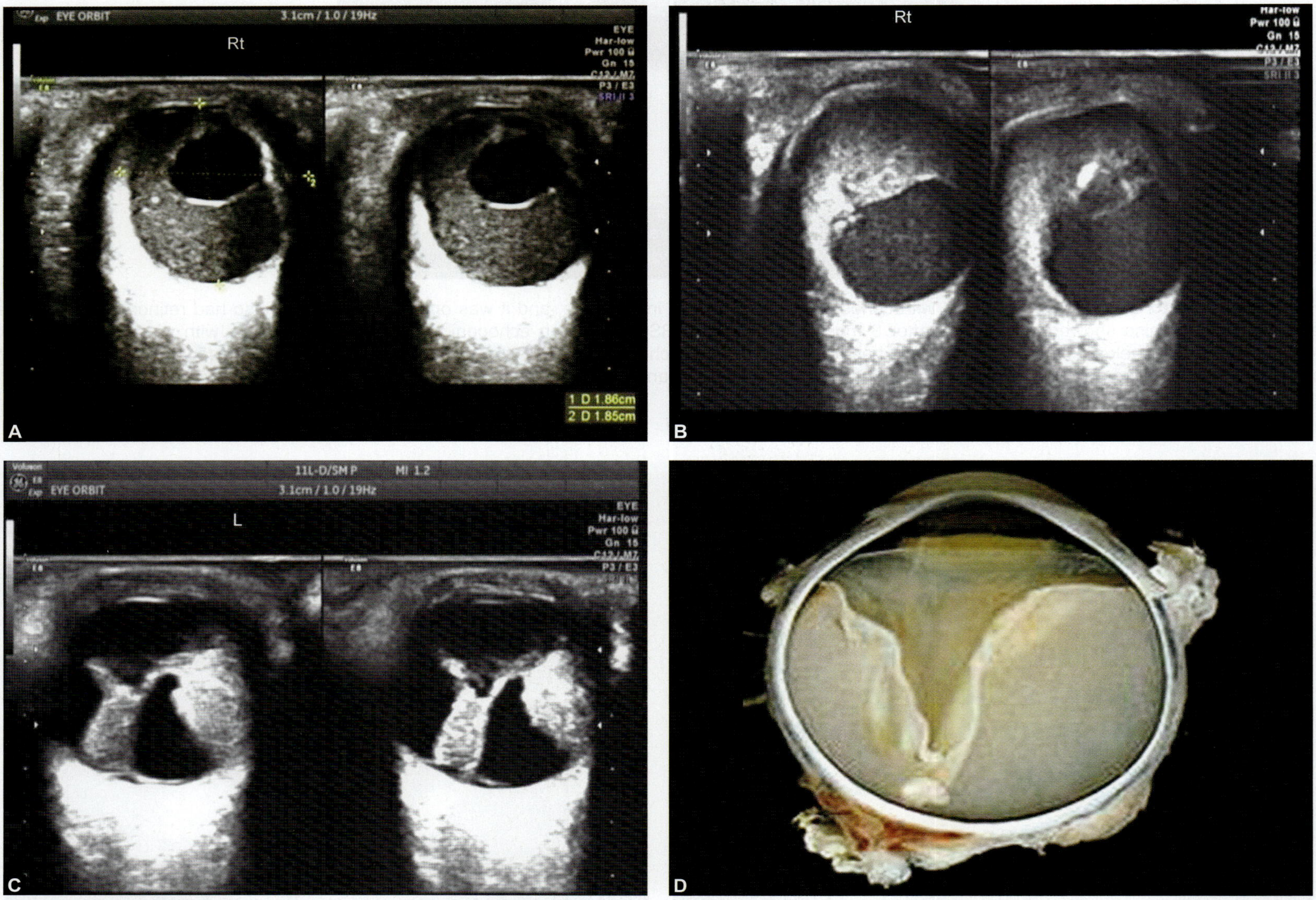

FIGURES 1.39A to D: Coat's disease. A young child presented with white eye reflex in both eyes. HRSG shows thick echogenic membranous shadows in the posterior segment of the eye. Exudative deposition is seen on the membrane suggestive of exudative retinal detachment (Coat's Disease). Figure D shows cuts section of the eye confirming the diagnosis.

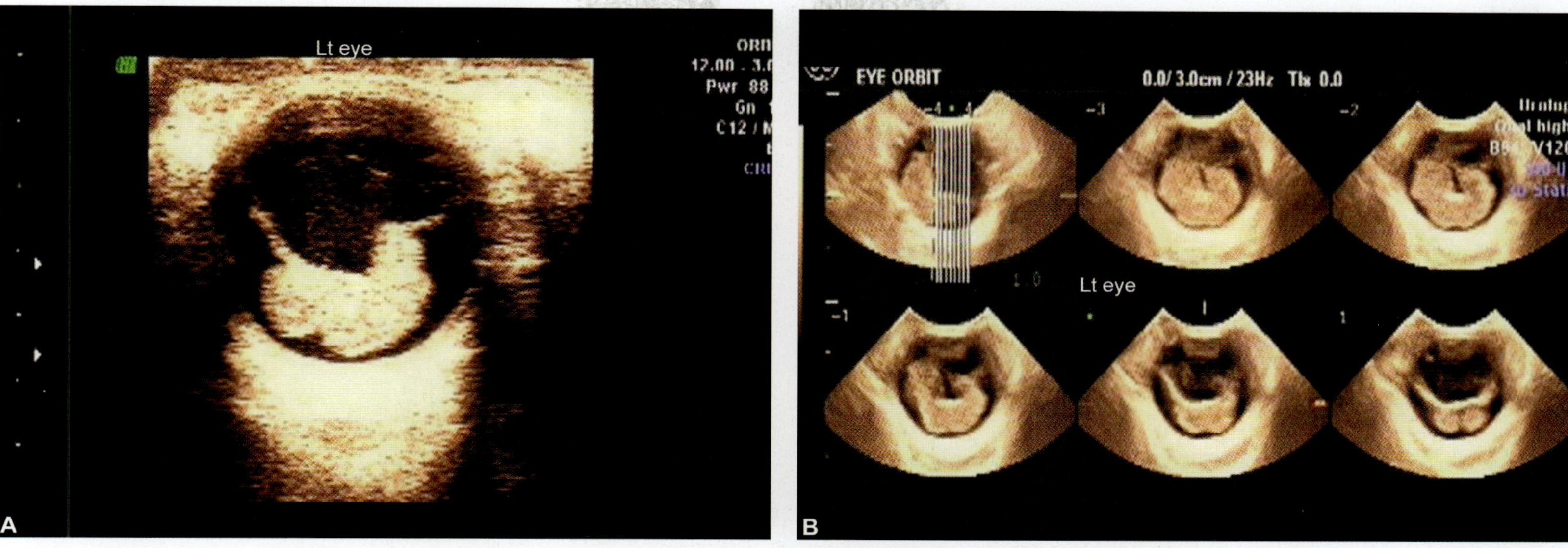

FIGURES 1.40A and B: Exudative retinal detachment. HRSG shows thick membranous shadows in the posterior segment of left eye in a patient presented with white eye reflex. Thick exudative deposits are seen on retina suggestive of Coat's disease.

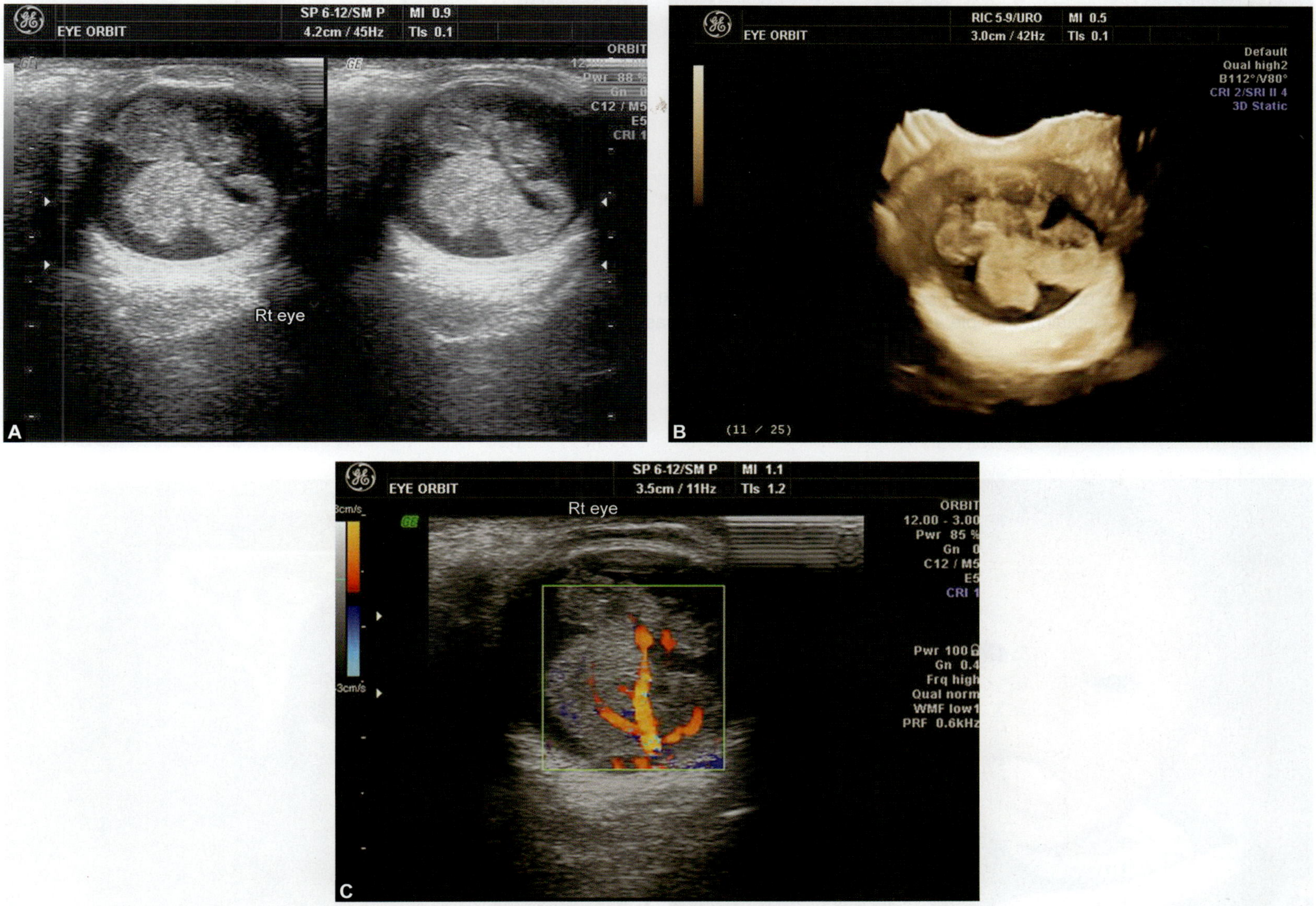

FIGURES 1.41A to C: Coats's disease with retinal artery. HRSG shows thick echogenic membranous shadow in the posterior segment of right eye in a patient presented with white eye reflex. The thick membrane shows folding of retina with exudative deposits. On color flow imaging, the retinal artery is seen pulled up in the membrane suggestive of Coat's disease.

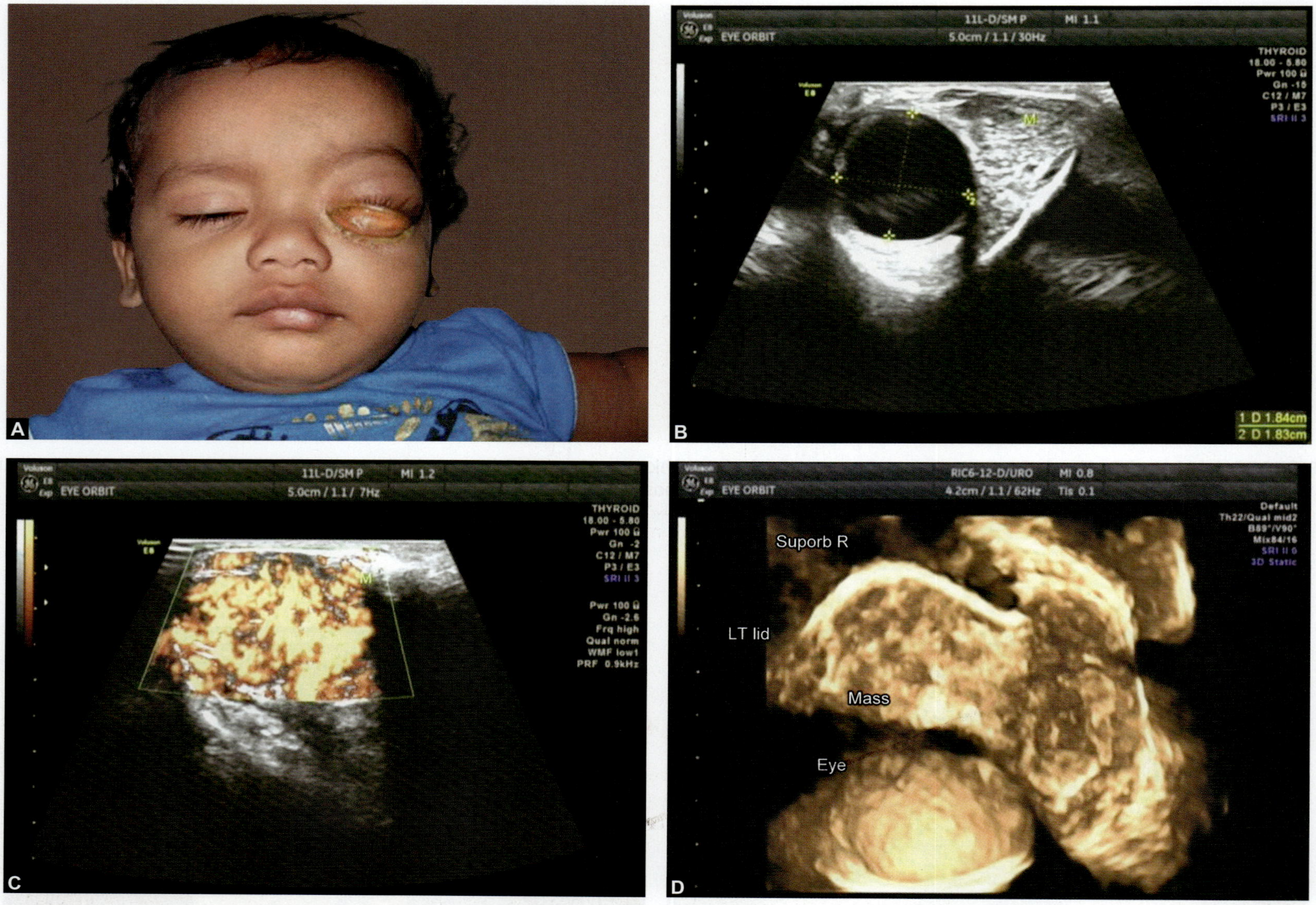

FIGURES 1.42A to D: A baby is born with soft tissue swelling over the left lower lid of left eye. HRSG shows a soft tissue membranous shadow over the left lid. On color flow imaging, multiple vessels are seen feeding the mass. However, the eye is normal. The mass appears to be hemangiomatous mass.

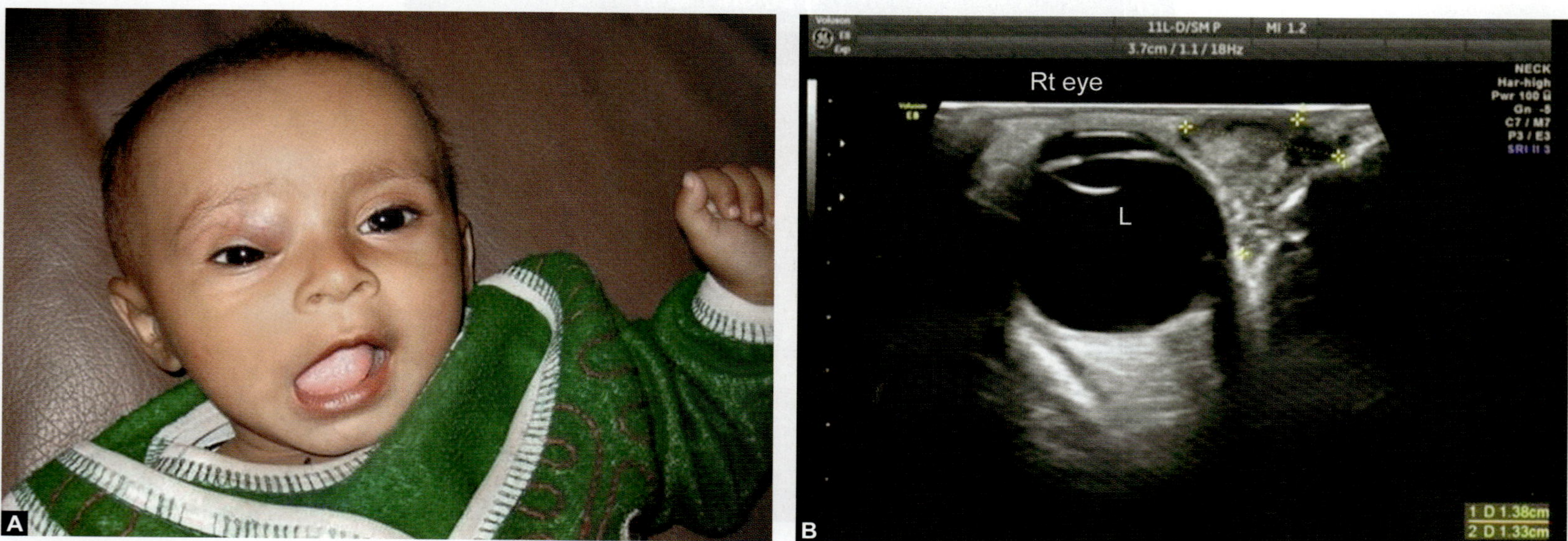

FIGURES 1.43A and B

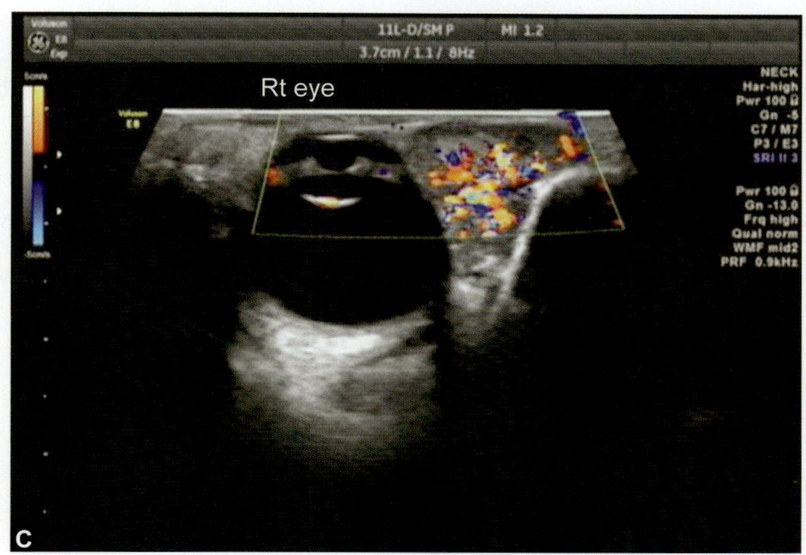

FIGURE 1.43C

FIGURES 1.43A to C: An 8-month-old baby presented with soft tissue swelling over right upper inner orbit. HRSG shows a homogeneous mass in the medial side of orbit. No calcification or cystic degeneration is seen in the mass. On color flow imaging, multiple vessels are seen feeding the mass suggestive of vascular mass. However, the eye is normal.

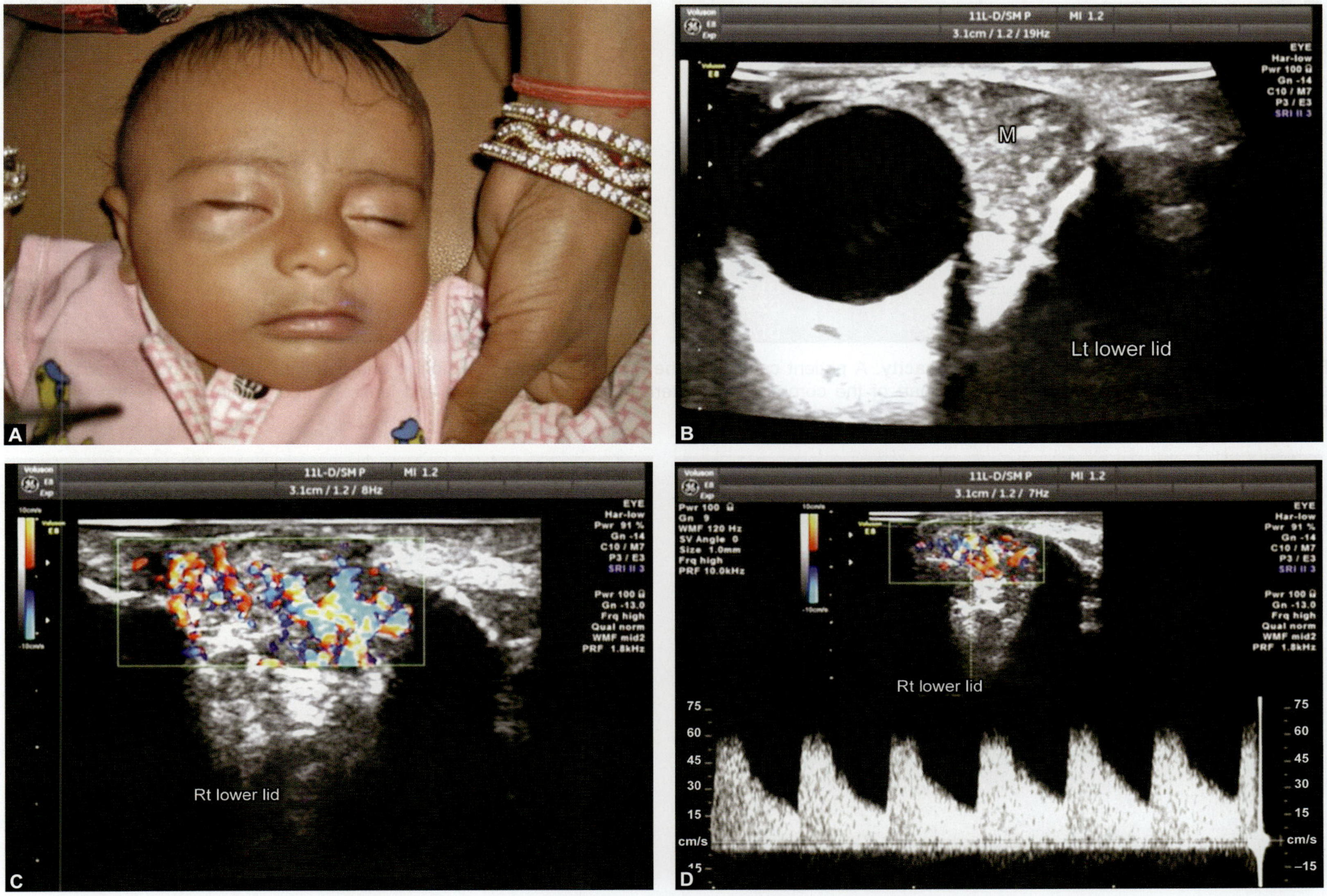

FIGURES 1.44A to D: A 3-month-old baby presented with soft tissue swelling over right lower lid. Multiple vessels are seen feeding the mass. On spectral Doppler tracing, moderate arterial flow is seen in the mass suggestive of highly vascular mass.

Acquired Pathologies

All the pathological conditions where direct ophthalmoscopy is not possible are the indications for HRSG. They are grouped as under.

Opaque Ocular Media

Anterior segment: The anterior segment can be very well evaluated with high-resolution sonography. Following are the main conditions, which can be easily evaluated on HRSG:

i. Corneal opacification
ii. Hyphema or hypopyon
iii. Miosis
iv. Cataract
v. Pupillary or retrolental membrane

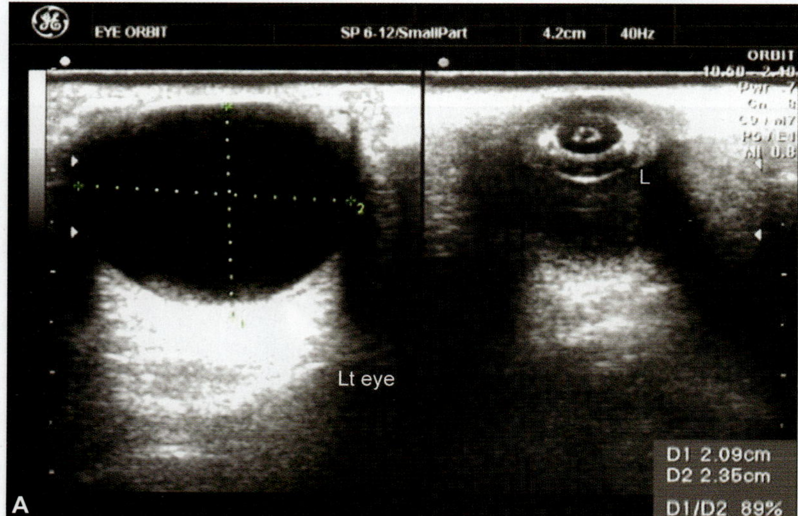

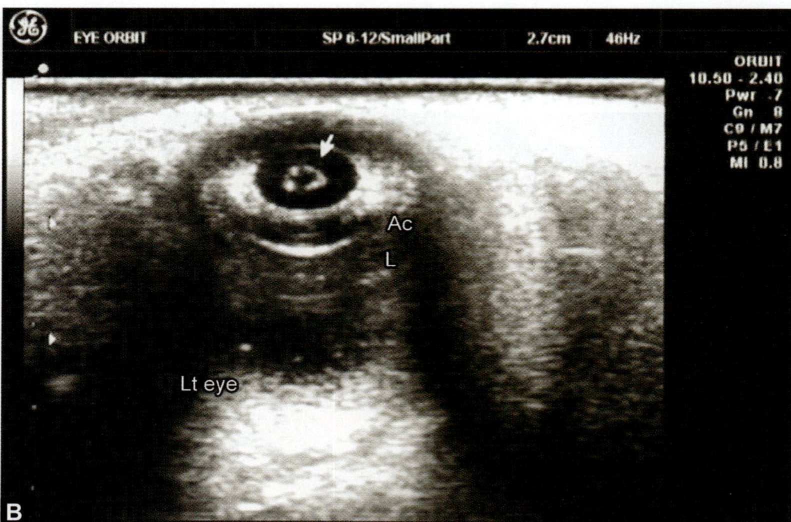

FIGURES 1.45A and B: Central corneal opacity. A patient came with the marked diminished vision in one eye with central corneal opacity. HRSG shows an echogenic shadow in the central part of the cornea. The posterior segment of the eye and lens are free. 3D imaging of the eye shows final details of the corneal opacity.

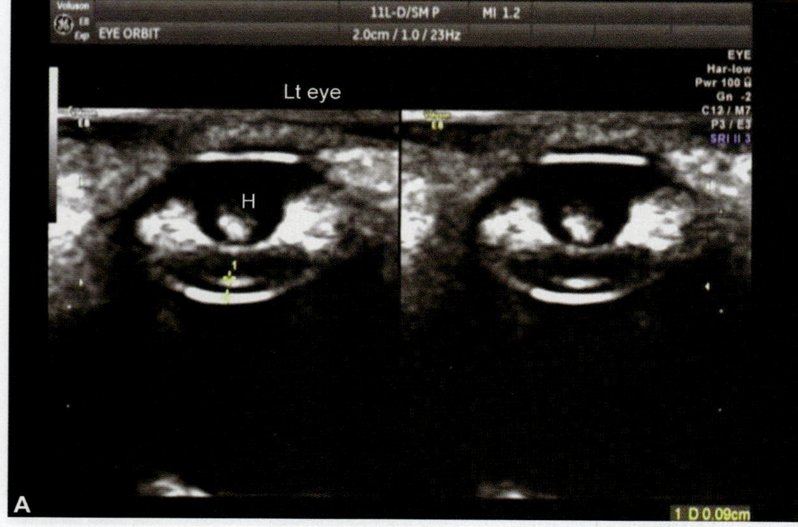

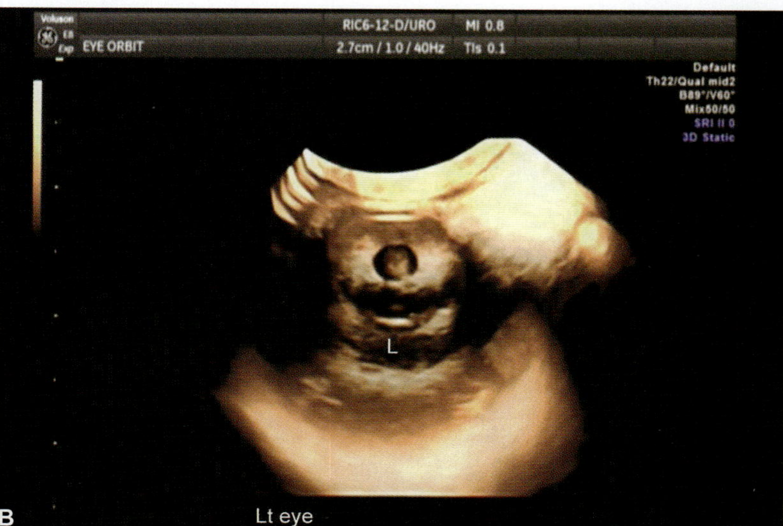

FIGURES 1.46A and B

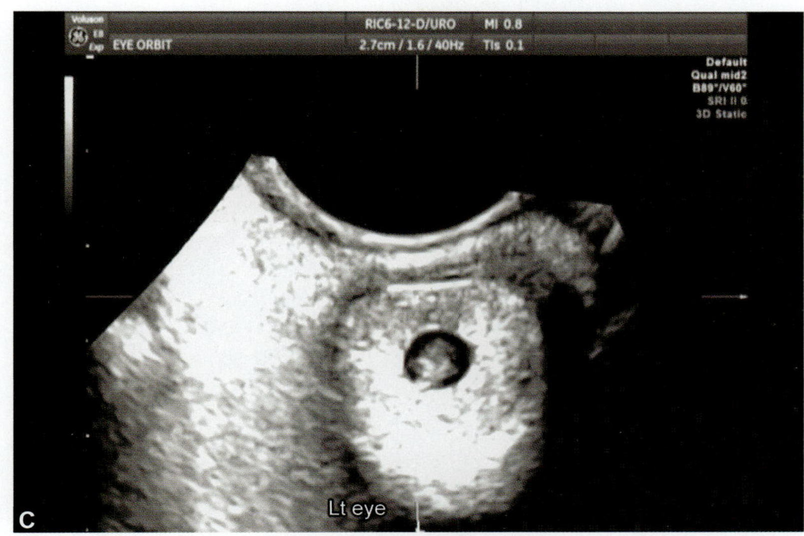

FIGURE 1.46C

FIGURES 1.46A to C: Anterior chamber hyphema. A patient presented with blurring of vision. HRSG shows echogenic collection in the anterior chamber suggestive of anterior chamber hyphema. 3D imaging shows the hemorrhage in the anterior chamber. Early thickening of the lens is also seen.

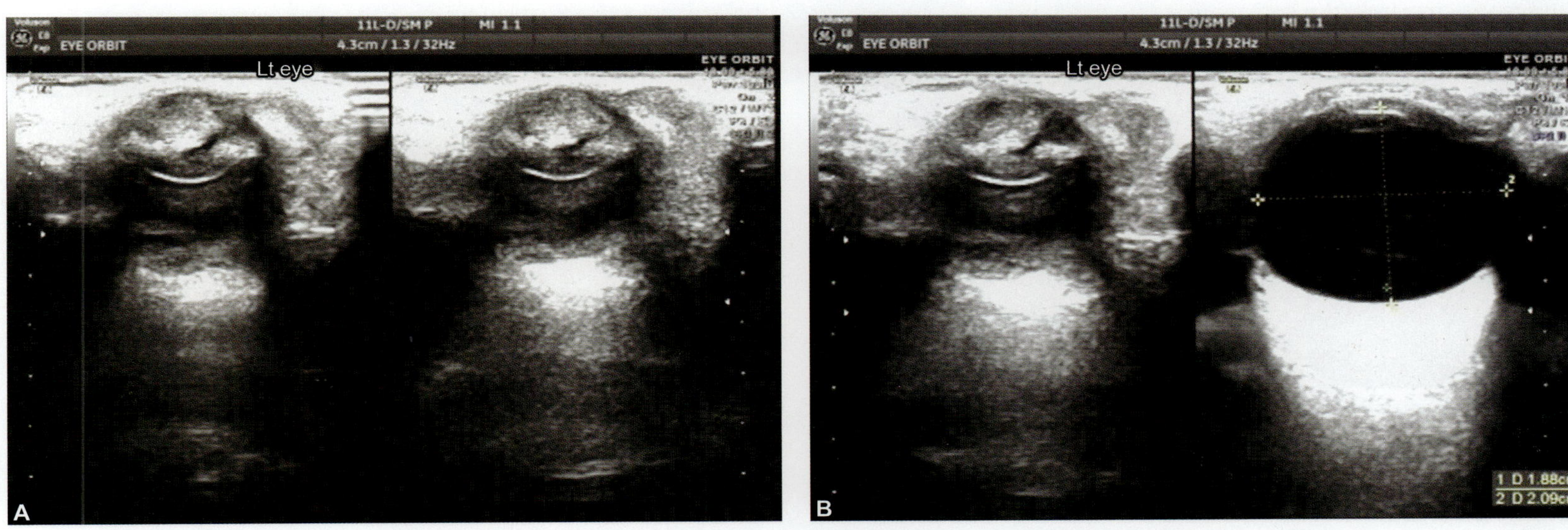

FIGURES 1.47A and B: Anterior chamber hyphema. HRSG shows hemorrhagic blood in the anterior chamber of left eye. It is echogenic in texture suggestive of fresh hemorrhage.

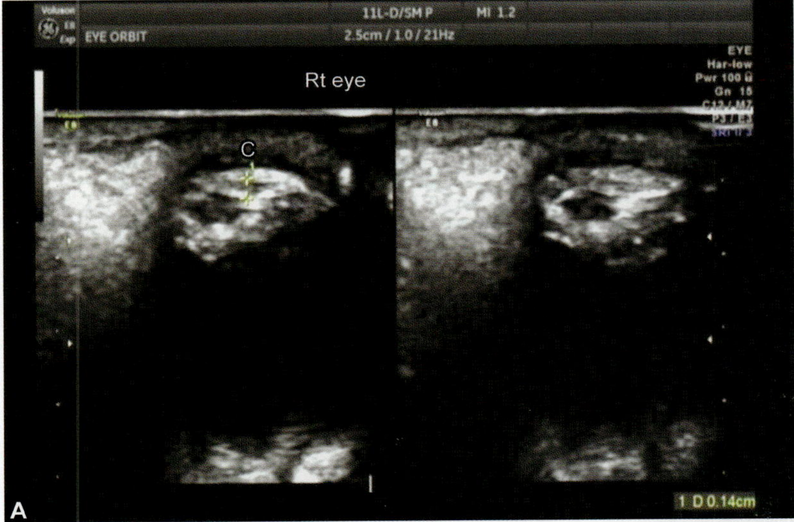

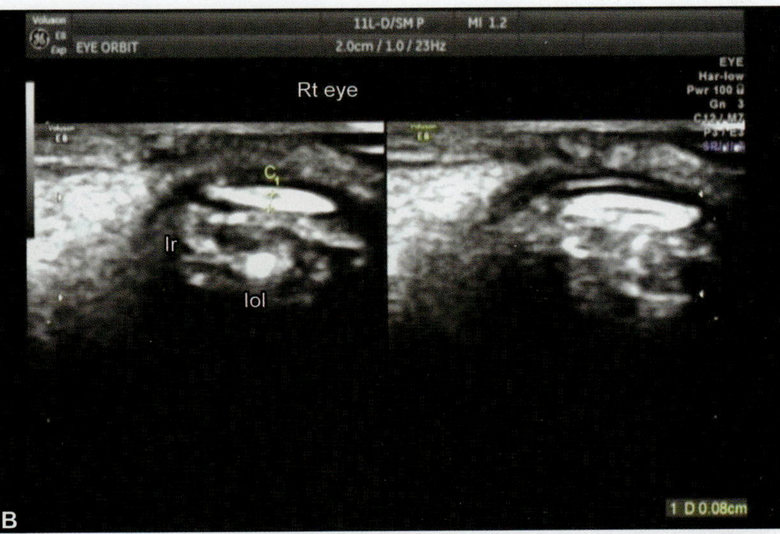

FIGURES 1.48A and B

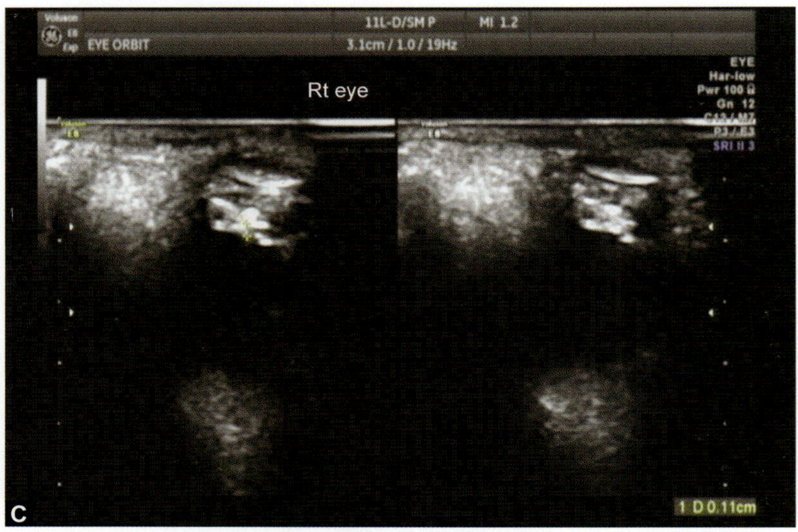

FIGURE 1.48C

FIGURES 1.48A to C: Thickened opaque cornea. HRSG shows thickened opaque cornea in the right eye. The intraocular lens (IOL) is seen as an echogenic shadow posterior to the cornea. The Iris is also thickened and irregular in outline. However, posterior segment of the eye is free.

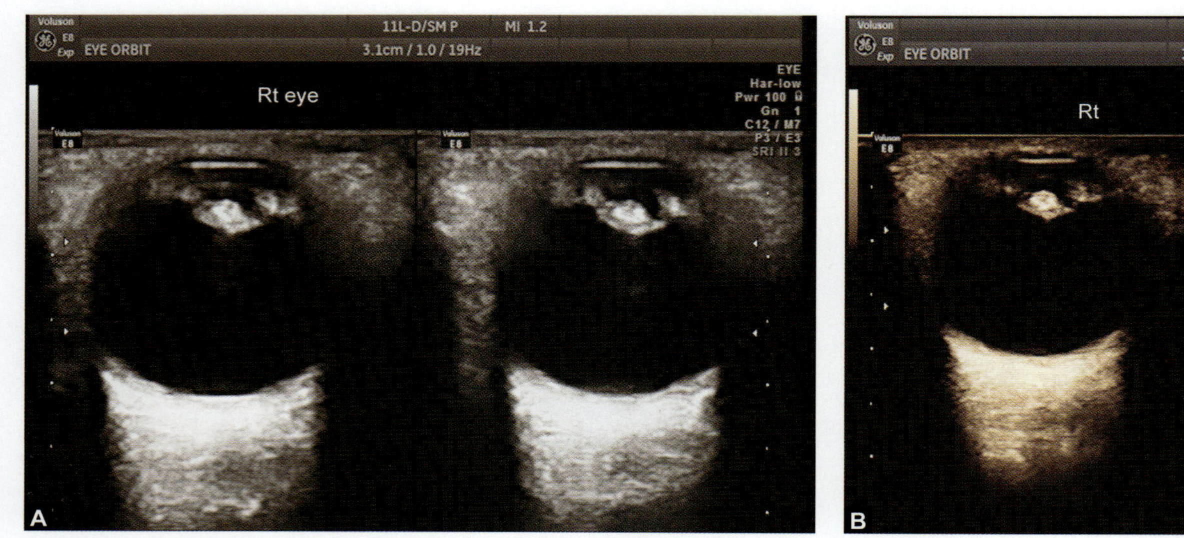

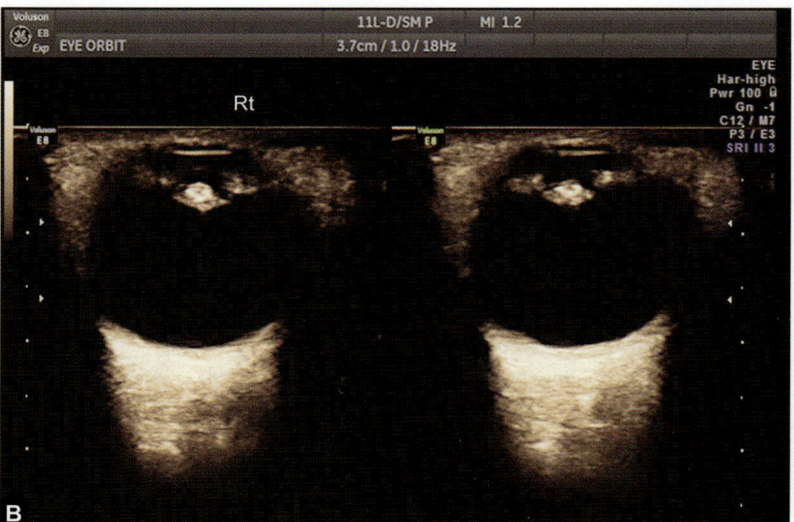

FIGURES 1.49A and B: Congenital cataract. A young child presented with white eye reflex. HRSG shows thickened opaque lens in the eye. The nucleus is calcified. The posterior segment of the eye is free.

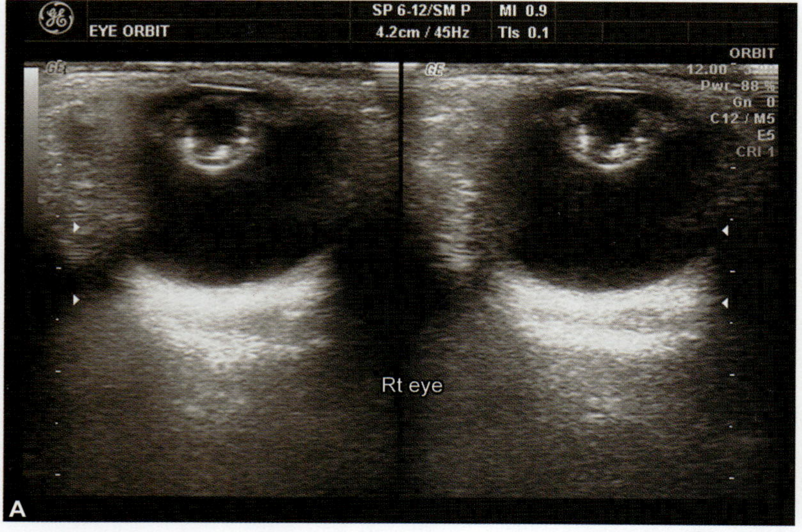

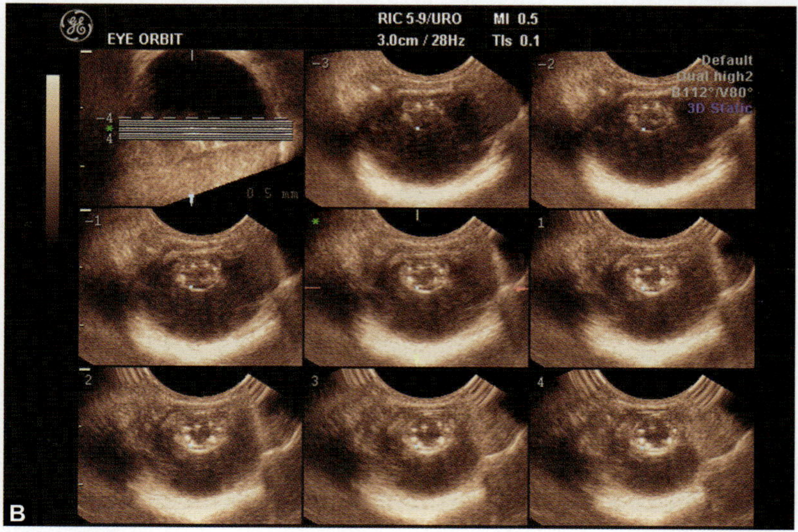

FIGURES 1.50A and B

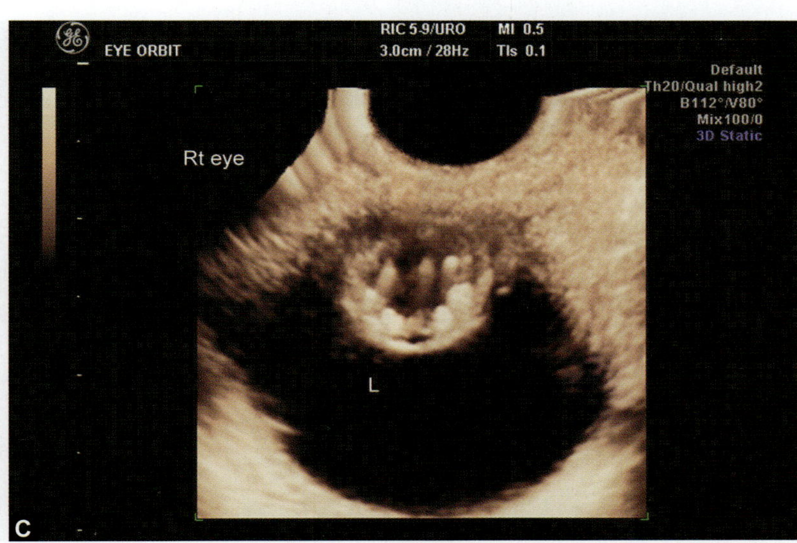

FIGURE 1.50C

FIGURES 1.50A to C: Congenital cataract. A young child presented with thickened opaque lens in right eye. The lens is markedly thickened. Multiple calcified specks are seen in the lens. On 3D imaging, detail of calcification is seen beautifully. Posterior segment of the eye is free.

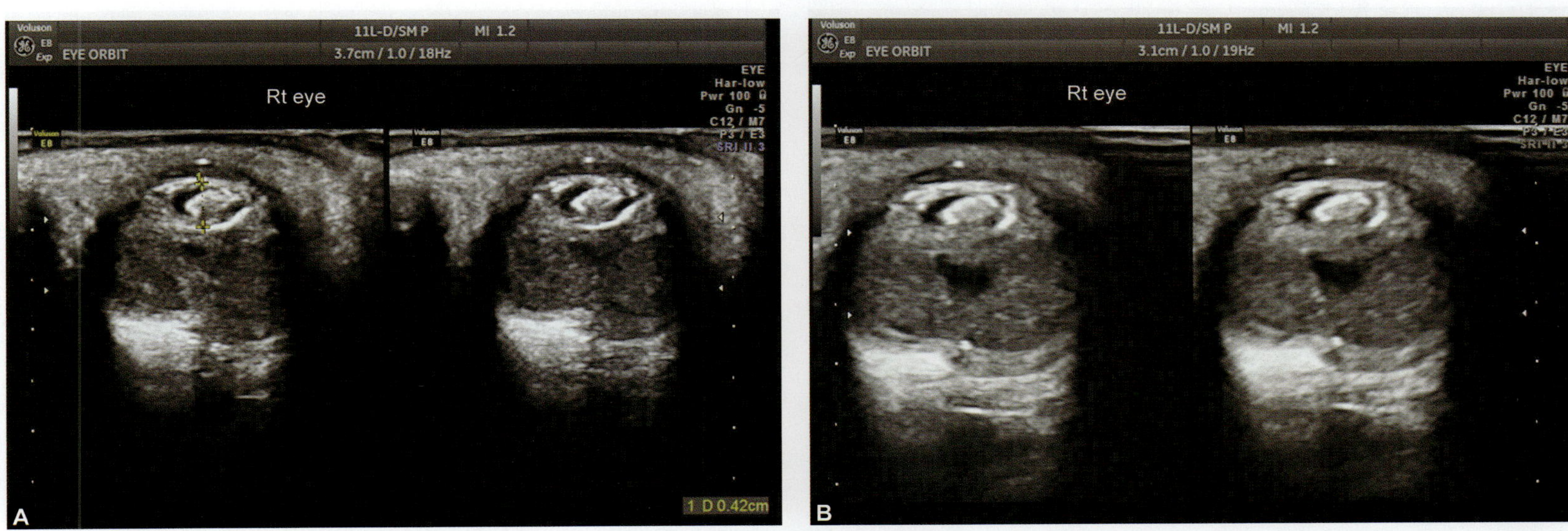

FIGURES 1.51A and B: Calcification of the nucleus. A young child presented with a loss of vision after injury to the eye. HRSG shows thickened opaque lens with densely calcification nucleus. It is highly echogenic. Posterior segment of the eye also shows intragel collection suggestive of intragel hemorrhage. The eye coat is edematous.

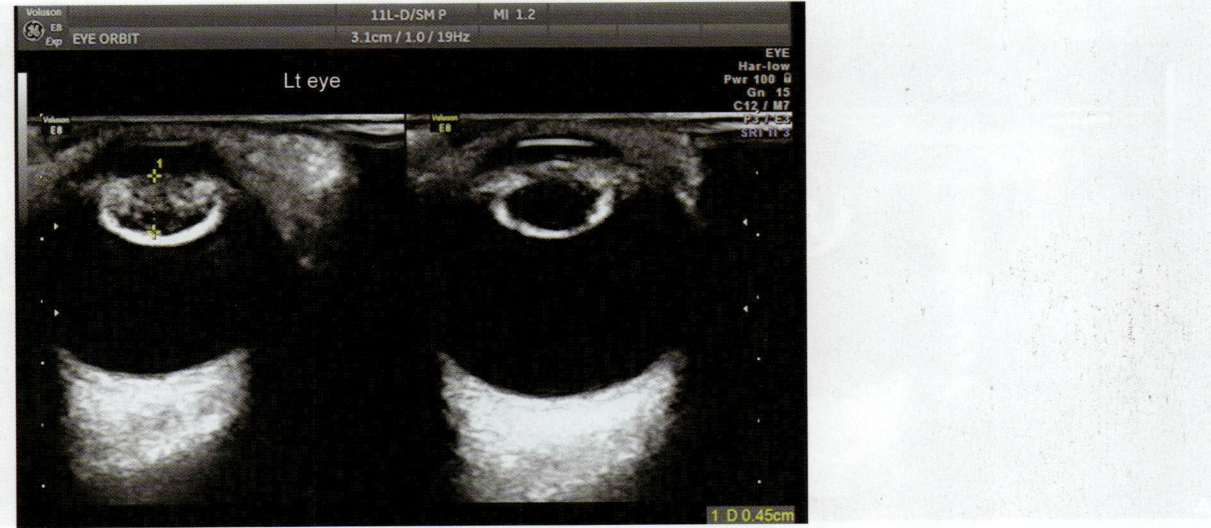

FIGURE 1.52: Mature cataract. An 18-year-old boy presented with grossly diminished vision. HRSG shows markedly thickened lens. It is 4.5 mm in thickness. Internal echoes are seen in the lens suggestive of mature cataract.

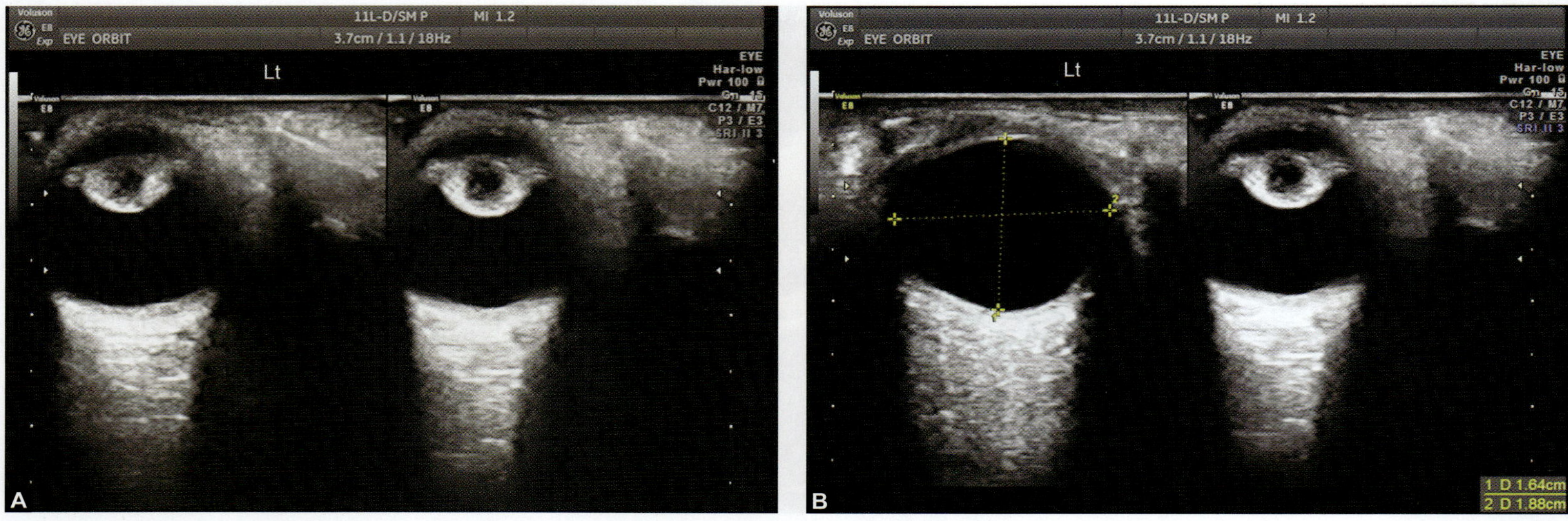

FIGURES 1.53A and B: Mature congenital cataract. A 1-year-old baby presented with white eye reflex. HRSG shows markedly thickened opaque lens with swollen capsule. However, posterior segment of the eye is free.

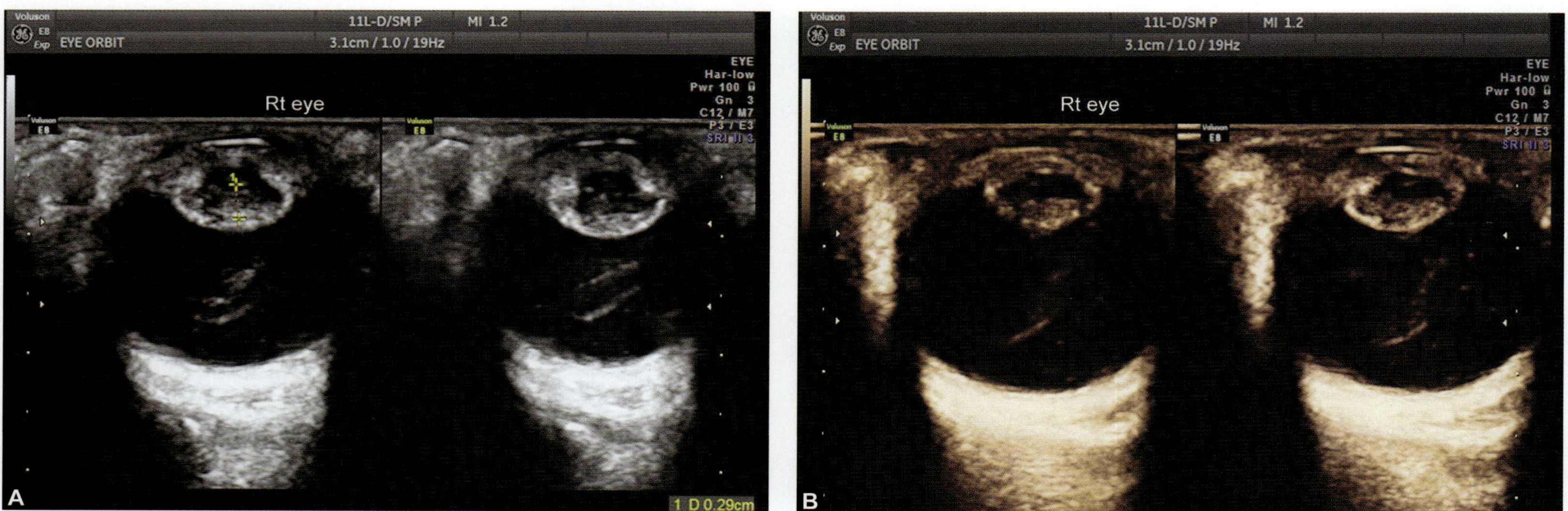

FIGURES 1.54A and B: Thickened opaque lens with swollen nucleus. HRSG shows markedly thickened opaque lens in a 6-year-old child. The nucleus shows tumefaction. Posterior segment of the eye shows low level intragel opacities suggestive of subtle intragel haemorrhage.

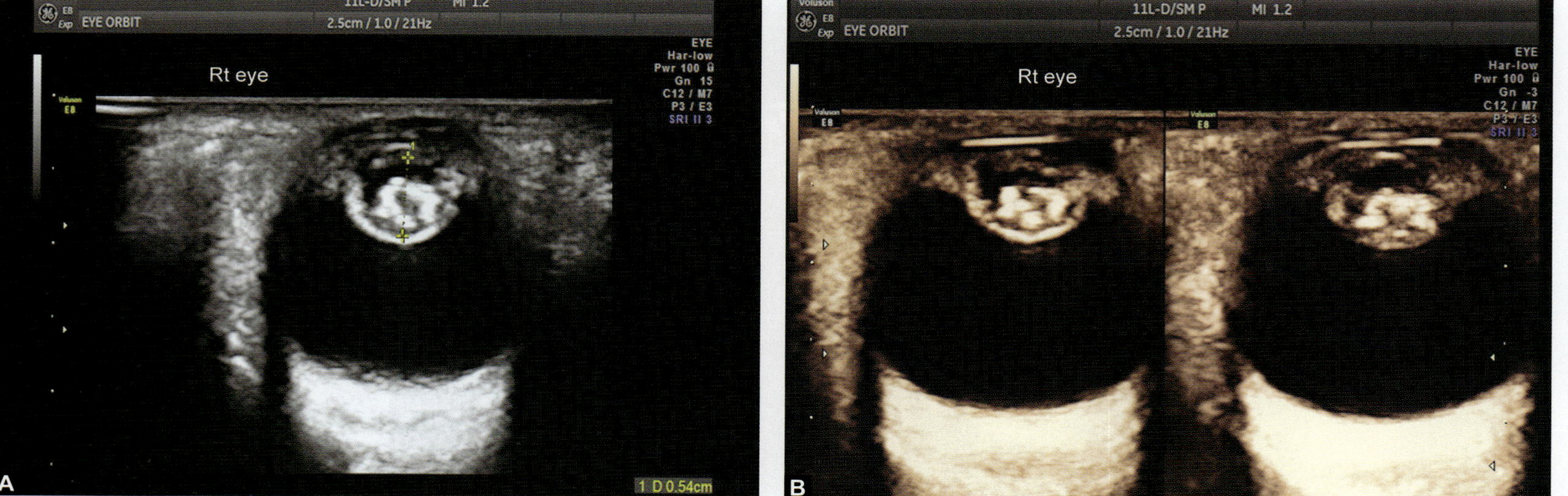

FIGURES 1.55A and B: Congenital cataract. Densely calcified nucleus. A 1-year-old baby girl presented with markedly thickened opaque lens. The nucleus is markedly calcified and multiple calcified specks are seen in nucleus. However, posterior segment of the eye is free. No intragel pathology is seen.

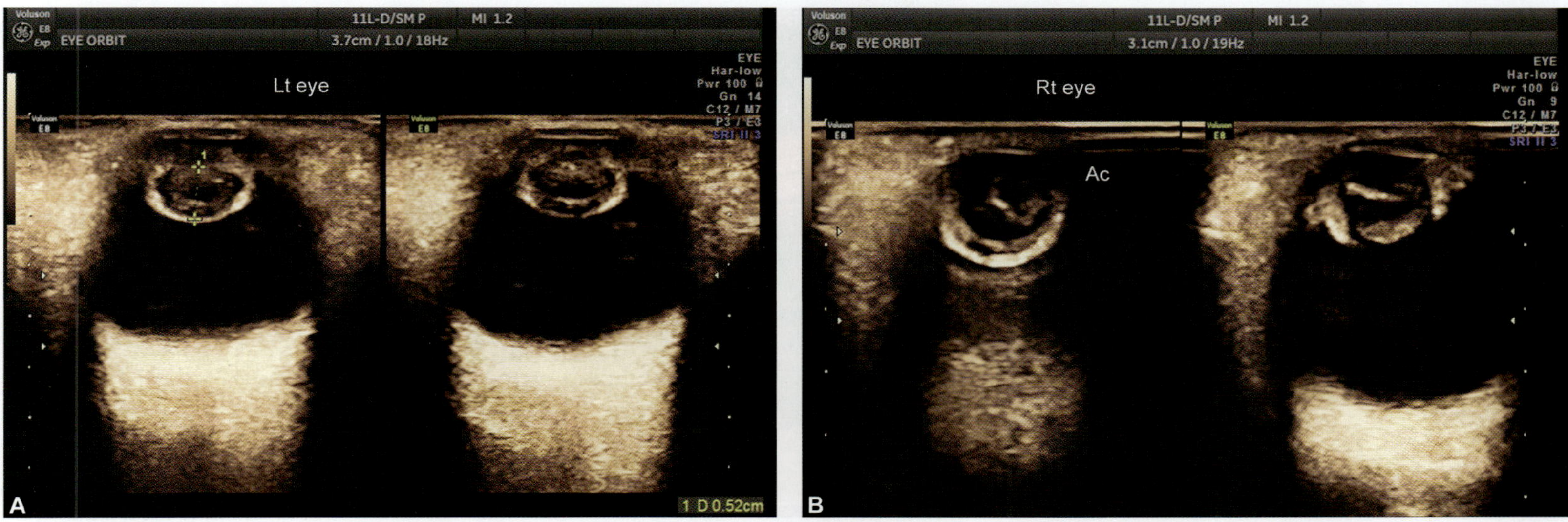

FIGURES 1.56A and B: Hypermature cataract. A 60-year-old lady presented with loss of vision. HRSG shows markedly thickened lens with calcification of anterior and posterior capsule of the lens. FIGURE A shows hypermature cataract in 7-year-old child. The anterior chamber also shows echogenic shadows suggestive of anterior chamber hyphema.

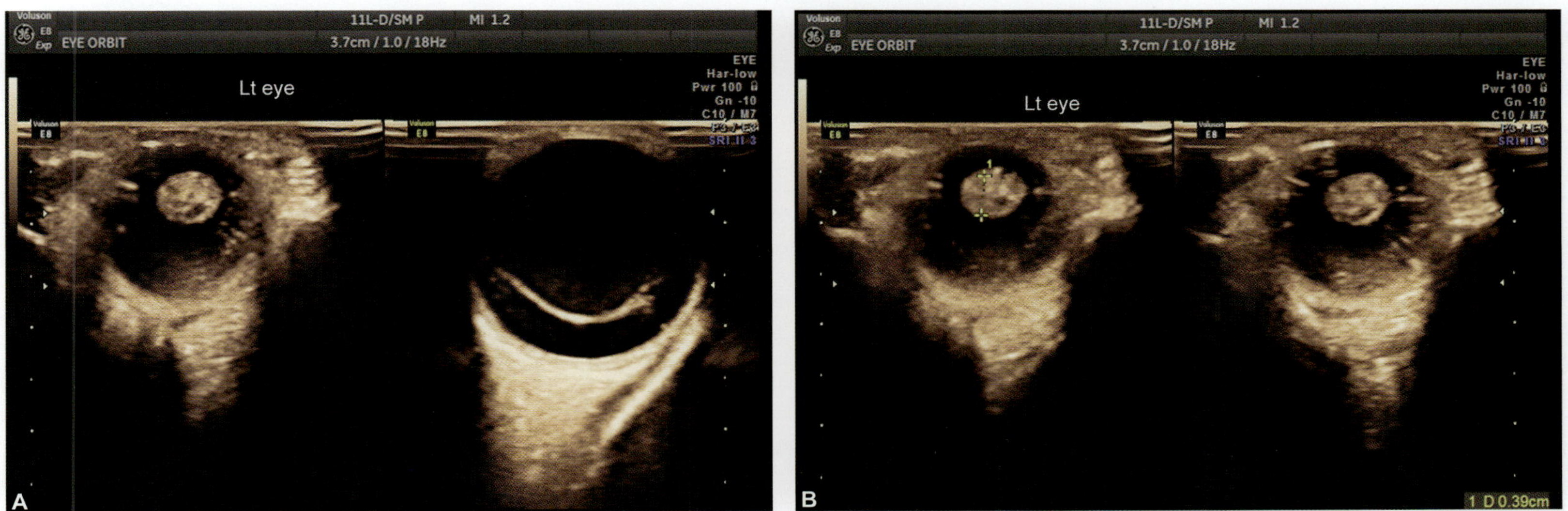

FIGURES 1.57A and B: Hypermature cataract with retinal detachment (RD). A 4-month-old baby presented with white eye reflex. HRSG shows markedly thickened lens which shows dense echoes. Posterior segment of the eye shows a thick membrane seen detached from its surface suggestive of total retinal detachment.

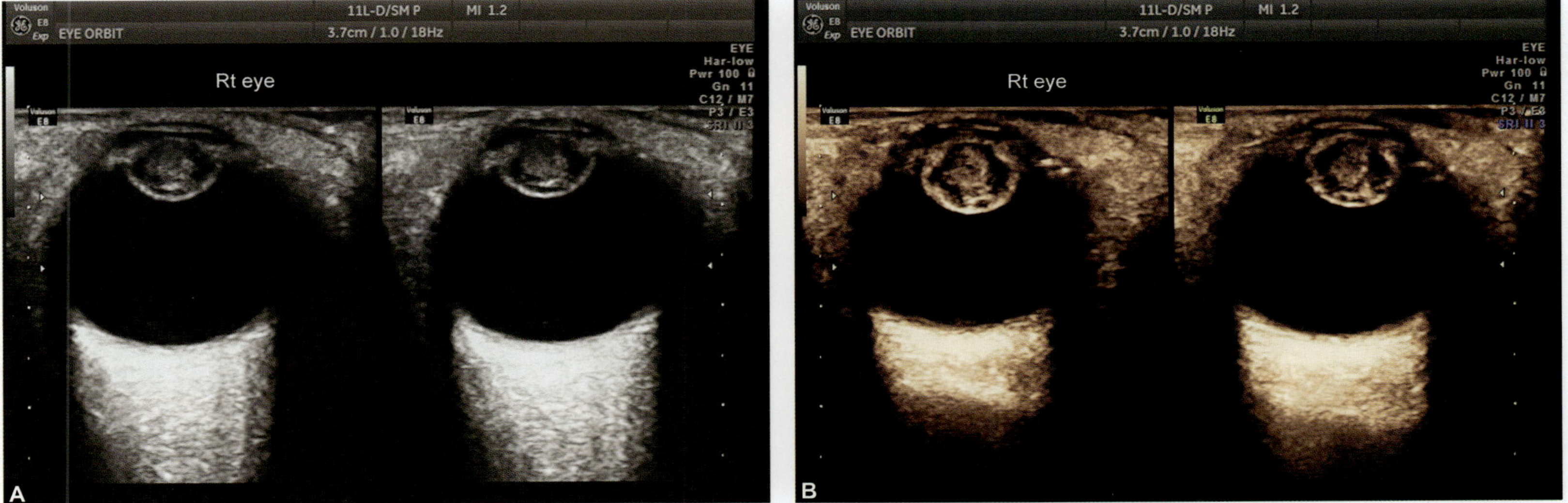

FIGURES 1.58A and B

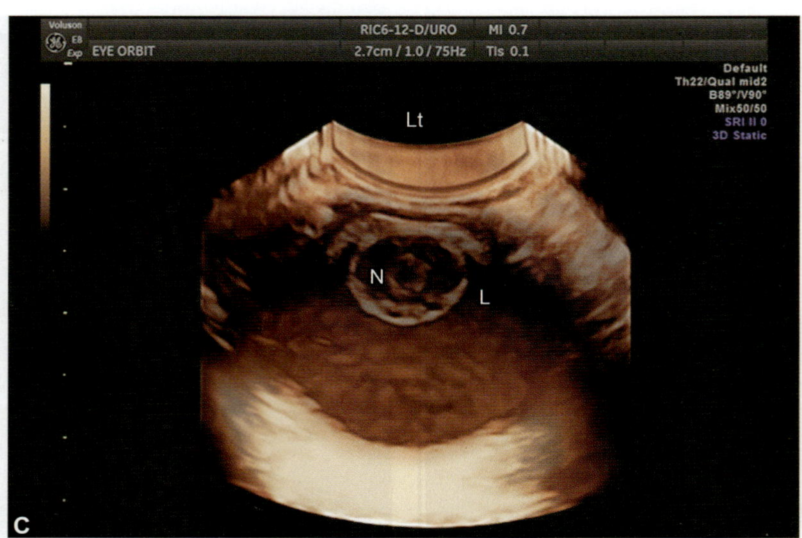

FIGURE 1.58C

FIGURES 1.58A to C: Post-traumatic cataract. A 20-year-old girl presented with eye trauma with loss of vision. HRSG shows markedly thickened opaque lens. Tumefaction of the lens is also seen, which is clearly seen on 3D imaging in Figure C.

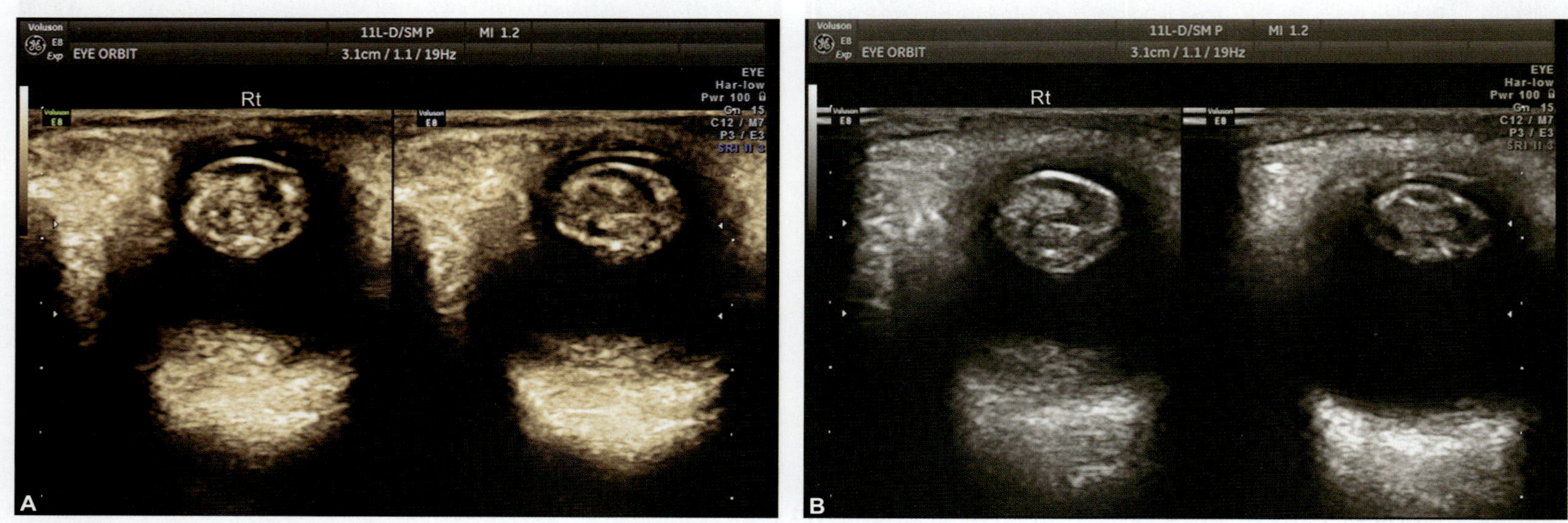

FIGURES 1.59A and B: Hard calcified lens. HRSG shows markedly thickened opaque lens in a 17-year-old girl. Calcified specks are also seen in the lens. The posterior segment of the eye shows intragel collection suggestive of intragel hemorrhage.

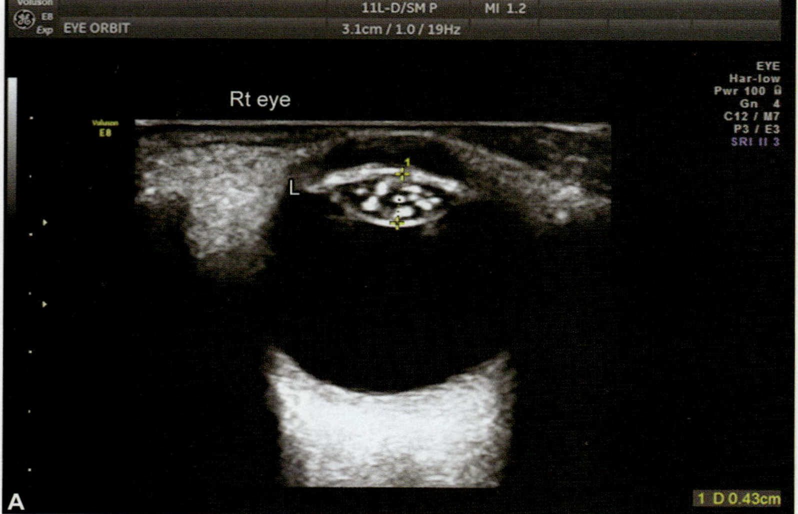

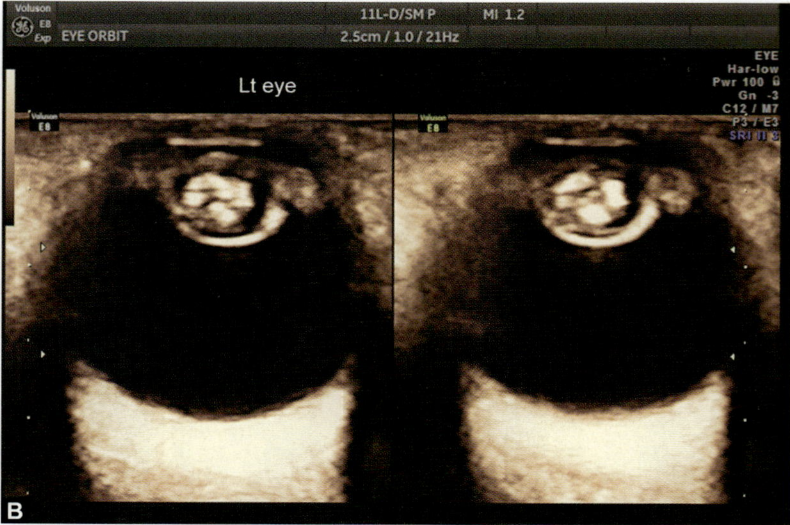

FIGURES 1.60A and B

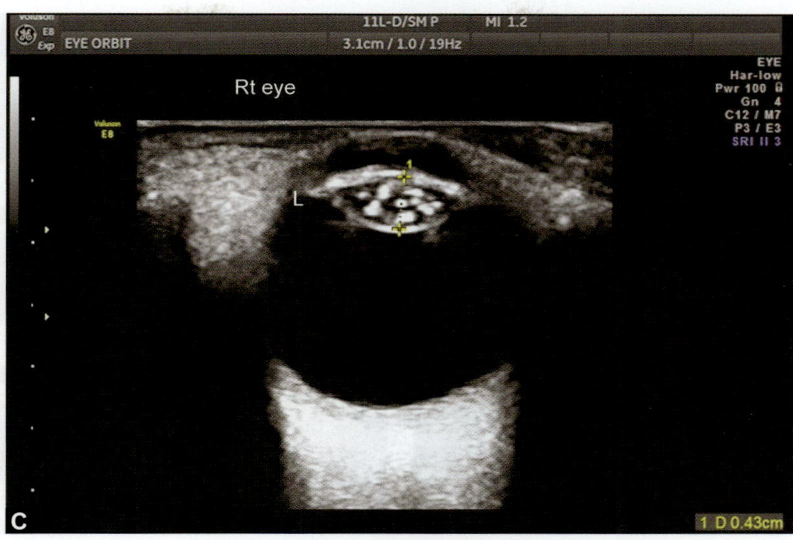

FIGURE 1.60C

FIGURES 1.60A to C: Dense calcified cataract. HRSG shows a thickened opaque lens. The lens is 4.3 mm in thickness. Multiple echogenic calcified specks are seen in the substance of the lens suggestive of hypermature cataract.

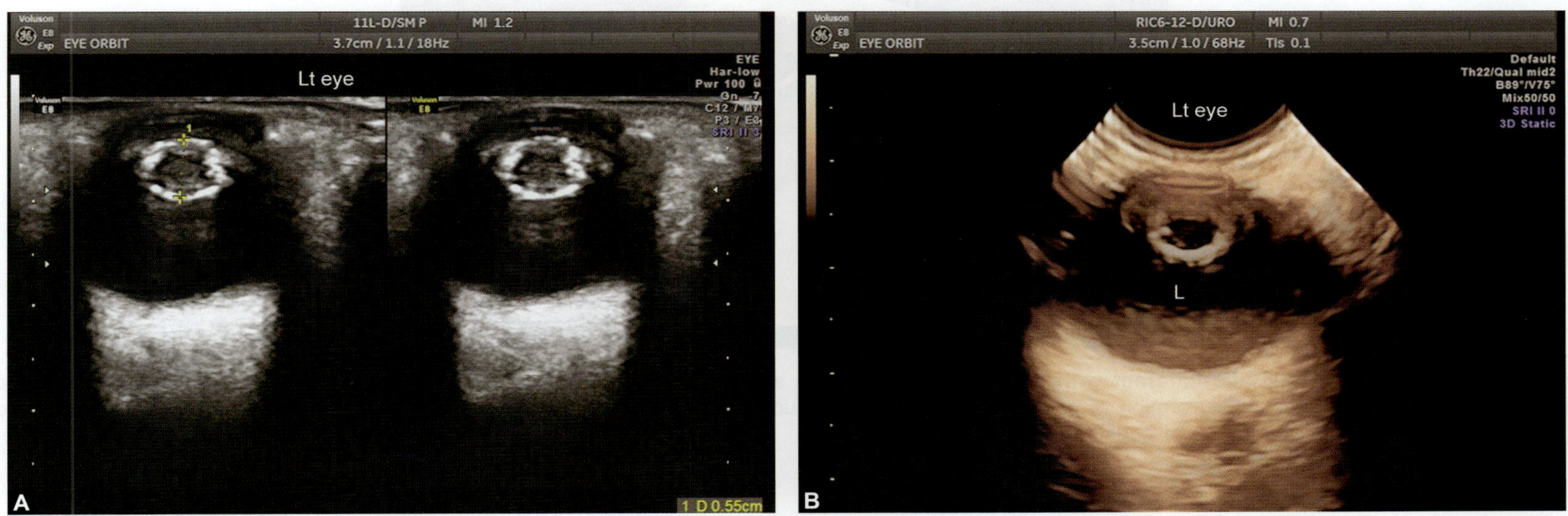

FIGURES 1.61A and B: Dense peripheral calcification. HRSG shows dense calcification in the capsule of the lens seen as an echogenic rim. 3D imaging shows the calcified rim beautifully.

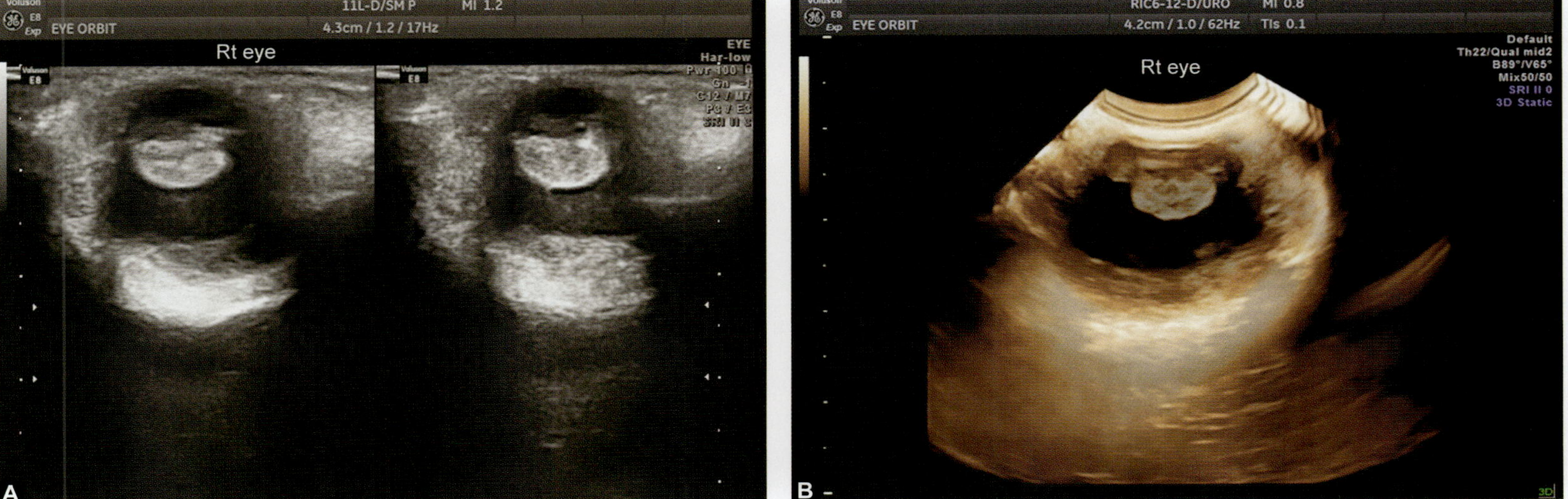

FIGURES 1.62A and B: Densely calcified lens. HRSG shows densely calcified lens in a 10-year-old girl after sustaining trauma. The posterior segment of the eye shows associated intragel hemorrhage.

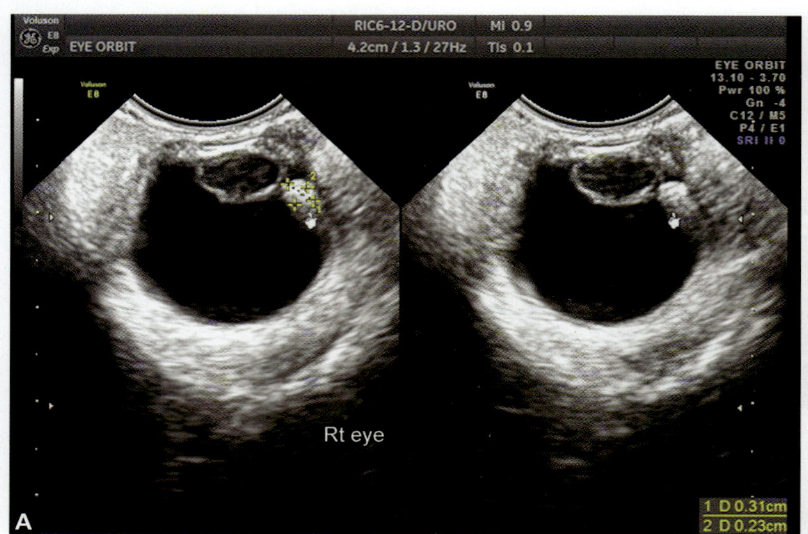

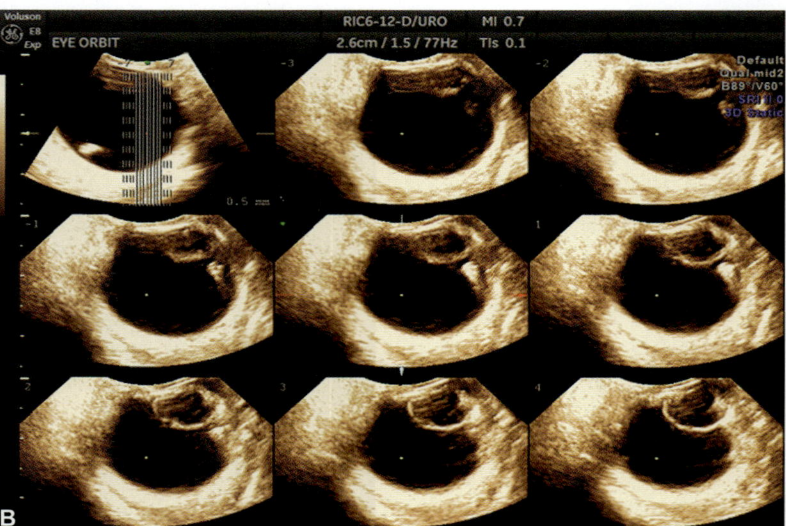

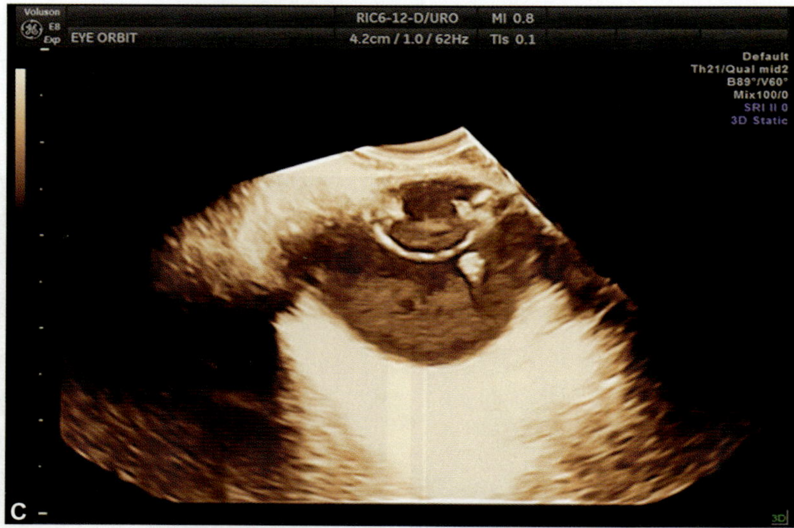

FIGURES 1.63A to C: Traumatic cataract with perforation of capsule and prolapse of nucleus. HRSG shows post-traumatic thickened opaque lens. There is also evidence of perforation of capsule and prolapse of nucleus seen on nasal side. The tomographic ultrasound imaging (TUI) and 3D imaging clearly show perforation of capsule and prolapse of nucleus.

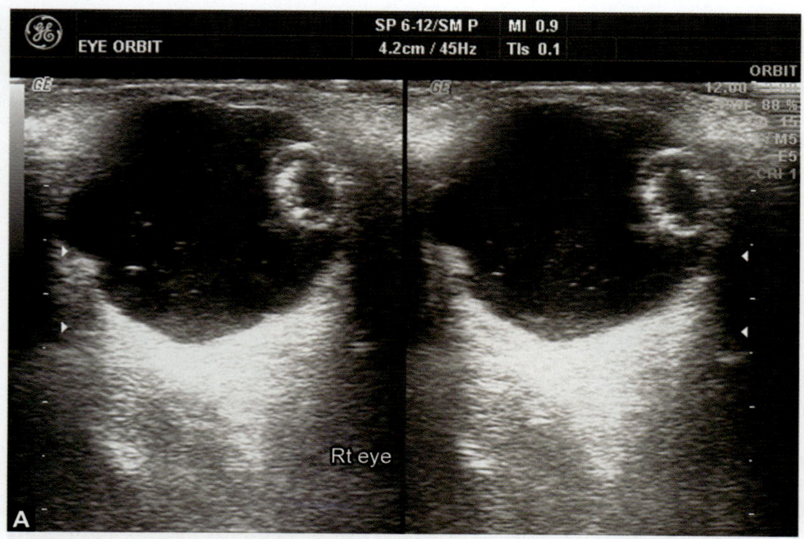

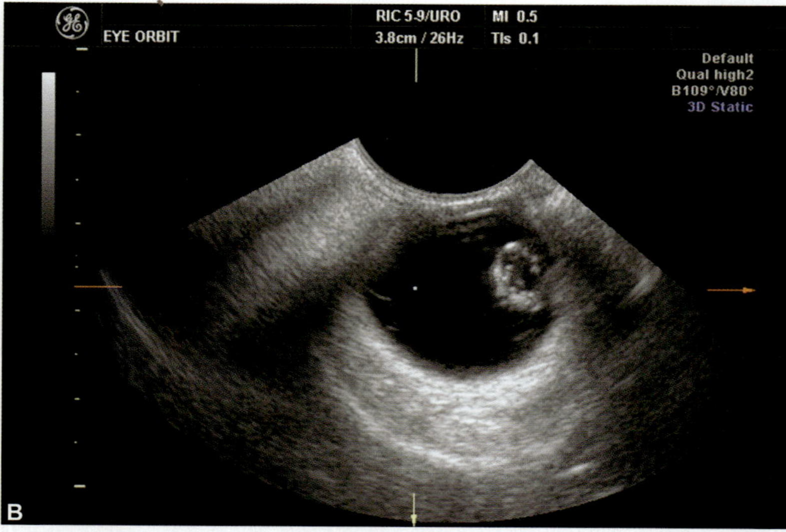

FIGURES 1.64A and B: Traumatic lens with subluxation. HRSG shows thickened opaque lens after sustaining trauma. The lens is also seen subluxated.

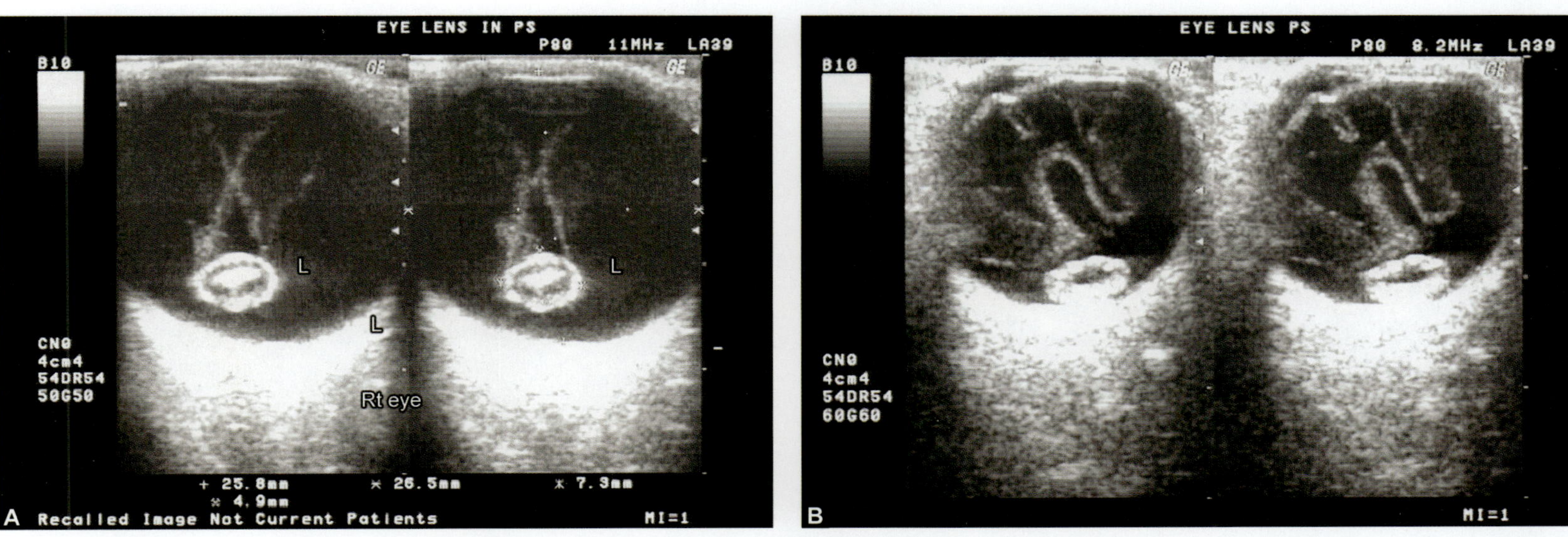

FIGURES 1.65A and B: Lens in the posterior segment. HRSG shows thickened opaque lens dislocated in the posterior segment of the eye after sustaining trauma. The nucleus is calcified. Post-traumatic intragel hemorrhage is also seen in the posterior segment.

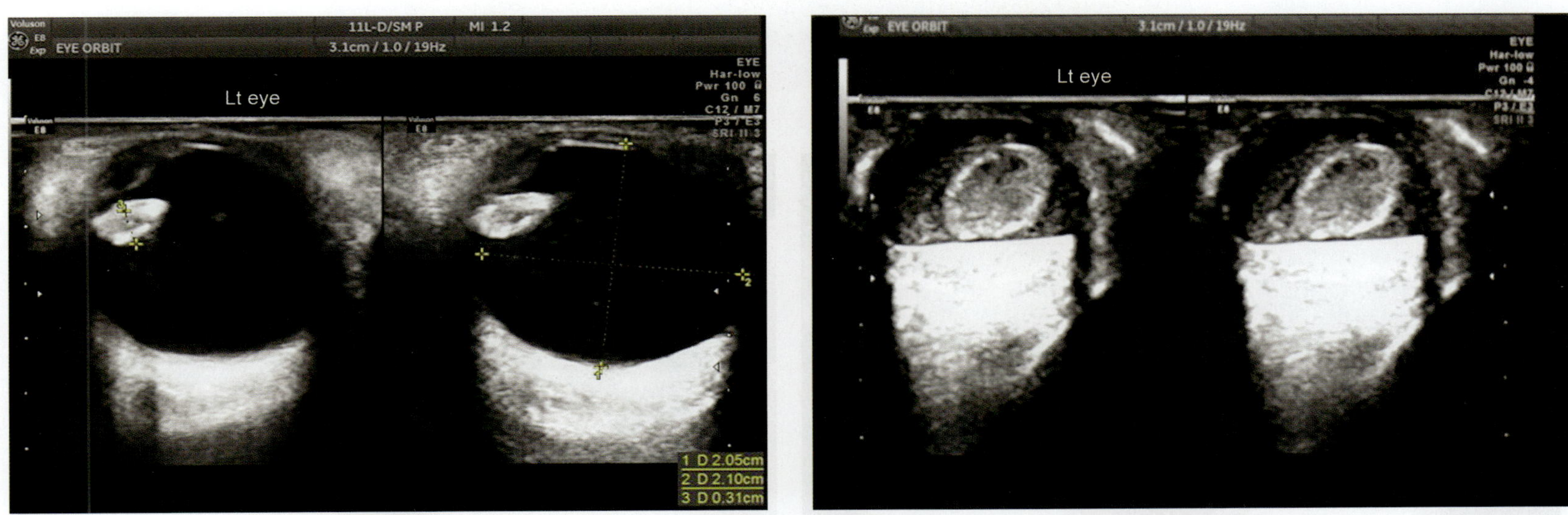

FIGURE 1.66

FIGURE 1.67

FIGURES 1.66 and 1.67: Dislocated lens in the posterior segment. HRSG shows dislocated thickened opaque lens in the posterior segment of the eye. The lens shows tumefaction.

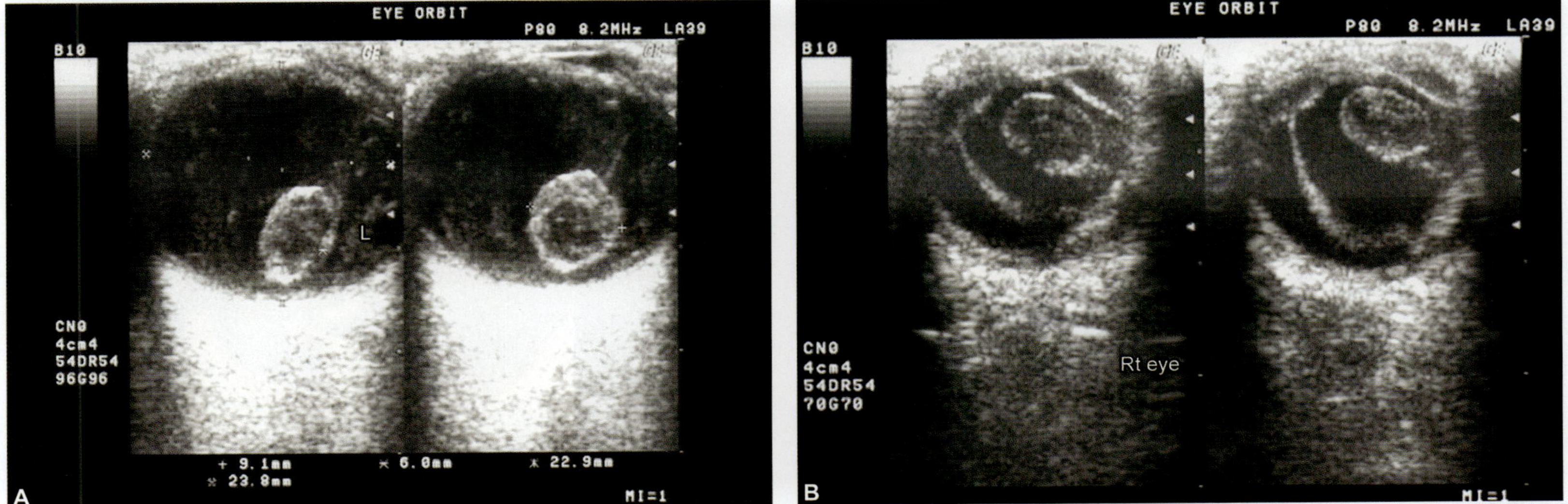

FIGURES 1.68A and B: Post-surgical trauma with dislocation of lens. HRSG shows thickened opaque lens in posterior segment of eye after cataract surgery. The lens is seen dislocated. Associated intragel hemorrhage is also seen with retinal detachment.

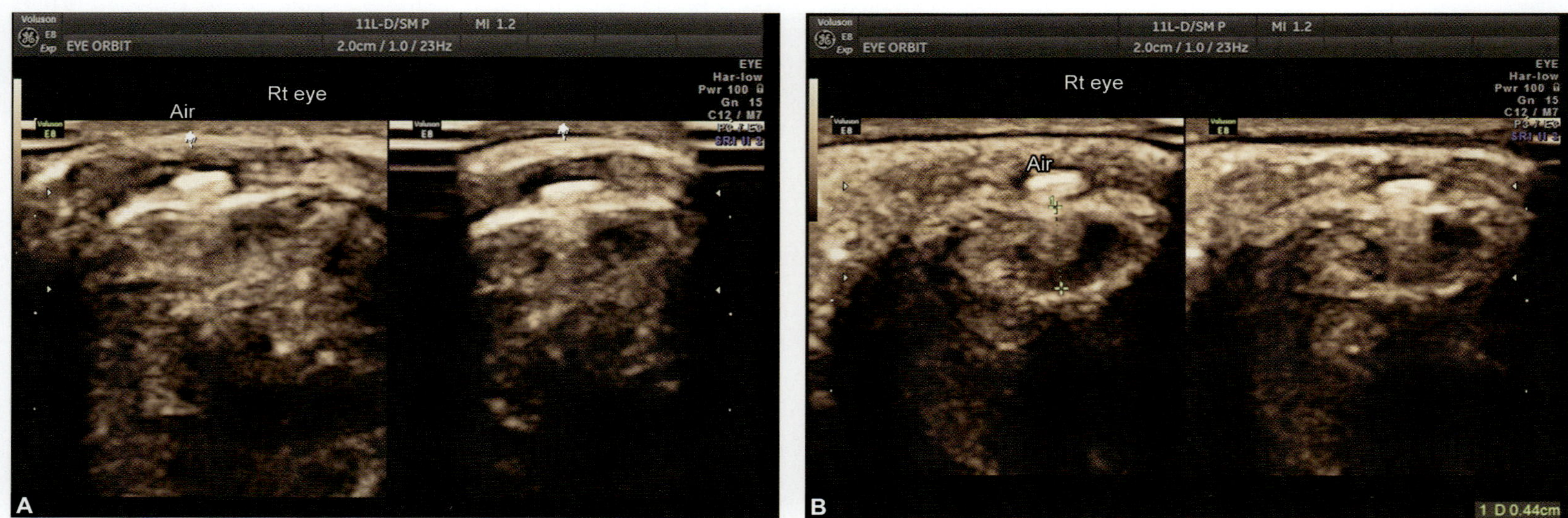

FIGURES 1.69A and B: Corneal ulcer with air. A patient presented with intense pain in the eye. HRSG shows an irregular crater in the cornea. Air is seen entrapped in the ulcer crater. It shows movements on dynamic scanning. The underlined lens is also thickened and opaque.

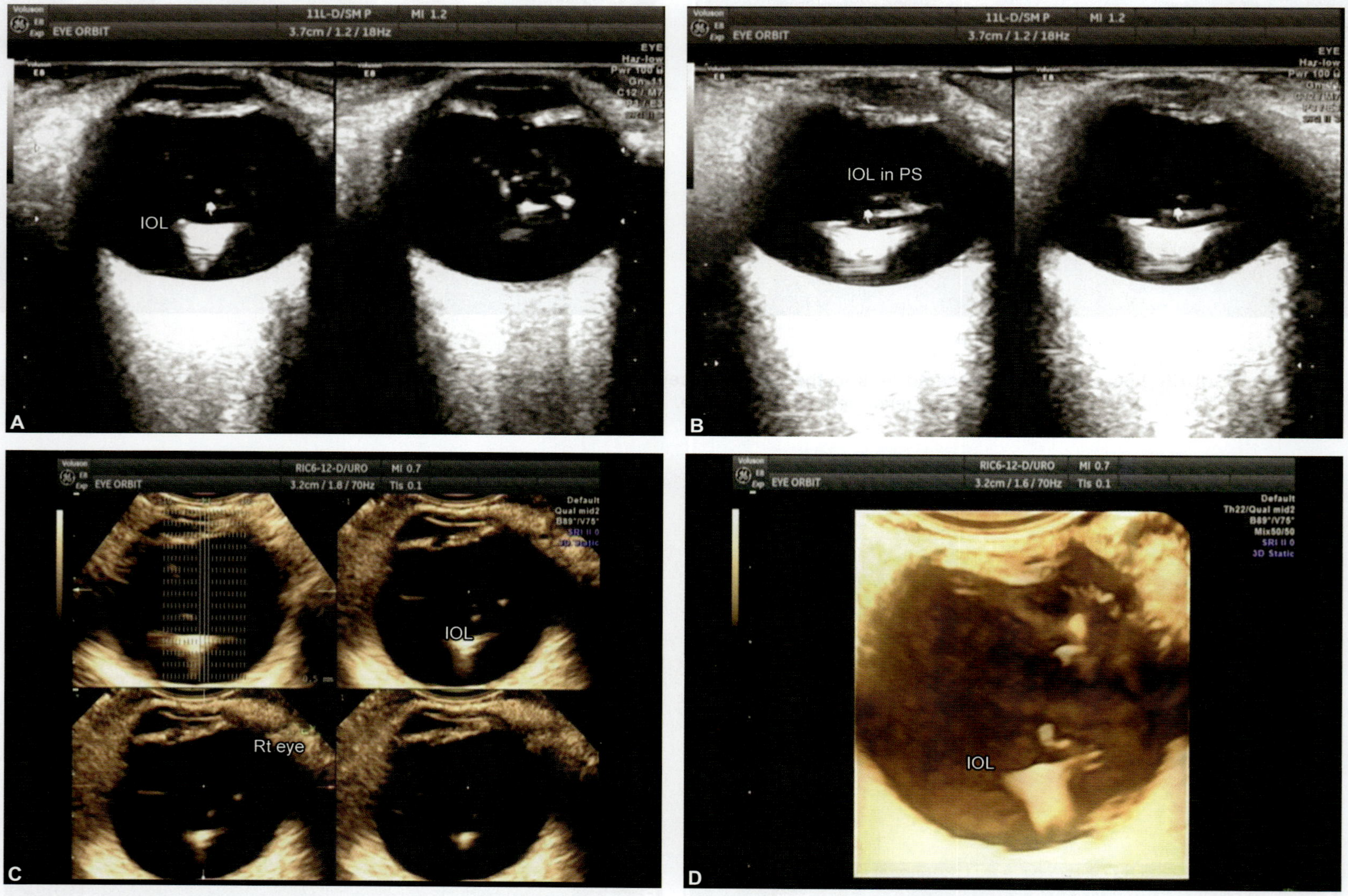

FIGURES 1.70A to D: IOL in posterior segment. A patient presented with loss of vision after cataract surgery. A hyperreflective echogenic curvilinear shadow is seen in the posterior segment suggestive of IOL in posterior segment. Strong artifacts are seen posterior to IOL. 3D with TUI imaging shows details of IOL.

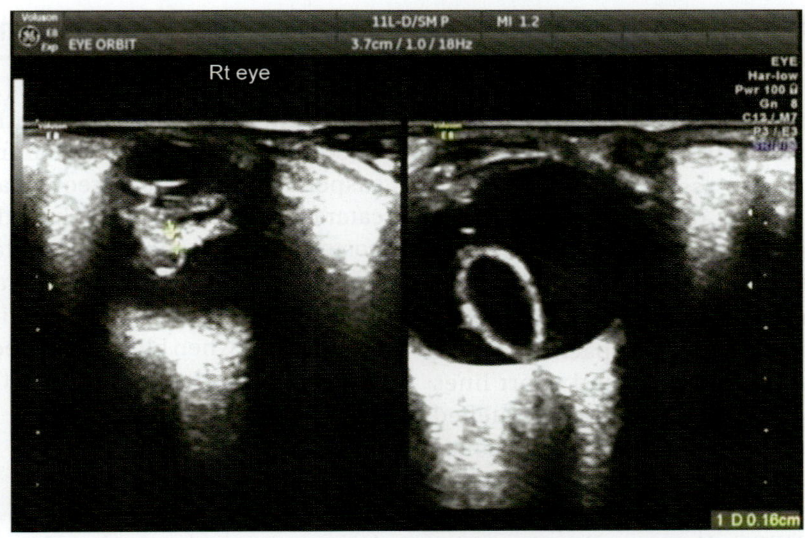

FIGURE 1.71: IOL with RD. A patient presented with loss of vision after cataract surgery. HRSG shows IOL in position. However, the posterior segment of the eye shows intragel collection. A thick membrane is seen detached in the posterior segment suggestive of retinal detachment.

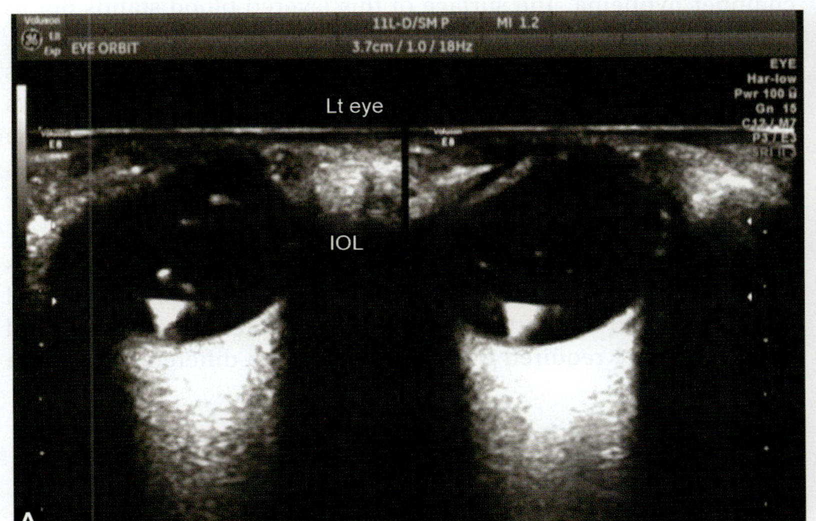

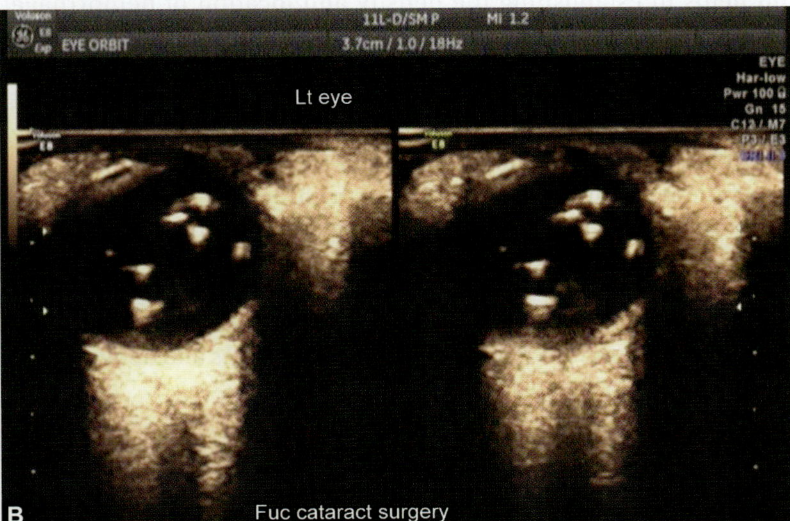

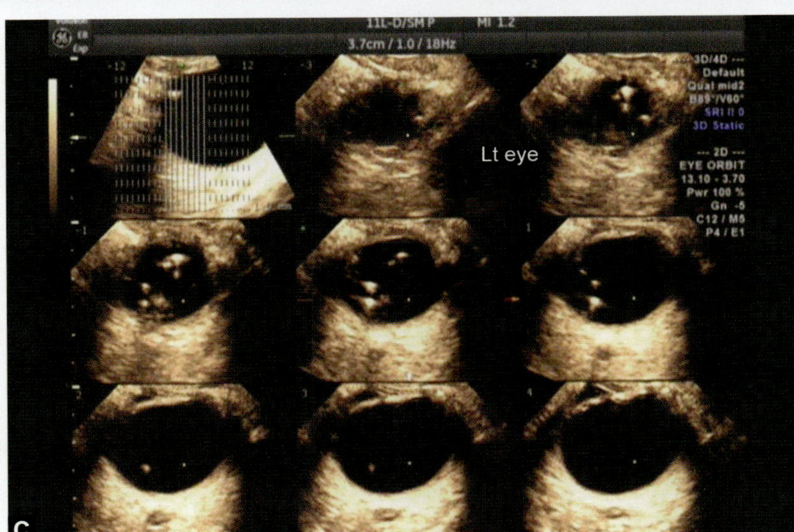

FIGURES 1.72A to C: Broken IOL in posterior segment. A patient presented with loss of vision after cataract surgery. HRSG shows dislocated IOL in posterior segment. Multiple echogenic fragments of broken IOL seen in posterior segment.

EXAMINATION OF VITREOUS

The vitreous is a transparent gel. It does not produce any echo on B-scanning in normal conditions. However, scattered opacities of low density may be noted in aging eye due to degenerative changes. The vitreous evaluation should include assessment of vitreous body, posterior hyloid, subvitreal space, retina, choroid, sclera and optic disk. The anterior segment should also be examined in cases of hyphema lens, cataract and for lesions of pupil and cilliary body. As stated earlier, normal vitreous is an echo-free cavity on HRSG. It should be evaluated for the presence of opacities, bands and membrane. Vitreous opacities produce dots and short lines on 'B' scanning. These opacities may be originated from liquefied vitreous, hemorrhage, inflammation, infections or calcium soaps (asteroid hylosis). In vitreous hemorrhage, the bright echoes of dots are produced due to clump or cells having blood. Small, subtle hemorrhage is difficult to see on HRSG. However, low intensity echoes are seen on high gain setting. Medium to dense level echoes are seen in vitreous hemorrhage depending upon the severity of hemorrhage. Vitreous hemorrhage is second most common cause of opaque ocular media after cataract. It is associated with a number of conditions. The most common causes are trauma, diabetic retinopathy, macular degeneration, vein occlusion, retinal tear and intraocular tumors. Ultrasonography is a useful tool to examine it and helps in establishing the density and location of hemorrhage and cause of hemorrhage, which is not clinically explained. In fresh hemorrhage, dense echogenic collection is seen in posterior segment. Layering of collection is noted in organization of the hemorrhage. Dense interfaces are formed due to layering. They stand out clearly on HRSG. Pseudomembranes are also formed. Posterior vitreous detachment commonly takes place with vitreous hemorrhage.

The asteroid hylosis is senile degenerative condition of unknown etiology. It is usually unilateral in 75% of the cases. It is possible to diagnose it on HRSG. The findings are quite typical. Calcium soaps from asteroid bodies which are scattered throughout the vitreous. These bodies show multiple bright echogenic echoes and demonstrate considerable movements.

Posterior Vitreous Detachment

Posterior vitreous detachment (PVD) may be focal or diffuse. It is most commonly associated with synchysis senilis a degenerative disorder. The gel loses it volume and becomes hypermobile. It remains suspended from the vitreous base. It is also seen associated with cataract eye. The posterior hyloid may separate completely from the posterior pole. It may remain attached at optic disk giving a funnel-shaped appearance. Vitreoretinal adhesions may also be noted in areas of retinal tear. On "B" scan imaging, PVD is usually smooth and may be thick when blood is layered posteroinferiorly. Real-time HRSG shows an undulating movement in PVD. This differentiates it from retinal detachment.

Subvitreal Hemorrhage

At times vitreous hemorrhage is associated with subvitreal hemorrhage. It may also present alone. In mild subvitreal hemorrhage, very high gain setting is required to detect it. Subvitreal blood usually does not clot. Therefore, it is of reflectivity and mobile even in chronic cases.

Posterior Hyphema

Subvitreal hemorrhage has the tendency to layer out similar to anterior chamber hyphema. The surface of this layered blood stands out as smooth, dense echogenic membrane on "B" scans. With the kinetic movements of eye, this hyphema normally slides across the fundus surface of eye. In sitting upright position, this hyphema changes its position in the eye. The probe position should not be changed while changing the position of patient from lying to sitting position. This change of position also excludes underlying retinal detachment or retinochoroid layer thickening.

The characteristic motion of vitreous and retina normally differentiates their pathologies. However, if posterior hyloid surface is thickened and attached to the optic nerve head, very careful monitoring and observation are required dynamic scanning to differentiate it from detached retina.

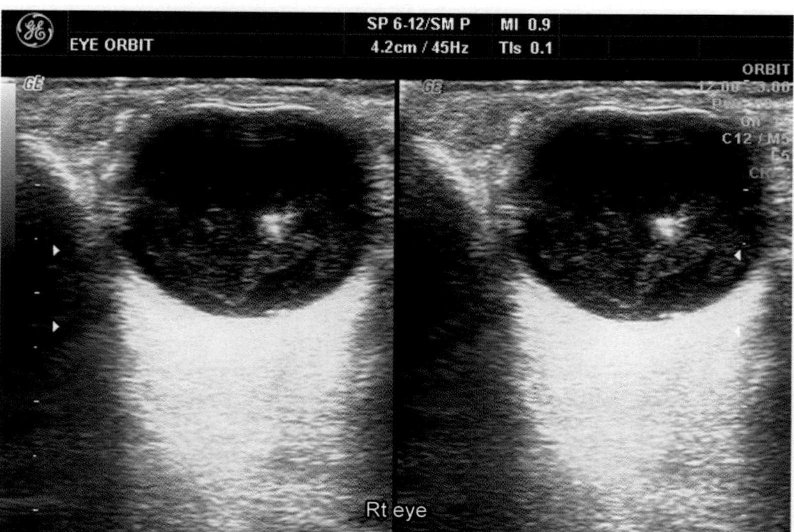

FIGURE 1.73: Subtle intragel hemorrhage. HRSG is very sensitive in picking of intragel hemorrhage. Low level echoes are seen in the posterior segment of eye suggestive of subtle intragel hemorrhage.

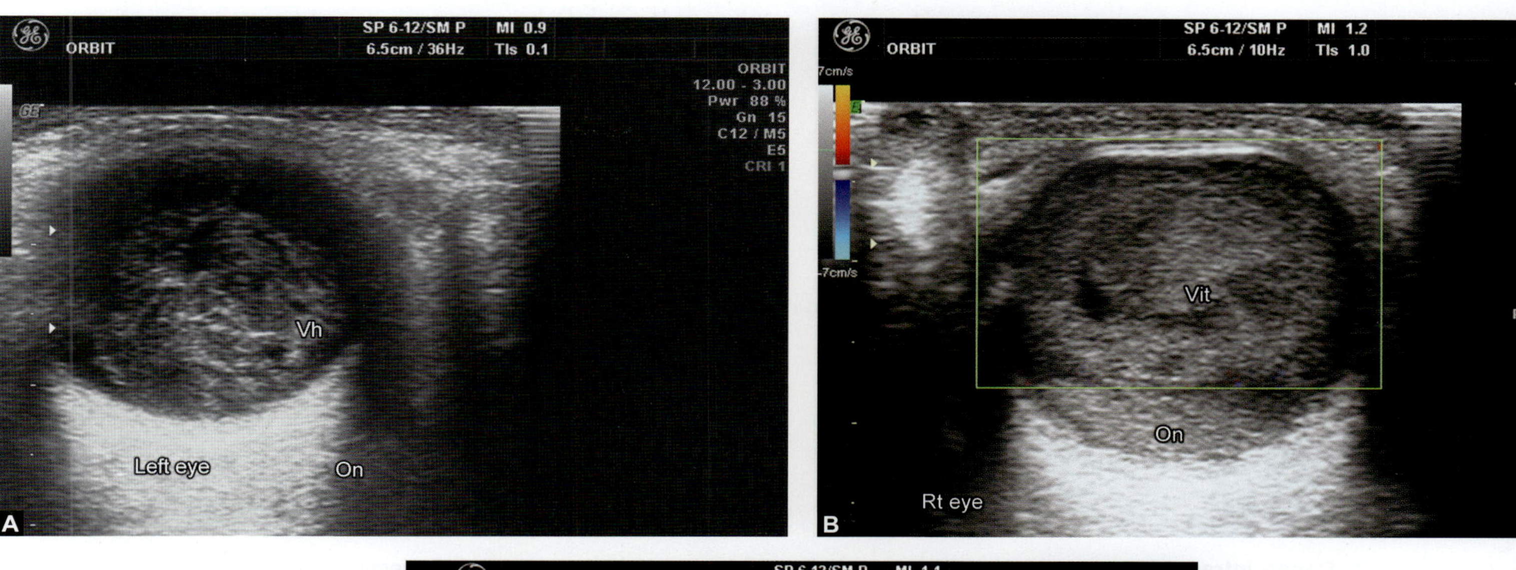

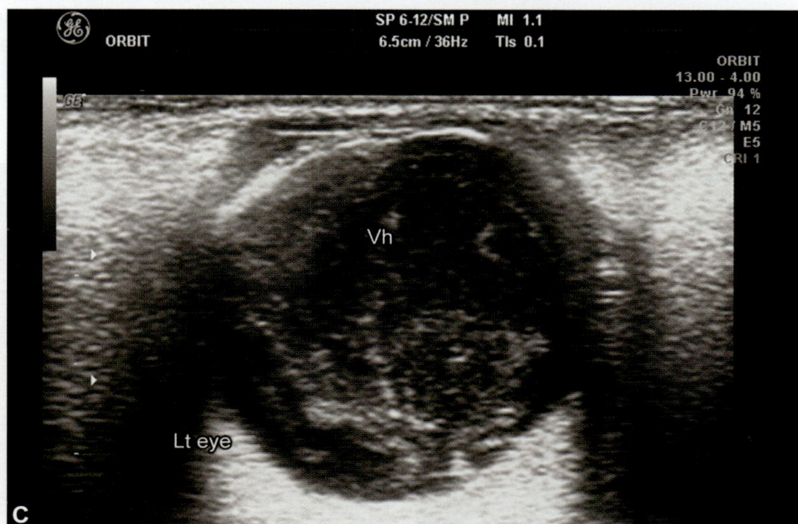

FIGURES 1.74A to C: Dense intragel hemorrhage. A young child presented with trauma. The eye is enlarged. The eye coat is edematous. Dense intragel collection is seen in the posterior segment of the eye suggestive of dense intragel hemorrhage. But no foreign body is seen. No retinal detachment is seen.

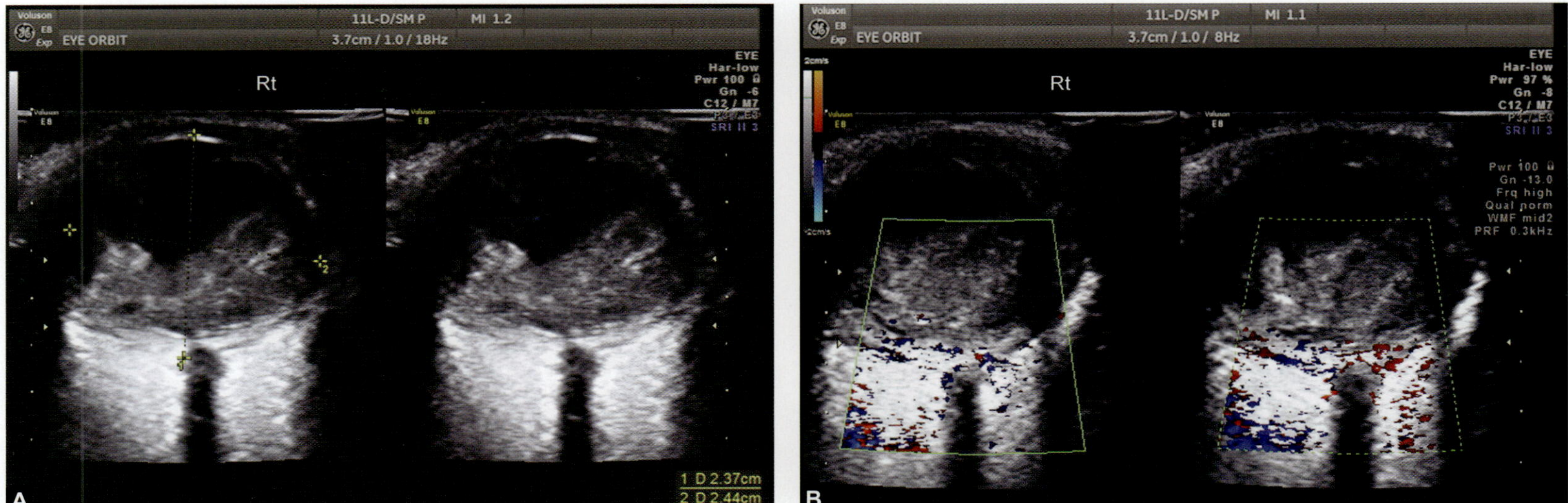

FIGURES 1.75A and B: Blunt trauma to eye with intragel hemorrhage. A patient presented with loss of vision after sustain blunt trauma. The eyecoat is thickened and edematous. Dense intragel hemorrhage is seen in the posterior segment of the eye. Echogenic sustaining are seen in the posterior segment suggestive of fresh hemorrhage.

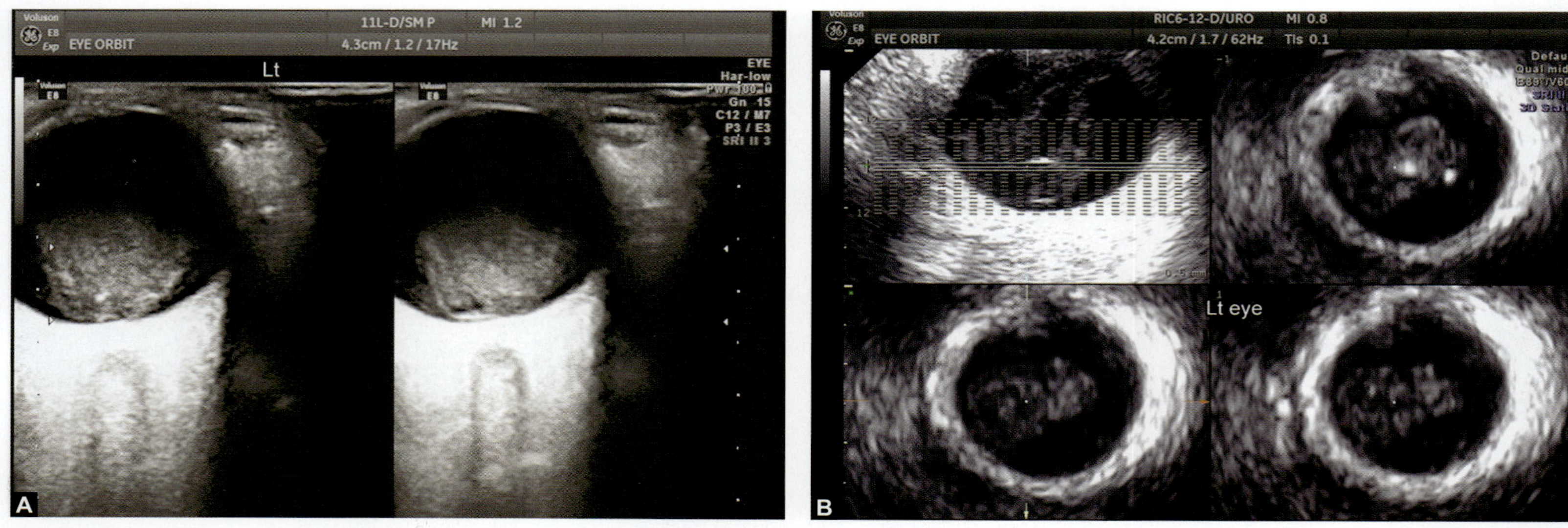

FIGURES 1.76A and B: Dense intragel hemorrhage with TUI imaging. HRSG shows dense echogenic collection in the posterior segment of the eye suggestive of intragel hemorrhage. The TUI imaging shows the hemorrhage is confined to the posterior segment. No evidence of any rupture of eyecoat is seen.

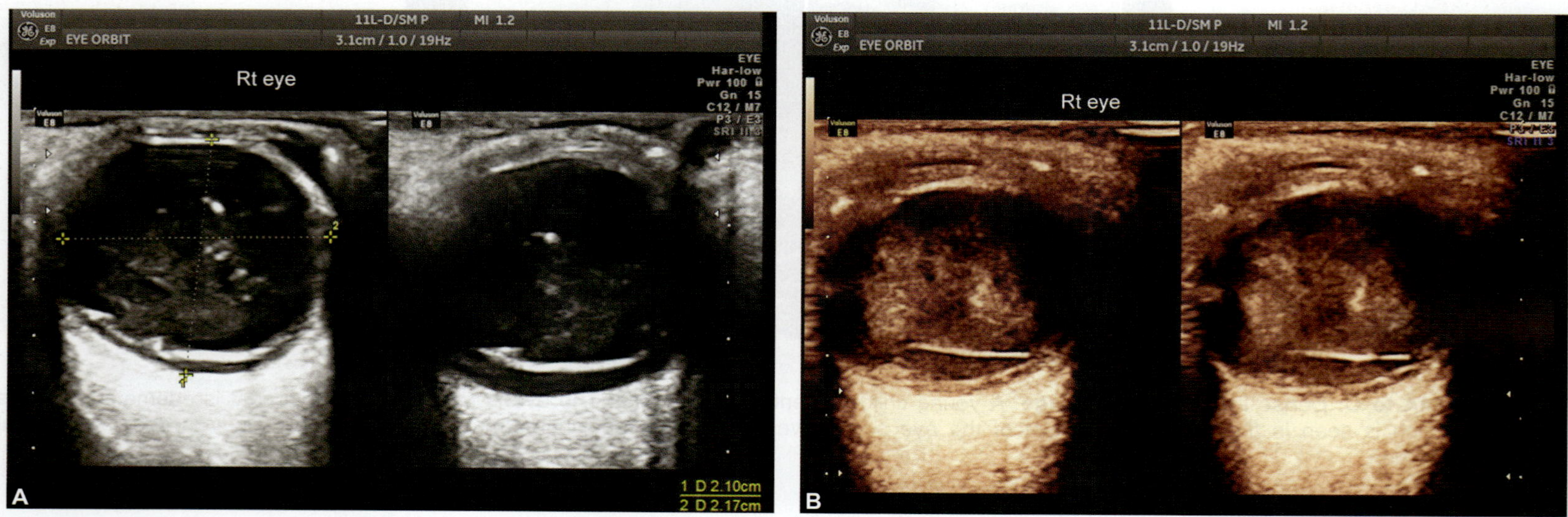

FIGURES 1.77A and B: Intragel hemorrhage with posterior vitreous detachment. HRSG shows dense intragel hemorrhage in the posterior segment of eye. An echogenic membrane is seen detached in the posterior segment suggestive of posterior vitreous detachment. Collection is also seen posterior to the membrane suggestive of subhyloid hemorrhage.

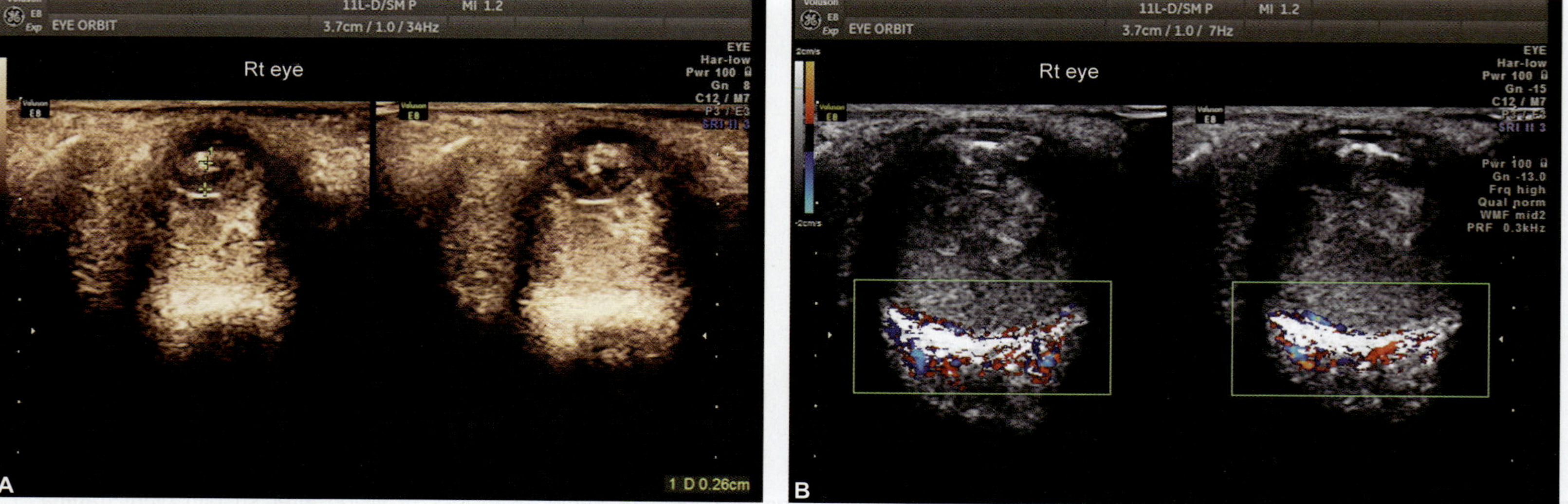

FIGURES 1.78A and B: Post-traumatic cataract with intragel hemorrhage. A patient presented with blunt trauma to the eye. HRSG shows thickened opaque lens. Posterior segment of the eye shows intragel hemorrhage filling the posterior segment.

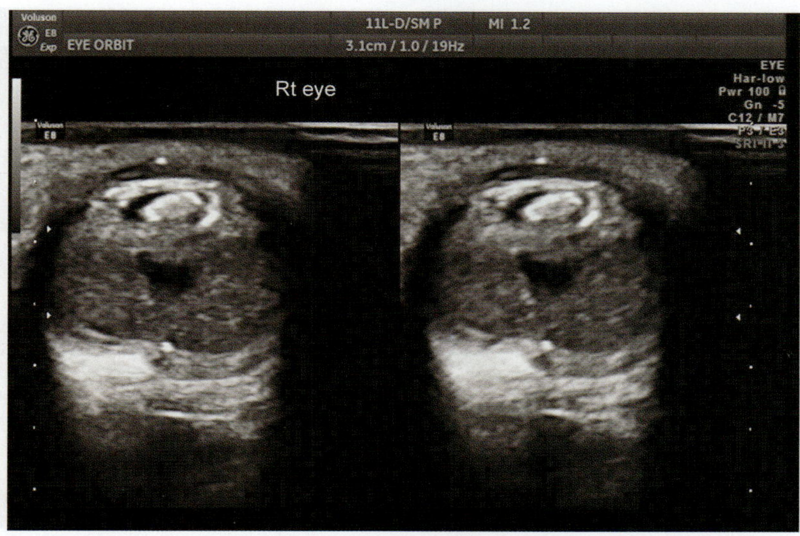

FIGURE 1.79: Post-traumatic cataract with intragel hemorrhage. A young girl presented with trauma to the eye. The lens is thickened and opaque. The nucleus is calcified. The eye coat is edematous. Dense intragel hemorrhage is seen in the posterior segment of the eye.

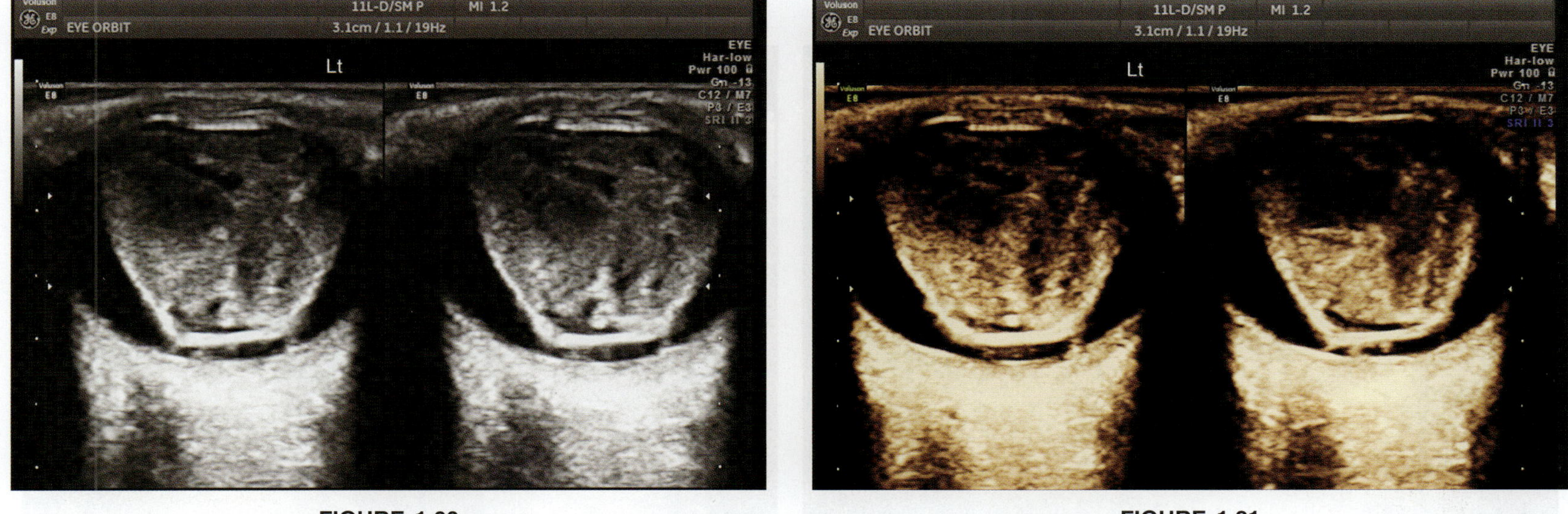

FIGURE 1.80 **FIGURE 1.81**

FIGURES 1.80 and 1.81: Fresh intragel hemorrhage with posterior vitreous detachment (PVD). A patient presented with loss of vision after sustaining trauma. HRSG shows dense intragel collection. The collection is seen limited by a membrane suggestive of PVD. But no retinal detachment is seen.

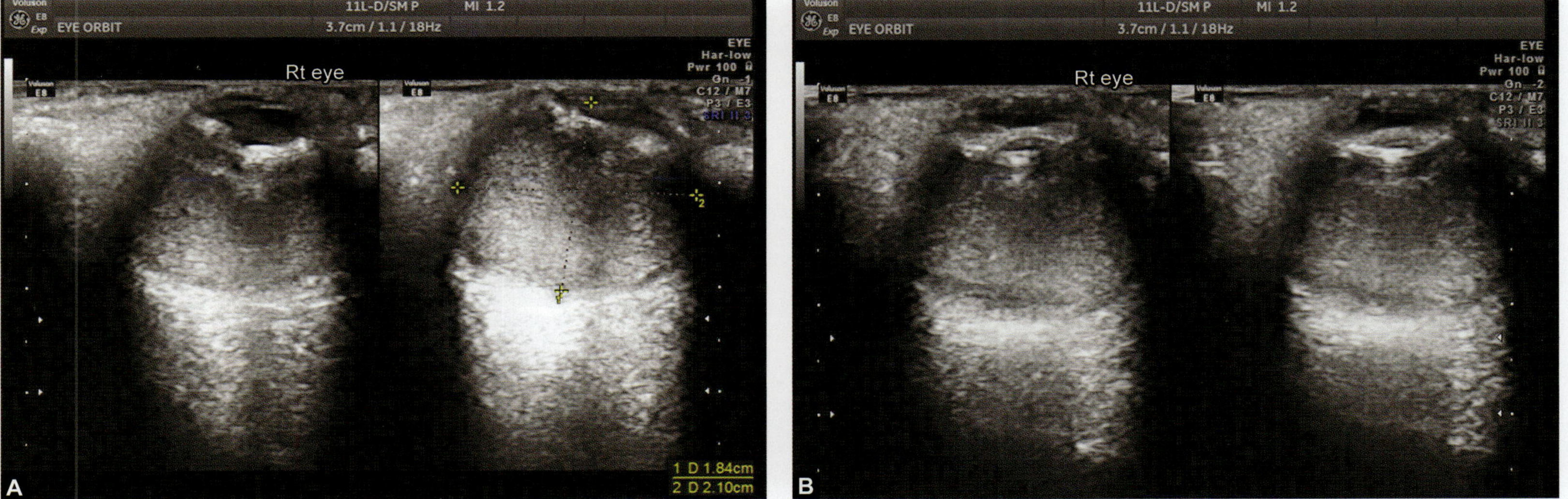

FIGURES 1.82A and B: Hemorrhagic cystic eye. Dense echogenic collection is seen in posterior segment of eye after postcataract surgery. The hemorrhage is highly echogenic suggestive of fresh blood. However, IOL is seen in position.

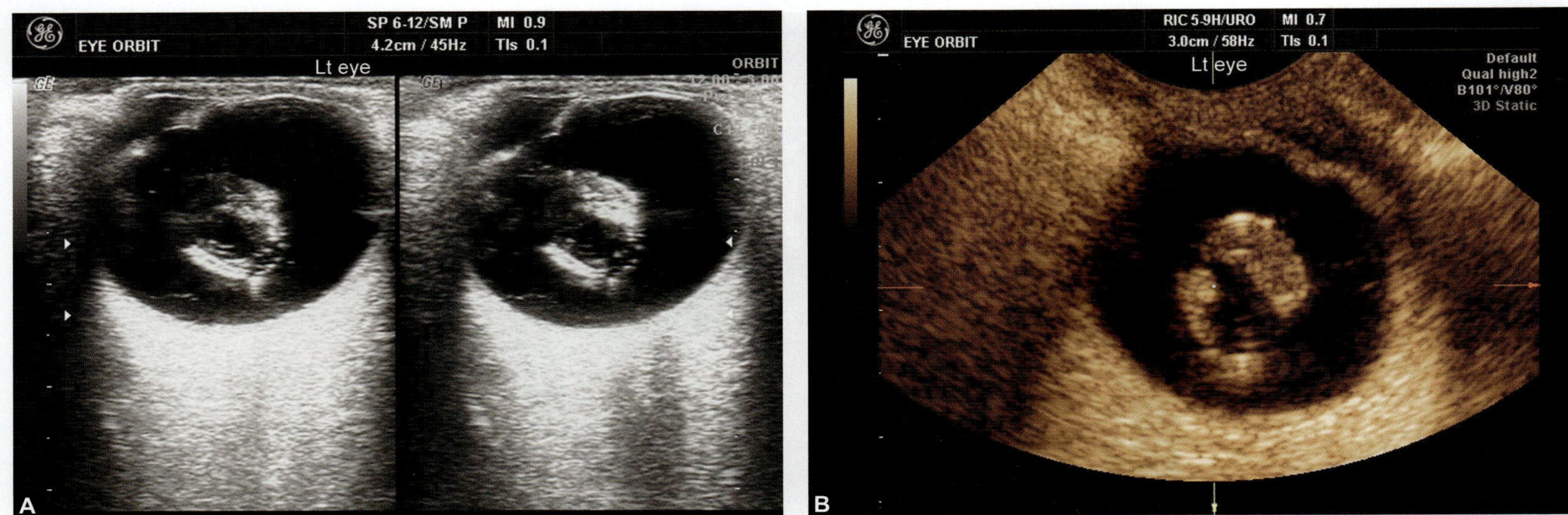

FIGURES 1.83A and B: Intragel hemorrhage with retraction of vitreous. HRSG shows echogenic membranous shadows in the posterior segment of the eye. The hemorrhage shows retraction and hemorrhagic clot is seen in center in the posterior segment of eye.

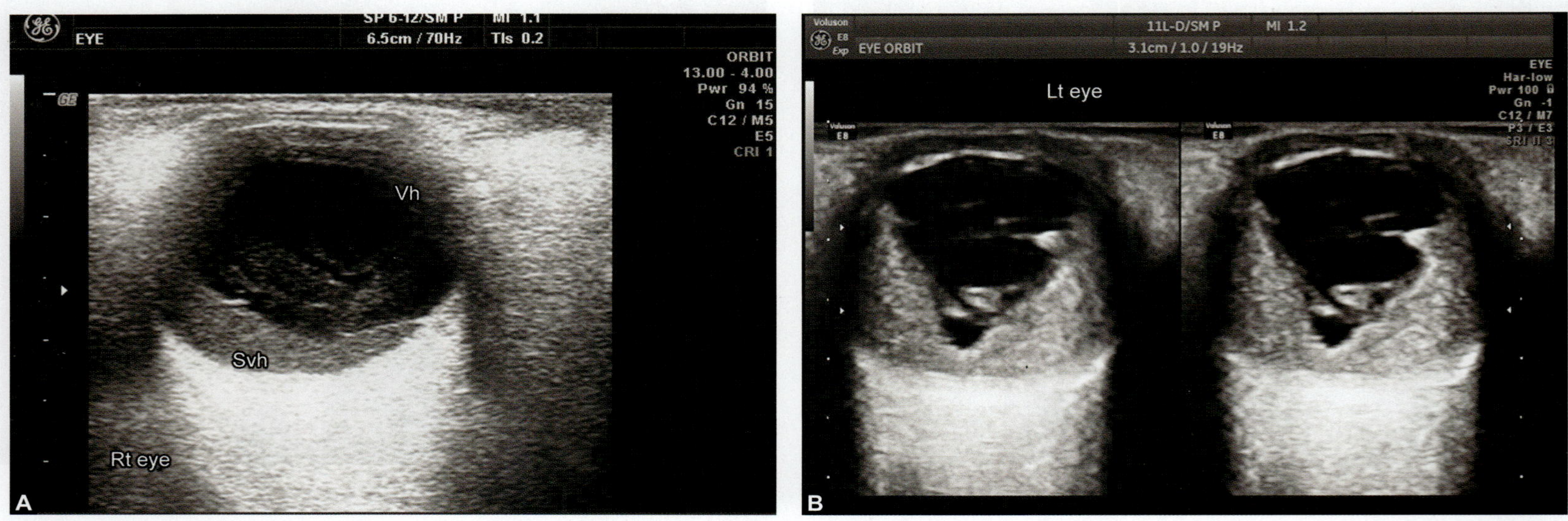

FIGURES 1.84A and B: Subvitreal hemorrhage. A patient presented with loss of vision. HRSG shows intragel hemorrhage. The hemorrhage is seen limited by a membrane suggestive of subhyloid hemorrhage. Figure B shows the vitreous membrane seen going to the equator and hemorrhagic collection is seen under the membrane.

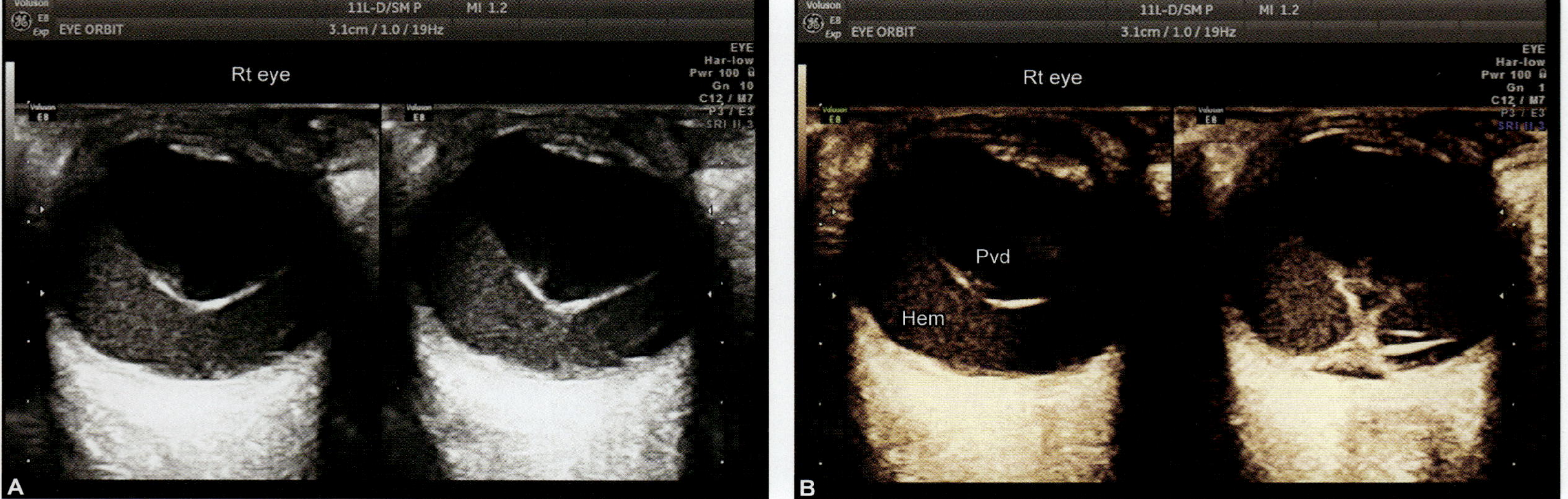

FIGURES 1.85A and B

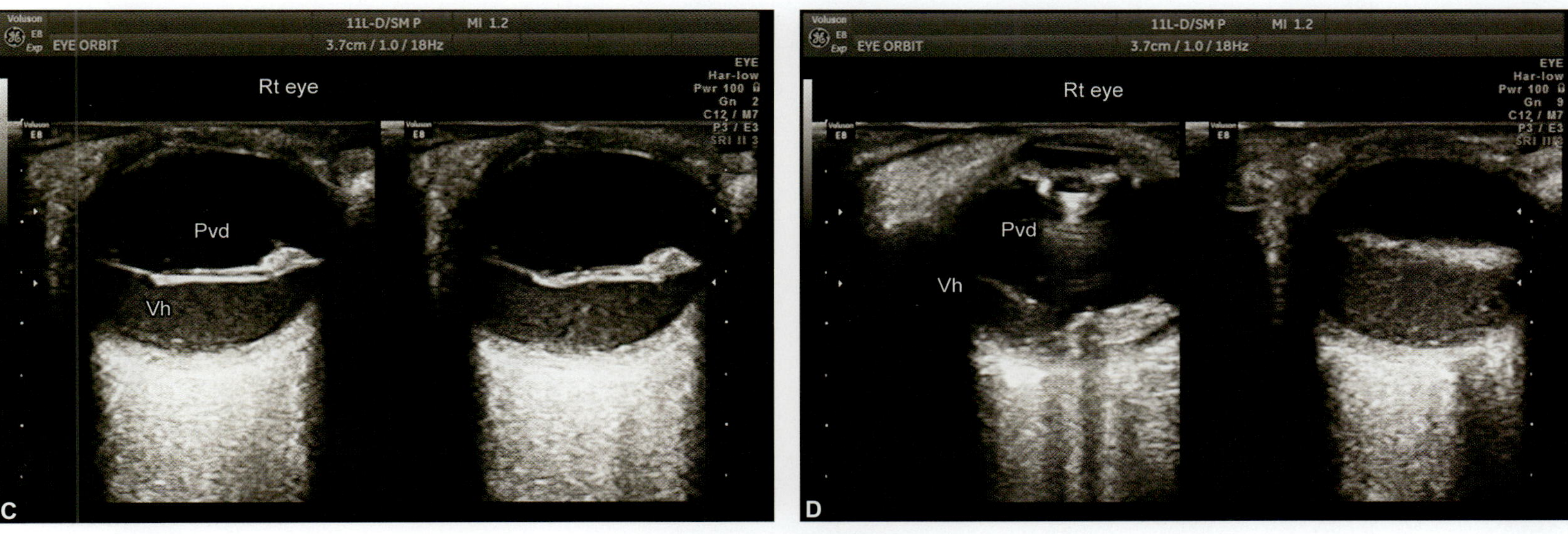

FIGURES 1.85C and D

FIGURES 1.85A to D: Subvitreal hemorrhage with vitreoretinal bands. HRSG shows intragel hemorrhage in the posterior segment of the eye, which is seen limited by an echogenic membrane suggestive of posterior vitreous detachment. However, there is evidence of multiple bands seen going to the posterior pole from vitreous membrane suggestive of vitreoretinal bands.

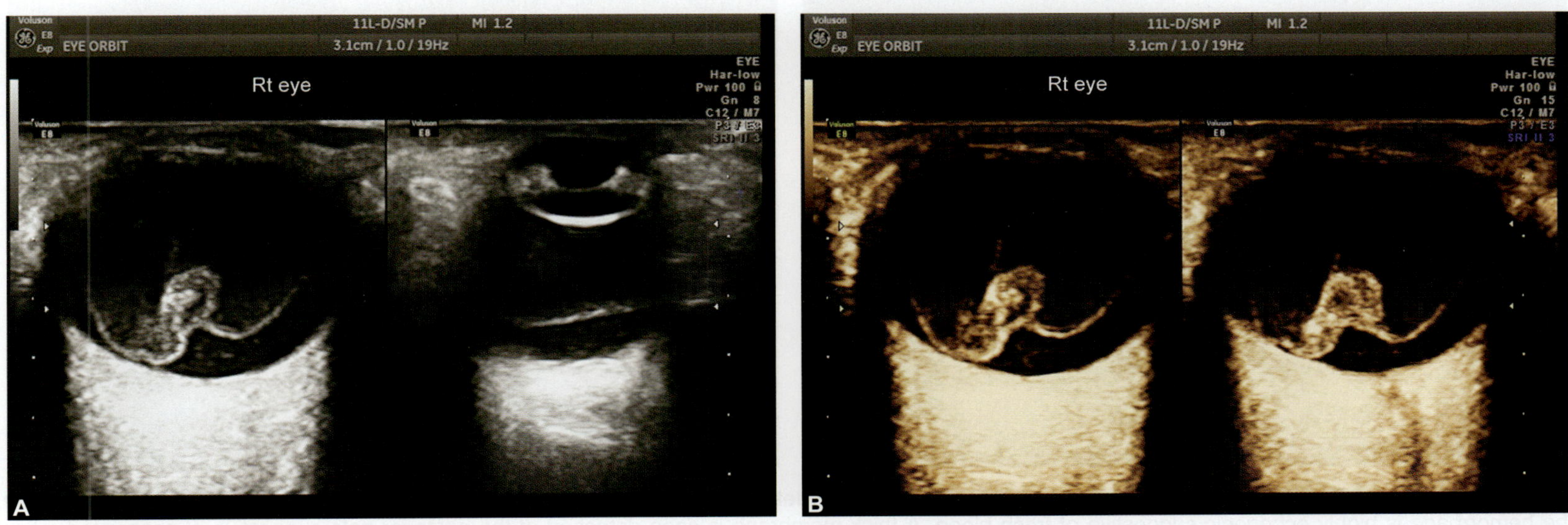

FIGURES 1.86A and B: Posterior vitreous detachment with hemorrhage. HRSG shows isolated posterior vitreous detachment associated with vitreal haemorrhage. Folding of vitreal membrane is seen on HRSG.

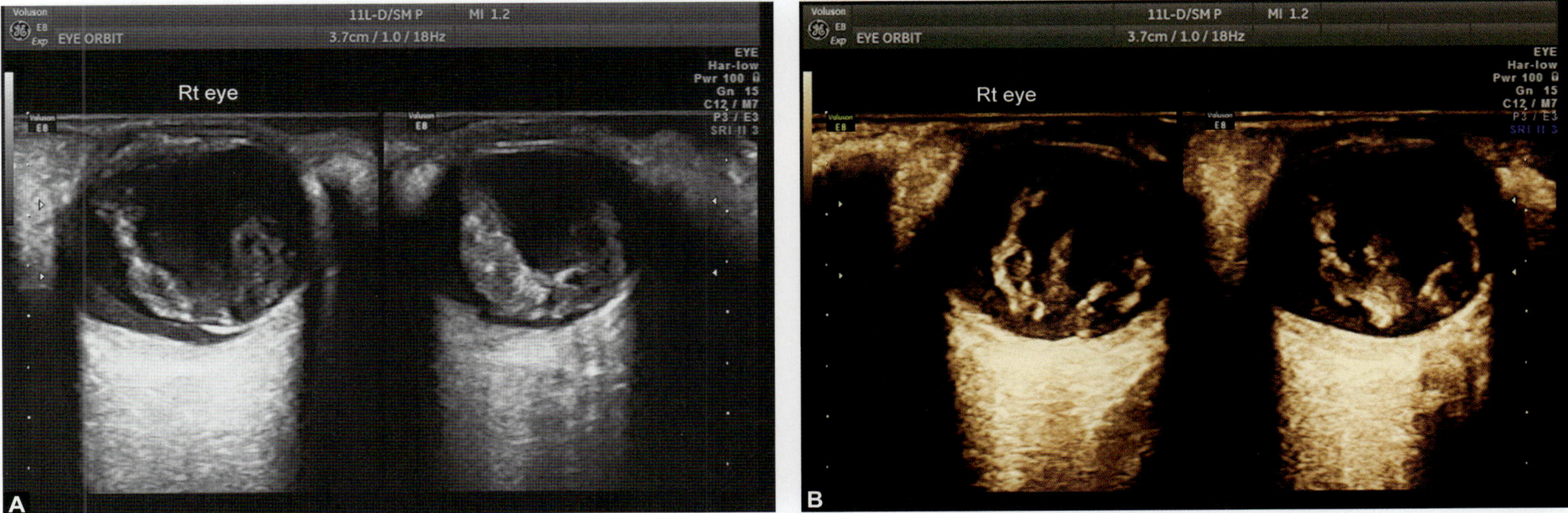

FIGURES 1.87A and B: Posterior vitreous detachment with vitreal band formation. HRSG shows dense intragel hemorrhage in right eye after sustaining trauma. The vitreal membrane shows multiple folds. Echogenic collection is seen in posterior segment suggestive of hemorrhage.

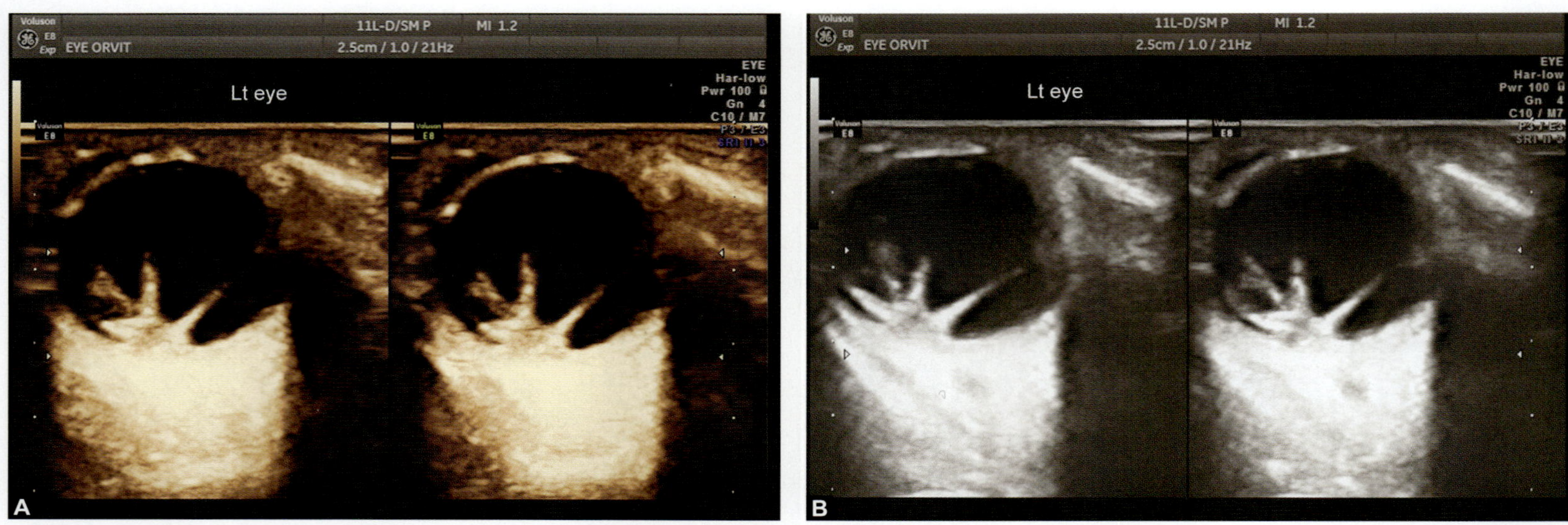

FIGURES 1.88A and B: Vitreous hemorrhage with vitreoretinal bands. A 2-month-old baby presented with white eye reflex. HRSG shows intragel collection suggestive of intragel haemorrhage. Multiple bands are seen going from the collection to the posterior pole suggestive of vitreo retinal bands.

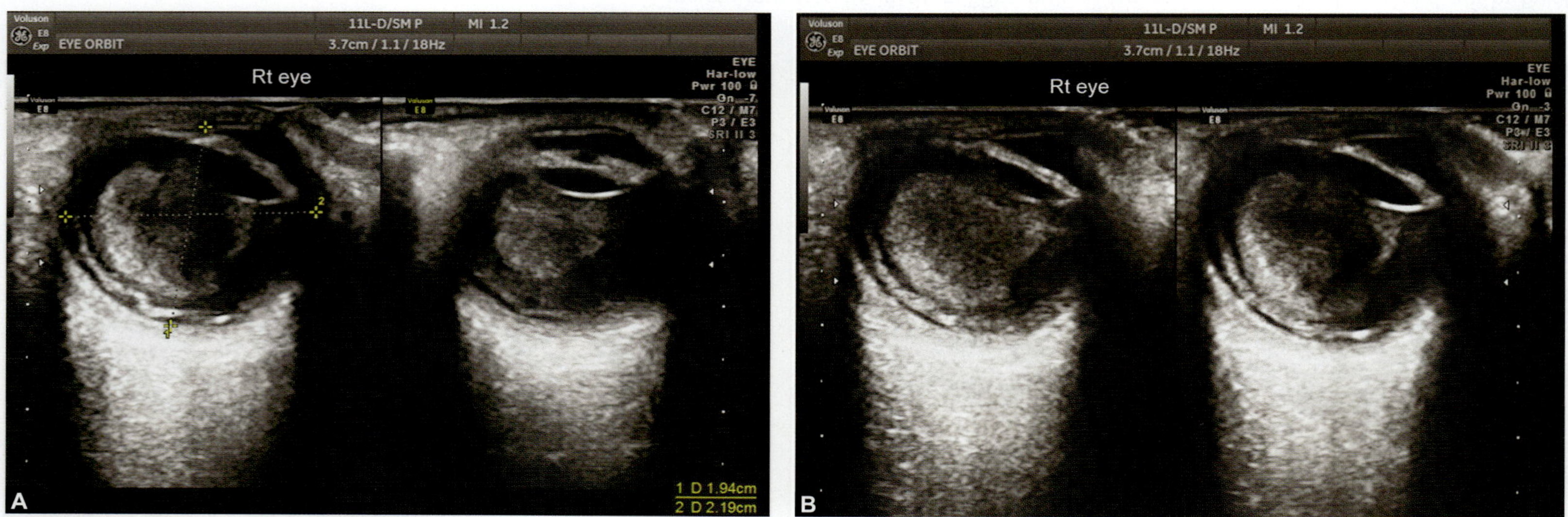

FIGURES 1.89A and B: Intragel hemorrhage with associated retinal detachment. HRSG shows dense intragel hemorrhage in posterior segment. The hemorrhage is highly echogenic suggestive of fresh bleed. A thick membrane is seen detached at the posterior pole suggestive of associated retinal detachment.

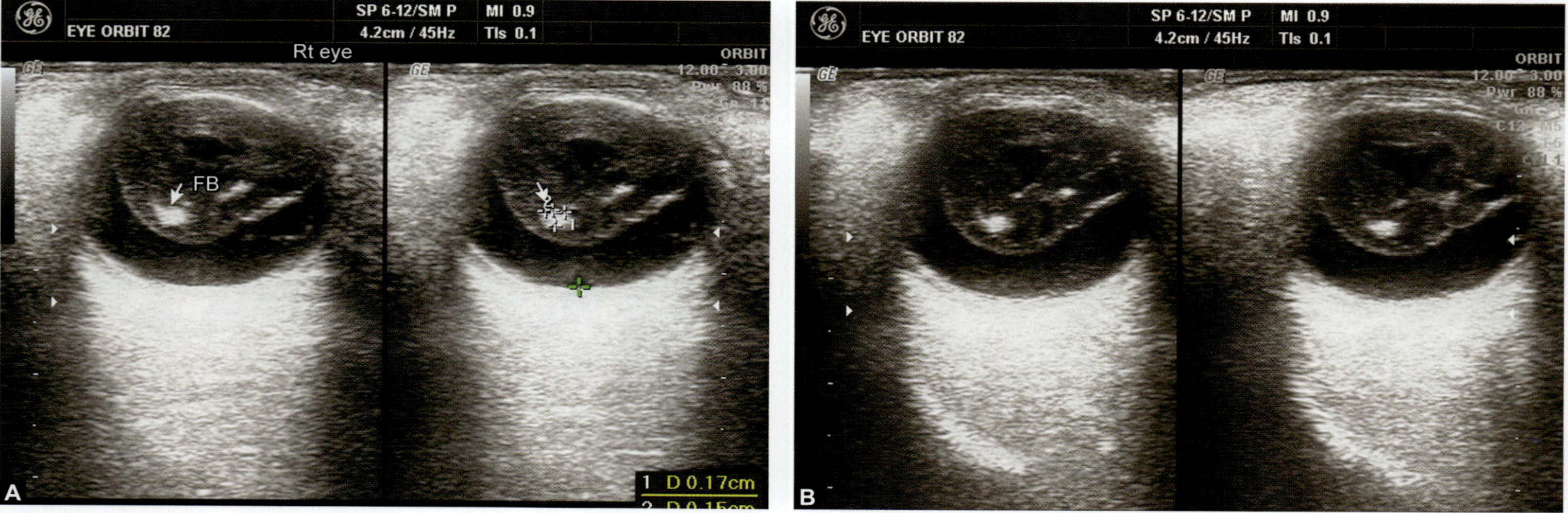

FIGURES 1.90A and B

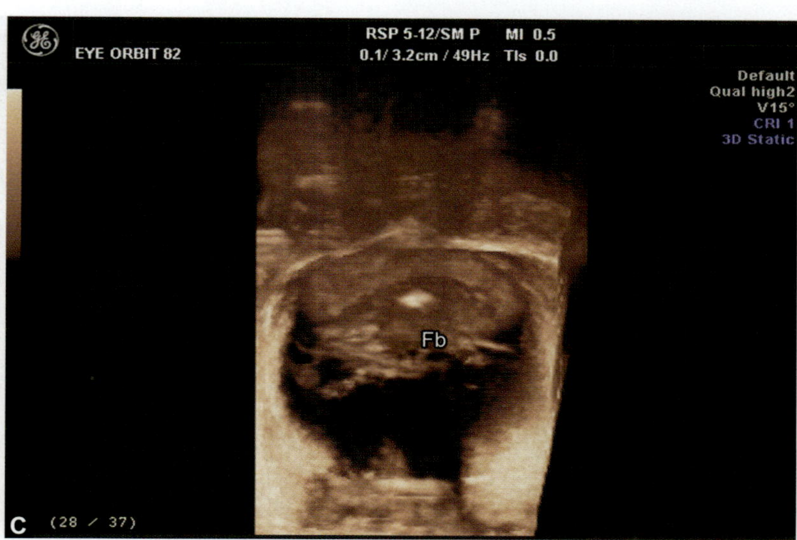

FIGURE 1.90C

FIGURES 1.90A to C: Foreign body with hemorrhage. A patient presented with painful right eye after sustaining penetrating trauma. HRSG shows a highly echogenic shadow in the posterior segment suggestive of a foreign body. Figure 1.90C shows 3D imaging of the eye, which shows the foreign body clearly. Associated intragel hemorrhage is also seen.

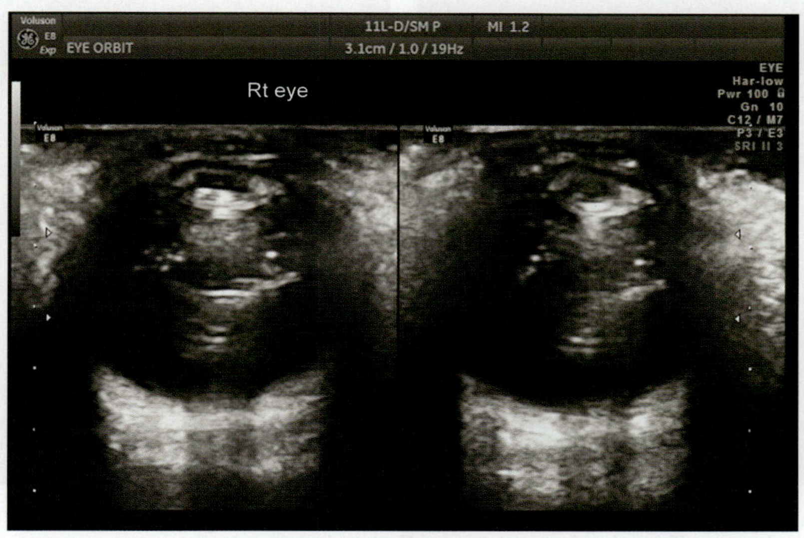

FIGURE 1.91: Postsurgery intragel hemorrhage. HRSG shows intragel hemorrhage after cataract surgery. Echogenic IOL is seen in position. Dense intragel collection is seen in the posterior segment.

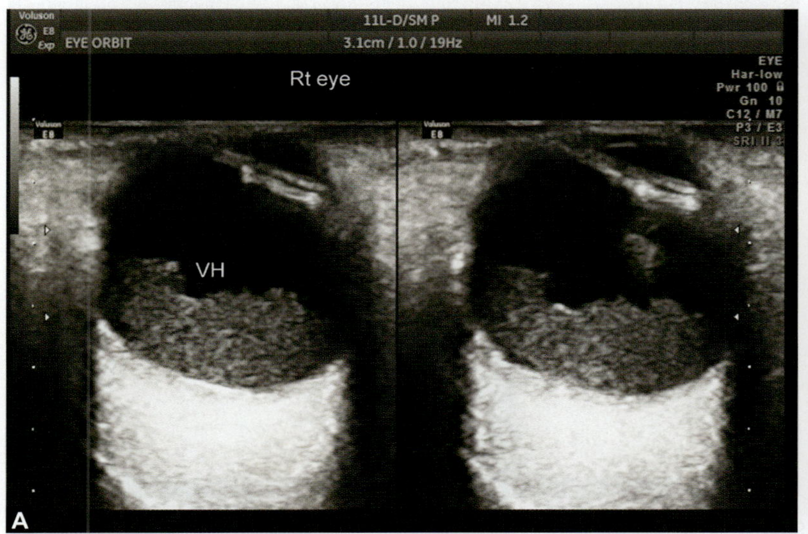

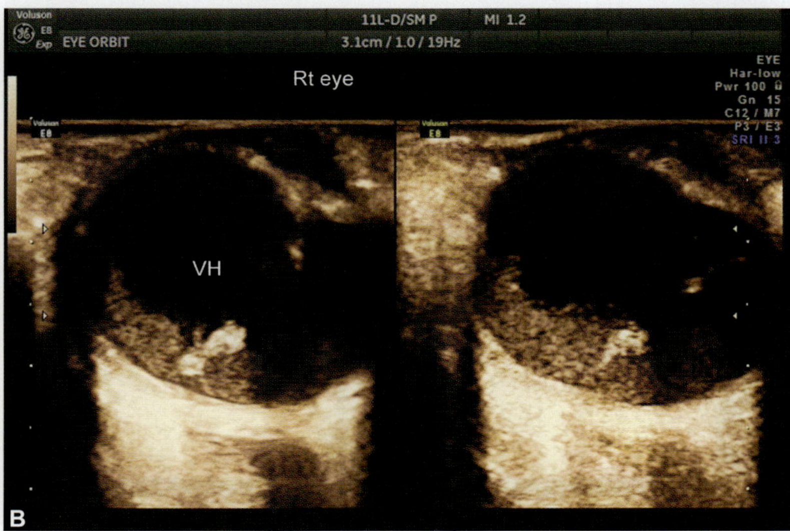

FIGURES 1.92A and B: Postsegment with hemorrhage. A patient presented with loss of vision after cataract surgery. HRSG shows dense intragel hemorrhage in posterior segment. An echogenic shadow is seen in the posterior segment suggestive of broken dislocated IOL in posterior segment.

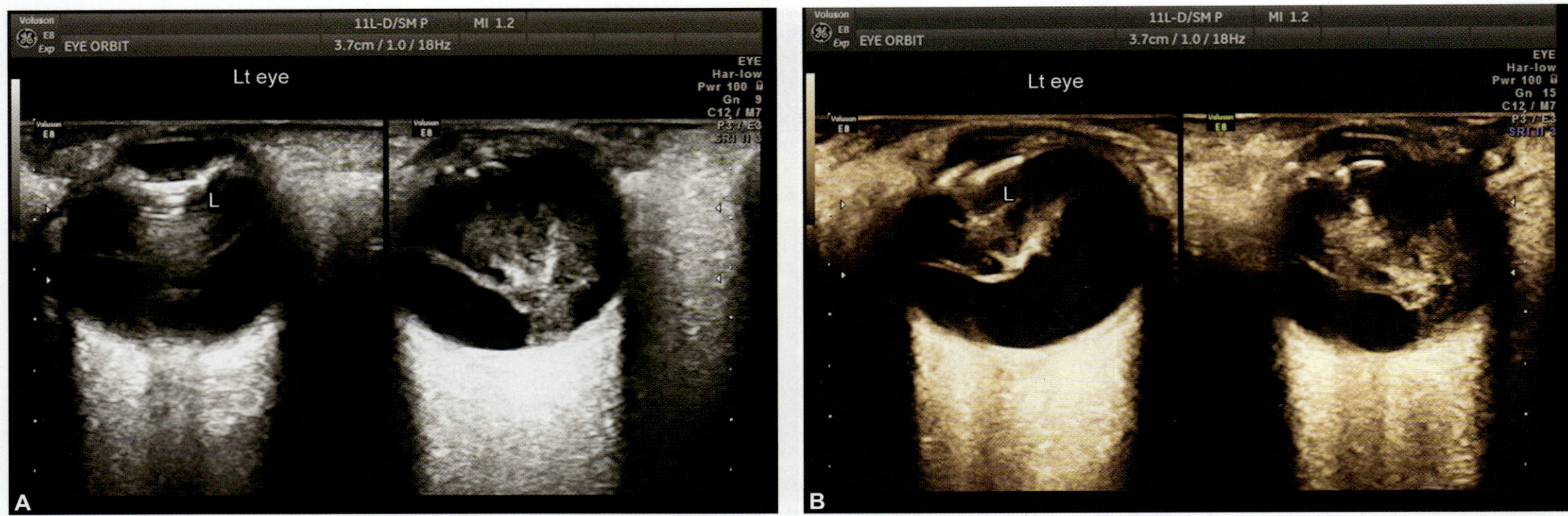

FIGURES 1.93A and B: Postsurgery hemorrhage. A patient underwent cataract surgery and complaint of loss of vision. HRSG shows IOL in position. However, dense intragel hemorrhage is seen in posterior segment. Retraction of vitreous is also seen with a pseudomembrane formation.

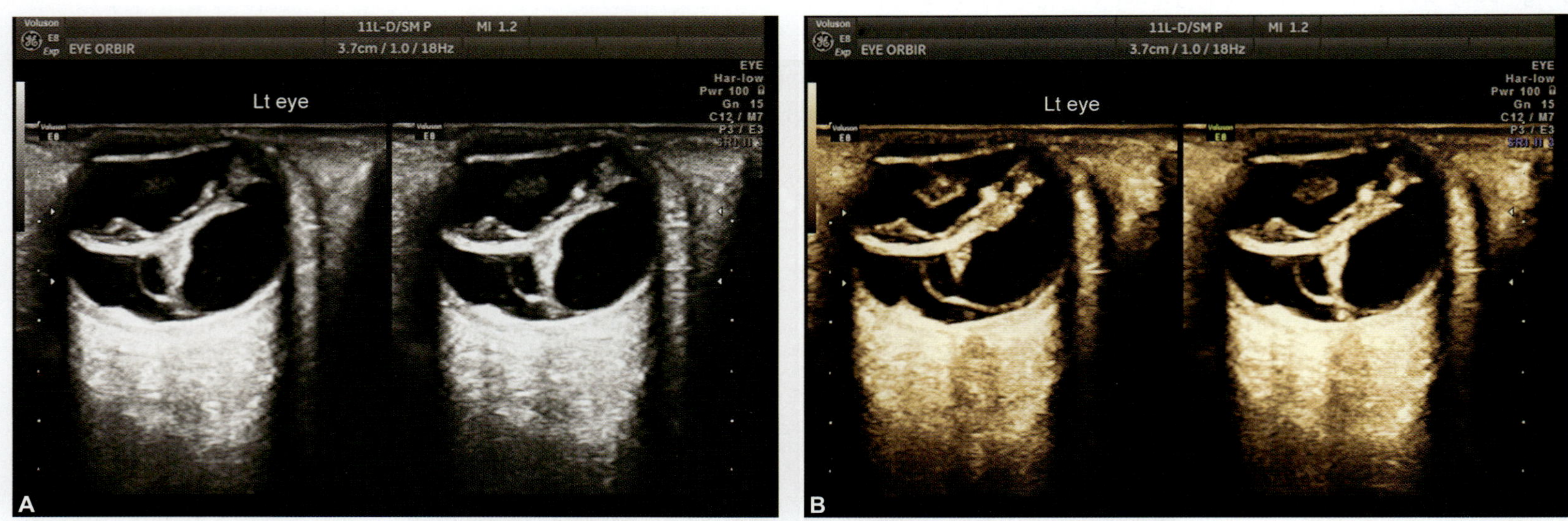

FIGURES 1.94A and B: Proliferative vitreoretinopathy. A patient presented with loss of vision. Lens is thickened and opaque. Posterior segment of the eye shows thick echogenic membranes. Triangle sign is positive. Retinal bands are also seen suggestive of proliferative vitreoretinopathy.

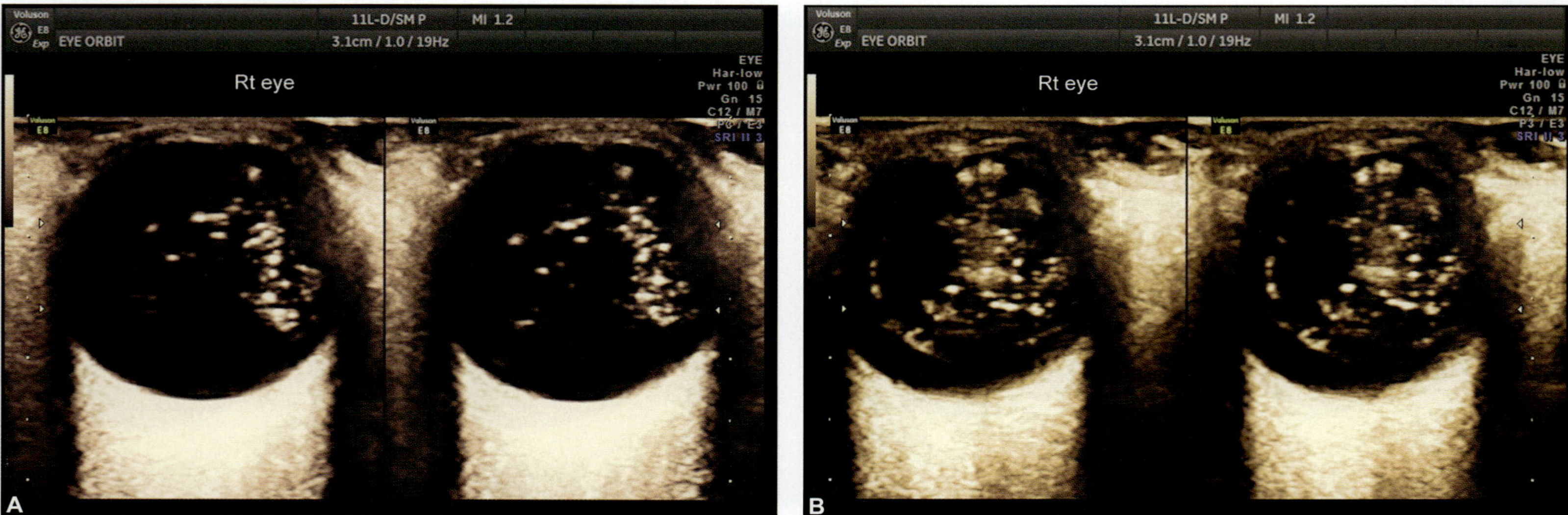

FIGURES 1.95A and B

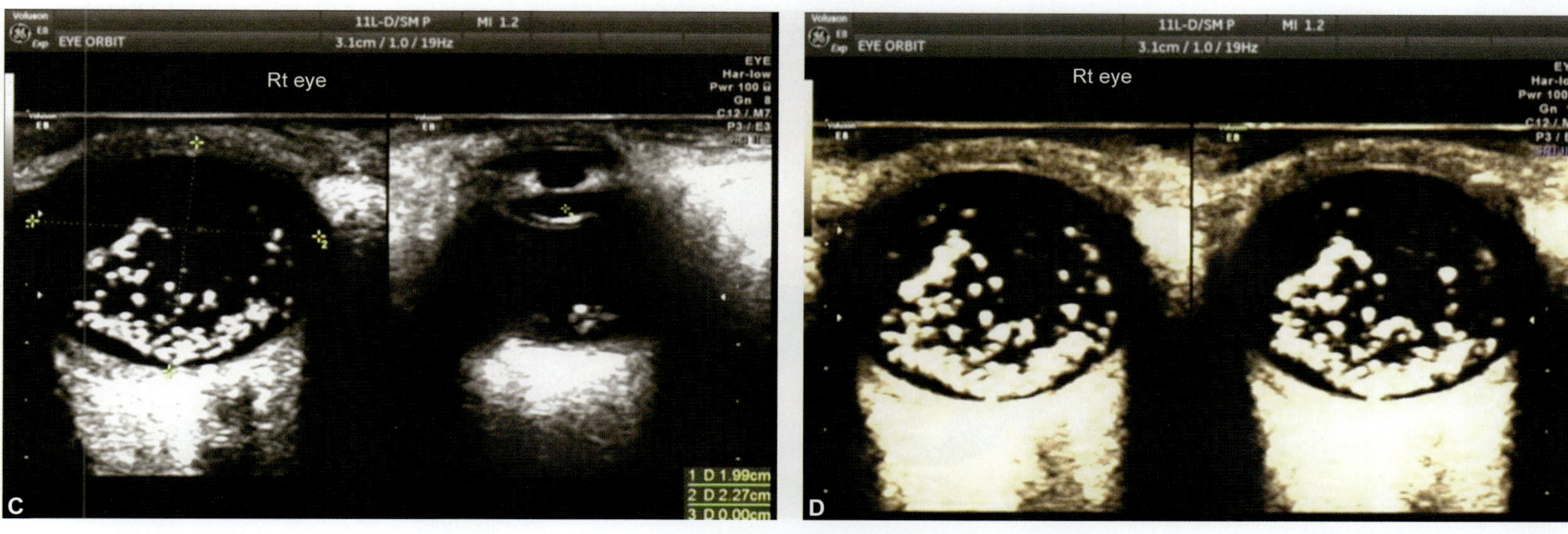

FIGURES 1.95C and D

FIGURES 1.95A to D: Asteroid hylosis. HRSG shows multiple bright echogenic dots in posterior segment of right eye. They look like shiny stars in sky suggestive of starry eye appearance. It is typical finding of asteroid hylosis. The lens is normal.

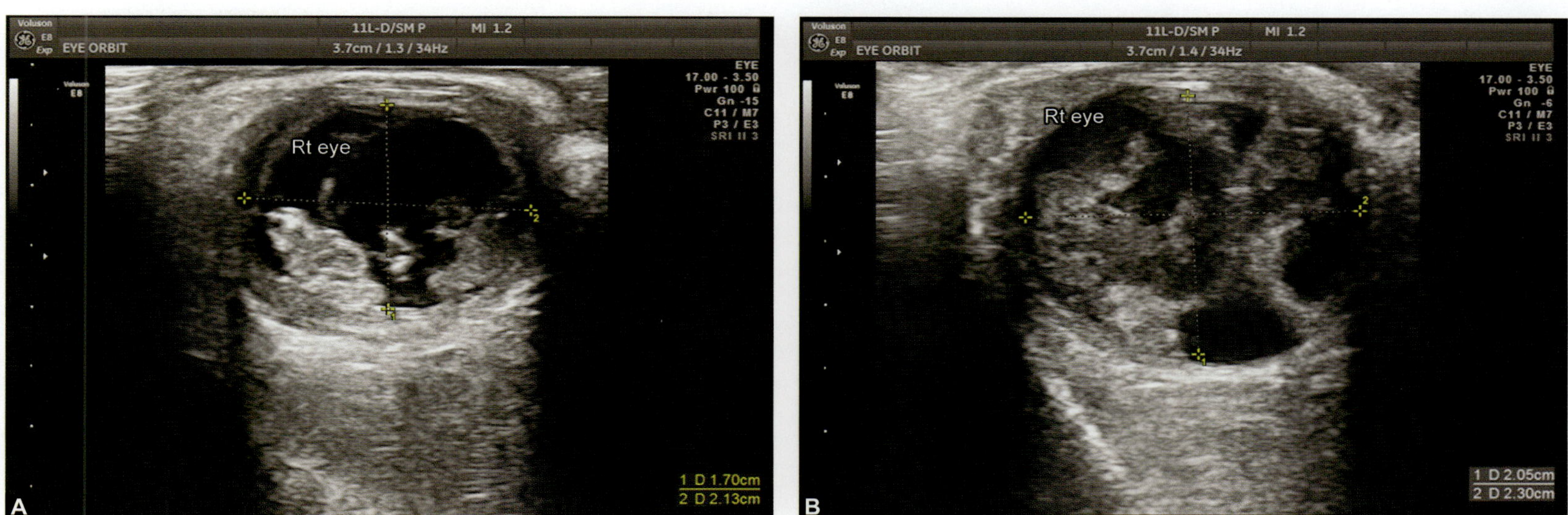

FIGURES 1.96A and B: Collapsed right eye. A patient presented with a soft eye after sustaining trauma. HRSG shows markedly thickened eye coat. The eye coat is irregular in outline and it is edematous. Normal anatomy is distorted. The dome shaped membranes are seen at the periphery suggestive of choroid detachment. Echogenic shadows are seen under the choroidal membrane suggestive of subchoroidal hemorrhage.

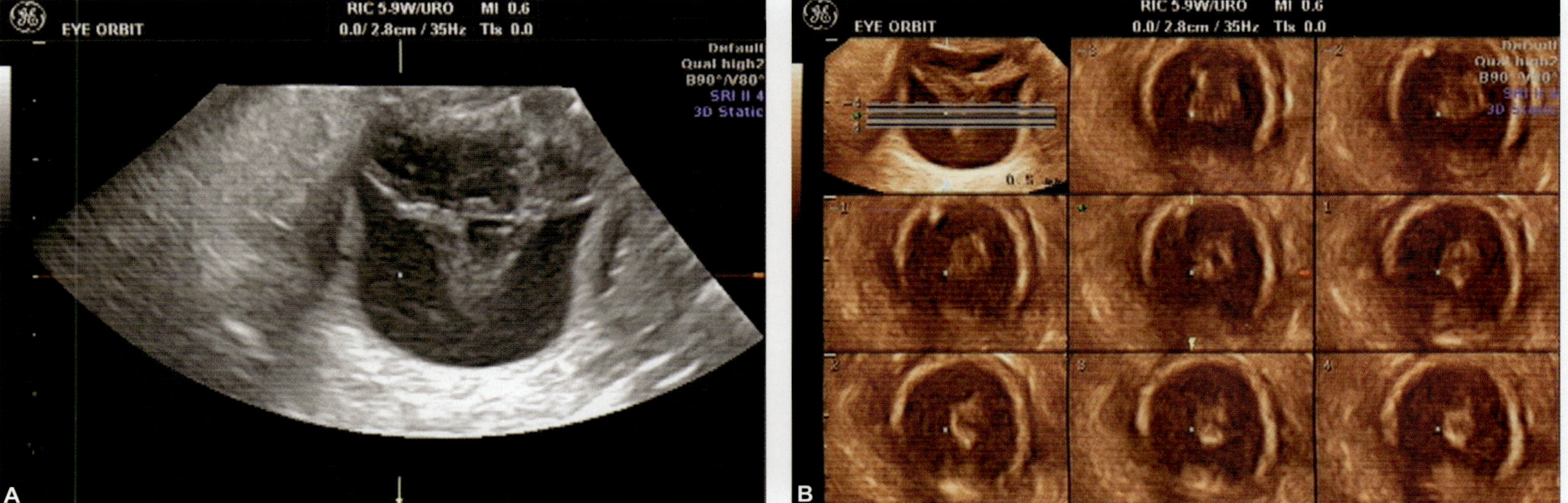

FIGURES 1.97A and B

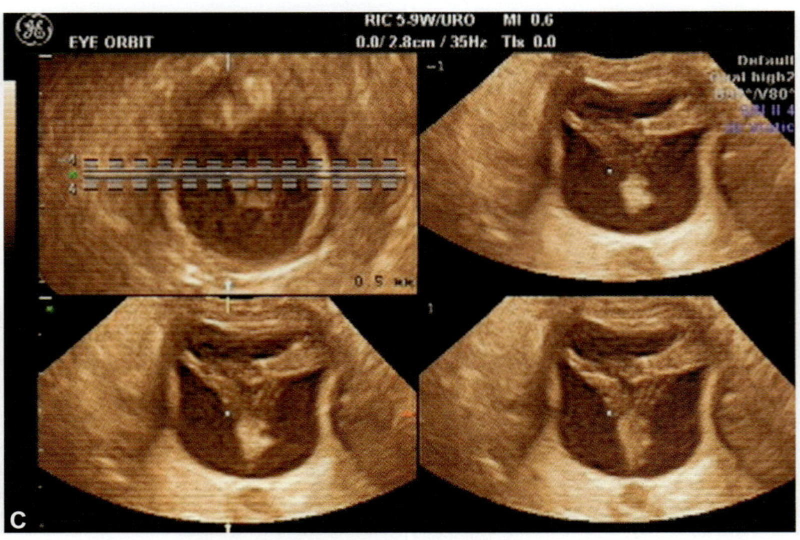

FIGURE 1.97C

FIGURES 1.97A to C: Choroid detachment with PVR. HRSG shows a deshaped eye. Thick dome shaped membranes are seen at periphery suggestive of choroidal detachment. Triangle sign is positive. Retina is seen collapsed and detached forming a funnel suggestive of proliferative vitreoretinopathy. The 3D and TUI imaging show clearly choroidal detachment with proliferative vitreoretinopathy (PVR).

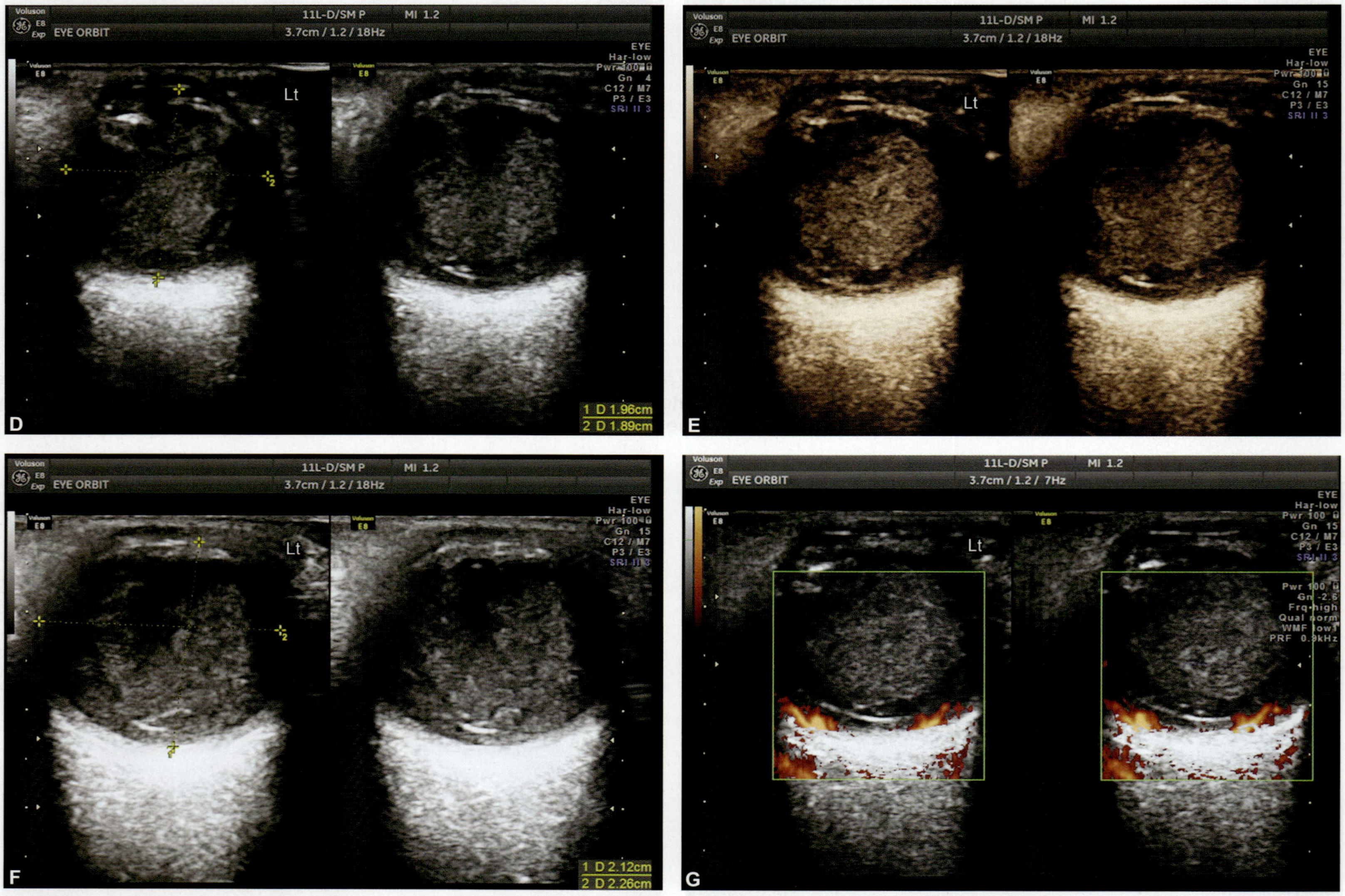

FIGURES 1.97D to G: Pyoophthalmos. A young child presented with red swollen edematous Rt eye. HRSG shows edematous right eye coat. The eye is enlarged. Lens shows early thickening. Posterior segment of eye shows homogeneous low level echo collection. It shows slow movements on dynamic scanning. Sedimentation is seen in the collection suggestive of exudative collection due to pyoophthalmos.

RETINA

One of the most important roles of HRSG is in evaluating the pathology of retina in opaque ocular media like retinal tears, retinal detachments, retinoschisis and other disorders.

Retinal tears and retinal detachments can be easily evaluated on HRSG. Small retinal tears show flappy movements on dynamic scanning. They are usually present in superior peripheral fundus. They may be associated with posterior vitreous detachment but giant retinal tears show varied presentation and usually associated with severe injury to eye. When an unusual insertion of membrane is seen on HRSG possibility of giant retinal tear is to be kept.

Retinal Detachment

Retina is closely applied to choroid. It is firmly attached at optic nerve head and ora serrata. Retinal detachment (RD) typically produces a bright continuous normally folded membrane on 'B' scan. It is usually attached at optic nerve head and ora serrata giving a funnel-shaped appearance. The RD shows little or more restricted movement than posterior vitreous detachment. Extensive detachment may present as funnel-shaped membrane which may be open or closed type. Long-standing retinal detachment may develop retinal cyst. It may be partially calcified and cholesterol debris may accumulate in subretinal space. Three main types of retinal detachments are seen:

1. *Rhegmatogeneous retinal detachment:* It is caused due to the brake in the continuity of retina due to the weakness in the peripheral retina due to degeneration as in myopia, diabetic retinopathy or vitreoretinal traction in detached vitreous.
2. *Nonrhegmatogeneous retinal detachment:* It is further devided into two types:
   a. Tractional RD—it is caused due to fraction of detached vitreous pulling the retina from the pigmented epithelium through vitreoretinal resulting into angular or fix retinal detachment.
   b. Exudative retinal bands detachment—It is caused due to collection of fluid in the subvitreal space due to inflammation-uveal effusion or tumors.
3. *Exudative retinal detachment (Coat's disease)*: Coat's disease is a unilateral condition mainly found in children, usually presents in first decade of life. It is more common in males than females. It is to be differentiated from retinoblastoma, retinopathy of prematurity, toxocara and PHPV.

Proliferative Vitreoretinopathy

In proliferative vitreoretinopathy (PVR), thin membranes are formed on inner retinal surface and posterior hyloid interface. Contraction of the membrane leads to gel retraction, retinal traction and hemolization. In moderate PVR, HRSG shows flappy movements of retina. But in a severe PVR funnel like retina is seen at postequatorial retina. A fibrous membrane is seen stretching across the anterior retina giving a classical triangle appearance. It is an important indication in a poor surgical in prognosis.

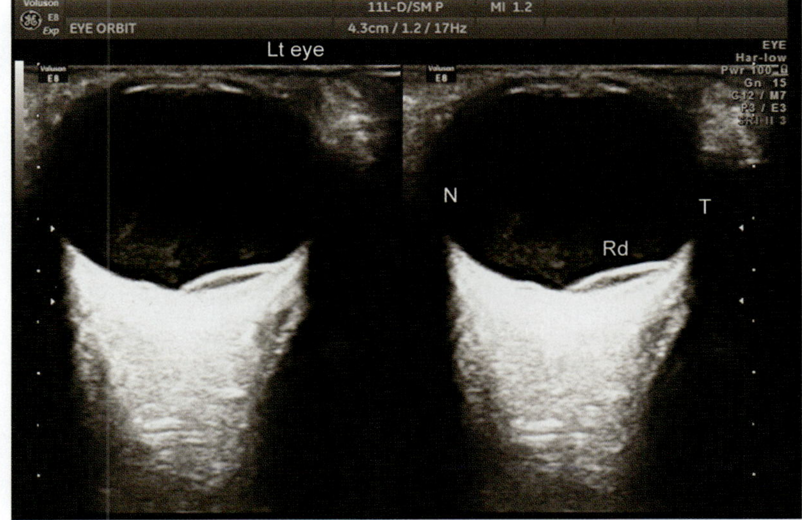

FIGURE 1.98

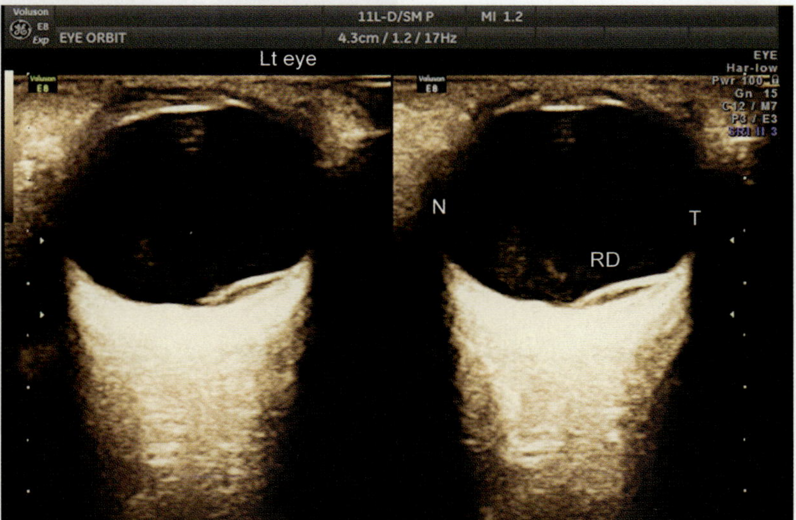

FIGURE 1.99

FIGURES 1.98 and 1.99: Retinoschisis. HRSG shows a thin dome-shaped membrane in the temporal inferior quadrant. It is more focal, smooth and thin in outline and not seen inserting at the optic nerve head suggestive of retinoschisis. In this condition retina splits into two thin layers. One layer is lifted up and another layer is seen down in relation to the choroid. HRSG shows a thin echogenic membrane lifted up in the inferiotemporal quadrant of eye. It is smooth in outline suggestive of retinoschisis.

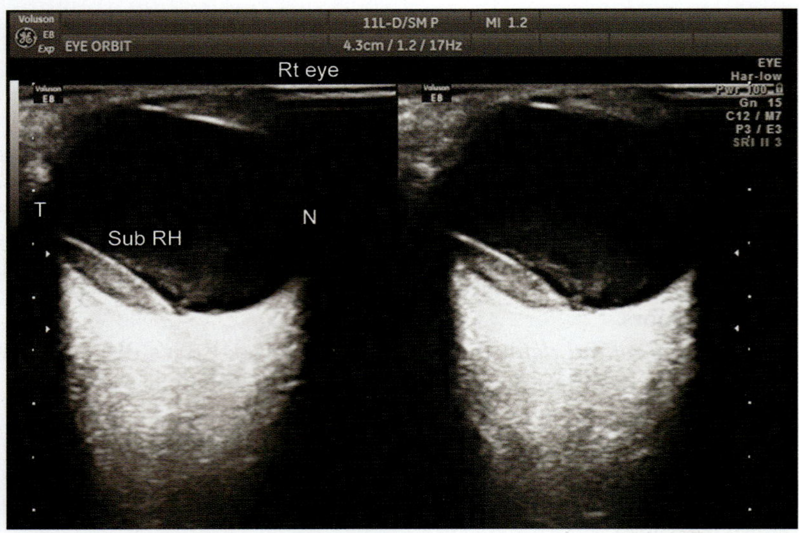

FIGURE 1.100

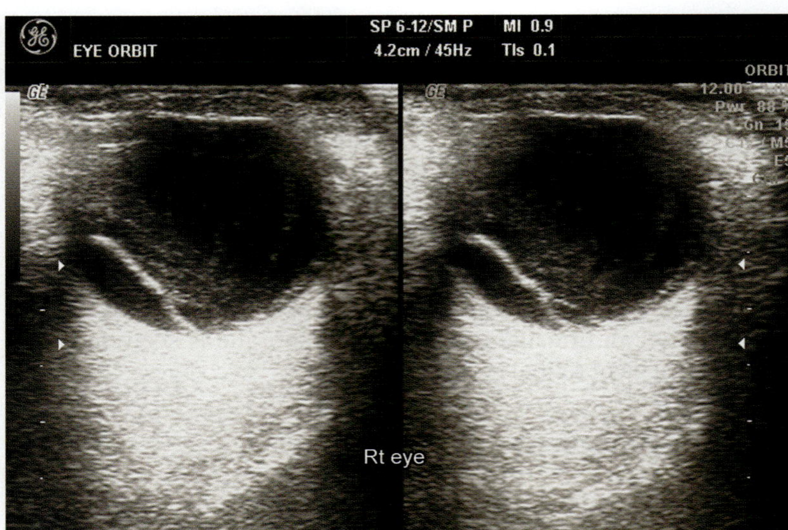

FIGURE 1.101

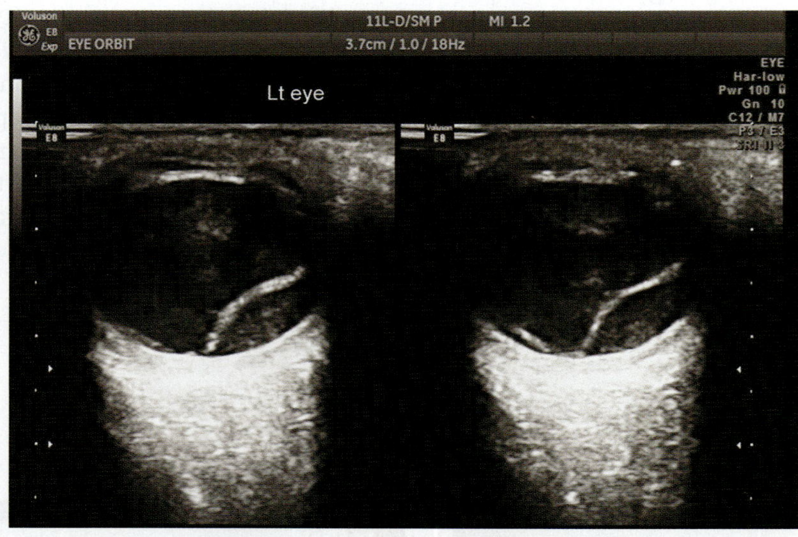

FIGURE 1.102

FIGURES 1.100 to 1.102: Subretinal hemorrhage. HRSG shows partial lifting of retina at the posterior pole suggestive of partial retinal detachment. Echogenic collection is seen under the retina suggestive of subretinal hemorrhage.

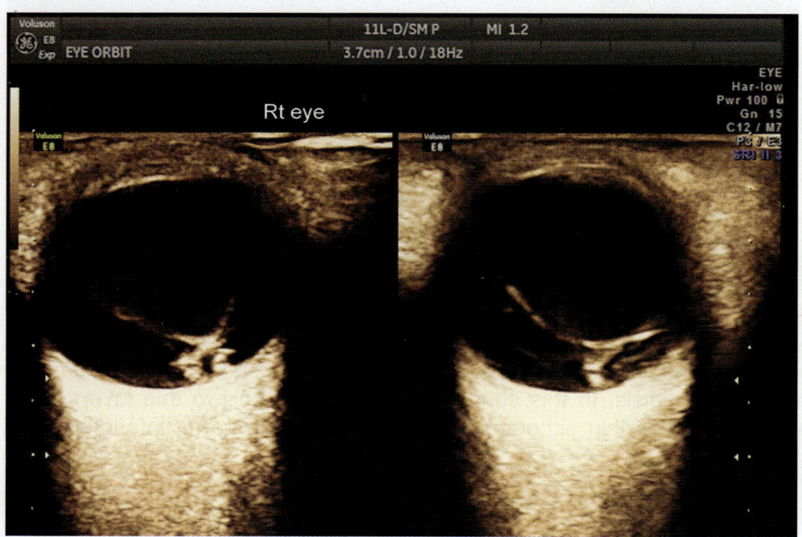

FIGURE 1.103

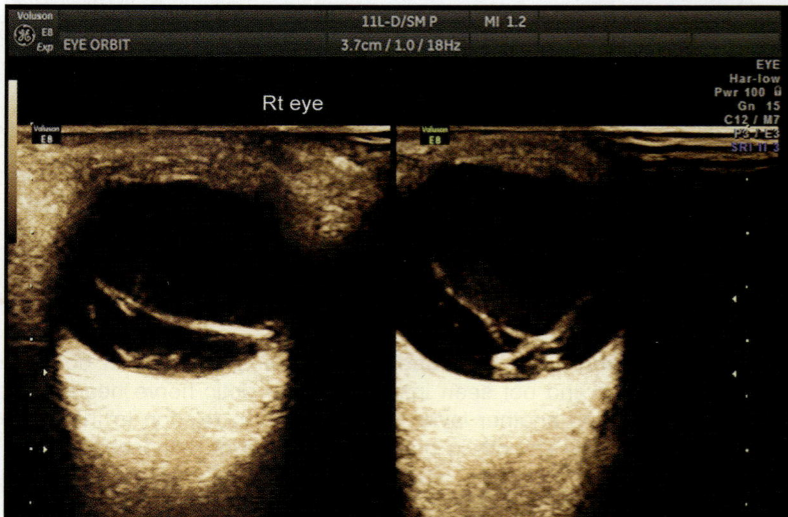

FIGURE 1.104

FIGURES 1.103 and 1.104: Tractional retinal detachment. A patient presented with partial loss of vision. HRSG shows intragel hemorrhage with PVD. Vitreoretinal bands are also seen. The vitreal band are seen partially lifting the retina suggestive of tractional retinal detachment.

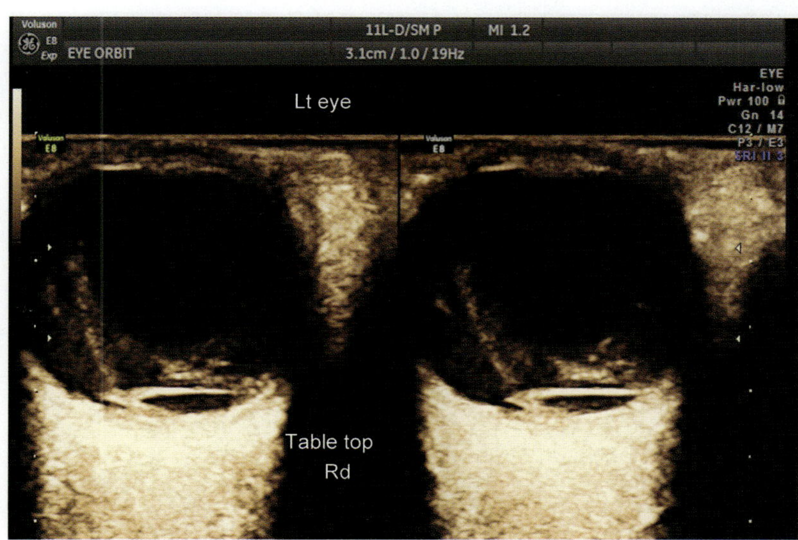

FIGURE 1.105

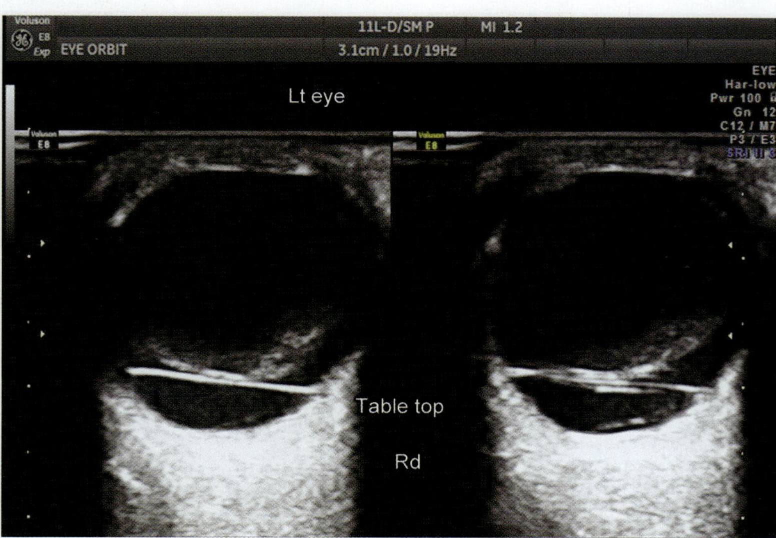

FIGURE 1.106

FIGURES 1.105 and 1.106: Tabletop retinal detachment. A patient presented with partial loss of vision. HRSG shows intragel hemorrhage with vitreoretinal bands. The retina is seen lifted up in a flat manner with a wide base suggestive of tabletop retinal detachment.

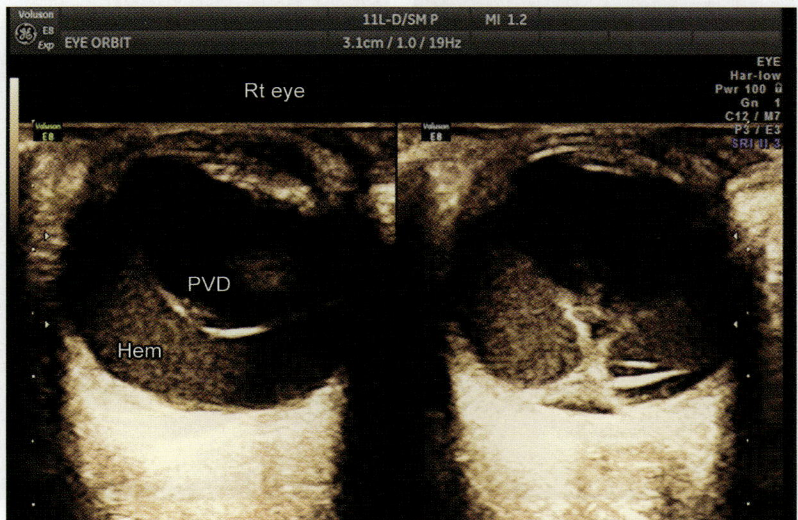

FIGURE 1.107

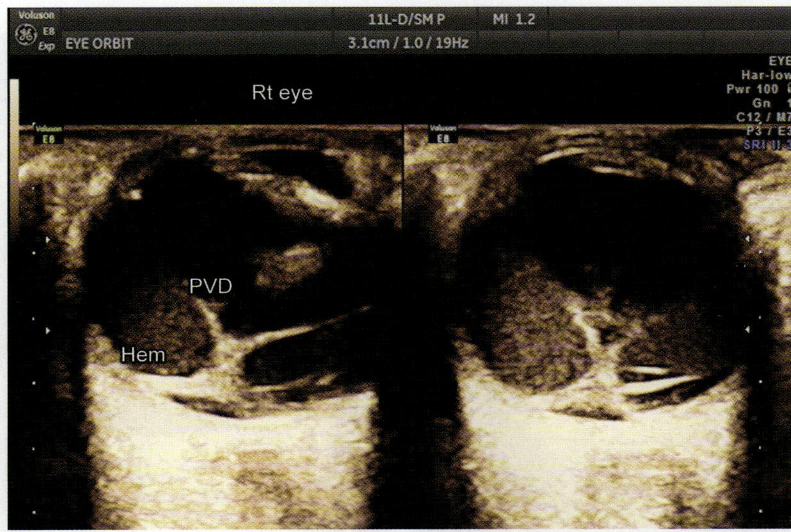

FIGURE 1.108

FIGURES 1.107 and 1.108: Tractional retinal detachment. HRSG shows multiple vitreoretinal bands in a patient presented with loss of vision. Intragel hemorrhage is also seen. Tractional retinal detachment is also seen because of vitreoretinal bands.

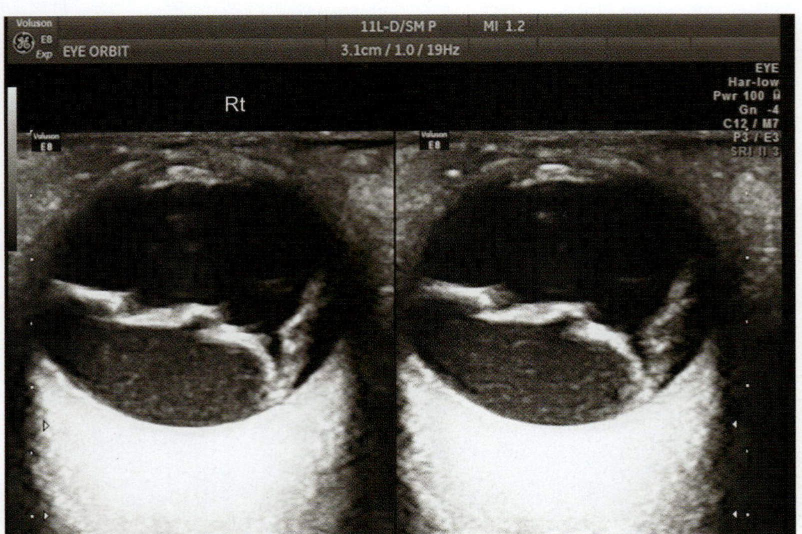

FIGURE 1.109

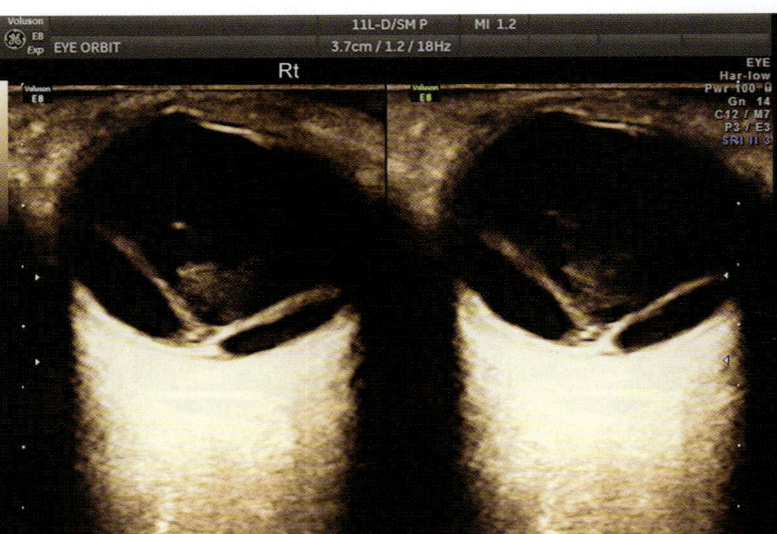

FIGURE 1.110

FIGURES 1.109 and 1.110: Extensive retinal detachment. A patient presented with loss of vision. HRSG shows a thick membrane detached in posterior segment. It is seen attached at optic nerve head and ora-serrata. On dynamic scanning, it shows limited movements suggestive of retinal detachment.

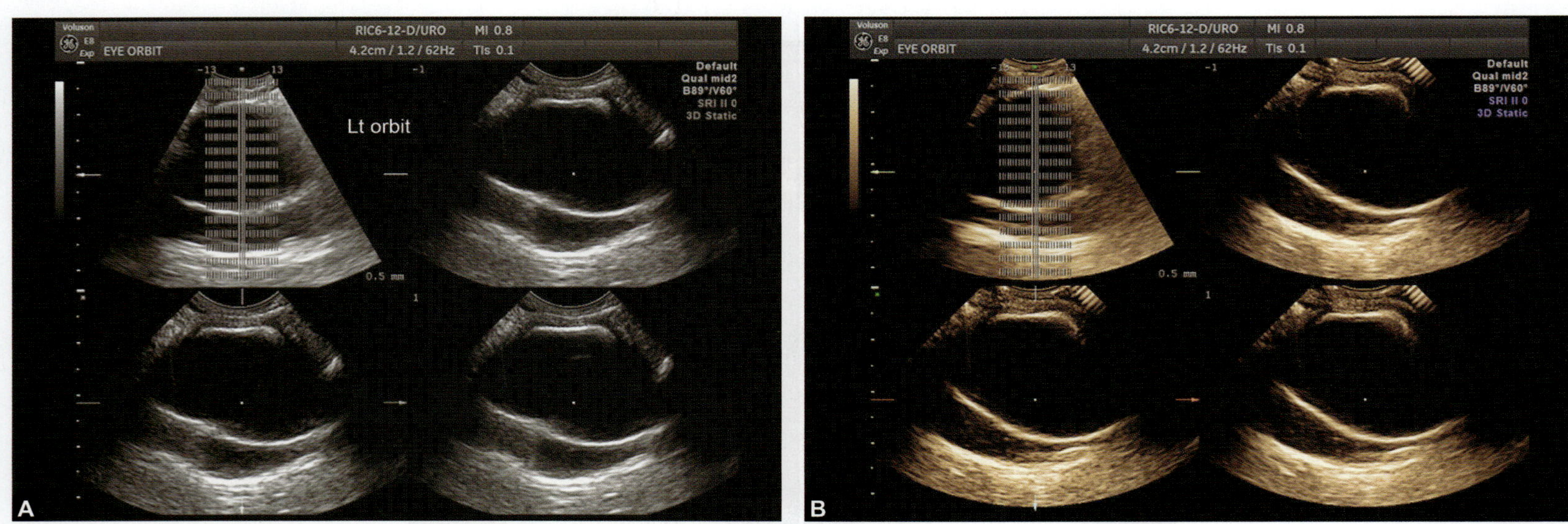

FIGURES 1.111A and B: Subretinal hemorrhage. An 18-year-old boy presented with loss of vision. HRSG shows a thick membrane seen detached in the posterior segment, which shows limited movement. On TUI imaging, echogenic collection is seen under the membrane suggestive of subretinal hemorrhage.

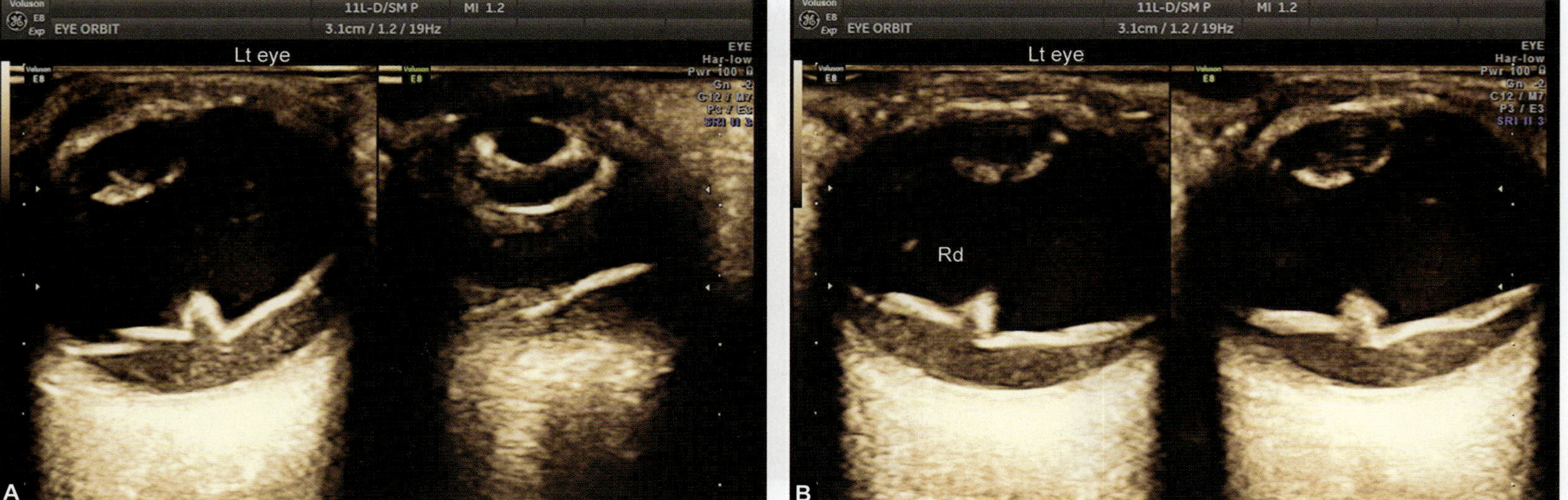

FIGURES 1.112A and B: Retinal detachment with subretinal hemorrhage. A patient presented with sudden loss of vision. HRSG shows thickened opaque lens. A dense echogenic shadow is seen in the posterior segment suggestive of retinal detachment. Echogenic collection is seen under the retina suggestive of subretinal hemorrhage.

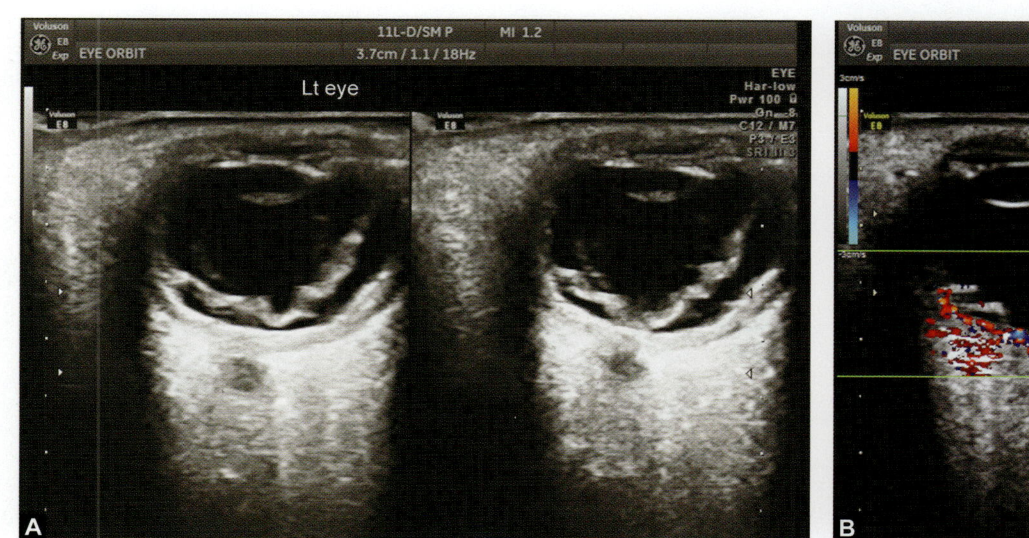

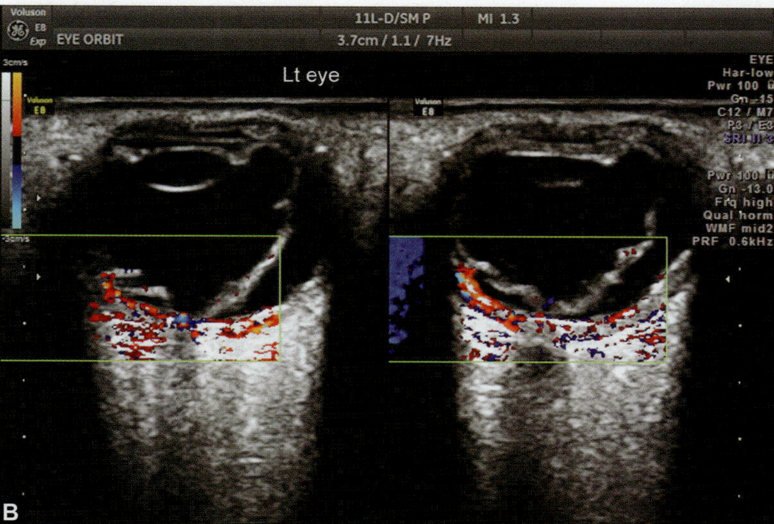

FIGURES 1.113A and B: Total retinal detachment. A patient presented with loss of vision. HRSG shows early thickening of the lens. Posterior segment of the eye shows a thick membrane detached from all sides suggestive of total retinal detachment. On color flow imaging, few vessels are seen dragged with detached retina.

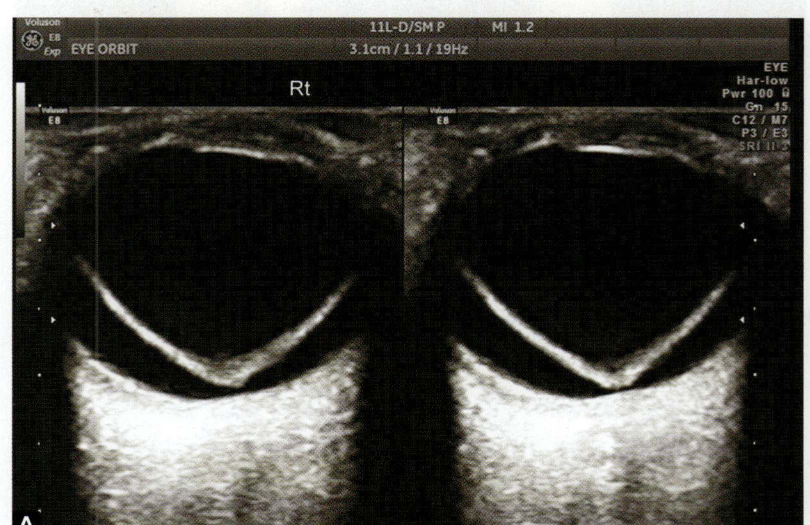

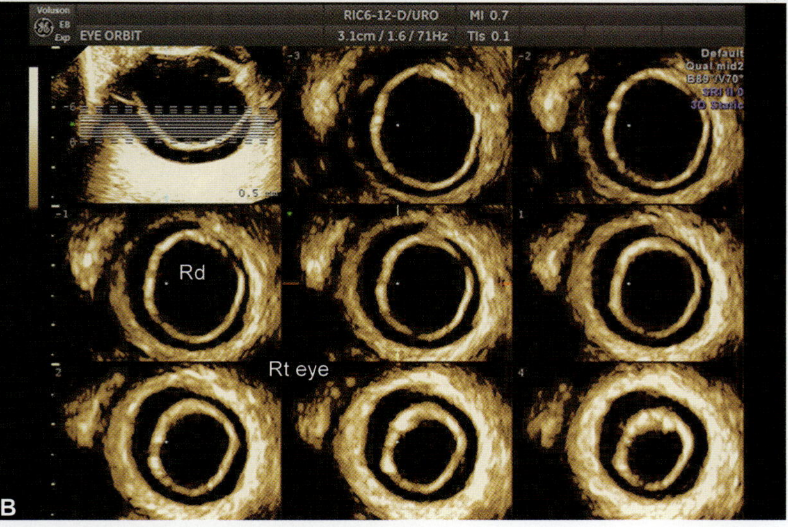

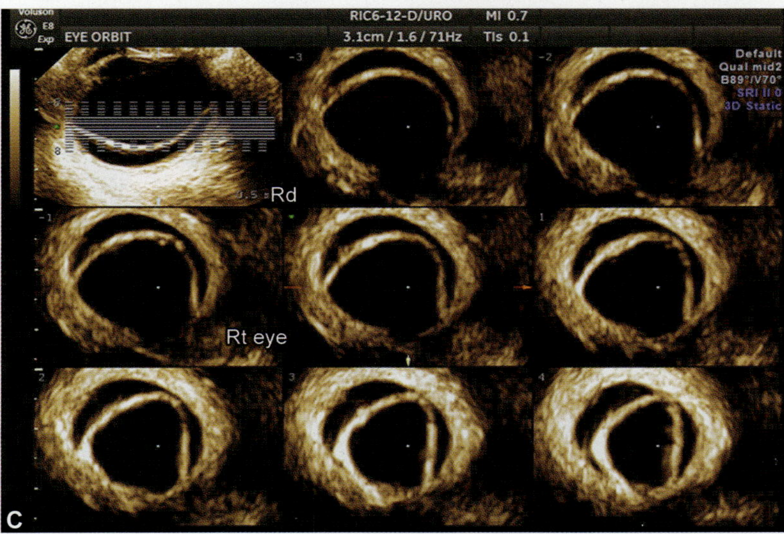

FIGURES 1.114A to C: Total retinal detachment with TUI imaging. A patient presented with sudden loss of vision. HRSG shows total retinal detachment in right eye. The 3D TUI imaging shows total retina seen detached from all sides of globe.

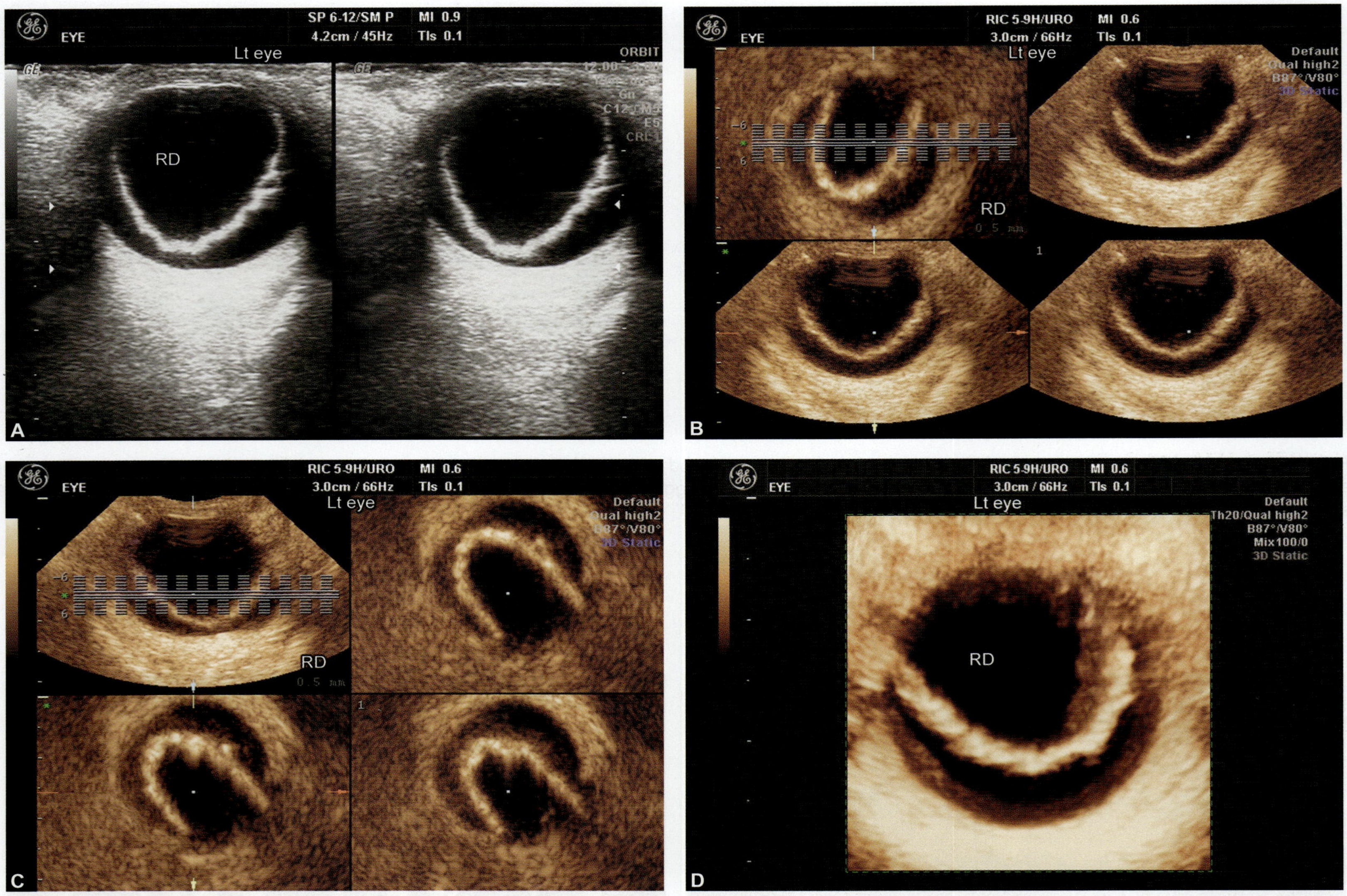

FIGURES 1.115A to D: Total retinal detachment with 3D and TUI imaging. HRSG shows total retinal detachment in a patient presented with loss of vision. The 3D and TUI imaging shows beautifully the detached retina.

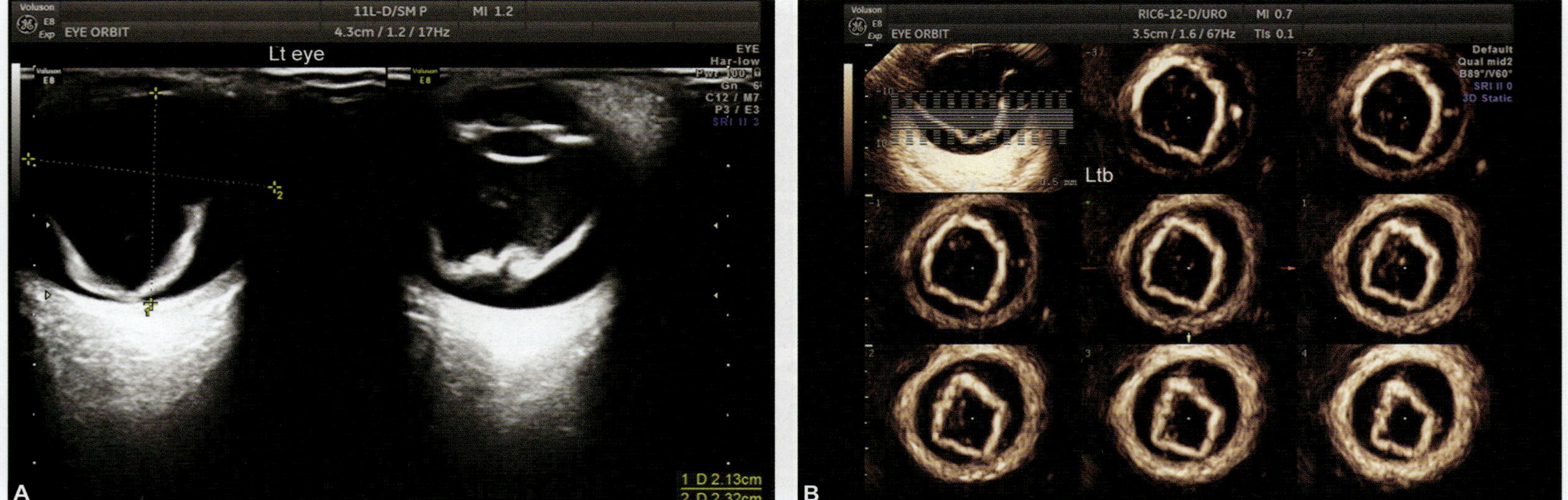

FIGURES 1.116A and B: Total retinal detachment. A 13-year-old child presented with loss of vision after sustaining trauma. HRSG shows total retinal detachment. On TUI imaging, the retina is seen detached from all sides of the globe.

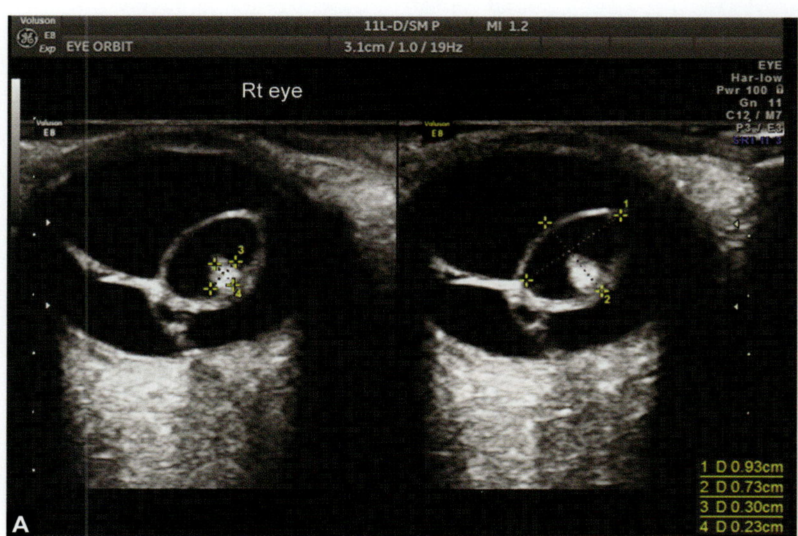

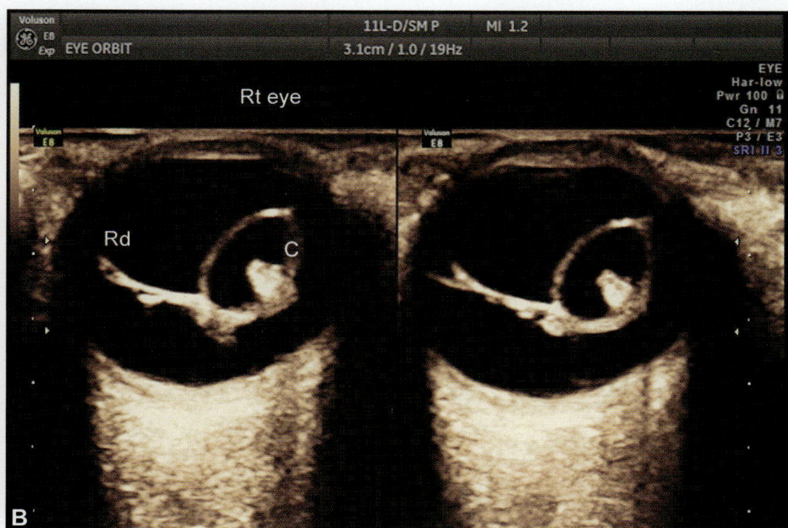

FIGURES 1.117A and B: Retinal detachment with cysticercus cyst. A patient presented with acute pain in eye with sudden loss of vision. HRSG shows a well defined cyst in the posterior segment. An echogenic nidus is seen fixed with the inner wall of cyst suggestive of cysticercus cyst. The cyst is seen attached at retina and retina is seen detached from its surface suggestive of retinal detachment.

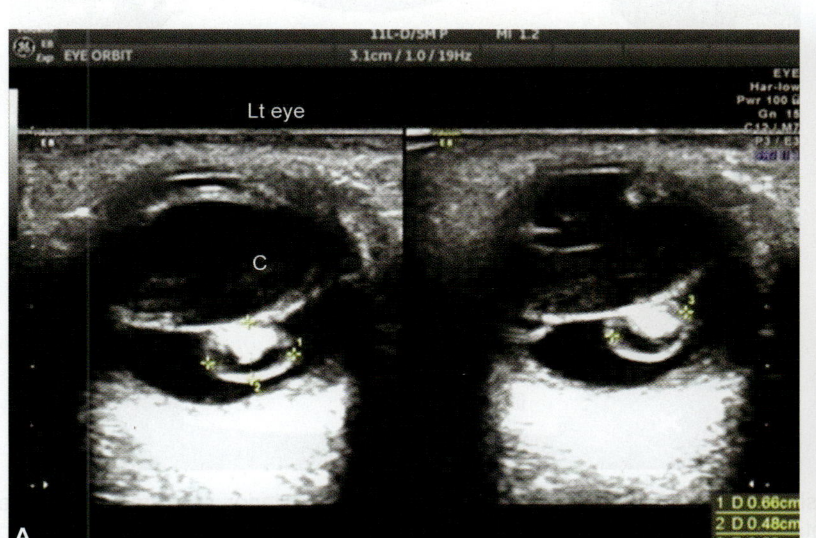

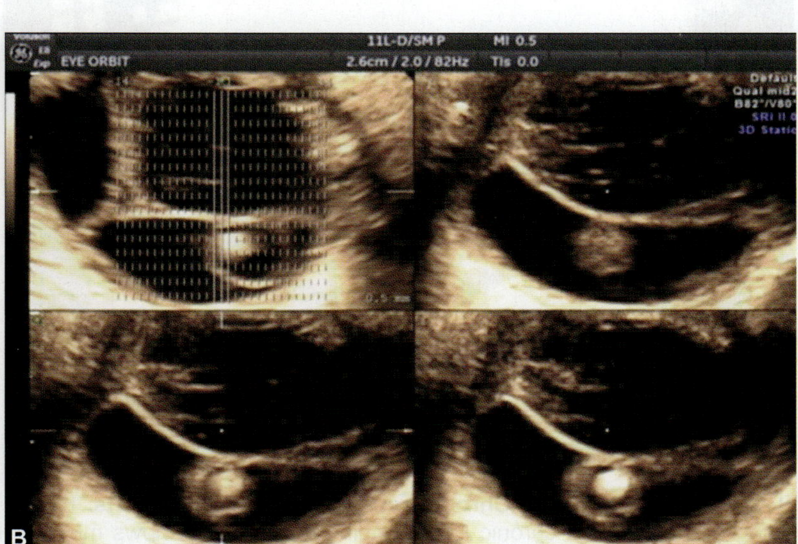

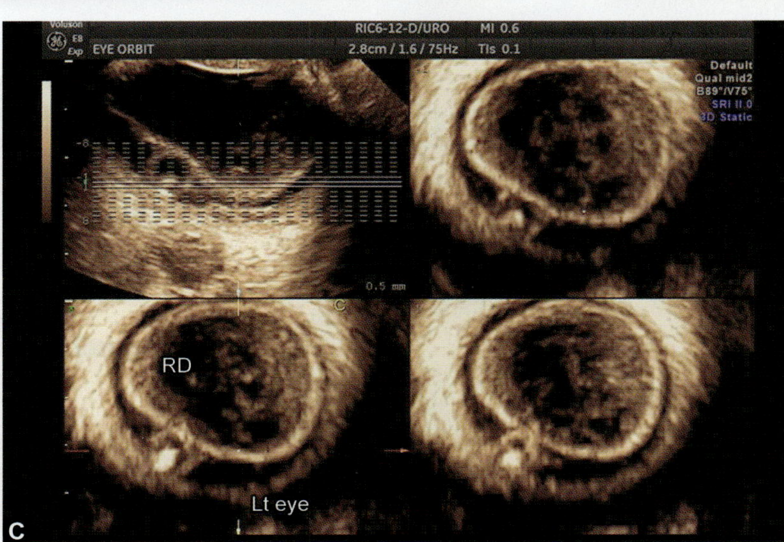

FIGURES 1.118A to C: Retinal detachment with cysticercus cyst. A patient presented with sudden loss of vision. HRSG shows a well-defined cyst in subretinal space. The cyst shows echogenic nidus fixed with inner wall of cyst. The cyst results into lifting of retina causing total retinal detachment. On 3D TUI imaging, the total retinal detachment with cyticercus cyst is seen in the subretinal space clearly.

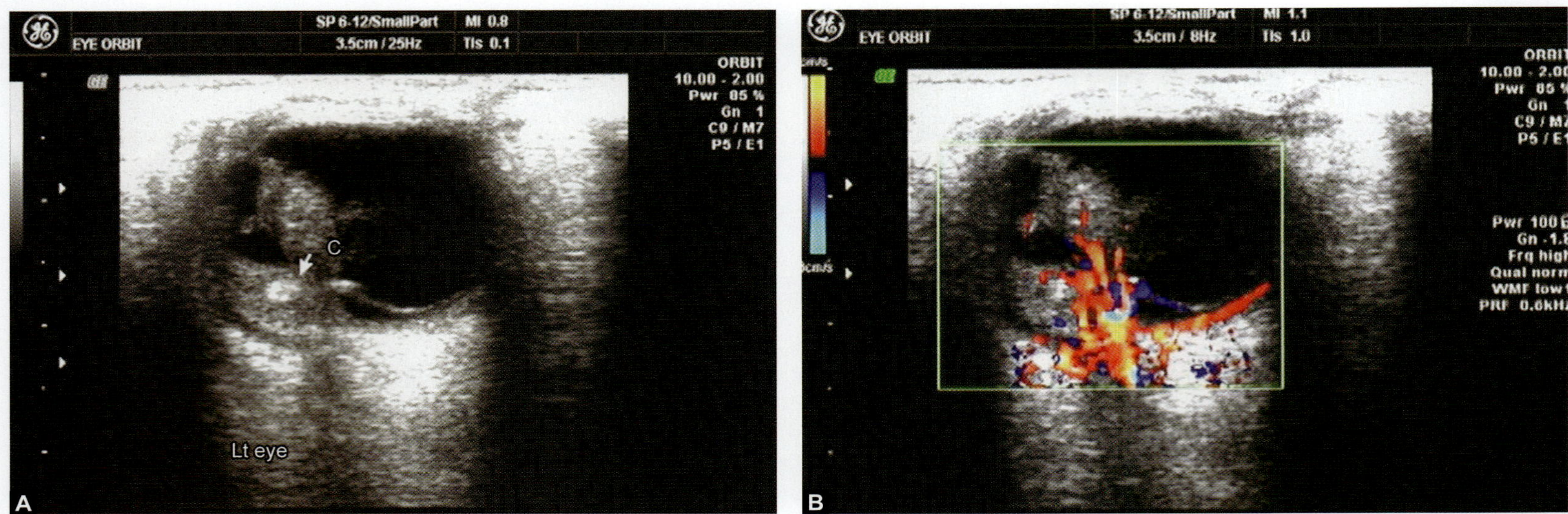

FIGURES 1.119A and B: Ruptured cysticercus cyst. A patient presented with sudden loss of vision and acute pain in eye. HRSG shows a low level echo complex mass in the subretinal space. An echogenic nidus is seen in it. The retina is seen lifted up. Associated intragel hemorrhage is also seen. On color flow imaging, increased flow is seen in it suggestive of intense inflammatory reaction. Findings are suggestive of ruptured cysticercus cyst with retinal detachment with intragel hemorrhage.

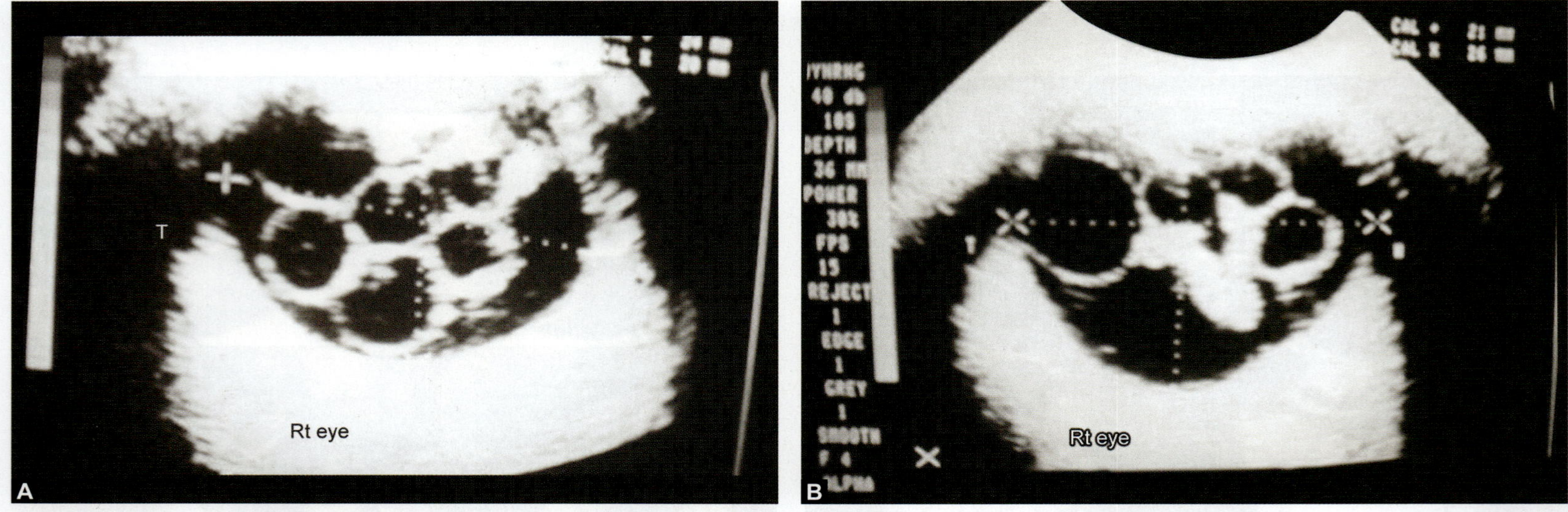

FIGURES 1.120A and B: Chronic retinal tear or retinal cysts. HRSG shows multiple retinal cysts formation in the posterior segment due to the folding of the retina in chronic long-standing tear. HRSG shows multiple retinal cysts formed in chronic retinal tear with calcification of retina are also seen in the posterior segment.

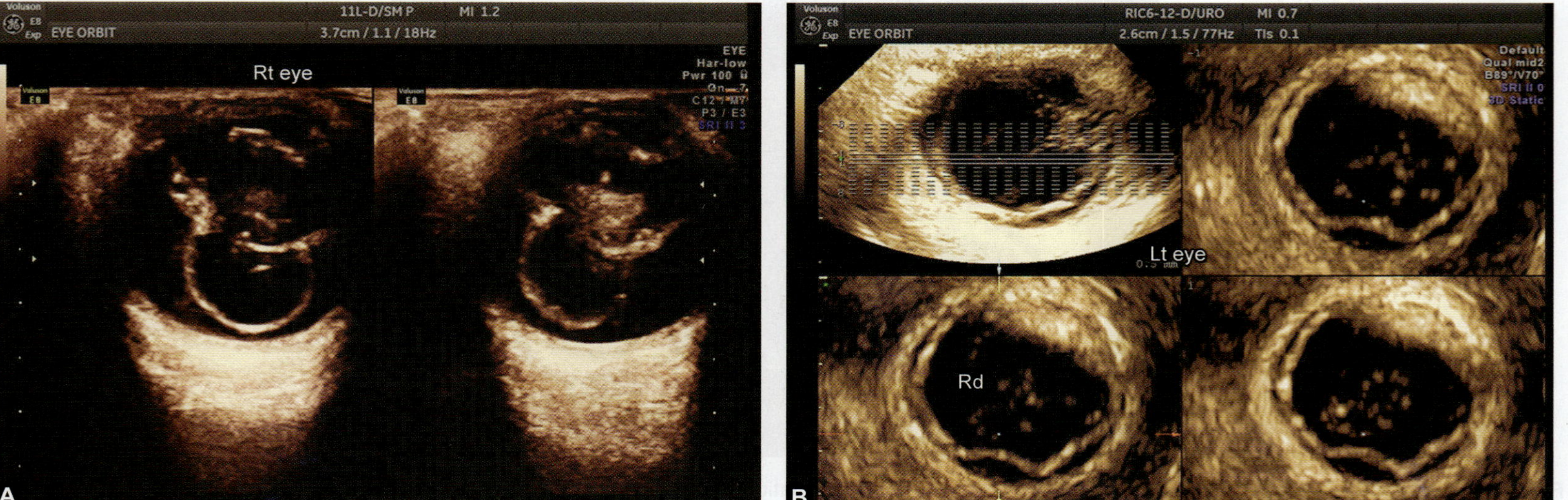

FIGURES 1.121A and B

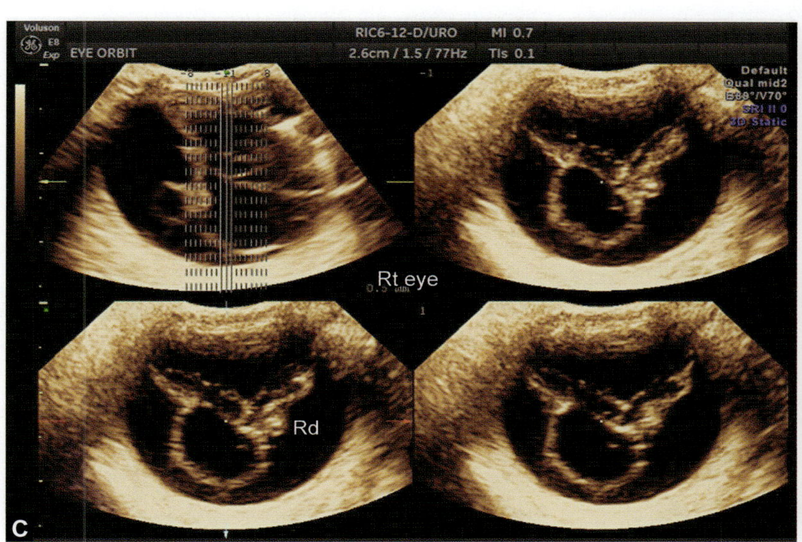

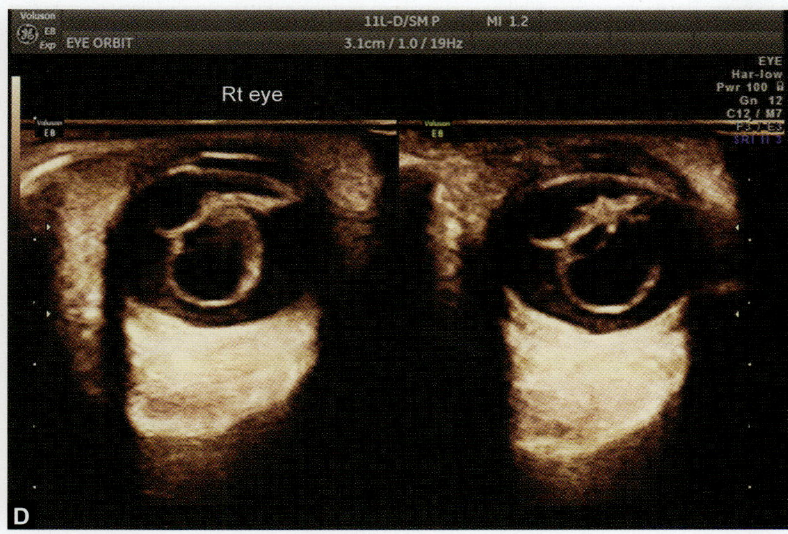

FIGURES 1.121C and D

FIGURES 1.121A to D: Giant retinal tear. HRSG shows a giant retinal tear in the right eye. The total retina is seen detached from all sides. Folding of retina is seen suggestive of retinal cyst formation.

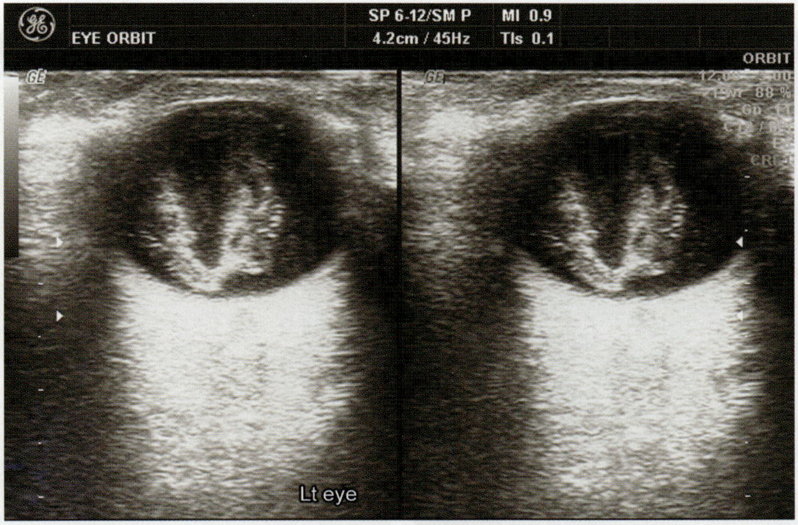

FIGURE 1.122: Giant retinal tear. A patient presented with loss of vision. HRSG shows a thick membrane seen detached from all sides. It shows flattening. Open funnel sign is positive suggestive of giant retinal tear. Associated intragel hemorrhage is also seen.

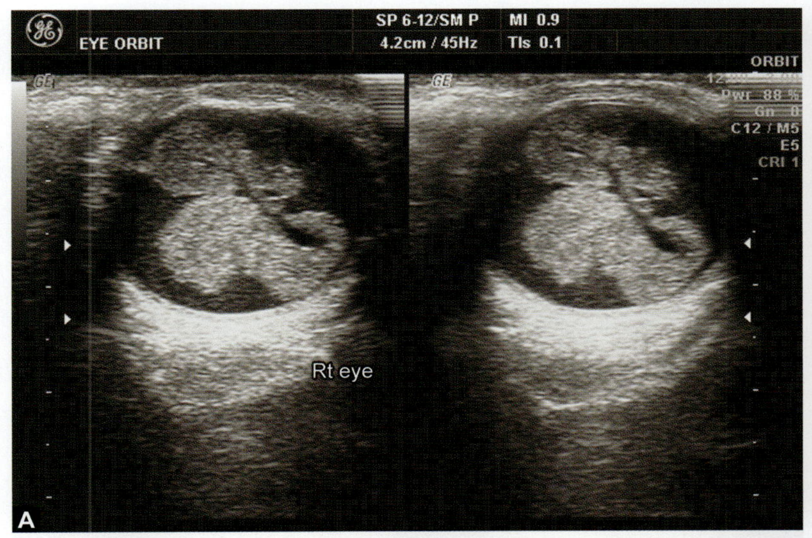

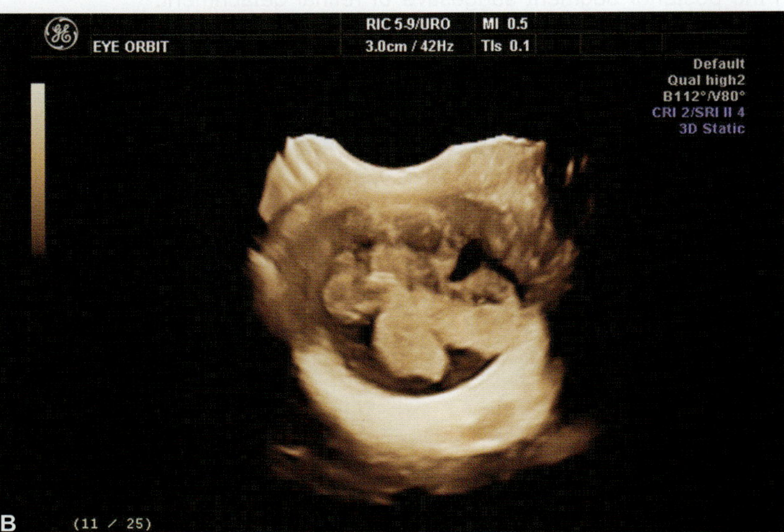

FIGURES 1.123A and B

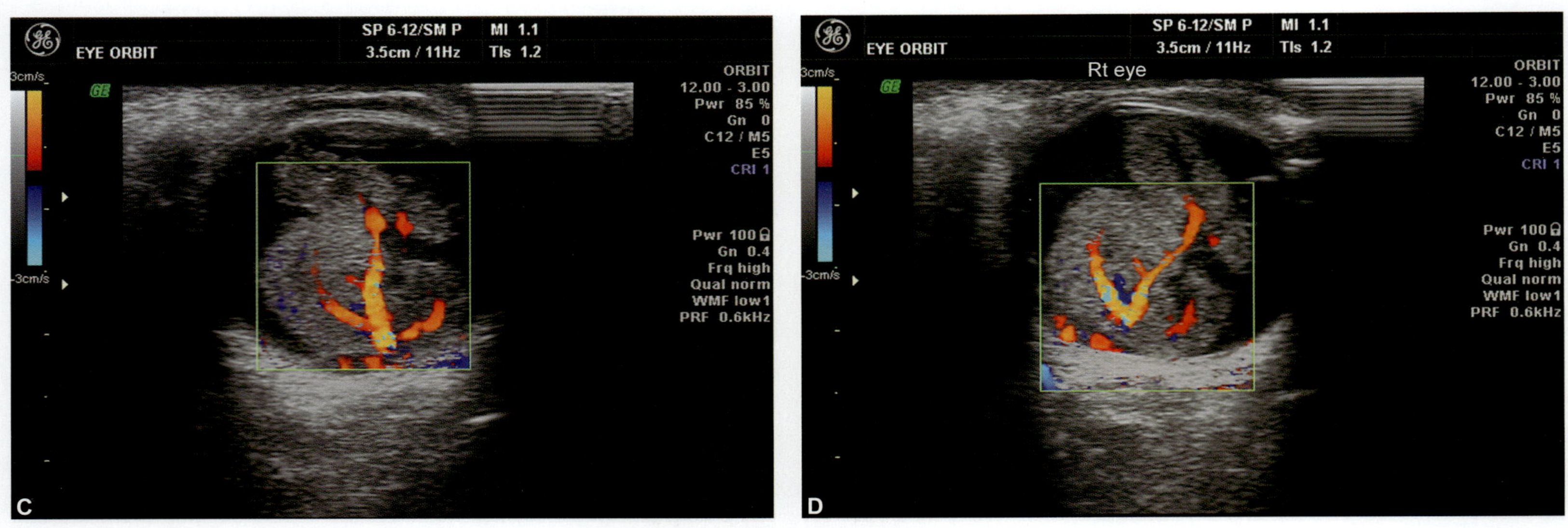

FIGURES 1.123C and D

FIGURES 1.123A to D: Coat's disease. A baby of 3.5 years age presented with white eye reflex. HRSG shows a thick membrane seen detached in the posterior segment. It shows multiple folds. Thick exudation is seen in the membrane. But no calcification is seen. On color flow imaging, retinal artery is seen dragged in the membrane. The 3D imaging of the eye shows the thick membrane confined in the posterior segment. The findings are highly suggestive of Coat's disease.

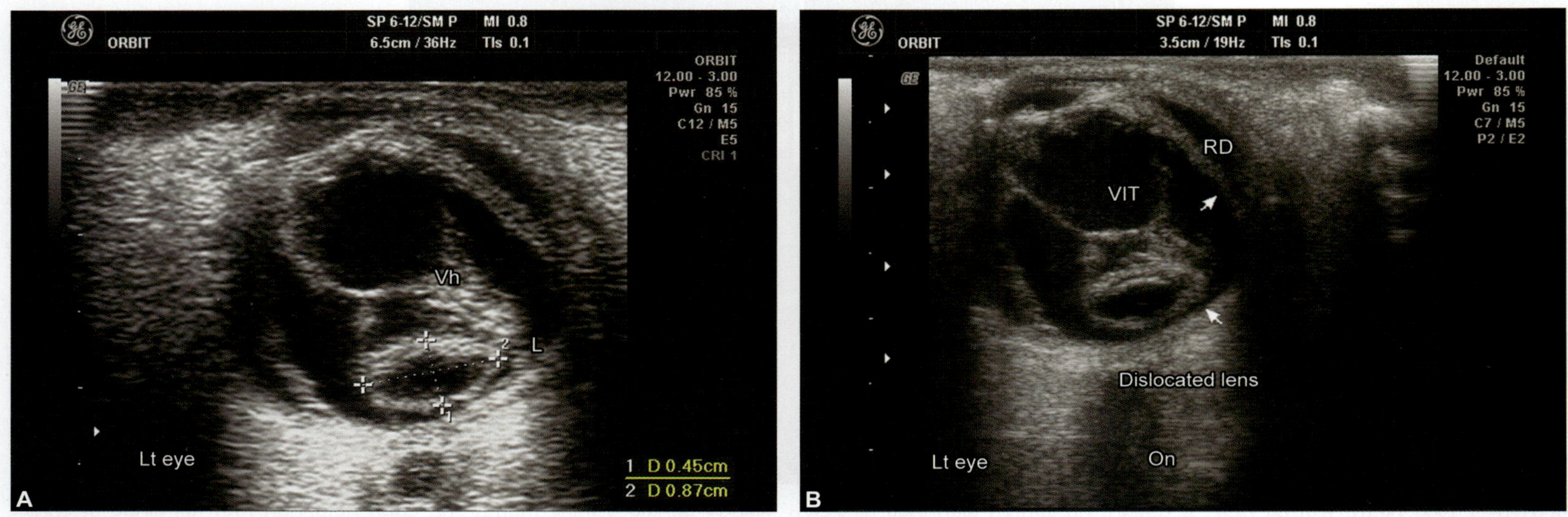

FIGURES 1.124A and B: Postsurgical retinal detachment with IOL in position. A patient presented with loss of vision with soft eye after cataract surgery. HRSG shows cataractous lens dislocated in posterior segment. Associated intragel hemorrhage is also seen. A thick membrane is also seen in the posterior segment suggestive of retinal detachment.

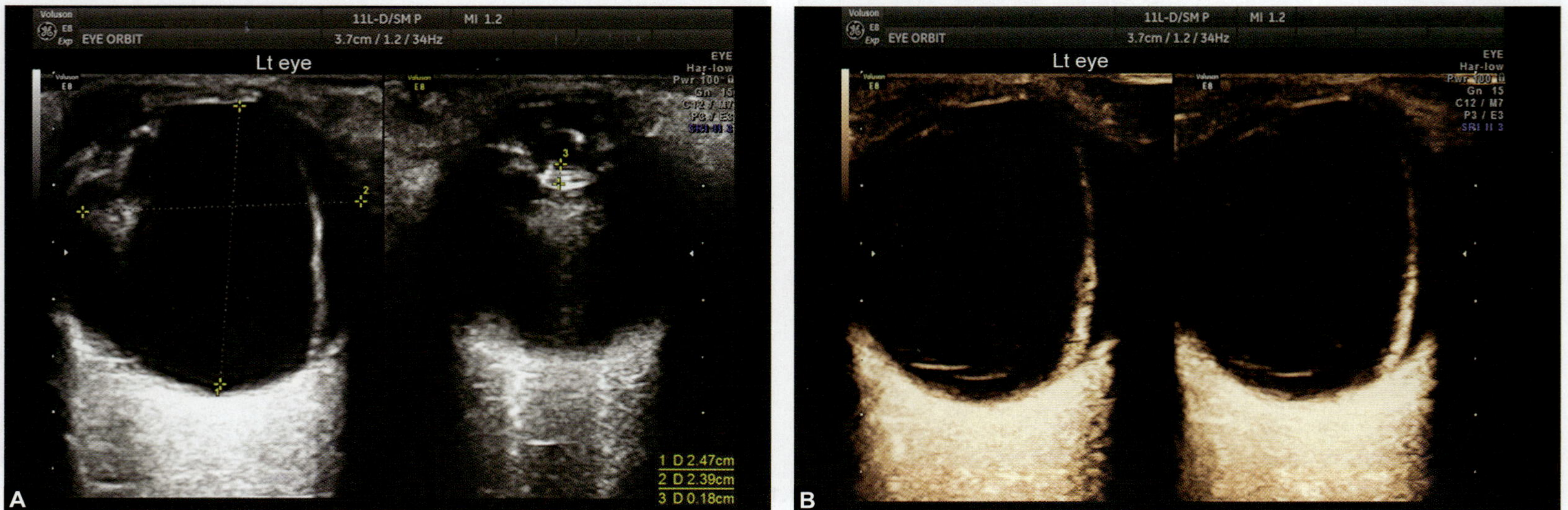

FIGURES 1.125A and B

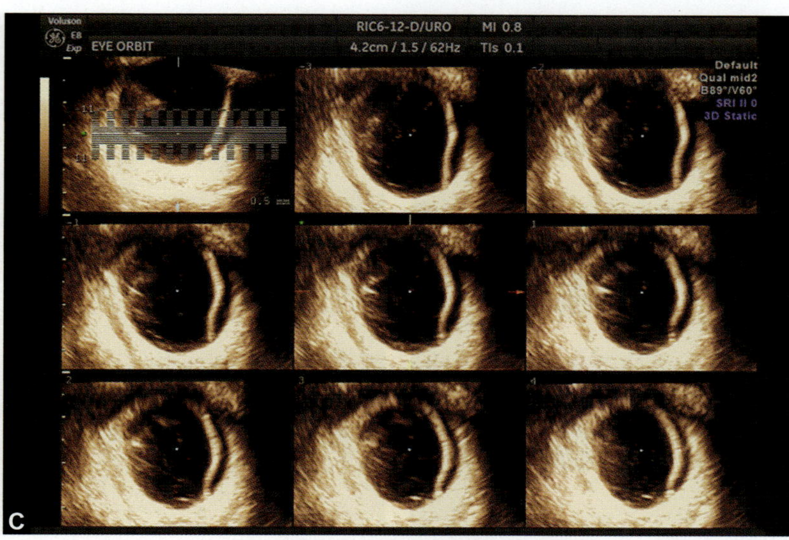

FIGURE 1.125C

FIGURES 1.125A to C: RD with intragel oil instillation. A patient presented with retinal detachment after cataract surgery. Intraocular oil was instilled in the eye for apposition of retina. HRSG shows focal retinal detachment on temporal side. It is seen as a thick echogenic band.

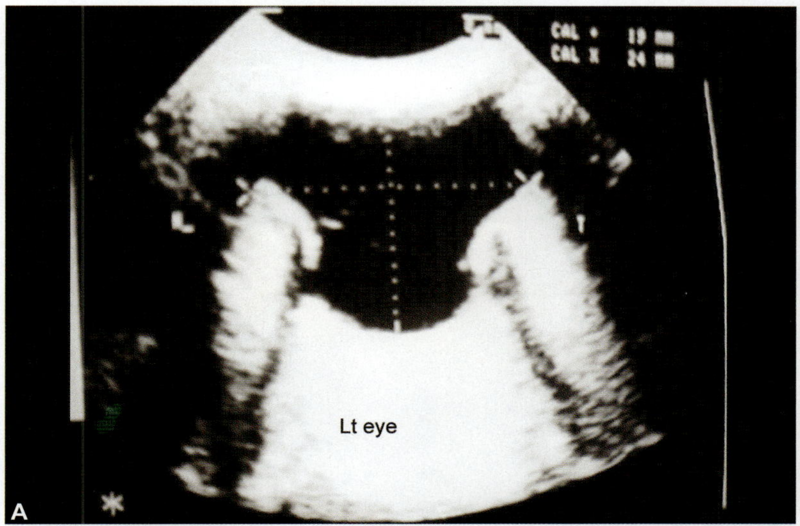

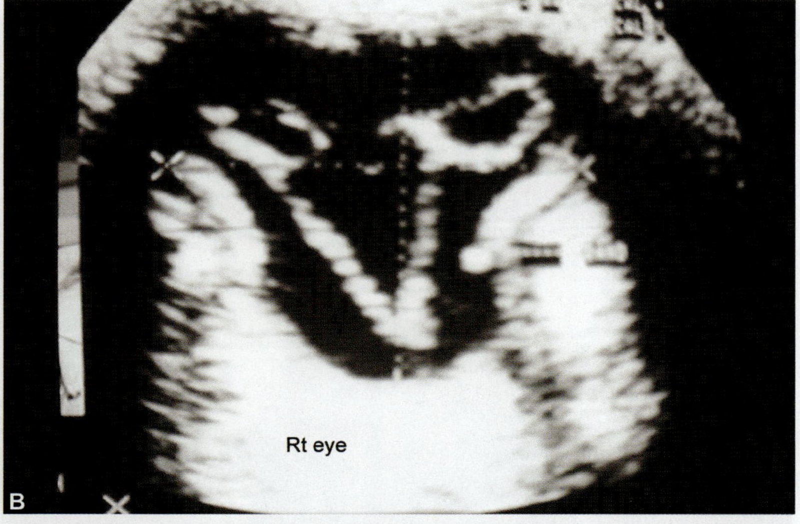

FIGURES 1.126A and B: Retinal buckle applications in a case of retinal detachment. HRSG shows buckle application at the equator in a case of retinal detachment. The buckles are seen in position and also keeping the retina close to the choroid. HRSG is a valuable investigation for the evaluation of success of post surgical treatment of retinal detachment. Slipping out of the retina under buckles. HRSG shows slipping out retina from the buckle in a case of failed surgical treatment of retinal detachment. The slipped retina is seen as a 'V' shaped membrane and folding of the retina is also seen at the base. The buckles are seen in position at the equator as echogenic bands applied at the equator.

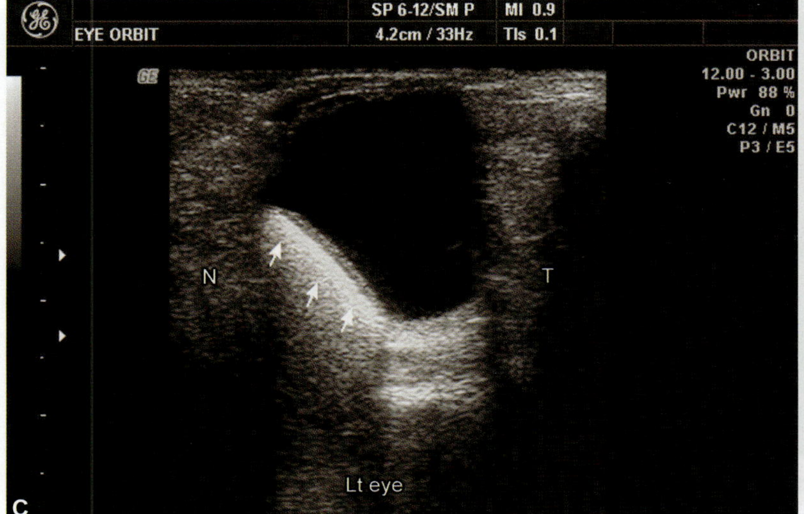

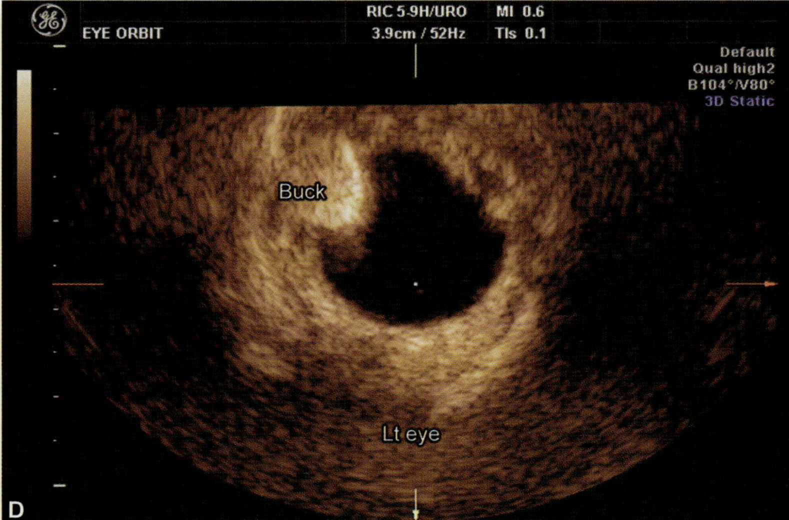

FIGURES 1.126C and D

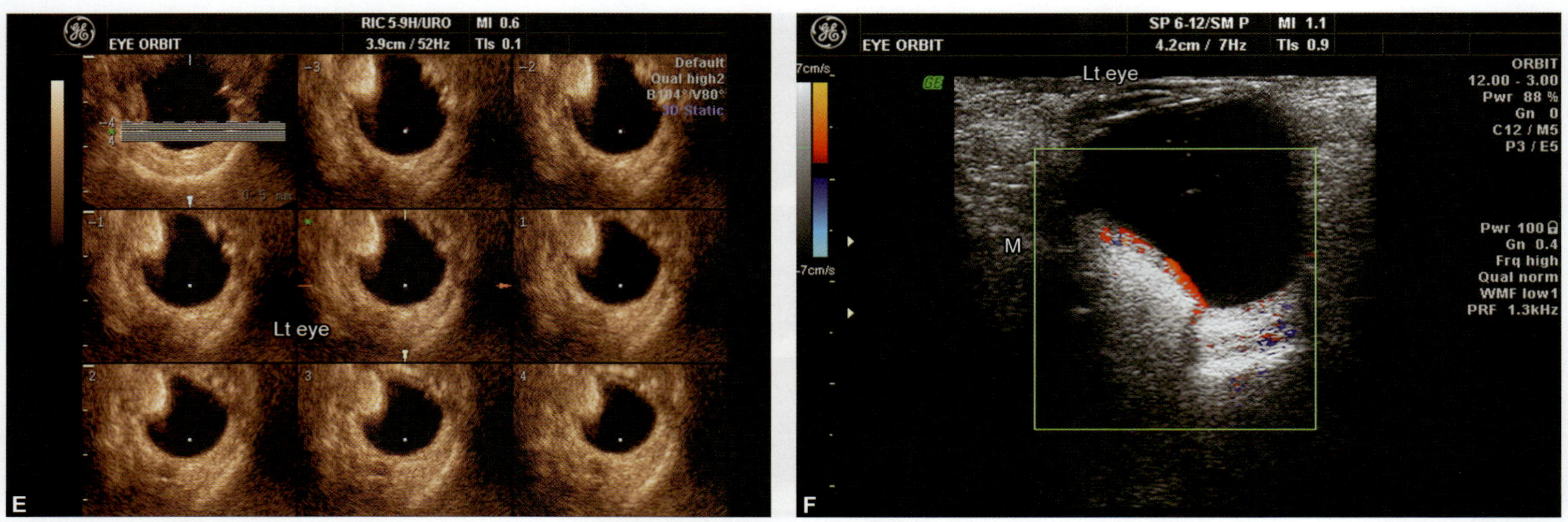

FIGURES 1.126E and F

FIGURES 1.126C to F: Retinal buckle. A patient underwent surgery for retinal detachment with placement of buckle for apposition of retina. Focal laxity of buckle is seen at nasal side on superior pole of eye resulting into a focal bulge. The 3D ultrasound with TUI imaging shows the bulge of the buckle very clearly. However, the buckle is seen in position in the lower medial quadrant of the eye, and it is seen as a hyperreflective band. On color flow imaging, the artery is seen going anterior to the buckle.

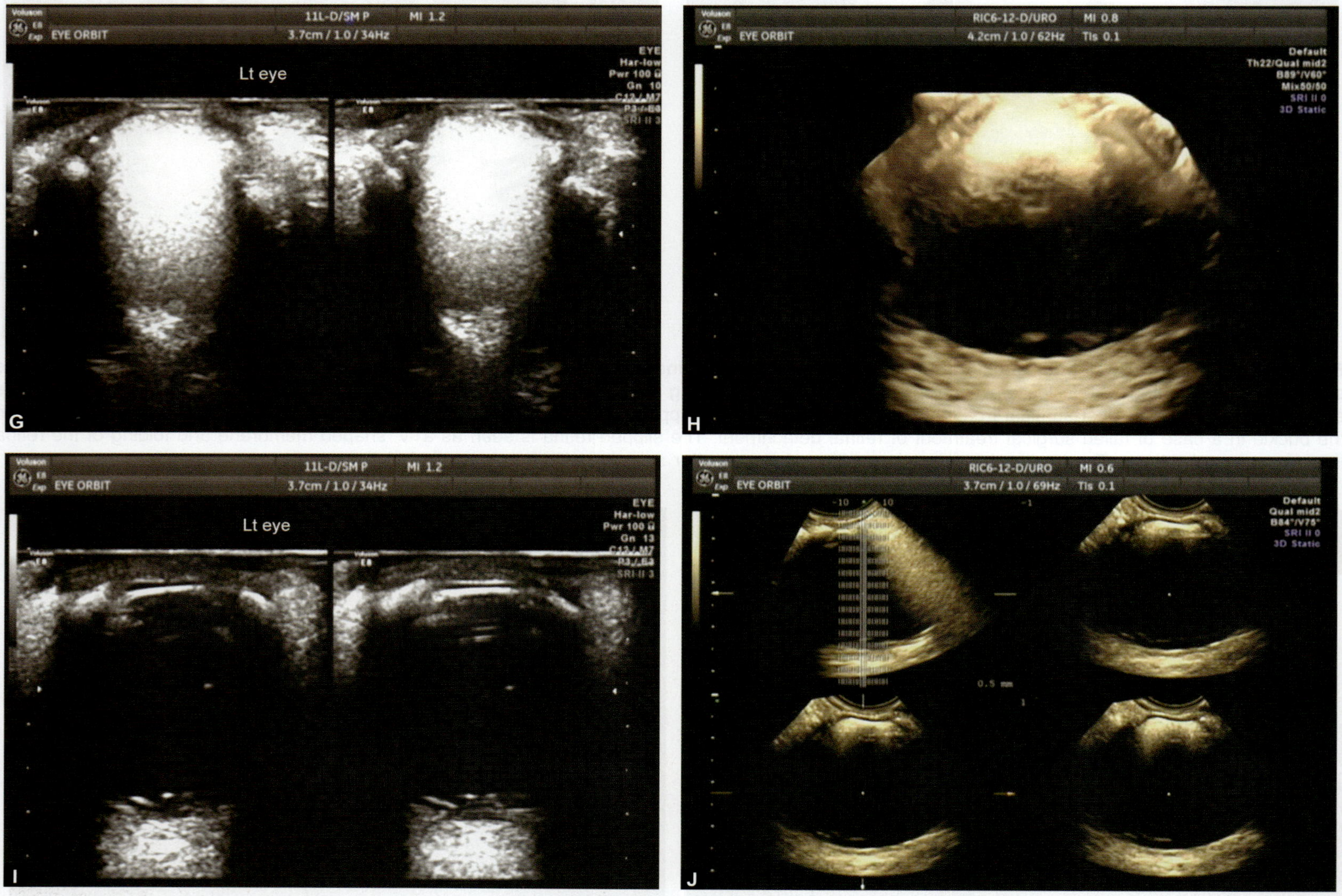

FIGURES 1.126G to J

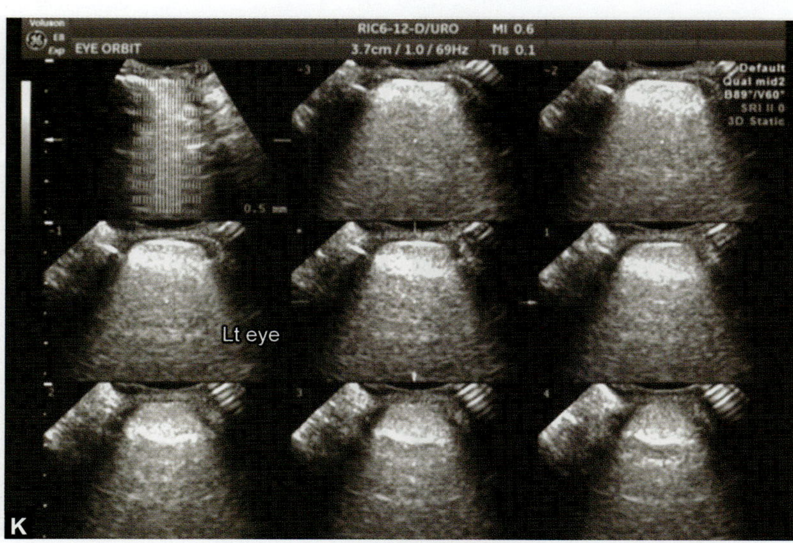

FIGURE 1.126K

FIGURES 1.126G to K: Oil in the anterior segment. A patient underwent surgery for retinal detachment in left eye. However, there is evidence of a highly echogenic collection seen in the anterior segment of eye, which casts strong artifacts. Posterior segment of the eye is not seen on clinical examination. However, HRSG shows clear posterior segment with retina in position. But echogenic oil is seen in anterior segment.

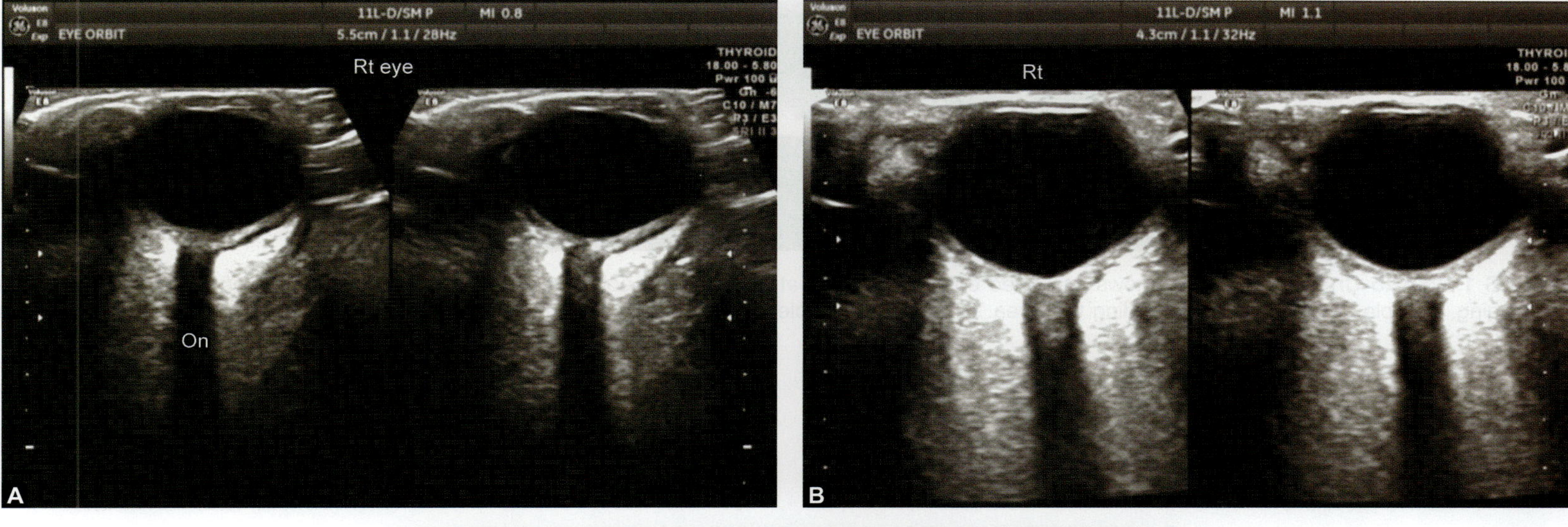

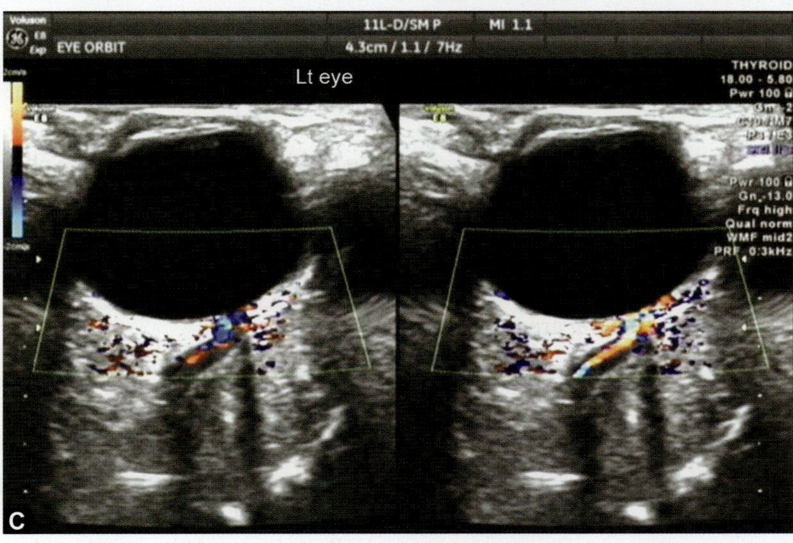

FIGURES 1.127A to C: Uveitis. A patient presented with diminished vision. HRSG shows markedly thickened edematous uvea. The edema is also seen in the optic nerve. "T" sign is positive suggestive of uveitis. On color flow imaging, increased flow is seen in uvea.

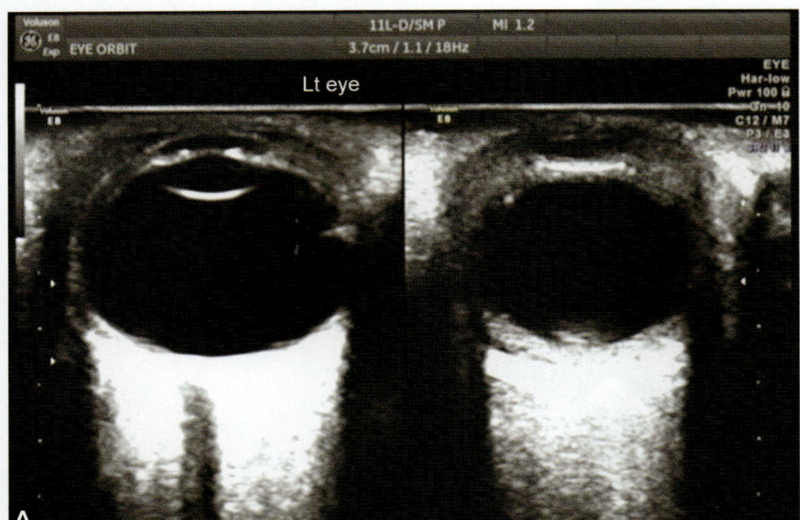

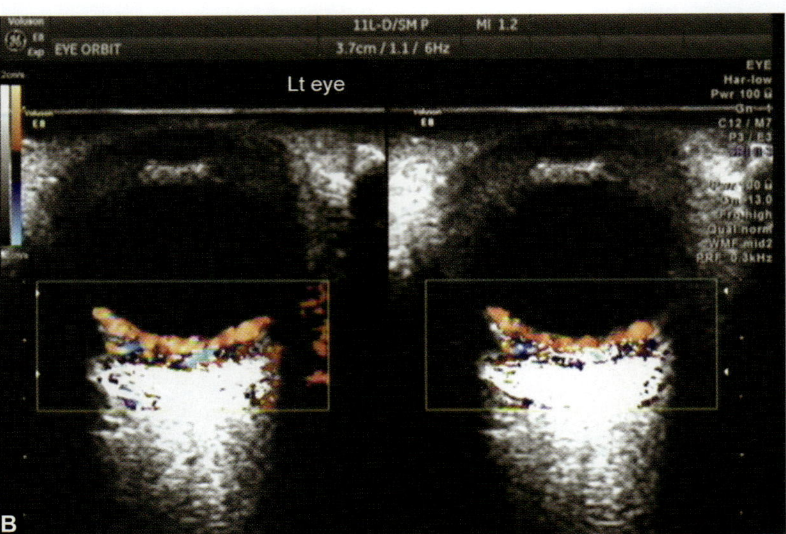

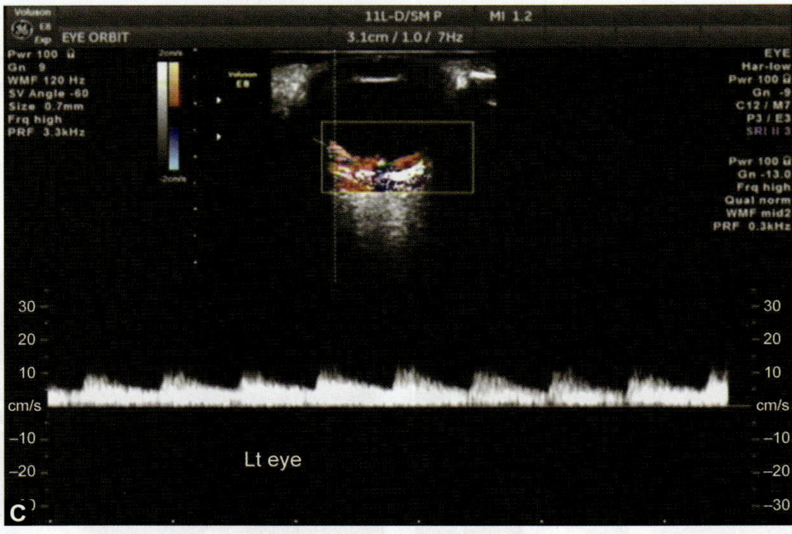

FIGURES 1.128A to C: Uveitis. HRSG shows thickened edematous uvea at the posterior pole of the eye. Marked edema is seen in the uvea. On color flow imaging, multiple vessels are seen feeding the uvea. On spectral Doppler tracing, moderate arterial flow is seen in uvea suggestive of inflammation.

EXAMINATION OF CHOROID

Choroid

Choroidal thickening may be focal or diffuse. It is associated with many conditions. It can be due to swelling or edema. Following are the main causes of choroidal swelling or edema:

1. Hypotoni of ocular muscles.
2. Vascular congestion
3. End ophthalmitis.
4. Uveitis.
5. Scleritis.

HRSG shows a highly reflective or low to medial reflective band in choroidal thickening. However, small choroidal tumors are difficult to be differentiated from it like choroidal melanomas, metastatic deposit or lymphomas.

Choroidal Detachment

The choroidal detachment may take place due to trauma, post surgery or spontaneously. HRSG findings are characteristic in choroidal detachment (CD) on B scanning. It presents as a smooth dome-shaped thick echogenic membrane in the periphery. It shows little or no movement on dynamic scanning. In shallow CD, it is more flat than dome shape. Extensive choroidal detachment shows classical kissing bullae sign on 'B' scanning. Anterior choroidal detachment extends to ciliary body and known as ciliochoroidal detachment.

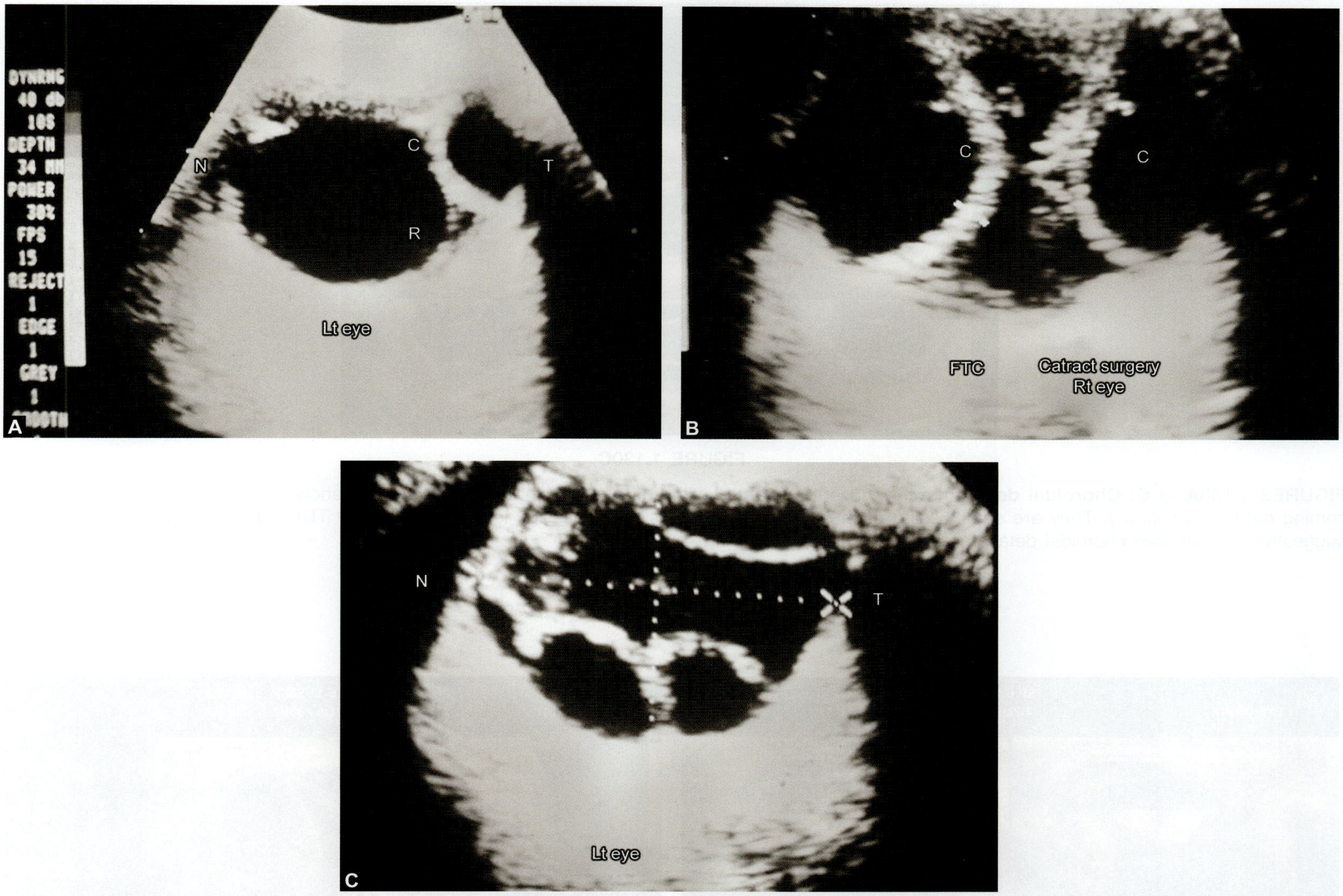

FIGURES 1.129A to C: Choroidal detachment. HRSG shows a thick echogenic membrane due to trauma in the upper temporal quadrant of the left eye. It is smooth in outline and dome shaped seen at the periphery. No movement is seen on dynamic imaging. **Postsurgical choroidal detachment**. Patient complaints of sudden loss of vision after the surgery for cataract. HRSG shows two well-defined thick echogenic dome shaped membranes seen detached on both temporal and nasal side at the periphery. They are seen coming into the center and give a kissing bullae sign. Associated intragel haemorrhage is also seen. Multiple choroidal detachment- HRSG shows multiple thick echogenic dome-shaped membranous shadows seen at the periphery in the posterior pole, upper pole and nasal side of the left eye with smooth outline suggestive of multi focal choroidal detachment following trauma. Associated intragel haemorrhage is also seen.

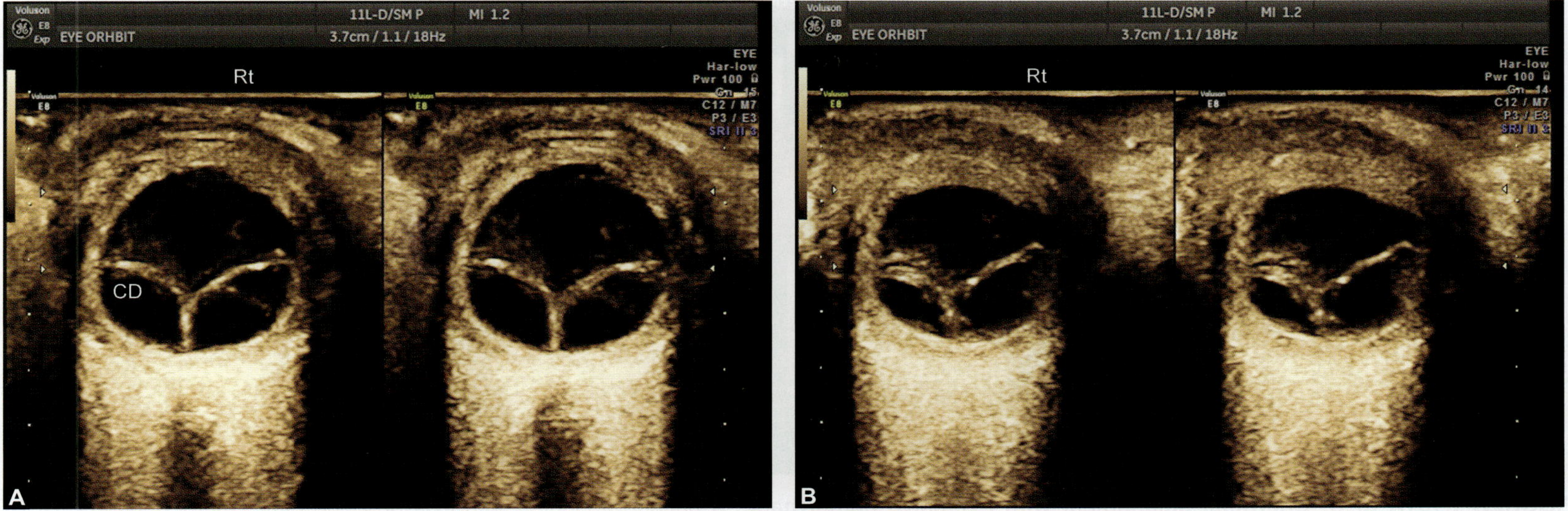

FIGURES 1.130A and B

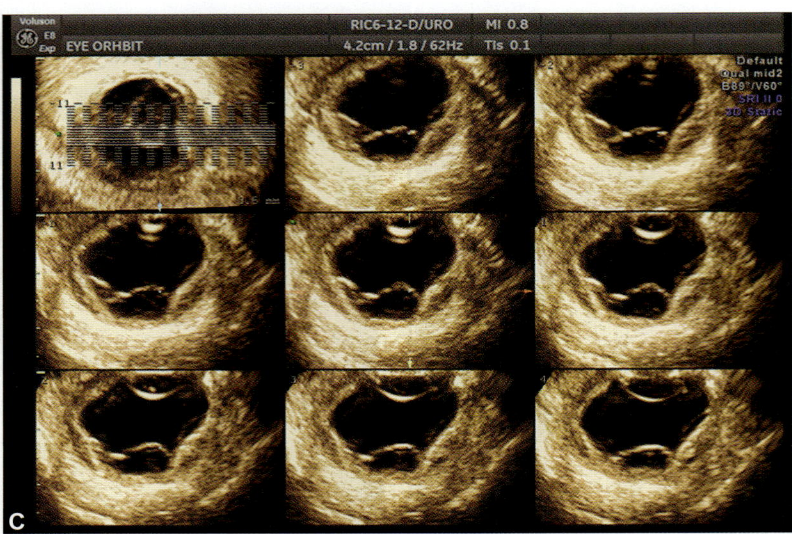

FIGURE 1.130C

FIGURES 1.130A to C: Choroidal detachment. A patient presented with soft eye and loss of vision. HRSG shows thick dome-shaped membranes coming out from periphery. They are seen kissing each other in center. Kissing bullae sign is positive. The 3D TUI imaging show the deshaped eye suggestive of extensive choroidal detachment.

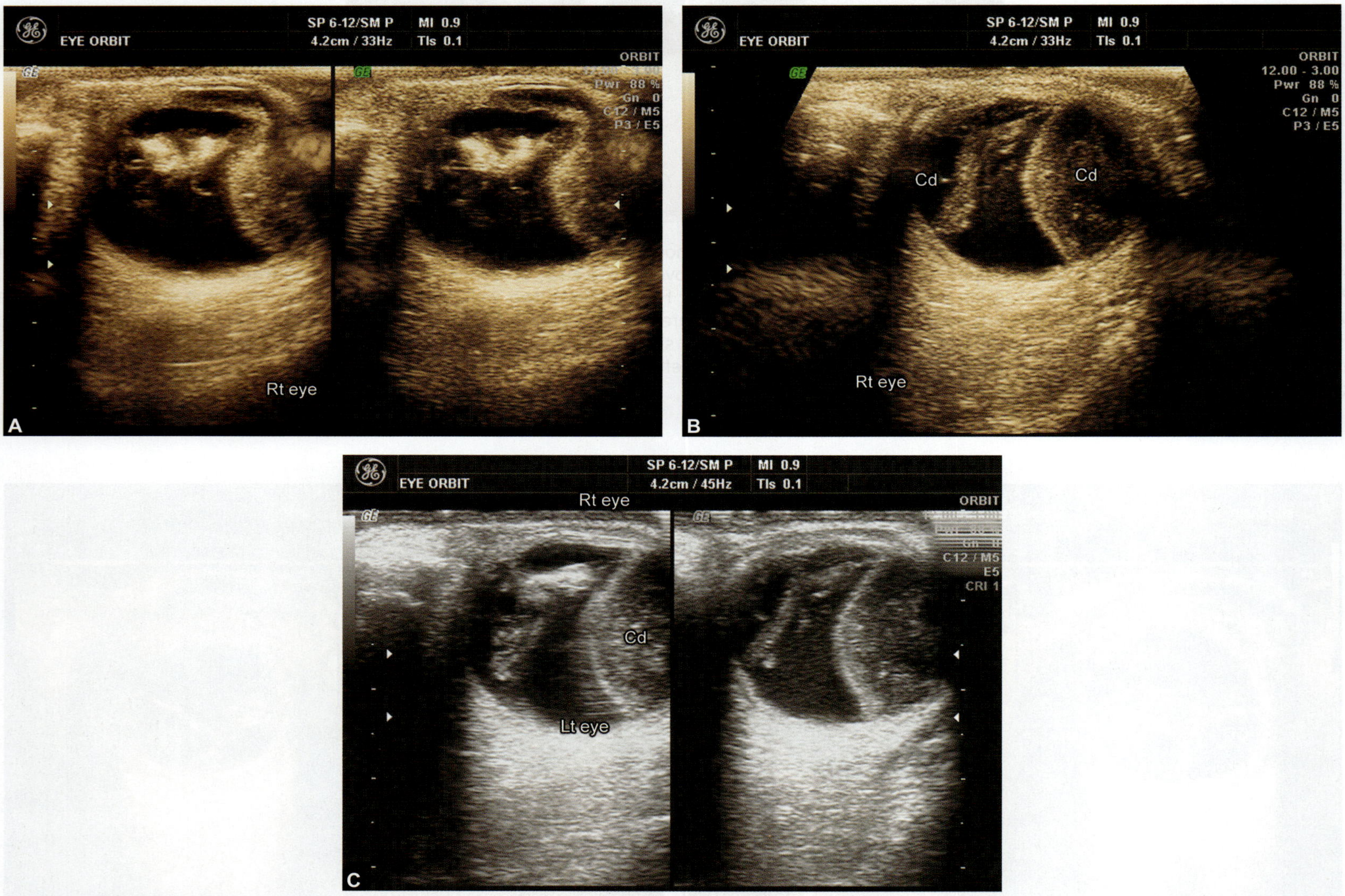

FIGURES 1.131A to C: Choroidal detachment with expulsive hemorrhage. A patient presented with loss of vision after cataract surgery. HRSG shows IOL in position. Thick dome-shaped membranes are seen detached from the periphery on either side. Echogenic collection is seen under the dome shaped membrane suggestive of choroid detachment with expulsive hemorrhage.

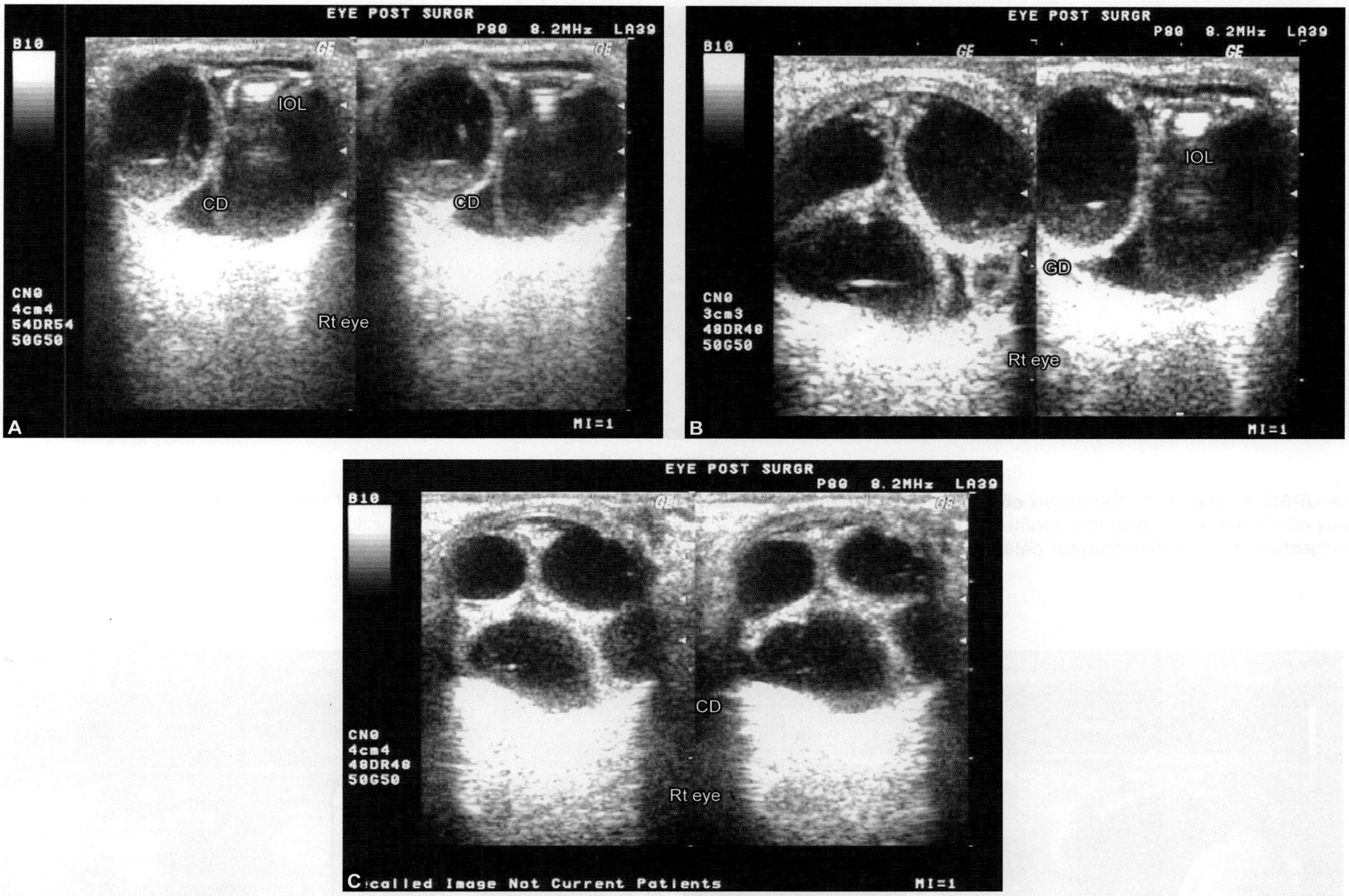

FIGURES 1.132A to C: Postsurgical choroidal detachment following surgery. HRSG shows well-defined dome-shaped echogenic membranous shadows coming into the center from the periphery suggestive of choroidal detachment. An echogenic hyper reflective shadow is seen at the junction of anterior and posterior segment suggestive of intraocular lens in position. Figure C shows multifocal choroidal detachments. Thick-dome shaped membranes are seen bulging from periphery and meeting each other in center suggestive of kissing bully sign.

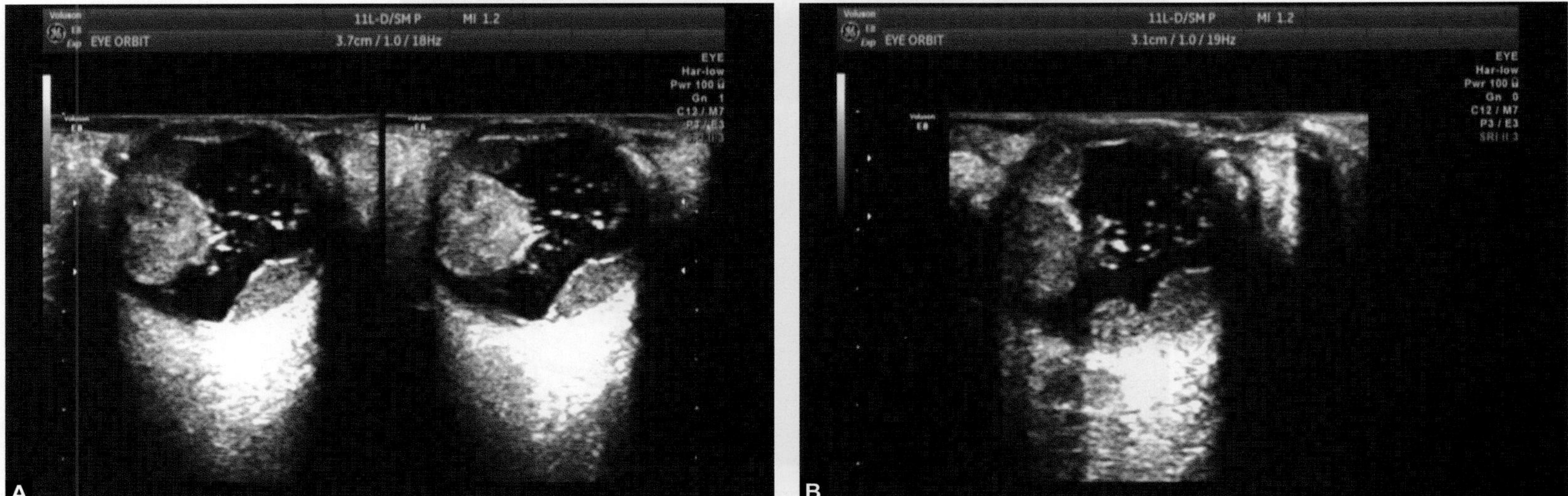

FIGURES 1.133A and B

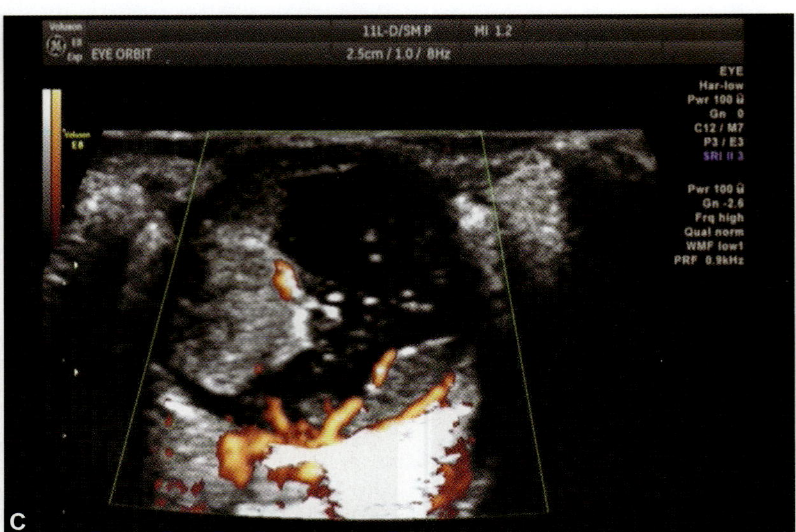

FIGURE 1.133C

FIGURES 1.133A to C: Expulsive choroidal detachment with fresh bleed. A patient presented with loss of vision. HRSG shows multiple dome-shaped masses in the posterior segment. Thick echogenic collection is seen under the masses. But on color flow imaging, no flow is seen the masses suggestive of multifocal choroidal detachment with organized subchoroidal hematomas.

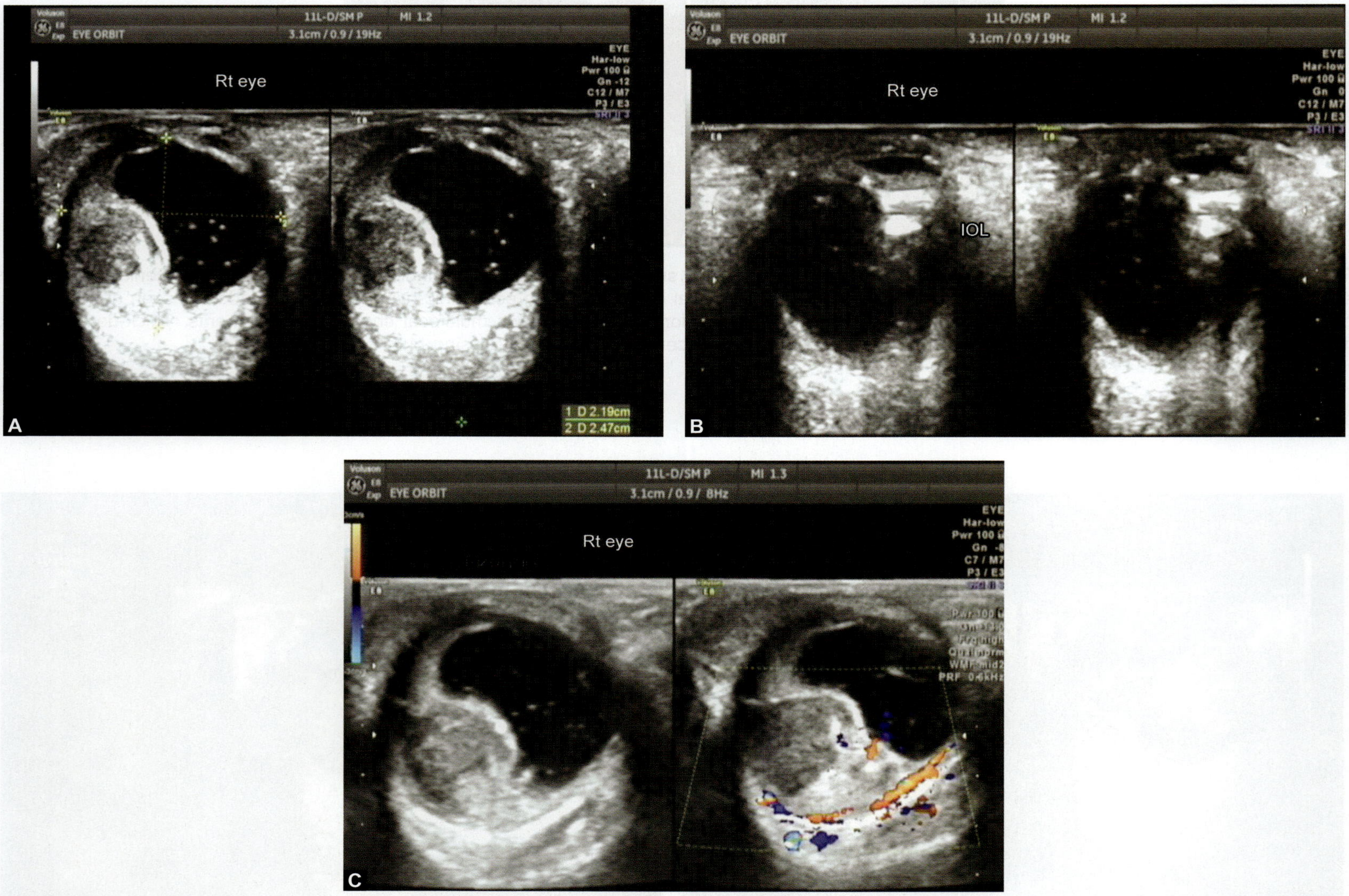

FIGURES 1.134A to C: Postsurgical choroidal detachment. A patient presented with loss of vision after cataract surgery. HRSG shows echogenic HRSG shows echogenic IOL in position. However, the posterior segment of the eye shows multiple dome-shaped humps. They are covered by thick membranes show little movements. Thick echogenic collection is seen in the humps suggestive of postsurgical choroidal detachment with hematoma formation.

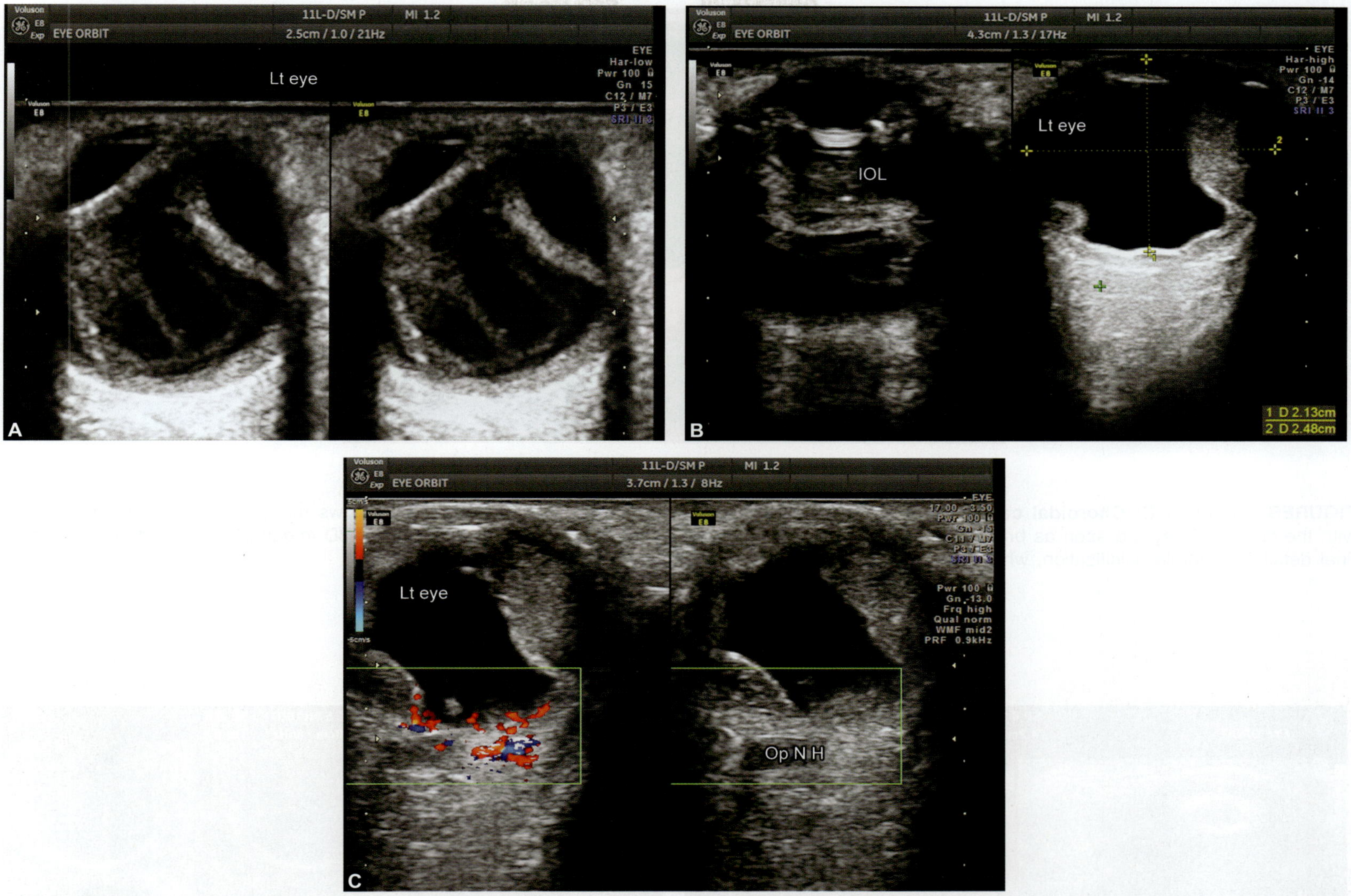

FIGURES 1.135A to C: Extensive choroidal detachment with soft eye and deformed eyeball after cataract surgery. A patient presented with acute pain with loss of vision in the eye after cataract surgery. HRSG shows IOL in position. Thick dome-shaped shadows are seen from periphery. Echogenic collection is seen under the membrane suggestive of choroidal detachment with expulsive hemorrhage. The membranes are seen kissing each other in entire globe resulting into soft eye coat and deformed shape of the eye.

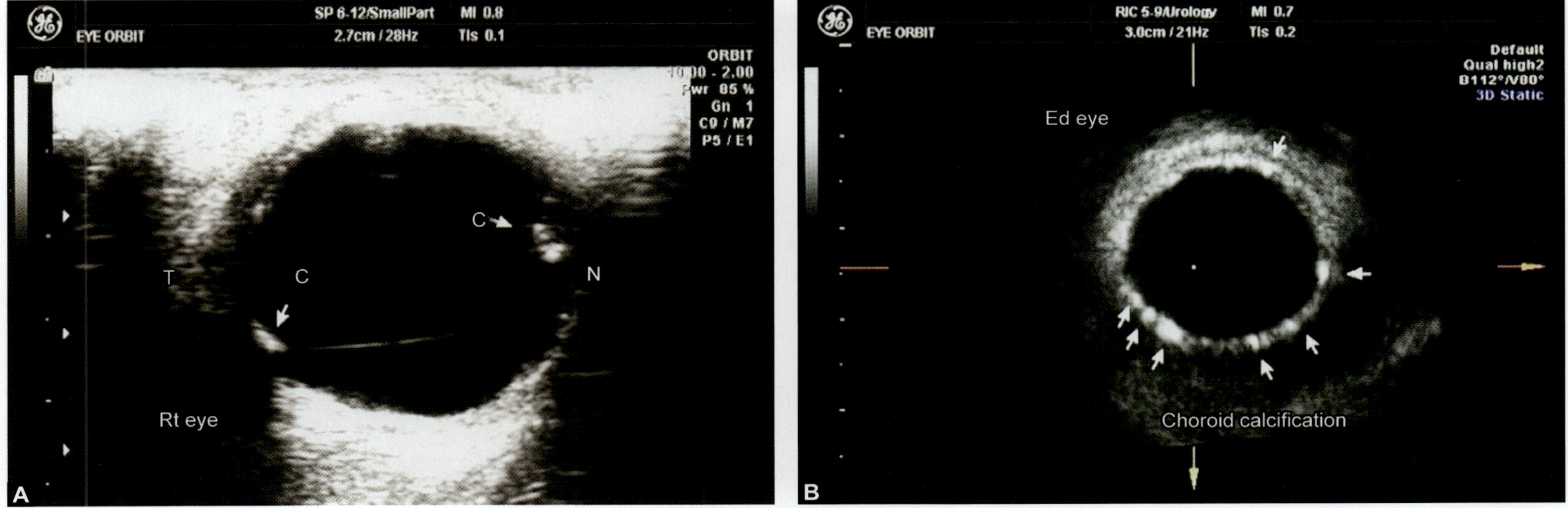

FIGURES 1.136A and B

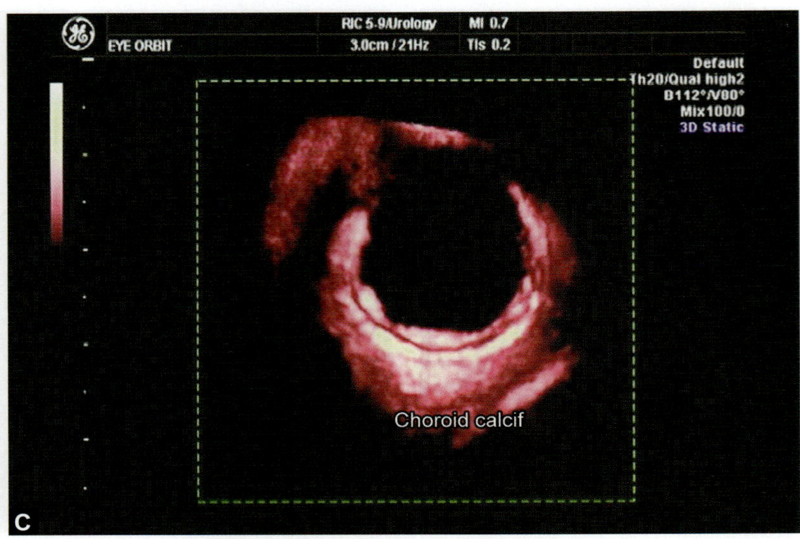

FIGURE 1.136C

FIGURES 1.136A to C: Choroidal calcification. A patient presented with gradual loss of vision. HRSG shows multiple fine calcified specks fixed with the choroid. They are seen as bright echogenic spots in choroid. **3D imaging of choroid calcification.** 3D imaging of the same patient shows final details of choroid calcification, which are seen embedded in the choroidal layer.

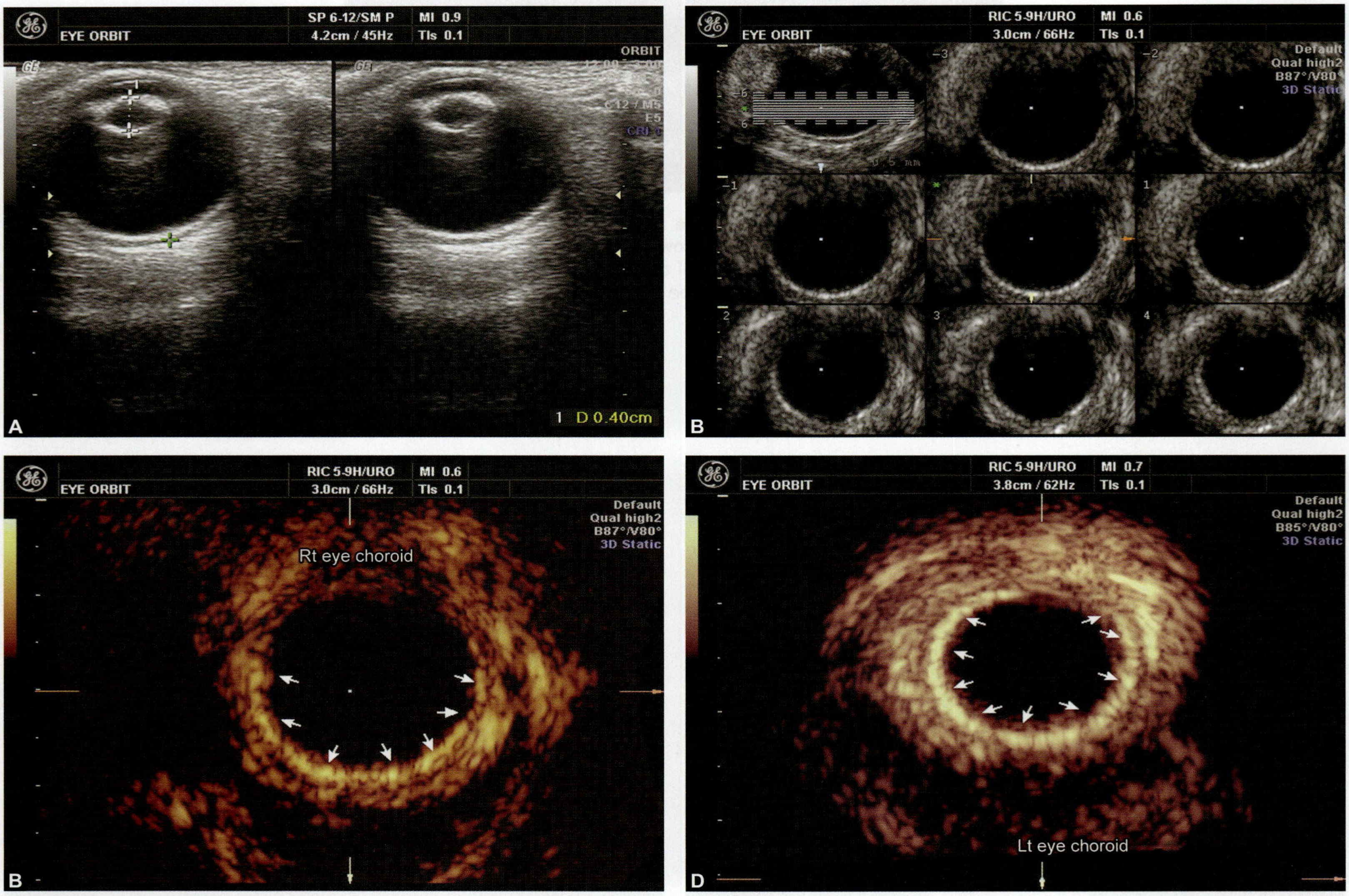

FIGURES 1.137A to D: Choroidal calcification. A patient presented with gradual loss of vision. HRSG shows thickened opaque lens. Multiple calcified specks are seen in the choroid. On 3D ultrasound with TUI imaging, a dense calcified rim is seen in the choroid suggestive of calcification in the choroid.

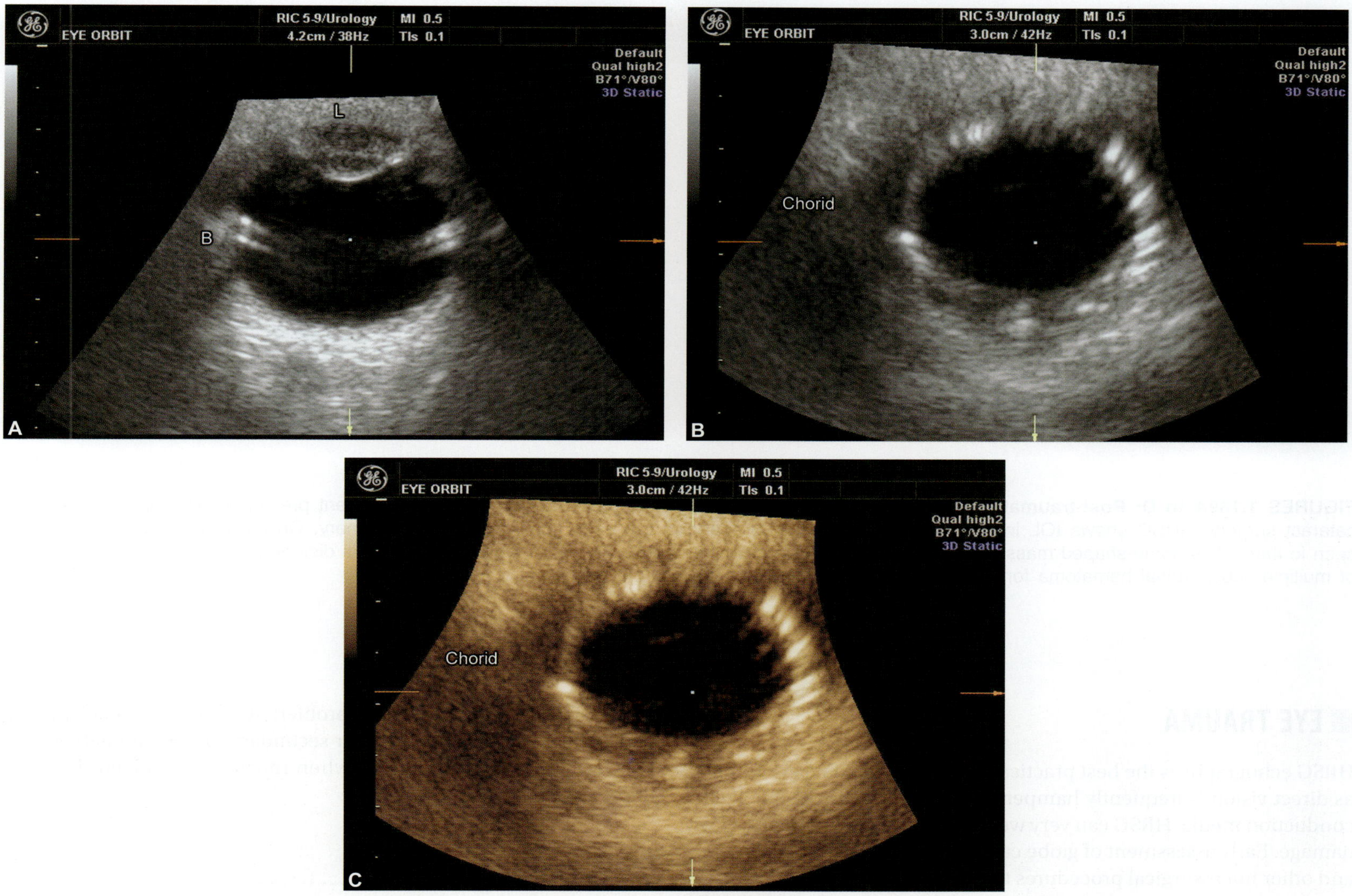

FIGURES 1.138A to C: Choroidal calcification with 3D imaging. HRSG shows thickened opaque lens in eye. On 2D imaging, calcified specks are seen at equator. On 3D ultrasound imaging, multiple calcified specks are seen in the choroid suggestive of degenerative changes in the choroid.

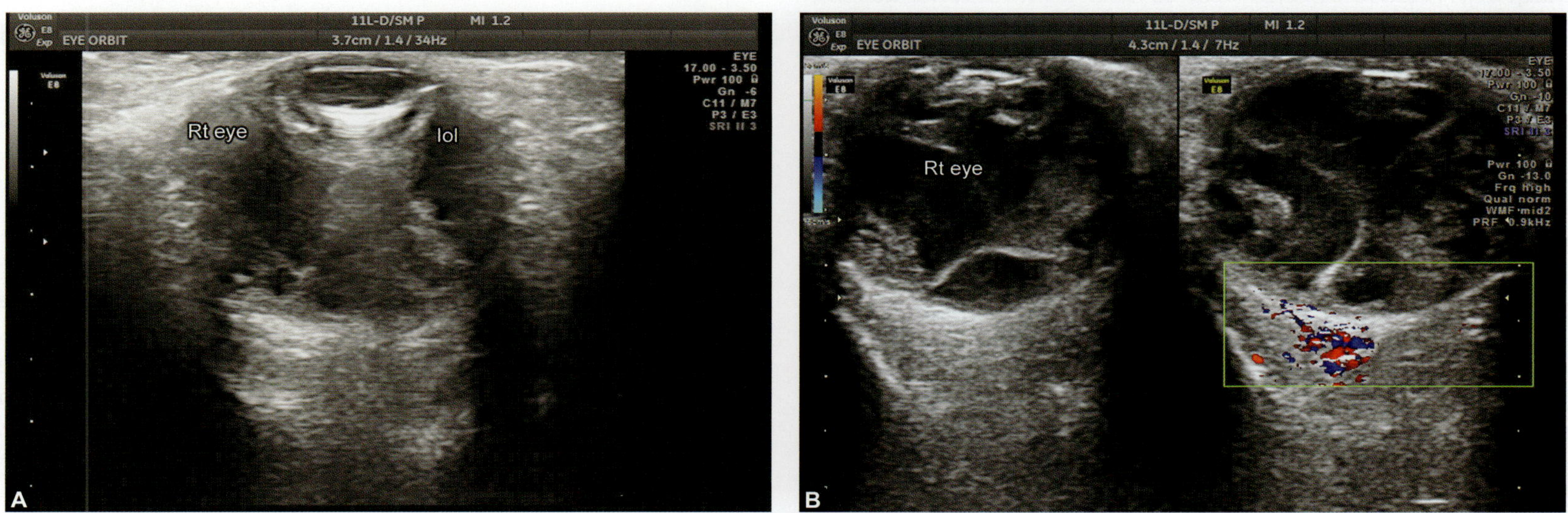

FIGURES 1.139A and B

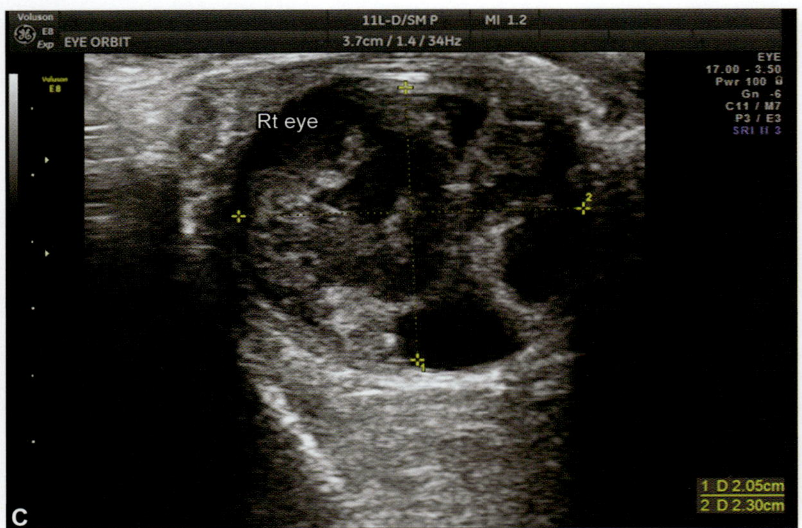

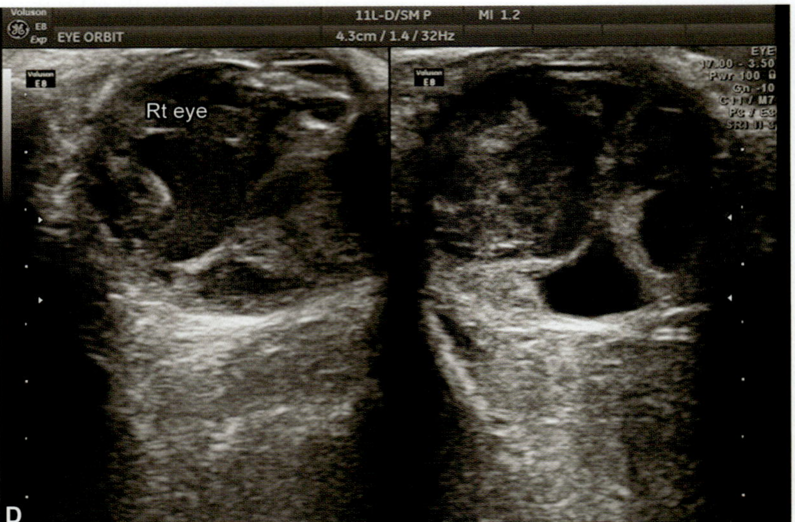

FIGURES 1.139C and D

FIGURES 1.139A to D: Post-traumatic choroidal detachment with big subchoroidal hemorrhage. A patient presented with loss of vision after cataract surgery. HRSG shows IOL in position. Big dome-shaped shadows are seen coming out from periphery. On color flow imaging, no flow is seen in them. The dome-shaped masses are seen covered with thick membrane. Normal anatomy of the eye is distorted. The findings are suggestive of multiple subchoroidal hematoma formation covered with dome-shaped choroid membranes.

EYE TRAUMA

HRSG echography is the best practical method to evaluate eye trauma as direct vision is frequently hampered after trauma by opaque light-conduction media. HRSG can very well assess the extent and degree of damage. Early assessment of globe can result into early surgical repair and other microsurgical procedures to save the eye.

Severe blunt trauma to eye leads to sudden compression of the eyeball anteroposteriorly and corresponding expansion of the equatorial plane. It may lead to rupture of globe at equator with collapse of the eyeball. Retraction of gel with retinal tearing or dialysis can take place. This traumatic dialysis can take place anywhere, but it s more common in upper nasal quadrant of globe.

Anterior Segment Trauma

Anterior segment trauma can be better evaluated with immersion technique. This is important in corneal opacification or anterior chamber hyphema. HRSG can very well display the blood clot and depth of anterior chamber. Even status of lens can be assessed. The trauma can also injure lens. Although mild cataractous changes are difficult to appreciate, but moderately dense post-traumatic cataract can easily be picked up of HRSG. Location of lens or subluxation of lens can be detected on HRSG. This helps in the proper management in restoring the vision.

Posterior Segment Trauma

Eye trauma can lead to many posterior segment abnormalities including vitreous hemorrhage, PVD, retinal detachment and retinal tears. The findings are already described in various heads. Penetrating ocular trauma may lead to retinal detachment in almost one-fifth cases. Small or subtle hemorrhage in vitreous is difficult to detect. However, with high gain setting, it can be picked up on HRSG. Hemorrhage may be confined to vitreous gel, retrohyloid space or including both. Dynamic scanning reveals vitreoretinal adhesions. Long-standing post-traumatic retinal detachment may lead to proliferative vitreoretinopathy (PVR). Thickening of retinochoroid layer secondary to posttraumatic edema can lead to severe visual loss when macula is involved. It can be demonstrated by HRSG.

Posterior Scleral Rupture

Severe blunt trauma can lead to posterior scleral rupture which may be difficult to detect clinically. The patient usually presents with normal intraocular pressure but with marked hemorrhage chemosis and vitreous hemorrhage. On HRSG, the sclera in the area of rupture shows moderately irregular contour and low echogenicity. There may be indirect signs of rupture seen on HRSG. They are as follows:

Indirect Signs of Scleral Rupture

1. Vitreous incarceration into fundus with vitreous hemorrhage and PVD.
2. Thickening or detachment of surrounding retina or choroid.
3. Hemorrhage in the episcleral space.
4. Vitreous traction towards the site of incarceration.

Rupture of the Globe

Severe blunt trauma may lead to rupture of globe. It usually takes place at equator. The eye looses its normal shape and loss of ocular volume. Associated intravitreal hemorrhage and intraocular air are also seen. The eye gets separated form the orbital wall and shrinks. Air may be seen in globe if associated blowout fracture of ethmoid is present with eye injury.

Pyo-ophthalmos

Acute infection of the eyeball results into enlarged, swollen painful eye. The eye size increases in acute stage. The eyeball is filled with low-level homogeneous echoes suggestive of pus collection. It can be very well appreciated on HRSG. Ultimately this eye goes into endophthalmitis due to pyogenic process.

Endophthalmitis

Endophthalmitis may result due to an endogenous infection presenting elsewhere in body. However, it most commonly occurs following surgical trauma or penetrating injury to eye. HRSG is highly useful in evaluating endophthalmitis. On "B" scan imaging. Dense opacities are seen in the posterior segment. Thick echogenic exudative collection is seen in endophthalmitis. Diffuse thickening of retinochoroid layer as well as tractional or exudative retinal detachment can occur.

Expulsive Hemorrhage

Expulsive hemorrhage is most devastating complication or intraocular surgery. Massive subchoroidal hemorrhagic detachment fills the vitreous cavity. This may include only one or two quadrant of eye in few cases. HRSG is also very helpful in detecting delayed expulsive hemorrhage. In most of the cases, delayed hyperechoic dots can present in subchoroidal space. On following scan these clots diminish in size and also become less reflective.

Lens Material

Normal lens appears as a highly reflective concave shadow on HRSG. It is seen sitting over the vitreous gel. However, cataract lens is seen as thickened biconvex reflective body. HRSG can very well delineate the intralenticular constituents and also accurately measures the thickness of cataract lens. Lens material may be lost in vitreous cavity during surgery. Dislocated lens may adhere to retina and does not move on dynamic scanning unlike a dislocated intact lens.

Intraocular Lens

Intraocular lens creates strong artifacts, which makes evaluation of posterior segment difficult. The smooth very highly reflective surface of lens produces numerous signals producing strong artifacts. Therefore, for proper evaluation the probe should be kept peripheral to limbus.

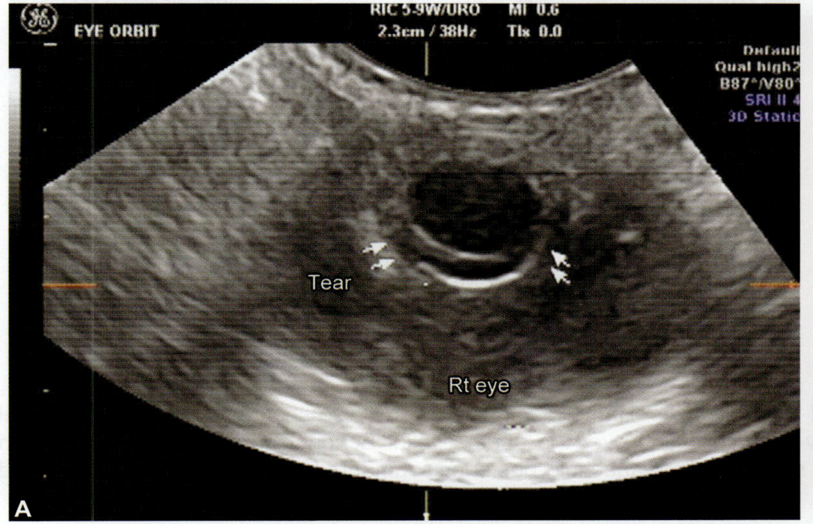

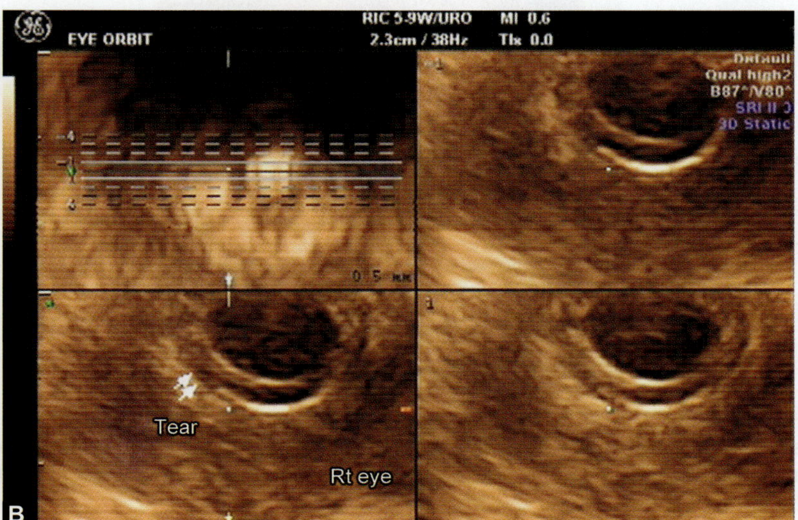

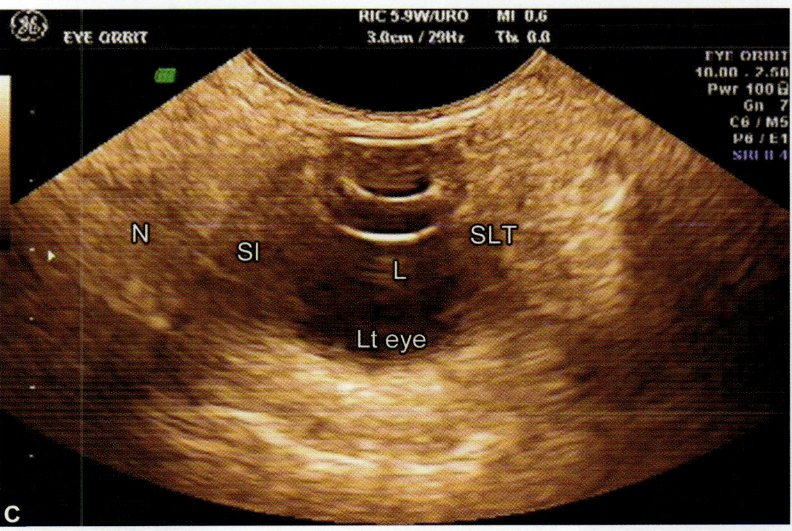

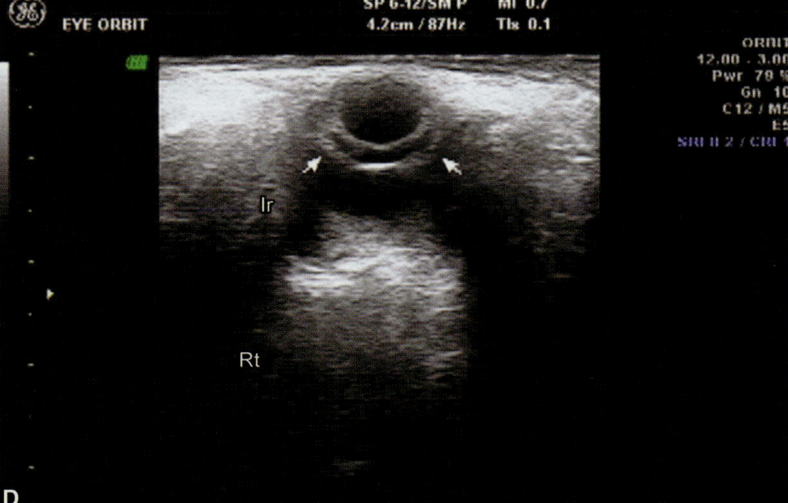

FIGURES 1.140A to D: Subtle trauma of the eye suspensary ligament tear. A patient presented with distorted vision. HRSG shows tear of suspensary ligament of the lens on right side. Discontinuity of the ligament is seen on right side. The left eye shows intact suspensary ligament on both sides. The posterior segment of the eye is free. No intragel pathology is seen.

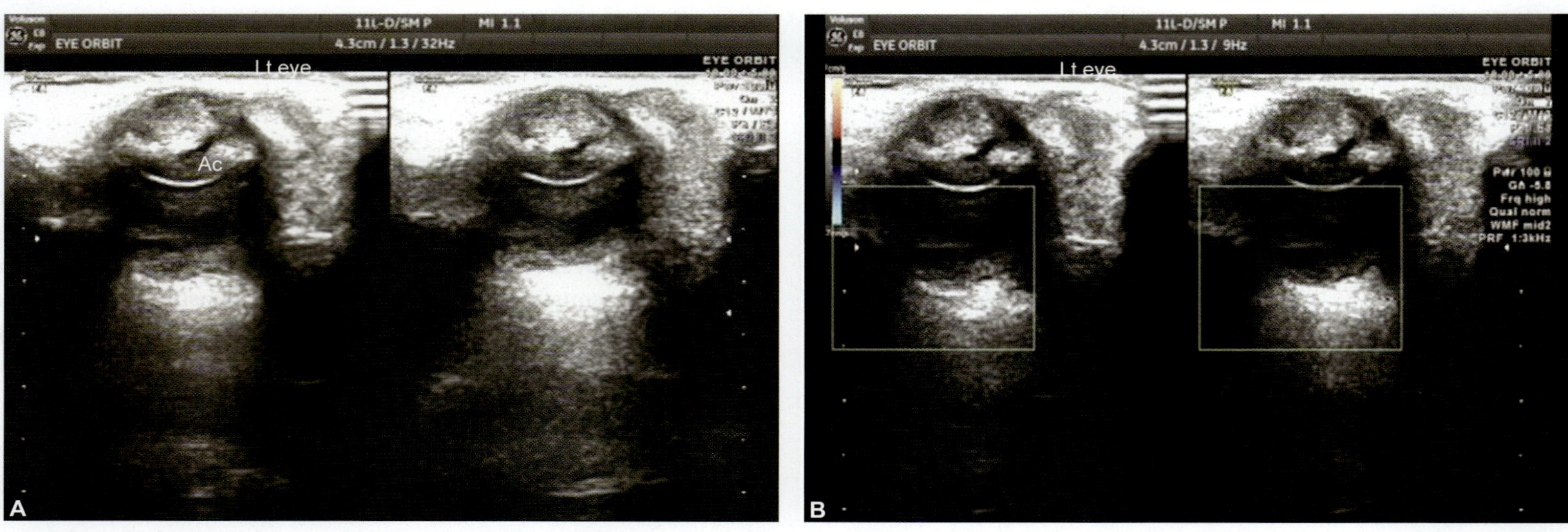

FIGURES 1.141A and B: Anterior chamber hyphema. A patient presented with loss of vision after sustaining trauma. HRSG shows highly echogenic collection in the anterior chamber of eye suggestive of anterior chamber hyphema.

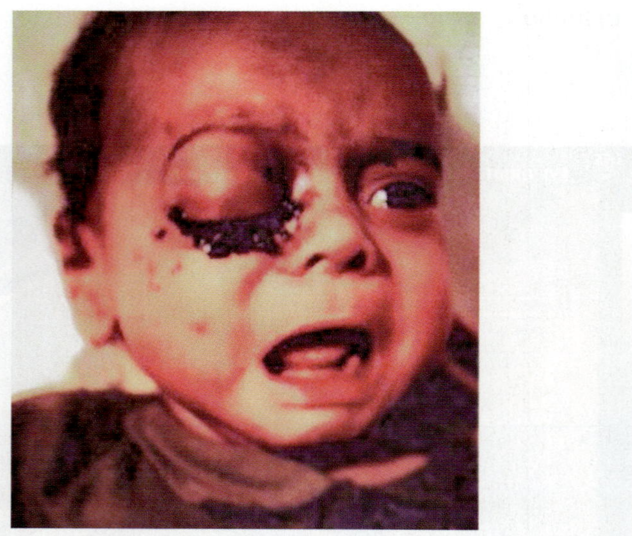

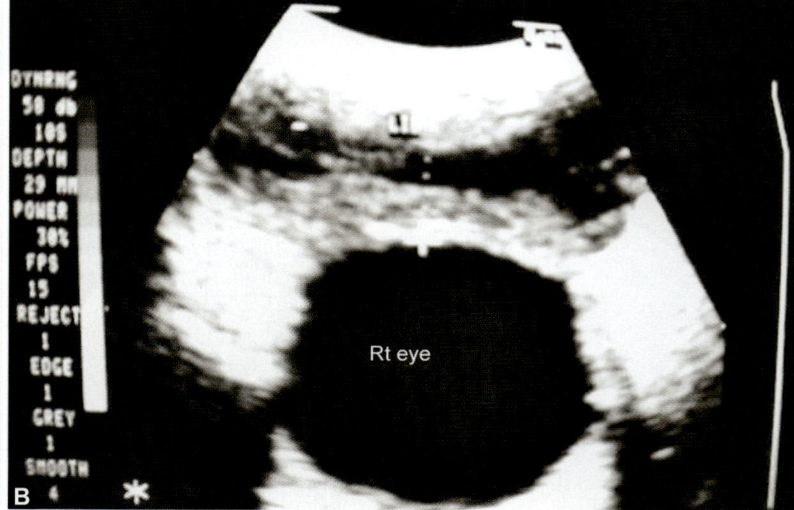

FIGURES 1.142A and B: A young child came with markedly swollen eyelid with chymosis. Hemorrhagic specks are also seen over the eyelid. Clinical examination was not possible due to marked lid edema. HRSG shows low-level collection over the upper eyelid. Echogenic shadows are also seen in the collection suggestive of hematoma formation. However, the eyeball shows normal anechoic posterior segment. Although, it has been pushed down by the edematous eyelid.

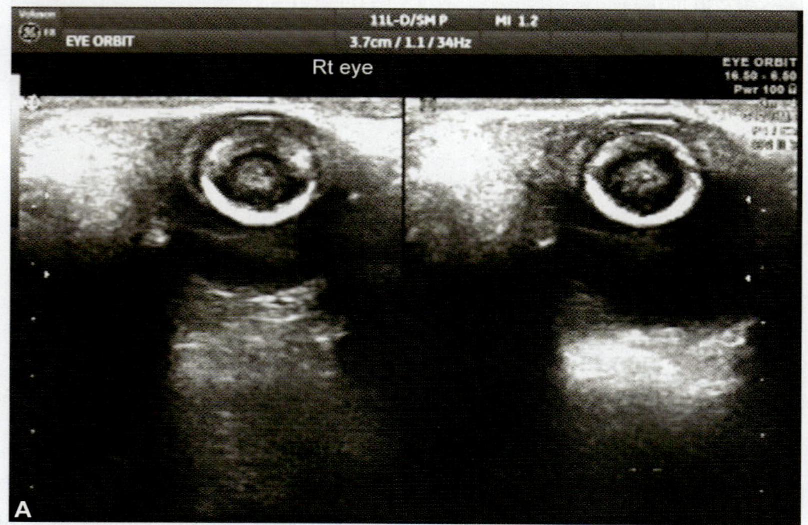

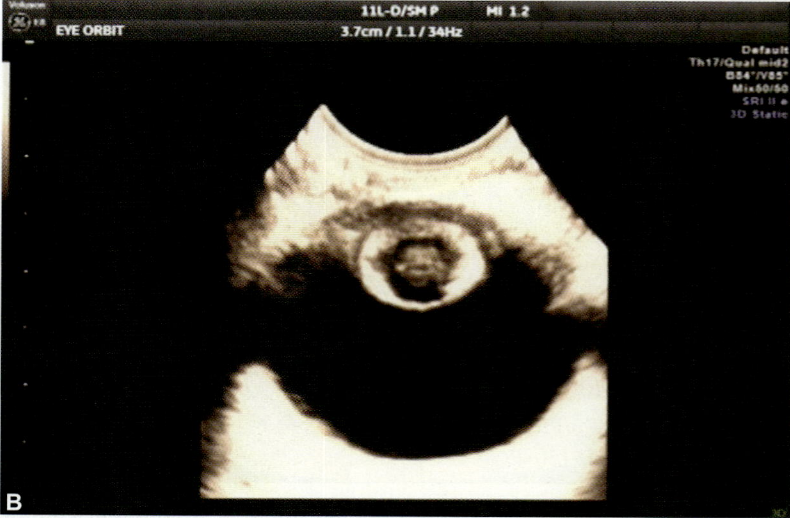

FIGURES 1.143A and B: Post-traumatic cataract. A lady presented with markedly diminished vision after sustaining trauma. HRSG shows grossly thickened opaque lens. The nucleus is seen calcified in the center. However, the posterior segment of the eye is free.

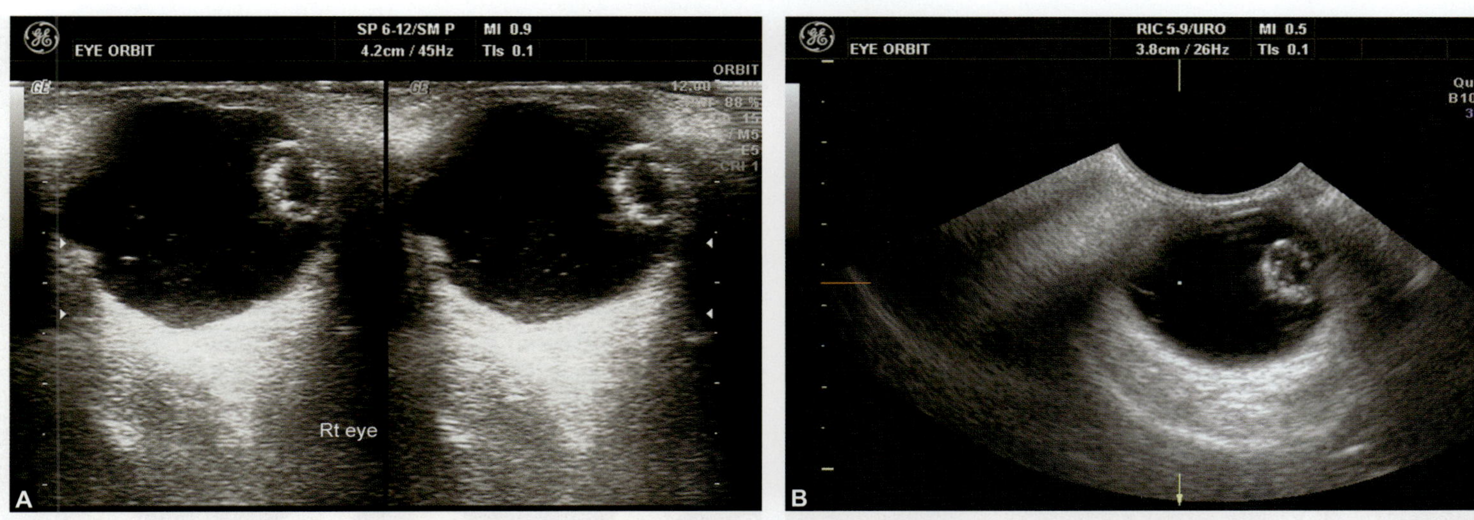

FIGURES 1.144A and B: Post-traumatic cataract with subluxation of lens. HRSG shows thickened opaque lens after sustaining trauma. The lens is not seen in normal position and it is seen subluxated to the nasal side.

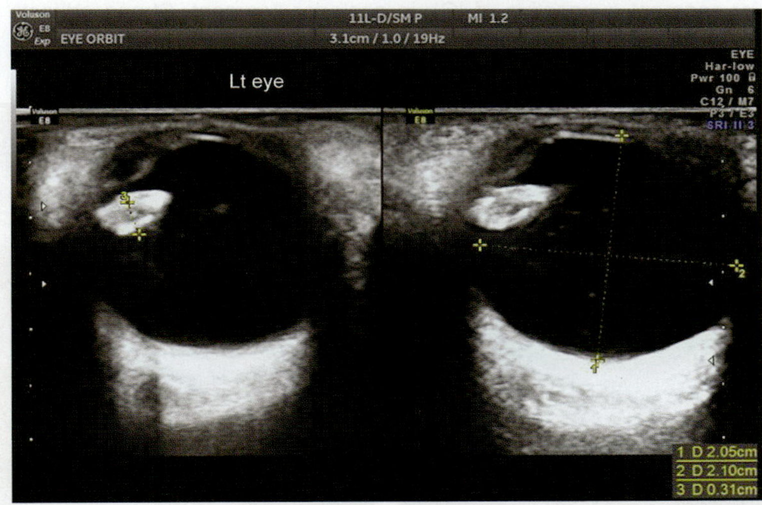

FIGURE 1.145: Post-trauma dislocated lens in posterior segment. A young child presented with diminished vision after sustaining trauma. HRSG shows cataractous lens in the posterior segment.

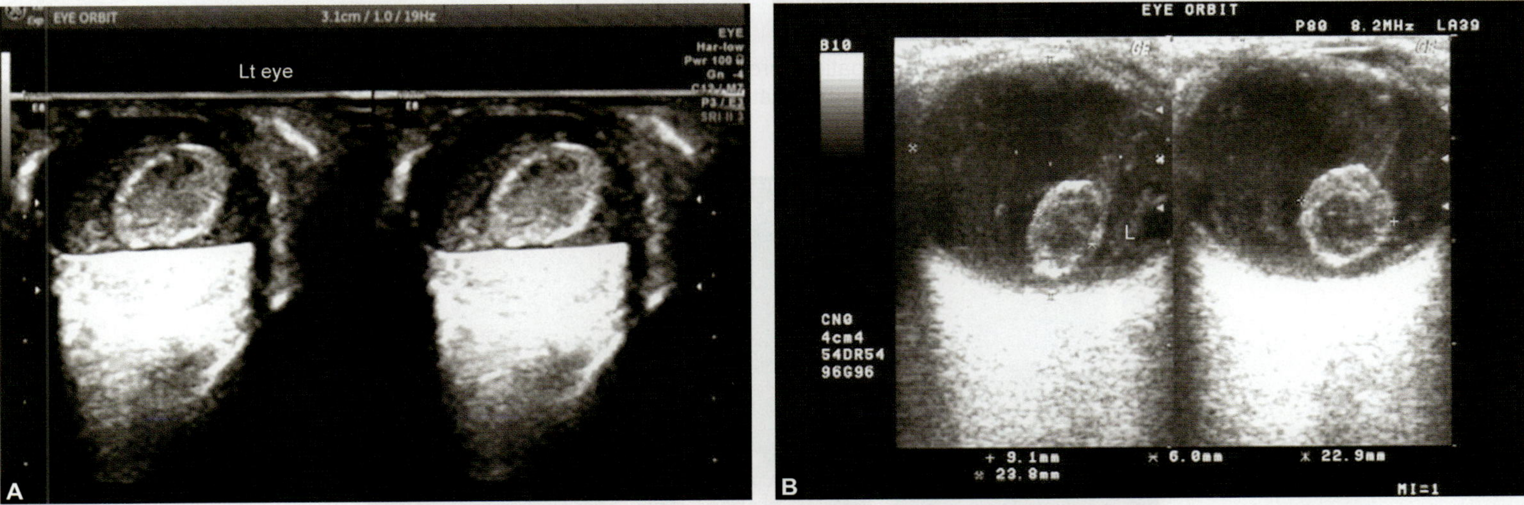

FIGURES 1.146A and B: Cataractous lens dislocated in posterior segment. HRSG shows thickened opaque lens dislocated in posterior segment of eye after sustaining trauma. The lens shows tumefaction. Associated intragel pathology is also seen.

EYE TRAUMA FOREIGN BODIES

Intraocular foreign bodies in most of the cases can be easily located on HRSG. Even when the foreign body (FB) is previously localized by X-ray or computed tomography (CT), ultrasonographic examination should be performed for more precise location of FB and to determine the extent of intraocular damage. Further if FB is lying near to sclera, CT does not identify if it lies just within or just outside the globe. Most Foreign bodies are detectable on HRSG. Small FB as metal, glass fragments, etc. traveling at high-speed causes penetrating injury to eye. Metals, glass and stones are highly reflective masses and can be picked up easily. They may cast acoustic shadowing. HRSG is highly sensitive even in picking up the track of traveling of FB outlining trajectory of the object. The entry of exist sites of FB may cause vitreous incarceration. Air bubbles are also seen in globe associated with FB. They stand out as highly reflective spots, which show rapid movements. Associated vitreous hemorrhage, retinal tears and scleral rupture can be well assessed on HRSG.

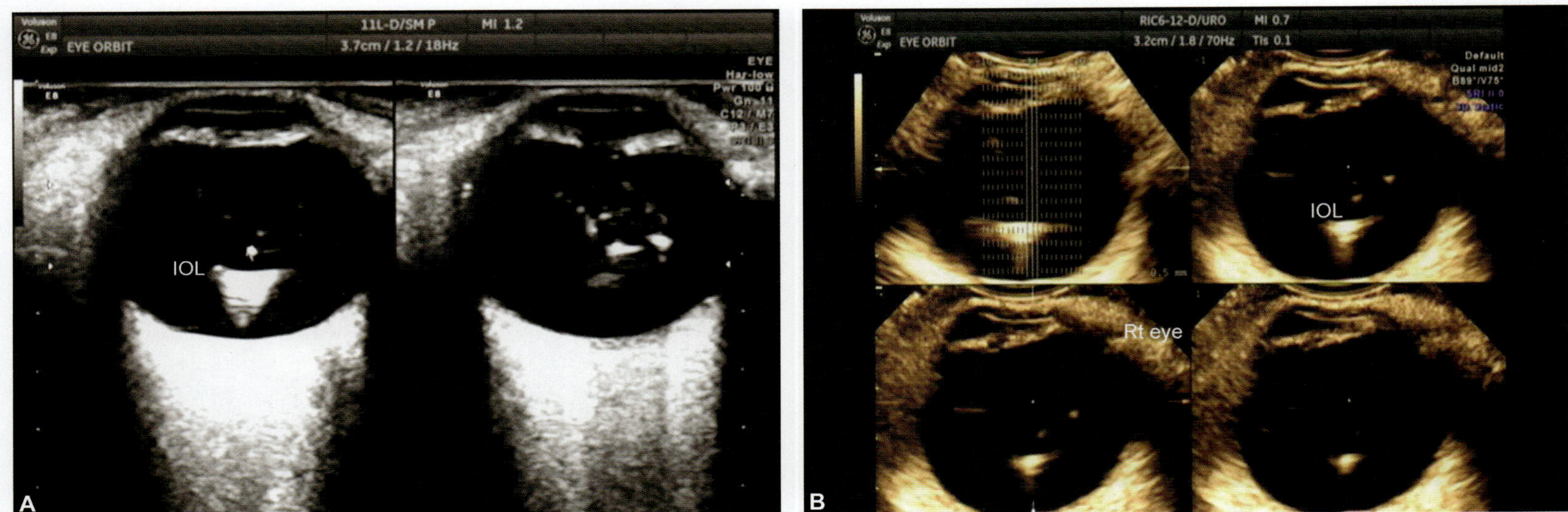

FIGURES 1.147A and B: IOL in posterior segment. A patient presented with loss of vision after cataract surgery. A hyper reflective echogenic curvilinear shadow is seen in the posterior segment suggestive of IOL in posterior segment. Strong artifacts are seen posterior to IOL. 3D with TUI imaging shows details of IOL.

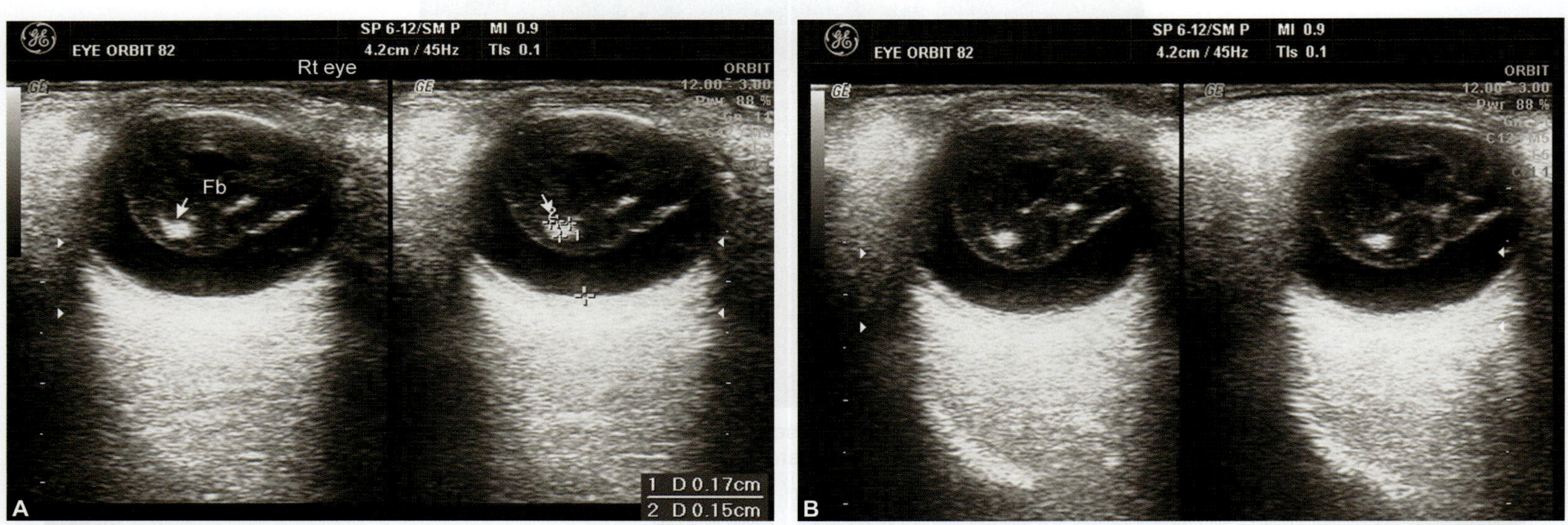

FIGURES 1.148A and B: Foreign body with hemorrhage. A patient presented with painful right eye after sustaining penetrating trauma. HRSG shows a highly echogenic shadow in the posterior segment, suggestive of a foreign body.

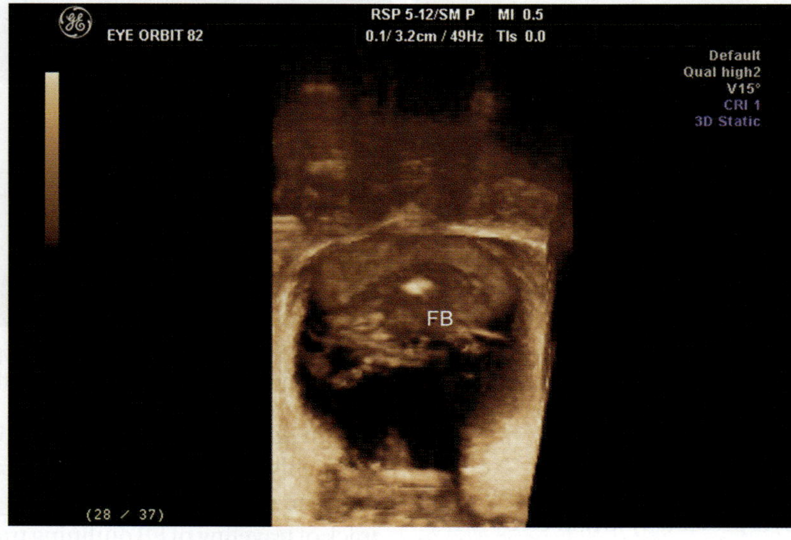

FIGURE 1.149: Foreign body with hemorrhage. 3D imaging of the eye shows the foreign body clearly. Associated intragel hemorrhage is also seen.

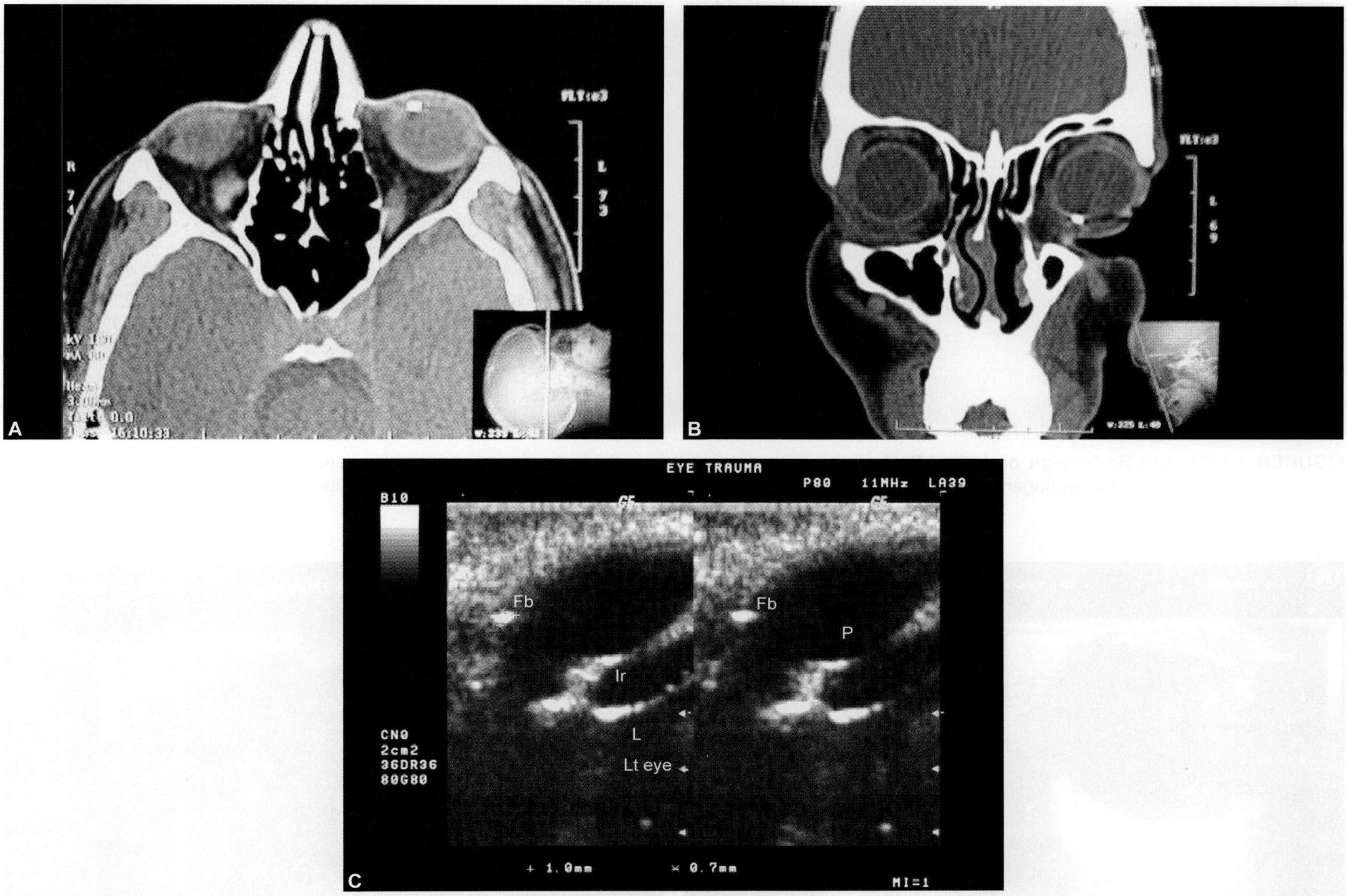

FIGURES 1.150A to C: CT scan axial and coronal cut shows a hyperdense foreign body in the orbital socket. However, it is not confirmed whether it is lying in the eye or outside the eye. HRSG clearly shows that the foreign body is lying outside the eyeball. It is confined to the just in the conjunctiva.

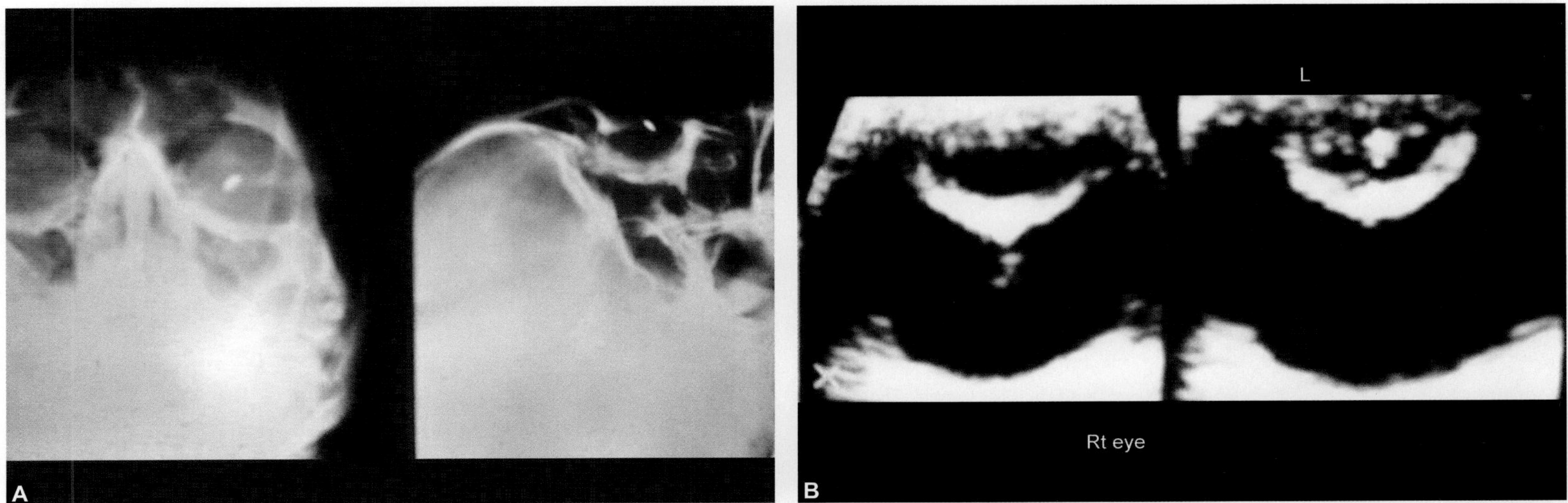

FIGURES 1.151A and B: Foreign body in anterior chamber. X-ray of the patient shows a radio-dense shadow in the orbit. However, exact location of the foreign body could not be determined. HRSG of the same patient shows an echogenic hyperreflective shadow in the anterior chamber. It is accompanied with acoustic shadowing.

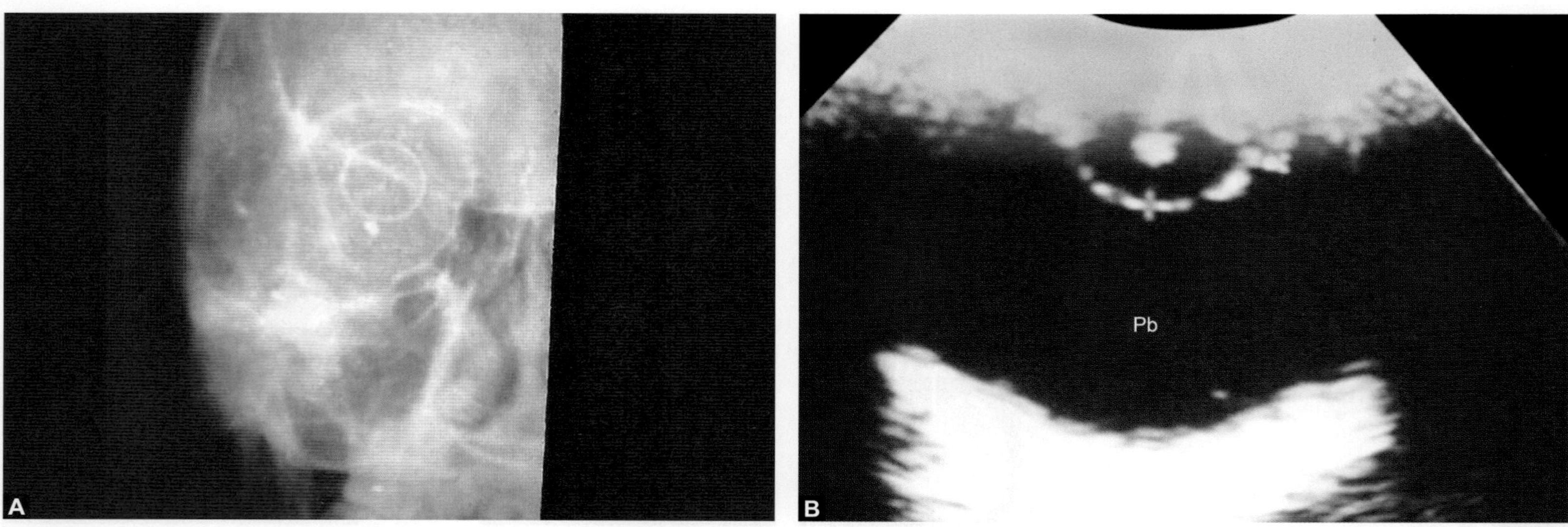

FIGURES 1.152A and B: Foreign body in AC. X-ray of the patient shows radio-dense opacity of metallic density in orbit. HRSG shows a hyper-dense echogenic foreign body confined in the anterior chamber. Posterior segment of the eye is free.

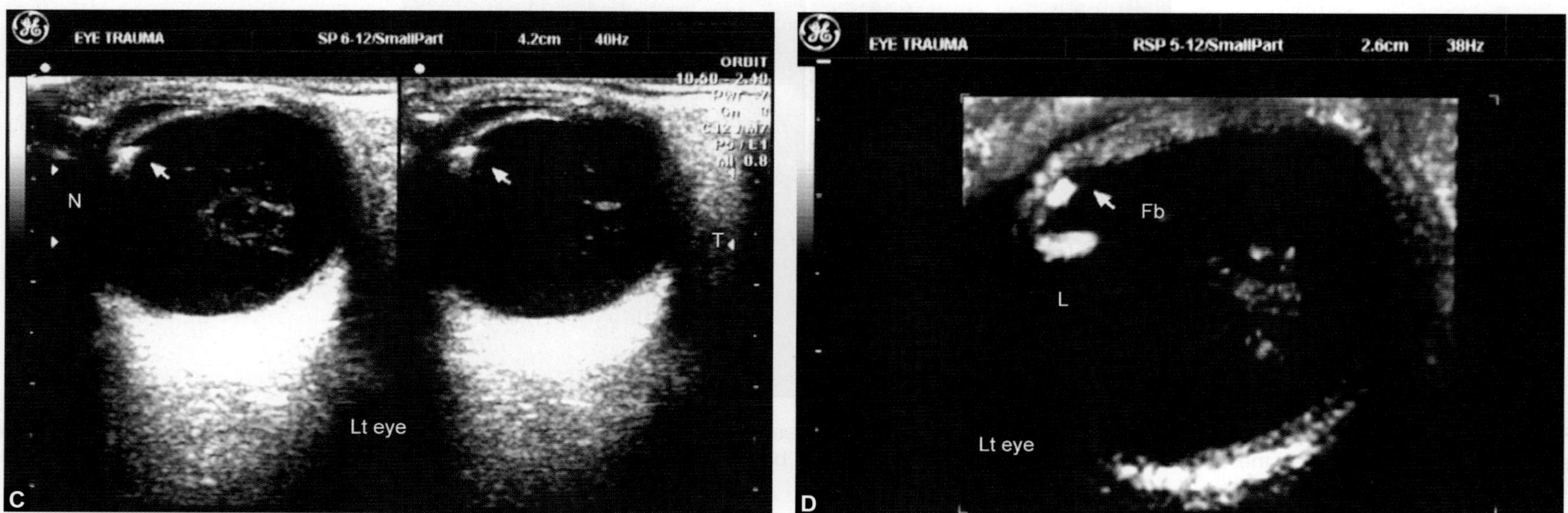

FIGURES 1.152C and D: Foreign body trauma. HRSG shows a small echogenic shadow in the anterior chamber in just near to the lens. It is difficult to differentiate from the lens on 2D imaging. 3D imaging of the same patient clearly shows the foreign body is lying away from the lens.

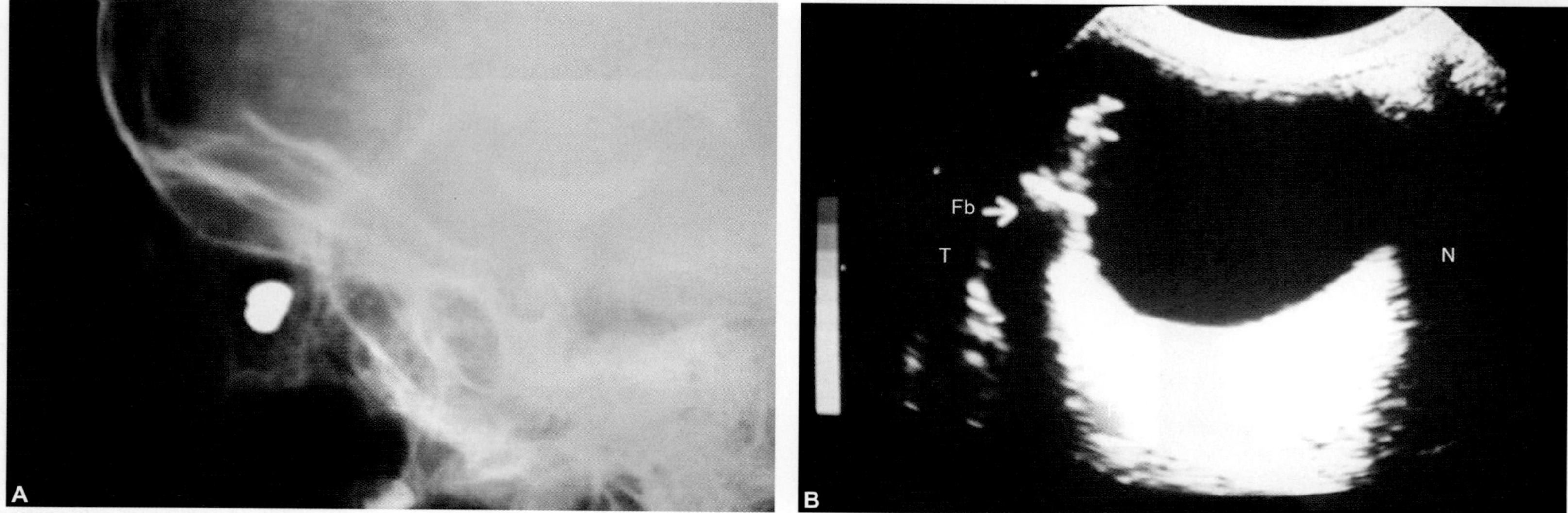

FIGURES 1.153A and B: Penetrating injury to the eye. X-ray of the patient shows a hyper-dense metallic shadow lodged in the orbital socket. The shape of the shadow is suggestive of a bullet. HRSG shows a hyper-dense echogenic body lodged in the episcleral space. However, no intragel hemorrhage is seen. No retinal detachment is seen.

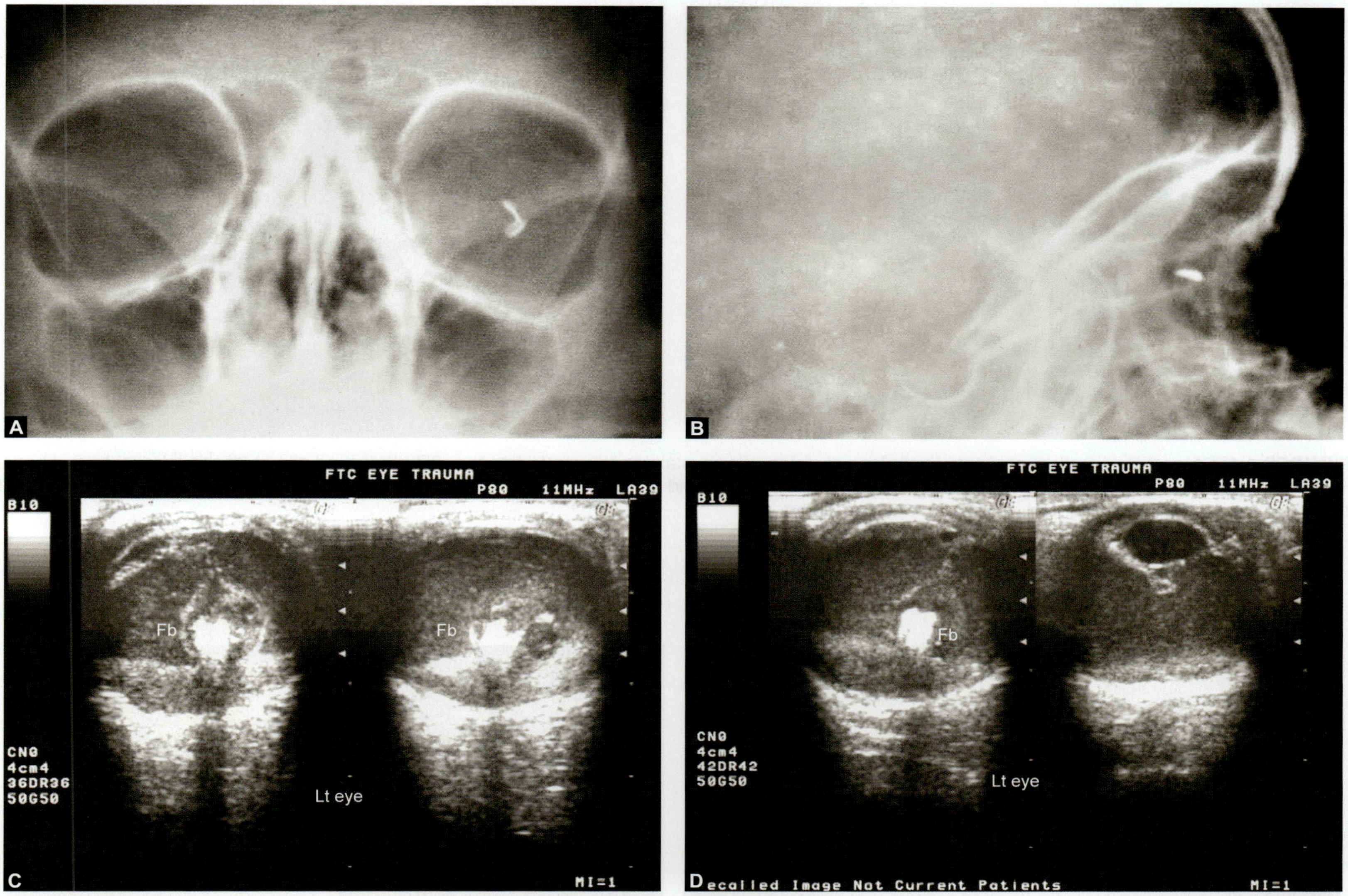

FIGURES 1.154A to D: Penetrating injury to the eye. X-ray of the patient shows radio-opaque foreign body of metallic density lodged in the posterior segment. HRSG of the same patient shows a hypo-dense echogenic foreign body lodged in the posterior segment with irregular shape. It is accompanied by acoustic shadowing. Associated dense intragel hemorrhage is also seen filling the posterior segment.

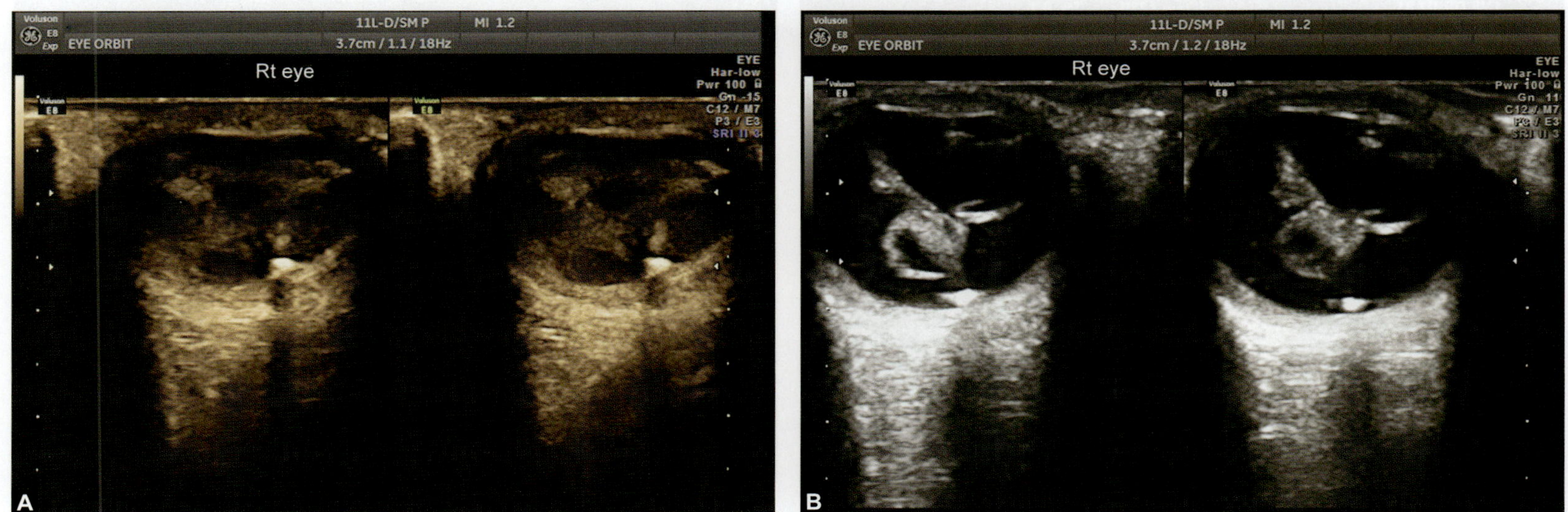

FIGURES 1.155A and B: Penetrating trauma with foreign body. A patient presented with penetrating foreign body trauma with loss of vision. HRSG shows a highly echogenic small shadow lodged in the posterior segment. It is of metallic density. Dense intragel hemorrhage is also seen with associated retinal detachment.

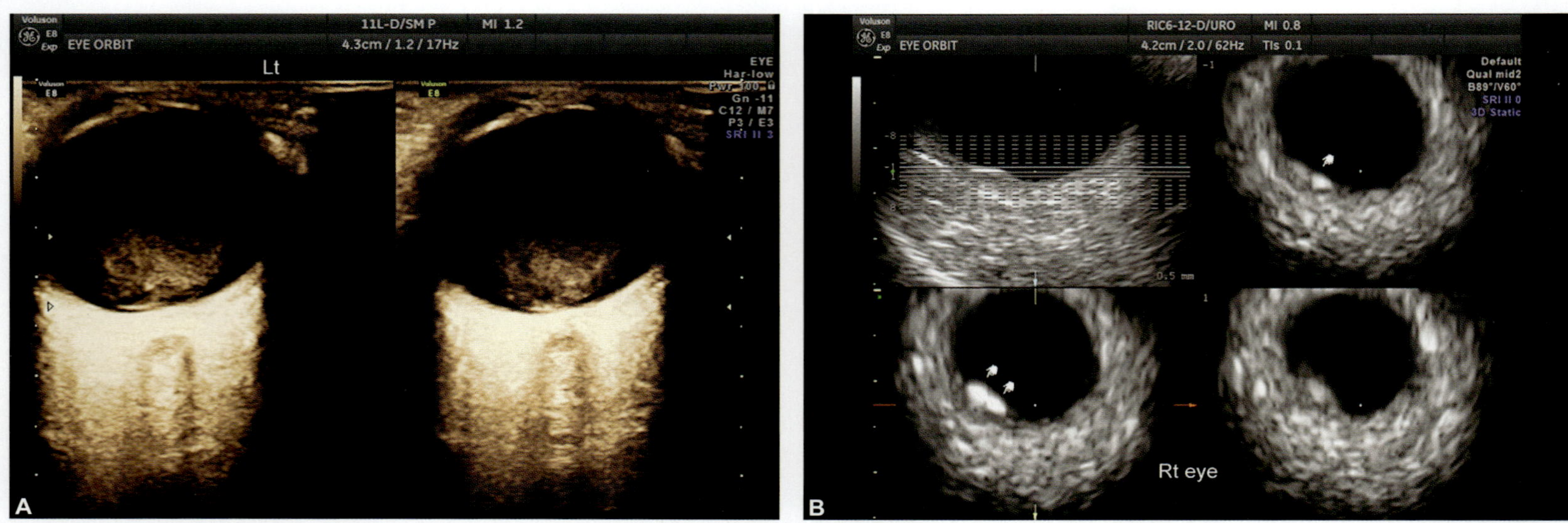

FIGURES 1.156A and B: A patient presented with loss of vision after sustaining trauma to the eye. 2D ultrasound shows dense intragel hemorrhage. However, no foreign body is seen on 2D ultrasound. But on 3D ultrasound with TUI imaging, shows a hyperreflective body in the posterior segment of the eye embedded in sclera. But no scleral rupture is seen.

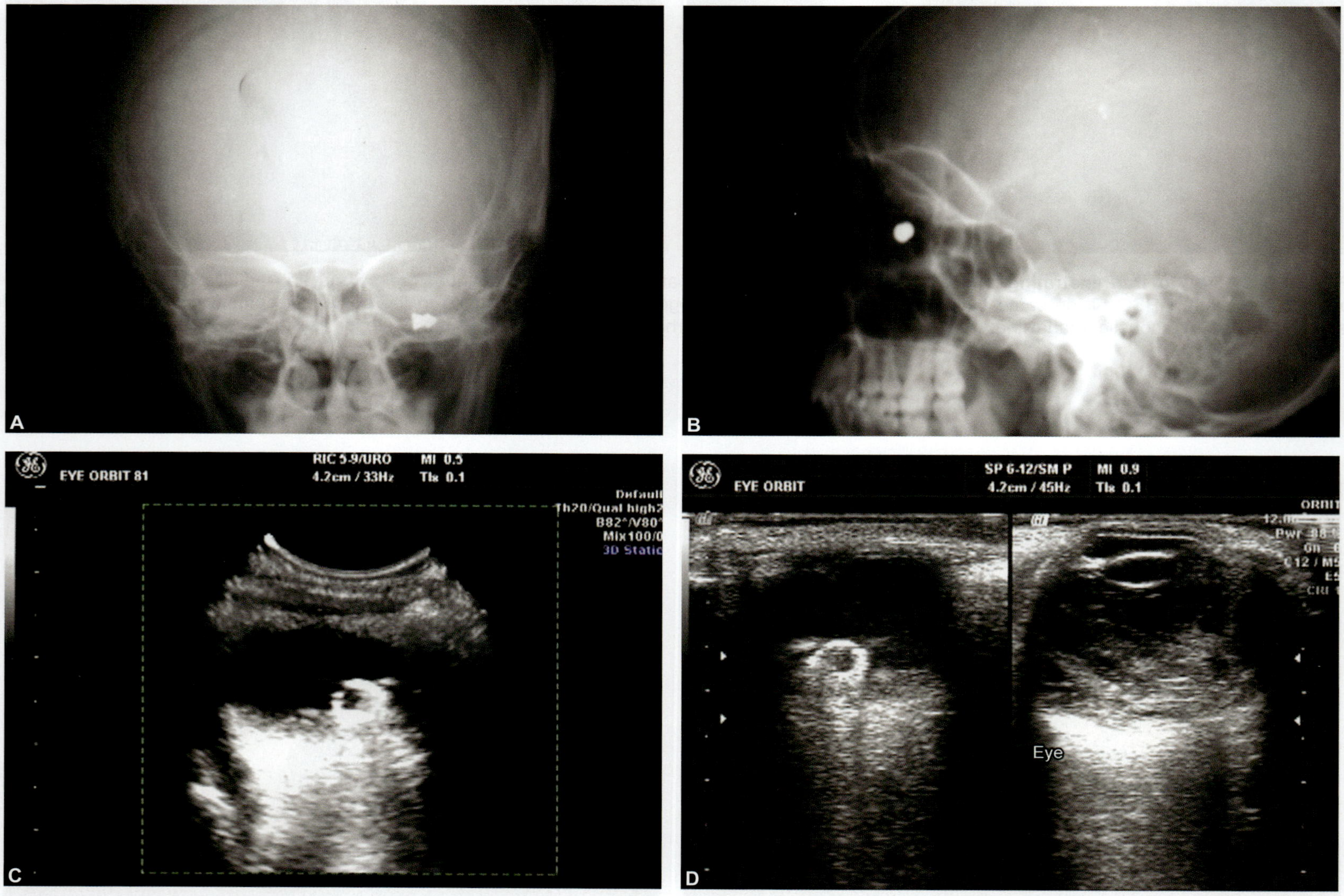

FIGURES 1.157A to D: Penetrating trauma to the eye. A young boy presented with history of gunshot injury. Plane X-ray shows a palate seen lodged in the left orbit. HRSG shows a highly dense echogenic shadow in the posterior segment of the eye. Dense intragel hemorrhage is also seen. The eye is small and collapsed.

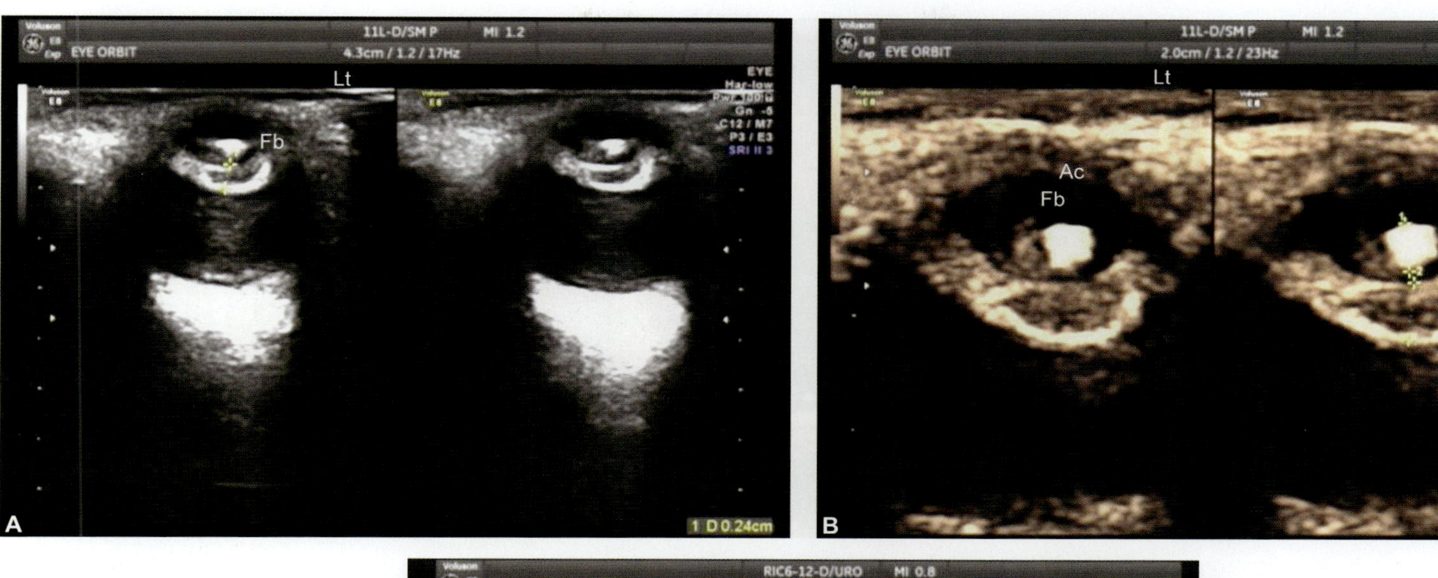

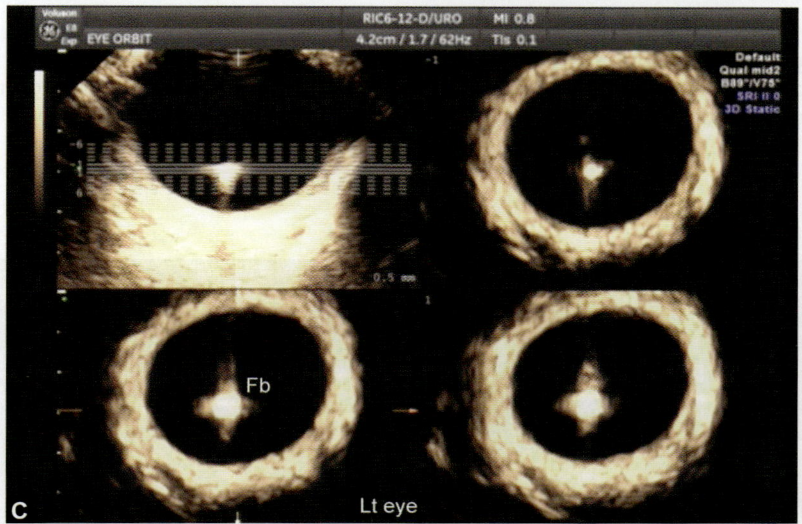

FIGURES 1.158A to C: Foreign body in the anterior segment. A young child presented with trauma to the eye. HRSG highly dense shadow of metallic density suggestive of foreign body in the anterior segment. The TUI imaging shows another foreign body in the posterior segment of the eye, which is not seen on 2D ultrasound.

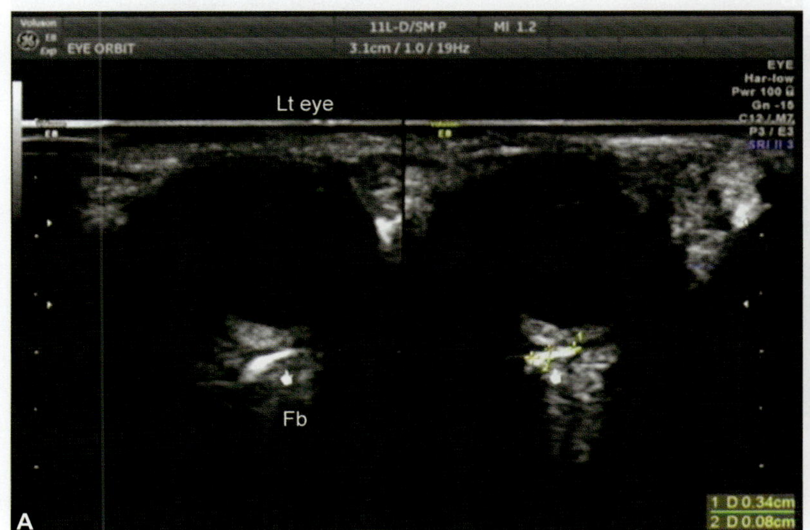

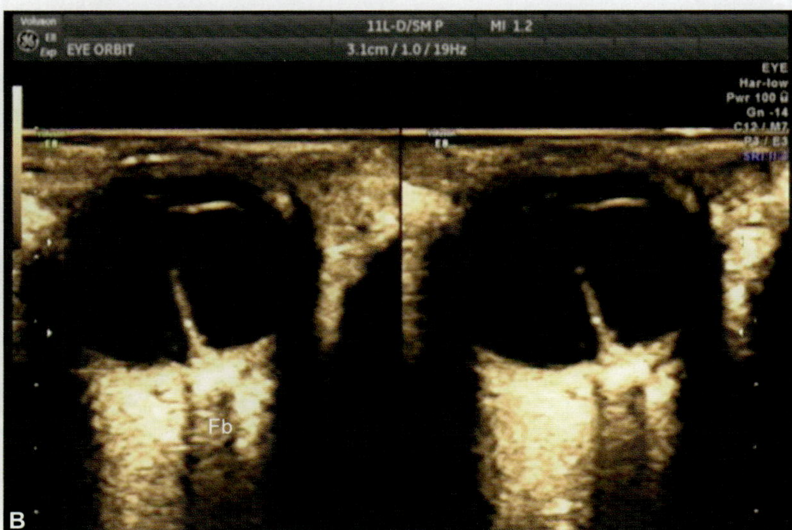

FIGURES 1.159A and B

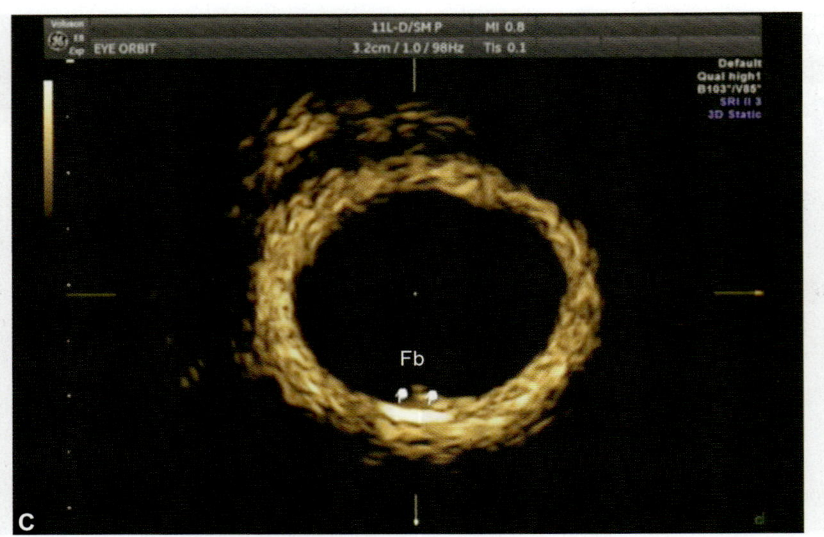

FIGURE 1.159C

FIGURES 1.159A to C: Foreign body lodged in sclera with scleral tear. A patient presented with history of penetrating trauma with loss of vision. HRSG shows a highly echogenic shadow lodged at the posterior pole of left eye. Dense intragel hemorrhage is seen. The trajectory of foreign body is also seen. On 3D ultrasound, the foreign body is seen lodged in the scleral coat with perforation of sclera.

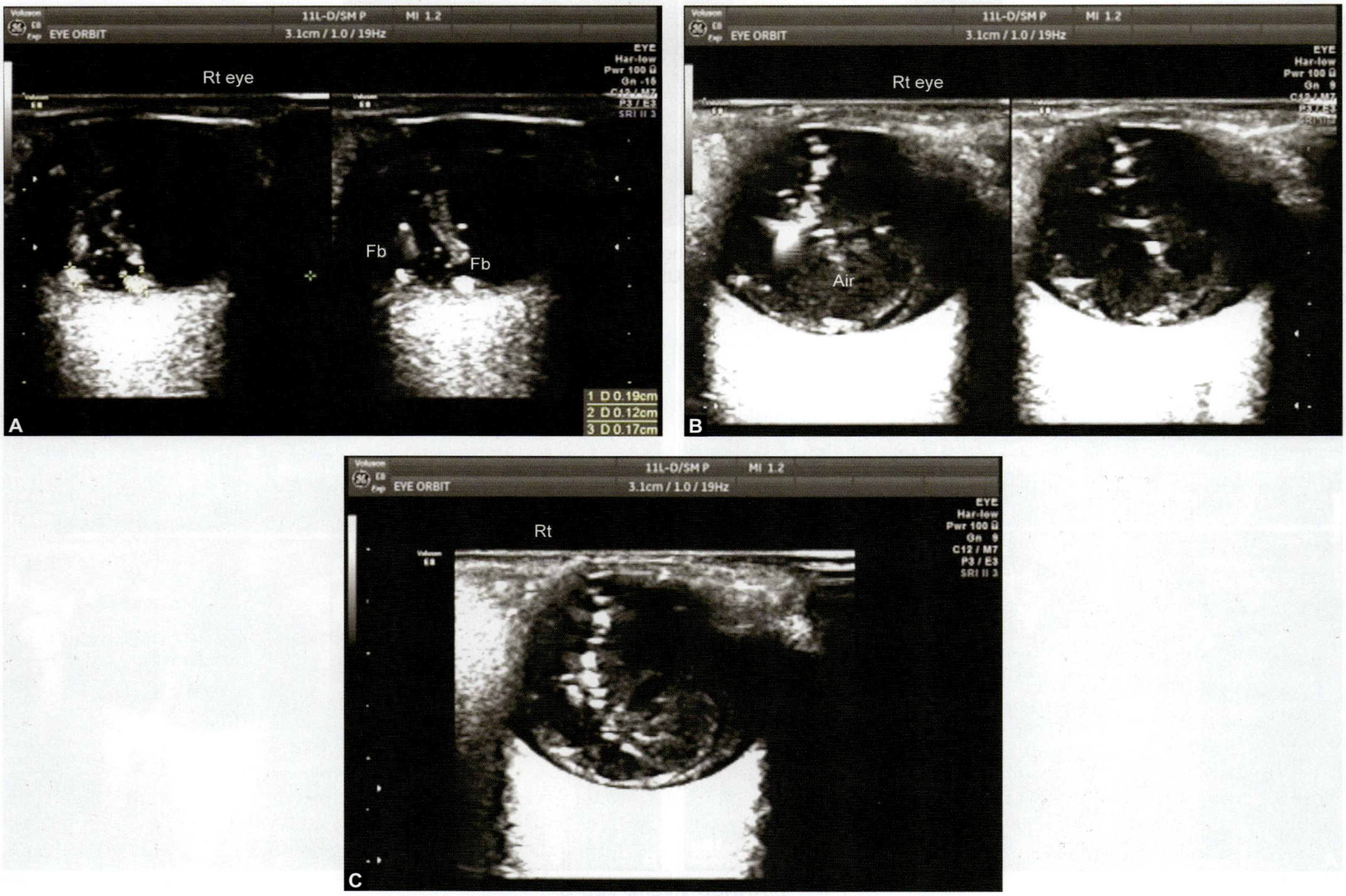

FIGURES 1.160A to C: Foreign body with trajectory. A patient presented with history of penetrating trauma. HRSG shows highly dense shadow lodged in the posterior segment of eye. It is of metallic density suggestive of foreign body. The echogenic air bubbles are seen floating in the trajectory of the foreign body. Dense intragel hemorrhage is also seen associated with trauma.

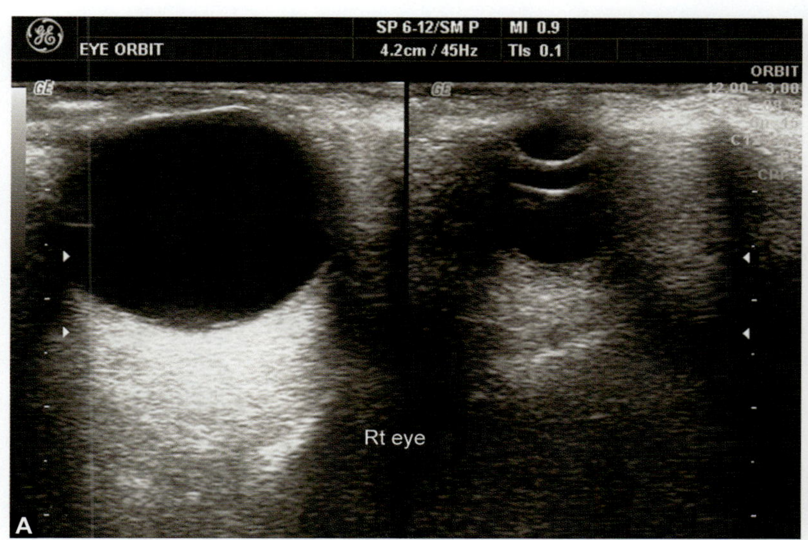

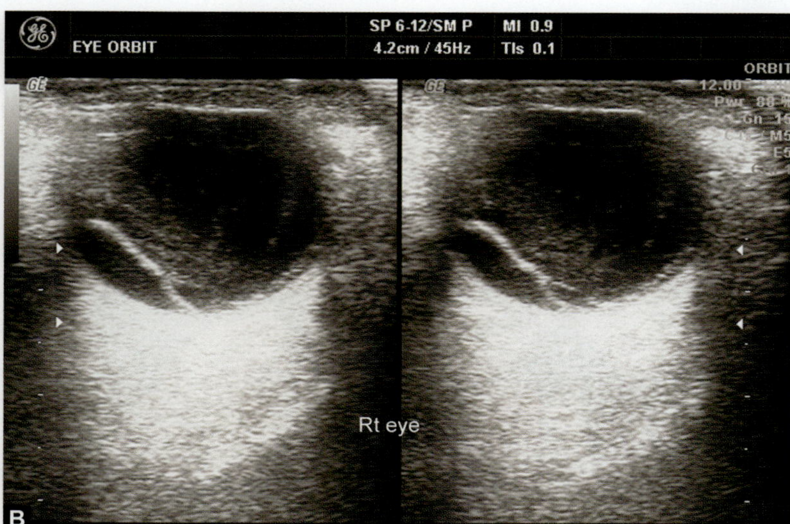

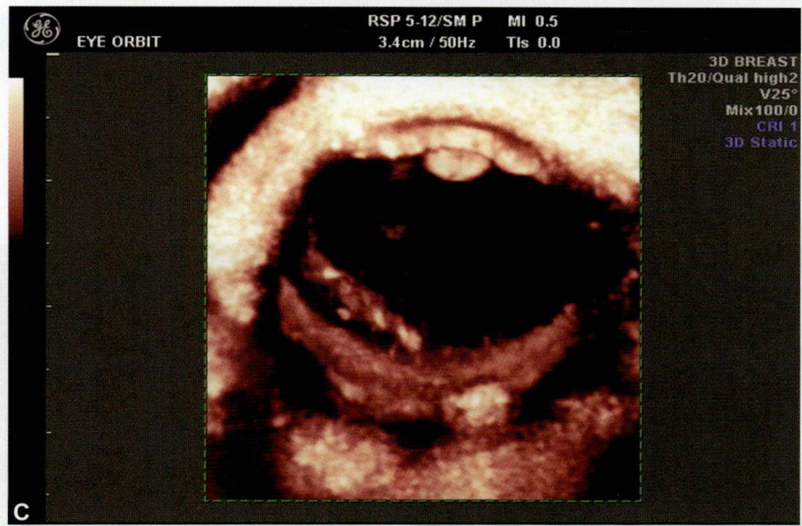

FIGURES 1.161A to C: Intragel hemorrhage with retinal detachment with foreign body in subretinal space. A patient presented with loss of vision after sustaining penetrating trauma. 2D ultrasound shows dense intragel hemorrhage in the posterior segment. A thick membrane is seen detached in the posterior segment suggestive of retinal detachment. However, no foreign body is seen on 2D ultrasound. But on 3D ultrasound, a highly echogenic shadow is seen in the subretinal space suggestive of a foreign body. The cataractous lens is also seen clearly on 3D ultrasound.

INTRAOCULAR TUMORS

HRSG has become one of the foremost investigations in evaluation of ocular tumors. It has also become the most important, noninvasive method to evaluate ocular tumors in the presence of clear ocular media. HRSG provides valuable assessment of size, shape, growth and regression of ocular tumor.

Sonographic Criteria

An intraocular tumor must have a minimum thickness or elevation before it can be picked up by HRSG. A lesion must have an elevation of minimum 8 mm before it can be picked up on HRSG. Choroidal tumors are more elevated than surrounding retinochoroid layer in order to be detected by HRSG. Ciliary body lesion need to be more elevated than choroidal lesion due to irregular surface of the ciliary body. A lesion, as small as 3 mm, can be easily picked up on HRSG. Other criteria include reflectivity of lesions. Hypoechoic lesions are easily picked up than echogenic lesions. HRSG can tell about base, diameter, extra ocular extension of the growth and solid and cystic nature of the mass.

Tumors of Anterior Chamber

HRSG is important investigation for evaluation of tumors of the anterior chambers like iris tumors, anterior ciliary body tumors, vascular masses of sclera.

Medulloepithelioma (Diktyoma)

Medulloepithelioma or diktyoma is a rare tumor of ciliary body. It is seen in children. The tumor presents as a whitish mass within the ciliary body. These tumors may be associated with iris cysts or free floating cysts within the anterior chamber or vitreous cavity. The tumors may be echogenic or shows moderate echogenicity. On color flow imaging, moderate flow is seen in them. The teratoid variant of the tumor shows heterogeneous texture due to cartilage.

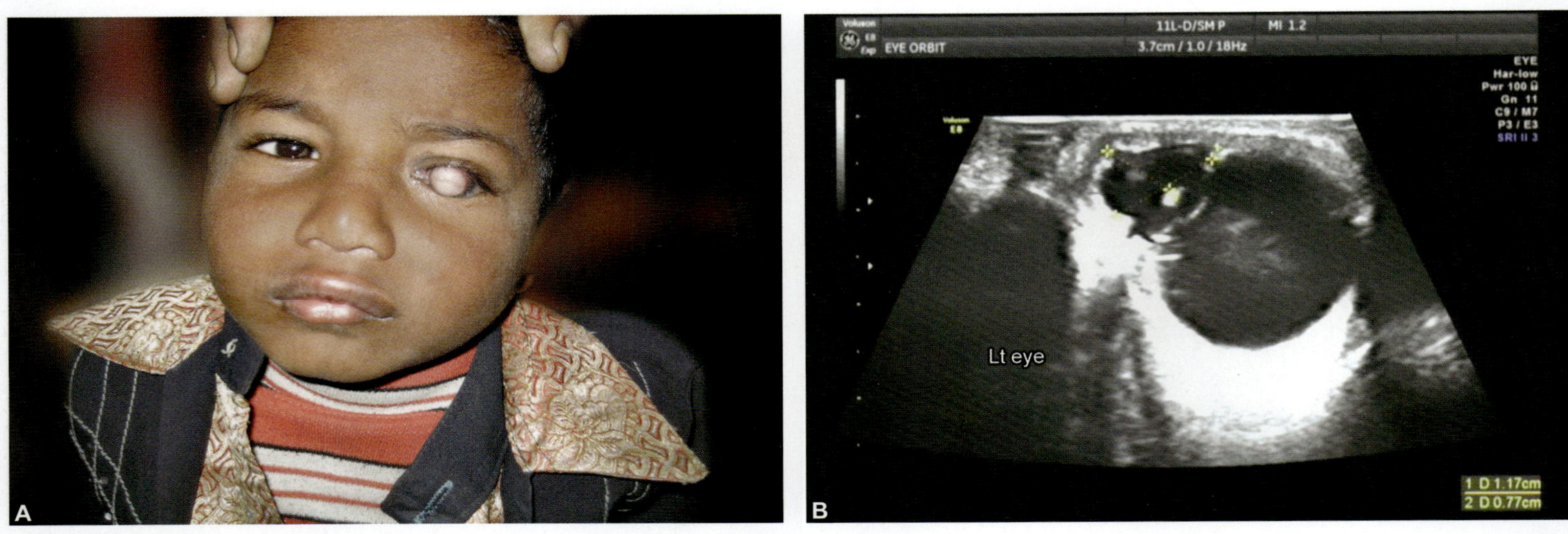

FIGURES 1.162A and B: Anterior staphyloma with adherent lens. A young child presented with soft tissue swelling over the left eye. HRSG shows a well-defined cystic shadow seen coming out from the Iris suggestive of anterior staphyloma. Echogenic lens is seen embedded in the cyst suggestive of embedded lens. Posterior segment of the eye is free.

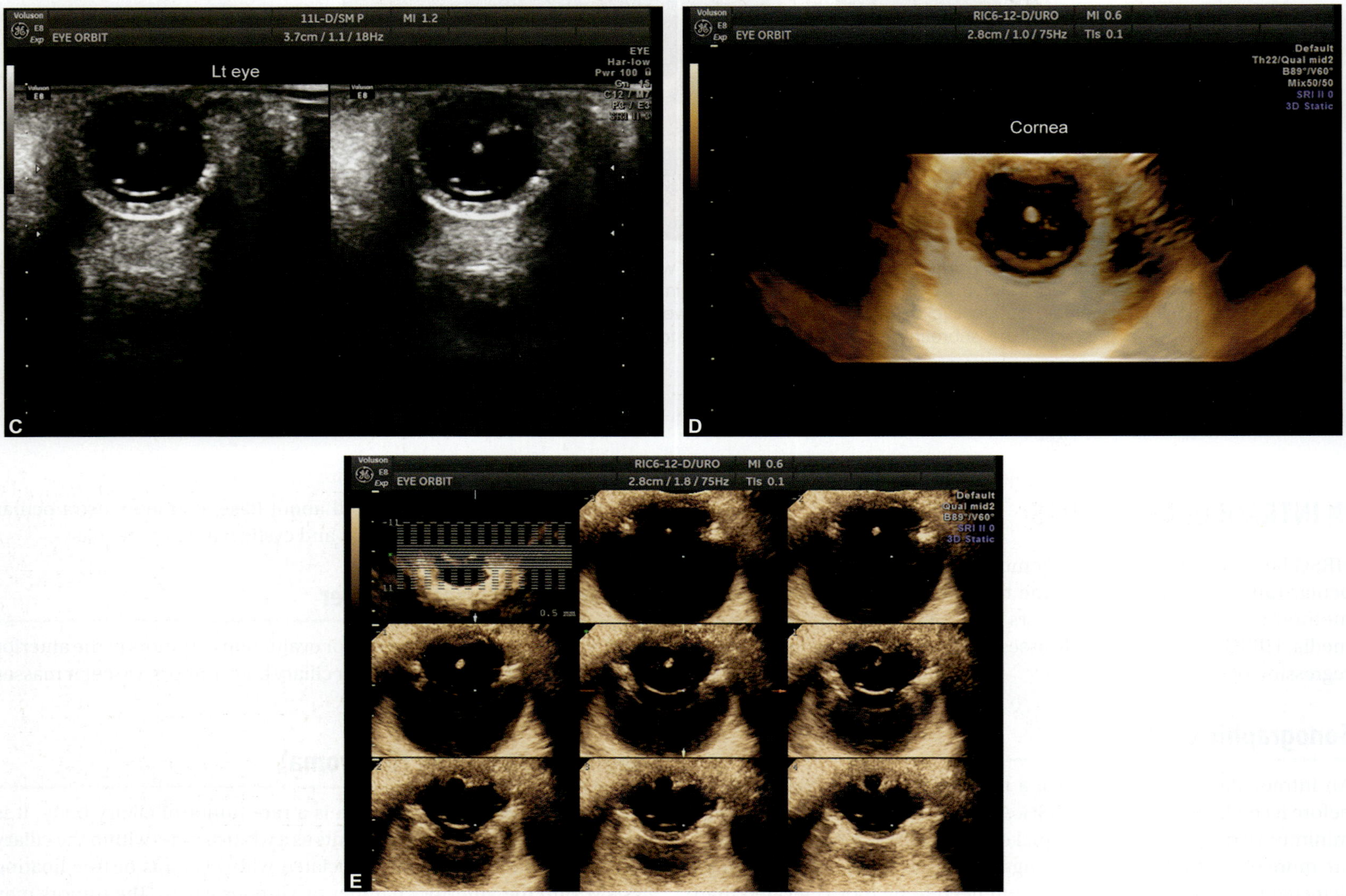

FIGURES 1.162C to E: Anterior staphyloma. A young girl presented with soft tissue swelling over the left eye. HRSG shows a well-defined cyst in the anterior segment of the eye. An echogenic shadow is seen in the cyst. It is separate from the lens and appears to be coming out from iris suggestive of anterior staphyloma.

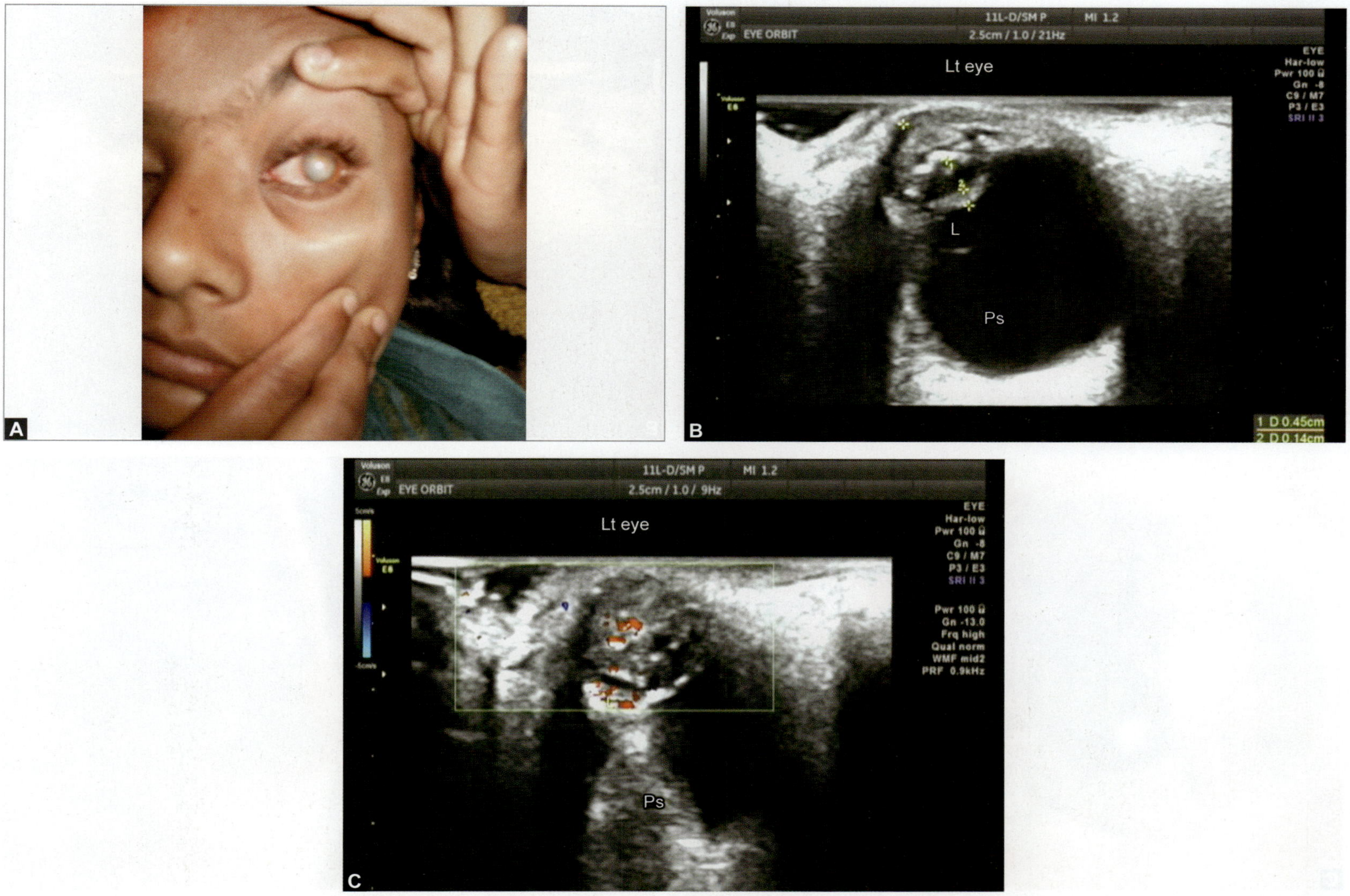

FIGURES 1.163A to C: Anterior staphyloma with adherent lens. A young girl presented with soft tissue mass coming out from cornea. HRSG shows an echogenic mass bulging out from iris. It shows soft tissue shadows. Calcification is also seen in it. On color flow imaging, few vessels are seen feeding it. The lens is thickened and opaque. It is adherent with the mass suggestive of anterior staphyloma with adherent lens.

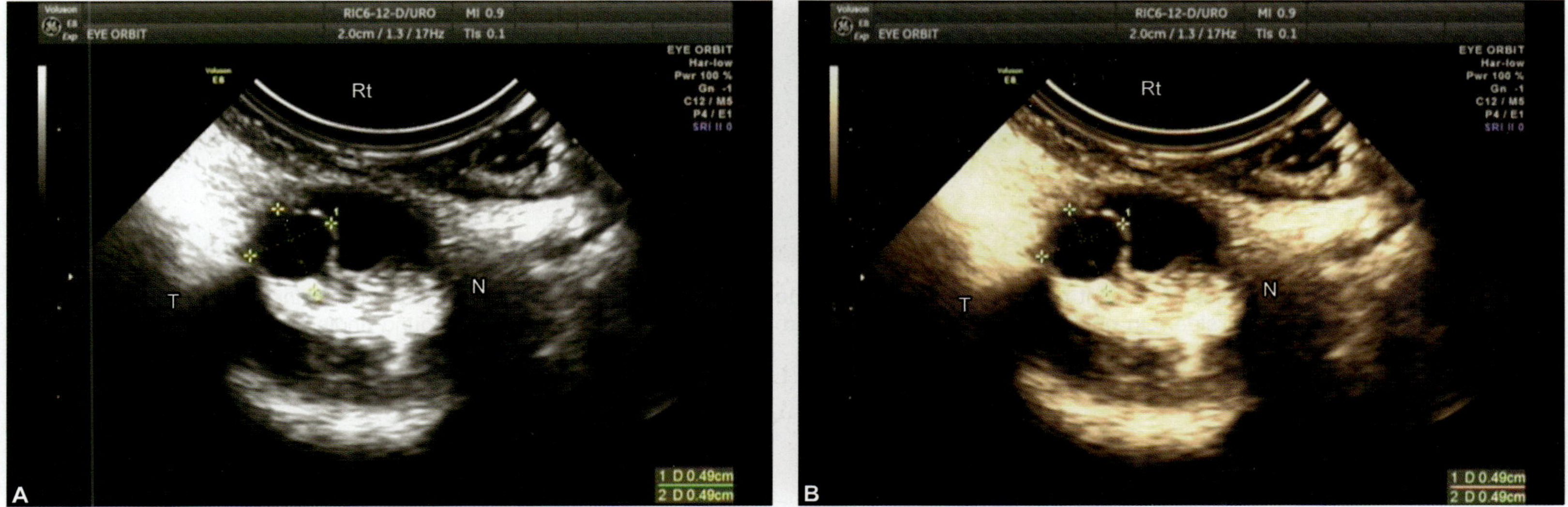

FIGURES 1.164A and B: Iris cyst. A patient presented with cystic shadow in the anterior segment. A cystic mass is seen coming out from the iris on temporal side suggestive of iris cyst. The lens is also thickened and opaque with evidence of cataractous changes in the lens.

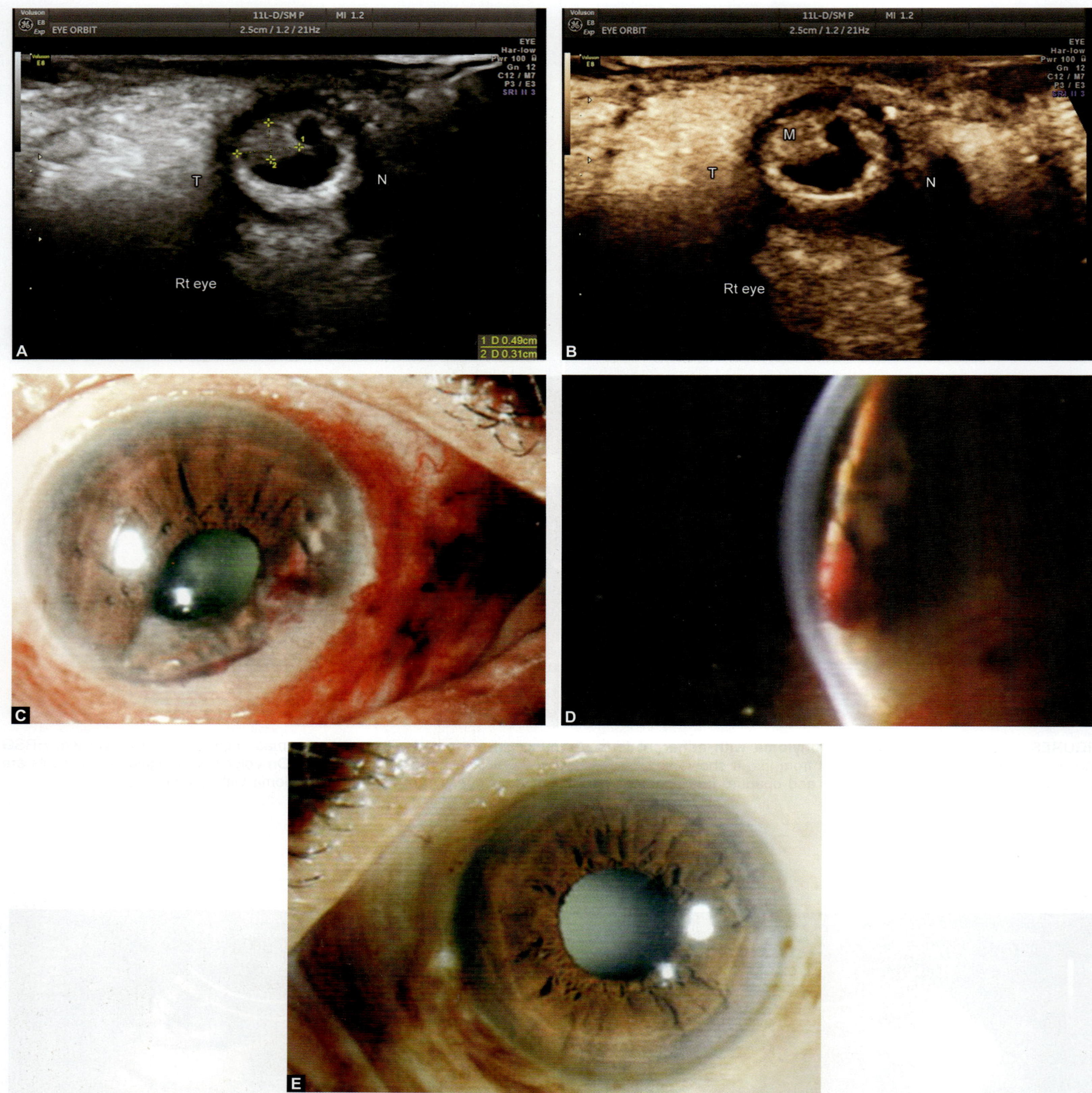

FIGURES 1.165A to E: Iris mass. A patient presented with a soft tissue mass over the Iris. HRSG shows a well defined mass coming out from the iris on temporal side. On ophthalmoscopy and ultrasound biomicroscopy (UBM), the ultrasound findings are confirmed.

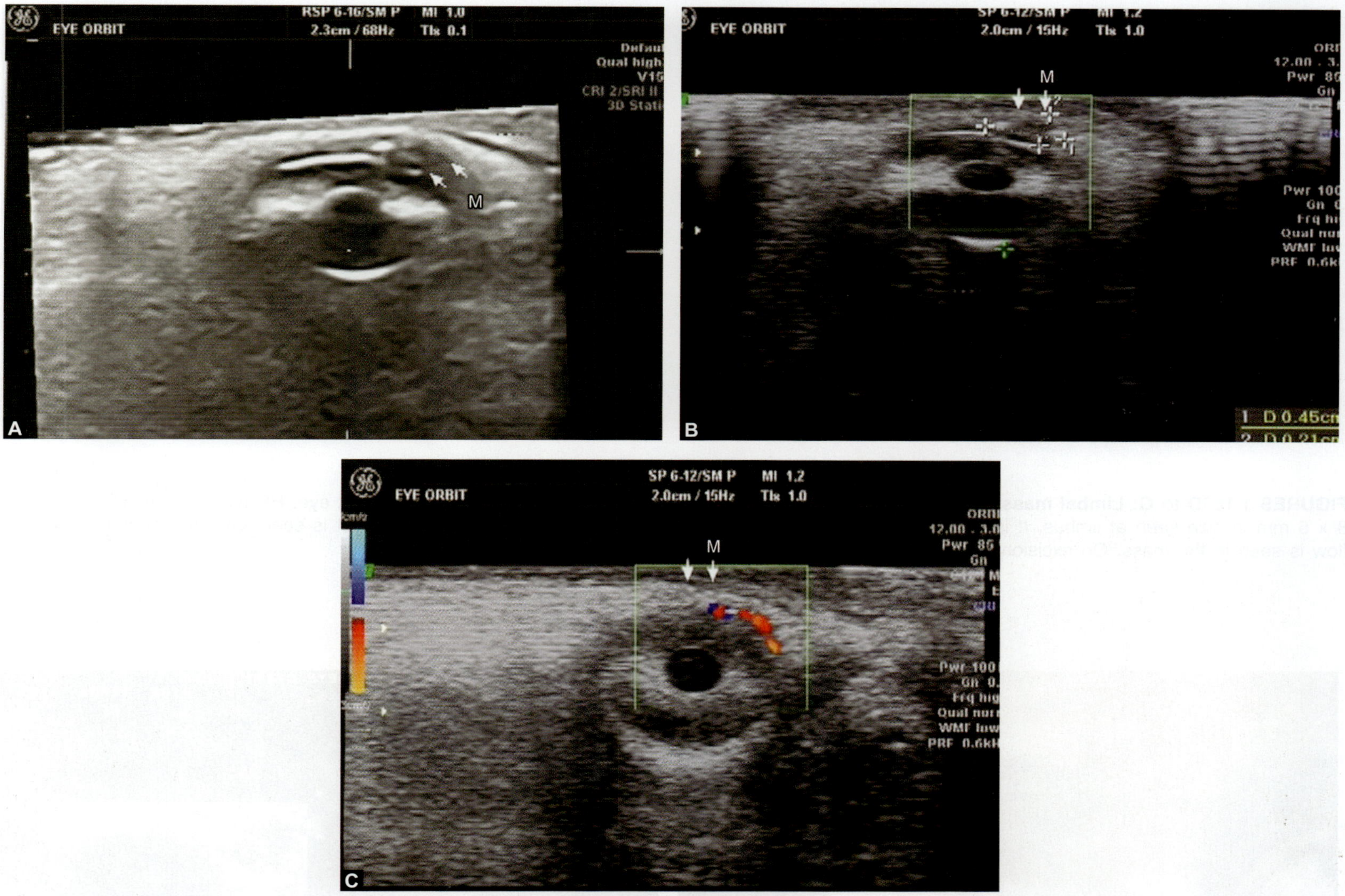

FIGURES 1.166A to C: Limbal mass. A lady presented with superficial mass at the limbus. The mass is seen at the limbus area and measures 4.5 × 2.1 mm in size. On color flow imaging, few vessels are seen feeding the mass.

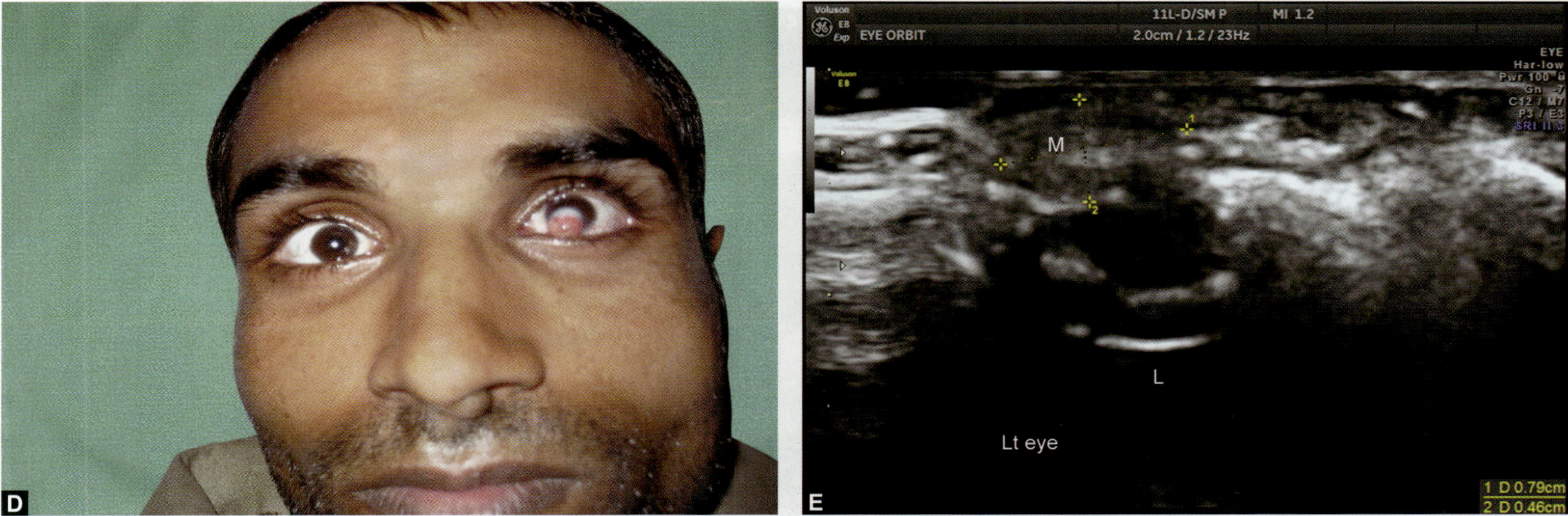

FIGURES 1.166D and E

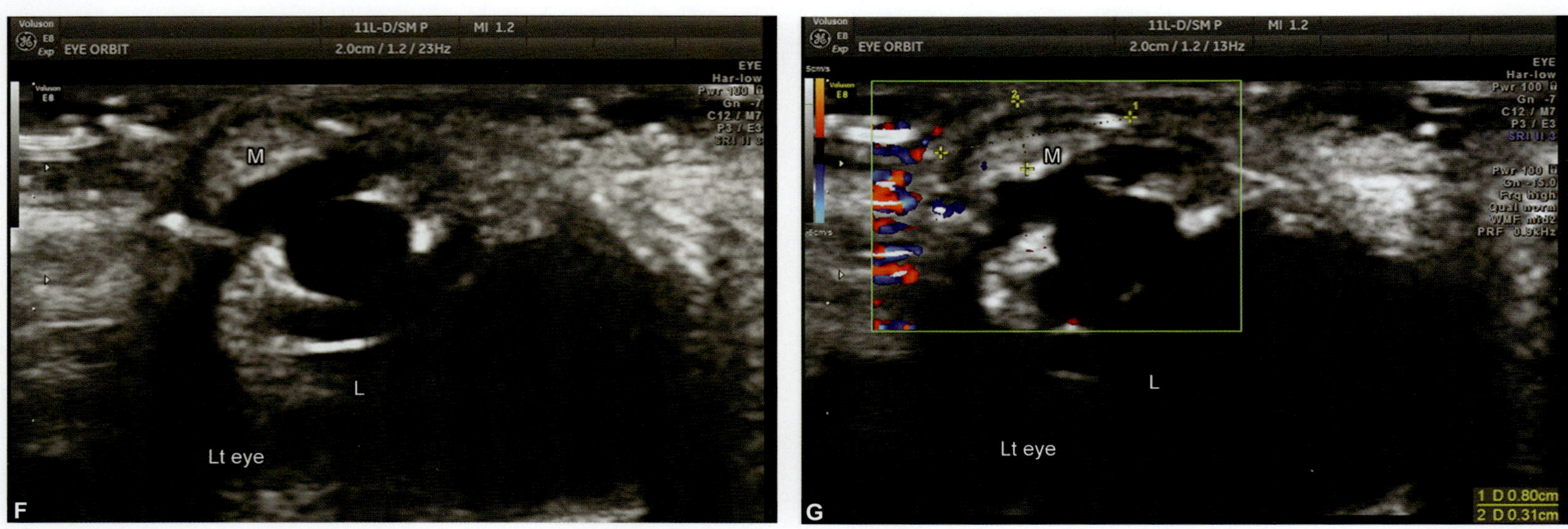

FIGURES 1.166F and G

FIGURES 1.166D to G: Limbal mass. A patient presented with soft tissue mass coming out from limbus of left eye. HRSG shows a soft tissue mass 8 x 5 mm in size seen at limbus. It is homogeneous in texture. No calcification is seen in the mass. No cyst is seen. On color flow imaging, poor flow is seen in the mass. On excision and biopsy, it came out to be low-grade hemangiomatous mass.

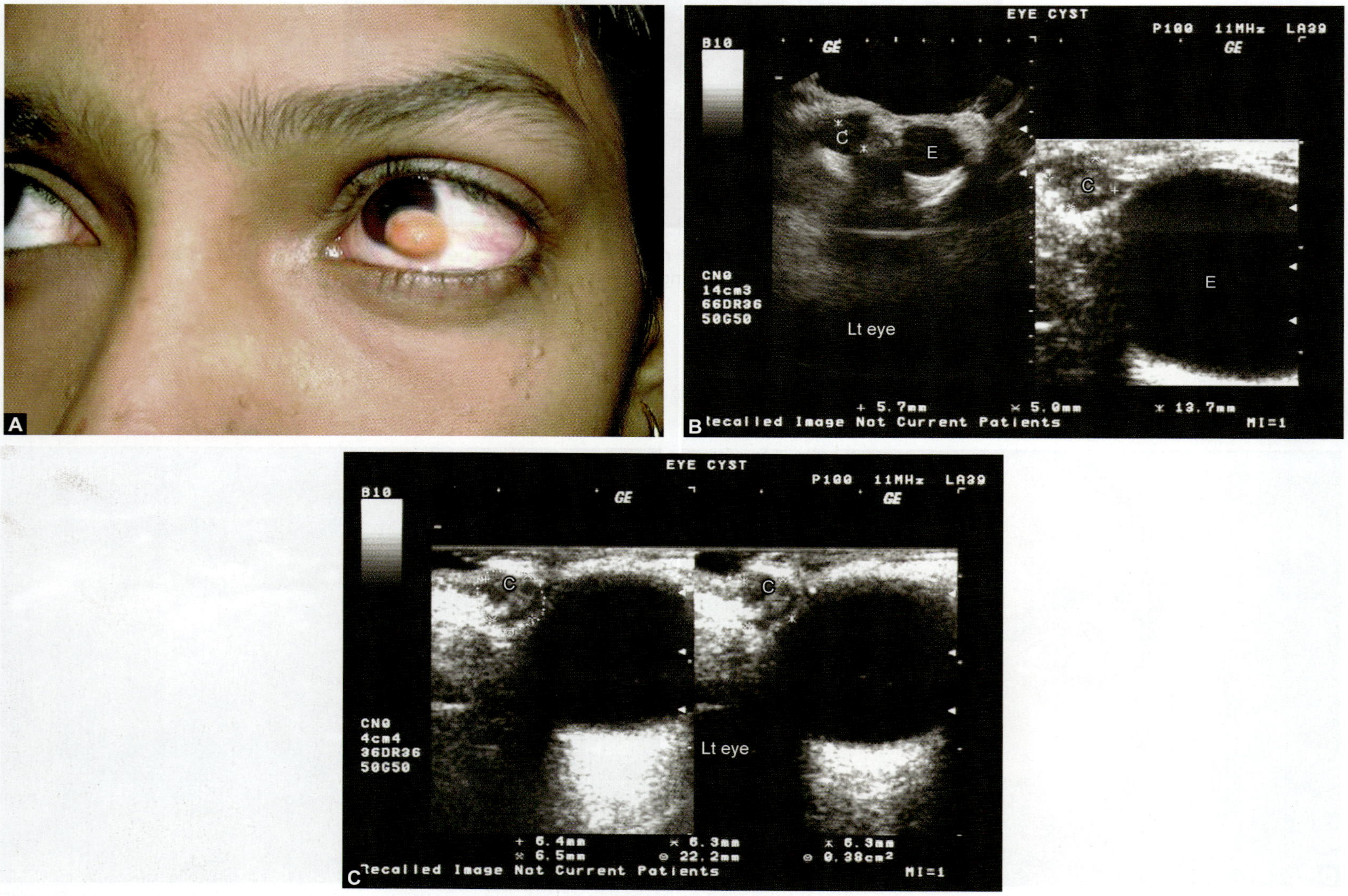

FIGURES 1.167A to C: A well-defined mass with sharp seen over the left eye encircling the pupil and hampering vision at cornea. HRSG shows a well-defined cyst coming out from corneoscleral junction: and also involving the IRIS. Multiple thick echoes are seen in it with: thick wall due to keratirization. Part of the inner cyst is seen involving the iris on nasal side. However, the eyeball shows normal posterior segment.

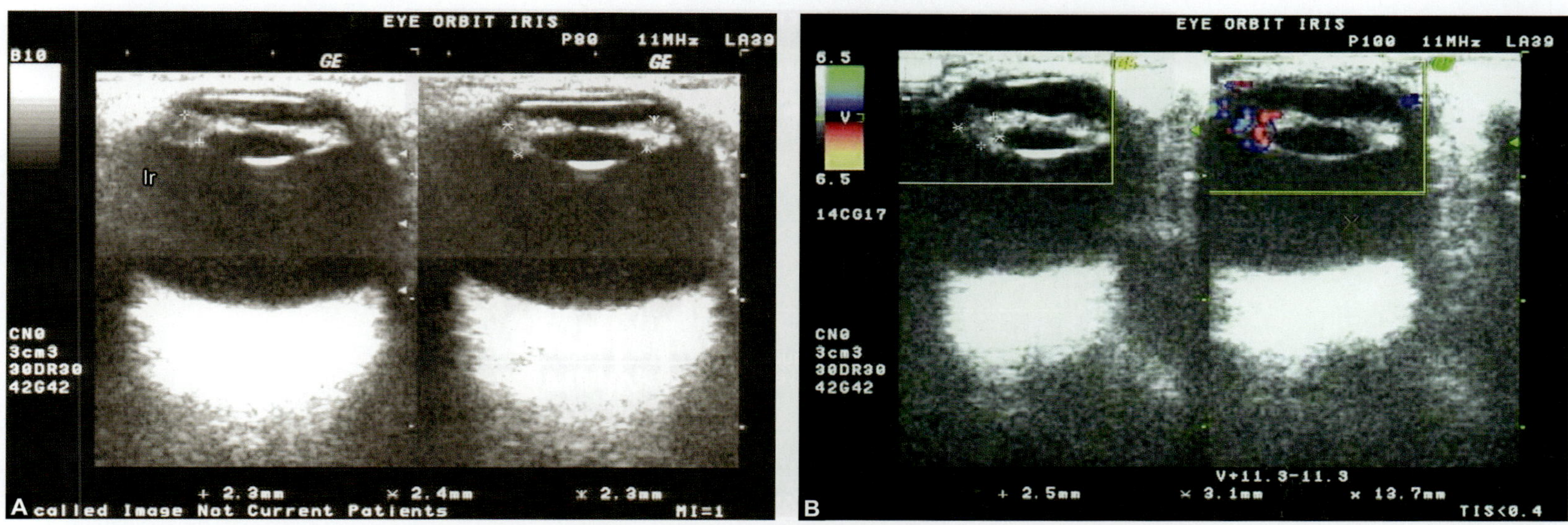

FIGURES 1.168A and B: Iris mass. Epithelioma HRSG shows an irregular hyperechoic mass in the iris in a 4-month-old child. On color Doppler, study the mass shows increased vascularity. Biopsy showed epithelioma.

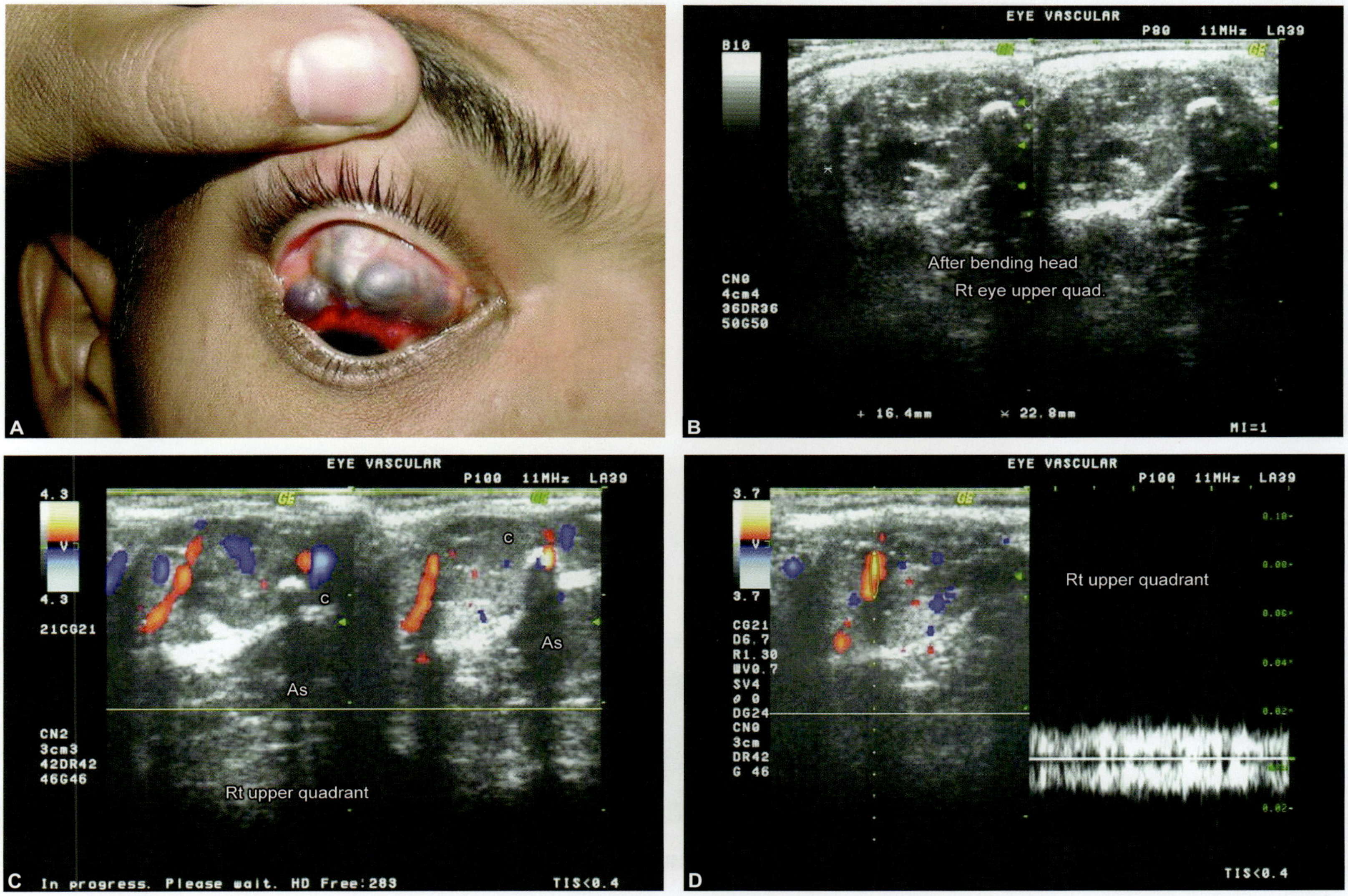

FIGURES 1.169A to D

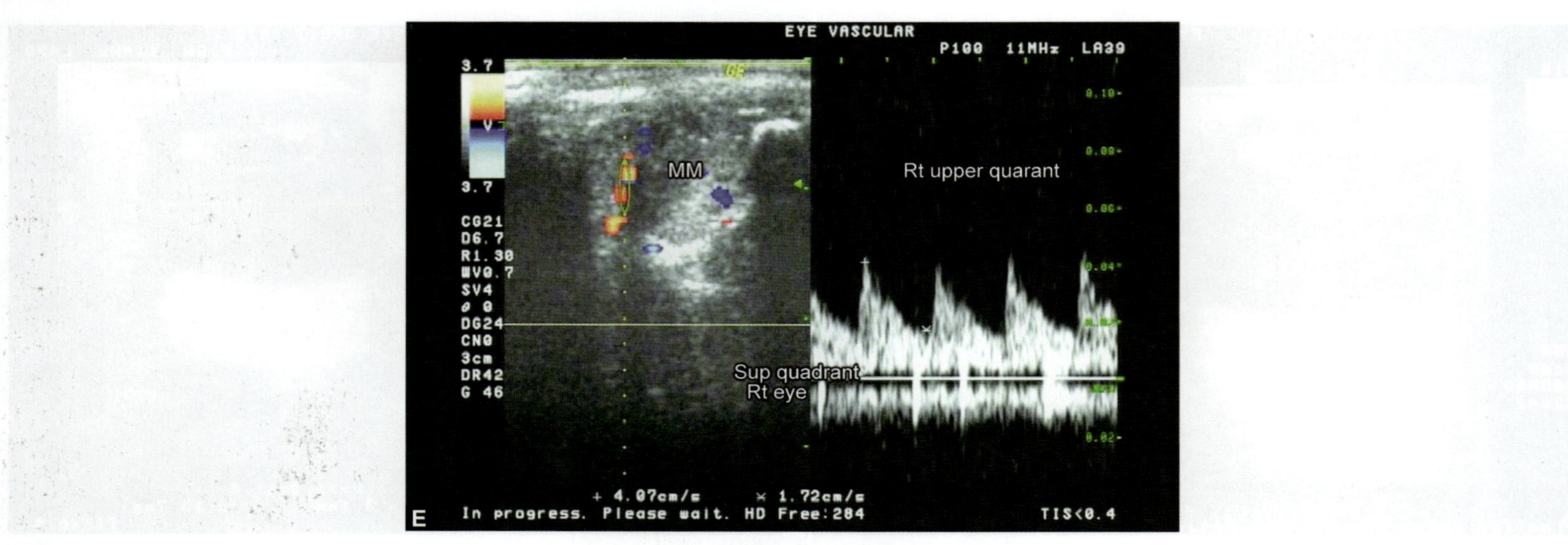

FIGURE 1.169E

FIGURES 1.169A to E: Cavernous hemangioma. A young man presented with mass having multiple dilated vessels in upper part of right eye. HRSG shows a soft tissue mass with multiple dilated vessels. Echogenic calcified shadows are also seen in the mass. They are associated with acoustic shadowing suggestive of phlebolith. On color Doppler flow study, low flow is seen in the blood vessels with venous flow pattern. Color Doppler tracing shows venous and arterial flow in the mass.

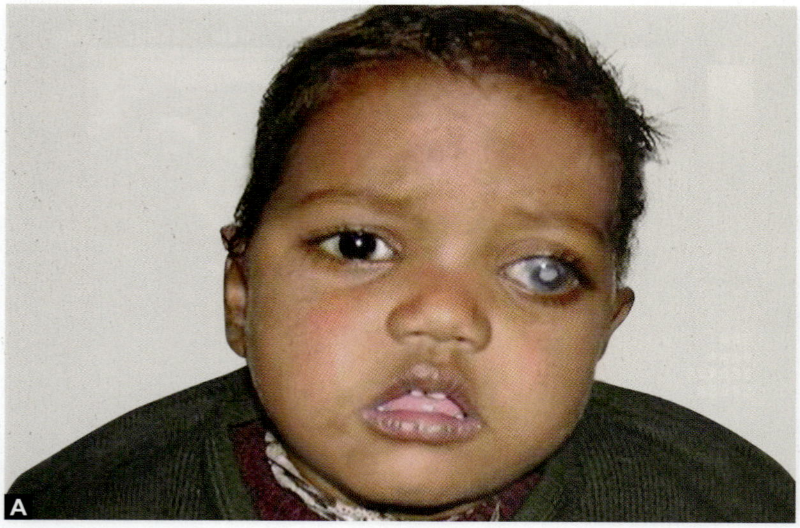

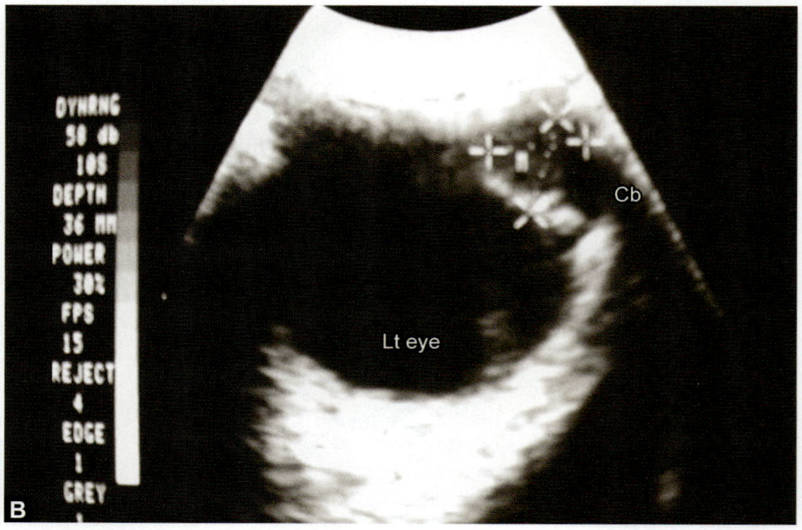

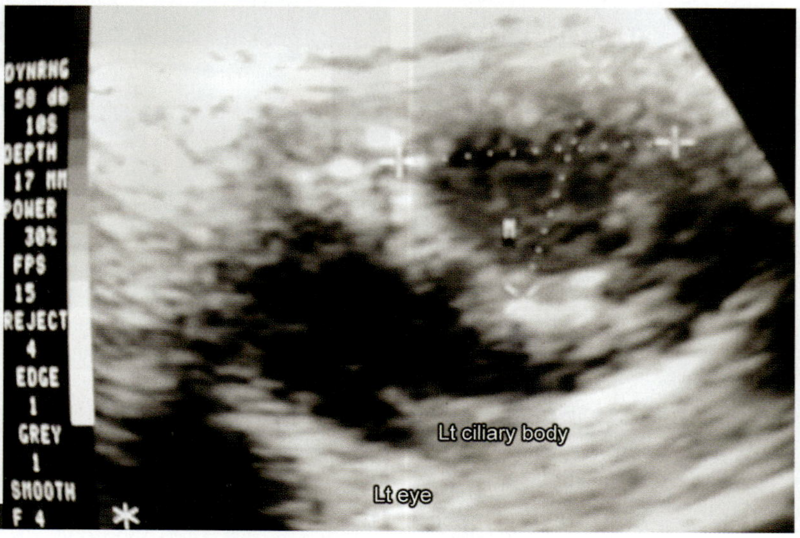

FIGURES 1.170A to C: A young boy presented with leukoria and loss of vision in left eye. Diktyoma. HRSG shows a hypodense well-defined mass coming out from left ciliary body. A linear calcification is seen in the mass. The ciliary body has been destroyed by the mass.

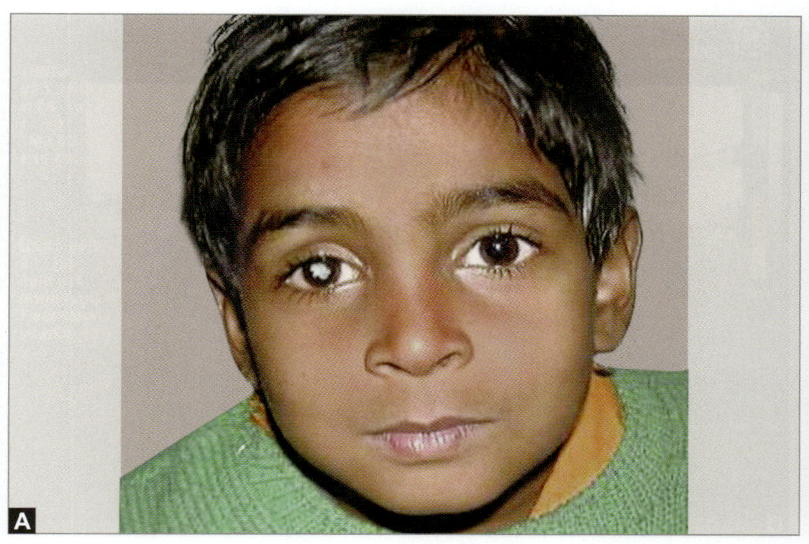

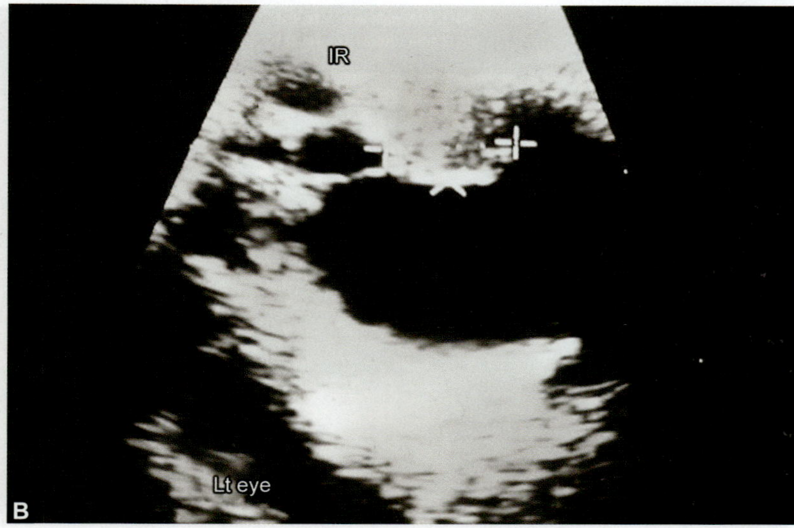

FIGURES 1.171A and B: Diktyoma. A young girl presented with white eye reflex and diminished vision on clinical examination. HRSG shows a well defined echogenic mass coming out from the ciliary body and extending into the vitreous cavity. No cystic degeneration is seen in the mass. It came out to be diktyoma on biopsy.

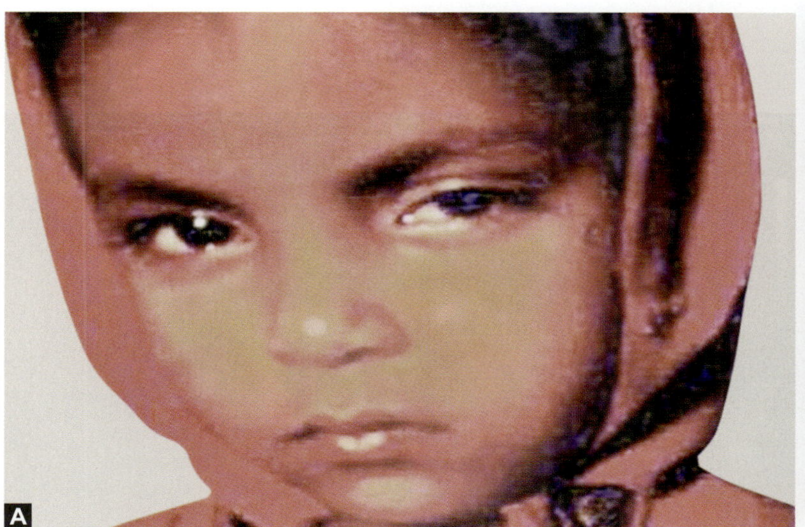

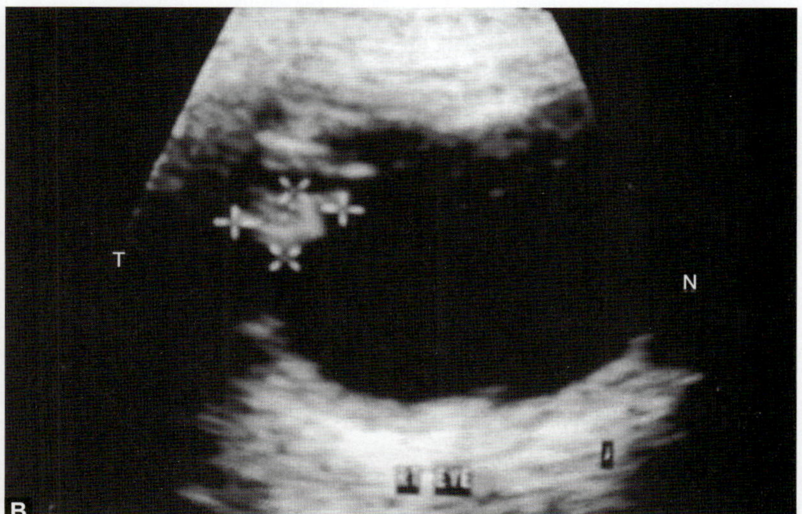

FIGURES 1.172A and B: Diktyoma. A young girl presented with white eye reflex and a mass in anterior chamber on clinical examination. HRSG shows a well-defined homogeneous mass coming out from the ciliary body and confined to the anterior chamber. The sonographic findings are suggestive of diktyoma or medulloepithelioma.

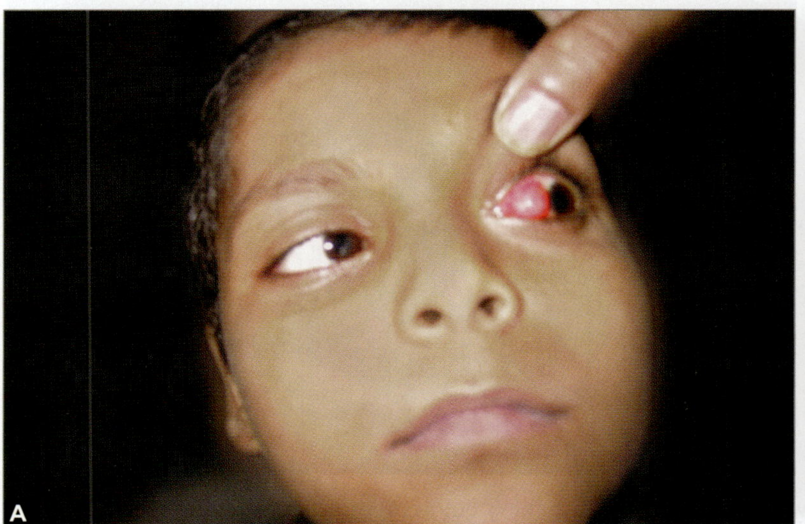

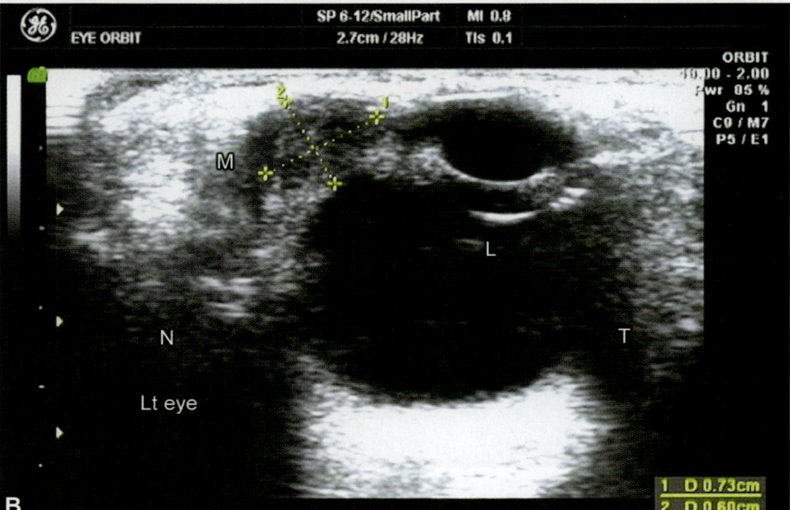

FIGURES 1.173A and B

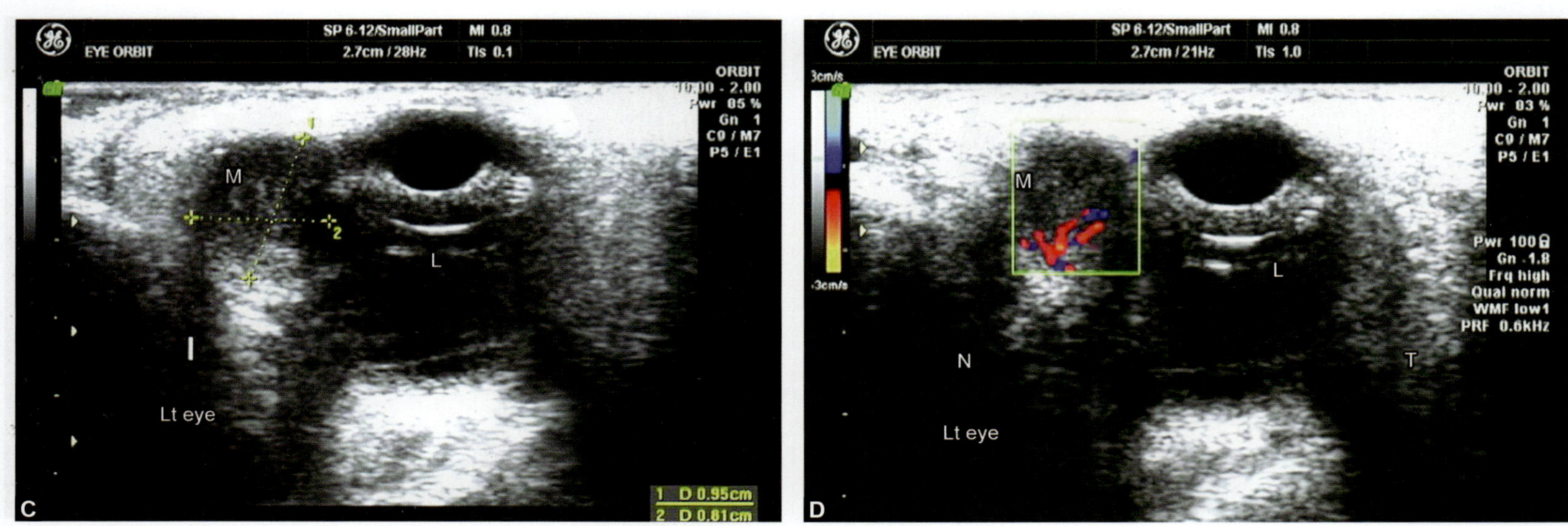

FIGURES 1.173C and D

FIGURES 1.173A to D: A young girl presented with soft tissue mass coming out from medial side of eye and reaching up to cornea. HRSG shows a medium level soft tissue mass coming out from sclera. It is homogeneous in texture. On color flow imaging, multiple vessels are seen feeding the mass. The 3D imaging shows, the mass is separate from the limbus. Excision and biopsy of the mass shows a vascular mass.

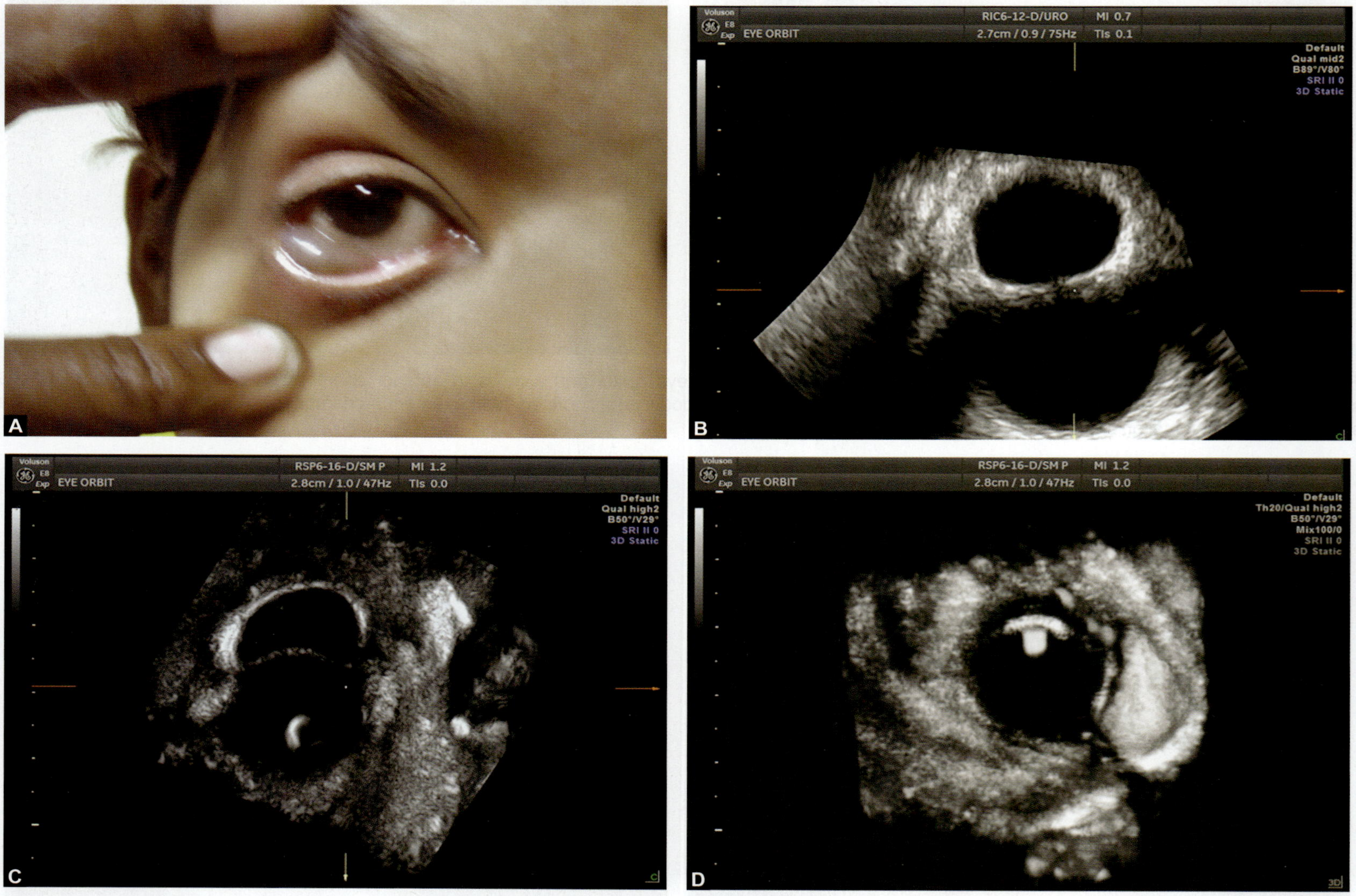

FIGURES 1.174A to D: Conjunctival cyst. A 20-year-old girl presented with soft tissue mass coming out from lower part of eye. HRSG shows a well defined cyst coming out from conjunctiva. On 3D imaging, the cyst is seen separate from the eye. The lens is normal.

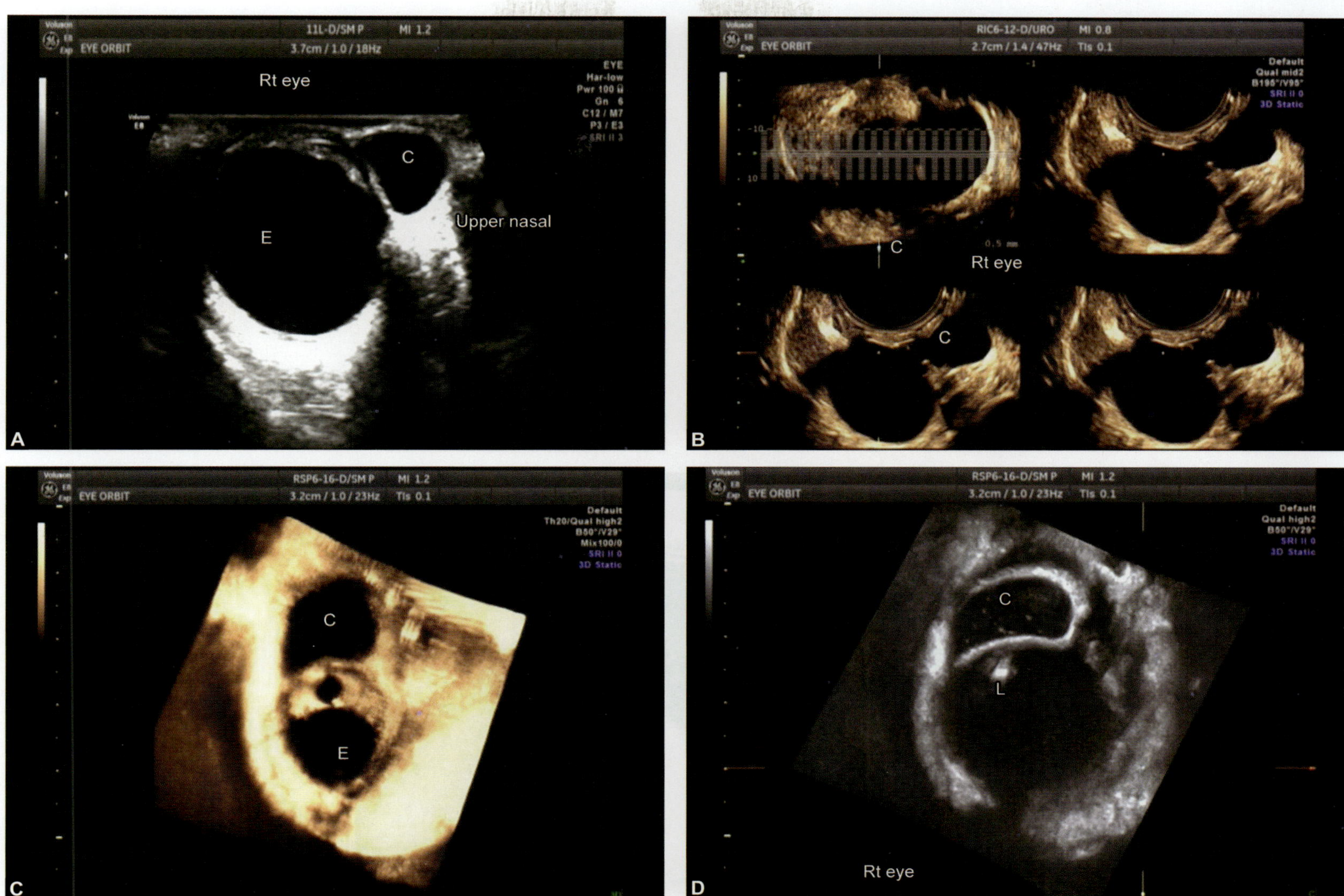

FIGURES 1.175A to D: Conjunctival cyst. A young boy presented with soft tissue swelling in the upper nasal quadrant of right eye. HRSG shows a well-defined cyst coming out from upper medial quadrant. The cyst is seen over the limbus. However, on 3D imaging, it is separated from the eyeball. No septation or calcification is seen in the cyst. The eye is normal.

Retinoblastoma

Retinoblastoma is the most common intraocular tumor in infant and children up to the age of 6 years. It comprises about 30% of all ocular tumors. It may be unilateral, bilateral, focal or multifocal and frequently presents as white eye reflex or cat eye reflex in the children. The tumor can grow either anteriorly from inner surface of the retina towards the vitreous (endophytic), or posteriorly from the posterior surface of retina towards the choroid (exophytic).

Sonographic Features

Sonographically, the tumor can have smooth dome-shaped appearance when it is small in size. However, it is frequently having heterogeneous and irregular texture. Calcium deposit is the hallmark of retinoblastoma. Usually, it comes out from one surface of retina, however, in unusual case it involves retina from its entire surface known as retinoblastoma circumference. The tumor usually grows anteriorly and fills the vitreous cavity. However, it can invade the choroid and grows posteriorly in the retrobulbar space. HRSG can clearly assess the retrobulbar extension of tumor growth and its excavation in the choroid. HRSG is also very useful and noninvasive tool to monitor the treatment response of the tumor or to asses regression of tumor growth. The tumor is radiosensitive, and rapid regression takes place after radiotherapy and chemotherapy. The differential diagnoses of tumor are Coat's disease or exudative retinal detachment, persistent hyperplastic primary vitreous (PHPV), retrolental fibroplasia and Toxocara, a worm infestation caused by ingestion of intestinal worm. In ocular Toxocara, the most common ocular lesions are ocular endophthalmitis or a posterior pole granuloma.

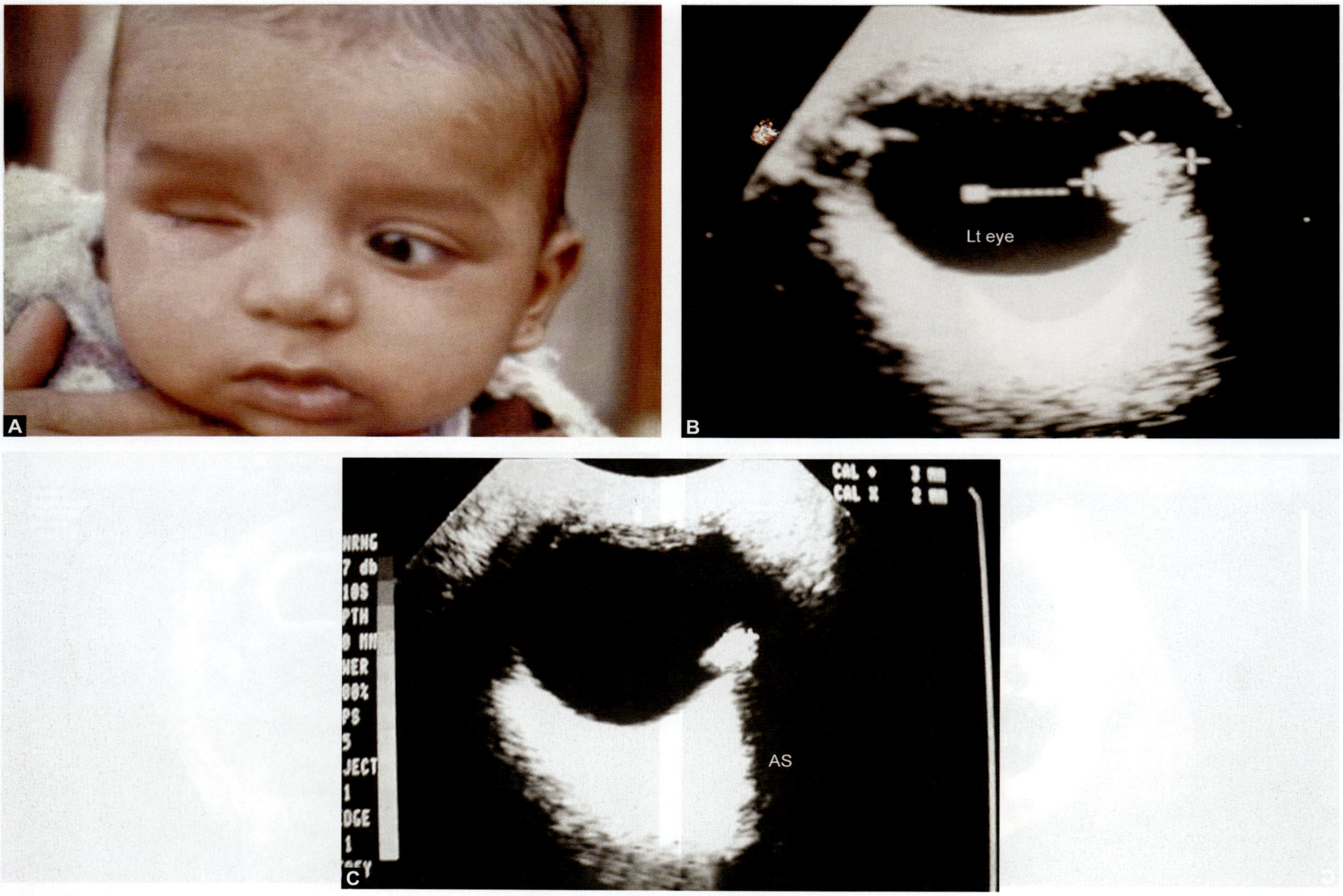

FIGURES 1.176A to C: An infant presented with congenital retinoblastoma in right eye, and it was operated. His father also had retinoblastoma in one eye. Another eye also showed white reflex after 3 months of his birth. HRSG shows an echogenic mass on temporal side with wide base typical of retinoblastoma. Post-teleradiotherapy—The mass has regressed in size. Echogenic calcification is seen at the base of the mass. HRSG is an excellent modality to evaluate treatment response. It is noninvasive, cost effective and does not require any sedation.

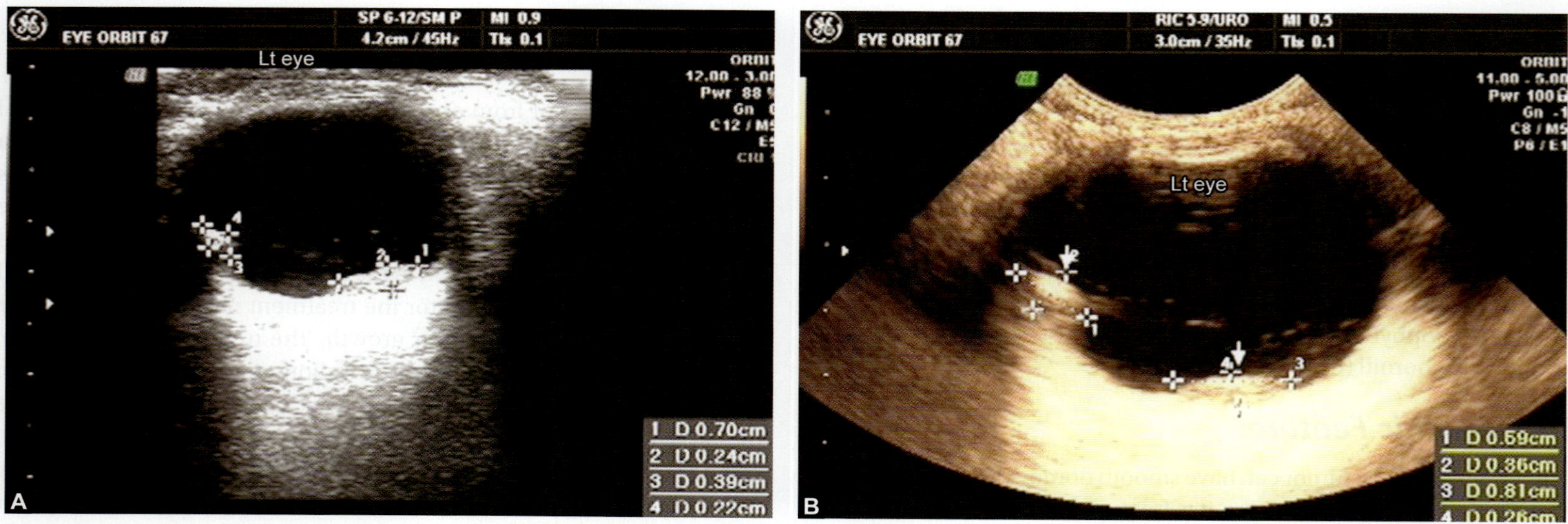

FIGURES 1.177A and B

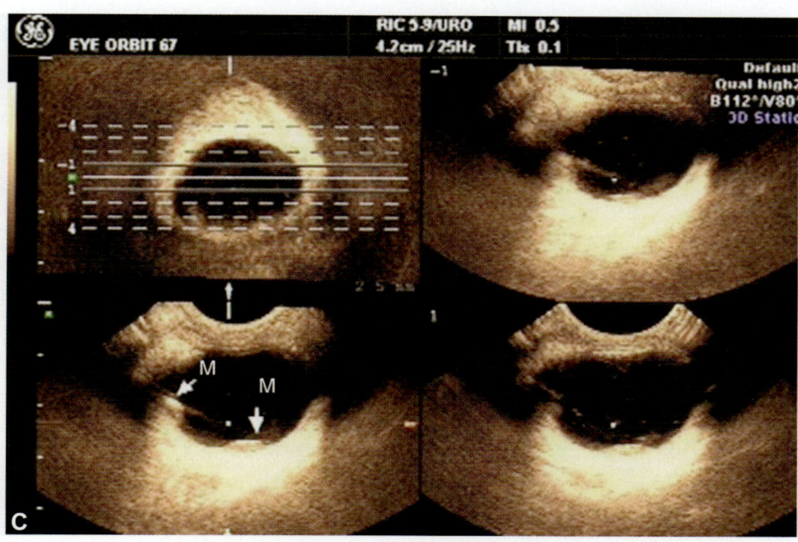

FIGURE 1.177C

FIGURES 1.177A to C: Multifocal retinoblastoma. A young girl presented with white eye reflex. HRSG shows echogenic soft tissue masses in the posterior segment of the eye. The masses show dense calcification suggestive of retinoblastoma. On TUI imaging, they are confined to the Coat. No choroidal excavation is seen.

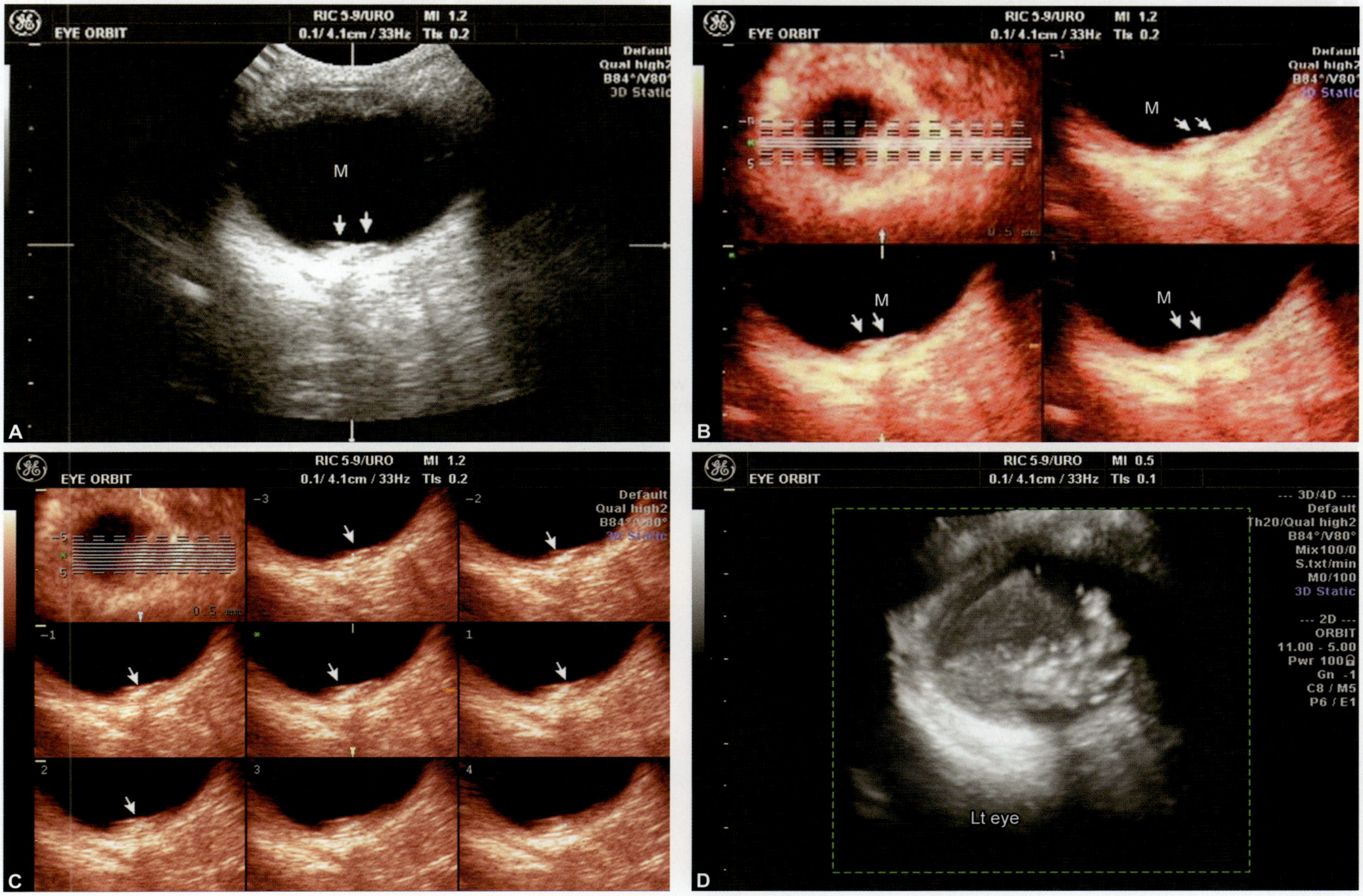

FIGURES 1.178A to D

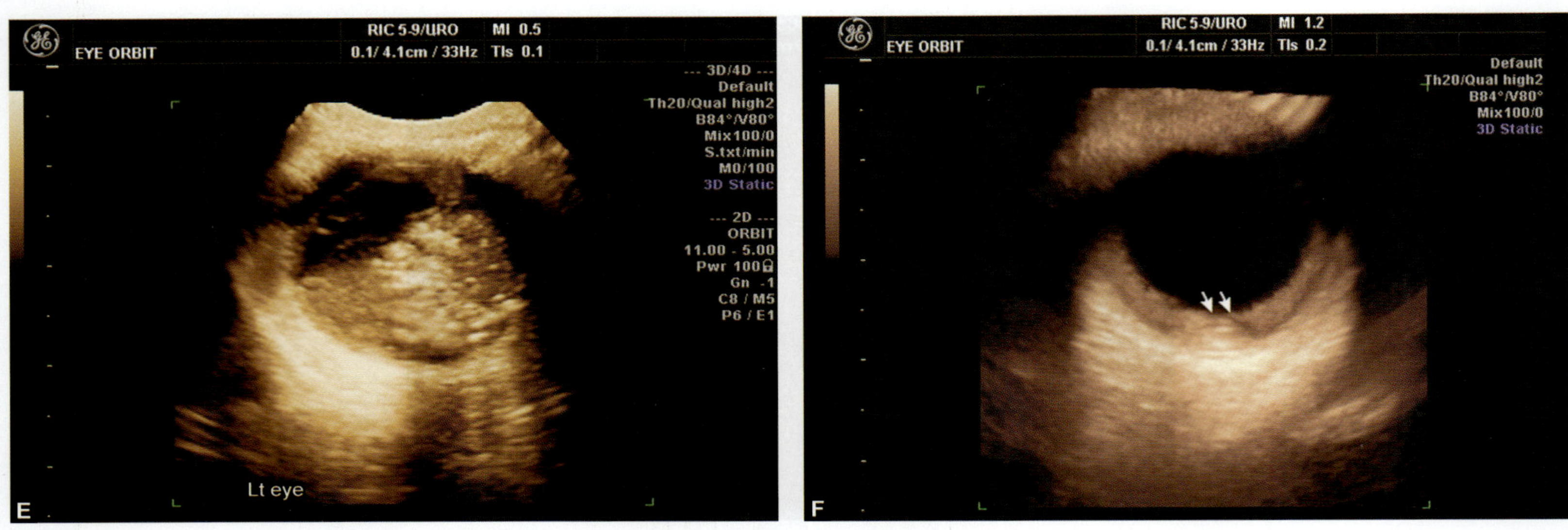

FIGURES 1.178E and F

FIGURES 1.178A to F: Bilateral retinoblastoma. A young child presented with white eye reflex in both eyes. The right eye shows small tumor fixed with posterior wall. Dense echogenic calcification is seen in it. On TUI imaging, the mass is clearly defined. No choroidal excavation is seen in the mass. The left eye shows a big tumor mass filling the posterior segment. Dense echogenic calcification is seen in the mass. But no choroidal excavation is seen. On 3D imaging, Figure F shows the mass in the right eye coming out from retina sitting over choroid. However, the choroid shows smooth outline.

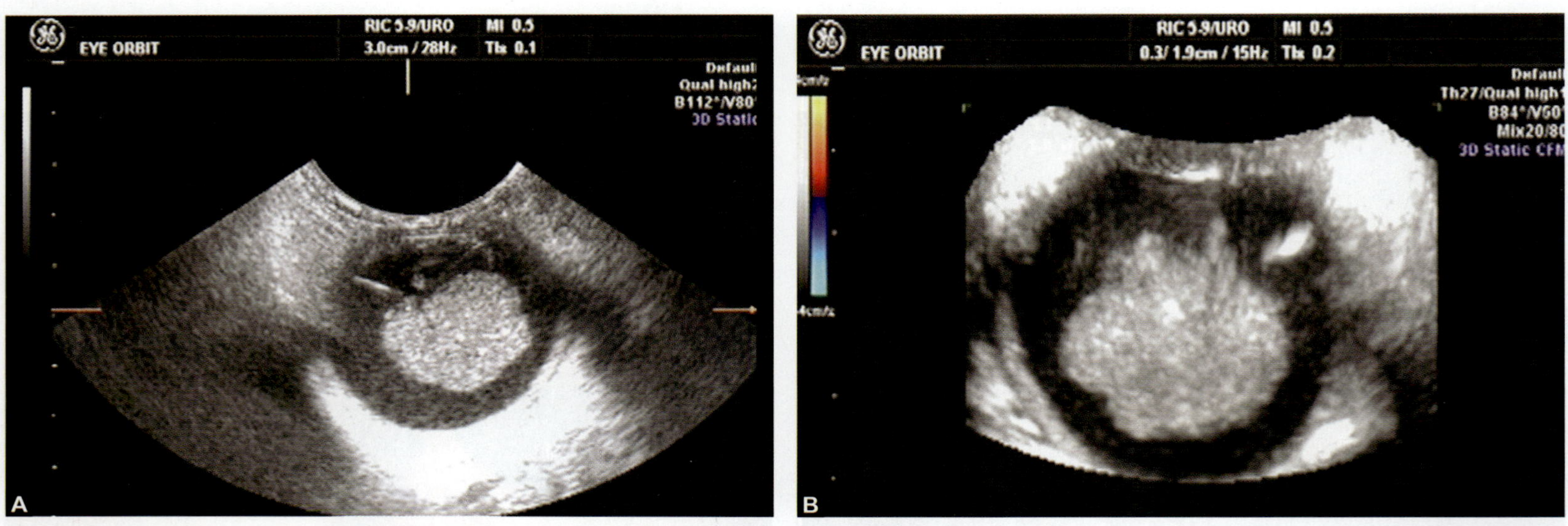

FIGURES 1.179A and B: Retinoblastoma. A young child presented with white eye reflex. HRSG shows a soft tissue mass in the posterior segment of the eye. The mass is seen confined to the globe. Echogenic calcified specks are seen in the mass suggestive of retinoblastoma.

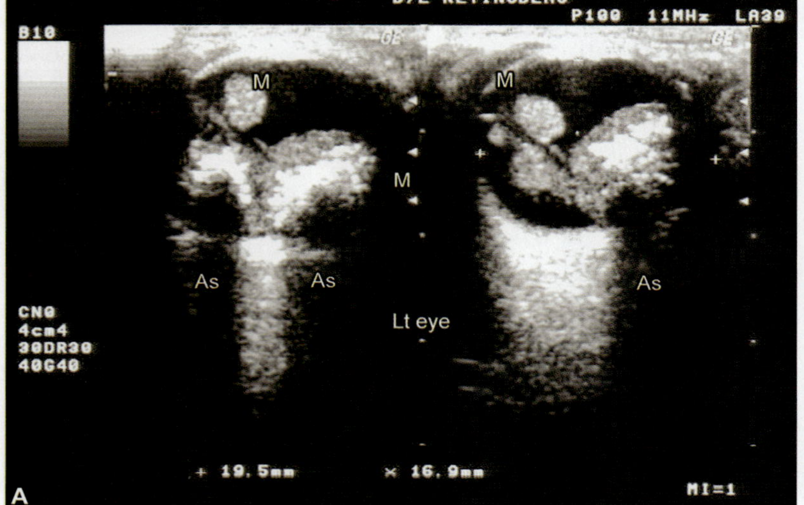

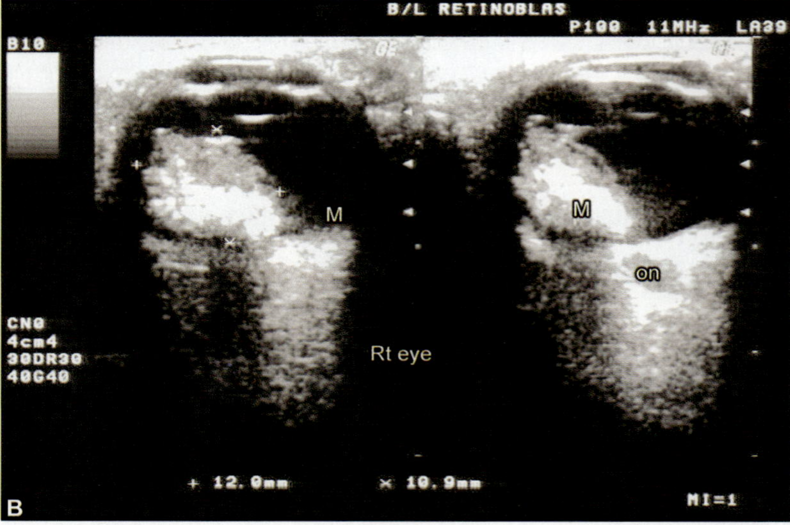

FIGURES 1.180A and B: Multifocal retinoblastoma. HRSG shows multifocal retinoblastoma invading whole of eye ball. Dense echogenic calcification is seen in the tumors. Right eye of the same patient also shows a big tumor with dense calcification.

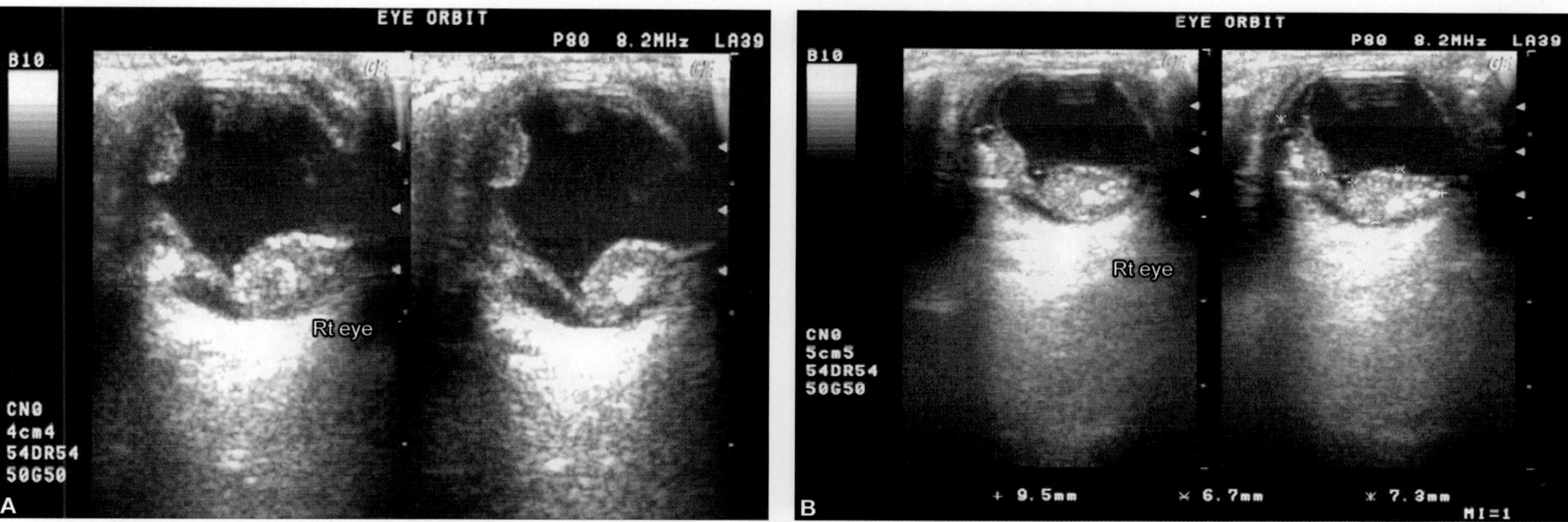

FIGURES 1.181A and B: Multifocal retinoblastoma. HRSG shows multiple tumor masses coming out from the retina in the posterior segment of eye. Fine calcified specks are seen in the masses. Associated subretinal hemorrhage is also seen.

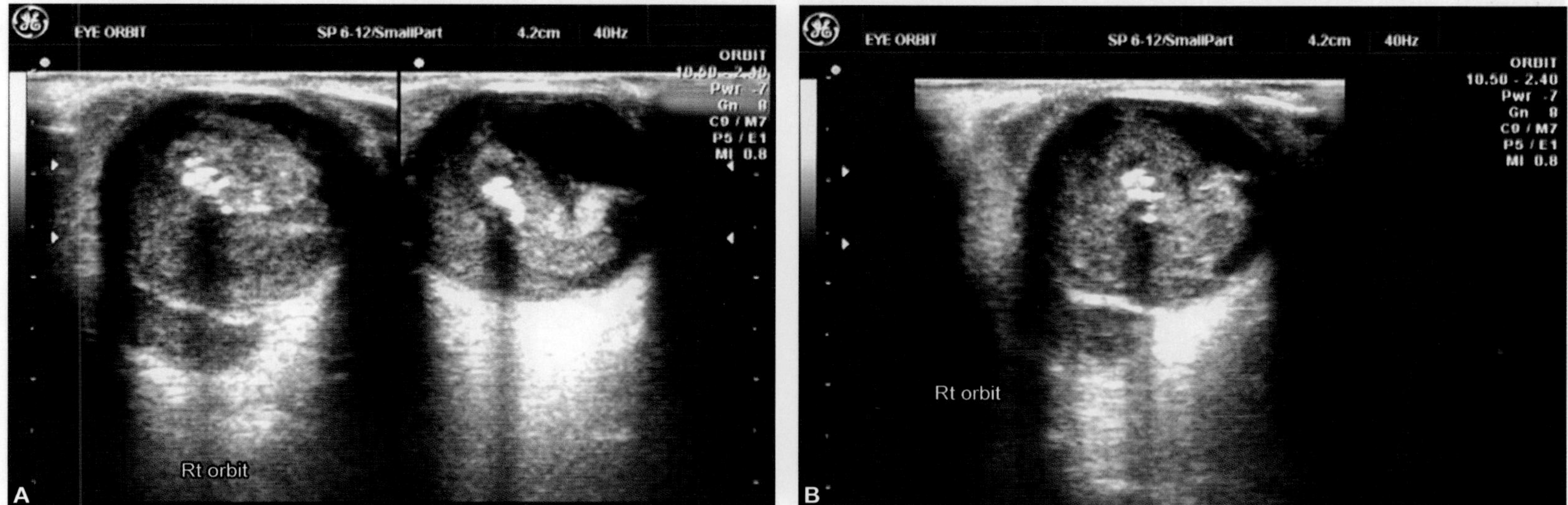

FIGURES 1.182A and B: Retrobulbar extension of retinoblastoma. Big retinoblastoma is seen invading the sclera and also extending in retrobulbar space. The tumor has caused pressure over optic nerve.

Differential Diagnosis of Retinoblastoma

Retinoblastoma presents with white eye reflex. However, there are other conditions of eye, which present with white eye reflex mimicking retinoblastoma. They are mainly persistent hypetrophic primary vitreous (PHPV), retinopathy of prematurity, *Toxocara*, Coat's disease, intraocular cysticercus cyst, coloboma of eye and endophthalmitis.

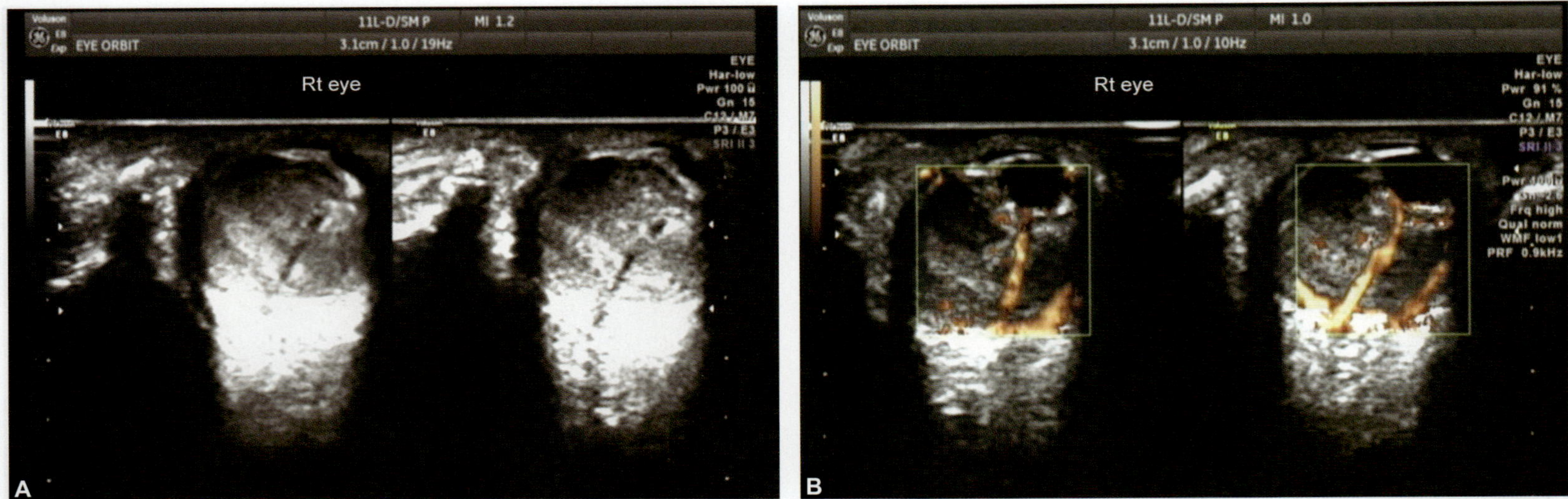

FIGURES 1.183A and B: PHPV. An infant presented with white eye reflex. HRSG shows small right eye. Echogenic soft tissue shadows are seen in the eye. A hypoechoic vascular band is seen passing through the mass. On color flow imaging, an artery is seen in it suggestive of posterior hyloid artery. The findings are suggestive of PHPV

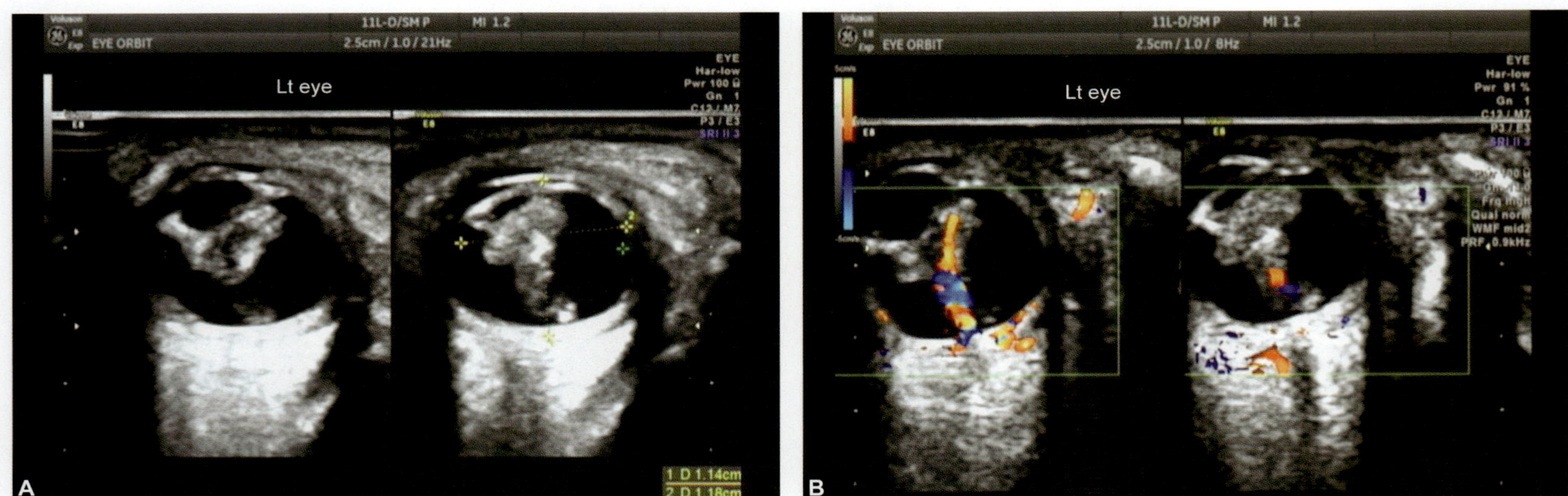

FIGURES 1.184A and B: PHPV mimicking retinoblastoma. Another case of PHPV mimicking retinoblastoma seen in the left eye in 12 days old baby. HRSG shows a soft tissue mass in the posterior segment of eye. A thick membrane is seen going from the posterior pole. On color flow imaging, persistent hyloid artery is seen in this band suggestive of PHPV.

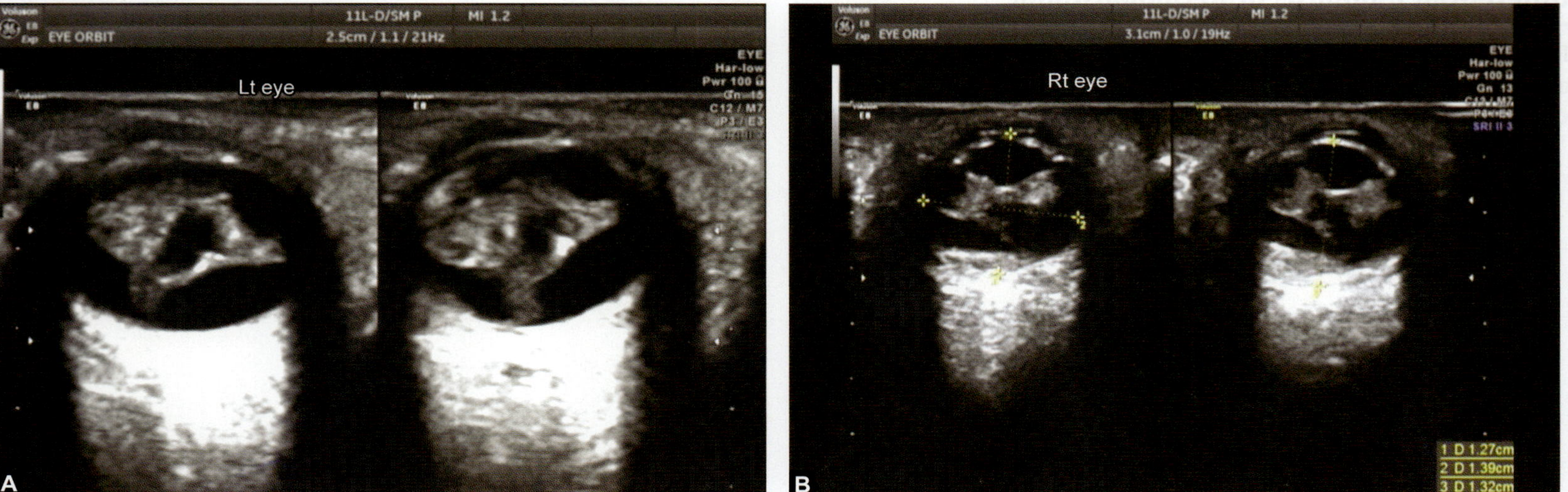

FIGURES 1.185A and B

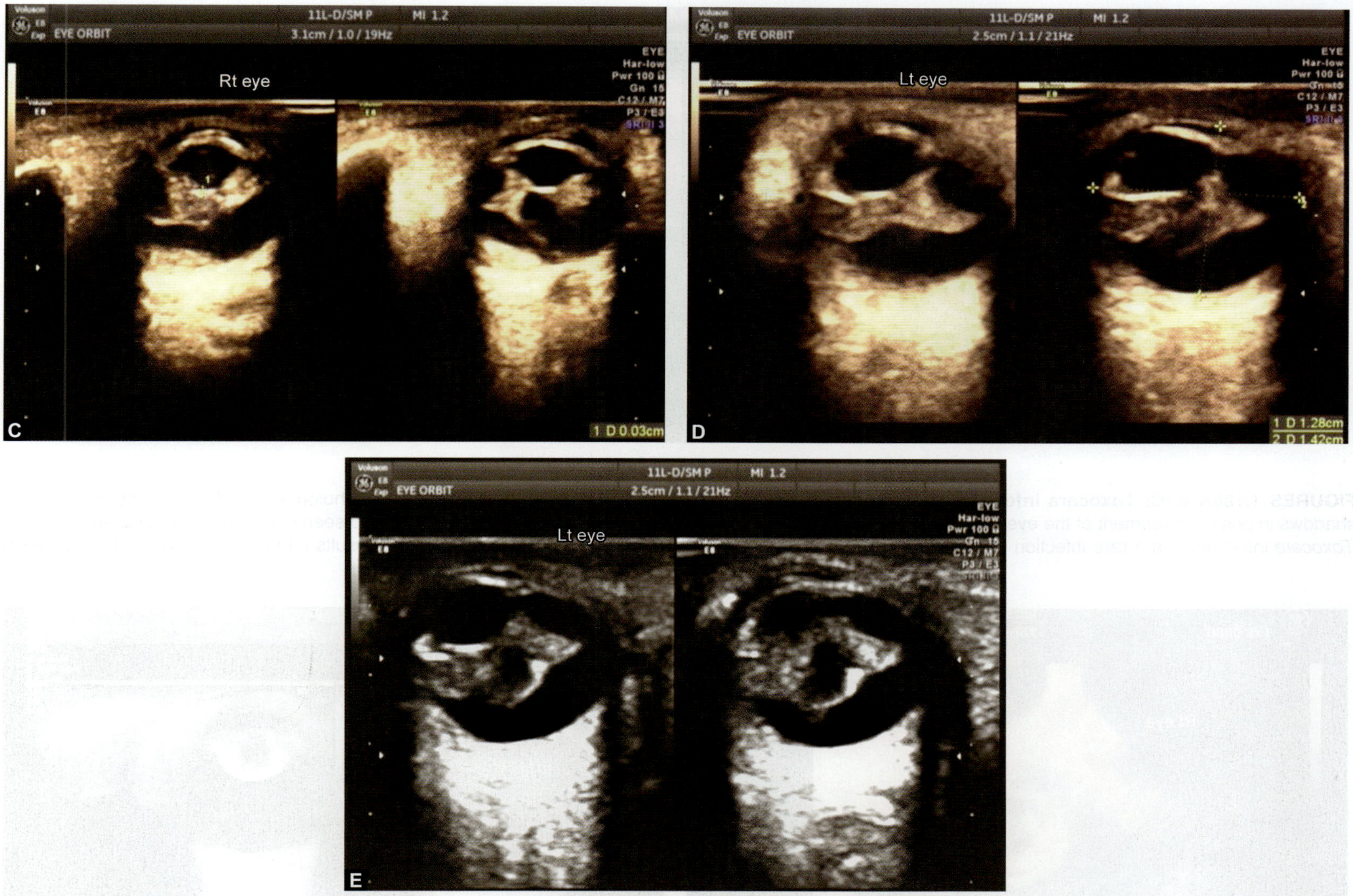

FIGURES 1.185C to E

FIGURES 1.185A to E: Retinopathy of prematurity. A 9-month-old baby presented with white reflex in both the eyes. HRSG shows bilateral small eyes. Membranous shadows are seen in the posterior segment. No calcification is seen in the membranes. Small cyst formation is also seen. Findings are suggestive of retinopathy of prematurity in both the eyes.

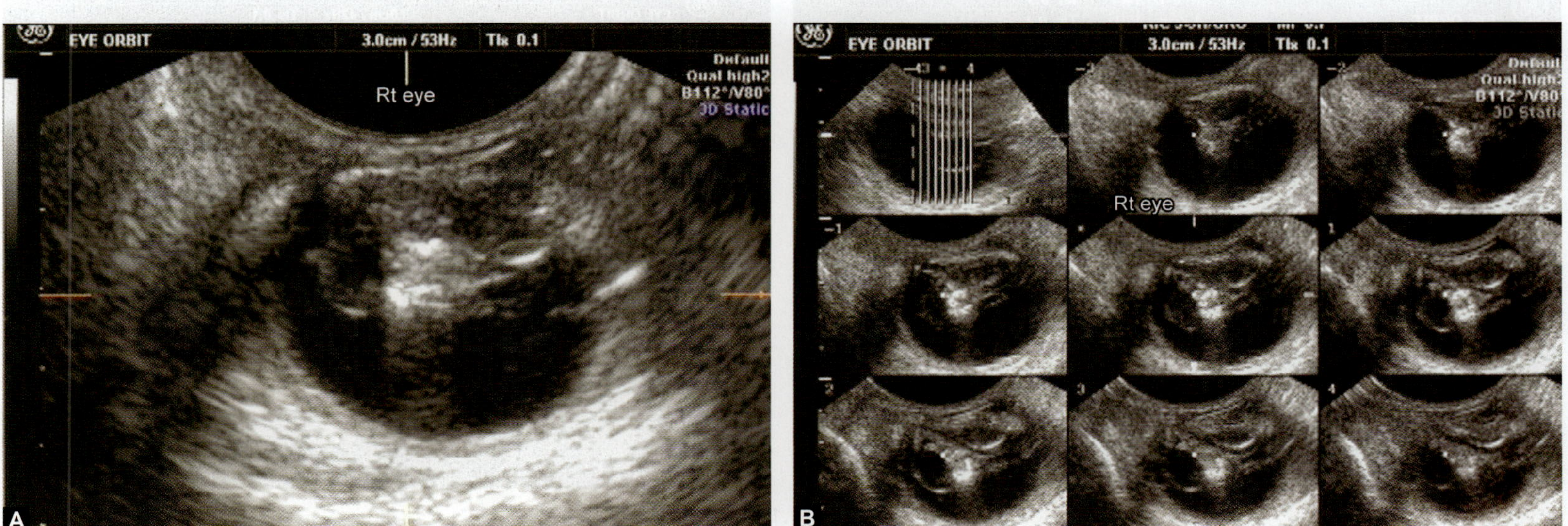

FIGURES 1.186A and B

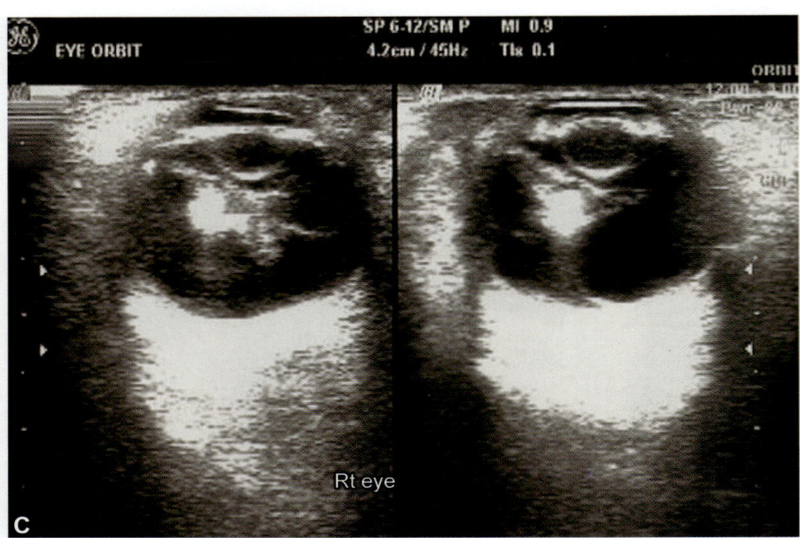

FIGURE 1.186C

FIGURES 1.186A to C: Toxocara infection. A young boy presented with white eye reflex with reduced vision, photophobia. HRSG shows membranous shadows in posterior segment of the eye. The retina shows multiple granulomatous changes. Echogenic foci are also seen in it. The patient was suffering from *Toxocara* infection. It is a rare infection caused by *Toxocara* parasite, *Toxocara canis* and *Toxocara cati*, which results into granulomatous endophthalmitis.

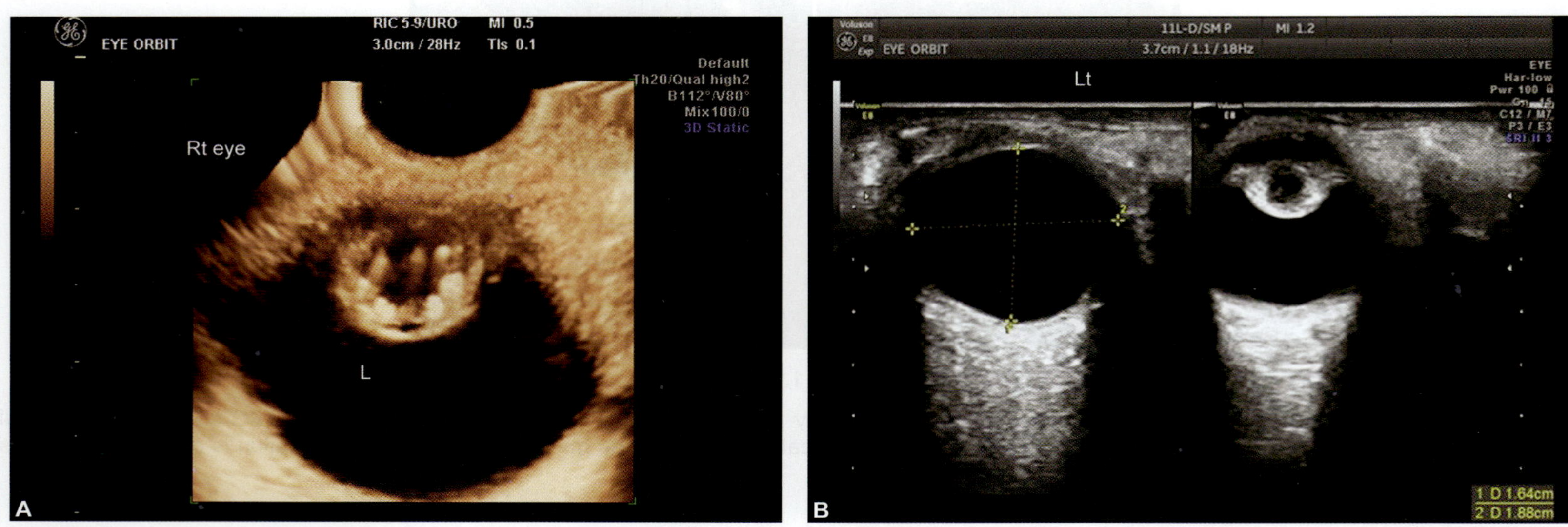

FIGURES 1.187A and B: Hypermature cataract presented as white eye reflex. The hypermature calcified lens also presents as white eye reflex. HRSG shows thickened opaque lens with multiple calcified foci. However, the posterior segment of the eye is free suggestive of calcified lens.

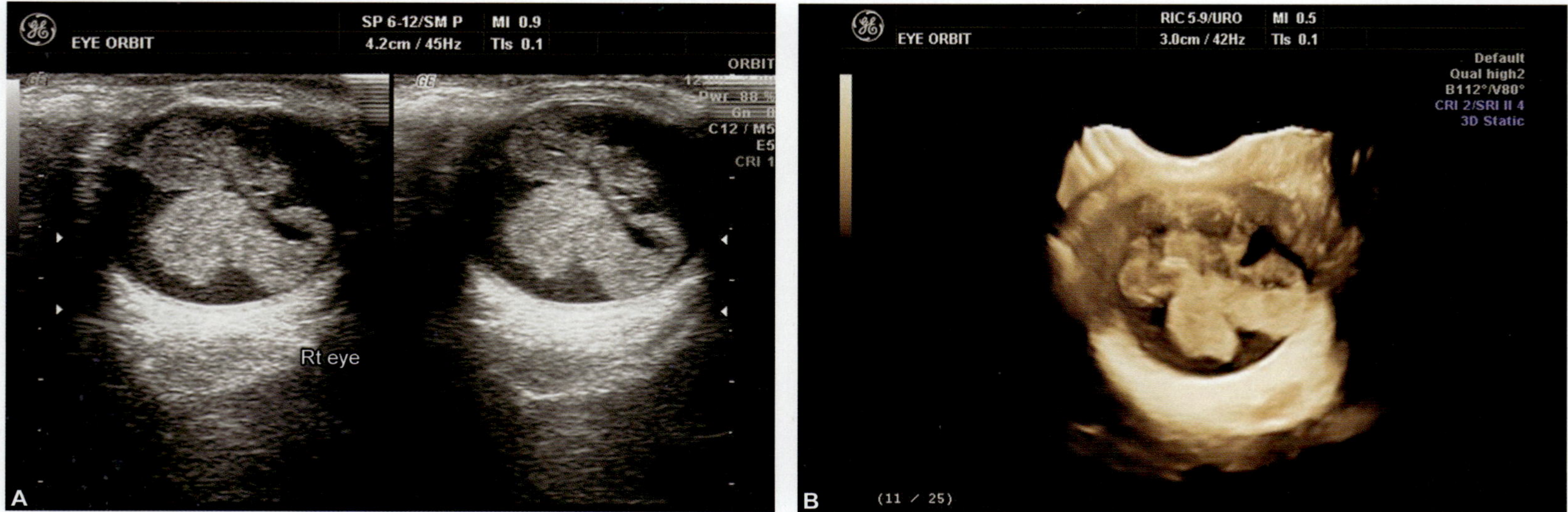

FIGURES 1.188A and B

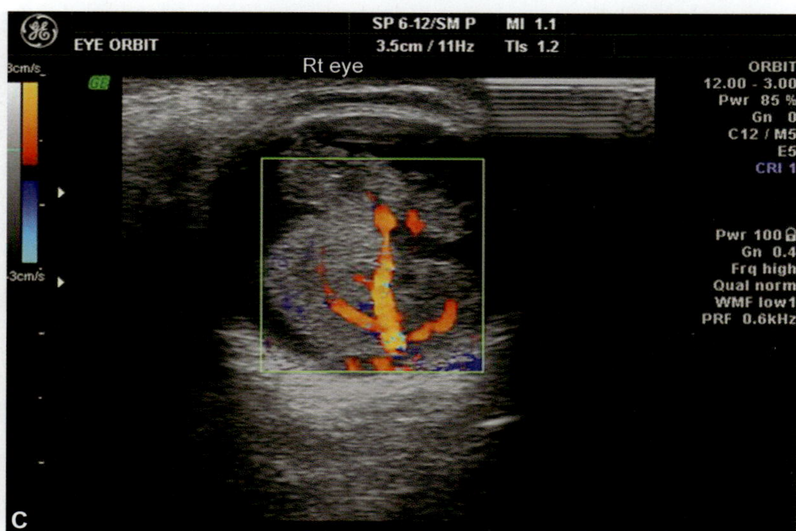

FIGURE 1.188C

FIGURES 1.188A to C: Coat's disease. A baby of 3.5 years age presented with white eye reflex. HRSG shows a thick membrane seen detached in the posterior segment. It shows multiple folds. Thick exudation is seen in the membrane. But no calcification is seen. On color flow imaging, retinal artery is seen dragged in the membrane. The 3D imaging of the eye shows the thick membrane confined in the posterior segment. The findings are highly suggestive of Coat's disease.

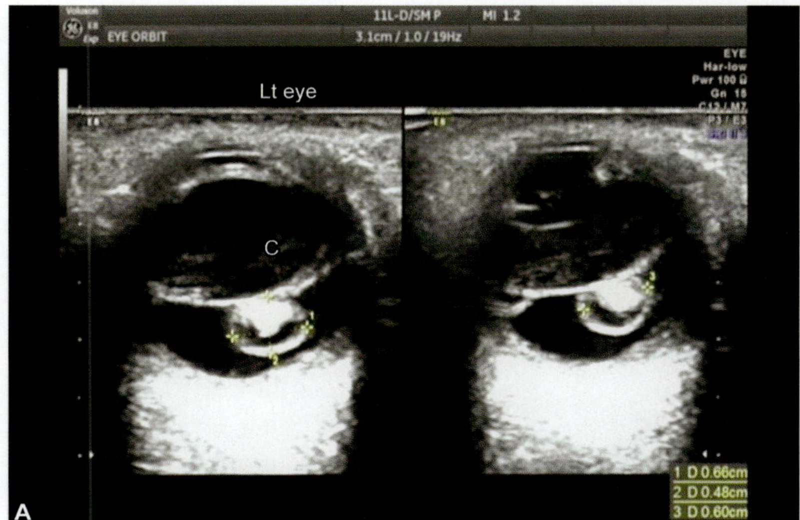

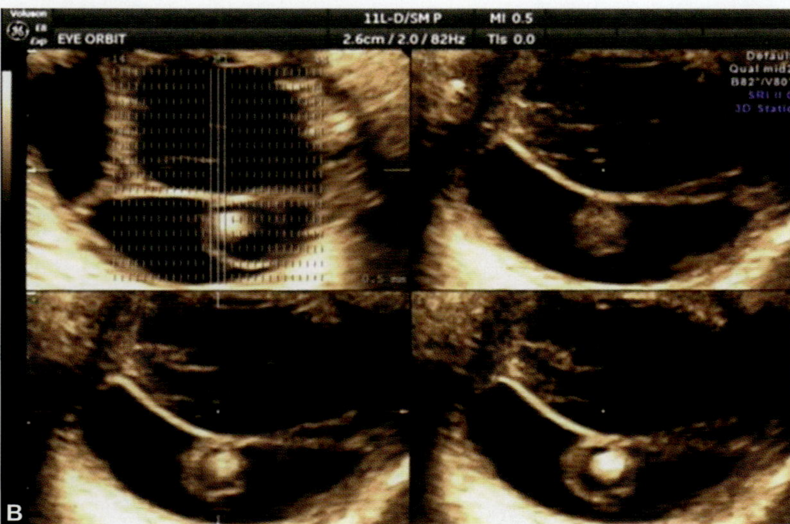

FIGURES 1.189A and B: Retinal detachment with cysticercus cyst. A patient presented with acute pain in eye with sudden loss of vision. HRSG shows a well-defined cyst in the posterior segment. An echogenic nidus is seen fixed with the inner wall of cyst suggestive of cysticercus cyst. The cyst is seen attached at retina and retina is seen detached from its surface suggestive of retinal detachment.

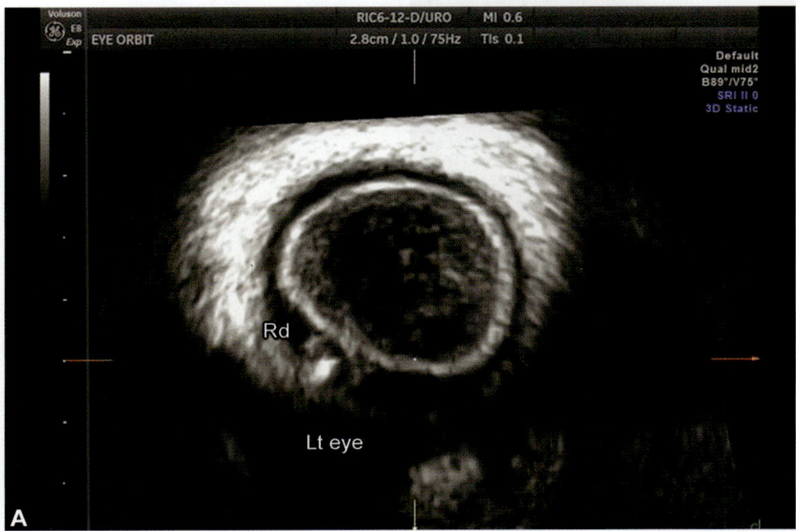

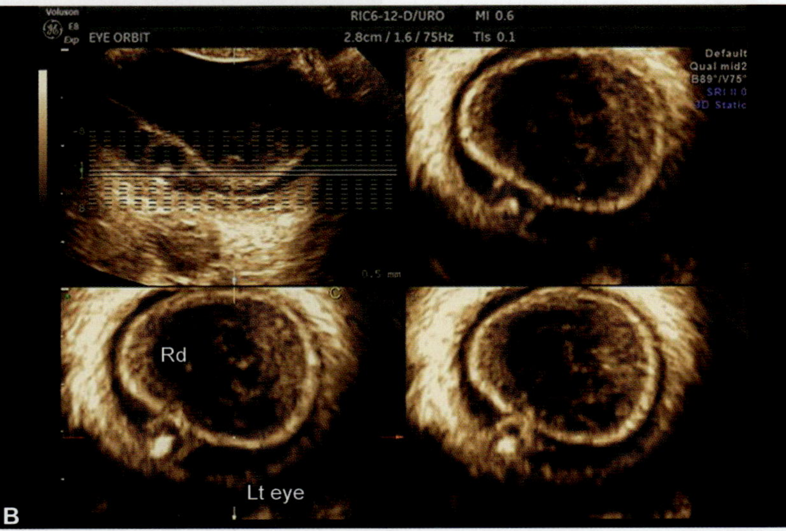

FIGURES 1.190A and B: Retinal detachment with cysticercus cyst. A patient presented with sudden loss of vision. HRSG shows a well-defined cyst in subretinal space. The cyst shows echogenic nidus fixed with inner wall of cyst. The cyst results into lifting of retina causing total retinal detachment. On 3D and TUI imaging, the total retinal detachment with cysticercus cyst is seen in the subretinal space clearly.

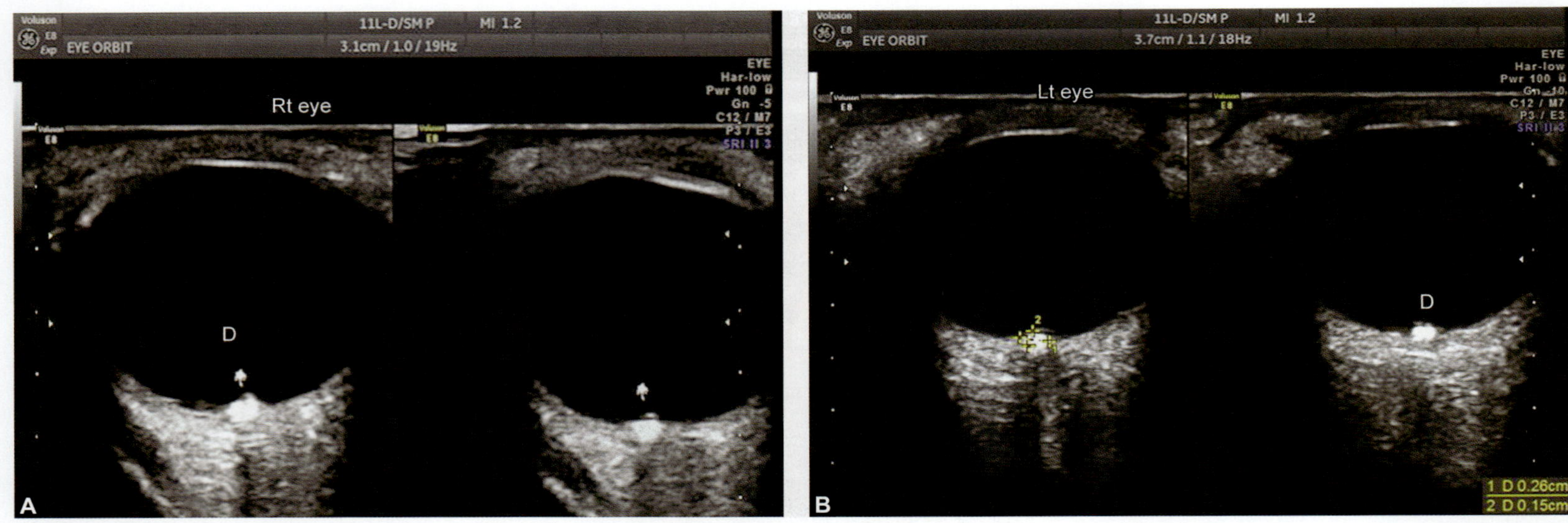

FIGURES 1.191A and B: Drusen body. Drusen body is calcification of optic nerve head because of deposition of globules of mucoproteins, which calcify with the time. It may mimic as retinoblastoma. HRSG shows dense calcified specks only confined to optic nerve head.

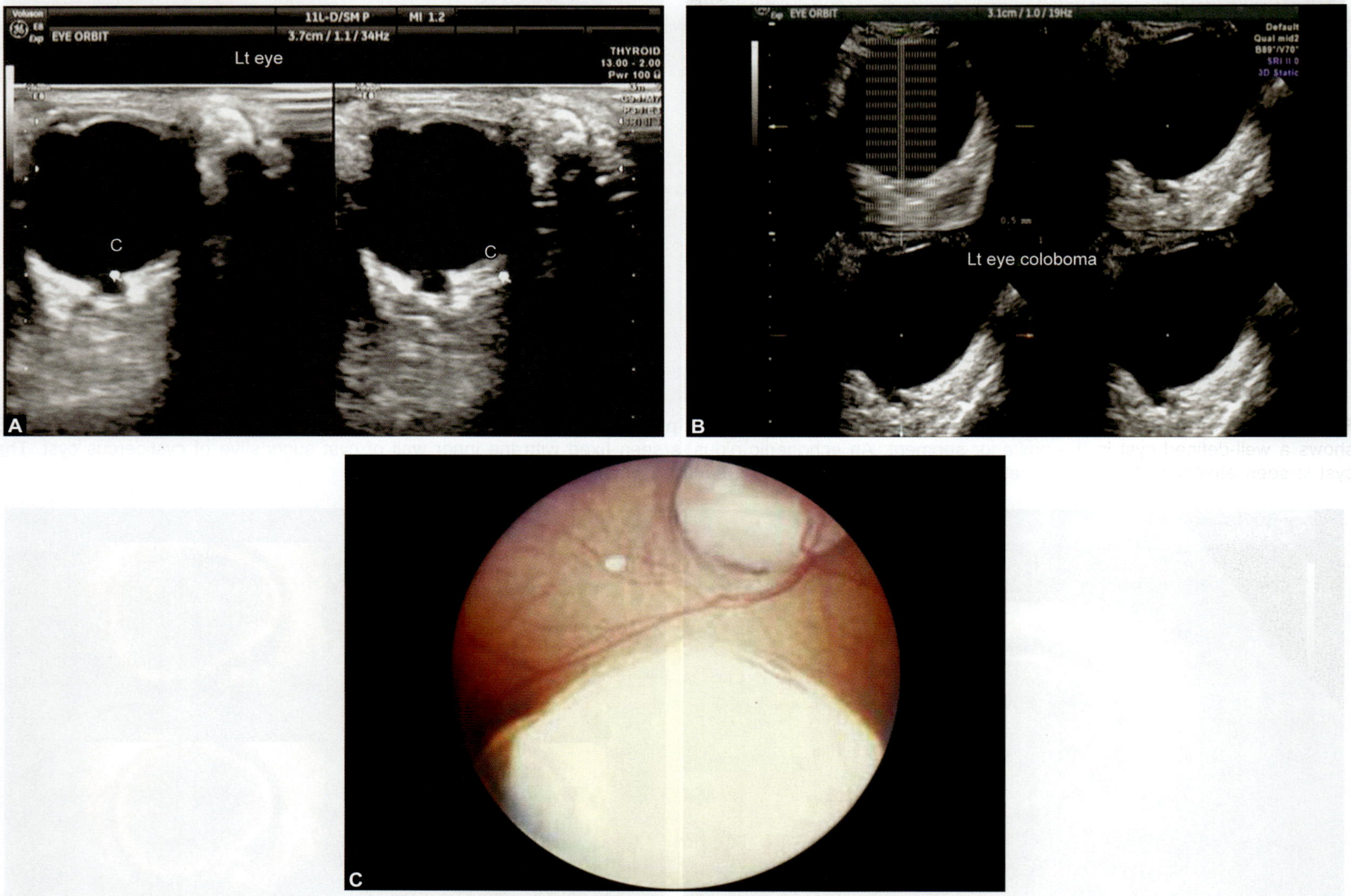

FIGURES 1.192A to C: Coloboma eye. A patient presented with white eye reflex. HRSG shows defect in the eye coat suggestive of coloboma. Figure 1.192C shows defect on direct ophthalmoscopy.

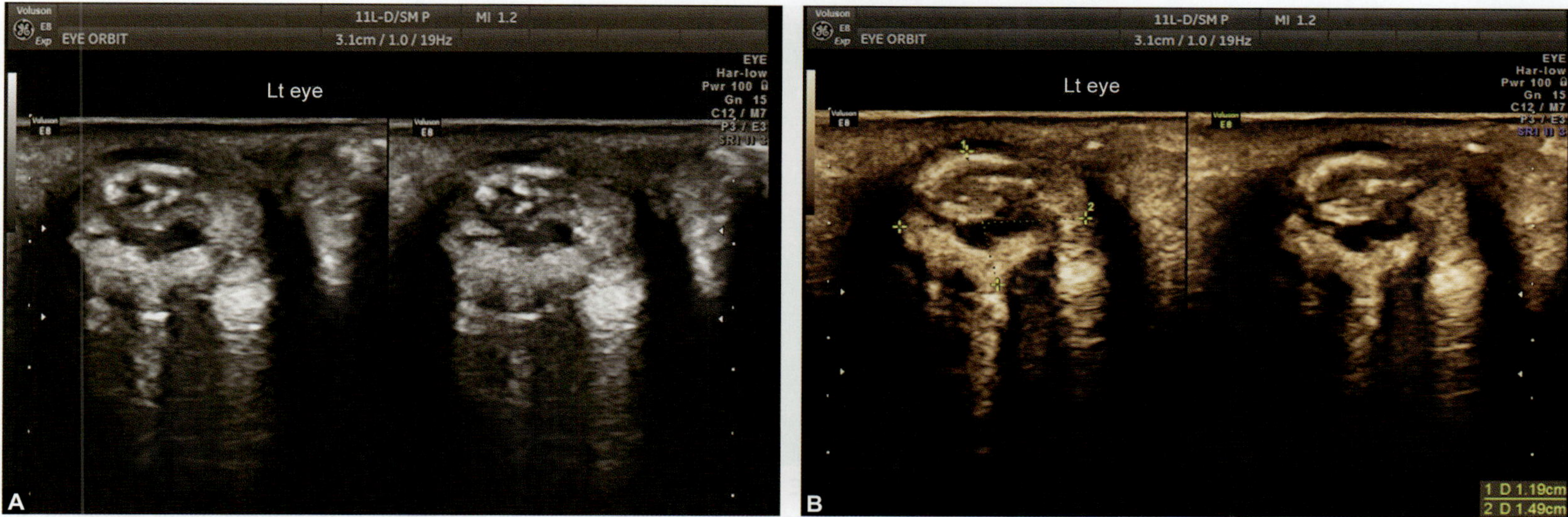

FIGURES 1.193A and B: Endophthalmitis. A 15-year-old girl presented with small eye with white eye reflex. HRSG shows small collapsed deshaped eye. Dense echogenic calcified specks are seen in the eye. Normal anatomy is distorted suggestive of endophthalmitis.

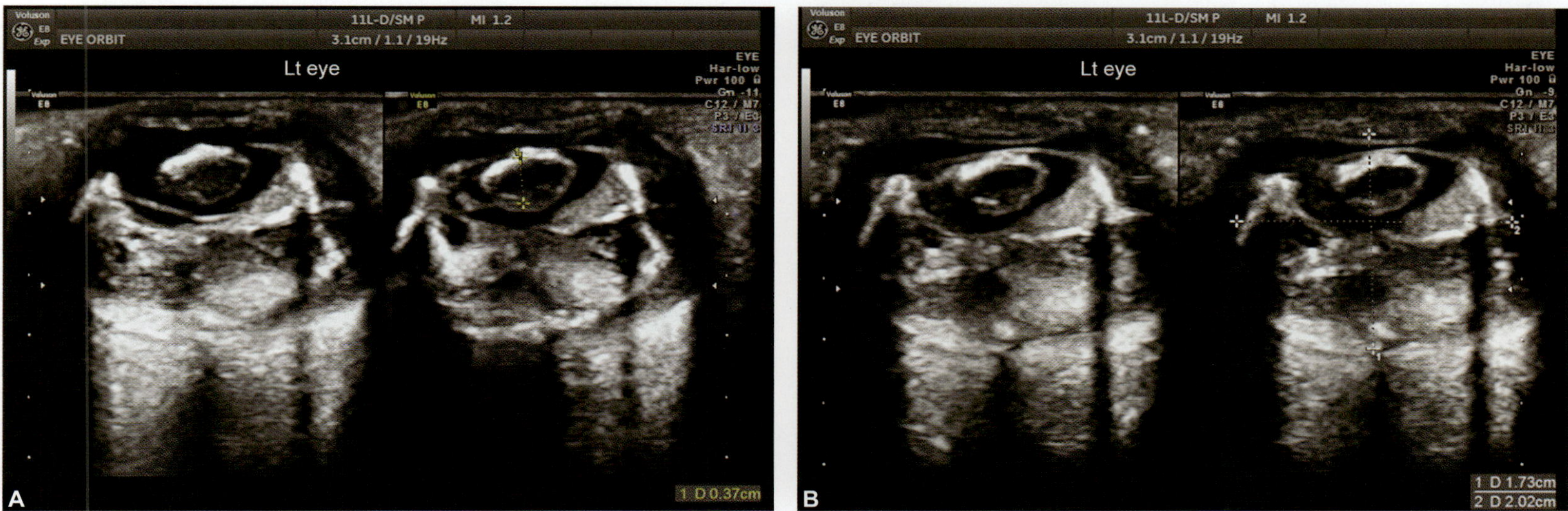

FIGURES 1.194A and B: Endophthalmitis with dense calcification. A patient presented with white eye reflex. HRSG shows densely echogenic shadows filling the posterior segment. Dense echogenic rim calcification is seen around it. Lens is also thickened and opaque. Normal anatomy is distorted suggestive of chronic endophthalmitis.

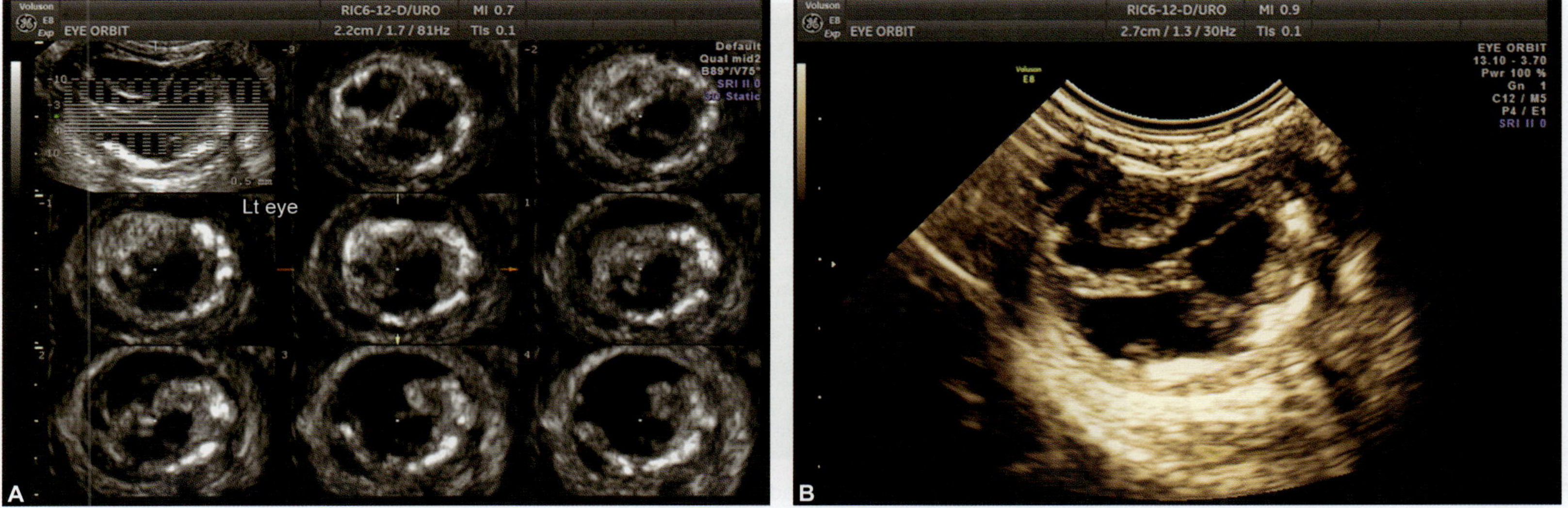

FIGURES 1.195A and B

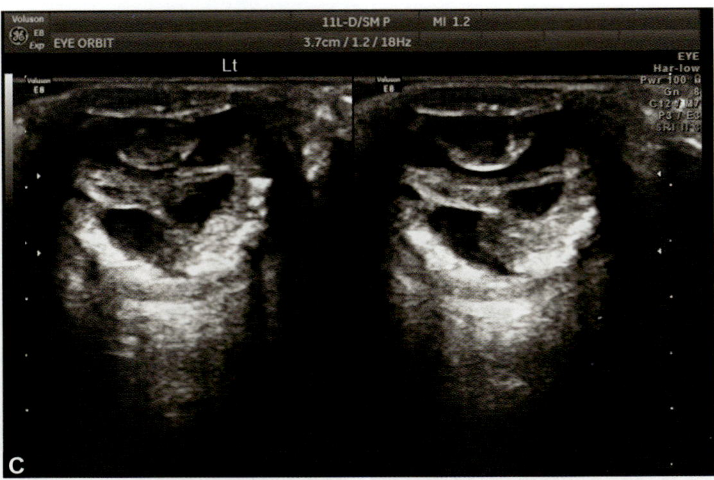

FIGURE 1.195C

FIGURES 1.195A to C: Endophthalmits with white eye reflex. A young boy presented with white eye reflex. HRSG shows small shrunken eye. Dense calcification is seen in the retinochoroid layer. Lens is also thickened. On TUI imaging, rim calcification is seen around it. Soft tissue shadows are also seen in it suggestive of chronic endophthalmitis.

Ocular Melanoma

Ocular melanomas are the most common tumors in adults. It comprises about 40% of all ocular tumors. An 85% of the melanomas arise from choroid and remaining 15% arise from ciliary body. Melanomas most commonly occur in fifth and sixth decades of life and rarely occur before third decade and after eighth decade of life. The tumors are most common in white skin people and rare in blacks. HRSG is highly sensitive in evaluating the size, shape, growth and extent of the tumor, which are important prerequisites prior to surgery. Typical sonographic features are seen on HRSG in ocular melanomas.

Sonographic Features

On ultrasound, melanomas are typically dome-shaped, collar button appearance with smooth surface. They have low reflectivity with medium echoes. They are homogenous in texture.

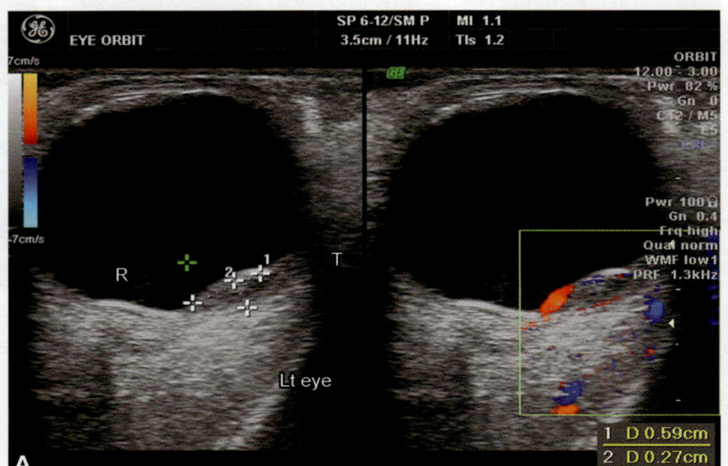

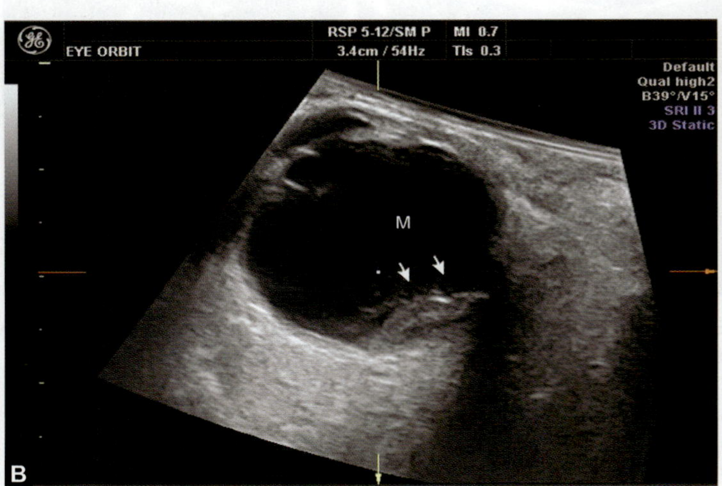

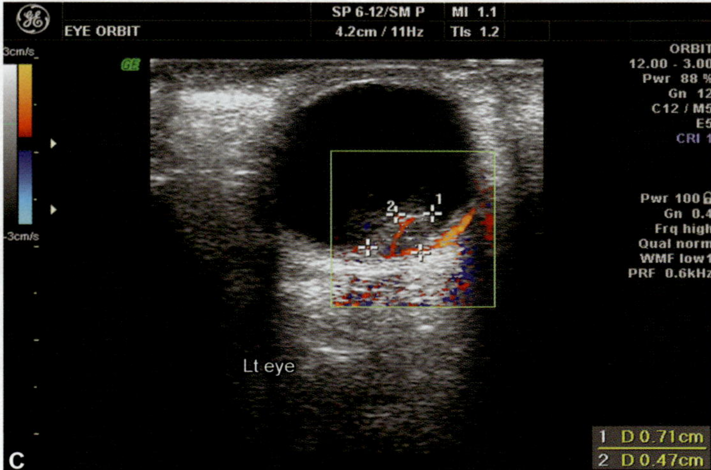

FIGURES 1.196A to C: Discoid melanoma. A 71-year-old male presented with diminished vision. HRSG shows a well-defined discoid mass on the temporal side lateral to the optic nerve head. It is smooth in outline and homogeneous in texture. No calcification is seen in it. On color flow imaging, an artery is seen feeding it suggestive of discoid melanoma.

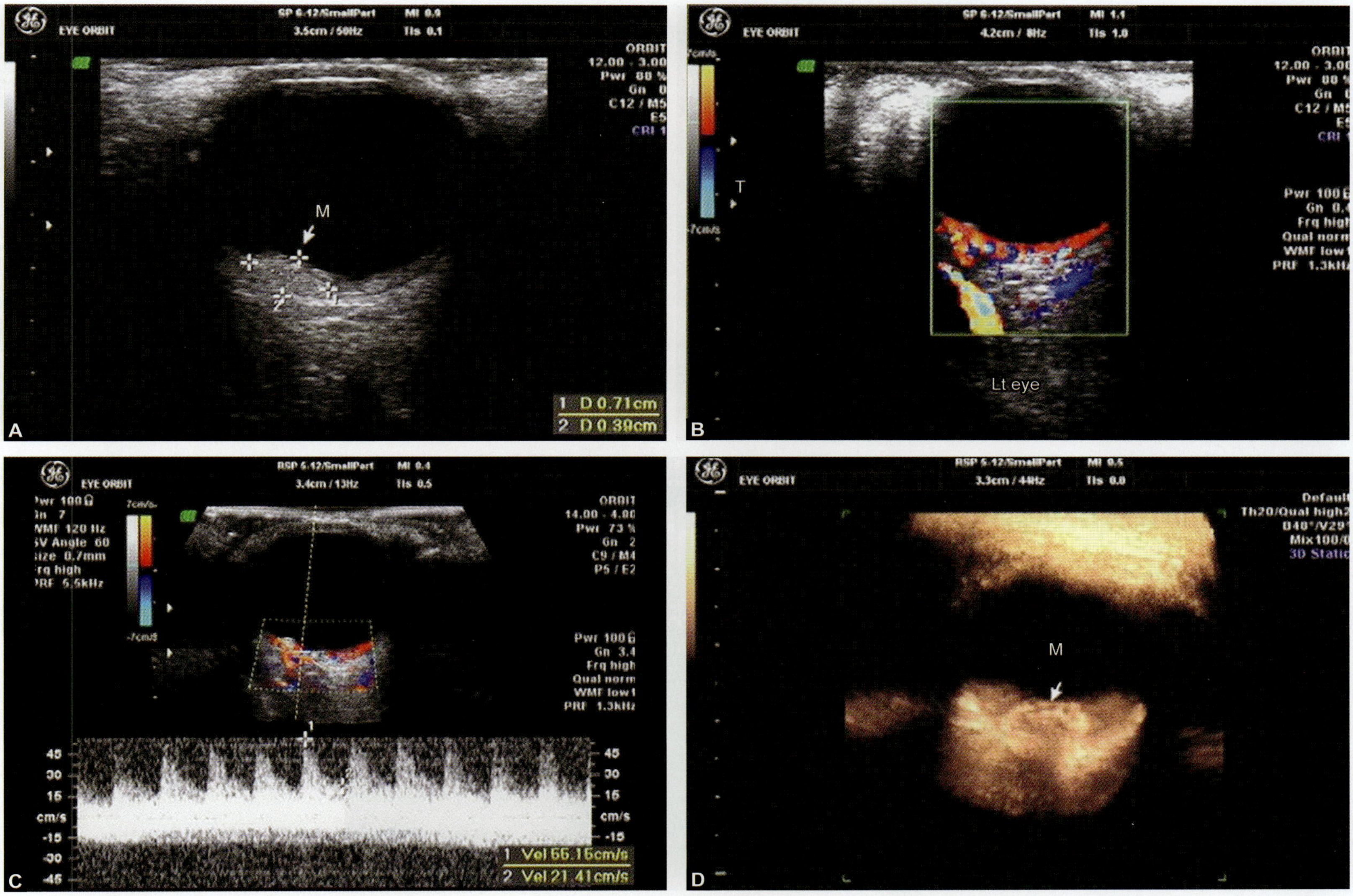

FIGURES 1.197A to D: Discoid melanoma. A patient presented with decreased vision with painful eye. HRSG shows a well-defined soft tissue mass coming out from choroid. It is smooth in outline with homogeneous in texture. On color flow imaging, multiple vessels are seen feeding it. On spectral Doppler tracing, moderate arterial flow is seen in it. Figure D shows 3D of tumor, which clearly shows its relation with choroid.

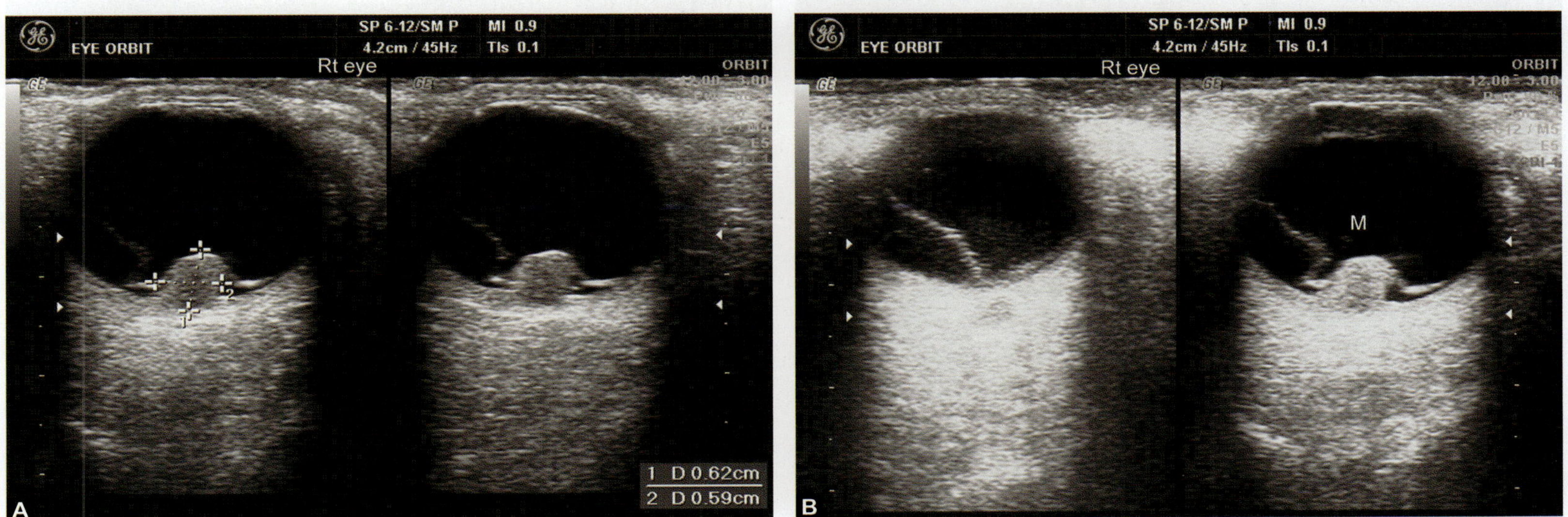

FIGURES 1.198A and B

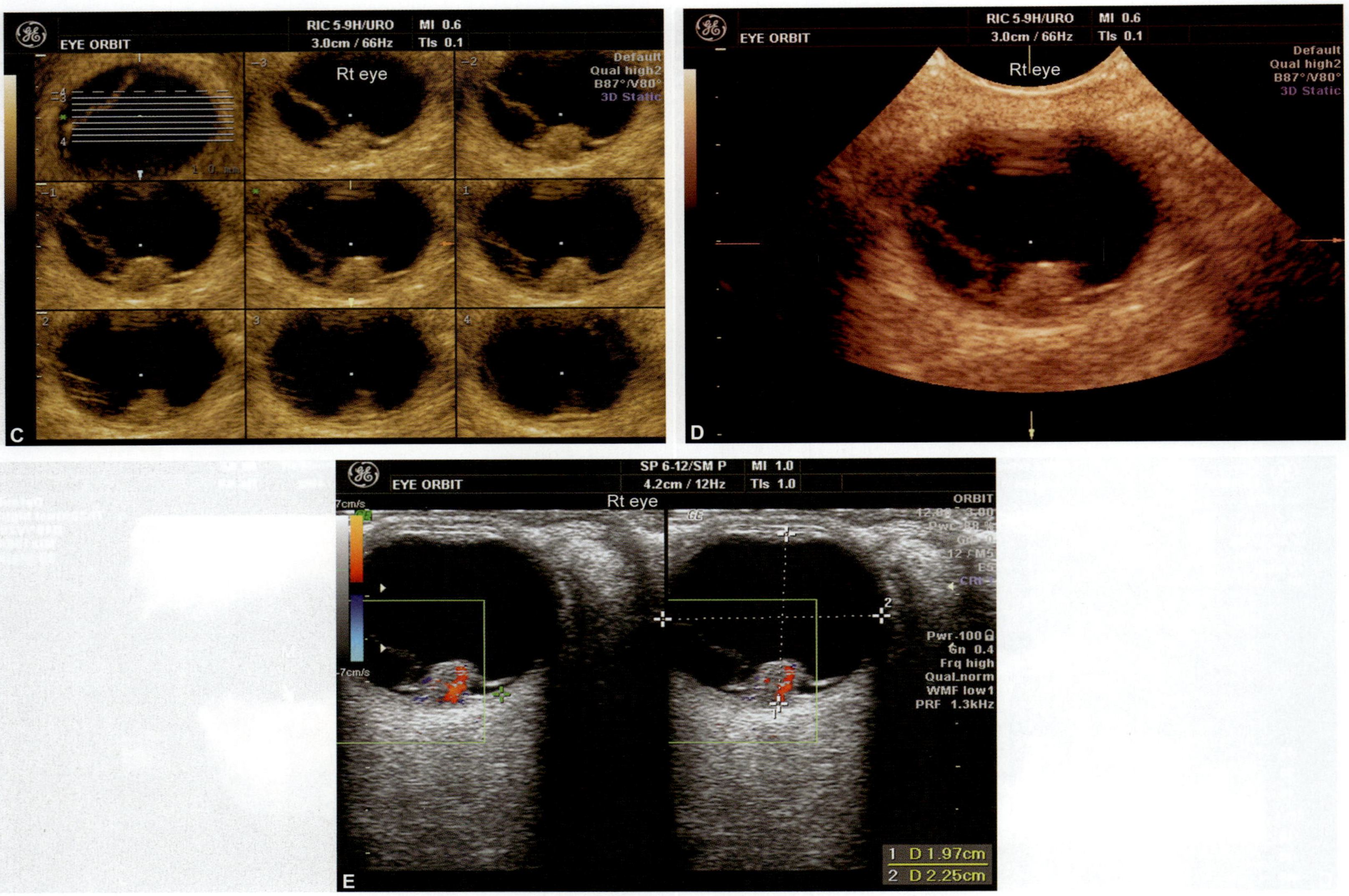

FIGURES 1.198C to E

FIGURES 1.198A to E: Collor button melanoma. A patient presented with decreased vision. HRSG shows a well-defined soft tissue mass, which is seen elevated from choroid. It is seen bulging in the posterior segment. On 3D TUI imaging, the mass is seen coming out from choroid. Associated retinal detachment is also seen in the posterior segment of the eye. The retina is seen passing over the mass. Figure E shows a vessel feeding the mass.

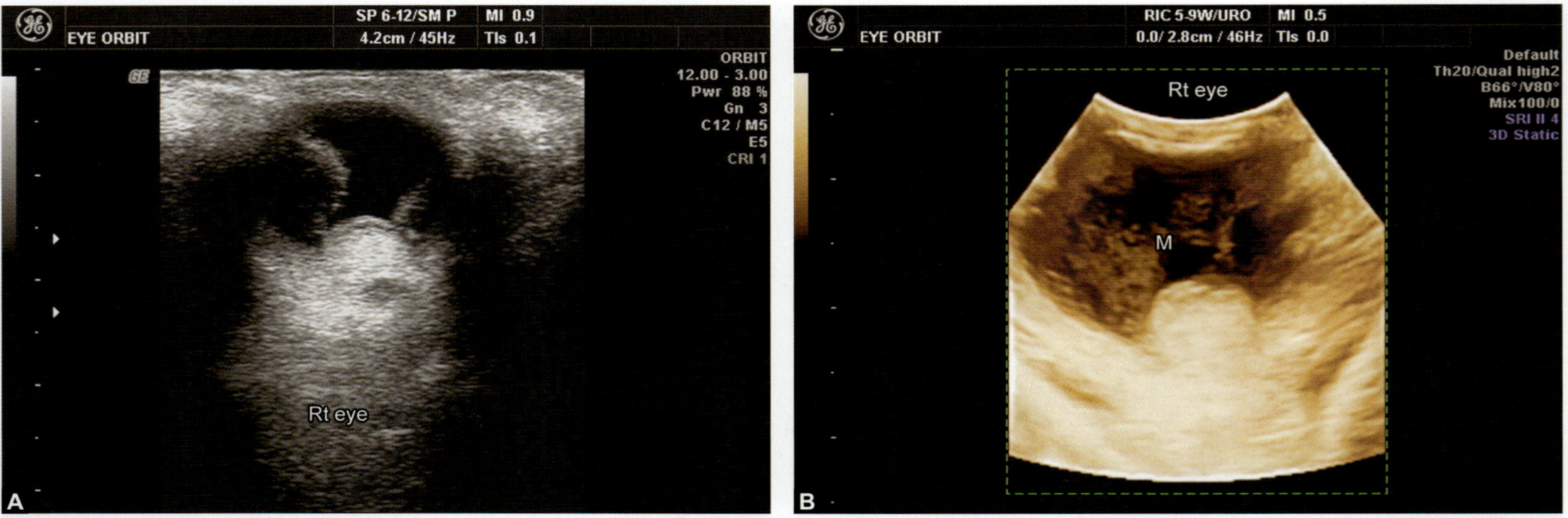

FIGURES 1.199A and B: A patient presented with loss of vision. HRSG shows a well-defined soft tissue mass, which is homogeneous in texture suggestive of melanoma. On 3D imaging, intragel hemorrhage is also seen with retinal detachment.

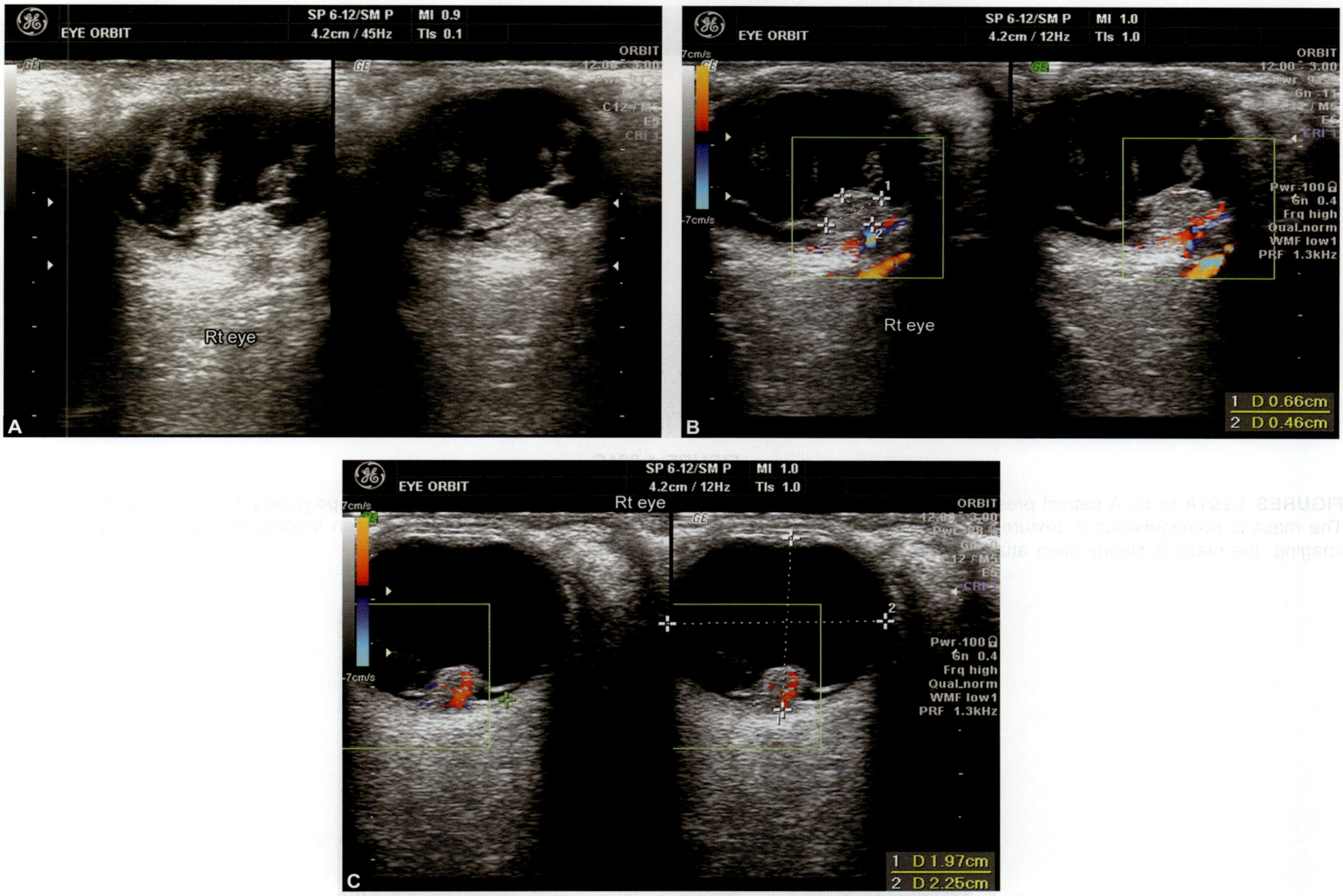

FIGURES 1.200A to C: Intragel hemorrhage masking the melanoma. A patient presented with loss of vision. HRSG shows intragel hemorrhage in the eye. However, there is also evidence of a well-defined soft tissue mass seen in the posterior segment of the eye coming out from choroid. It is homogeneous in texture. A vessel is seen feeding the mass suggestive of melanoma which has been masked by a hemorrhage.

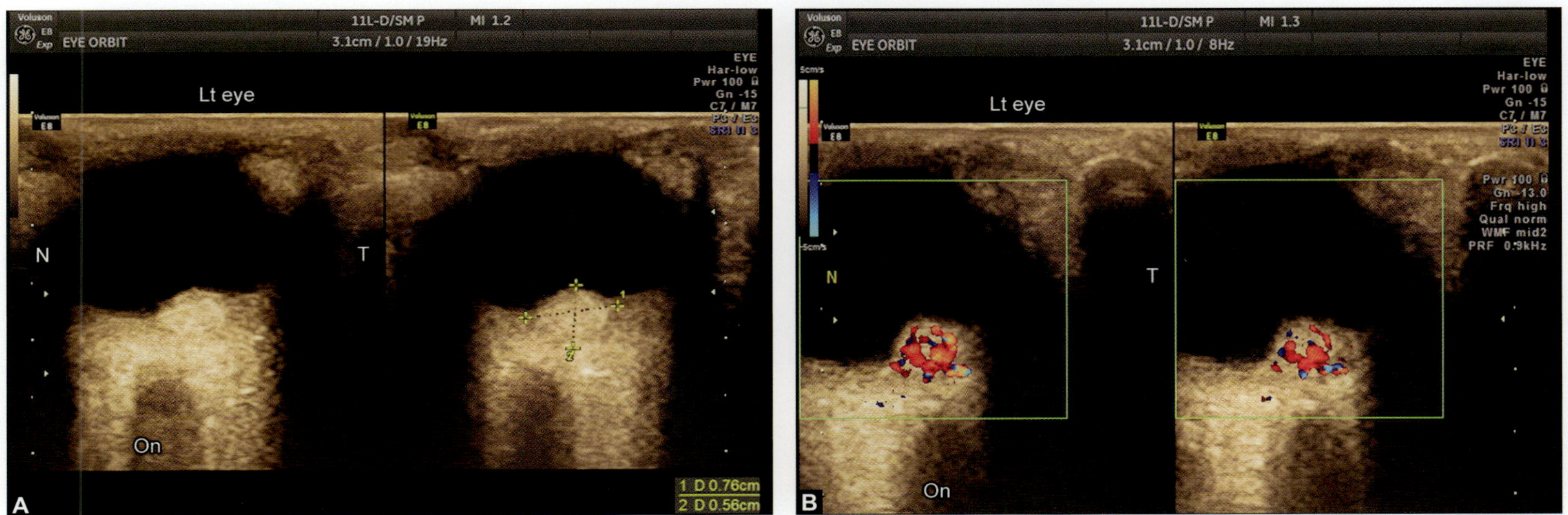

FIGURES 1.201A and B

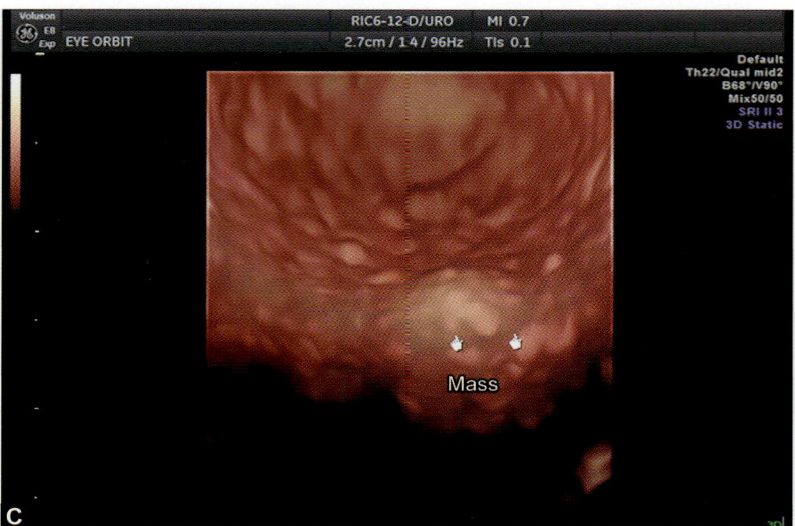

FIGURE 1.201C

FIGURES 1.201A to C: A patient presented with decreased vision. HRSG shows a well-defined homogeneous polypoidal mass fixed with the choroid. The mass is homogeneous in texture and smooth in outline. On color flow imaging, multiple vessels are seen feeding the mass. On 3D ultrasound imaging, the mass is clearly seen attached with choroid.

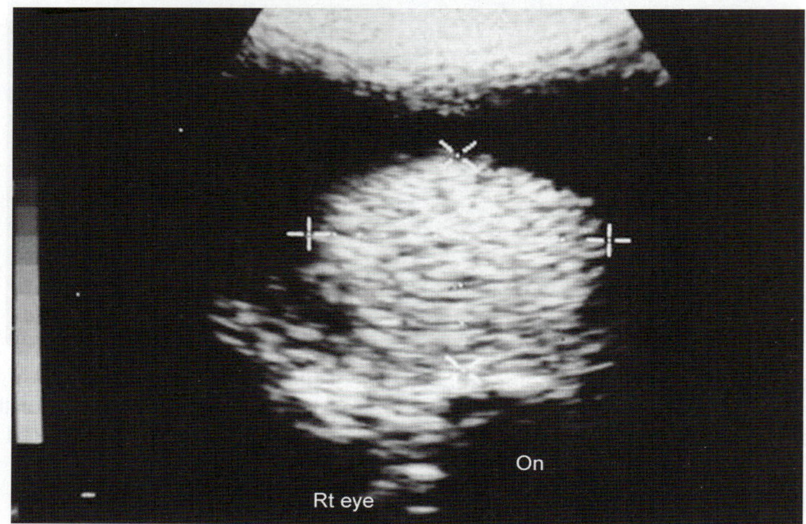

FIGURE 1.202: Collar button melanoma. HRSG shows well-defined collar button-shaped tumor with homogeneous texture. Fine interfaces are seen in the tumor mass suggestive of tightly packed tumor cells.

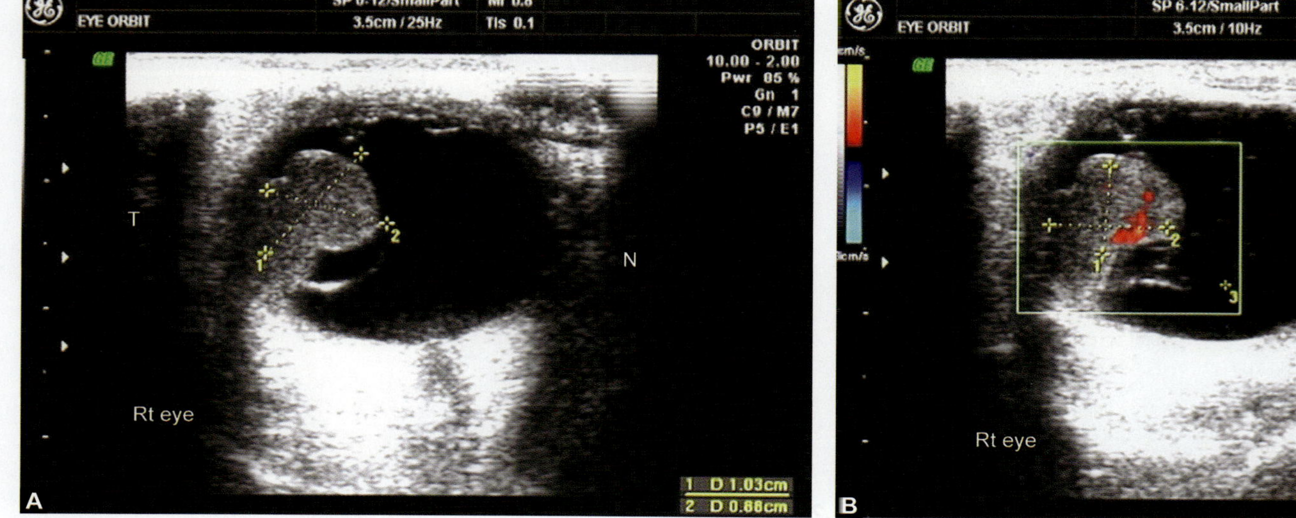

FIGURES 1.203A and B: Cillary body melanoma. A big mass is seen coming out of the right cilliary body. It is club-shaped and projecting in the posterior segment. Color Doppler spectral imaging shows low flow in the vessel supplying the tumor mass.

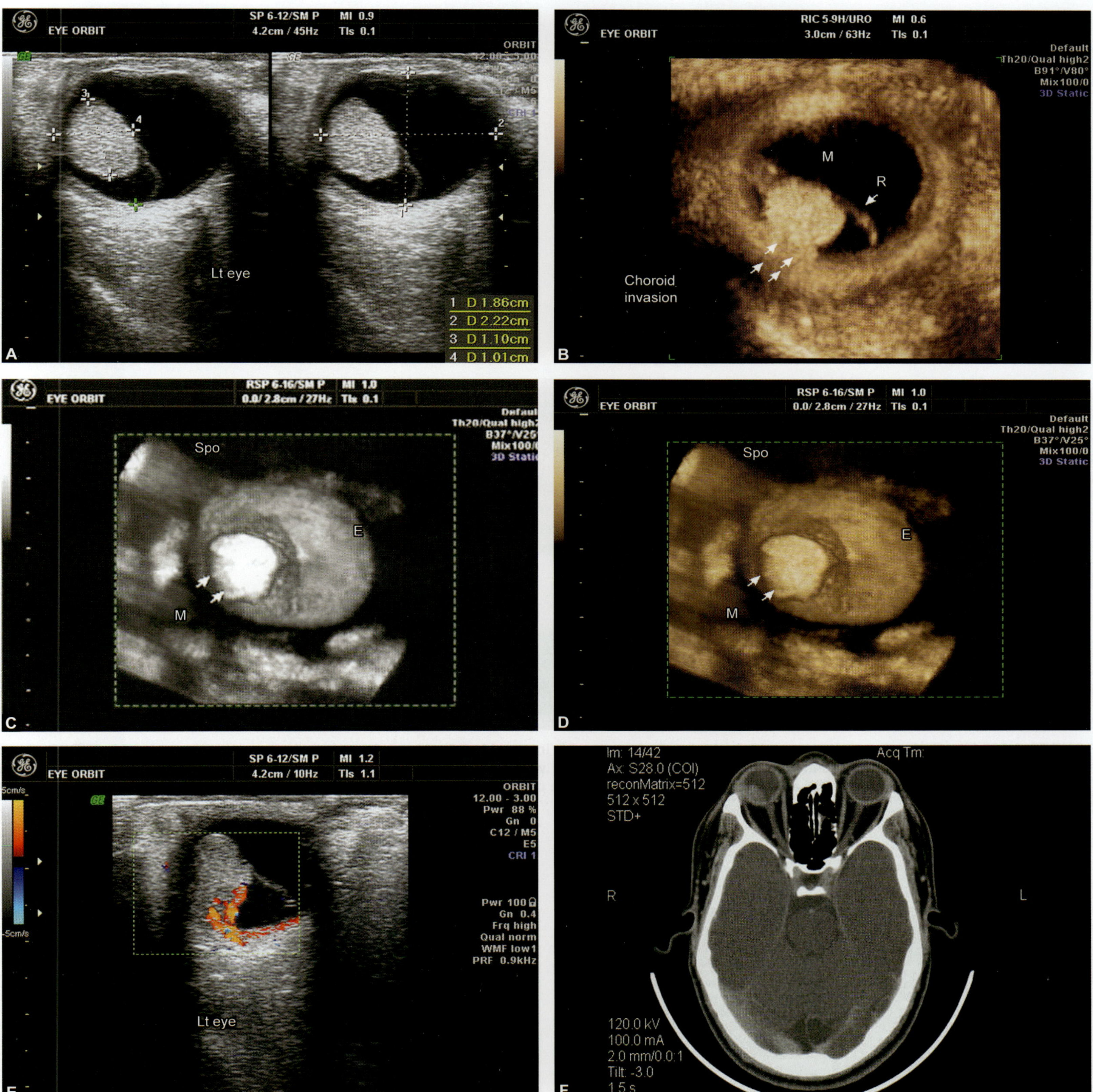

FIGURES 1.204A to F: Ciliary body melanoma. HRSG shows a well-defined soft tissue mass seen coming out from ciliary body on nasal side. It is homogeneous in texture. The retina is seen detached and seen anterior to the mass. On 3D ultrasound, the mass is seen invading the choroid. In Figure B, the volume contrast 3D imaging clearly shows the mass relation with choroid. On color Doppler imaging, multiple vessels are seen feeding the mass. CT scan of the same patient confirms the diagnosis. However, USG with 3D imaging give much more information than CT scan.

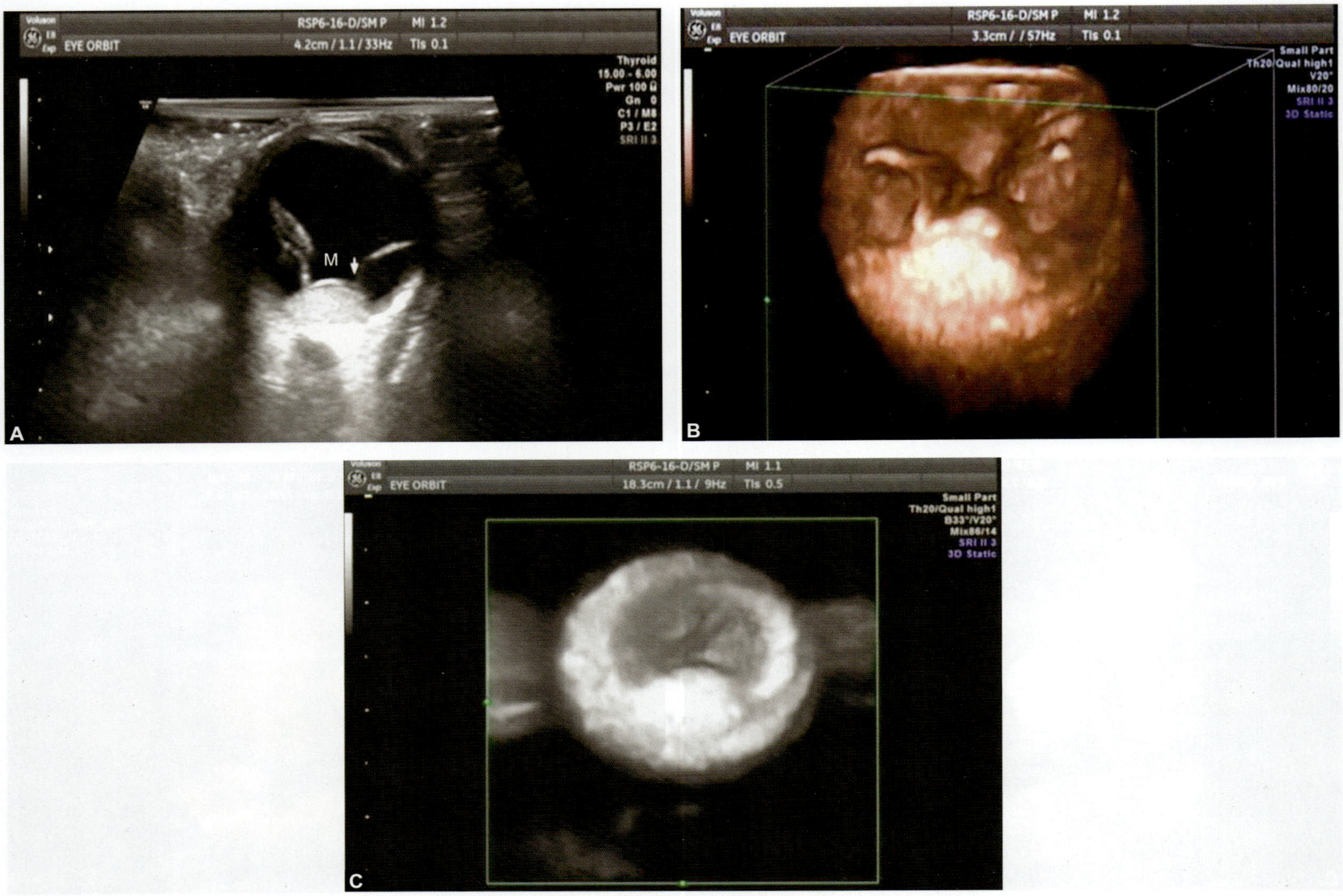

FIGURES 1.205A to C: Ocular melanoma with retinal detachment with intragel hemorrhage. A patient presented with loss of vision. HRSG shows intragel hemorrhage in eye. Retinal detachment is also seen. However, a well-defined soft tissue mass is seen in the posterior segment of the eye. The mass is not seen due to hemorrhage. The 3D ultrasound with volume contrast imaging clearly shows the mass, which is confined to the choroid.

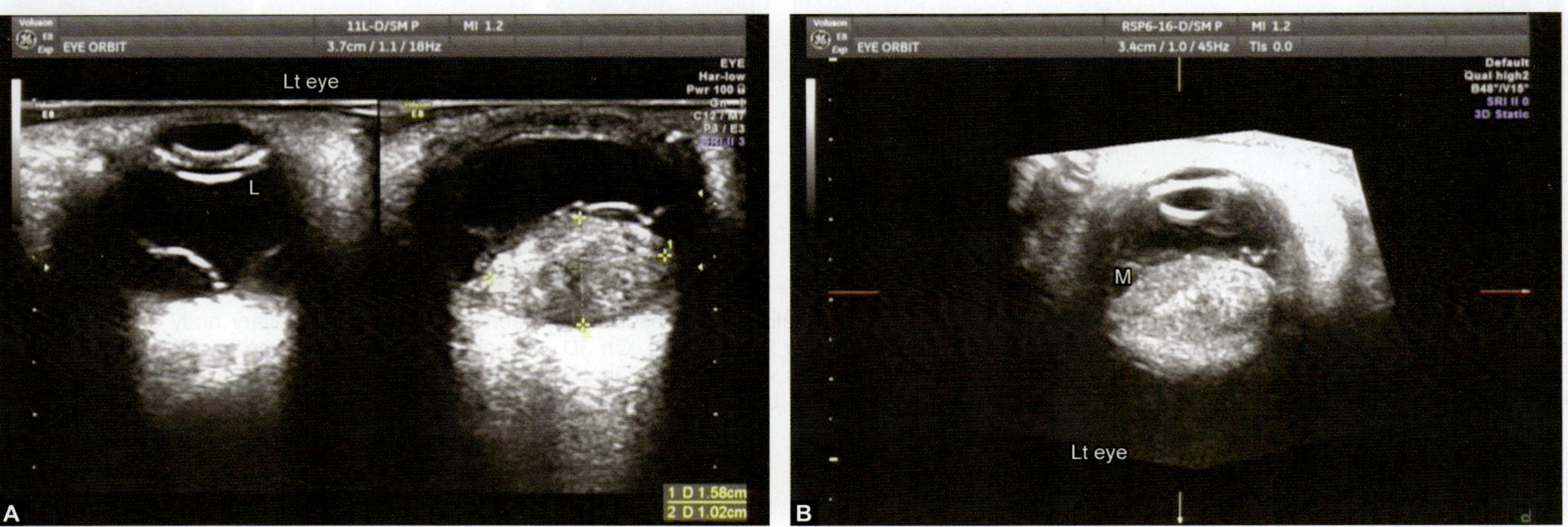

FIGURES 1.206A and B

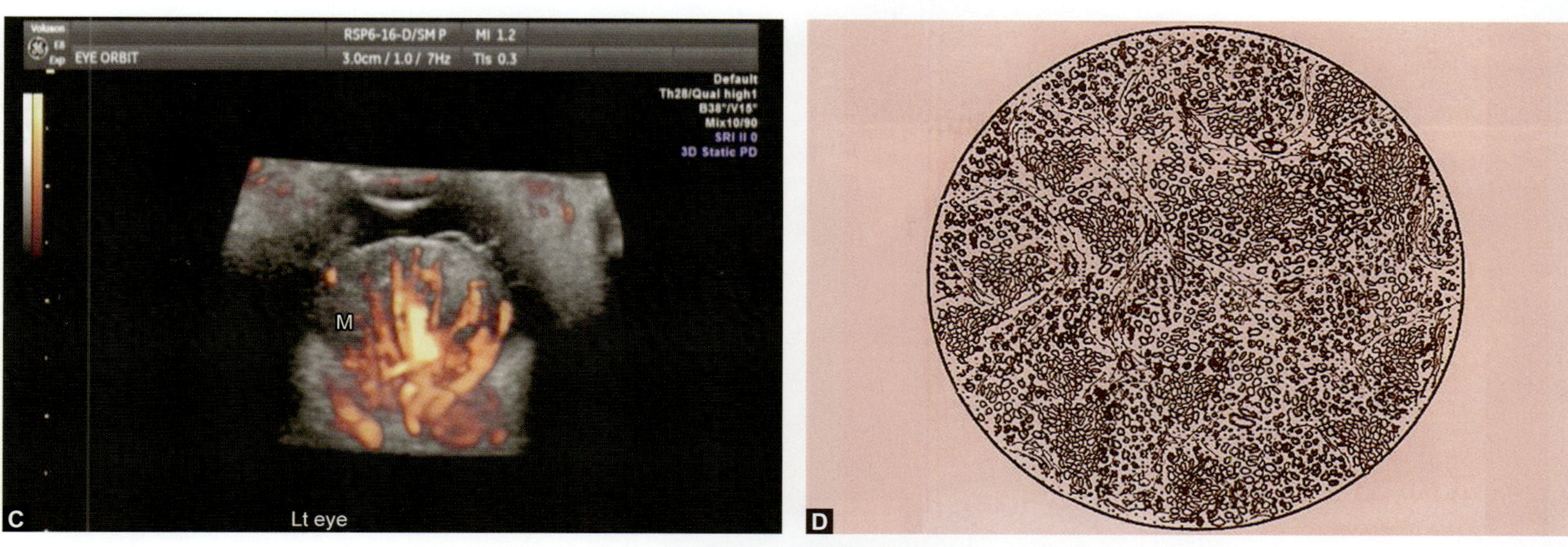

FIGURES 1.206C and D

FIGURES 1.206A to D: A patient presented with sudden loss of vision in left eye. HRSG shows a big mass in the posterior segment of eye. It is smooth in outline and homogeneous in texture. On color flow imaging, multiple vessels are seen feeding the mass. Figure D shows the uniform cell nature of the mass (Melanoma).

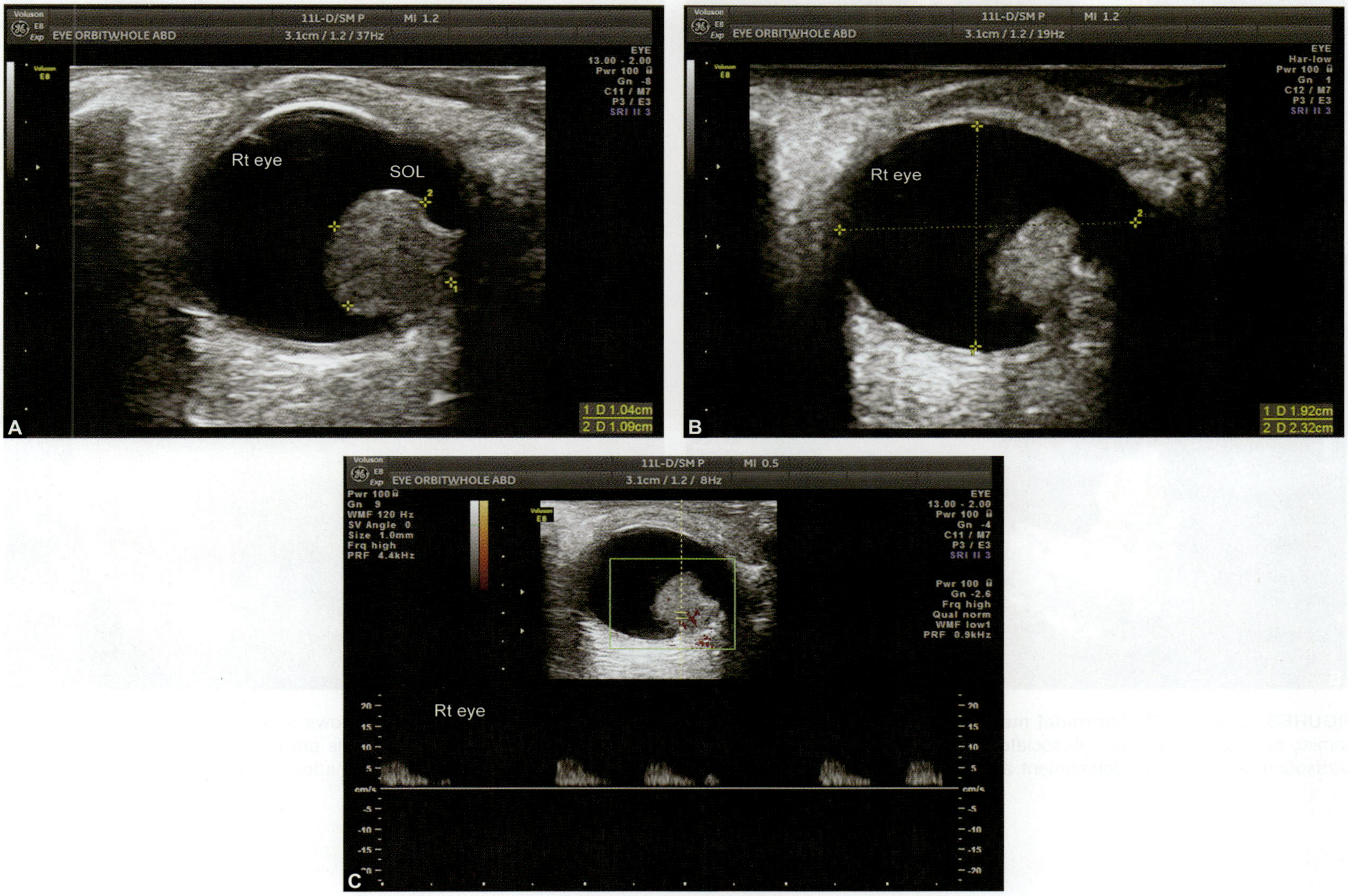

FIGURES 1.207A to C: Melanoma with choroidal excavation. A well-defined soft tissue mass is seen coming out from the nasal side of right eye. The mass is seen excavating the choroid. It is mushroom shaped. On color flow imaging, low arterial flow is seen in the mass.

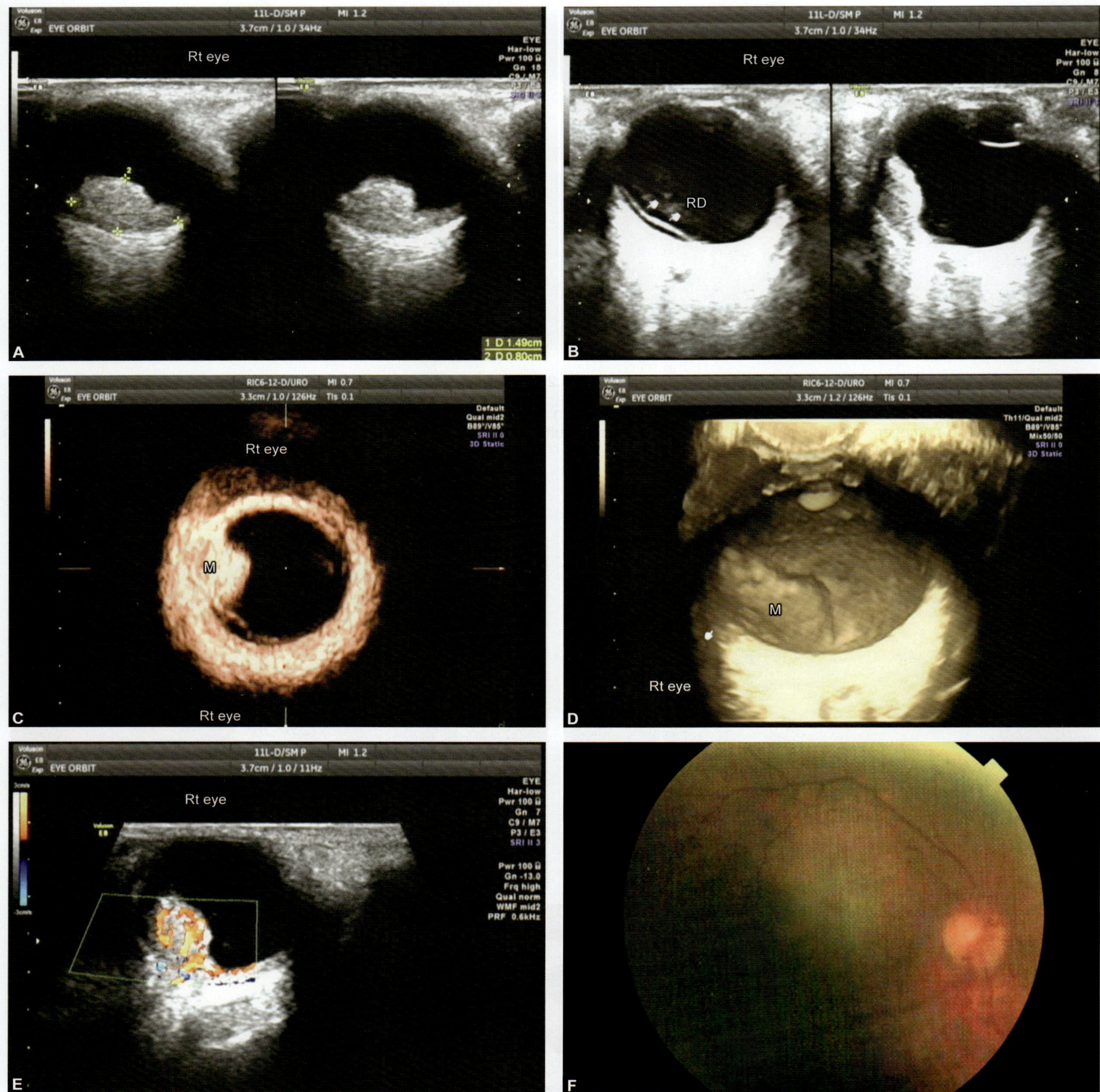

FIGURES 1.208A to F: Choroidal melanoma. A lady presented with loss of vision in the right eye. HRSG shows a homogeneous soft tissue mass coming out from the choroid. Associated retinal detachment is also seen. On color flow imaging, multiple vessels are seen feeding the mass. The 3D ultrasound shows retinal detachment and the mass clearly. The direct fundoscopy shows bulging soft tissue shadow in the choroid.

DIFFERNTIAL DIAGNOSIS OF MELANOMA

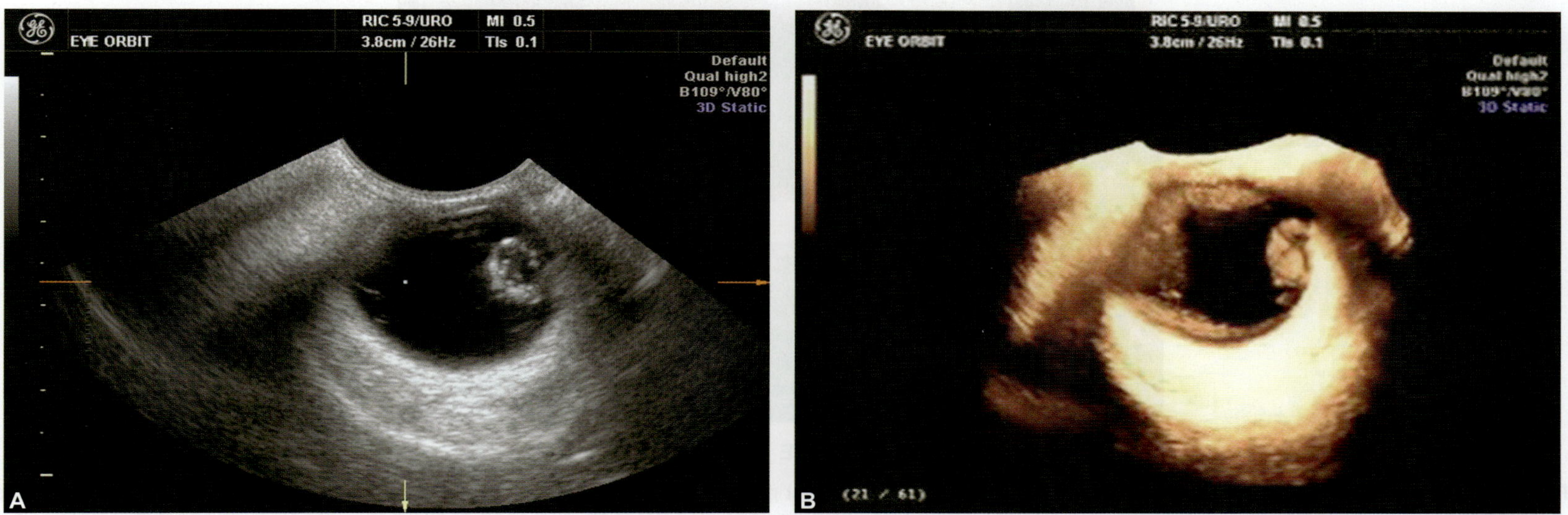

FIGURES 1.209A and B: Dislocated cataractous lens in posterior segment. HRSG shows a dislocated cataractous lens in posterior segment of eye on temporal side, which may mimic as melanoma.

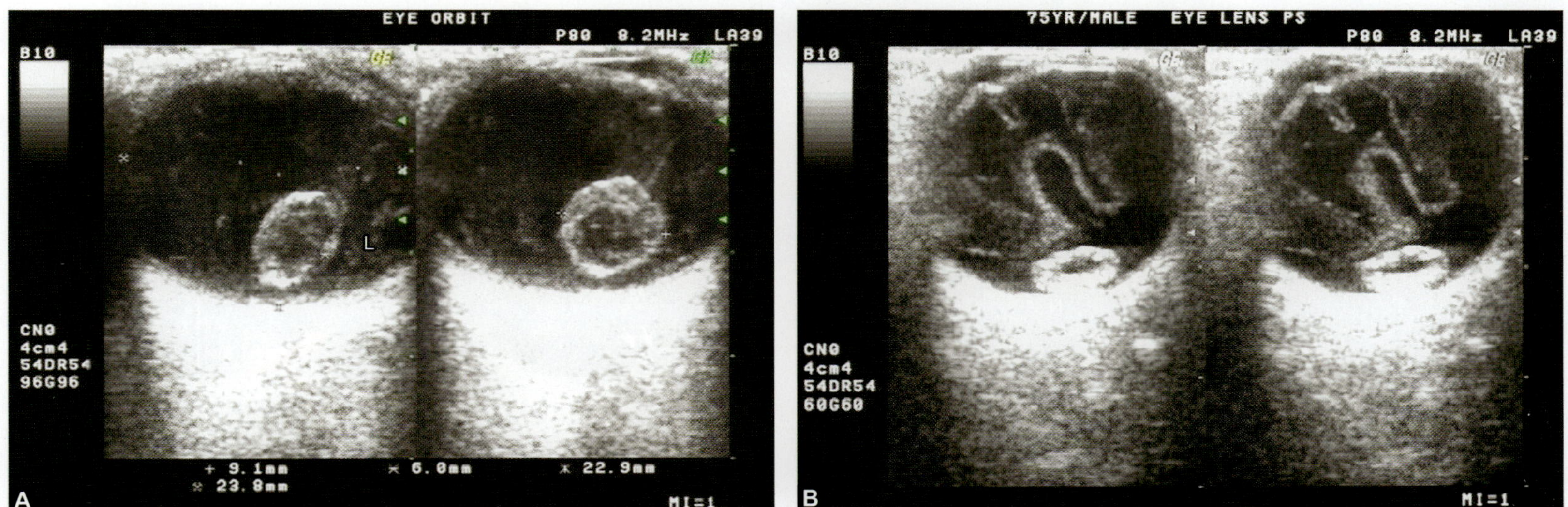

FIGURES 1.210A and B: Dislocated cataractous lens in posterior segment. HRSG shows cataractous lens dislocated in the posterior segment of eye. Associated intragel hemorrhage is also seen. It may be mistaken as melanoma.

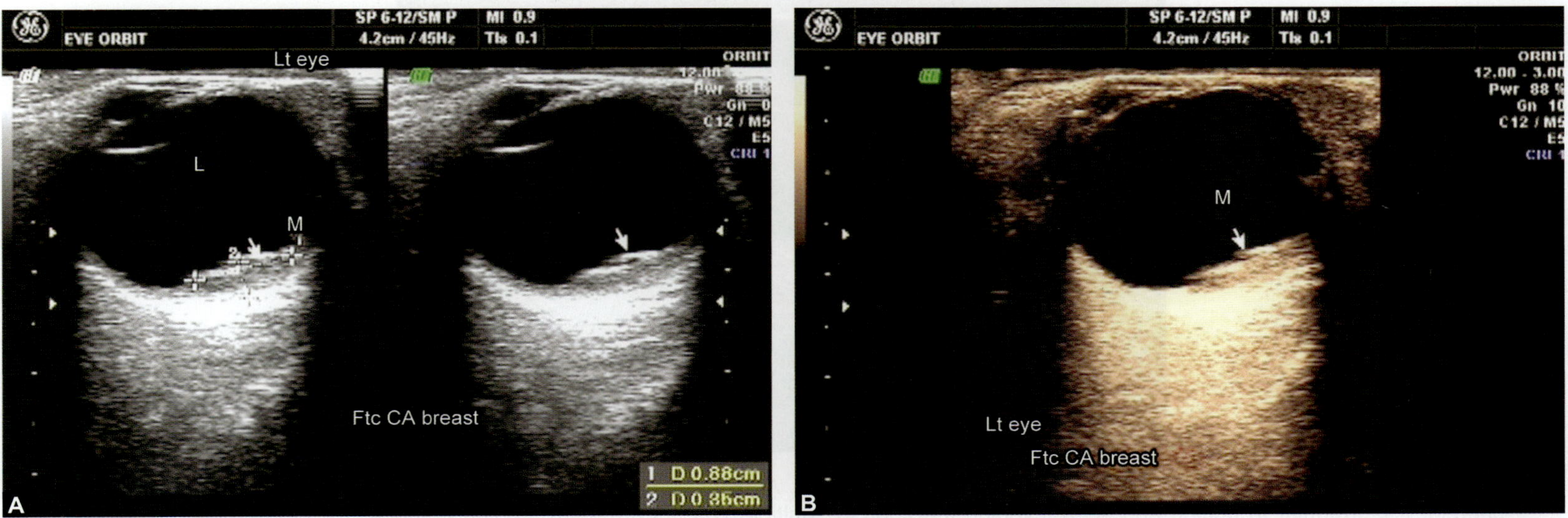

FIGURES 1.211A and B

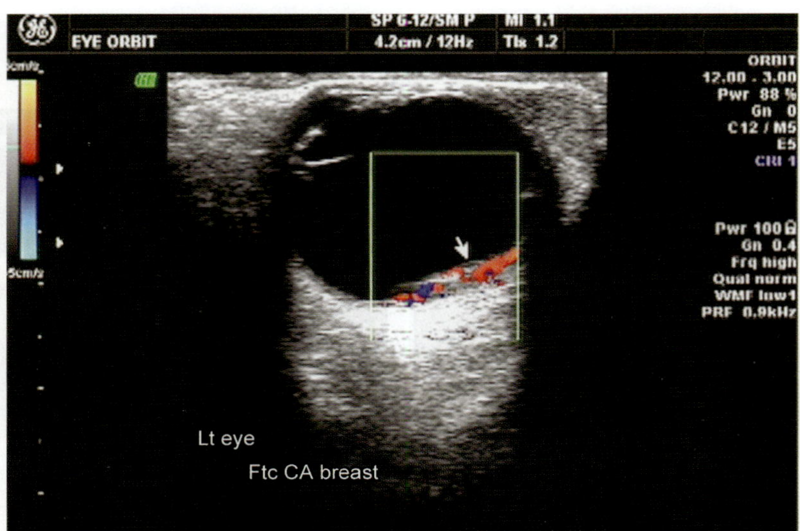

FIGURE 1.211C

FIGURES 1.211A to C: Choroidal metastasis. A known case of CA breast presented with pain in eye and diminished vision. HRSG shows a soft tissue mass in the choroid, which shows homogeneous texture. On color flow imaging, few vessels are seen feeding it suggestive of choroidal metastasis.

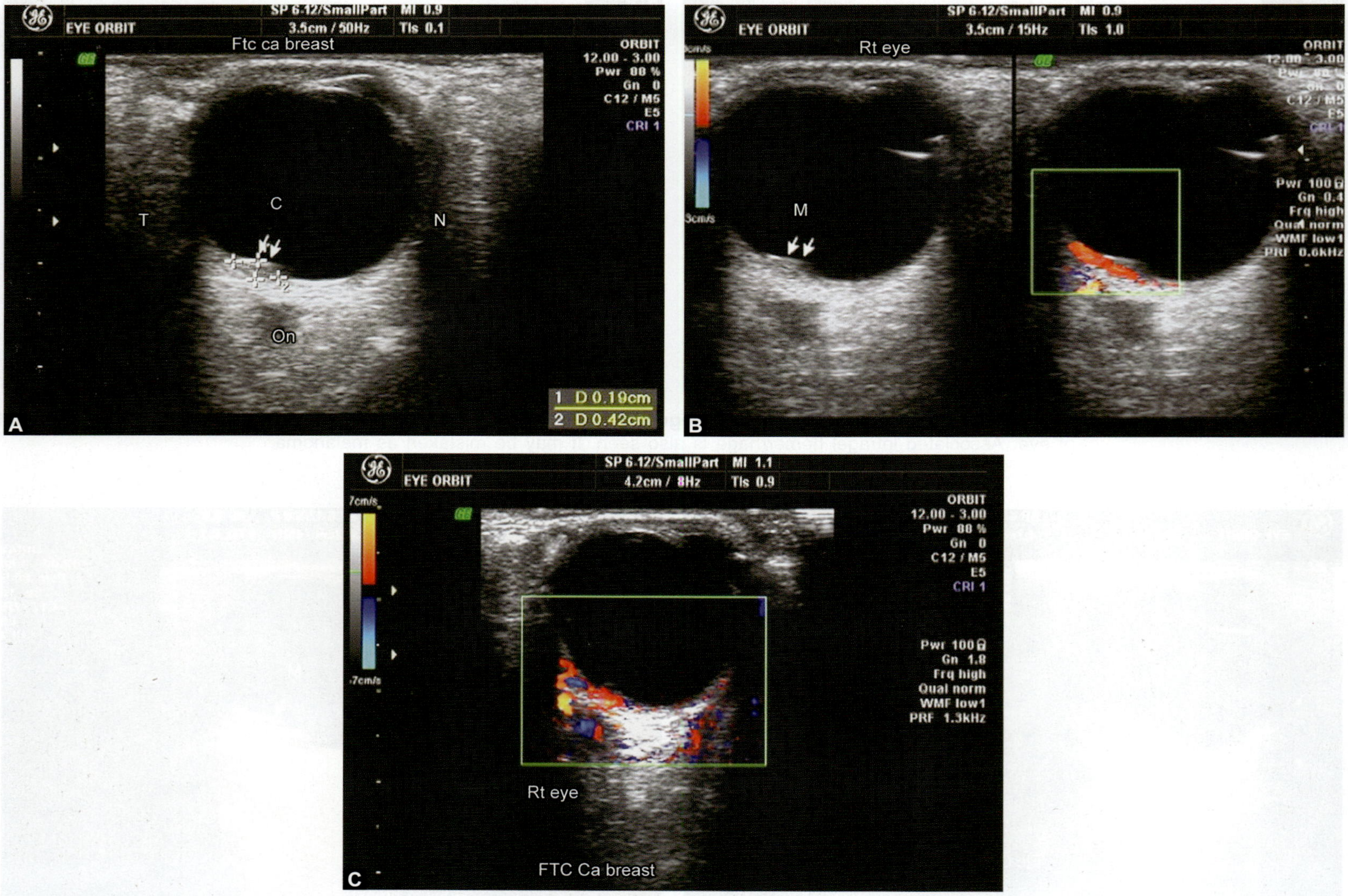

FIGURES 1.212A to C: Choroidal metastasis with choroid invasion. Another case of carcinoma breast shows soft tissue mass fixed with the choroid. It is irregular in outline and seen invading the choroid. Multiple vessels are seen feeding it suggestive of choroidal metastasis.

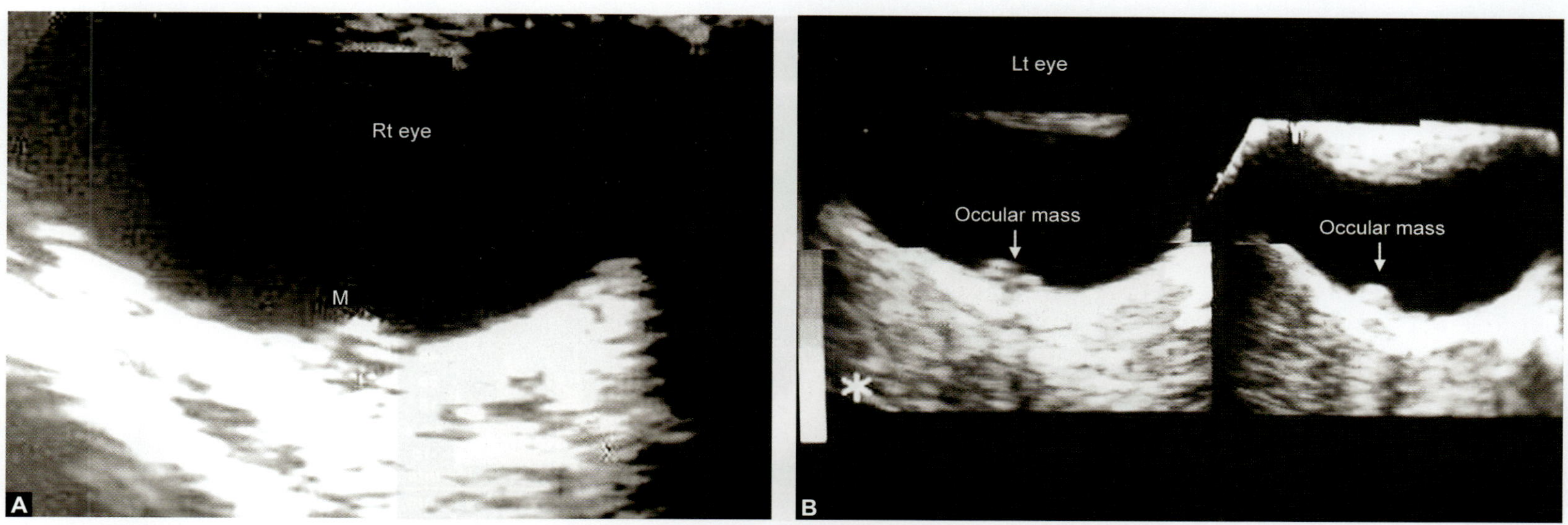

FIGURES 1.213A and B: Differential diagnosis of melanoma—Choroidal metastasis. A young child of acute lymphatic leukemia presented with diminished vision and painful eye. HRSG shows metastatic deposit in choroid. Associated retrobulbar deposit also seen as a hypodense irregular focus in retrobulbar fat.

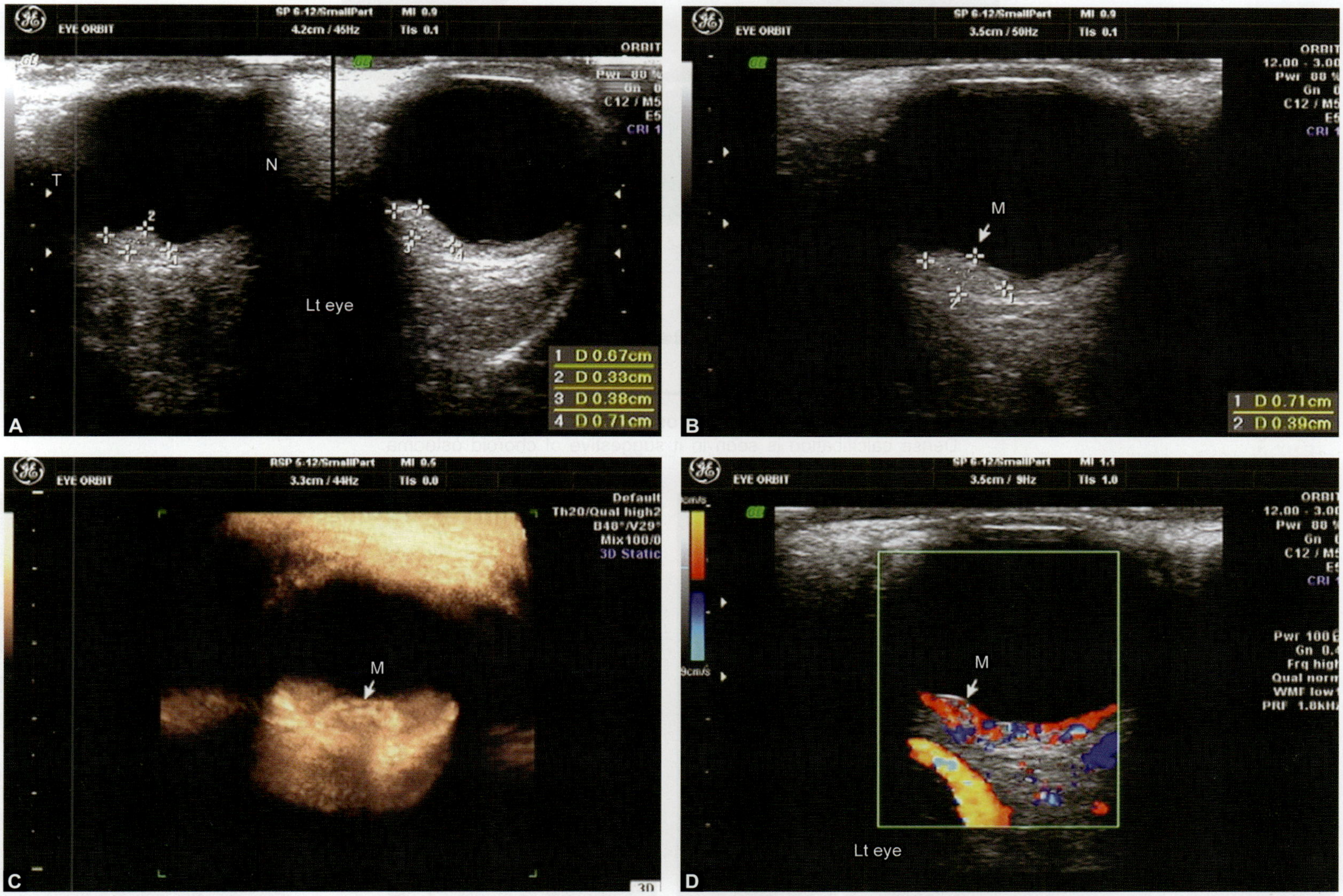

FIGURES 1.214A to D

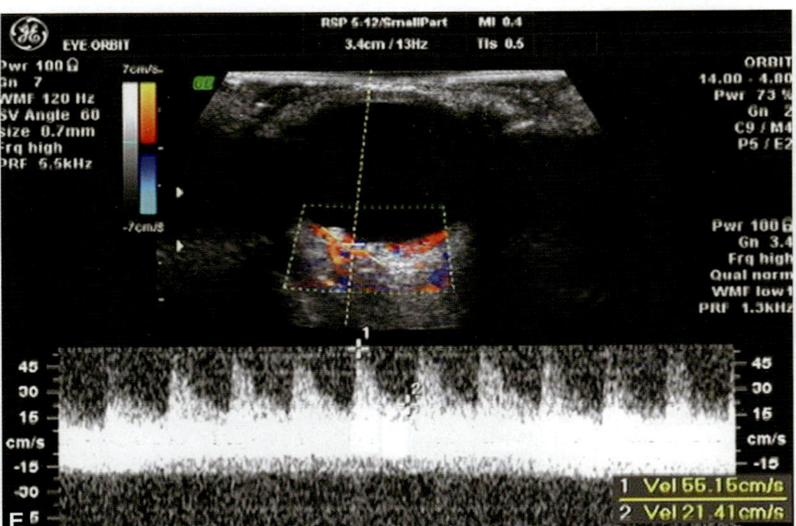

FIGURE 1.214E

FIGURES 1.214A to E: Choroidal angioma. A patient presented with painful eye. HRSG shows a well defined mass homogeneous in texture fixed with choroid. On color flow imaging, multiple vessels are seen feeding the mass. On spectral Doppler tracing, moderate arterial flow is seen in the mass suggestive of choroidal angioma.

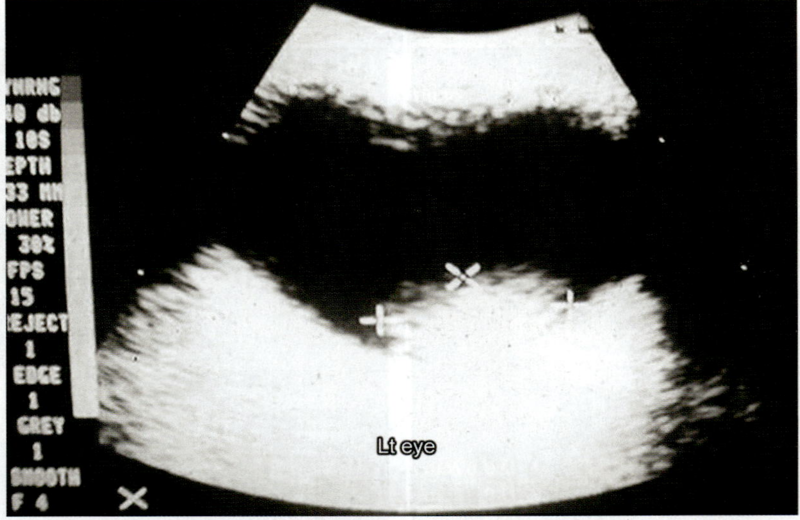

FIGURE 1.215: Differential diagnosis of melanoma—Choroidal osteoma. HRSG shows a highly echogenic mass fixed with choroid. Dense calcification is seen in it suggestive of choroid osteoma.

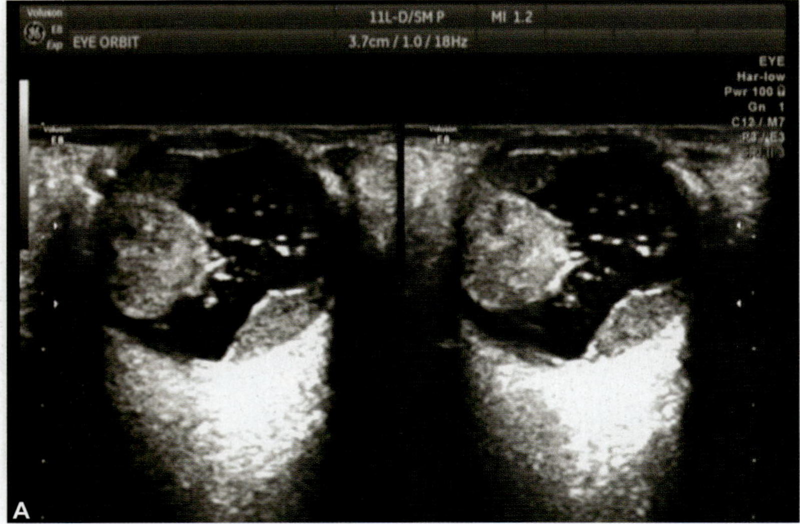

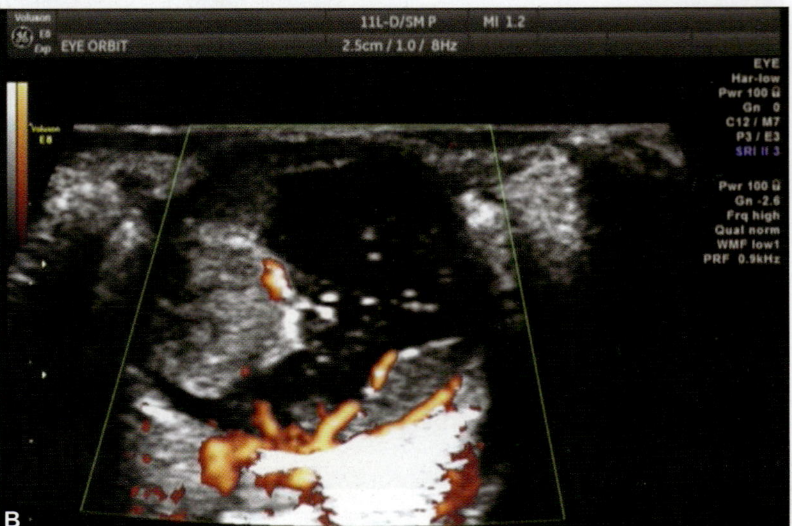

FIGURES 1.216A and B: Expulsive choroidal detachment with fresh bleed. A patient presented with loss of vision. HRSG shows multiple dome shaped masses in the posterior segment. Thick echogenic collection is seen under the masses. But On color flow imaging, no flow is seen the masses suggestive of multifocal choroidal detachment with organized subchoroidal hematomas. Subchoroidal hematomas may mimic as choroidal melanomas.

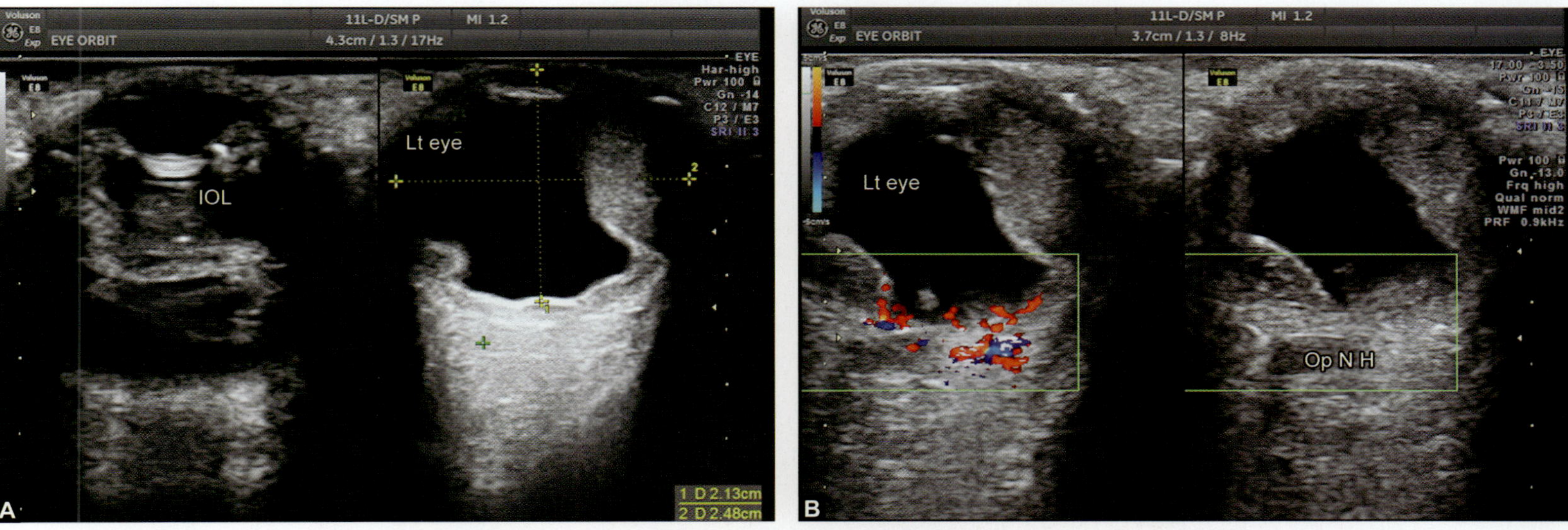

FIGURES 1.217A and B: Extensive choroidal detachment with soft eye and deformed eyeball after cataract surgery. A patient presented with acute pain with loss of vision in the eye after cataract surgery. HRSG shows IOL in position. Thick dome-shaped shadows are seen from periphery. Echogenic collection is seen under the membrane suggestive of choroidal detachment with expulsive hemorrhage. The membranes are seen kissing each other in entire globe resulting into soft eye coat and deformed shape of the eye.

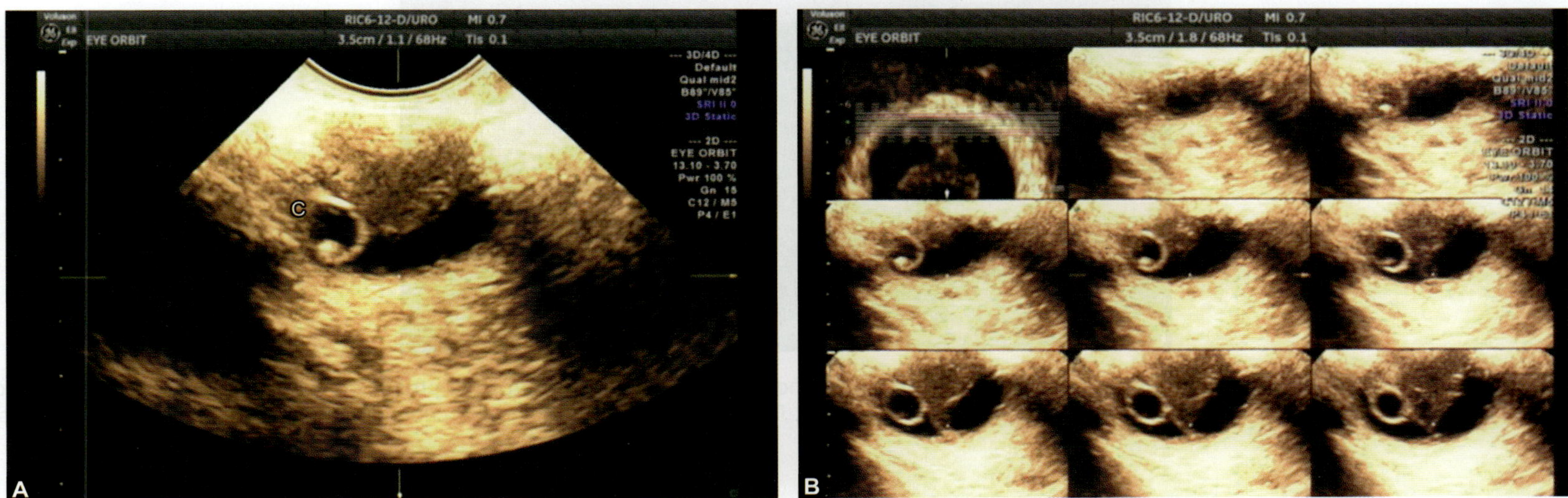

FIGURES 1.218A and B: Cysticercus cyst with hemorrhage. The intraocular cysticercus cyst may mimic as ocular melanoma. HRSG shows intraocular cyst with echogenic nidus in the eye suggestive of cysticercus cyst. Associated intragel hemorrhage is also seen in it, which has masked the cyst.

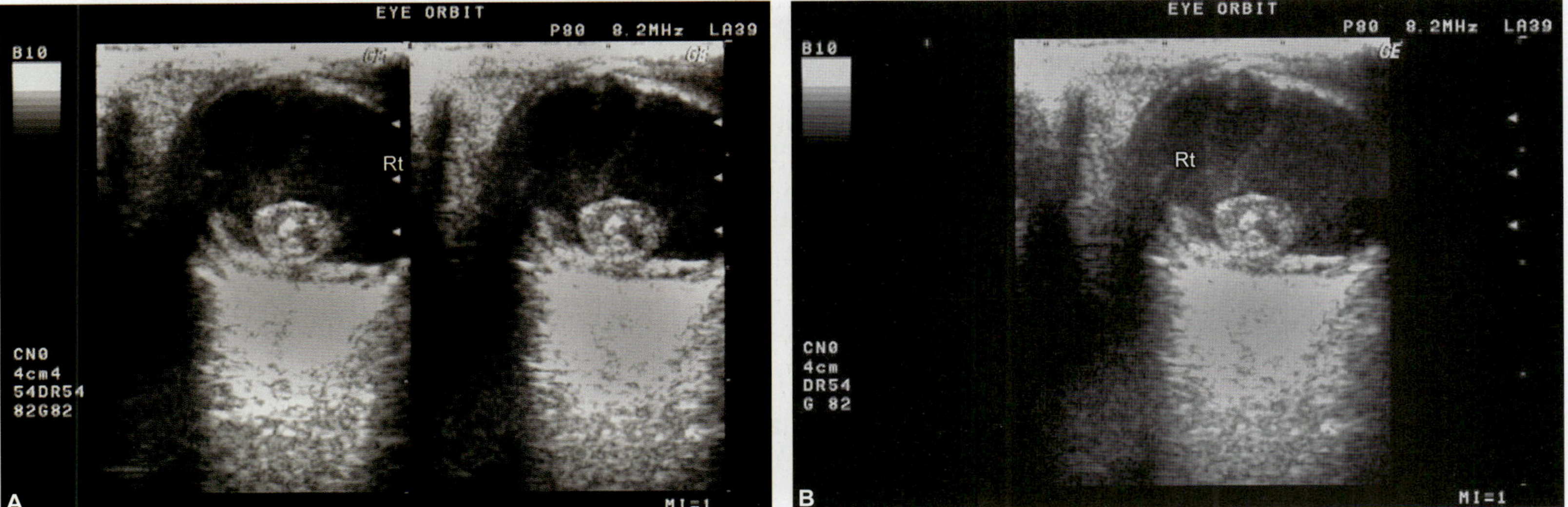

FIGURES 1.219A and B: Ruptured cysticercus cyst. The ruptured cysticercus cyst may present as intraocular mass mimicking ocular melanoma. HRSG shows ruptured cysticercus cyst in the posterior segment. Dense intragel hemorrhage is also seen in the posterior segment masking the cysticercus cyst.

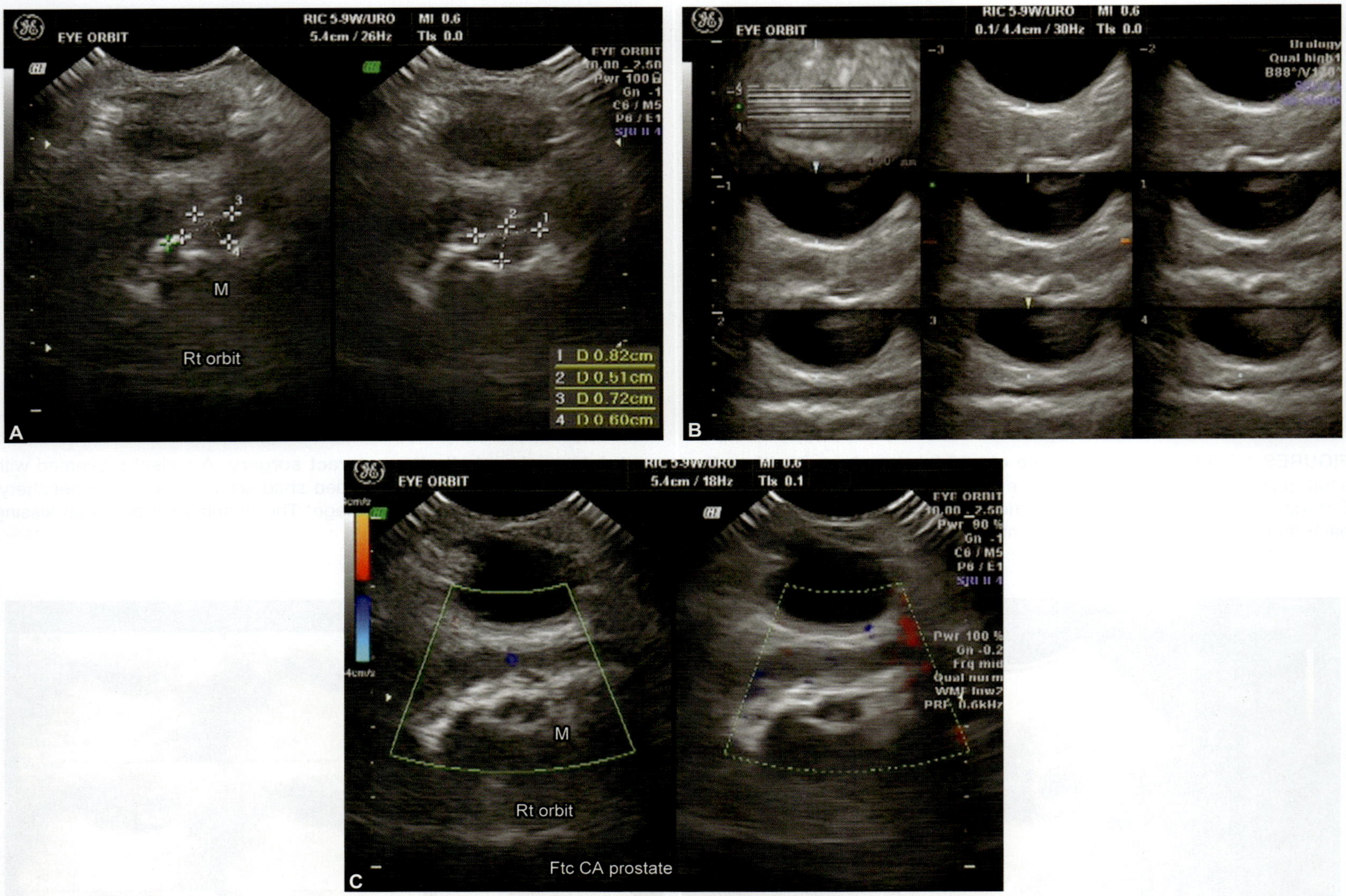

FIGURES 1.220A to C: Choroidal metastasis carcinoma prostate. A known case of carcinoma prostate presented with painful eye with decreased vision. HRSG shows an irregular ill-defined mass in the retrobulbar space. The mass is seen invading the choroid suggestive of choroidal metastasis.

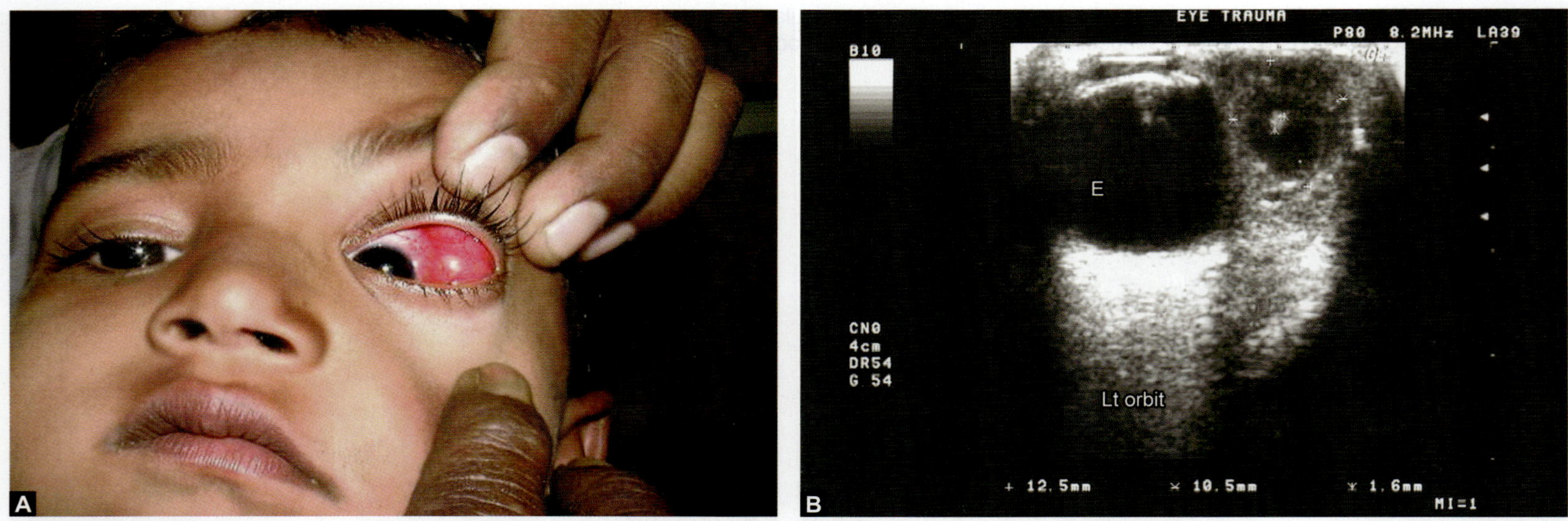

FIGURES 1.221A and B

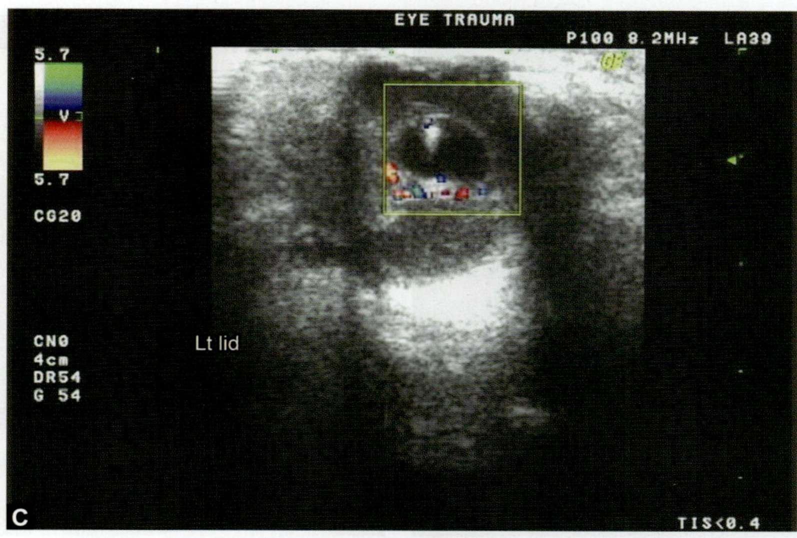

C

FIGURE 1.221C

FIGURES 1.221A to C: Ocular cysticercosis. Lateral canthus cysticercus. A young child presented with left lateral canthus swelling. HRSG shows a well defined cystic mass coming out from the lateral canthus. An echogenic nidus is seen fixed with the inner wall of the cyst typical of cysticercus cyst. Color Doppler imaging of the cyst shows cyst wall hyperemia.

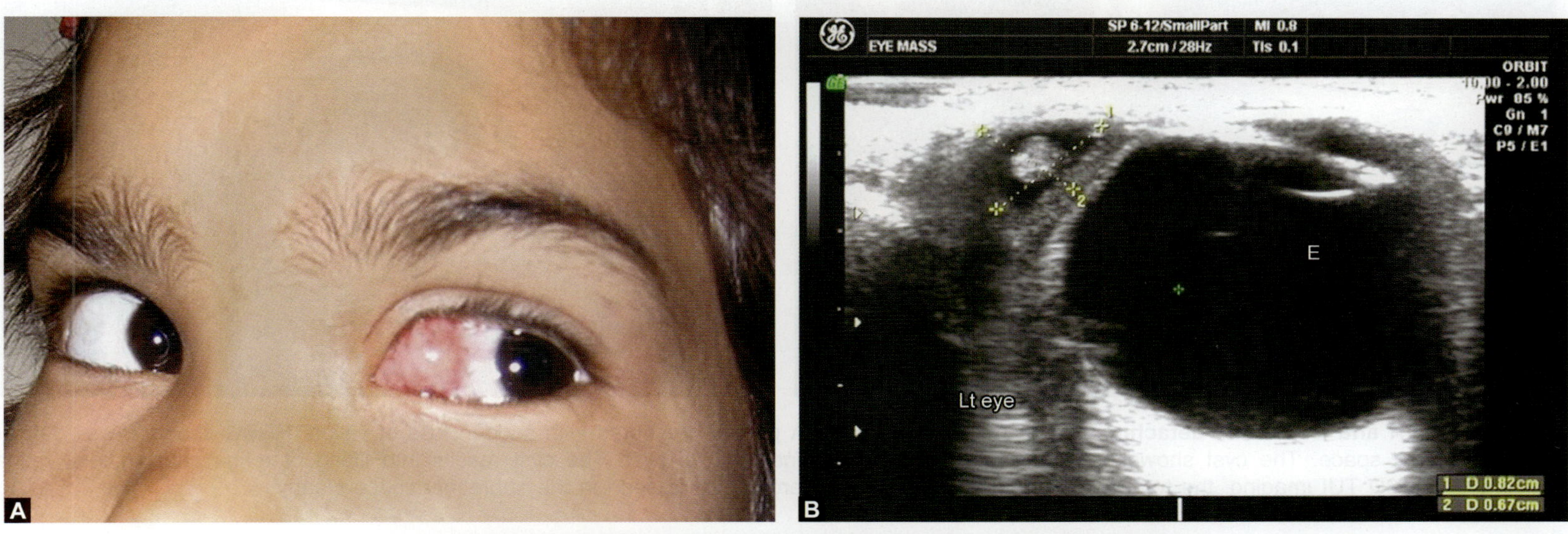

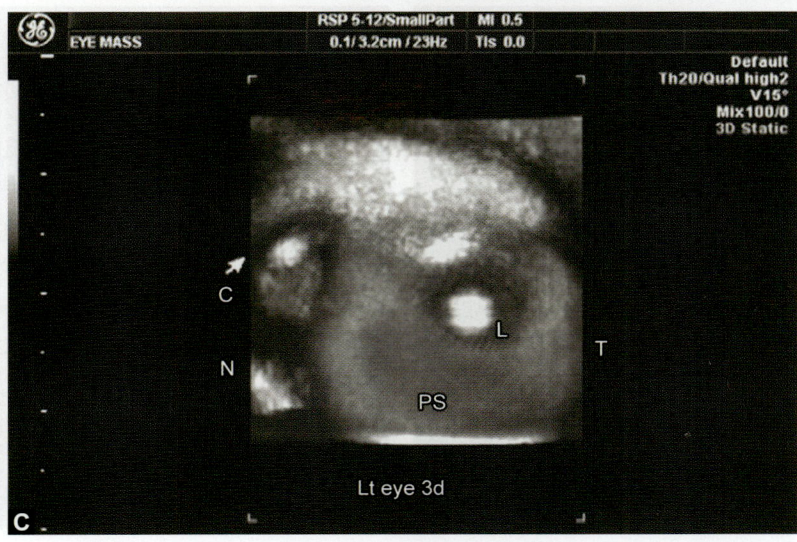

FIGURES 1.222A to C: Medial canthus cysticercosis. A young girl presented with cystic mass over the medial canthus. HRSG shows a well-defined cyst having an echogenic nidus fixed with inner wall of the cyst typical of cysticercus cyst. Color Doppler imaging shows no flow in the cyst. 3D imaging of the cyst shows the finer details of the cyst. It is seen confined to the sclera.

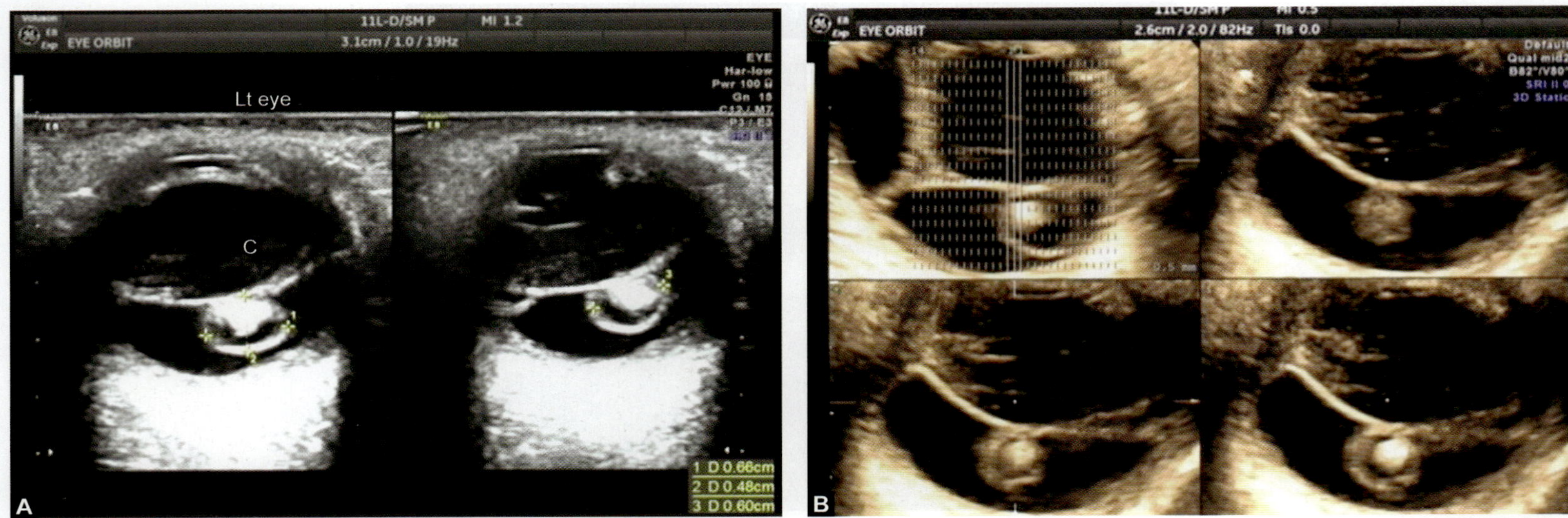

FIGURES 1.223A and B: Retinal detachment with cysticercus cyst. A patient presented with acute pain in eye with sudden loss of vision. HRSG shows a well defined cyst in the posterior segment. An echogenic nidus is seen fixed with the inner wall of cyst suggestive of cysticercus cyst. The cyst is seen attached at retina and retina is seen detached from its surface suggestive of retinal detachment.

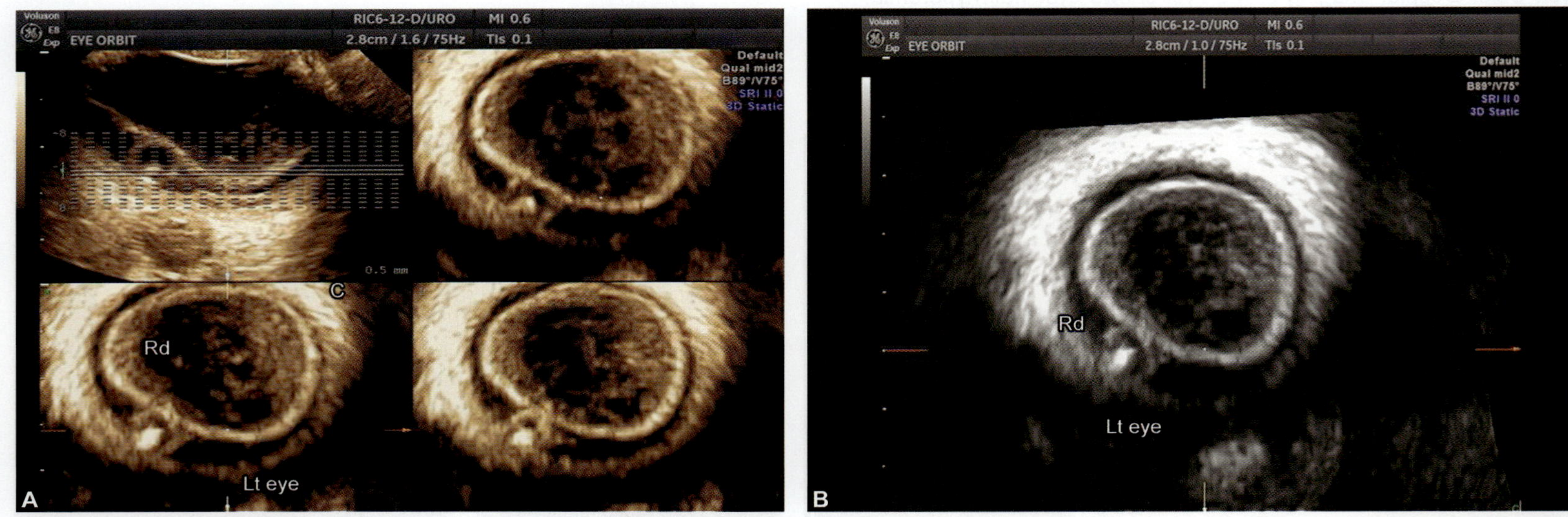

FIGURES 1.224A and B: Retinal detachment with cysticercus cyst. A patient presented with sudden loss of vision. HRSG shows a well defined cyst in subretinal space. The cyst shows echogenic nidus fixed with inner wall of cyst. The cyst results into lifting of retina causing total retinal detachment. On 3D TUI imaging, the total retinal detachment with cysticercus cyst is seen in the subretinal space clearly.

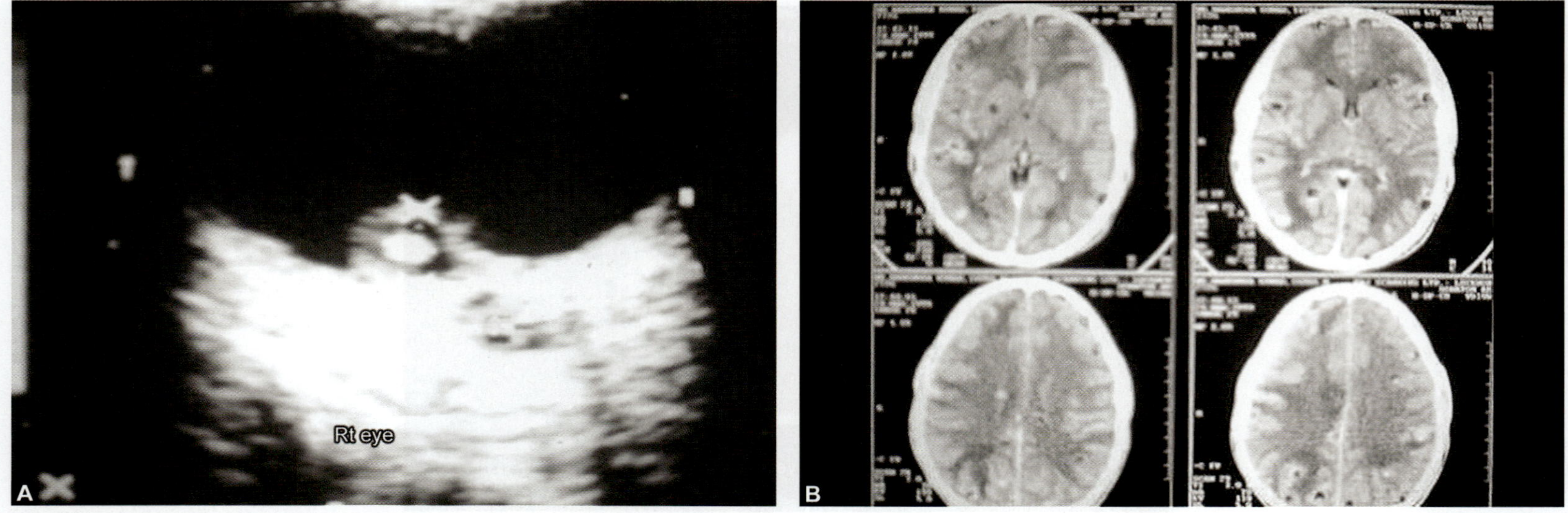

FIGURES 1.225A and B: Intraocular cysticercosis. The patient came with the history of painful eye with blurred vision and dementia. HRSG shows a well-defined cyst fixed above the optic nerve head with an echogenic nidus fixed with the inner wall of the cyst, typical sonographic feature of cysticercus cyst. CT scan head of the same patient shows multiple hypodense dot like shadows in the brain showing diffuse intracranial cysticercus cysts and it was the cause of dementia.

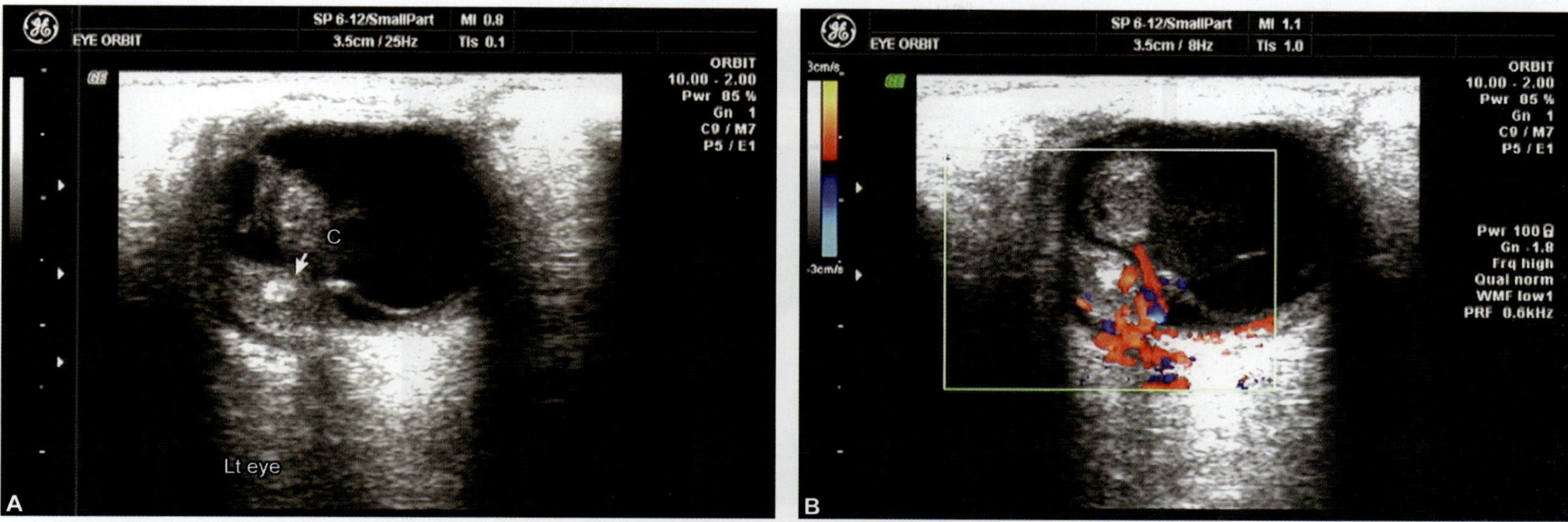

FIGURES 1.226A and B: Ruptured cysticercus cyst and subvitreal space. A patient presented with sudden loss of vision with painful eye. HRSG shows a ruptured cysticercus cyst in subvitreal space with associated intragel hemorrhage. On color flow imaging, increased hyperemia is seen in the ruptured cyst suggestive of recent rupture of the cyst.

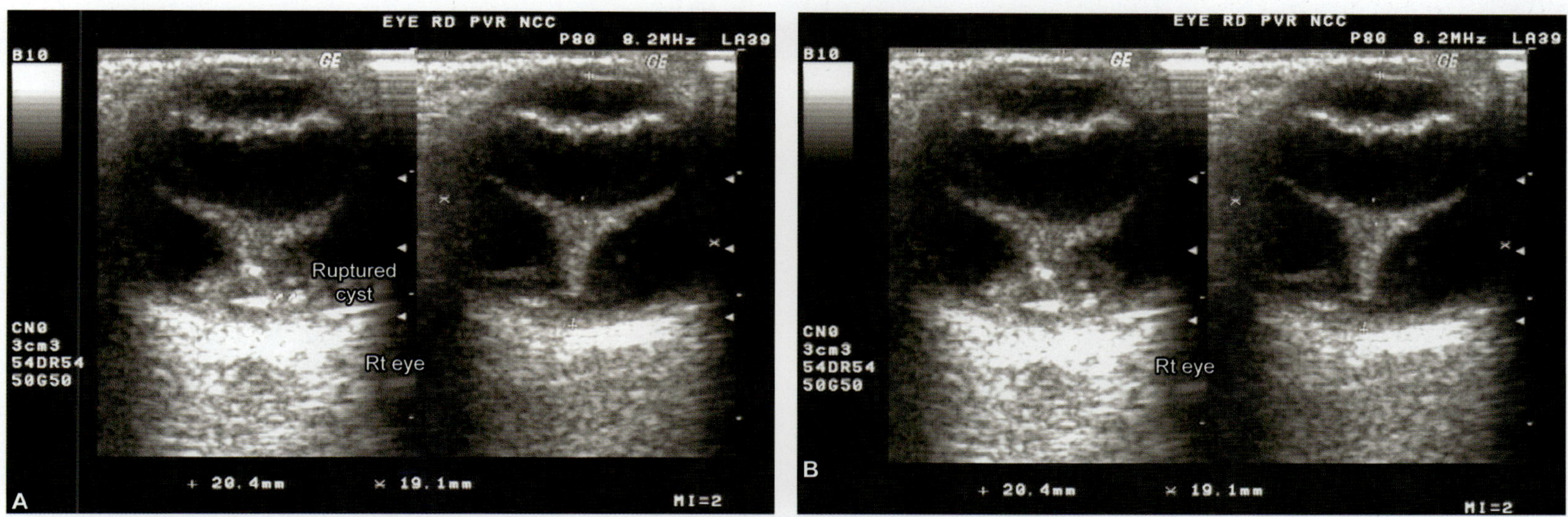

FIGURES 1.227A and B: HRSG shows collapsed flattened cyst with vitreoretinal bands in the same patient. Color flow imaging shows dragging of the vessels along the retinal membranes.

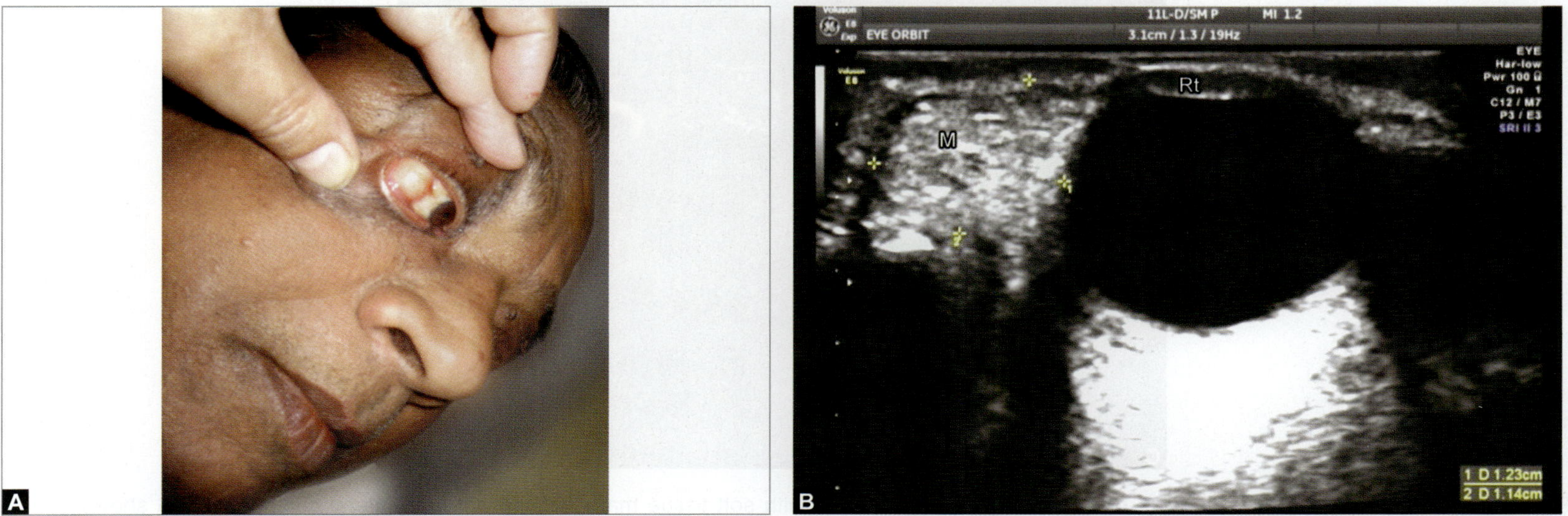

FIGURES 1.228A and B

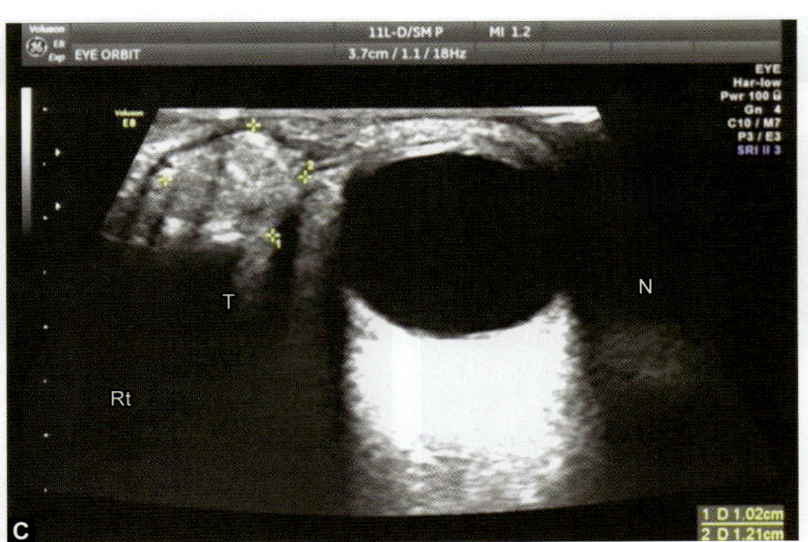

FIGURE 1.228C

FIGURES 1.228A to C: Lateral canthus dermoid. A patient presented with soft tissue swelling coming out from lateral canthus. HRSG shows a highly echogenic mass coming out from lateral canthus. It shows echogenic texture similar to the fat. Echogenic foci are also seen in it suggestive of dermoid cyst.

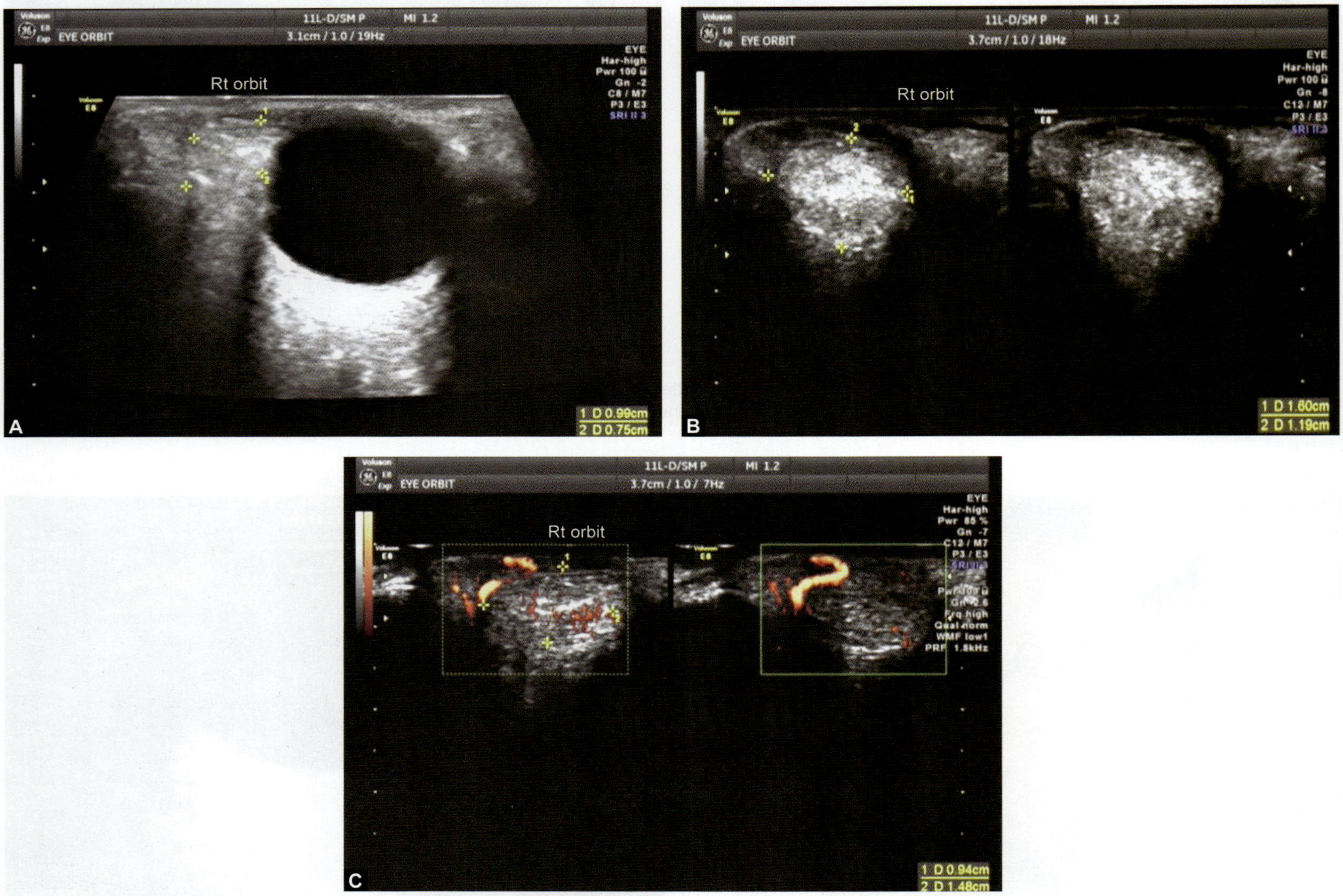

FIGURES 1.229A to C: Lateral canthus dermoid. A patient presented with soft tissue mass coming out from lateral canthus. HRSG shows a highly echogenic mass seen coming out from superior orbital quadrant on the left side. It shows echogenic fat in it. On color flow imaging, no flow is seen in it. However, a small vessel is seen encircling it suggestive of dermoid cyst.

EXAMINATION OF ORBIT

Introduction

Standardized high-resolution sonography (HRSG) of orbit is highly sophisticated and accurate method for detecting and differentiating orbital lesions. HRSG is rapid noninvasive screening method to examine orbital lesions. Dynamic examination of lesion by HRSG is the added advantage on other imaging modalities. However, computed tomography (CT) is the investigation of choice for orbital lesions, as it produces excellent tissue details of surrounding structures with clear delineation of anatomy. But, the major disadvantage of CT is time-consuming; delivering of radiation dose to eye and costly investigation. Ultrasonography has advantage of rapidity and easy accessibility. With its ability to identify the orbital walls, retrobulbar fat, ocular muscles, optic nerve and orbital mass, it is a useful first line of investigation in orbital diseases and proptosis.

The aim of orbital imaging is to demonstrate an orbital lesion, determine its position and extent within the orbit. At times, it becomes difficult to predict the pathological nature of lesion, as most of ultrasonographic features are nonspecific; therefore, clinical history is important.

Examination Technique

Short focus high-frequency transducers with frequency ranging from 5 MHz to 10 MHz are the ideal probes to examine the orbit. Direct contact method is the ideal technique. The examination is carried out in both transocular and paraocular approaches. The orbit is examined in transverse, axial and longitudinal views. Transocular method clearly delineates mid and posterior orbital masses. The paraocular approaches clearly demonstrate anterior lesions and relationship to the globe and orbital wall. The paraocular approach is used in both transverse and longitudinal directions. The orbit is examined in all four directions: superior, inferior, medial (nasal) and lateral (temporal).

Orbital Anatomy

The orbit is a bony socket, which contains eyeball, extrinsic muscles and optic nerve embedded in fat with vessels and nerves innervating the eyeball. The two eyeballs are the dominant structures in the orbit, which are not lying along the axis of orbit. They face forward and lie parallel to each other. The optic nerve is echo poor in texture, which lies freely in the retrobulbar fat which is highly echogenic. Intraorbital part of optic nerve length is around 25 mm, whereas orbital length is around 18 to 20, thus allows free movement of eye. HRSG can show the whole length of optic nerve in the orbit with careful examination. It can be seen longitudinally and transversely as oval hypoechoic shadow. The four recti muscles arise from a tendinous ring at the apex broaden out to form a cone of muscles around the eyeball.

The orbital muscles are seen as thin, echo poor straps. These tendons are narrowed anteriorly and muscle belly is more fusiform in shape. The medial and lateral recti are seen best in horizontal planes and superior and inferior recti are seen in vertical planes. The inferior oblique muscle is seen behind the globe just below the macula. The superior oblique is seen in superomedial part of the orbit. Its sonoappearance is similar to the recti muscle appearance.

Proptosis

Anterior displacement of the eyeball due to retrobulbar pathology can be easily evaluated on HRSG. The retrobulbar masses, which can be detected well on HRSG are grouped as under.

i. Muscle hypertrophy in thyroid disease.
ii. Pseudotumors-inflammatory orbital disease.
iii. Vascular tumors
   1. Hemangioma
   2. AV malformations
   3. Orbital varix
   4. Lymphangioma
   5. Dilated superior ophthalmic vein.
iv. Parasitic infestations
   1. Cysticercosis
   2. Hydatid cysts.
v. Optic nerve tumors-glioma
   1. Meningioma
   2. Optic nerve cyst
   3. Optic nerve glioma.
vi. Rhabdomyosarcoma.
vii. Lymphoproliferative masses.
viii. Lymphoma.
ix. Metastatic deposits in the orbit.
x. Orbital trauma.
   1. Orbital hematoma.

Pseudoproptosis

Increased axial length of the eye ball in congenital and acquired conditions is seen in pseudoproptosis.

Vascular Tumors of Orbit

Many vascular tumors are found in the orbit. It is one of the most common causes of proptosis. HRSG is excellent modality to diagnose vascular tumors. Color Doppler flow study can easily differentiate between venous or arterial nature of the tumor mass.

Hemangiomas

Orbital hemangioma (cavernous type) are common in adult. They are benign in nature. They occur in second to fifth decade of life. Clinically, they are characterized with slowly progressive swelling of eyeball with unilateral proptosis. HRSG shows a highly reflective echogenic mass in retrobulbar space which is seen located in the muscle cone. The multiple interfaces of dilated capillary walls produce an echogenic mass. Doppler examination gives a good account of blood flow in the mass.

Arteriovenous Fistulae

These may develop after trauma or spontaneously. They are often missed clinically. Therefore, HRSG is useful investigation to diagnose them. Doppler examination is helpful in diagnosing small fistulae.

Orbital Varices

These are usually diagnosed clinically. They often exacerbate with bending of head or valsalva maneuver. These patients ultimately land up in endophthalmitis most likely due to fat necrosis.

Lymphangioma

These are mostly detected in children or young adults. These lesions grow slowly and causing proptosis. They may present as acute onset due to spontaneous secondary hemorrhage. These tumors can be small or large enough to fill the orbital space. On HRSG, multiple dilated septate lymph-filled spaces are seen in retrobulbar areas. A multiloculated multiseptate mass is seen with echogenic septa. If hemorrhage is present in the tumor, low to medium level echoes are seen in the dilated spaces. Decompression of lymphangioma at times becomes necessary and "B" scan imaging is used to guide the aspiration needle.

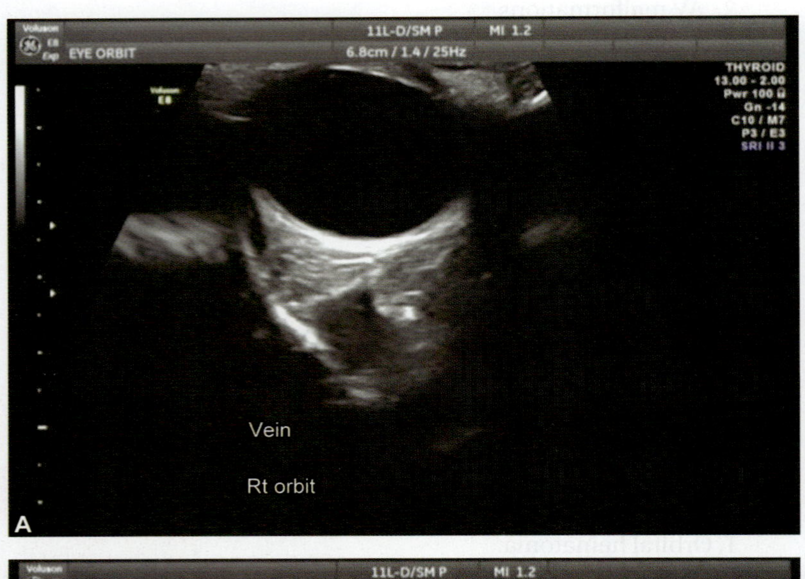

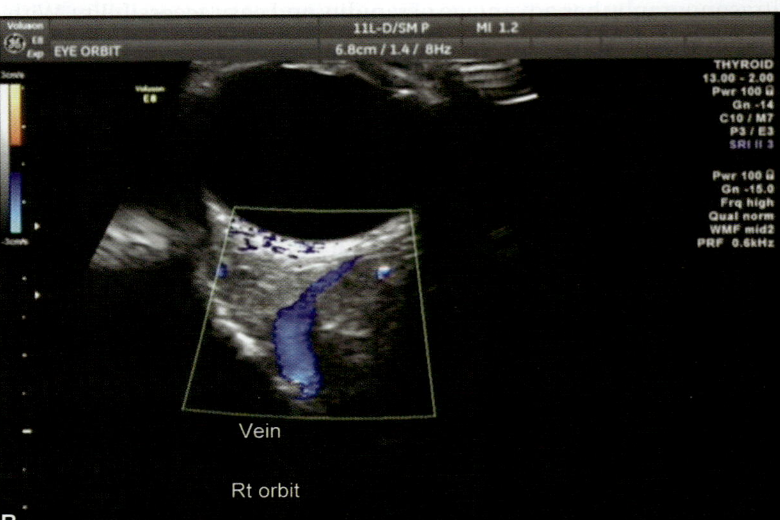

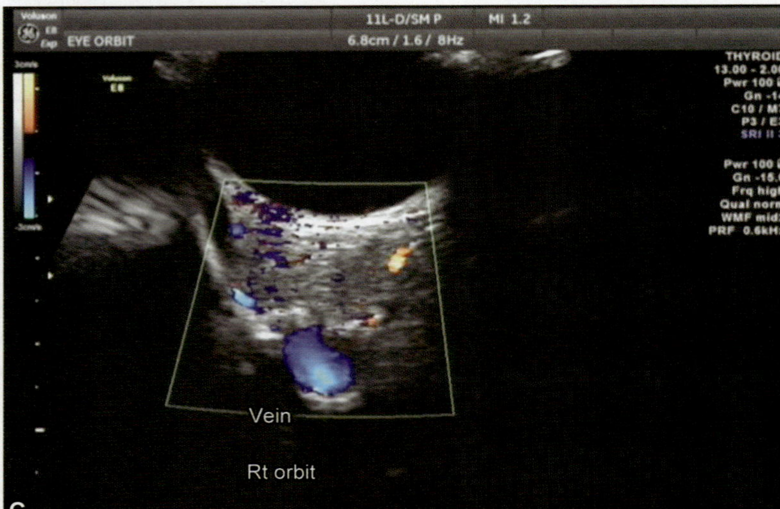

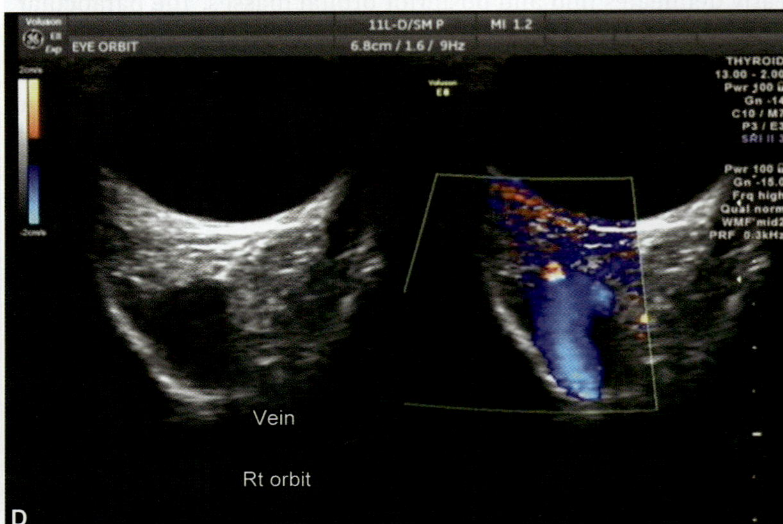

FIGURES 1.230A to D

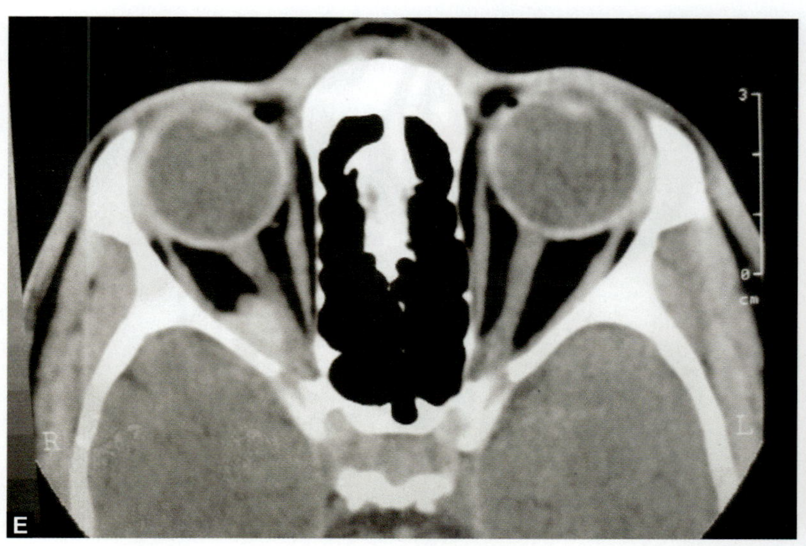

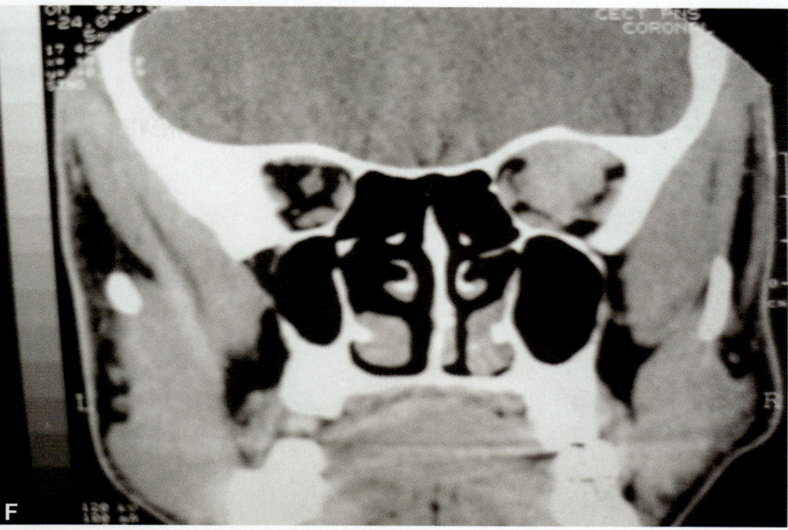

FIGURES 1.230E and F

FIGURES 1.230A to F: Dilated ophthalmic vein. A patient presented with proptosis and discomfort in right eye. HRSG shows a dilated vein in the intraconal part of orbit. On color flow imaging, it is dilated superior ophthalmic vein. The contrast CT scan of the same patient confirms the ultrasound findings.

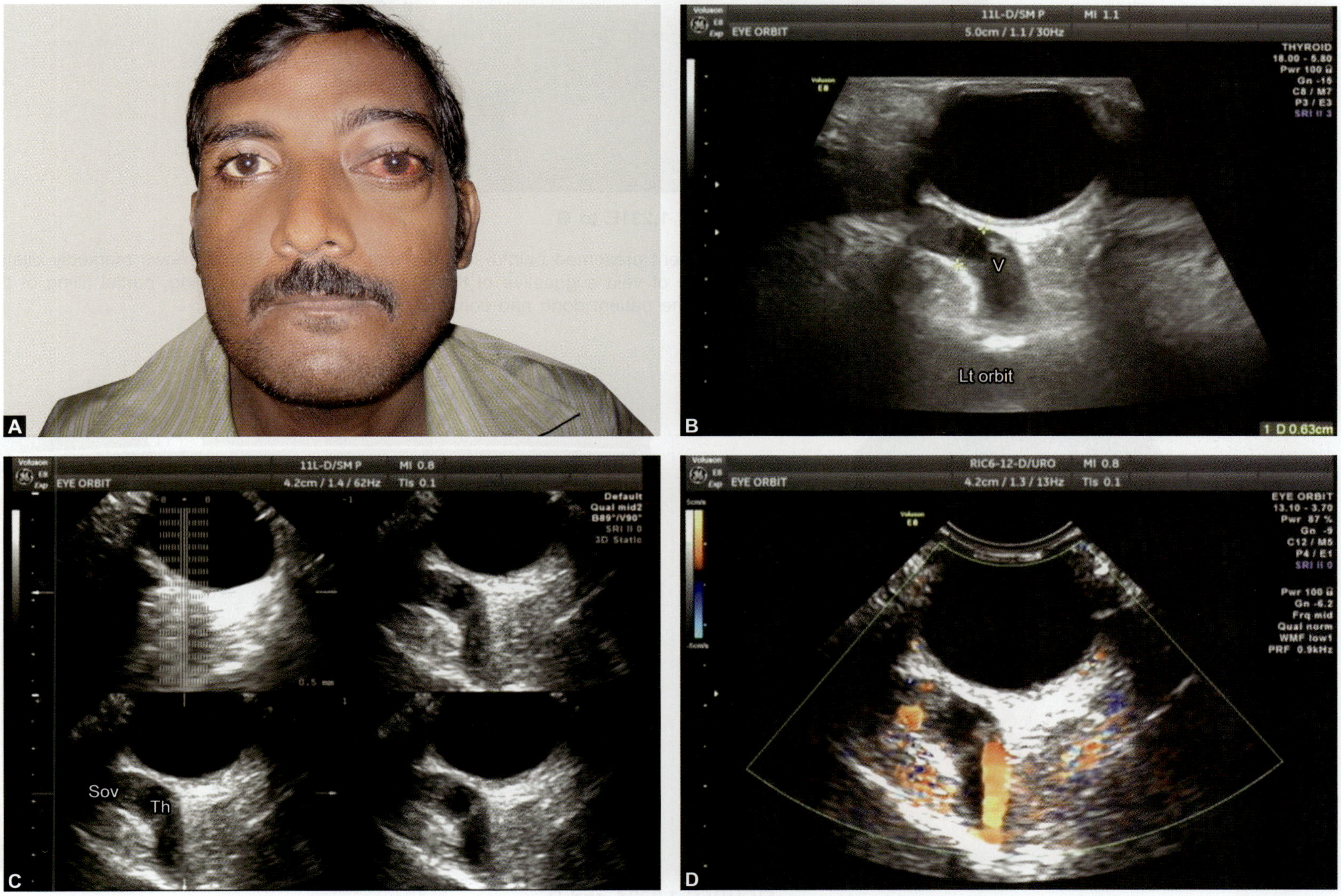

FIGURES 1.231A to D

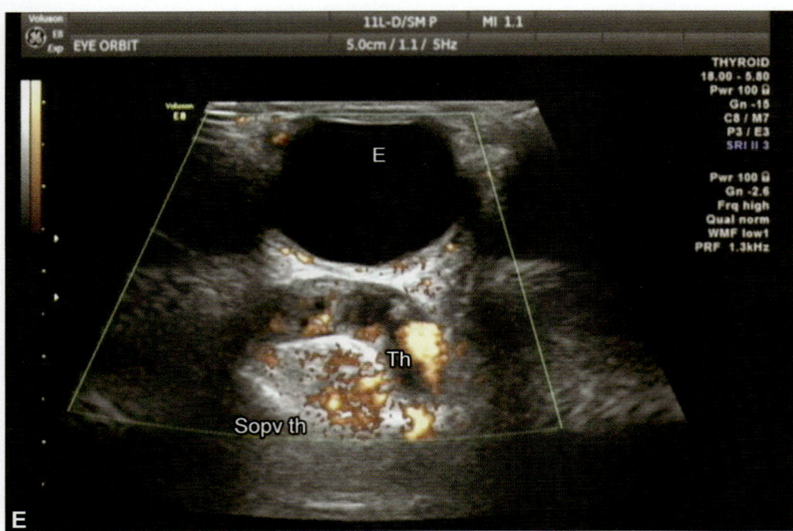

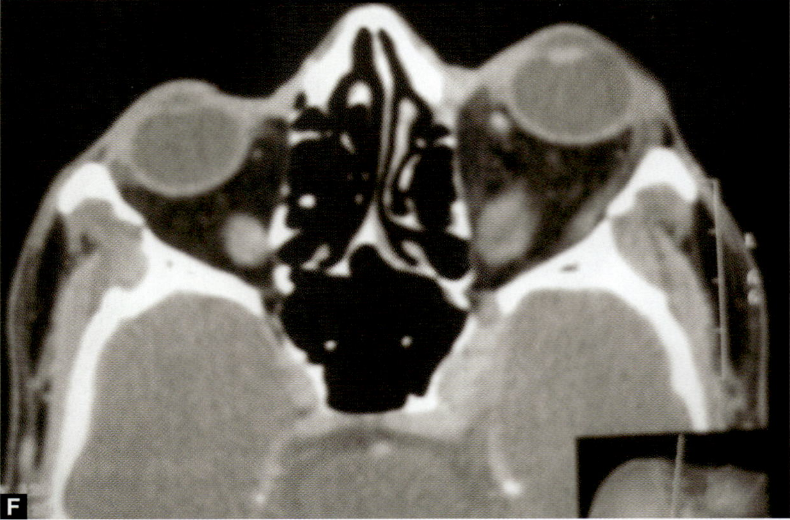

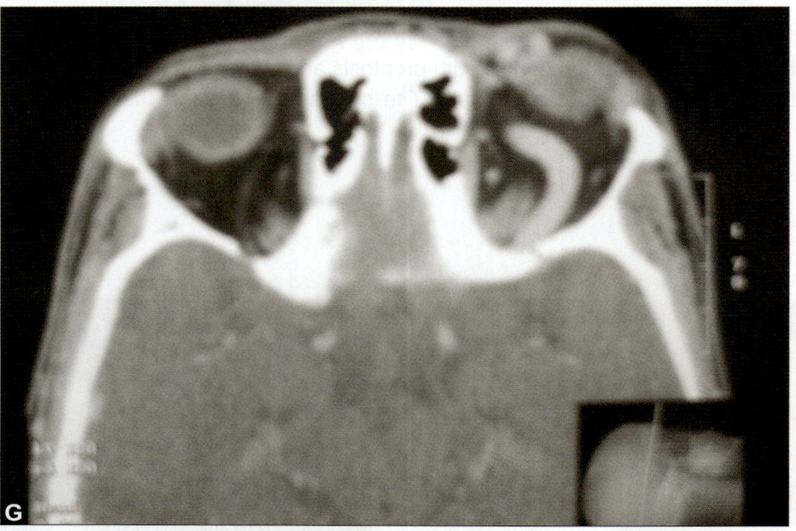

FIGURES 1.231E to G

FIGURES 1.231A to G: Superior ophthalmic vein thrombosis. A patient presented painful left eye with proptosis. HRSG shows markedly dilated superior ophthalmic vein. Echogenic shadows are seen filling the lumen of vein suggestive of thrombus. On color flow imaging, partial filling of the lumen is seen because of the thrombus in the vein. CT scan of the same patient done and confirms the ultrasound findings.

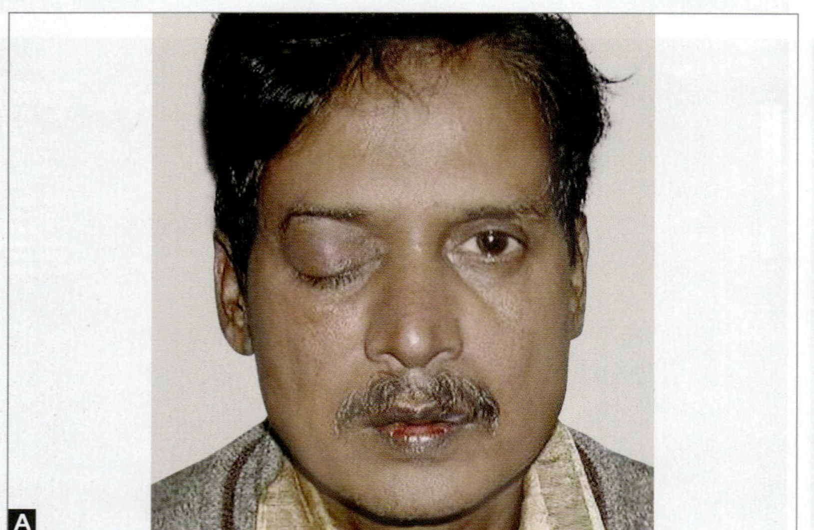

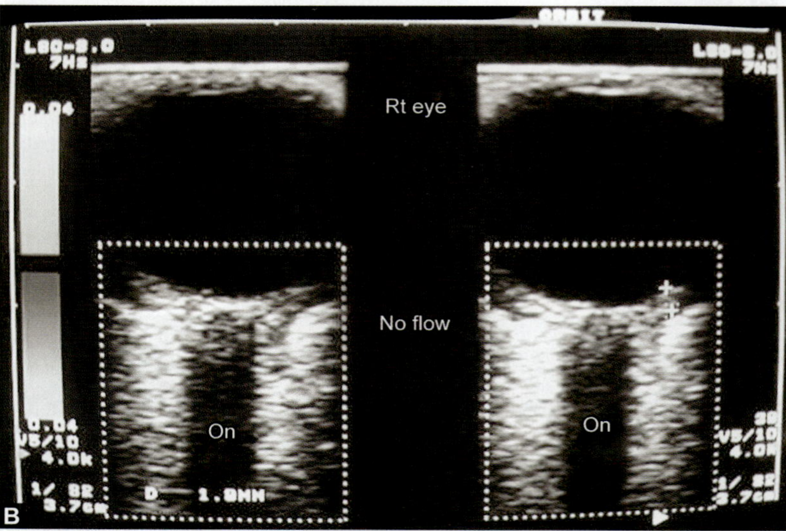

FIGURES 1.232A and B

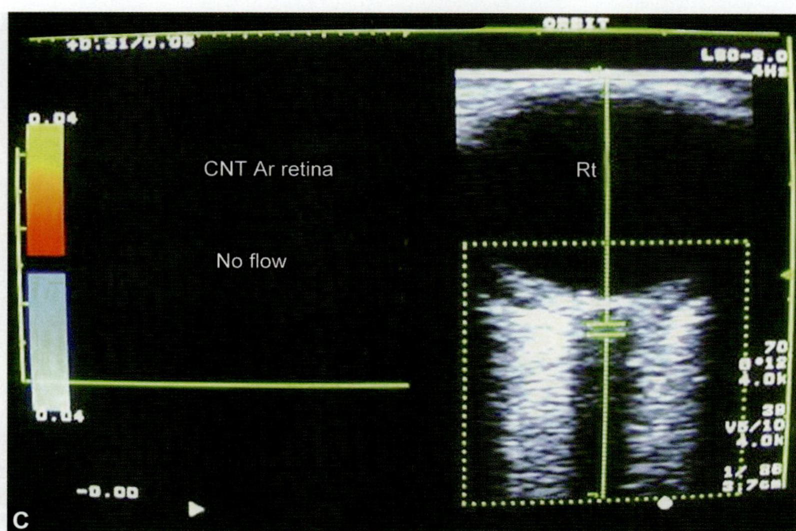

FIGURE 1.232C

FIGURES 1.232A to C: Central artery retina thrombosis. A middle-aged man presented with sudden lose of vision and painful swollen right eye. HRSG and color flow imaging show hypoechoic edematous optic nerve with no flow seen in central artery of retina suggestive of: central artery of retina occlusion. It is confirmed on Duplex Doppler study. Color Doppler study shows no flow in left orbit no flow in right central artery of retina. However, normal flow is seen in left central artery retina.

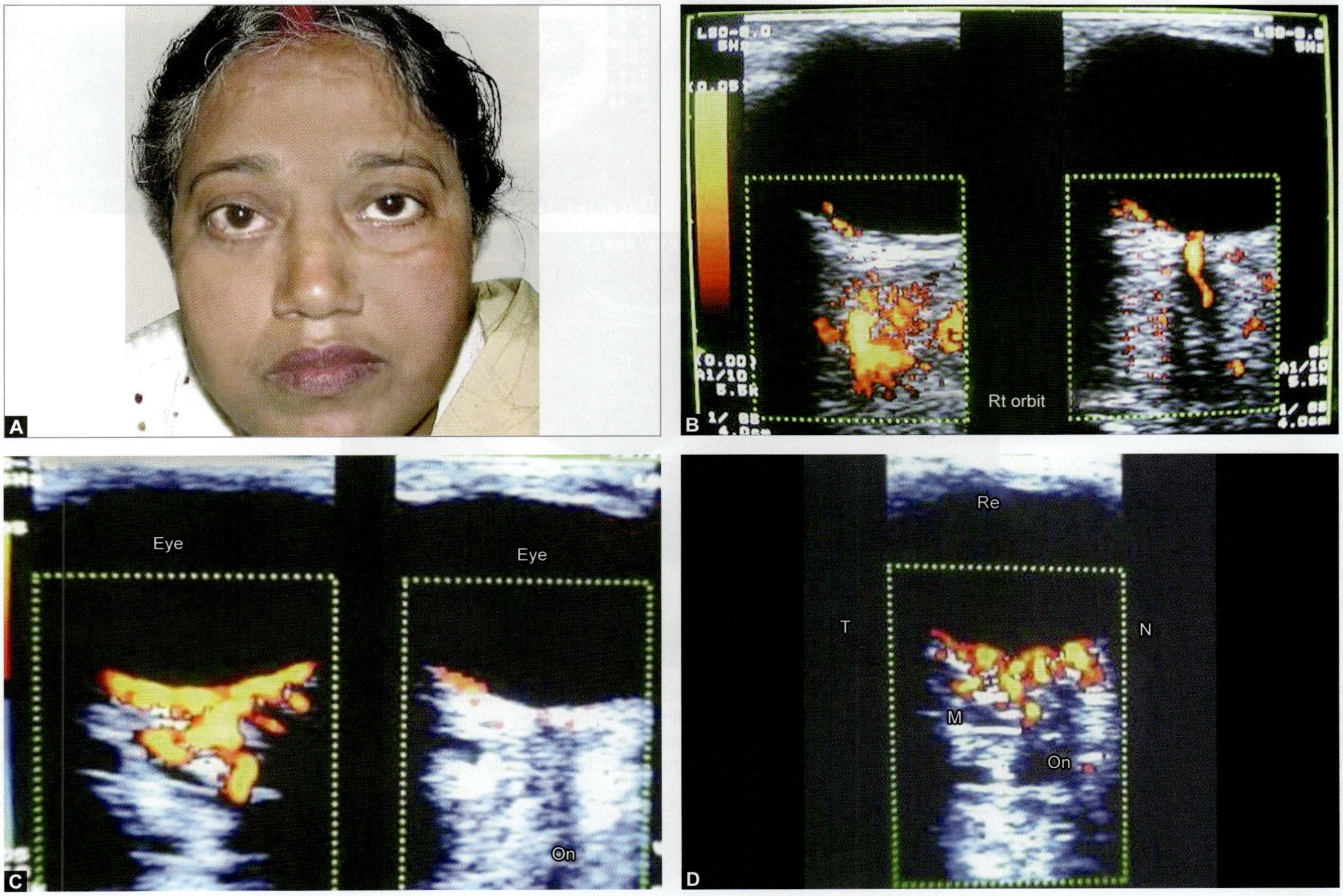

FIGURES 1.233A to D: Orbital varix. Multiple-detailed vessels are seen in retrobulbar intraconal area suggestive of orbital varix. On color Doppler flow, low venous flow is seen in them. Multiple-dilated vessels are seen in right retrobulbar space in a patient with the history of proptosis on persistent bending of the head. Color Doppler shows multiple dilated vessels distended on drooping of the head. Confirms orbital varices.

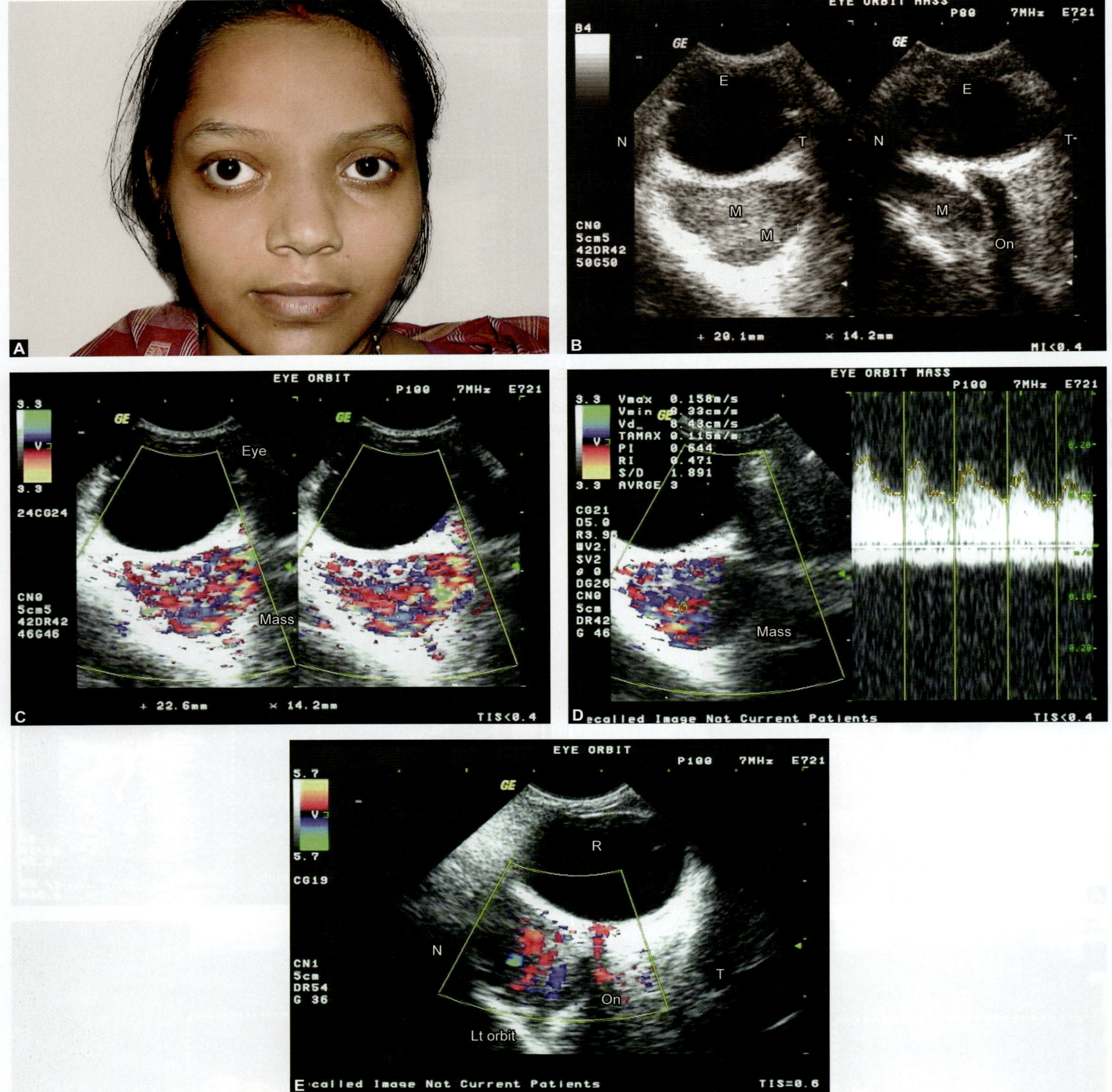

FIGURES 1.234A to E: Cavernous hemangioma. A young lady came with the history of proptosis in right eye with blurring of vision. HRSG shows a low-level echo complex mass in intraconal part of right orbit. Multiple fine thin interfaces are seen in the mass. The mass is seen pressing over the optic nerve and displacing it to the opposite side. a smooth indentation is seen over the nerve. No evidence of any calcification is seen in the mass. Color Doppler flow imaging show multiple dilated vessels seen in the mass with high flow pattern. Spectral Doppler flow shows high flow with arterial pulsation in the mass suggestive of cavernous hemangioma.

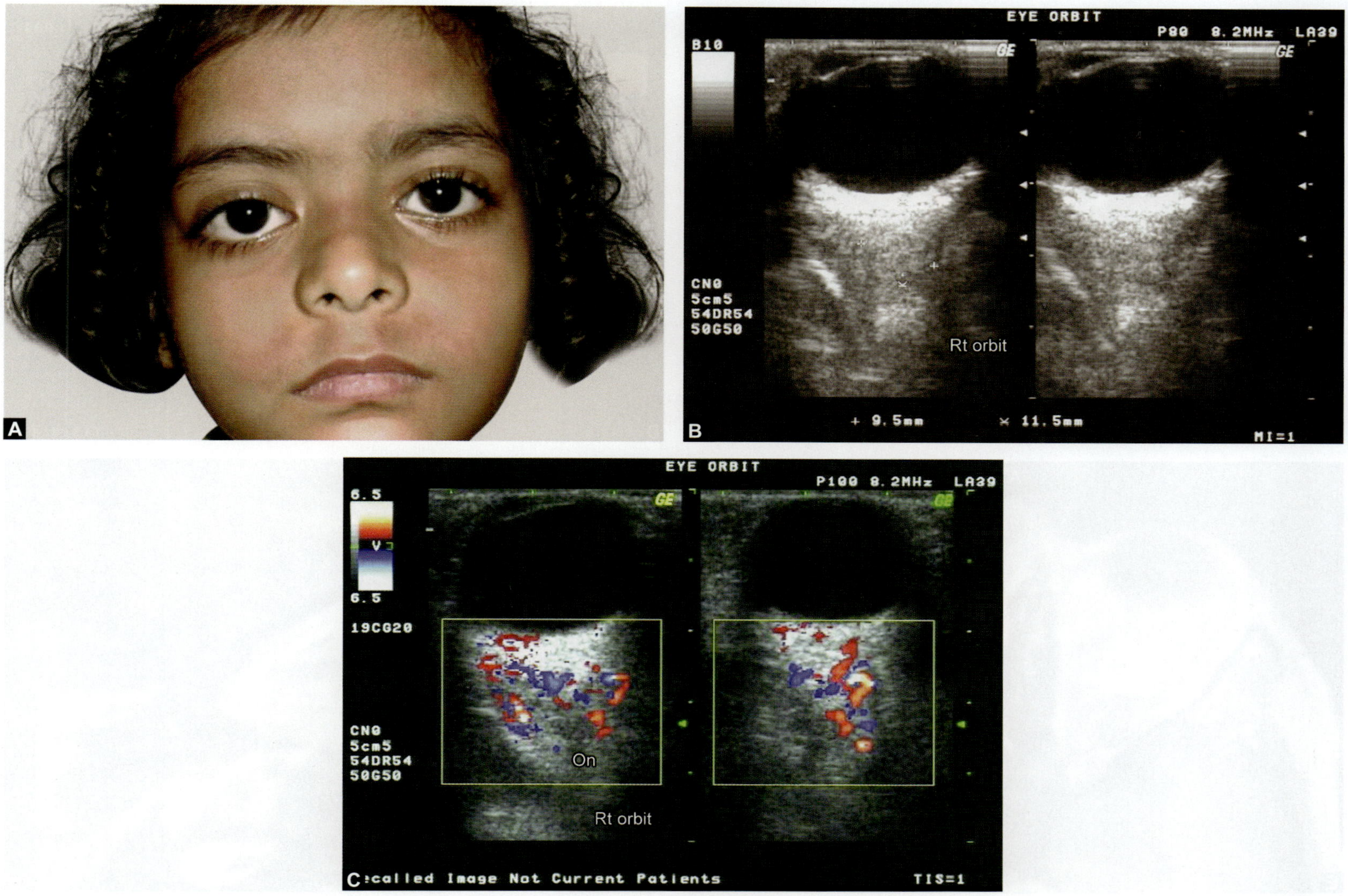

FIGURES 1.235A to C: Young girl complains of proptosis left eye with no pain but diplopia. HRSG shows well-defined intraconal mass with homogeneous texture. On color flow imaging moderate flow is seen in the mass suggestive of hemangioma.

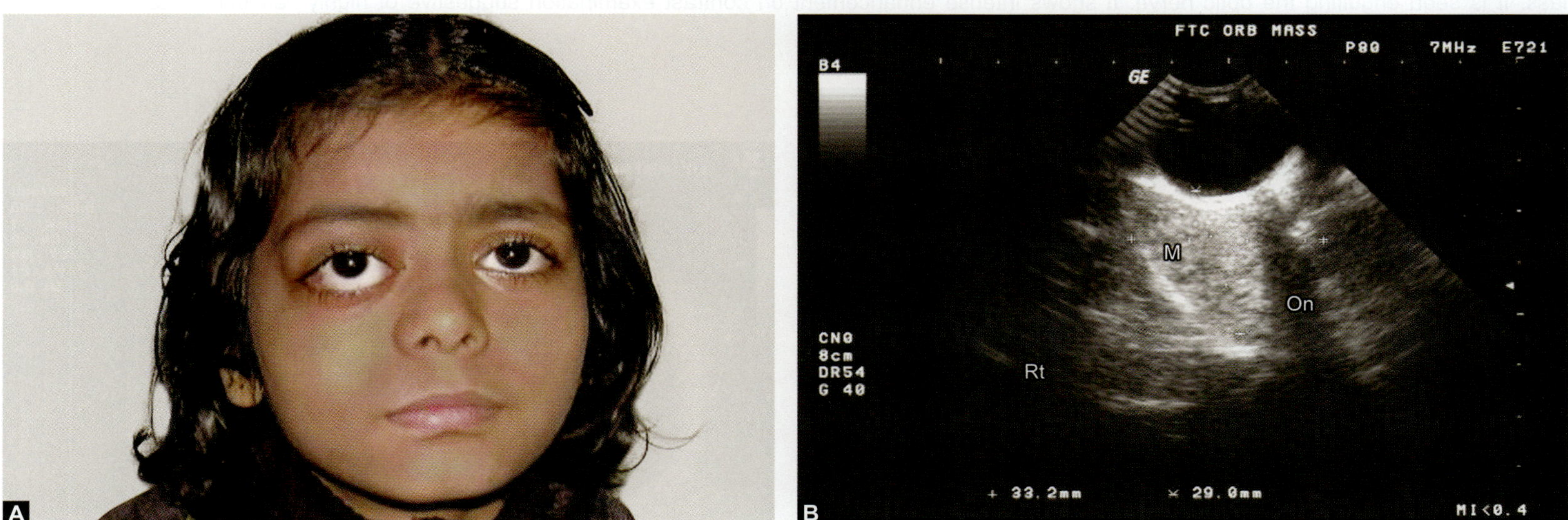

FIGURES 1.236A and B

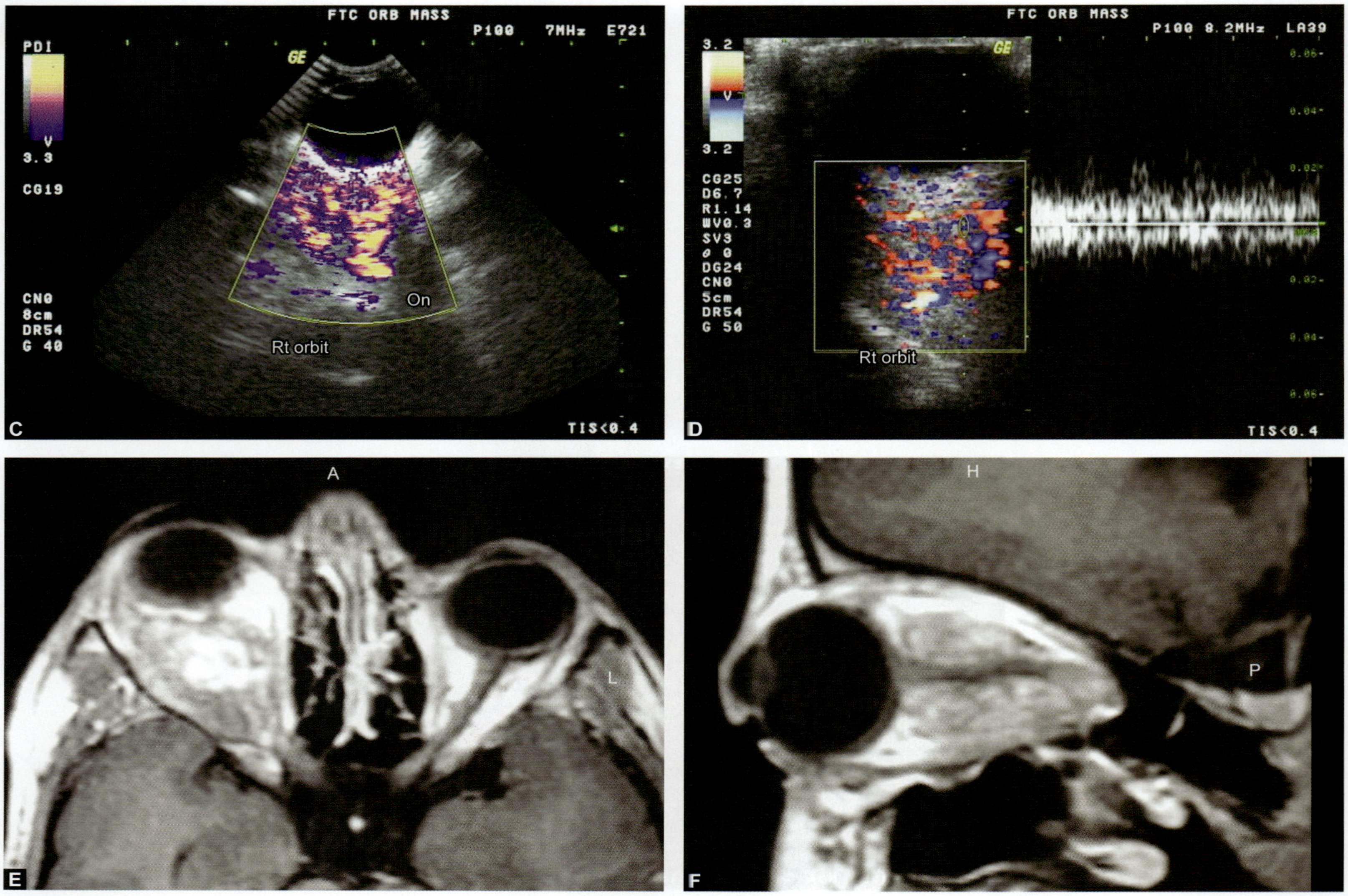

FIGURES 1.236C to F

FIGURES 1.236A to F: The same girl after 3 years presented with persistent proptosis with diplopia. HRSG shows echogenic mass in the intraconal part of the orbit. It is seen pressing and displacing the optic nerve. On color Doppler imaging multiple small vessels are seen in the mass suggestive of highly vascular mass. On spectral Doppler tracing low flow is seen in the mass. Contrast enhanced MRI of the same patient shows intraconal mass. It is seen engulfing the optic nerve. It shows intense enhancement on contrast examination suggestive of highly vascular mass.

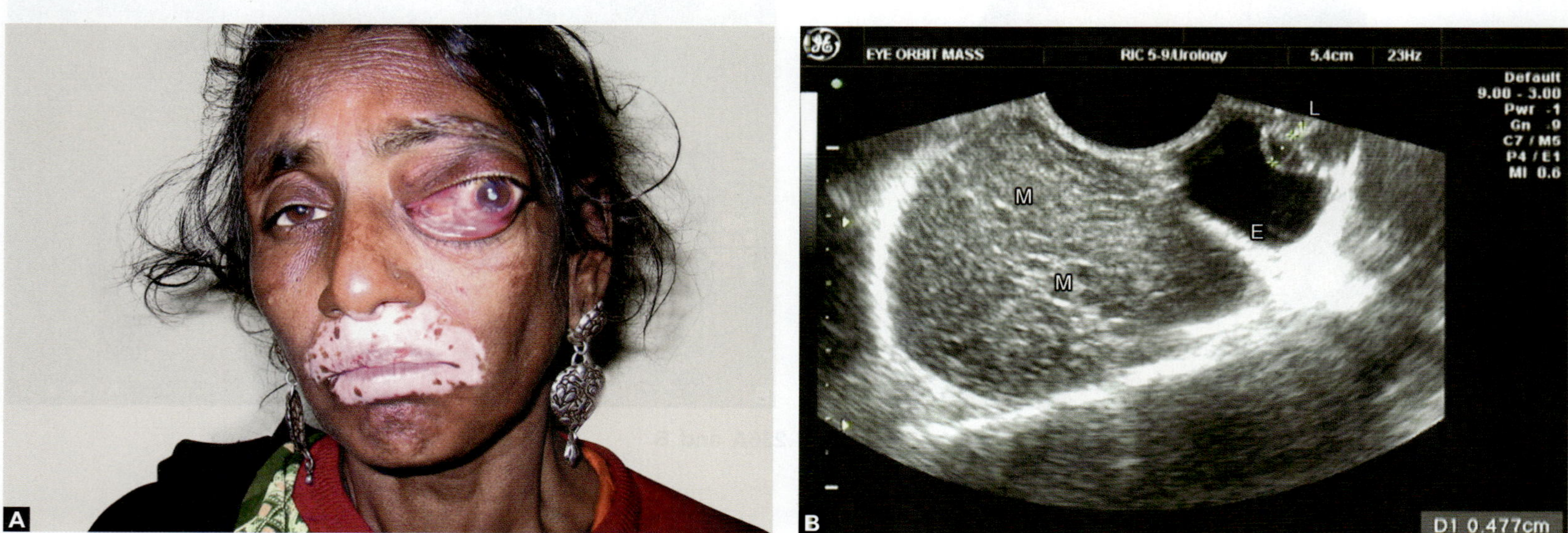

FIGURES 1.237A and B

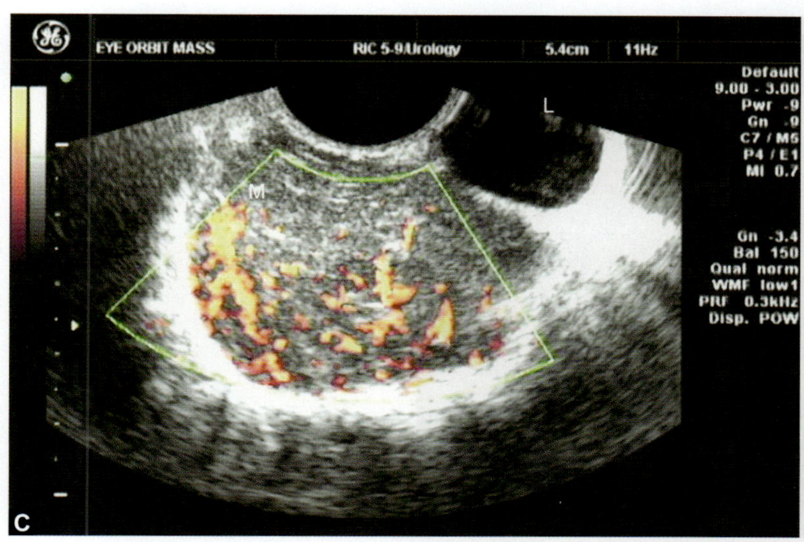

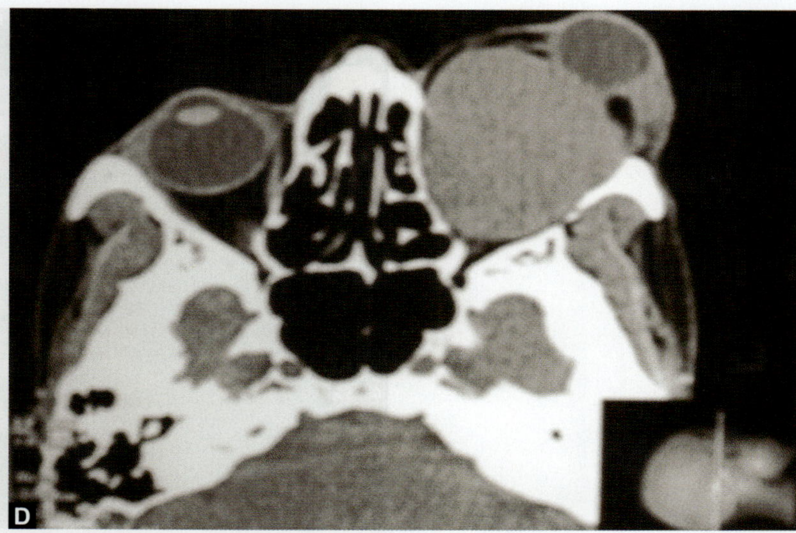

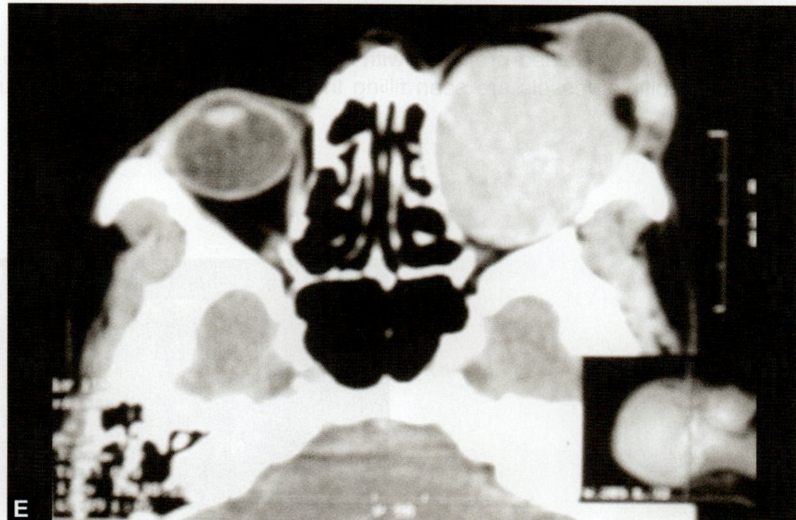

FIGURES 1.237C to E

FIGURES 1.237A to E: Big vascular mass. A middle-aged lady presented with marked proptosis with lateral displacement of left eye. HRSG shows a big mass with medium level echoes in the retrobulbar space of the left eye. The mass is seen pressing and displacing of the eyeball. It is also seen extending in to extra conal space. Multiple small cystic areas are seen in the mass. On color flow imaging, multiple vessels are seen feeding the mass they are running to the mass suggestive of vascular mass. CT scan of the same patient shows a big homogeneous hypodense mass in the left retrobulbar space. The mass shows intense enhancement on contrast examination confirming the vascular nature of the mass.

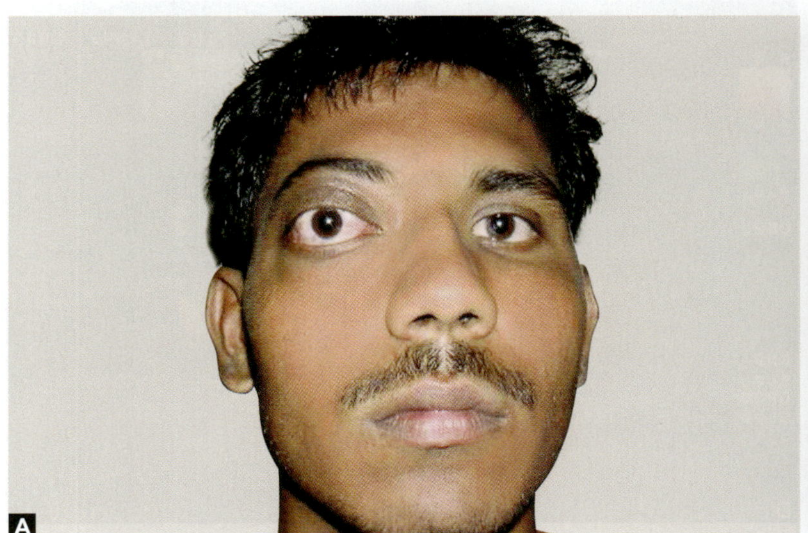

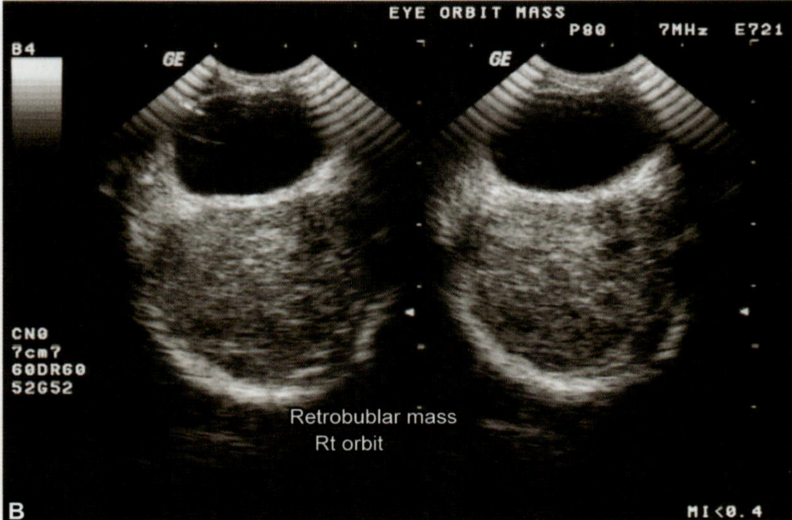

FIGURES 1.238A and B

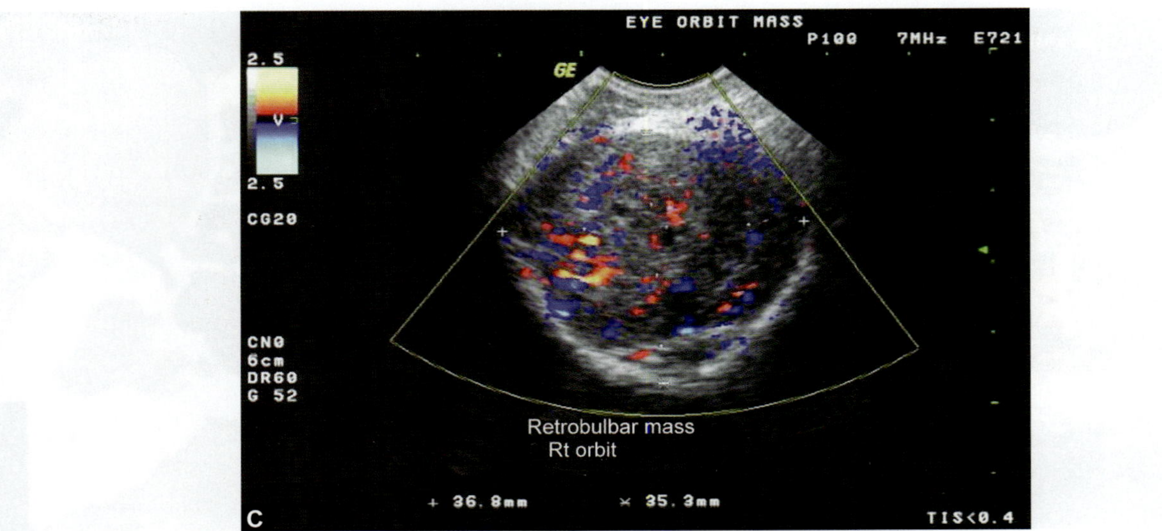

FIGURE 1.238C

FIGURES 1.238A to C: A young man presented with right-sided proptosis with diplopia. HRSG shows a big low-level echo complex mass filling whole of the retrobulbar space. On color flow imaging, multiple vessels are seen filling the mass suggestive of vascular nature of the mass big hemangioma.

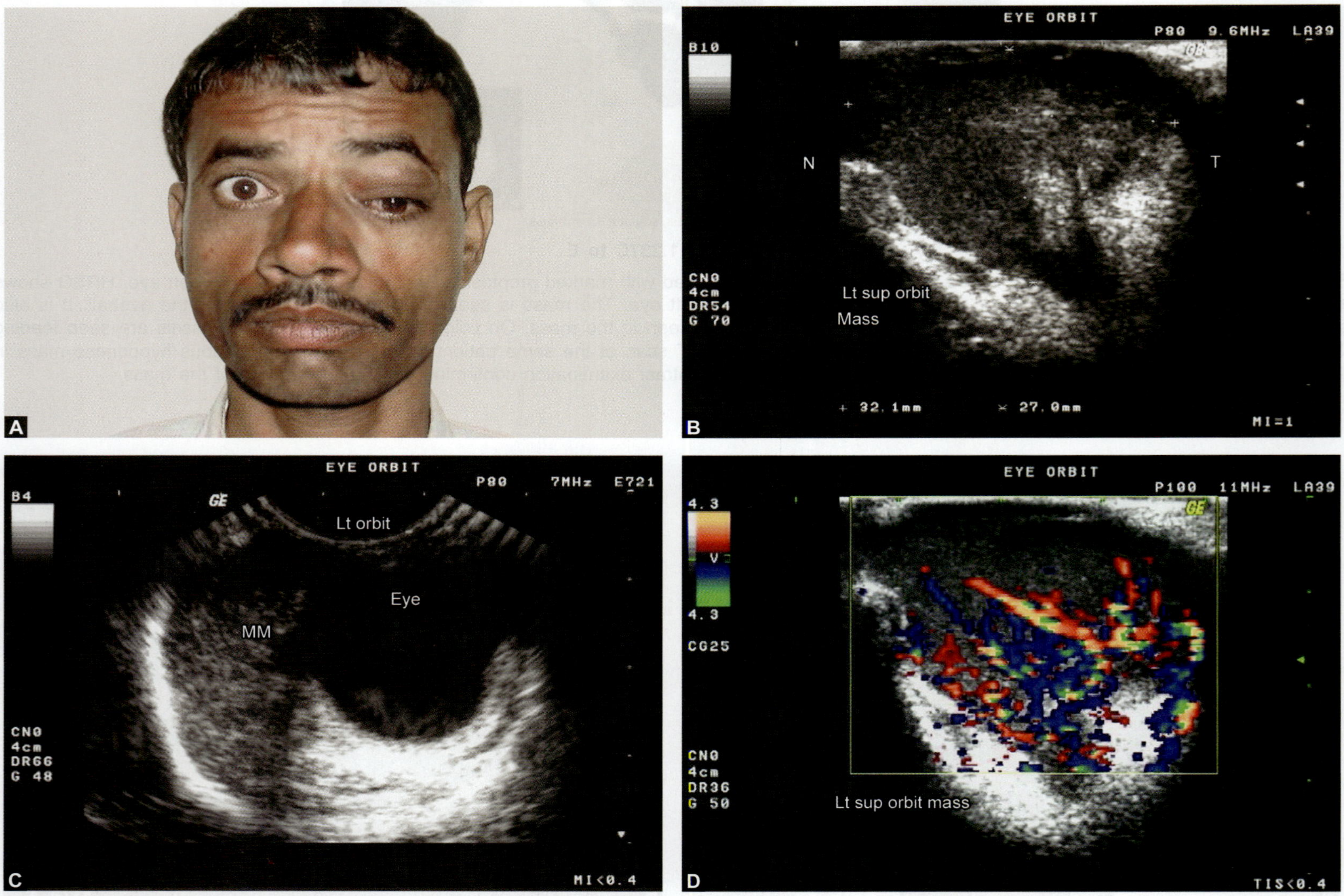

FIGURES 1.239A to D

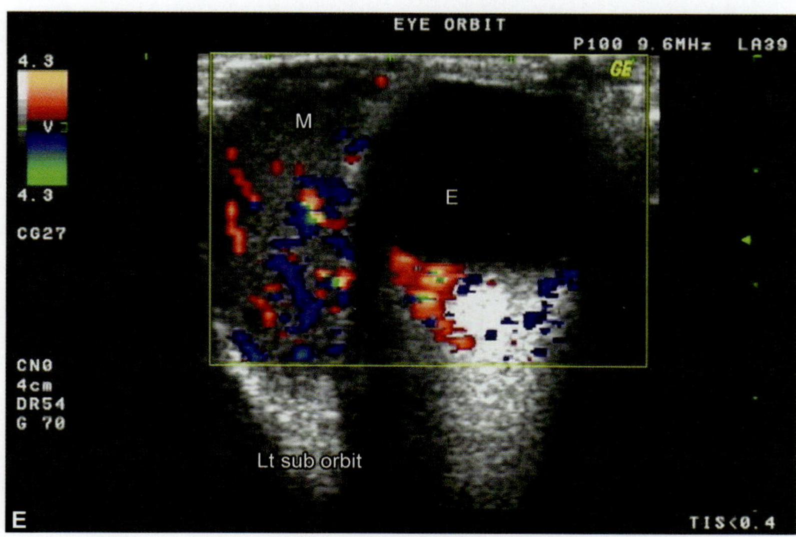

FIGURE 1.239E

FIGURES 1.239A to E: A man presented with soft tissue mass coming out from the superior part of the left orbit with downward displacement of the left eye. HRSG shows a low-level echo complex mass coming out from the superior quadrant of the left orbit. It shows homogeneous echoes and small tiny cysts. On color flow imaging, multiple vessels are seen feeding the mass suggestive of vascular nature of the mass.

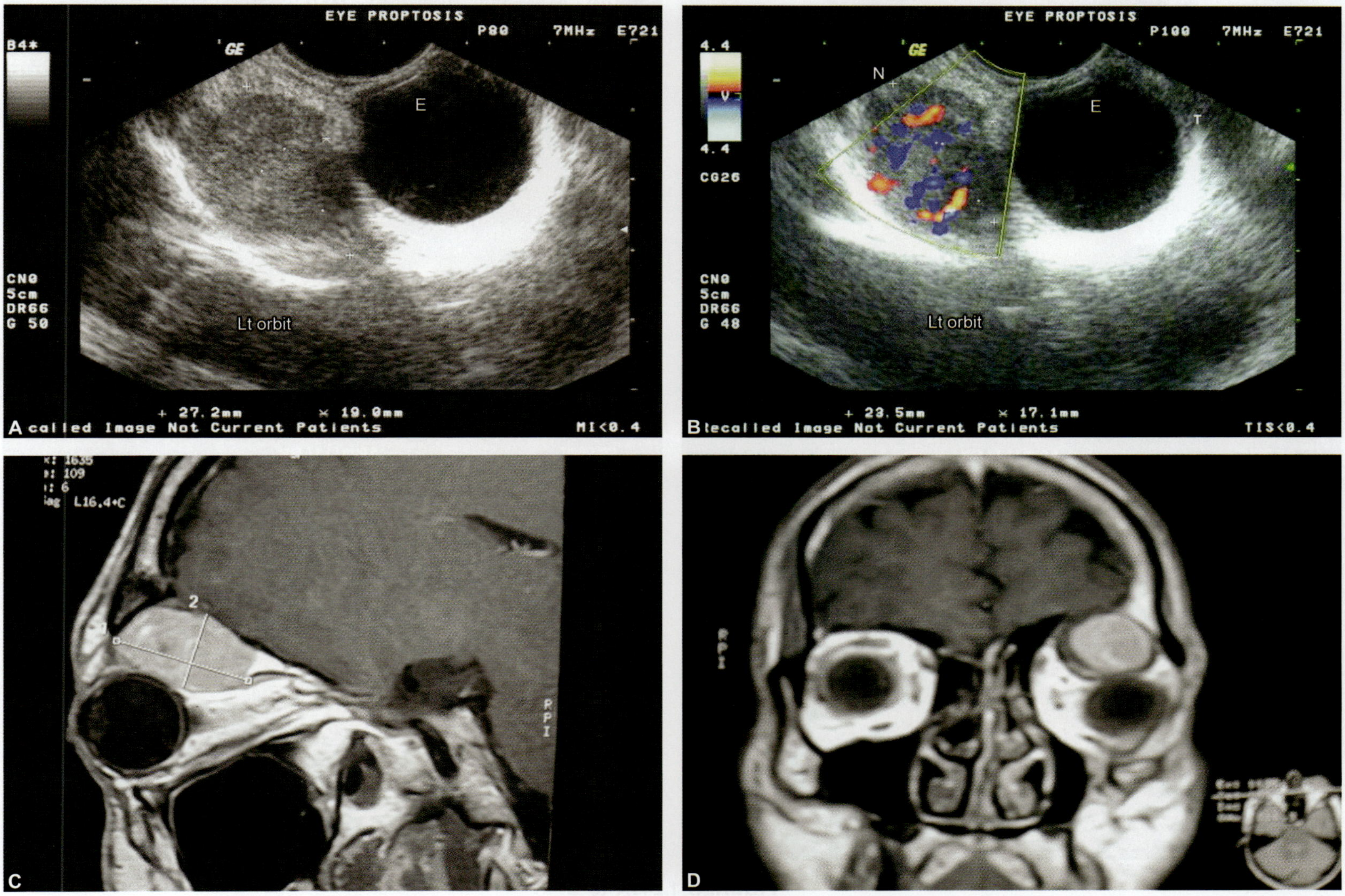

FIGURES 1.240A to D

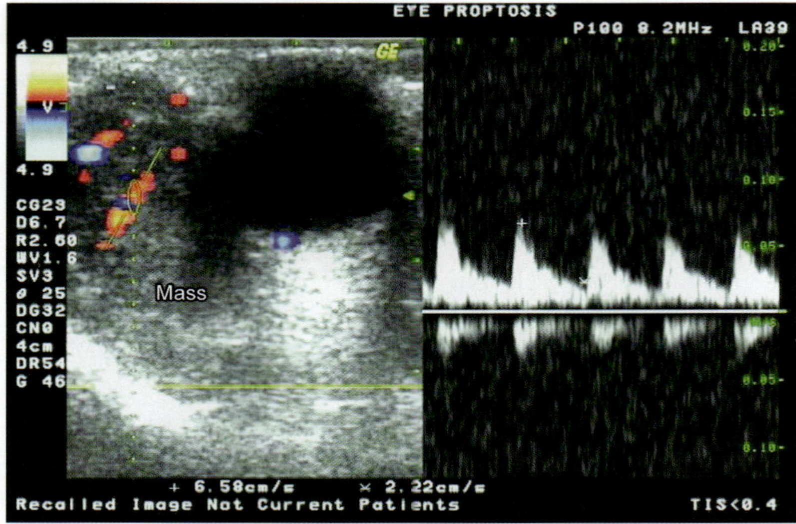

FIGURE 1.240E

FIGURES 1.240A to E: Retrobulbar vascular mass. HRSG shows well-defined lobulated mass seen coming out from superior quadrant of left orbit with down ward displacement of eyeball. On color flow imaging moderate flow is seen in the mass. MRI of the same patient shows homogeneous mass in superior quadrant. Spectral Doppler tracing shows arterial flow in the mass.

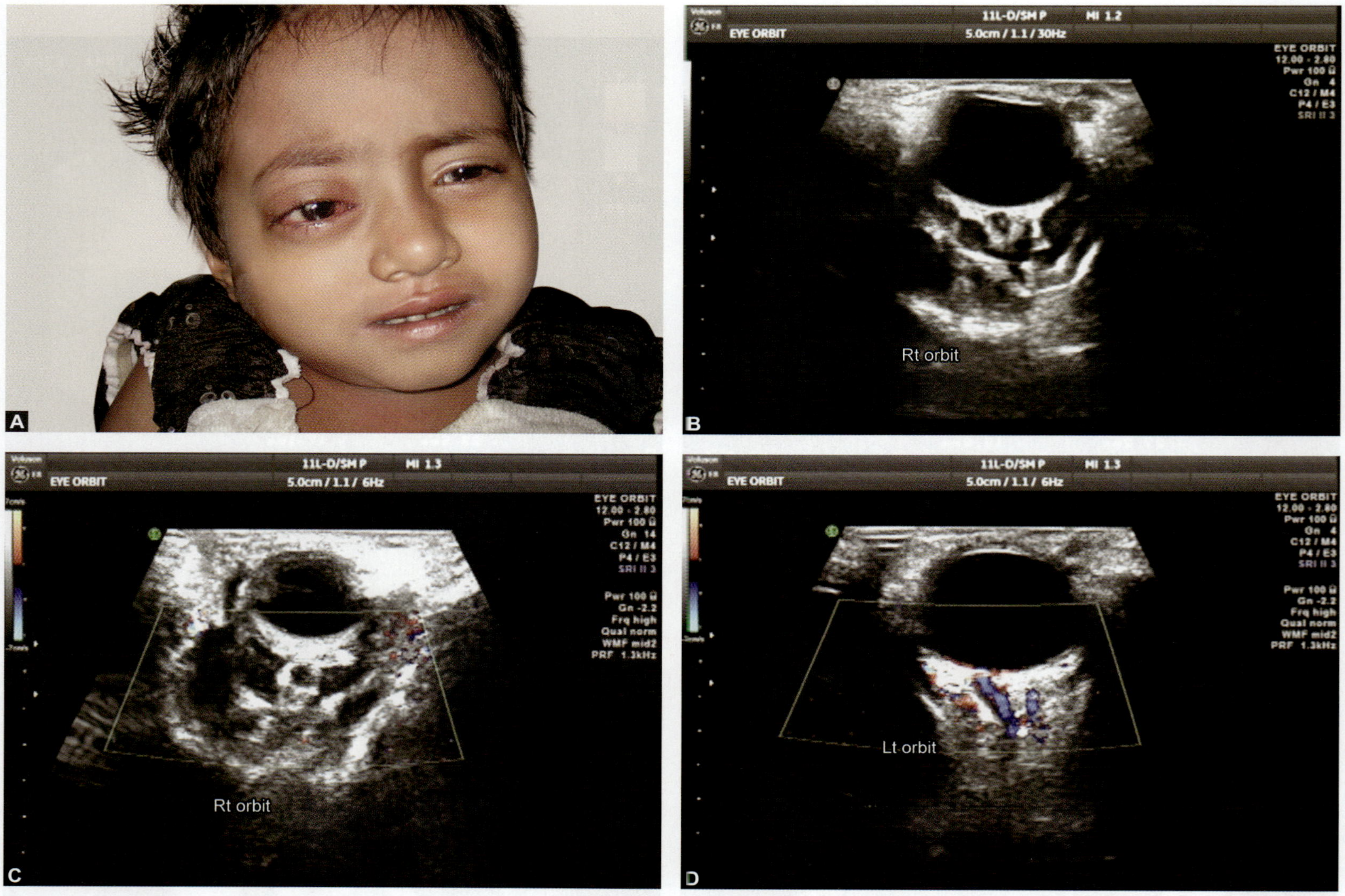

FIGURES 1.241A to D

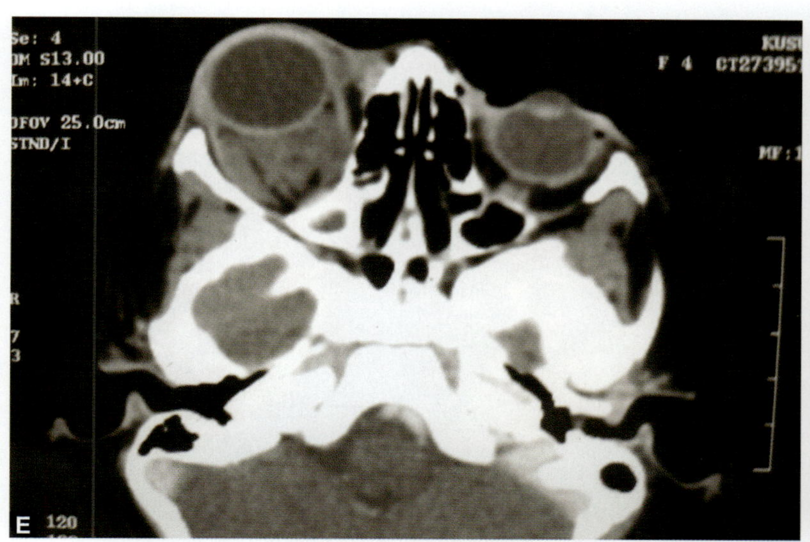

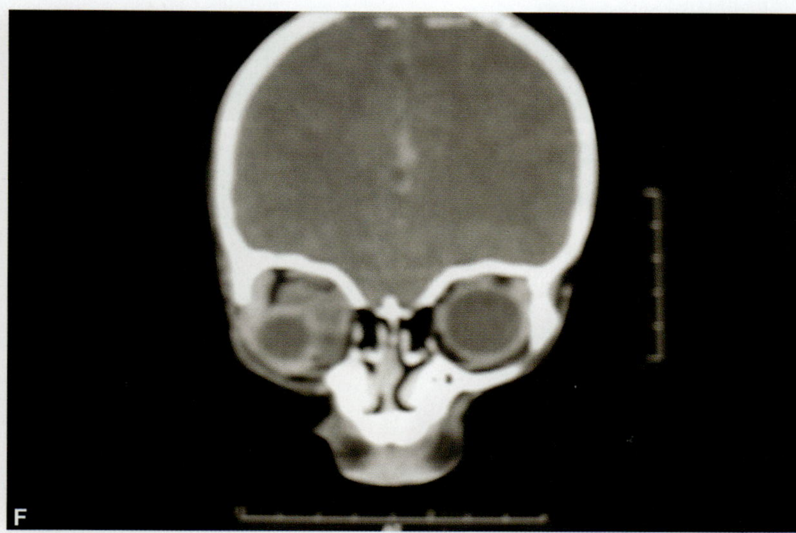

FIGURES 1.241E and F

FIGURES 1.241A to F: Lymphangioma. A young child presented with right eye proptosis. HRSG shows multiloculated cystic mass in the posterior segment of the eye. The mass shows multiple septa. Thick echoes are seen in the mass. On color flow imaging, poor flow is seen in it. The mass is seen confined in the intraconal part of the orbit. It is seen pushing the eye anteriorly and downward. The optic nerve is not engulfed by the mass. However, the pressure is seen on orbital vessels. Findings are suggestive of retrobulbar lymphangioma. CT scan of the same patient confirms ultrasound findings.

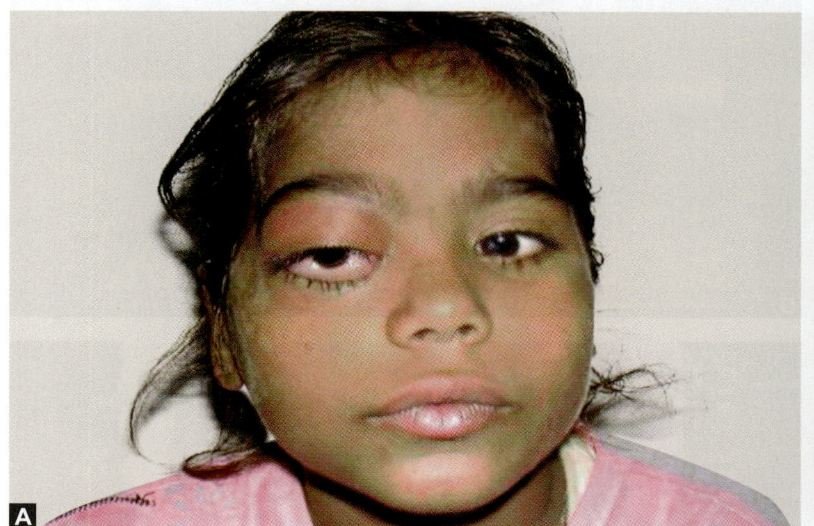

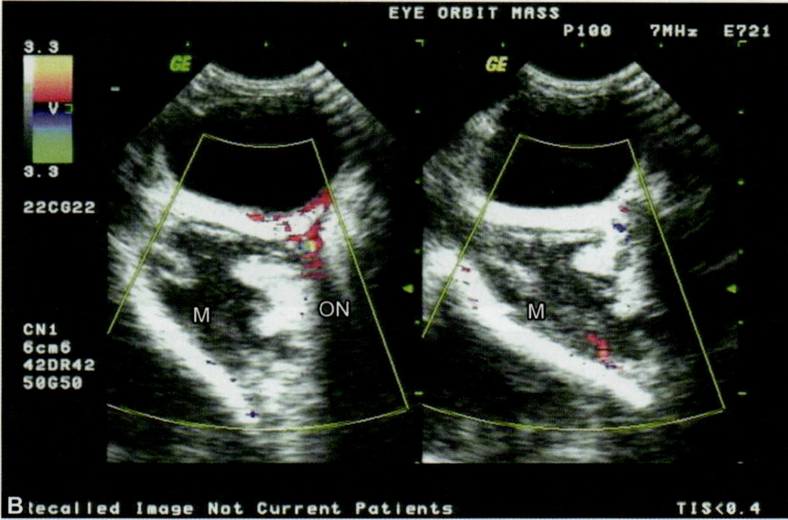

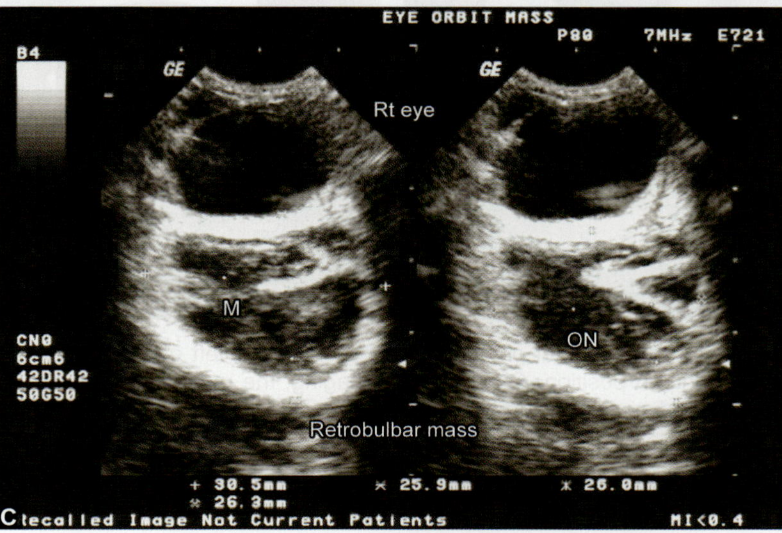

FIGURES 1.242A to C: Lymphangioma. A young girl presented with slowly increasing proptosis of right eye with drooping of upper eyelid and blurred vision. Cystic mass with thick echogenic septa is seen filling the retrobulbar space. Poor flow is seen in the mass on color flow. Biopsy proved lymphangioma.

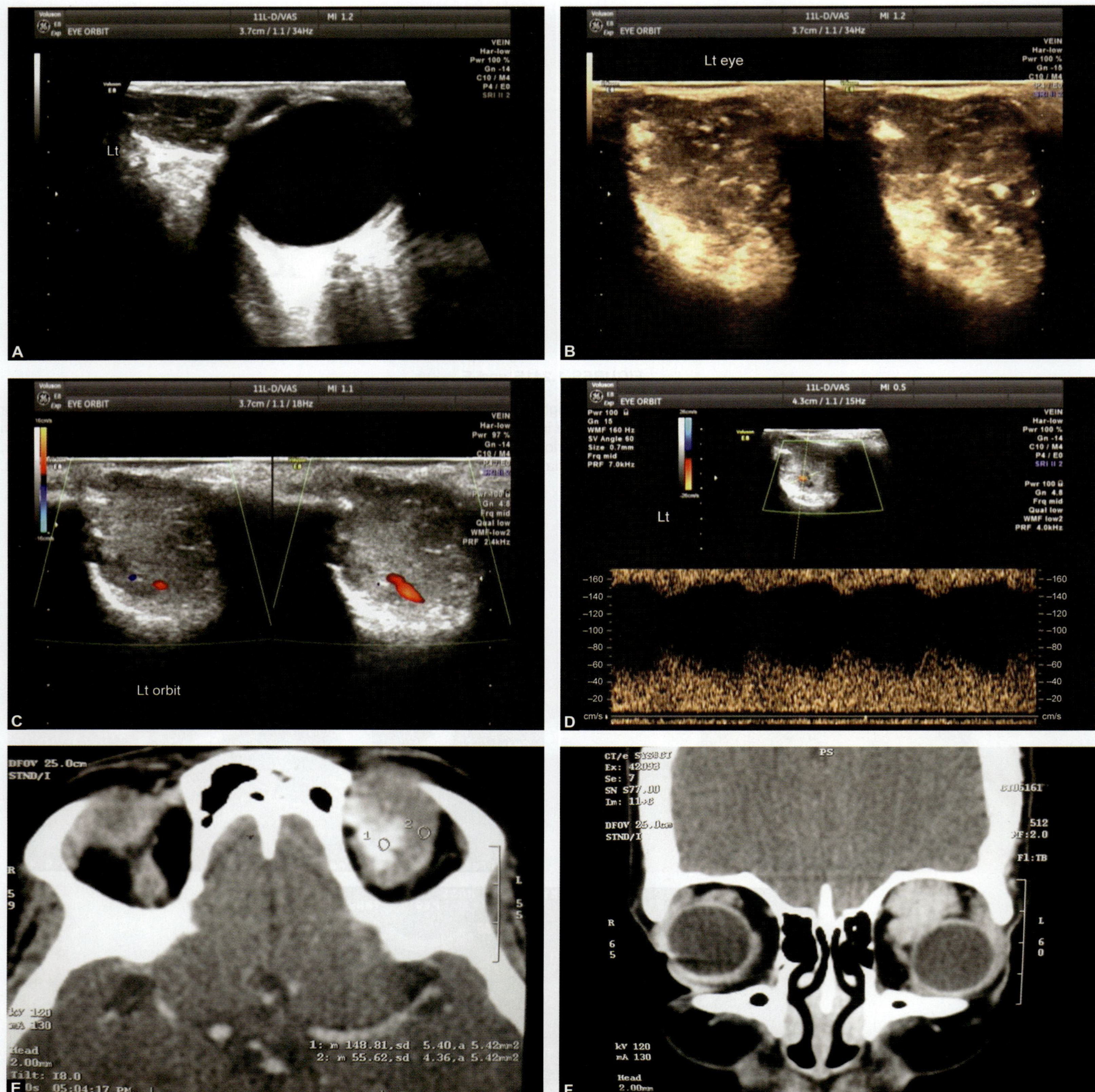

FIGURES 1.243A to F: Retrobulbar hemangioma. A patient presented with proptosis in left eye. HRSG shows an echogenic mass in the orbit. Low level echoes are seen in the mass. It is intraconal in position. On color flow imaging, the mass shows low arterial flow suggestive of hemangiomatous mass. Contrast CT scan of the same patient confirms ultrasound findings.

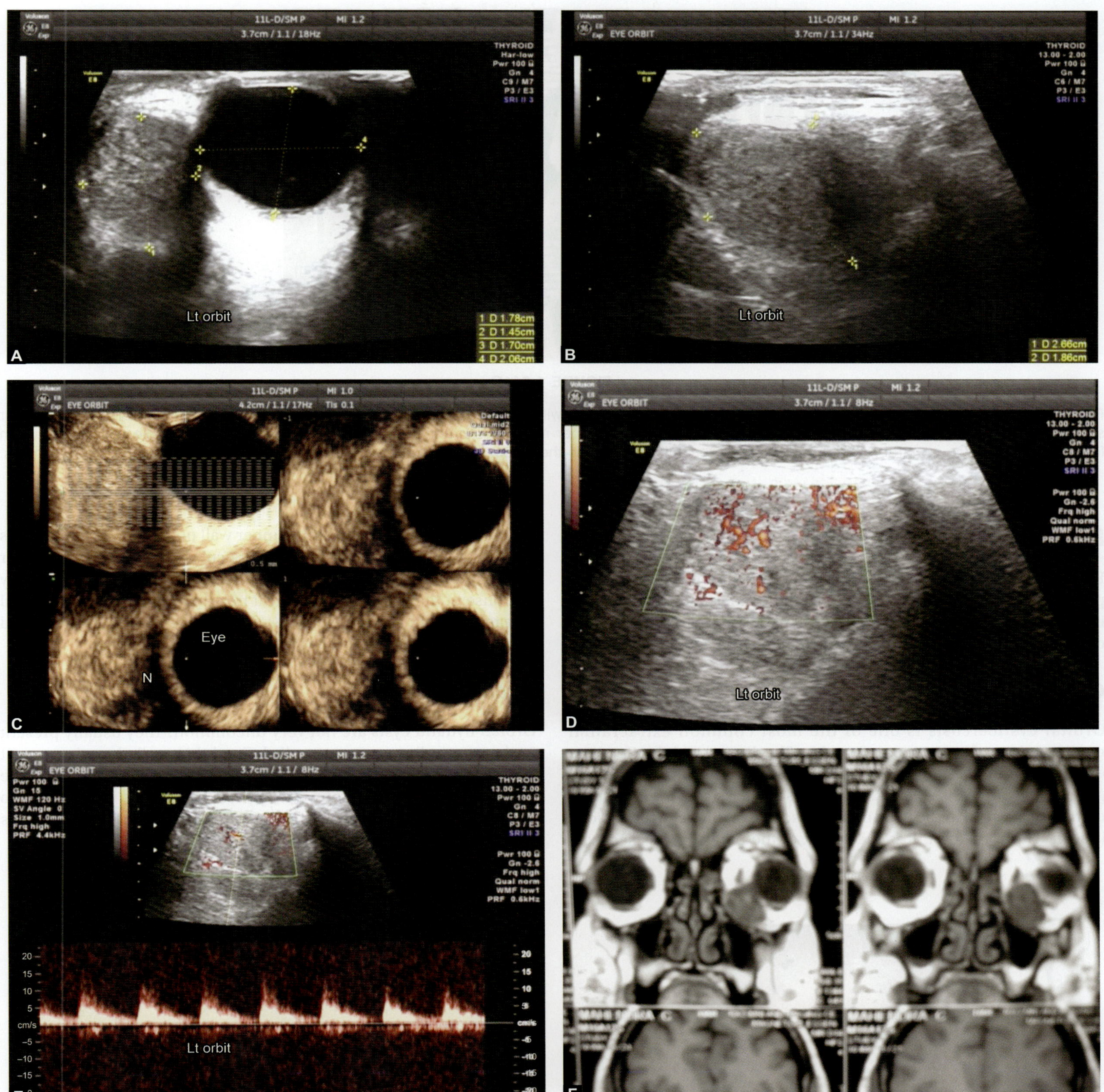

FIGURES 1.244A to F

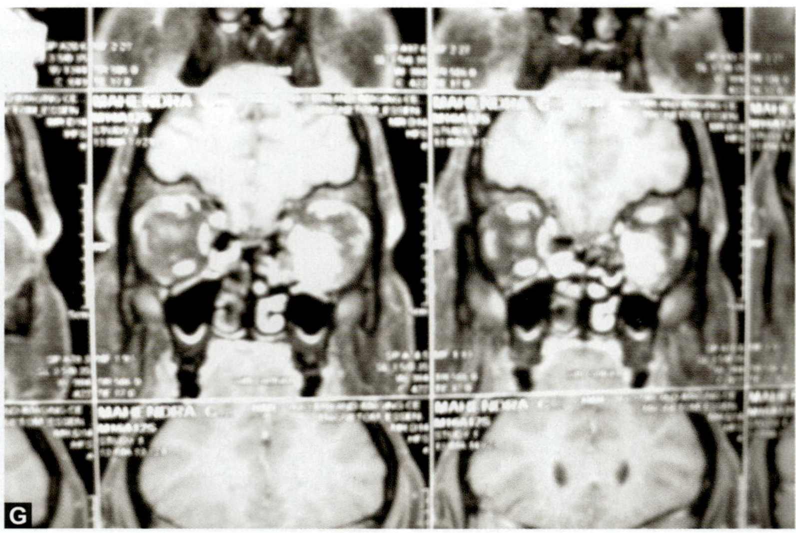

FIGURE 1.244G

FIGURES 1.244A to G: Retrobulbar hemangioma. A patient presented with proptosis in left eye. HRSG shows a soft tissue mass in the retrobulbar space. The TUI imaging shows the mass is seen coming out from upper medial quadrant of eye. On color flow imaging, multiple vessels are seen feeding the mass. On spectral Doppler tracing, low arterial flow is seen in the mass. MRI of the same patient also confirms the hemangiomatous mass.

Retrobulbar Parasitic Infestation

High resolution ultrasound is very good modality for evaluation of parasitic infestation of orbit. The most common infestation is cysticercus infesting the ocular muscles. However, in occasional cases, the hydatid cysts are also seen in the orbit, but the incidence is not that common.

Orbital Cysticercosis

Orbital cysticercosis is one of the most common extracranial manifestations of cysticercus infestation. The disease mainly affects the extraocular muscles and mainly the recti. It presents as painful slowly progressing proptosis. The HRSG findings are classical. A well-defined cystic mass is seen in the belly of the muscle. A highly echogenic nidus is seen within the cyst. It is the scolex of the parasite. This scolex is echo dense and present near the inner wall of the cyst. Echography is the choice of investigation in orbital or ocular cysticercosis. It is better than CT of MRI. It is also a very good tool to evaluate the post-therapy response of the disease. On medical treatment, the parasite dies and cyst regresses in size and vanishes. The muscle belly shows localized thickening, which can be well appreciated on HRSG.

Hydatid Cyst

Orbital hydatid cysts are not very uncommon. They usually present in the retrobulbar area as a well-defined thin walled cystic mass. It stands out very clearly on HRSG. At times thin septa are seen in the cyst making the loculations and septation. The eye is displaced to opposite side by the pressure effect of the cyst and associated proptosis is also present.

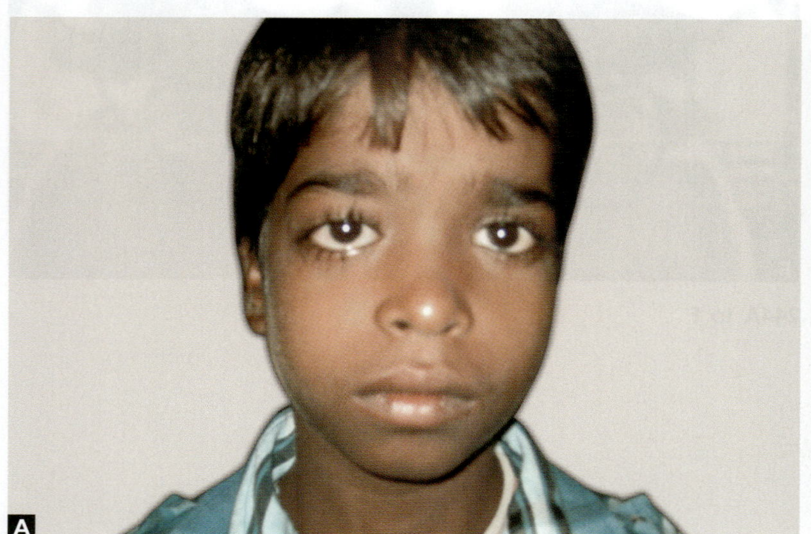

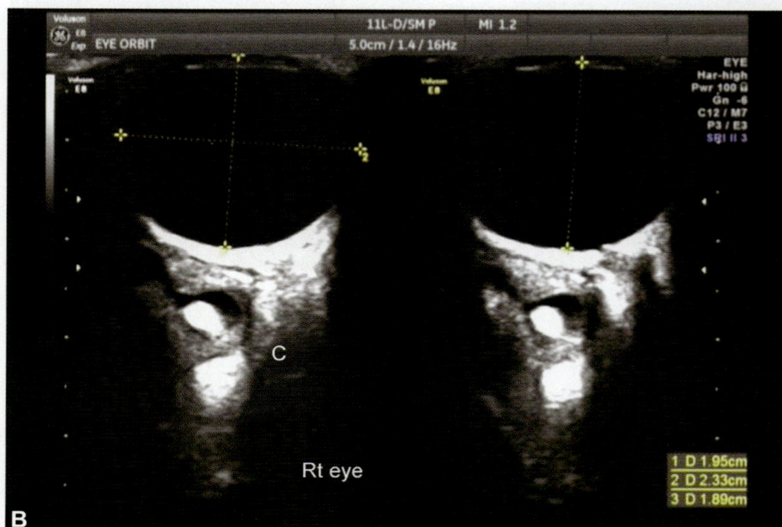

FIGURES 1.245A and B

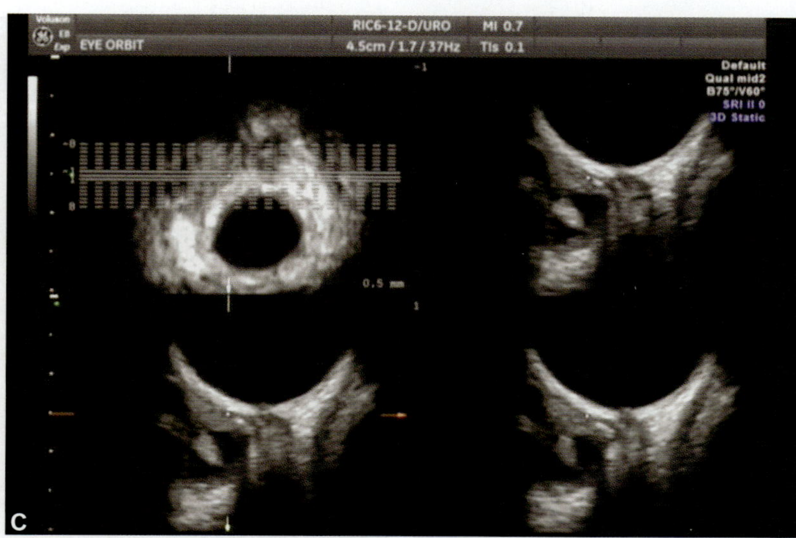

FIGURE 1.245C

FIGURES 1.245A to C: Retrobulbar cysticercus. A young boy presented with proptosis in right eye. HRSG shows a well-defined cystic mass in the inferior rectus muscle of the eye. An echogenic nidus is seen fixed with the inner wall of cyst suggestive of cysticercus cyst. The TUI imaging clearly shows cysticercus cyst.

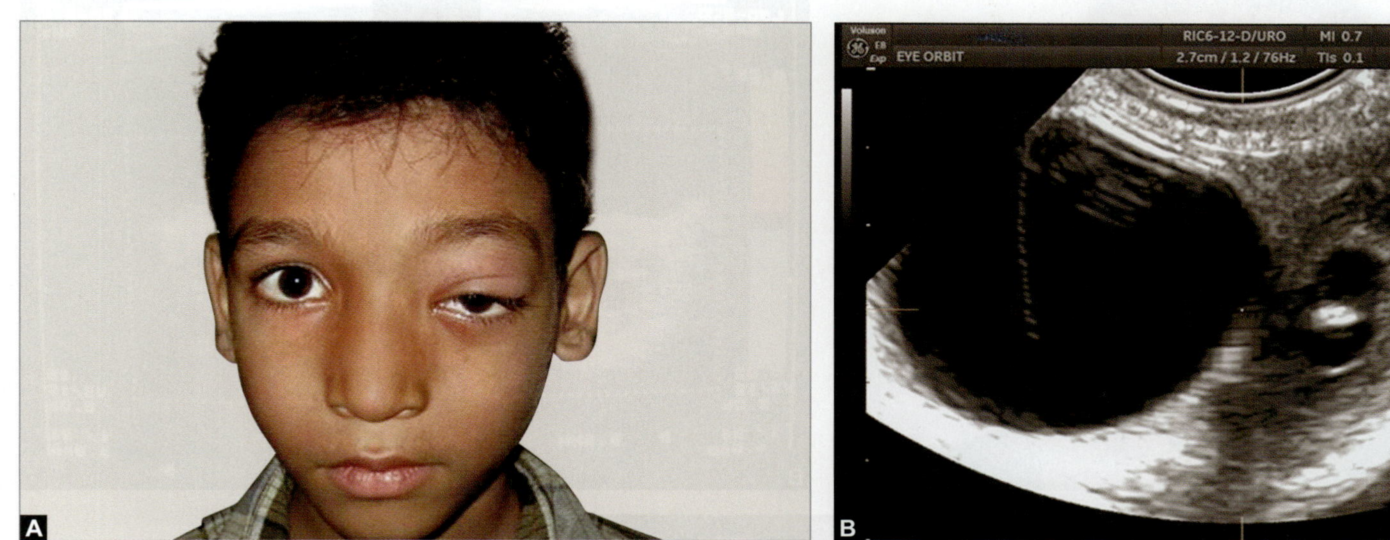

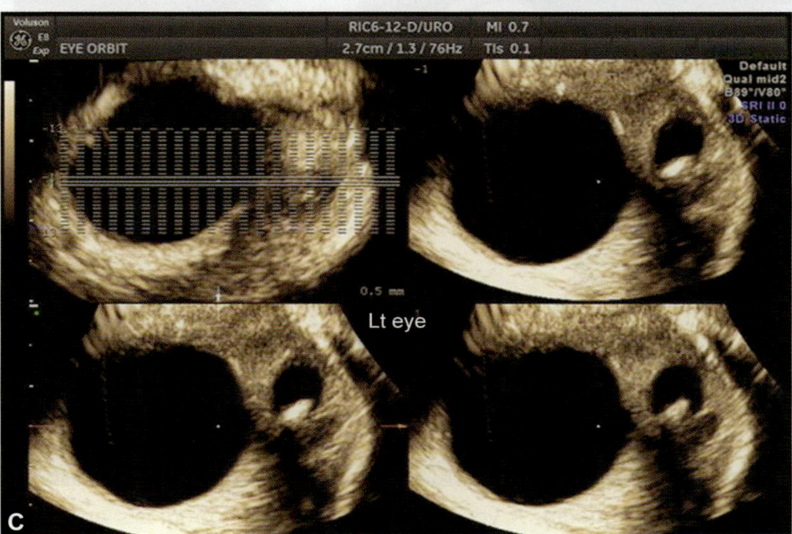

FIGURES 1.246A to C: Superior rectus cysticercus cyst. A young boy presented with left side proptosis with inferior displacement of eyeball. HRSG shows thickened belly of superior rectus muscle. A well-defined cyst is seen in the muscle. An echogenic nidus is seen fixed with the inner wall of cyst suggestive of cysticercus cyst. But no evidence of any intraocular extension is seen. On color flow imaging, no flow is seen in the cyst.

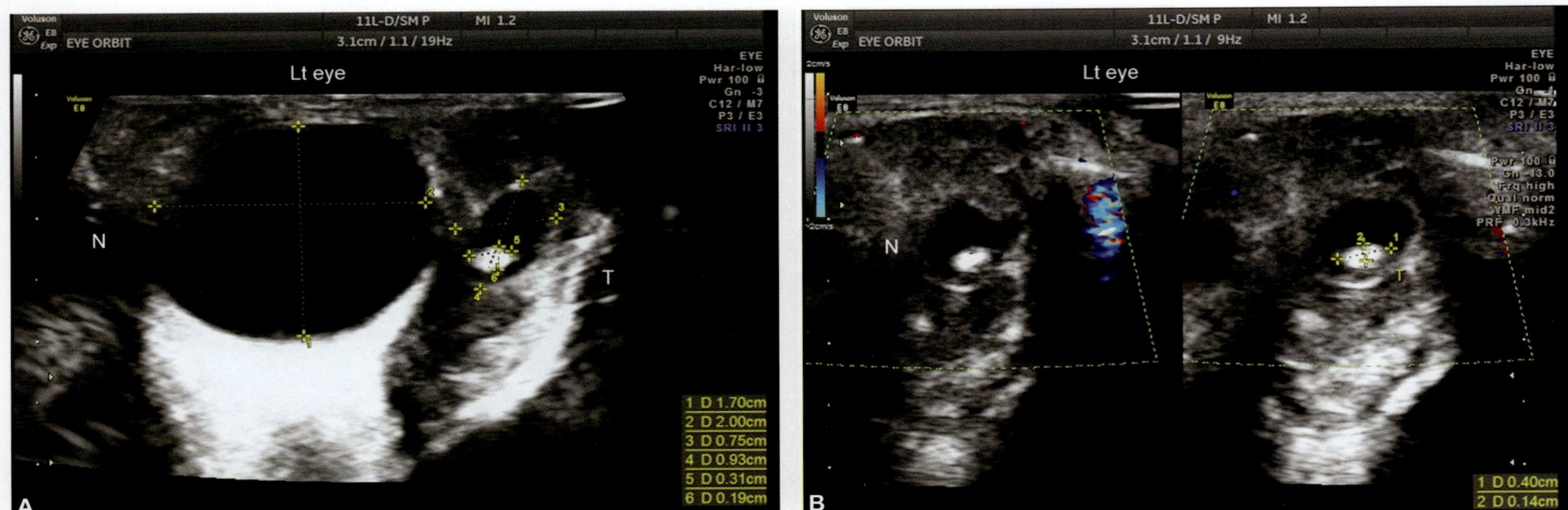

FIGURES 1.247A and B: Superior rectus cysticercus. A young lady presented with proptosis of right eye. HRSG shows diffuse thickening of superior rectus muscle. A big cyst is seen in the belly of superior rectus muscle. An echogenic nidus is seen fixed with the inner wall of cyst. 3D ultrasound shows the cyst clearly coming out from the superior rectus muscle.

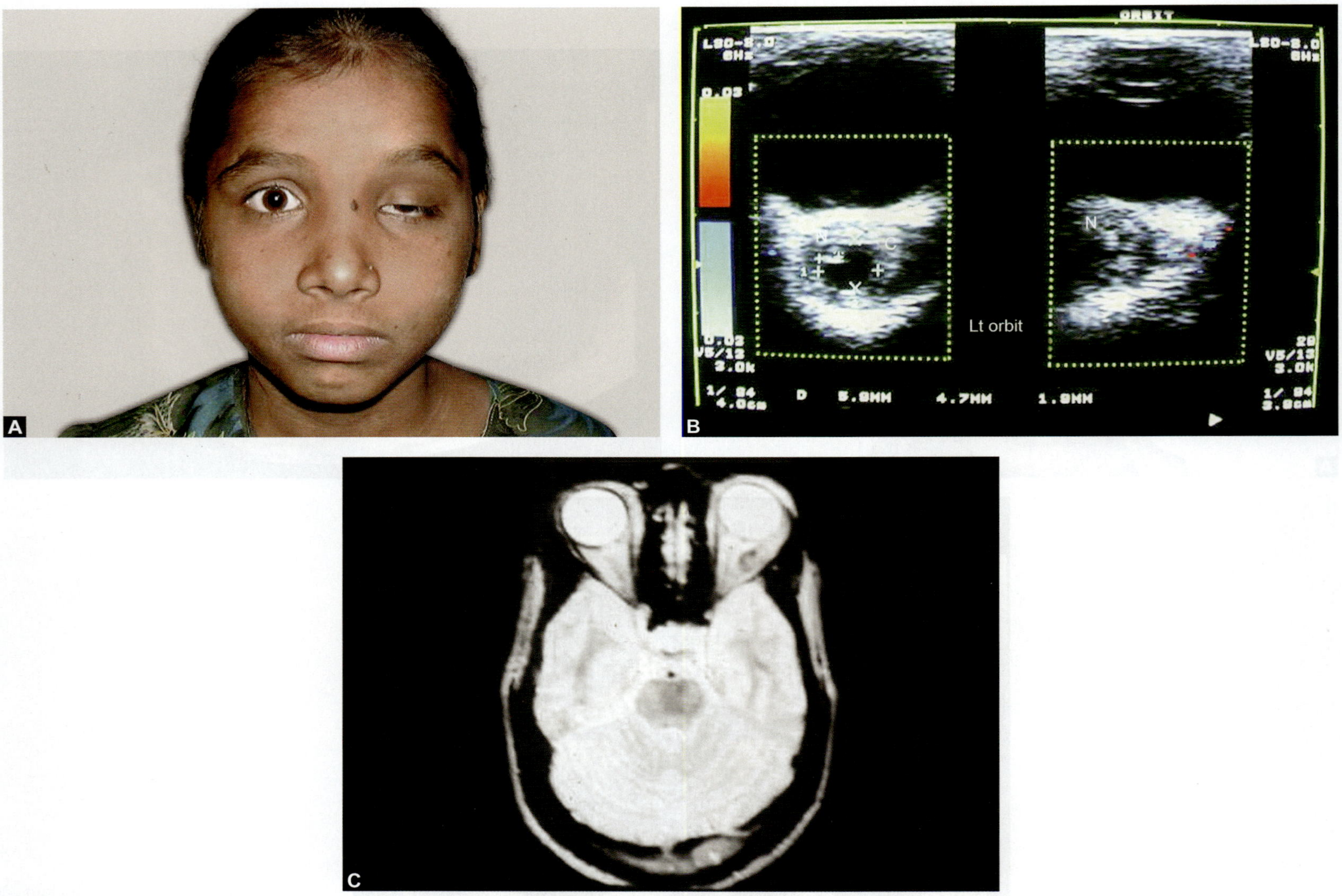

FIGURES 1.248A to C: Cysticercosis lateral rectus muscle. A young girl presented with proptosis and dropping of left eyelid and painful left eye. HRSG shows inflamed superior rectus muscle with a well-defined cyst. An echogenic nidus is seen fixed with inner wall of the cyst is scolex. MRI shows an ill-defined hypodense mass in belly of lateral rectus muscle.

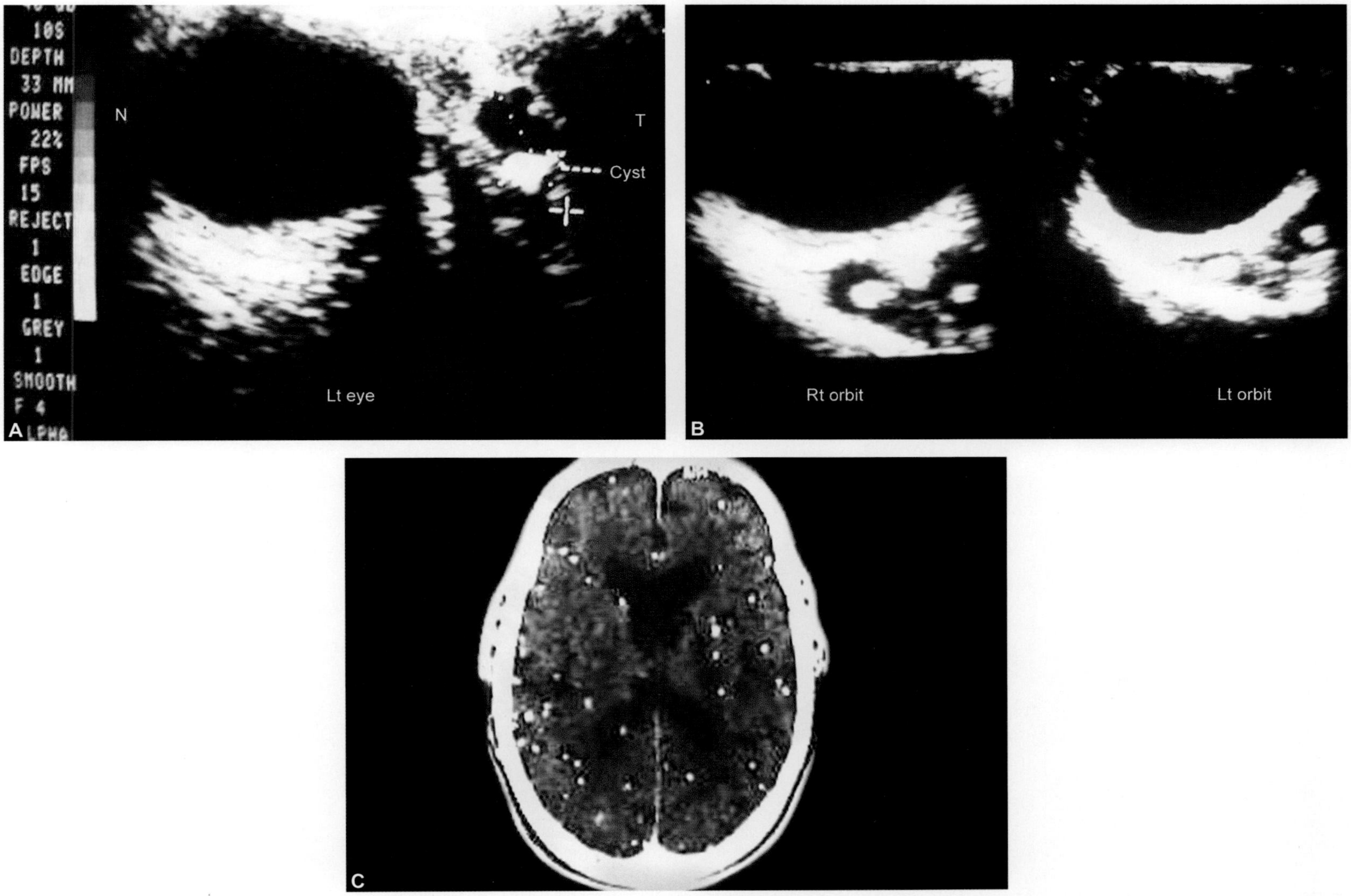

FIGURES 1.249A to C: HRSG shows a well-defined cyst with an echogenic nidus fixed with inner wall of the cyst typical of cysticercus cyst.: HRSG shows thick-walled cysts in both side lateral recti with scolex fixed with inner wall of cyst as echogenic nidus. CT head of the same patient shows multiple hyperdense dot shadows diffuse in distribution in wide spread neurocysticercosis.

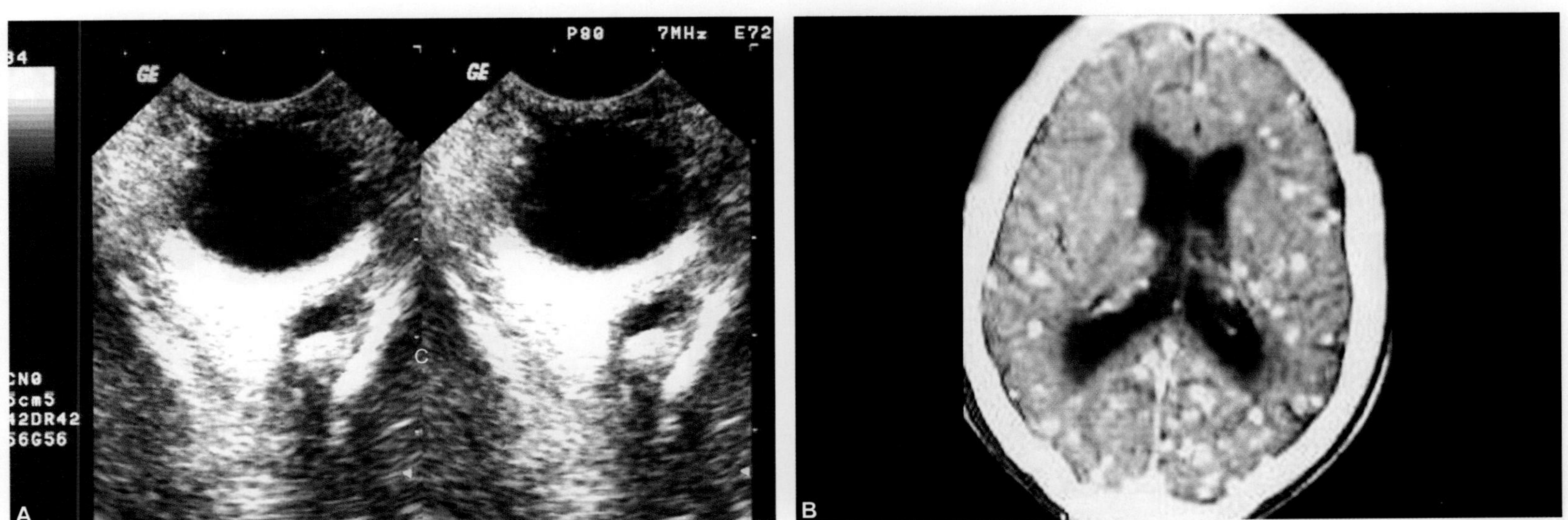

FIGURES 1.250A and B: Lateral rectus cysticercosis. Well-defined cyst in lateral rectus with a hyperdense echogenic nidus fixed with inner wall of the cyst. CT head of the same patient shows gross impregnation of brain parenchyma with neurocysticercosis.

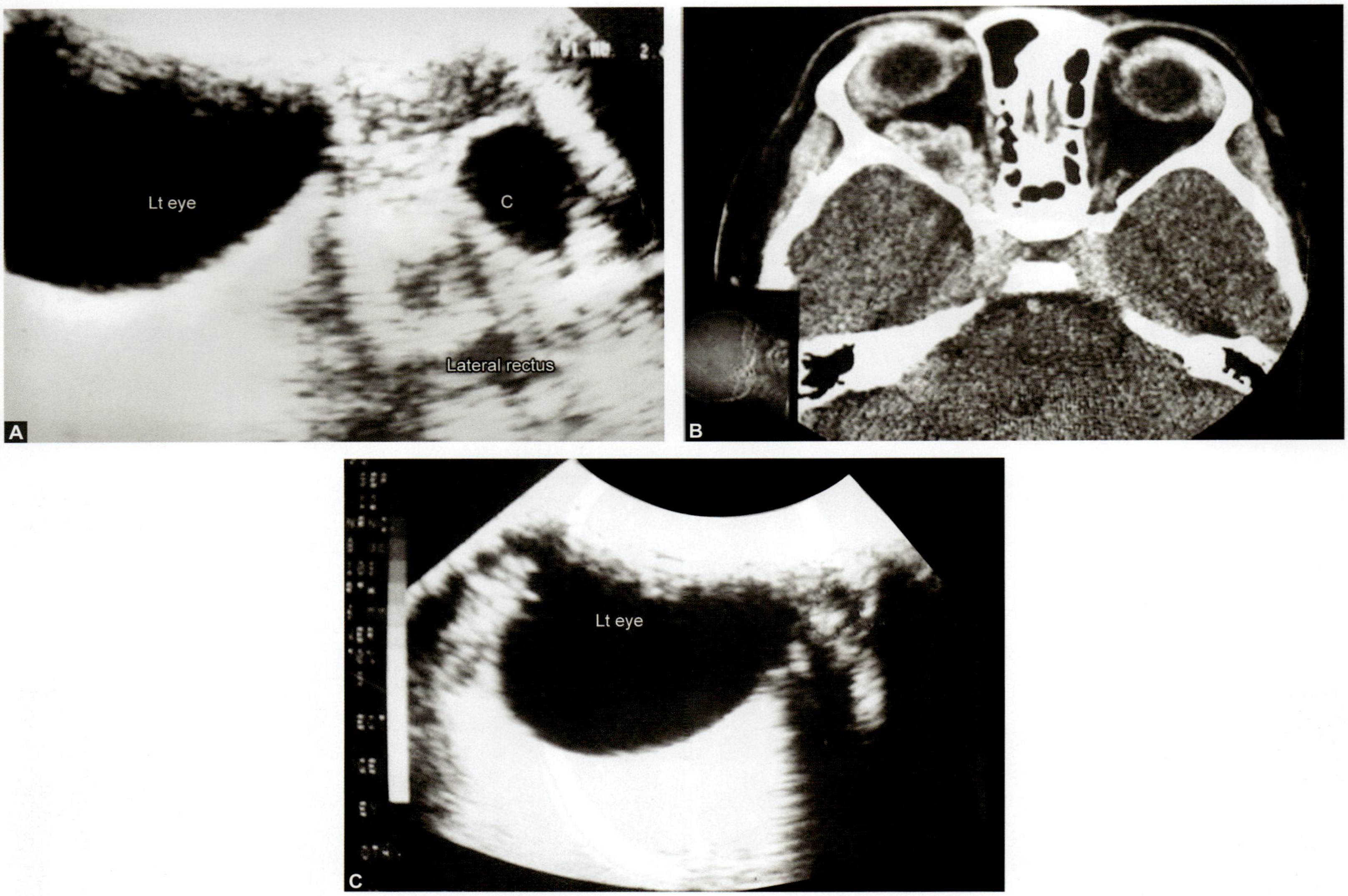

FIGURES 1.251A to C: CT of a young girl shows irregular thickening of lateral rectus muscle with a hypodense area. HRSG of the same patient shows well-defined cyst in lateral rectus with an echogenic nidus suggestive of cysticercus cyst. Post-treatment: HRSG shows localized thickening of lateral rectus muscle with collapse of the cyst after medical treatment in the same patient. HRSG is very good to assess the treatment response of the therapy.

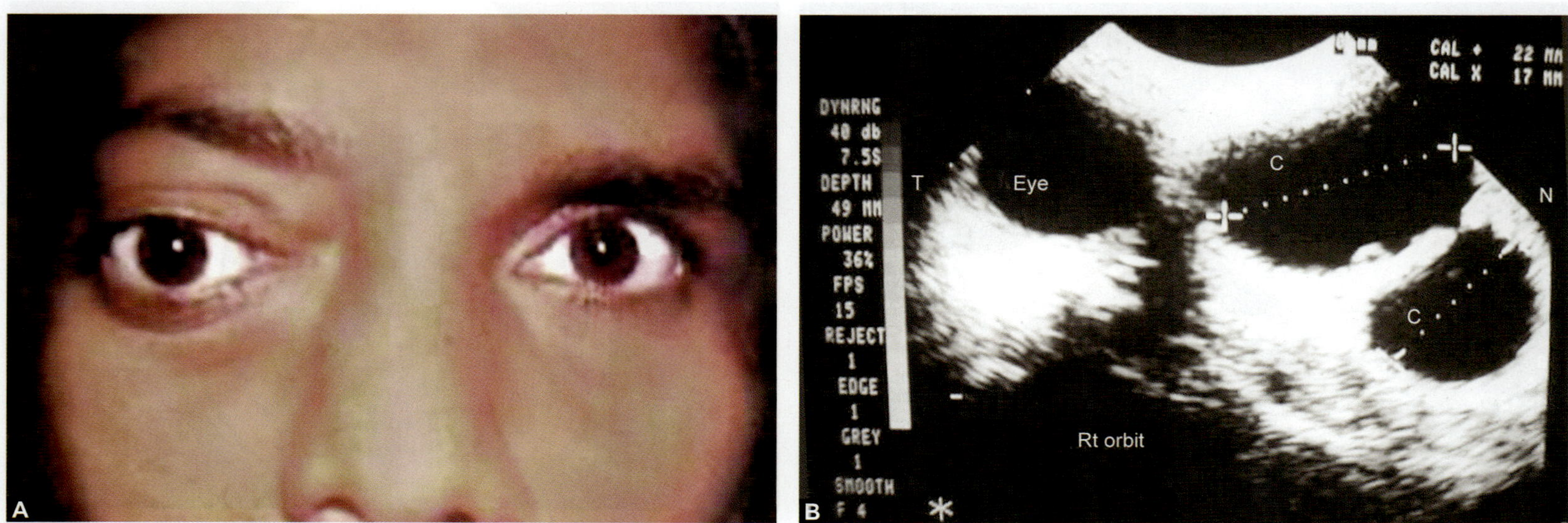

FIGURES 1.252A and B

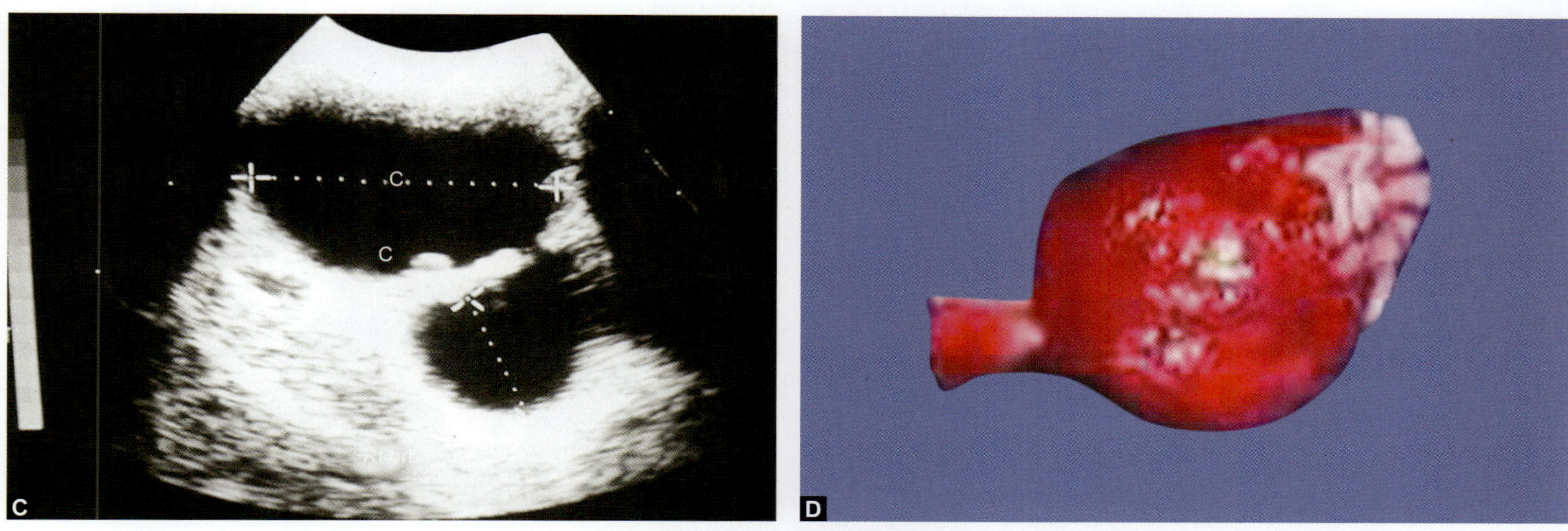

FIGURES 1.252C and D

FIGURES 1.252A to D: Hydatid cyst orbit. A middle-aged woman presented with right eye proptosis with diplopia. HRSG shows a bilobed cystic mass in retrobulbar space of right orbit. The big cyst shows another small daughter cyst fixed with its wall and anterior displacement of eyeball. Typical findings of the Hydatid cyst. The gross post-operated specimen of the same patient shows the cyst in gross.

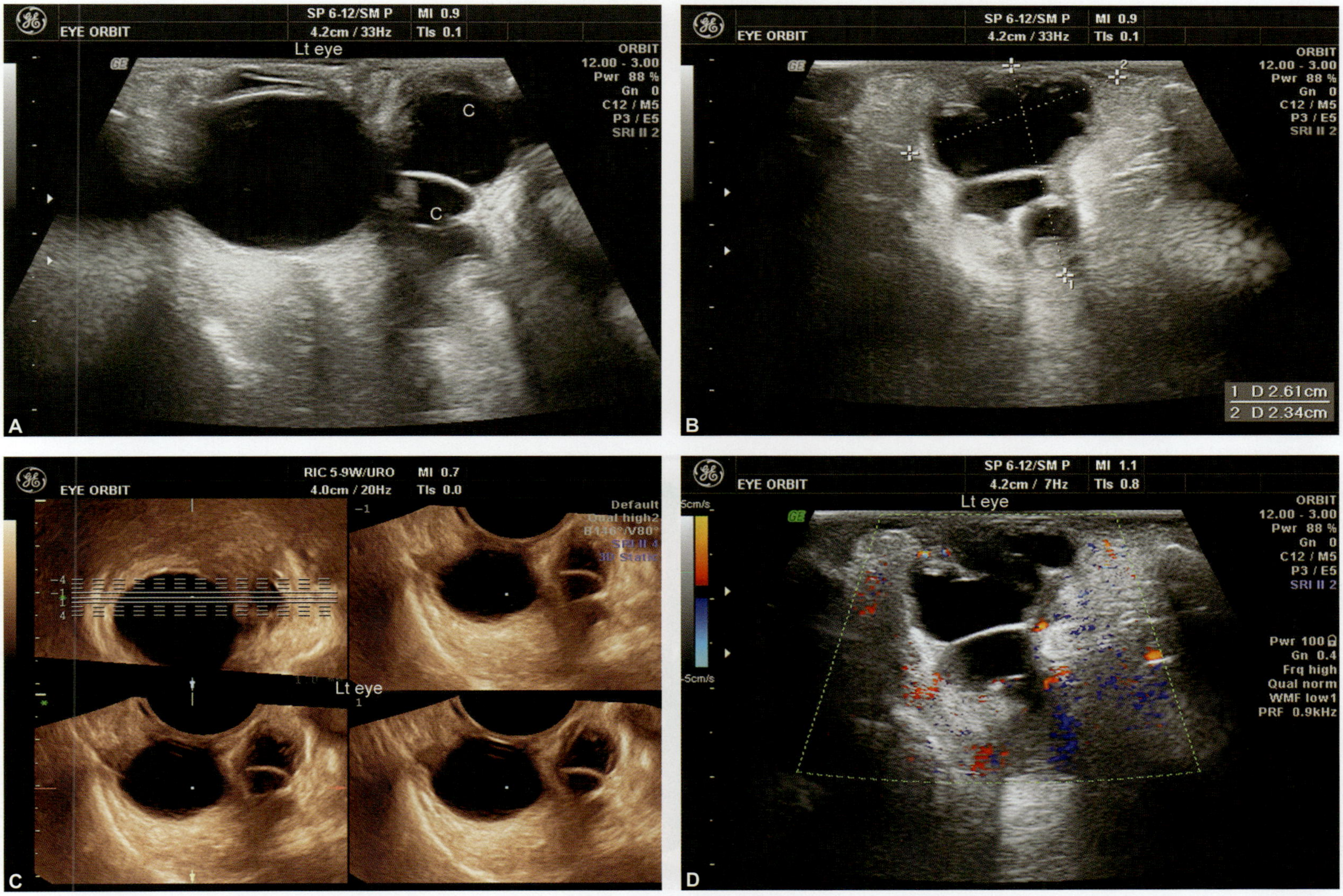

FIGURES 1.253A to D: A man presented with proptosis of left eye. HRSG shows lobulated cystic mass in left orbit. A big cyst is seen in it. Another is also seen in big cyst. The TUI imaging shows the cyst clearly. On color flow imaging, poor flow is seen in the cyst. The findings are suggestive of orbital hydatid cyst.

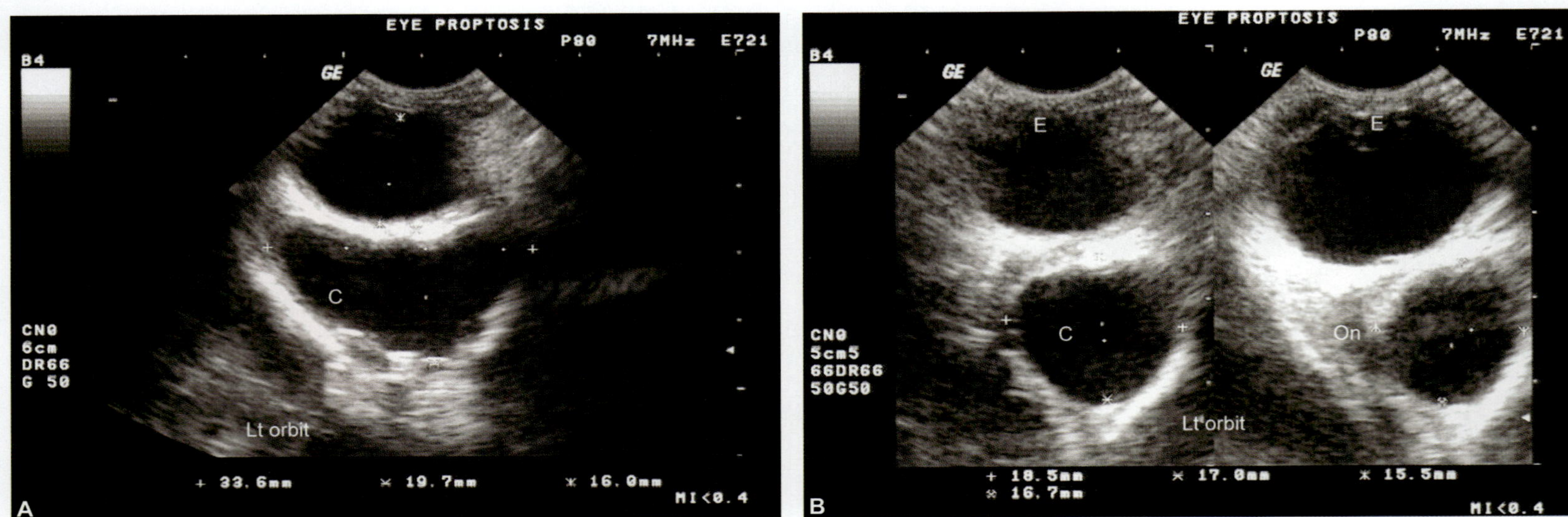

FIGURES 1.254A and B: Retrobulbar hydatid cyst. A young boy presented with left eye proptosis. HRSG shows a thick walled cyst in retrobulbar space. Cyst wall also shows calcification, typical finding of hydatid cyst. However no daughter cyst is seen.

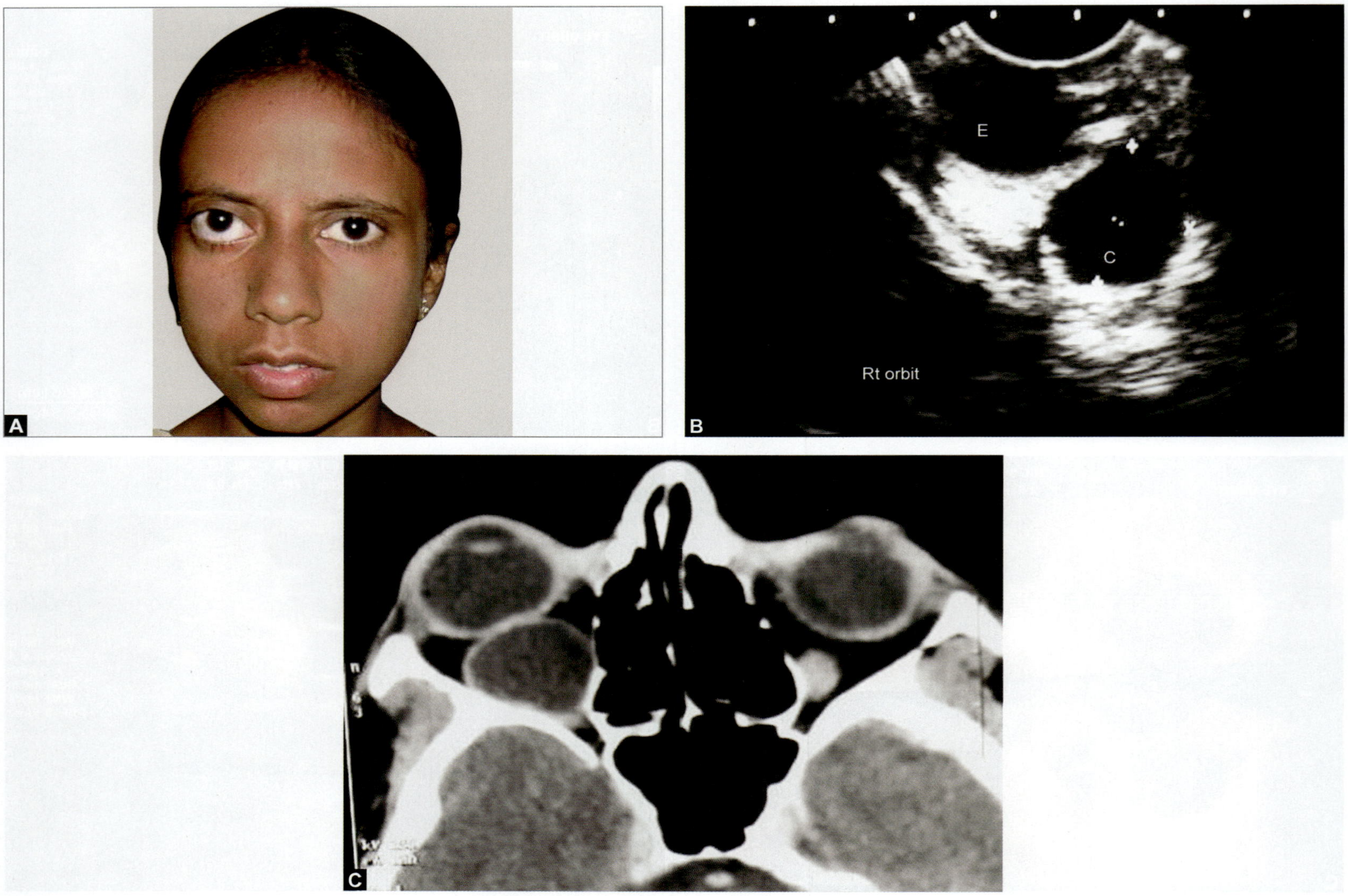

FIGURES 1.255A to C: Retrobulbar cystic dermoid. A young girl presented with right-sided proptosis. HRSG shows a thick-walled cystic mass in the retrobulbar space. Echogenic calcification is seen in it. CT scan of the same patient shows well defined cyst in the retrobulbar intraconal space. Biopsy of the cyst was dermoid cyst.

INFLAMMATORY MASSES

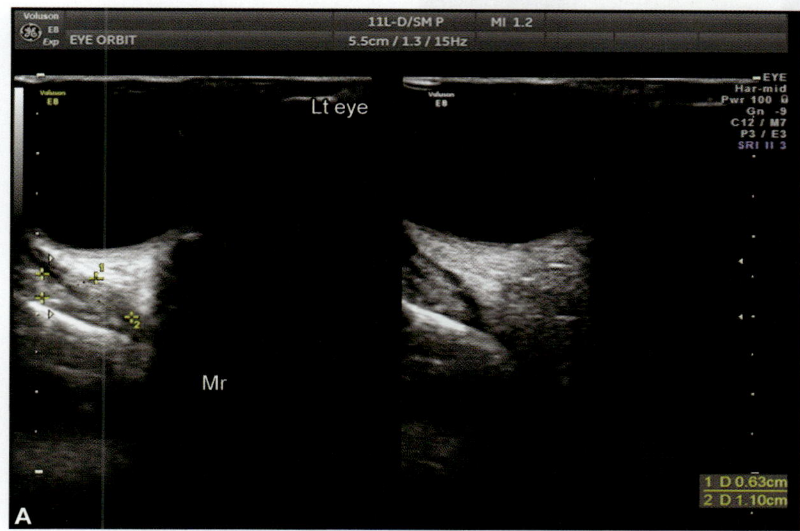

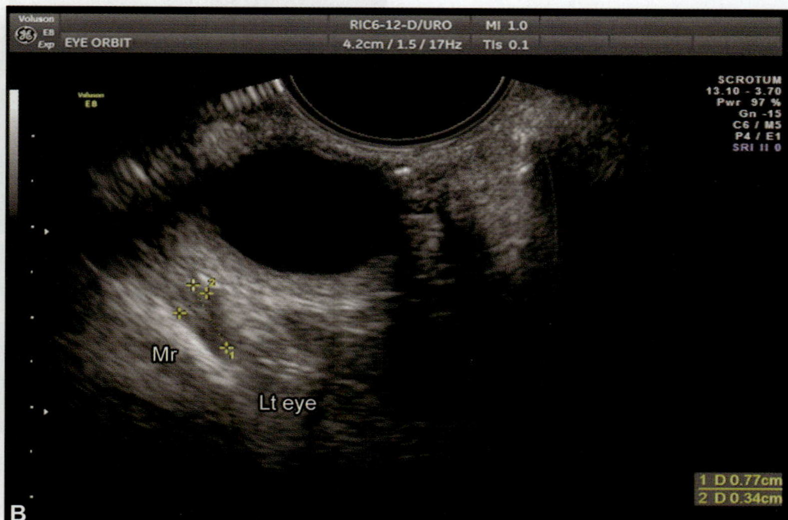

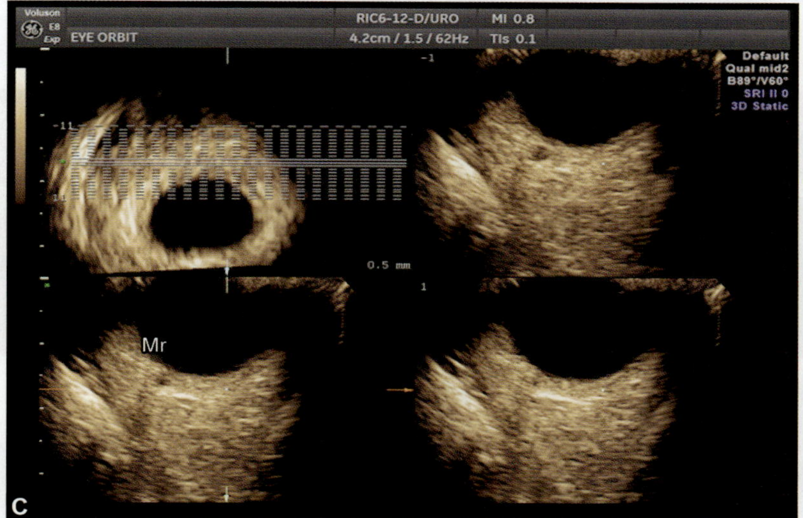

FIGURES 1.256A to C: A patient presented with proptosis of left eye. HRSG shows diffuse thickening of medial rectus muscle. It is 6 mm in thickness (normal < 3 mm). But it is homogeneous in texture suggestive of myositis.

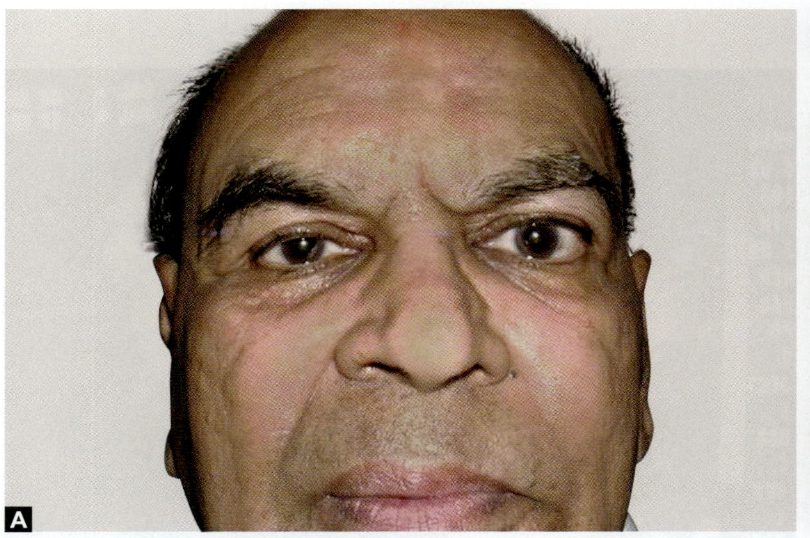

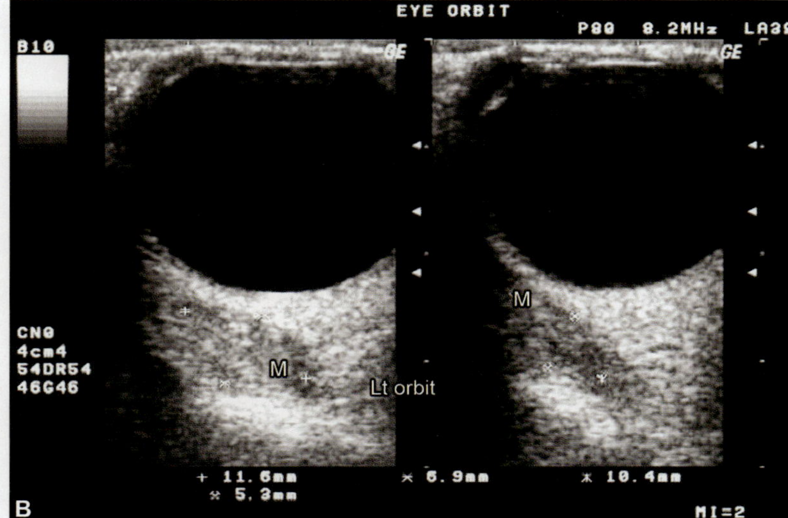

FIGURES 1.257A and B

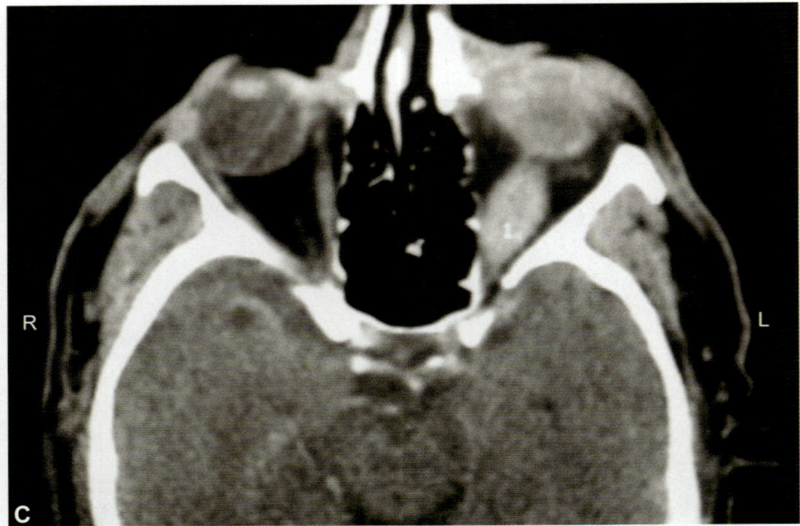

FIGURE 1.257C

FIGURES 1.257A to C: Myositis superior rectus muscle. An old man presented with proptosis of the left eye. HRSG shows well-defined thickening of superior rectus muscle with homogeneous texture. CT of the same patient also shows the same findings.

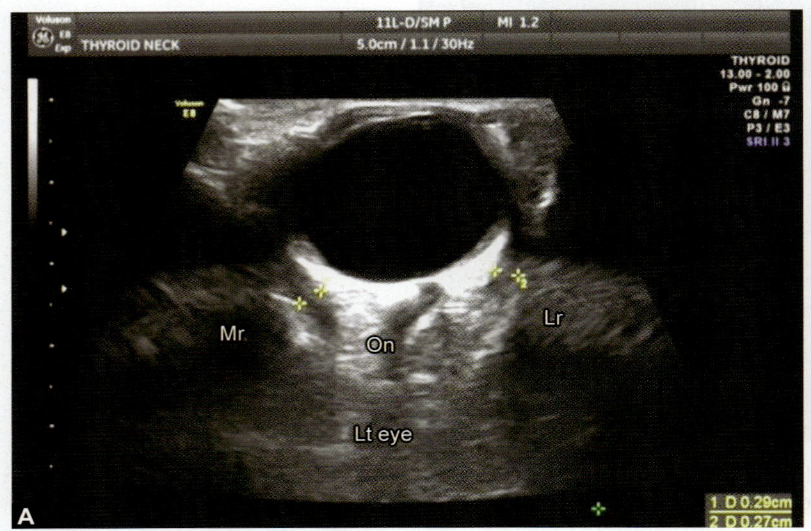

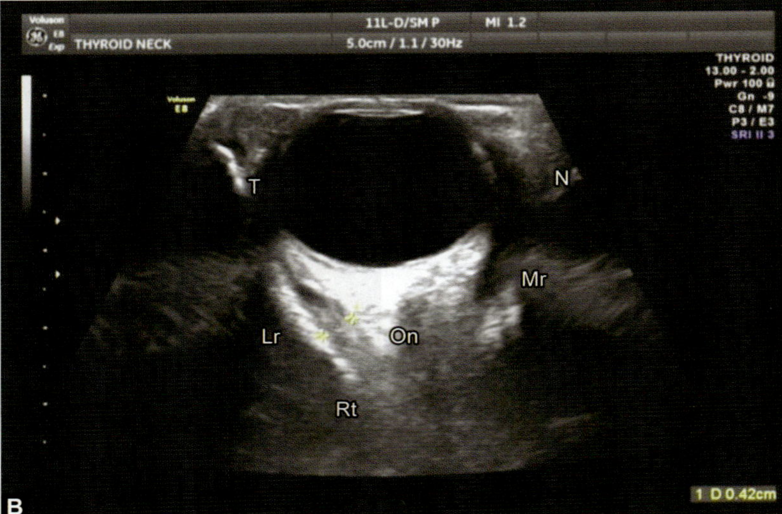

FIGURES 1.258A and B: Normal recti muscles. HRSG shows normal medial and lateral rectus muscle. The medial rectus is 2.7 mm in thickness and lateral rectus muscle 2.1 mm in thickness. Echo texture is homogeneous.

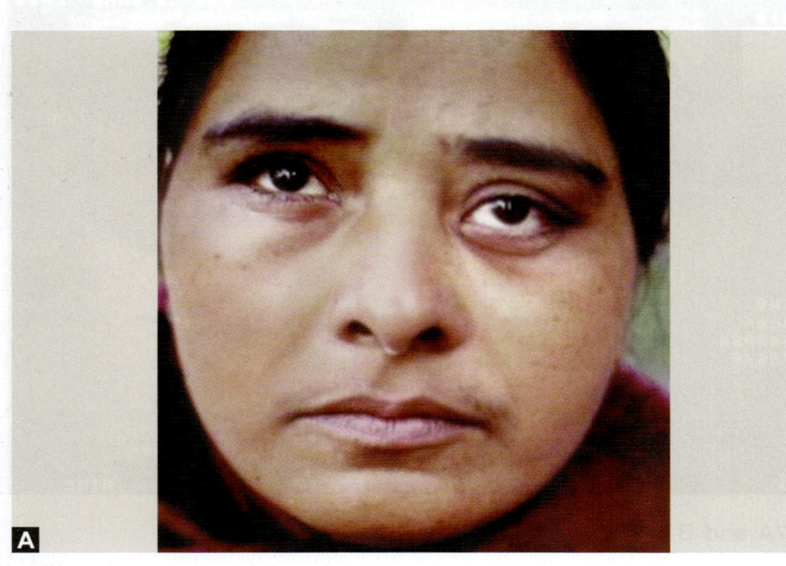

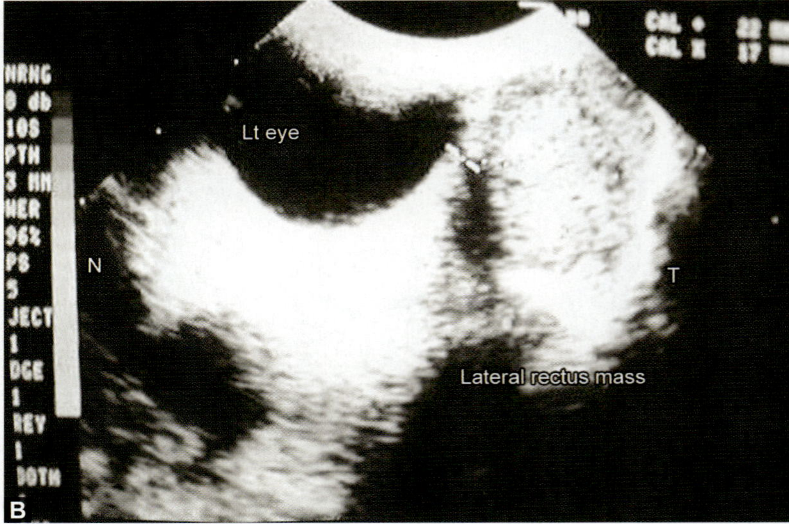

FIGURES 1.259A and B

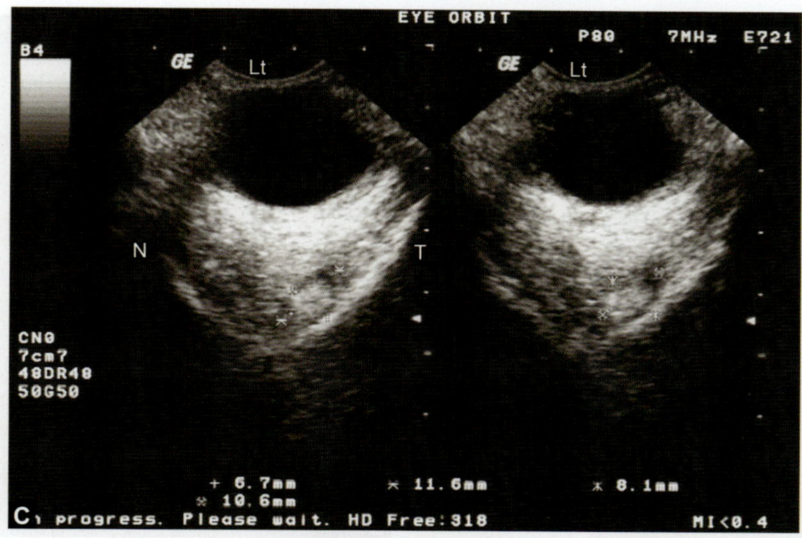

FIGURE 1.259C

FIGURES 1.259A to C: Pseudotumor orbit. Patient presented with unilateral proptosis with diplopia. Well defined homogeneous lobulated mass in lateral rectus muscle. The mass regressed in size on corticosteroid therapy.

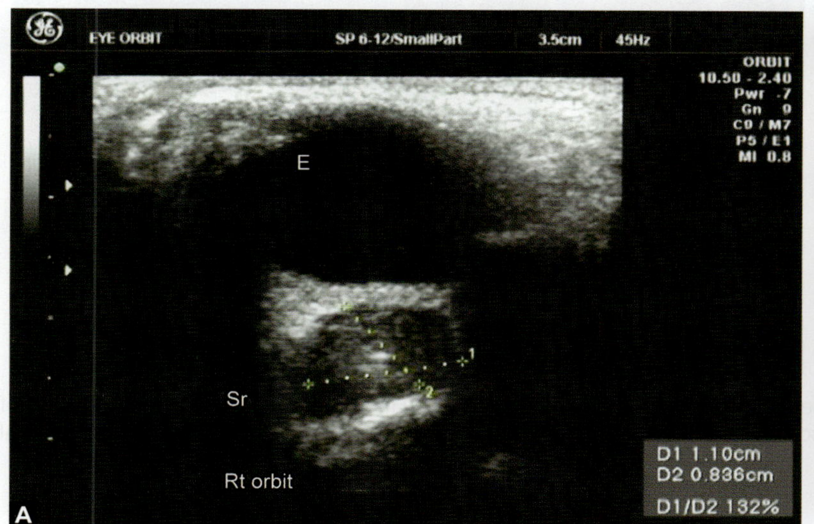

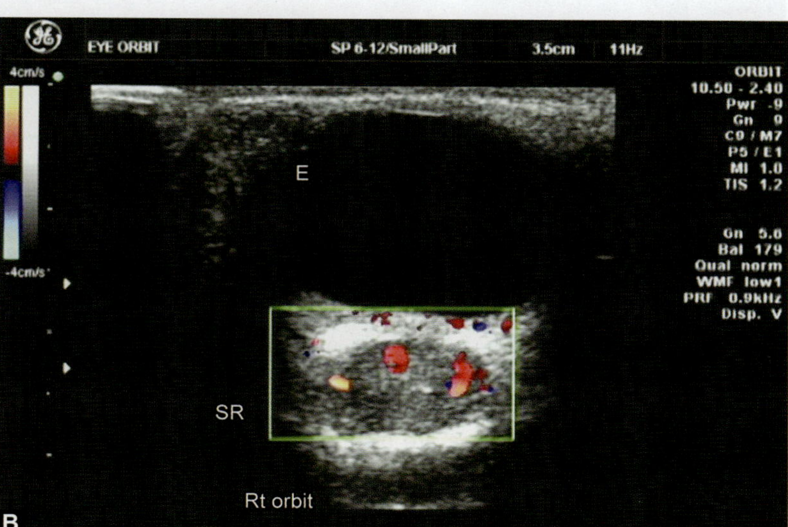

FIGURES 1.260A and B: Myositis of superior rectus muscle. HRSG shows marked thickening of superior rectus muscle in a patient presented with proptosis. Color Doppler imaging shows increased flow in thickened muscle.

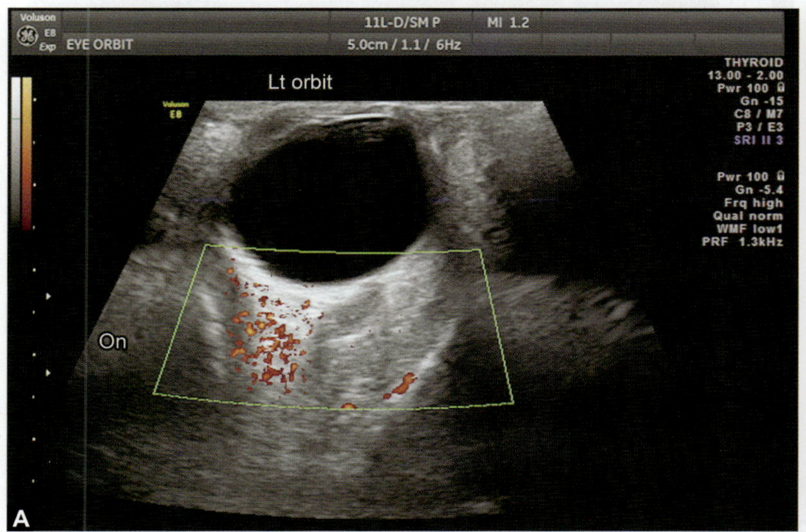

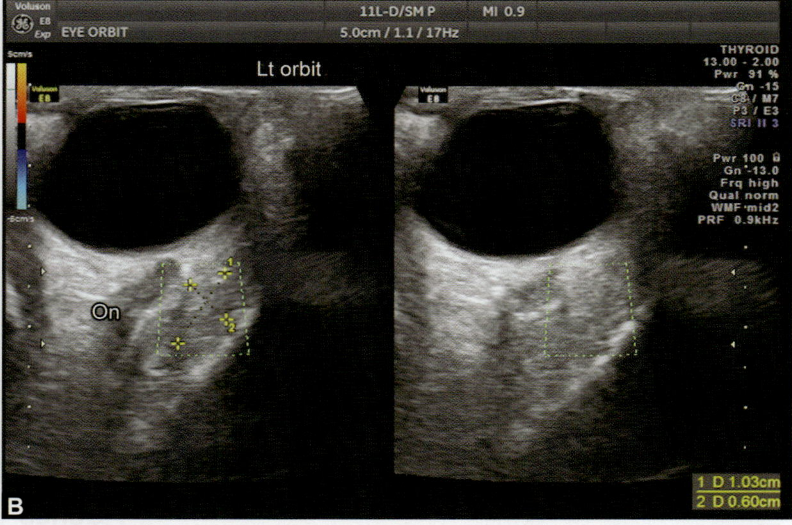

FIGURES 1.261A and B: Pseudotumor. A patient presented with proptosis of left orbit. HRSG shows fusiform thickening of lateral rectus muscle. It is smooth in outline. No calcification is seen in it. On color flow imaging, poor flow is seen in it suggestive of pseudotumor.

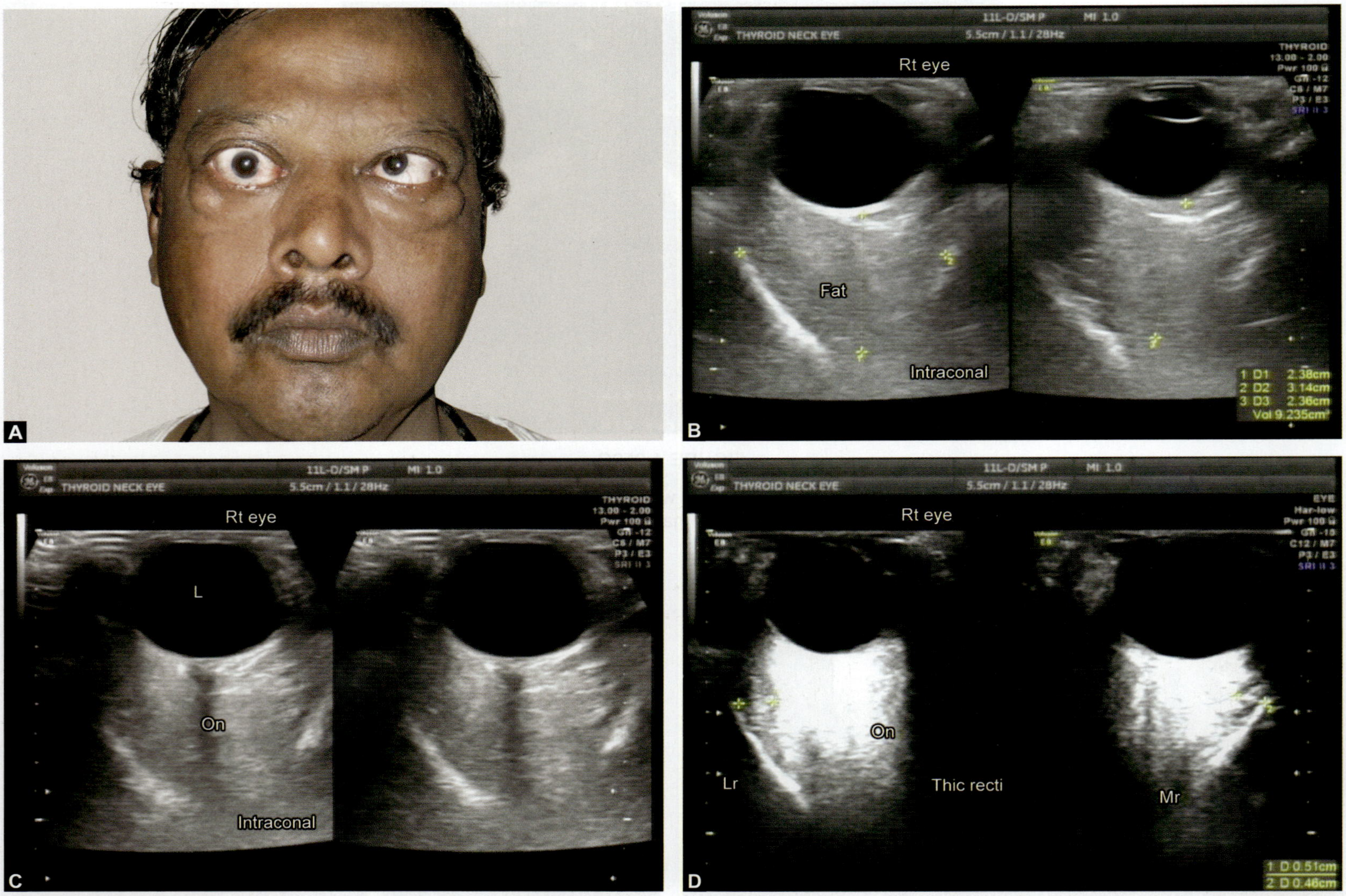

FIGURES 1.262A to D: Graves' disease. A patient of Graves' disease presented with bilateral exophthalmos. HRSG shows increased deposition of intraconal fat. The recti muscles are also thickened. The lateral rectus muscle is 5.1 mm in thickness and medial rectus 4.2 mm in thickness (normal muscle thickness < 3 mm).

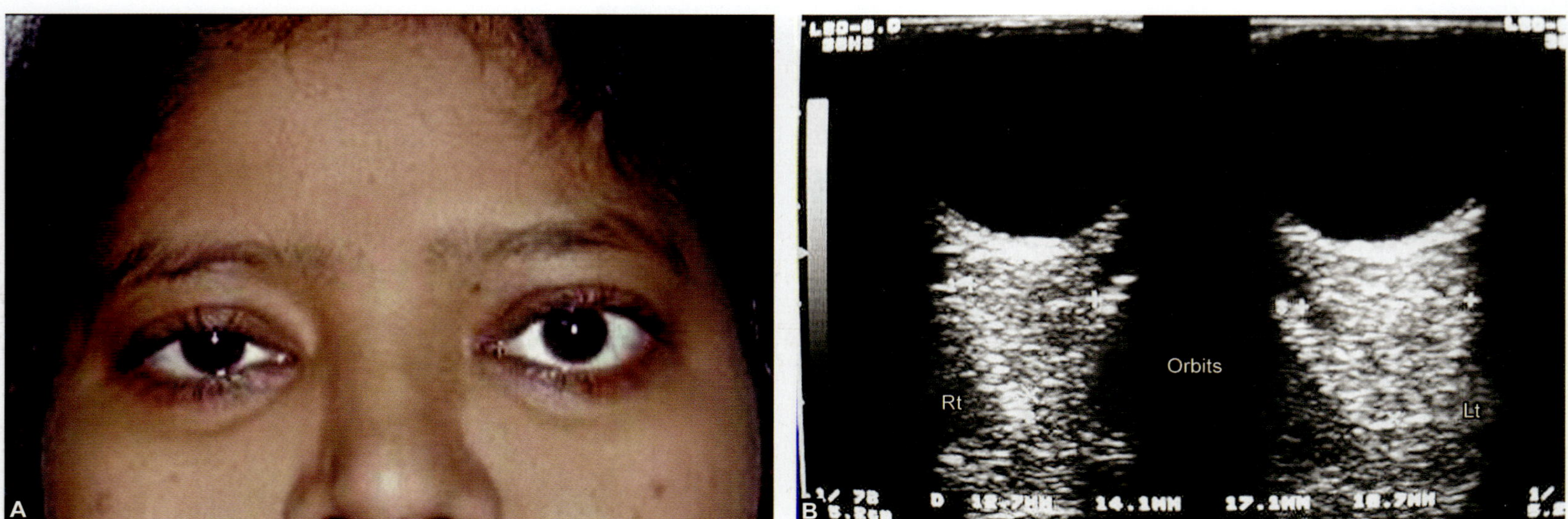

FIGURES 1.263A and B

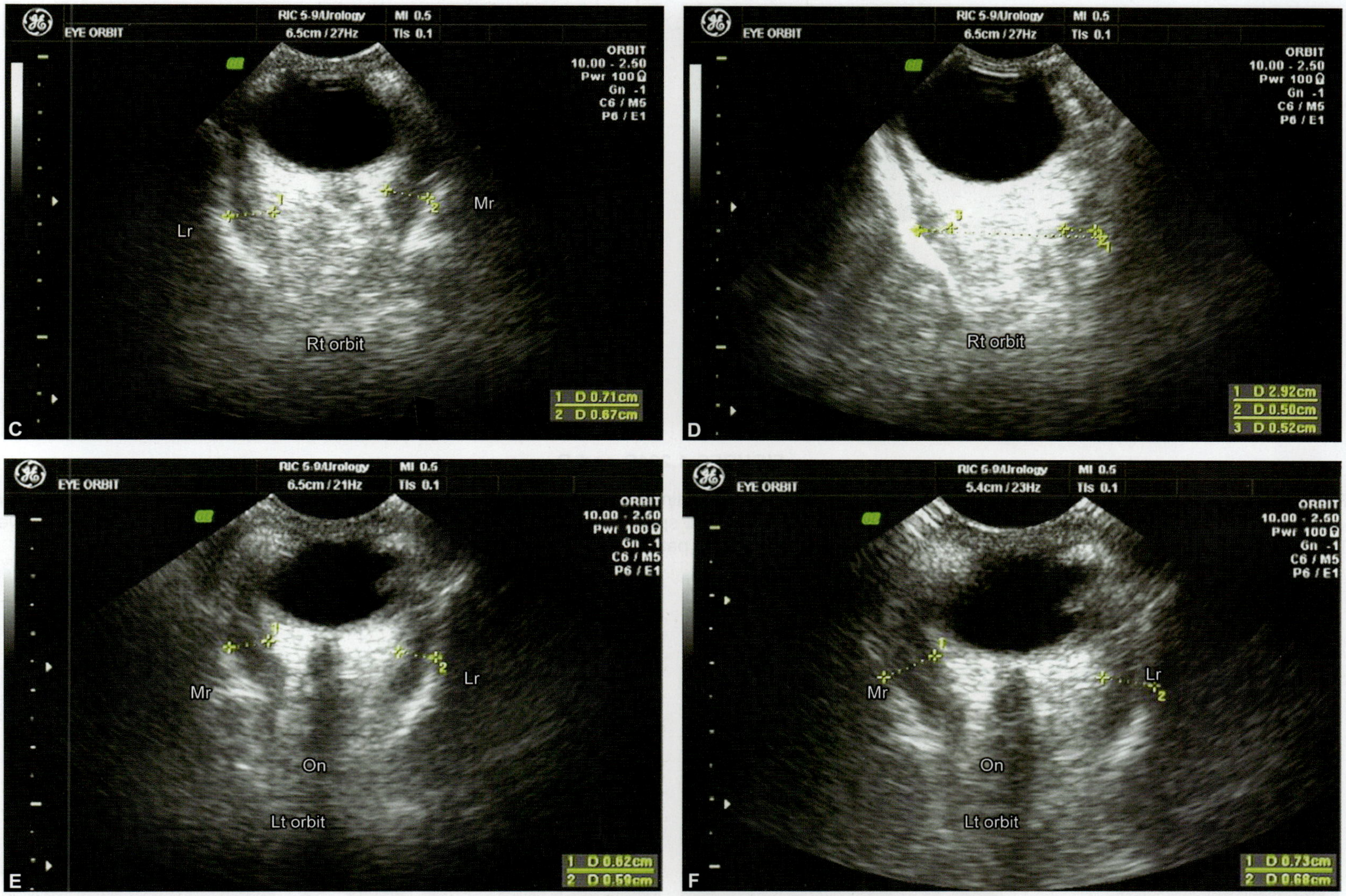

FIGURES 1.263C to F

FIGURES 1.263A to F: Thyrotoxicosis. Patient presented early proptosis left eye. HRSG shows increased amount of retrobulbar fat in left orbit coming early proptosis. A patient presented with bilateral orbital proptosis. HRSG shows marked thickening of the recti muscles in the orbit. The lateral and medial recti muscles are 7 and 6 mm in thickness (normal <3 mm). Increased amount of intraconal fat is also seen typical feature of thyrotoxicosis. Left eye also shows thickened recti muscles. They are 7 and 6mm in thickness (normal < 3 mm).

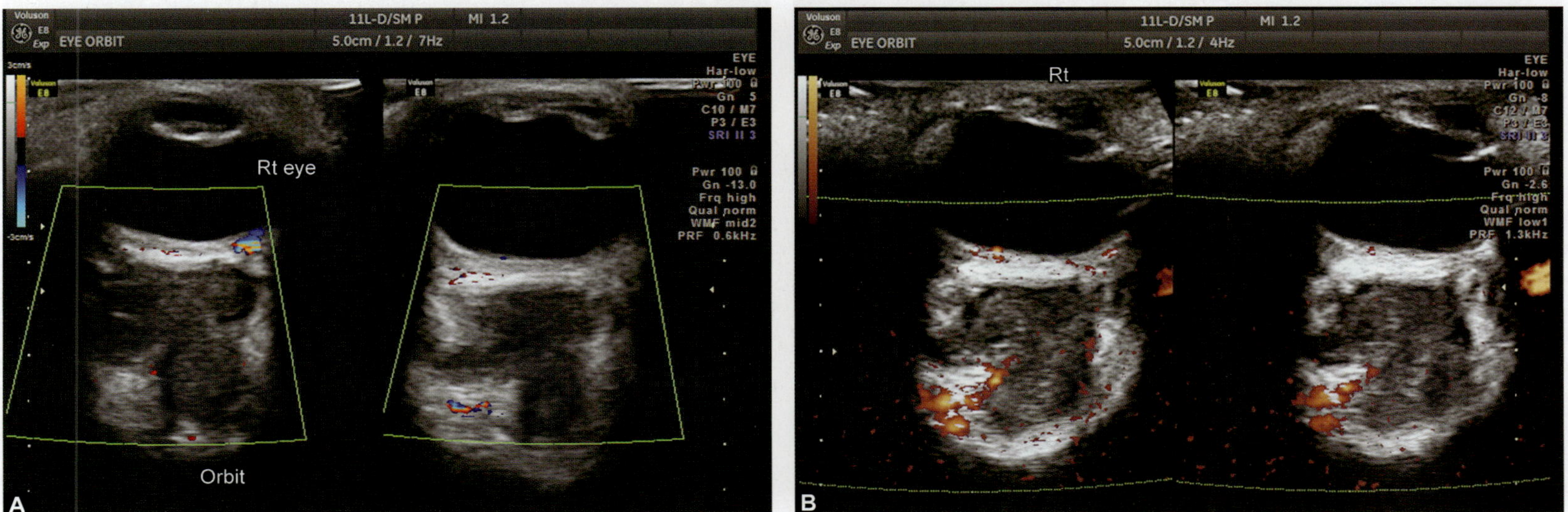

FIGURES 1.264A and B

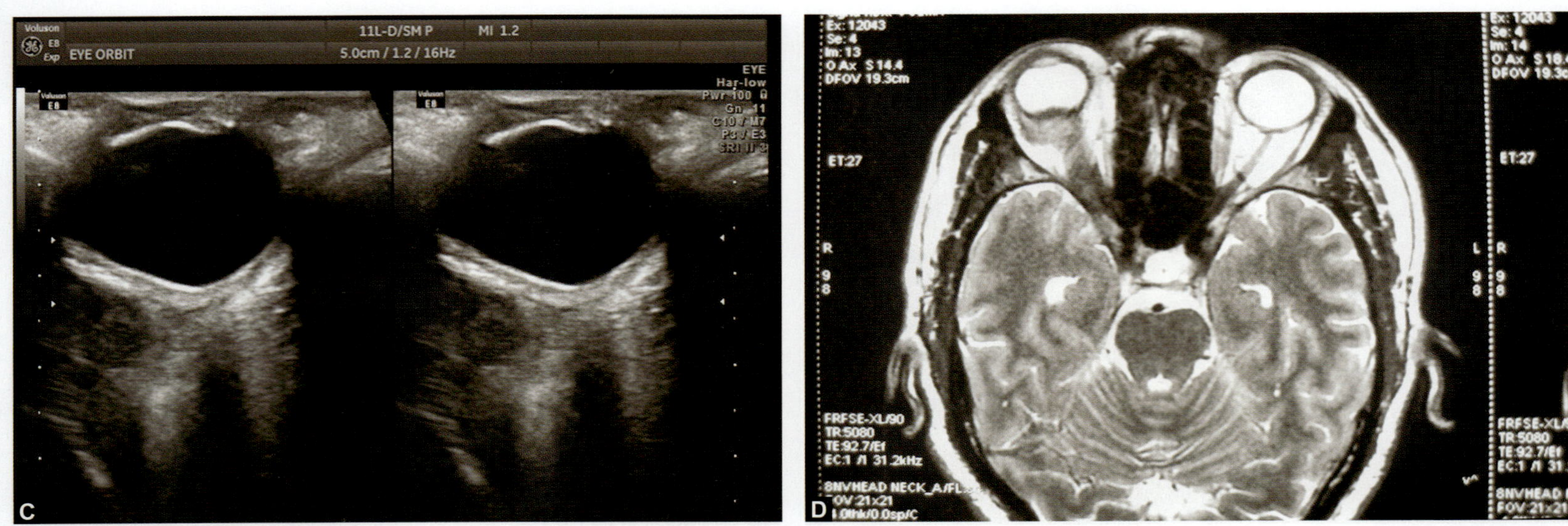

FIGURES 1.264C and D

FIGURES 1.264A to D: Retrobulbar abscess. A man presented with painful proptosis of right eye with limited movements. HRSG shows thick low level echo collection in the retrobulbar space. It is seen in the intraconal space suggestive of an abscess. Pressure is also seen on the optic nerve. The uveal coat is also thickened and edematous. The MR of the same patient confirms USG findings.

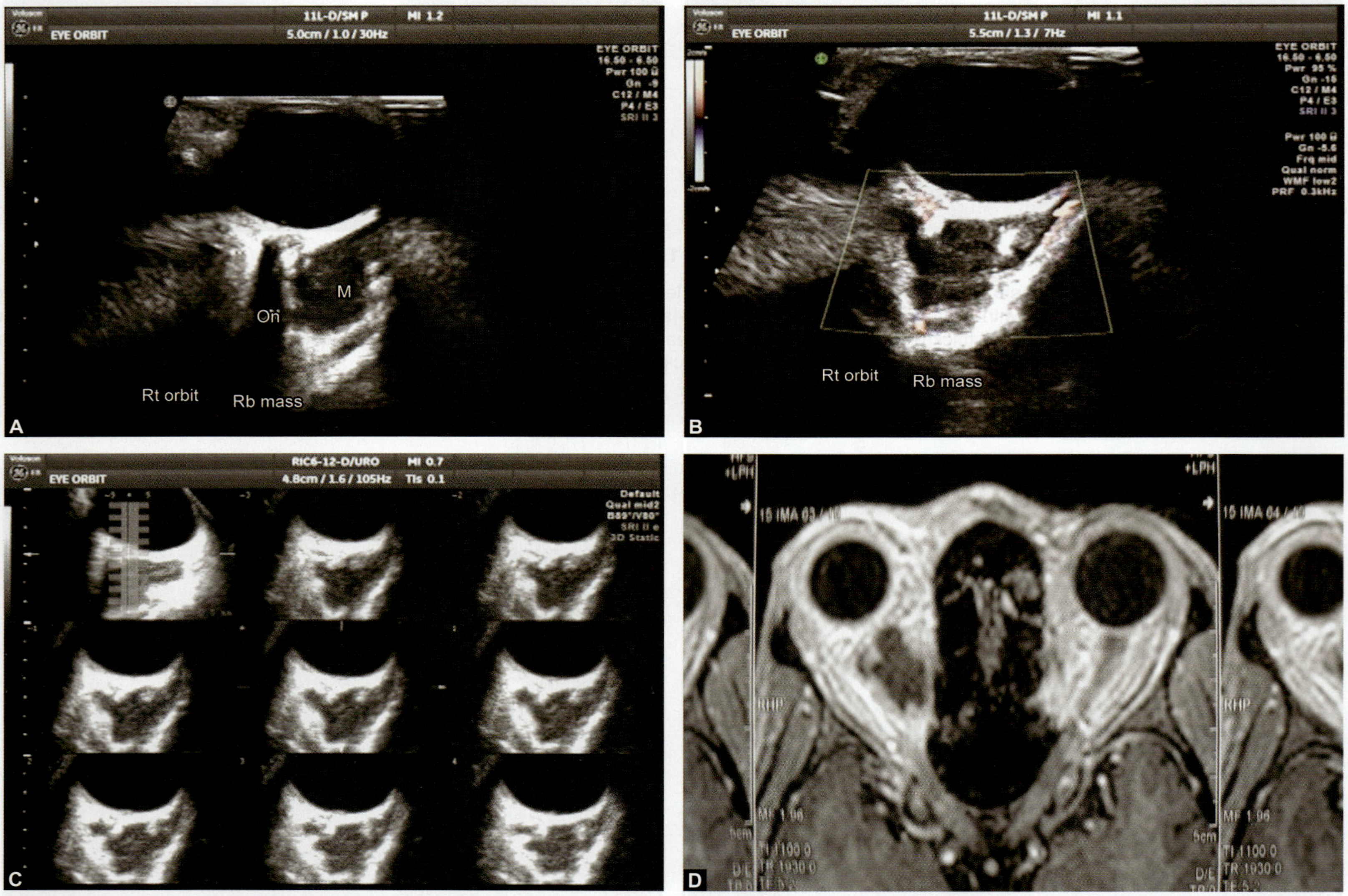

FIGURES 1.265A to D: Retrobulbar abscess. A patient presented with painful proptosis of the right eye. HRSG shows thick pocket of collection in the retrobulbar space. It is seen pressing and displacing the optic nerve suggestive of an abscess. On color flow imaging, no flow is seen in it. MR of the same patient shows the similar findings.

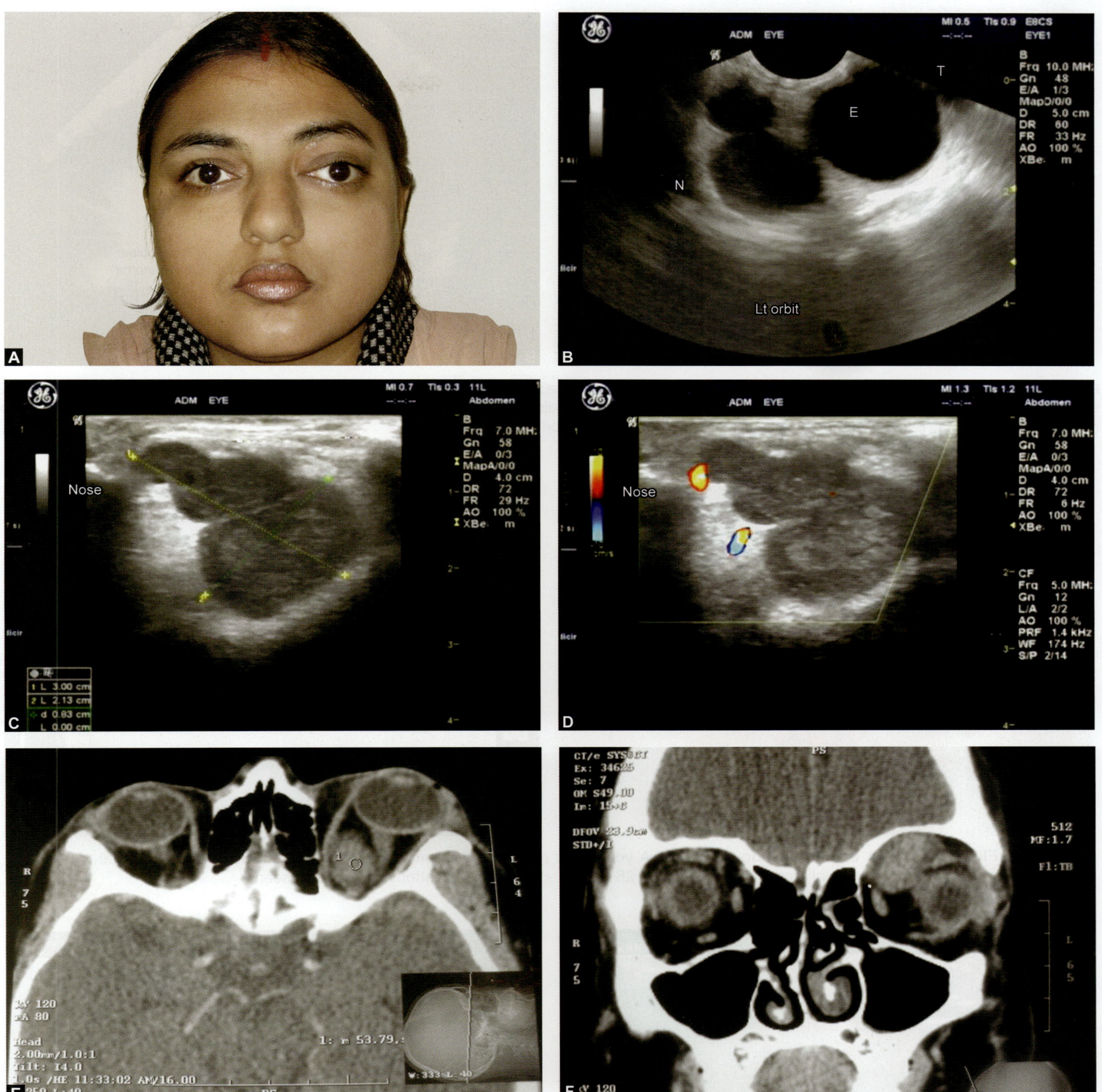

FIGURES 1.266A to F: Organized abscess. A young girl presented with proptosis of left eye with swelling of the medial side in the infraorbital region. HRSG shows a lobulated pocket of thick collection coming out from the upper medial quadrant of the orbit. Thick echoes are seen in it suggestive of an abscess. On color flow imaging, no flow is seen in it. CT scan of the same patient shows the organized collection in the retrobulbar space. USG-guided aspiration confirms organized pus collection.

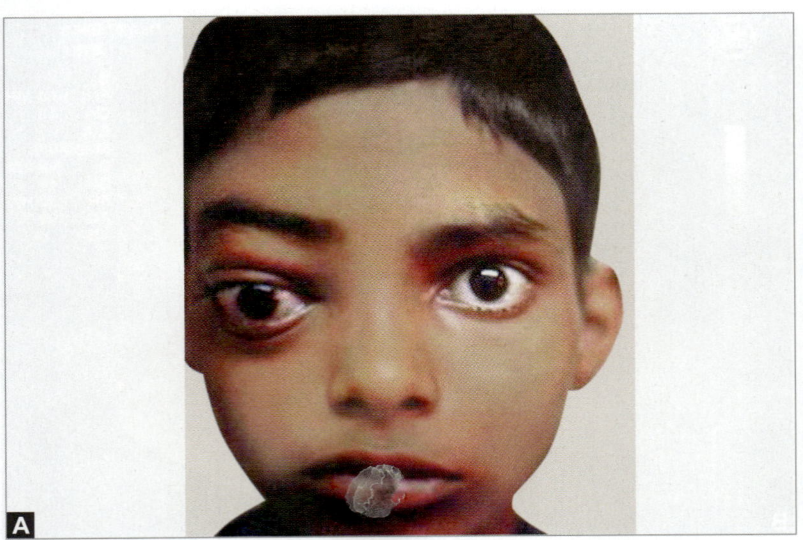

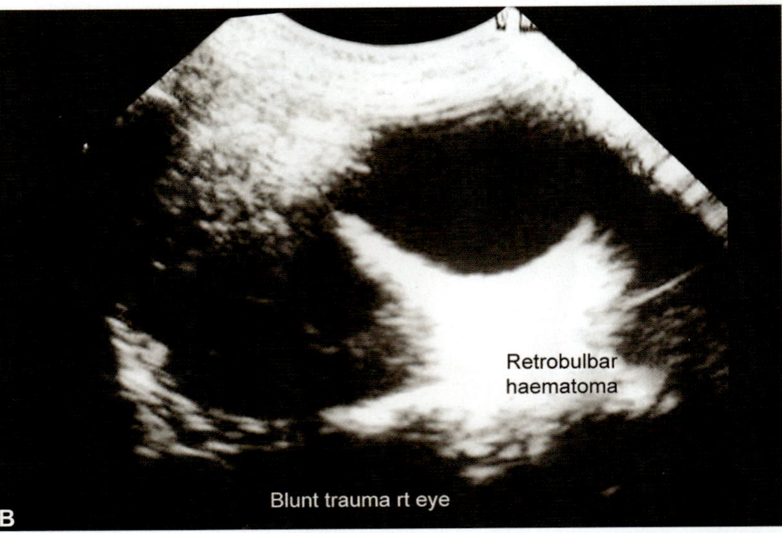

FIGURES 1.267A and B: Retrobulbar hematoma. A young boy sustained blunt injury to eye and presented with proptosis with painful eye. HRSG shows low-level echo complex mass in retrobulbar space with anterior displacement of eyeball. Few internal echoes are seen in it suggestive of retrobulbar hematoma. Eye was normal. Patient responded to compression bandage.

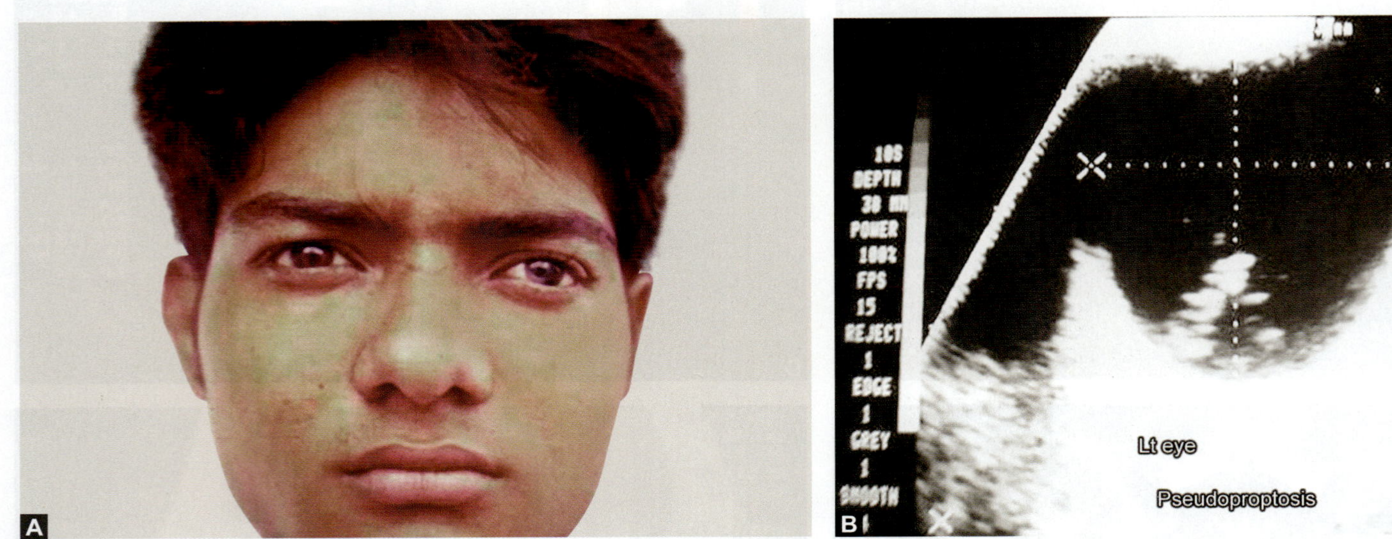

FIGURES 1.268A and B: Pseudo-proptosis. A young boy presented with proptosis of left eye. HRSG shows increased axial length of left eye. It is 26 mm (N < 24 mm). No retrobulbar mass is seen.

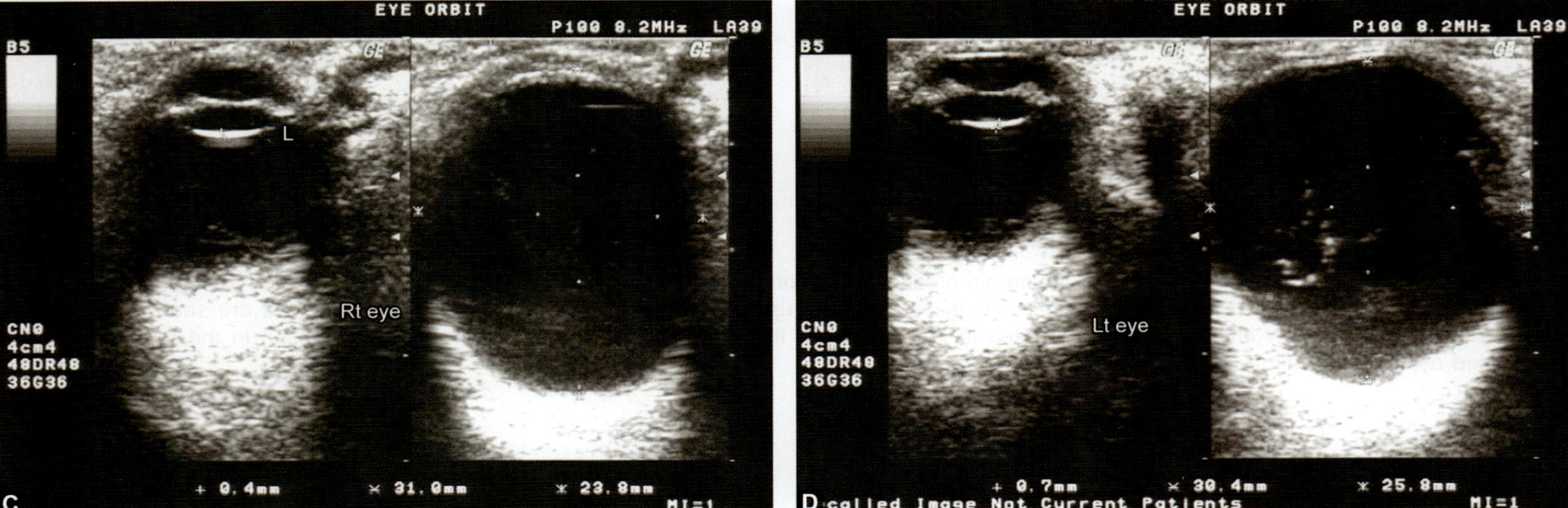

FIGURES 1.268C and D: Posterior staphyloma. Both eyeballs are oblong in shape with increased axial length. Right eye is 30 mm and left eye 30.4 mm, presented as bilateral proptosis. The staphyloma is an abnormal protrusion of the uveal tissue because of thinning of outer white coat of the eye sclera. Posterior staphyloma is most congenital or an manifestation of more extreme form of myopia.

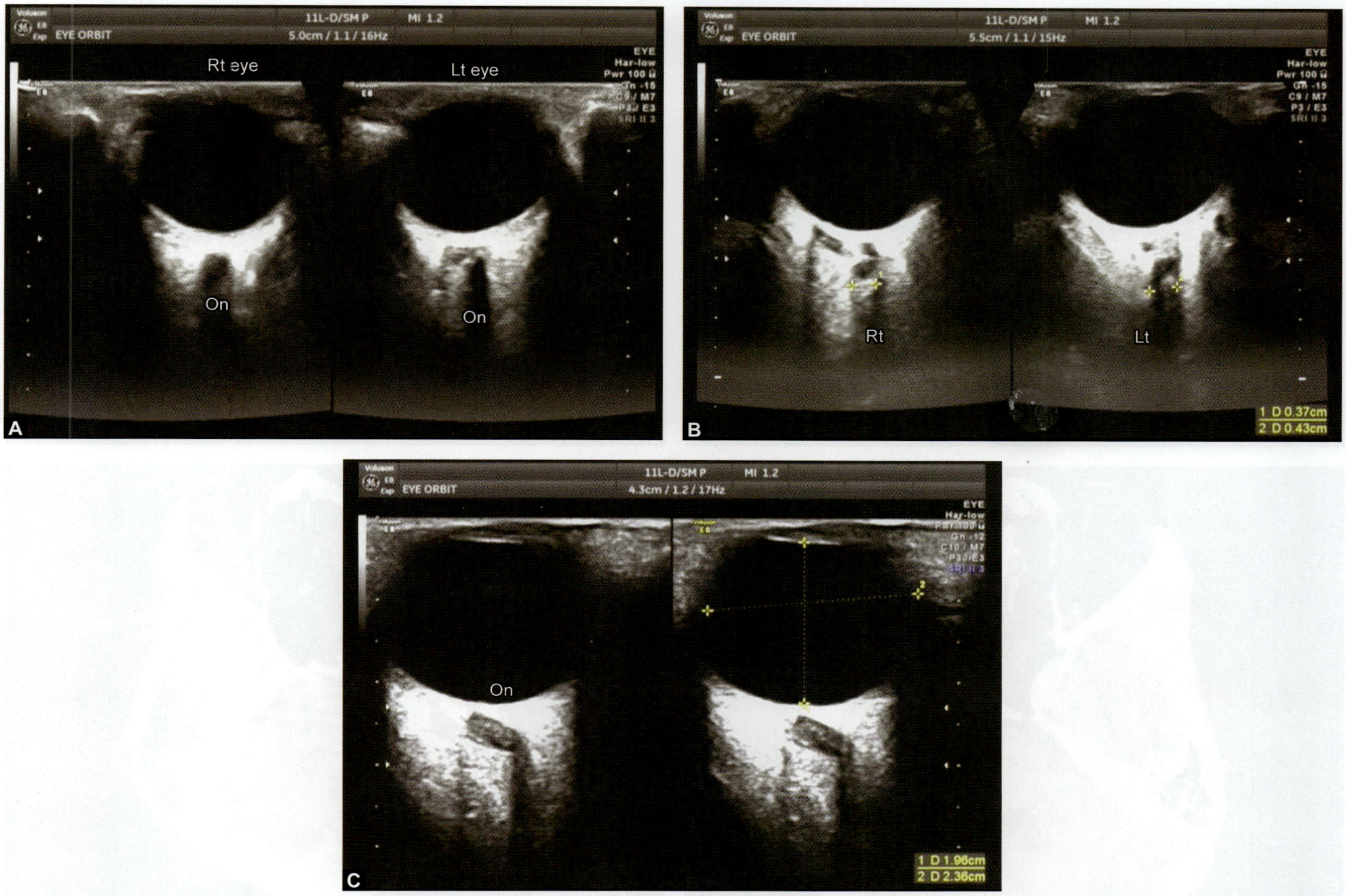

FIGURES 1.269A to C: Optic nerve edema. A patient presented with blurring of vision. HRSG shows diffuse edema of the optic nerve. Left optic nerve is thickened than the right and edematous suggestive of neuritis. On 30° rotation of the eye the fluid seeps along the optic nerve sheath and nerve becomes normal in thickness.

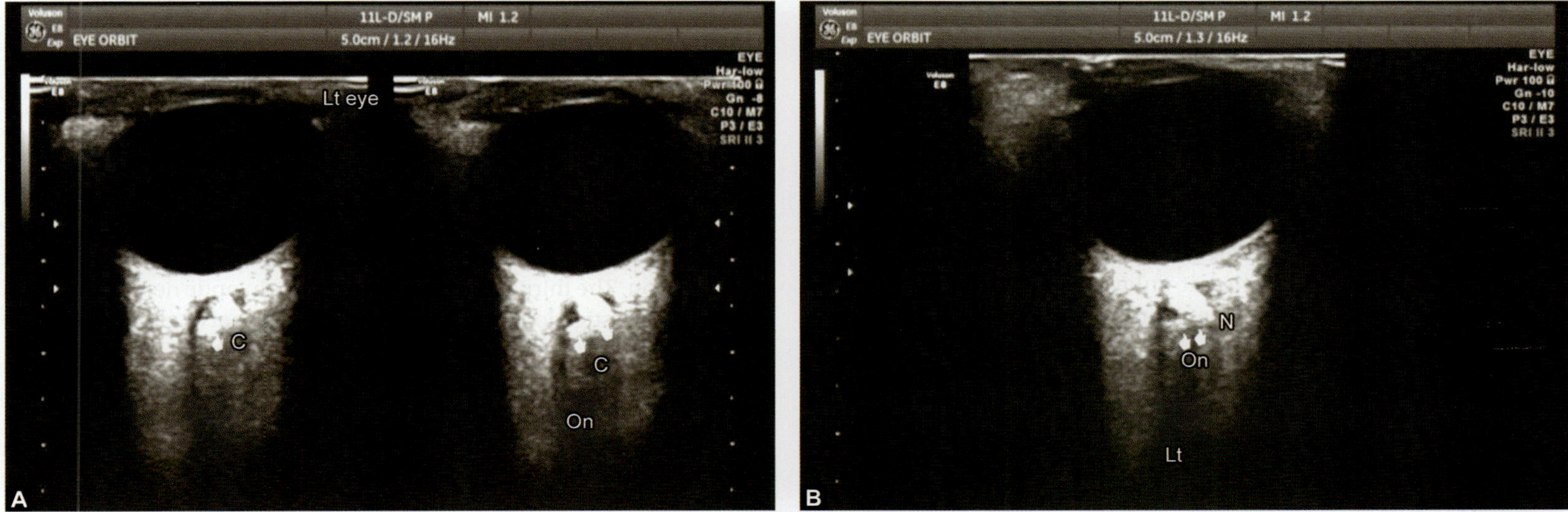

FIGURES 1.270A and B

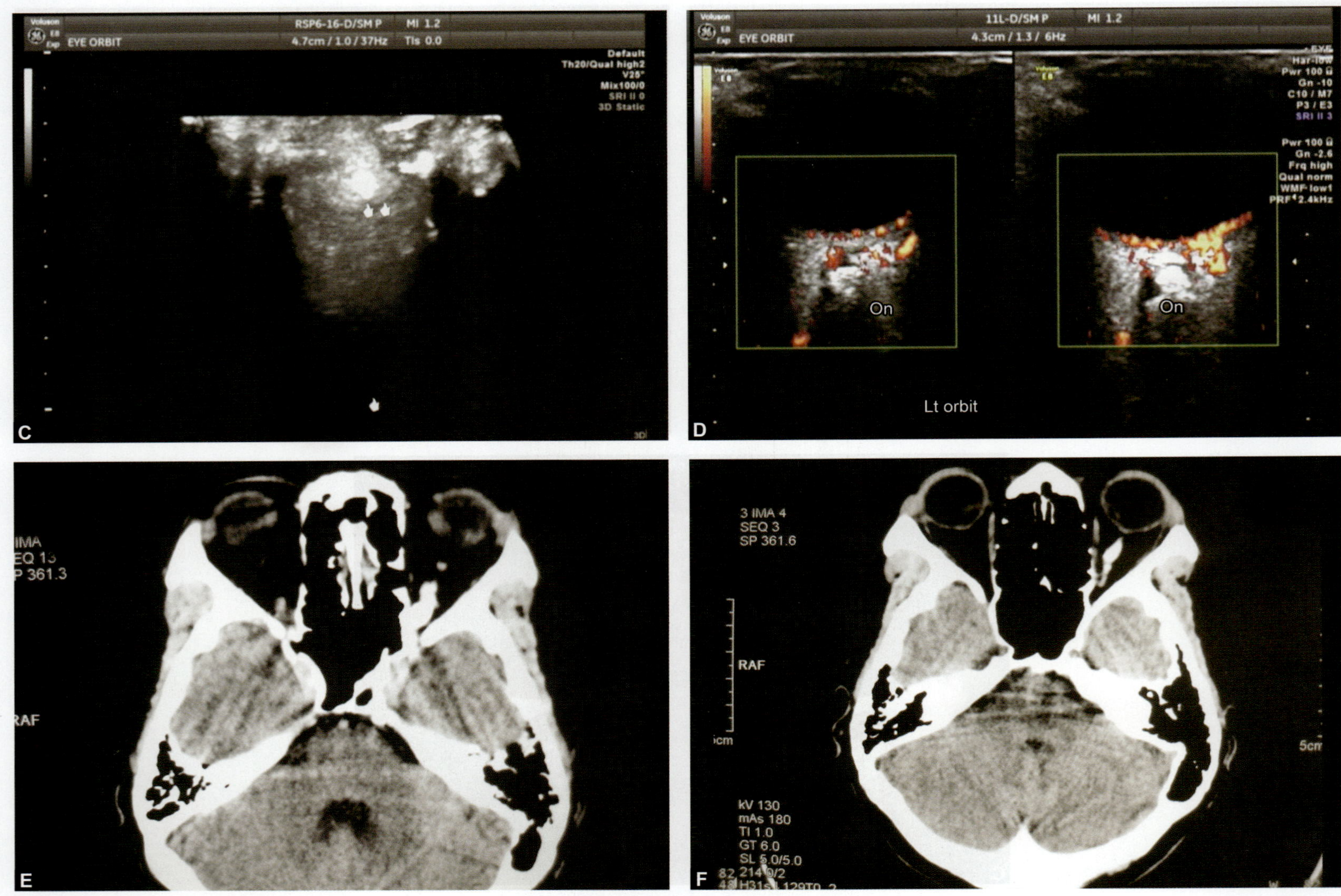

FIGURES 1.270C to F

FIGURES 1.270A to F: Chronic optic neuritis with nerve calcification. A patient presented with gradual loss of vision in left eye. HRSG shows dense echogenic calcification in the optic nerve. Punctate calcification is seen in the optic nerve. On color flow imaging, no flow is seen in the nerve sheath suggestive of chronic neuritis with calcification. CT scan of the same patient shows calcified nerve in the left orbit.

Optic Nerve Tumors

Meningioma

Meningiomas are optic nerve sheath tumors. They present as slowly developing proptosis and unilateral in origin. Vision impairment is associated with the tumor when it enlarges and ruptures through the duramater, it occupies the retrobulbar space. They are highly reflective masses and calcification may present in optic nerve sheath or in tumor.

Optic Nerve Glioma

Optic nerve glioma are smooth, fusiform or ovoid mass which replace the normal optic nerve. The lesion is poorly reflective and shows poor acoustic transmission. The thirty-degree test is negative in optic nerve glioma. CT is a better investigation for the diagnosis of optic nerve glioma.

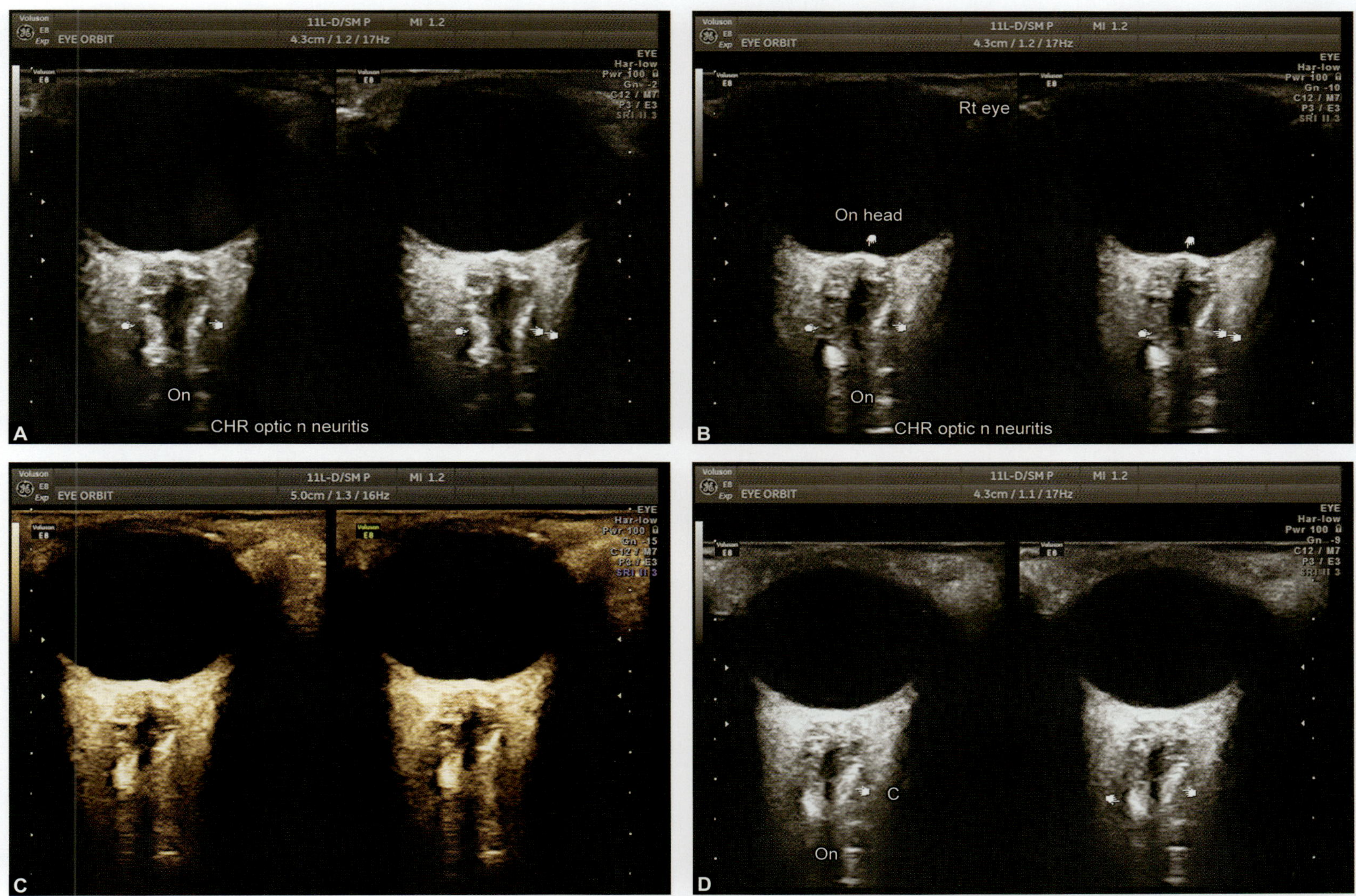

FIGURES 1.271A to D: A patient presented with gradual loss of vision in both eyes. HRSG shows dense echogenic calcification in the nerve sheath of optic nerve on both sides. The optic nerve head also shows calcification. The calcified specks are seen distributed along the nerve sheath suggestive of chronic optic neuritis.

Neurilemmoma

Neurilemmomas are rare tumors. They arise from proliferation of Schwann cells. They are hypoechoic nodular masses and seen in the superior orbit. They may be present in muscle cone of in extraconal compartment.

Optic Neuritis

In optic neuritis, the optic nerve is enlarged due to fluid collection in perineural sheath. Therefore, the optic nerve gets thickened. The thirty-degree test is the valuable test to differentiate between optic nerve tumor or inflammation. The test is carried out in fixed primary gaze position, and the patient is asked to rotate his eye to 30 degree towards to probe. In case of fluid collection, the fluid redistributes itself along the optic nerve sheath as the nerve stretches and the swelling subsides. However, the swelling persists on rotation of eye to 30 degree in case of tumor of optic nerve.

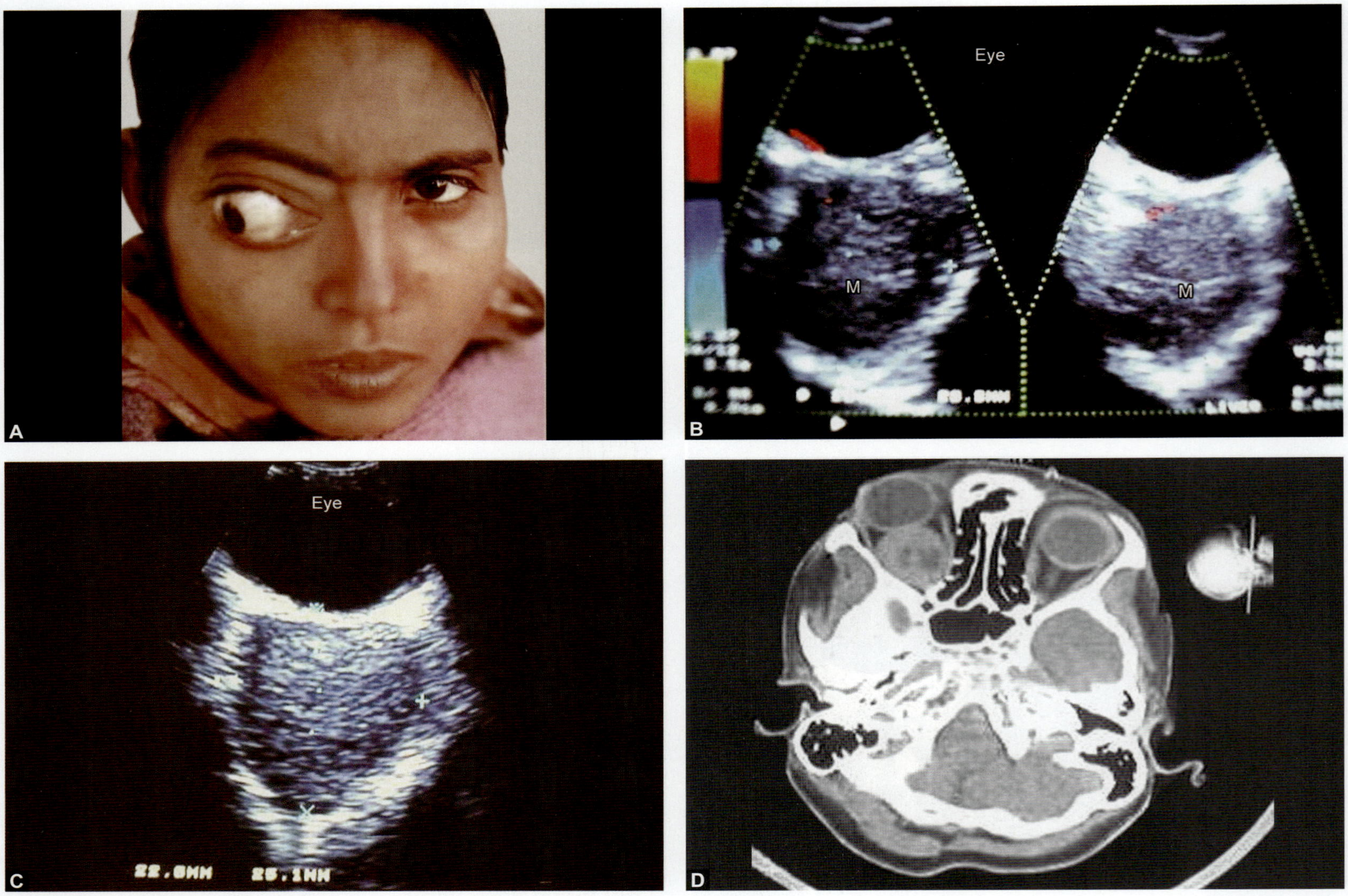

FIGURES 1.272A to D: Optic nerve meningioma. A women presented with proptosis and, diminished vision. HRSG shows well-defined fusiform soft tissue mass coming out from the optic nerve. Echogenic calcification is seen in it. On Color flow Doppler poor flow is seen in it. Biopsy shows optic nerve meningioma. CT shows a heterogeneous intraconal mass with area of necrosis. HRSG show a highly heterogeneous mass occupying whole intraconal space. No nerve is seen. Biopsy showed optic nerve glioma.

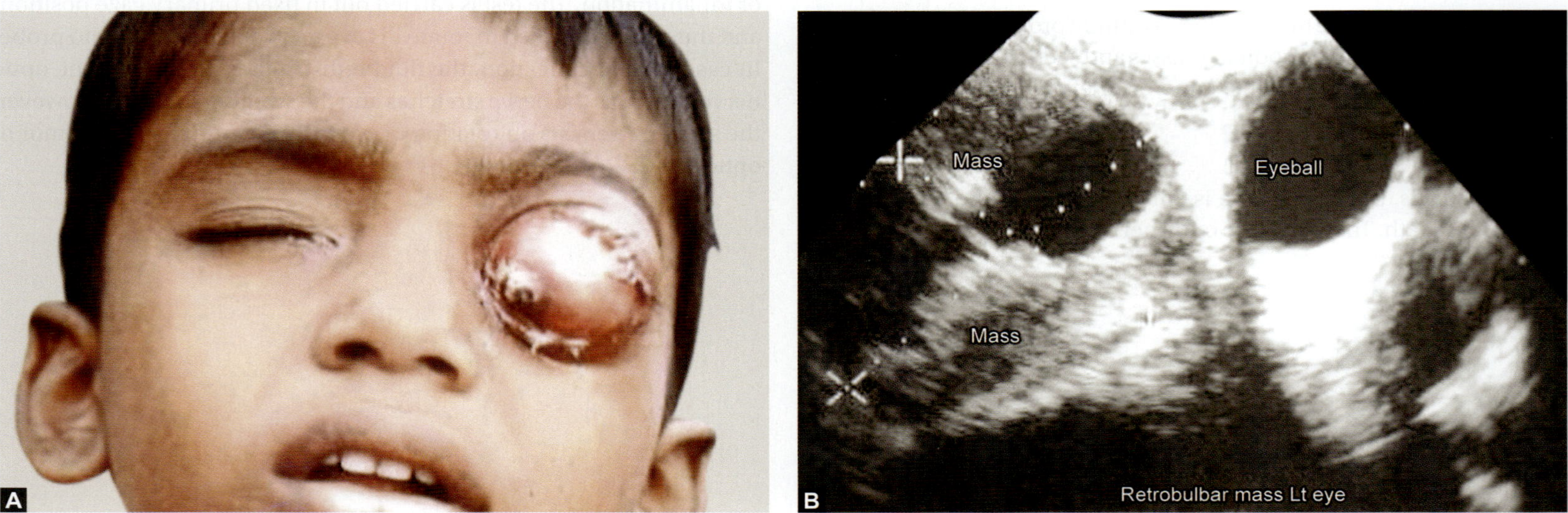

FIGURES 1.273A and B: A young boy presented with proptosis, loss of vision with exposure keratitis. HRSG shows a heterogeneous cystic mass in retrobulbar space. Biopsy showed cystic glioma of optic nerve.

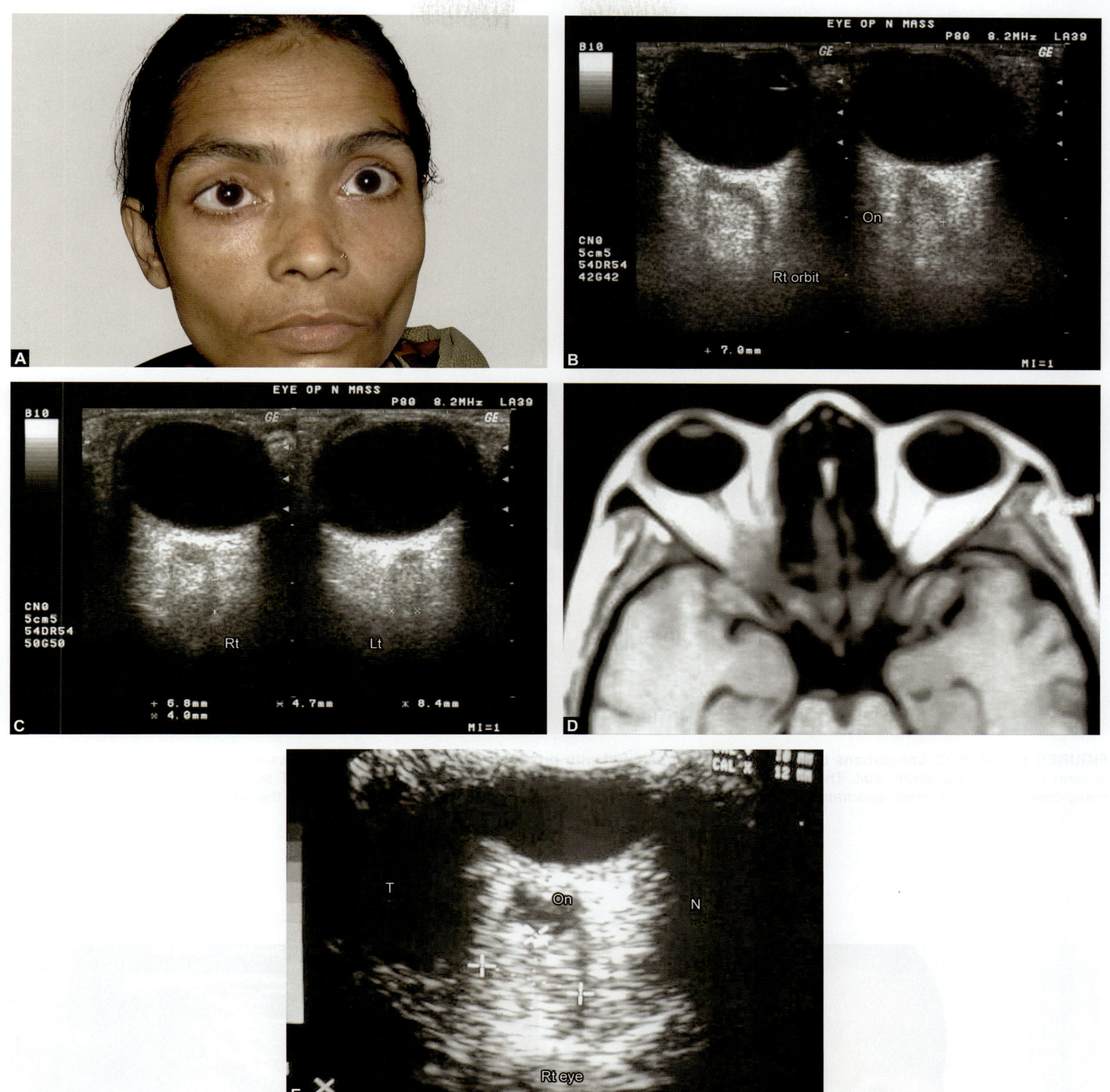

FIGURES 1.274A to E: A young lady presented with loss of vision with proptosis right eye. HRSG shows fusiform widening of optic nerve with echogenic mass in the nerve suggestive of optic nerve tumor. MRI of the same patient shows fusiform mass coming out from the optic nerve with expansion of apex of the cone. Biopsy showed optic nerve glioma. HRSG shows smooth widening of optic nerve. Expansion of the sheath is seen with a fusiform mass seen in the upper part of optic nerve. In a patient came with history of loss of vision. Sonographic features are suggestive of optic nerve tumor. Biopsy of the tumor show optic nerve glioma.

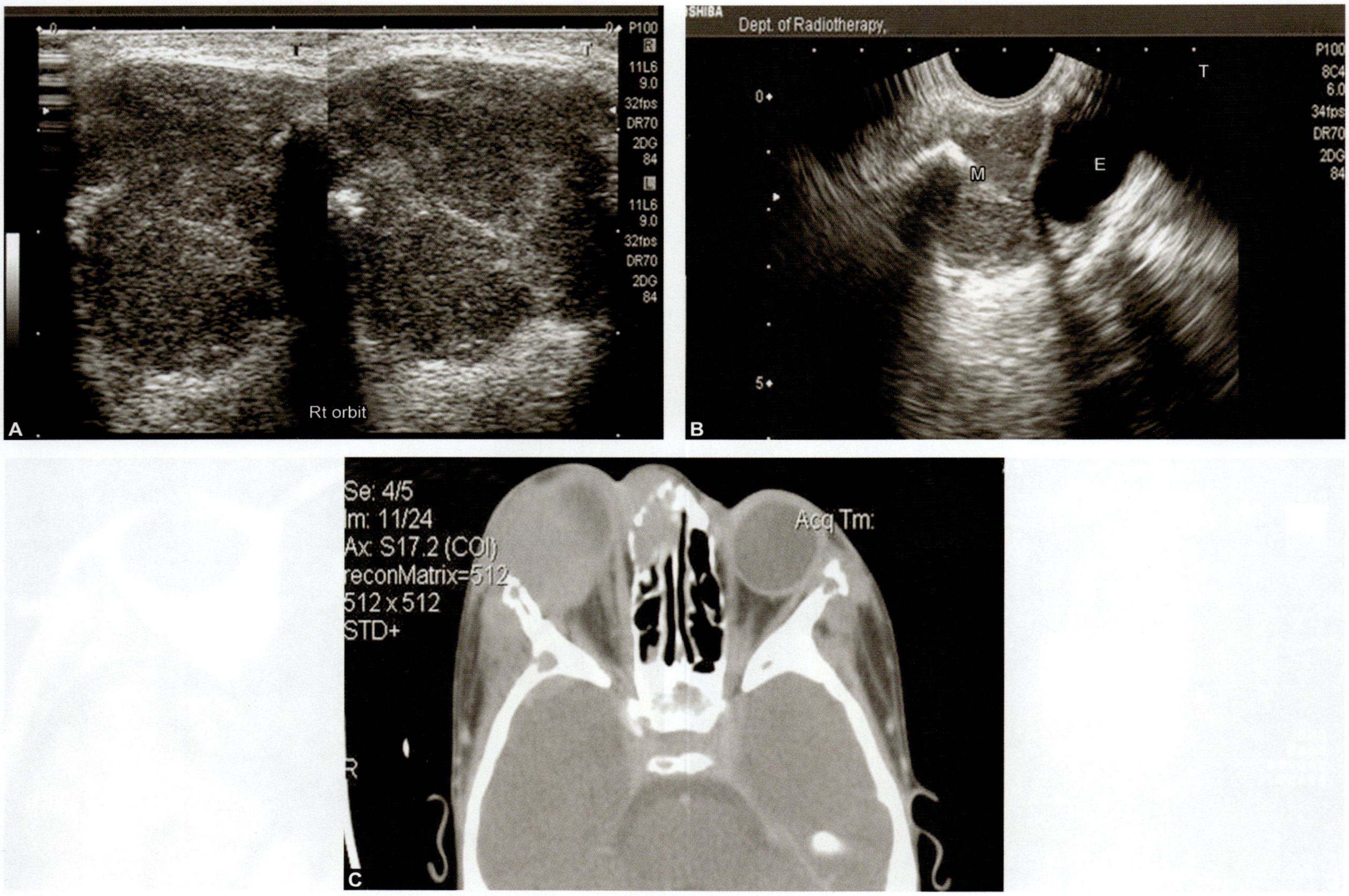

FIGURES 1.275A to C: Langerhans cell histiocystosis presented with proptosis. HRSG shows a big soft tissue mass in the right orbit. The mass is seen occupying the whole orbit. The eyeball is also seen adherent with the mass and it is compressed. CT scan of the same patient shows the mass coming out from lateral quadrant of the orbit and invading the eyeball. It is also seen extending outside the orbit.

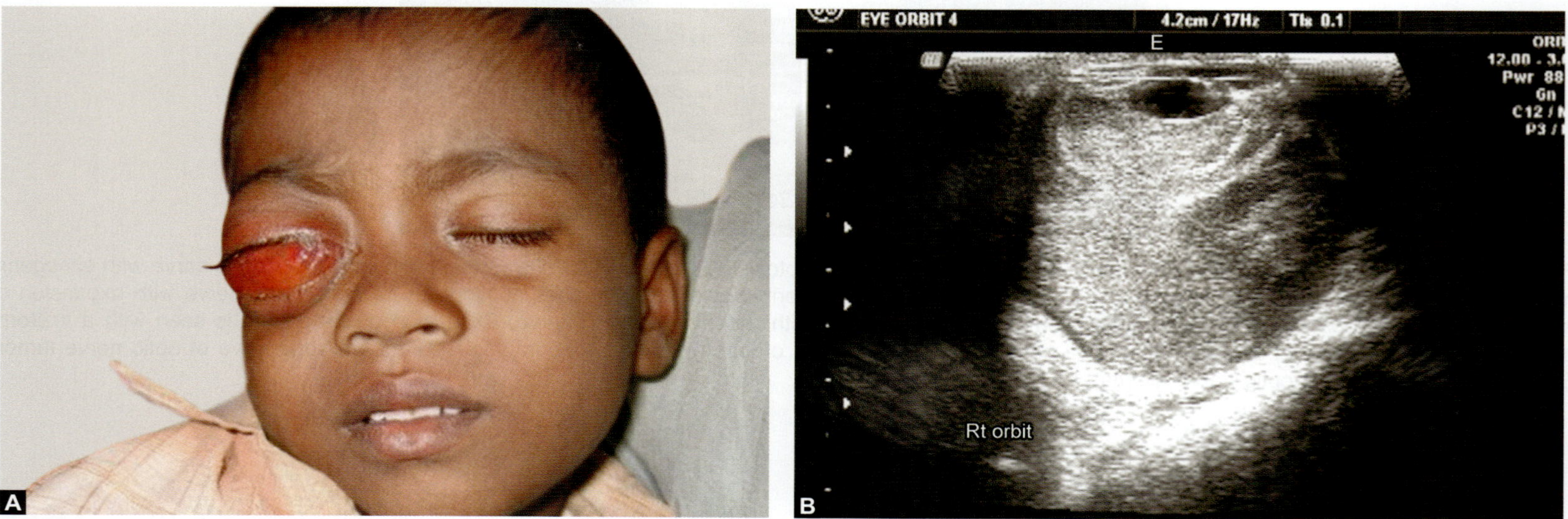

FIGURES 1.276A and B

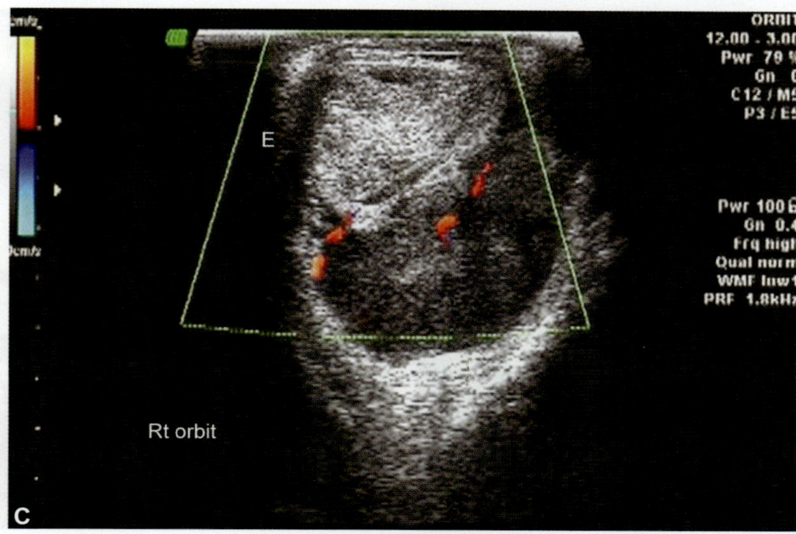

FIGURE 1.276C

FIGURES 1.276A to C: Congenital rhabdomyosarcoma. A young child presented with marked proptosis with bulging eye from the orbit. HRSG shows a huge mass in retrobulbar space. It is seen invading the eyeball. Normal anatomy is distorted. The biopsy of the mass confirms rhabdomyosarcoma.

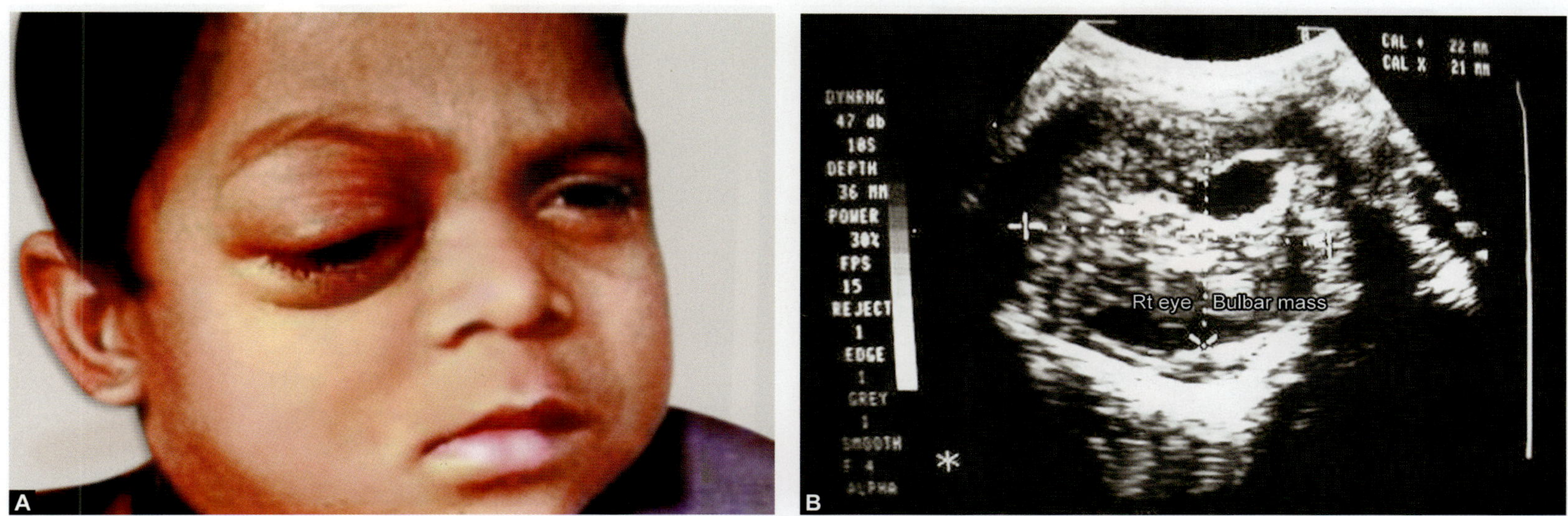

FIGURES 1.277A and B: Rhabdomyosarcoma muscle. A boy presented with proptosis and loss of vision.: Big tumor is seen filling the orbit engulfing the eyeball and invaded it. Biopsy rhabdomyosarcoma.

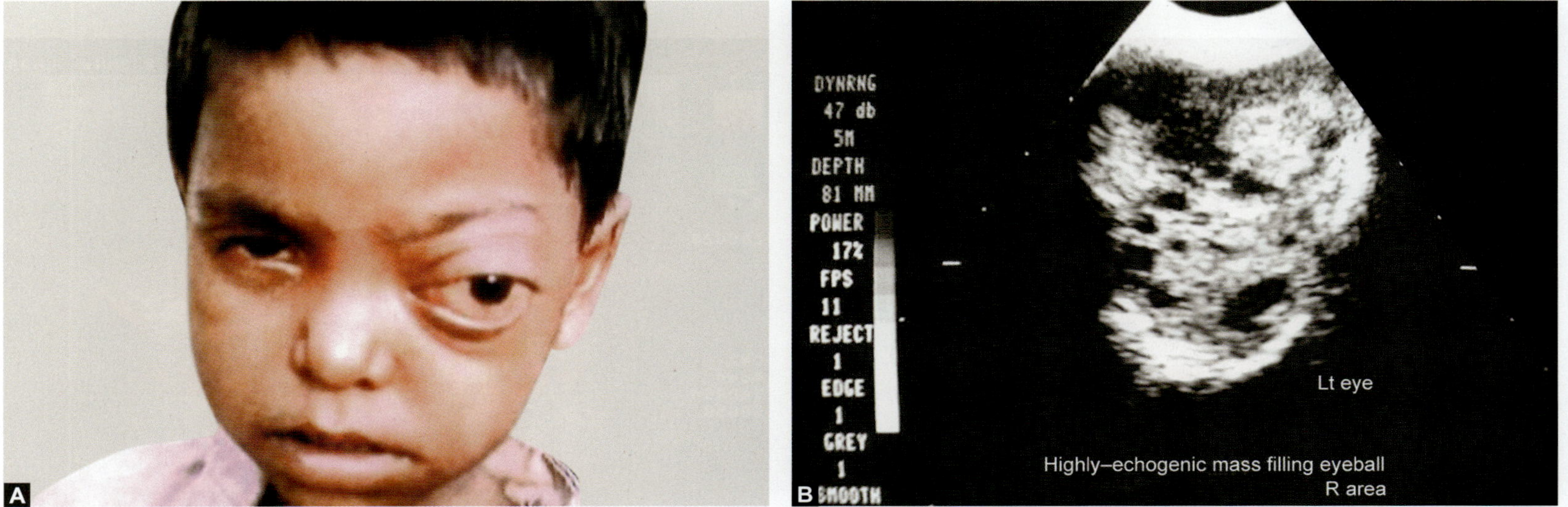

FIGURES 1.278A and B: Leukemic deposits. Known case of acute lymphatic leukemia presented with proptosis and loss of vision. HRSG show highly heterogeneous mass giving the whole of retrobulbar area. It has destroyed normal anatomy and also invaded optic nerve area of necrosis also been in the mass.

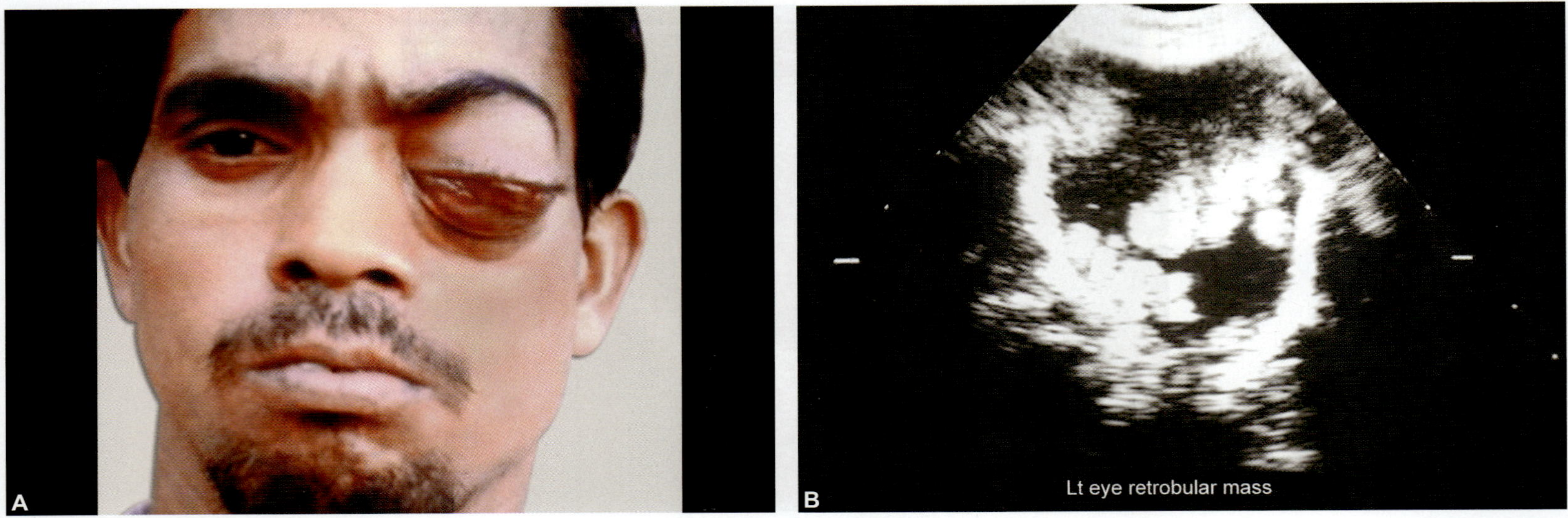

FIGURES 1.279A and B: FTC-operated lymphoma. A patient operated for lymphomatous deposits presented with recurrence and soft tissue mass filling the orbit suggestive of lymphoid tumor filling the orbit area of necrosis also seen in the mass.

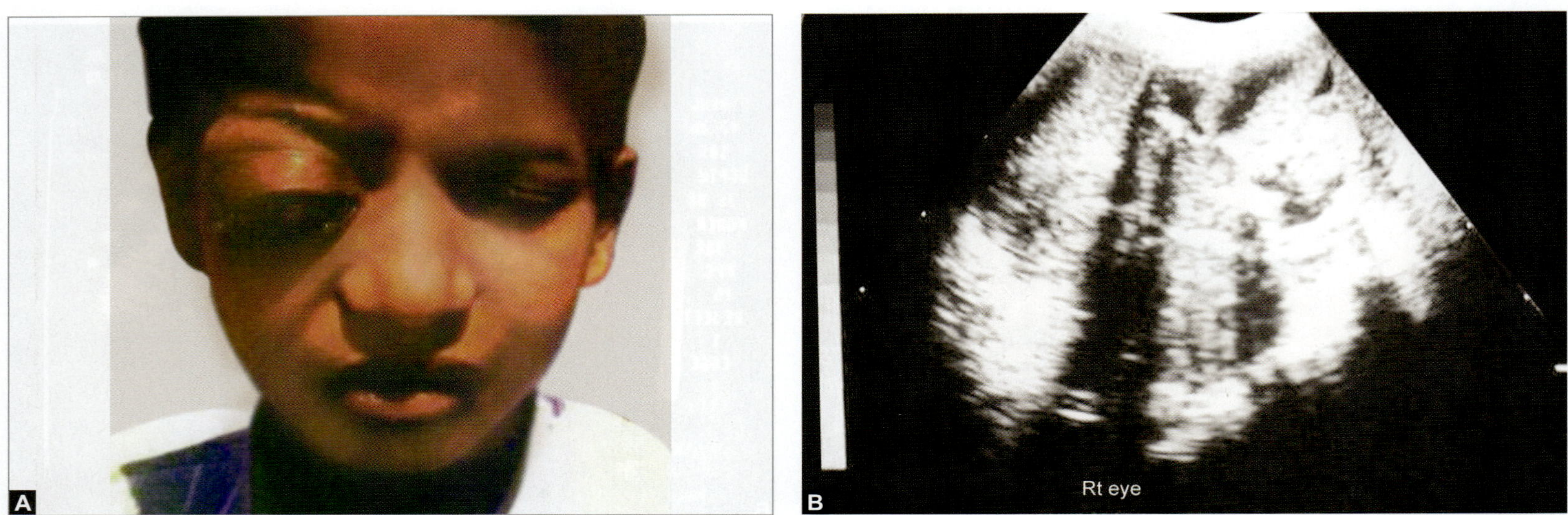

FIGURES 1.280A and B: Orbital lymphoma: Heterogeneous mass seen filling the orbit and also invaded the eyeball. The eye coat is broken by the mass and tumor is seen in the eyeball.

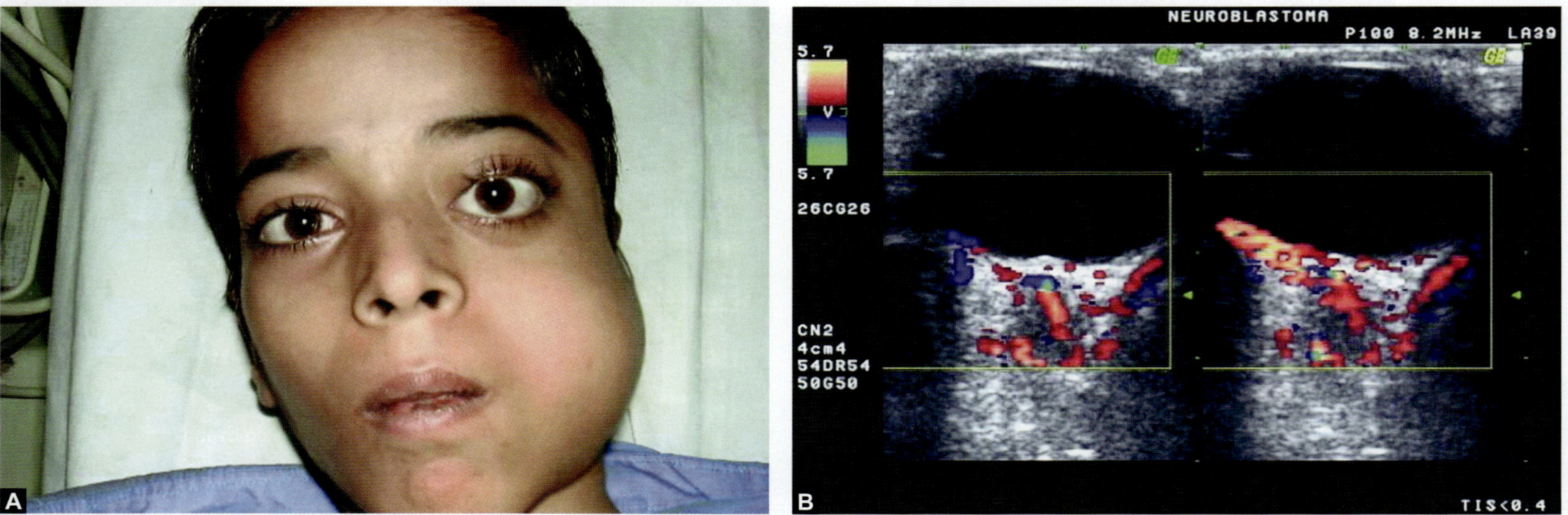

FIGURES 1.281A and B

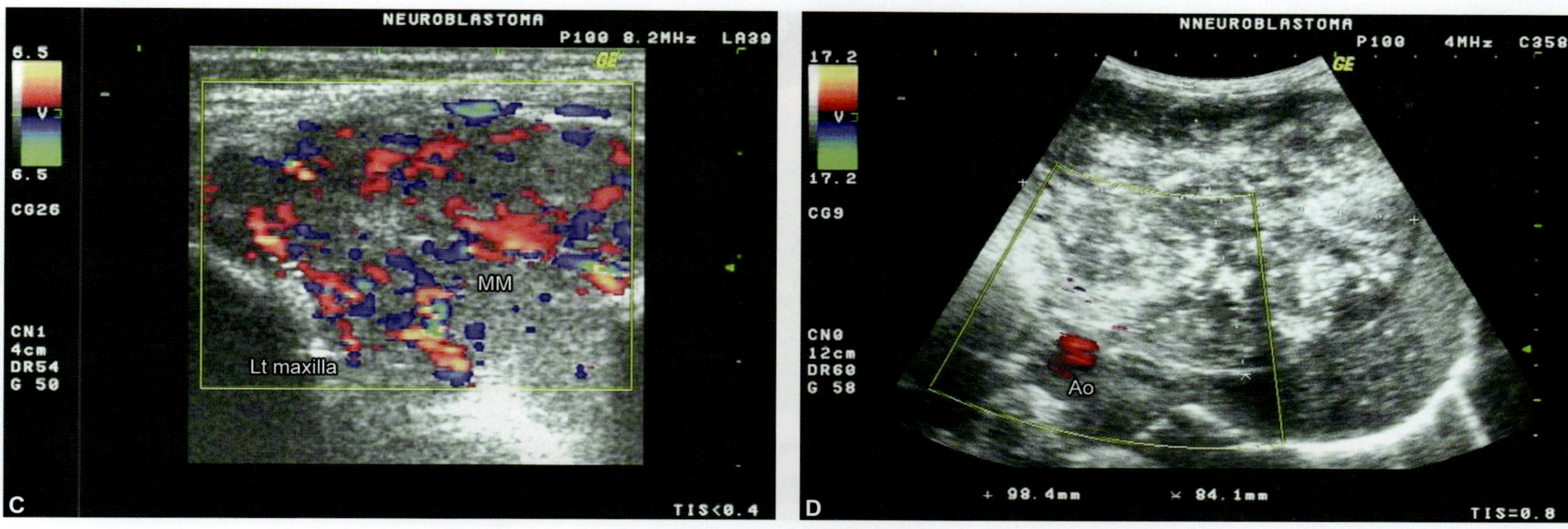

FIGURES 1.281C and D

FIGURE 1.281A to D: Metastatic deposits from neuroblastoma. A young boy presented left proptosis with swelling of the left jaw. Highly vascular soft tissue mass in left orbit metastatic deposit from the tumor. Highly vascular mass invading left maxilla and eaten up the bone metastatic deposit of suggestive of metastatic deposits. The primary tumor neuroblastoma was seen in abdomen. A big heterogeneous mass seen in left suprarenal area crossing the mid line. HRSG shows the mass—Biopsy proved neuroblastoma.

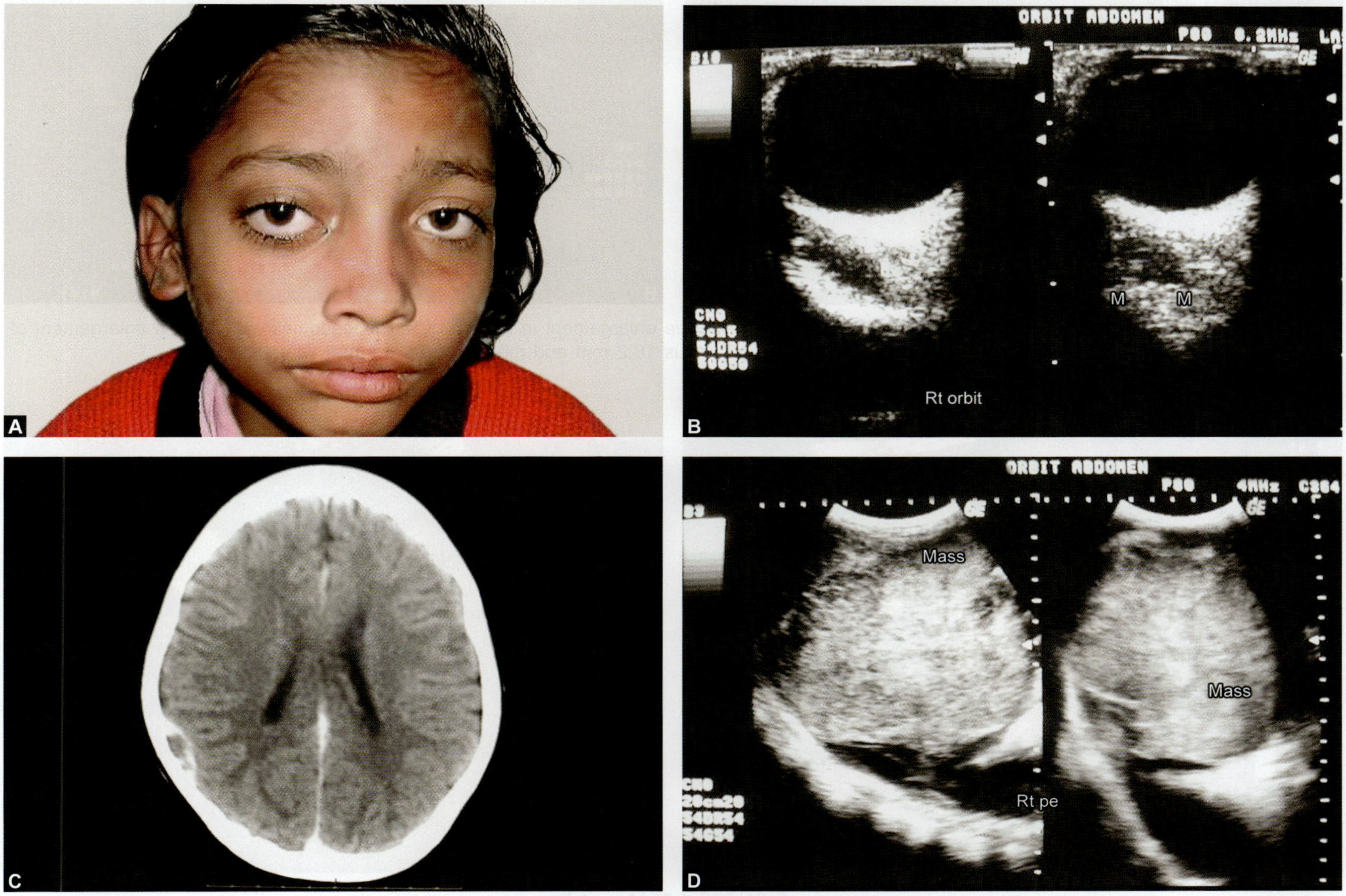

FIGURES 1.282A to D

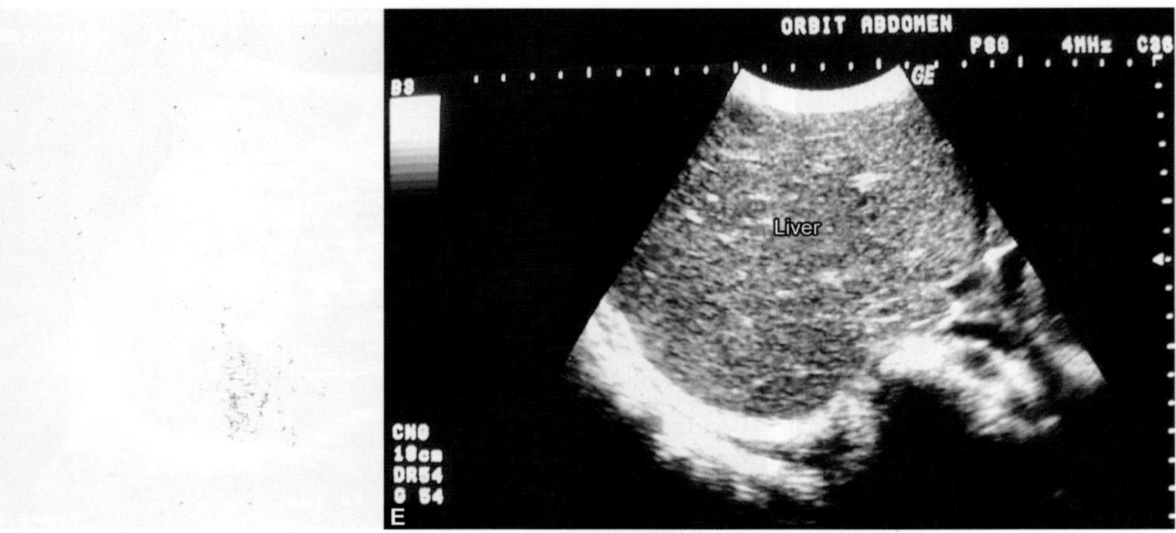

FIGURE 1.282E

FIGURES 1.282A to E: Primary neuroblastoma metastasis in the orbit. A young girl presented with proptosis right eye with painful eye. HRSG shows retrobulbar deposit. A hypodense mass is seen in intraconal region of the right orbit. CT of the same patient shows bony metastasis of the right parietal bone. Abdominal USG shows heterogeneous mass in right suprarenal area with liver deposits and right sided pleural effusion.

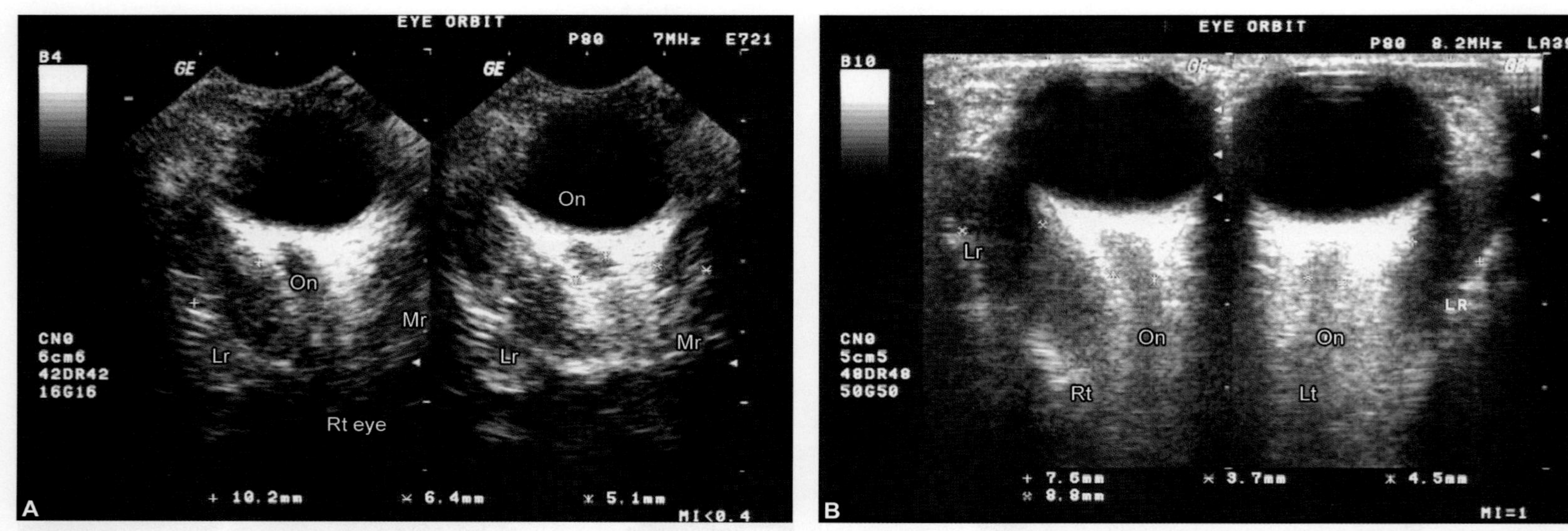

FIGURES 1.283A and B: Reticuloendotheliosis. Bilateral rectus muscle enlargement in a case of reticuloendotheliosis. Smooth enlargement of medial and lateral rectus muscles is seen. Lateral rectus 10.2 mm and medial rectus 6.4 mm (Normal <3 mm).

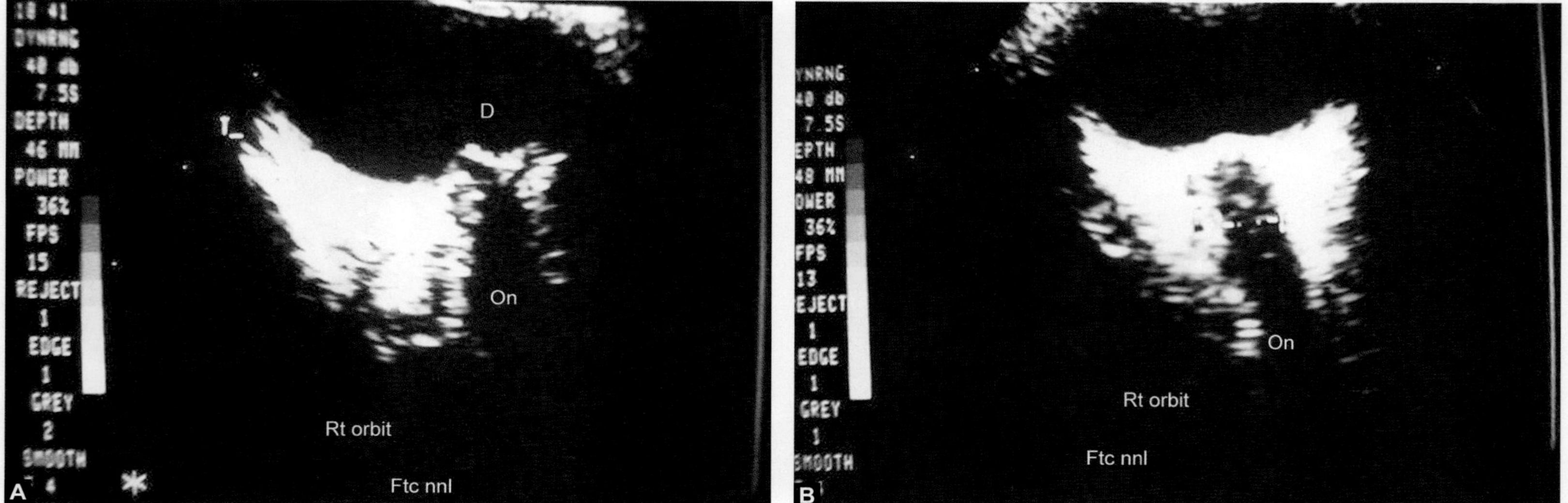

FIGURES 1.284A and B

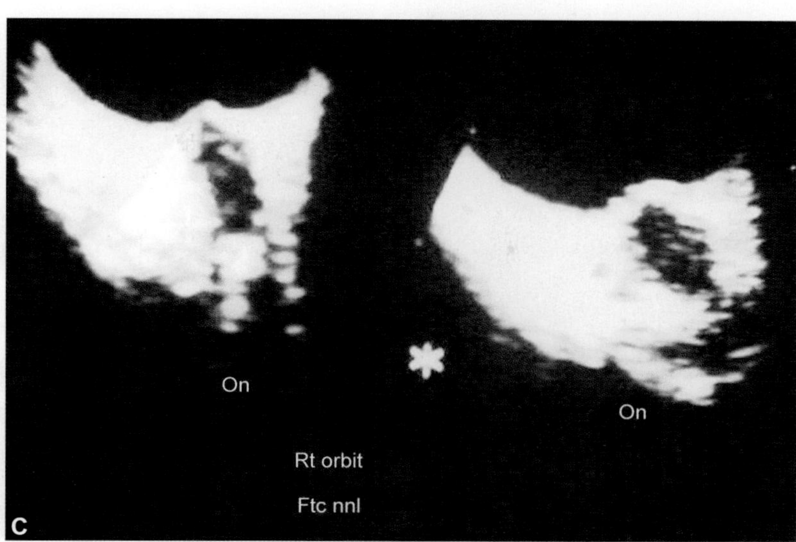

FIGURE 1.284C

FIGURES 1.284A to C: Metastasis of non-Hodgkin lymphoma. A known case of NHL presented loss of vision and pain in right eye. HRSG shows irregular mass invading optic nerve, optic nerve head. Calcification is also seen at optic nerve head accompanied with shadowing.

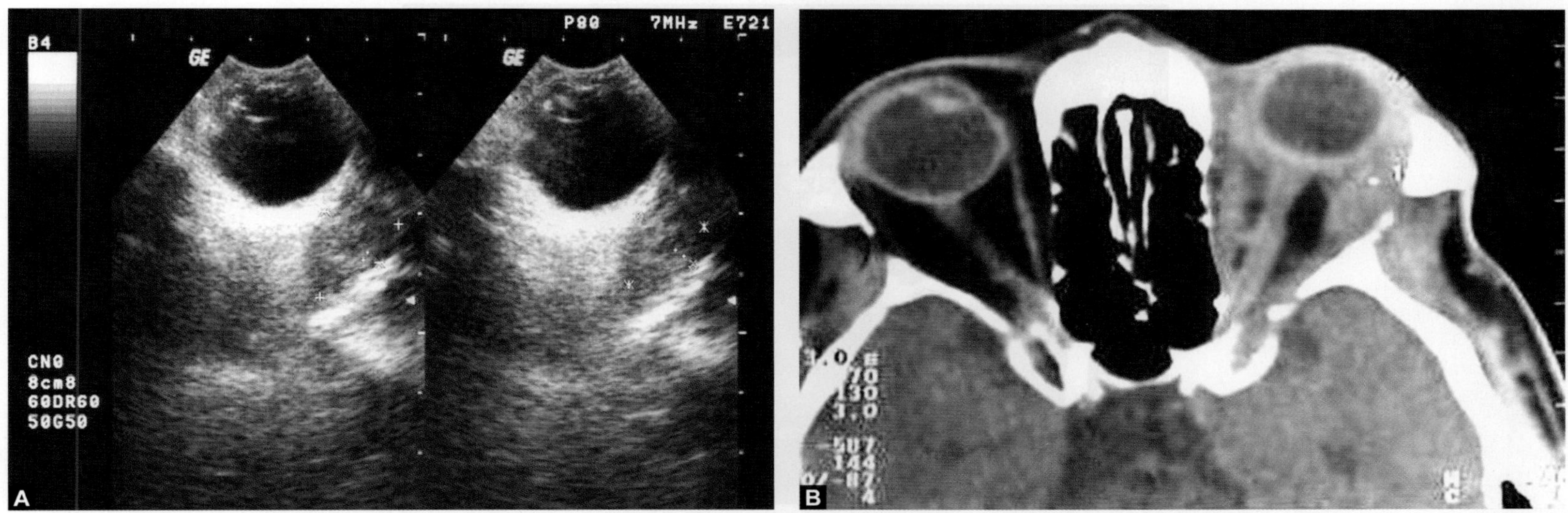

FIGURES 1.285A and B: Metastatic deposit—adenocarcinoma. Patient presented with swelling over lateral side of left orbit. HRSG showed irregular nodular mass in the lateral quadrant of orbit displacing the eyeball—open Biopsy–Metastatic deposit from adenocarcinoma. CT of the same patient shows the deposit mass in outer upper quadrant of left orbit.

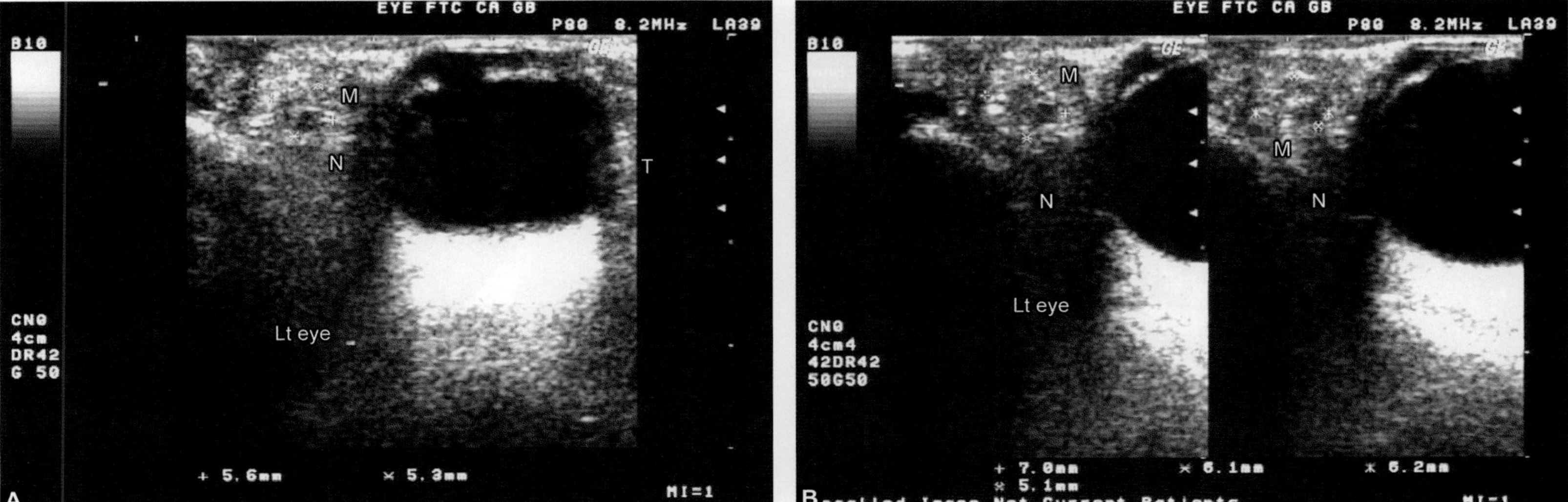

FIGURES 1.286A and B: Metastasis from carcinoma GB. A known case of carcinoma GB presented with mass in upper medial quadrant of left eye. HRSG shows heterogeneous nodular mass in upper medial part of left orbit. Biopsy proved metastasis carcinoma GB.

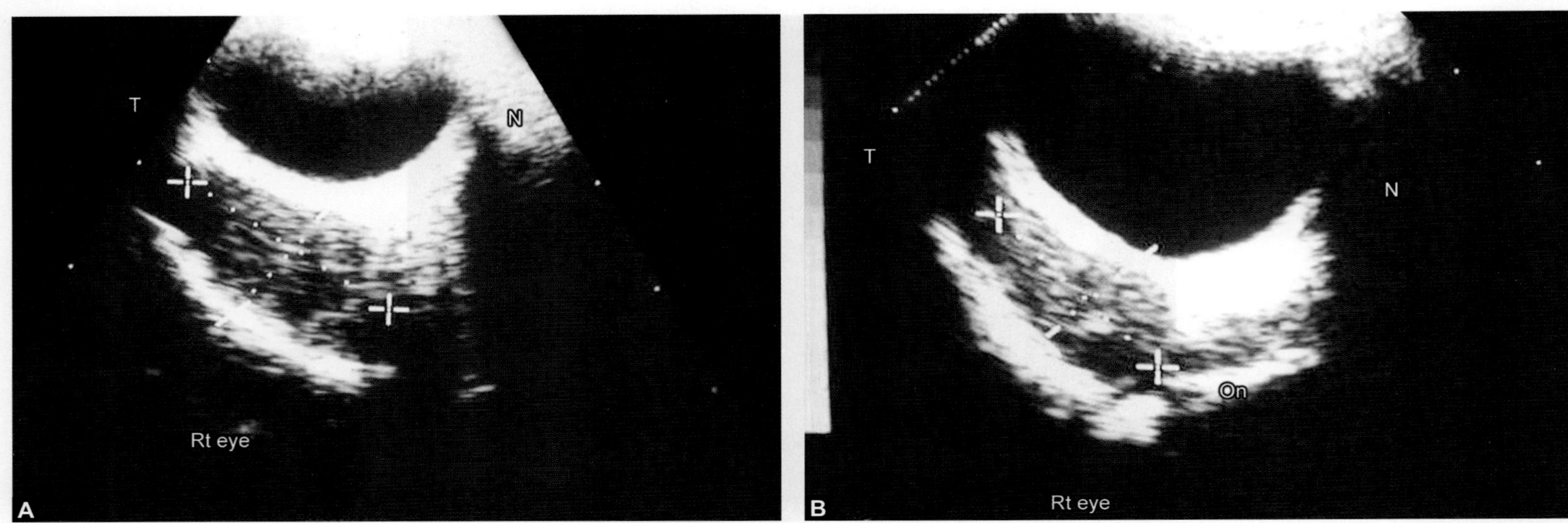

FIGURES 1.287A and B: Metastatic deposits osteosarcoma tibia. A known case of osteosarcoma of tibia presented with right eye proptosis and painful eye. HRSG shows hypoechoic metastatic deposit in retrobulbar area. Osteosarcoma is not known to metastasize to orbit. This was an unusual finding.

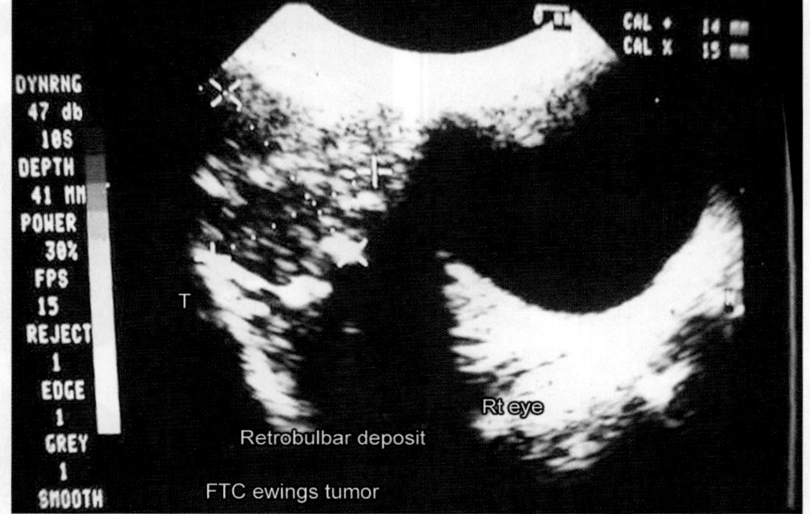

FIGURE 1.288: Metastatic deposit Ewing sarcoma. A young boy of 12 years of age known case of Ewing's tumor complained of diminished vision and right eye proptosis. HRSG shows a retrobulbar deposit in right upper outer quadrant. A heterogeneous mass was seen in upper outer quadrant.

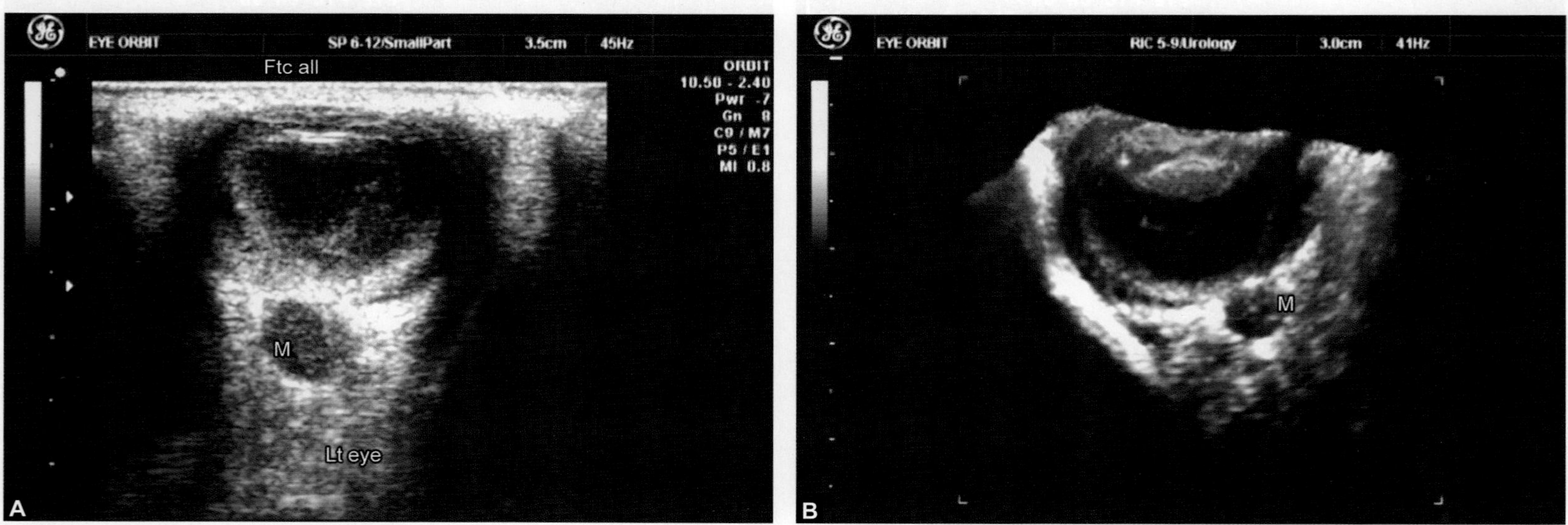

FIGURES 1.289A and B

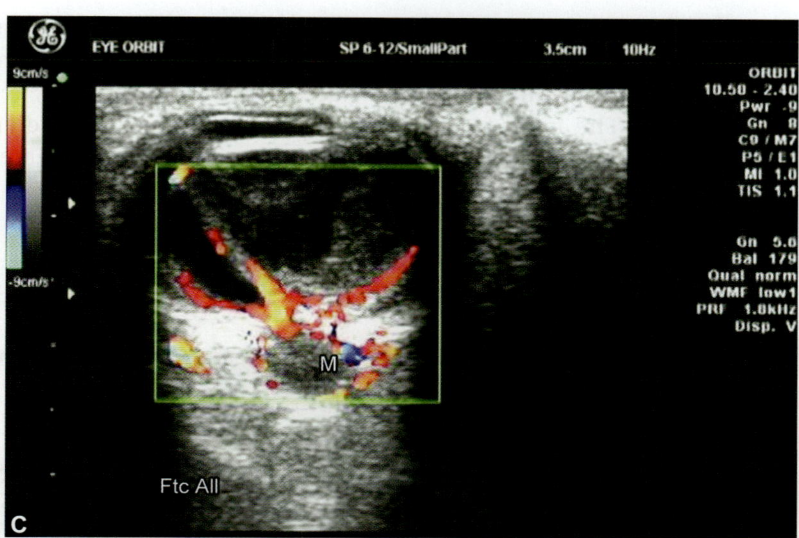

FIGURE 1.289C

FIGURES 1.289A to C: Metastasis deposit of acute lymphatic leukemia (ALL). A young child known case of ALL presented with sudden loss of vision. HRSG shows a hypoechoic deposit in the retrobulbar space. Eye also shows associated subchoroidal hemorrhage with collapsed eye. 3D imaging of the eye shows details of the deposit and subchoroidal hemorrhage. Color Doppler imaging shows increased flow in the metastasis and also in the membranes.

Periorbital Masses

HRSG is highly sensitive to evaluate periorbital masses like abscess, dermoid cyst, mucoceles, lid tumors and other periorbital pathologies.

Lacrimal Gland Tumors

HRSG is a good tool to evaluate tumors present in lacrimal fossa. Since large varieties of tumors can occur in lacrimal fossa, the differentiation is difficult. HRSG can very well identify the nature of the mass, whether it is solid, cystic or mixed echo-complex in nature. The lesions most commonly found in this area include inflammatory or lymphoid origin, primary lacrimal gland epithelial tumors and cyst. Normal lacrimal gland and surrounding soft tissues are highly reflective. Therefore, the gland cannot be separately delineated on HRSG. The most common lacrimal gland tumors are adenoid cystic carcinoma, mucoepidermoid carcinoma and pseudotumors and lymphoma.

Periorbital Abscess

A periorbital abscess is a painful swelling in the periorbital space which may push the eyeball to other side. HRSG shows a thick-walled low-level collection with week sound transmission. It is also helpful in the guided needle aspiration of the abscess. In the thick abscess, areas of necrosis are also noted in the abscess cavity.

Dermoid Cyst

The most common orbital and periorbital cysts are dermoid cysts. They usually present superotemporally or superonasally. They may be present with the lids, at the orbital rim, near outer canthus, on the conjunctiva or within the orbit. They most commonly occur in infants and children. They are usually heterogeneous in texture and different sound characteristics are seen in dermoids. Some attenuates the sound beam and other thoroughly transmits the sound. Homogeneous low-level echoes are seen in HRSG. They may contain keratins, sebaceous materials, hair follicles or inflammatory cells. When they are present deep in the orbit, it becomes difficult to differentiate them from the benign mixed tumors.

Mucoceles

Mucoceles are formed due to blockage in the sinus drainage openings. This leads to enlargement. This may bulge into the orbit. On HRSG, a mucocele looks like a low reflective, homogeneous nonvascular cystic mass, which is most commonly present in the supranasal quadrant (frontoethmoidal). This may cause outward and downward displacement of the globe.

Lid Tumors

Lid tumors arising from meibomian cells or tarsal glands are rare tumors. They are seen well-encapsulated homogeneous low-level echo complex mass on HRSG. The eyeball is pushed down and covered by the tumor mass. HRSG can clearly depict the involvement of eyeball or invasion of it by the tumor infiltration. It the tumor is well encapsulated and not involving the eyeball, it can be very well excised.

Lacrimal Ductal Cysts (Dacryops)

HRSG shows multiple small cysts in the upper left lid involving palpebral part of lacrimal duct. Tiny echogenic calcified specks are also seen in them suggestive of ductal ectasia of lacrimal duct also known as dacryops. It is a rare condition of lacrimal duct caused due to obstruction and ectasia of lacrimal gland duct.

Carcinoma of Lid

Carcinoma of lid is the malignant tumor. It is highly heterogeneous in texture and rapidly growing tumor. The tumor can invade the eyeball and infiltrate the sclera which can be very well appreciated on HRSG. The tumor is seen invading the conjunctiva, sclera and muscle coat of the eyeball. The lid is firmly attached and it is not retractable. Therefore, direct examination of eye is not possible in adherent tumor of the lid.

Orbital Biometry

Ocular measurement can be accurately carried out by using standardized "A" scanning and 2D imaging. The most frequent measurements are required prior to cataract surgery for intraocular lens implantation. The measurements required are axial length of the eyeball and corneal curvature. The high myopic eye shows proptosis. The other measurements, which can be taken on HRSG, are thickness of cornea, retina, choroid, sclera or size, shape, elevation and base diameters of intraocular tumors. For anterior chamber depth measurement, immersion technique is used for proper evaluation.

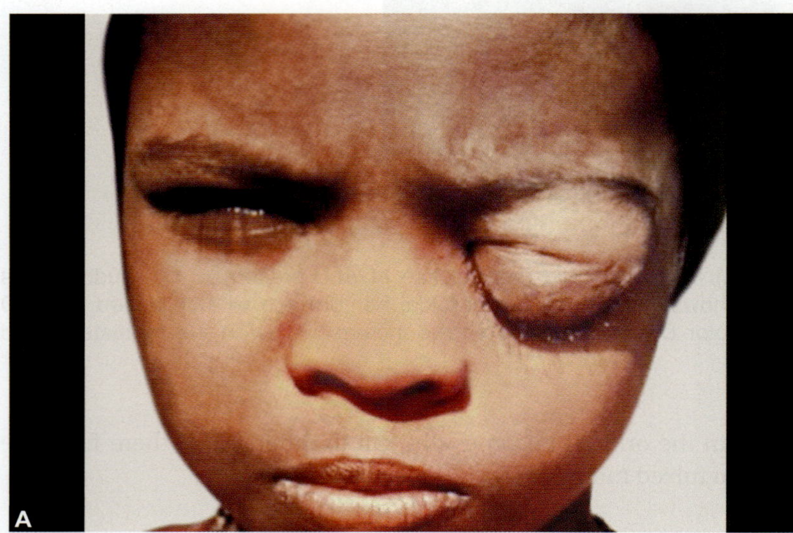

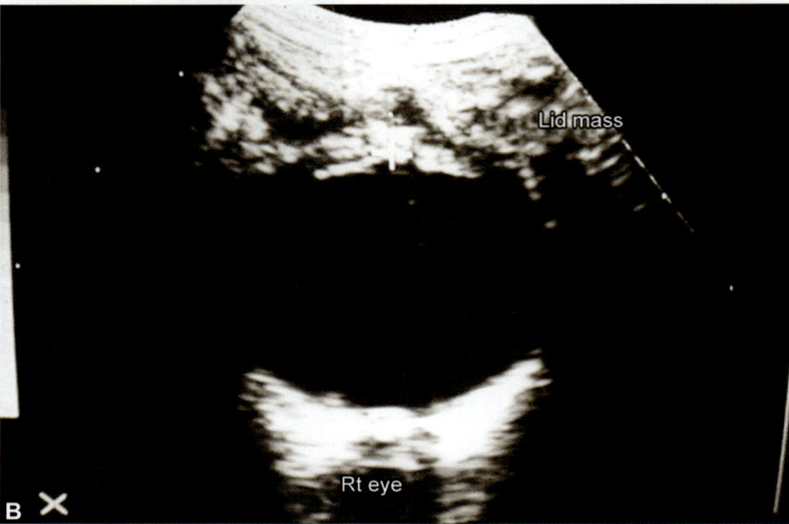

FIGURES 1.290A and B: Neurofibroma lid. A young girl presented with very soft tissue mass over the left upper eyelid covering the eyeball. HRSG shows a soft tissue mass with homogenous texture and covering the eyelid. It is not seen invading the eyeball. Eye is spared. The biopsy proved neurofibroma.

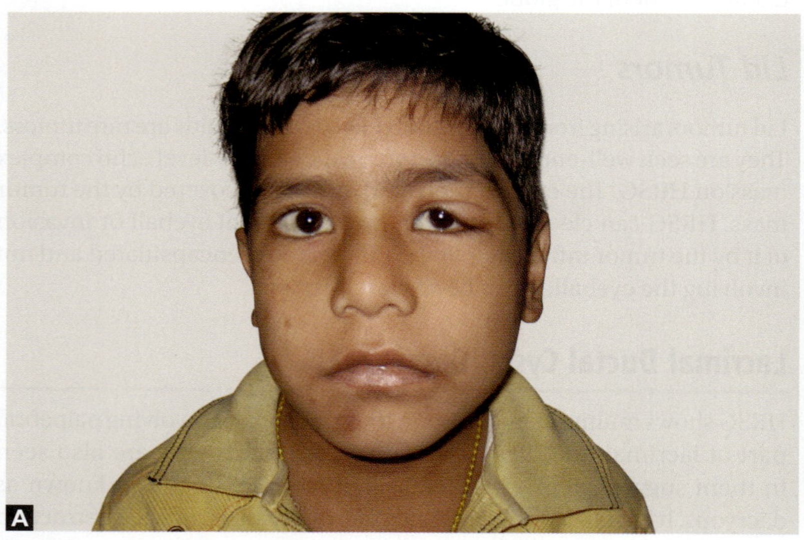

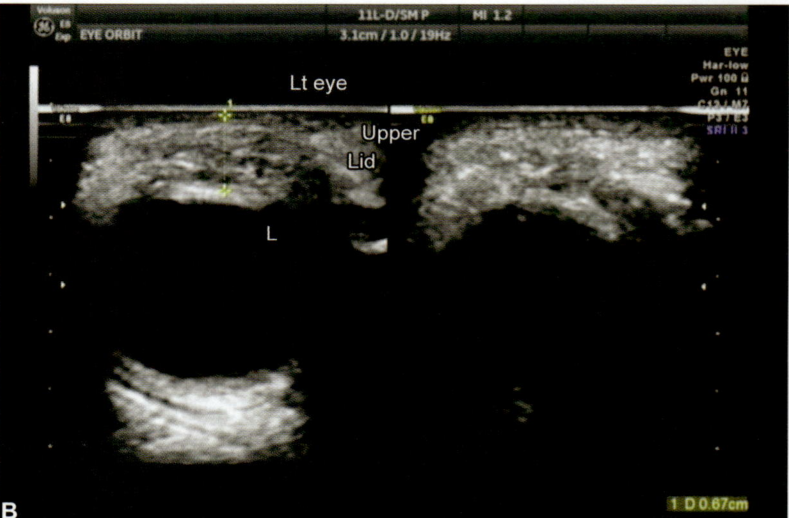

FIGURES 1.291A and B

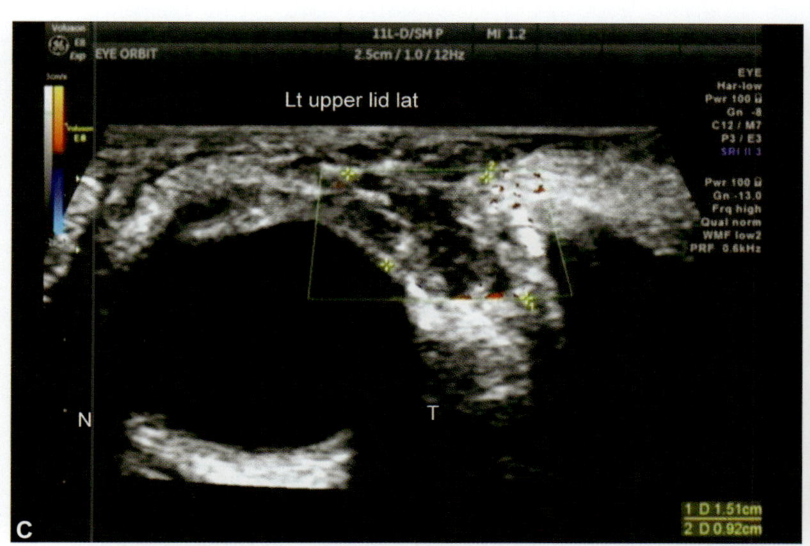

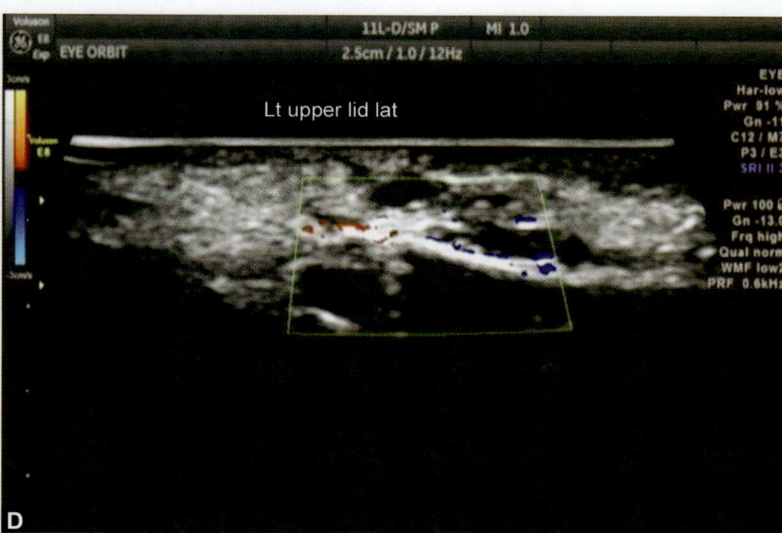

FIGURES 1.291C and D

FIGURES 1.291A to D: A young boy presented with soft tissue swelling over the left upper lid. HRSG shows a diffuse fusiform swelling over the left upper lid, which shows homogeneous texture. No calcification or cyst is seen in it. On color flow imaging, no flow is seen in it. Biopsy of the mass confirms neurofibroma.

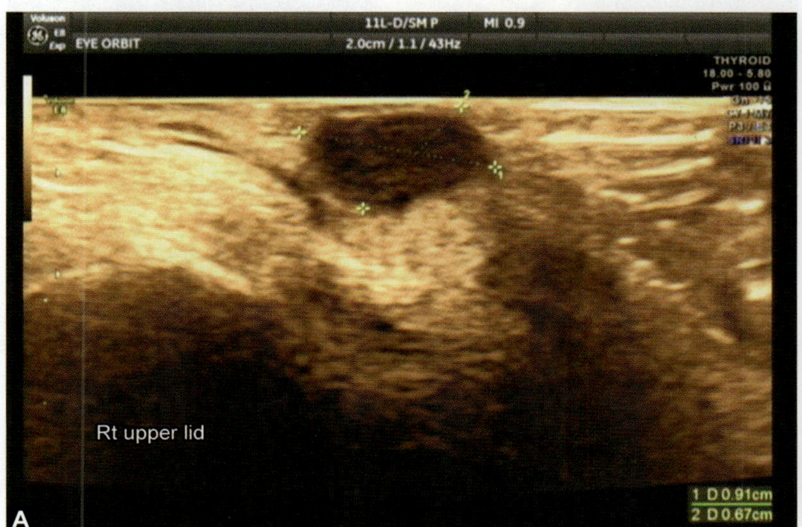

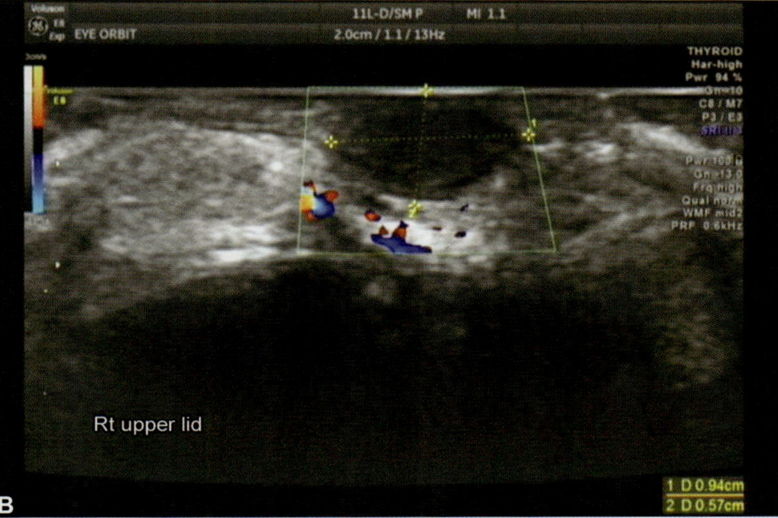

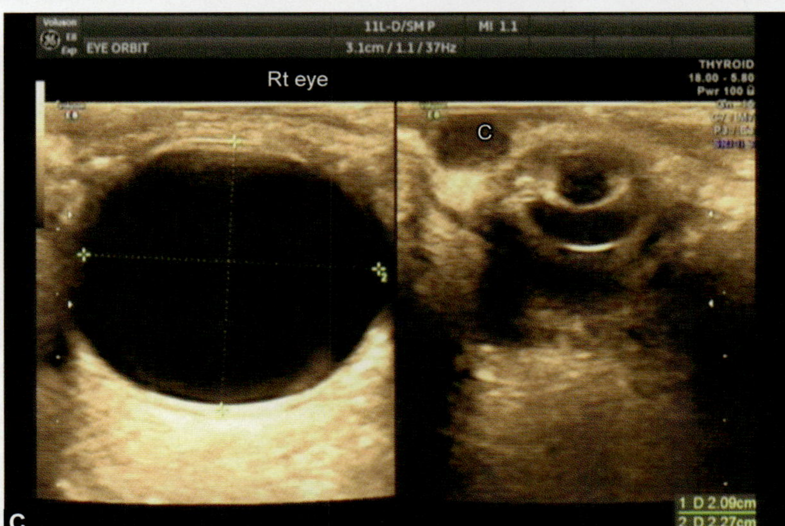

FIGURES 1.292A to C: Cyst in the lid. A patient presented with soft cystic swelling in the right upper lid. HRSG shows a well defined cystic mass in the cyst. The margins are smooth. No calcification is seen in it. On color flow imaging, no flow is seen in it. On aspiration biopsy, simple cyst is seen.

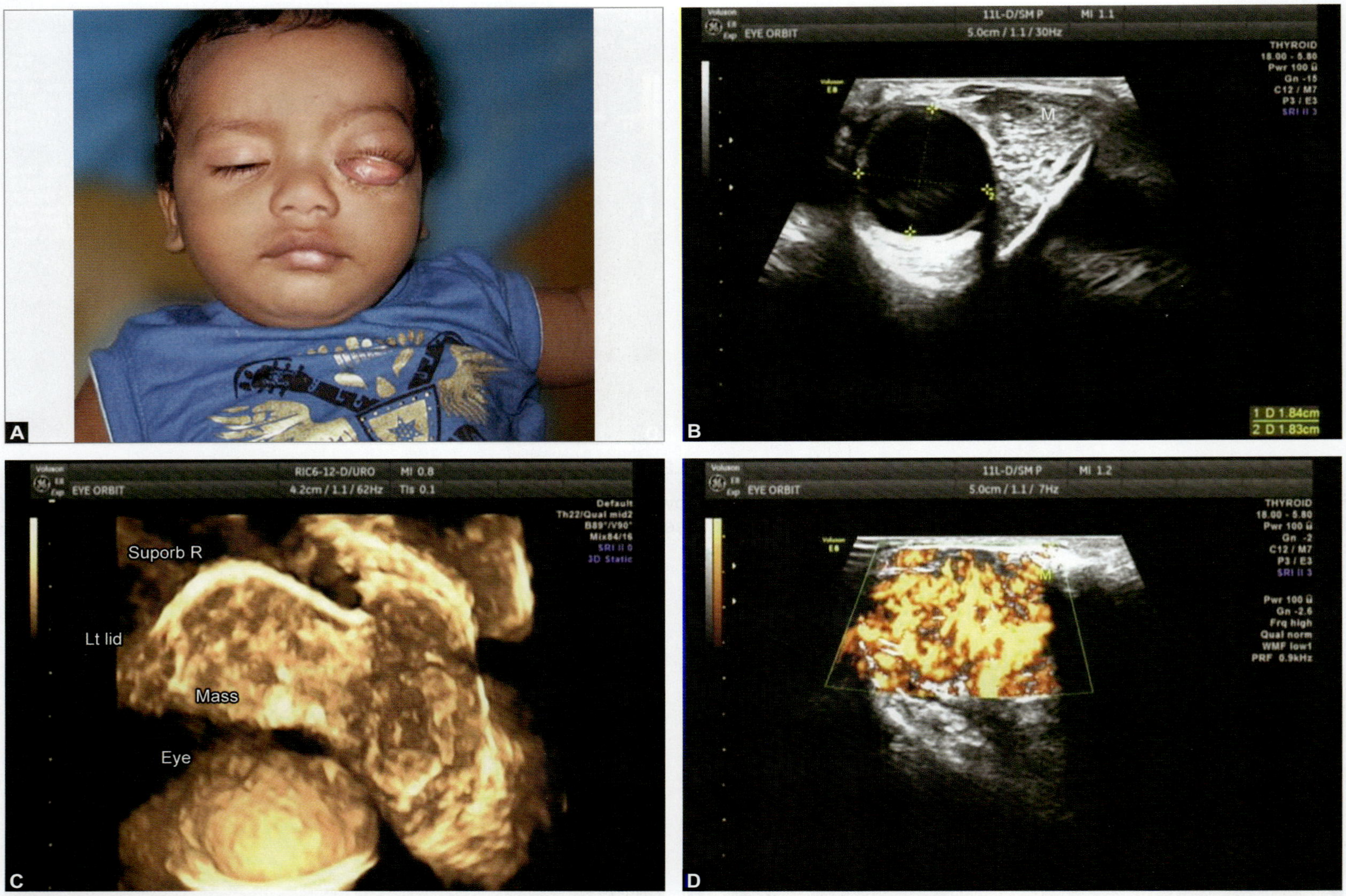

FIGURES 1.293A to D: A baby is born with soft tissue swelling over the left lower lid of left eye. HRSG shows a soft tissue membranous shadow over the left lid. On color flow imaging, multiple vessels are seen feeding the mass. However, the eye is normal. The mass appears to be hemangiomatous mass.

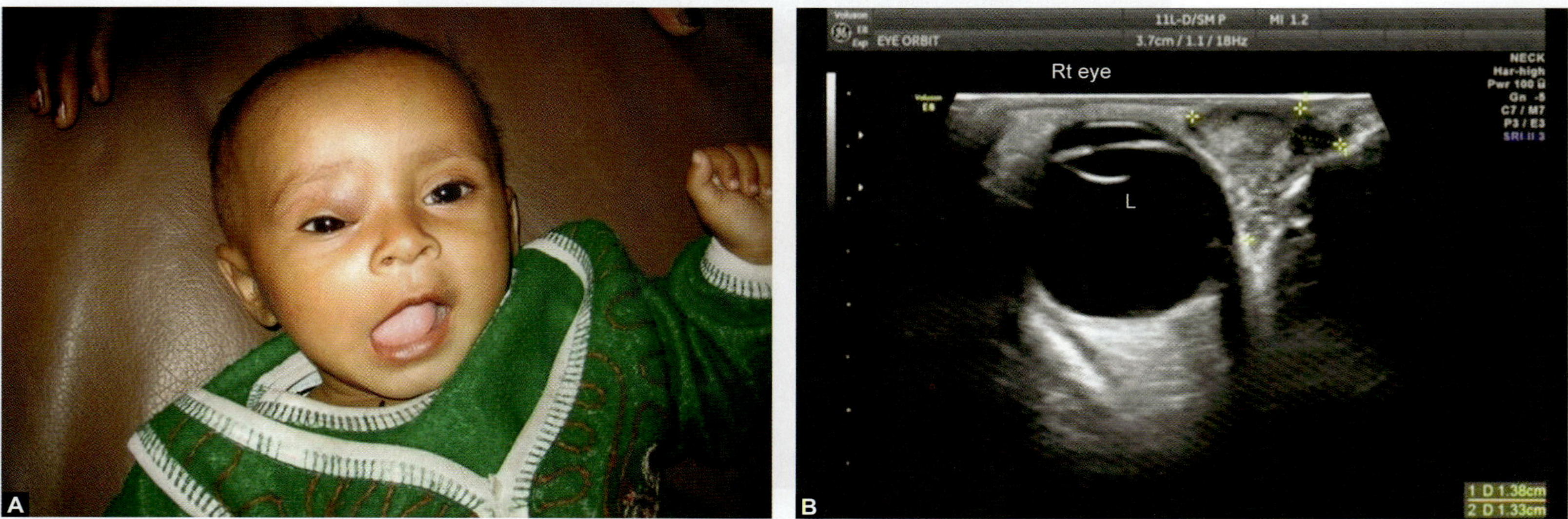

FIGURES 1.294A and B

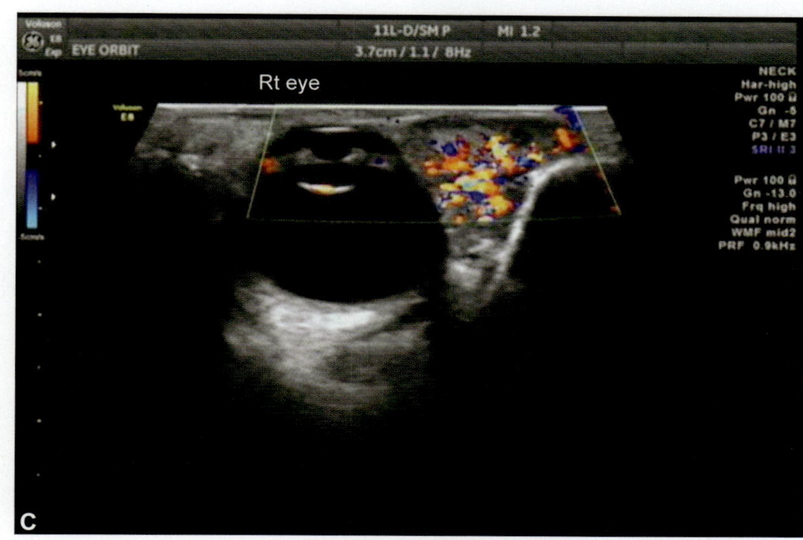

FIGURE 1.294C

FIGURES 1.294A to C: An 8-month-old baby presented with soft tissue swelling over right upper inner orbit. HRSG shows a homogeneous mass in the medial side of orbit. No calcification or cystic degeneration is seen in the mass. On color flow imaging, multiple vessels are seen feeding the mass suggestive of vascular mass. However, the eye is normal.

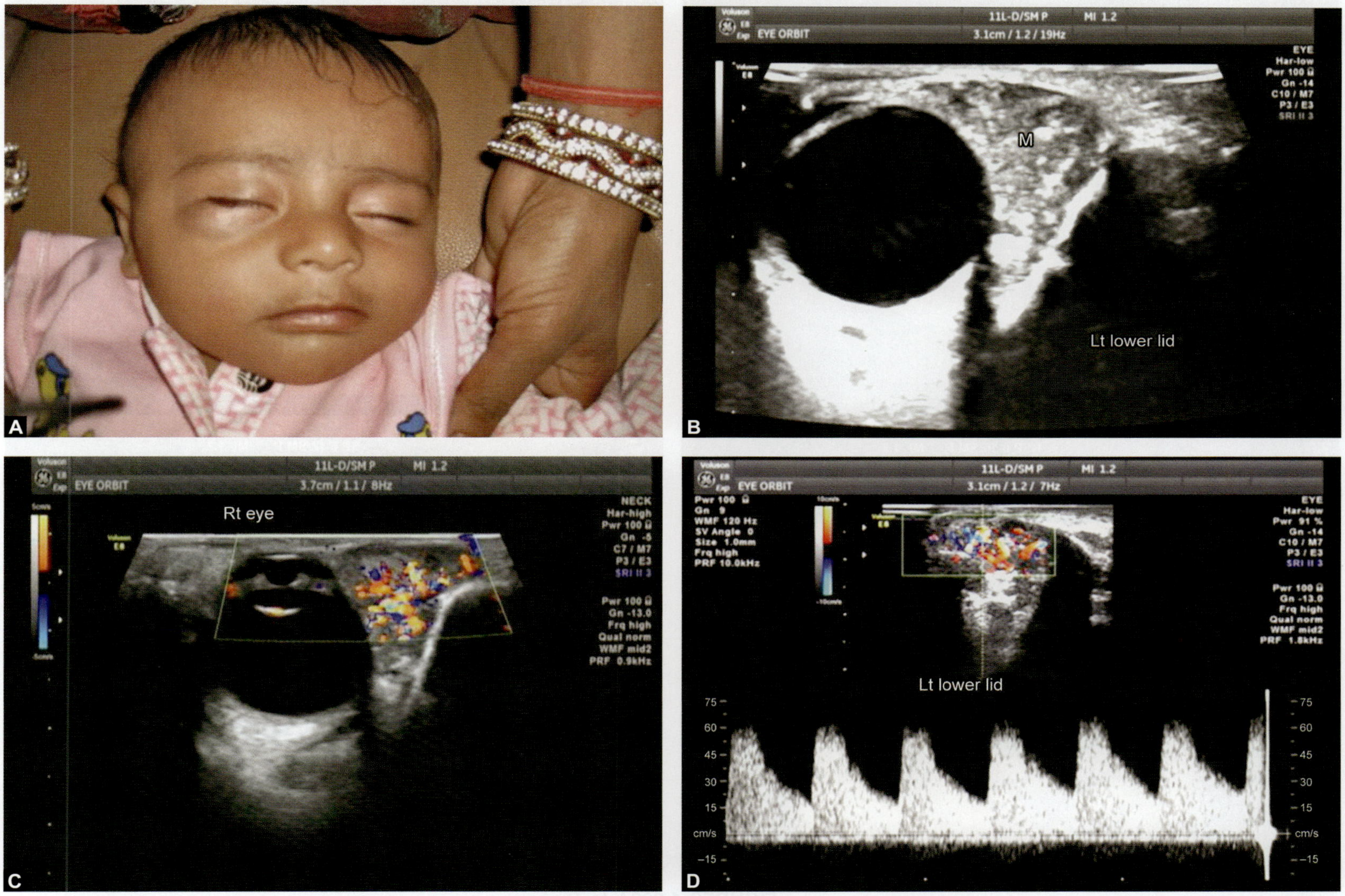

FIGURES 1.295A to D

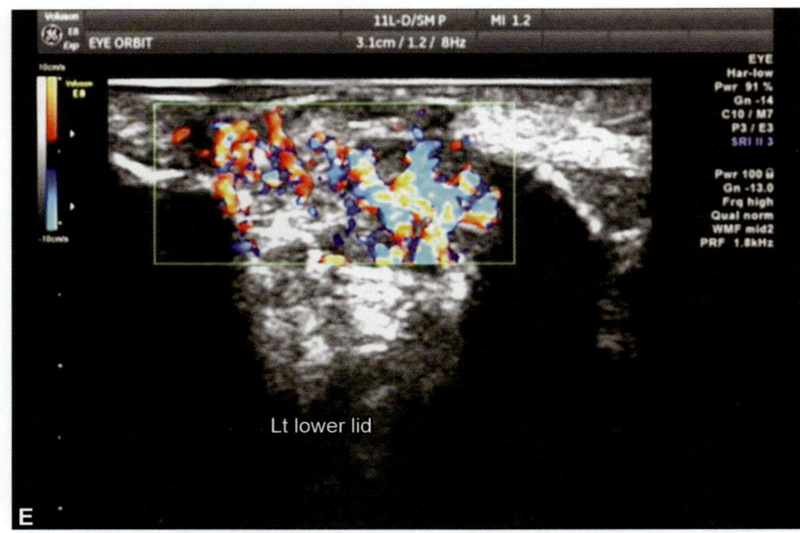

FIGURE 1.295E

FIGURES 1.295A to E: A 3-month-old baby presented with soft tissue swelling over right lower lid. Multiple vessels are seen feeding the mass. On spectral Doppler tracing, moderate arterial flow is seen in the mass suggestive of highly vascular mass.

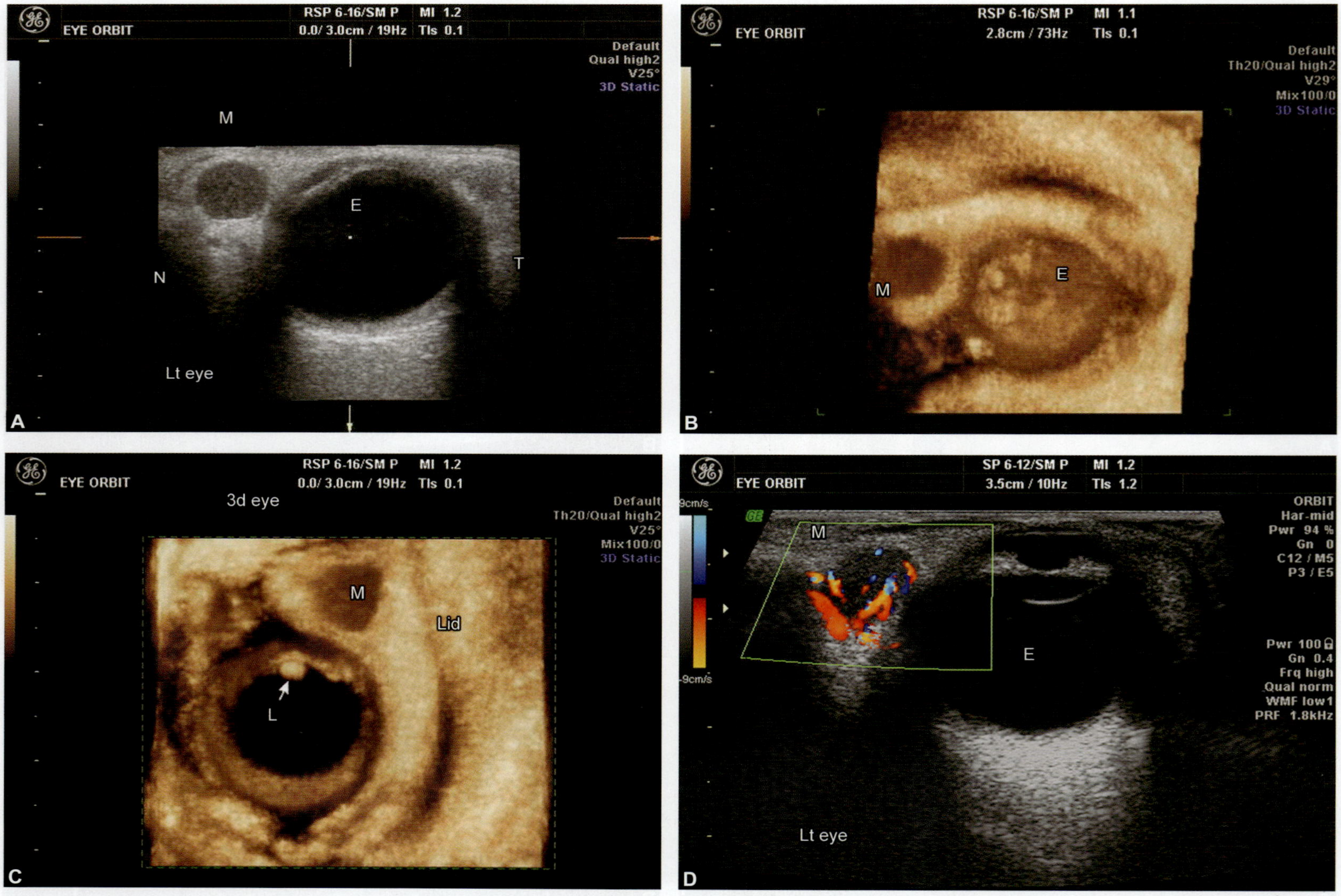

FIGURES 1.296A to D

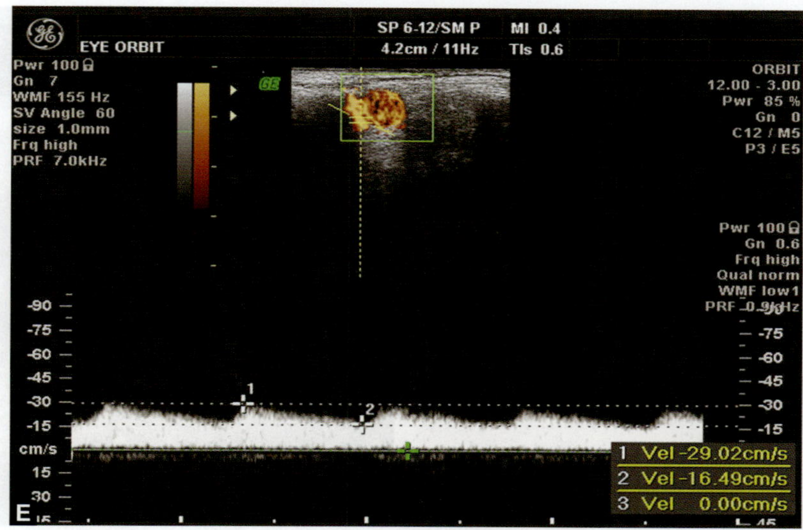

FIGURE 1.296E

FIGURES 1.296A to E: Vascular mass. A patient presented with painful swelling in the left lid. HRSG shows a hypoechoic soft tissue mass over the medial side of upper lid. The mass is confined in the upper medial part of lid. The 3D imaging clearly shows the mass. On color flow imaging, the mass shows increased vascularity. On spectral Doppler tracing, moderate arterial flow is seen in the mass suggestive of vascular mass.

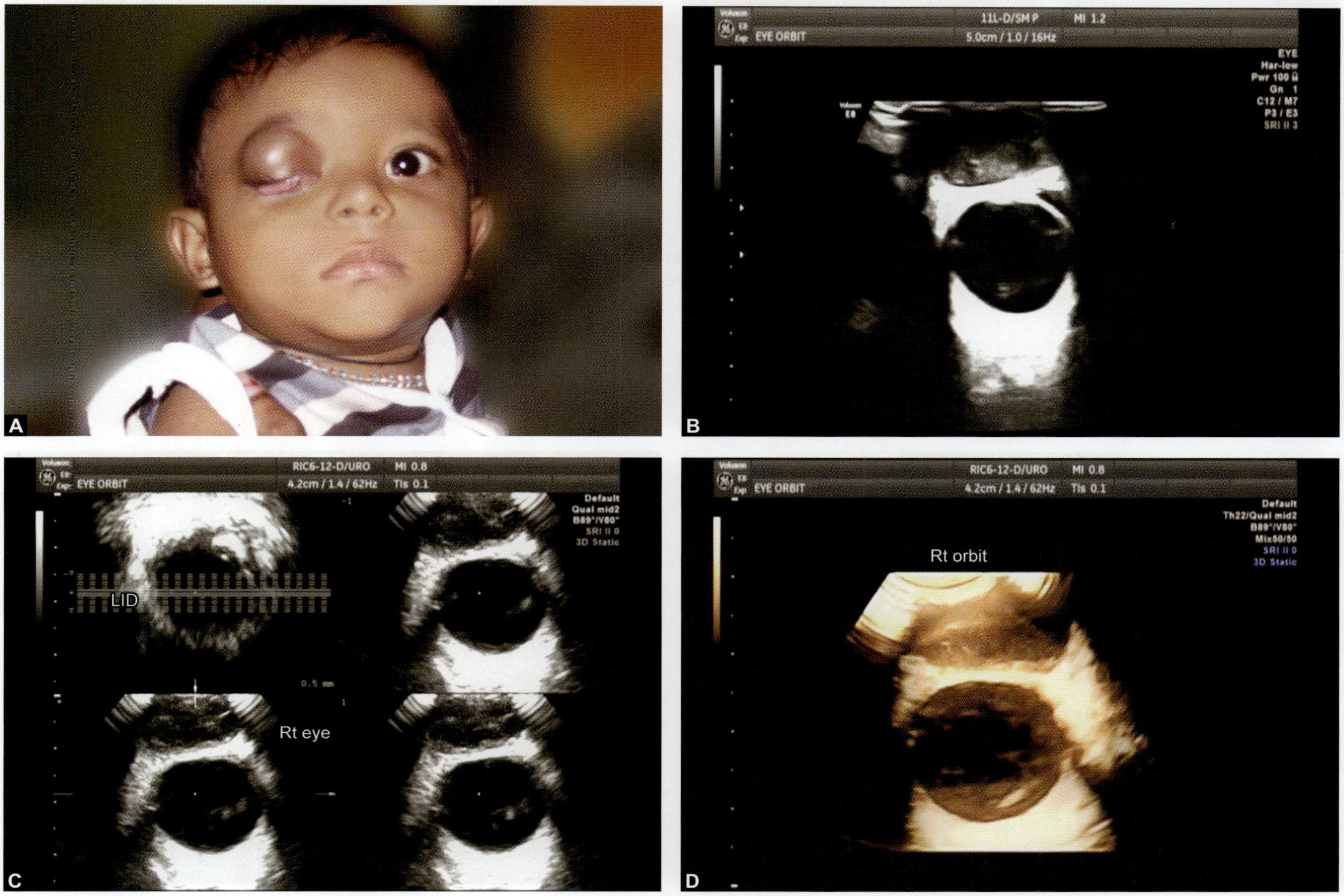

FIGURES 1.297A to D: Lid abscess. An 8-month-old baby presented with painful swelling over the right orbit. It is tense. HRSG shows a thick echo complex mass in the right upper lid. On 3D imaging, the mass is seen confined in the lid. Layering sign is positive suggestive of an abscess.

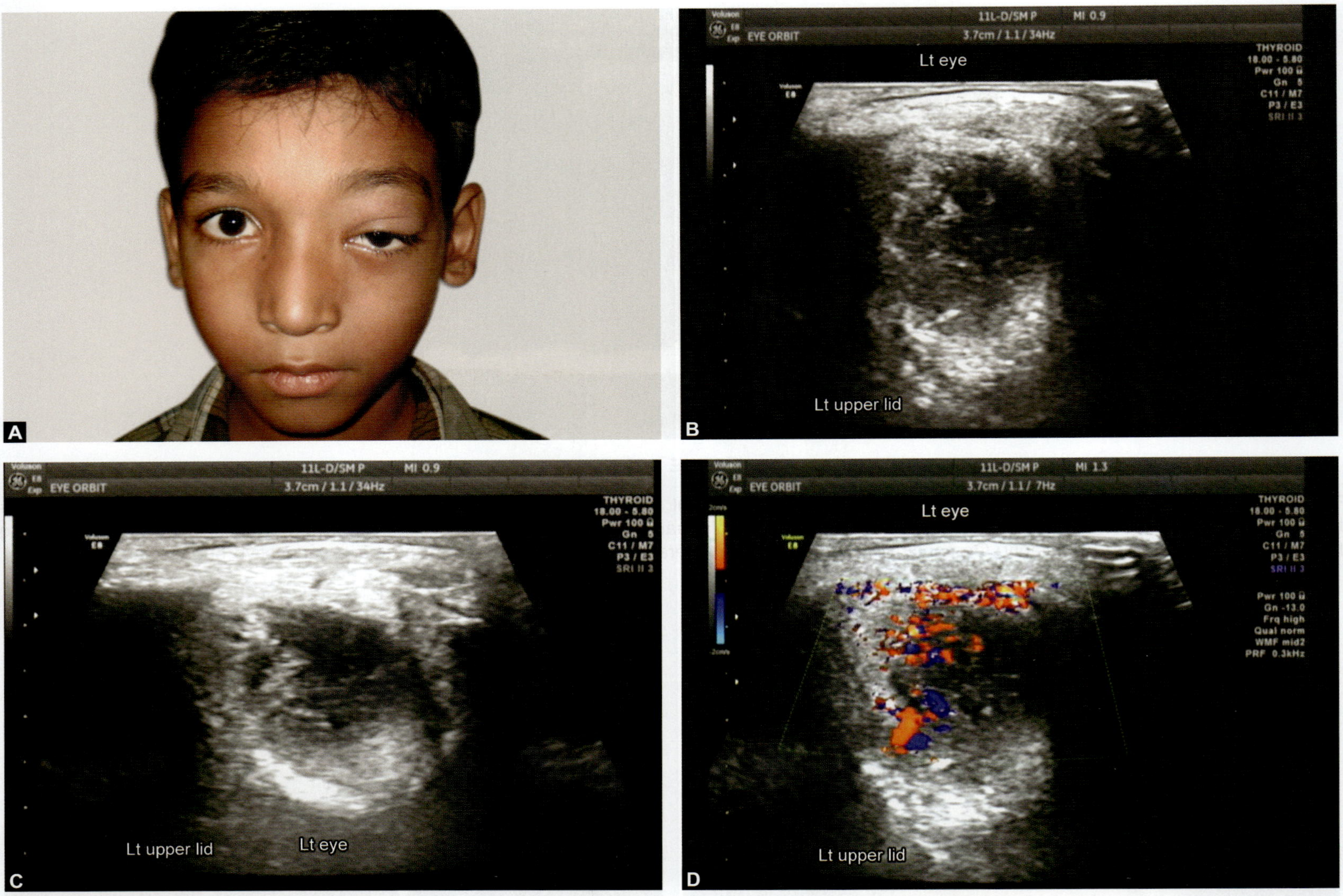

FIGURES 1.298A to D: Lid abscess. A young boy presented with painful swelling in left upper lid. HRSG shows thick echo complex mass over the left upper lid. Perifocal edema is present. On color flow imaging, poor flow is seen in it. Fine needle aspiration confirms the chronic inflammatory abscess.

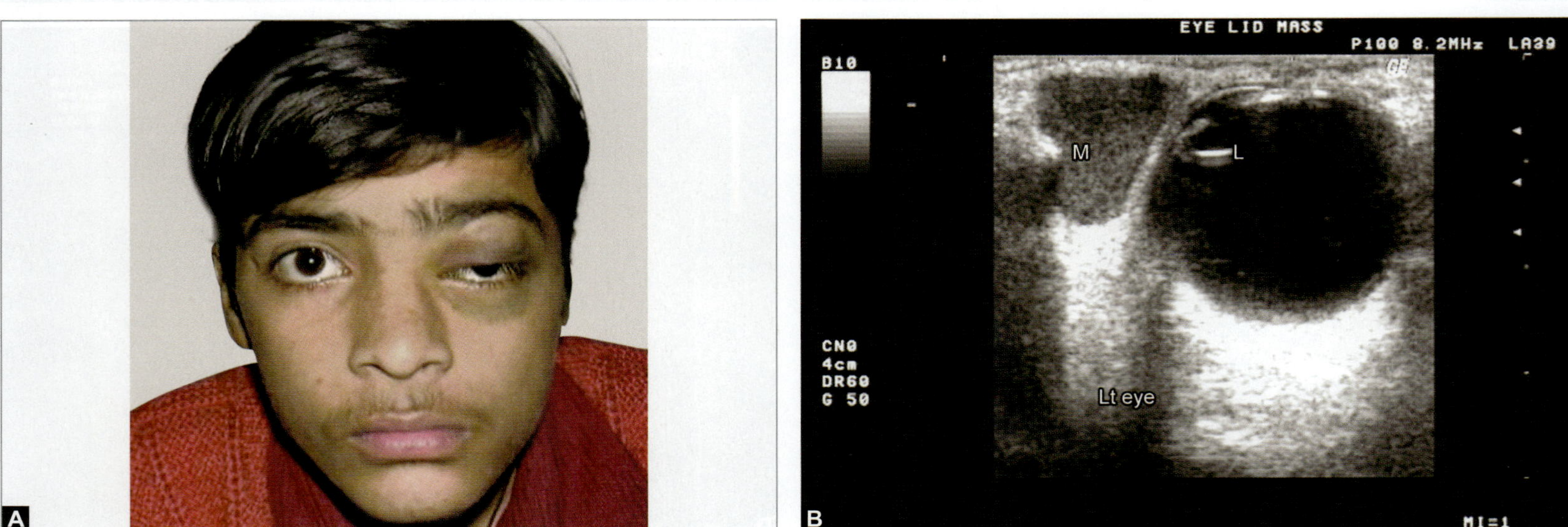

FIGURES 1.299A and B

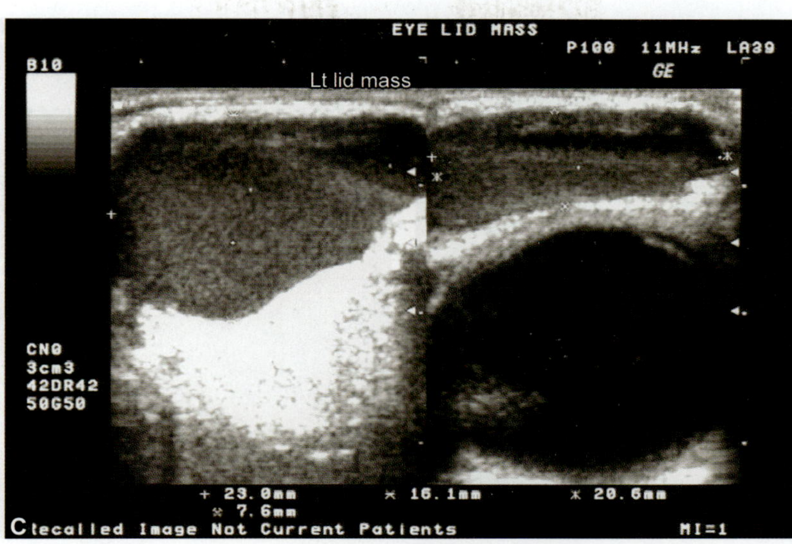

FIGURE 1.299C

FIGURES 1.299A to C: Upper lid abscess. A young boy presented with painful lid swelling with chymosis. HRSG shows low-level echo complex mass in upper lid with homogeneous echoes. Echogenic collection is also seen sedimented at the lower side. The eyeball is normal. The findings are suggestive of lid abscess. The abscess is seen going down laterally.

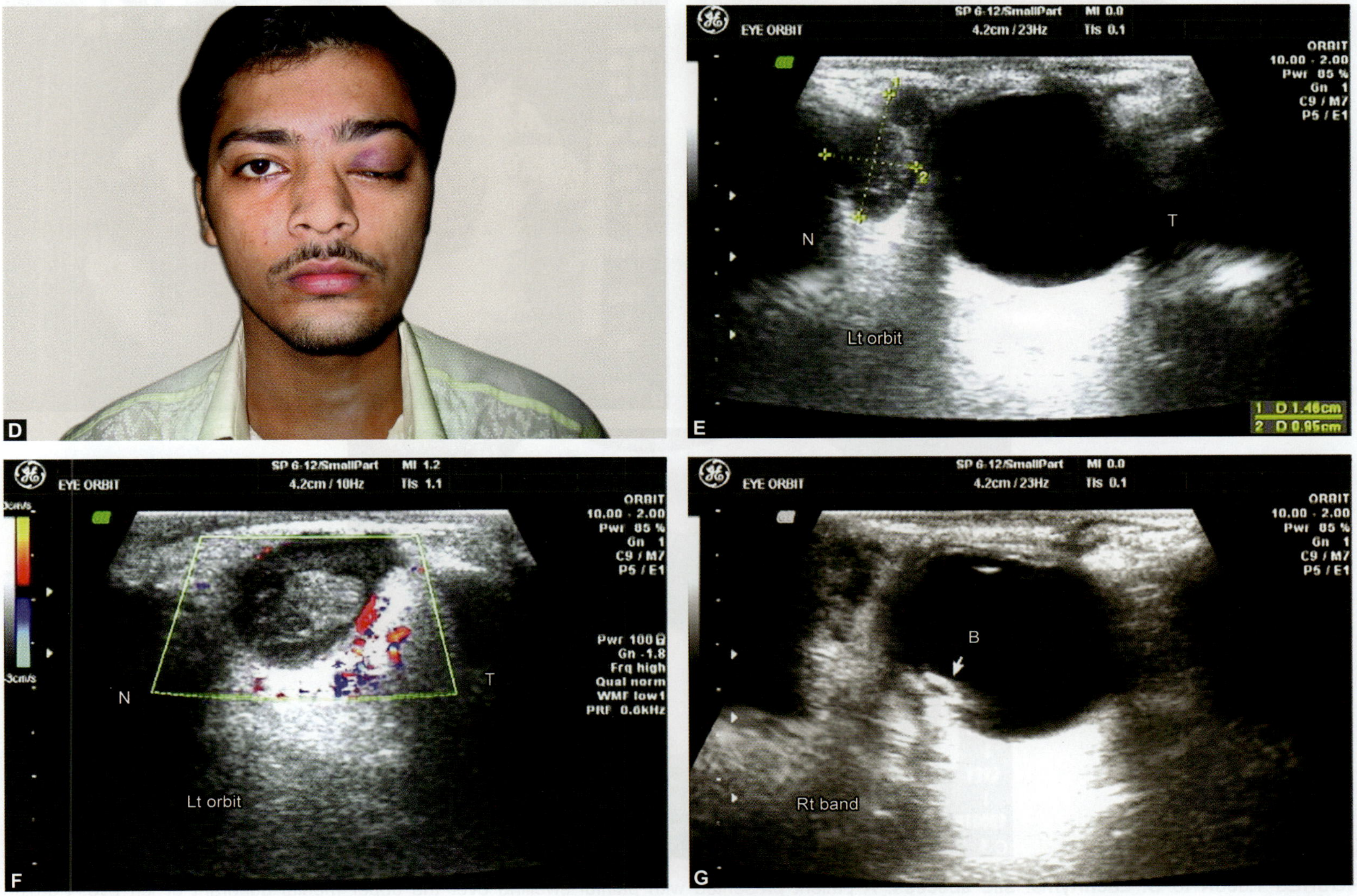

FIGURES 1.299D to G

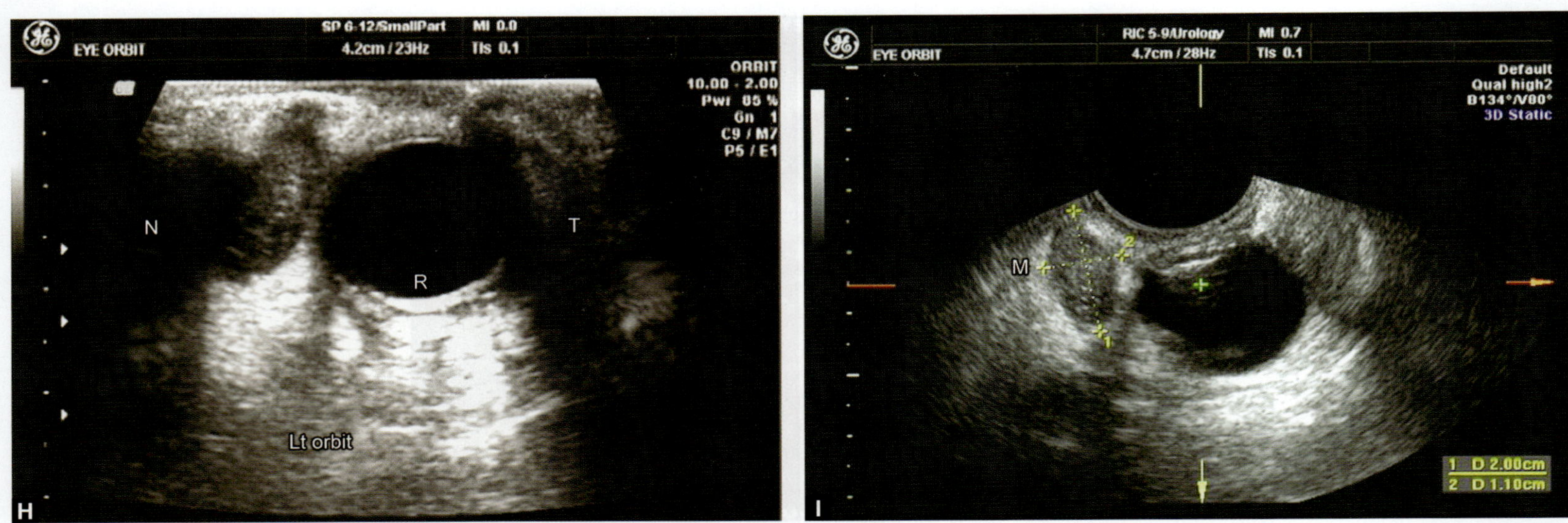

FIGURES 1.299H and I

FIGURES 1.299D to I: The same patient after 3 years, presented with drooping of the eye lid with lateral displacement of the eye ball. HRSG shows a thick walled low-level echo complex mass coming out from medial side of the orbital wall. Thick echoes are seen in it suggestive of periorbital abscess. HRSG shows associated retinal buckle placed in position for associated retinal detachment. The retina is seen in place.

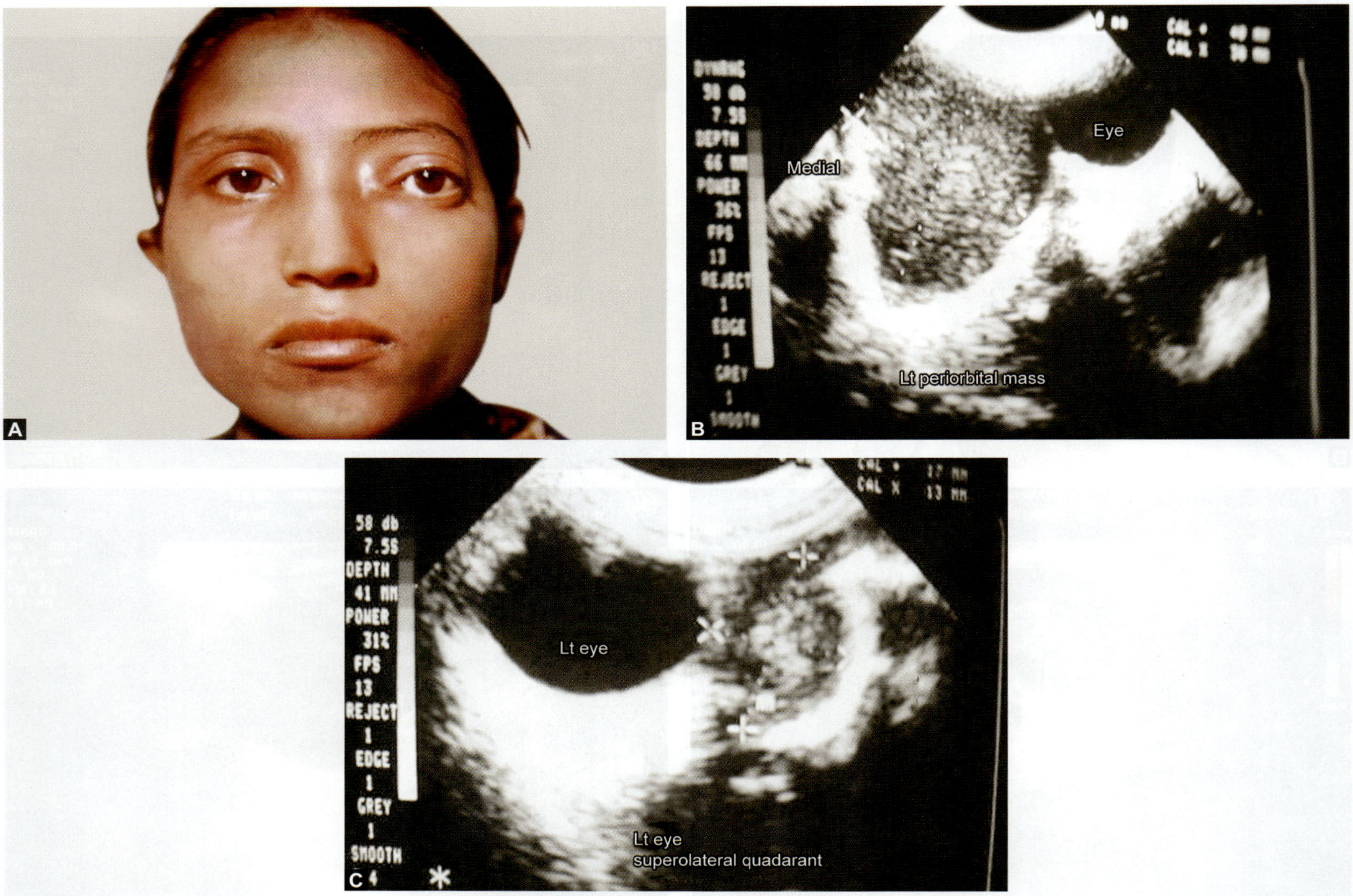

FIGURES 1.300A to C: Lachriymal sac abscess. A patient presented with painful swelling over the upper medial quadrant of left eye. Purulent discharge through the nose was coming out. HRSG shows a thick walled low-level echo complex mass seen in left upper medial quadrant of orbit. The mass is seen having homogenous collection pushing eyeball laterally. It is typical lacriymal sac abscess. The eyeball is normal. **Periorbital abscess:** HRSG show well encapsulated thick walled cystic mass in left superolateral part of orbit. The mass shows thick echoes suggestive of pus. It was a lachriymal gland abscess. Eyeball is normal but pushed medially and dome.

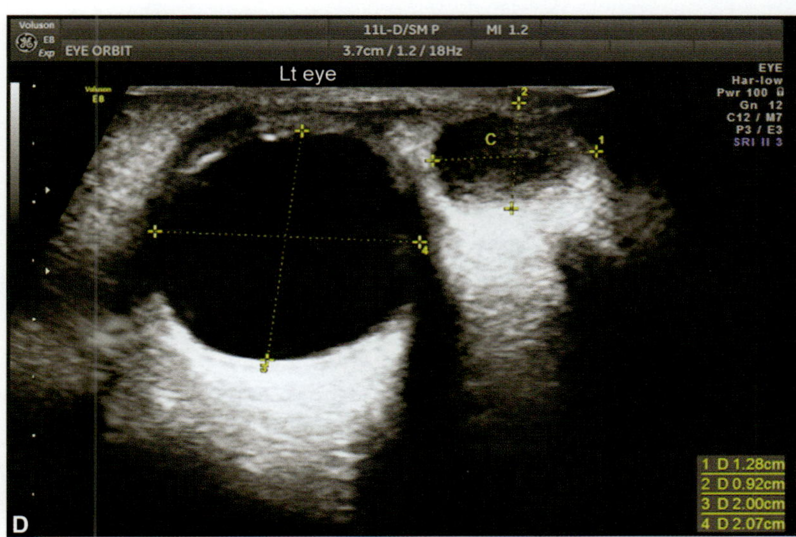

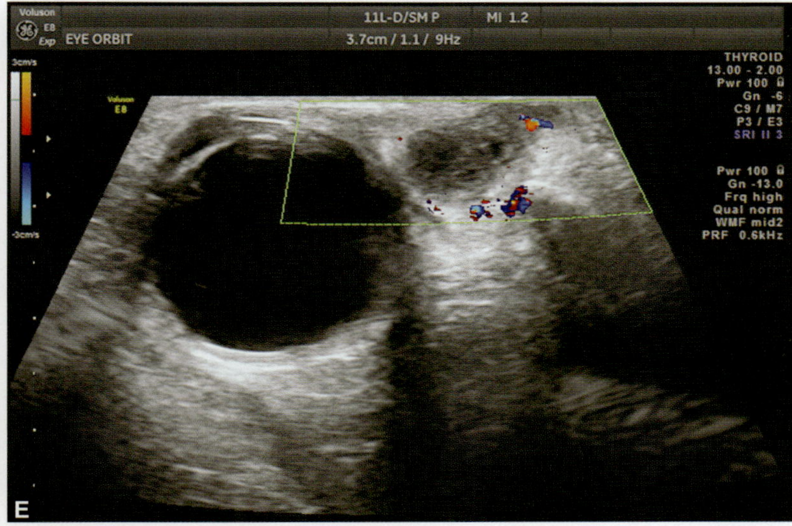

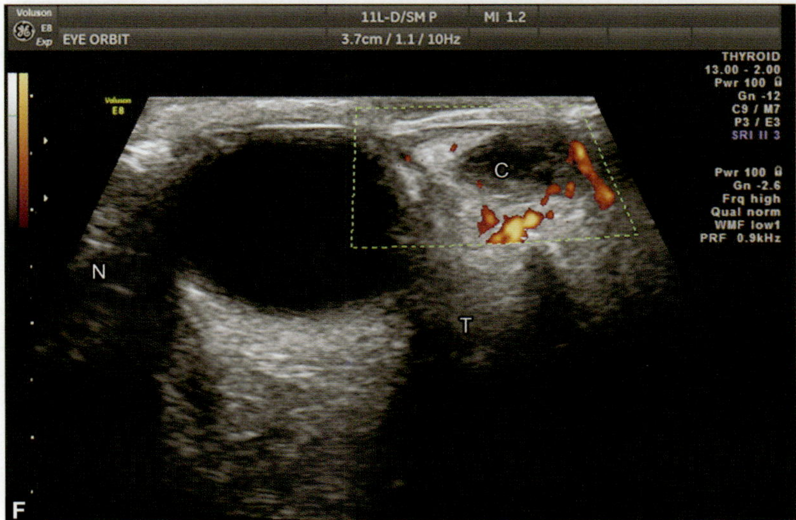

FIGURES 1.300D to F: Lachriymal gland abscess. A young boy presented with soft tissue swelling over the lateral side of left orbit. HRSG shows a pocket of thick collection in the lachriymal gland. Thick echoes are seen in it. On color flow imaging, no flow is seen in it. Aspiration biopsy confirms lachriymal gland abscess. However, the eyeball was normal.

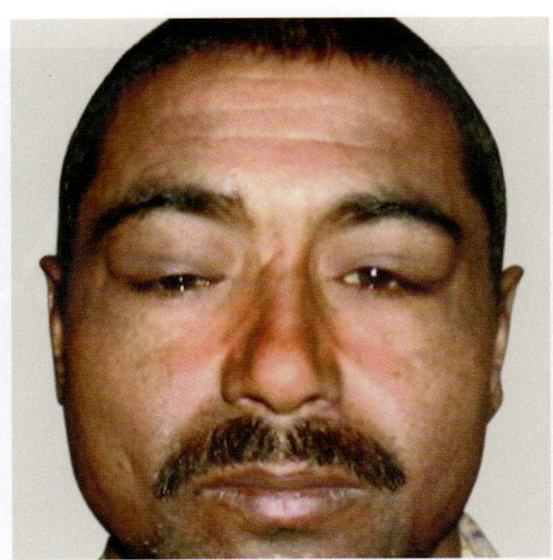

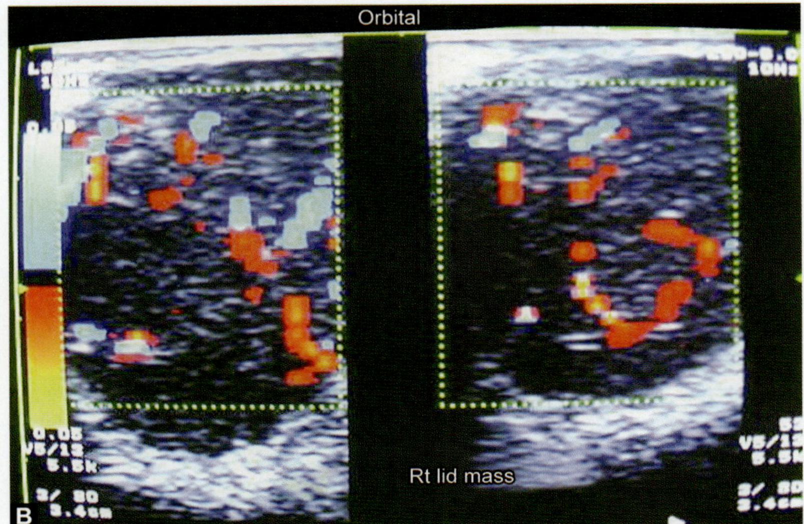

FIGURES 1.301A and B

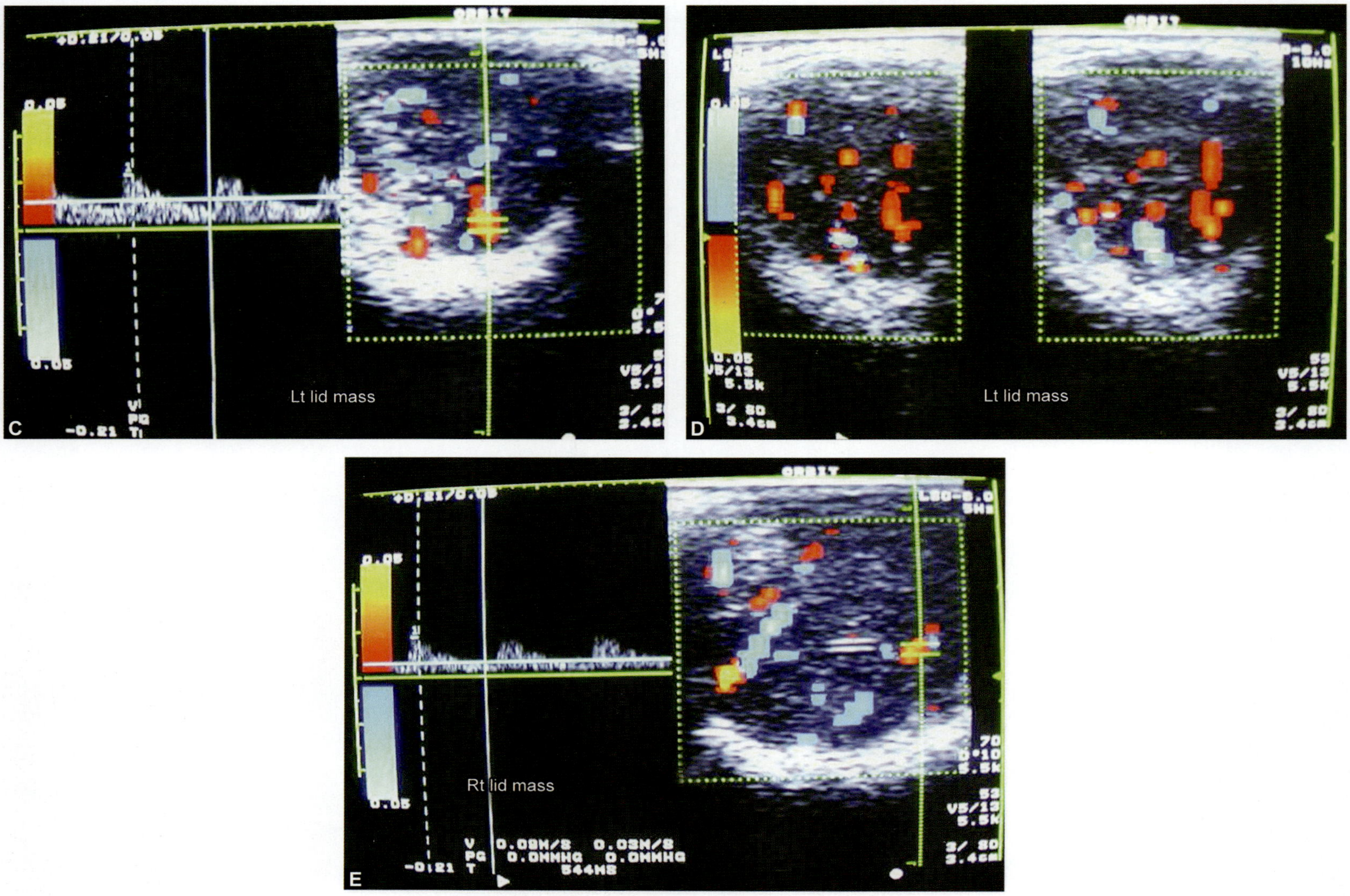

FIGURES 1.301C to E

FIGURES 1.301A to E: Neurofibroma of both lids. A middle-aged man presented with bilateral swelling of lid with dropping eyelids. He finds difficulty in opening the lid. HRSG shows low-level echo masses in right lid. On color Doppler imaging, multiple dilated vessels are seen in the mass. Spectral Doppler tracing of the mass shows low flow. The lid mass came out to be neovascularization in neurofibroma. The same HRSG findings were noted in left lid mass with multiple dilated vessels. Neovascularization of neurofibroma in left lid.

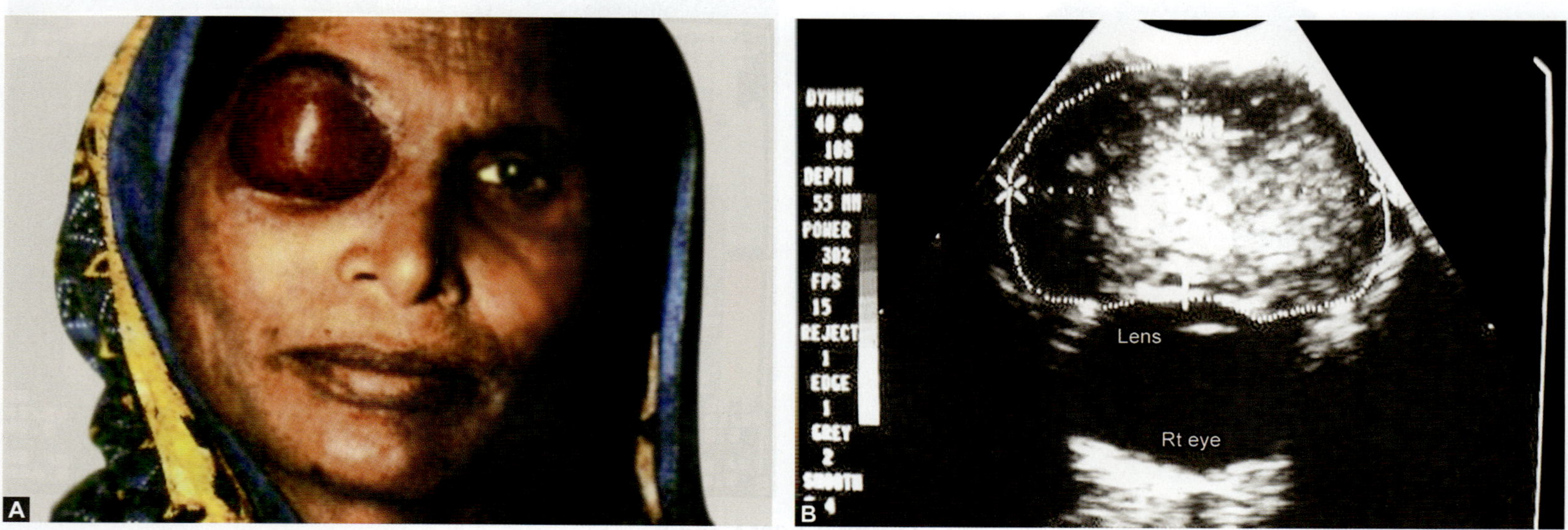

FIGURES 1.302A and B: Mebobian cell tumor right lid. A woman presented with soft tissue mass over right eyelid. The mass was covering the eyeball and it was semi hard in consistency. HRSG shows a well-defined echogenic mass over the eyelid covering the eyeball. Multiple bright echoes are seen in the mass. No cystic degeneration is seen. The mass is seen pushing the eyeball down. Lens is normal. Posterior segment of the eye is free. Biopsy of the mass showed mebobian cell tumor of tarsal plate.

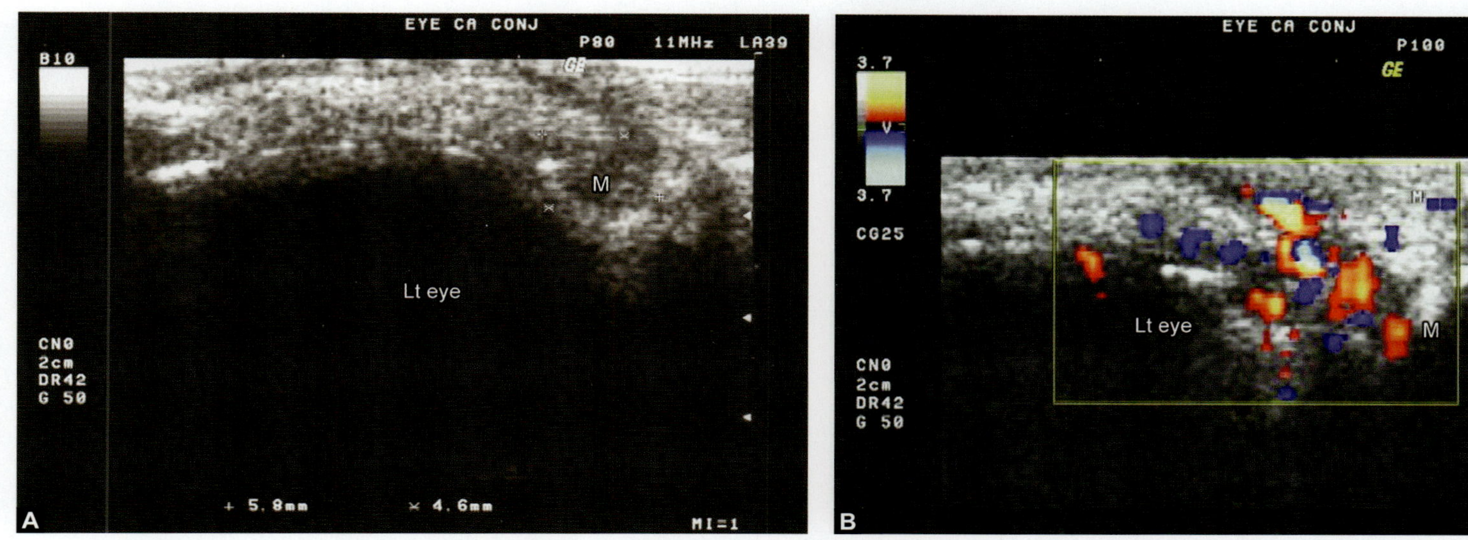

FIGURES 1.303A and B: Carcinoma conjunctiva. A patient presented with a soft tissue mass over the lateral side of the eyeball coming of from conjunctiva. HRSG shows a heterogeneous irregular soft tissue mass on the lateral of the eye. It is seen invading the conjunctiva and also invading the sclera. On color flow imaging, multiple vessels are seen invading the sclera.

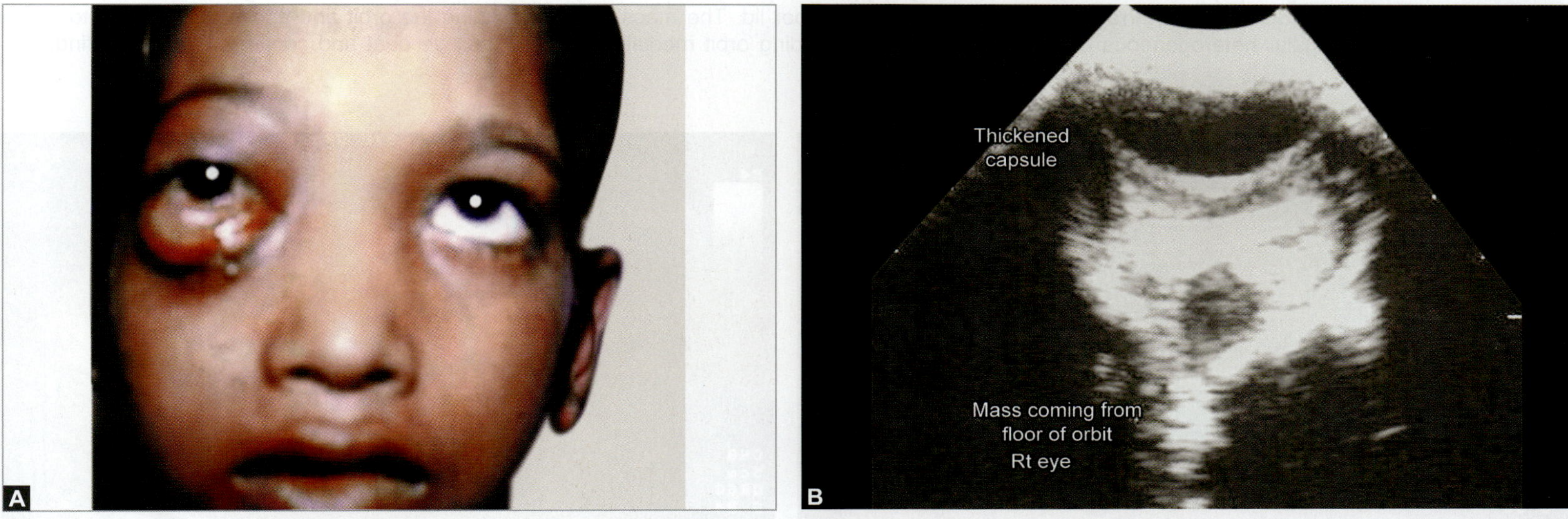

FIGURES 1.304A and B: Carcinoma maxilla invading orbital floor. A young boy presented with soft tissue mass of lower lid with proptosed eyeball and diminished vision. HRSG shows a soft tissue mass coming out from floor of orbit invading the sclera coat and pushing the eyeball anteriorly. Biopsy proved infiltrating carcinoma of right maxilla.

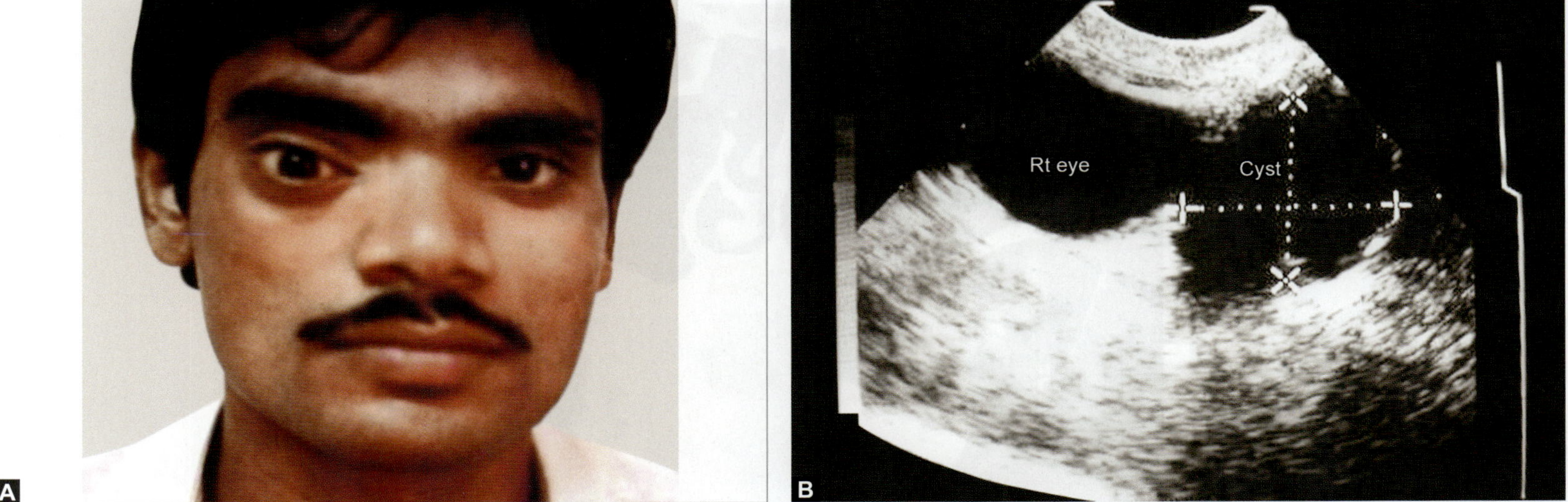

FIGURES 1.305A and B

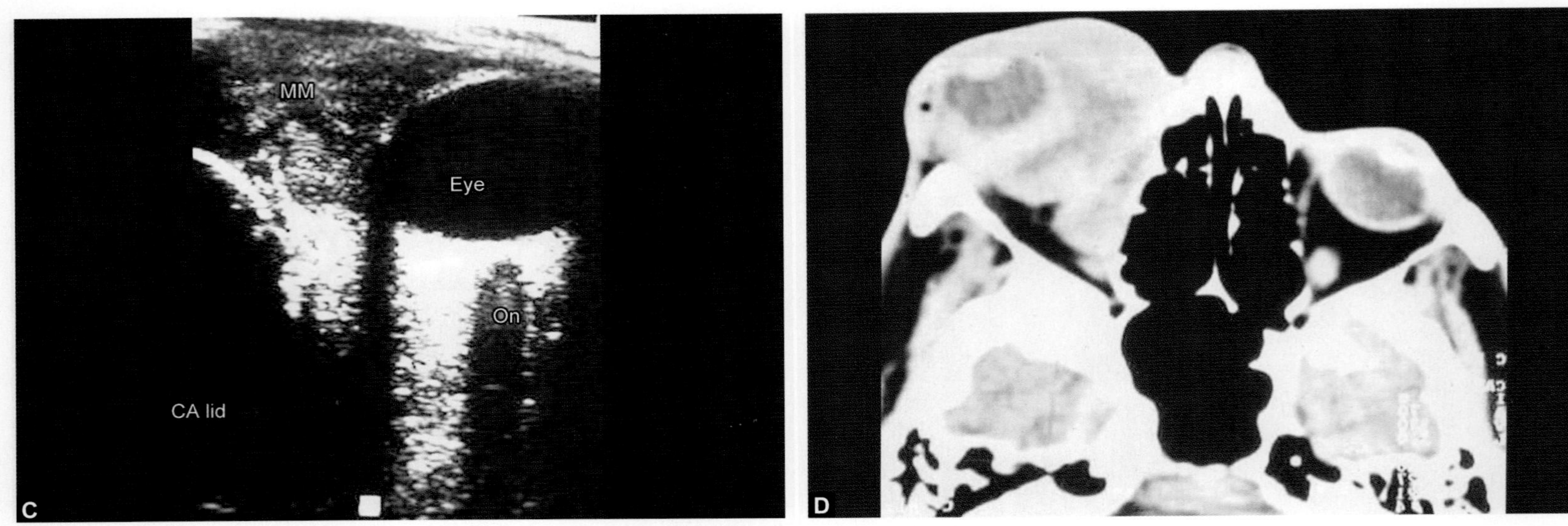

FIGURES 1.305C and D

FIGURES 1.305A to D: Carcinoma maxilla invading orbit. A young man presented with mild proptosis of right eye with diplopia. Fullness of right maxilla is also seen on clinical examination. HRSG shows an irregular cystic mass in retrobulbar space coming out from the floor of orbit. The mass appears to be anechoic and pushing the eyeball anteriorly. However, eye appears to be spared. Biopsy proved maxillary carcinoma cystic variant. **Squamous cell carcinoma of Lid**: HRSG shows an irregular mass over the right upper lid. The mass is seen invading the orbit and above the sclera into broken wall. CT scan shows irregular heterogeneous mass over the right lid-invading orbit medially and also the eye coat and confirms the HRSG findings.

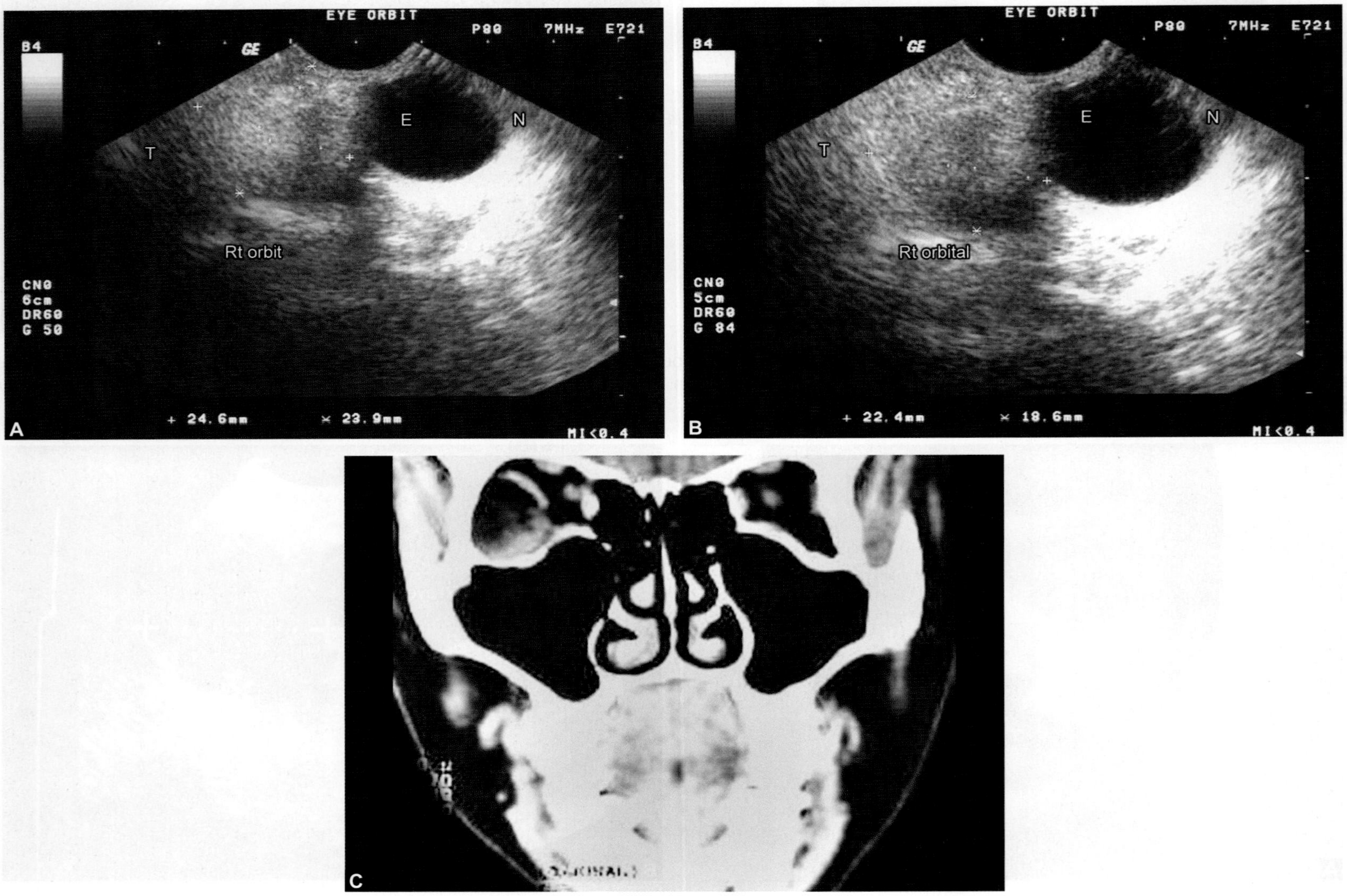

FIGURES 1.306A to C: A homogeneous well-defined soft tissue mass. Multiple fine homogeneous echoes are seen in the mass pushing the eye to medial side suggestive of a dermoid cyst. CT scan of the same patient shows a well defined soft tissue mass predominantly having fat contents confirms HRSG findings.

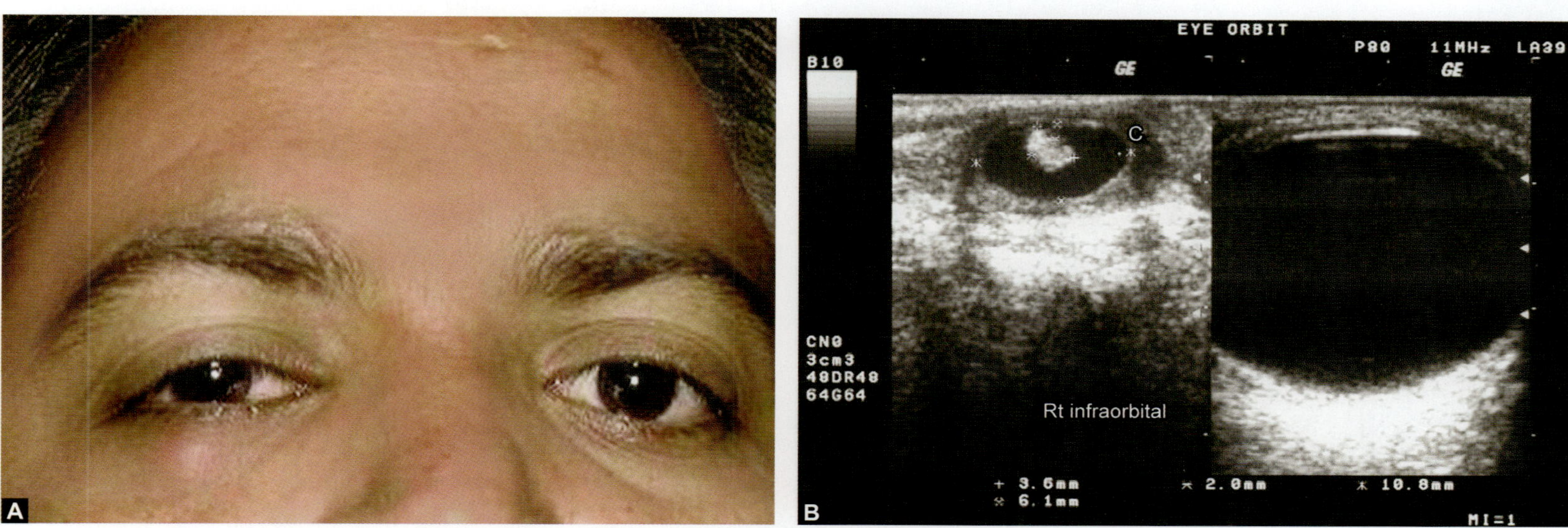

FIGURES 1.307A and B: Infraorbital cysticercosis. A patient presented with soft tissue nodular shadow below the right lower orbital margin. HRSG shows a well defined cystic mass. An echogenic nidus is seen fixed with inner wall of the cyst suggestive of cysticercosis.

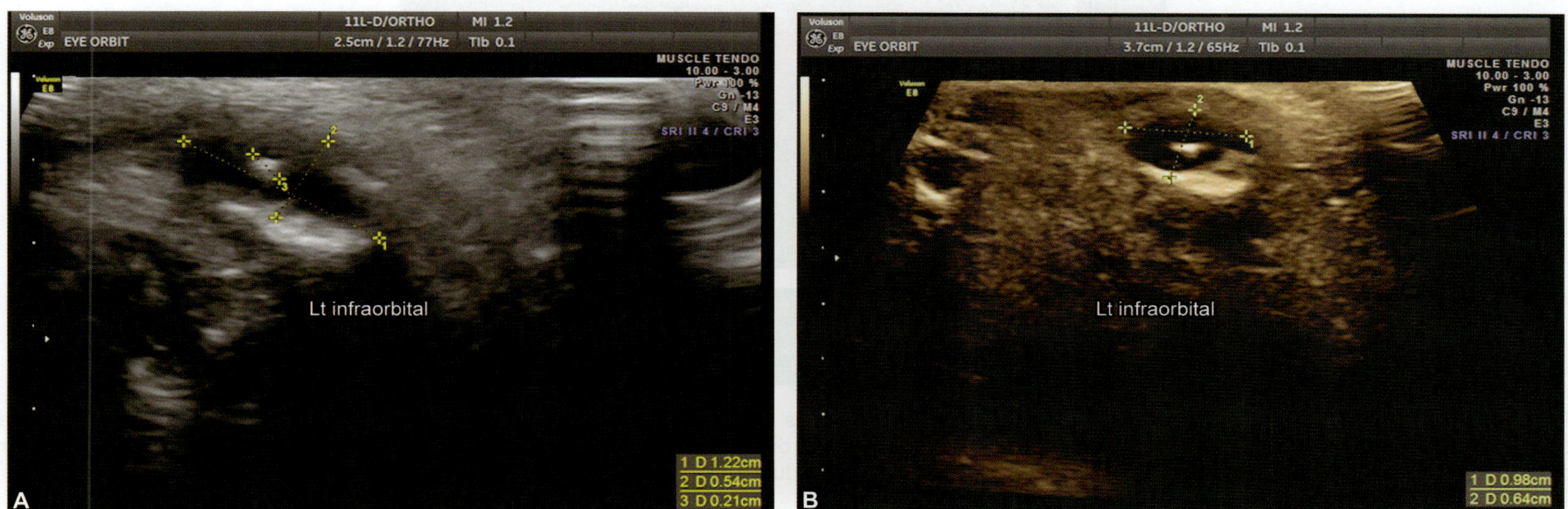

FIGURES 1.308A and B: Infraorbital cysticercus. A patient presented with soft tissue swelling in the left infraorbital region. HRSG shows a thick walled cystic mass in the infraorbital region. An echogenic nidus is seen in the cyst suggestive of cysticercus cyst.

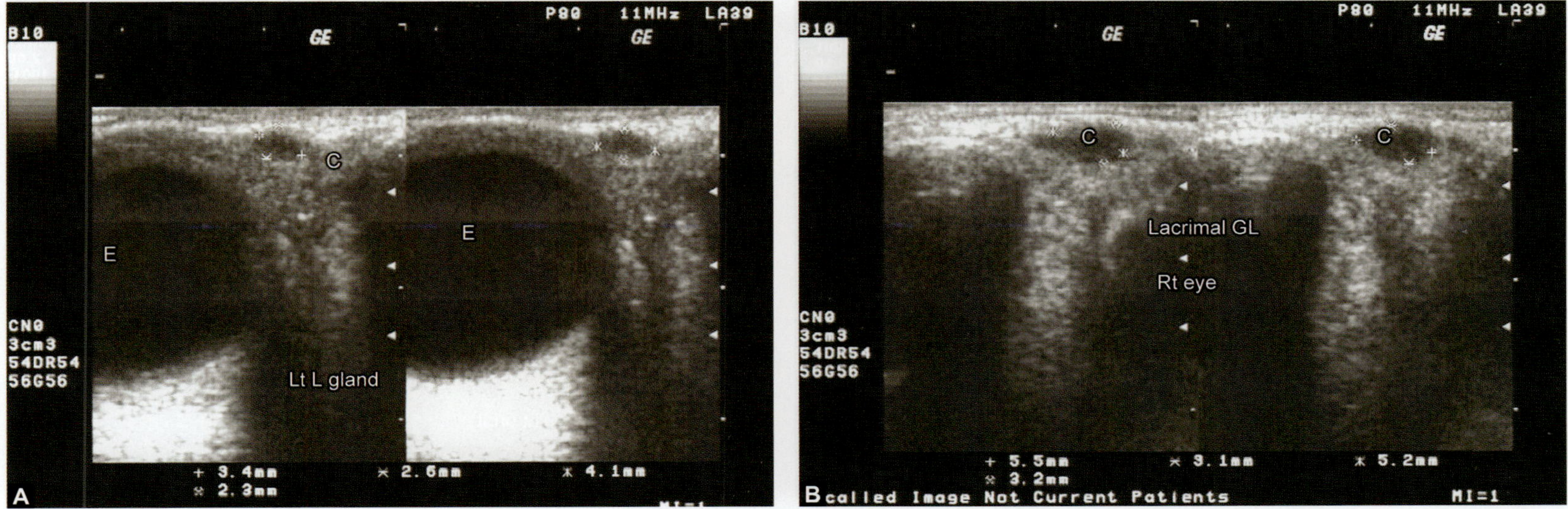

FIGURES 1.309A and B: Lacrimal gland cysts. HRSG shows well-defined thin walled cysts in both lacrimal glands on either side. No internal debris is seen in the cyst. No septation is seen. Eyeballs are normal.

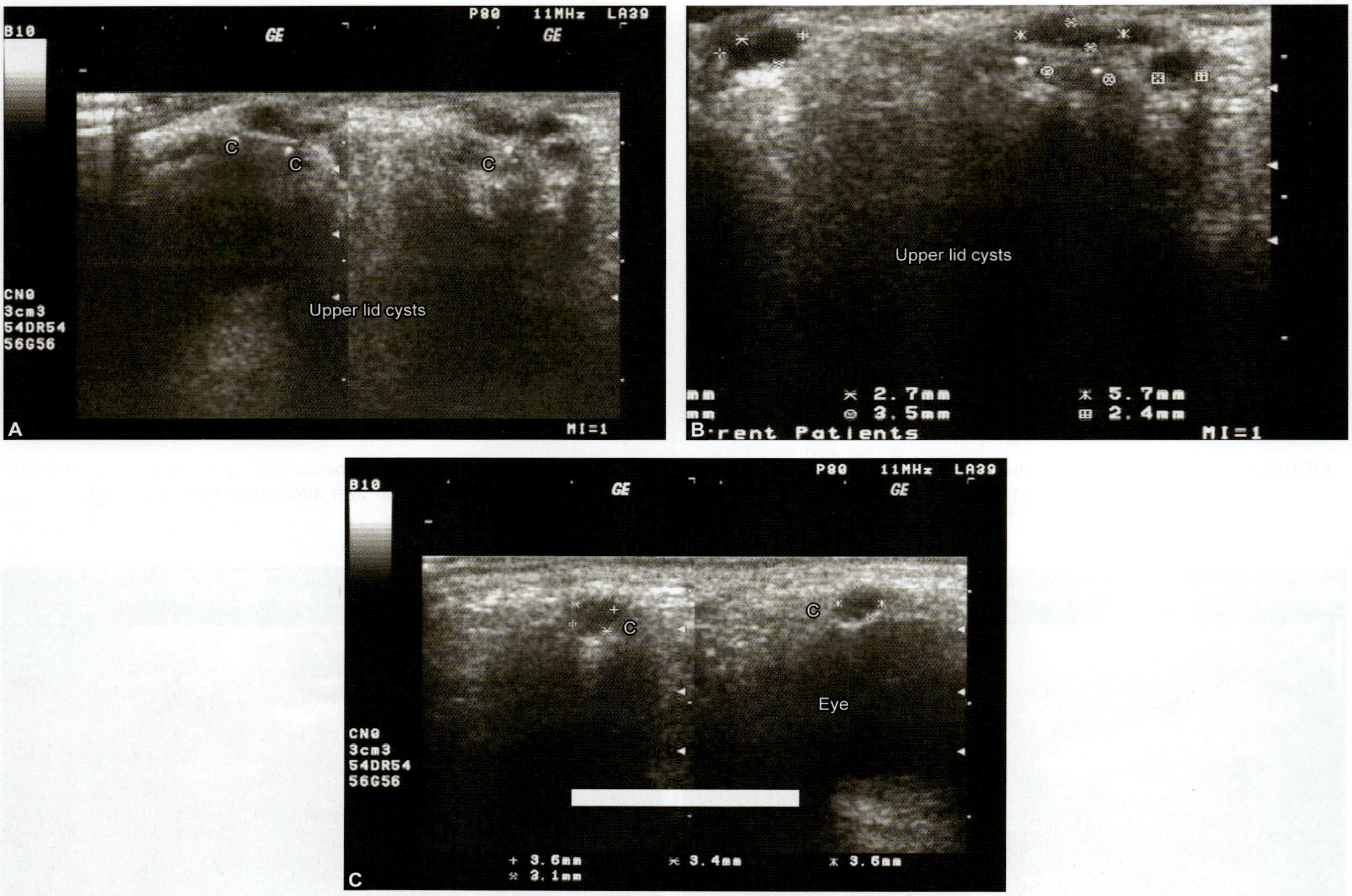

FIGURES 1.310A to C: Lacrimal ductal cysts (Dacryops). HRSG shows multiple small cysts in the upper left lid involving palpebral part of lacrimal duct. Tiny echogenic calcified specks are also seen in them suggestive of ductal ectasia of lacrimal duct also known as dacryops. It is a rare condition of lacrimal duct caused due to obstruction and ectasia of lacrimal gland duct.

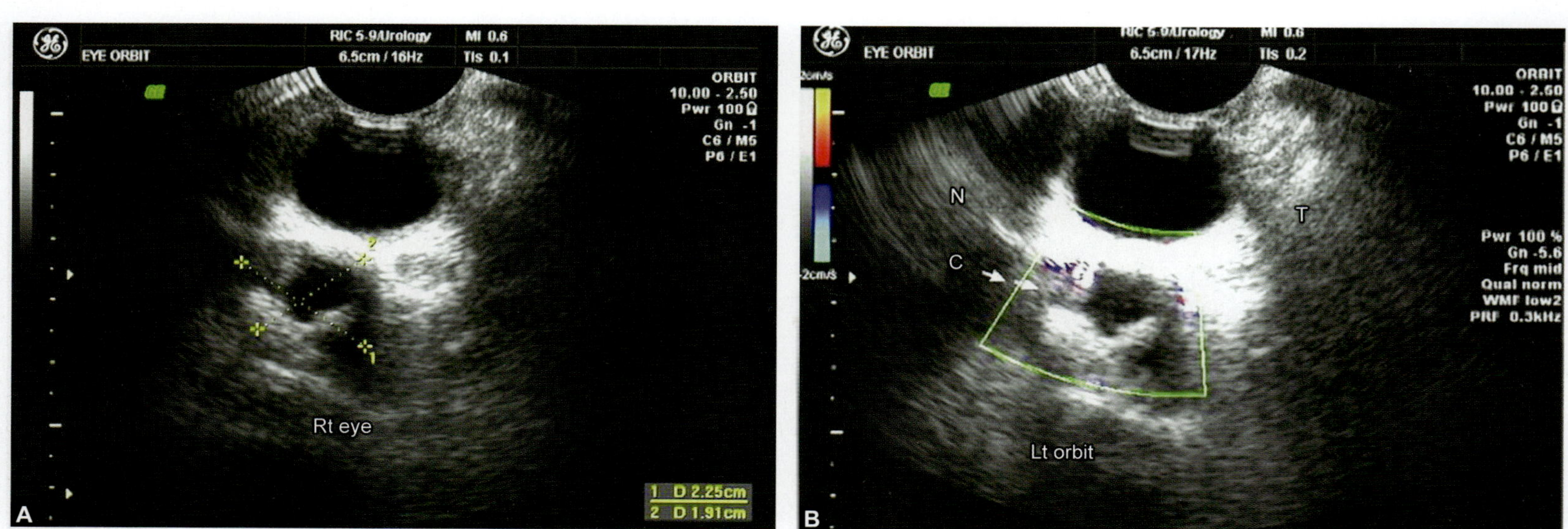

FIGURES 1.311A and B

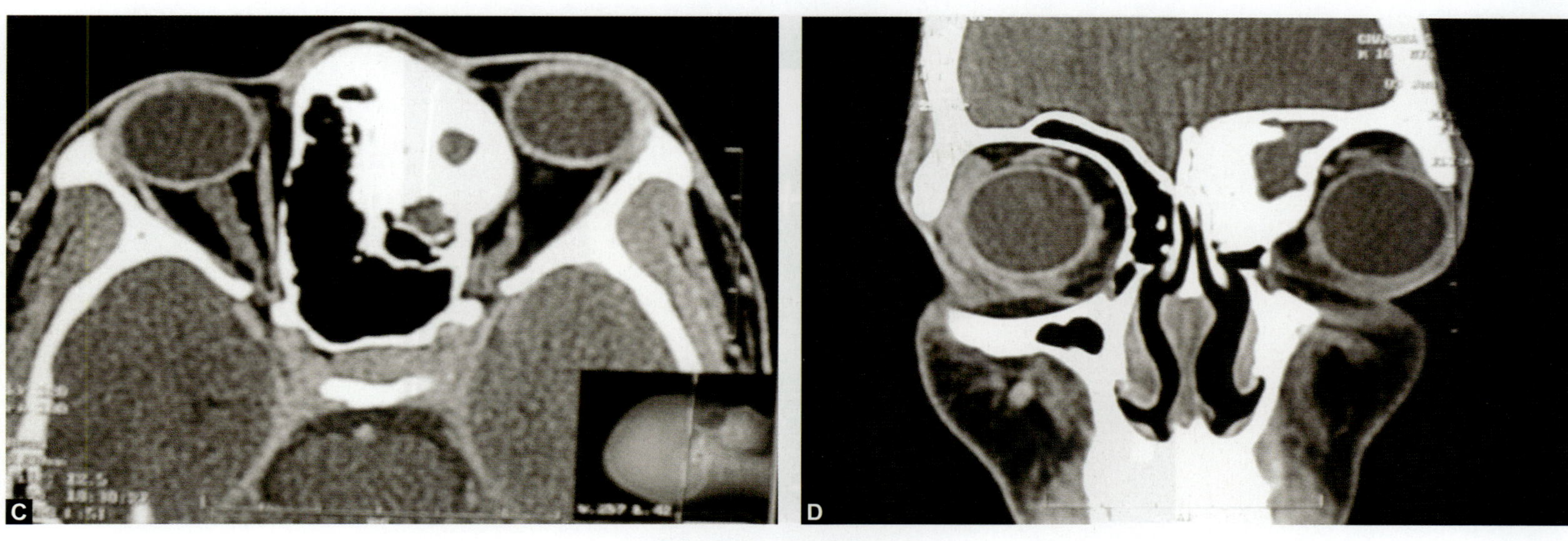

FIGURES 1.311C and D

FIGURES 1.311A to D: Nasal mass protruding in orbit. A young boy presented with lateral displacement of the eye ball with proptosis. HRSG shows a complex cystic mass coming out from the medial side of the orbit wall. Echogenic thick septa is seen in it. Multiple internal echoes are seen in it. The eye appears to be normal. CT scan of the same patient shows highly enhancing mass seen coming out from the nasal cavity. It is seen eroding the medial wall of the left orbit and invading the retrobulbar space.

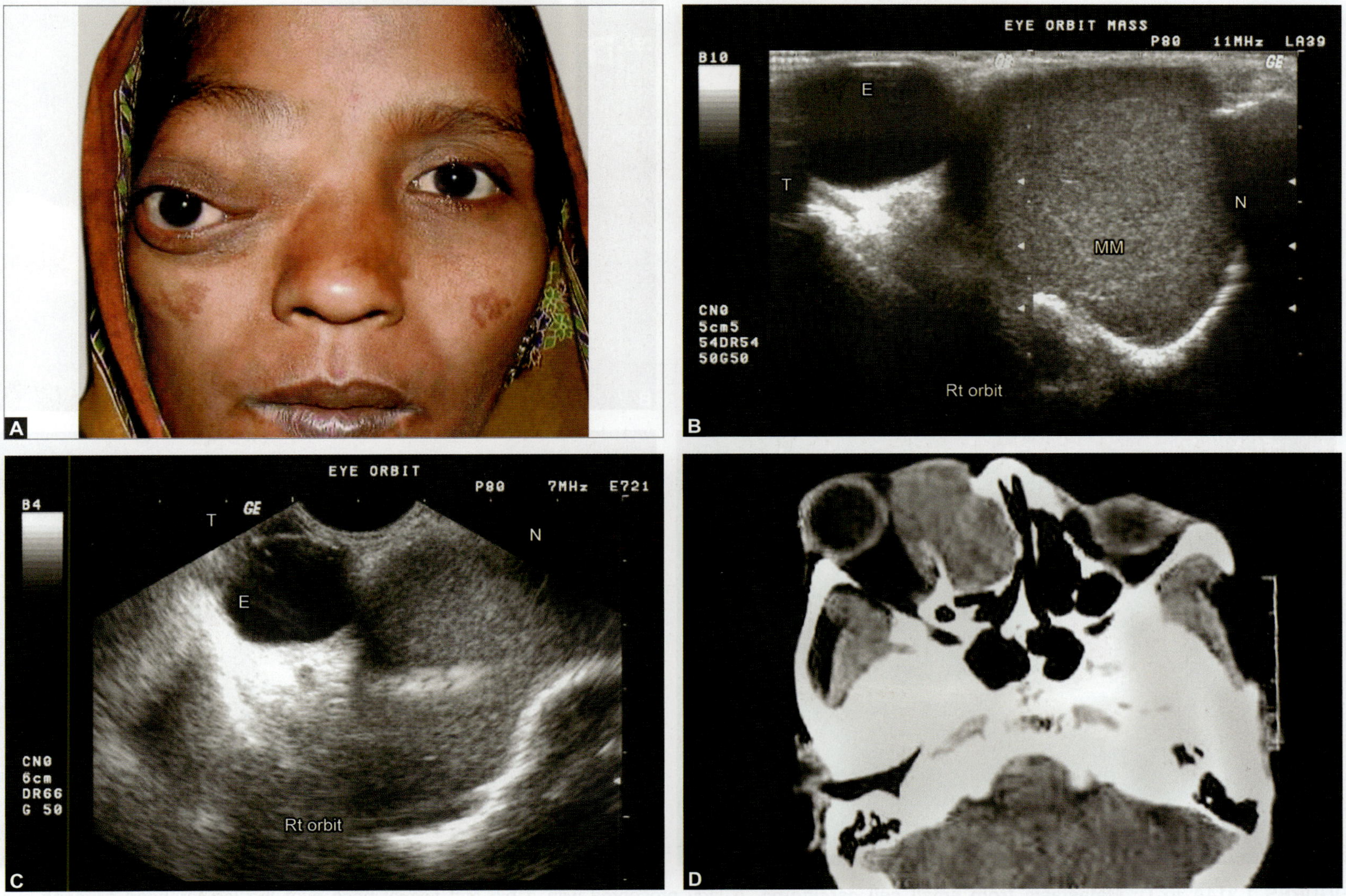

FIGURES 1.312A to D: Mucocele invading the right orbit. A lady patient presented with swelling over the medial side of the eye with lateral displacement. HRSG shows a thick echo complex mass coming out from the nasal cavity and pressing over the right orbit displacing the eye ball down. Thick echoes are seen in it suggestive of mucocele. CT of the same patient shows a hypoechoic dense mass seen coming out from the right nasal cavity eroding the medial wall of the orbit and invading the retrobulbar space.

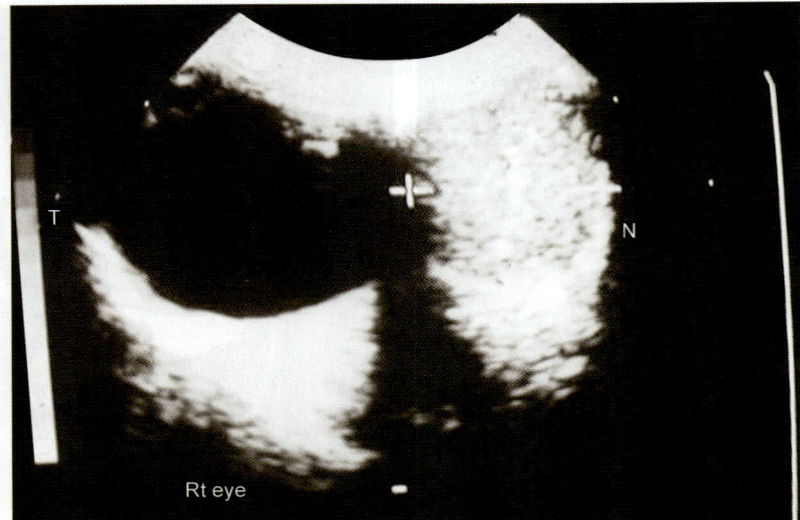

FIGURE 1.313: HRSG shows a well-defined echogenic mass in right upper medial quadrant. Fine echogenic interfaces are seen in the mass. Thick capsule is also seen. Biopsy shows dermoid cyst.

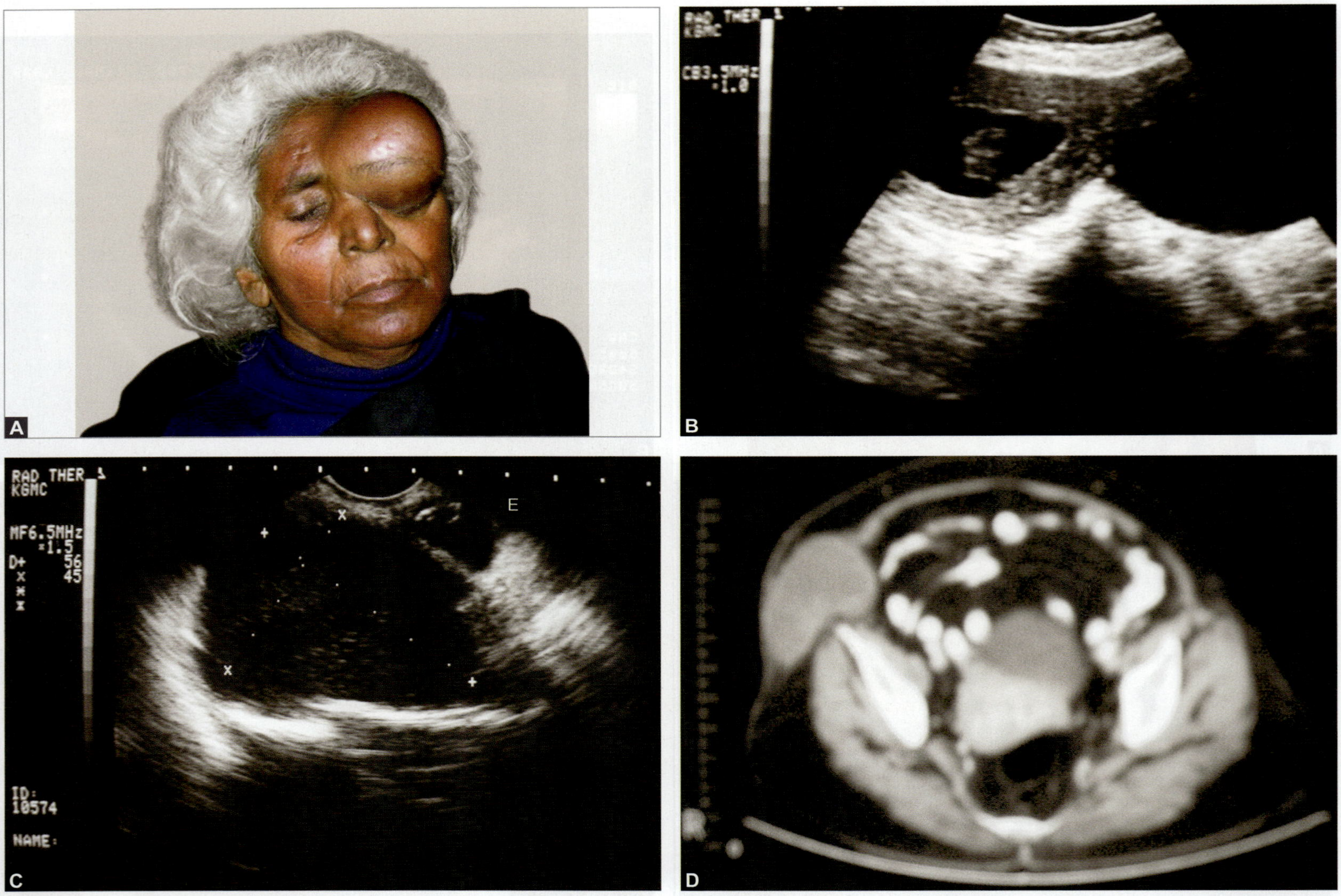

FIGURES 1.314A to D: Metastasis from small cell carcinoma. A lady presented with a big soft tissue mass over the left forehead covering over the left orbit. HRSG shows a big thick walled cystic mass over the left orbit. It is seen pressing and displacing the eye ball. However, the eye ball is separate from the mass and intact. CT abdomen of the same patient shows metastatic deposit also over the right side of the anterior abdominal wall.

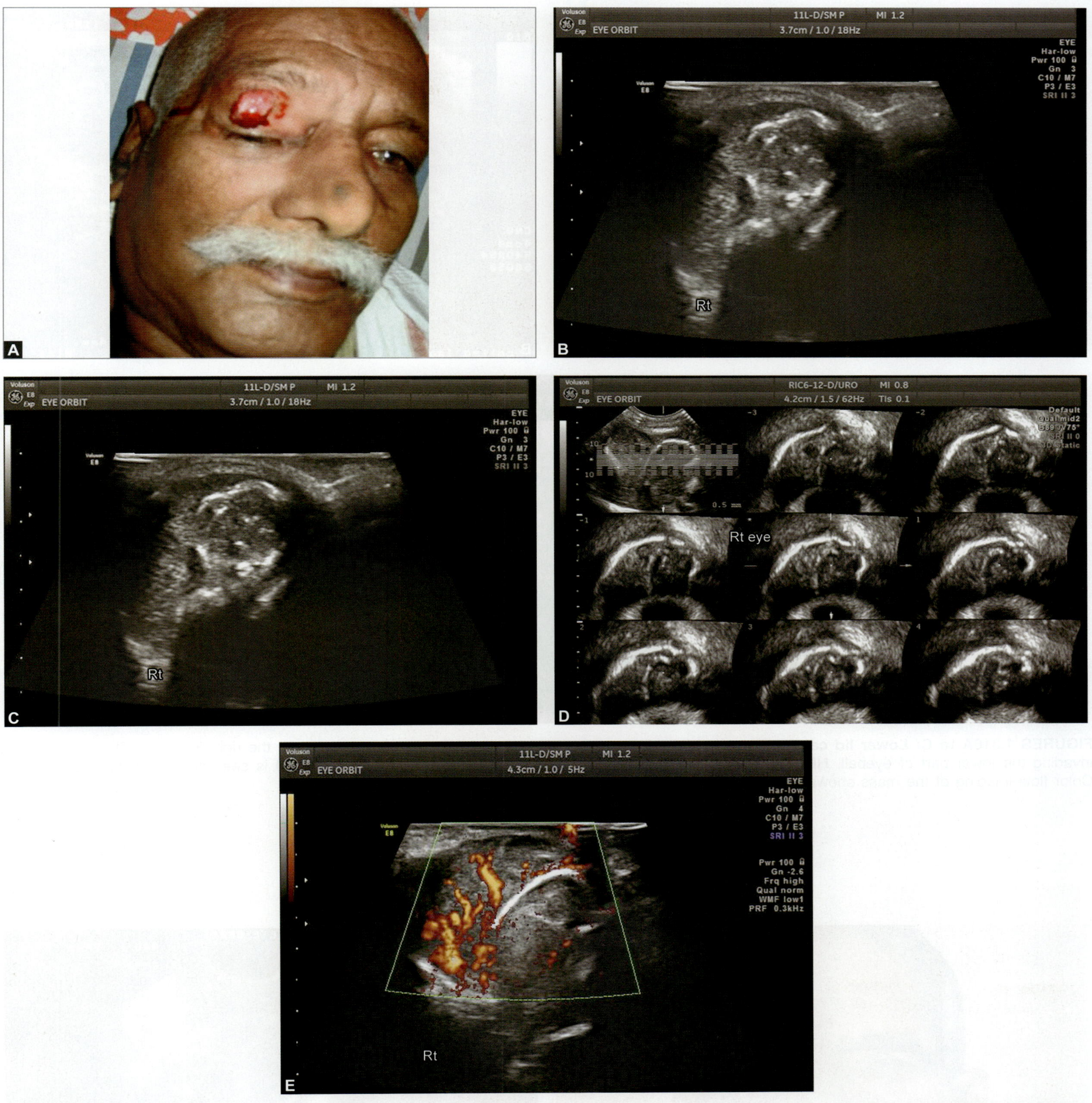

FIGURES 1.315A to E: Squamaus carcinoma of lid. An old man presented with heterogeneous soft tissue mass over the right lid. HRSG shows an irregular ill defined soft tissue mass over the lid. The mass is heterogeneous in texture. On 3D imaging, the superior orbital ridge is not seen invaded by the mass. On color flow imaging, increased flow is seen in the mass. However, the eyeball is spared by the mass. Biopsy of the mass confirms squamaus cell carcinoma.

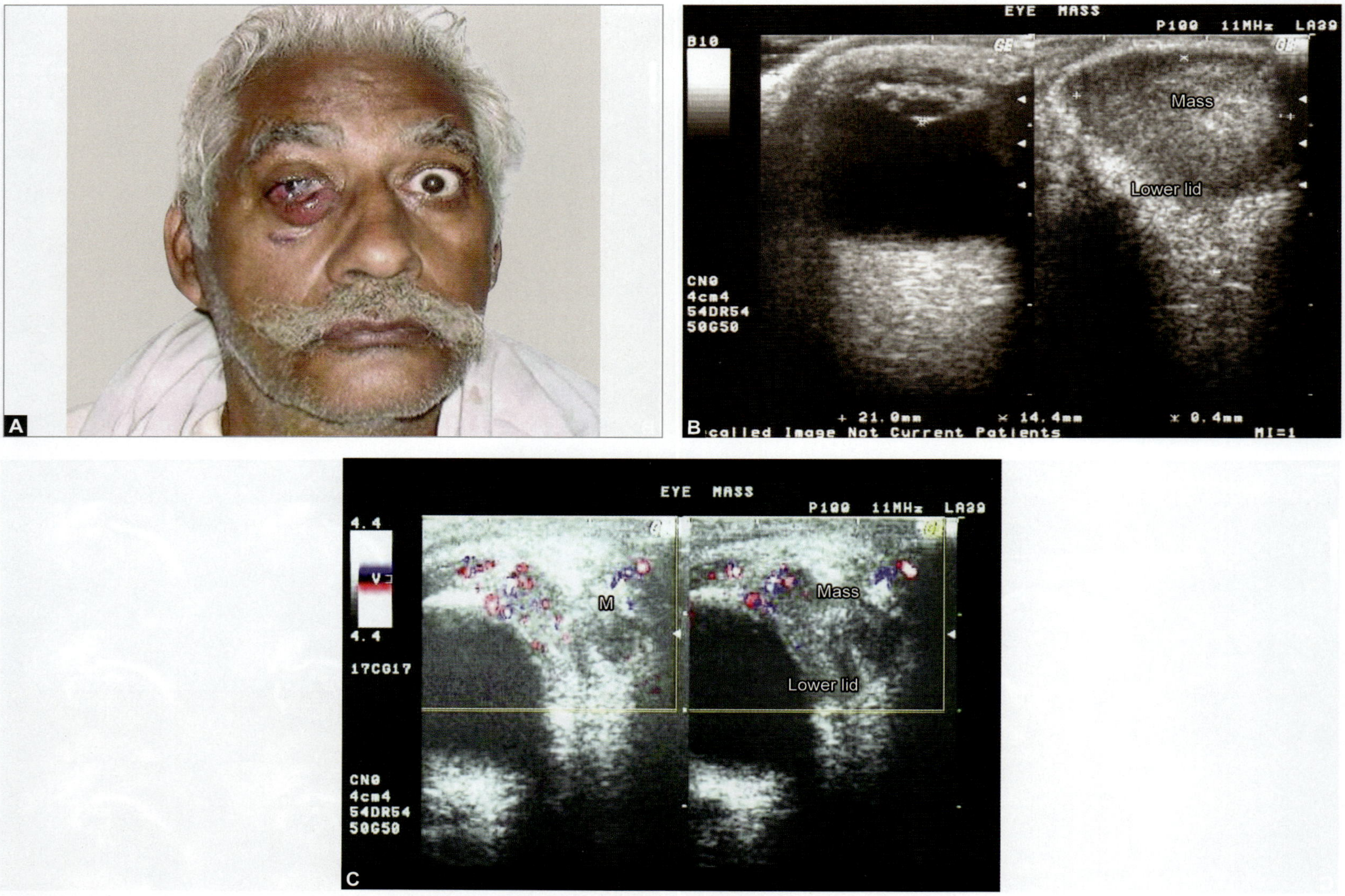

FIGURES 1.316A to C: Lower lid carcinoma. An old man presented with soft tissue mass coming out from the right lower lid. The mass is seen invading the lower part of eyeball. HRSG shows predominantly solid mass of lower eyelid. However, eyeball is seen spared at the time of study. Color flow imaging of the mass shows poor flow. Biopsy of the mass came out to be carcinoma lid.

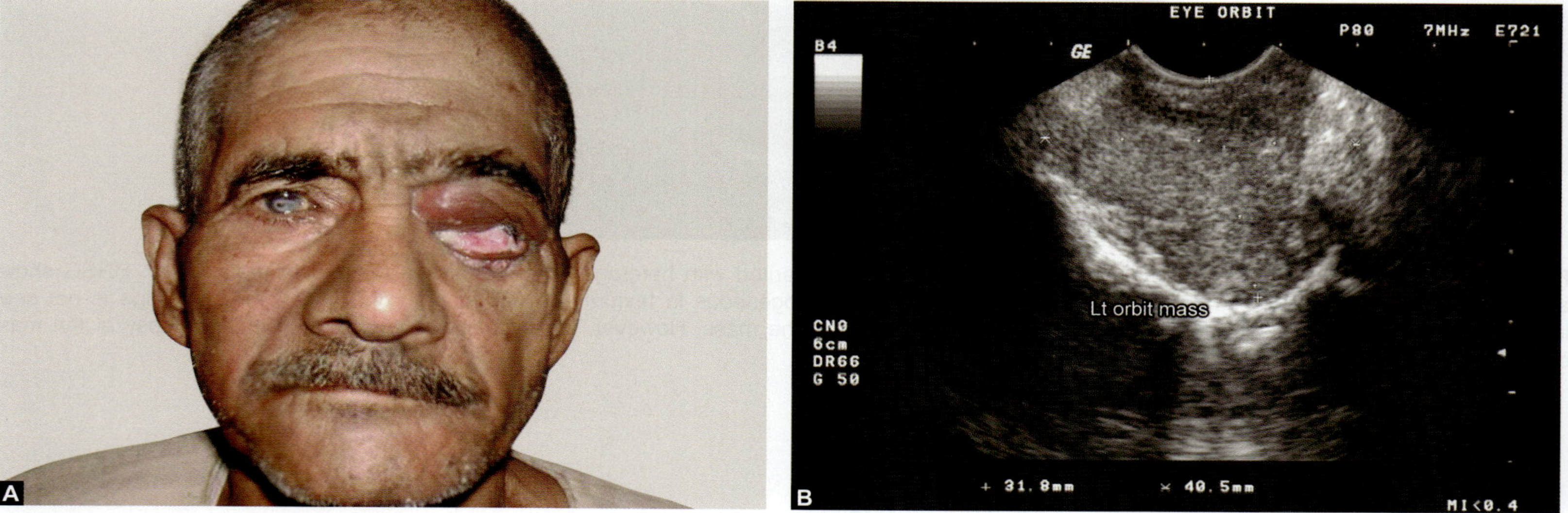

FIGURES 1.317A and B

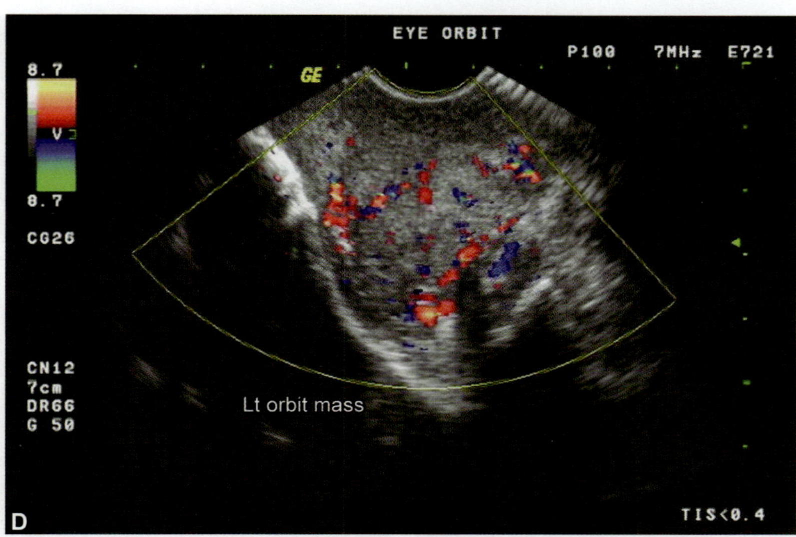

FIGURE 1.317C

FIGURES 1.317A to C: Carcinoma lower lid invading in the orbit. A patient presented with squamous cell carcinoma of lower lid of the left orbit. The lid was excised. HRSG shows the mass is seen invading the orbit. It is seen going posteriorly in the retrobulbar space and completely destroyed the normal orbital anatomy.

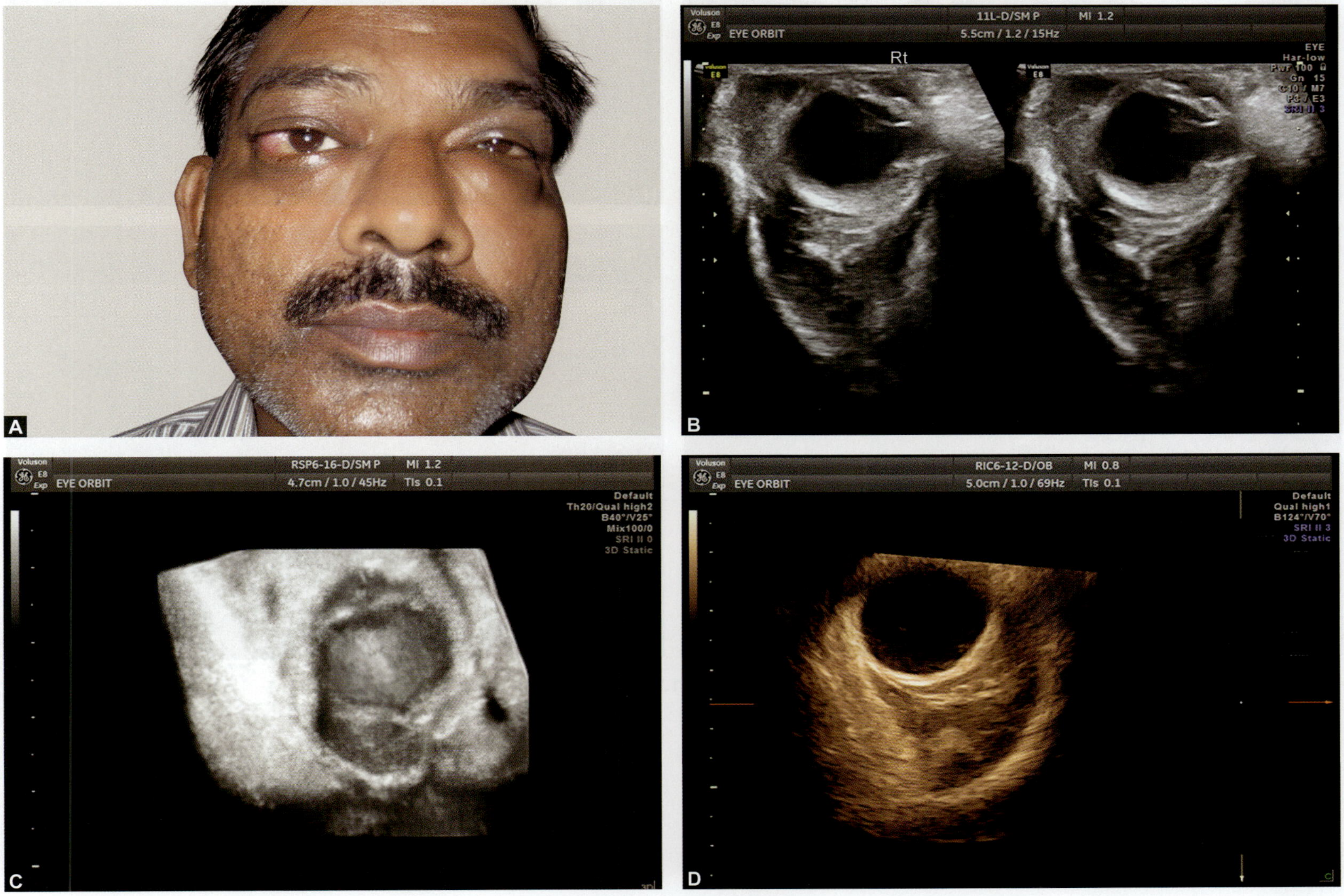

FIGURES 1.318A to D

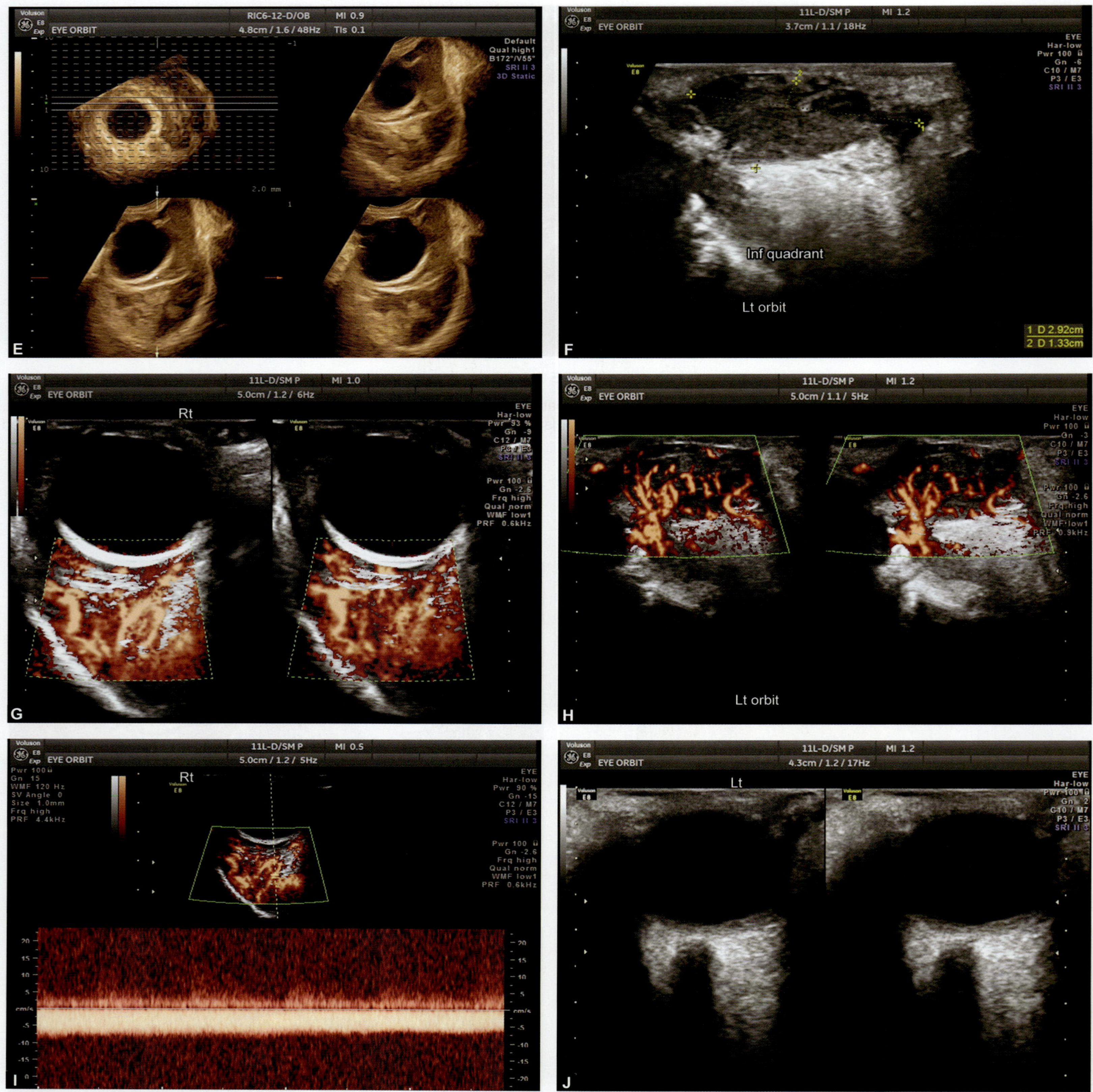

FIGURES 1.318E to J

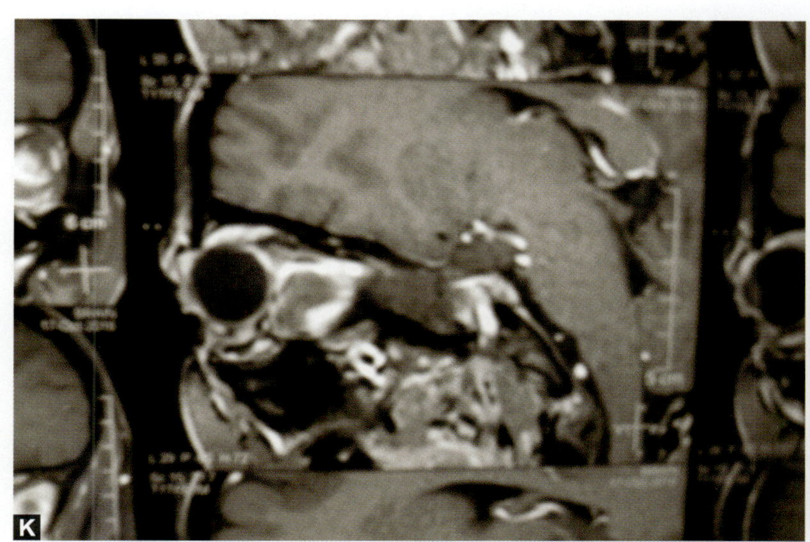

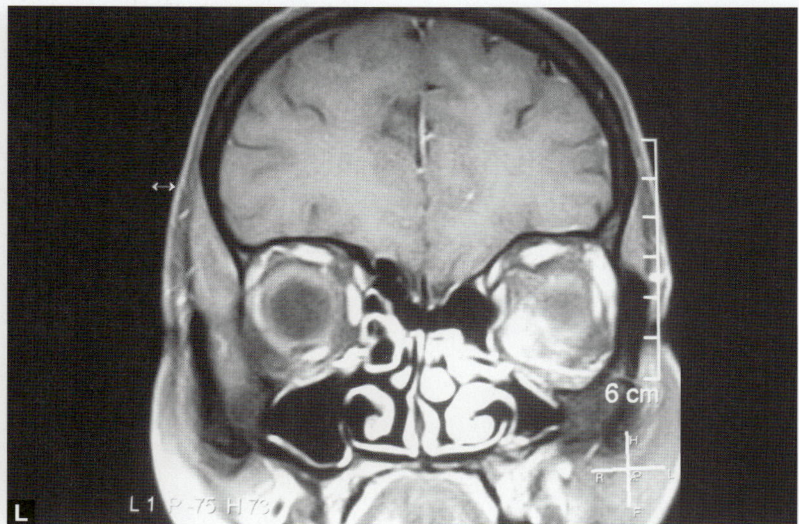

FIGURES 1.318K and L

FIGURES 1.318A to L: Bilateral orbital lymphoma. A patient presented with bilateral proptosis more marked on the right side. HRSG shows soft tissue intra conal mass in both the orbits. The right optic nerve is seen encased by the mass. The mass shows homogeneous echoes. No calcification or cystic changes seen in the mass on either side. It is more marked on Rt side. On color flow imaging, multiple vessels are seen feeding the mass in both the orbits. Moderate arterial flow is seen in the mass. However, no intra ocular extension is seen. MRI of the same patient also shows intra conal soft tissue mass in both the orbits. Findings are suggestive of intra orbital lymphoma.

CONCLUSION

High-resolution sonography is noninvasive multi-planer, widely available imaging modality for evaluation of eye and orbit. The tissue characterization of mass is better the CT. It is the only practical method of examining the eye, when light conducting media are opaque. For orbit, CT is better technique as it provides the global view. But HRSG is better to differentiate between solid and cystic masses.

The limitation of HRSG is limited field of view and extraorbital extension of the disease in the cranium, where CT is definitely superior than USG. The biggest advantage of ultrasonography over CT is its wide availability, rapidity of investigation and cost-effectiveness. Therefore, it is first line of investigation in orbital proptosis.

CHAPTER 2

Face

PK Srivastava

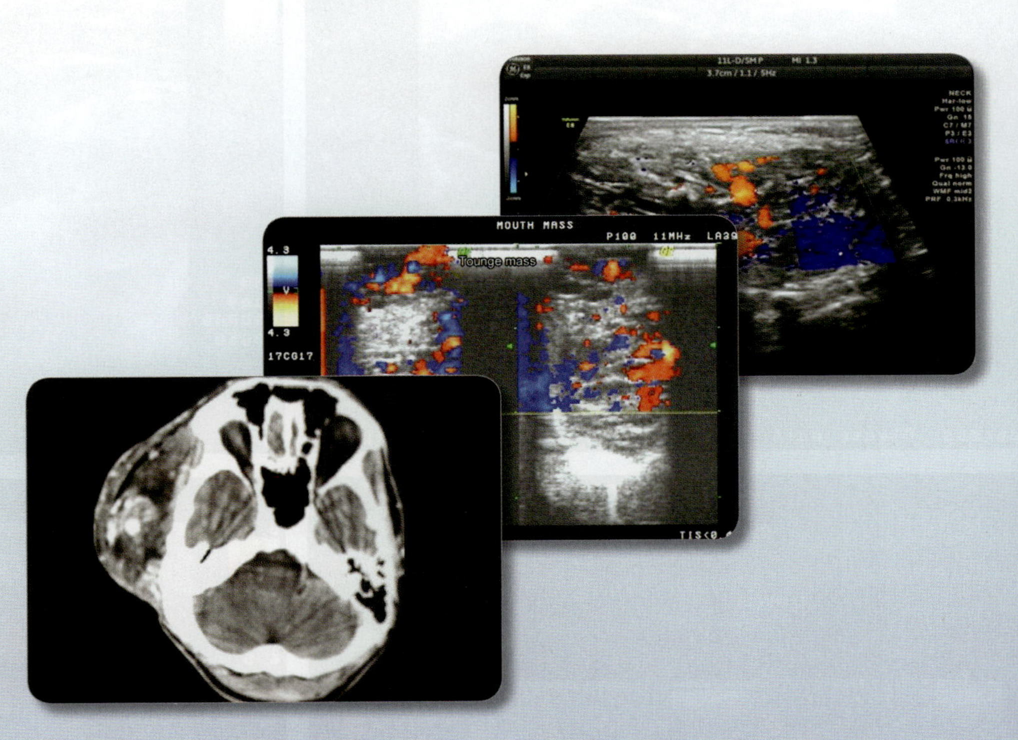

High-resolution ultrasound is a very good modality for evaluation of Human Face. It gives reliable information about various face masses resulting into disfigurement of face. It is also having great value in evaluating facial injuries causing disfigurement of face. The various parts of the face which can be easily evaluated by ultrasound are as under: -

1. Forehead Mass
2. Ocular and Orbital Masses
3. Masses in the Cheek
4. Nose
5. Lip
6. Chin
7. Muscles of the Face
8. Vessels
9. Bone and Cartilage
10. Tumors
11. Parasitic Infestations
12. Fascial Defects
13. Trauma
14. Post-surgical Trauma.

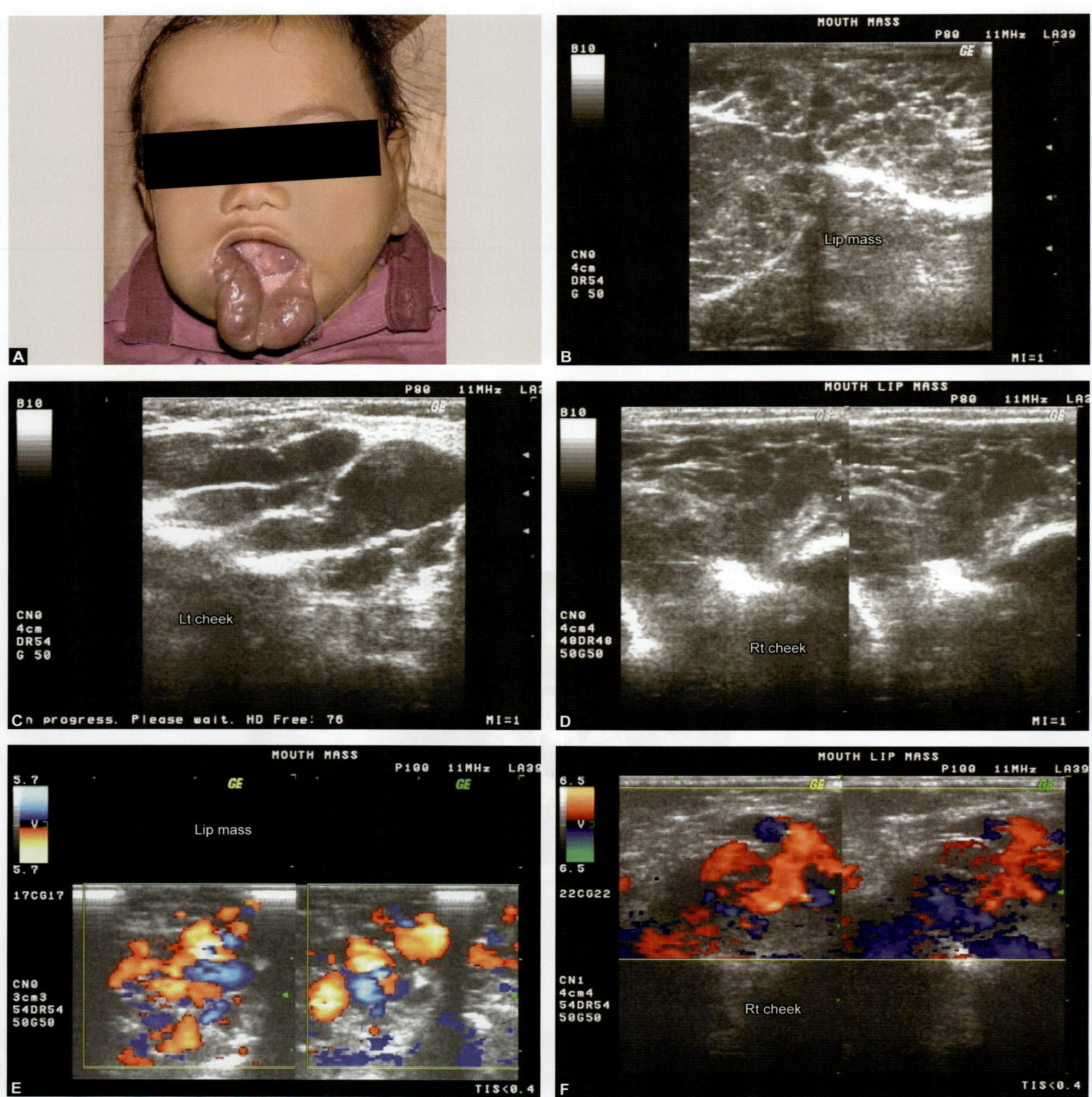

FIGURES 2.1A to F

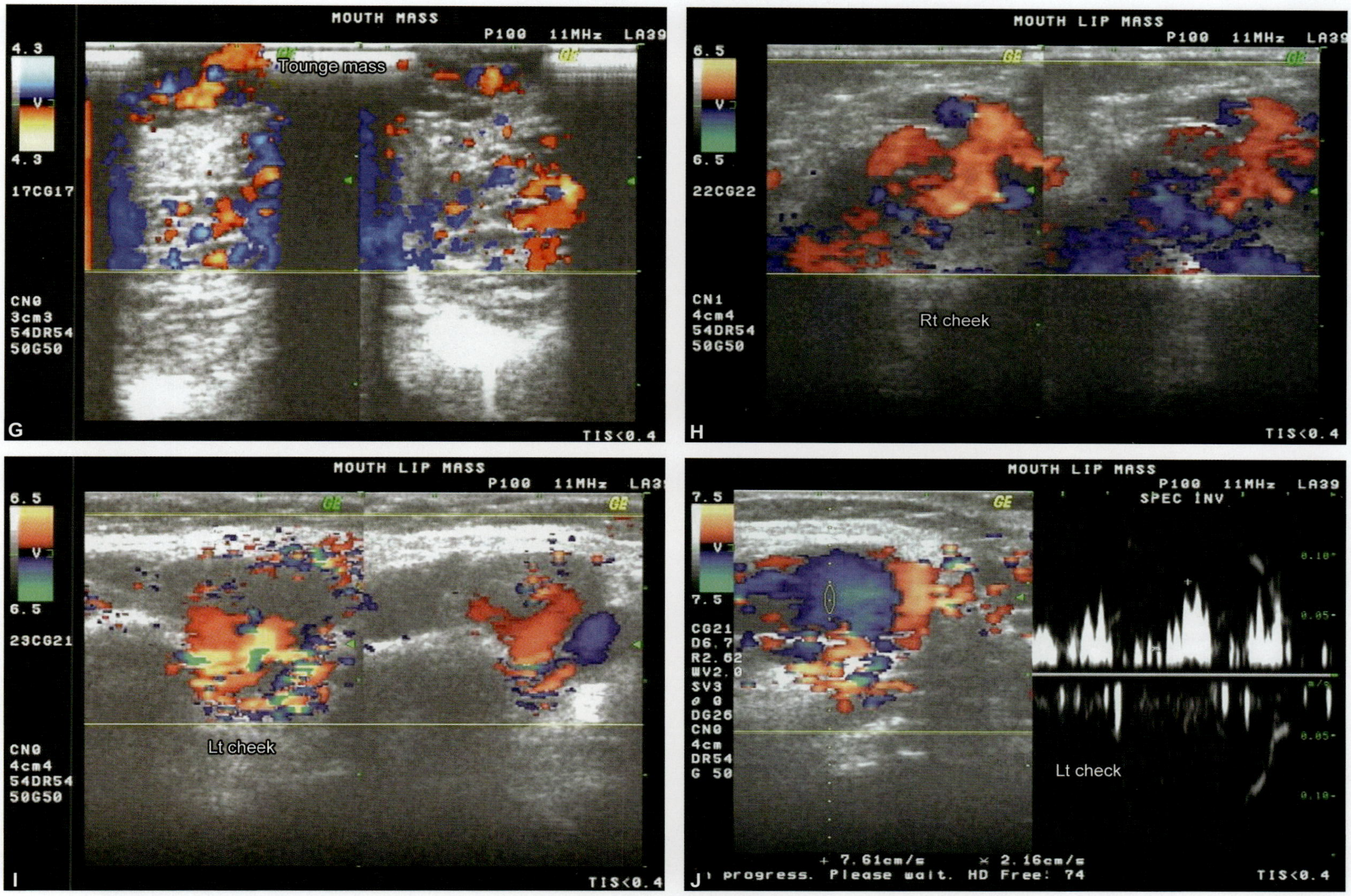

FIGURES 2.1G to J

FIGURES 2.1A to J: Arteriovenous malformation. A young child presented with marked lip hypertrophy with multiple bluish masses seen over the tongue and fullness of both cheek and the floor of the mouth. HRSG shows markedly hypertrophied lips with multiple dilated vessels seen in the lower lip. Few calcified specks are also seen in it. HRSG shows grossly dilated vessels in right and left cheeks. Color Doppler imaging shows high flow in the lip vessels with irregular pattern. HRSG shows multiple dilated vessels on the under surface of the tongue. Color Doppler imaging shows high flow in these vessels. Color flow imaging shows increased flow in the cheek vessels on either side. Spectral Doppler flow-tracing shows high flow in the vessels with arterial and venous flow pattern suggestive of arteriovenous malformation involving tongue, lower lip, both cheek and floor of the mouth.

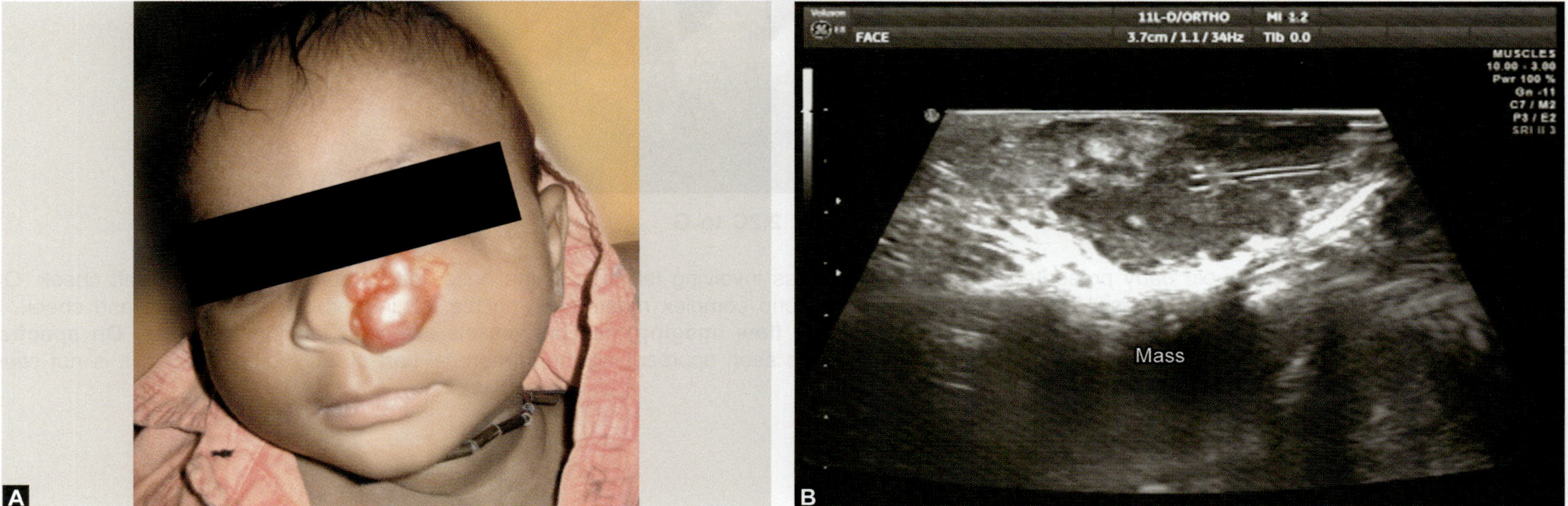

FIGURES 2.2A and B

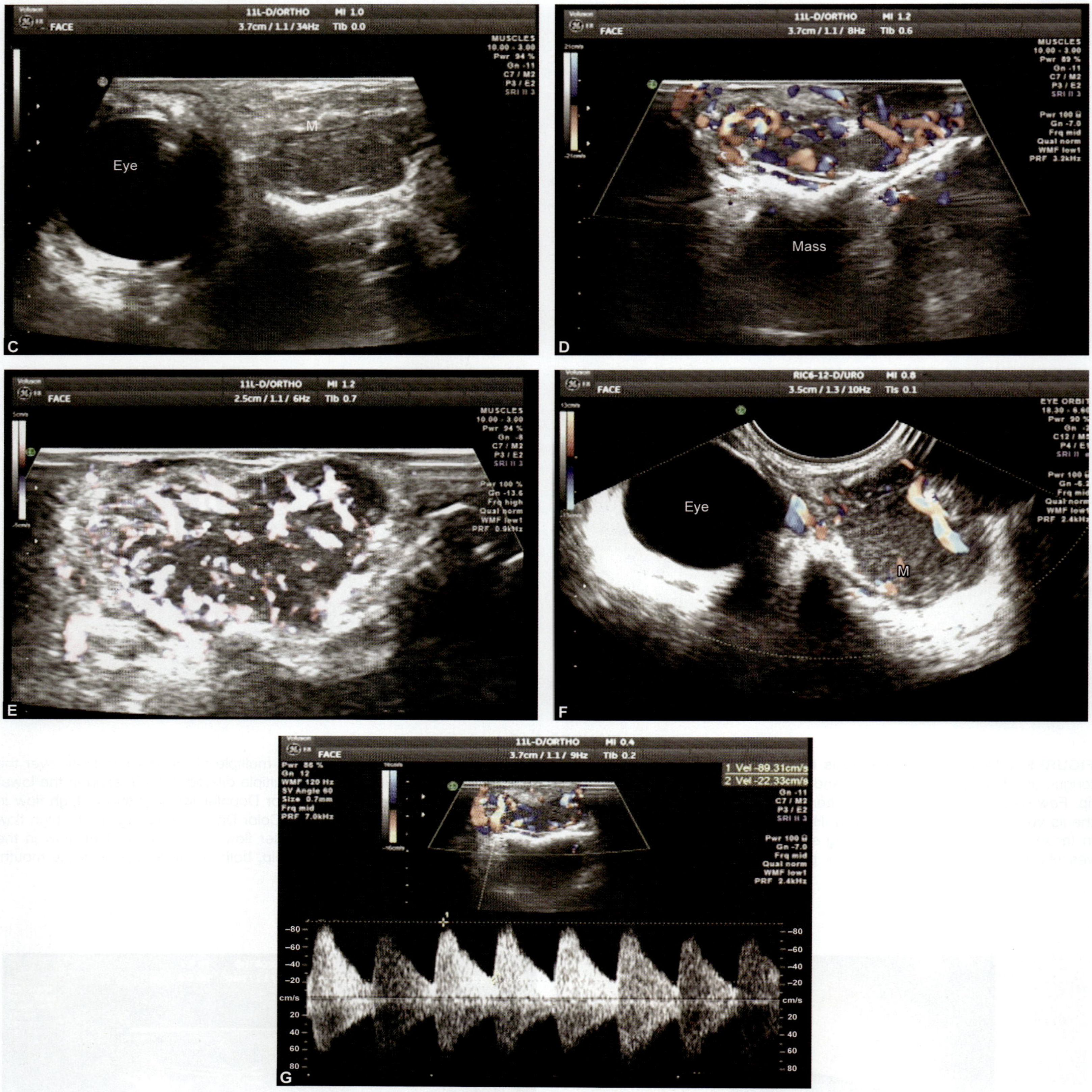

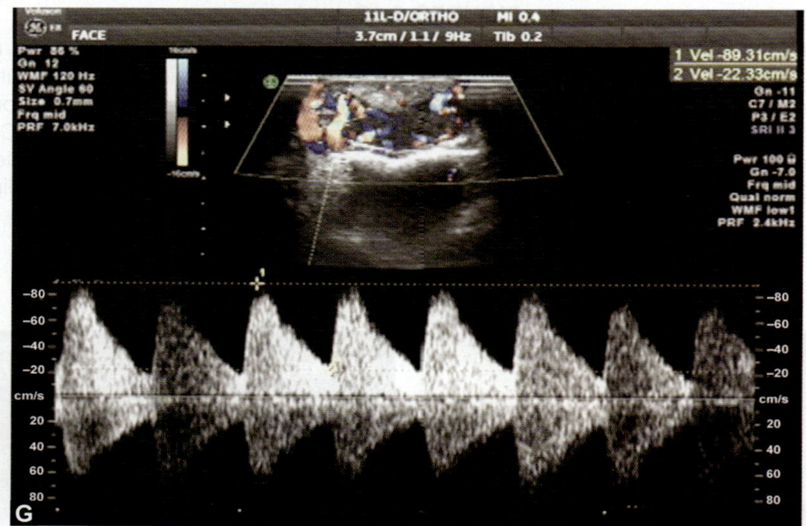

FIGURES 2.2C to G

FIGURES 2.2A to G: A 7-month-old baby presented with soft tissue mass involving left side of the nose, left infraorbital region and left cheek. On clinically, it appears to be a vascular mass. HRSG shows a low level echo complex mass involving the left infraorbital region, nose and cheek. It shows few echogenic foci. No septation is seen in the mass. **On color flow imaging,** multiple vessels are seen feeding the mass. **On spectral Doppler tracing,** moderate arterial flow is seen in the mass. The mass is seen approaching the infraorbital part of left orbit. However, it is not seen invading the left eye.

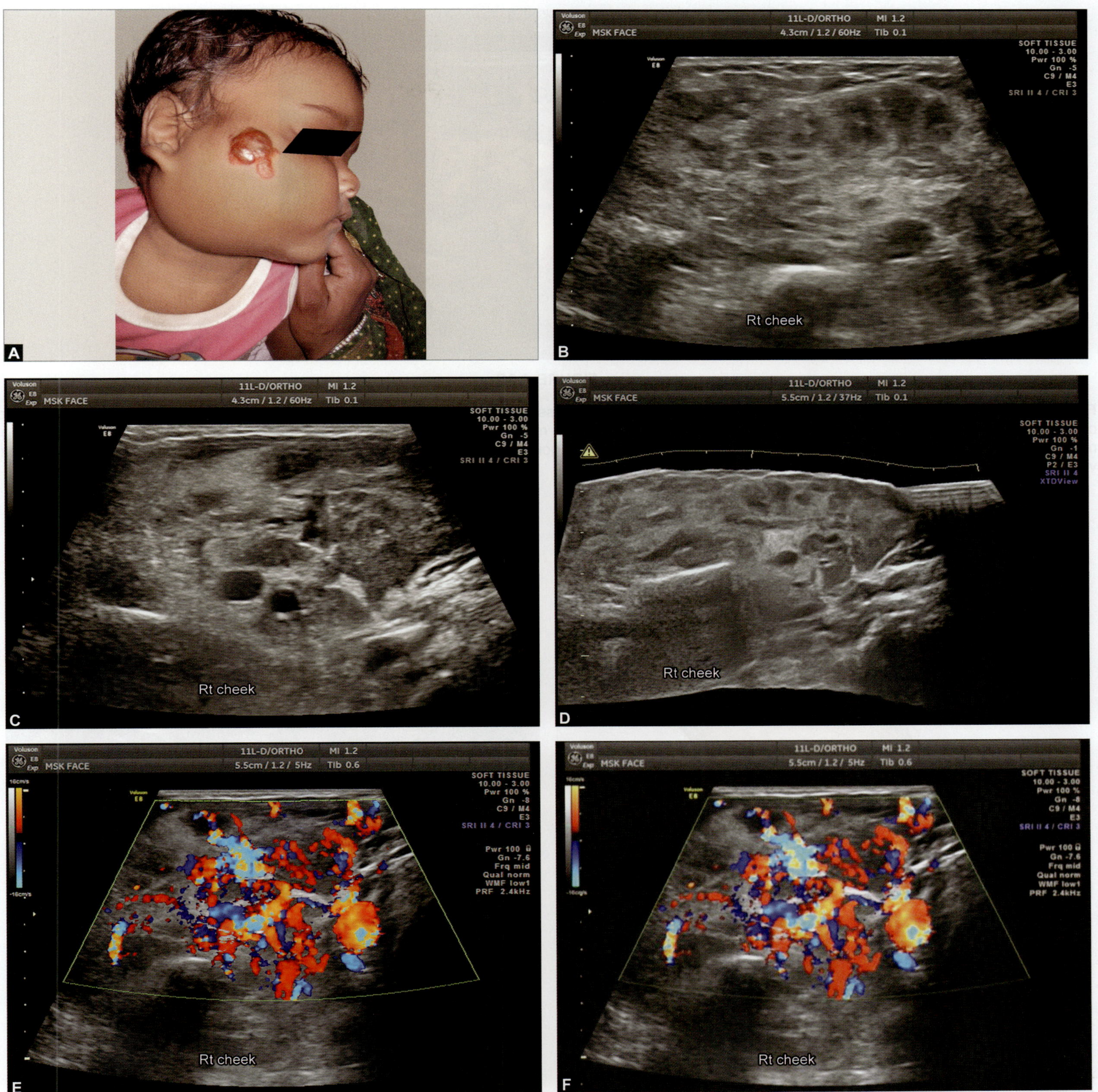

FIGURES 2.3A to F

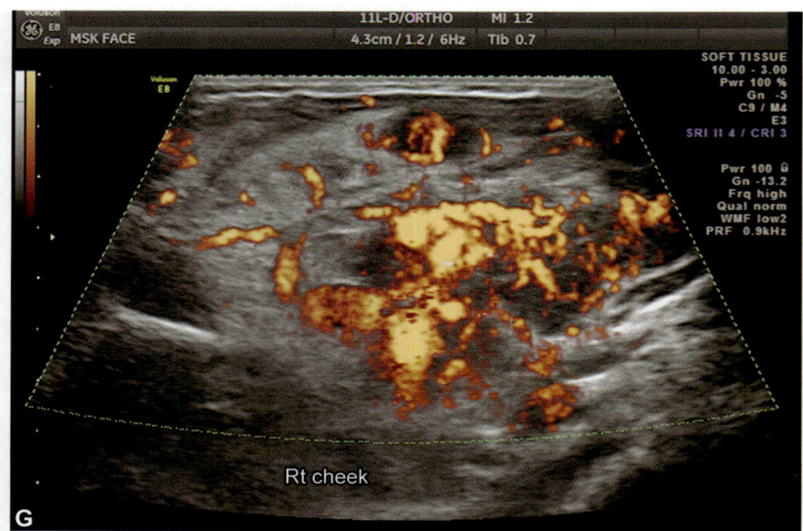

FIGURE 2.3G

FIGURES 2.3A to G: A 10-month-old baby presented with soft tissue mass over the right cheek. HRSG shows an irregular ill-defined low level echo complex mass involving the right cheek. The mass is seen invading the muscles. Multiple cystic shadows are seen in it. **On color flow imaging,** multiple vessels are seen feeding the mass. The vessels are also seen going deep in the muscles. **On spectral Doppler tracing,** moderate arterial venous flow is seen in the mass suggestive of hemangiomatous mass.

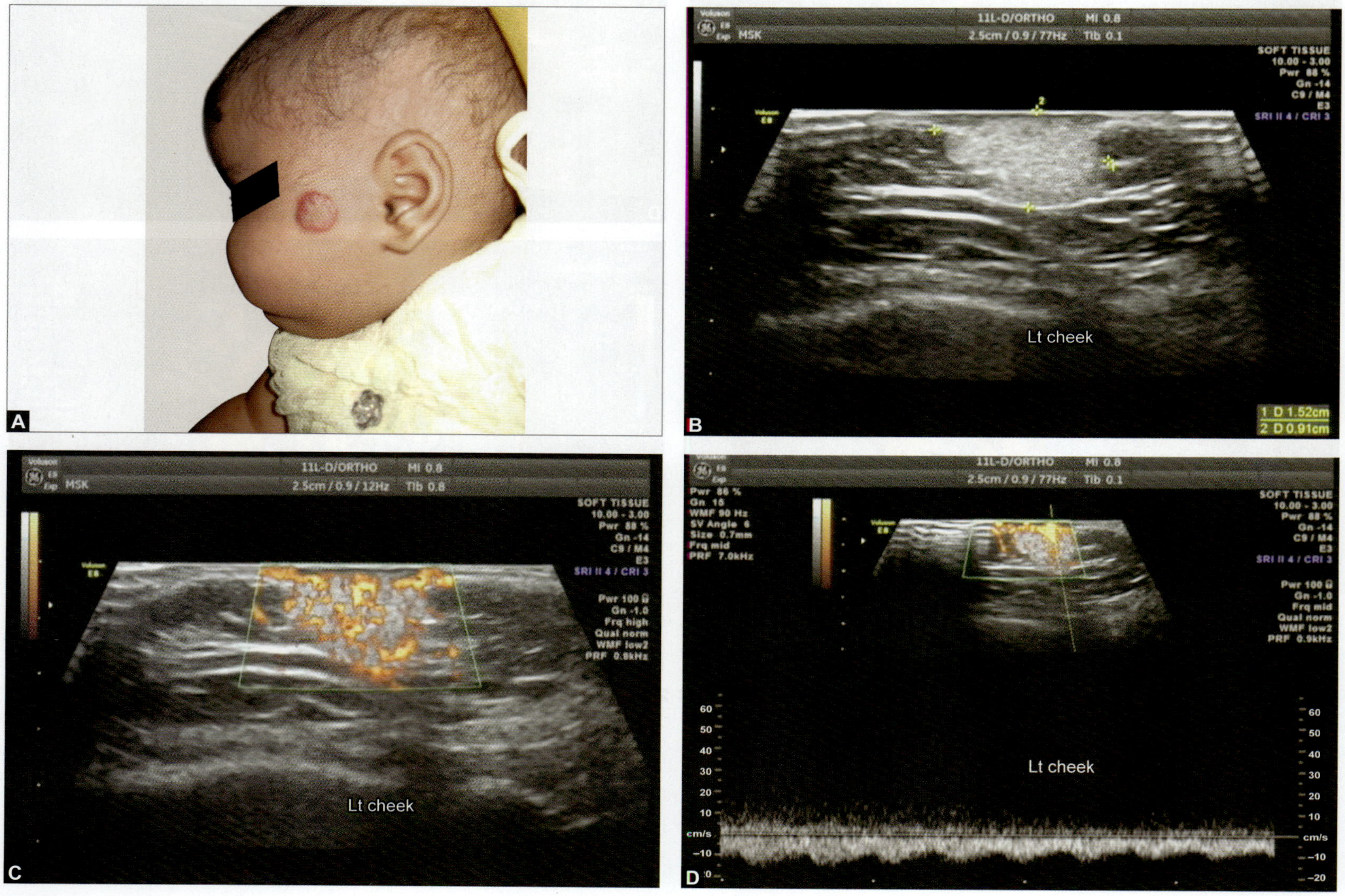

FIGURES 2.4A to D: A 6-month-old baby presented with soft tissue mass over the left cheek. HRSG shows an echogenic mass in left subcutaneous plane. It is homogeneous in texture. It is confined to the subcutaneous tissue. **On color flow imaging,** multiple vessels are seen feeding the mass. **On spectral Doppler tracing,** low arterial flow is seen in it suggestive of hemangioma.

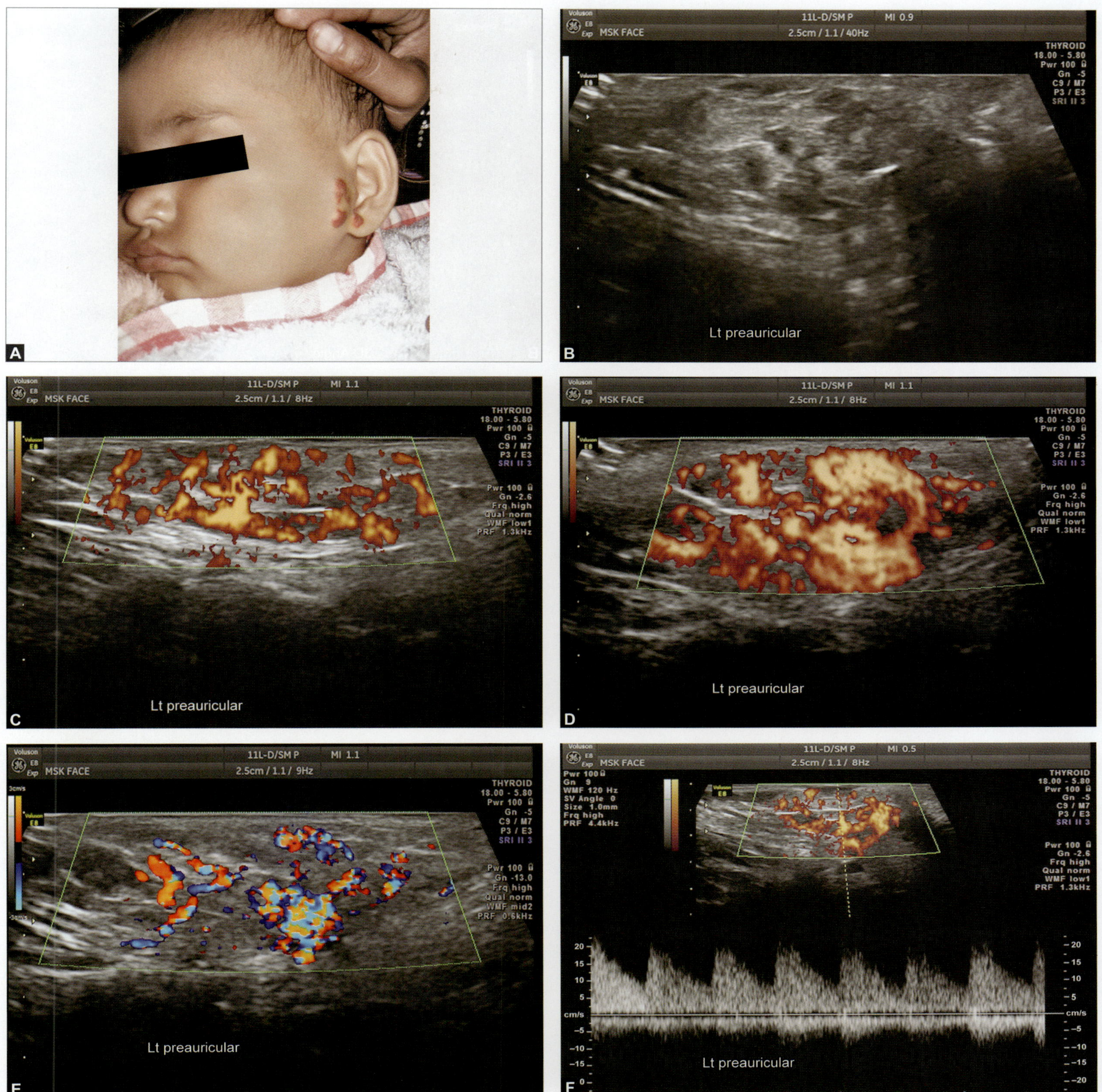

FIGURES 2.5A to F: A 1.5-year-old baby presented with soft tissue mass involving left preauricular region and lower part of the left lobe of the ear. HRSG shows an ill-defined inhomogeneous low level echo complex mass involving preauricular area. It is irregular in outline and confined to the subcutaneous tissue plane. **On color flow imaging,** multiple vessels are seen feeding the mass. **On spectral Doppler tracing,** low arterial flow is seen in it suggestive of hemangioma.

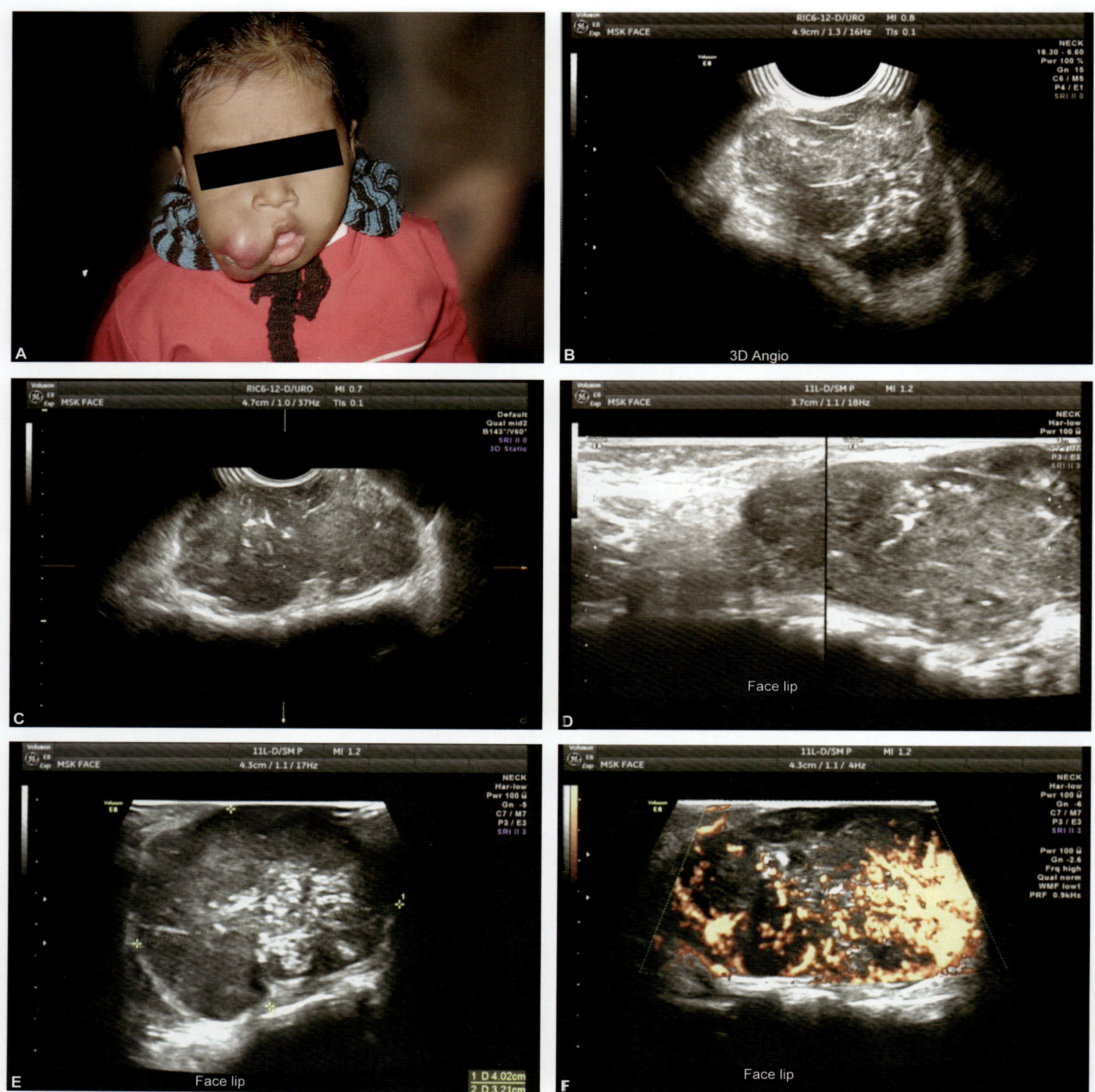

FIGURES 2.6A to F

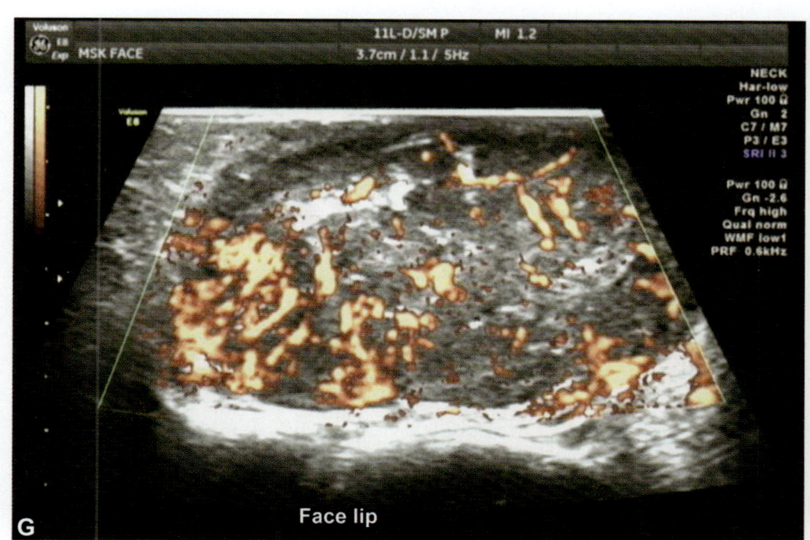

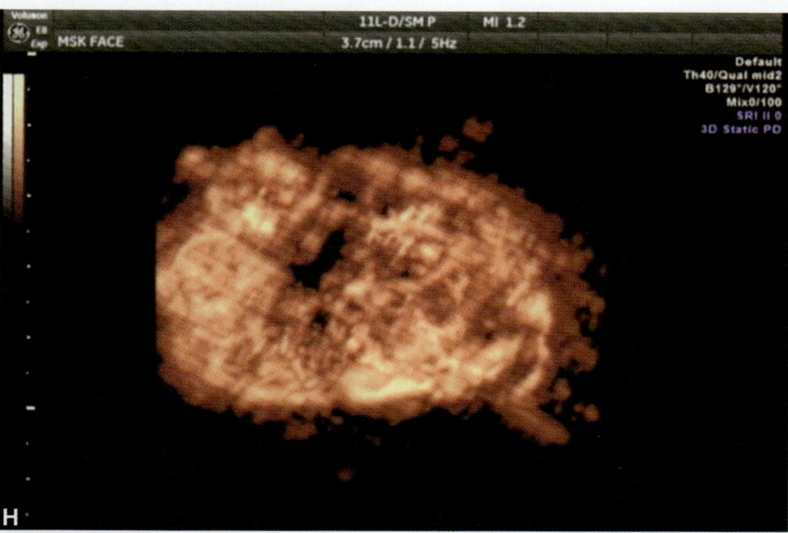

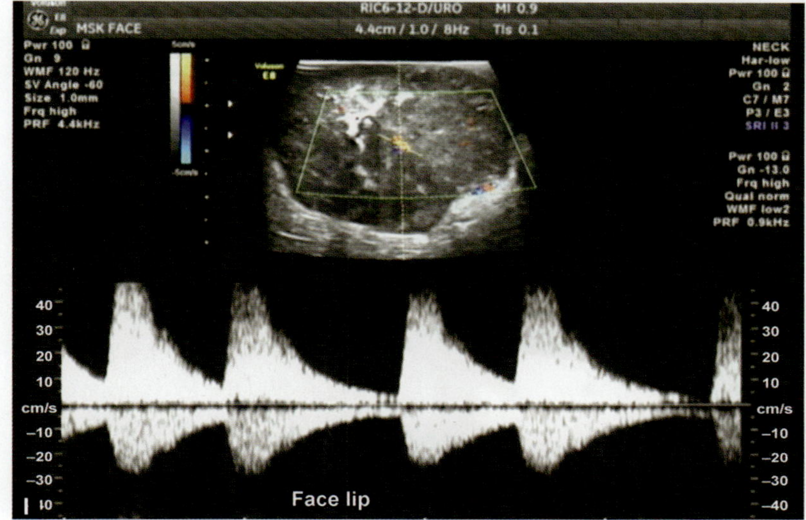

FIGURES 2.6G to I

FIGURES 2.6A to I: A 4-year-old girl presented with a soft tissue mass involving right cheek, right upper and lower lip and part of the right chin since birth. It shows progressive enlargement with the age. Diffuse hypertrophy of the soft tissue is seen and also involving right lower lip. **On color flow imaging,** a diffuse soft tissue mass is seen involving right cheek, right upper and lower lip and also right chin. Echogenic foci are also seen in the mass. But no cystic areas are seen in the mass. **On color flow imaging,** multiple vessels are seen feeding the mass. **On spectral Doppler tracing,** moderate arterial and venous flow is seen in the mass suggestive of vascular malformation.

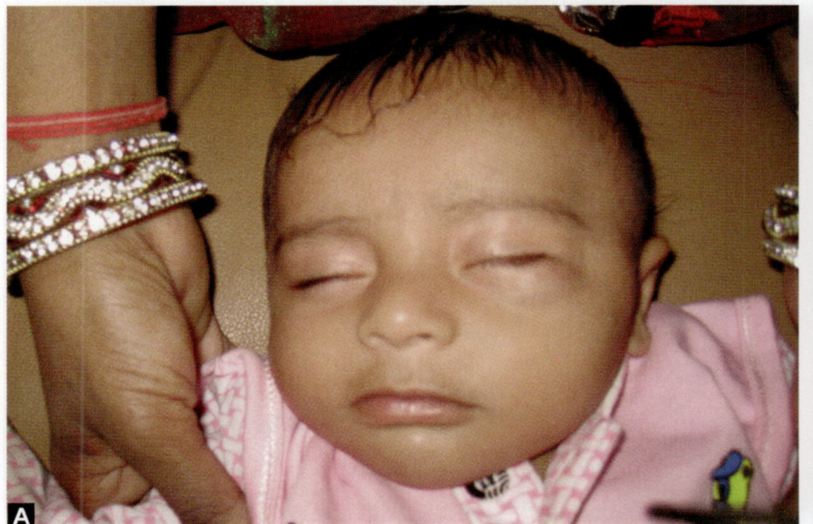

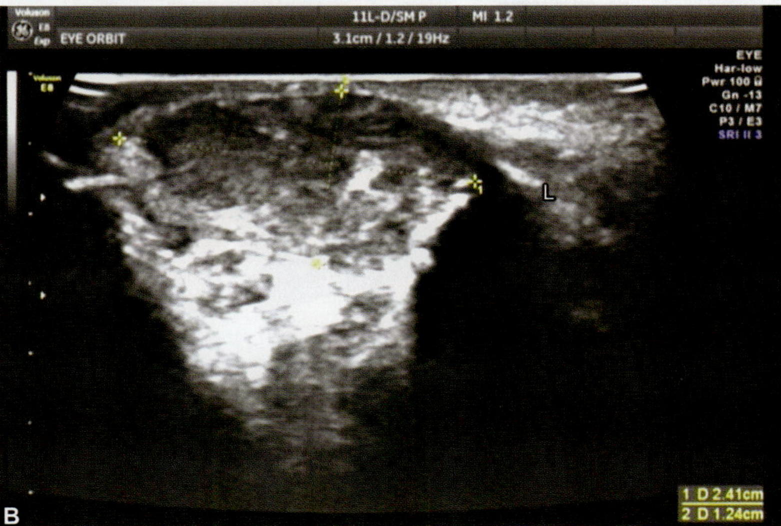

FIGURES 2.7A and B

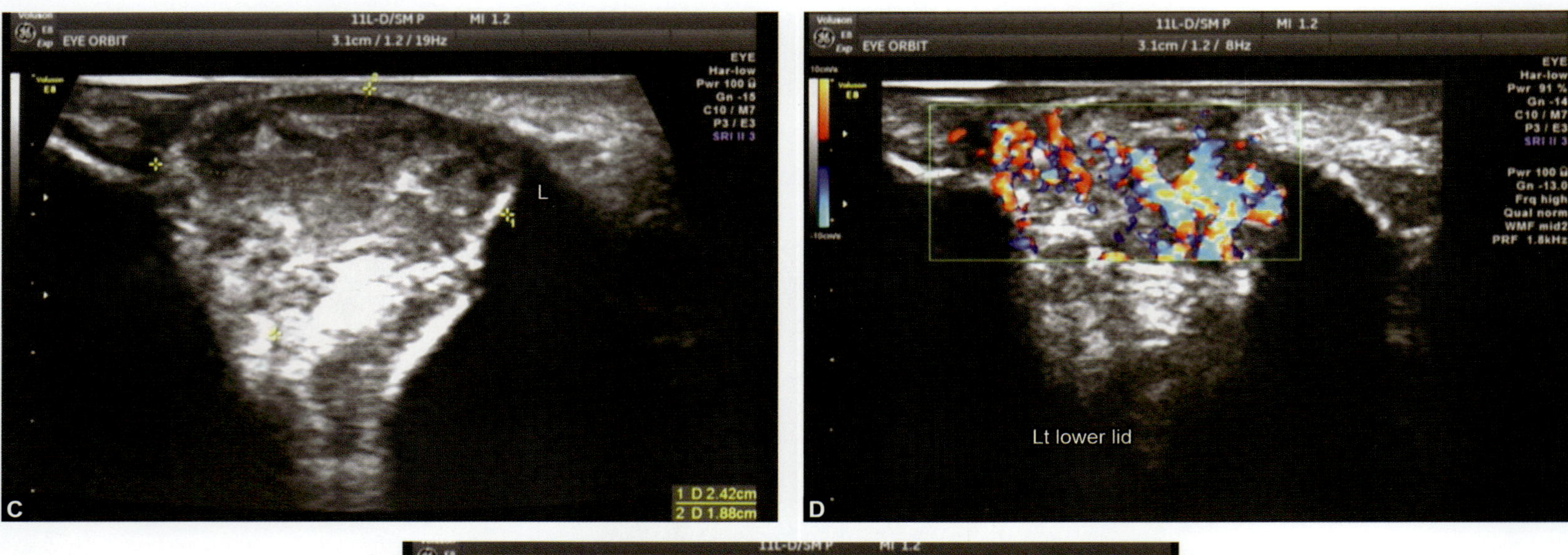

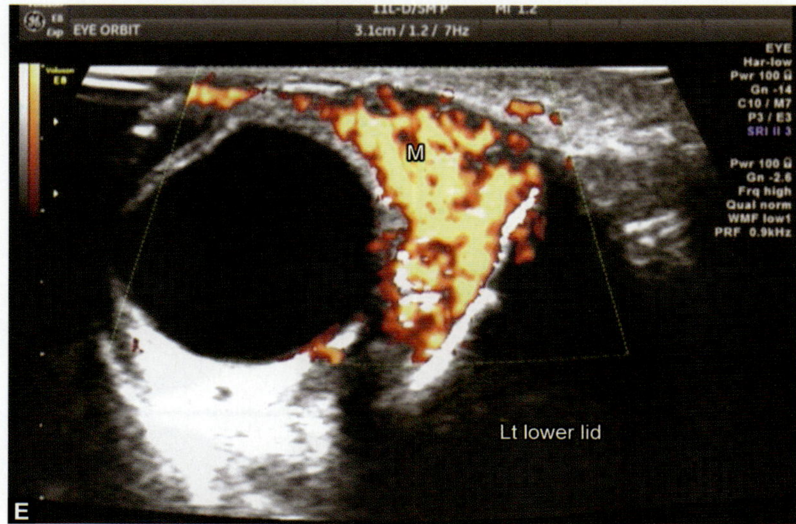

FIGURES 2.7C to E

FIGURES 2.7A to E: A 3-month-old baby presented with soft tissue swelling over left lower lid. Multiple vessels are seen feeding the mass. **On spectral Doppler tracing,** moderate arterial flow is seen in the mass suggestive of highly vascular mass.

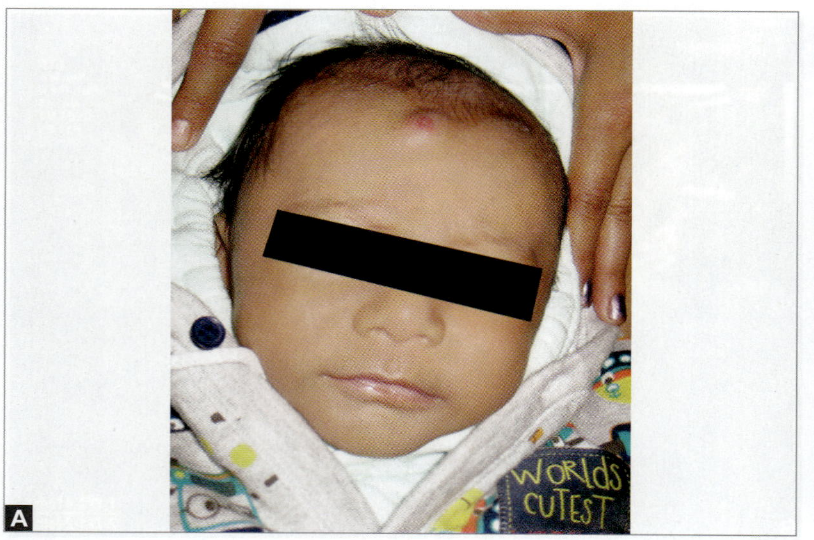

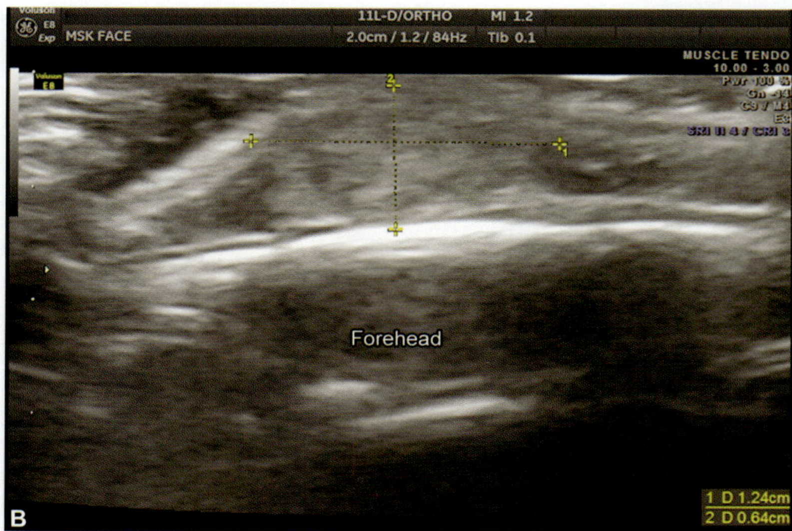

FIGURES 2.8A and B

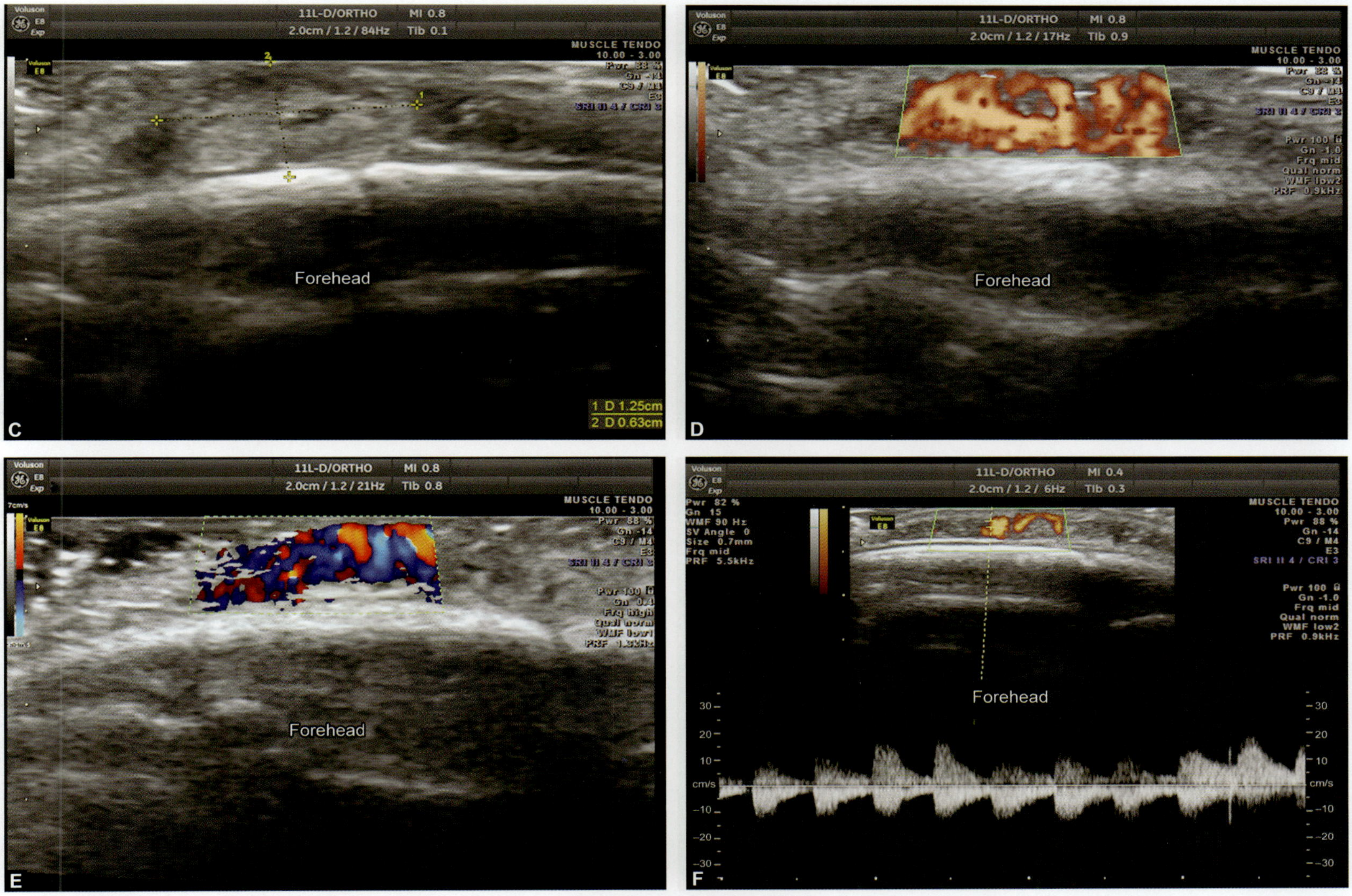

FIGURES 2.8C to F

FIGURES 2.8A to F: A 3-month-old baby presented with soft tissue mass over the forehead. High resolution sonography shows a well-defined homogeneous soft tissue mass over the forehead. The mass is homogeneous in texture. No calcification is seen in the mass. The mass is confined in the subcutaneous tissue plane. It is not seen invading the deeper tissue or skull table. **On color flow imaging,** multiple vessels are seen feeding the mass. **On spectral Doppler tracing,** low arterial flow is seen in the mass suggestive of hemangiomatous mass.

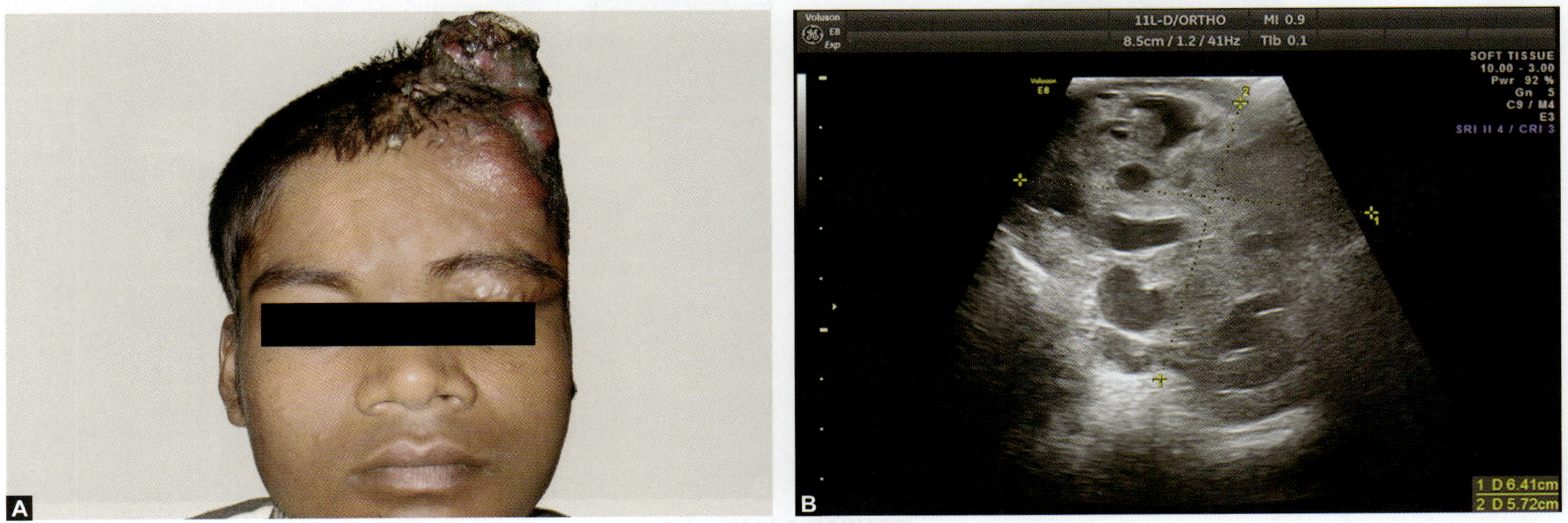

FIGURES 2.9A and B

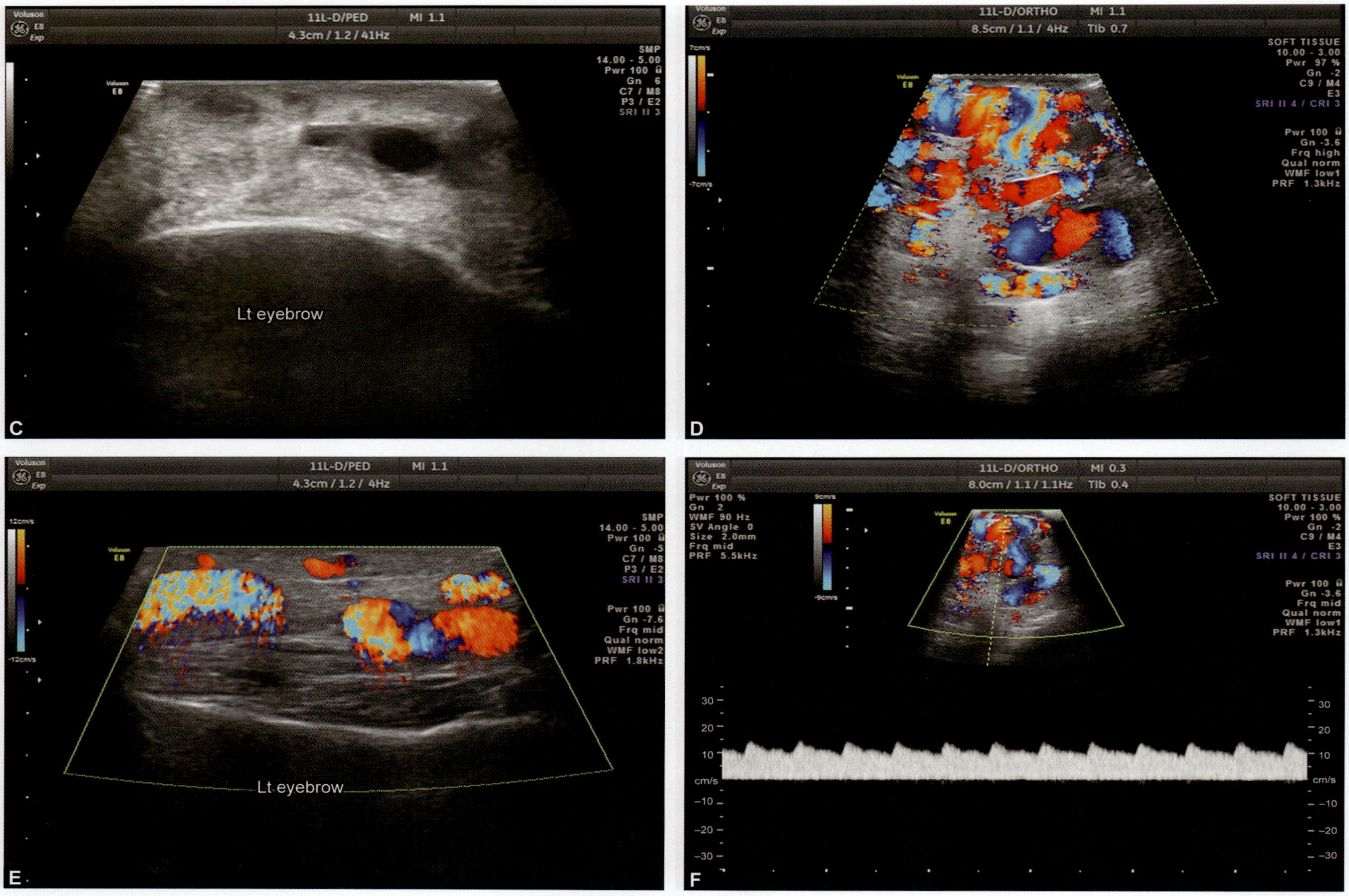

FIGURES 2.9C to F

FIGURES 2.9A to F: Scalp and forehead vascular mass: An 18-year-old boy presented with multiple nodular masses in left side of scalp, forehead, left supraorbital region and left upper lid. High resolution sonography shows a big irregular ill-defined heterogeneous mass involving left scalp, forehead, supraorbital region and left upper lid. Multiple vessels are seen feeding the mass. **On color flow imaging,** moderate arterial and venous flow is seen feeding the mass. The vessels are seen invading the skull table.

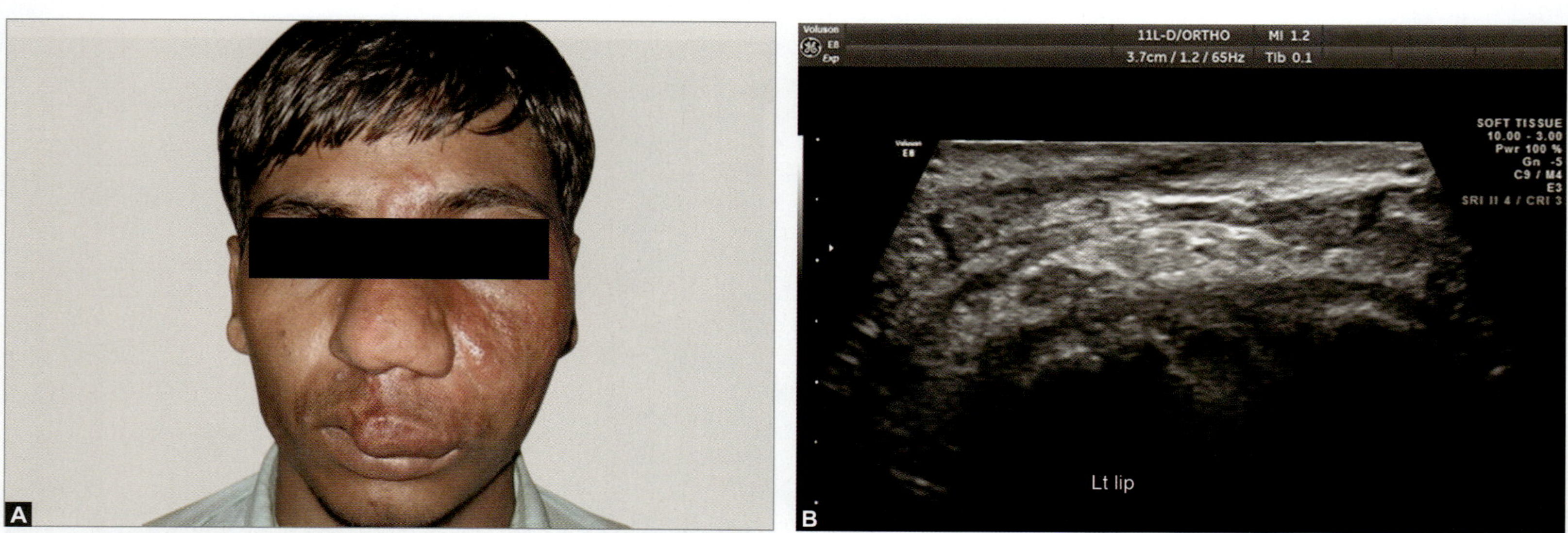

FIGURES 2.10A and B

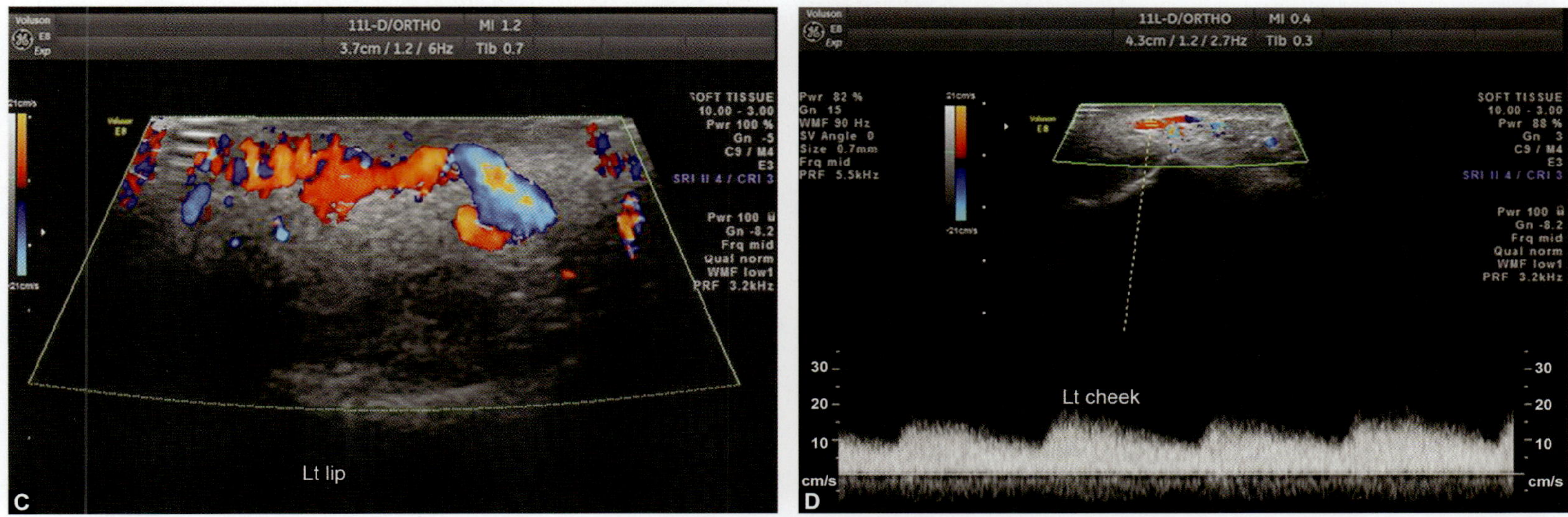

FIGURES 2.10C and D

FIGURES 2.10A to D: A man presented with diffuse hypertrophy of left side of face involving left forehead, left side of nose, left cheek and left upper lip. HRSG shows diffuse soft tissue hypertrophy of left hemi face. Multiple hypoechoic areas are seen in it. But no calcification is seen. No cystic degeneration is seen. **On color flow imaging,** multiple small vessels are seen feeding the soft tissue. **On spectral Doppler tracing,** low arterial flow is seen in the vessels suggestive of diffuse angiomatous malformation.

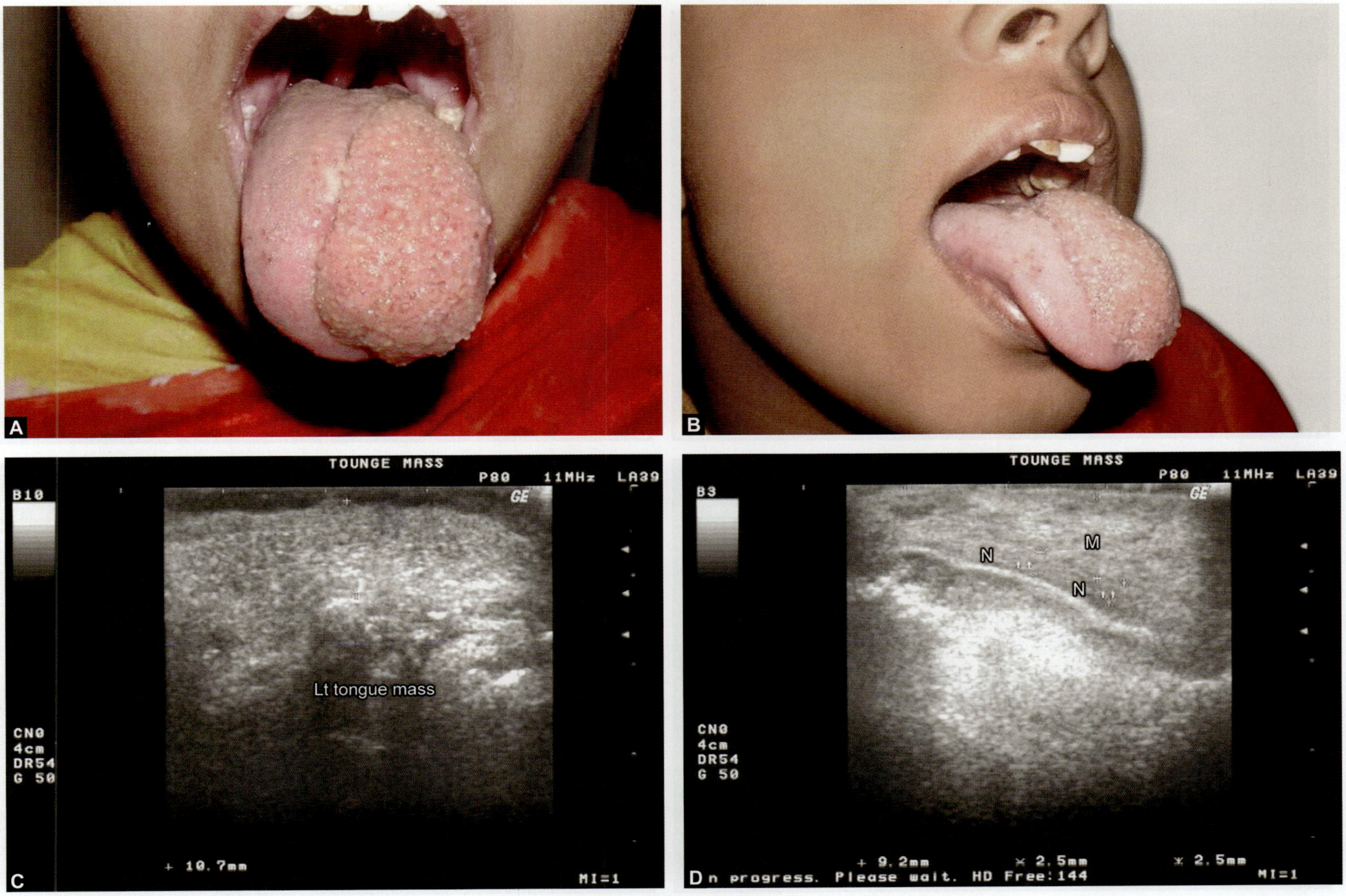

FIGURES 2.11A to D

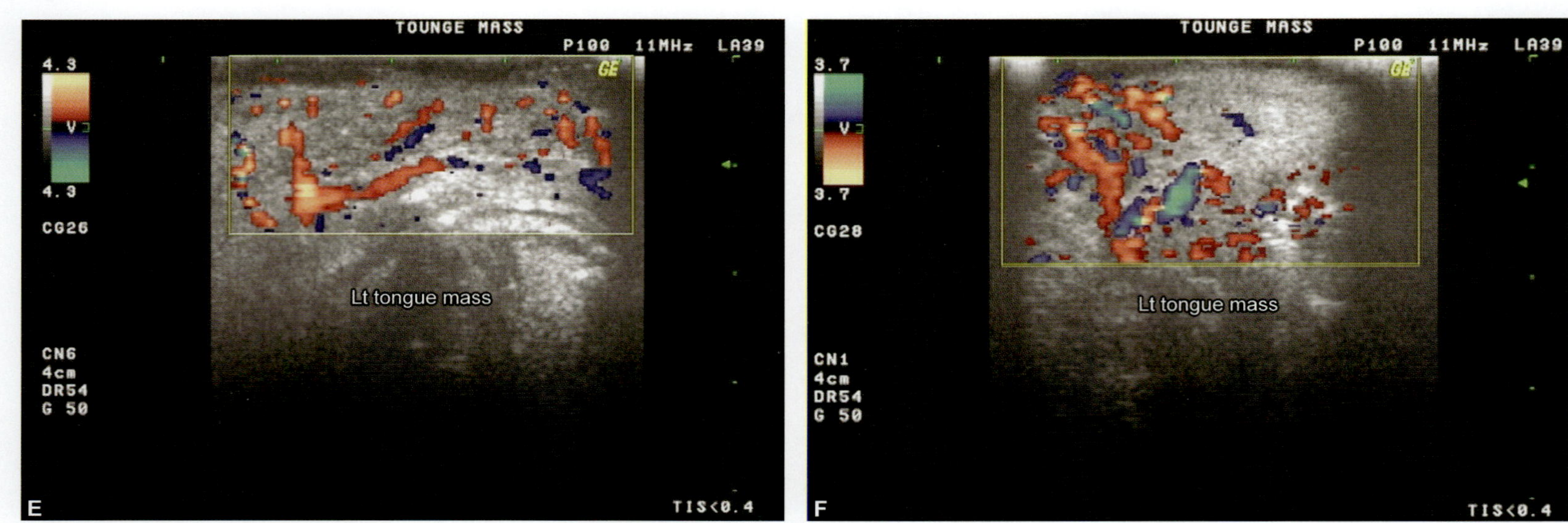

FIGURES 2.11E and F

FIGURES 2.11A to F: Papilloma tongue. A young girl presented with a well-defined homogeneous soft tissue mass over one half of the tongue. HRSG shows homogeneous soft tissue mass with smooth outline involving half of the tongue. No calcification, necrosis or cystic degeneration is seen in the mass. **On color flow imaging,** multiple vessels are seen feeding the mass. Biopsy confirmed papilloma of the tongue.

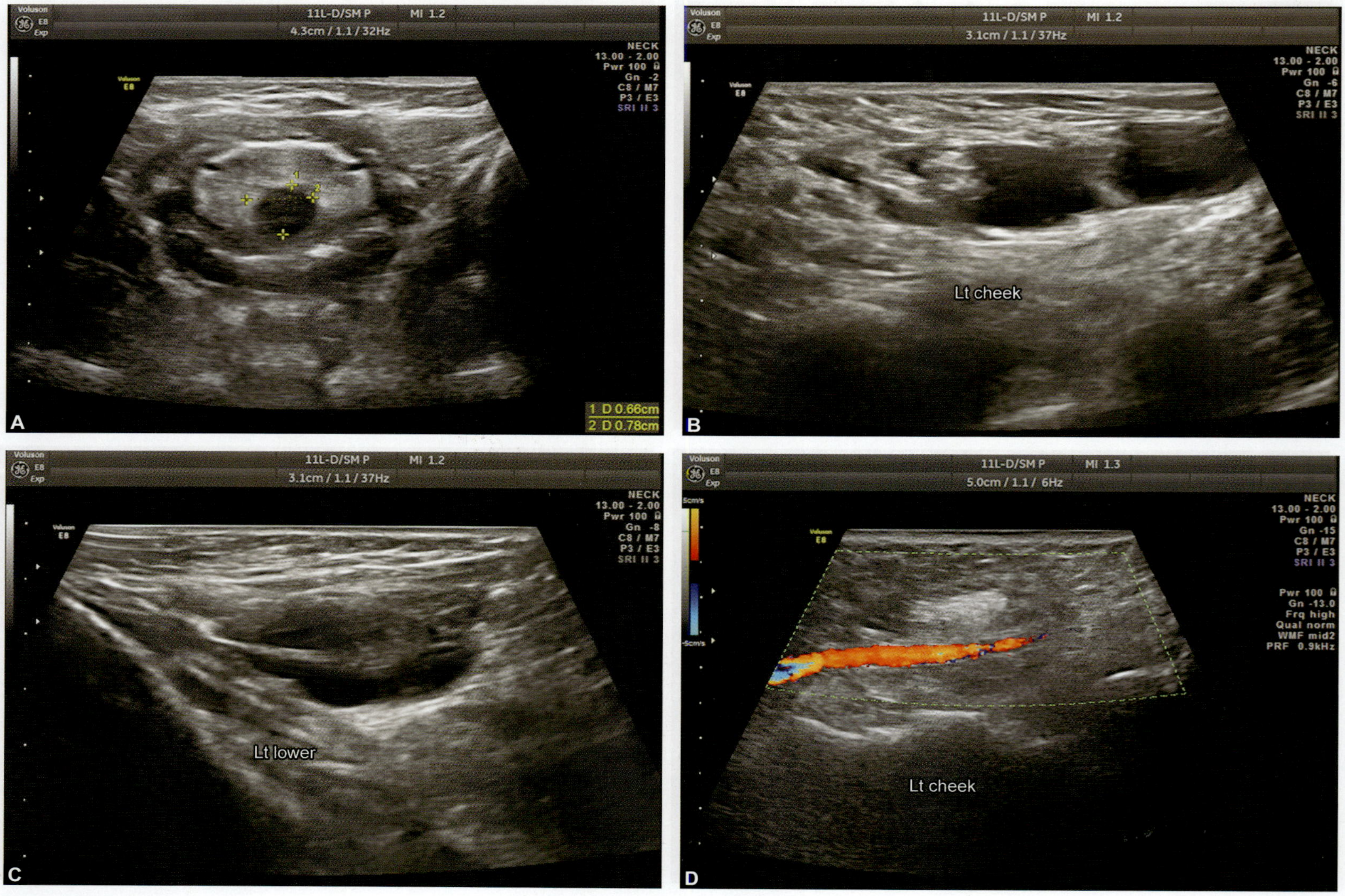

FIGURES 2.12A to D: An 8-month-old baby presented with soft tissue mass involving left cheek. High resolution sonography shows an irregular soft tissue mass in the left cheek. Multiple cystic areas are seen in it. **On color flow imaging,** low flow is seen in the mass. But no flow is seen in the cystic areas suggestive of lymphangioma.

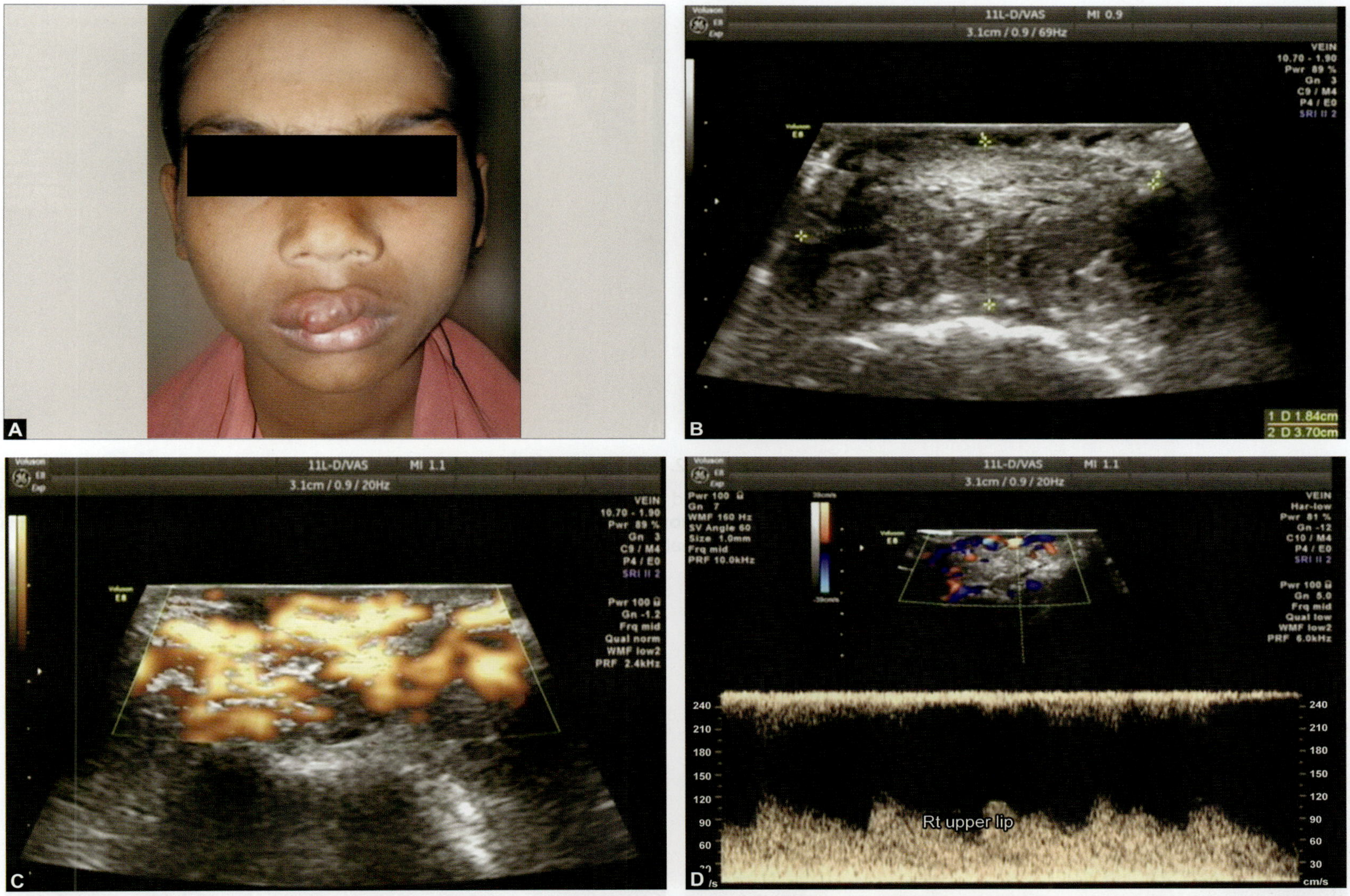

FIGURES 2.13A to D: A young girl presented with diffuse hypertrophy of upper lip. Multiple soft tissue nodules are seen in the lip. Diffuse hypertrophy of upper lip is seen. **On color flow imaging,** multiple vessels are seen feeding the soft tissue. **On spectral Doppler tracing,** moderate arterial flow is seen in it suggestive of vascular malformation.

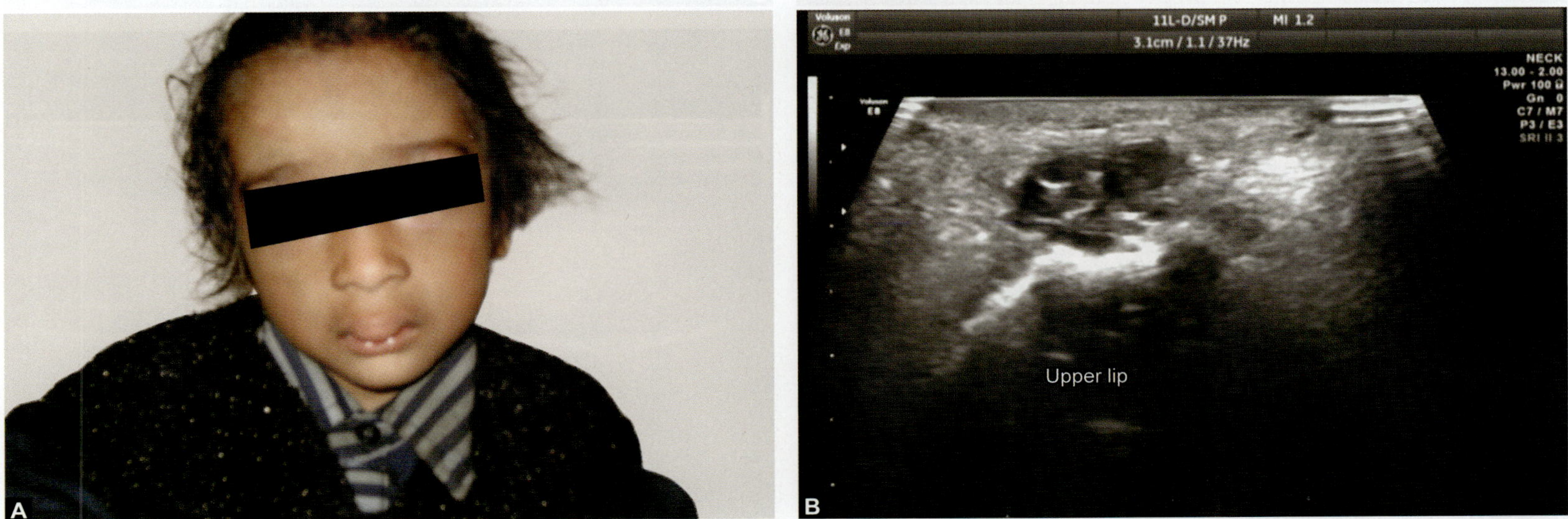

FIGURES 2.14A and B

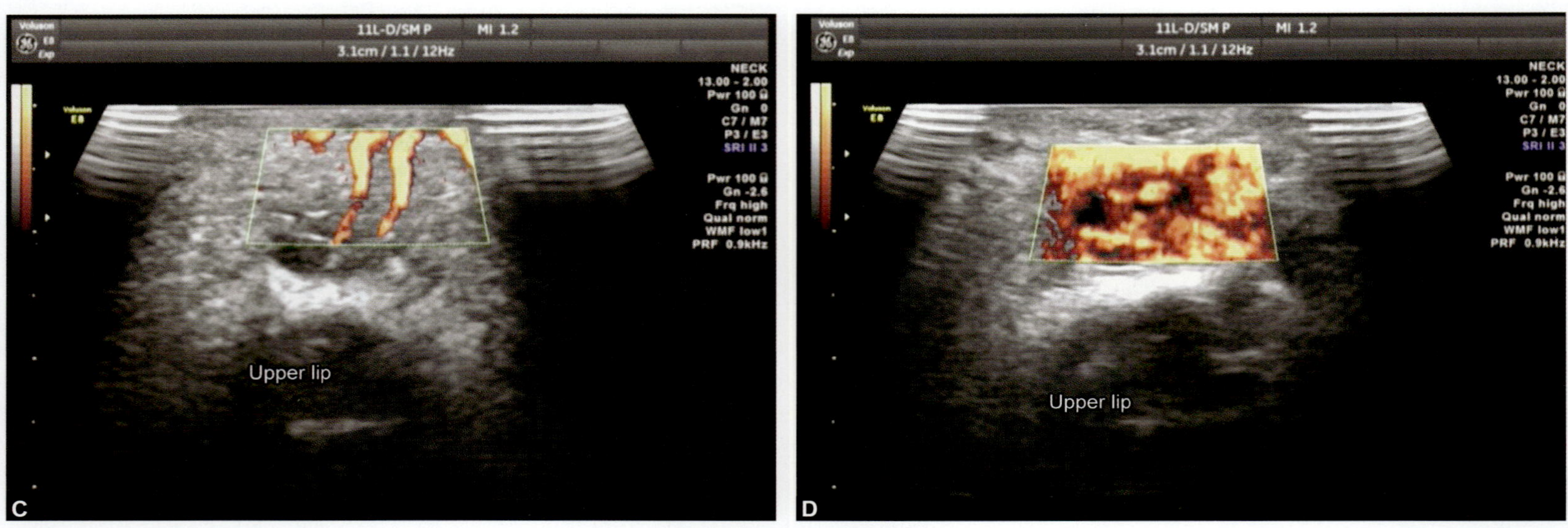

FIGURES 2.14C and D

FIGURES 2.14A to D: Diffuse hypertrophy of upper lip. A 2-year-old child presented with diffuse hypertrophy of upper lip. High resolution sonography shows a soft tissue low level echo complex mass in the upper lip. **On color flow imaging,** multiple vessels are seen feeding the mass. **On spectral Doppler tracing,** moderate arterial flow is seen suggestive of vascular malformation.

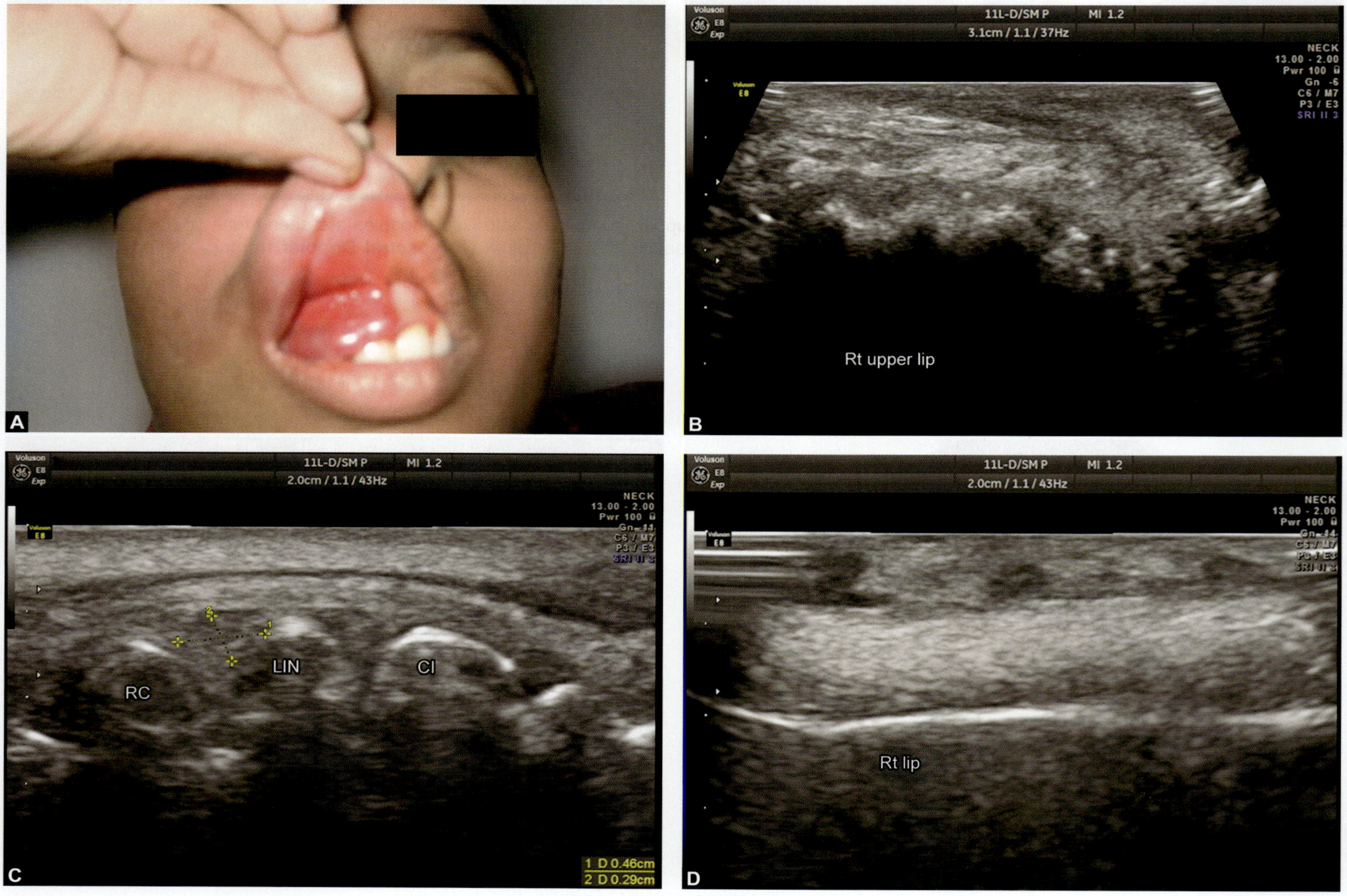

FIGURES 2.15A to D

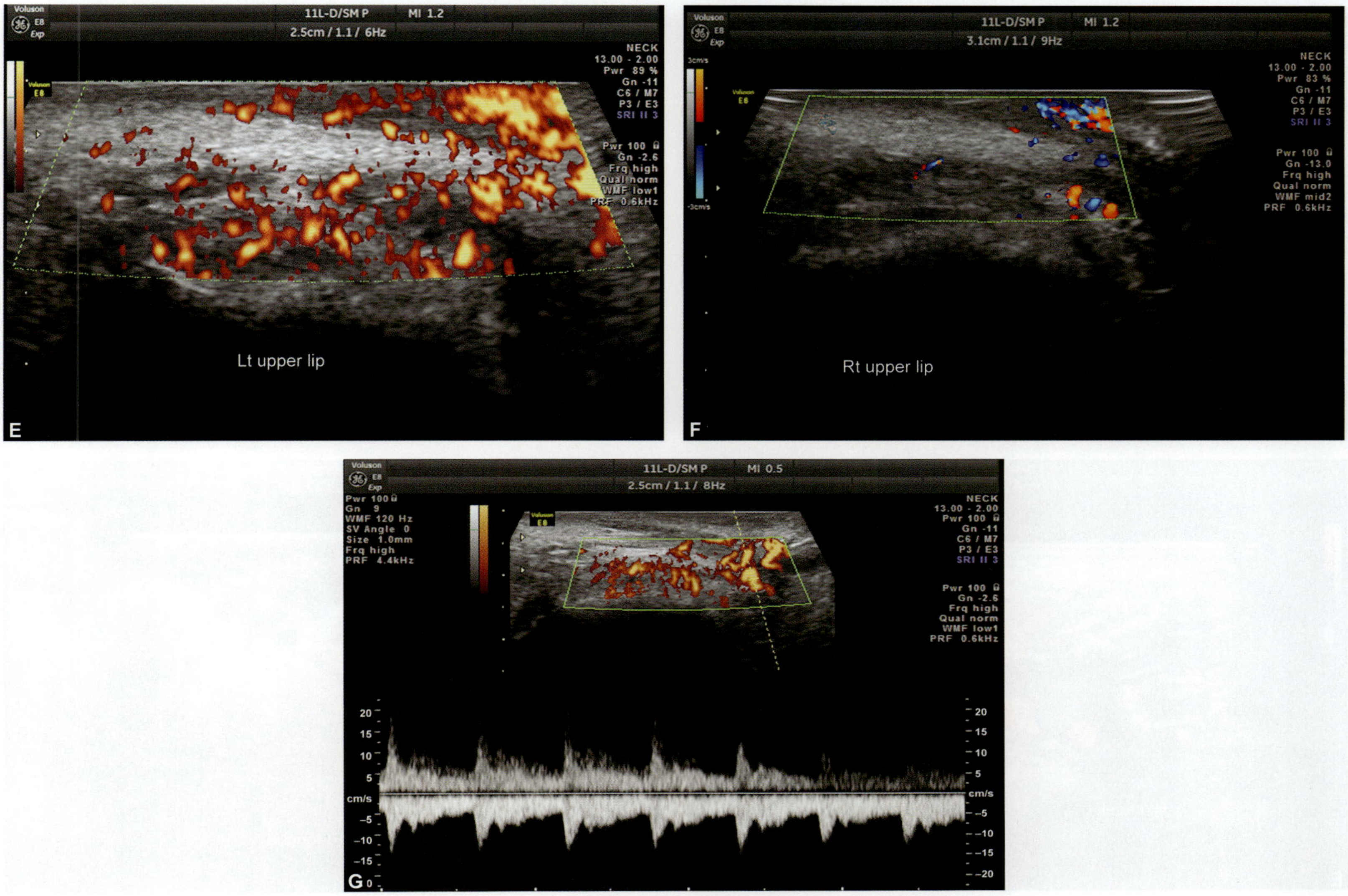

FIGURES 2.15E to G

FIGURES 2.15A to G: A young girl presented with upper lip hypertrophy and gingiva. HRSG shows diffuse hypertrophy of upper lip. The gingiva is also seen thickened. **On color flow imaging,** multiple vessels are seen feeding the upper lip and gingiva. No calcification is seen in the soft tissue of the upper lip.

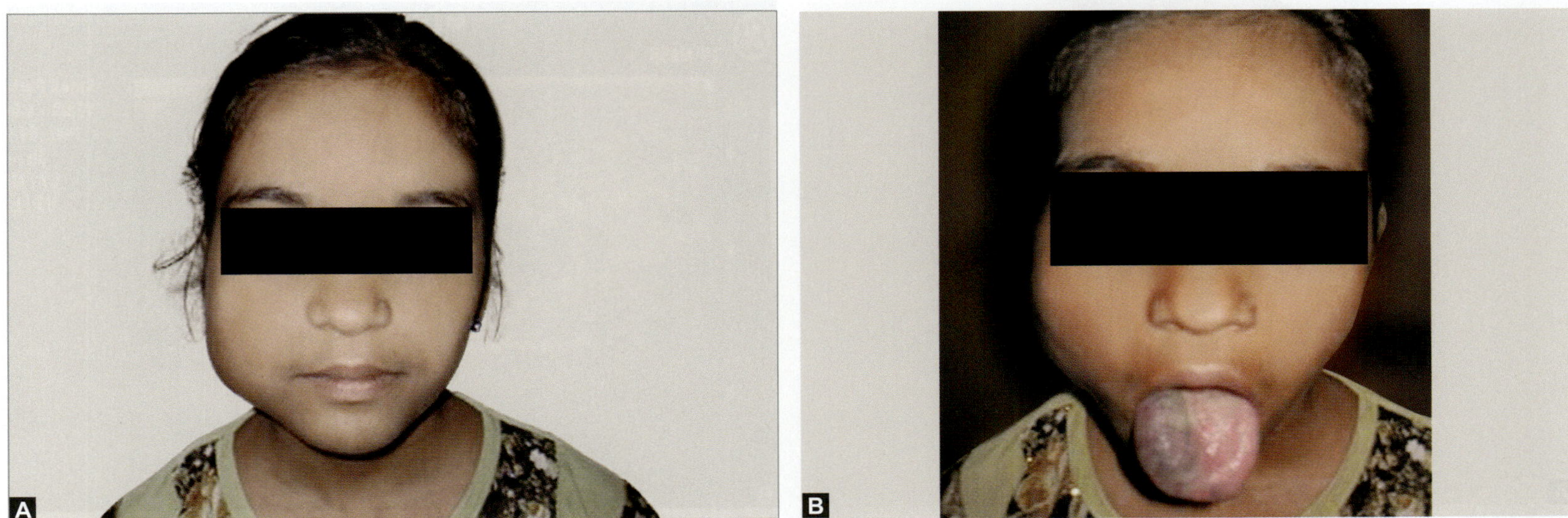

FIGURES 2.16A and B

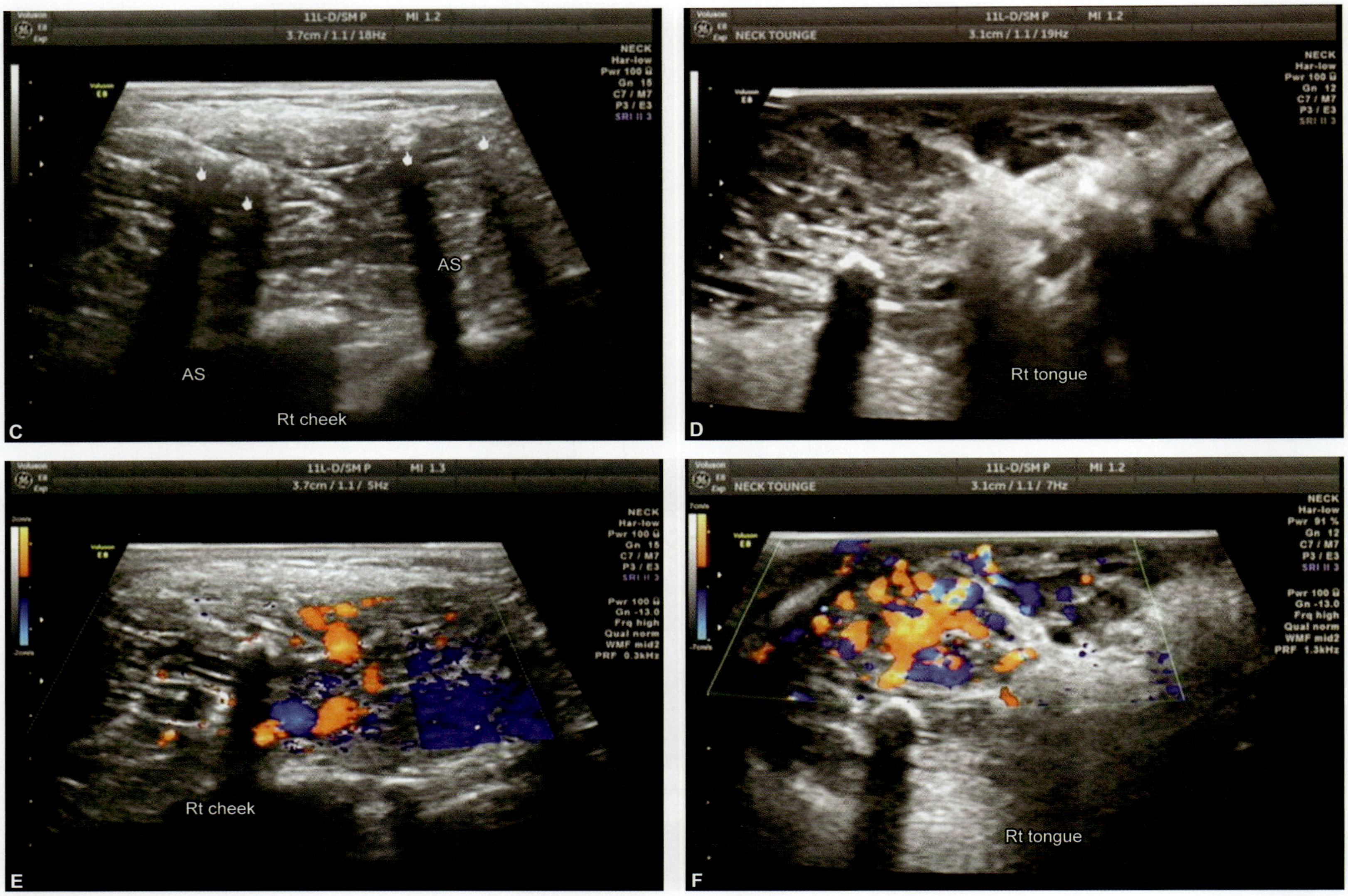

FIGURES 2.16C to F

FIGURES 2.16A to F: Vascular malformation of right cheek and right tongue. A young girl presented with diffuse soft tissue swelling over the right cheek. HRSG shows irregular ill defined inhomogeneous soft tissue mass over the right cheek. The mass is seen invading the deeper tissue. It is also seen involving the right half of the tongue. Multiple echogenic foci are seen in the mass, which are accompanied with acoustic shadowing. **On color flow imaging,** multiple vessels are seen feeding the mass. **On spectral Doppler tracing,** low arterial and venous flow is seen in the mass suggestive of vascular hemangiomatous AV malformation involving right cheek and right tongue.

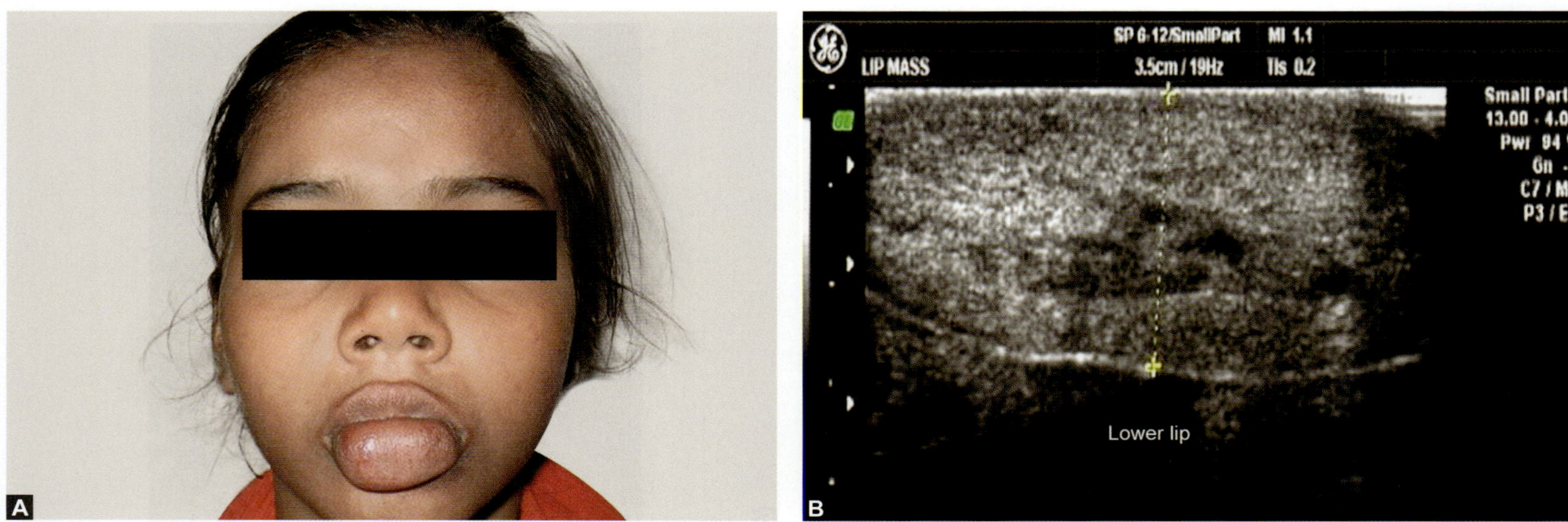

FIGURES 2.17A and B

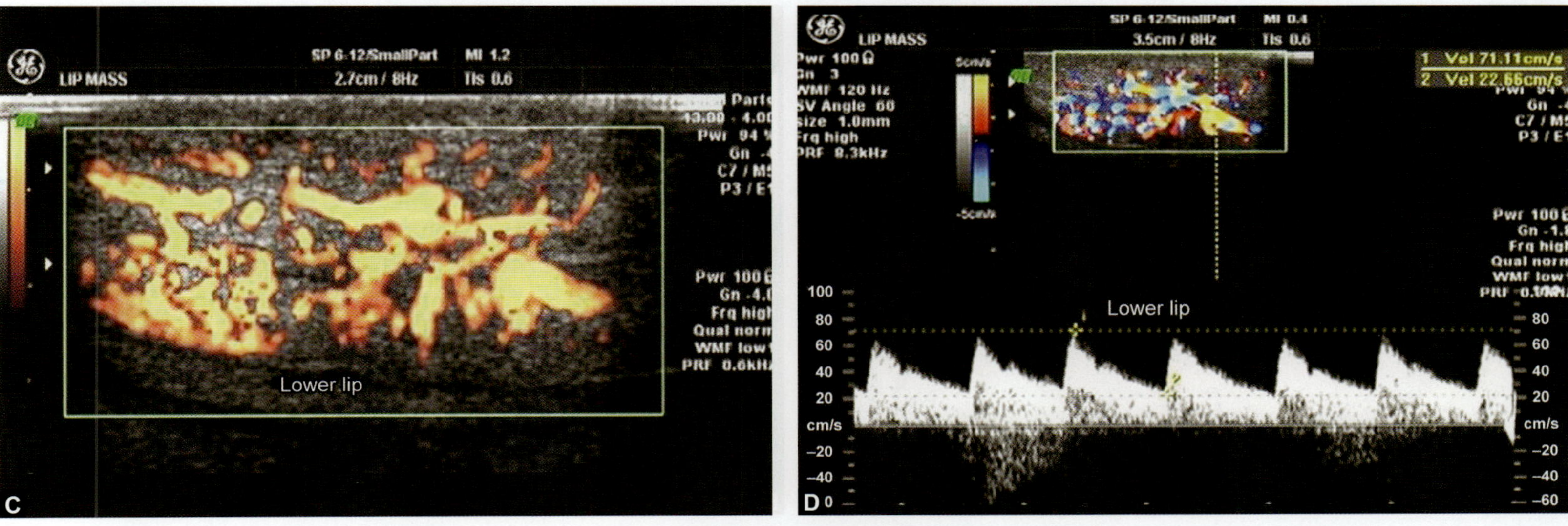

FIGURES 2.17C and D

FIGURES 2.17A to D: Traumatic AVM lower lip. A young girl presented with slowly increasing lower lip mass after sustaining trauma to the lip after a fall. HRSG shows soft tissue mass over the lower lip multiple dilated vessels are seen in the mass. **On color flow imaging,** multiple vessels are seen in the mass. Power Doppler also shows multiple vessels feeding the mass. Spectral Doppler Tracing shows predominantly arterial flow in the vessels. Sonographic findings were consistent with AVM.

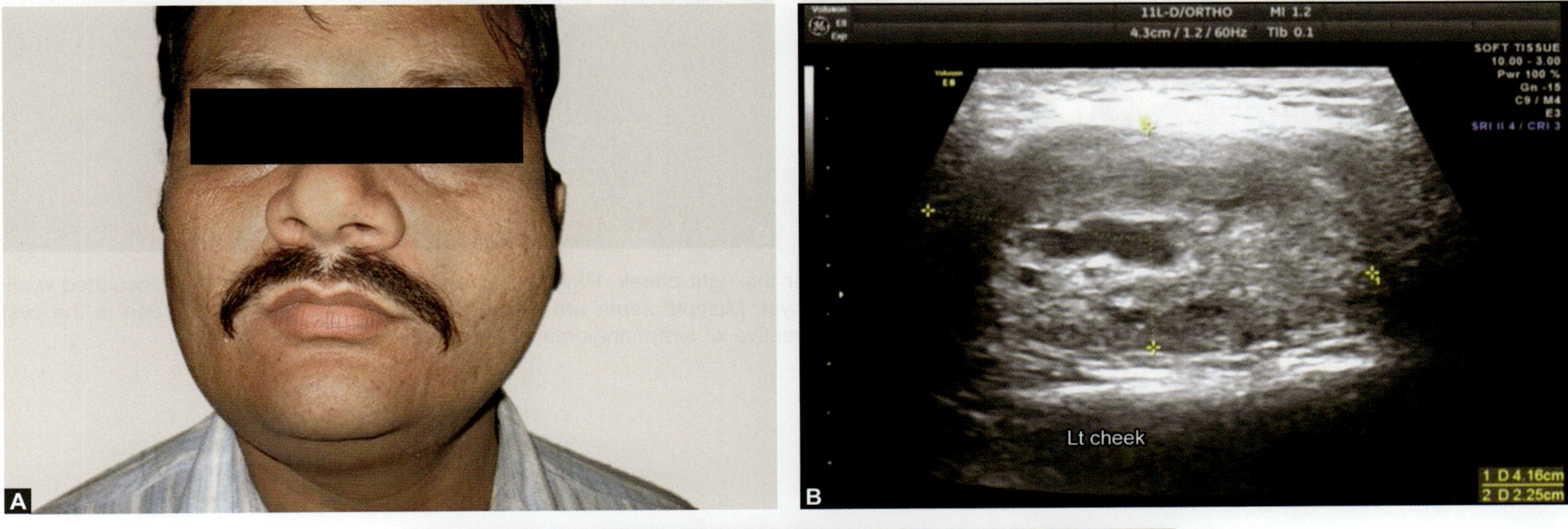

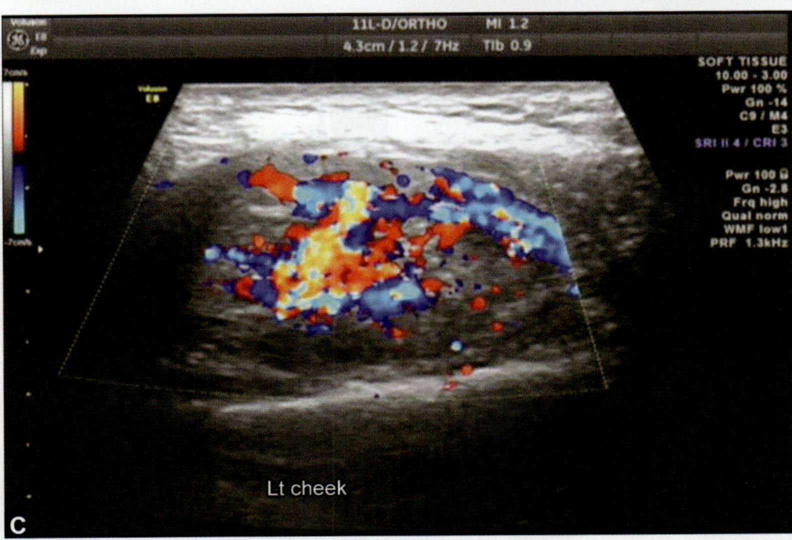

FIGURES 2.18A to C: A 36-year-old man presented with fullness of the left cheek. High resolution sonography shows a soft tissue mass in the left cheek. The mass shows heterogeneous texture. Multiple dilated vessels are seen in the mass. **On color flow imaging,** arterial and venous flow is seen in the mass suggestive of hemangiomatous mass.

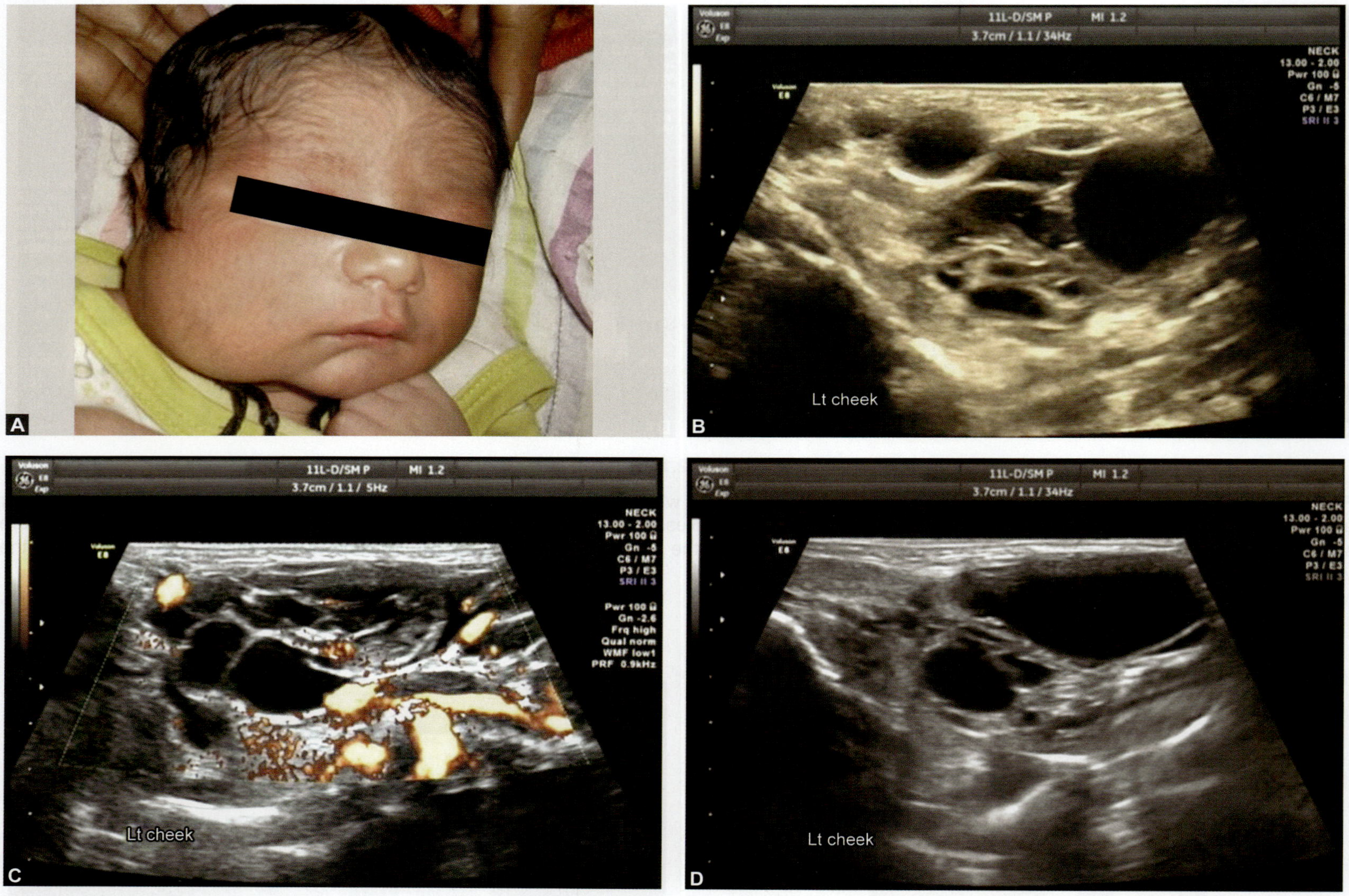

FIGURES 2.19A to D: A baby is born with diffuse soft tissue swelling over the right cheek. High resolution sonography shows a multiloculated cystic mass involving the right cheek. Low level echo collection is seen in the cyst. Multiple septa are also seen in it. No calcification is seen in the cyst. **On color flow imaging,** low flow is seen in the septa. Findings are suggestive of lymphangioma of the cheek.

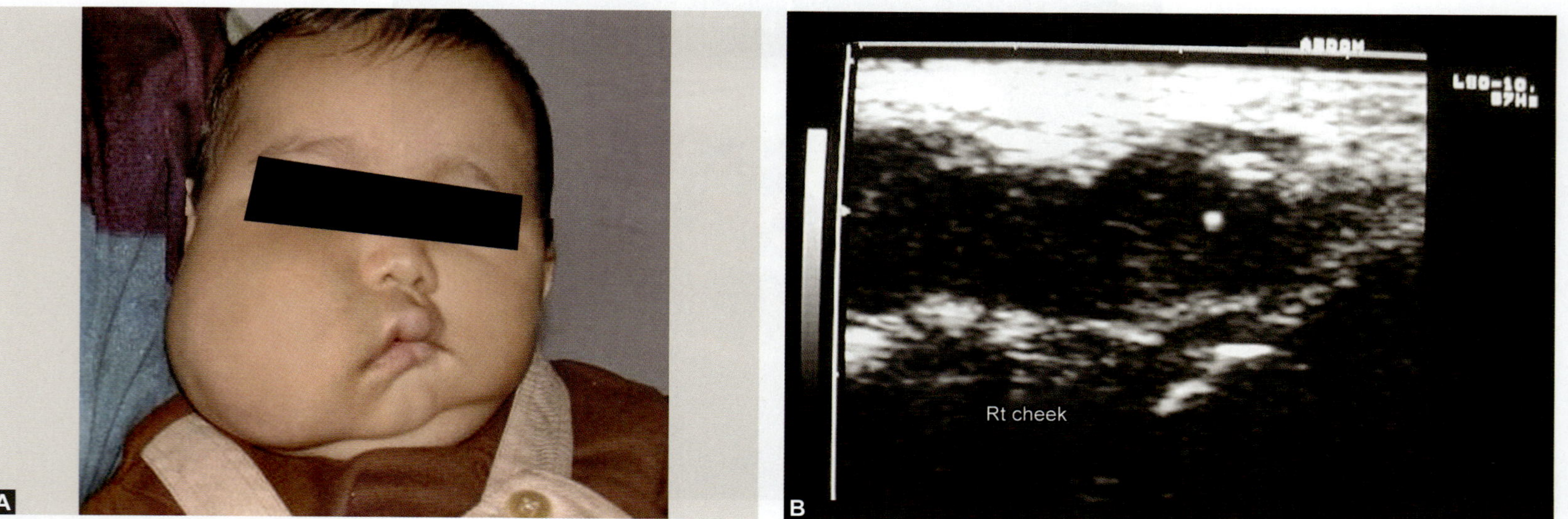

FIGURES 2.20A and B

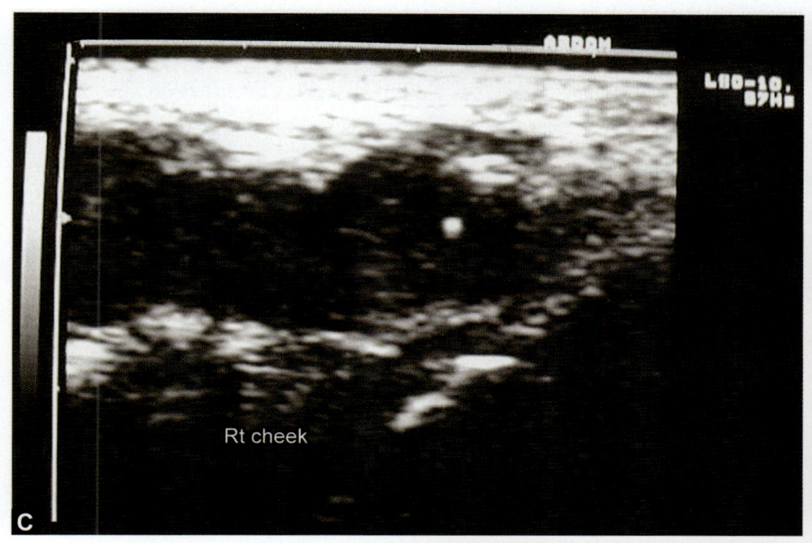

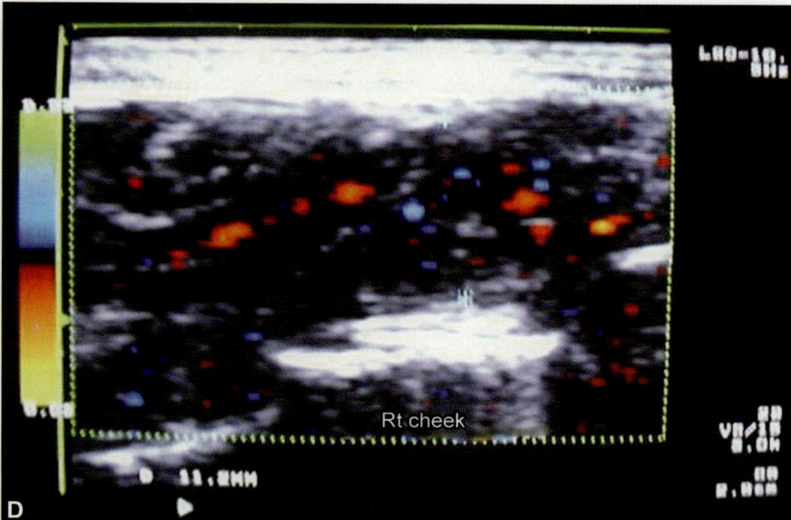

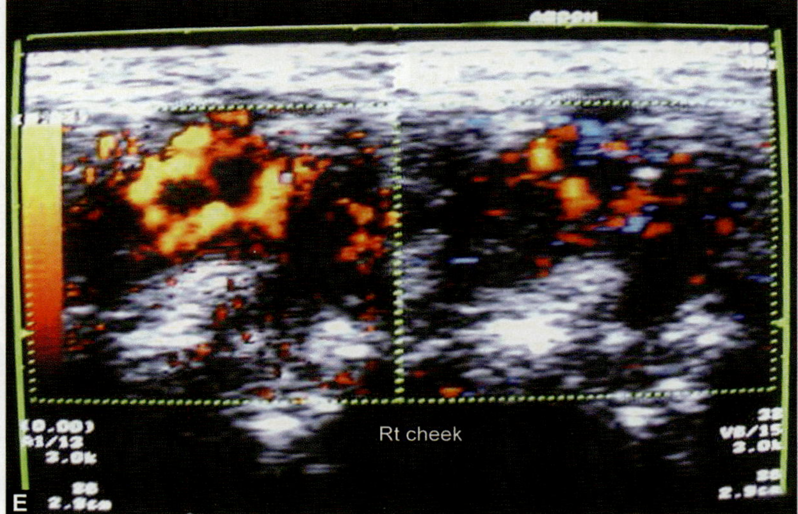

FIGURES 2.20C to E

FIGURES 2.20A to E: Lymphangioma. A 4-month-old boy presented with big large mass over the right cheek and part of the right cheek hanging down involving part of the chin. HRSG shows a multi loculated cystic mass. Dilated vessels are also seen in it. Color Doppler flow study shows little flow in the mass. However, few blood vessels are seen feeding the mass. Power Doppler imaging shows better visualization of the vessels showing blood flow in the vessels. Post-operative findings confirmed lymphangioma.

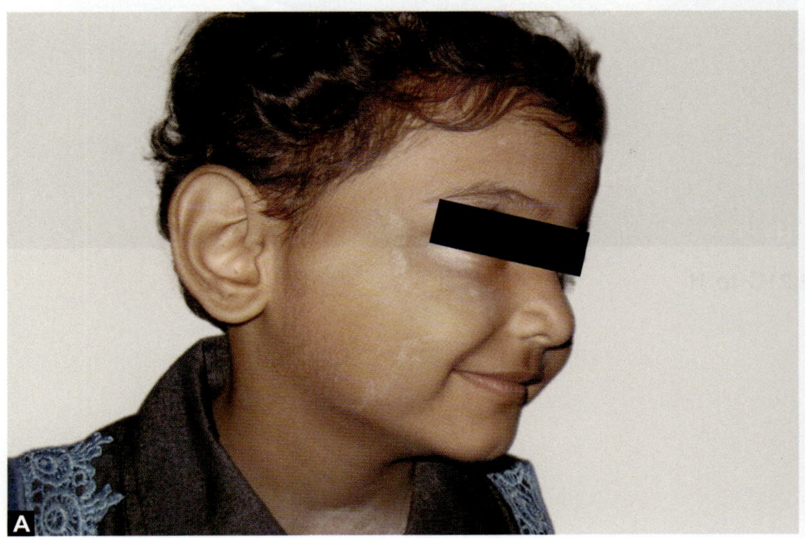

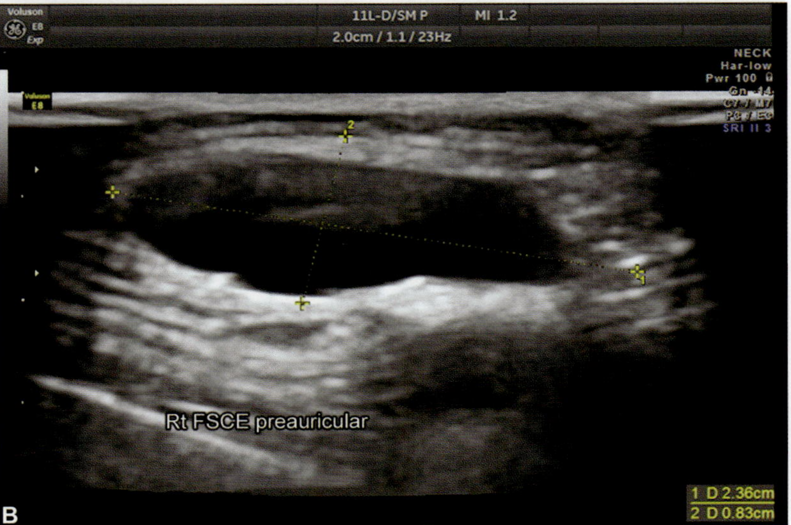

FIGURES 2.21A and B

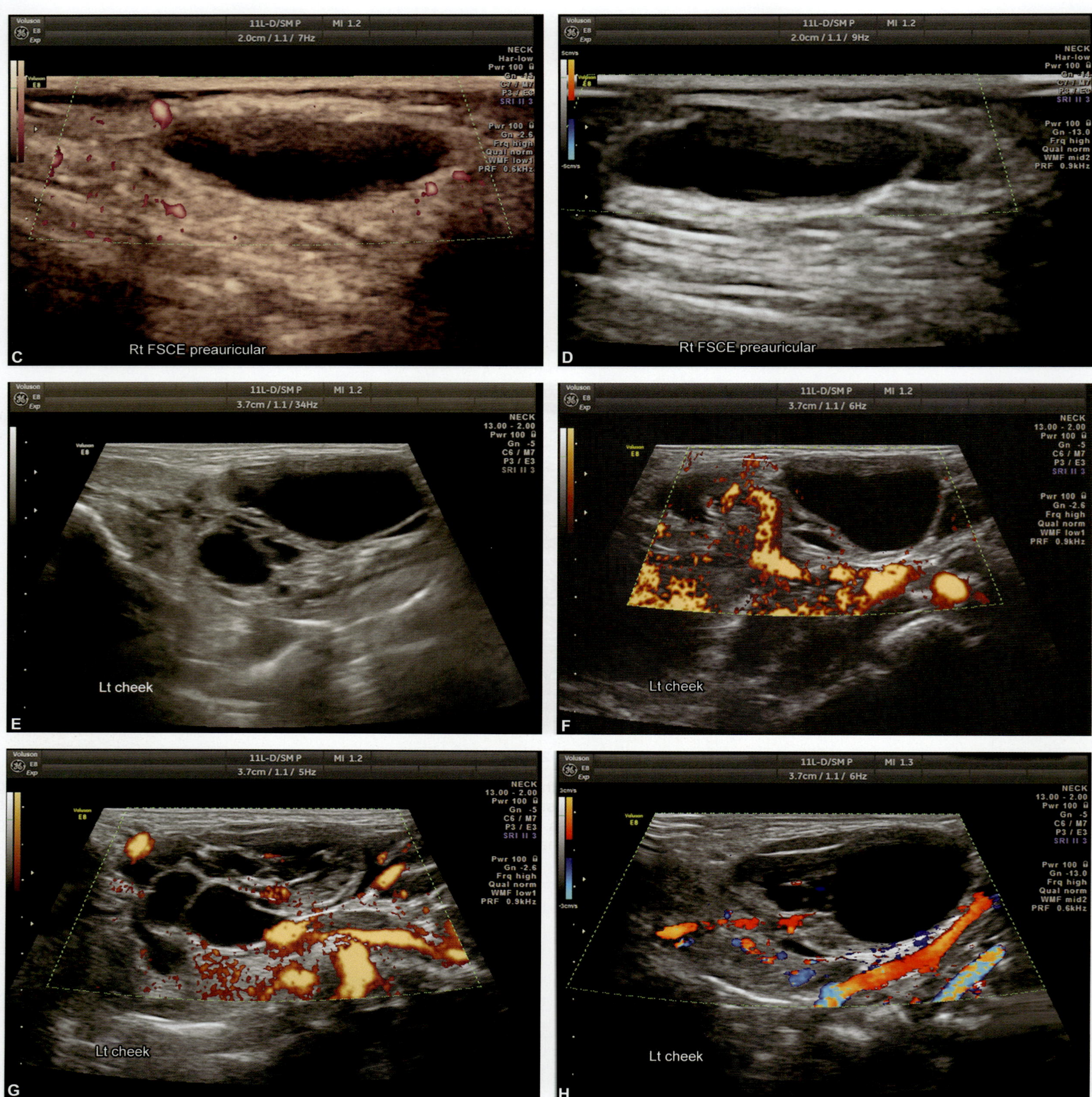

FIGURES 2 21C to H

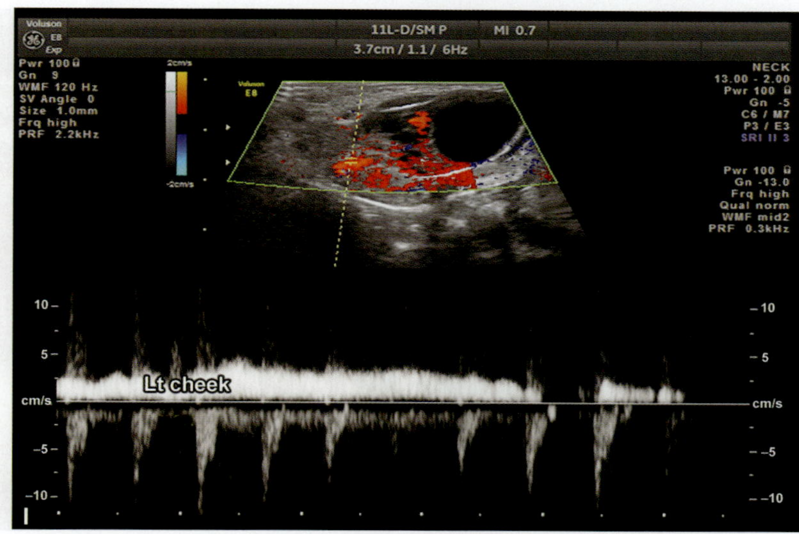

FIGURE 2.21I

FIGURES 2.21A to I: Lymphangioma of cheek. A 5-year-old girl presented soft tissue mass over the right cheek. The mass is seen extending from preauricular region to the right cheek. Multiple cystic areas are seen in it. Thick septa are also seen in it. **On color flow imaging,** moderate flow is seen in the septa suggestive of lymphangioma.

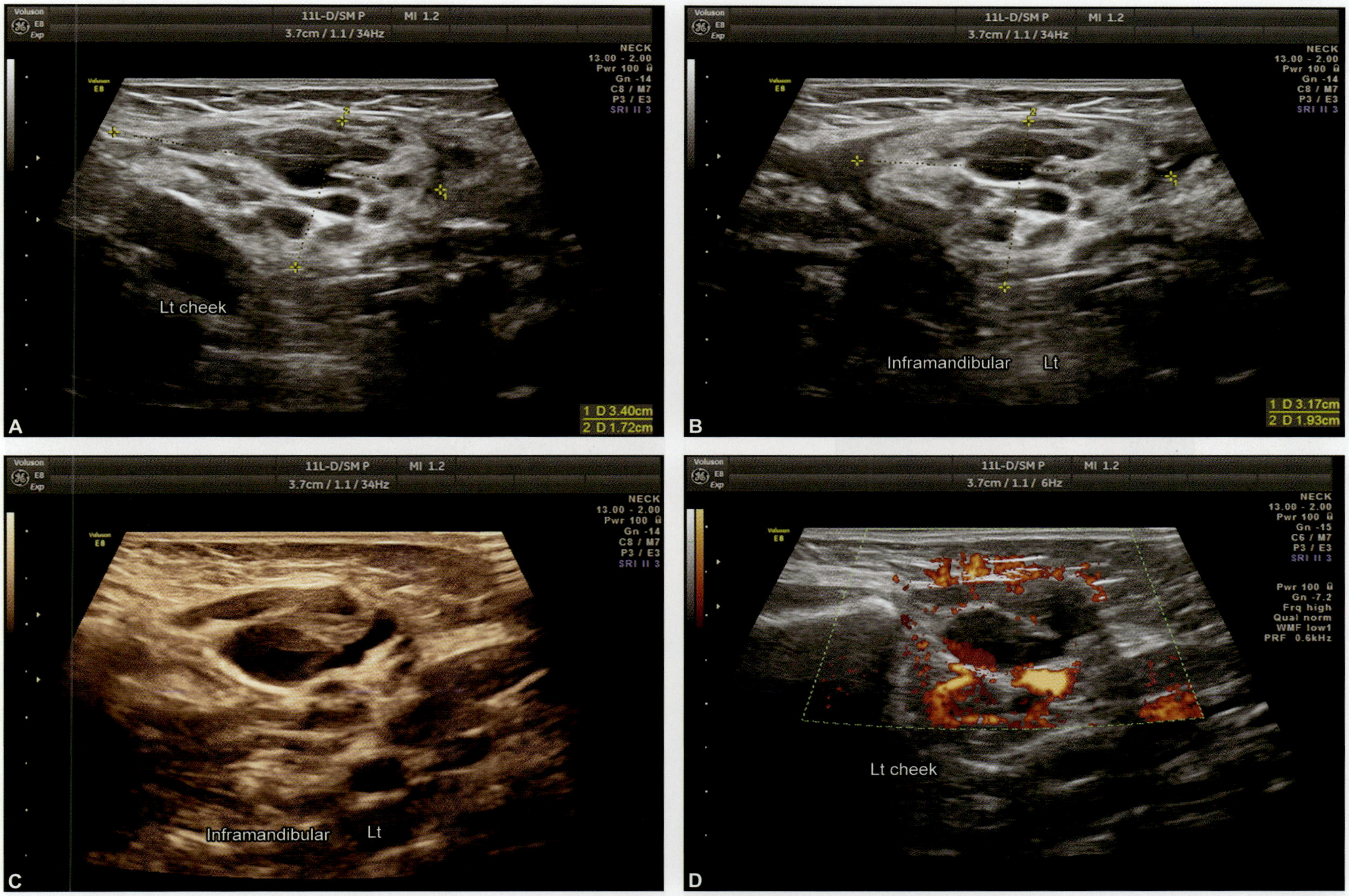

FIGURES 2.22A to D

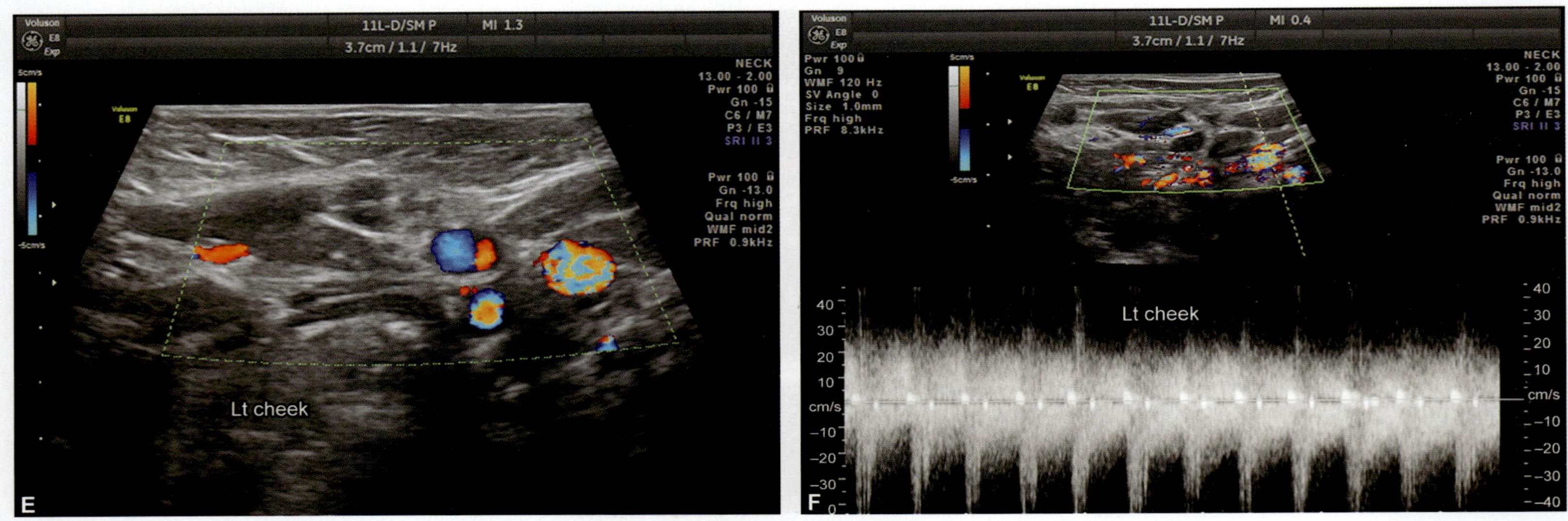

FIGURES 2.22E and F

FIGURES 2.22A to F: An 8-month-old baby presented with soft tissue mass involving the left cheek. It is also seen extending to inframandibular region. High resolution sonography shows multiloculated cystic mass in the left cheek. Thick septa are seen in it. **On color flow imaging,** poor flow is seen in the septa. Findings are consistent with lymphangioma.

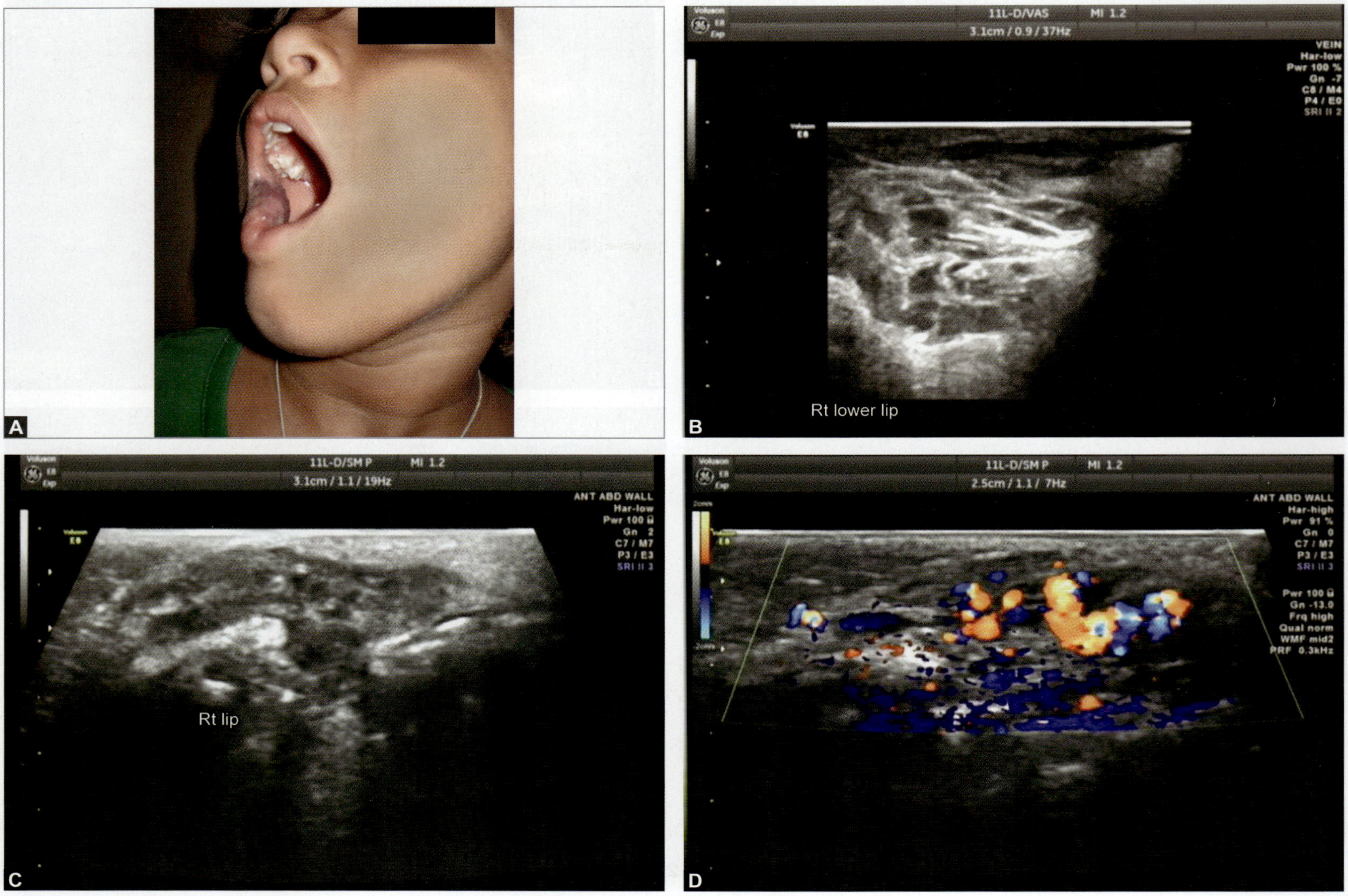

FIGURES 2 23A to D

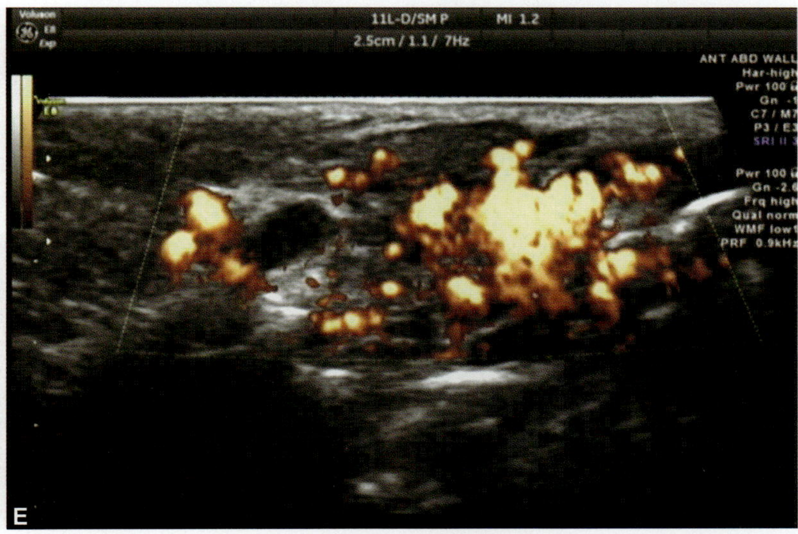

FIGURE 2.23E

FIGURES 2.23A to E: A 10-year-old girl presented with soft tissue mass involving right side of lower lip. Clinically it appears to be vascular mass. High resolution sonography shows a diffuse irregular heterogeneous soft tissue mass involving the lip. It is also seen extending the deeper tissue. **On color flow imaging,** multiple vessels are seen feeding the mass suggestive of hemangiomatous mass.

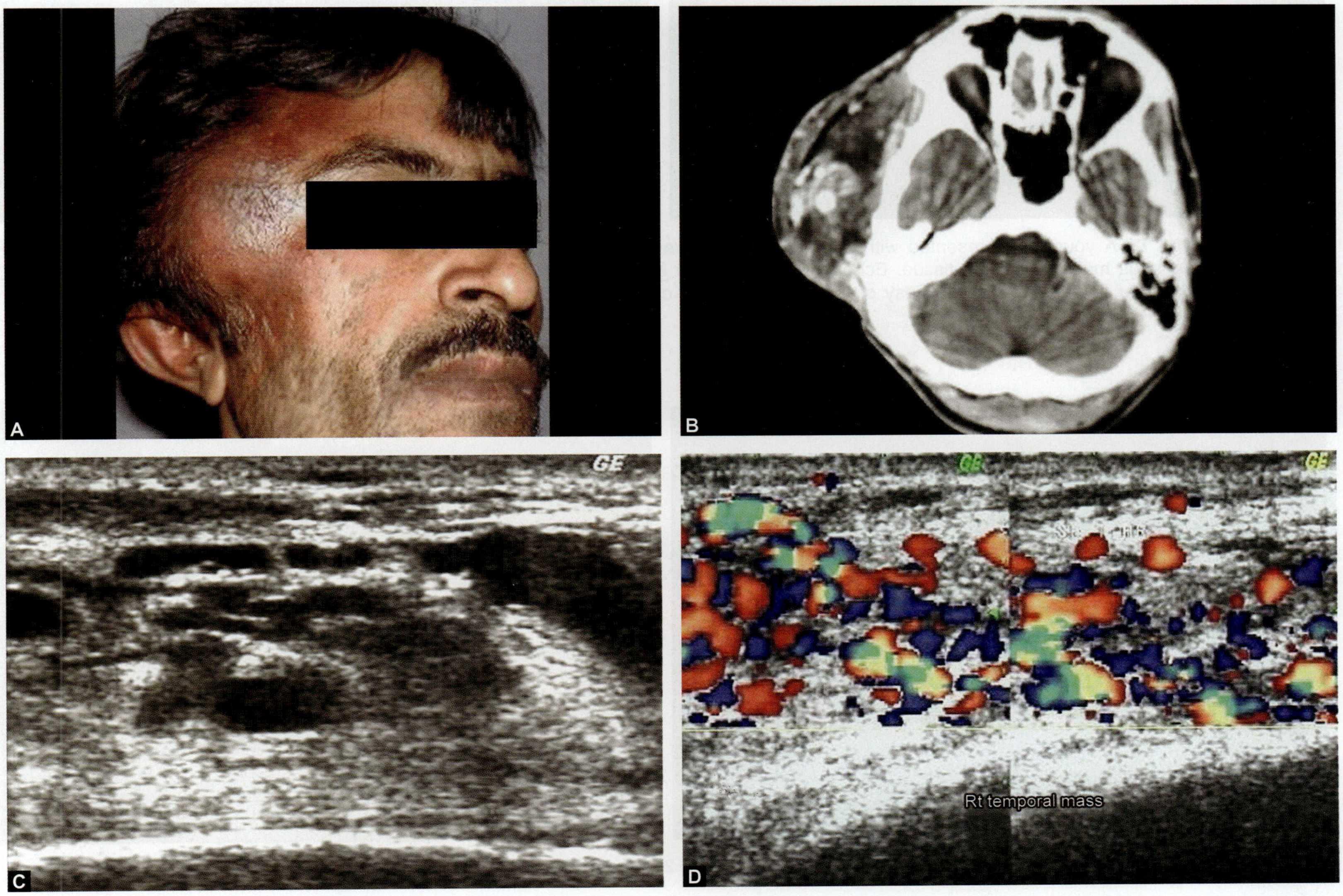

FIGURES 2.24A to D: AVM right temporal region. A patient presented with increasing swelling over the right temporal region. CT scan of the same patient shows enhancing soft tissue mass in the right temporal region. High resolution sonography shows multiple dilated vessels in the right temporal region. **On color flow imaging,** high flow is seen in the vessels. Spectral Doppler tracing shows increased arterial flow pattern suggestive of AVM of superficial temporal artery.

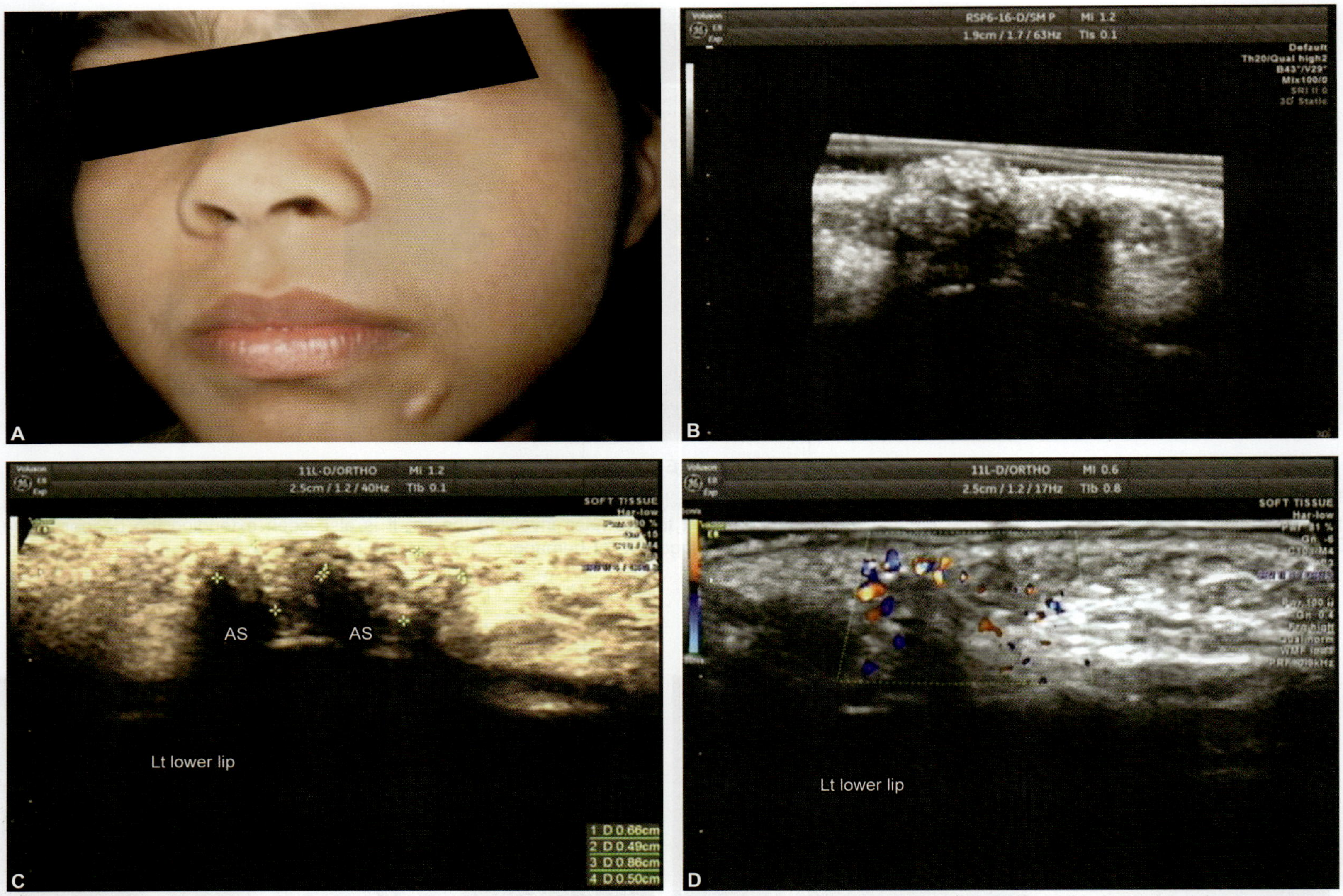

FIGURES 2.25A to D: A young girl presented with soft tissue mass over the left chin below the left side of lower lip. High resolution sonography shows a heterogeneous mass in the soft tissue. Echogenic calcified foci are seen in it, which are accompanied with dense acoustic shadowing. On color flow imaging, poor flow is seen in it. Biopsy of the mass suggests chronic granulomatous mass.

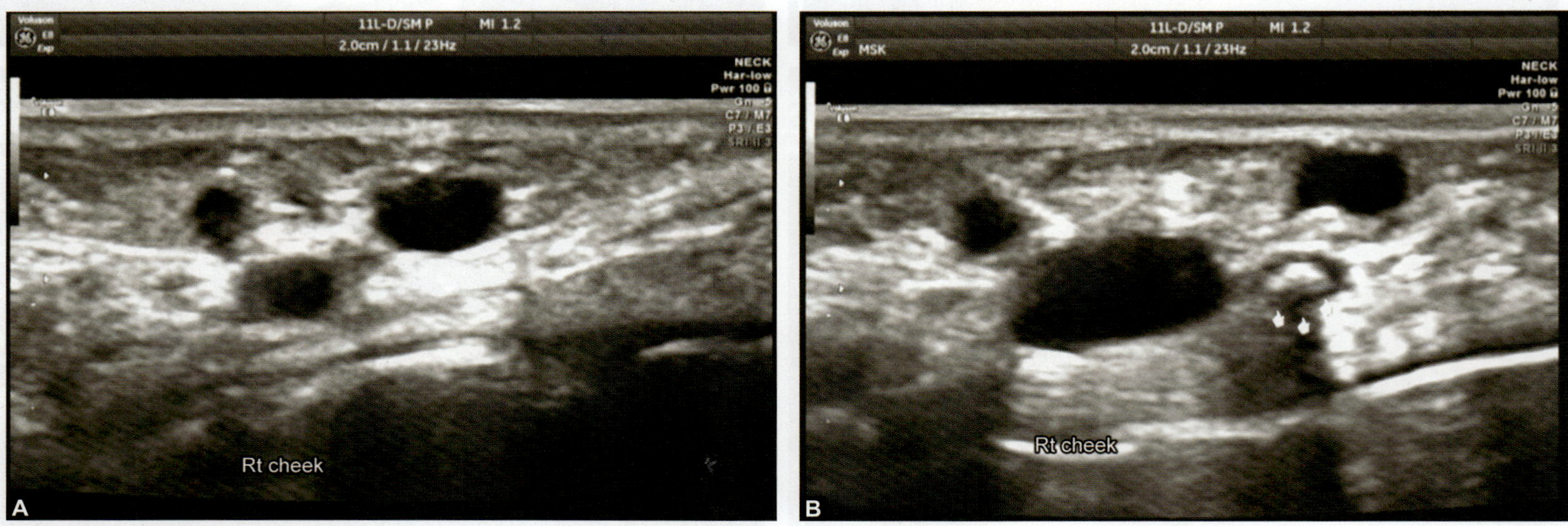

FIGURES 2.26A and B

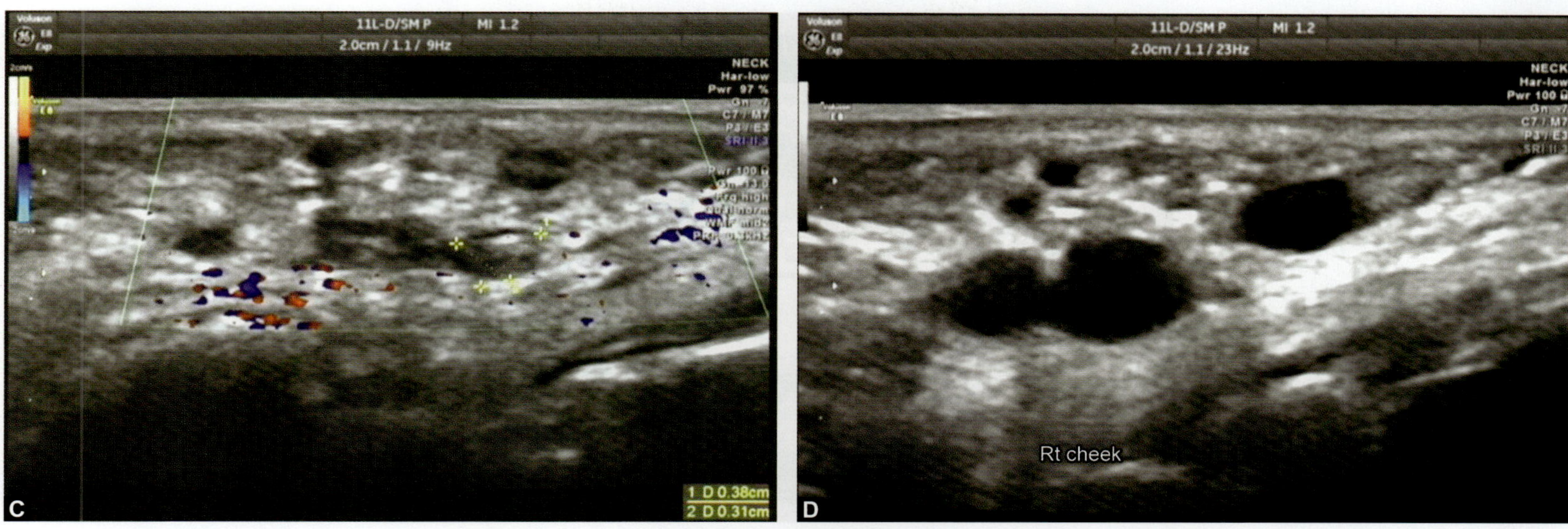

FIGURES 2.26C and D

FIGURES 2.26A to D: Cheek cyst. A patient presented with soft tissue swelling over the left cheek. High resolution sonography shows multiple cysts in the left cheek. They are well defined. Few cysts show echogenic foci suggestive of calcification. **On color flow imaging,** poor flow is seen in them.

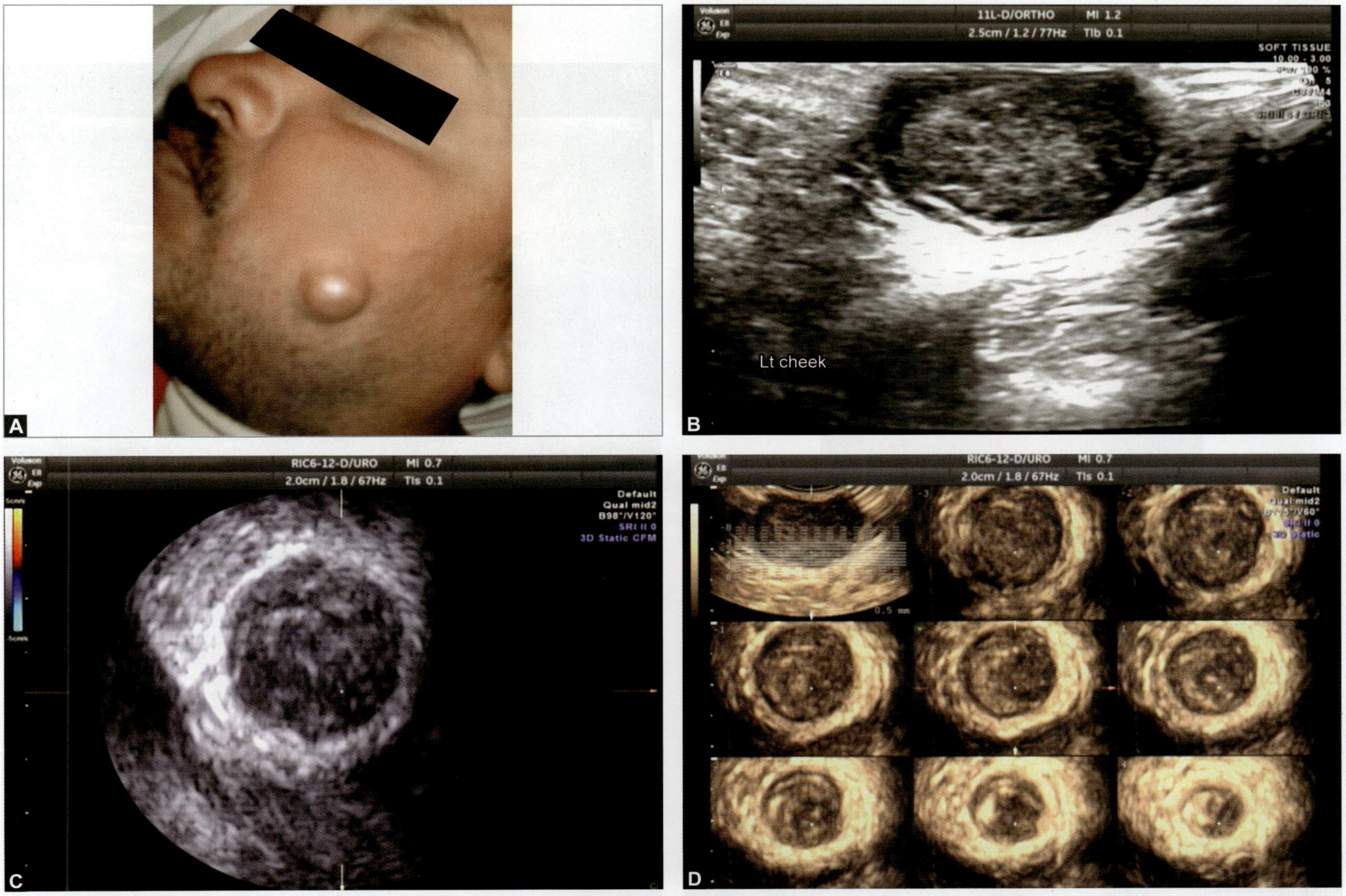

FIGURES 2.27A to D

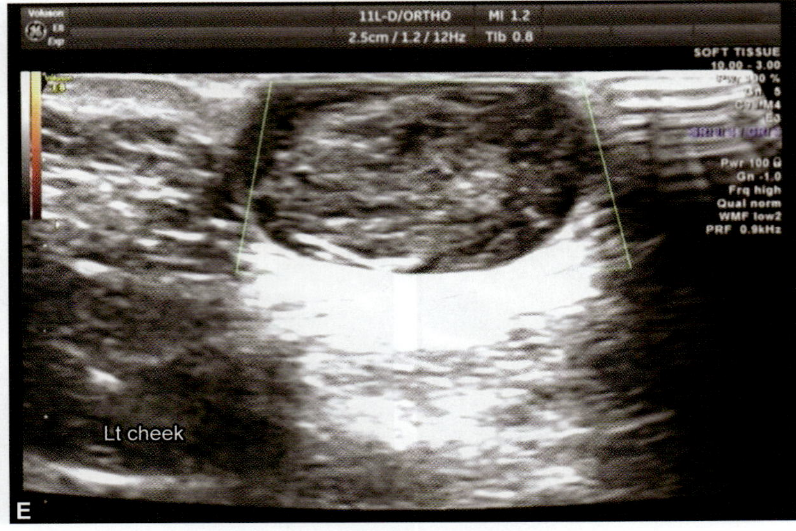

FIGURE 2.27E

FIGURES 2.27A to E: A man presented with soft tissue swelling over the left cheek. High resolution sonography shows a well-defined thick walled cystic mass involving the left cheek. Thick echo collection is seen in it. Small echogenic foci are also seen in it. 3D imaging clearly shows content of the cyst. **On color flow imaging,** poor flow is seen in the cyst suggestive of dermoid cyst.

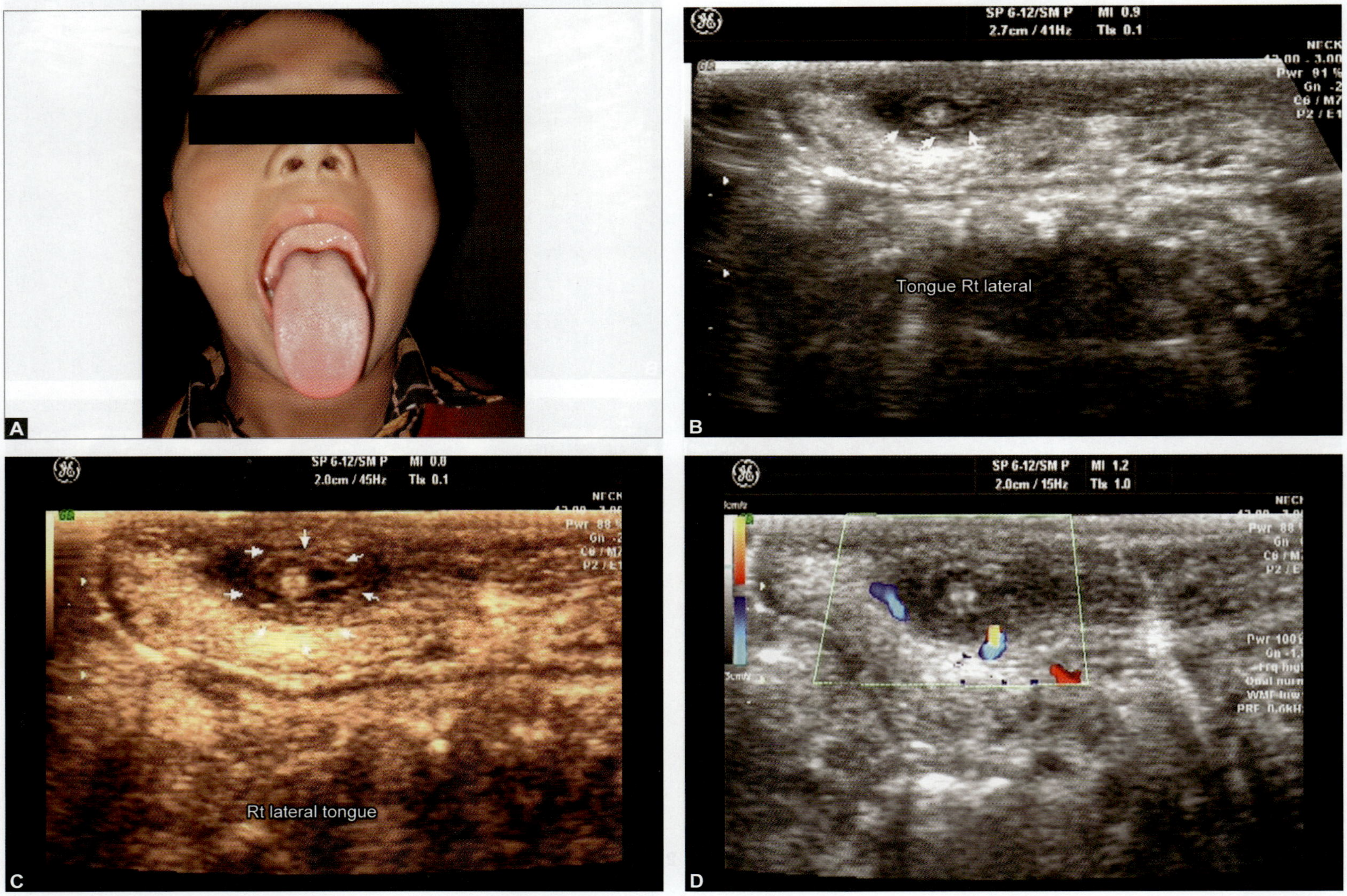

FIGURES 2.28A to D

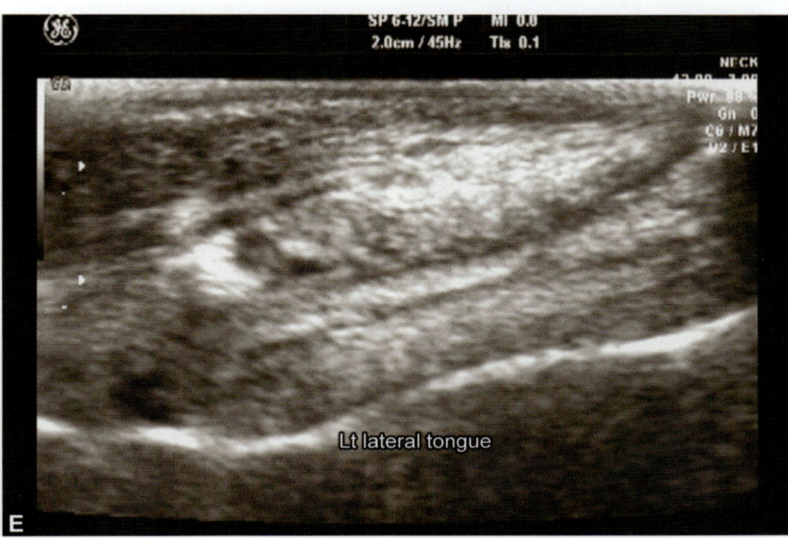

FIGURE 2.28E

FIGURES 2.28A to E: Tongue cysticercus. A young boy presented with soft tissue swelling over the anterior part of the tongue. High resolution sonography shows a well-defined cystic mass in the tongue. An echogenic nidus is seen in the cyst. Poor flow is seen around the cyst suggestive of cysticercus cyst.

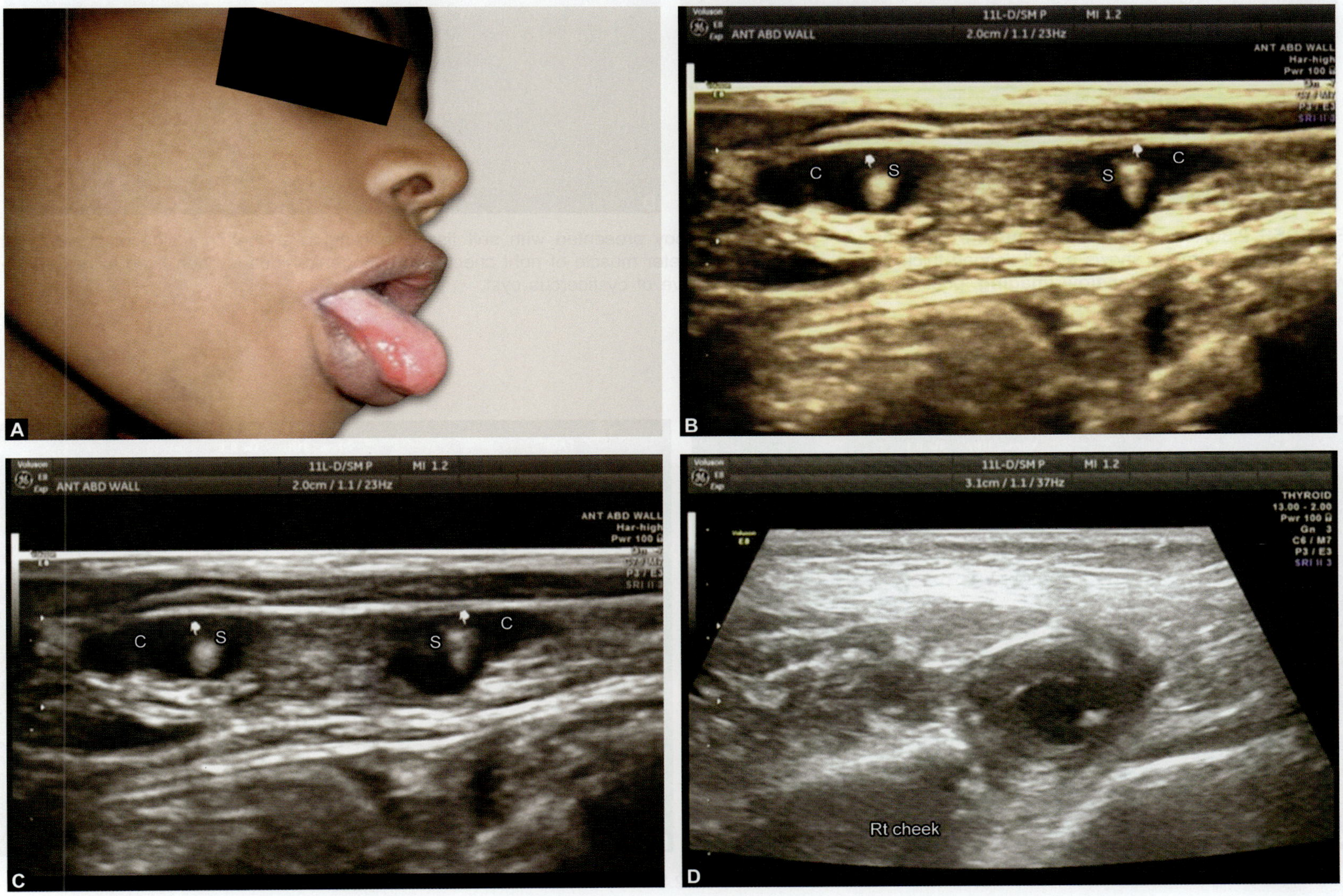

FIGURES 2.29A to D: Tongue and anterior abdominal wall cysticercus. A girl presented with soft tissue swelling over the right lateral aspect of tongue. HRSG shows multiple cystic masses in the tongue. Echogenic nidus is also seen in the cyst suggestive of cysticercus cyst. The anterior abdominal wall also shows multiple cysts with echogenic nidus suggestive of diffuse cysticercus cyst.

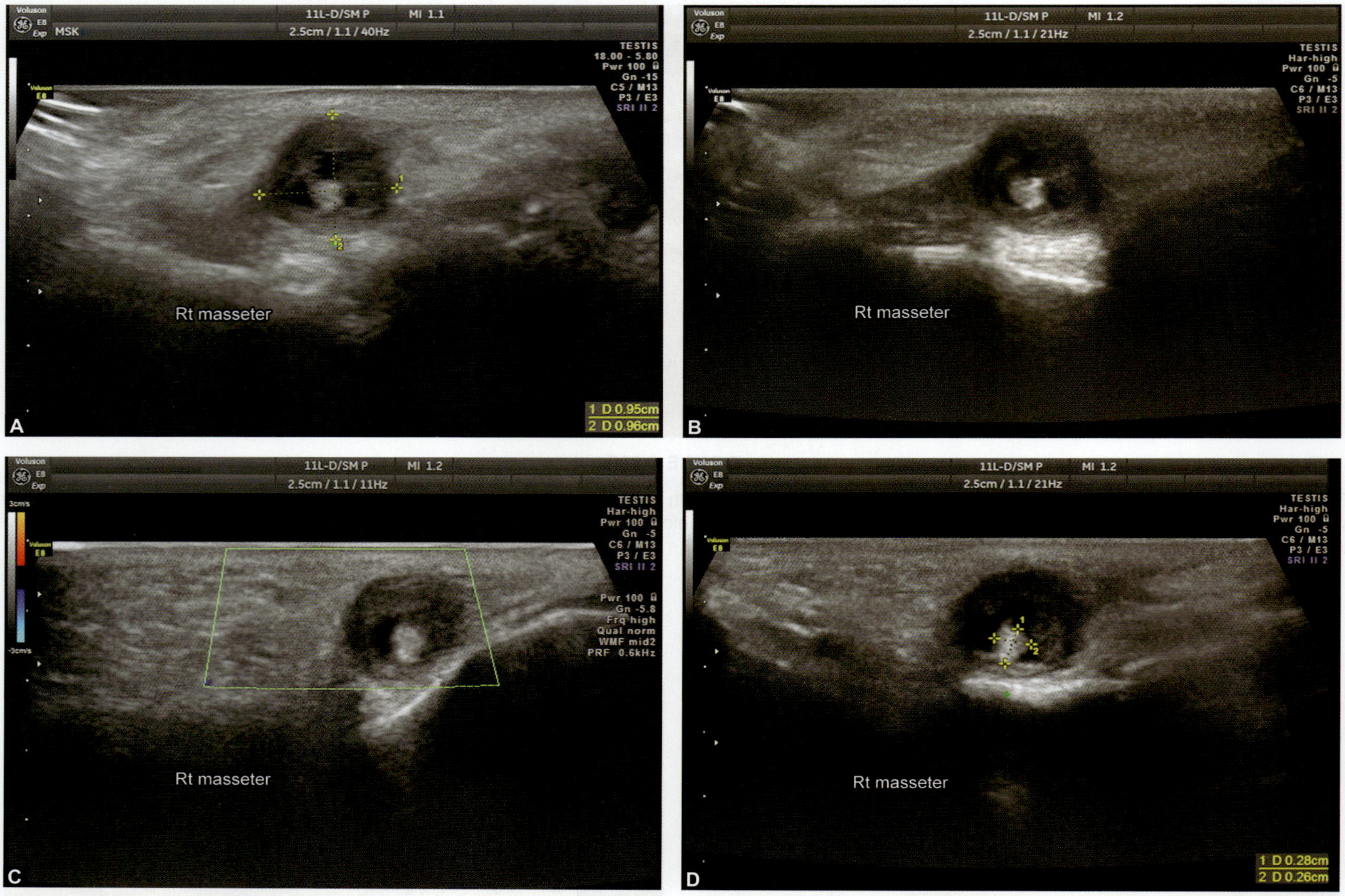

FIGURES 2.30A to D: Masseter muscle cysticercus cyst. A young boy presented with soft tissue swelling over the right side of cheek. High resolution sonography shows a well-defined thick walled cyst in the masseter muscle of right cheek. An echogenic nidus is seen fixed with the inner wall of the cyst. **On color flow imaging,** poor flow is seen in it suggestive of cysticercus cyst.

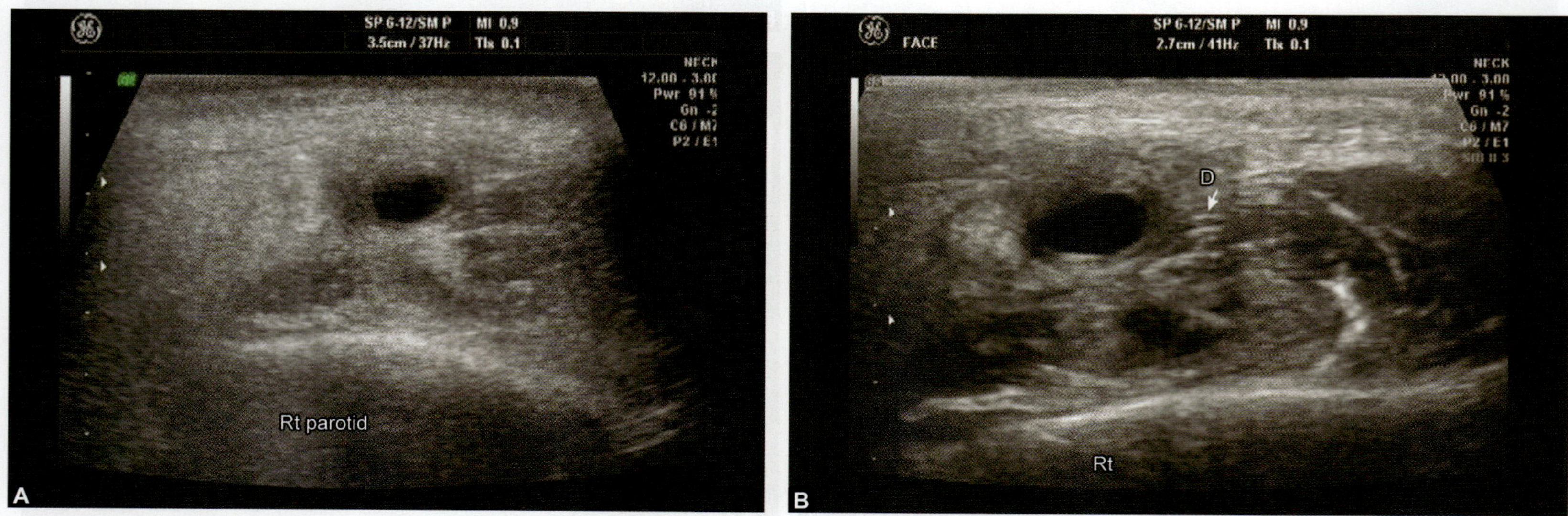

FIGURES 2.31A and B

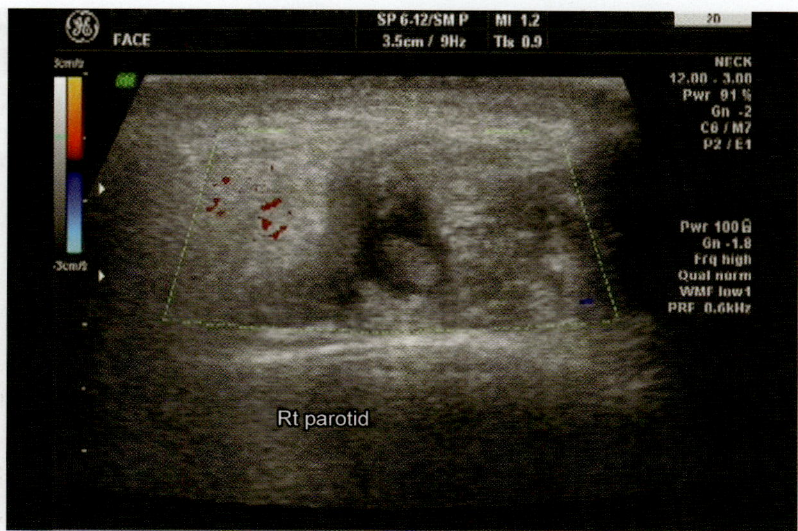

FIGURE 2.31C

FIGURES 2.31A to C: Parotid abscess. A patient presented with soft tissue swelling over the right parotid, which was tender on palpation. High resolution sonography shows a complex echo mass in the superficial lobe of right parotid. It shows perifocal edema. Central area of necrosis is also seen in it. **On color flow imaging,** poor flow is seen in it. Biopsy of the mass confirmed tuberculosis.

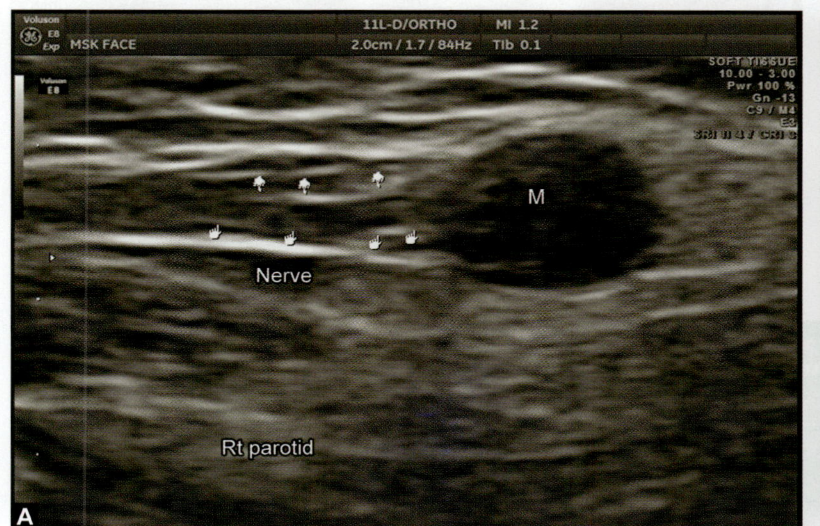

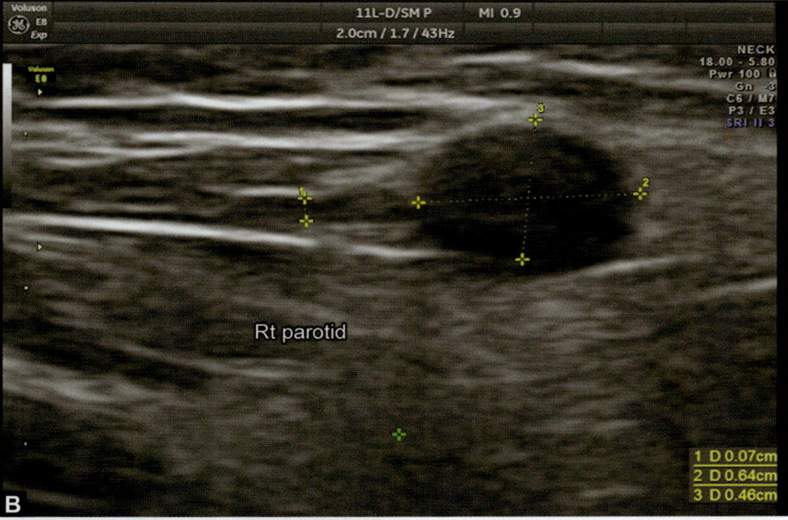

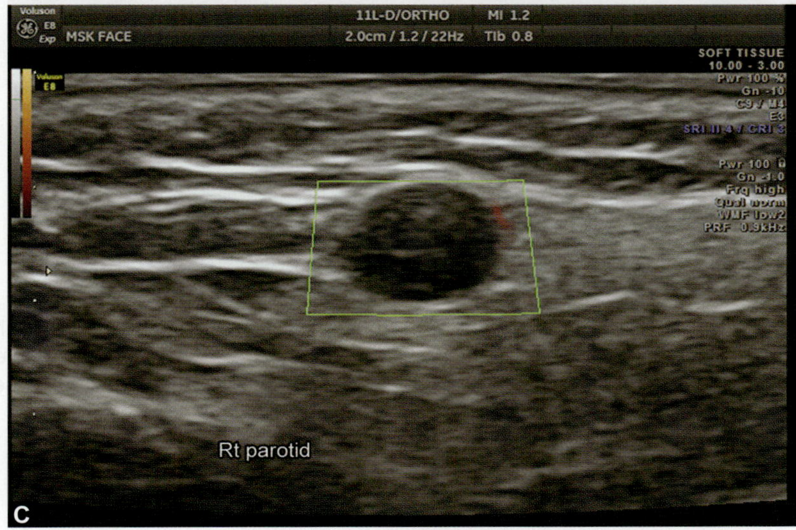

FIGURES 2.32A to C: Fasciaeo nerve tumor. A patient presented with a palpable nodule in the right side of face in the region of parotid gland. HRSG shows a well-defined homogeneous hypoechoic nodular shadow in the right side of face. It is seen in relation to the facial nerve. It is smooth in outline and eccentric in position. No calcification is seen in it. No cystic degeneration is seen. **On color flow imaging,** poor flow is seen in it. Findings are consistent with fascial nerve schwannoma.

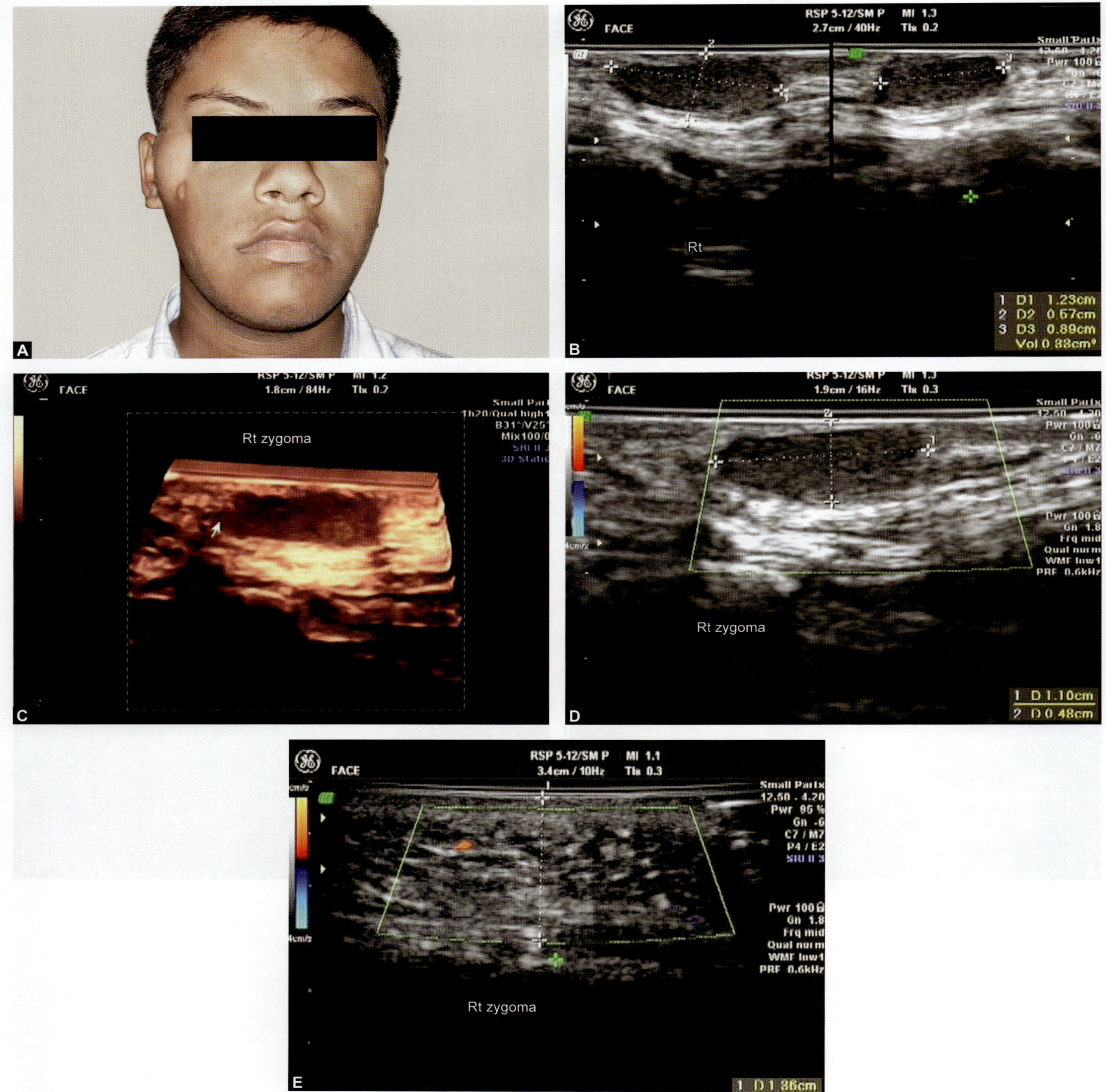

FIGURES 2.33A to E: Dermoid cyst of face. A young boy presented with soft tissue swelling over the right preauricular region. It is also seen extending to right infraorbital region. High resolution sonography shows a well defined low level echo complex mass in the preauricular region. It shows homogeneous echoes. No septation or calcification is seen in it. **On color flow imaging,** poor flow is seen in it. Biopsy of the mass confirms dermoid cyst.

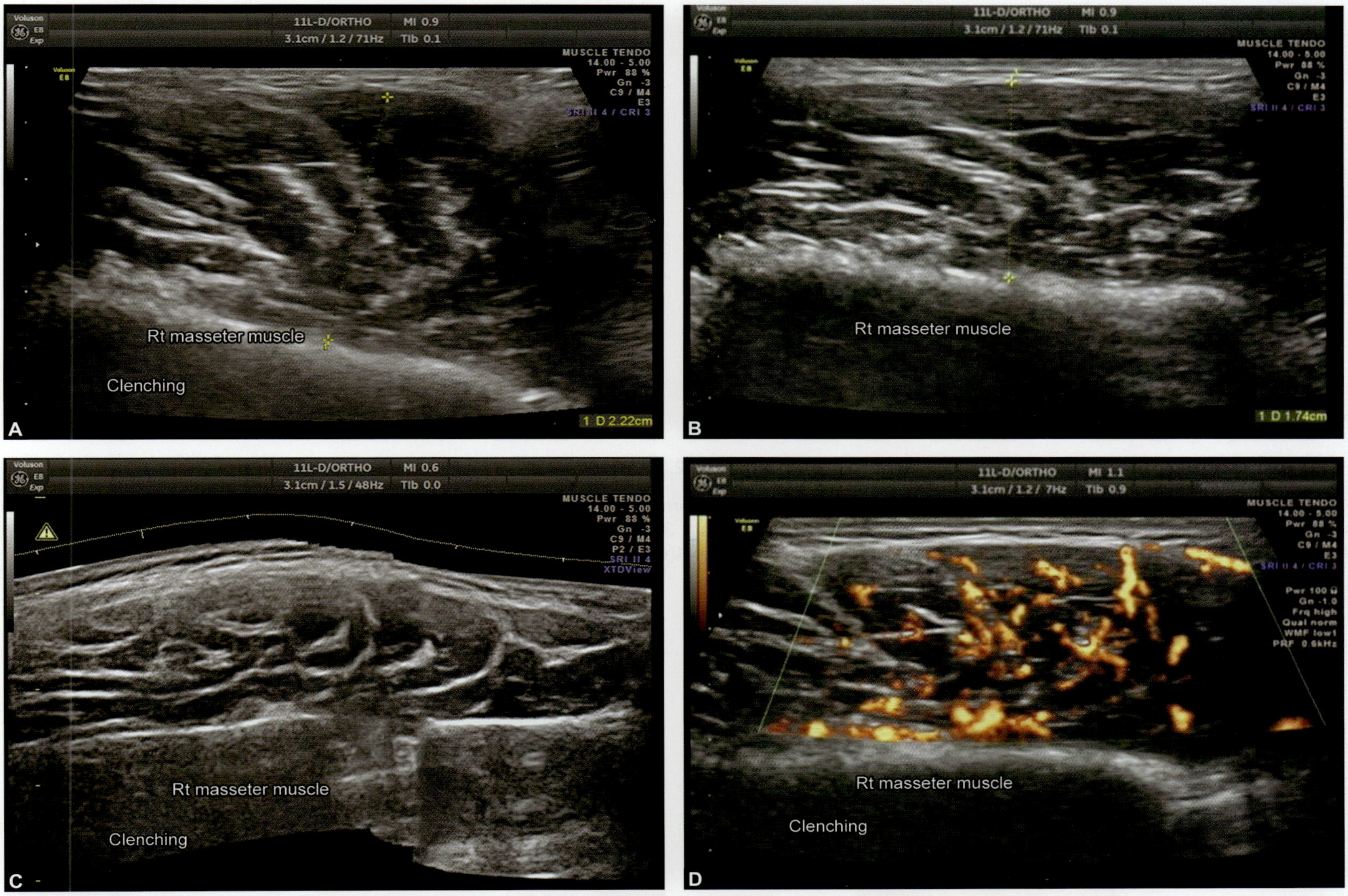

FIGURES 2.34A to D: Masseter muscle hypertrophy. A girl presented with soft tissue swelling on the right side of cheek. High resolution sonography shows diffuse hypertrophy of masseter muscle, which is 2.2 mm in thickness, whereas left masseter muscle is 1.7 mm in thickness. However, the muscle texture is intact. No focal mass is seen in the muscle. **On color flow imaging,** low flow is seen in the muscle suggestive of diffuse muscle hypertrophy.

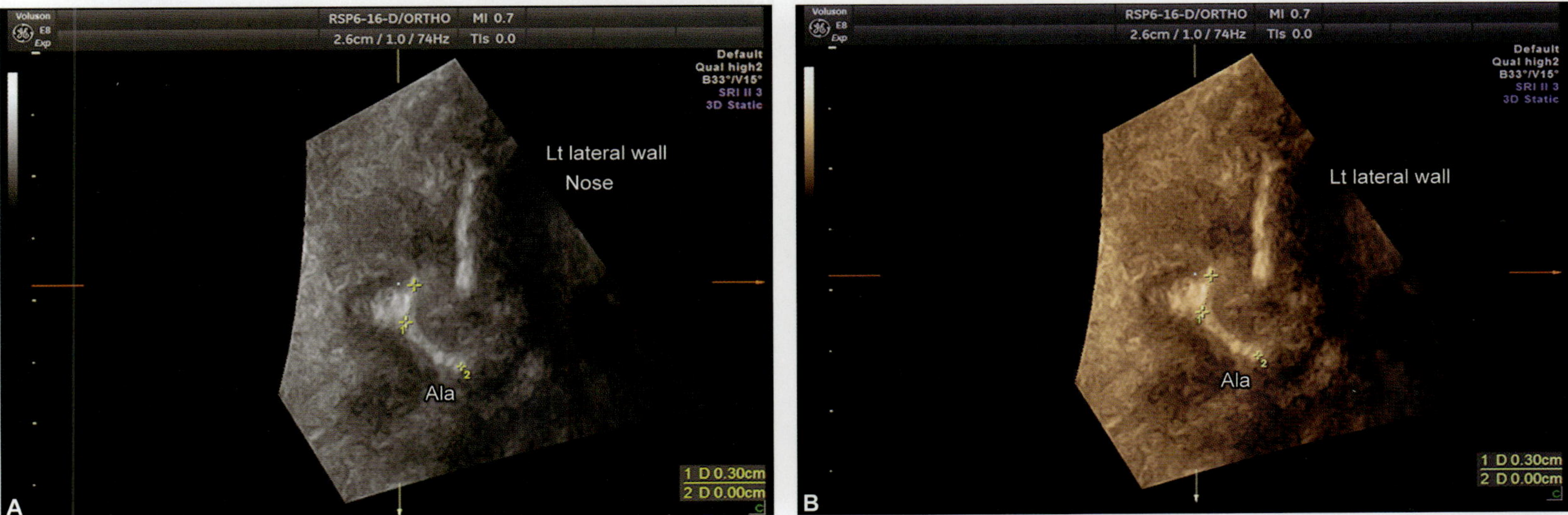

FIGURES 2.35A and B

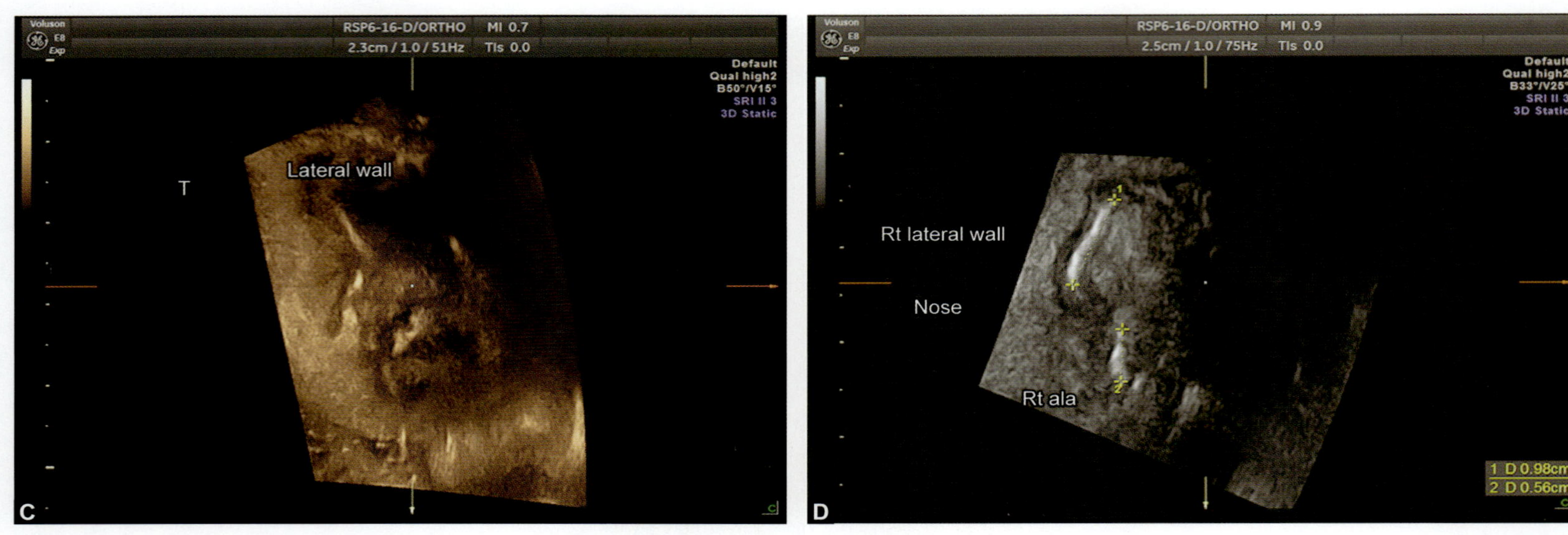

FIGURES 2.35C and D

FIGURES 2.35A to D: Hypertrophy of cartilage of nose. A young girl presented with asymmetrical enlargement of left ala of nose. High resolution sonography shows diffuse thickening of cartilage of left ala of the nose. 3D imaging clearly shows diffuse hypertrophy of the cartilage and diffuse thickening of the soft tissue of lateral wall of the nose. HRSG is excellent modality of evaluation of cartilage pathology.

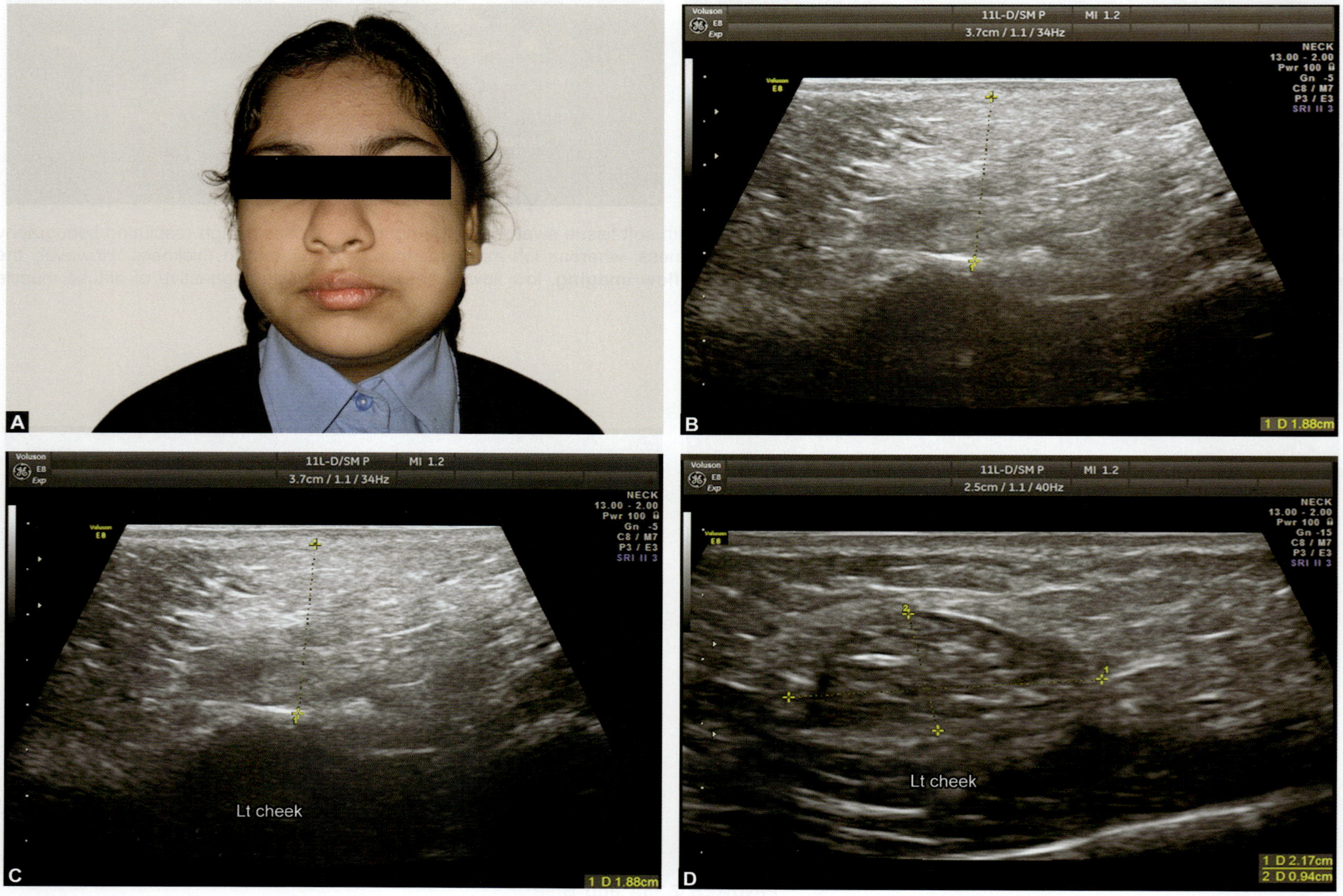

FIGURES 2.36A to D

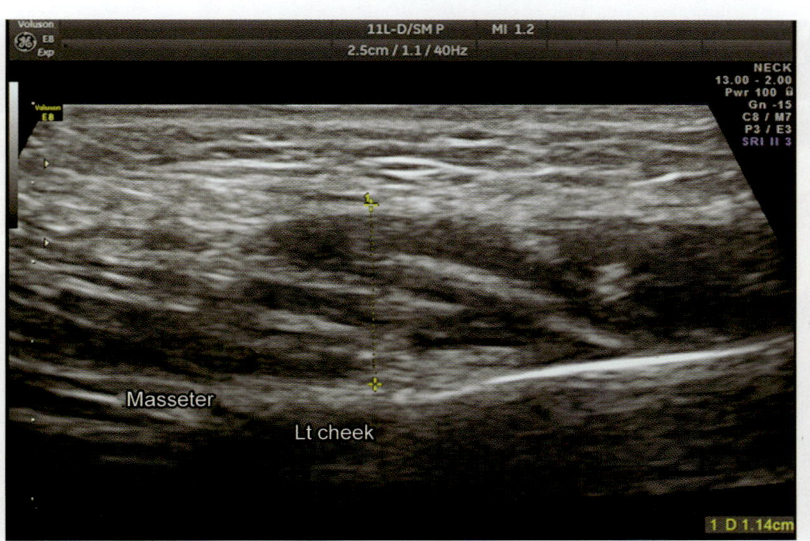

FIGURE 2.36E

FIGURES 2.36A to E: Pad of fat in the left cheek. A young girl presented with asymmetrical enlargement of left cheek. HRSG shows an echogenic soft tissue mass in the left cheek. It is homogeneous in texture and it is of fat density suggestive of increased pad of fat. right side of the cheek does not show any mass.

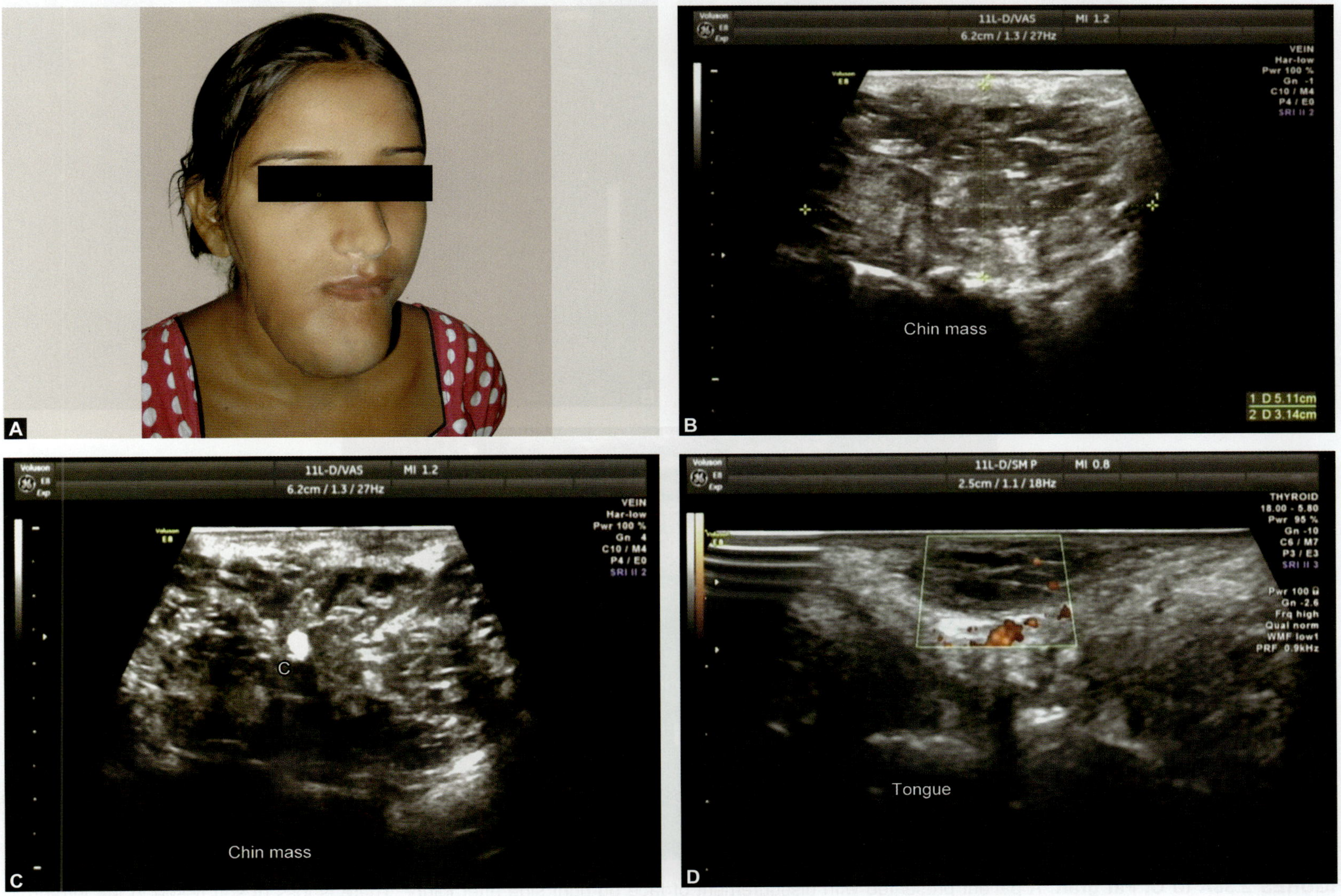

FIGURES 2.37A to D

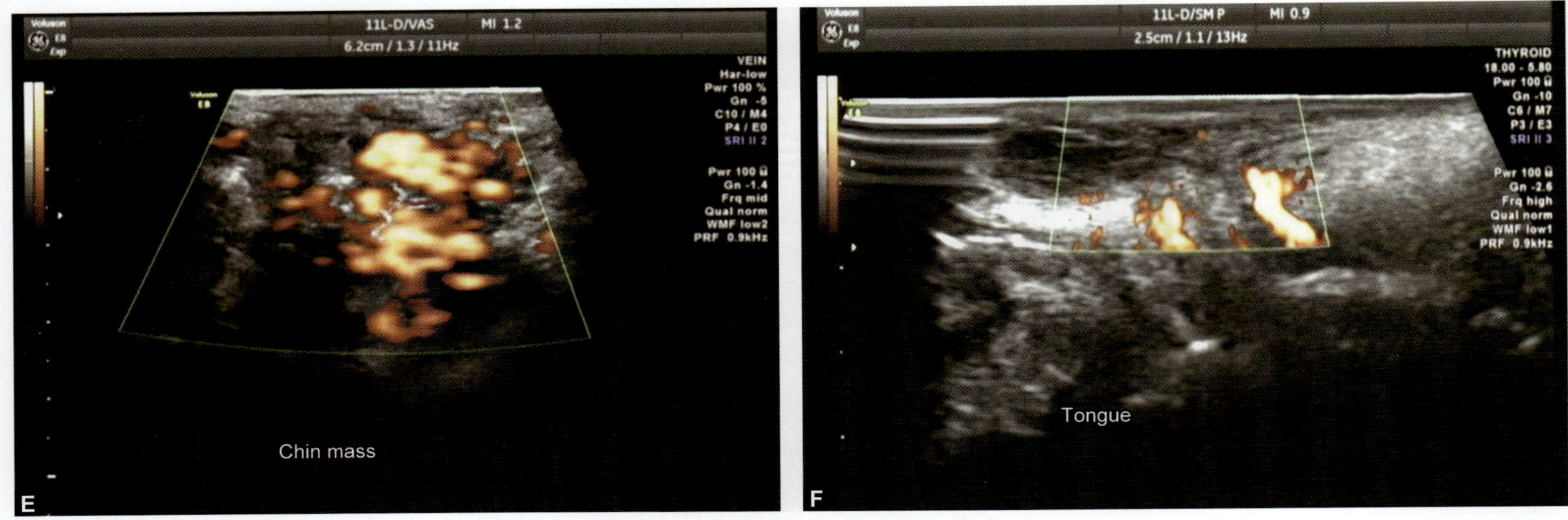

FIGURES 2.37E and F

FIGURES 2.37A to F: A young girl presented with soft tissue mass over the chin. HRSG shows a big heterogeneous soft tissue mass over the chin. Multiple echogenic shadows are seen in the mass suggestive of calcified foci. The mass is also seen involving the floor of the mouth and under surface of tongue. **On color flow imaging,** multiple vessels are seen feeding the mass. Findings are suggestive of vascular hemangiomatous mass.

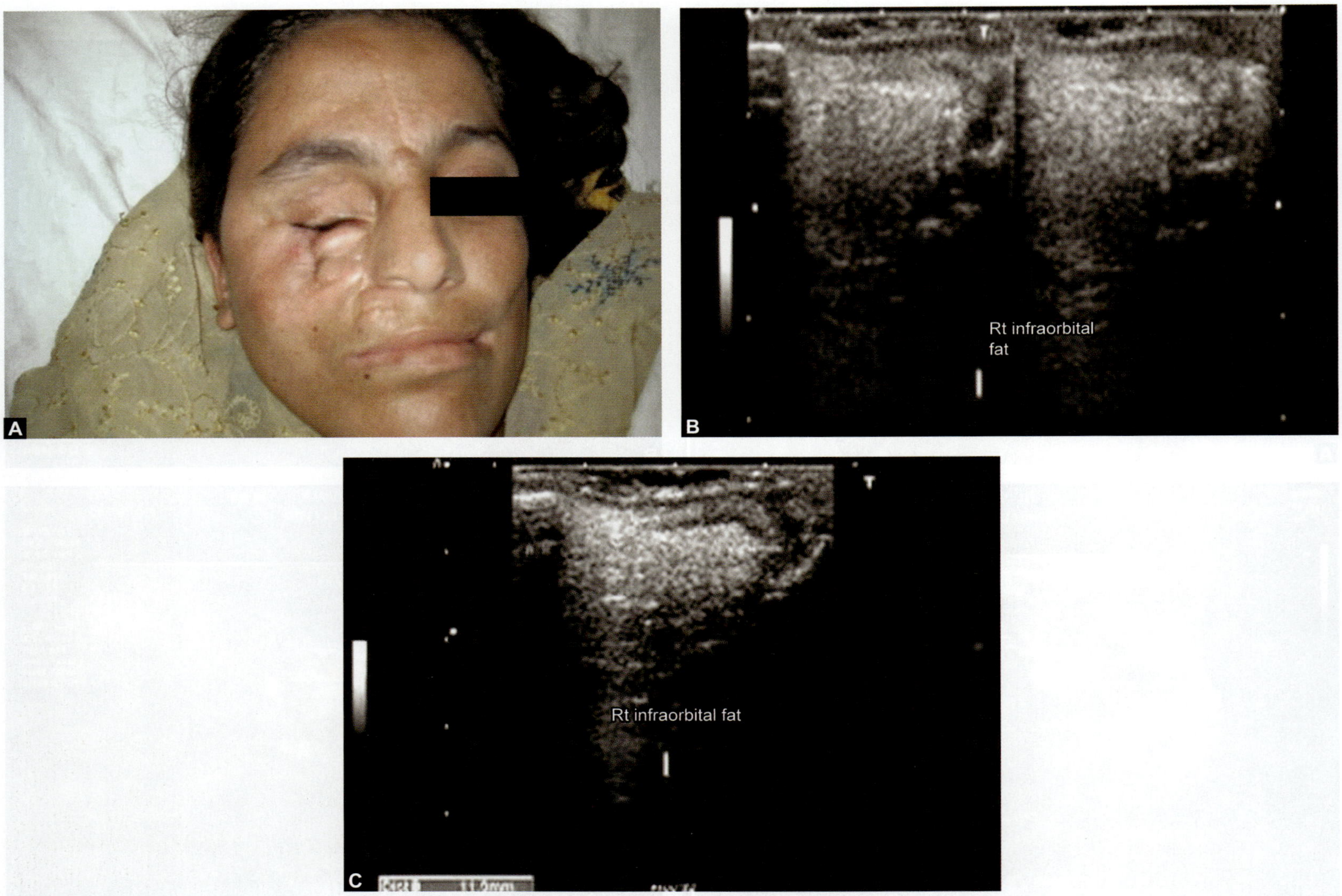

FIGURES 2.38A to C: Fat graft. A patient presented with disfigurement of face on right side after injury. There is loss of soft tissue in the infraorbital region. A pad of fat was grafted in the infraorbital part to fill the gap. HRSG shows echogenic fat pad graft in the infraorbital part of the face.

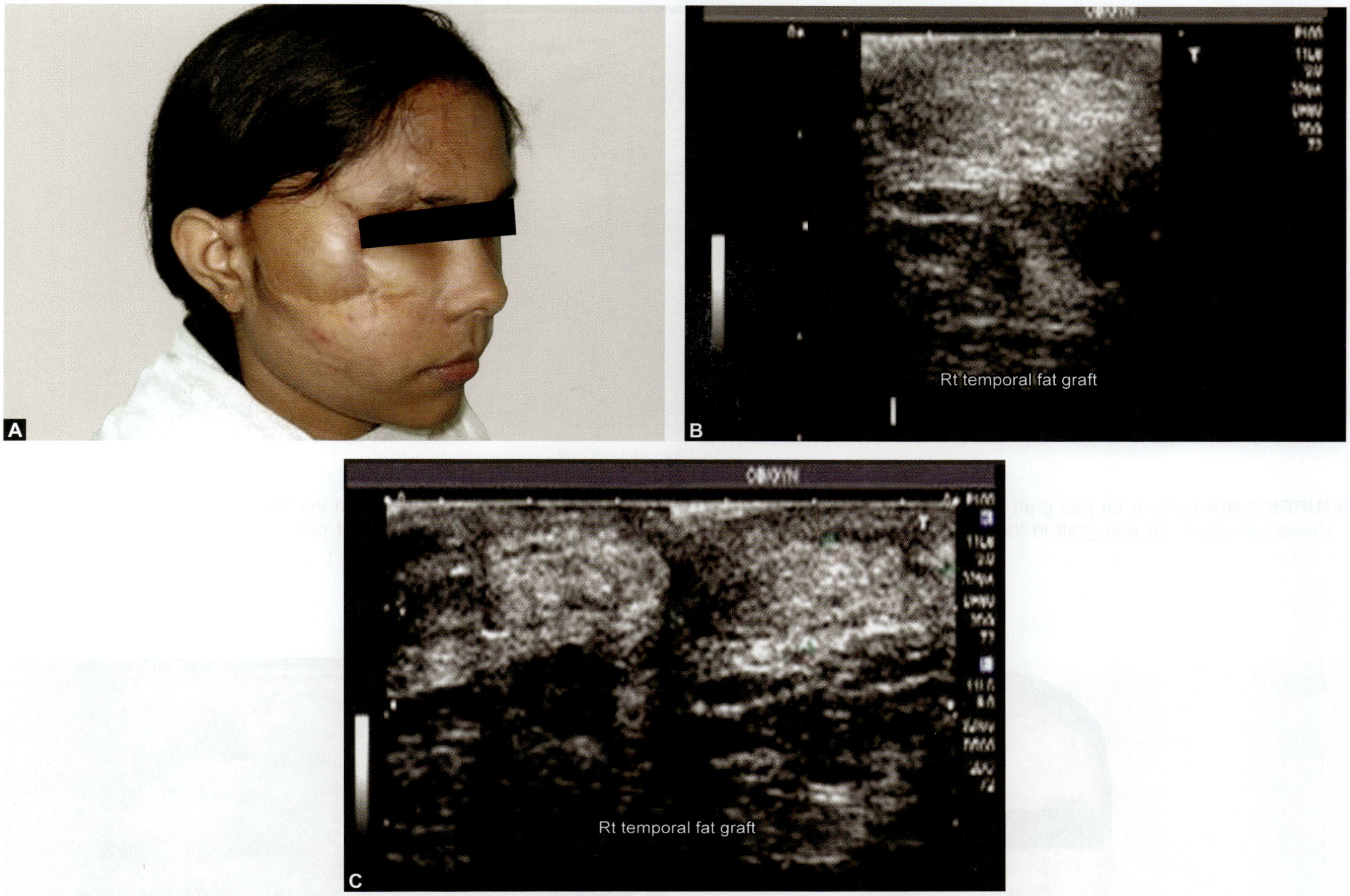

FIGURES 2.39A to C: Right temporal fat graft. A patient sustained injury over the face with loss of soft tissue in the temporal region. A fat pad graft was put under the skin to fill the gap. HRSG clearly shows the fat pad graft under the skin in temporal region.

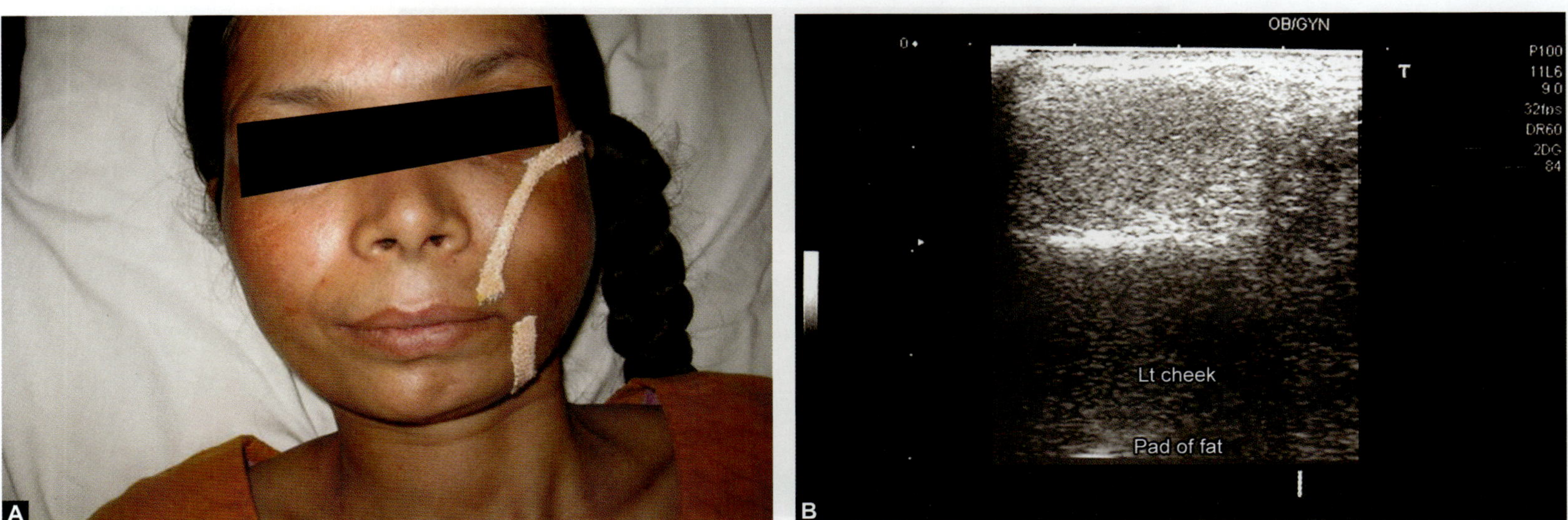

FIGURES 2.40A and B

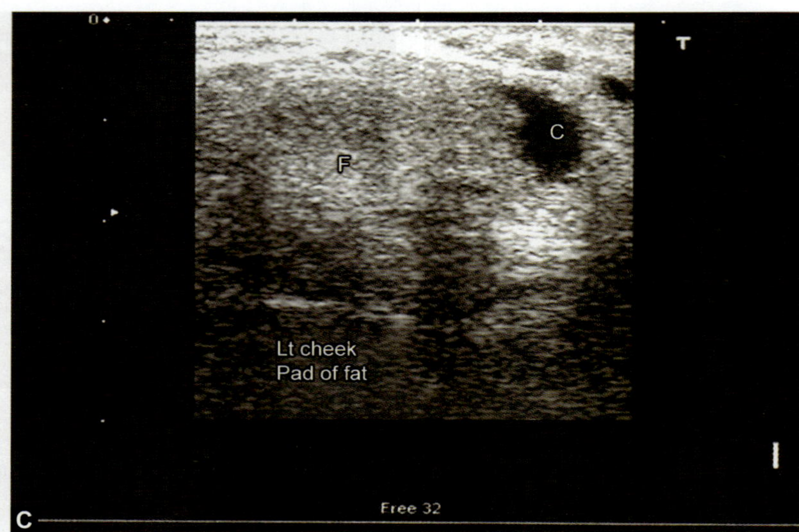

FIGURE 2.40C

FIGURES 2.40A to C: A fat pad graft was put in the left cheek to fill the gap in a lady, who sustained trauma in the face. High resolution sonography shows echogenic fat pad graft in the left cheek. However, there is cystic degenaration taken place in the fat pad graft due to necrosis marked.

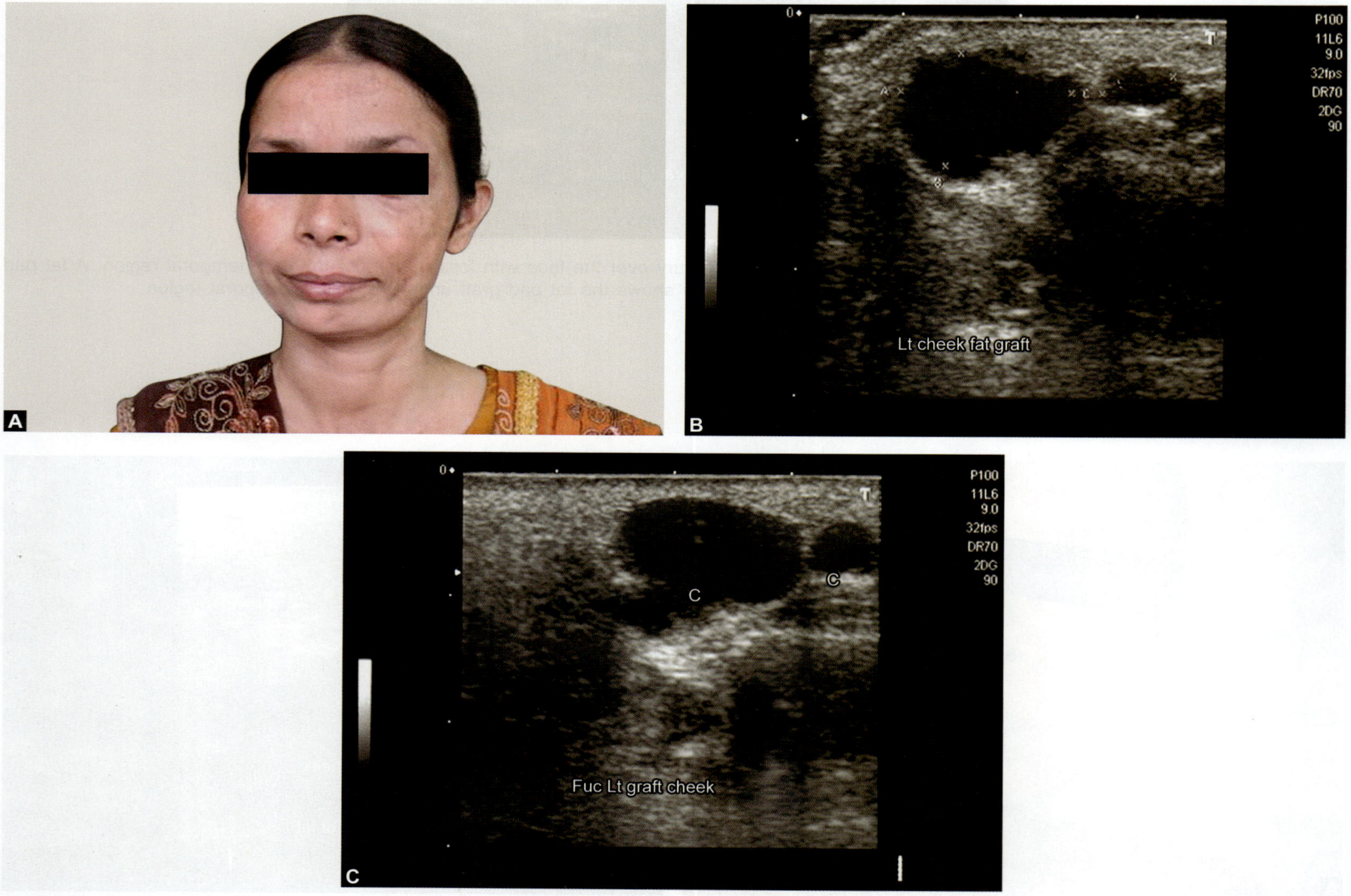

FIGURES 2.41A to C: The cystic degeneration increased in the same patient in the fat pad graft over the period of time. Liquefaction has taken place in the fat pad graft resulting into cyst formation. High resolution sonography has beautifully shown the cystic degeneration in fat pad graft.

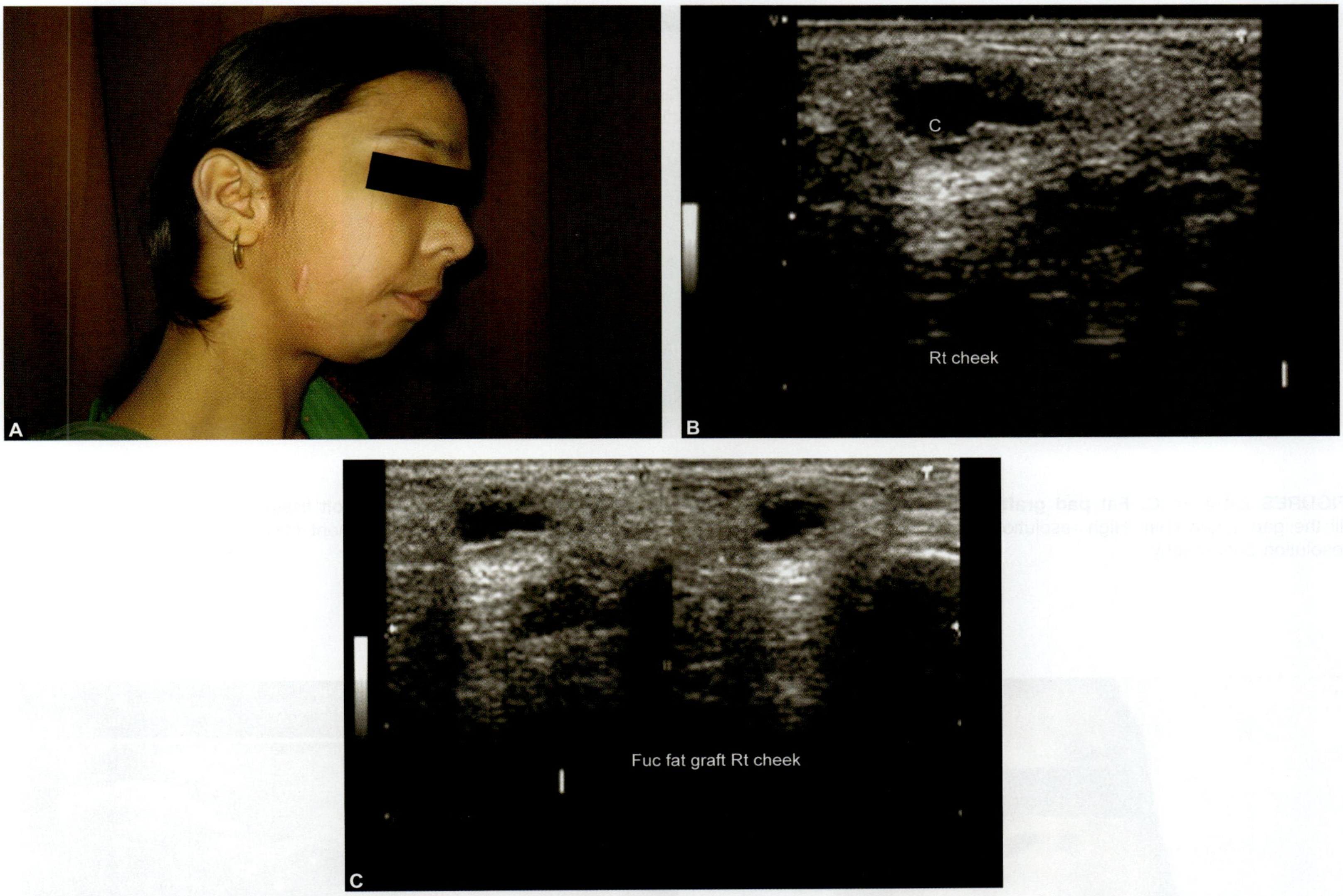

FIGURES 2.42A to C: Fat pad graft degeneration. A young girl underwent fat pad grafting to fill the gap in the right cheek. However, the graft shows loss of shape and volume due to cystic degeneration. High resolution sonography clearly shows the cystic degeneration in the fat pad graft.

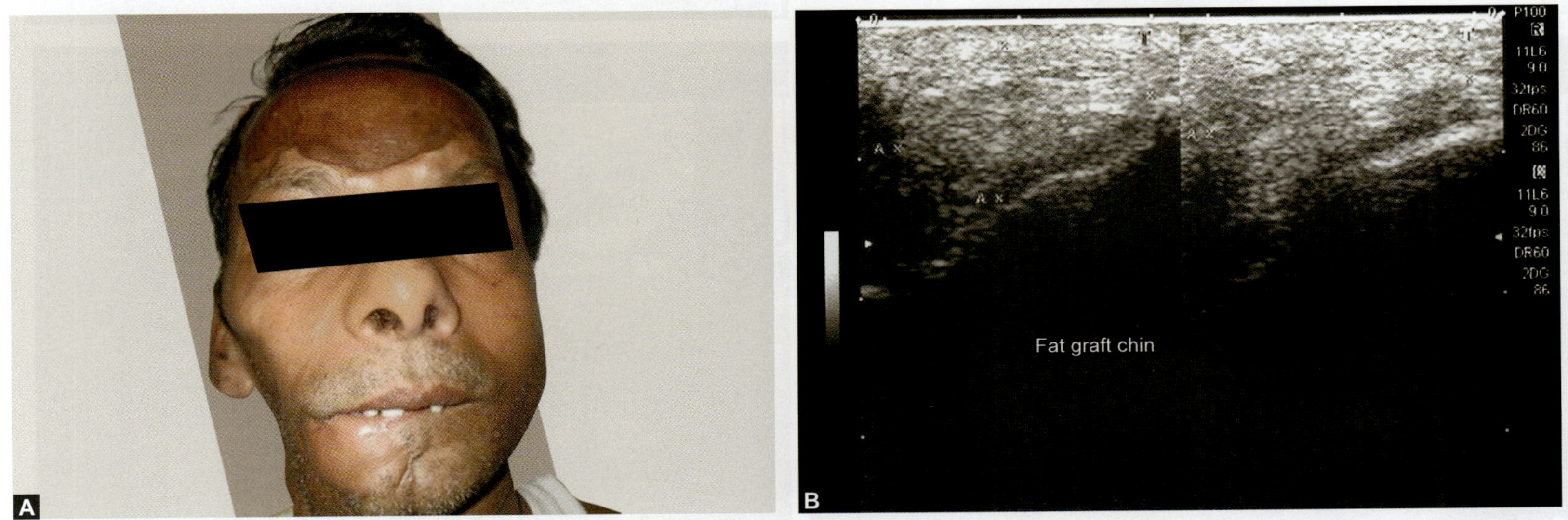

FIGURES 2.43A and B

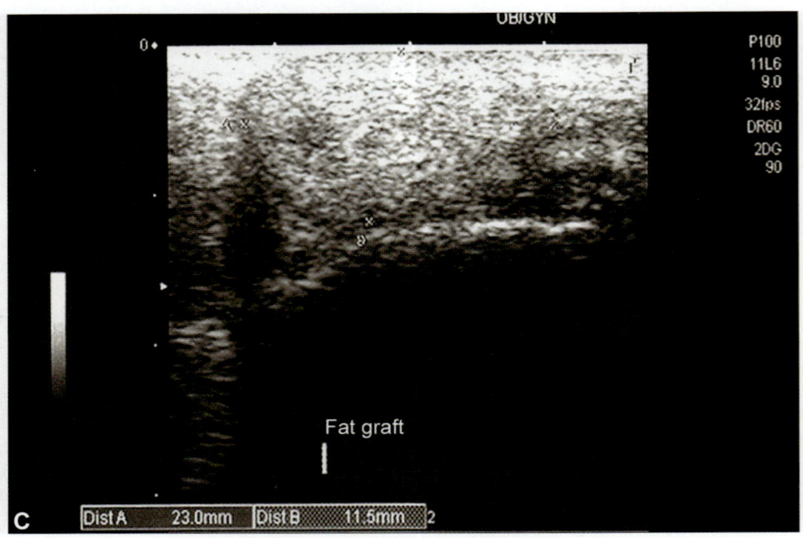

FIGURE 2.43C

FIGURES 2.43A to C: Fat pad graft in the chin. A patient presented with injury to the chin with loss of soft tissue. The fat pad was grafted to fill the gap in the chin. High resolution sonography shows echogenic fat pad in passion and proper assessment of the fat pad was done on High resolution sonography.

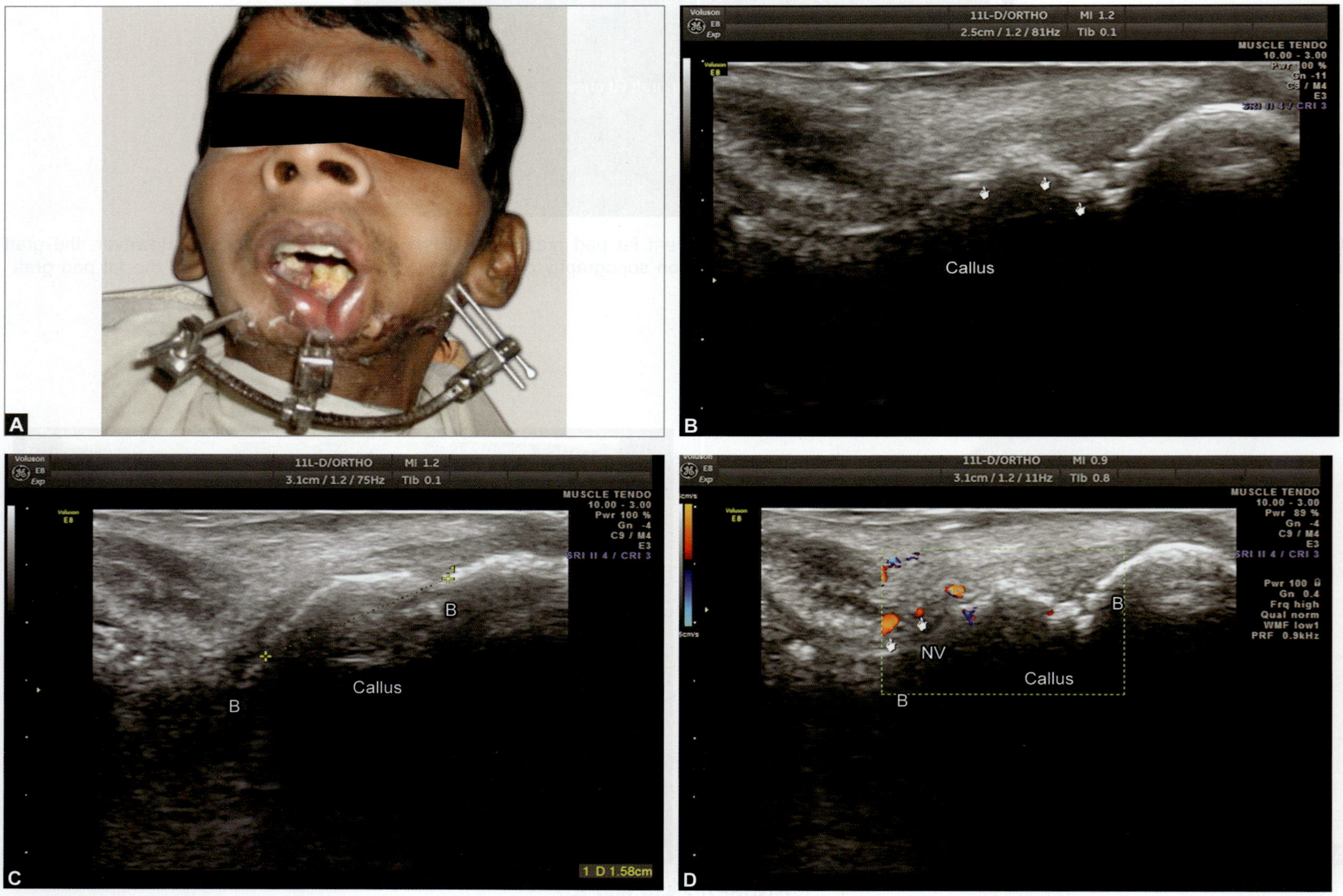

FIGURES 2.44A to D

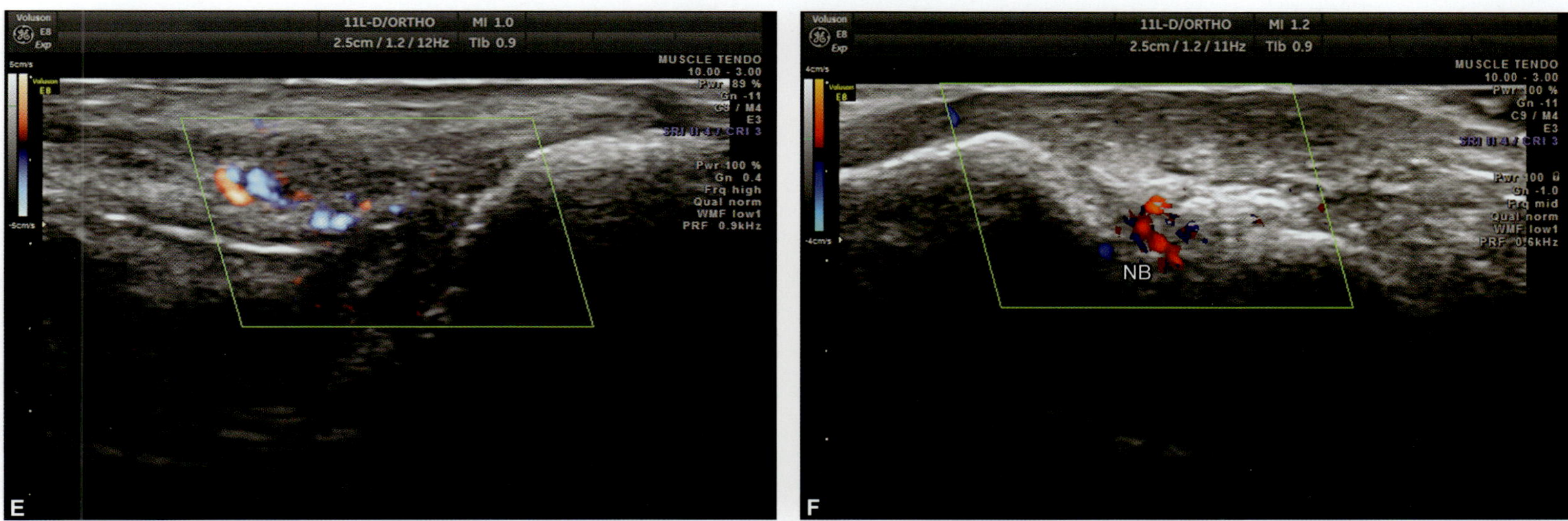

FIGURES 2.44E and F

FIGURES 2.44A to F: New callus formation in mandible. A man presented with fracture of mandible with loss of bone after sustaining trauma. Distraction operation was done with fixator application for callus formation. High resolution sonography clearly shows the new callus formation along the fractured bone as a bright echogenic line. **On color flow imaging,** multiple vessels are seen around the callus suggestive of neovascularisation. The new bone formation is soft in texture and it is not visible on X-ray. High resolution sonography is an excellent modality for evaluation of new bone formation.

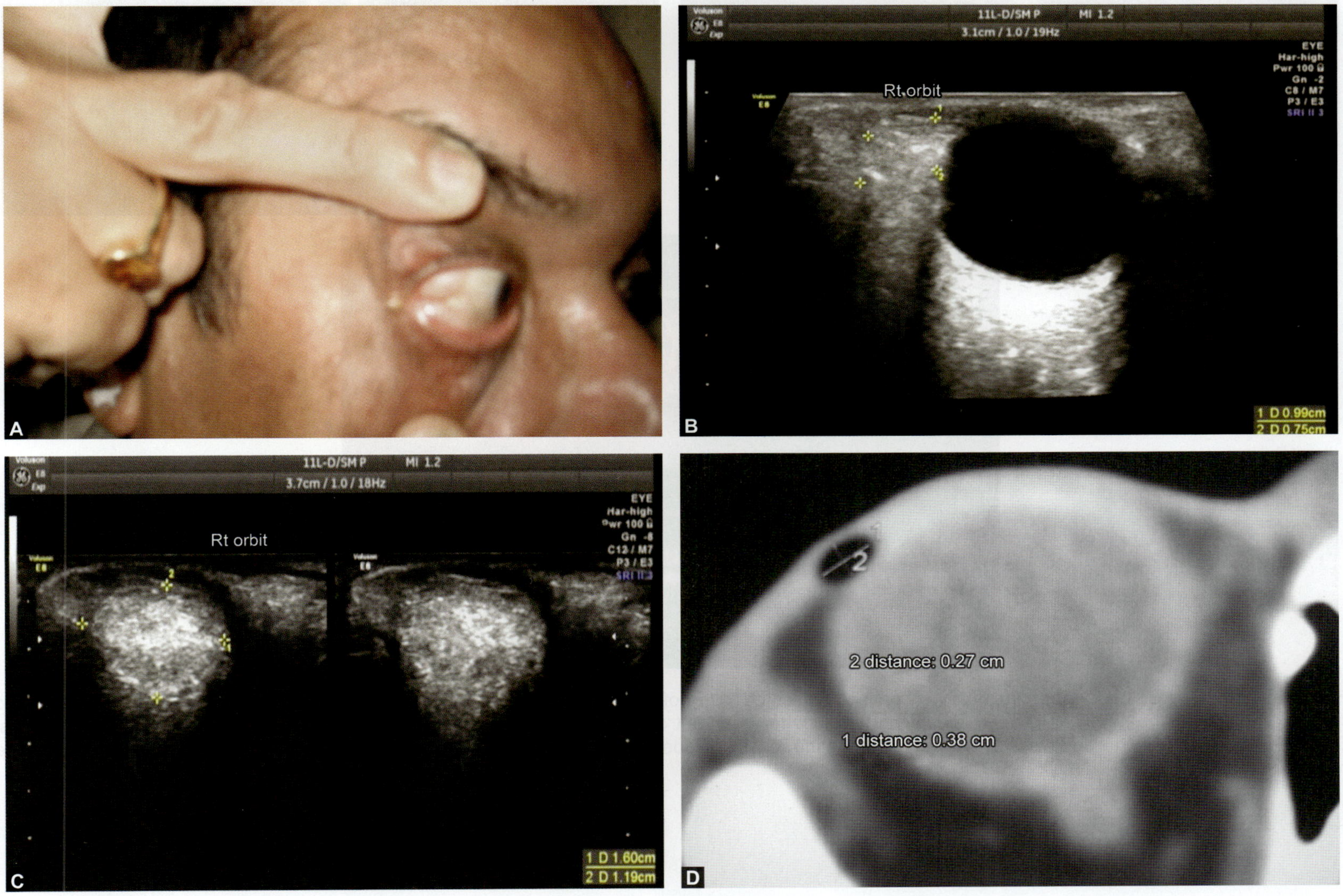

FIGURES 2.45A to D: Dermoid at the lateral canthus of right eye. a patient presented with a soft tissue swelling at the lateral canthus of right eye. HRSG shows an echogenic mass at the lateral canthus of right eye. The mass is seen filled with echogenic shadows similar to fat suggestive of a dermoid. CT scan of the eye of the same patient shows a cystic mass having fat in it confirming ultrasound findings.

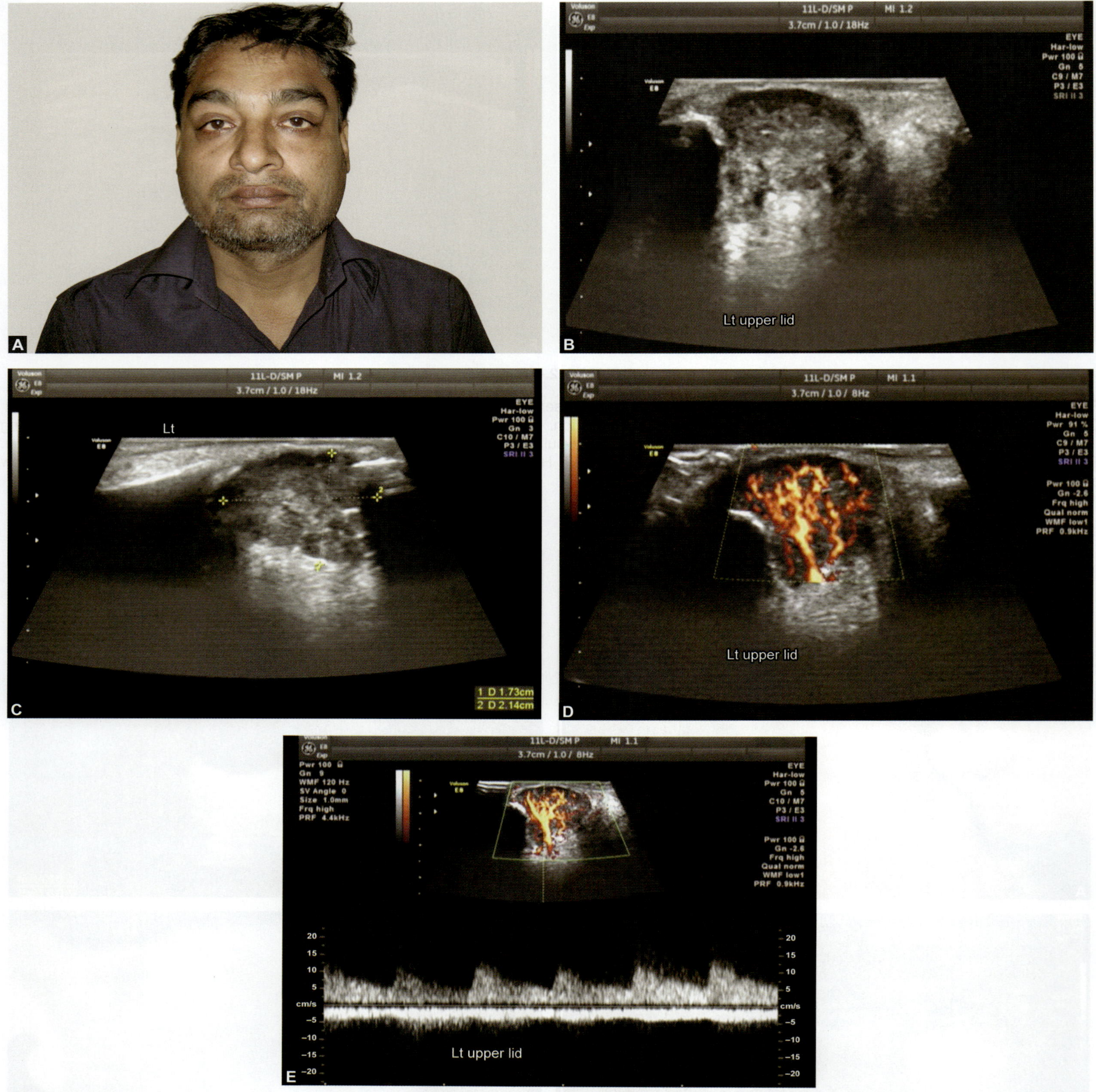

FIGURES 2.46A to E: Left upper lid mass. A patient presented with soft tissue swelling over the right upper lid. HRSG shows a low level echo complex mass over the left lid. It is seen occupying the superior quadrant over the orbit. No calcification or cystic degeneration is seen in the mass. **On color flow imaging,** multiple vessels are seen feeding the mass. On spectral Doppler tracing, moderate arterial flow is seen in the mass suggestive of vascular mass.

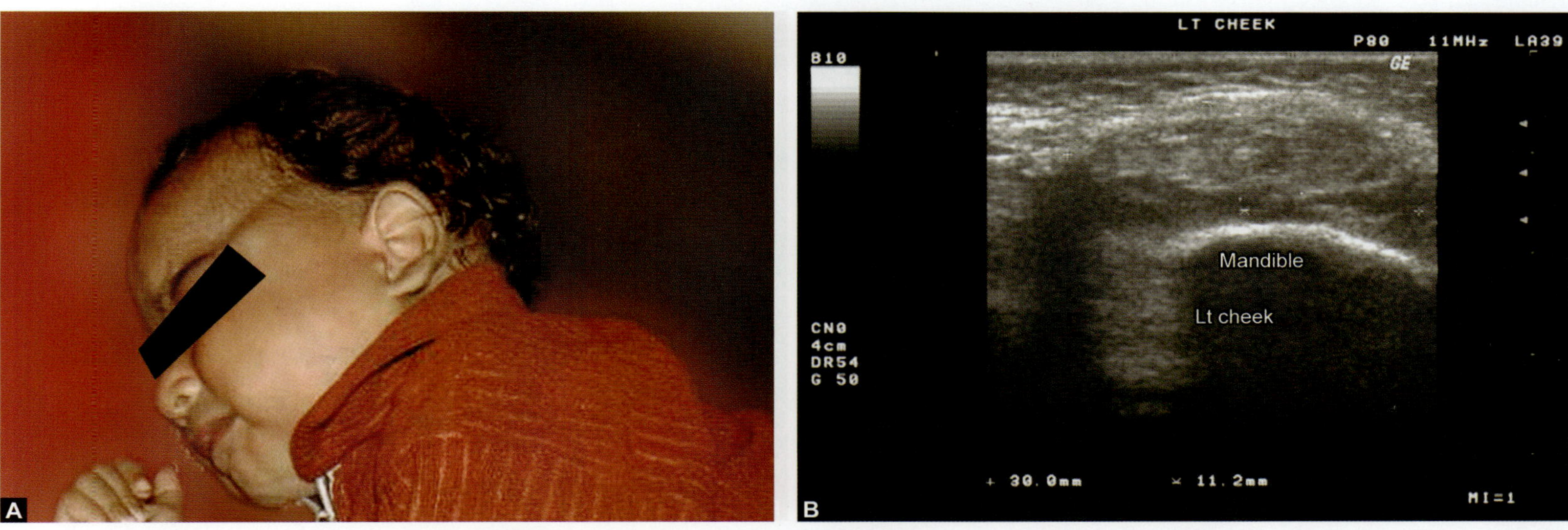

FIGURES 2.47A and B: Tumor of the masseter muscle. A child presented with soft tissue mass over the left masseter muscle. It is irregular in outline. No calcification is seen in it. No cystic degeneration is seen. FNAC confirmed masseter muscle mass. The mass is not seen invading the bone. FNAC confirmed a myosarcoma.

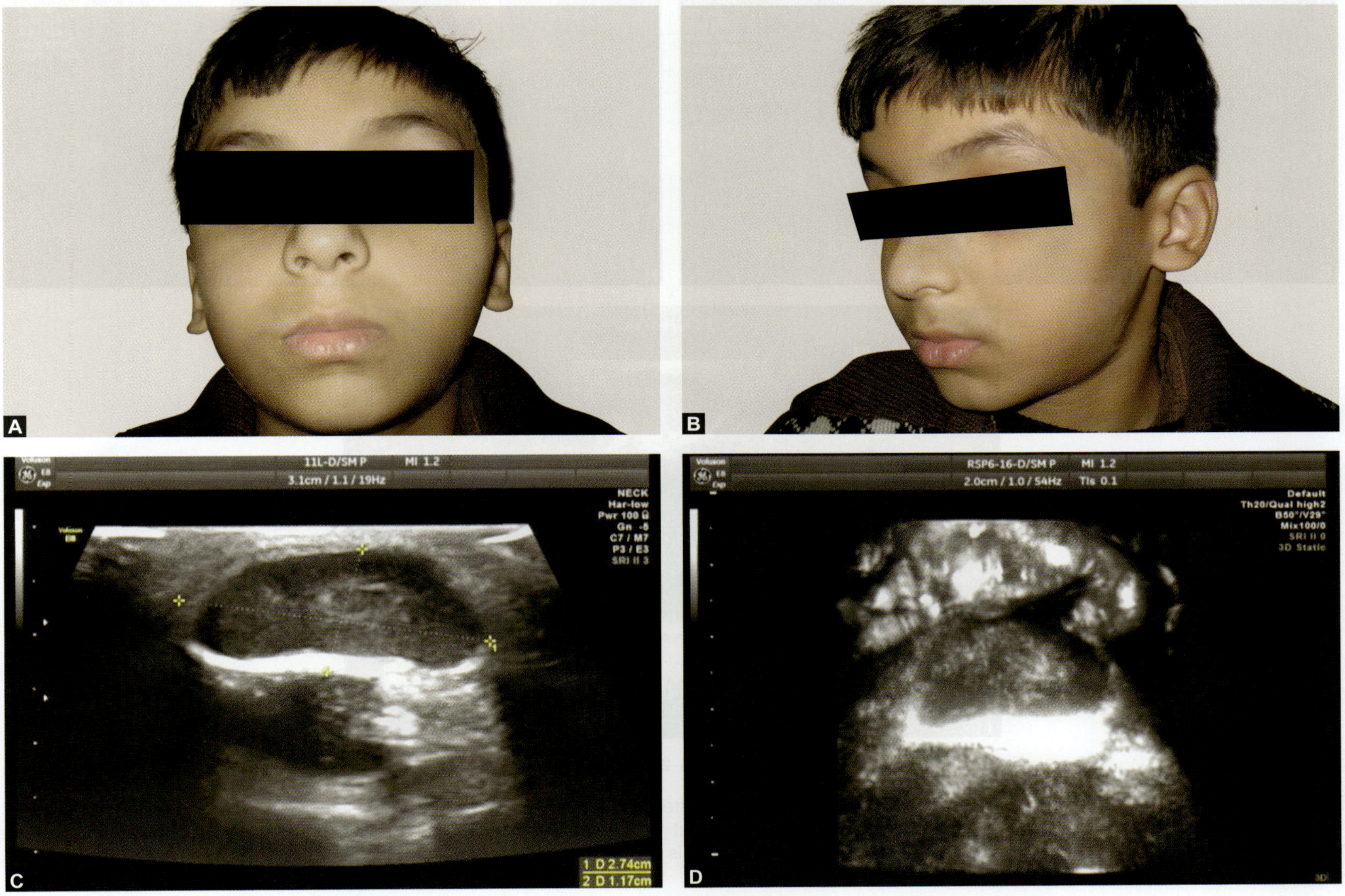

FIGURES 2.48A to D

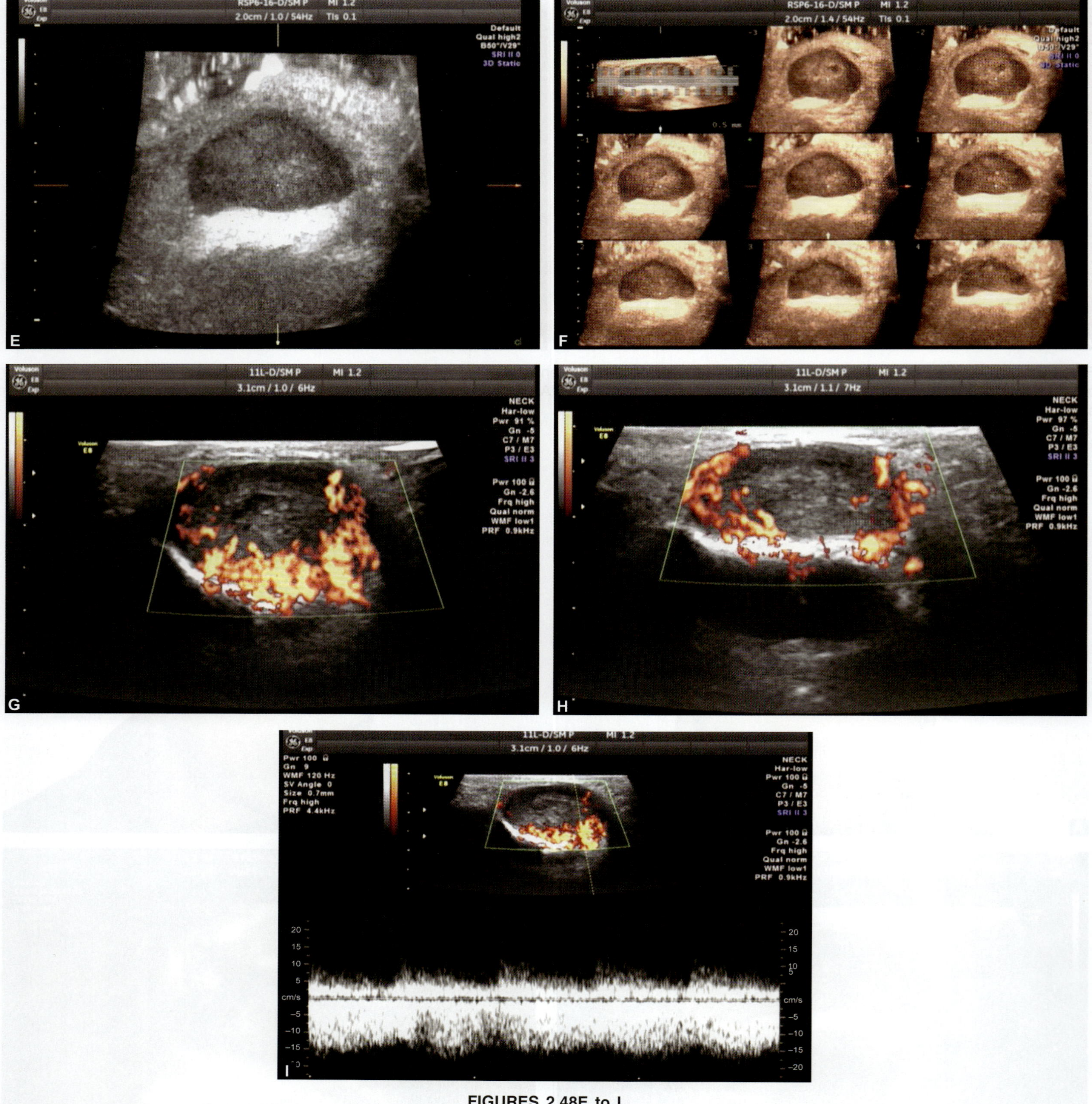

FIGURES 2.48E to I

FIGURES 2.48A to I: Ewing sarcoma of maxilla. A young boy presented with soft tissue swelling in the left cheek and infraorbital region. High resolution sonography shows a low level echo complex mass coming out from ramus of left maxilla. It is predominantly solid. On 3D imaging, the mass shows invading the maxilla. **On color flow imaging,** multiple vessels are seen feeding the mass. Biopsy of the mass confirms Ewing sarcoma.

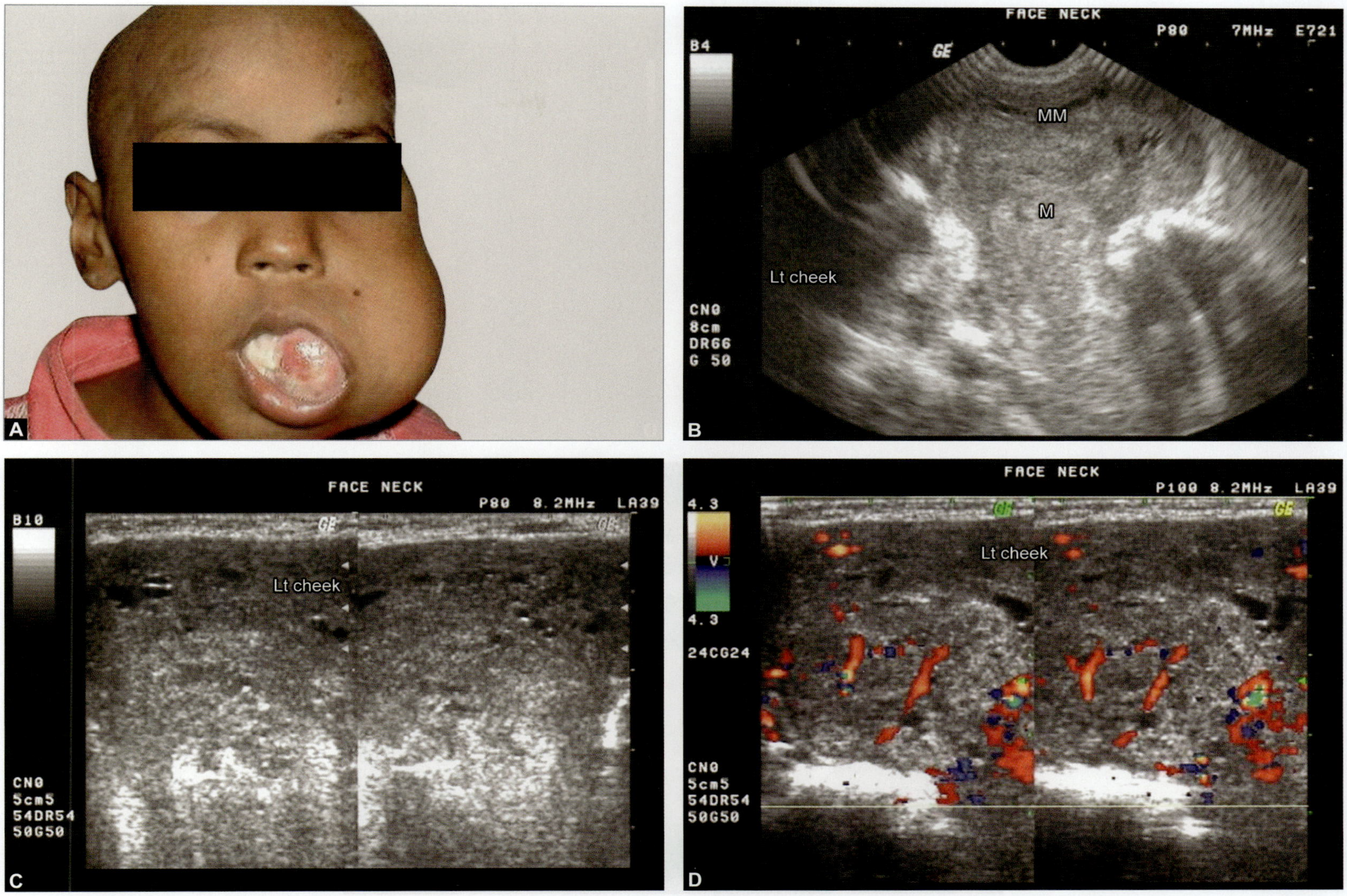

FIGURES 2.49A to D: A young boy presented with soft tissue mass in oral cavity. It is almost occupying whole of the oral cavity. He could not close the mouth. HRSG shows a big heterogeneous mass in the oral cavity. The mass is coming out from the cheek and going inside the oral cavity. It is also seen invading the maxilla. The bone erosion is also seen. Normal anatomic relations are distorted. The mass is predominantly solid. No cystic degeneration is seen in the mass. **On color flow imaging,** low flow is seen in the mass. Biopsy of the mass confirms Rhabdomyosarcoma coming out from the muscle.

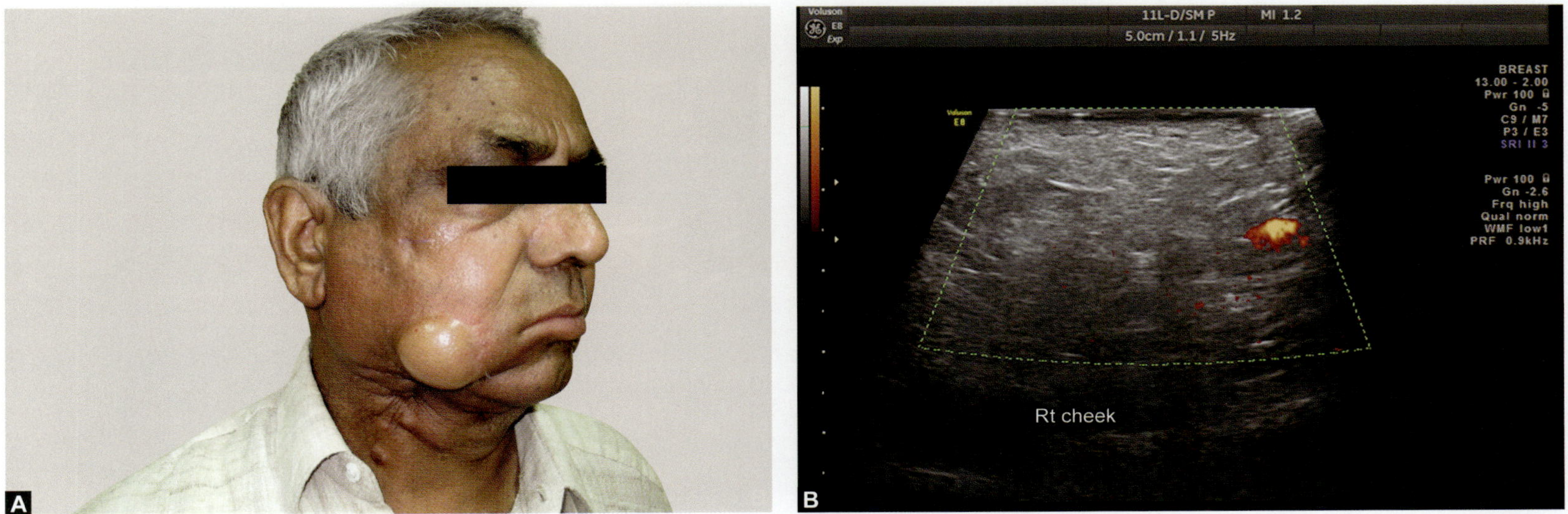

FIGURES 2.50A and B

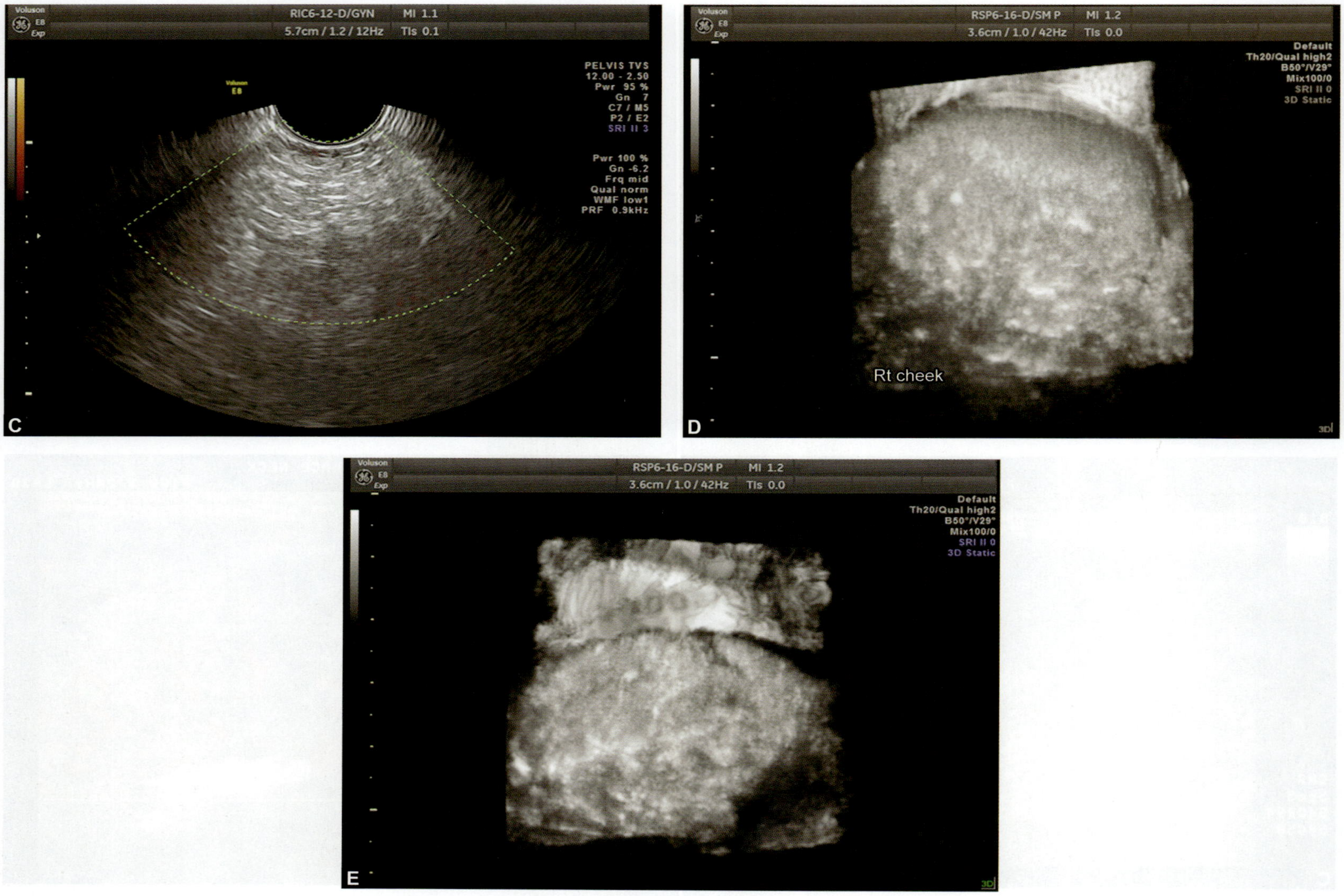

FIGURES 2.50C to E

FIGURES 2.50A to E: Recurrence of Ca cheek. A patient case of operated Ca cheek presented with soft tissue swelling over the right cheek. HRSG shows a heterogeneous predominantly solid mass over the right cheek. On 3D imaging, the mass is clearly seen invading the soft tissue. No calcification or cystic degeneration is seen in the mass. **On color flow imaging,** poor flow is seen in it suggestive of recurrence of growth.

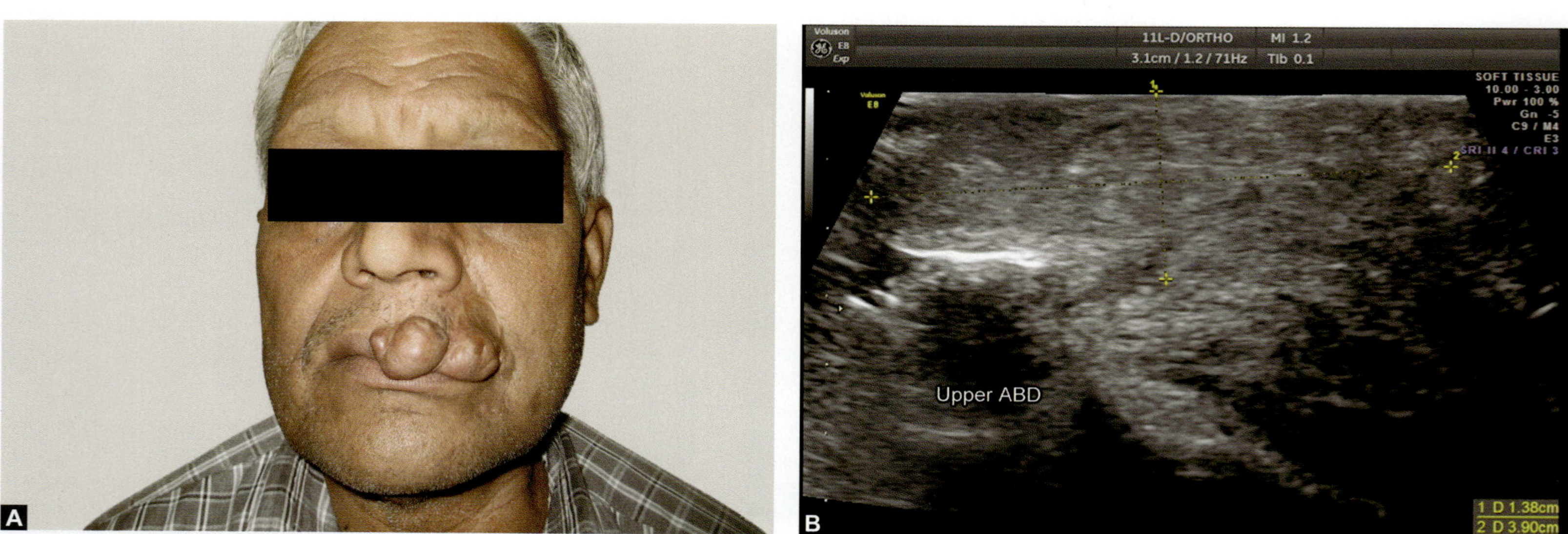

FIGURES 2.51A and B

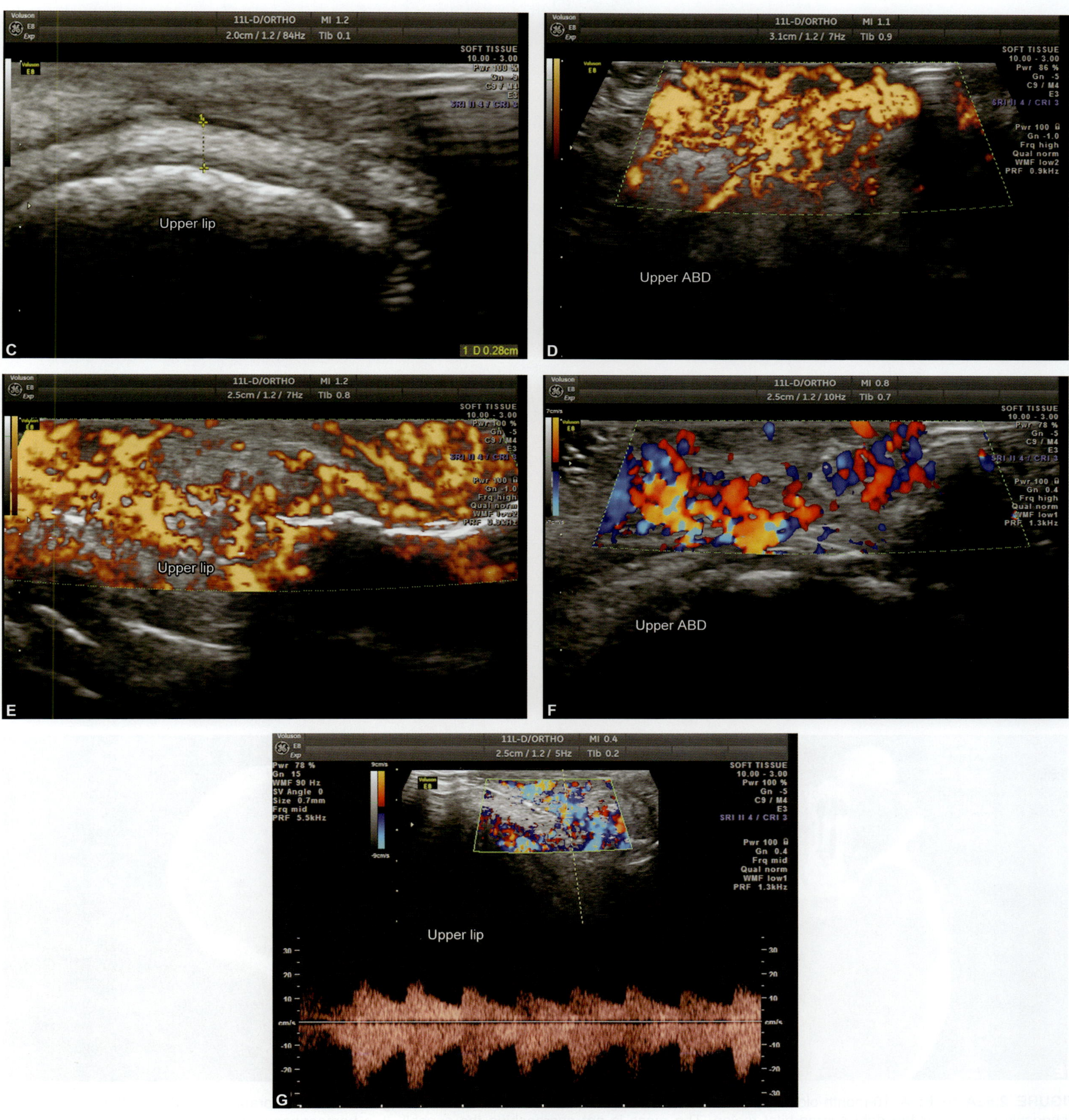

FIGURES 2.51C to G

FIGURES 2.51A to G: A patient presented with soft tissue nodular masses over the left side of upper lip. The masses are hard in consistency and increasing in size. High resolution sonography shows multinodular soft tissue masses over the upper lip. They are homogeneous in texture. No calcification is seen in them. Few hypoechoic areas are seen in them suggestive of dilated vessels. **On color flow imaging,** multiple vessels are seen feeding them. **On spectral Doppler tracing,** moderate arterial flow is seen in them. The gingiva is also thickened and shows hypertrophy. Findings are suggestive of angiomatous vascular malformation.

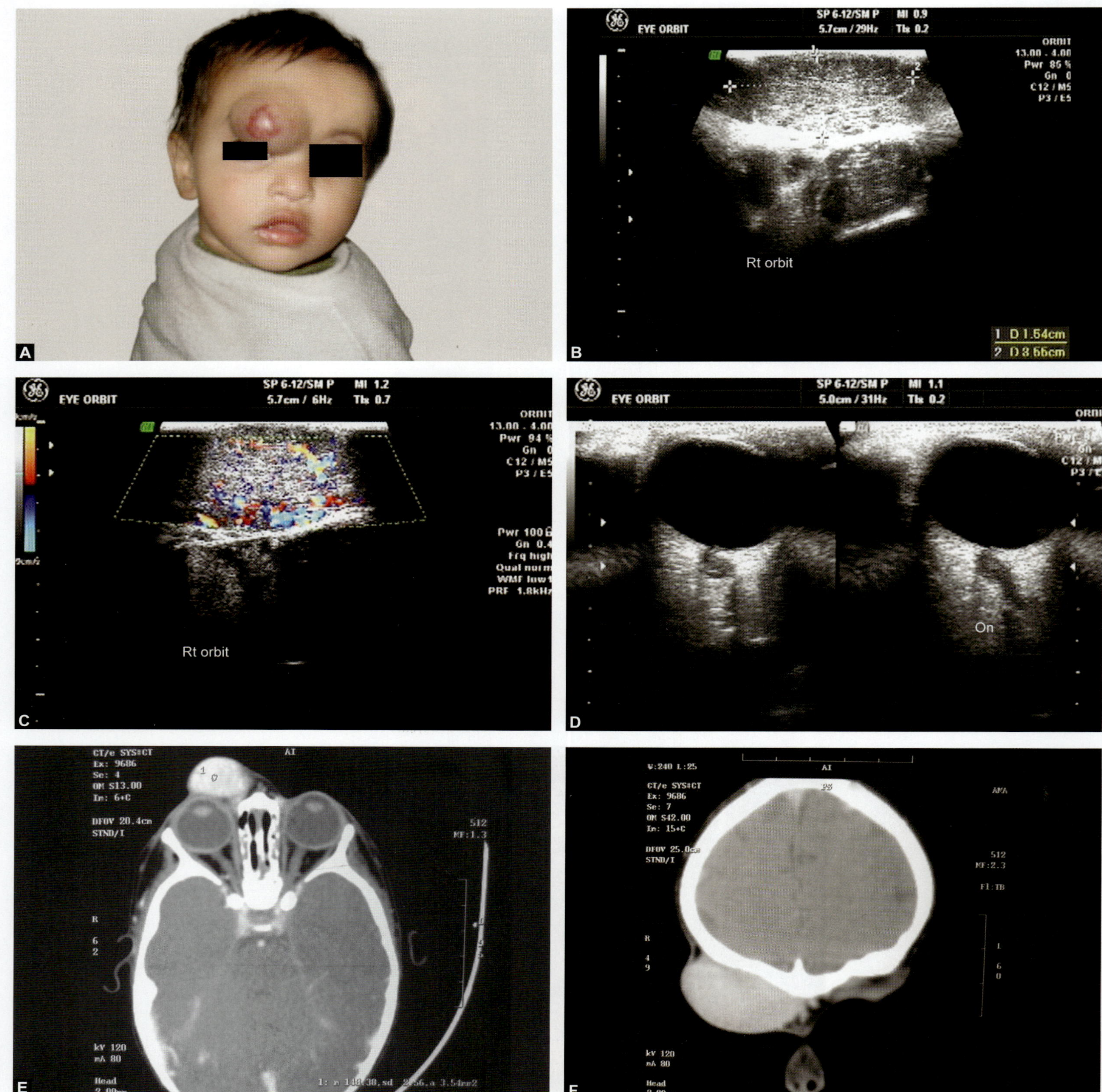

FIGURE 2.52A to F: A 10-month-old baby presented with big soft tissue mass over the right forehead supraorbital region. HRSG shows a big echogenic mass over the right supraorbital region. The mass is not encroaching the eyeball. It is homogeneous in texture. No calcification is seen in the mass. On color flow imaging, multiple vessels are seen feeding the mass suggestive of highly vascular mass. CT scan of same patient shows highly vascular mass showing intense on contrast examination. However, it is not seen invading the bone.

CHAPTER 3

Thyroid

PK Srivastava

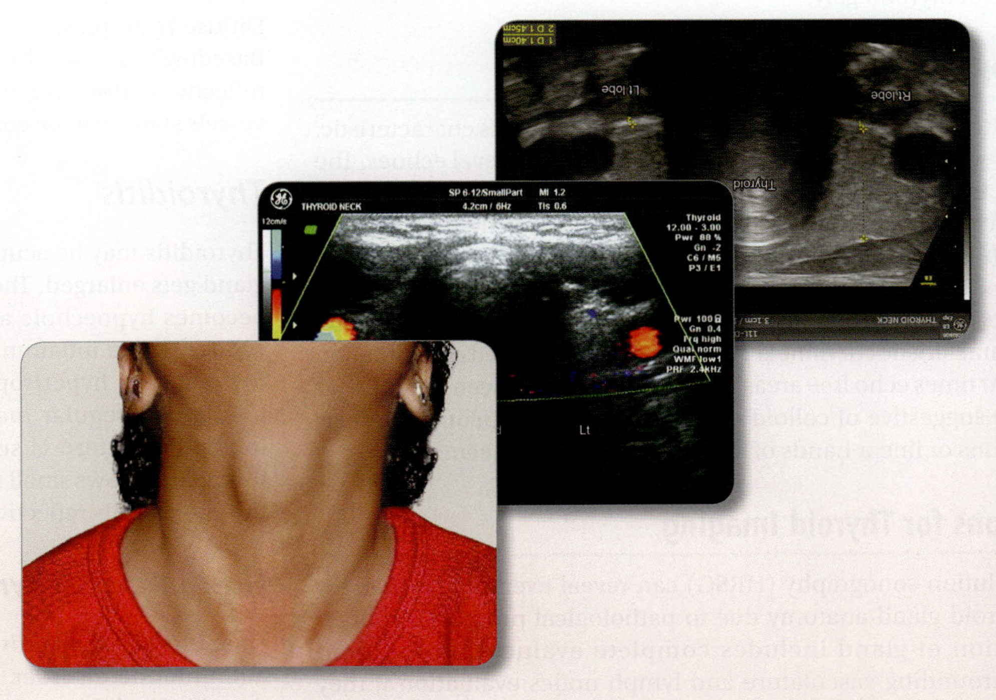

INTRODUCTION

High-resolution sonography (HRSG) has become an established imaging modality to evaluate thyroid gland and its diseases. Since, the gland is located superficially in anterior part of neck, it is an ideal organ to be imaged by HRSG. High-frequency transducers of 7.5 and 10 MHz are the ideal probes for thyroid imaging. However, in big thyroid mass, 5 MHz transducer is also required. Linear probes are preferred due to their wide contact surface.

Method

The patient is examined in supine position with extended neck with direct contact scanning technique. A thorough examination includes complete visualization of the thyroid gland, neck vessels, other adjoining structures and lymph node assessment, if they are enlarged. Subtle anatomic changes in thyroid gland and adjoining structures can be easily picked up on HRSG.

Normal Anatomy and Sono Appearance

The thyroid gland is situated in anterior part of the neck. The lateral lobes are situated on either side of trachea. They are connected with a band called isthmus. The lateral lobes are bounded laterally by great vessels, common carotid artery laterally and anteriorly. The recurrent laryngeal nerve lies in between carotid artery and jugular vein in a groove. Isthmus of gland lies anterior to trachea crossing it to both sides joining both lateral lobes. The normal gland measures more than 6–7 cm in length with thickness of 1–2 cm. The thickness of the gland is more reliable parameter than length and if it is more than 16 mm in thickness, it is suggestive of thyromegaly.

Sono Appearance

Normal ultrasonographic appearance of thyroid gland is characteristic. The gland shows homogeneous texture with medium level echoes. The echogenicity is more than the surrounding strap muscles. The gland is entrapped in thin highly reflective capsule. Vascular structures are seen piercing the glandular tissue mainly in upper parts. The strap muscles (sternohyoid and sternothyroid) are seen as sonolucent bands along the anterior surface of the thyroid gland. The air filled trachea in the midline gives a characteristic curvilinear reflection with associated reverberation artifacts. At times echo free areas of 2–3 mm in size are seen in the gland substance suggestive of colloid collection. In elderly people, nodular calcifications or linear bands of fibrous tissue may be seen.

Indications for Thyroid Imaging

High-resolution sonography (HRSG) can reveal even minor changes in the thyroid gland anatomy due to pathological process. A routine examination of gland includes complete evaluation of thyroid gland, surrounding vasculature and lymph nodes evaluation if they are enlarged. When thyroid is partly present in retrosternal area, additional scans should be taken from suprasternal notch to see the retrosternal extension of the gland. Any ultrasonographic assessment of thyroid pathology should first determine the nature of glandular involvement, whether it is diffuse parenchymal disease, multinodular disease or focal or solitary thyroid nodule. However, any combination of these appearances can occur. The thyroid nodule should be further evaluated on the basis of its reflectivity, presence of cyst, calcification, degeneration, margins and presence of echo-poor halo.

Diffuse Thyroid Disease

Diffuse thyroid disease includes thyroid hyperplasia which is most common pathology of thyroid gland. It may results due to iodine deficiency, may be familial or due to unilateral lobectomy. It may involve one or both lobes. When most of the gland is enlarged, it results into goiter. Diffuse hyperplasia may result in enlargement of one or both lobes. The gland size enlarges. The great vessels deviate laterally due to enlargement of gland. Pressure will be noted on trachea. However, tracheal walls are never infiltrated. The gland echotexture becomes inhomogeneous, but reflectivity remains the same. Nodular hyperplasia of thyroid gland shows multiple nodules in the gland. They vary in their size and numbers. They are seen studded in the normal parenchyma of the gland. HRSG can very well identify the multinodular status of the gland, which cannot be assessed clinically. HRSG can pick up nodule of even as small as 5 mm. A typical nodule has got the same reflectivity as normal gland. The nodules are isoechogenic. About 25% of these nodules show colloid or hemorrhagic degeneration. Calcification may also present as bright as echogenic foci in the nodules. They are accompanied with acoustic shadowing. Benign calcification is coarse and is seen scattered throughout the parenchyma. However, all visible nodules must be evaluated for possible malignancy, as 10–30% of the nodules may be malignant.

Basedow's Disease

Diffuse hyperplasia of thyroid with thyrotoxicosis is characteristic of Basedow's disease. The gland shows generalized enlargement with low reflectivity. However, nodules are absent and veins are enlarged. The vessels status can be confirmed on color flow imaging.

Thyroiditis

Thyroiditis may be acute, subacute or chronic. In early thyroiditis, the gland gets enlarged. The enlargement may be partial or diffuse. Gland becomes hypoechoic and coarse. Parenchyma shows medium level echoes. Acute inflammation may lead to abscess formation. Chronic thyroiditis in hypertrophic stage shows glandular enlargement with lobulated irregular margins. The echogenicity is reduced. Typical lobulated pattern is seen which is due to fibrotic bands. Atrophic thyroiditis shows small shrunken gland. It becomes difficult to identify the gland, as its reflectivity merges with the surrounding tissue.

Hashimoto's Thyroiditis

Hashimoto's thyroiditis or chronic lymphocytic thyroiditis is an autoimmune disorder. There is painless, diffuse enlargement of the thyroid gland. It may involve one lobe or both lobes. The gland shows typical sonographic features. It becomes enlarged. Echotexture becomes hypoechoic and coarse. However, it is homogeneous in texture. No normal parenchymal pattern is identified. At times discrete nodules may be seen in Hashimoto's thyroiditis.

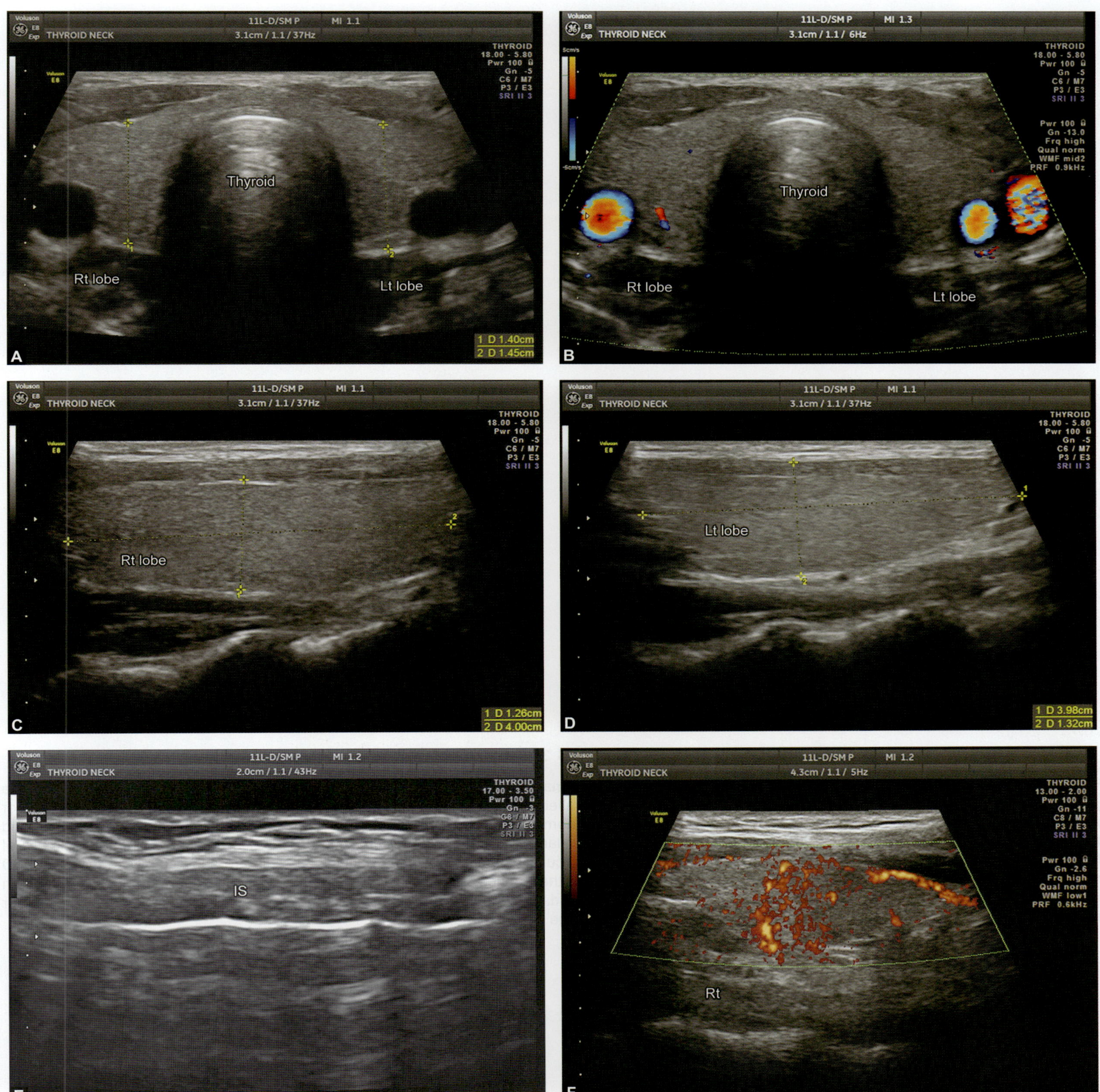

FIGURES 3.1A to F

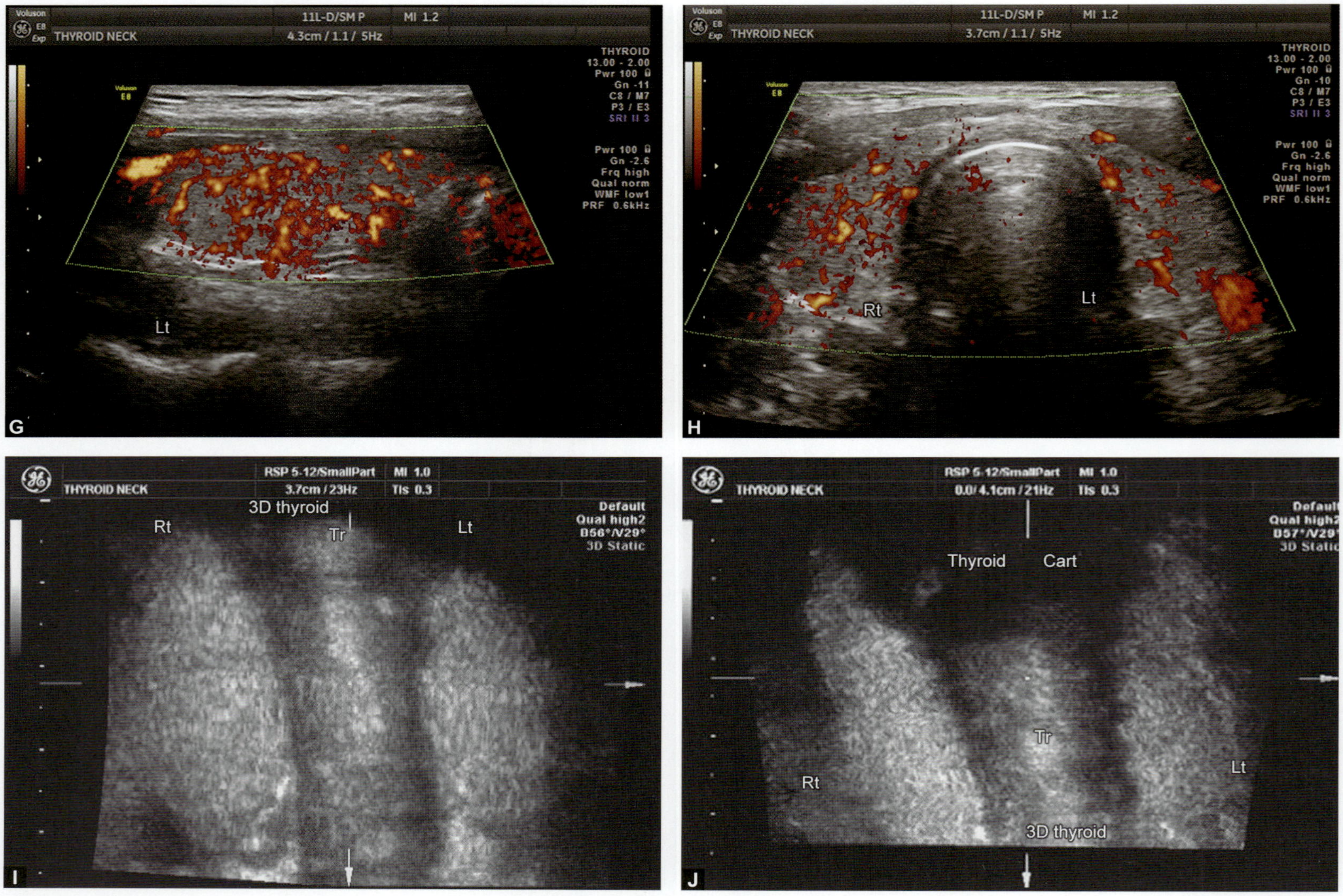

FIGURES 3.1G to J

FIGURES 3.1A to J: Normal thyroid and its relations. HRSG shows normal thyroid gland showing both the lobes, isthmus and the tracheal rings. The gland texture is homogeneous and shows medium level echoes. Highly reflective tracheal rings are seen as cresentric rings. Isthmus is seen a strap or band joint the lobes. The longitudinal images of the thyroid lobes show normal homogeneous gland in long axis. Isthmus is seen homogeneous band or strap joining the two lobes of thyroid. It shows normal echotexture similar to thyroid gland and crossing the trachea anteriorly. Normal thickness of the isthmus is 5 mm (upper limit). Color Doppler imaging shows high vascular nature of the gland. Multiple vessels are seen supplying the gland. 3D imaging of the thyroid gland in coronal plane shows gland in relation to the trachea. HRSG shows normal thyroid gland seen bounded by common carotid artery on either side. Homogeneous echoes are seen in the gland. Power Doppler color flow imaging of thyroid gland shows high vascular nature of the gland. Multiple small vessels are seen traversing through the parenchyma.

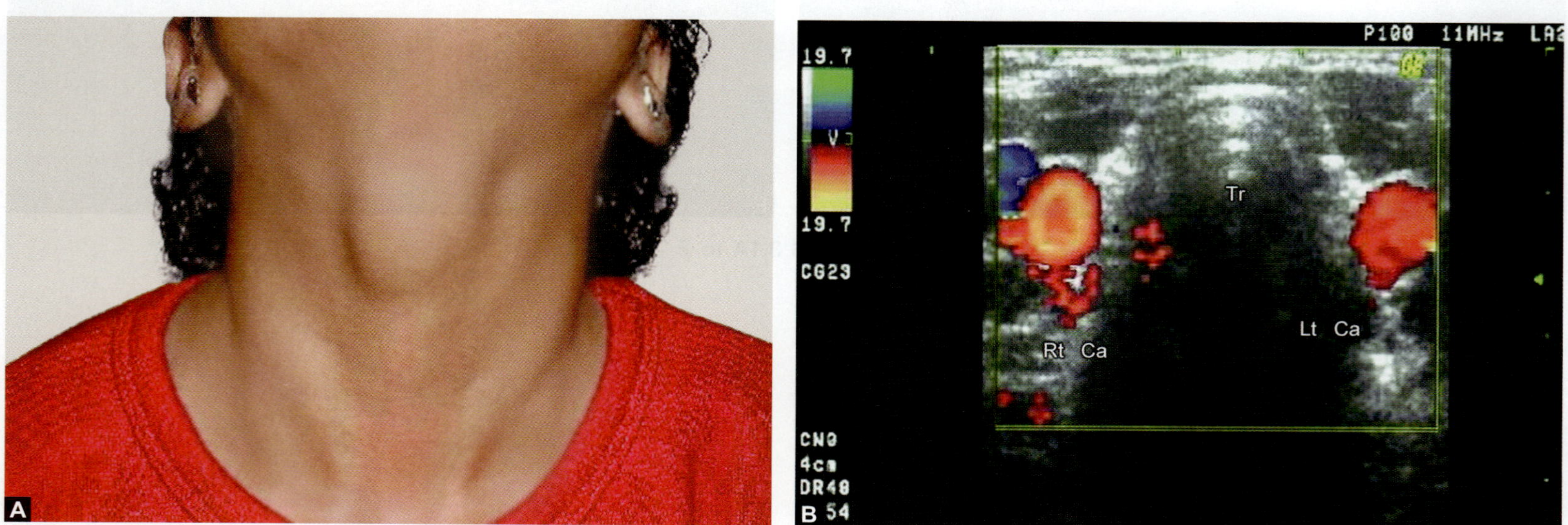

FIGURES 3.2A and B

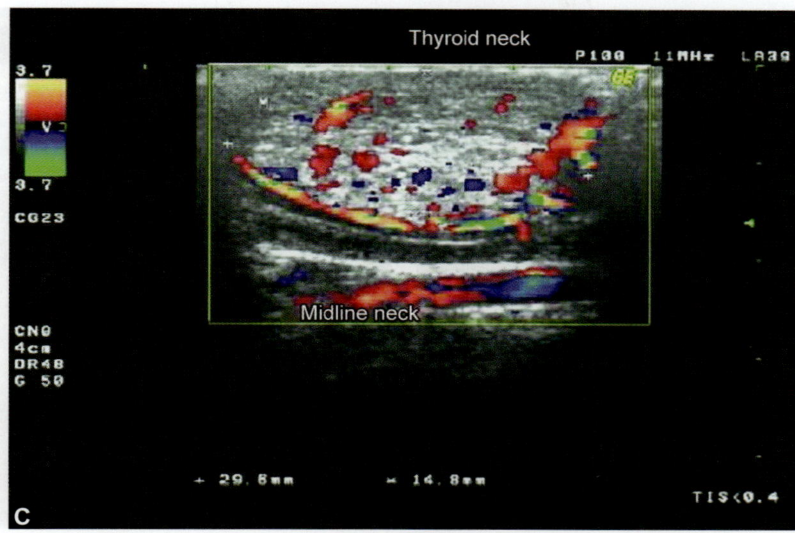

FIGURE 3.2C

FIGURES 3.2A to C: Ectopic thyroid. A young child presented with midline nodular mass. HRSG shows absence of thyroid gland on either side of the trachea in the thyroid fossa. A homogeneous nodular shadow similar to the thyroid gland is seen in the midline suggestive of ectopic thyroid. On color flow imaging it shows increased flow suggestive of rich vascular supply of the ectopic thyroid.

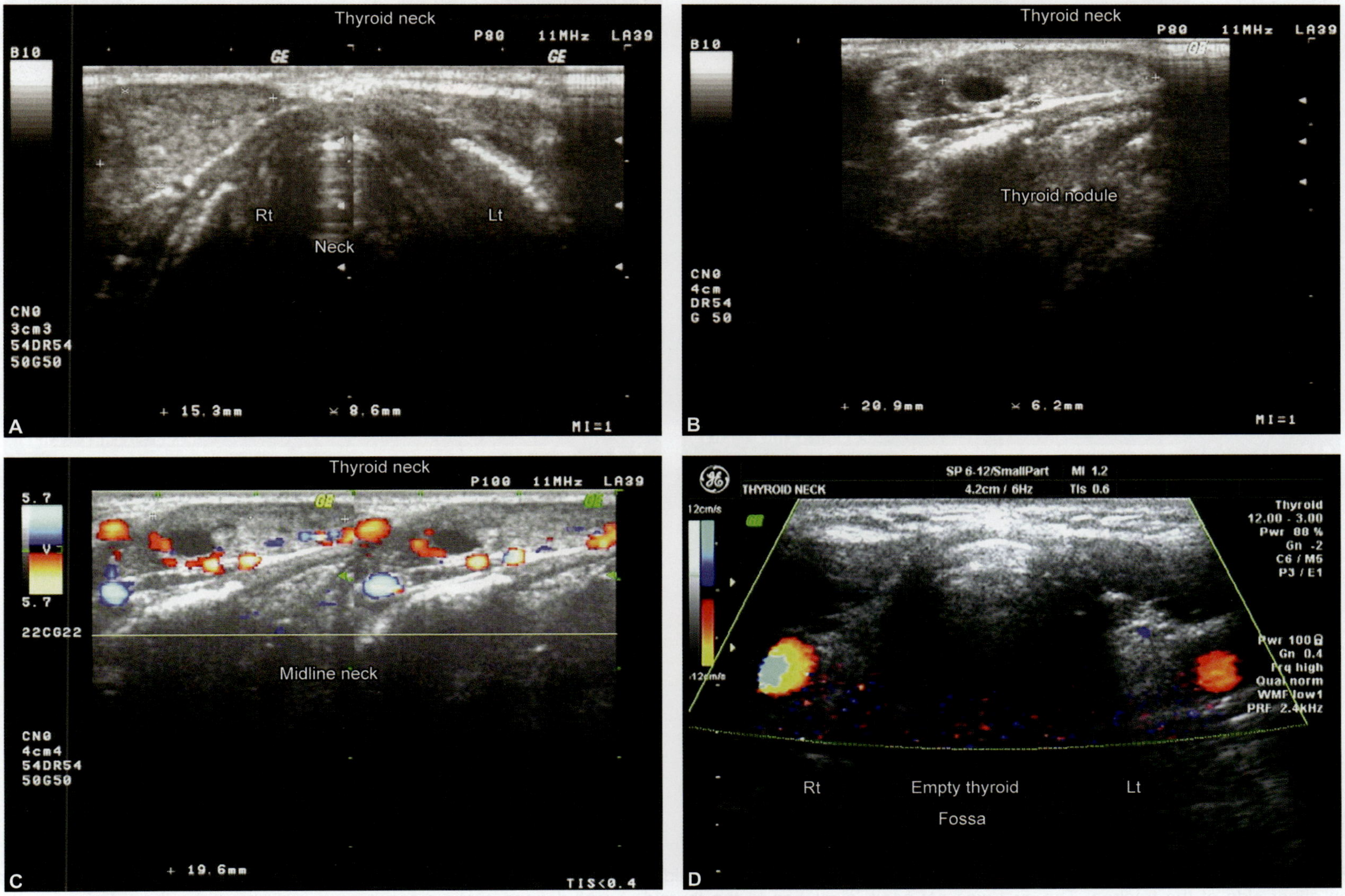

FIGURES 3.3A to D

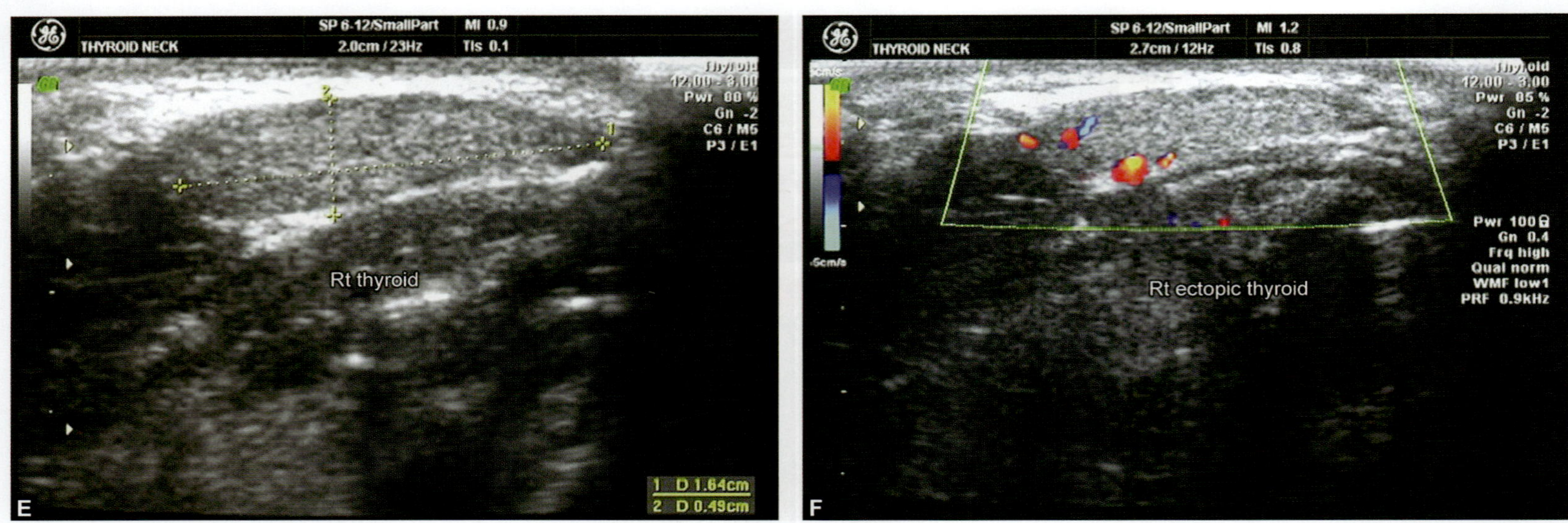

FIGURES 3.3E and F

FIGURES 3.3A to F: Ectopic thyroid. HRSG shows small normal thyroid glandular tissue in the right upper cervical region. Color Doppler imaging also shows rich flow in the gland. Normal thyroid gland is not seen in the thyroid fossa on either side. Same patient came after 2 years for repeat evaluation of the ectopic thyroid gland. HRSG shows the ectopic thyroid in the right upper cervical region as seen in the previous study. Normal thyroid gland was not seen in thyroid fossa.

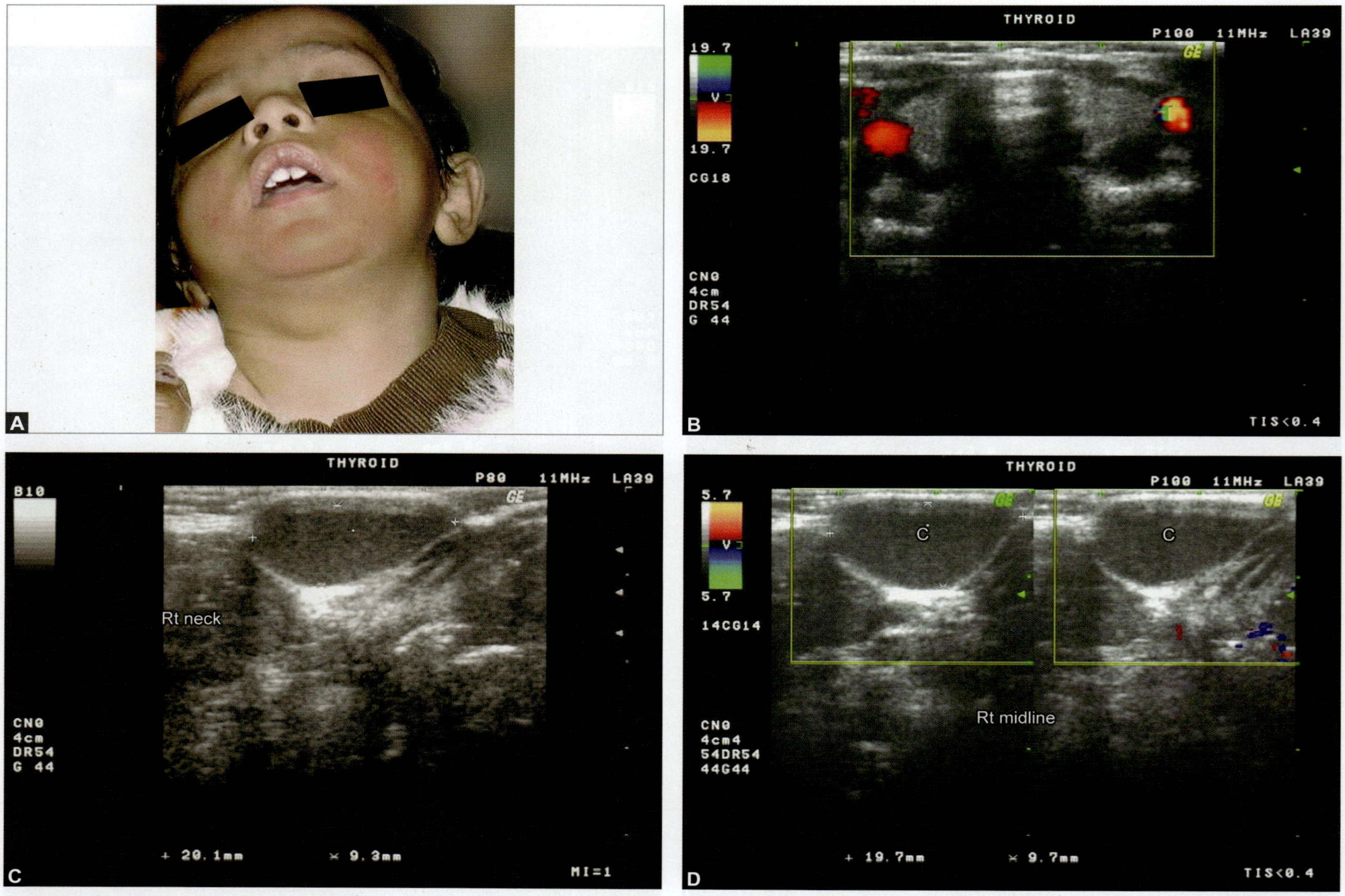

A B C D

Rt neck

Rt midline

FIGURES 3.4A to D: Thyroglossal cyst. A child was presented with midline cystic mass. HRSG shows normal thyroid gland in the thyroid fossa on either side of the trachea. The cyst was not seen in relation to the thyroid. A well-defined cystic mass is seen just above the thyroid gland in the midline. The cyst shows homogeneous anechoic texture. No evidence of any internal echo is seen in it suggestive of thyroglossal cyst.

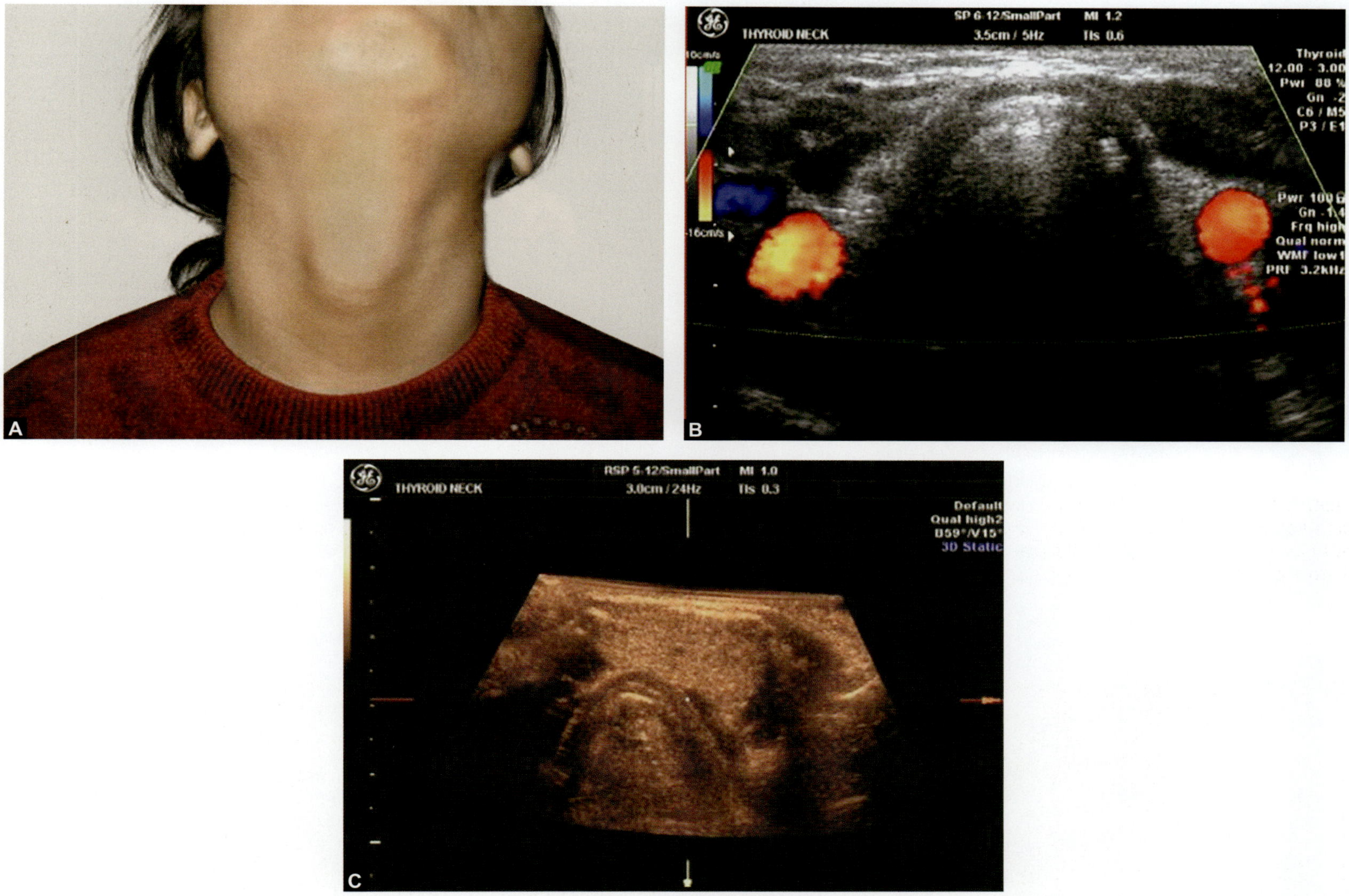

FIGURES 3.5A to C: Aberrant thyroid. A young girl presented with a soft tissue shadow in the midline. HRSG shows well-defined homogeneous nodular shadow seen in the neck upper mid cervical region. It measures 30 × 8 mm in size. Echotexture is similar to the thyroid gland. On color flow imaging, moderate flow is seen in it. No calcification seen. Normal thyroid gland is not seen in both thyroid fossa. Findings are suggestive of aberrant thyroid.

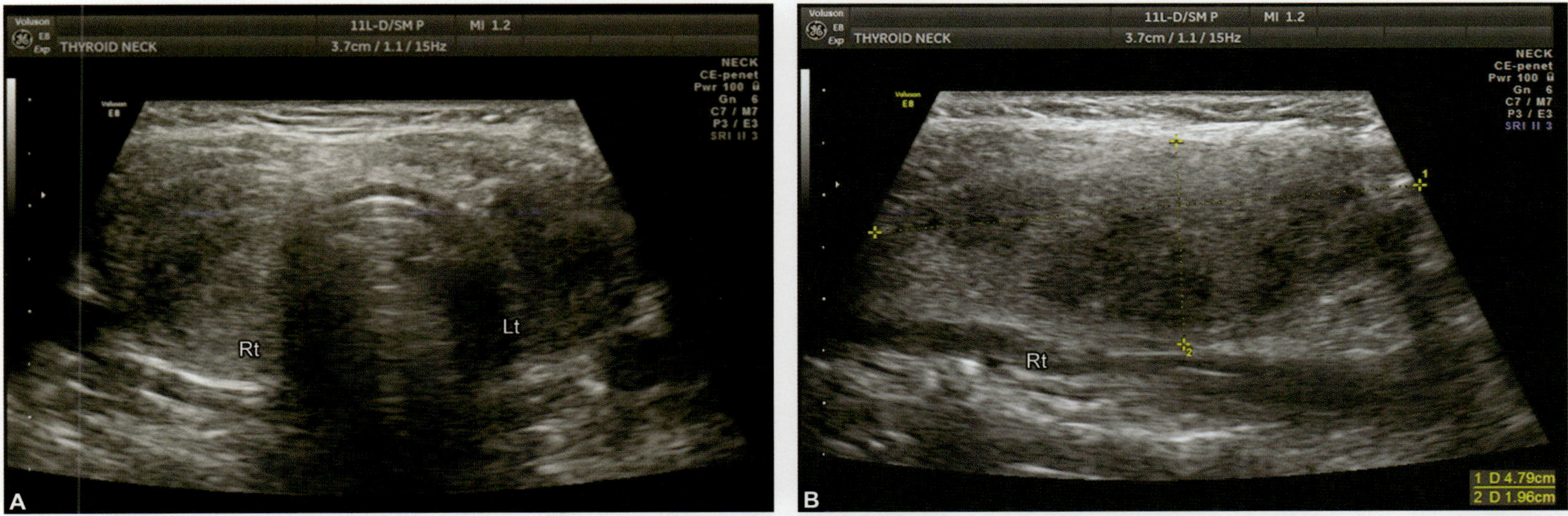

FIGURES 3.6A and B

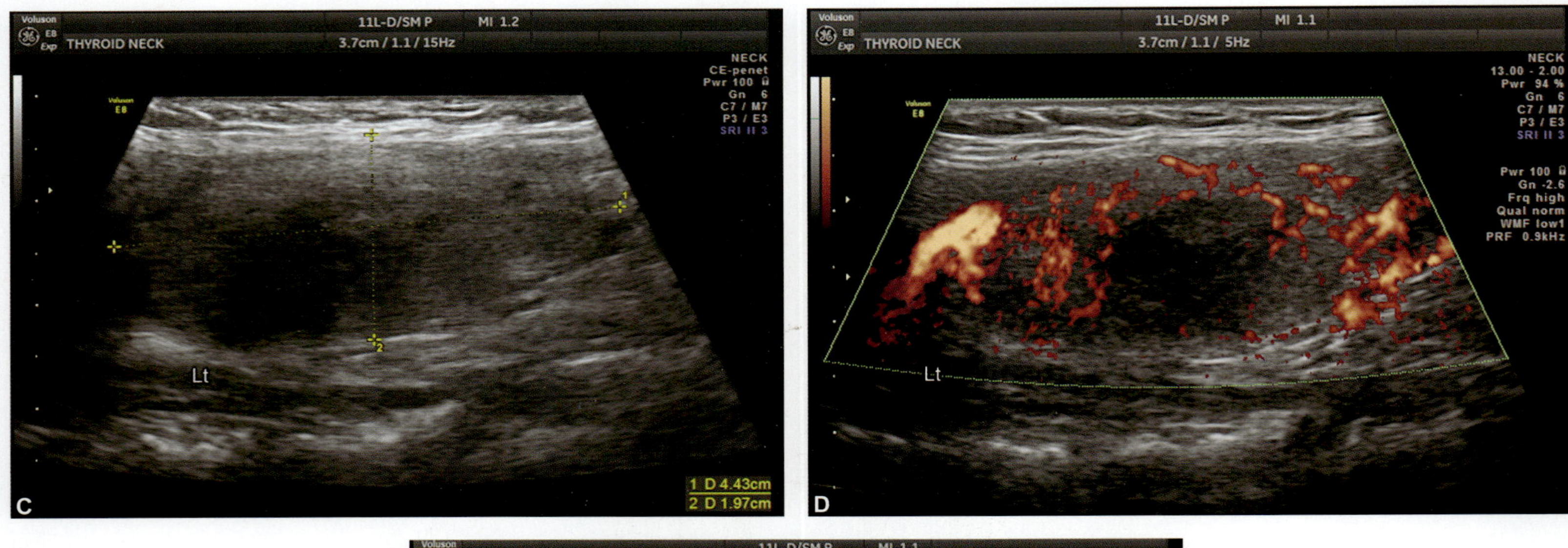

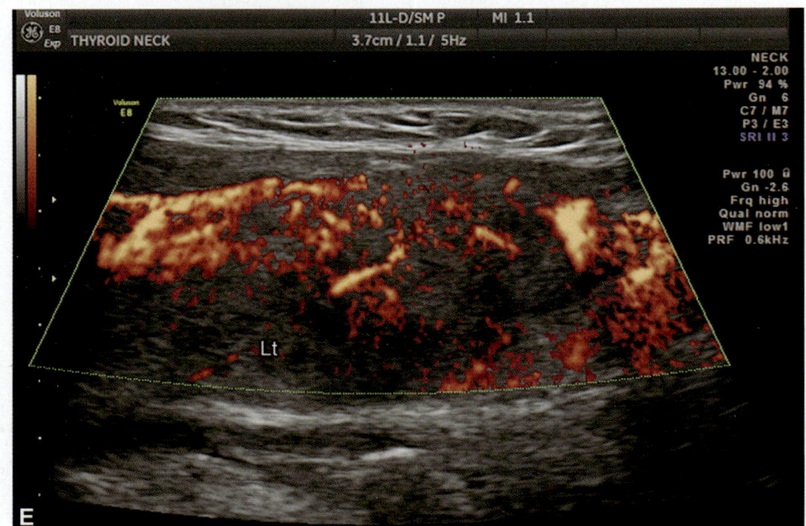

FIGURES 3.6C to E

FIGURES 3.6A to E: Acute thyroiditis. A lady presented with soft tissue painful swelling in the neck. HRSG shows enlarged both lobes of thyroid. They are edematous. Echotexture is normal. Right lobe measures 47 × 22 mm in size. Left lobe measures 45 × 2 mm in size. Irregular ill-defined inhomogeneous hypoechoic areas are seen in both the lobes. They are discrete in distribution. No calcification is seen in them. On color flow imaging, increased flow is seen in the gland on either side. Isthmus of the gland is normal. Findings are suggestive of acute thyroiditis.

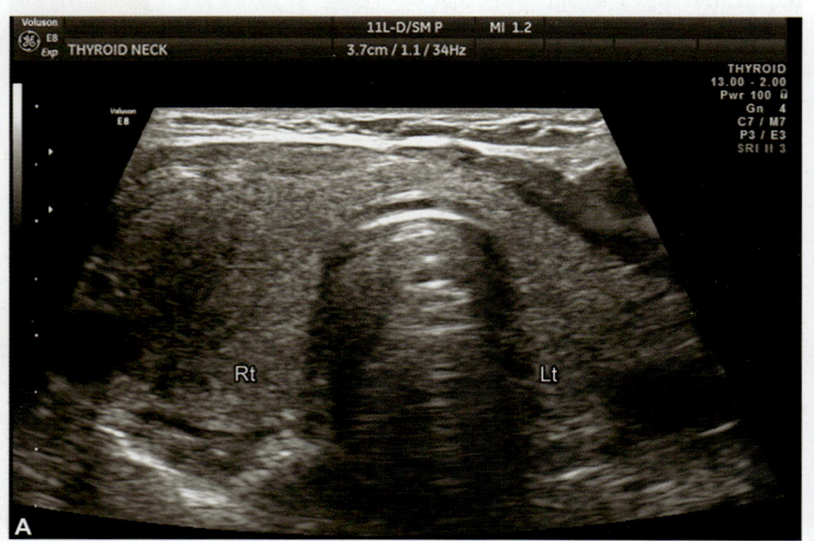

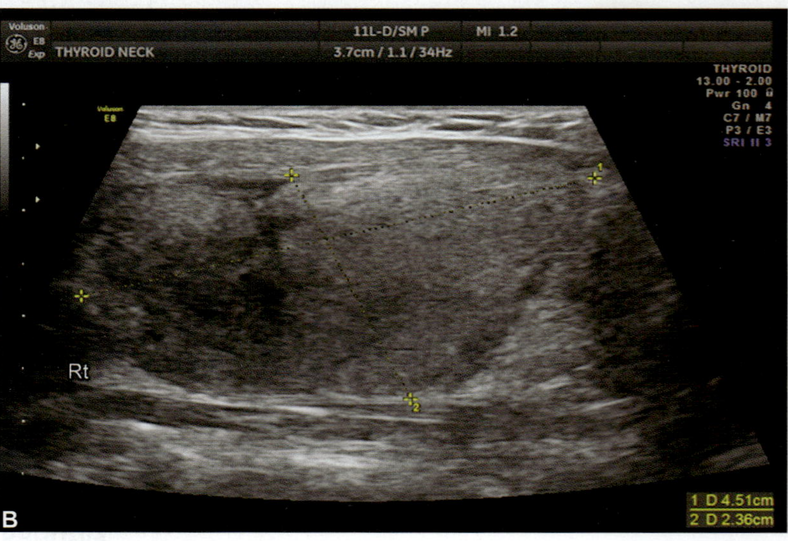

FIGURES 3.7A and B

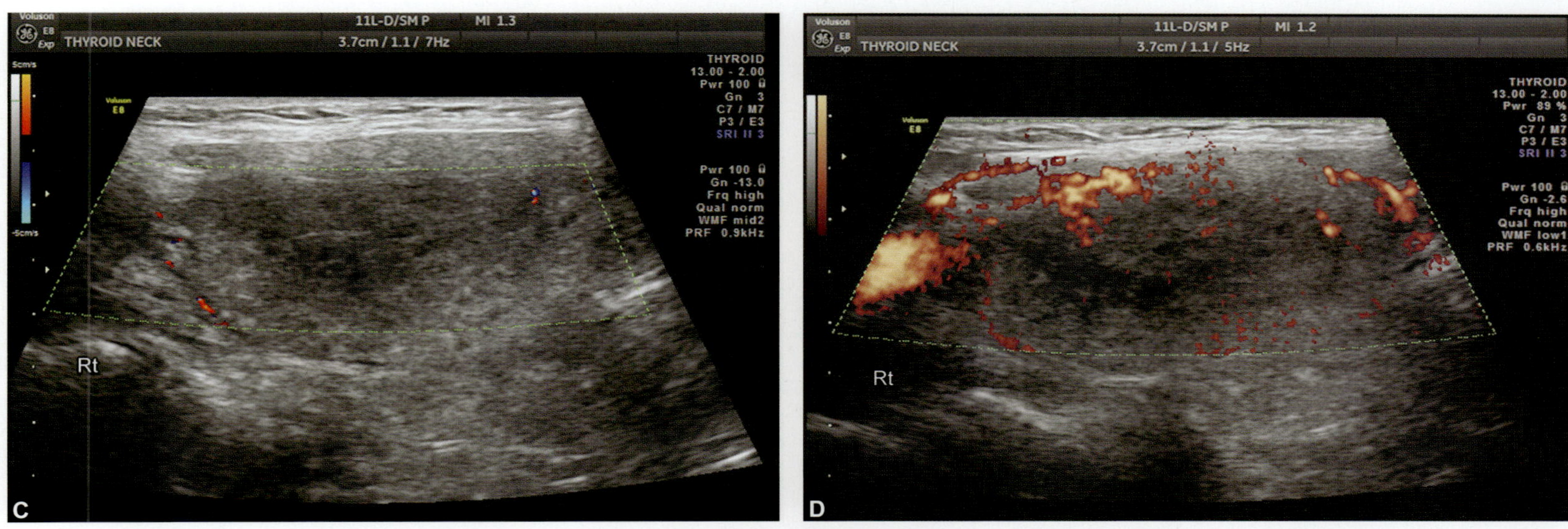

FIGURES 3.7C and D

FIGURES 3.7A to D: Acute thyroiditis. A patient presented with painful swelling in the right side of neck. HRSG shows diffuse enlargement of right lobe of thyroid. It is edematous and inhomogeneous in texture. It measures 45 × 23 mm in size. Hypoechoic areas are seen in the gland. On color flow imaging, capsular flow is seen in the gland. Findings are suggestive of acute thyroiditis.

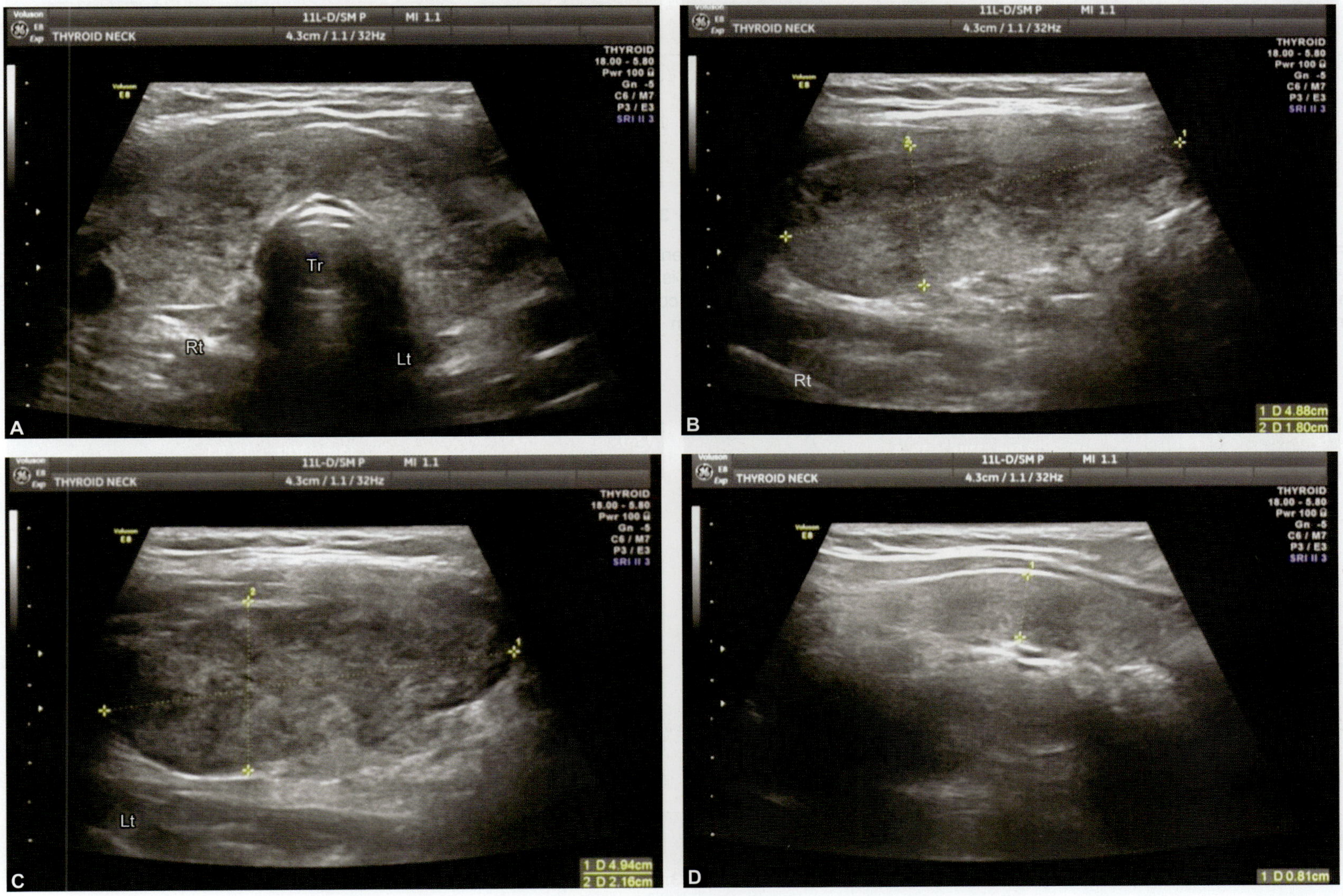

FIGURES 3.8A to D

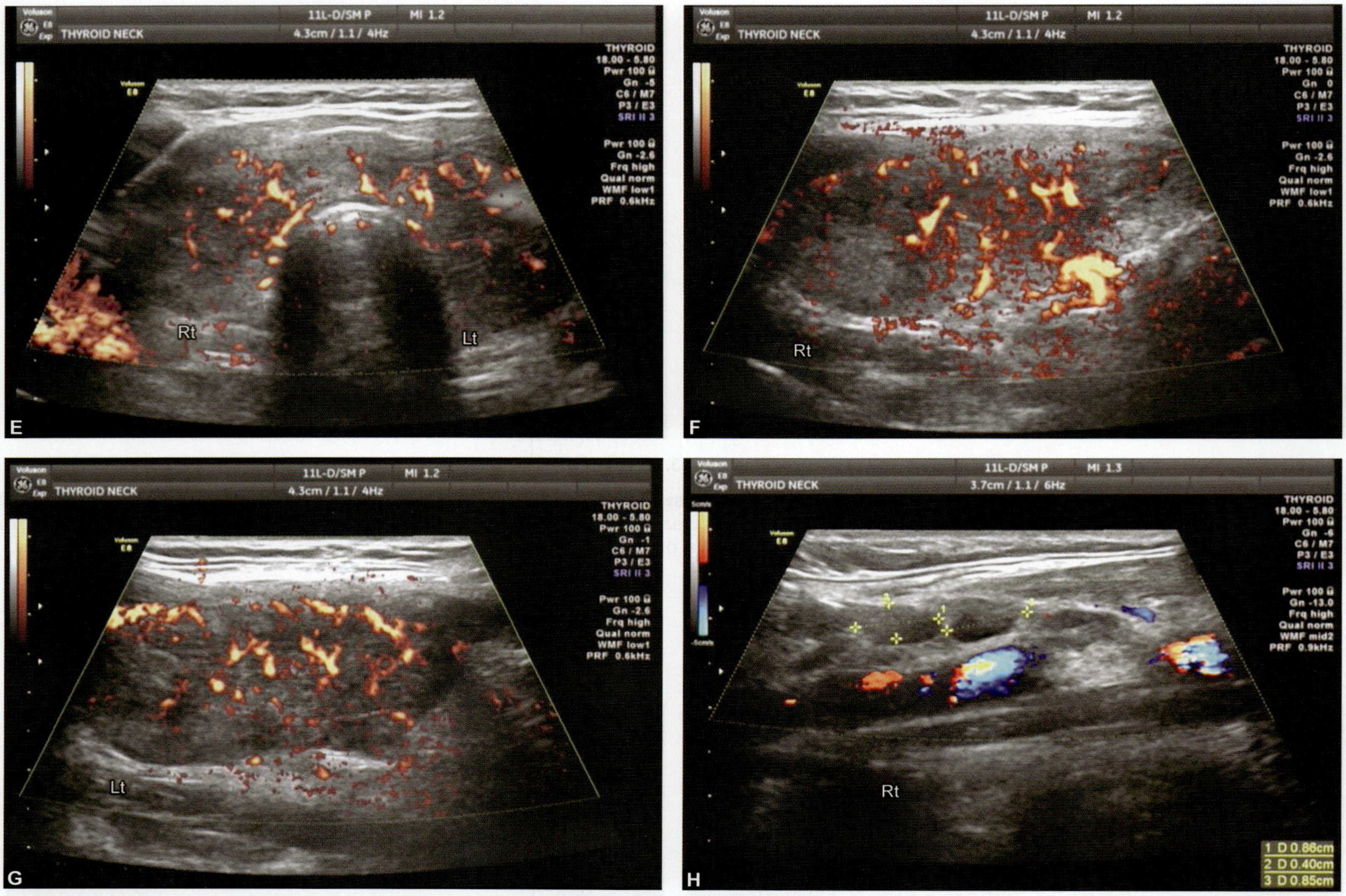

FIGURES 3.8E to H

FIGURES 3.8A to H: Acute thyroiditis involving both the lobes. A patient presented with acute thyroid swelling clinically the gland was tender. On HRSG diffuse enlargement of both lobes of thyroid is seen. The isthmus is also thickened. The texture of the gland is inhomogeneous. Hypoechoic areas are seen in the gland. But no focal mass is seen in the gland. On color flow imaging, increased flow is seen in the gland suggestive of acute inflammation of the thyroid. Few enlarged nodal shadows are also seen in right upper cervical region.

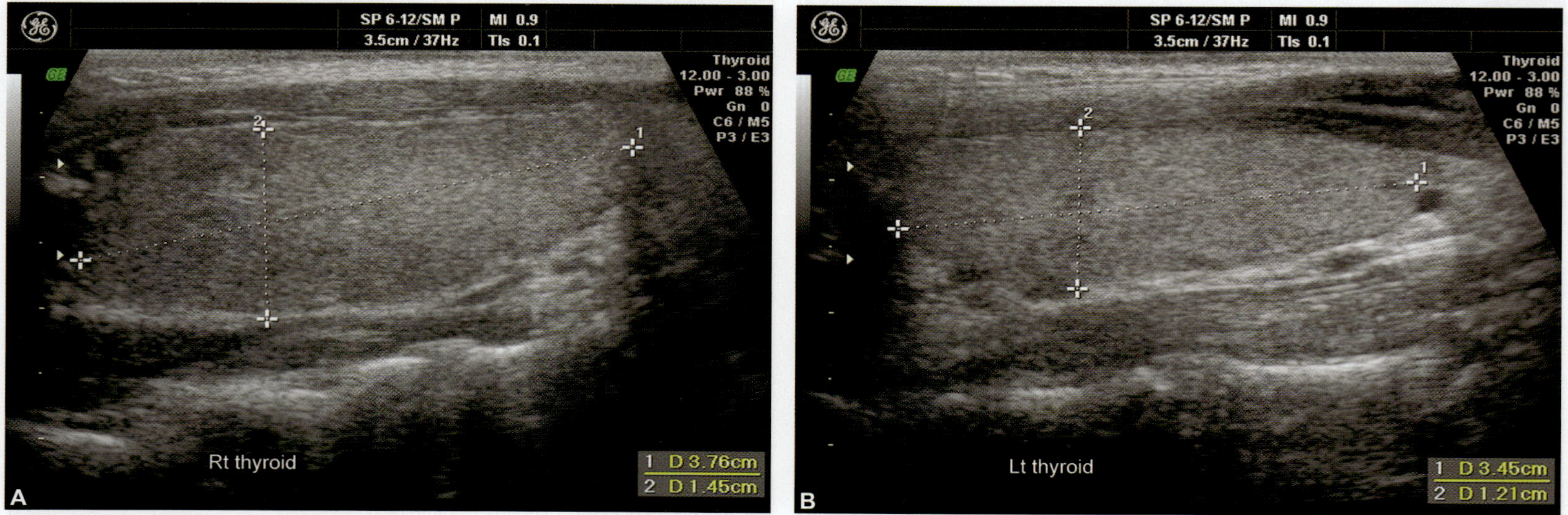

FIGURES 3.9A and B

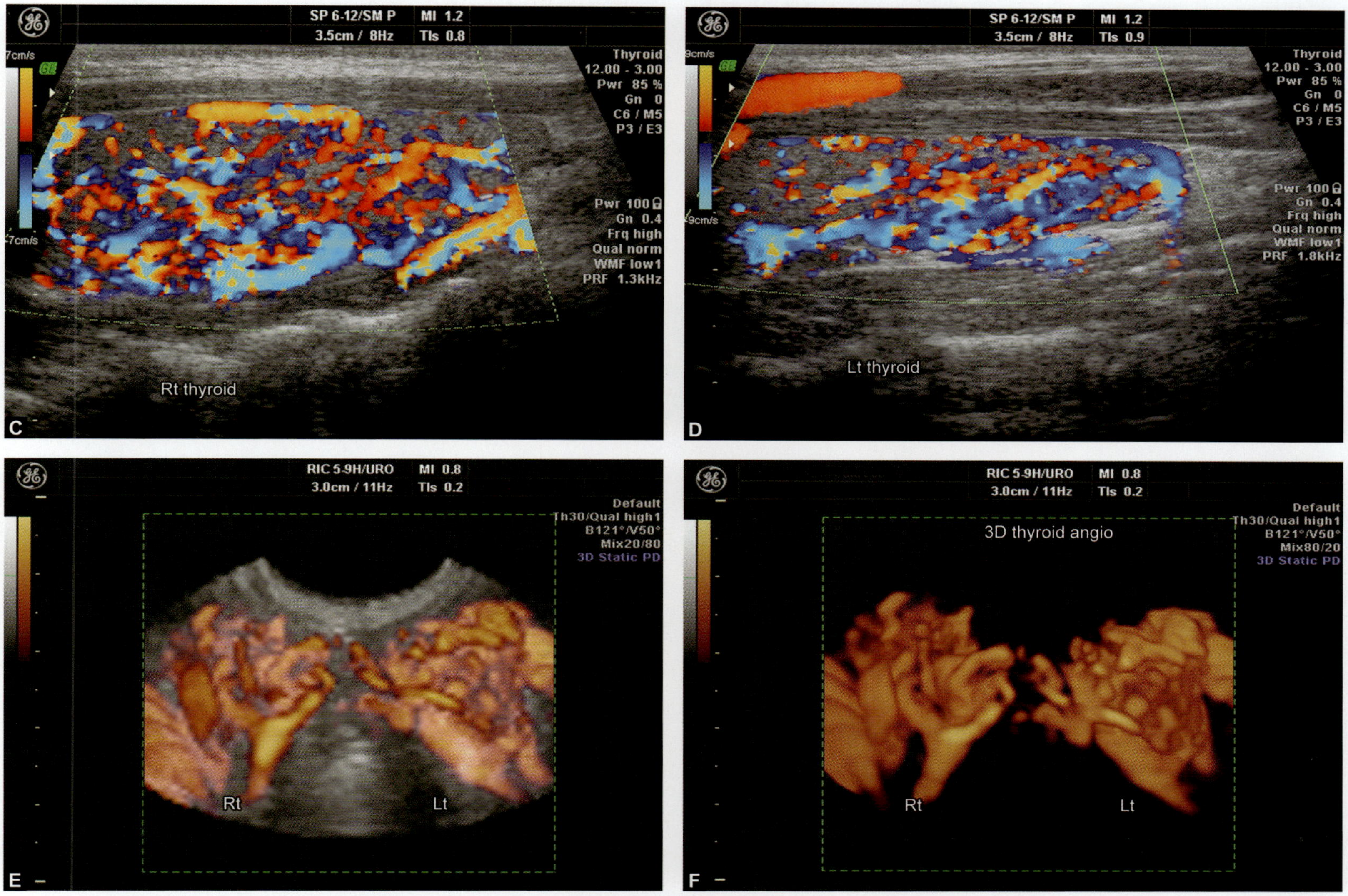

FIGURES 3.9C to F

FIGURES 3.9A to F: Thyrotoxicosis. A patient presented with soft tissue swelling in the neck. On HRSG both lobes of thyroid show hypoechoic texture. But no focal mass is seen in the gland. On color flow imaging, marked increased flow is seen in the thyroid. On power Doppler imaging, thyroid inferno sign is positive. 3D power Doppler angio shows multiple vessels feeding both lobes of thyroid suggestive of thyrotoxicosis.

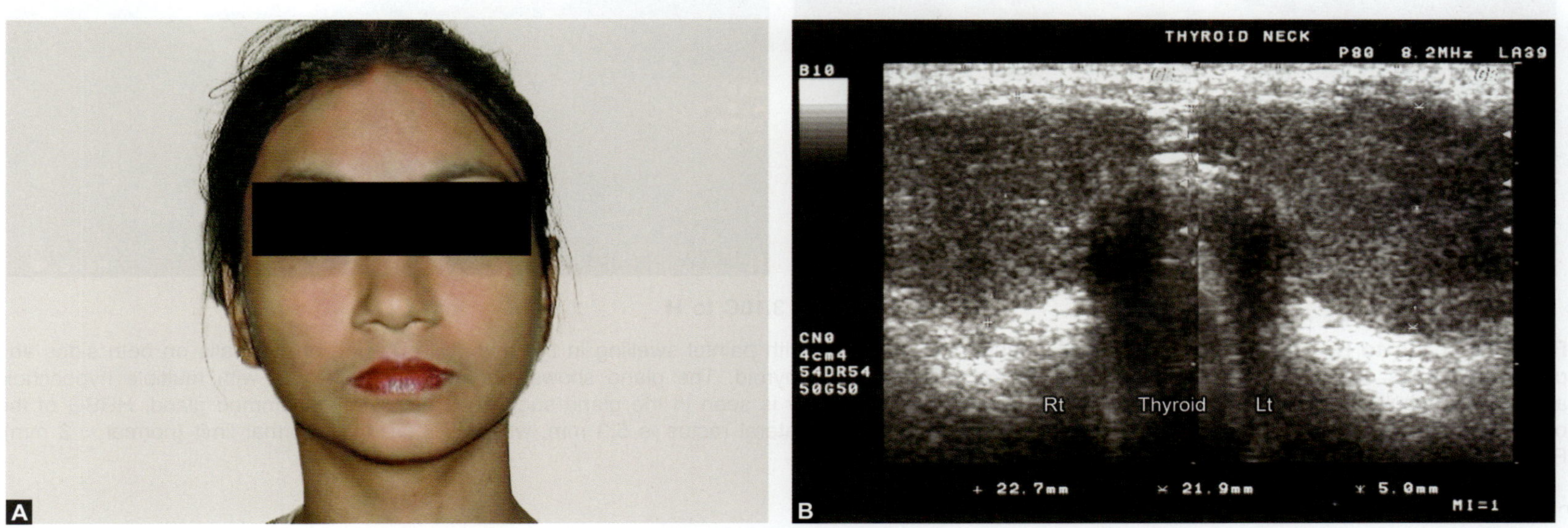

FIGURES 3.10A and B

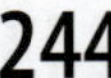

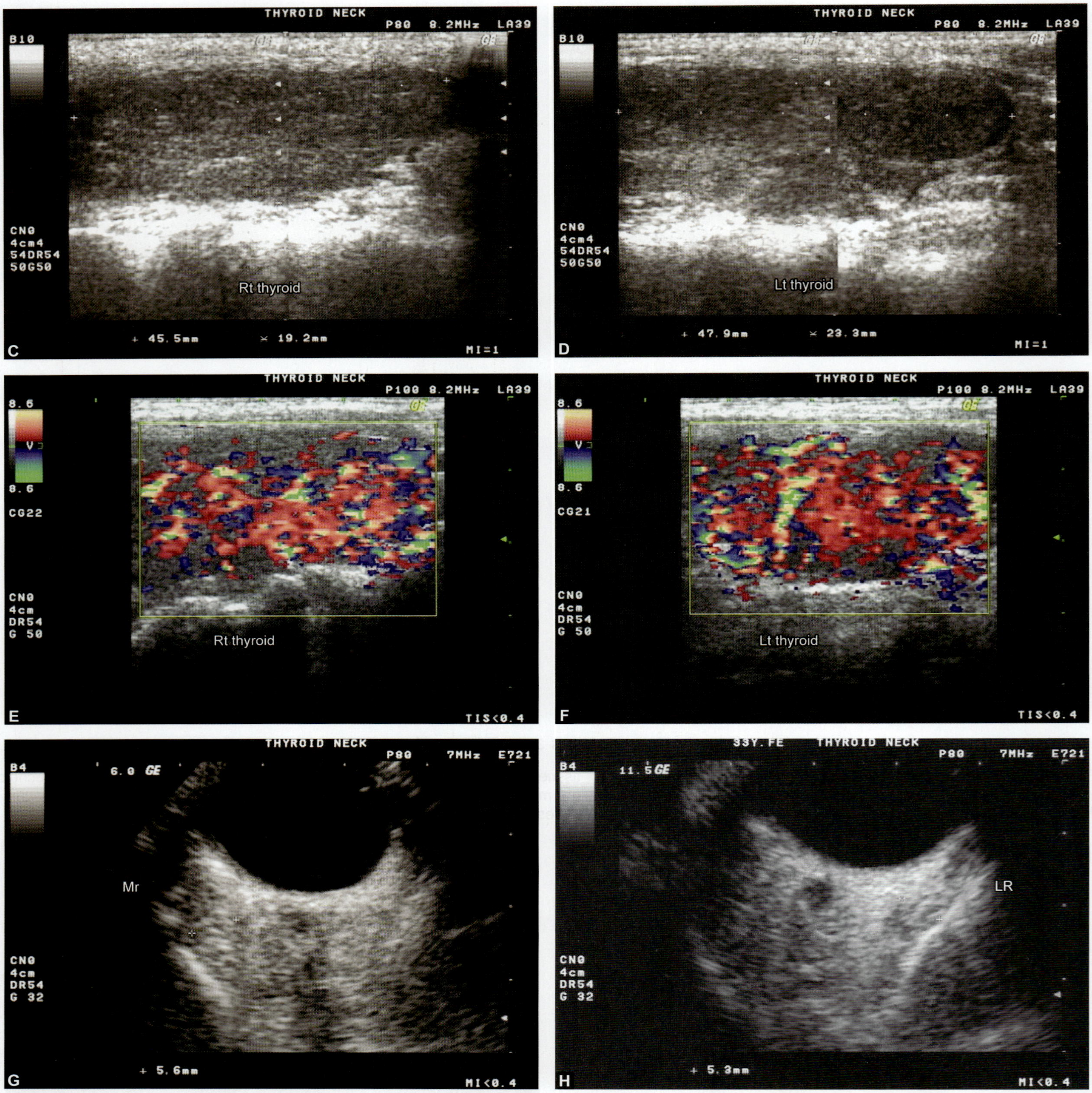

FIGURES 3.10C to H

FIGURES 3.10A to H: Acute thyrotoxicosis. A young lady presented with painful swelling in the neck with bulging of eye balls on both sides and pain in the eyes. HRSG shows diffuse enlargement of both lobes of thyroid. The gland shows inhomogeneous texture with multiple hypoechoic areas. Subcapsular edema is also seen. On color flow imaging, high flow is seen in the gland suggestive of acutely inflammed gland. HRSG of the orbit shows thickened recti muscles. The medial rectus is 5.6 mm and lateral rectus is 5.3 mm, which is more than normal limit (normal < 3 mm). Retrobulbar fat is also increased.

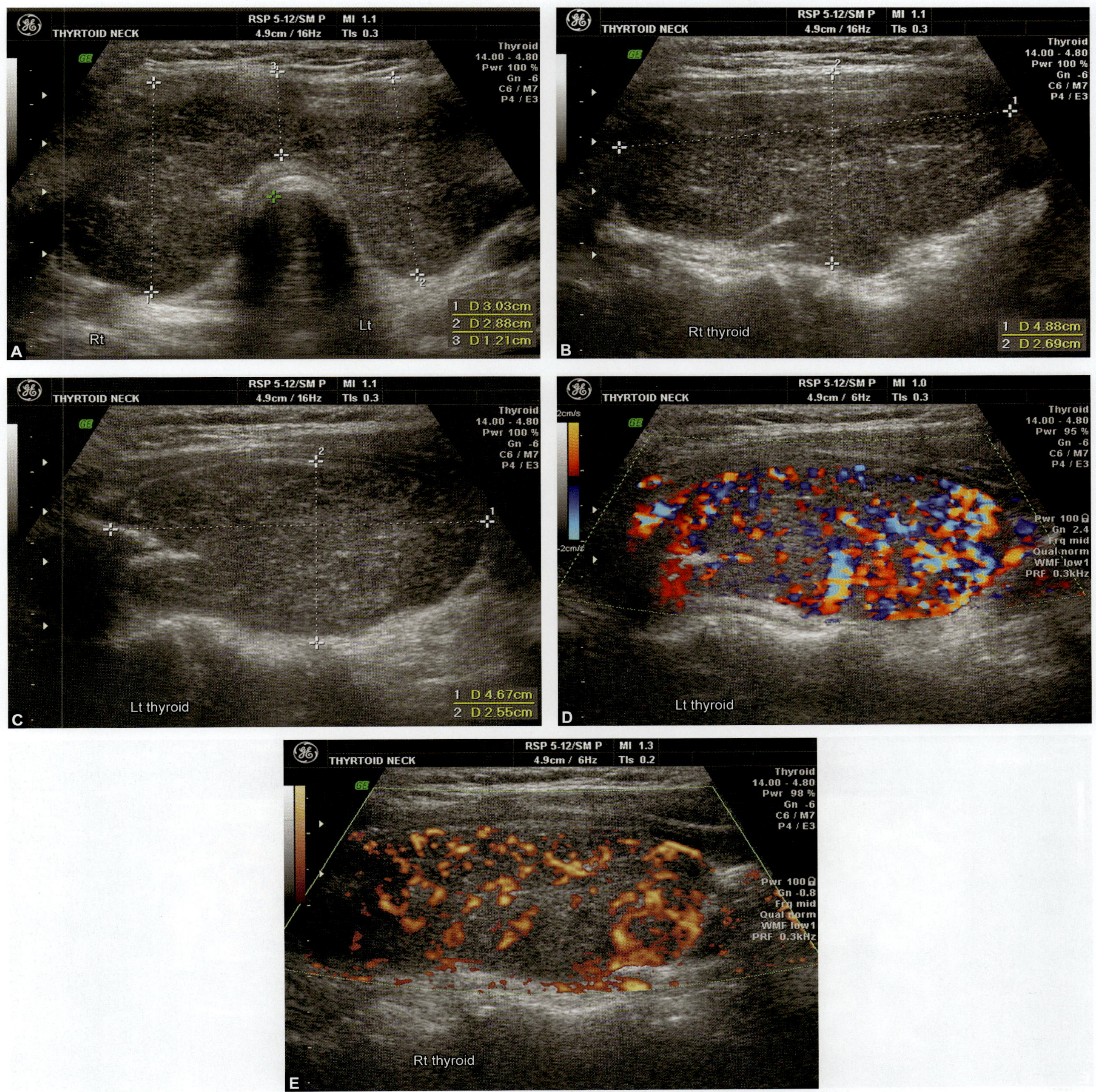

FIGURES 3.11A to E: Basedow's disease. HRSG shows diffuse enlargement of the thyroid gland involving both the lobes. The gland shows overall diffuse low reflectivity. However, it shows homogeneous texture. On color flow imaging, increased flow is seen in the gland. The veins show engorgement.

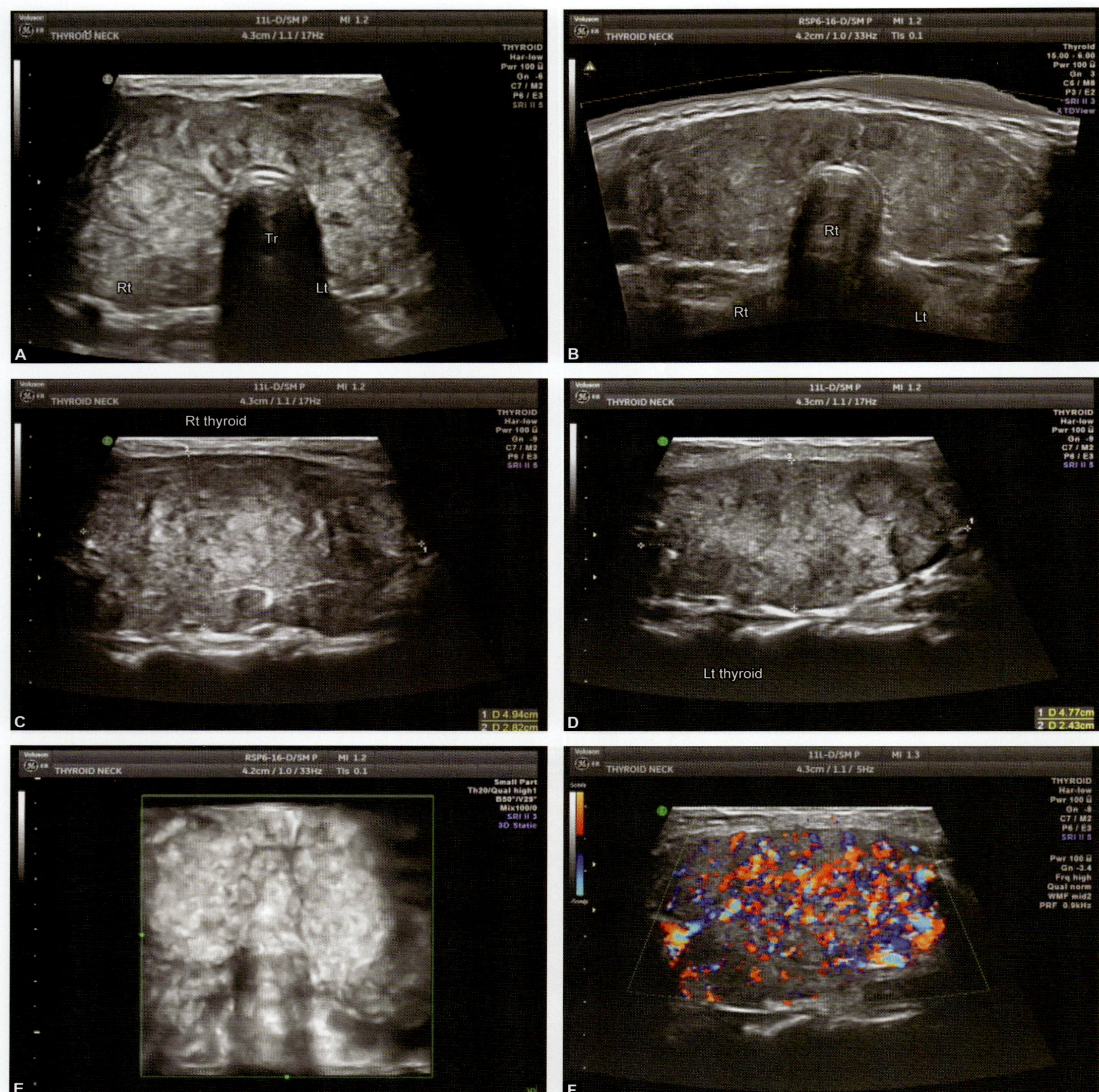

FIGURES 3.12A to F

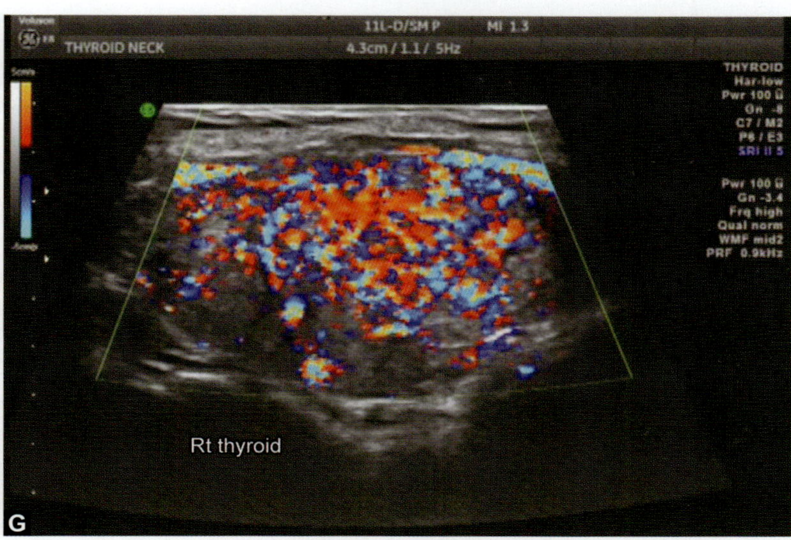

FIGURE 3.12G

FIGURES 3.12A to G: Diffuse thyroid enlargement. HRSG shows diffuse thyroid enlargement of both lobes of thyroid. Echotexture is inhomogeneous. Multiple small isoechogenic nodules are seen in both the lobes. On 3D imaging, the thyroid is seen wrapping around the trachea. But no calcification is seen in the gland. No cystic degeneration is seen. On color flow imaging, increased flow is seen in the gland.

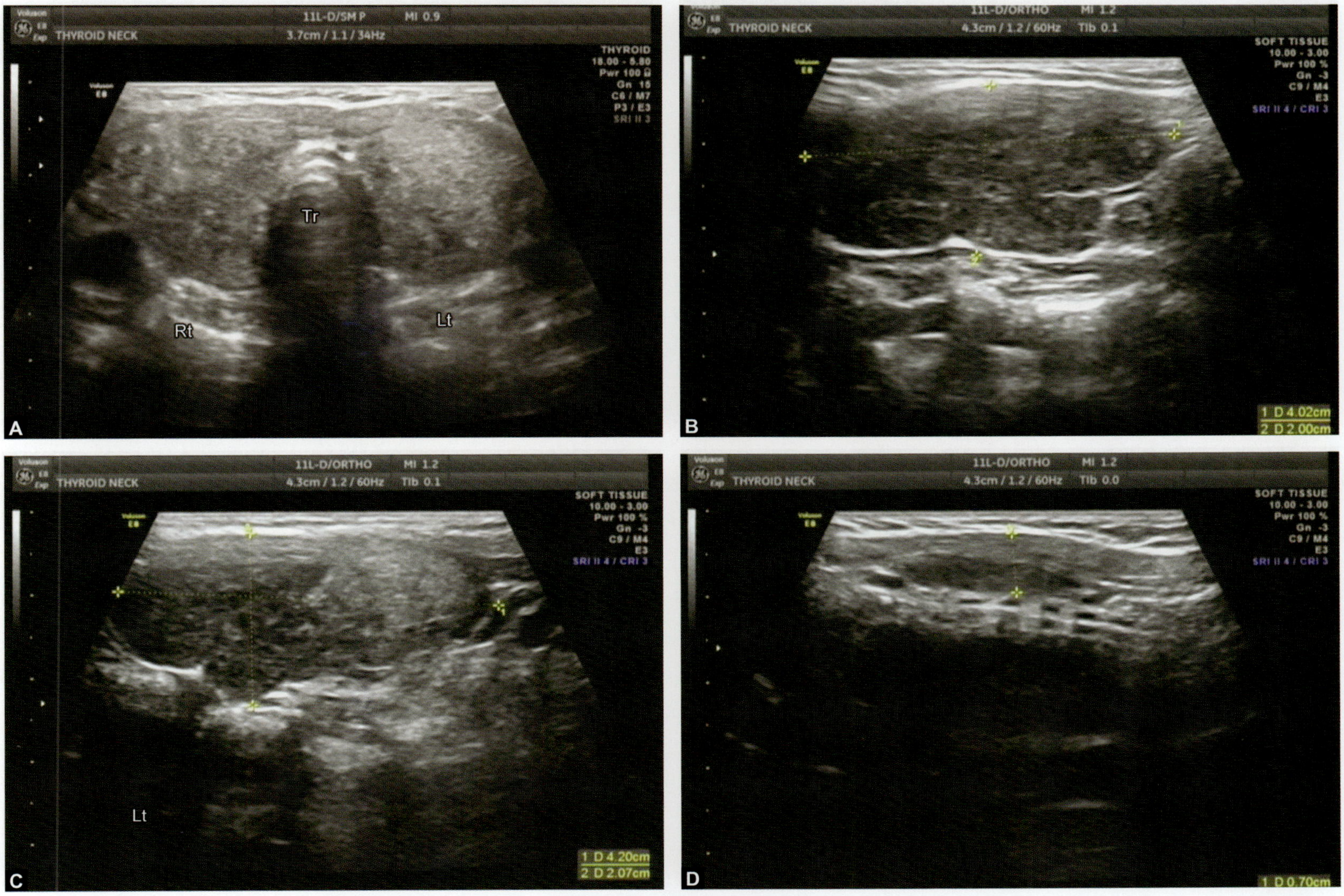

FIGURES 3.13A to D

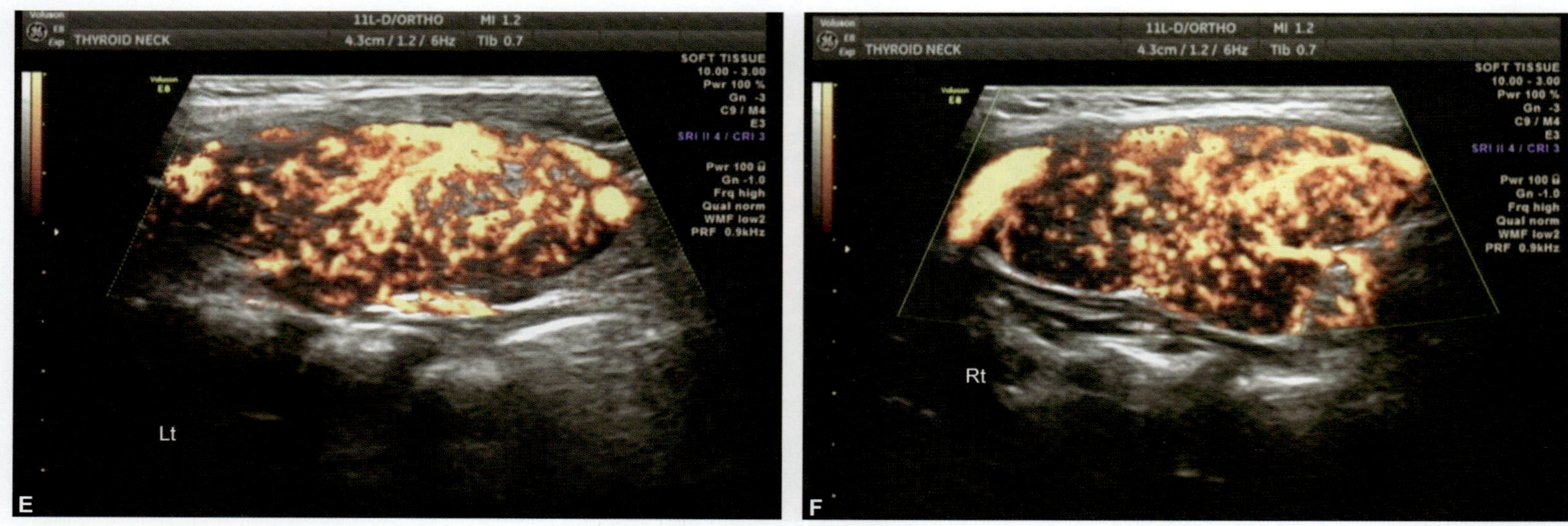

FIGURES 3.13E and F

FIGURES 3.13A to F: Acute thyroid enlargement in young girl. A 8-year-old girl presented with painful swelling in the neck. HRSG shows diffuse enlargement of both lobes of thyroid. The normal glandular texture is lost. The gland is hypoechoic in texture. Isthmus is also thickened. But no calcification or mass is seen in the gland. On color flow imaging, high flow is seen in the gland suggestive of acute parenchymal disease.

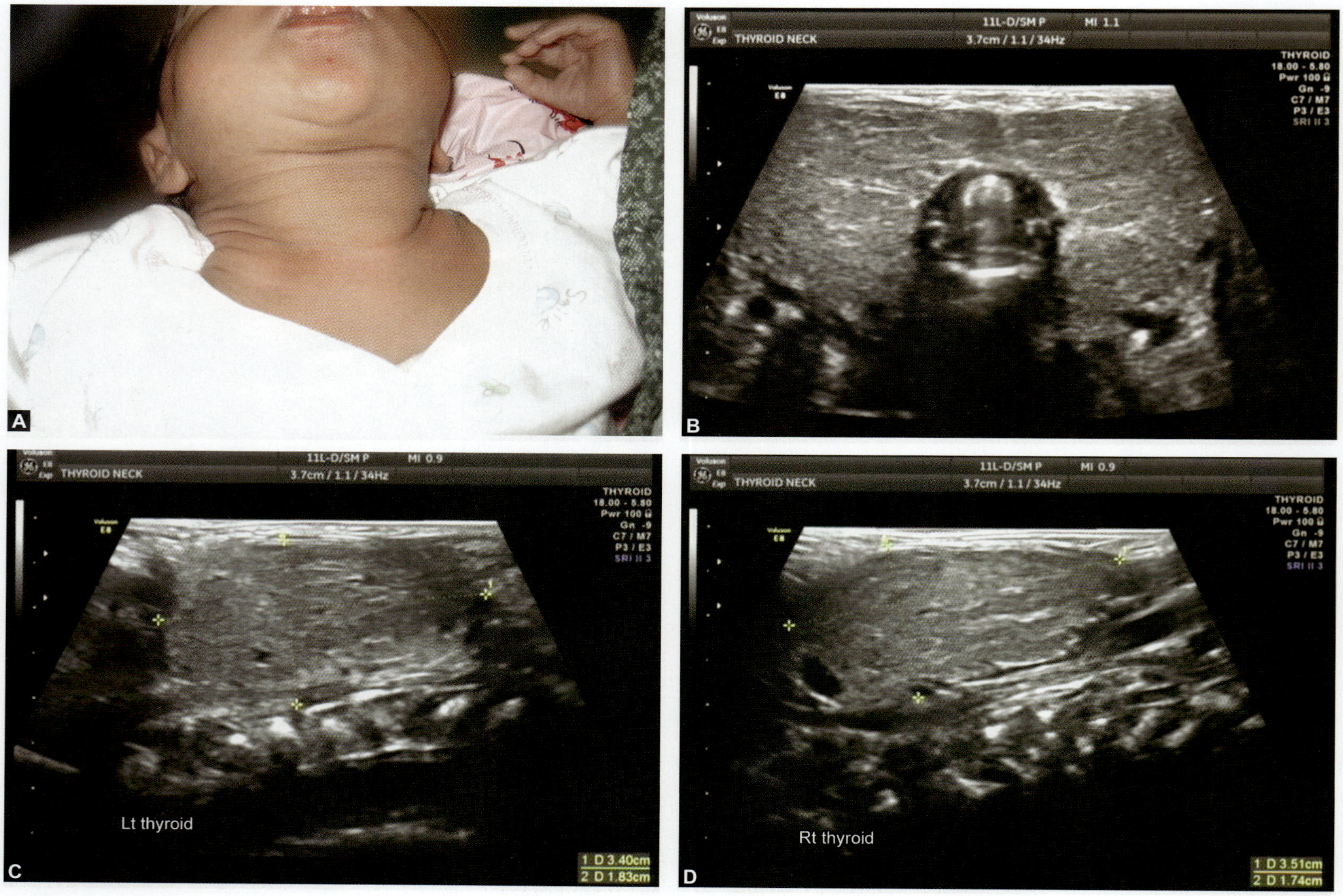

FIGURES 3.14A to D

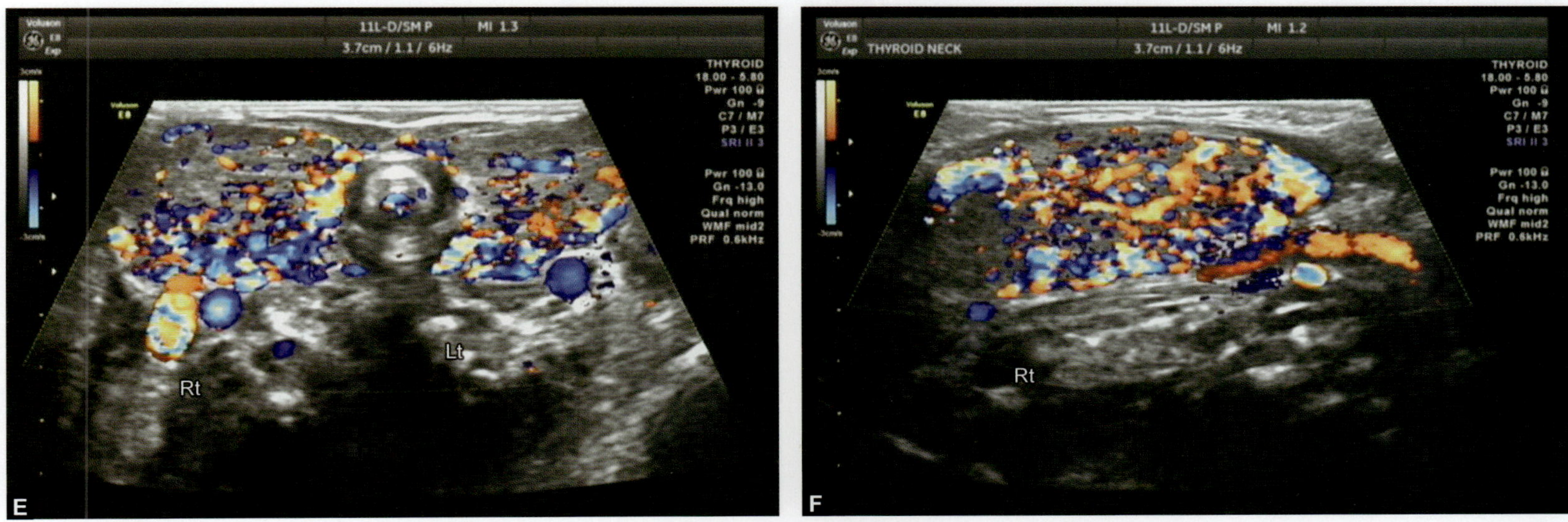

FIGURES 3.14E and F

FIGURES 3.14A to F: Diffuse thyroid enlargement in newborn. A 21days old newborn baby presented with diffuse swelling in the neck. HRSG shows marked enlargement of both lobes of thyroid. Normal glandular texture is lost. Isthmus is also thickened. But no focal mass is seen in the gland. On color flow imaging, marked increased flow is seen in the gland suggestive of acute parenchymal disease.

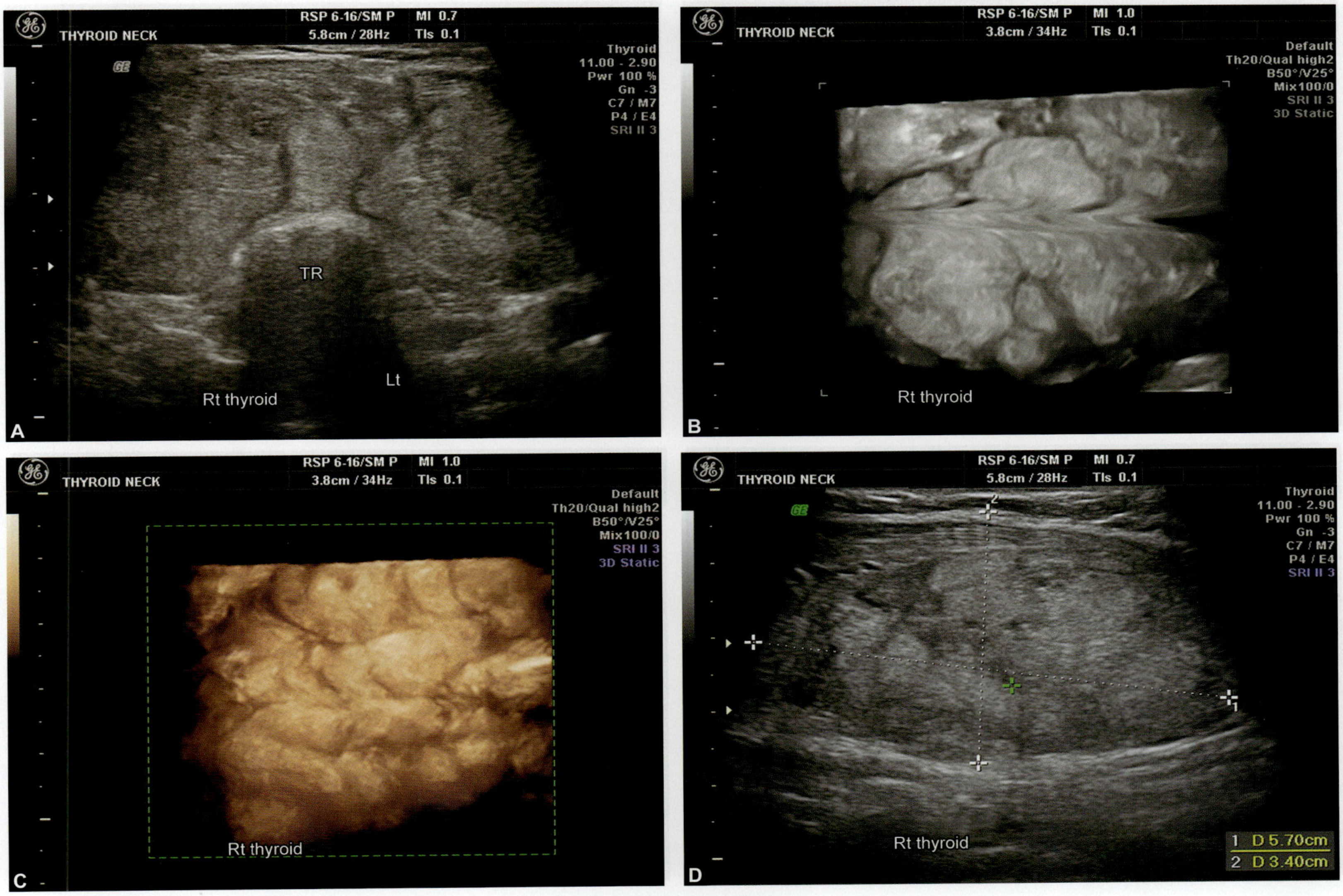

FIGURES 3.15A to D

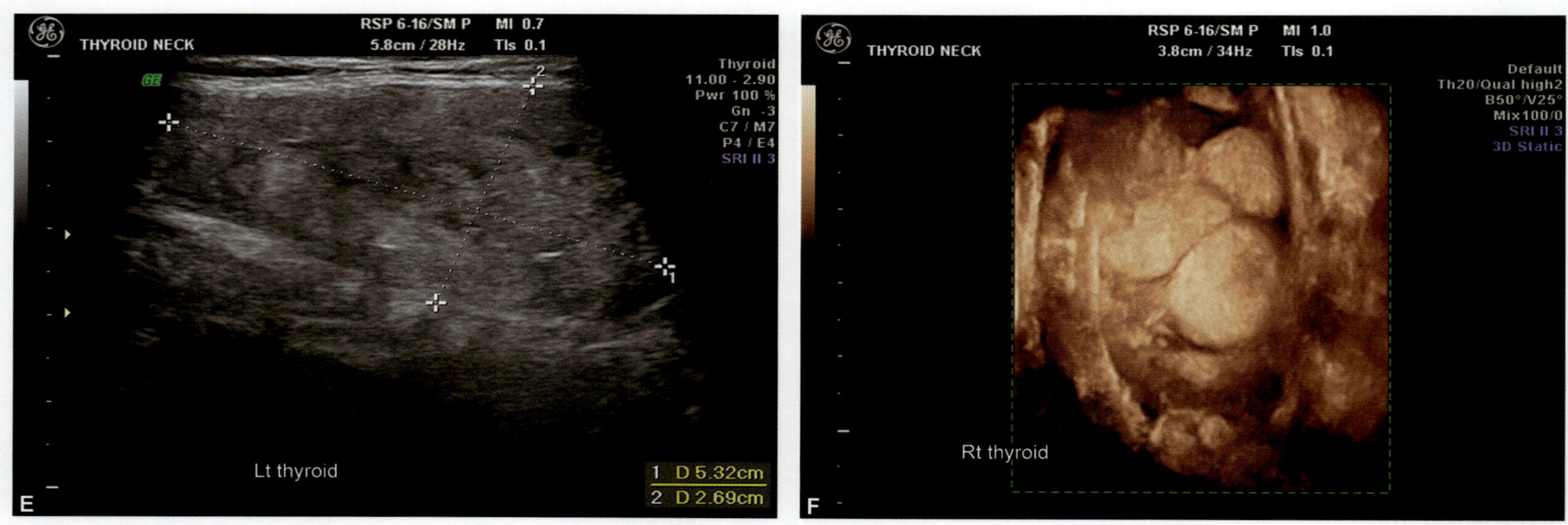

FIGURES 3.15E and F

FIGURES 3.15A to F: Multinodular goiter. A patient presented with grossly enlarged thyroid involving both the lobes. HRSG shows diffuse enlargement of thyroid on either side. Multiple isoechogenic nodules are seen in both the lobes, which are discrete in distribution. On 3D imaging, the nodules are seen clearly. No calcification is seen in the nodules. No cystic degeneration is seen. Findings are suggestive of multinodular hyperplasia of thyroid.

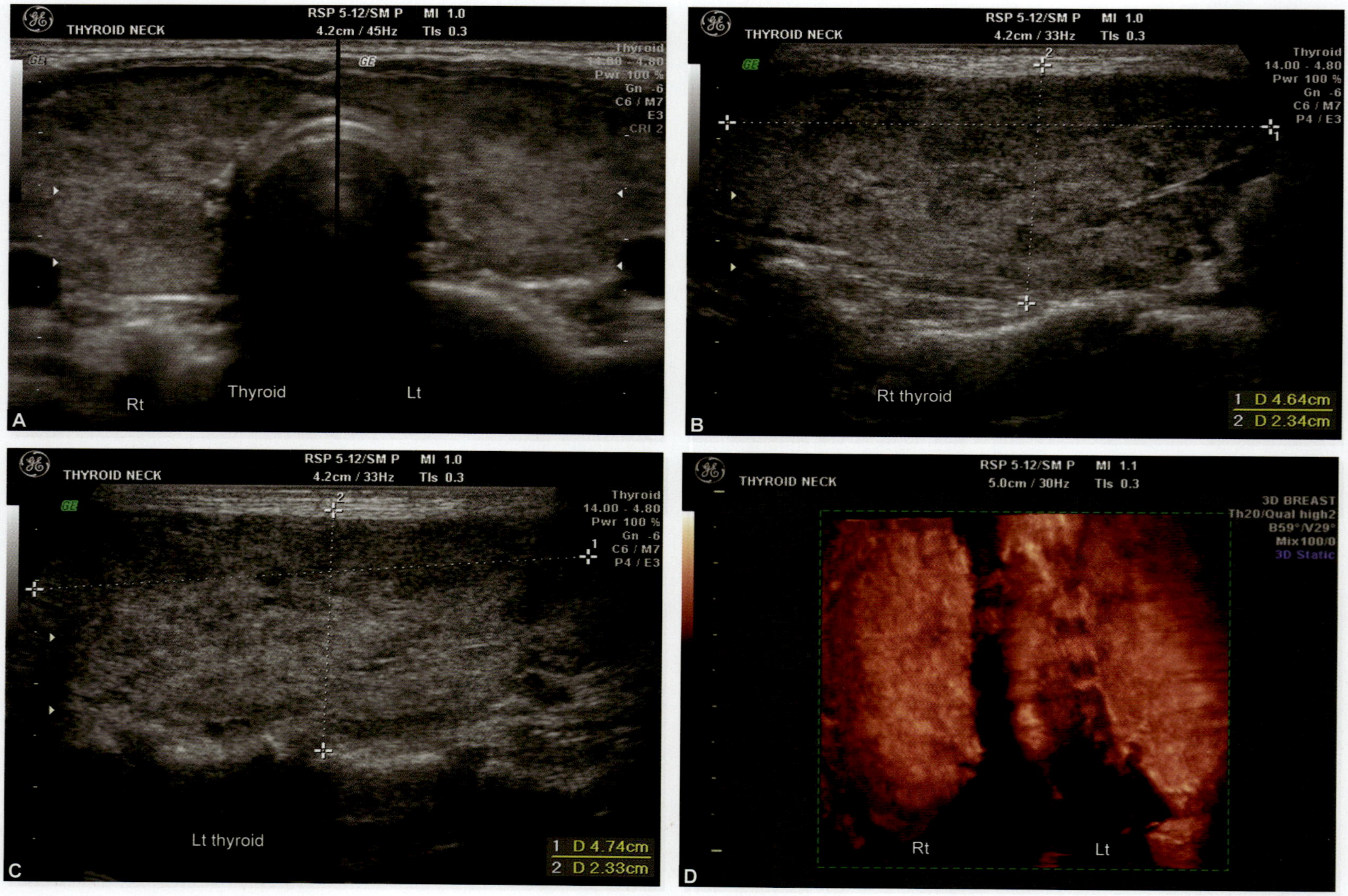

FIGURES 3.16A to D

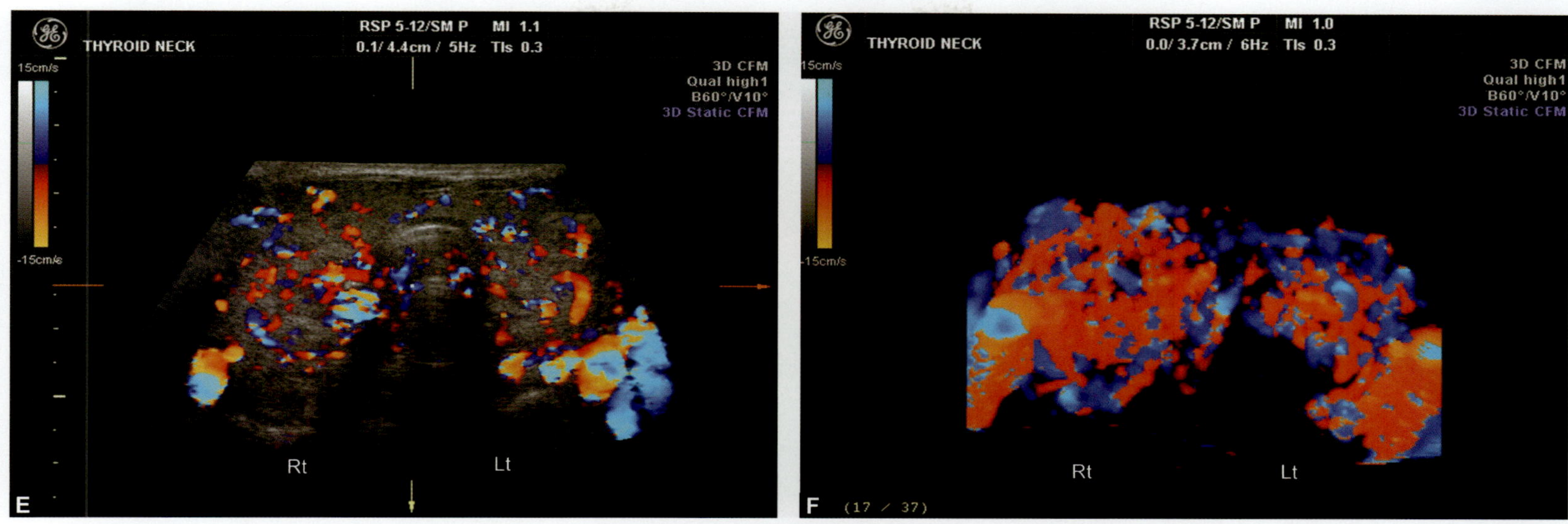

FIGURES 3.16E and F

FIGURES 3.16A to F: Multinodular hyperplasia with 3D imaging. HRSG shows diffuse enlargement of thyroid in both lobes in a lady. Multiple isoechogenic nodules are seen in both the lobes, which are discrete in distribution. 3D ultrasound shows the nodules clearly. On color flow and 3D power angio multiple vessels are seen feeding the mass suggestive of parenchymal disease.

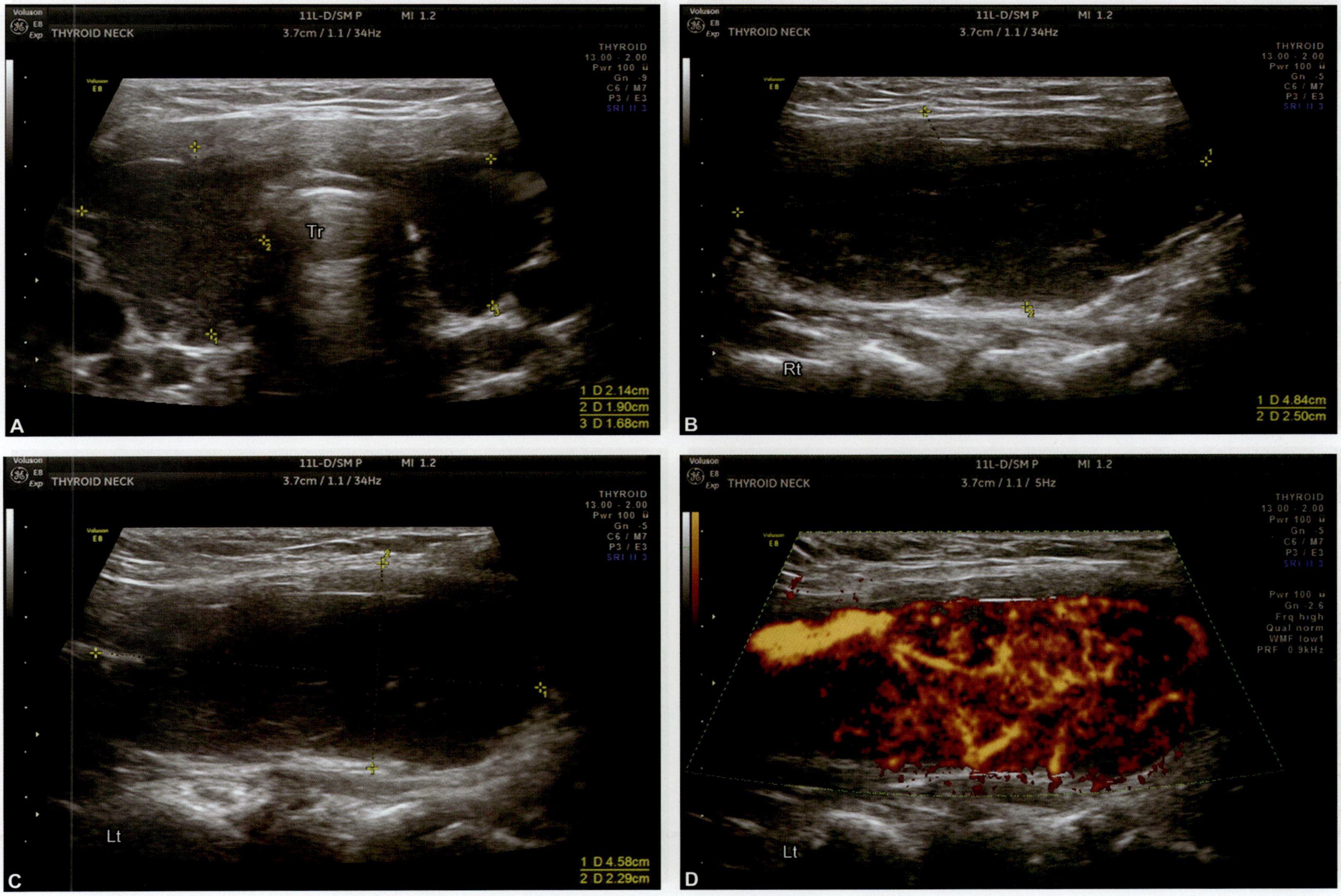

FIGURES 3.17A to D

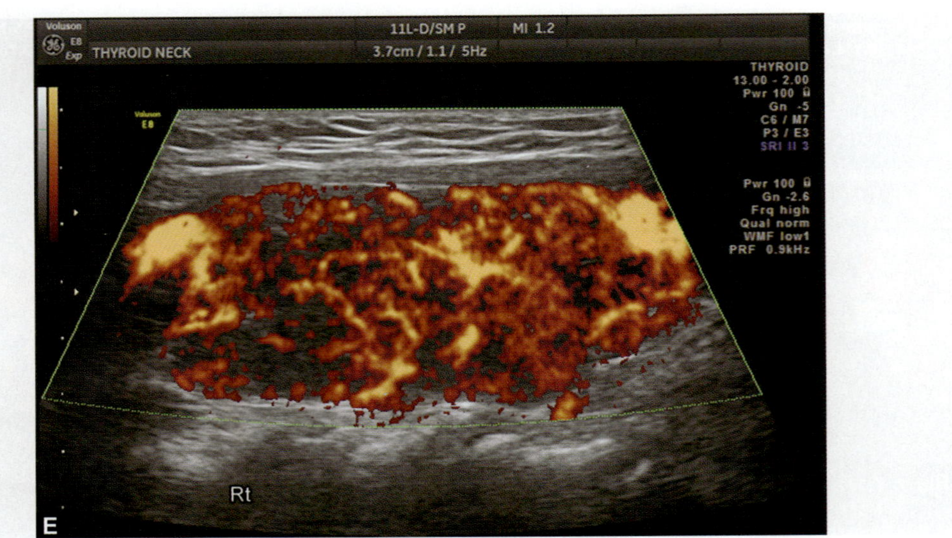

FIGURE 3.17E

FIGURES 3.17A to E: Hashimoto's thyroiditis. A lady presented with chronic thyroid dysfunction. HRSG shows enlarged both lobes of thyroid. Right lobe measures 50 × 25 mm in size. Left lobe measures 45 × 23 mm in size. Echotexture is inhomogeneous with coarse parenchyma. It is hypoechoic in texture. Thyroid inferno sign is positive. No evidence of any focal mass is seen in the gland on either side. On color flow imaging, high flow is seen in the gland on either side. Findings are suggestive of Hashimoto's thyroiditis.

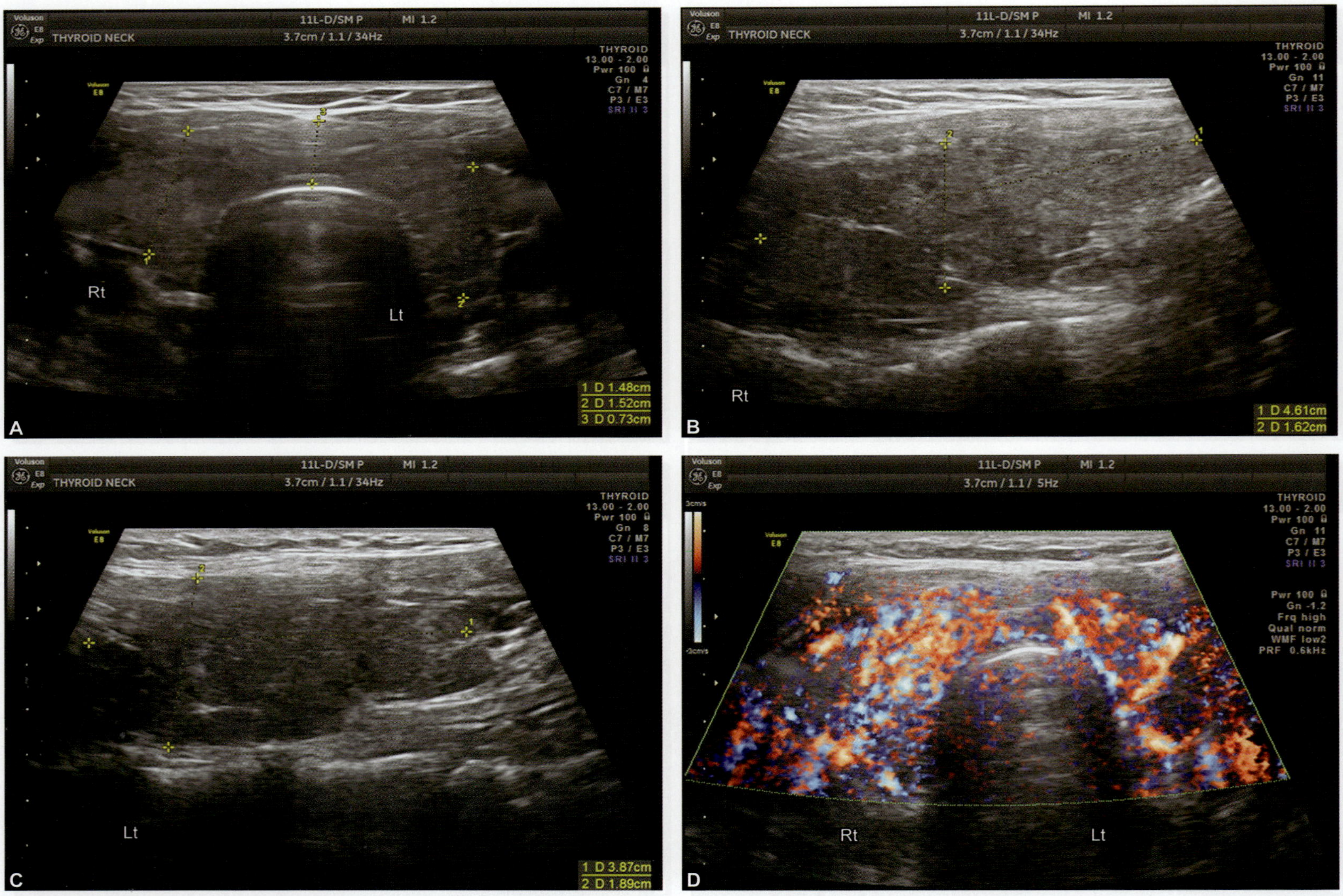

FIGURES 3.18A to D: Hashimoto's thyroiditis. HRSG shows normal size thyroid. However, normal glandular texture is lost. Hypoechoic areas are seen in the gland. But no mass or calcification is seen. On color flow imaging, moderate flow is seen in the gland. Biopsy of the thyroid confirms Hashimoto's thyroiditis.

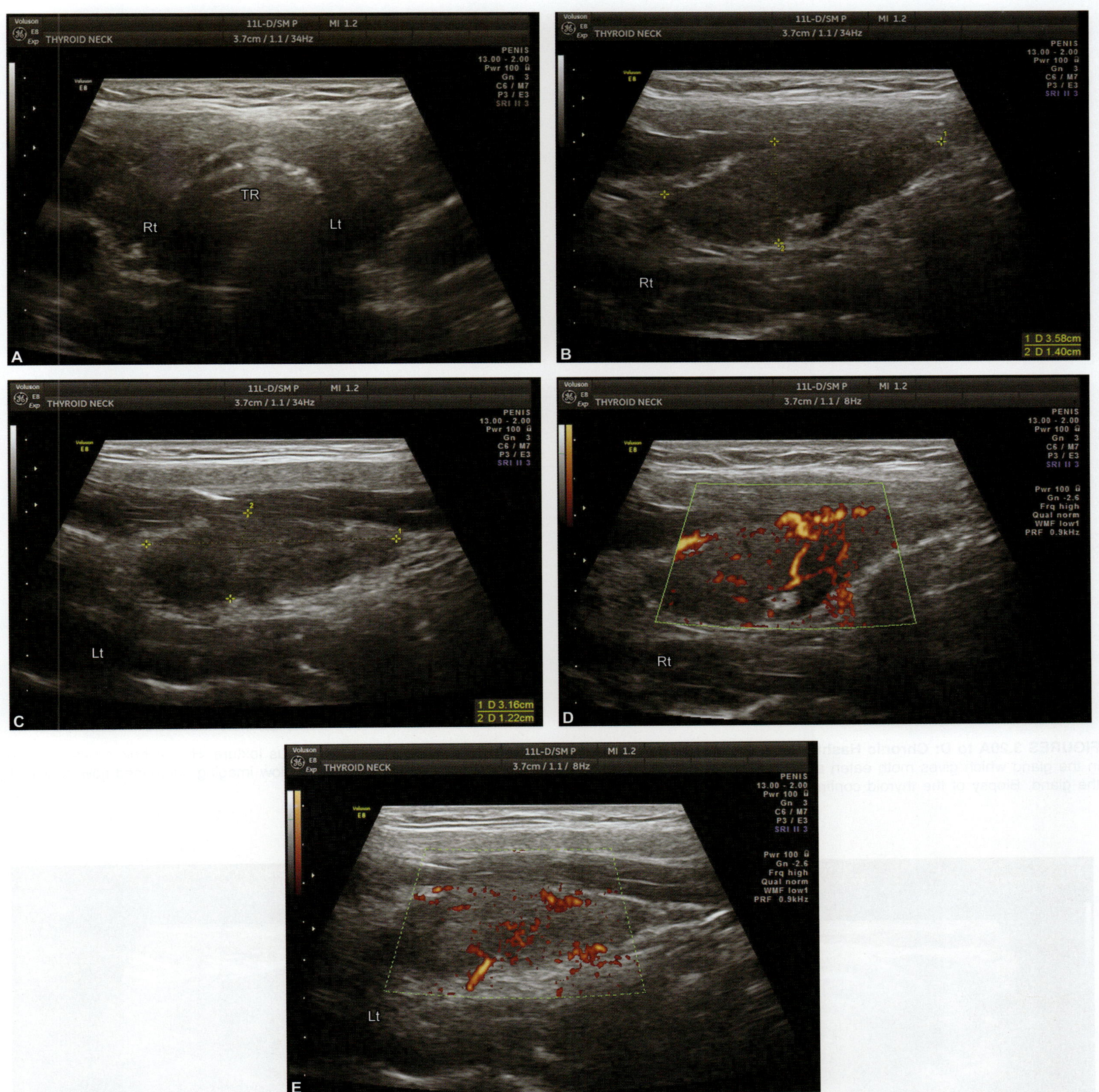

FIGURES 3.19A to E: Chronic thyroiditis. A patient presented with chronic dysfunction of thyroid. On HRSG both lobes of thyroid show grossly inhomogeneous texture. They are small in size. Normal glandular texture is lost. Rim calcification is seen around the capsule. But no focal mass is seen in the gland. On color flow imaging, low flow is seen in the gland suggestive of chronic thyroditis.

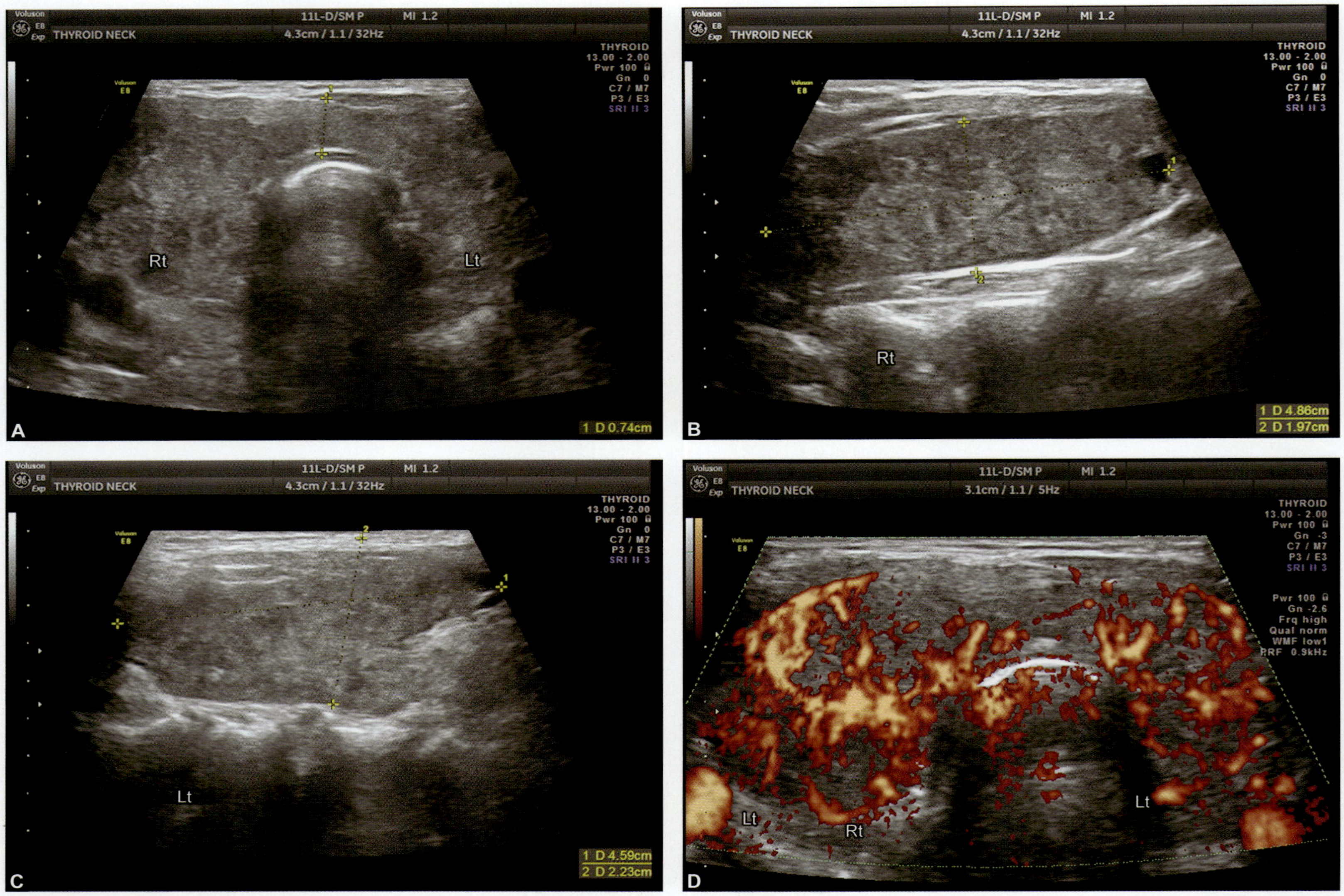

FIGURES 3.20A to D: Chronic Hashimoto's thyroiditis. Both lobes thyroid gland show grossly inhomogeneous texture. Hypoechoic areas are seen in the gland which gives moth eaten appearance. But no calcification or mass is seen in the gland. On color flow imaging, increased flow is seen in the gland. Biopsy of the thyroid confirms Hashimoto's thyroiditis.

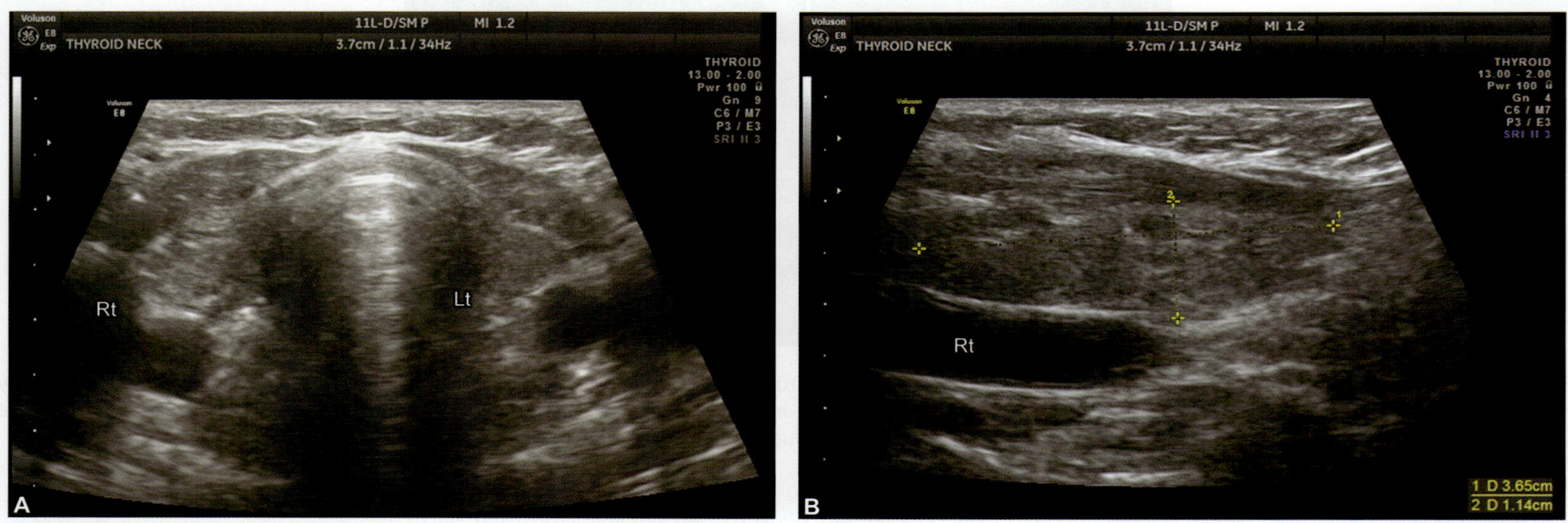

FIGURES 3.21A and B

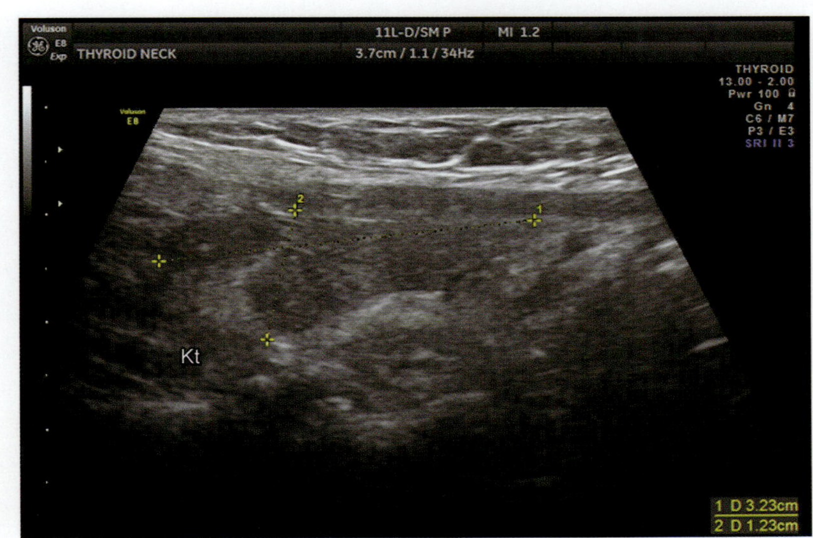

FIGURE 3.21C

FIGURES 3.21A to C: Chronic atrophic thyroiditis. On HRSG both thyroid glands are small in size. Echotexture is grossly inhomogeneous. Hypoechoic areas are seen in the gland. But no mass lesion is seen in the gland suggestive of chronic atrophic thyroiditis.

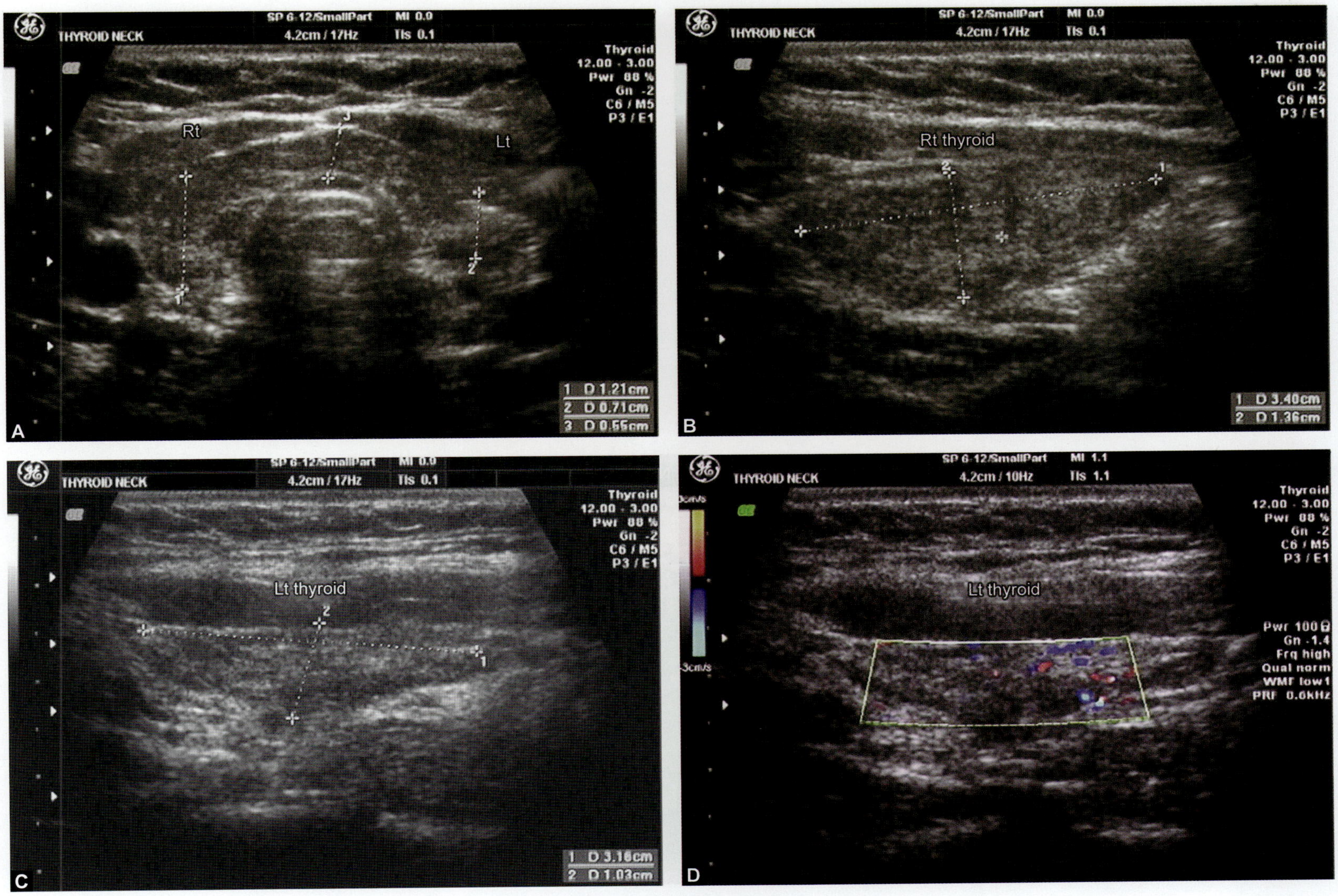

FIGURES 3.22A to D

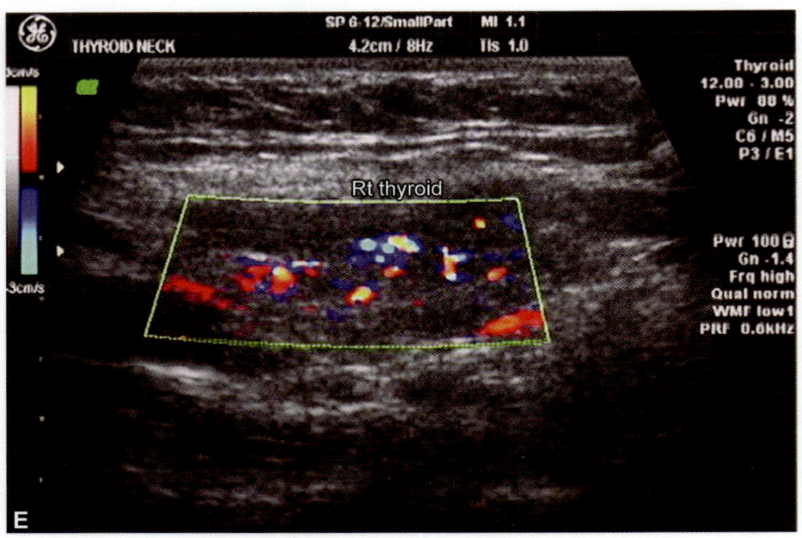

FIGURE 3.22E

FIGURES 3.22A to E: Chronic thyroiditis. HRSG shows a young child presented with chronic thyroid disease. HRSG shows small thyroid with inhomogeneous texture. Normal fine glandular texture is lost. HRSG shows diffuse parenchymal inhomogeneous texture with micronodularity. It shows typical "moth eaten" appearance. On color flow imaging the gland show low flow pattern due to loss of normal vascular glandular tissue.

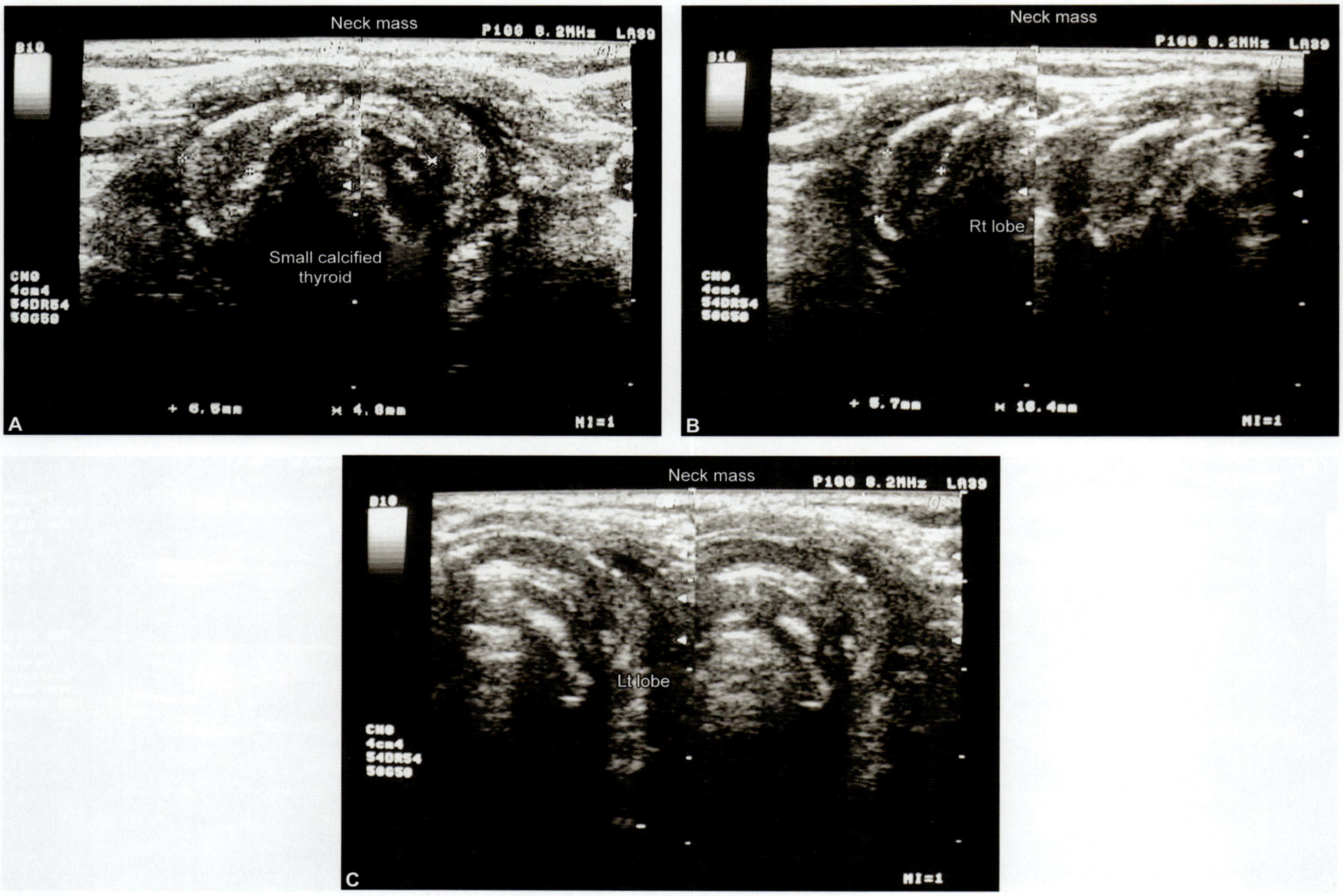

FIGURES 3.23A to C: Chronic calcific thyroiditis. HRSG of the neck shows irregular small atrophic both lobes of the thyroid with multiple calcified specks. The right lobe of the thyroid is small and measures 10 × 6 mm in size with multiple calcified shadows. Left lobe of the thyroid also shows small lobe with hypoechoic texture. Multiple calcified shadows are seen. Biopsy of the gland shows atrophic calcific thyroiditis.

SOLITARY THYROID NODULE

Solitary thyroid nodule is the most common manifestation of thyroid adenomas and carcinomas. About 25% of the nodules show malignant changes. They should be evaluated for malignancy by illustrating other signs of malignancy on HRSG.

Benign Thyroid Nodules

Benign thyroid nodules include follicular and non-follicular adenomas.

Follicular Adenoma

Follicular adenomas are most common than non-follicular adenomas. Usually, they are isoreflective. They present as homogeneous, well-defined isoechogenic nodule. They may undergo cystic degeneration or hemorrhage. The degenerative or hemorrhagic nodule shows low-level echoes on HRSG. The toxic adenomas usually are isoechogenic, and reflectivity of the nodule is same as of the gland. However, they are well-demarcated by a peripheral "halo". These nodules usually undergo cystic degeneration on medical treatment. HRSG is good to evaluate the response of medical treatment. These nodules show hypervascularity on color flow imaging than the adjacent normal glandular tissue.

Thyroid Cyst

True cysts of thyroid are not common. However, they are encountered as well-marginated cystic swelling in anterior part of neck. HRSG shows classical sono appearance of a cyst. They are well-defined with sharp margins, thin walled fluid-filled structures. No internal echo is seen in true cyst. No calcification is noted.

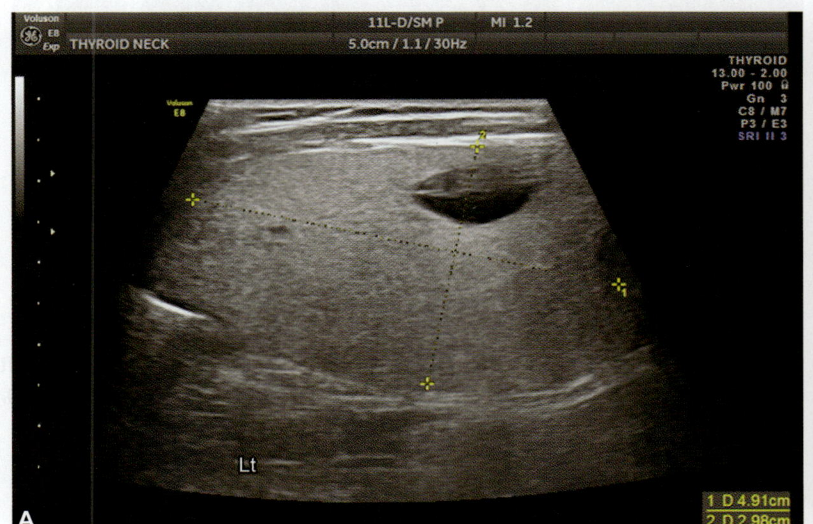

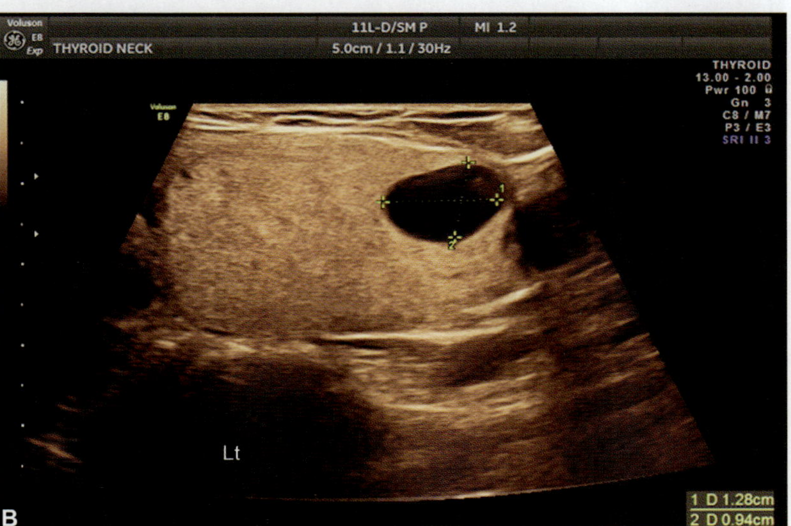

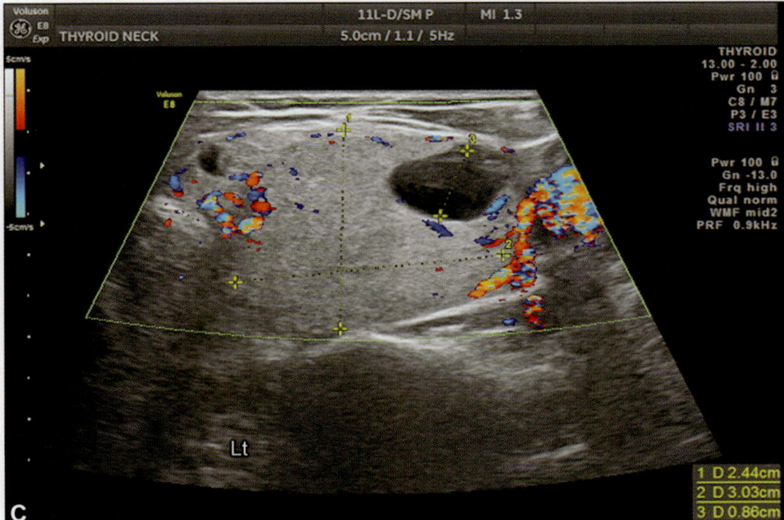

FIGURES 3.24A to C: Simple thyroid cyst. HRSG shows a well-defined cystic mass in the left lobe of thyroid. The cyst is anechoic. No septation or calcification is seen in the cyst. However, left lobe of thyroid shows diffuse enlargement in size.

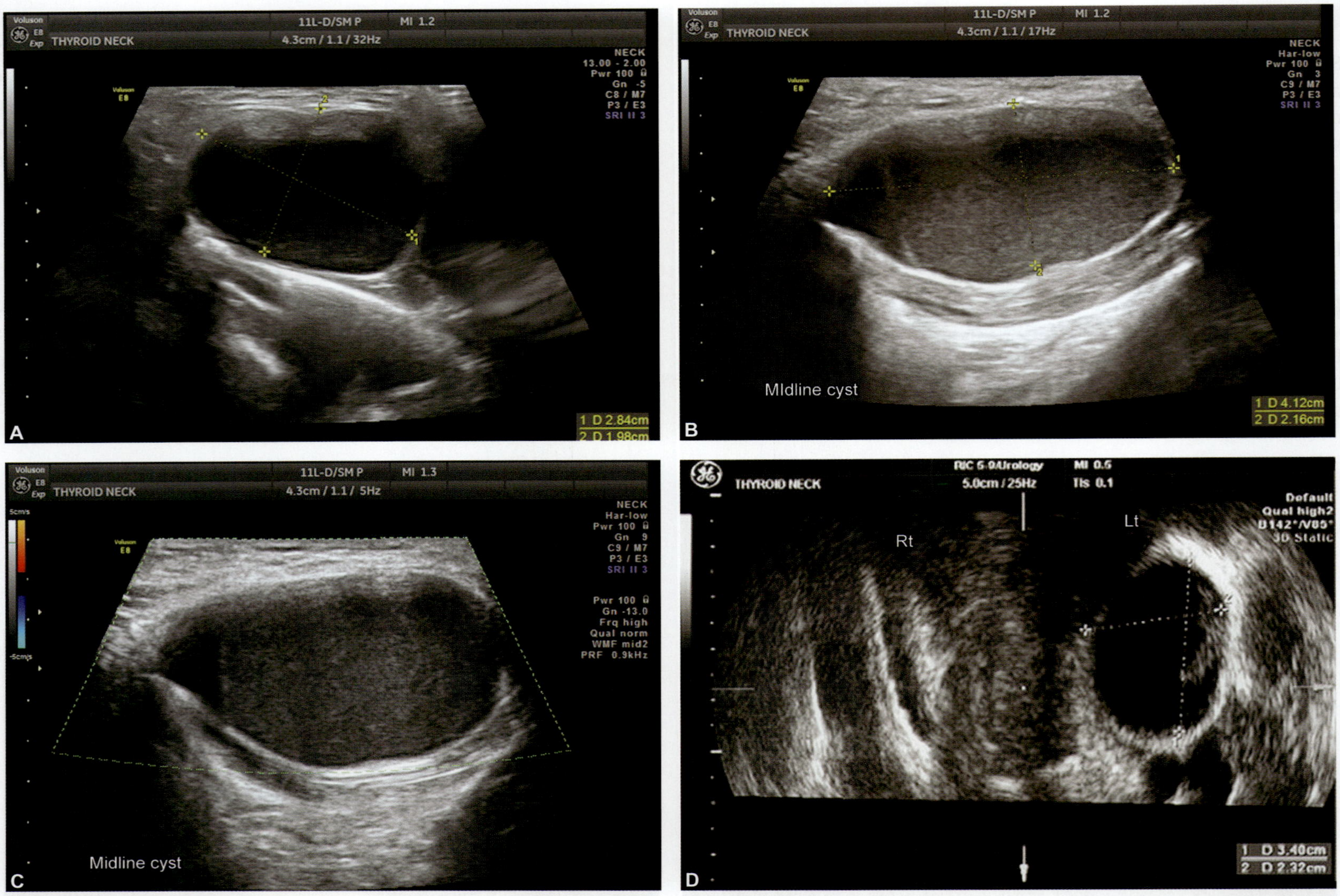

FIGURES 3.25A to D: Colloid cyst in thyroid. A patient presented with mass in the neck. HRSG shows a well-defined cystic shadow in the left lobe of thyroid. It is seen near the midline. It shows homogeneous echoes with ground glass appearance suggestive of colloid cyst. On 3D imaging, it is seen clearly confined to the left lobe.

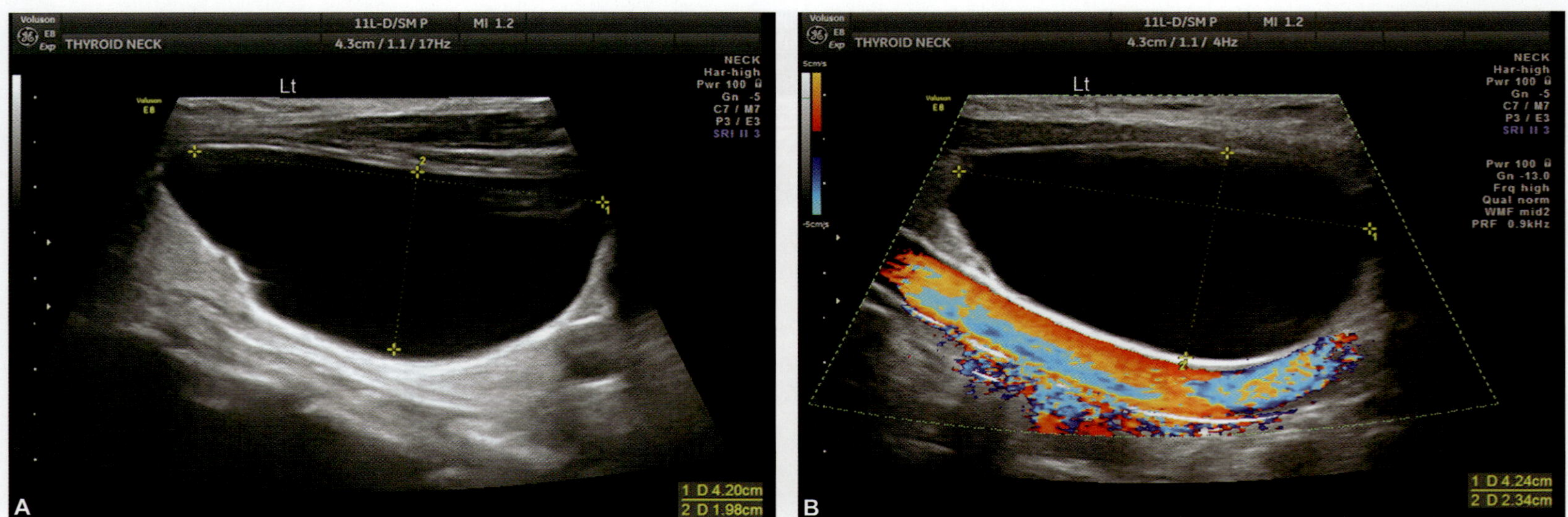

FIGURES 3.26A and B

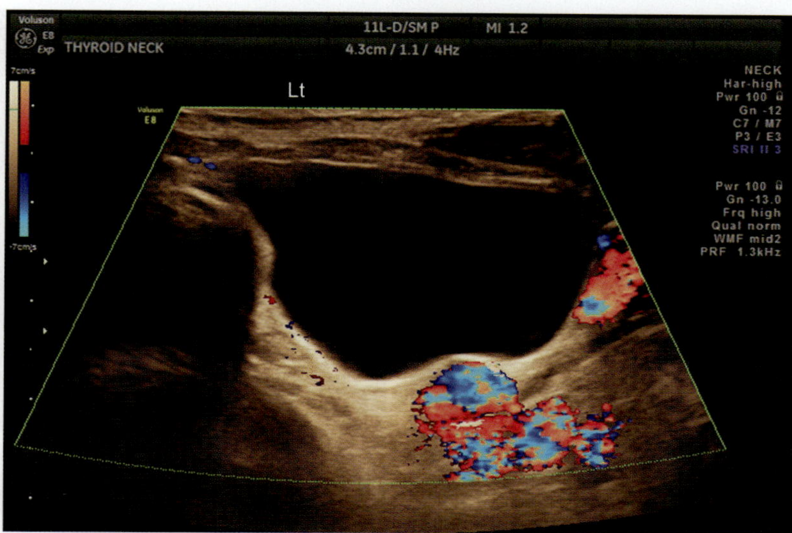

FIGURE 3.26C

FIGURES 3.26A to C: Simple thyroid cyst. HRSG shows a well-defined cystic shadow in the left lobe of thyroid. No internal echo seen in the cyst. No calcification is seen. On color flow imaging, no flow is seen in the cyst. On aspiration clear fluid was aspirated. Simple cyst of thyroid is not very common. However, they may present in thyroid.

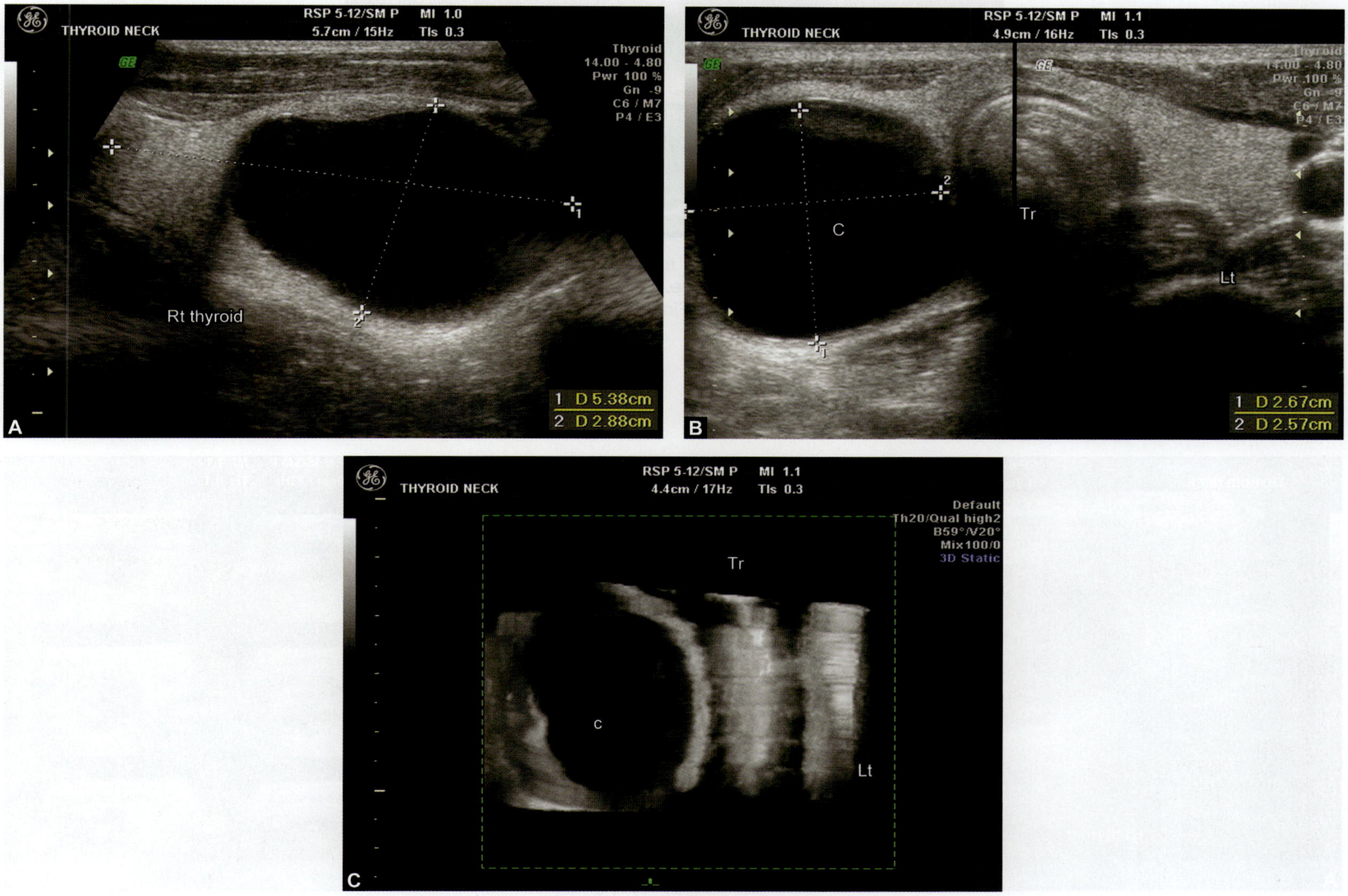

FIGURES 3.27A to C: A patient presented with soft tissue mass in the right thyroid. HRSG shows a big anechoic cystic shadow in the right lobe of thyroid. No septation or internal echo seen in it. The 3D imaging shows the cyst is confined in the right lobe of thyroid.

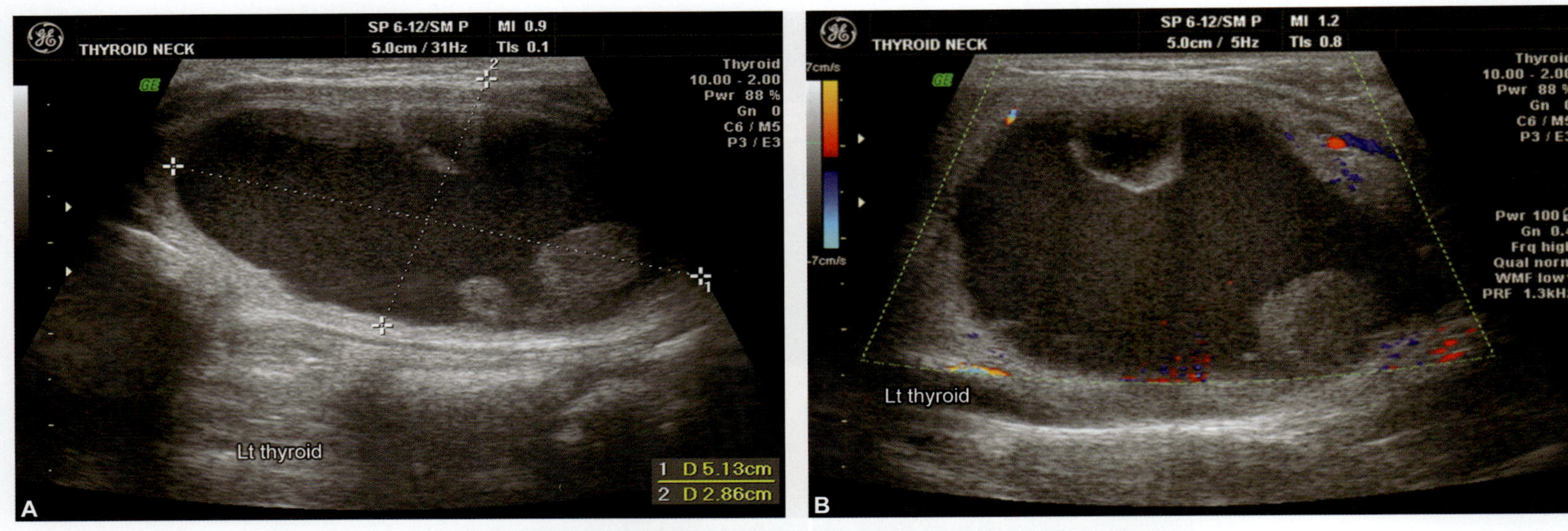

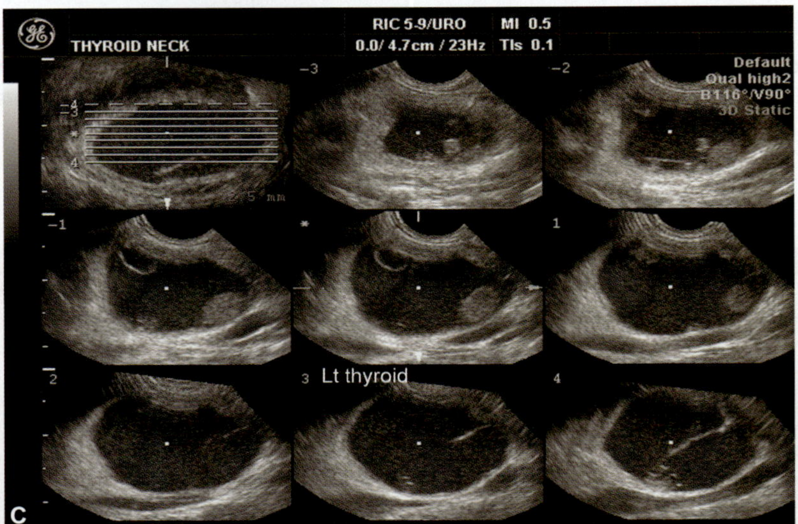

FIGURES 3.28A to C: Colloid cyst. A patient presented with soft tissue mass in the left lobe of thyroid. HRSG shows a big cystic mass in the left lobe. Homogeneous echoes are seen in it with ground glass appearance. Few isoechogenic nodules are also seen in the cyst. The TOI imaging shows the nodules very clearly. A thin septum is also seen in the cyst. Findings are suggestive of colloid cyst.

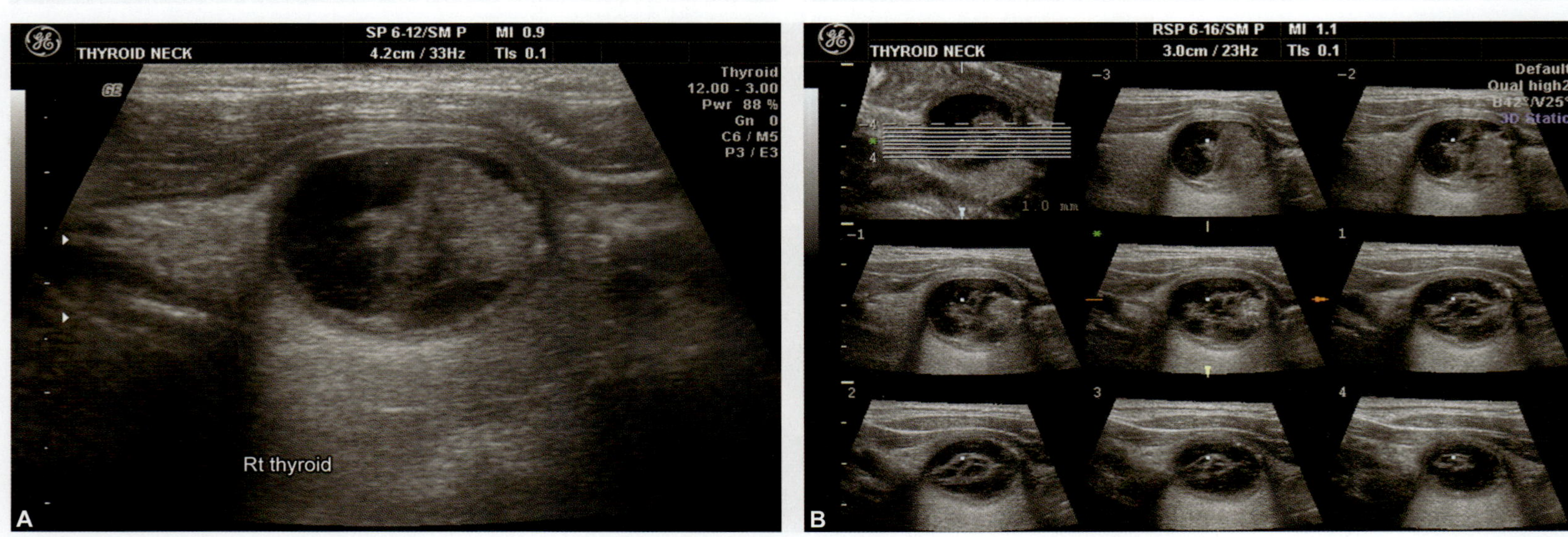

FIGURES 3.29A and B

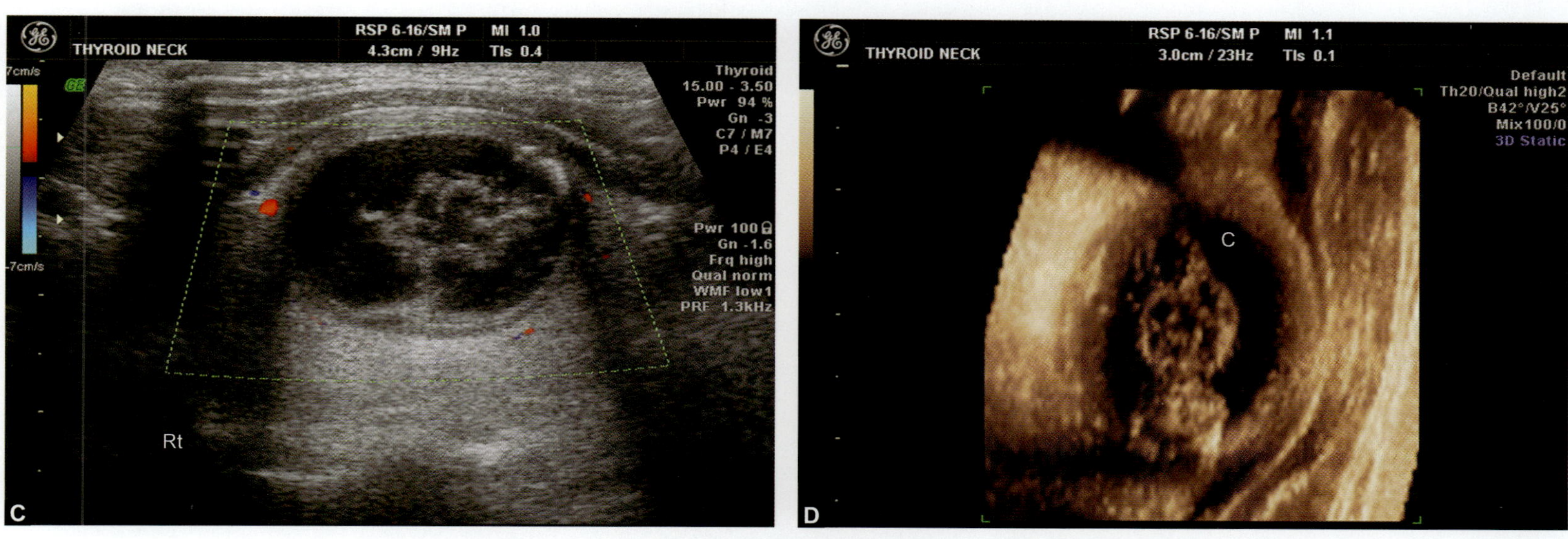

FIGURES 3.29C and D

FIGURES 3.29A to D: Colloid cyst. HRSG shows a complex cystic shadow in the right lobe of thyroid. The cyst wall is smooth in outline. However, soft tissue glandular shadow is seen in the cyst. The TOI imaging shows the soft tissue shadow clearly confined to the cyst. On color flow imaging, poor flow is seen in the cyst. Aspiration biopsy confirms colloid cyst.

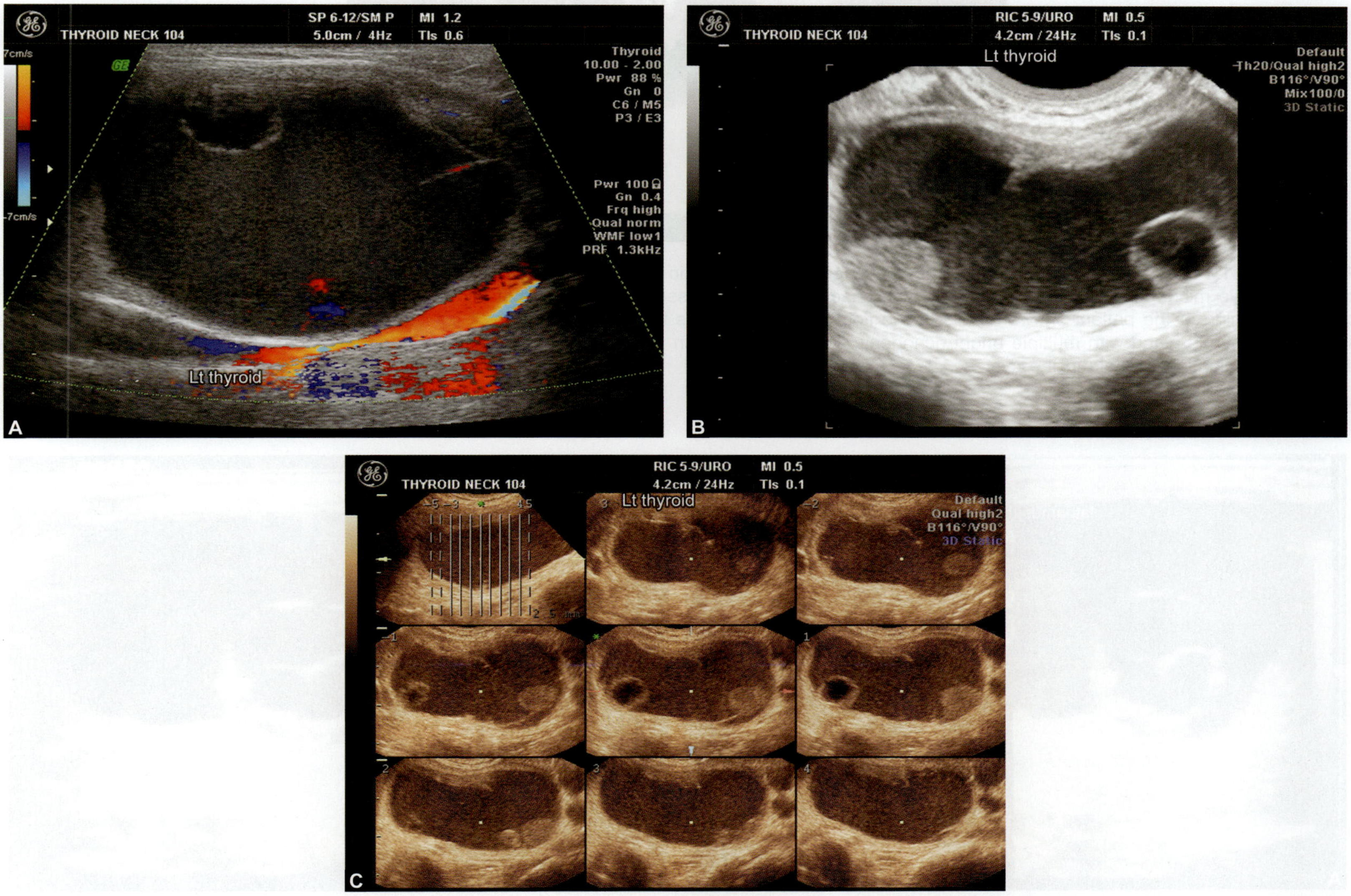

FIGURES 3.30A to C: Thyroid cyst with colloid nodule. A patient presented with big cystic mass in the left lobe of thyroid. HRSG shows well defined cyst in the left lobe. Echogenic nodules are also seen fixed with the inner wall of the cyst. On 3D ultrasound the nodules become prominent. Fine-needle aspiration cytology (FNAC) confirms colloid cyst.

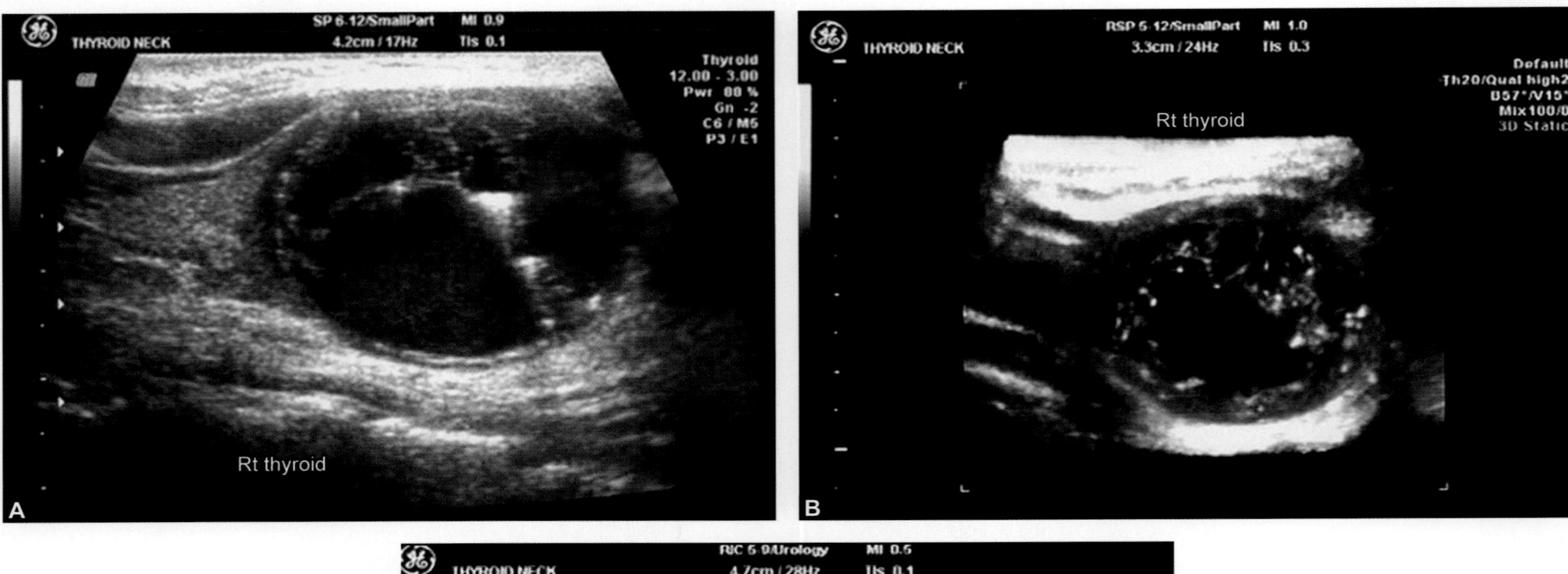

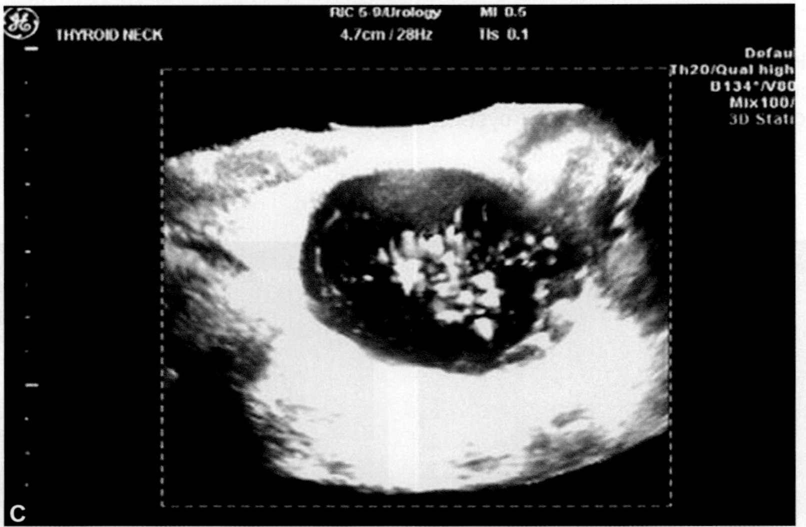

FIGURES 3.31A to C: Colloid cyst with comet tail sign. HRSG a cystic mass in the thyroid. Multiple echogenic tiny foci are seen floating in the cyst suggestive micro-colloid crystals. These floating shadows are seen associated with comet tail artifacts known as comet tail sign typical of colloid cyst. 3D imaging of the patient shows details of the floating micro crystals with evidence of thick jell-like colloid in the cyst. A thick wall cystic mass seen in the thyroid gland with multiple bright echogenic floating shadows in the cyst. They give starry sky appearance. 3D of the same patient shows details of the floating crystals in the cyst.

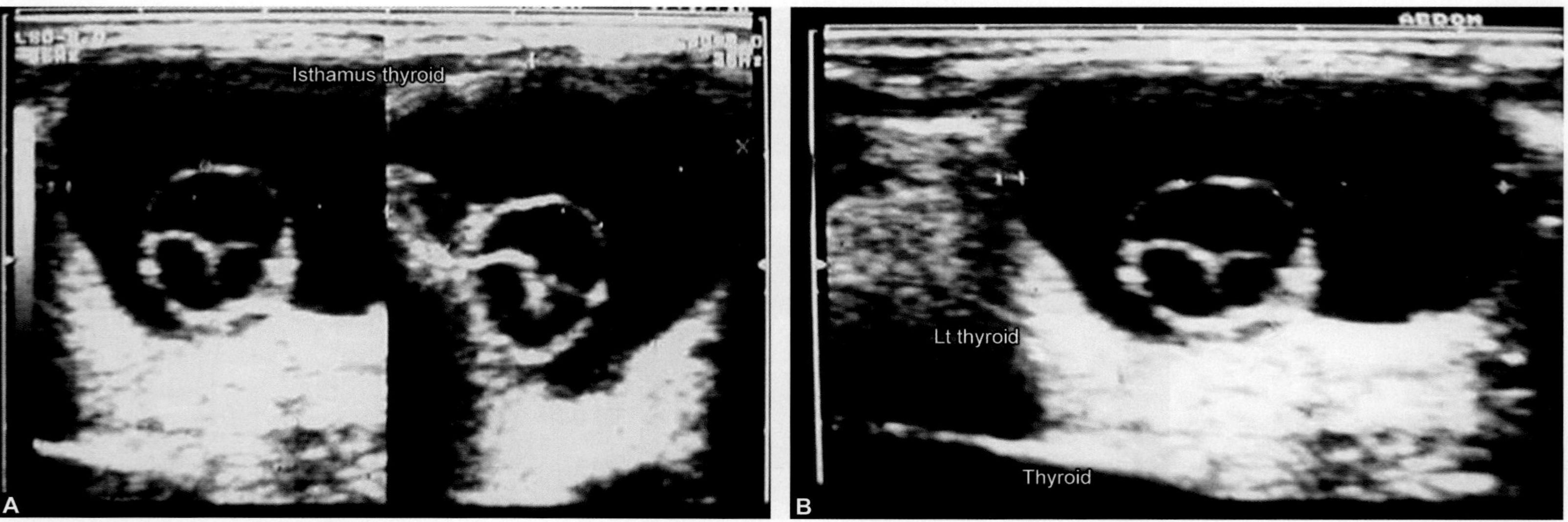

FIGURES 3.32A and B

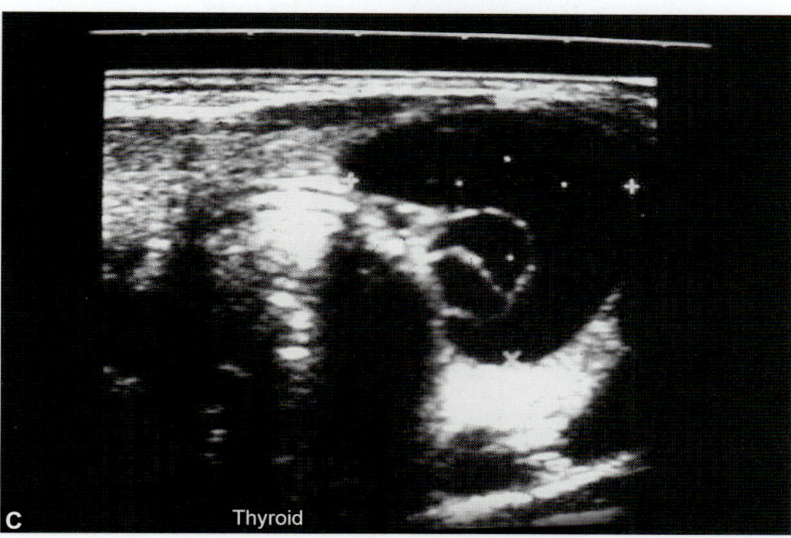

FIGURE 3.32C

FIGURES 3.32A to C: Hydatid cyst in the thyroid. HRSG shows a well-defined cystic in the left lobe of the thyroid. There is also evidence of a multi-loculated small cyst seen fixed with the inner wall of the cyst. Multiple small daughter cysts are seen in it typical feature of the hydatid cyst. Hydatid cysts are rare in thyroid. Well-defined multiloculated cystic mass is seen in the left lobe of thyroid. Multiple small daughter cysts are seen in the big cyst typical of the hydatid cyst. Aspiration biopsy confirmed the hydatid cyst.

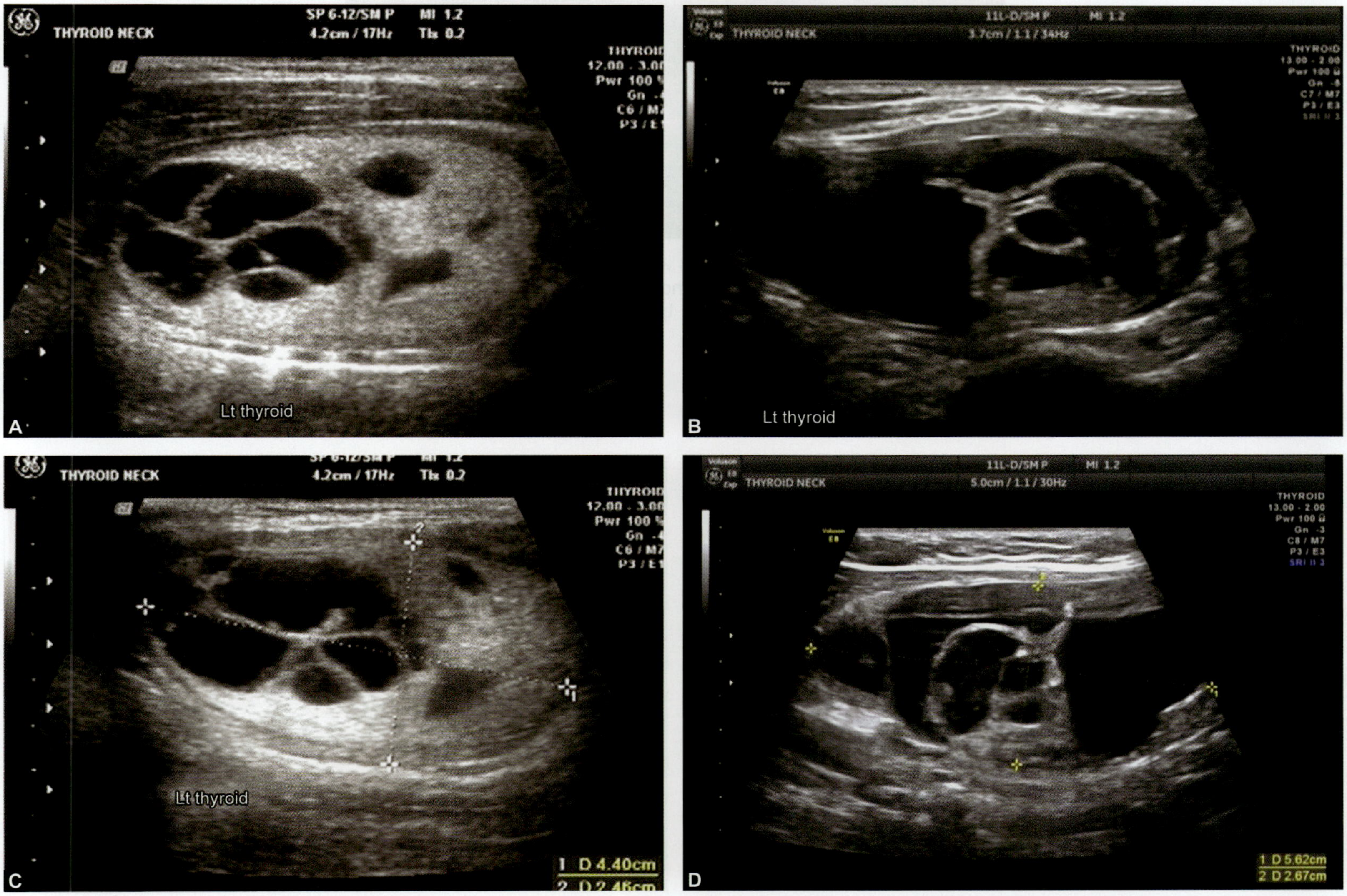

FIGURES 3.33A to D: Hydatid cyst thyroid. A patient presented with soft tissue mass in the left lobe of thyroid. HRSG shows a big cystic mass in the left lobe of thyroid. Multiple small cysts are seen in the big cyst. On real time imaging, septa are seen moving in the cyst suggestive of positive water lily sign. Findings are typical of hydatid cyst in thyroid.

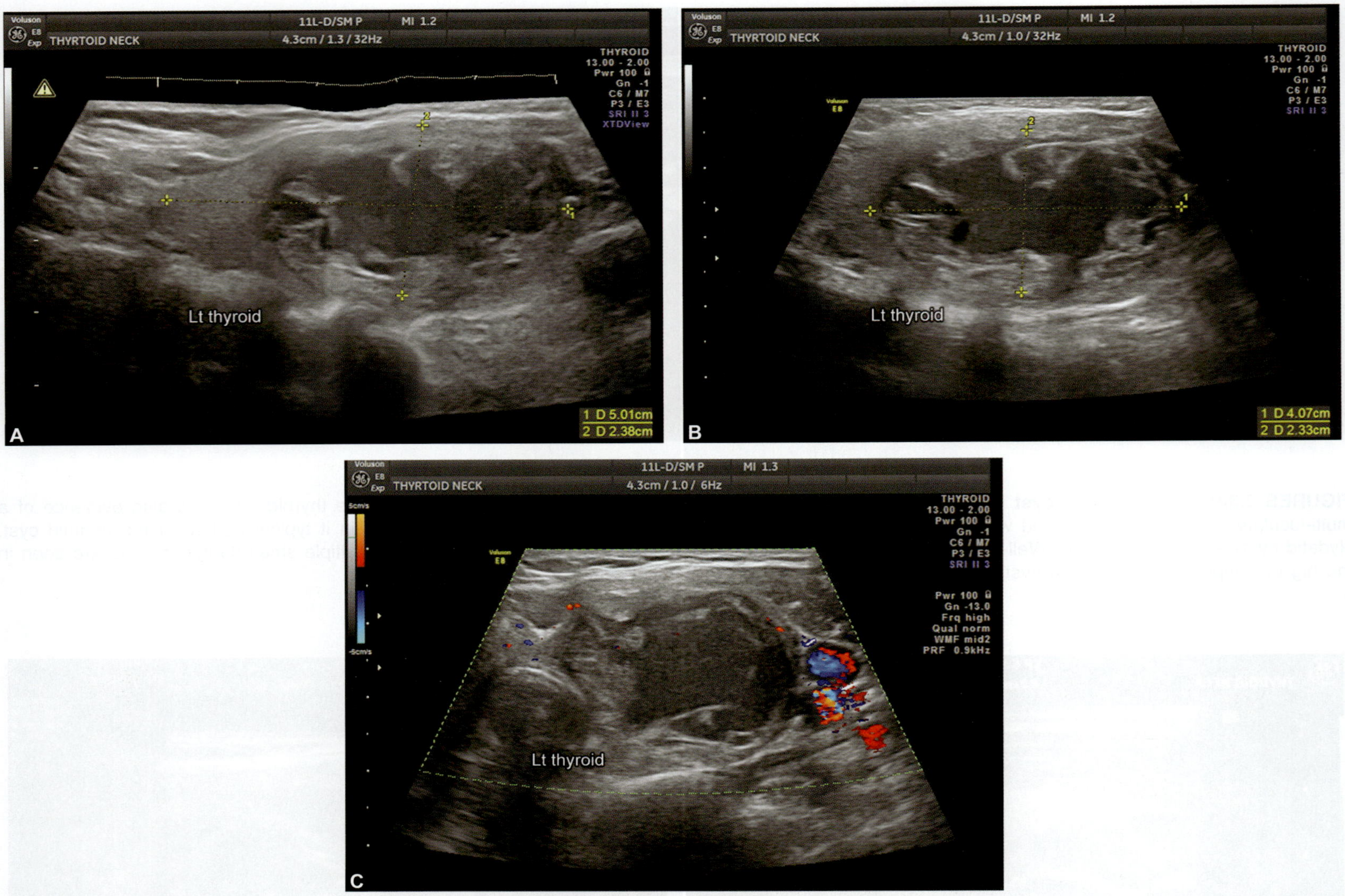

FIGURES 3.34A to C: Hemorrhagic cyst in thyroid. A patient presented with painful swelling in left lobe of thyroid. HRSG shows a complex cyst in the left lobe. Central area of hemorrhage is seen in the cyst. Low level echoes are seen in it. Perifocal edema is also present. On color flow imaging, no flow is seen in it suggestive of acute hemorrhage. On aspiration fresh blood was aspirated.

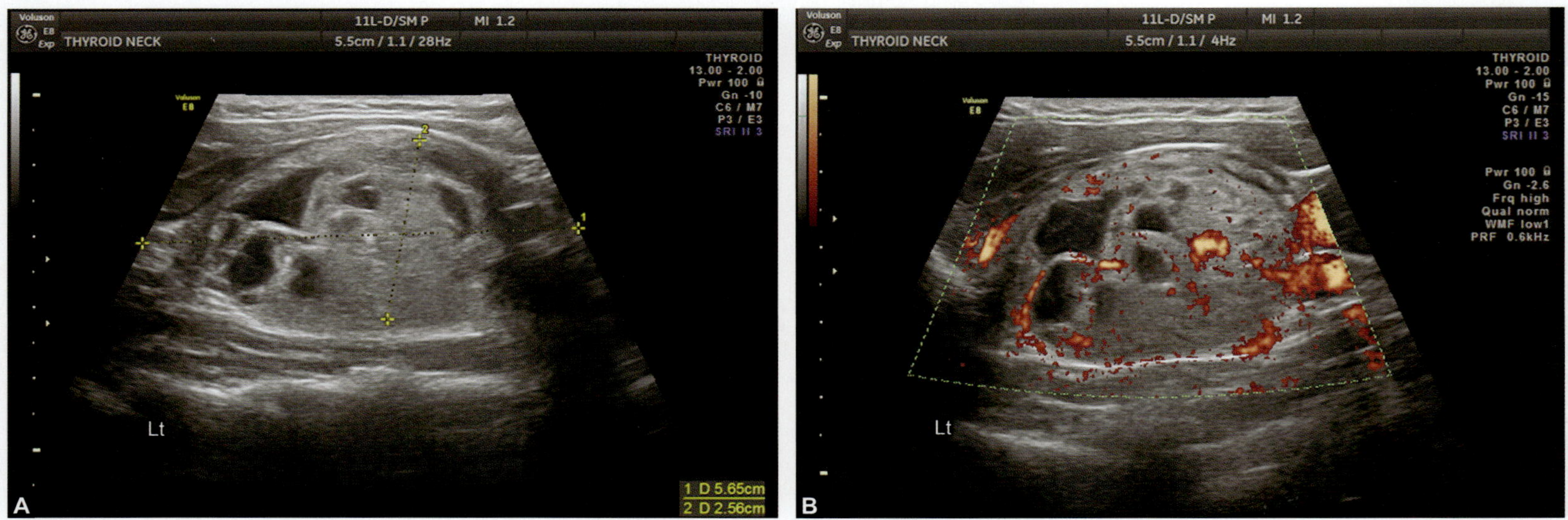

FIGURES 3.35A and B: Complex cyst in the thyroid. A patient presented with nodular swelling in the left side of neck. HRSG shows a complex cystic mass in the left side of neck. It shows solid cystic component. On color flow imaging, solid component shows blood flow. On aspiration biopsy it turns out to be follicular adenoma.

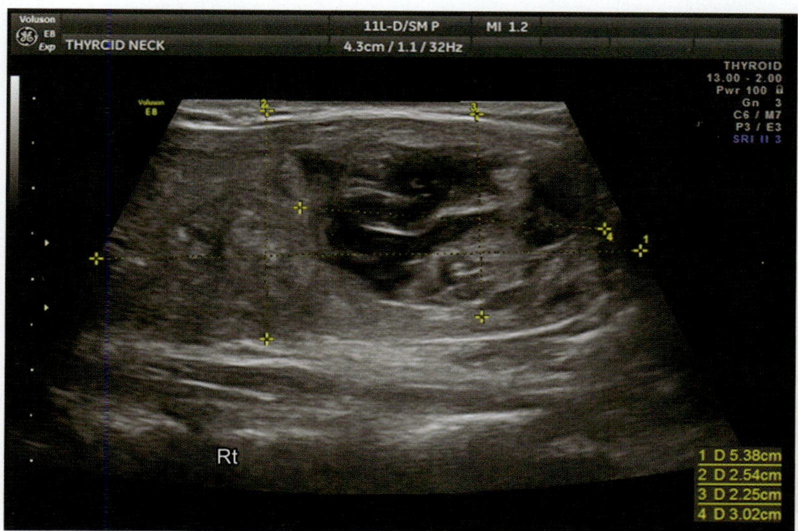

FIGURE 3.36

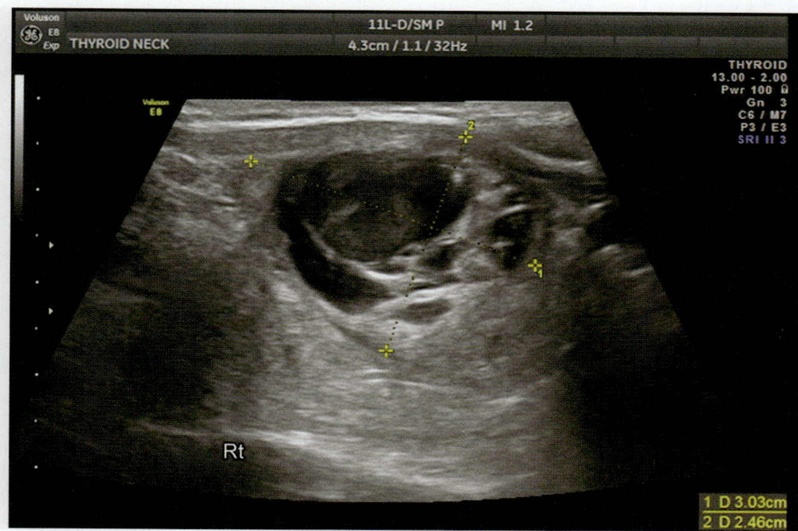

FIGURE 3.37

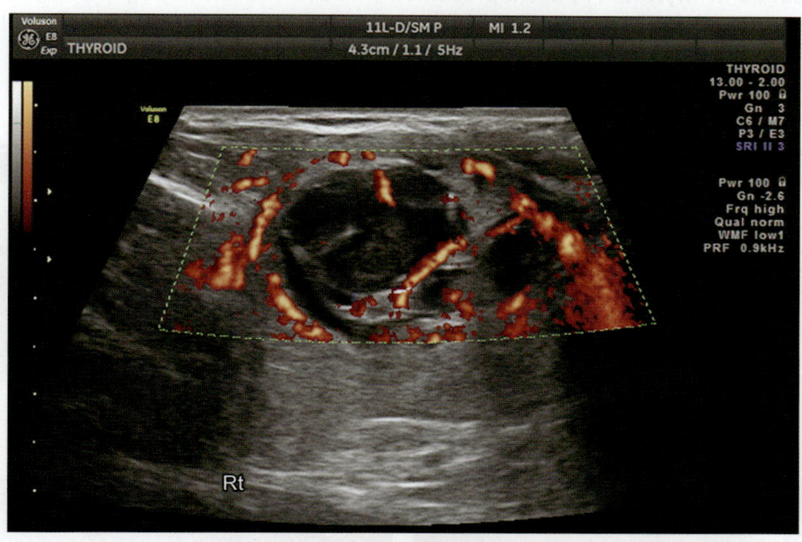

FIGURE 3.38

FIGURES 3.36 to 3.38: Complex nodular mass in the thyroid. A patient presented with diffuse enlargement of right lobe of thyroid. HRSG shows a complex echo mass in the left lobe. It is predominantly cystic. But solid components are also seen in the mass. On color flow imaging, moderate flow is seen in the solid tissue. Fine-needle aspiration cytology (FNAC) of the mass confirms a complex cyst.

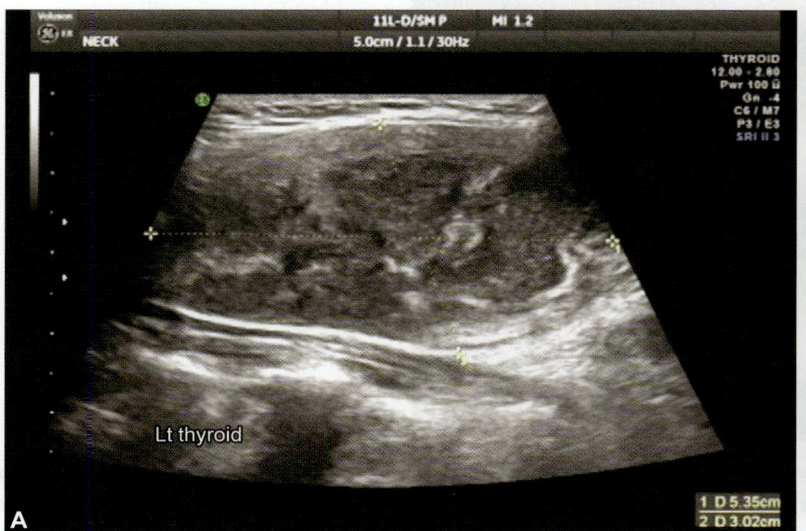

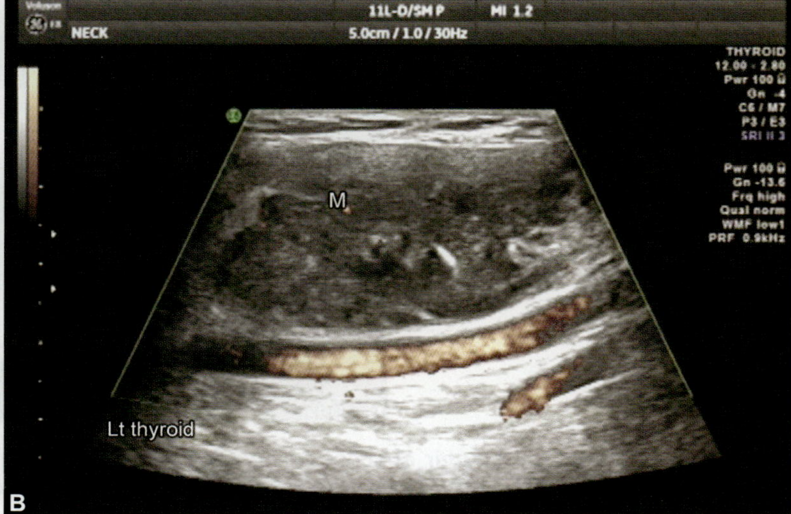

FIGURES 3.39A and B

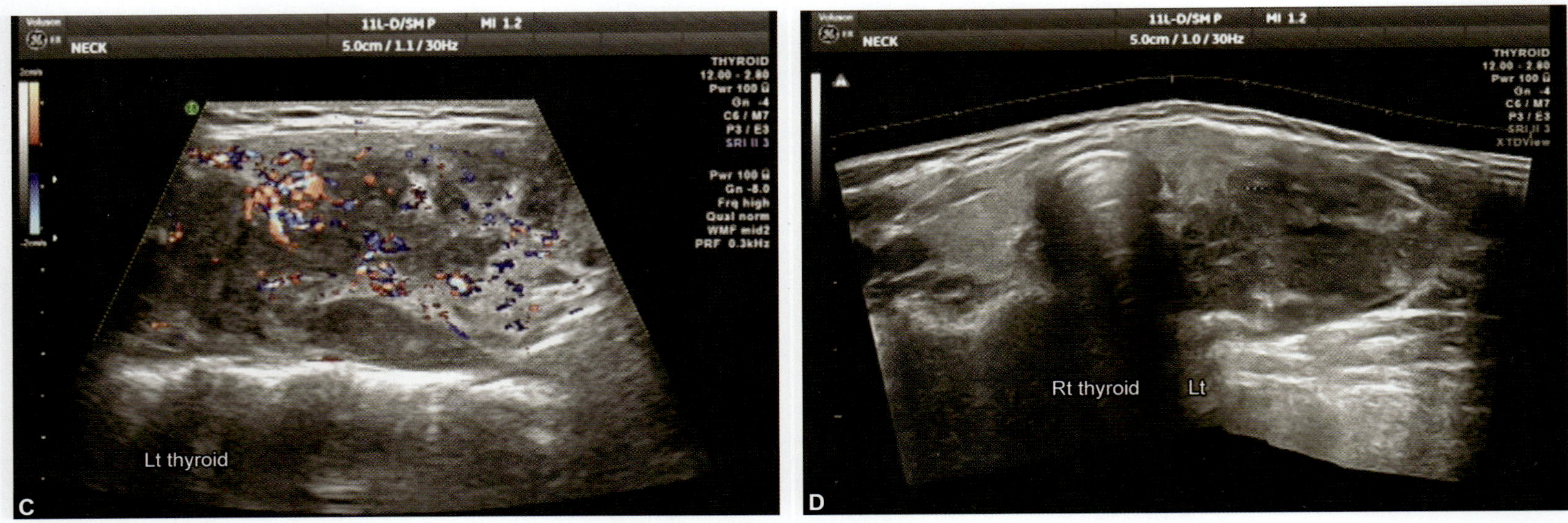

FIGURES 3.39C and D

FIGURES 3.39A to D: Tubercular abscess in thyroid. A patient presented with soft tissue swelling in the neck. HRSG shows a complex echo mass in the left lobe of thyroid. Thick echoes are seen in the mass. Few solid components are also seen in it. On color flow imaging, few vessels are seen feeding the solid component. Aspiration biopsy confirms tuberculosis thyroid.

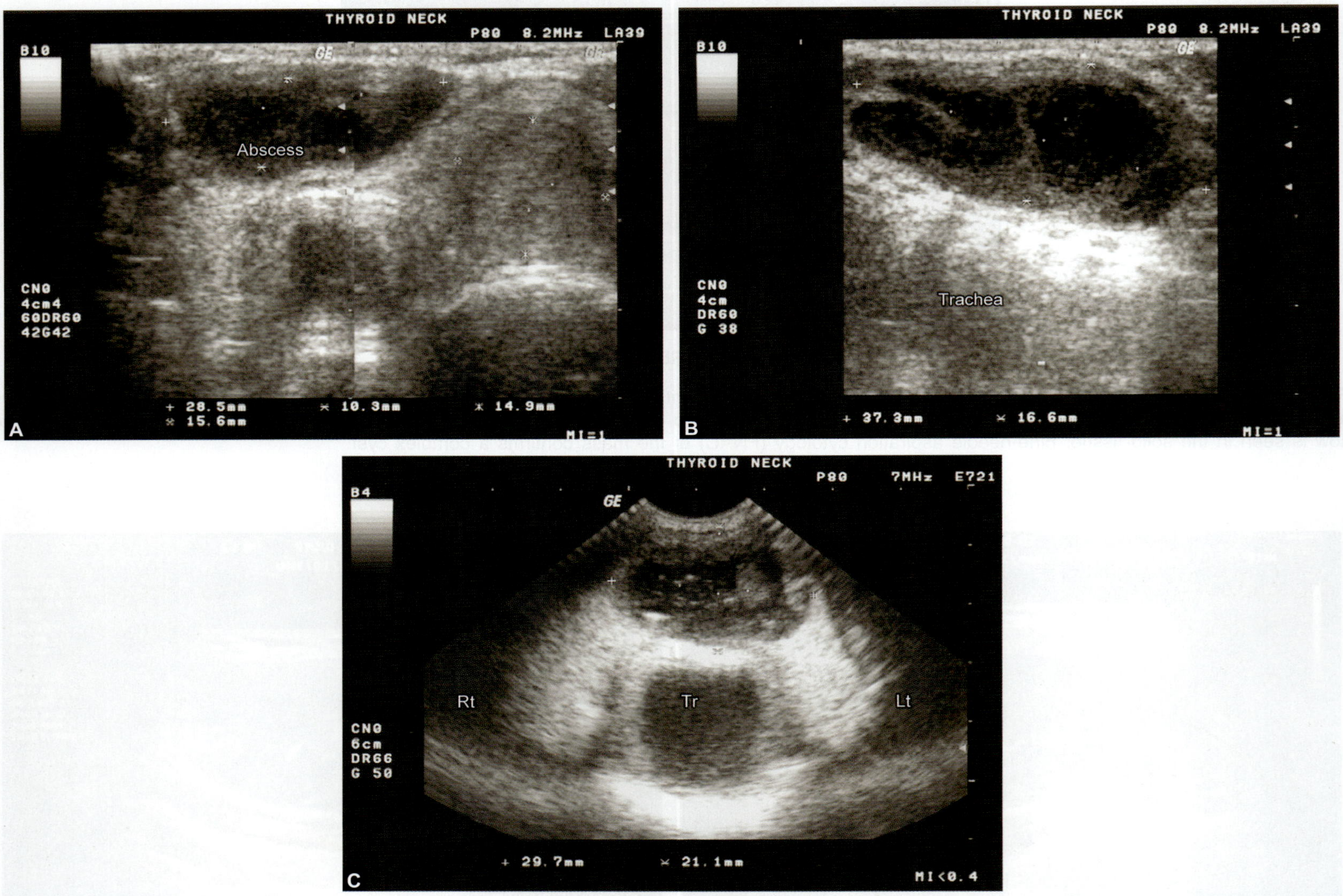

FIGURES 3.40A to C: Tubercular abscess in thyroid. A patient presented with painless soft tissue mass in the midline and right side of the neck in the region of the thyroid. HRSG shows a thick walled low level echo complex mass in the isthmus of the thyroid. Aspiration of the fluid confirmed tubercular abscess in the thyroid. Multiple enlarged nodes are also seen on right side of cervical region. HRSG shows the abscess was limited only in the isthmus pa right of the gland. The tracheal cartilage was intact. They are seen as echogenic bright shadows. Thick walled thick echo mass is seen in the isthmus of the gland. The mass shows multiple internal echoes. It was non-tender. Aspiration confirmed tubercular abscess.

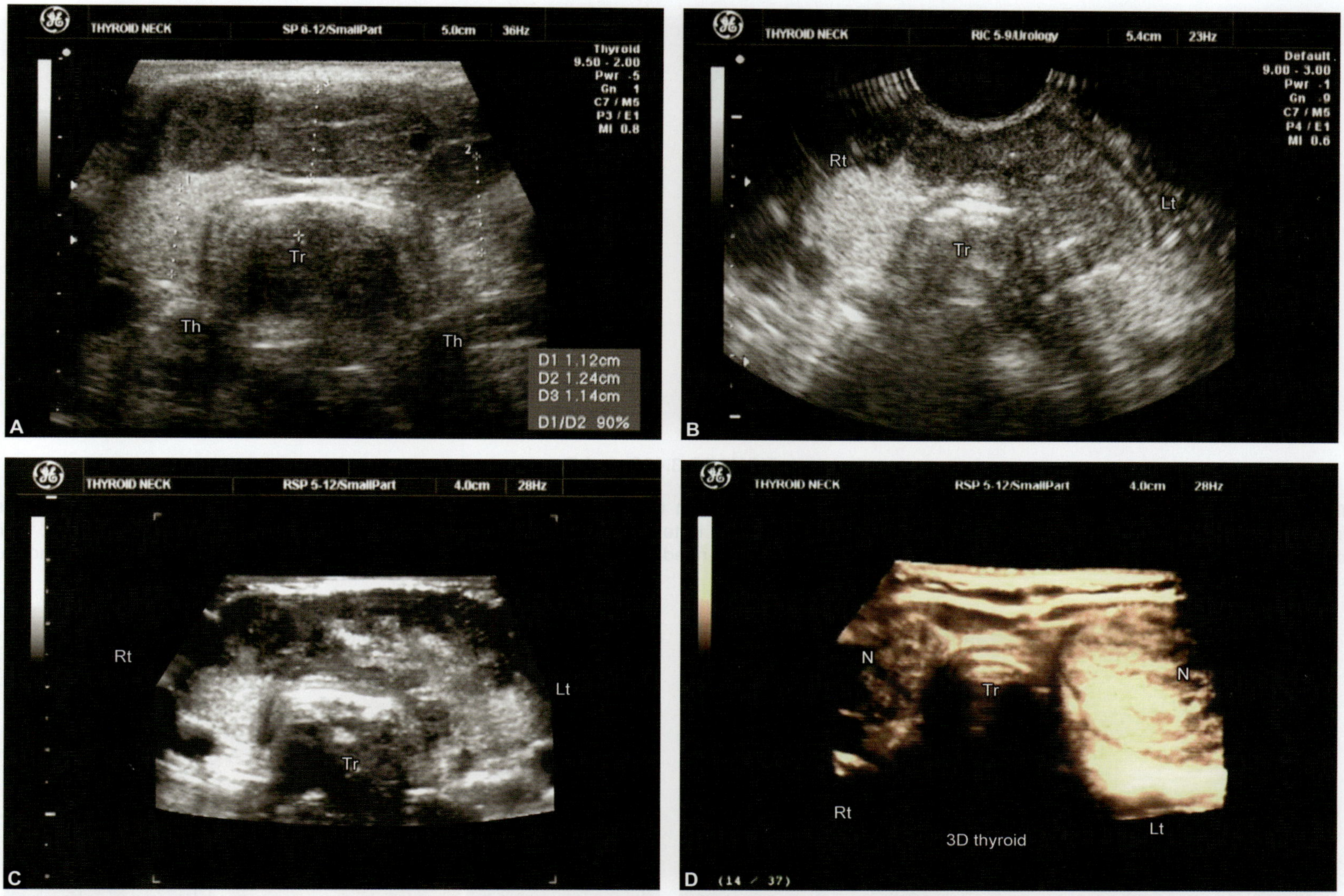

FIGURES 3.41A to D: Acute pyogenic abscess in thyroid. A patient presented with acutely painful thyroid with high fever. HRSG shows distorted texture of the thyroid involving isthmus and both upper lobes of the thyroid on either side. Diffuse necrosis of the gland is seen suggestive of acute pyogenic abscess. 3D imaging of the same patient shows the finer details of the necrosis in the gland. The debris is also seen in the gland.

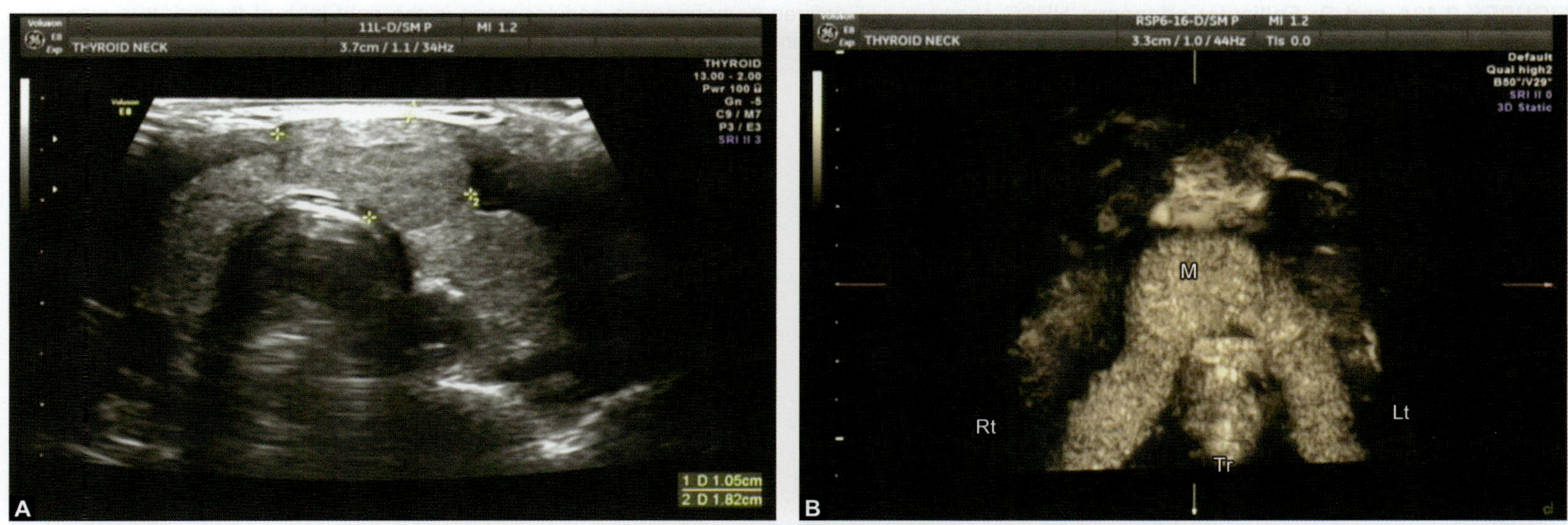

FIGURES 3.42A and B

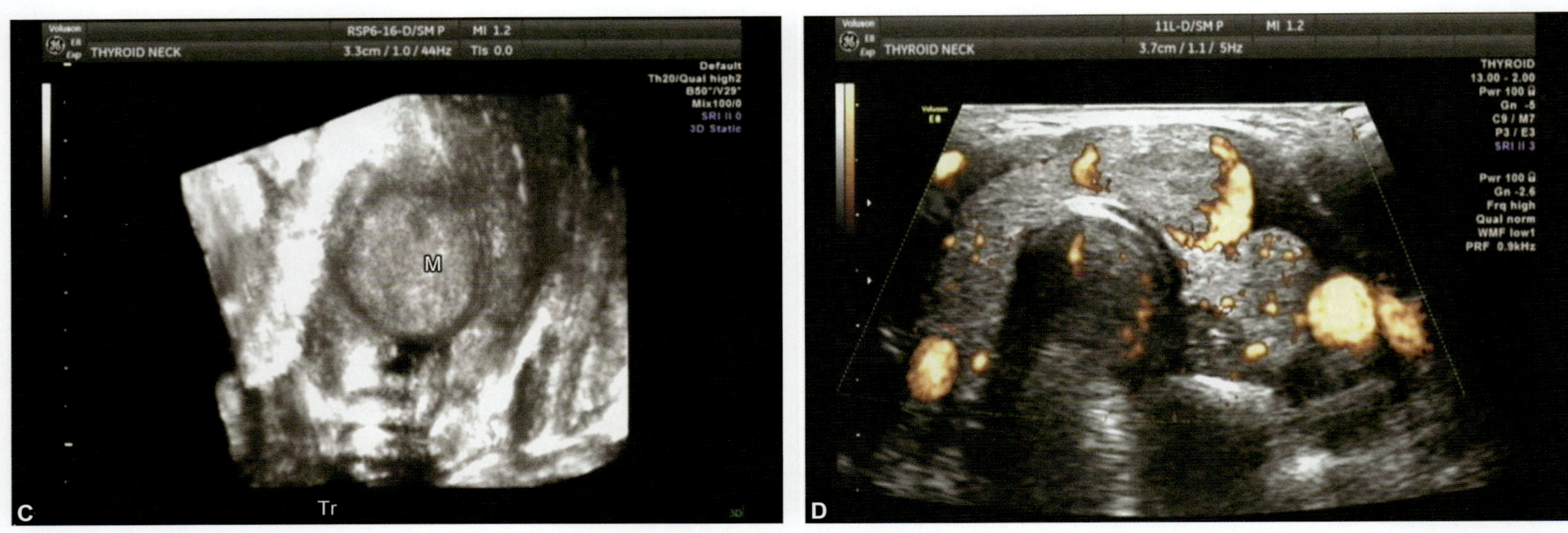

FIGURES 3.42C and D

FIGURES 3.42A to D: Isthmus adenoma. A patient presented with soft tissue swelling in the midline. HRSG shows a well-defined nodular mass in the isthmus of the gland. It is smooth in outline and homogeneous in texture. On 3D volume contrast imaging, it is seen clearly coming out from the isthmus. On color flow imaging, peripheral flow is seen in it. Fine-needle aspiration cytology (FNAC) from the mass confirms follicular adenoma.

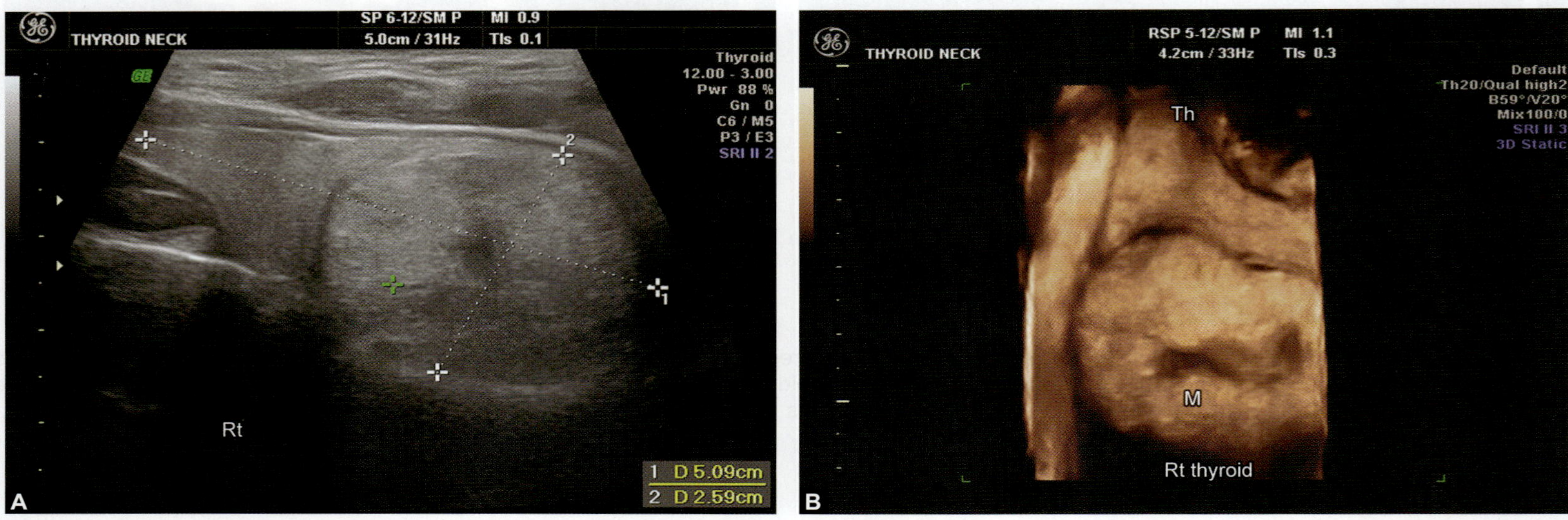

FIGURES 3.43A and B: Follicular adenoma. HRSG shows a well-defined homogeneous nodular mass in the right lobe of thyroid. It is smooth in outline with sharp margins. Perinodular halo is also seen. On 3D imaging fascial plane is well-maintain, the typical feature of benign adenoma.

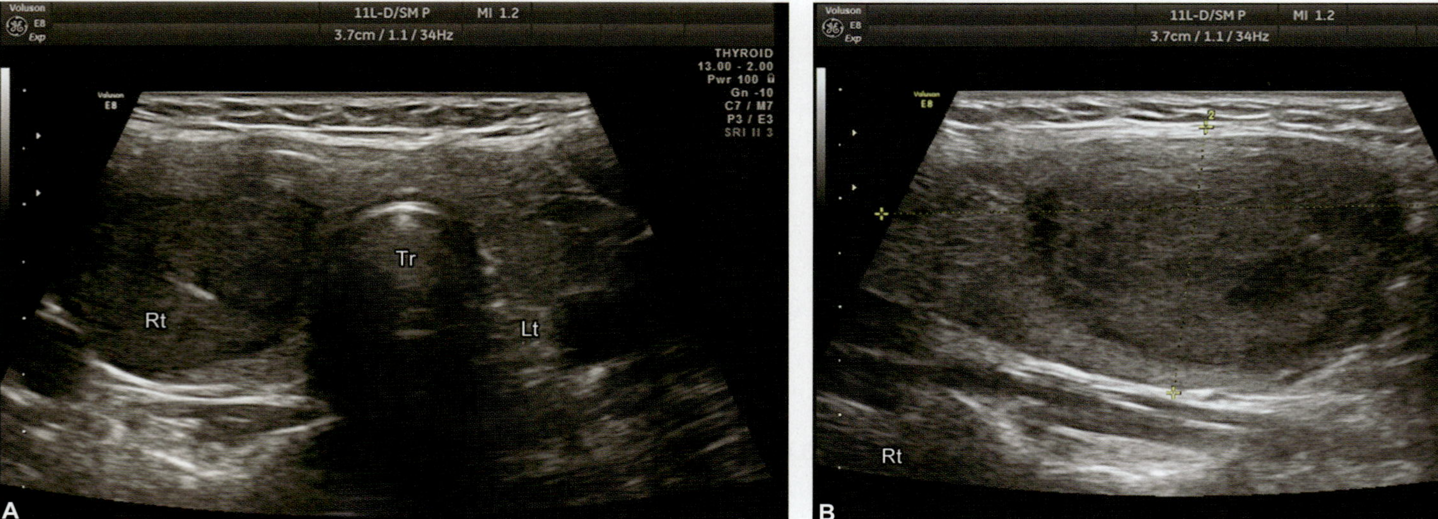

FIGURES 3.44A and B

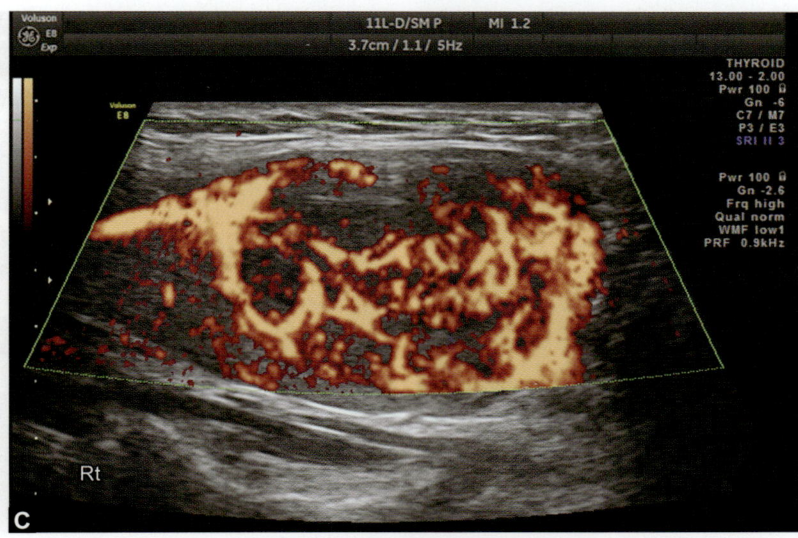

FIGURE 3.44C

FIGURES 3.44A to C: Follicular adenoma. HRSG shows a well-defined hypoechoic homogeneous nodular mass in the right lobe of thyroid. It shows perinodular halo. No calcification is seen in it. On color flow imaging, increased flow is seen in it, which is seen more in the periphery of the nodule suggestive of follicular adenoma.

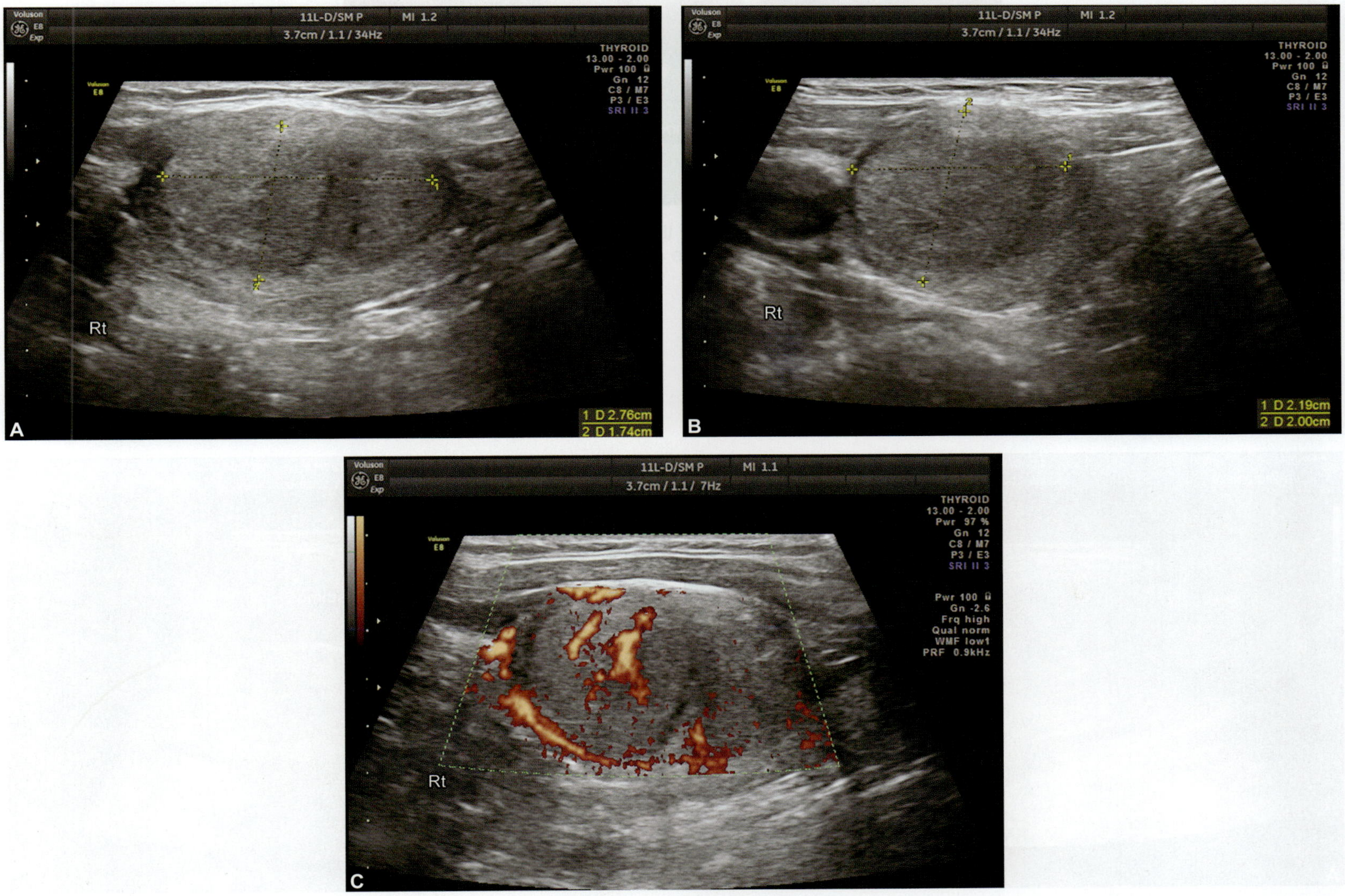

FIGURES 3.45A to C: Follicular adenoma. A well-defined isoechogenic nodular mass is seen in the right lobe of thyroid. Perinodular halo is seen around it. It is smooth in outline. No calcification is seen into it. On color flow imaging, flow is seen in the periphery of nodule suggestive of follicular adenoma.

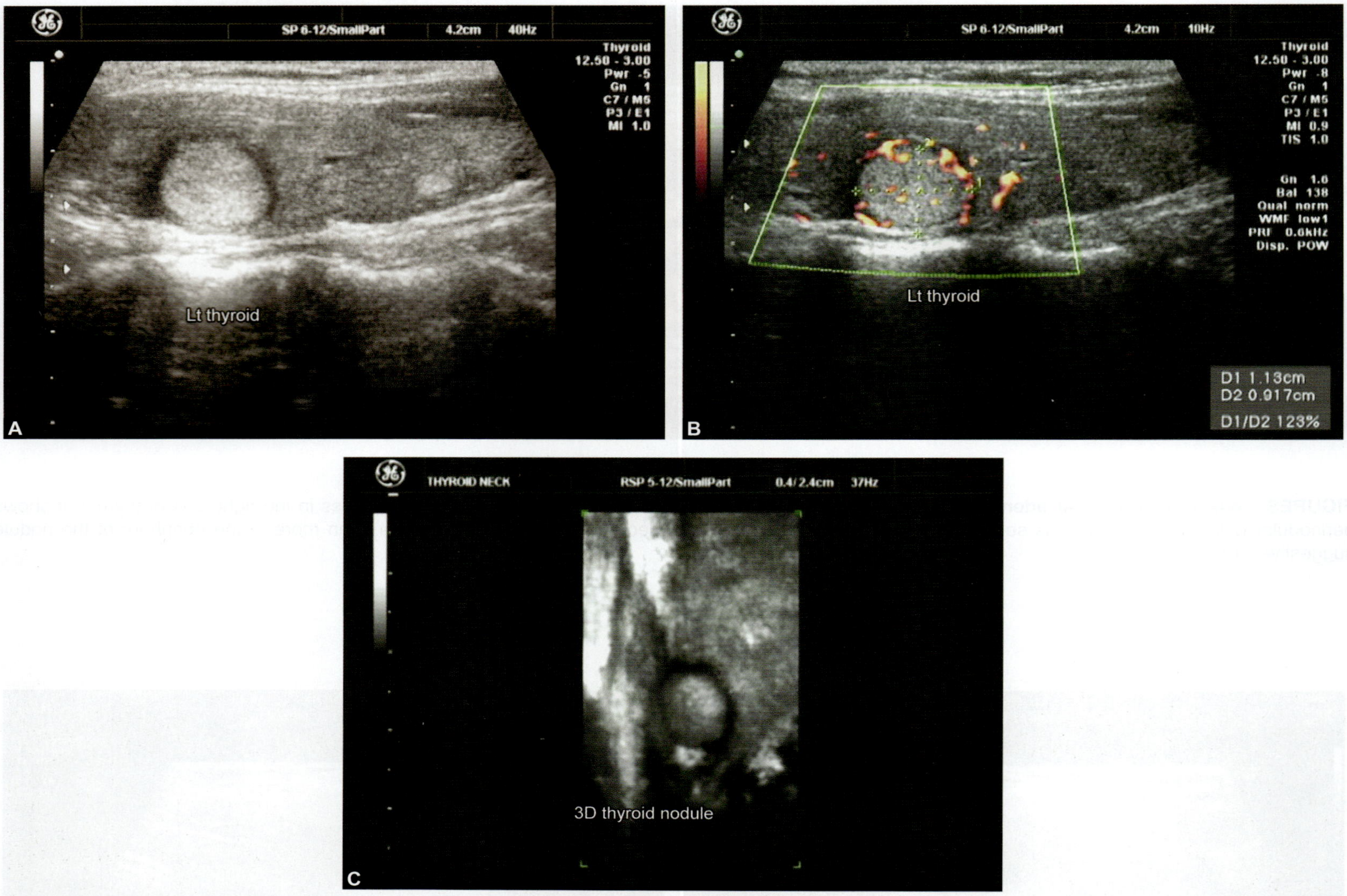

FIGURES 3.46A to C: On color flow imaging smooth flow is seen around the adenoma. Few vessels are also seen feeding the adenoma suggestive of follicular nature of the adenoma. 3D imaging of thyroid adenoma of the same patient shows better sonographic details of the adenoma with finer details of anatomical relationship.

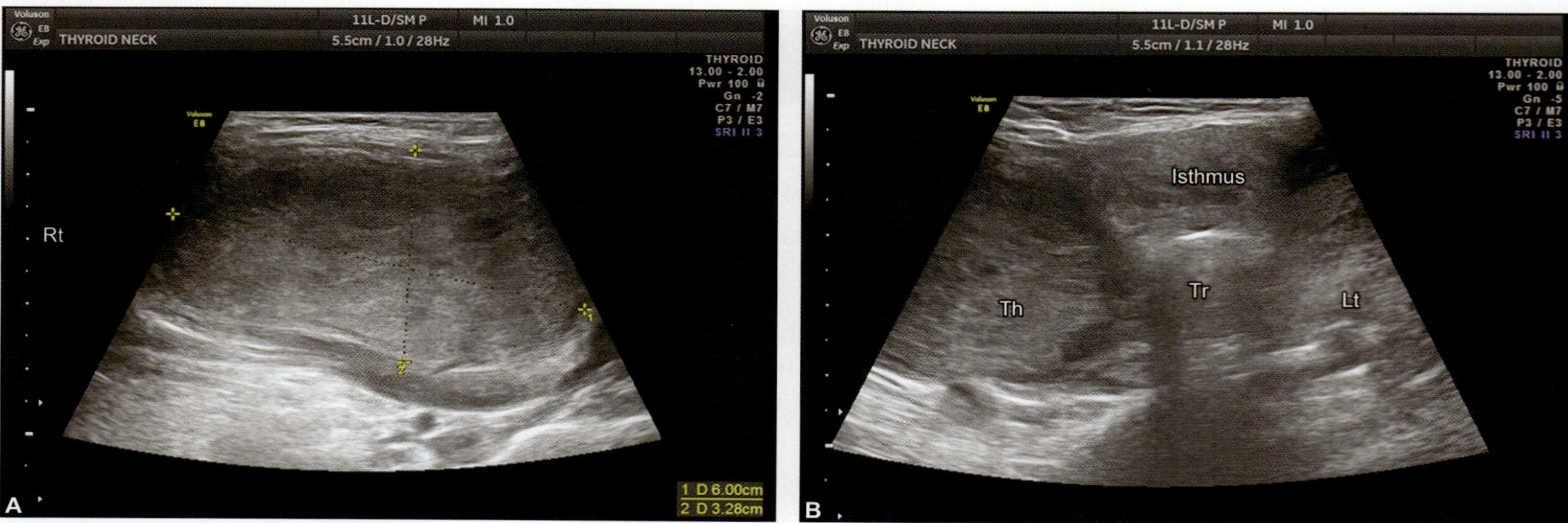

FIGURES 3.47A and B

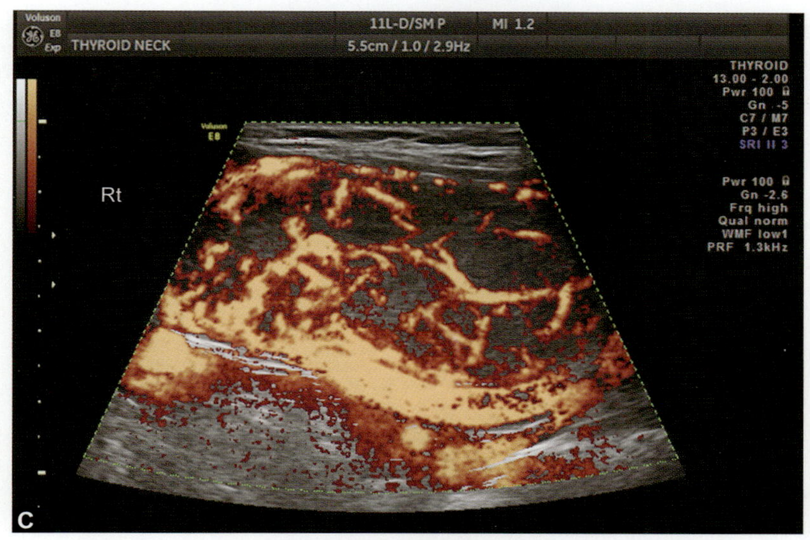

FIGURE 3.47C

FIGURES 3.47A to C: Big follicular adenoma. HRSG shows a big isoechogenic nodular mass in the right lobe of thyroid. Another nodular shadow is seen in the isthmus. They are smooth in outline. Perinodular halo is present. No calcification or cystic degeneration is seen in them. On color flow imaging, increased flow is seen in the periphery of the nodule. Biopsy of the mass confirms follicular adenoma.

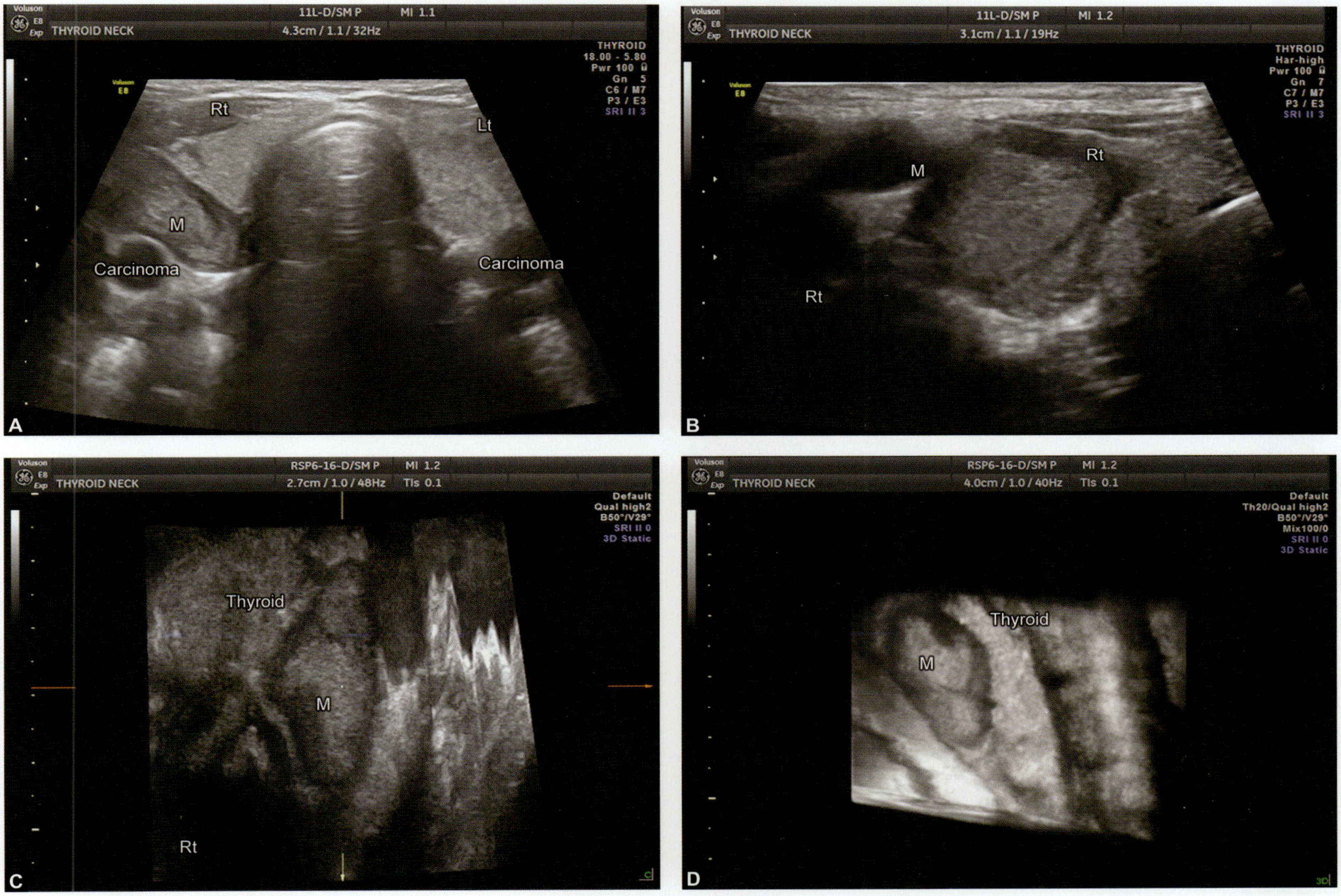

FIGURES 3.48A to D

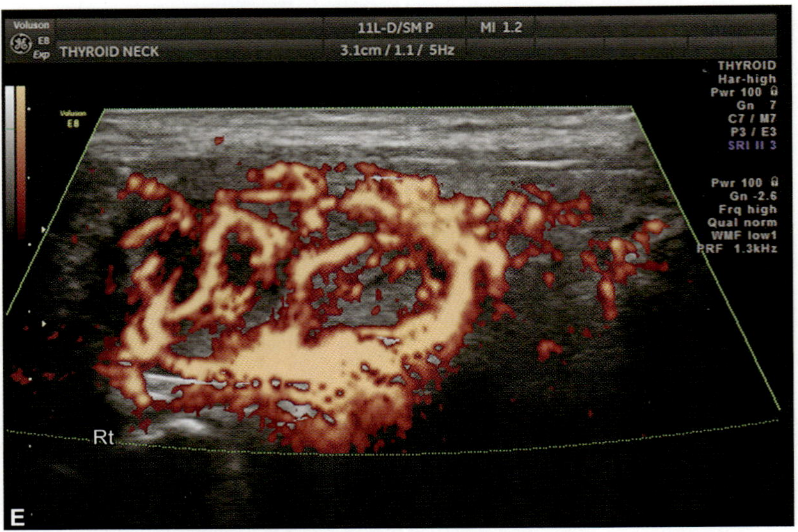

FIGURE 3.48E

FIGURES 3.48A to E: Parathyroid adenoma. A patient presented with soft tissue nodular mass in the neck. He was also having history of recurrent renal stone formation. HRSG shows a well-defined soft tissue mass at the inferior pole of the right lobe of thyroid. It is smooth in outline and homogeneous in texture. It is separate from the thyroid, which is clearly seen on 3D imaging. In volume contrast 3D imaging, the mass is clearly defined and separate from thyroid. On color flow imaging, it shows increased flow. Biopsy of the mass confirms parathyroid adenoma.

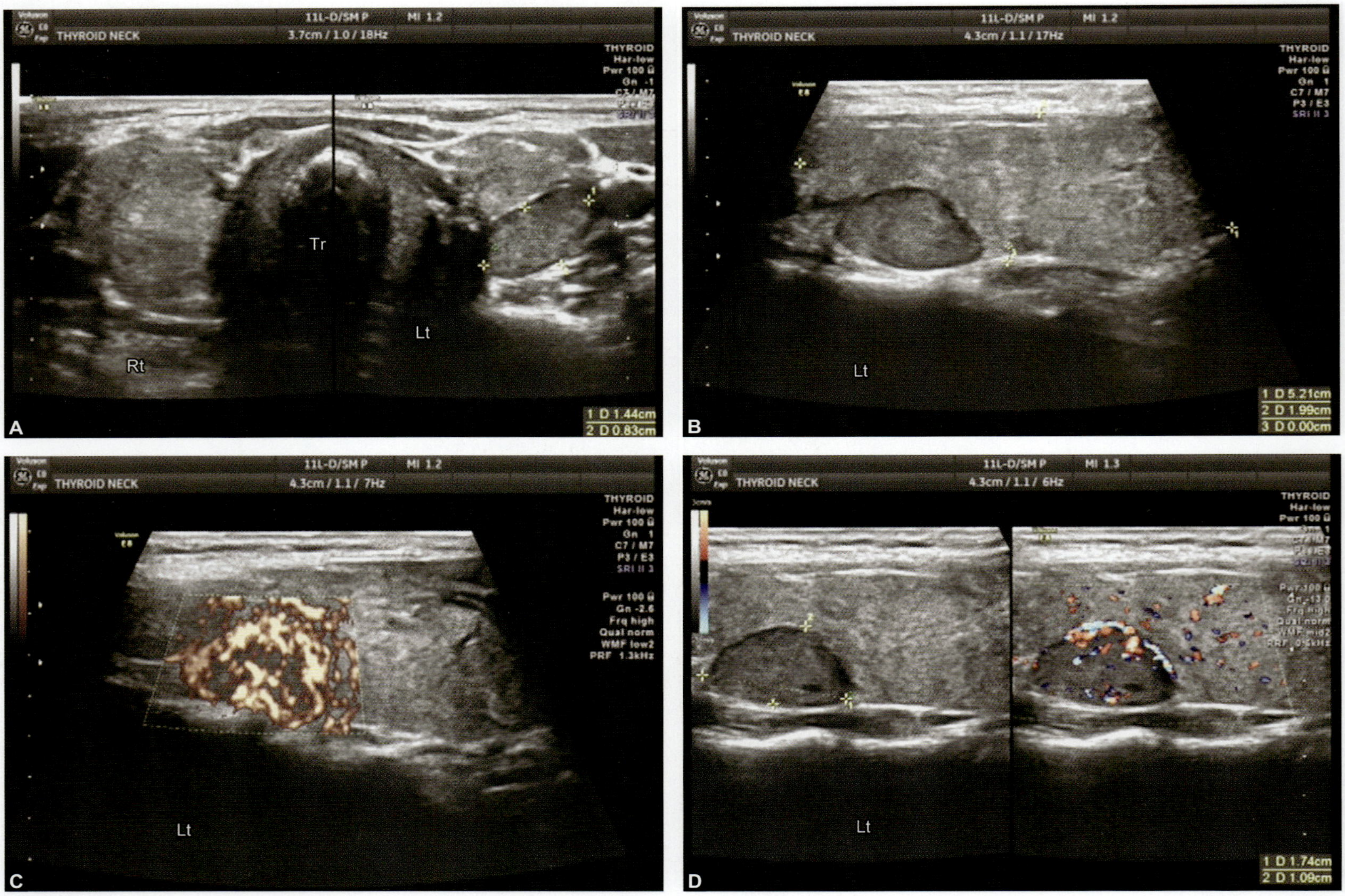

FIGURES 3.49A to D: Parathyroid adenoma. A well-defined homogeneous hypoechoic nodular mass seen in relation to lower pole of left lobe. Perinodular halo is seen around it. It is seen separate from the thyroid. No calcification or cystic degeneration is seen in it. On color flow imaging, increased flow is seen in the nodular mass. Biopsy of the mass confirms parathyroid adenoma.

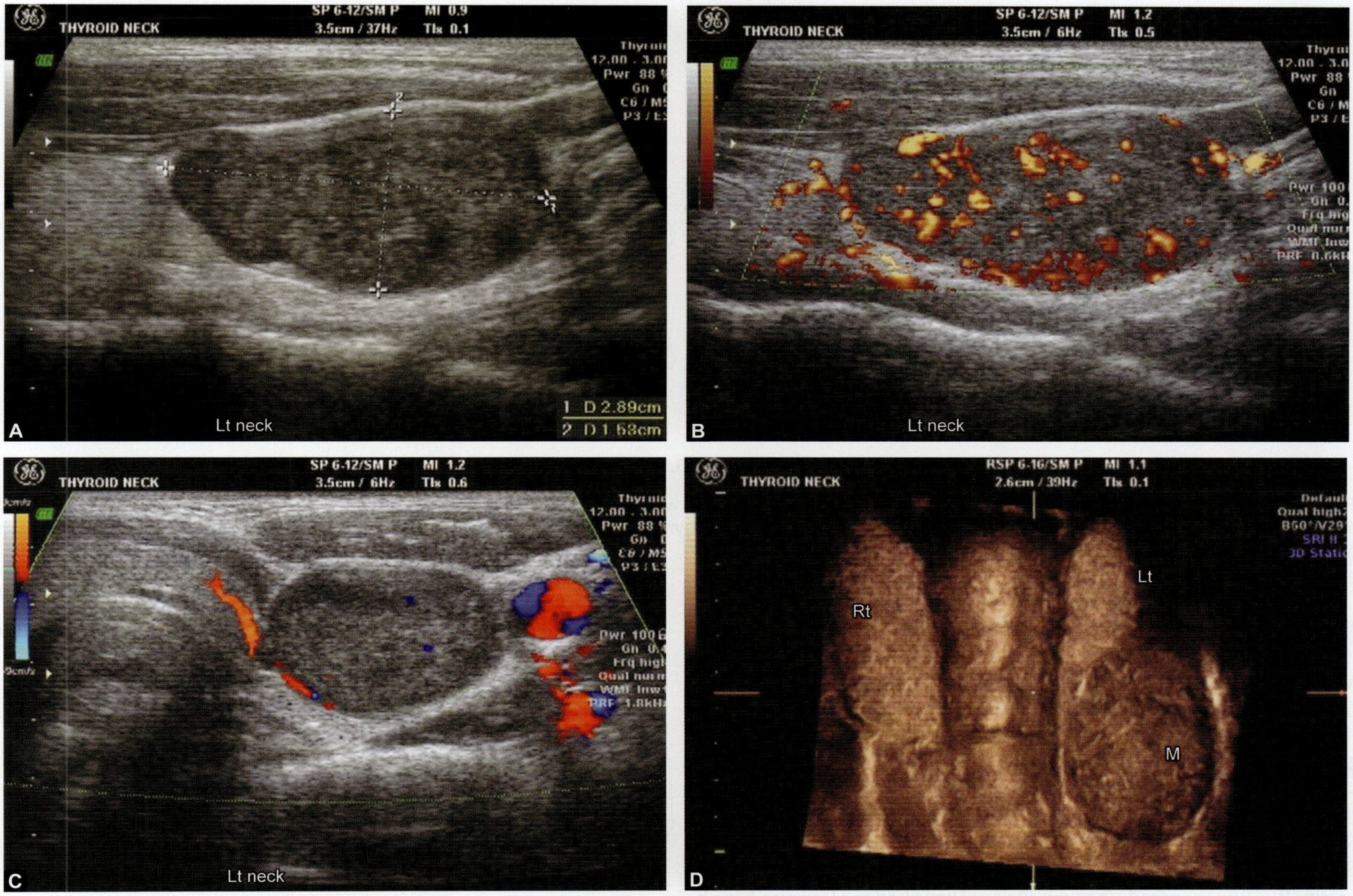

FIGURES 3.50A to D: Parathyroid adenoma. A patient presented with soft tissue mass in left side of the neck. HRSG shows a well-defined homogeneous hypoechoic lobulated mass. It is seen in relation to the inferior pole of the left thyroid. However, on 3D imaging, it is seen separate from the thyroid. No evidence of any calcification or cystic degeneration is seen in the mass. On color flow imaging, moderate flow is seen in it. Fine-needle aspiration cytology (FNAC) of the mass confirms parathyroid adenoma.

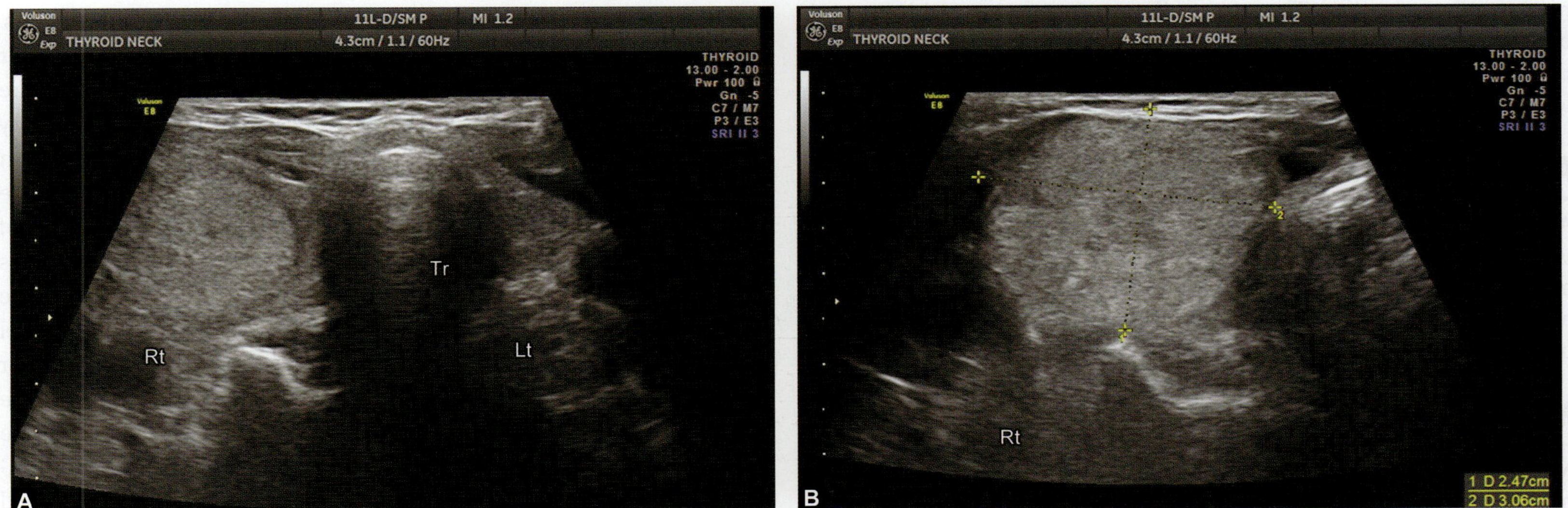

FIGURES 3.51A and B

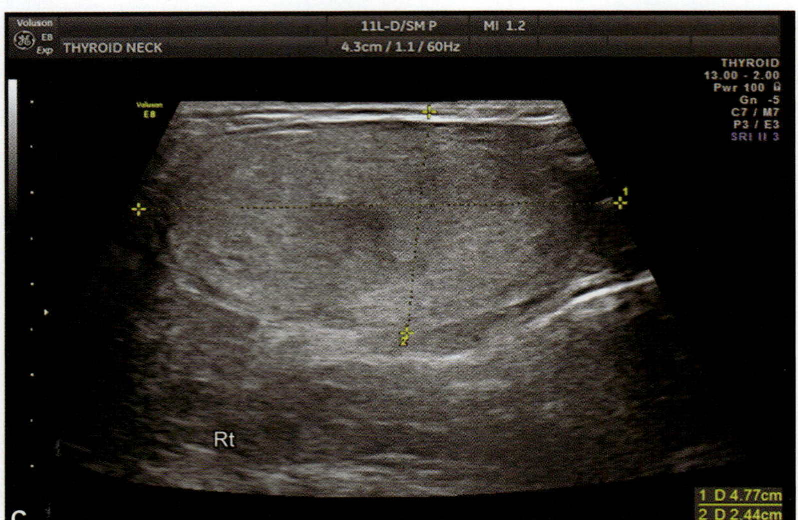

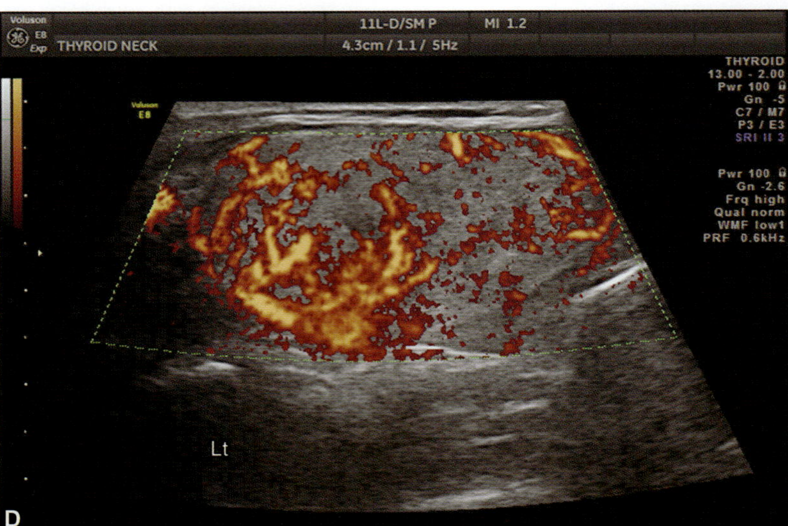

FIGURES 3.51C and D

FIGURES 3.51A to D: Big parathyroid adenoma. A patient presented with a big soft tissue mass in relation to the inferior pole of right lobe of thyroid. It is homogeneous in texture and it is seen separate from the thyroid. Perinodular halo is present. On color flow imaging, increased flow is seen in it. Biopsy of the mass confirms parathyroid adenoma.

MALIGNANT TUMORS OF THYROID

Malignant tumors of thyroid gland are not very common. They are present in 2–3 cases per 100,000. Thyroid neoplasms are grouped as follows.

Papillary Carcinoma

Papillary carcinoma is most common thyroid malignancy. It accounts for 60–65% of the total thyroid neoplasms. It is more common in females than males. The tumor incidence is high in young adults and elderly age group. This tumor spreads through regional lymphatics. However, lymph node involvement does not aggravate the prognosis. The prognosis is better in papillary neoplasms.

Follicular Carcinoma

Follicular carcinoma accounts for 15–20% of the thyroid neoplasms. It is more common in elder age group. It is well-differentiated from benign follicular adenoma on HRSG. The tumor spread is through hematonenous route. Therefore, distant metastases to lung and bones are more common in follicular neoplasm. Typical cannon ball metastases are found in lungs. However at times, poorly differentiated follicular neoplasms are also encountered.

Anaplastic Carcinoma

Anaplastic carcinoma is the most aggressive variety of thyroid cancer. It is found in 10–15% of total thyroid malignancy. It has worse prognosis, and 5-year survival is found only in 3–4% of the cases. The tumor presents as rapidly growing mass with surrounding tissue invasion. Therefore, it often presents as an inoperable mass.

Medullary Carcinoma

Medullary carcinomas are present in 5–10% of the thyroid cancers. They are derived from parafollicular or C cells. They secrete calcitonin hormone. It is used as serum tumor marker. The tumor is commonly familial. It is also an essential part of multiple endocrine neoplasia (MEN) type II syndrome. The tumor is multicentric and in about 90% cases involves both lobes of the gland. It spreads through lymph node metastasis. Prognosis of the disease is considered worse than follicular neoplasm.

Sonographic Features

Most of the time, thyroid malignant tumor presents as an echo poor nodule. However, no specific ultrasonographic pattern is described for thyroid malignancy. The tumor may present as isoreflective nodule in 25% cases, and mixed echo complex mass in about 10% cases. However, echogenic pattern of tumor is very rare. About 90% of the echo poor nodules are malignant tumors. Therefore, all the thyroid nodules require fine-needle aspiration cytology (FNAC) for confirmation. It can be done under ultrasonographic guidance. Cystic degeneration is also encountered both in malignant and benign nodule. Coarse calcification is a feature of benign mass, but it can be seen in malignant tumor. Microcalcification is the typical feature of malignant neoplasm. It is highly echogenic focus of less than 2 mm, which can be detected by 10 MHz probe. Cystic degeneration is also encountered. The margins are irregular and ill-defined. A peripheral halo is seen. However, it is also seen in benign mass. Therefore, it is not a reliable sign, but in malignant tumor, it is irregular and incomplete. The most reliable indications of thyroid malignancy are surrounding tissue invasion and lymph node involvement. HRSG is very sensitive tool to detect them when they are non-palpable. Big tumors can destroy the normal glandular pattern and surrounding tissue relations are frequently encountered in anaplastic carcinoma. Dynamic sonography of the mass during swallowing can show the fixity of mass to strap muscles anteriorly or longus colli muscle posteriorly. Vascular invasion of the tumor mass can be easily identified on HRSG. The most common vessel involved is internal jugular vein. The vein can be either infiltrated or thrombosed due to metastatic compression. Recurrent laryngeal nerve can be assessed on HRSG in 5–7% of the cases. Cervical lymph node involvement is found mainly in papillary or medullary carcinoma. HRSG is also valuable to assess post-surgery or post-irradiation status of thyroid malignancy. Recurrence of tumor or lymph node involvement is most easily picked up on HRSG, as surgical scarring and post-irradiation fibrosis make clinical examination difficult.

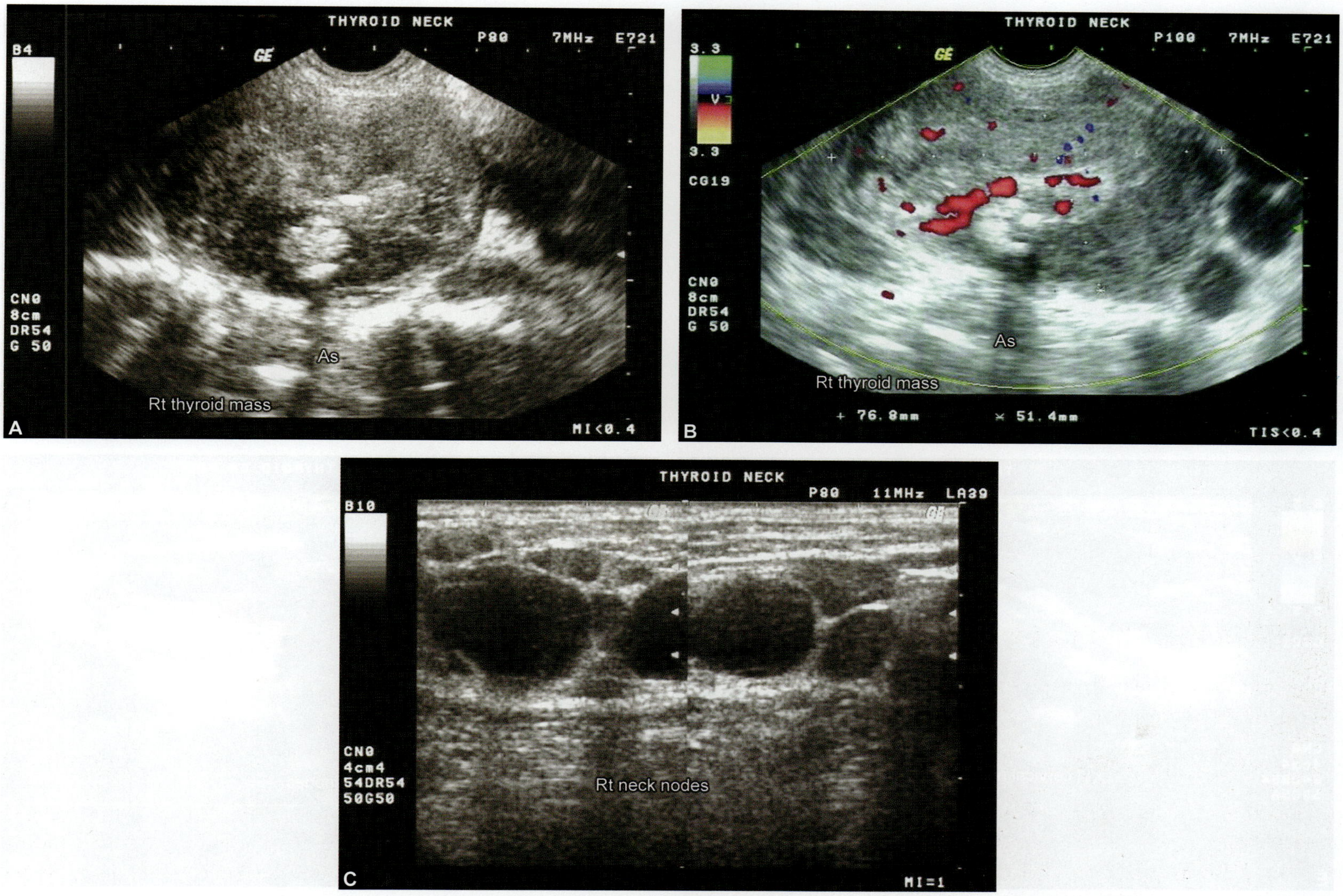

FIGURES 3.52A to C: Heterogeneous mass in thyroid. A big irregular heterogeneous mass was seen involving right lobe of the thyroid. The mass has destroyed normal glandular texture. Echogenic calcification is also seen in the mass. It is accompanied with acoustic shadowing. The mass was seen involving and invading the tracheal ring. Biopsy confirmed a poorly differentiated carcinoma of thyroid. Color Doppler imaging shows low flow in the mass suggestive of hypovascular nature of the mass. Multiple enlarged nodal shadows are seen in the neck suggestive of enlarged lymph nodes in the same patient. Normal nodal texture is lost with distorted hylum of the nodes. Biopsy confirmed metastatic nodes from adenocarcinoma.

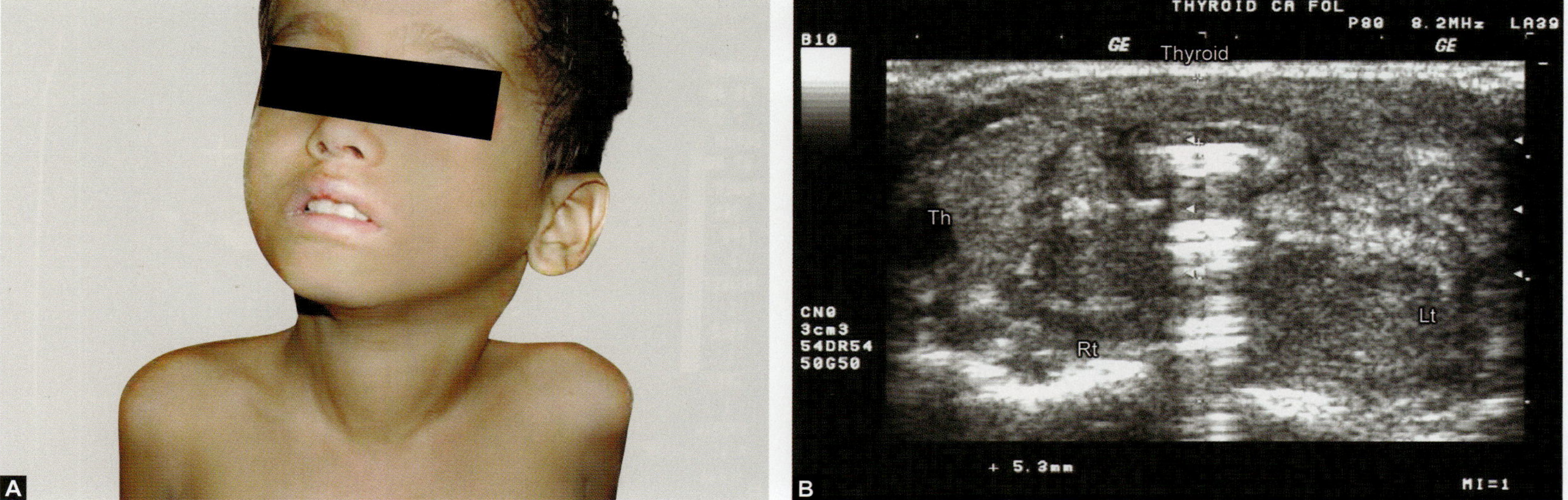

FIGURES 3.53A and B

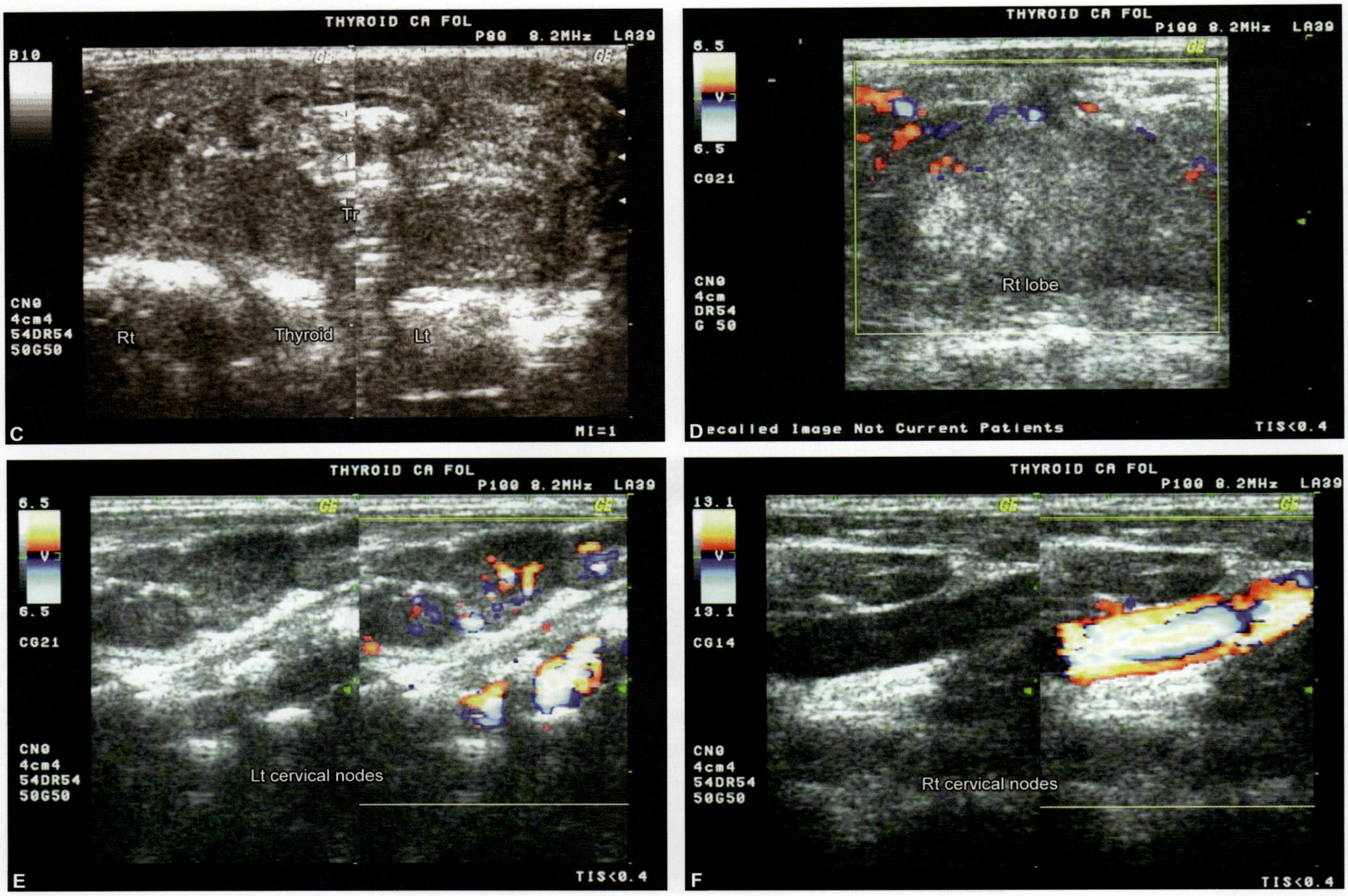

FIGURES 3.53C to F

FIGURES 3.53A to F: Invasive papillary carcinoma in a child. A young child presented with a soft mass swelling in the neck. The patient was presented with acute respiratory distress syndrome. HRSG shows a big irregular heterogeneous mass in young child of 5 years in both lobes of the thyroid. The mass has destroyed normal thyroid anatomy. It is seen invading the muscle planes and also the tracheal rings and pa right of trachea. Echogenic calcification is also seen in the mass. But no cystic degeneration is seen. Normal anatomy was destroyed. Color Doppler imaging of the mass shows poor flow suggestive of low vascularity, which was only confined to the periphery. HRSG also shows multiple enlarged irregular hypoechoic lymph node masses seen on either side of the neck with lost normal texture. Biopsy of the mass shows invasive papillary carcinoma with follicular predominance. Carcinoma of thyroid in children is rare and not reported below the age of 7 years. However, this was a rare case when invasive papillary carcinoma with follicular predominance was found in a young child of 5 years of age with local spread.

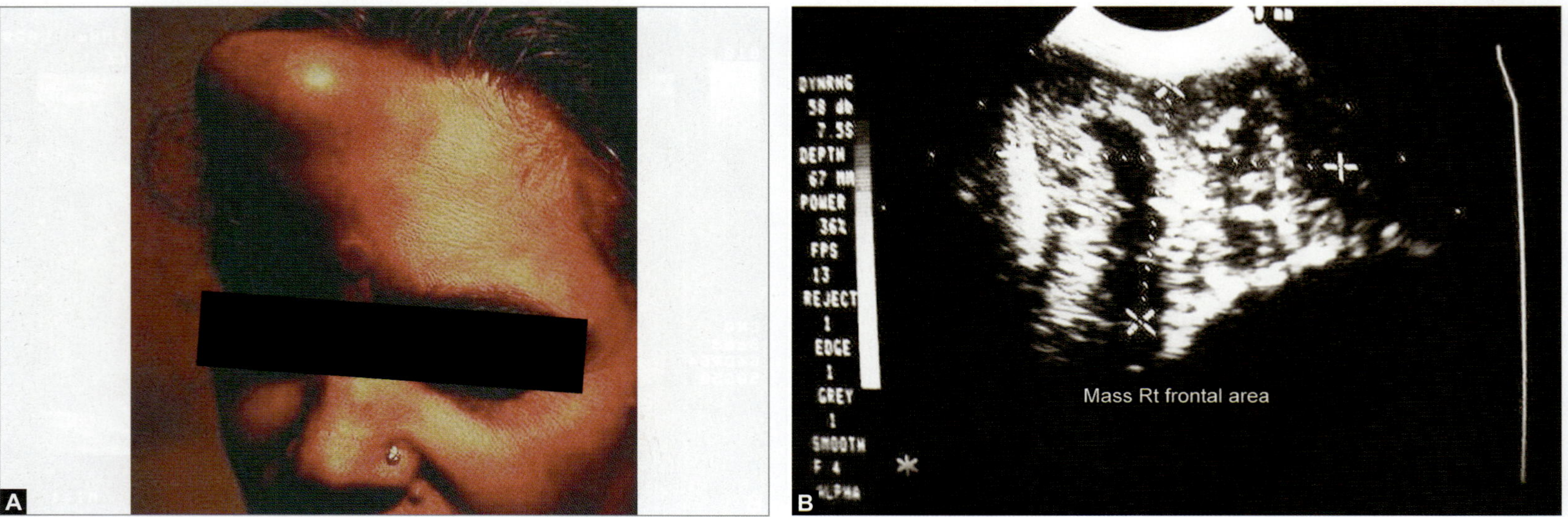

FIGURES 3.54A and B

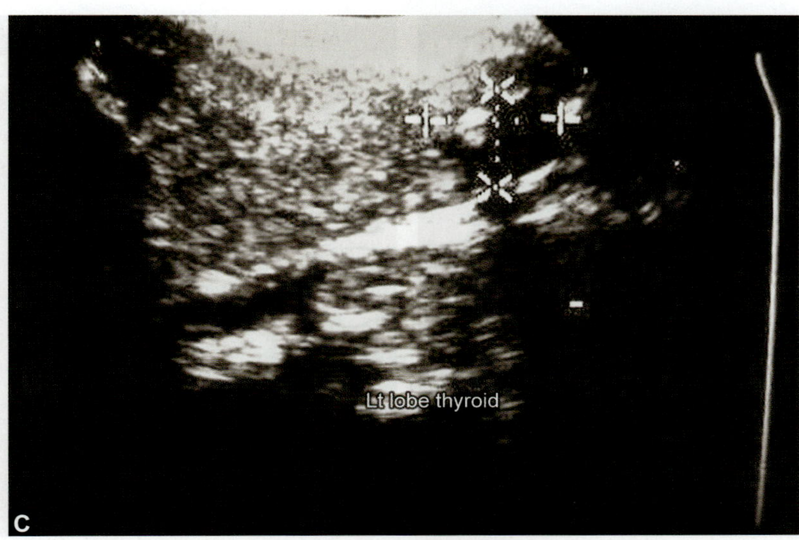

FIGURE 3.54C

FIGURES 3.54A to C: Occult papillary carcinoma in thyroid. A young lady was presented with a soft tissue mass over the frontal area. HRSG of the mass shows irregular heterogeneous mass with multiple hypoechoic areas. Biopsy of the mass shows metastatic deposits from adenocarcinoma. HRSG of the thyroid gland of the same patient shows small non-palpable irregular nodular mass in the left lobe of the thyroid measures 10 × 8 mm in size. Ultrasound guided fine-needle aspiration cytology (FNACA) of the mass shows papillary carcinoma.

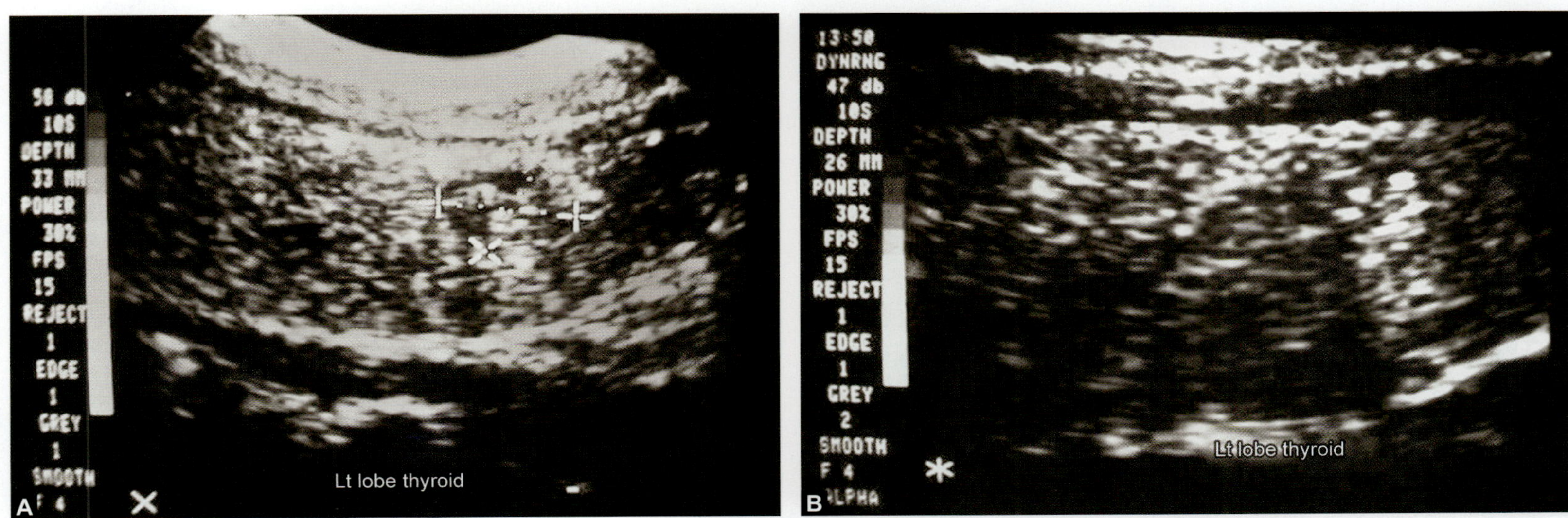

FIGURES 3.55A and B: Occult primary carcinoma of thyroid. A middle-aged man was presented with multiple metastatic nodes in the left side of the neck. Biopsy through metastasis of the adenocarcinoma HRSG of thyroid shows irregular heterogeneous nodular mass in the left lobe. Which was non-palpable in clinical examination. Ultrasound guided biopsy confirmed occu left primary in thyroid.

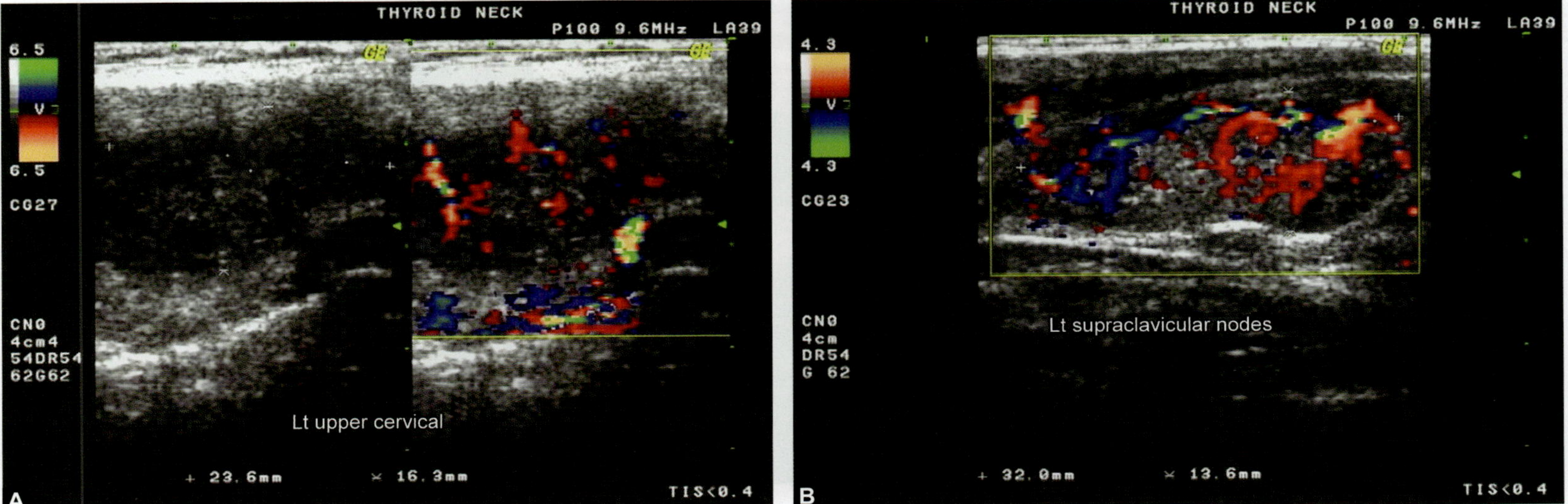

FIGURES 3.56A and B

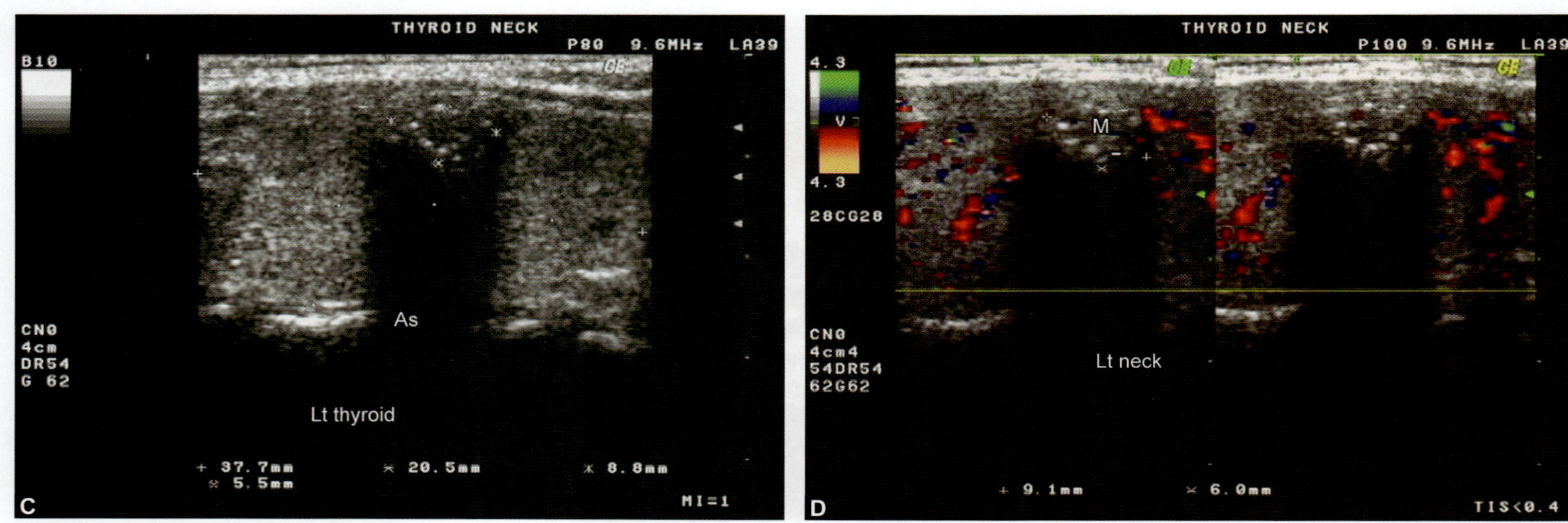

FIGURES 3.56C and D

FIGURES 3.56A to D: Invasive non-palpable papillary carcinoma thyroid. A young girl presented with multiple enlarged lymph nodes in the neck. HRSG shows irregular heterogeneous nodal masses in the neck. Biopsy of the nodes proved metastasis from adenocarcinoma. Color flow imaging shows high flow in the nodes. HRSG shows small heterogeneous nodular mass in the left lobe of thyroid gland. Echogenic punctate calcified specks are seen in it. Biopsy from the nodule confirmed invasive papillary carcinoma.

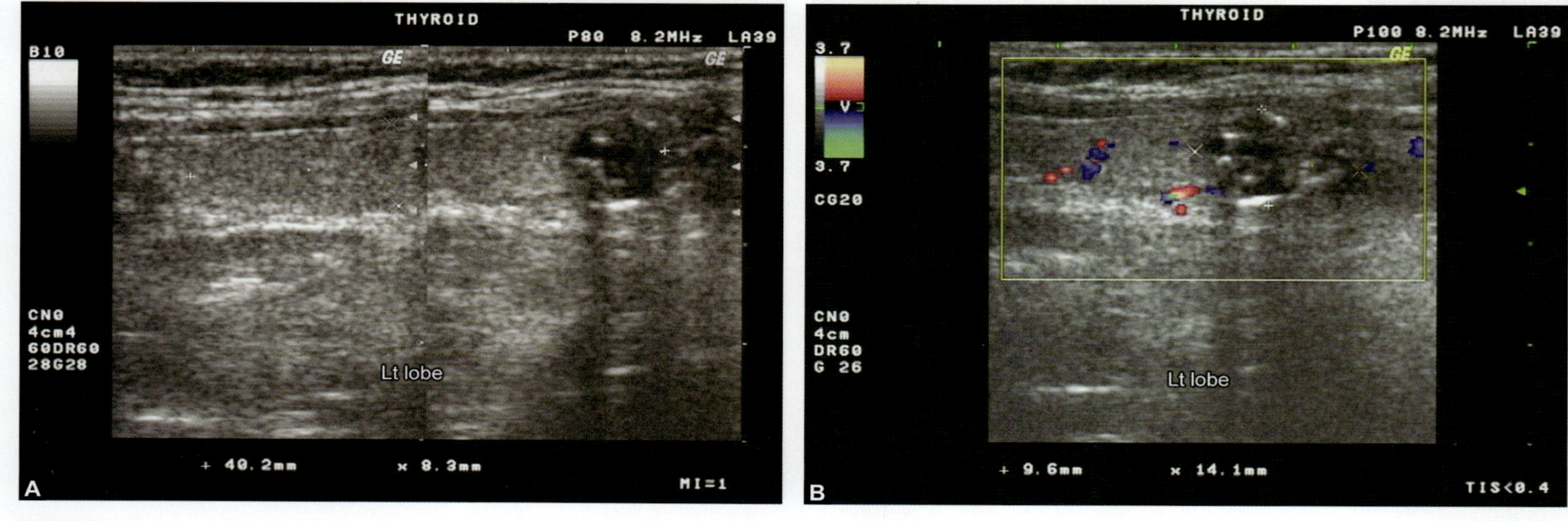

FIGURES 3.57A and B: Papillary carcinoma thyroid. A patient presented with heterogeneous non-palpable nodule in the left lobe of thyroid with microcalcification. HRSG guided fine-needle aspiration cytology (FNAC) confirmed papillary adenocarcinoma of thyroid.

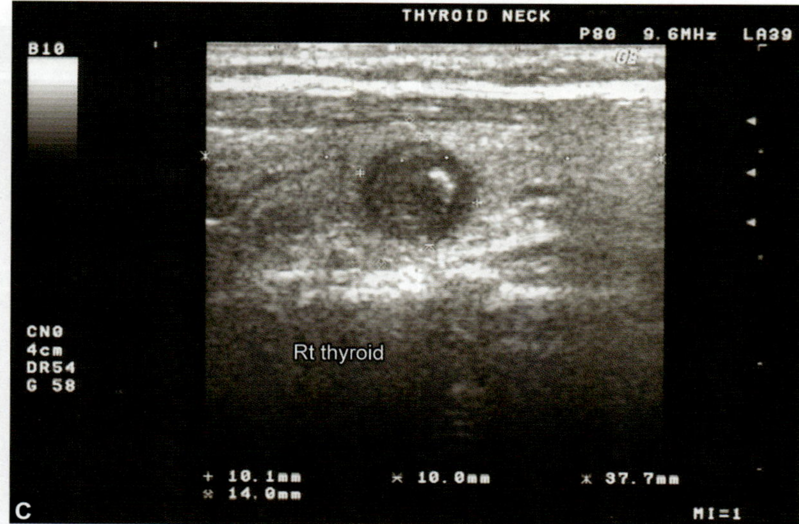

FIGURE 3.57C: Papillary adenocarcinoma thyroid. Longitudinal image of thyroid shows a hypoechoic nodular mass in the right lobe of the gland. Echogenic punctate calcification is seen in it. Biopsy showed papillary adenocarcinoma.

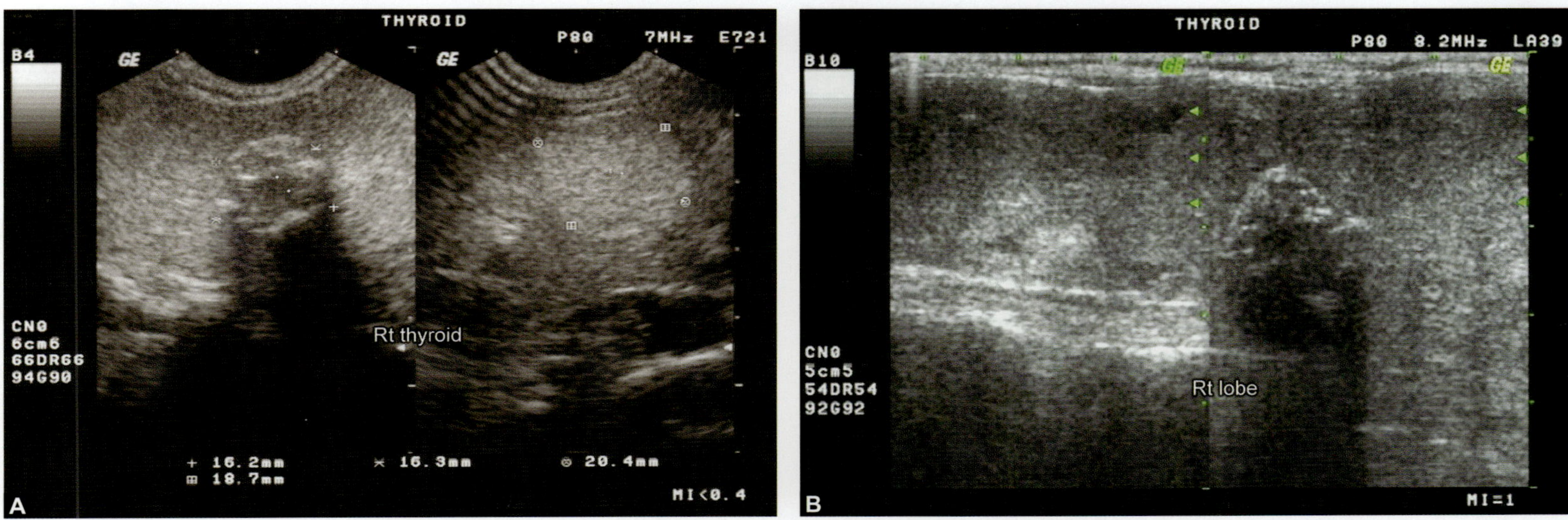

FIGURES 3.58A and B: Papillary carcinoma. A patient presented with multiple nodes in the neck. HRSG shows an irregular mass in the right lobe of the thyroid. Calcified rim is seen around the mass. Punctate calcification is also seen in the mass. No halo is seen. Biopsy proved papillary adenocarcinoma.

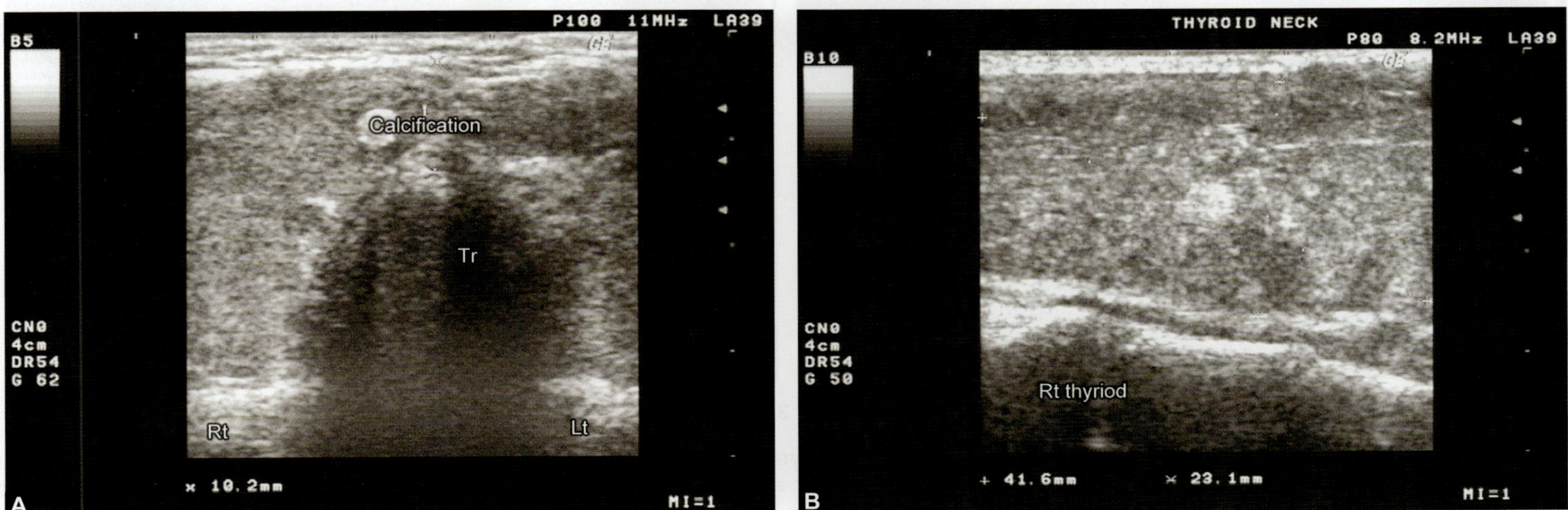

FIGURES 3.59A and B: Benign adenoma with macrocalcification. A hyperechoic non-palpable nodular mass is seen in the right lobe of thyroid. Dense echogenic macrocalcification is seen in it. Biopsy shows benign adenoma. This macrocalcification is different from the punctate microcalcification found in papillary adenocarcinoma.

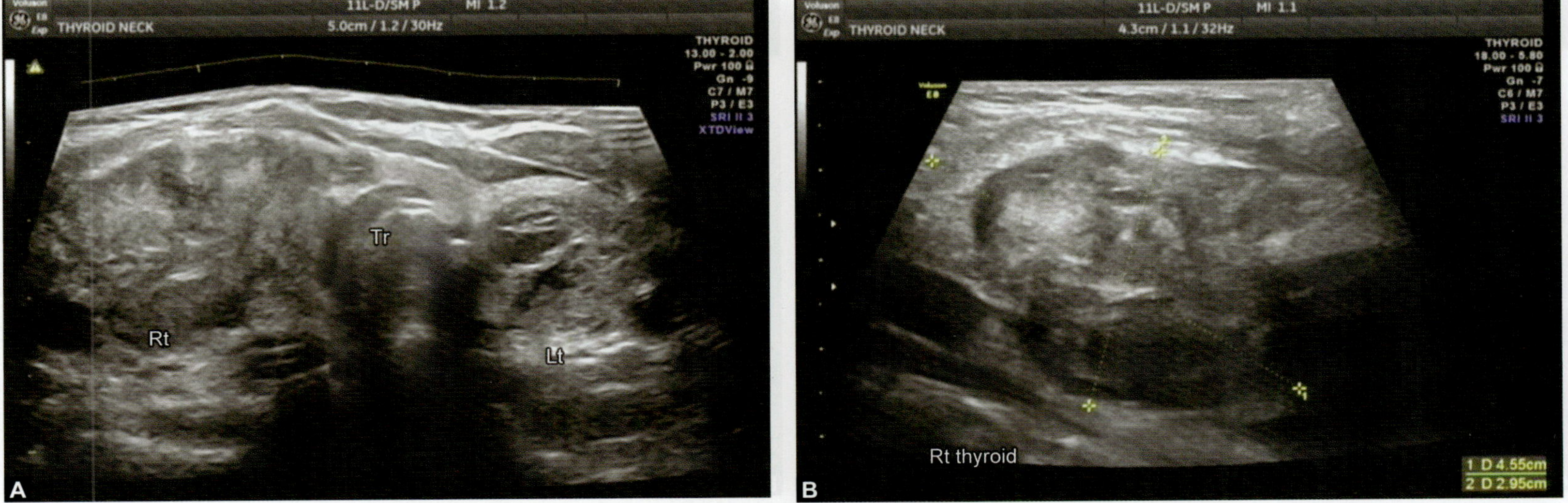

FIGURES 3.60A and B

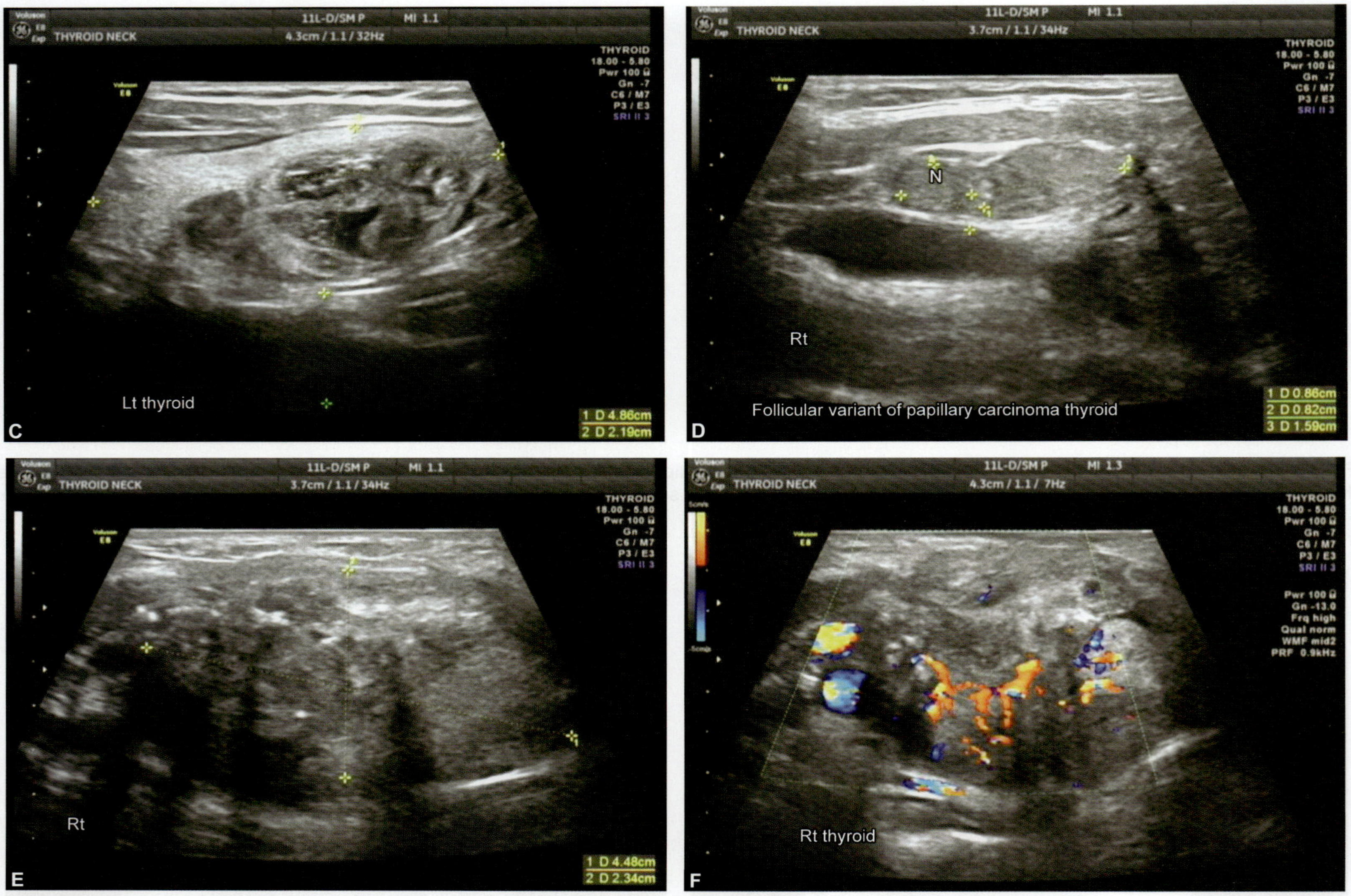

FIGURES 3.60C to F

FIGURES 3.60A to F: A known patient of operated papillary carcinoma thyroid presented with multiple masses in the neck. HRSG shows big irregular heterogeneous masses in the neck involving both lobes of thyroid. They are heterogeneous in texture. Multiple nodules are seen in them. But no cystic degeneration is seen. On color flow imaging, moderate flow is seen in the masses. Findings are suggestive of recurrence of the disease.

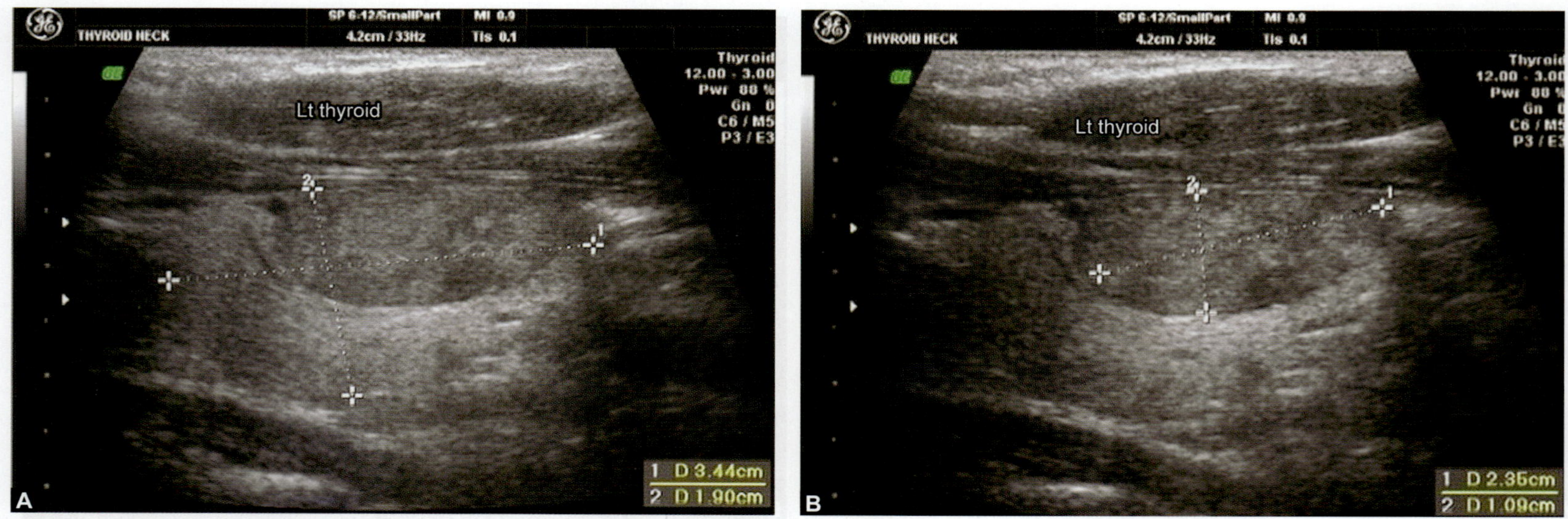

FIGURES 3.61A and B

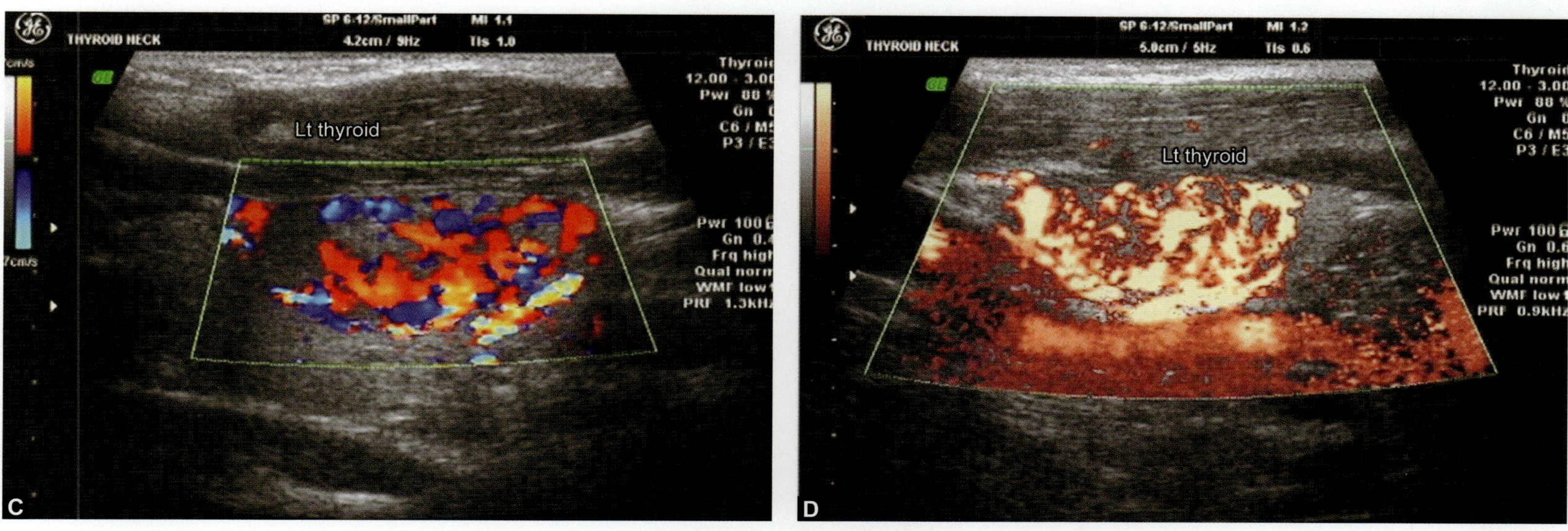

FIGURES 3.61C and D

FIGURES 3.61A to D: Follicular carcinoma with brain metastasis. A patient presented with nodular mass in the thyroid. HRSG shows an irregular ill-defined mass in the left lobe of thyroid. It shows heterogeneous texture. No perinodular halo is seen. On color flow imaging high flow is seen from center to periphery suggestive of malignant nature of the mass. Fine-needle aspiration cytology (FNAC) of the mass confirms follicular adenocarcinoma. The patient head seizures and CT scan of the head shows brain metastasis.

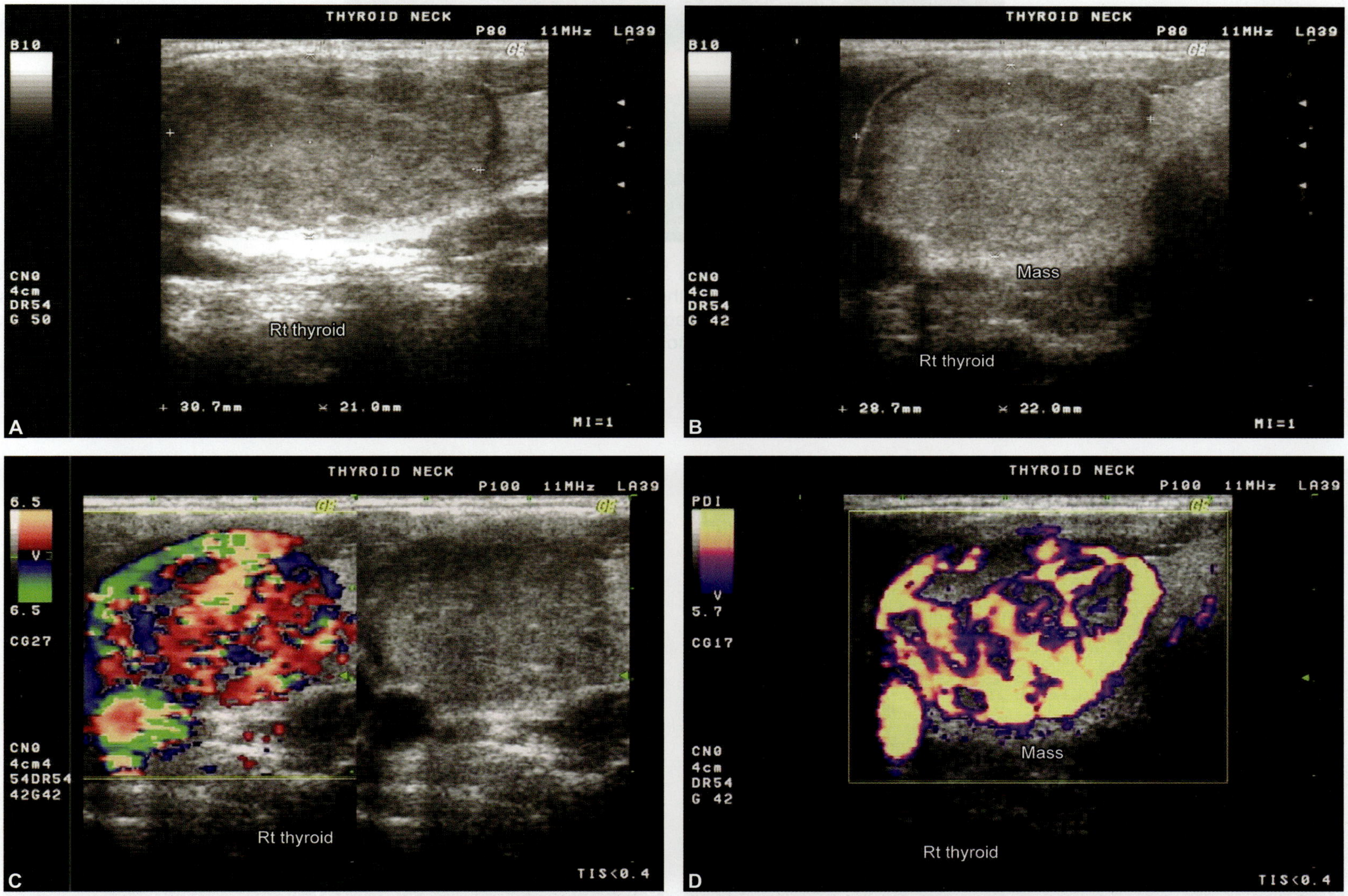

FIGURES 3.62A to D: Follicular adenocarcinoma. HRSG a hypoechoic ill-defined mass in the right lobe of thyroid. The mass shows bulging margins. No halo is seen around the mass. It is merging with the gland. However, it is homogeneous in texture. No calcification or necrosis is seen in the mass. On color flow imaging, very high flow is seen in the mass. Multiple vessels are seen feeding the mass in bizarre fashion. Biopsy proved follicular adenocarcinoma.

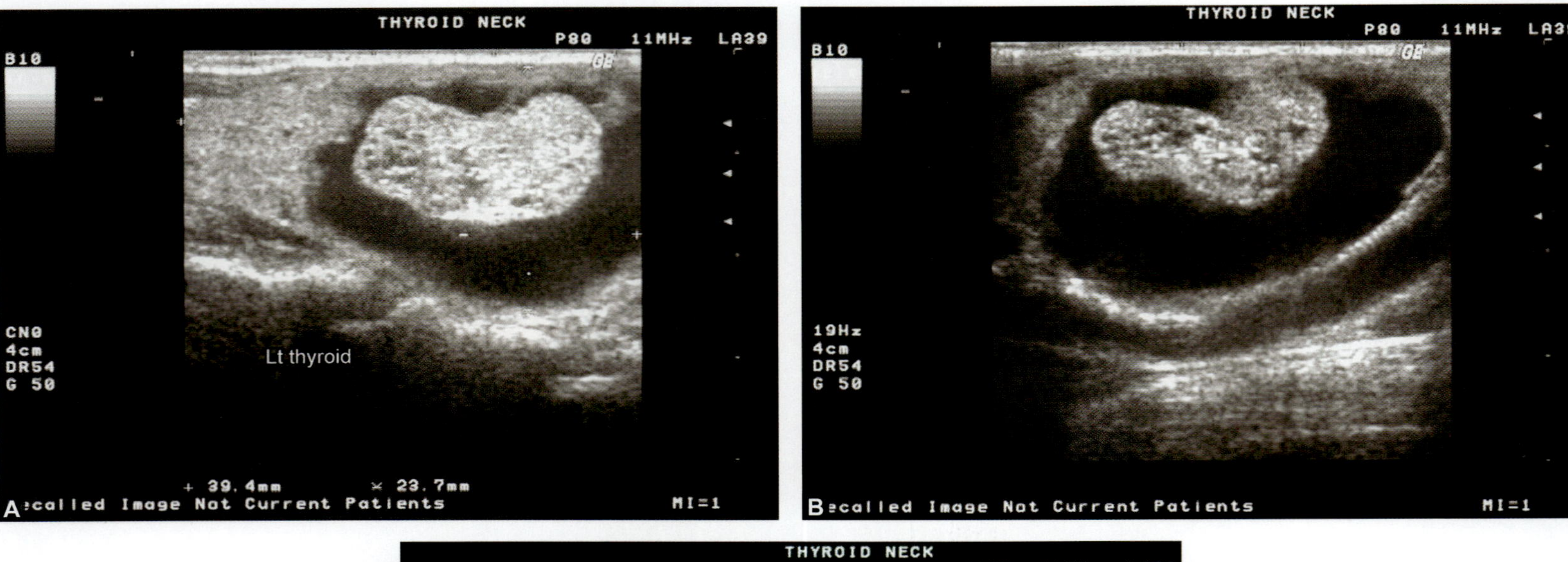

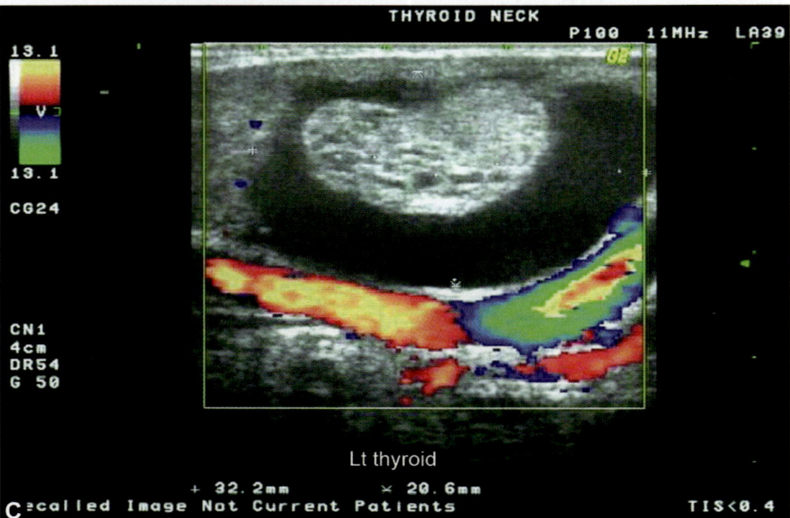

FIGURES 3.63A to C: Malignant cystic mass in thyroid. HRSG shows a heterogeneous cystic mass in the left lobe of the thyroid. The cyst was having an irregular heterogeneous soft tissue mass, which was fixed with the upper wall of the cyst. Multiple hypoechoic areas are seen in the mass. Irregular calcification was also seen in the solid mass. Color Doppler imaging the cyst in the mass shows poor flow. No evidence of any flow was seen in the soft tissue mass. Ultrasound guided fine-needle aspiration cytology and biopsy confirmed poorly differentiated adenocarcinoma.

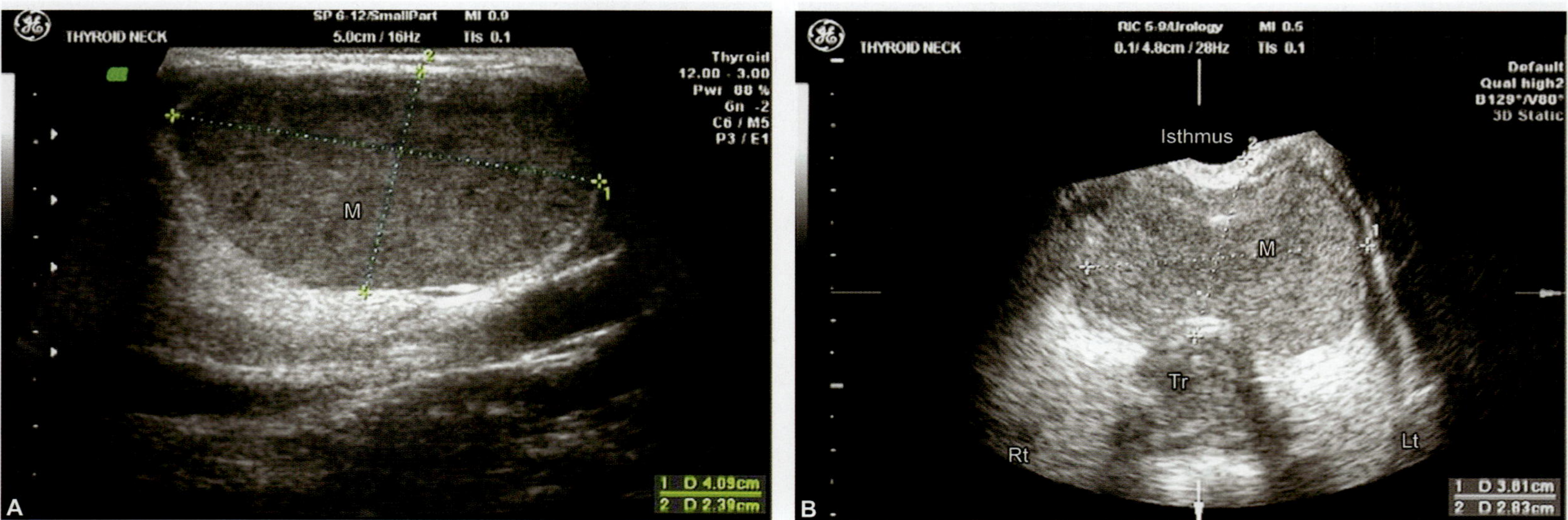

FIGURES 3.64A and B

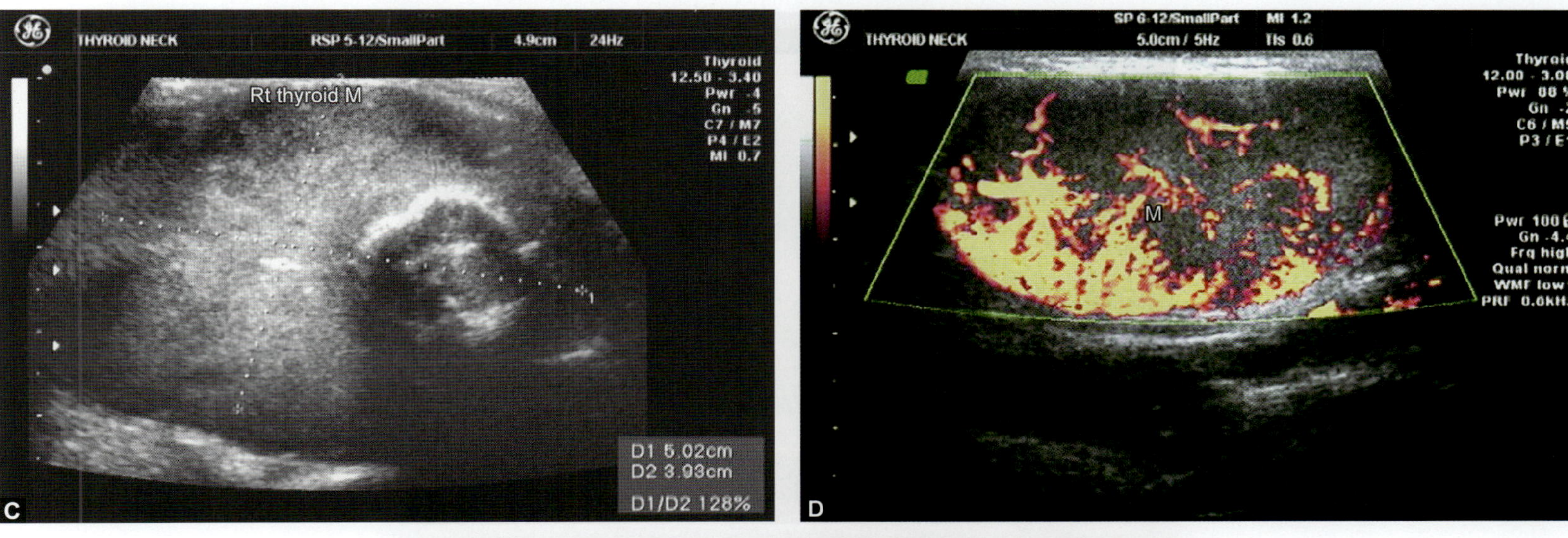

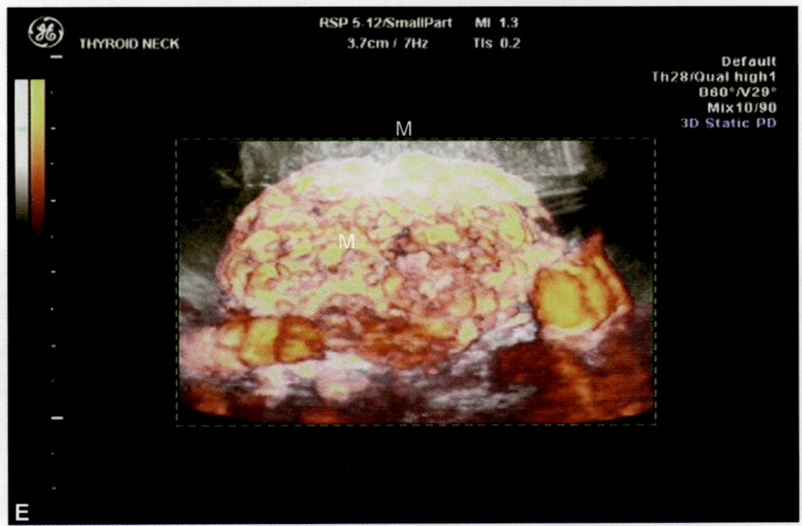

FIGURES 3.64C to E

FIGURES 3.64A to E: Follicular adenocarcinoma in the isthmus. A hypoechoic mass is seen in the isthmus of the gland. The mass shows homogeneous texture with scalloping of the margins. No peripheral halo is seen in the mass. On color flow imaging, very high flow is seen in it with bizarre pattern. Fine-needle aspiration cytology (FNAC) proved follicular adenocarcinoma. 3D of the same patient shows invasion of the tracheal ring by the mass. On 3D power angio multiple vessels are seen invading the tracheal ring.

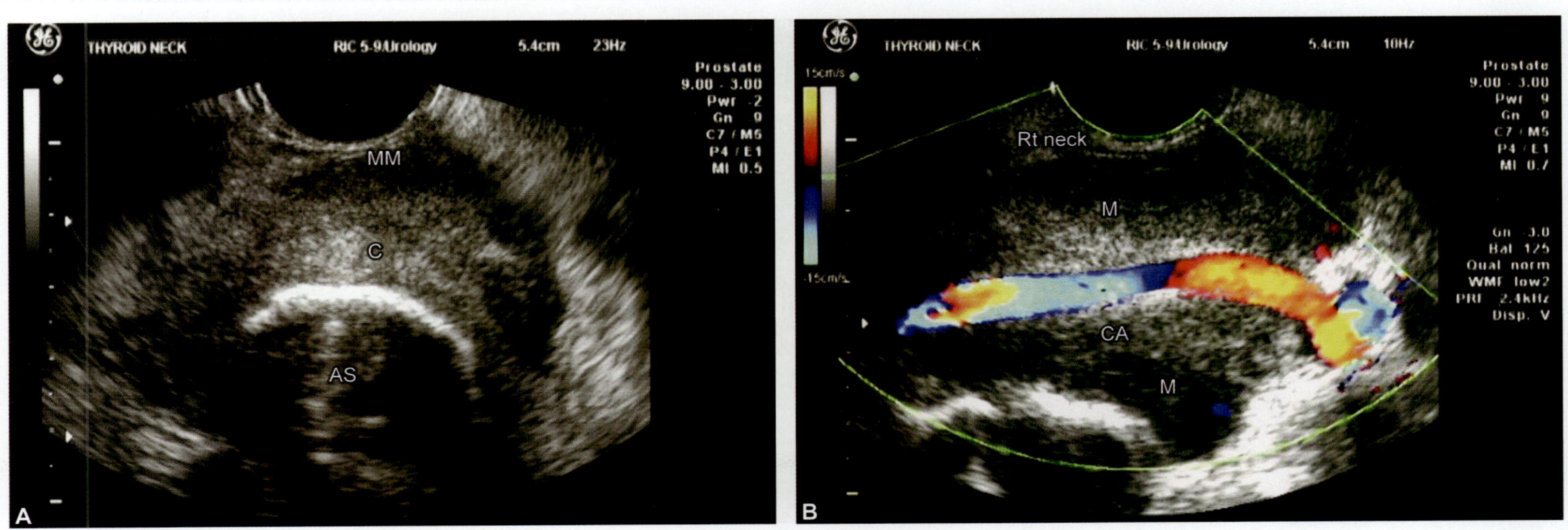

FIGURES 3.65A and B

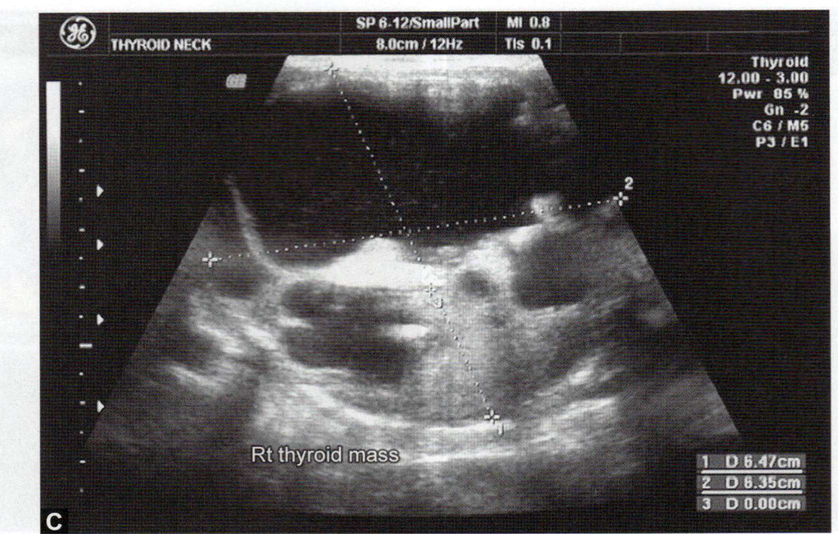

FIGURE 3.65C

FIGURES 3.65A to C: Invasive adenocarcinoma thyroid. A big heterogeneous mass is seen in the right lobe of thyroid. Normal glandular texture is lost. The mass shows dense calcification. It is seen invading the surrounding tissues. Normal anatomy is distorted. On color flow imaging, the mass is seen invading the neck vessels and going around the right common carotid artery. It is seen encasing the artery.

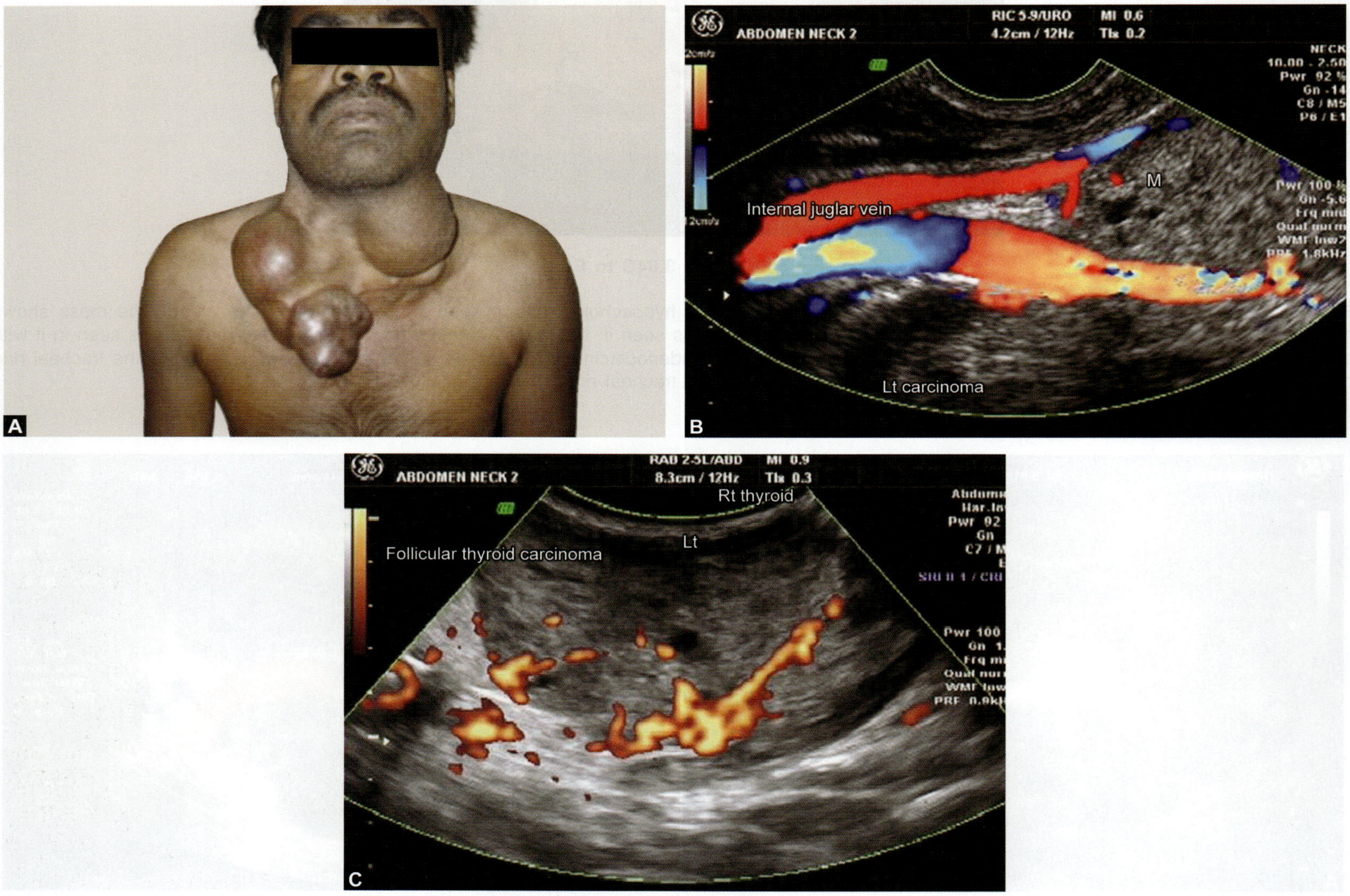

FIGURES 3.66A to C: A patient known case of medullary carcinoma presented with multiple masses in the neck and anterior chest wall. HRSG shows big irregular ill-defined masses in the neck and anterior chest wall. They are predominantly solid. No cystic degeneration is seen in them. On color flow imaging, increased flow is seen. The carotid vessels are also seen encased by the masses.

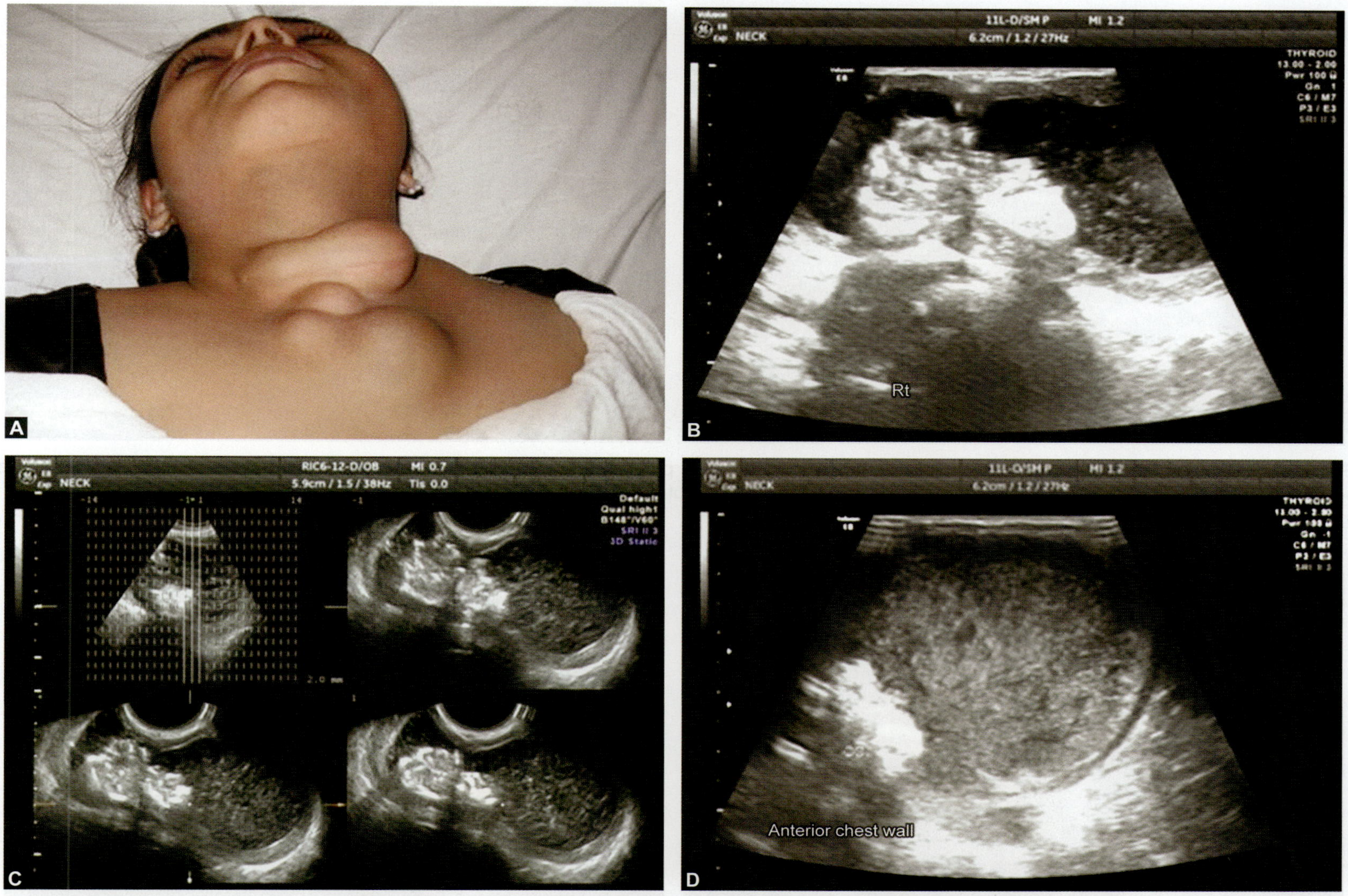

FIGURES 3.67A to D: Recurrence medullary carcinoma thyroid. A young girl and known case of medullary carcinoma thyroid presented with multiple masses in the neck and suprasternal region. HRSG shows big low level echo complex masses in the neck and suprasternal region. Cystic degeneration is also seen in them. Soft tissue shadows are seen in the masses. Normal anatomic relations are distorted. Aspiration biopsy confirms recurrence of disease.

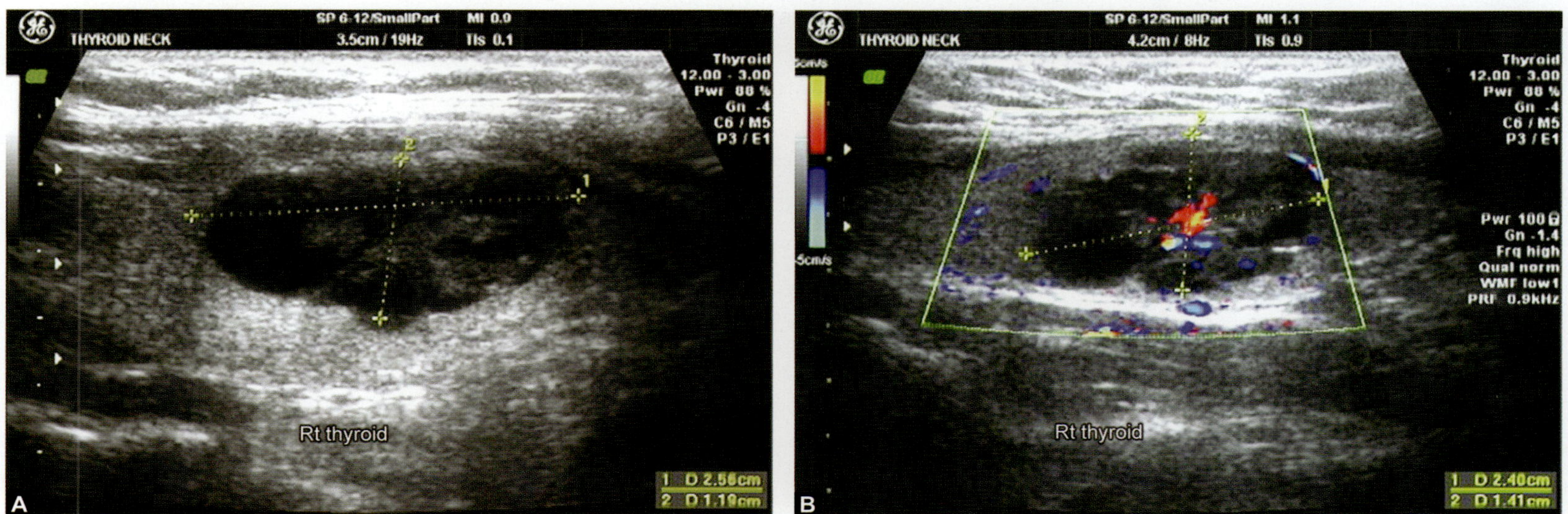

FIGURES 3.68A and B: Metastatic mass in thyroid. An irregular hypoechoic mass is seen in the right lobe of thyroid. The mass does not show any halo. Fine-needle aspiration cytology (FNAC) of the mass shows metastasis from carcinoma breast. The patient was known case of carcinoma breast operated in the past.

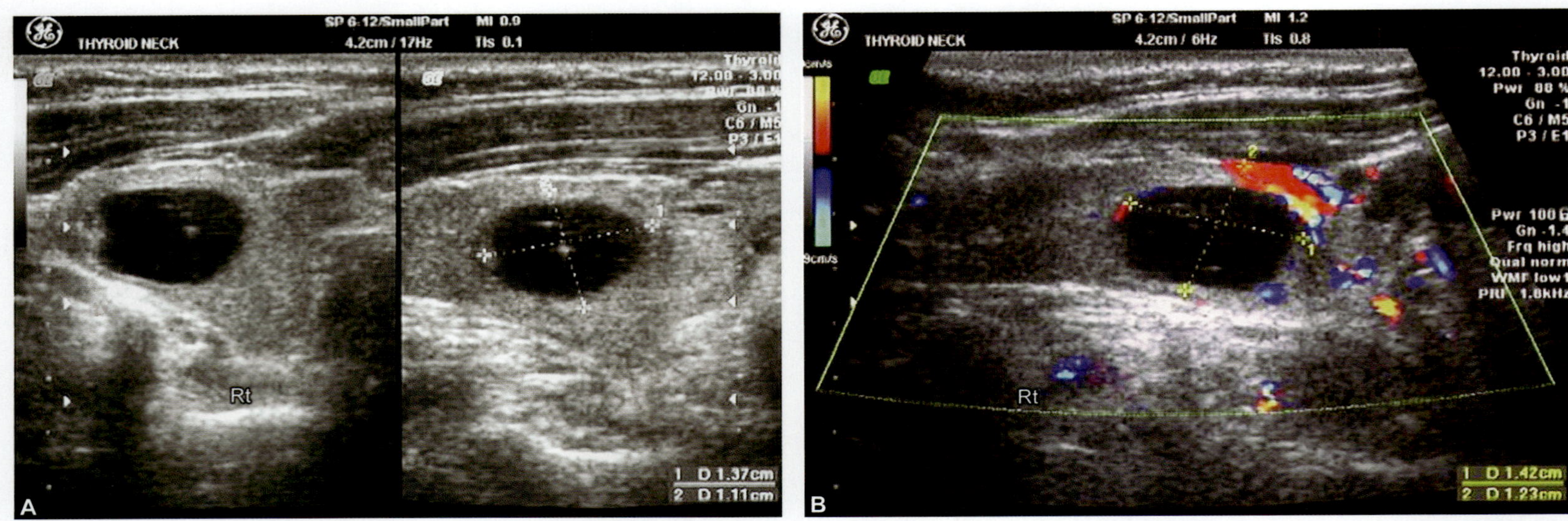

FIGURES 3.69A and B: Metastatic deposit of carcinoma bronchus. A patient presented with nodular mass in the thyroid. A hypoechoic mass is seen in the right lobe. Fine-needle aspiration cytology (FNAC) of the mass shows metastasis deposit from carcinoma bronchus.

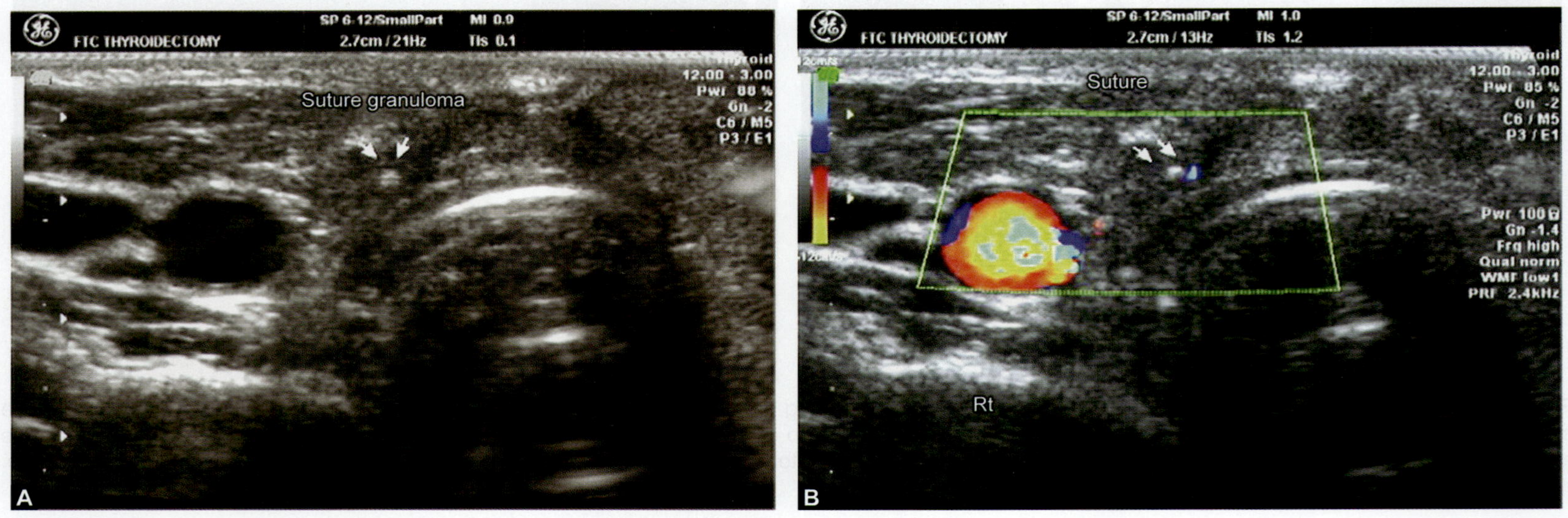

FIGURES 3.70A and B: Suture granuloma. A patient presented with palpable nodule in the right side of the neck after total thyrodectomy. HRSG shows the suture knot echogenic fibrous tissue is seen around it suggestive of suture granuloma.

CHAPTER 4

Neck

PK Srivastava

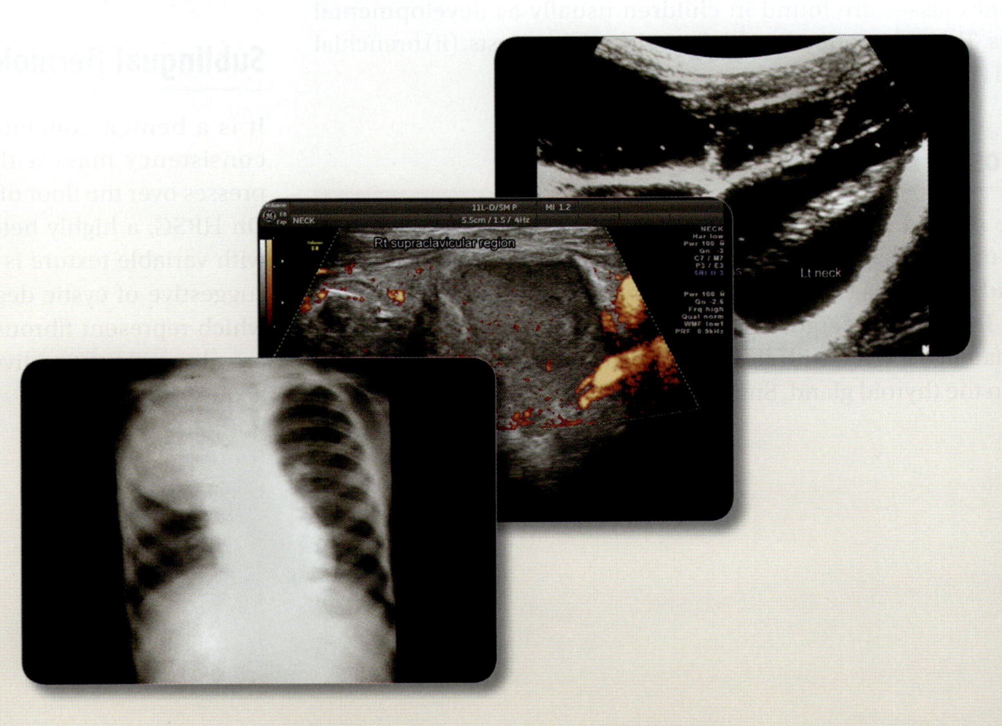

INTRODUCTION

High-resolution sonography (HRSG) is an excellent modality to examine the neck and neck masses. The excellent tissue details and anatomical landmarks in neck like thyroid cartilage; trachea, strap muscles and neck vessels have made assessment of neck masses a practical proposition. The neck masses have been divided into the following heads for convenience besides thyroid and parathyroid glands:

1. Cervical masses
2. Lymph node mass
3. Salivary glands

CERVICAL MASSES

Besides thyroid and parathyroid gland pathologies, other cervical masses are mainly present below hyoid bone in midcervical or lower cervical regions. They are mainly confined to anterior triangle of the neck; however, few masses are also seen in the posterior triangle of the neck like nerve tumors and abscess. The cervical masses are grouped as follows:

1. Congenital masses
2. Inflammatory masses
3. Vascular masses
4. Benign tumors
5. Malignant Tumors.

CONGENITAL MASSES

Congenital masses are found in children usually as developmental anomalies. They are grouped as: (i) thyroglossal duct cysts, (ii) branchial cysts, and (iii) cystic hygromas.

Thyroglossal Duct Cysts

These are formed due to remnant of the duct, which is filled due to secretion of epithelial cell rests. In normal embryological development, the thyroid gland descends down along thyroglossal duct to its normal position. The duct undergoes progressive atrophy. However, when it remains patent it is filled with clear fluid filled cystic mass in the midline anterior to the thyroid gland. Small cyst is difficult to differentiate from the reactive lymph node enlargement, which undergoes cystic necrosis. However, high frequency transducers of 13 to 15 MHz can differentiate them. Hemorrhage is common in the cyst. It can be seen as highly reflective mobile shadow in the dependent part of the cyst.

Branchial Cysts

These cysts arise from the branchial cleft usually from the second cleft. It is lateral in position. It is situated in the anterior triangle of neck along the anterior margins of sternocleidomastoid muscle. It is situated between suprahyoid and carotid spaces. These cysts are present in the childhood. The cyst is seen as a well-defined thin walled echo free mass on HRSG. It is round with sharp clear margins. It is clearly separated and demarcated with sternocleidomastoid muscle border. Secondary infection may take place in the cyst and low level echoes are noted on HRSG.

Cystic Hygromas

These are serous benign cystic masses arising from the lymphoid tissue. They are noncapsulated and usually confined to posterior triangle of the neck. When they are big they are seen reaching up to anterior part of neck or upper part of the superior mediastinum. They may also be seen reaching up to axilla. On HRSG, it appears to be multilocular cystic mass with echogenic fibrous septa with thin regular, smooth margins. The internal structures are usually free and anechoic. However, low amplitude echoes may be seen in the loculae representing fine jelly like consistency of cystic hygroma. Secondary hemorrhage is also encountered in cystic hygroma.

Sublingual Dermoid

It is a benign congenital condition. It is seen a medium to hard consistency mass with sharp margins on clinical examination. It presses over the floor of the mouth and pressure is seen on the tongue. On HRSG, a highly heterogeneous irregular mass with poor margins with variable texture is seen. Areas of low-level echoes are seen in it, suggestive of cystic degeneration. Echogenic shadows are also seen which represent fibrous element of the cyst. At times, echogenic foci are also seen suggestive of calcification. They are accompanied with acoustic shadowing.

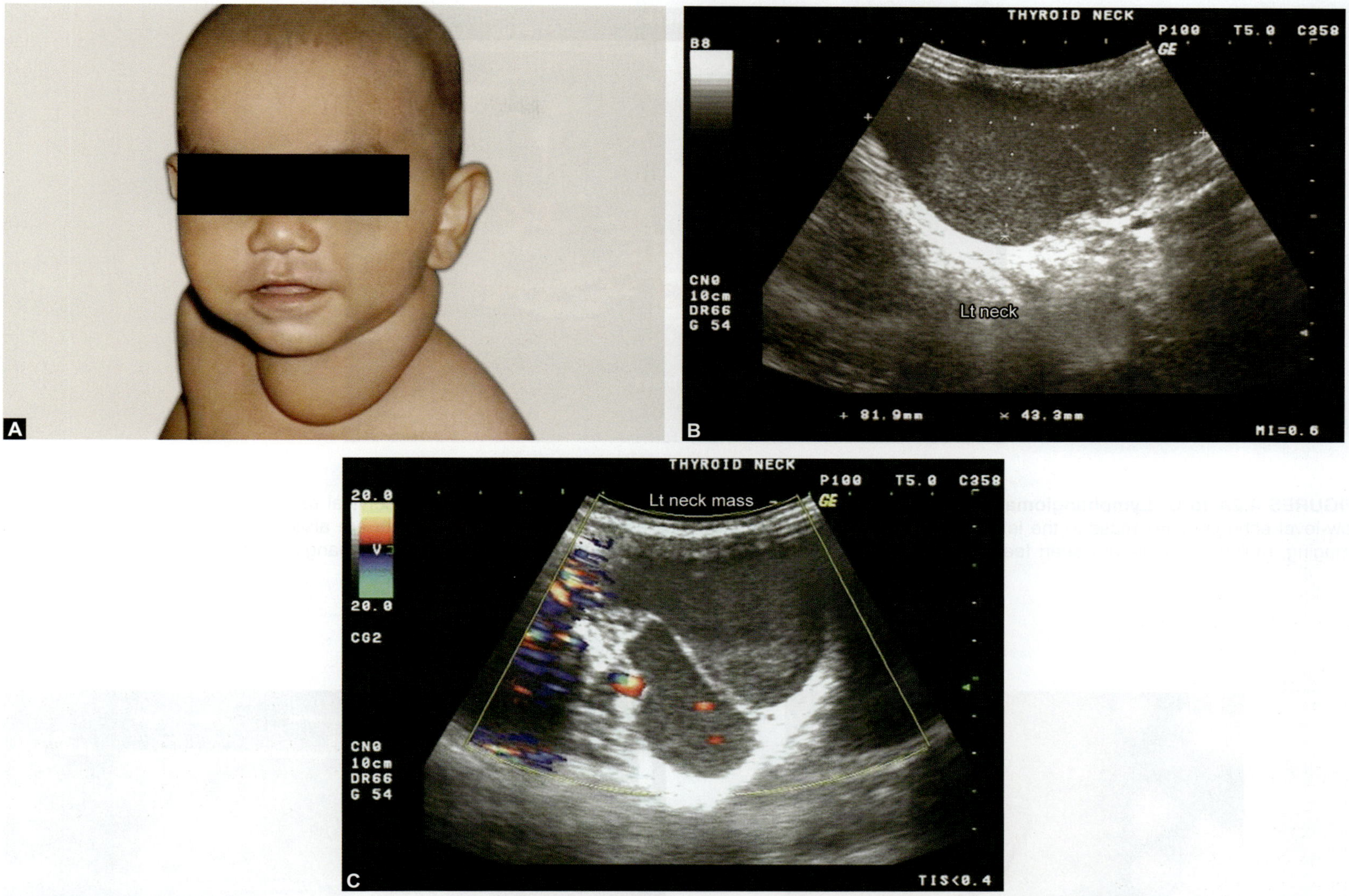

FIGURES 4.1A to C: Cystic hygroma. A young child presented with a soft tissue swelling in the neck. HRSG shows a multiloculated well-defined cystic mass in the left side of the neck. Echogenic septa are also seen in the mass. Low-level echo collection is seen in the cyst suggestive of serous collection. The margins are smooth, typical findings of a cystic hygroma.

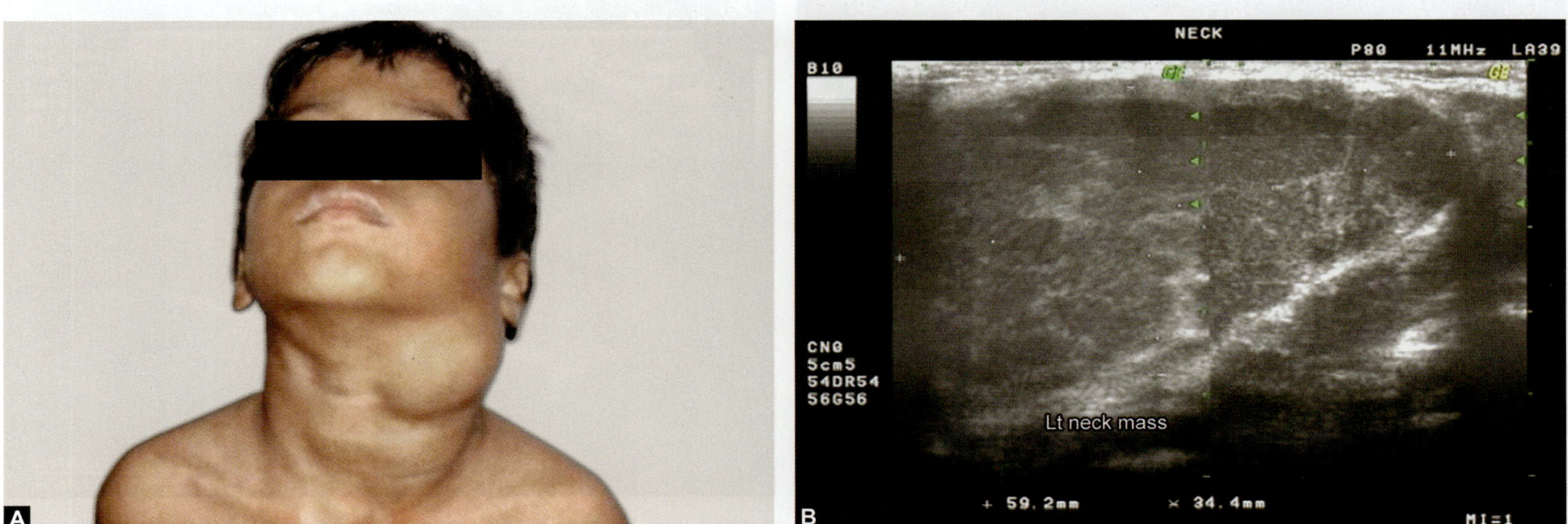

FIGURES 4.2A and B

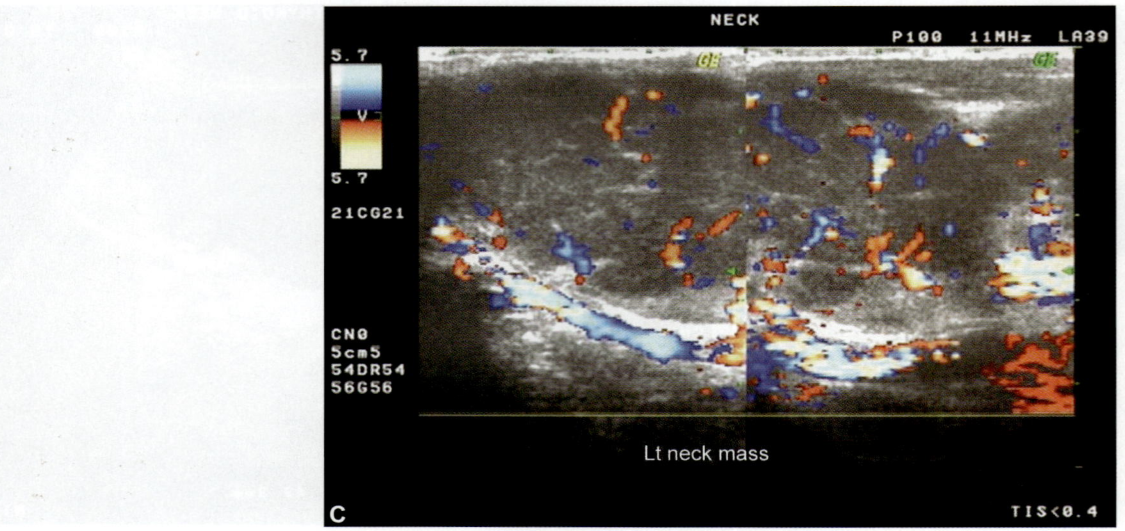

FIGURE 4.2C

FIGURES 4.2A to C: Lymphangioma neck. A young child presented with cystic mass in the left upper cervical region. HRSG shows a well-defined low-level echo complex mass in the left neck the mass shows low-level thick echoes. Thin echogenic septa are also seen in the mass. On color flow imaging, multiple vessels are seen feeding the mass. Fine needle aspiration cytology (FNAC) confirmed lymphangioma.

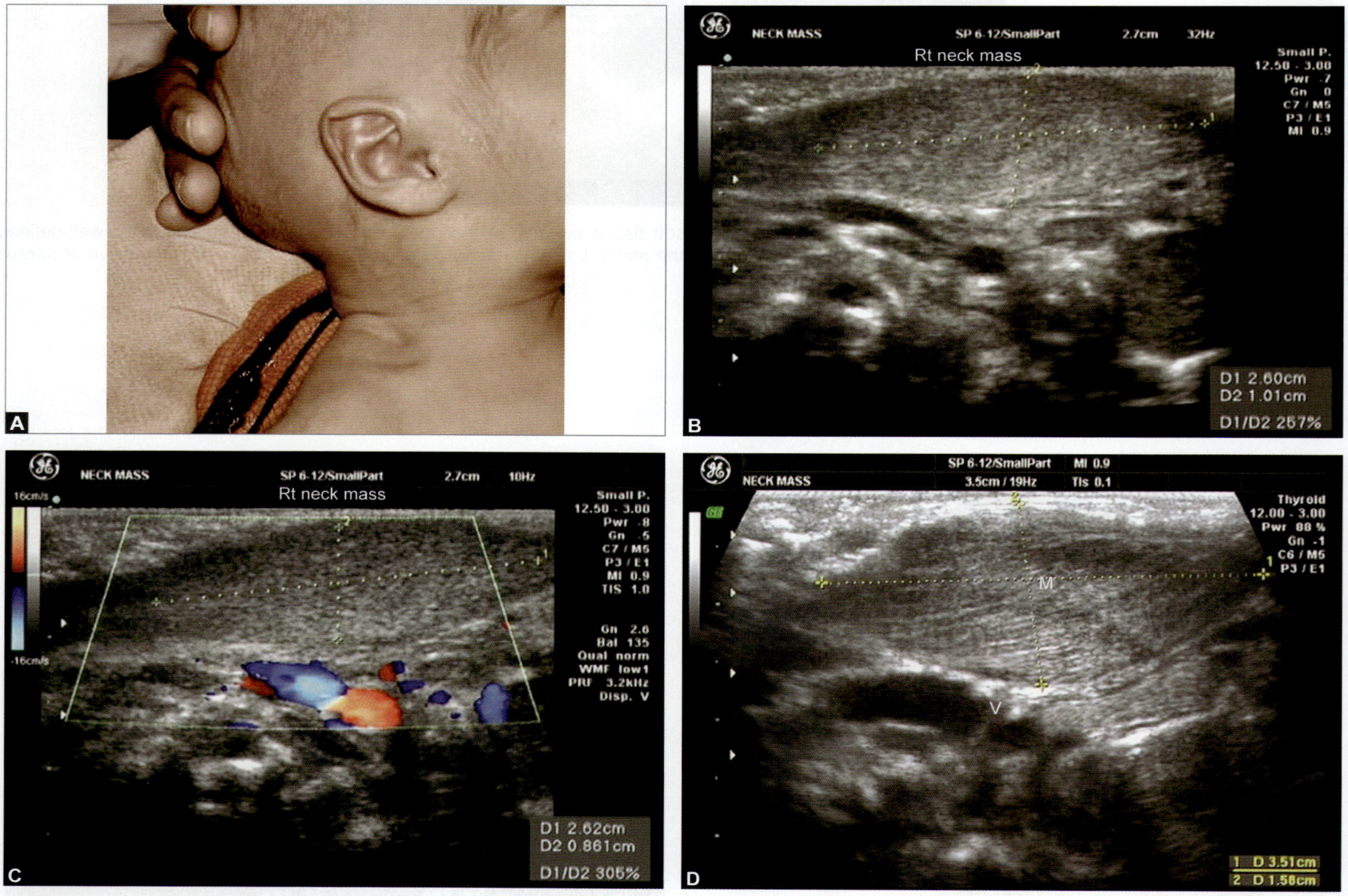

FIGURES 4.3A to D: Sternocleidomastoid tumor (SCM tumor). A young child was born with soft tissue swelling in the right side of the neck. HRSG shows a well-defined fusiform mass in the sternocleidomastoid muscle. It is homogeneous in texture. No calcification or necrosis is seen in it. On color flow imaging, no flow is seen in it.

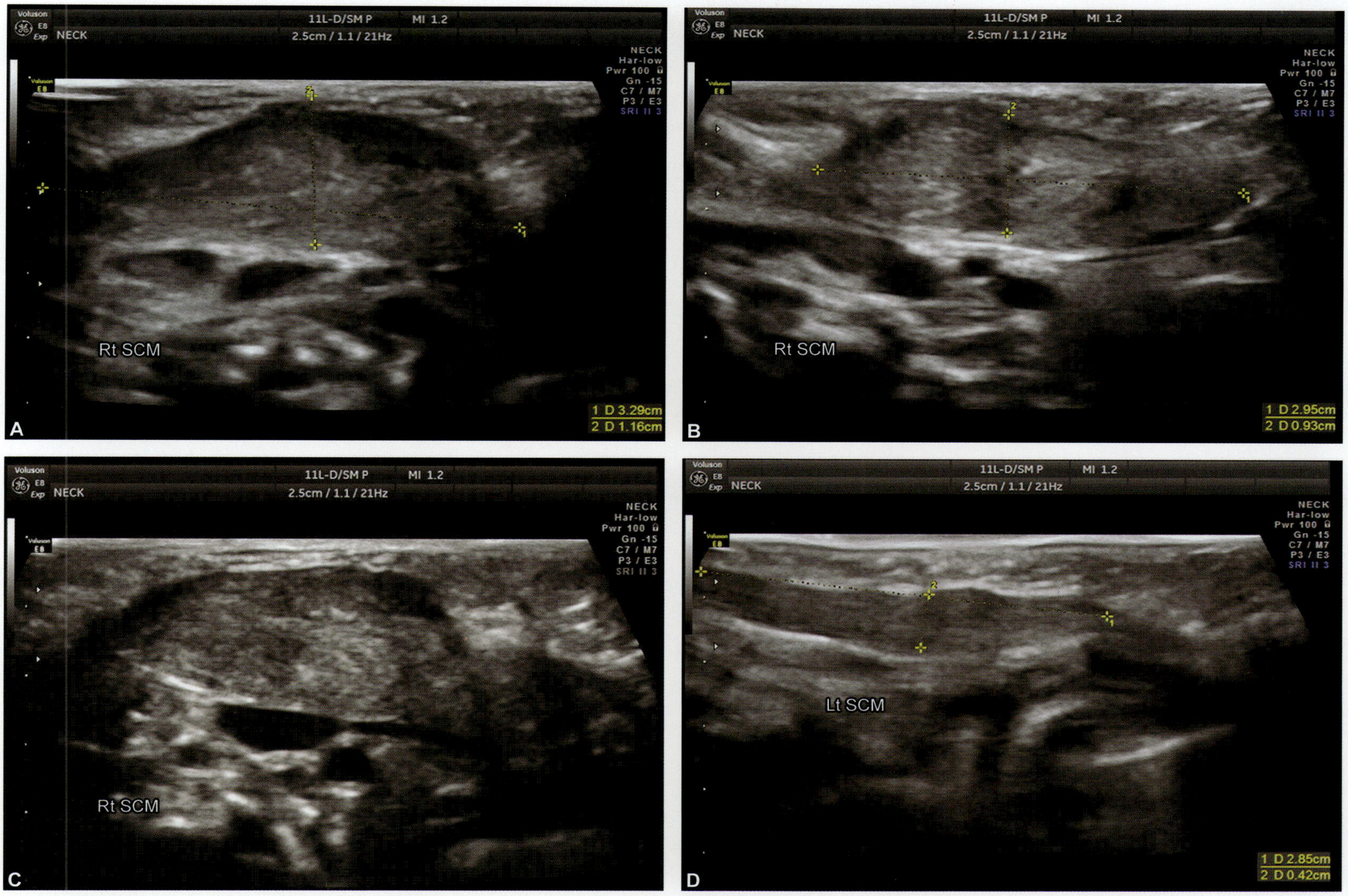

FIGURES 4.4A to D: Sternocleidomastoid (SCM) tumor. An infant girl was born with soft tissue mass in the neck. HRSG shows a well-defined mass in the sternocleidomastoid muscle. Fine muscle striations are also seen in the mass suggestive of SCM tumor. On color flow imaging, no flow is seen in it. Sternocleidomastoid tumor is also known as fibromatosis colli. The left SCM muscle shows normal texture with smooth outline.

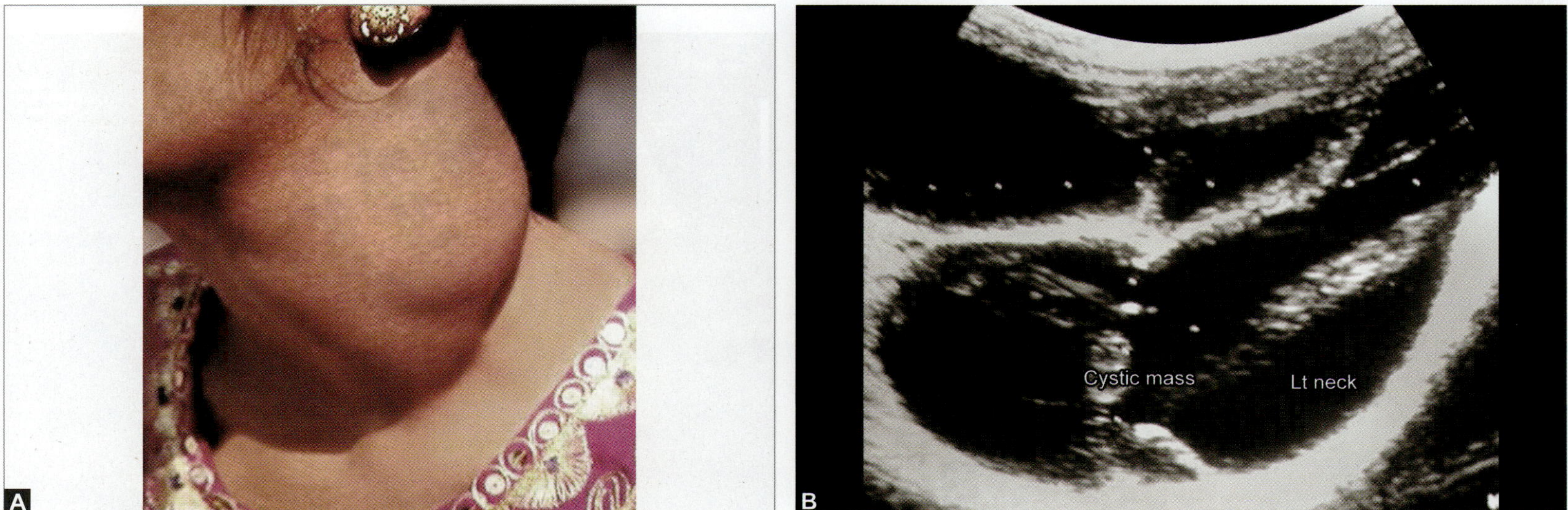

FIGURES 4.5A and B: Infected cystic hygroma. A young lady presented with a soft tissue mass swelling in the left side of the neck present since the birth. There was the history of intervention done in the cystic mass and serous fluid was aspirated. HRSG shows a big multiloculated cystic mass in the same patient. Multiple internal echoes are seen in the cyst. Few calcified specks are also seen. The cyst is seen low level echogenic collection at the base suggestive of debris. Biopsy of the cyst shows cystic hygroma.

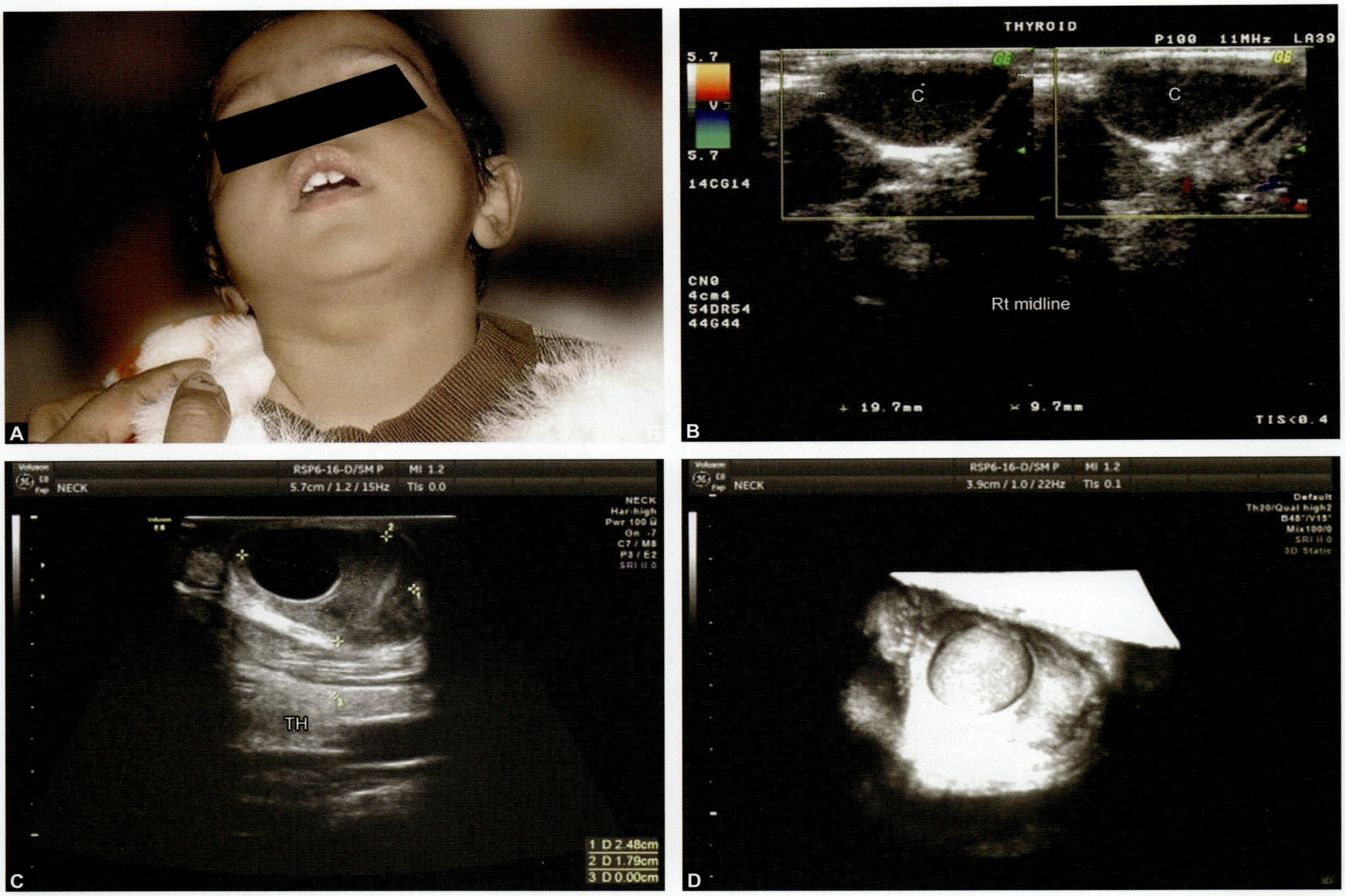

FIGURES 4.6A to D: Thyroglossal cyst. A child was presented with midline cystic mass. HRSG shows normal thyroid gland in the thyroid fossa on either side of the trachea. The cyst was not seen in relation to the thyroid. Three-dimensional (3D) volume contrast imaging shows the cyst very clearly.

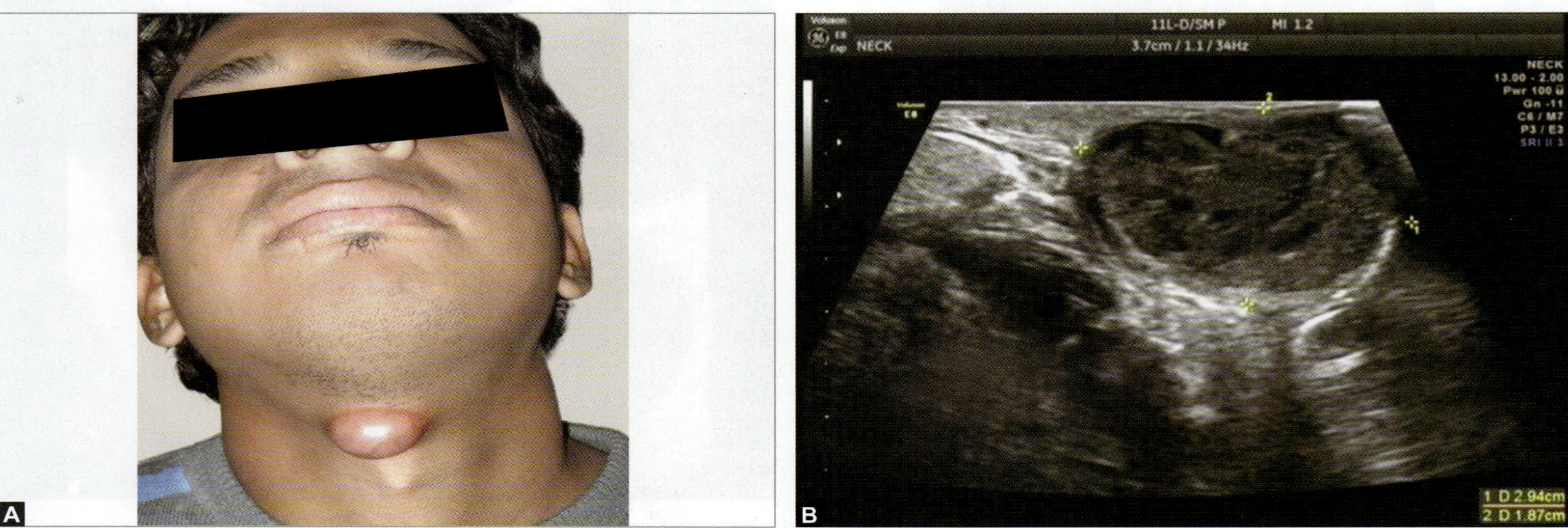

FIGURES 4.7A to B

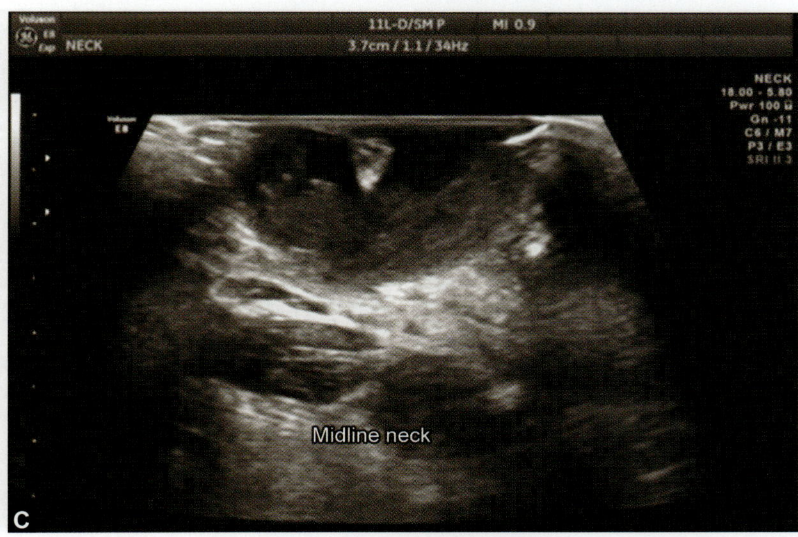

FIGURE 4.7C

FIGURES 4.7A to C: Infected thyroglossal duct cyst. A young man presented with midline soft tissue swelling in the neck, which was tensed and hot. HRSG shows a thick-walled well-defined cystic mass anterior to the thyroid gland in the midline of neck. Multiple internal echoes are seen in it suggestive of secondary infection. Fine needle aspiration confirms infected thyroglossal cyst.

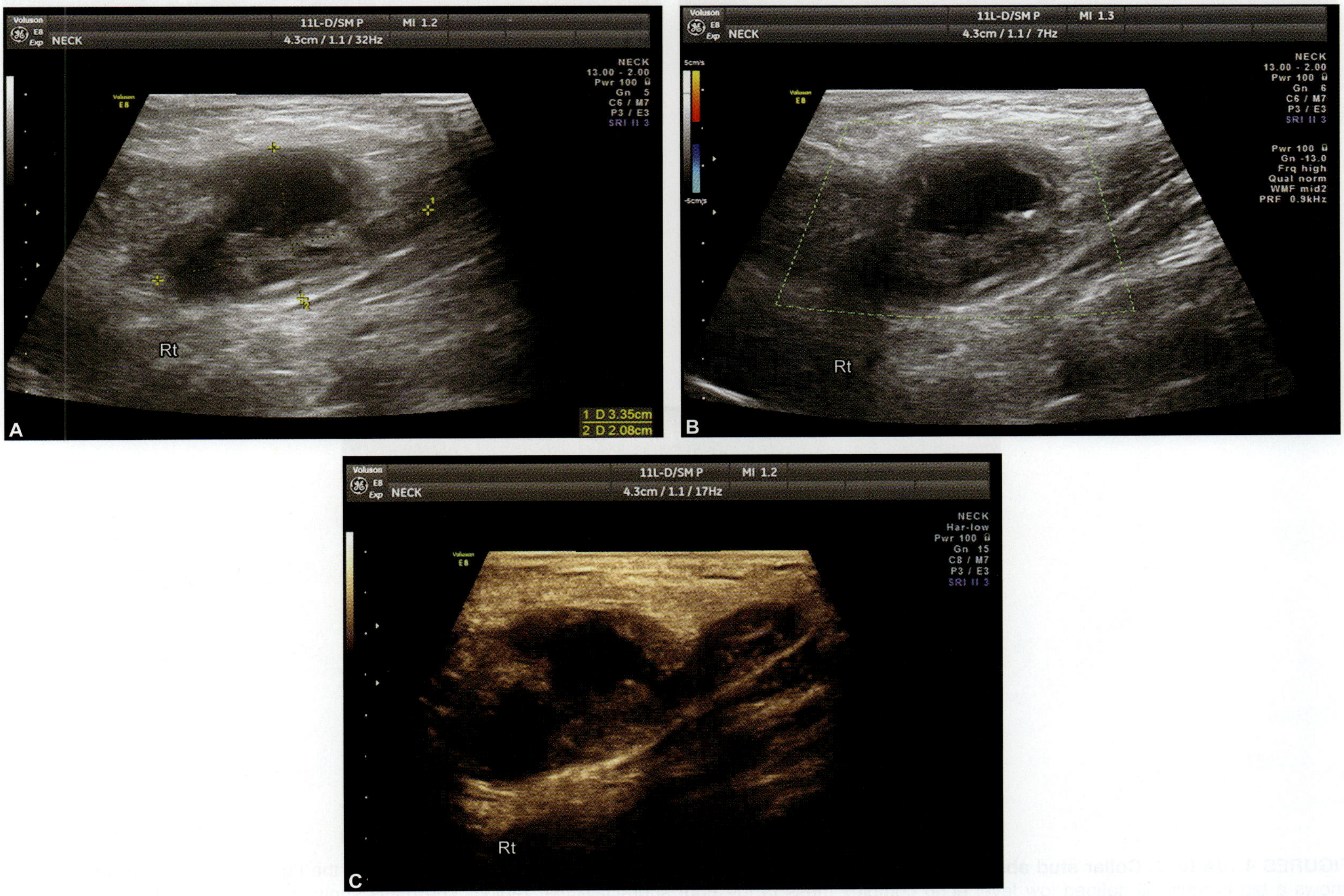

FIGURES 4.8A to C: Neck abscess. A lady presented with soft tissue mass in the right side of neck. It was tense and hot. Multiple internal echoes are seen in it. It is seen supraclavicular region. Central area of necrosis is seen in it. On color flow imaging, it shows poor flow. Findings are suggestive of pyogenic abscess in the neck.

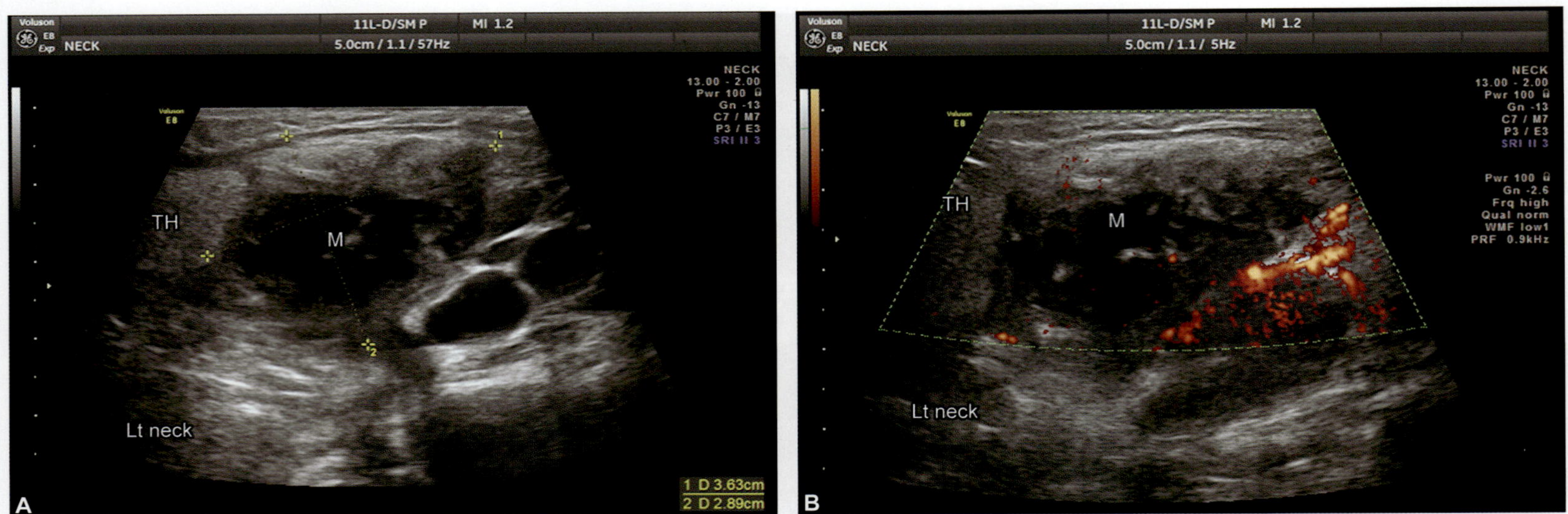

FIGURES 4.9A and B: Neck abscess. HRSG shows a big irregular ill defined low level echo complex mass in the left side of the neck in the mid cervical region. Margins are irregular. Central area of necrosis is seen into it. But no cystic degeneration is seen. It is separate from the left lobe of thyroid. On color flow imaging, no flow is seen in it. Few enlarged nodal shadows are also seen in the left side of neck.

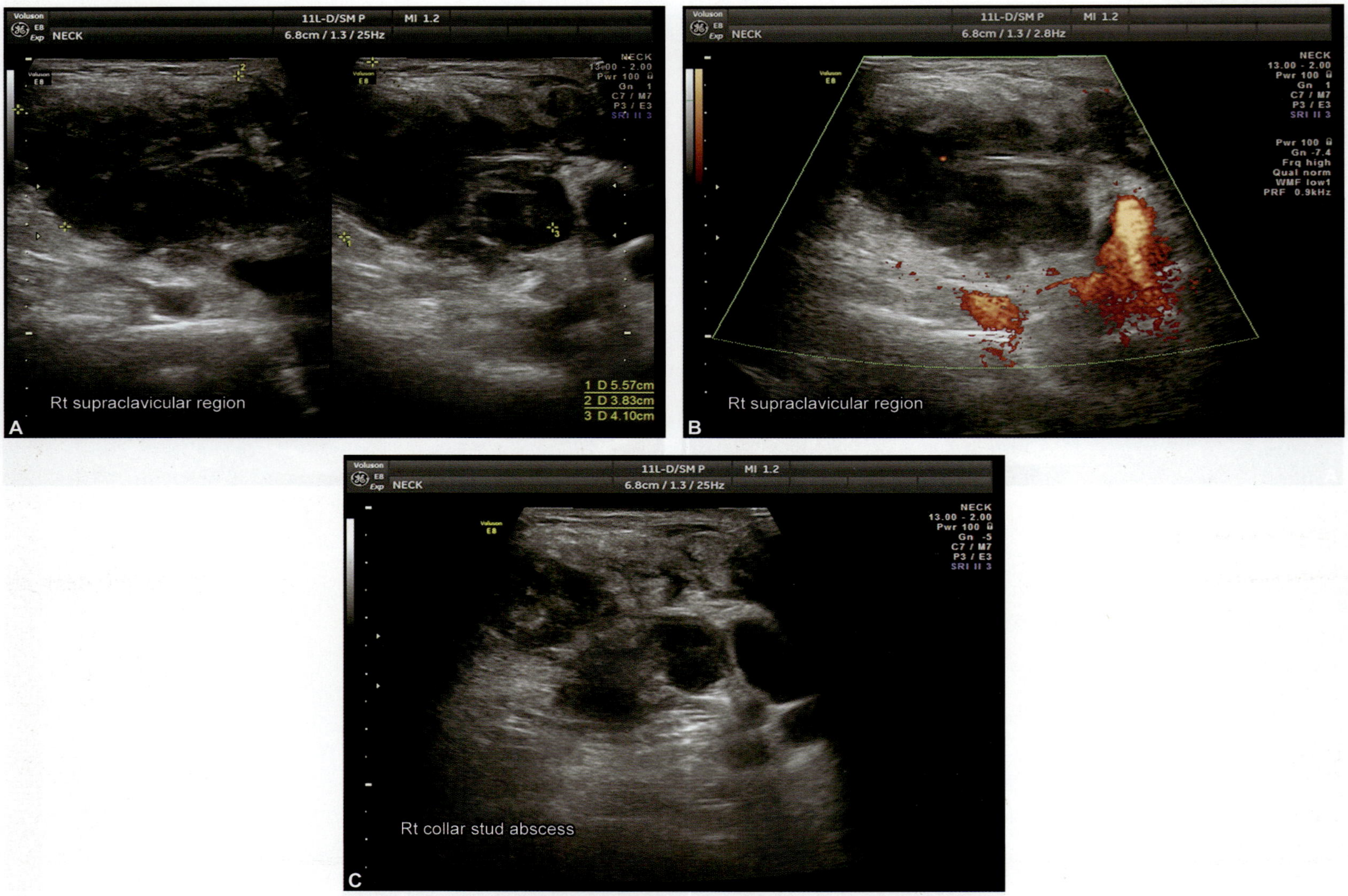

FIGURES 4.10A to C: Collar stud abscess with cellulitis. A patient presented with painful soft tissue mass in the right supraclavicular region. HRSG shows a big irregular ill defined low level echo complex mass in the right supraclavicular region. The mass shows hypoechoic texture. Thick cheesy collection is seen into it suggestive of an abscess. Marked perifocal edema is also present. Subcutaneous soft tissue edema is present in the mass. But no cystic degeneration is seen. On color flow imaging, no flow is seen in it. Enlarged nodal shadows are also seen in the neck suggestive of reactive nodal enlargement. Neck vessels are normal in appearance. However, pressure is seen in the neck vessels.

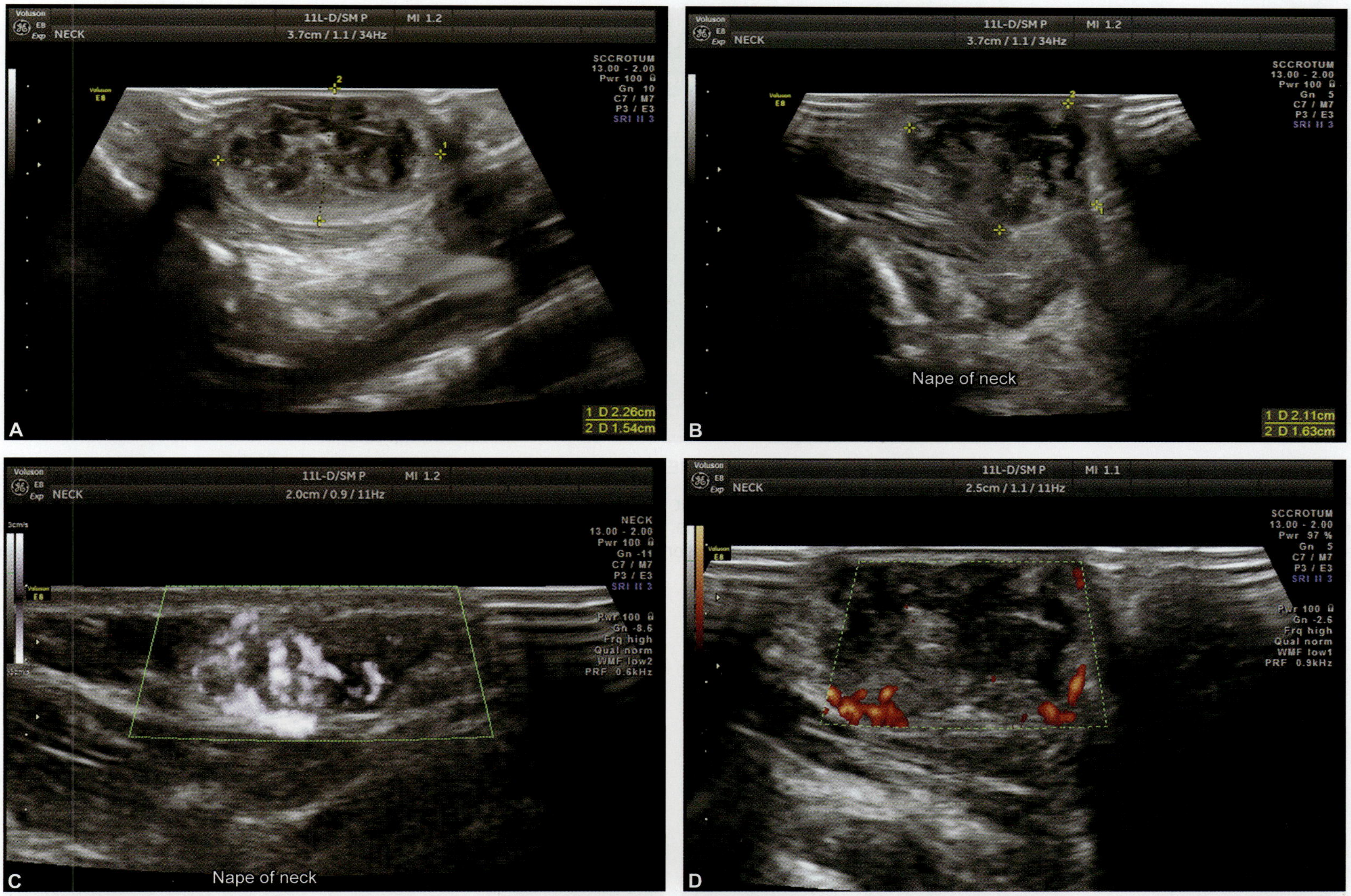

FIGURES 4.11A to D: Abscess at the nape with cellulitis. A newborn 15 days old baby presented with soft tissue swelling over the nape of neck. HRSG shows a thick walled mixed echo complex mass over the nape of the neck. Thick echoes are seen into it. But no cystic degeneration is seen. However, area of necrosis is seen in the mass. On color flow imaging, increased flow is seen around it. Associated soft tissue subcutaneous edema is also seen. The mass is not seen communicating with spinal cord. No intracranial extension of the mass is seen. Few enlarged nodal shadows are also seen in the posterior triangle.

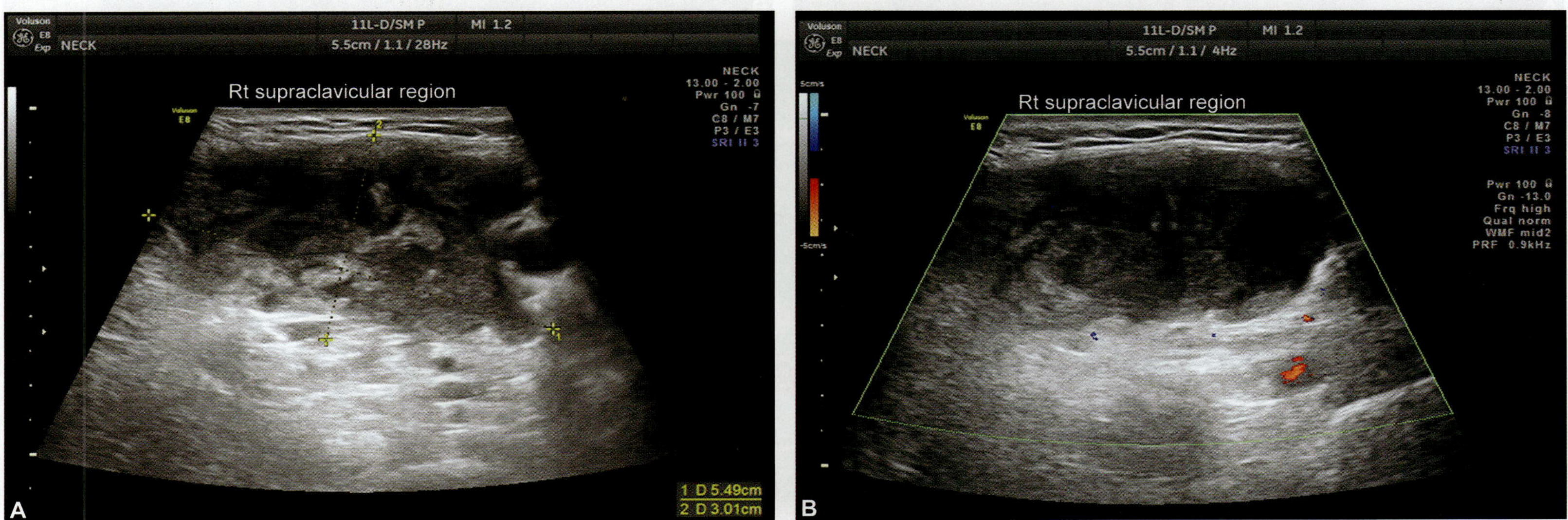

FIGURES 4.12A and B

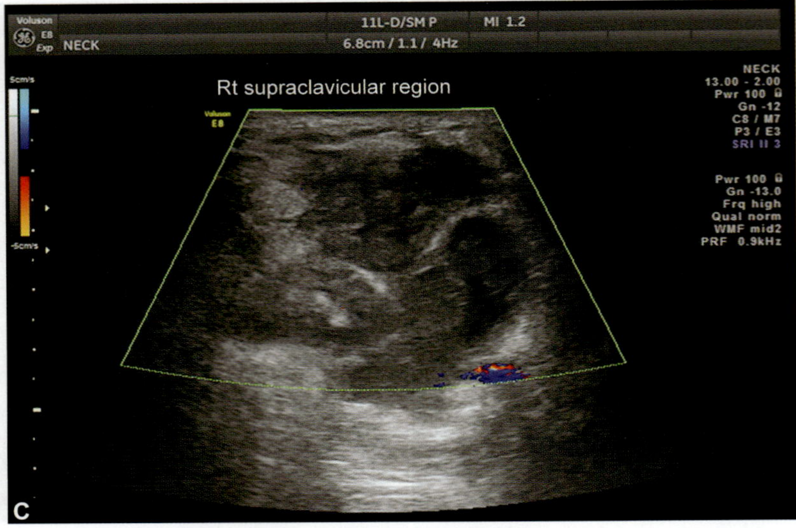

FIGURE 4.12C

FIGURES 4.12A to C: Collar stud abscess. HRSG shows a big irregular ill-defined inhomogeneous hypoechoic low level echo complex mass seen in the right supraclavicular region. It is seen extending to the posterior side. Walls are ill defined. Central area of necrosis is seen into it. Thick echoes are seen in it. On color flow imaging, no flow is seen into it. It is not seen pressing over the neck vessels. Enlarged nodal shadows are also seen in the right upper cervical region.

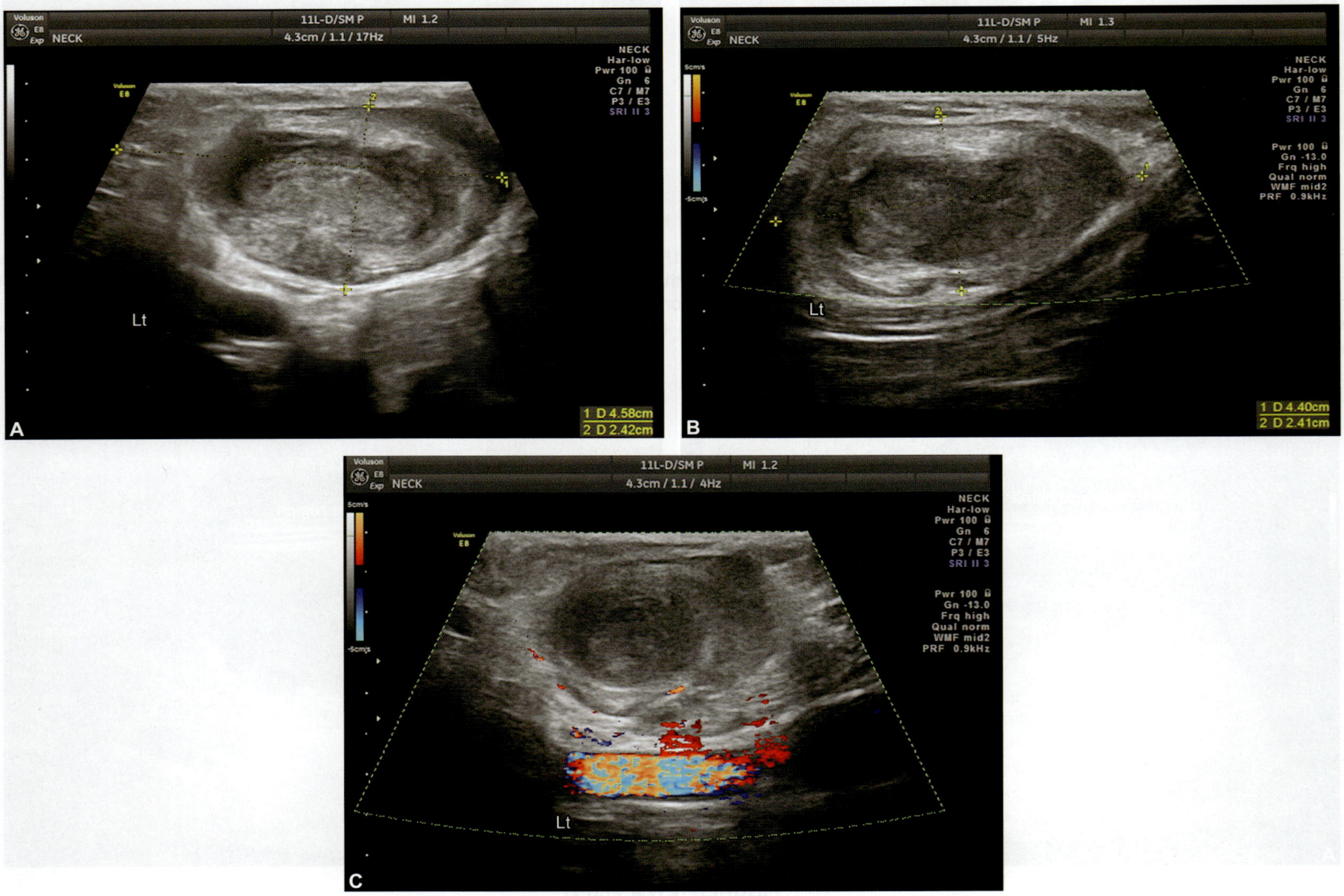

FIGURES 4.13A to C: Acute hemorrhage in the cyst. A patient presented with a painful soft tissue swelling with acute onset in the left side of neck. Clinically, it was thought to be thyroid mass. However, HRSG shows a thick-walled cystic mass in the left side of neck. It is seen in the superficial plane. Thick echoes are seen into it. But no calcification is seen. But no cystic degeneration is seen. On color flow imaging, no flow is seen into it. No pressure is seen on neck vessels.

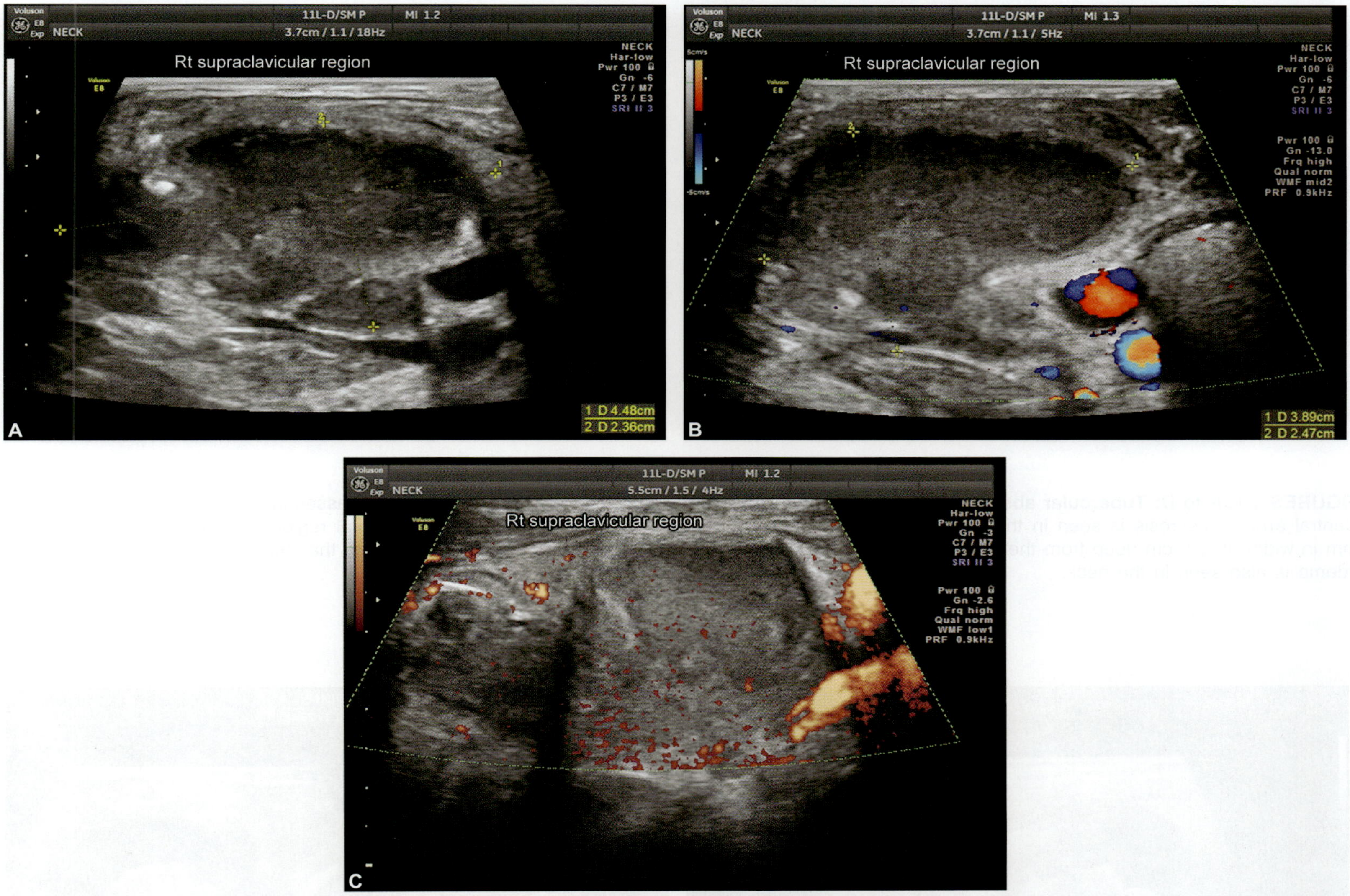

FIGURES 4.14A to C: Collar stud abscess. HRSG shows a thick-walled pocket of low level echo collection in the right supraclavicular region. Thick echoes are seen into it. It is seen extending below the clavicle collar stud abscess. Multiple enlarged nodes are also seen in right upper cervical and midcervical regions.

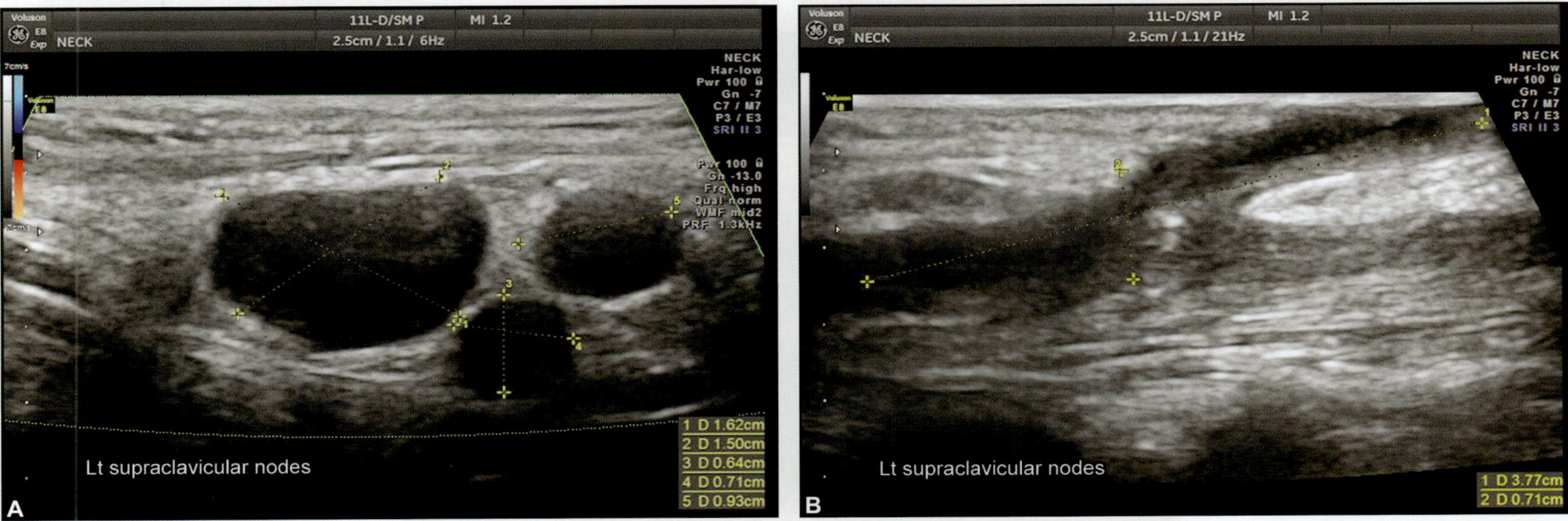

FIGURES 4.15A and B

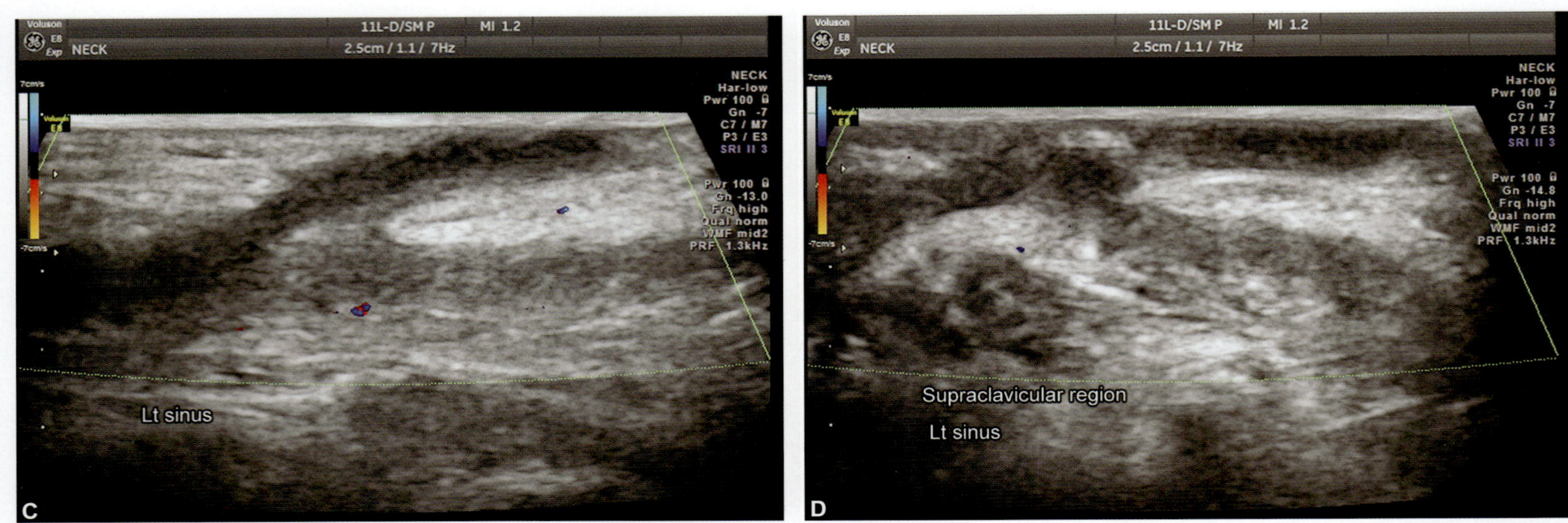

FIGURES 4.15C and D

FIGURES 4.15A to D: Tubercular abscess with sinus formation. HRSG shows multiple hypoechoic nodal masses in the left supraclavicular region. Central area of necrosis is seen in them. An obliquely running sinus tract is also seen in the left midcervical region. It is 40 mm in length and 5 mm in width. It is 2 cm deep from the skin. Small pocket of collection is seen in the neck communicating with the sinus tract. Associated soft tissue edema is also seen in the neck.

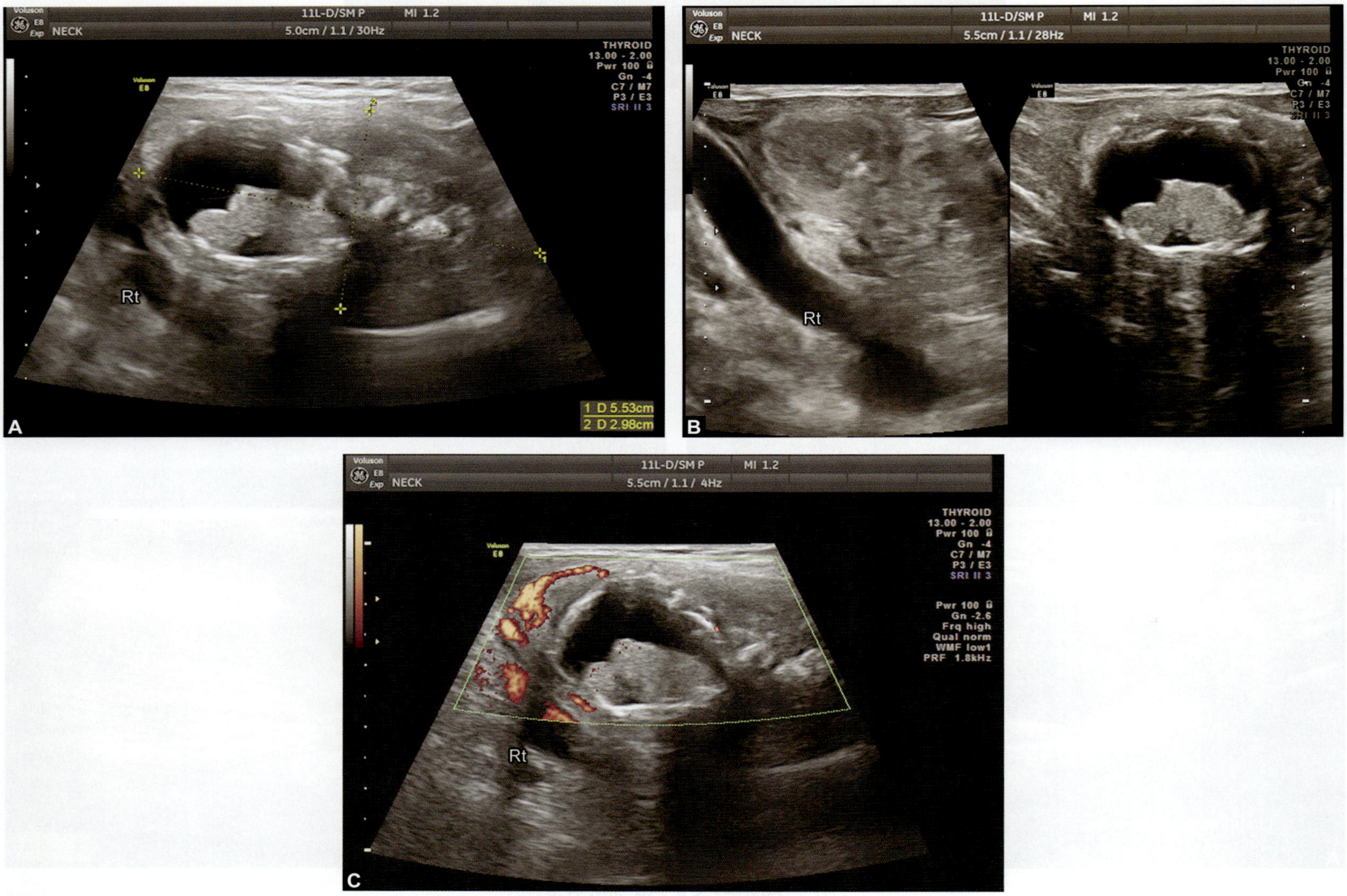

FIGURES 4.16A to C: A patient presented with soft tissue mass in the right side of neck. HRSG shows a heterogeneous mass in right lobe of thyroid. The mass is predominantly cystic. Echogenic soft tissue shadows are also seen. On color flow imaging, poor flow is seen. FNAC of the mass confirms cystic adenoma.

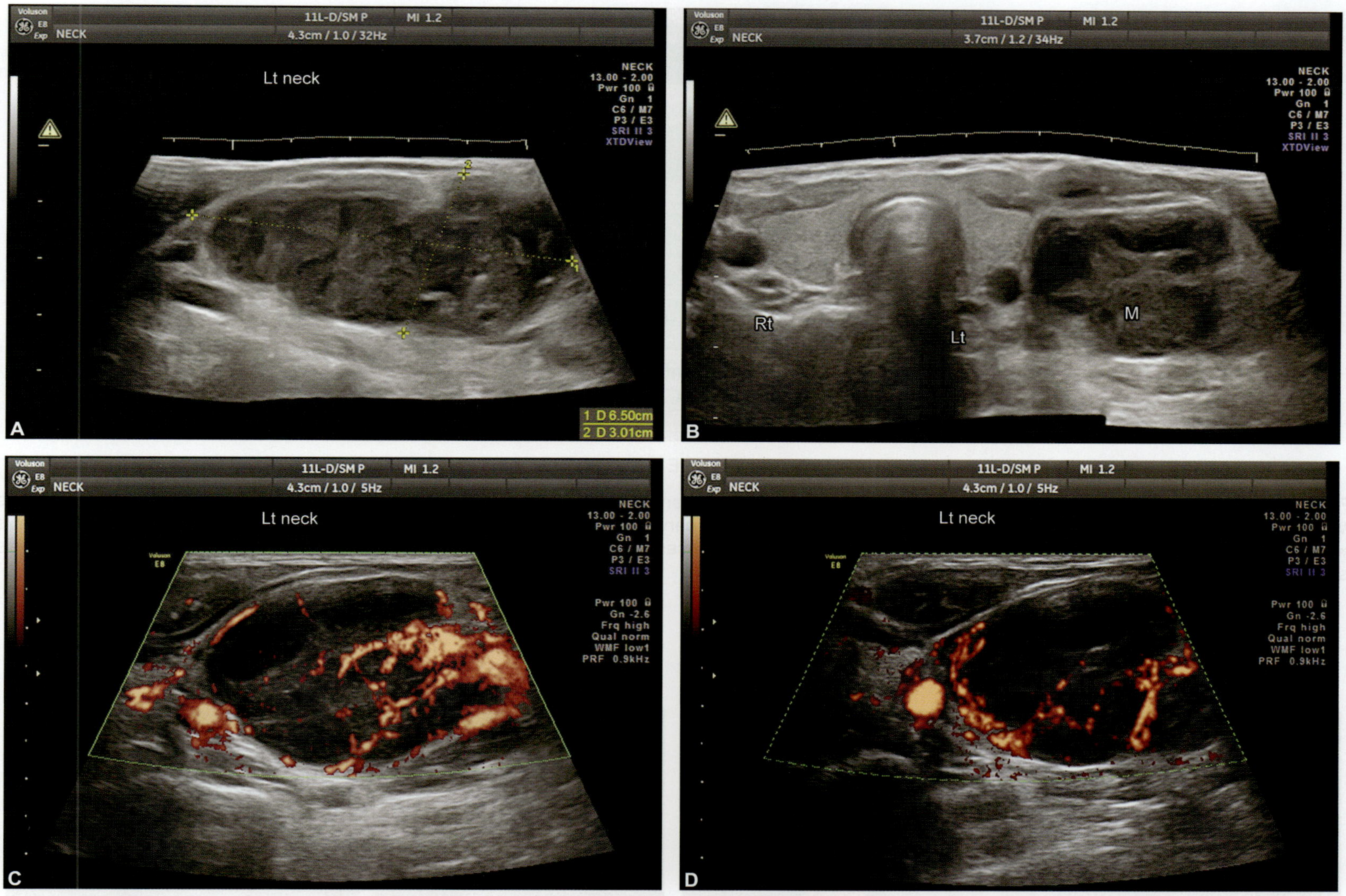

FIGURES 4.17A to D: Collar stud abscess. HRSG shows a big irregular low level echo complex mass in the left supraclavicular region. It is seen extending to the midcervical region. Low level echoes are seen into it. Thick echo collection is seen into it. But no cystic degeneration is seen. It is extending into the infraclavicular and retrosternal regions. On color flow imaging, moderate flow is seen in the mass. Enlarged nodal shadows are also seen into it in the posterior triangle. The abscess is seen pressing over the left lobe of thyroid. However, the fascial plane between left lobe of thyroid and the abscess is maintained.

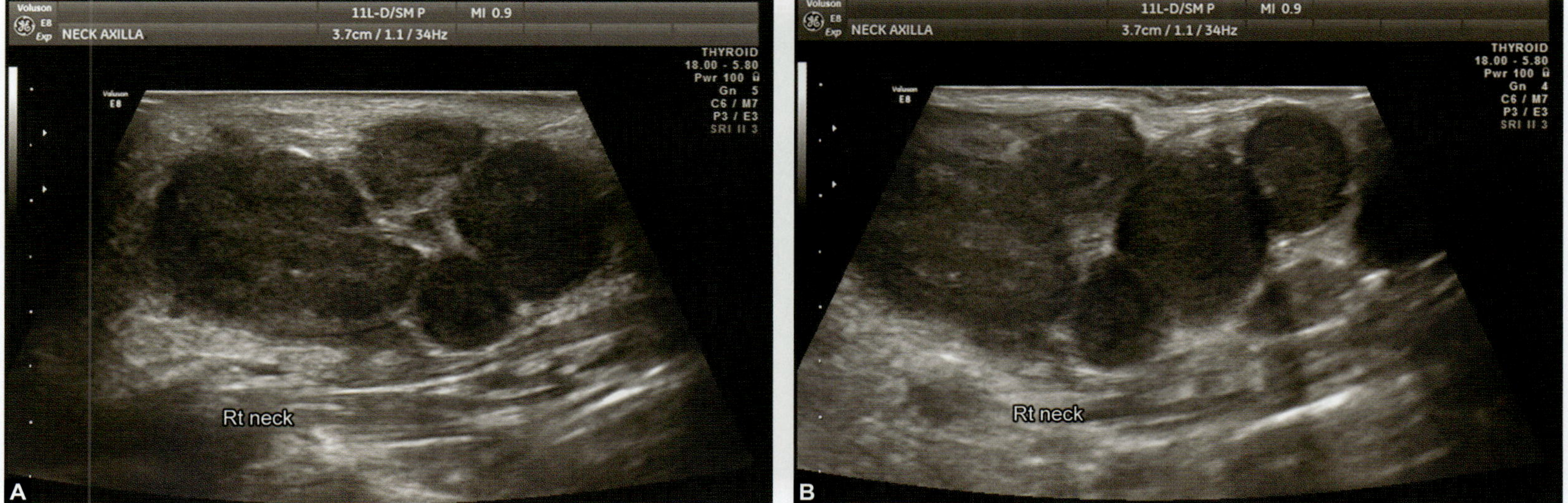

FIGURES 4.18A and B

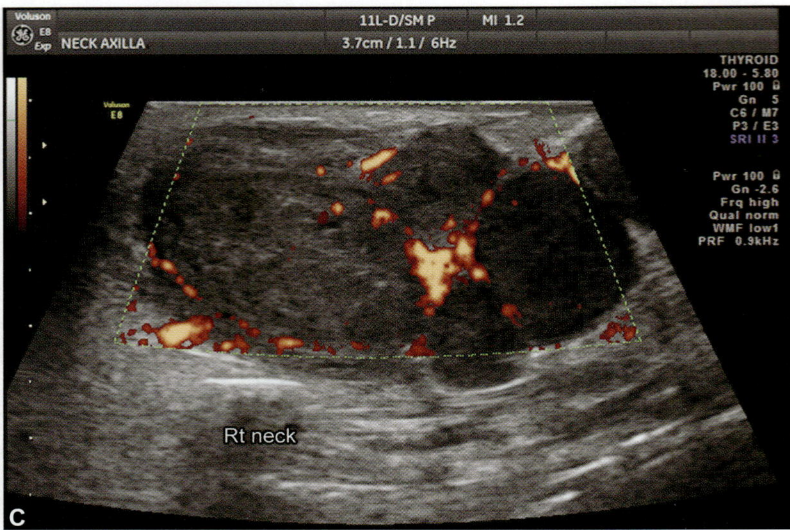

FIGURE 4.18C

FIGURES 4.18A to C: Non-Hodgkin lymphoma (NHL). A patient presented with nodular mass in the right side of neck. HRSG shows multiple well-defined lobulated soft tissue masses in right side of neck in upper cervical region. They are homogeneous in texture. No cystic degeneration is seen. They appear to be enlarged lymph node. Few enlarged nodal masses are also seen in left upper cervical and midcervical region. No necrosis is seen in them. No cystic degeneration is seen.

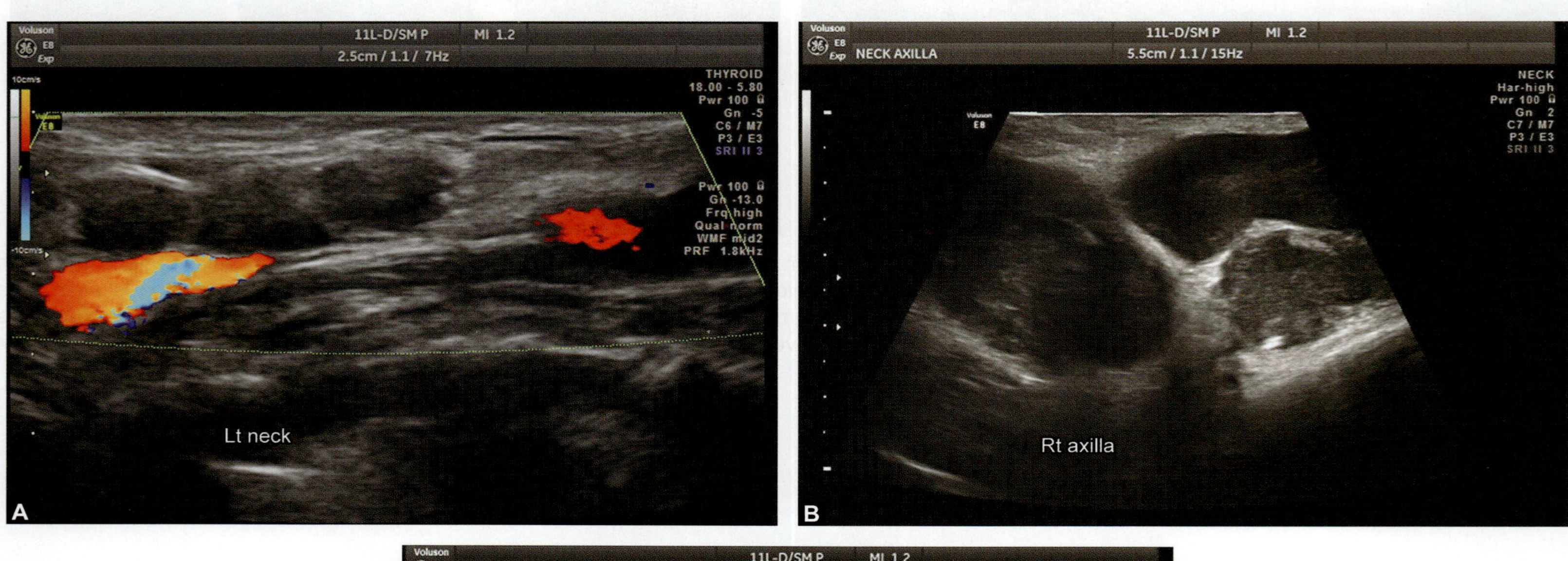

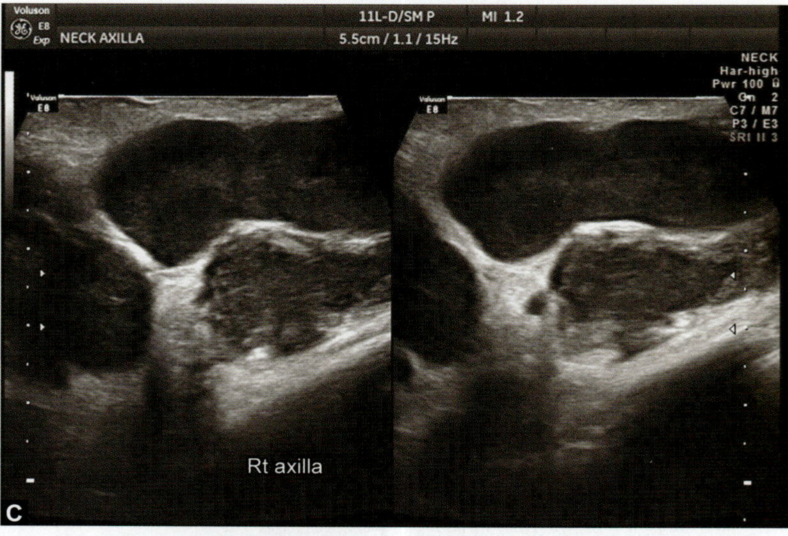

FIGURES 4.19A to C: The same patient shows multiple enlarged nodes in right axilla. No necrosis is seen. Lymph node hilum is seen destroyed. Few nodal masses show cystic degeneration. FNAC shows non-Hodgkin lymphoma.

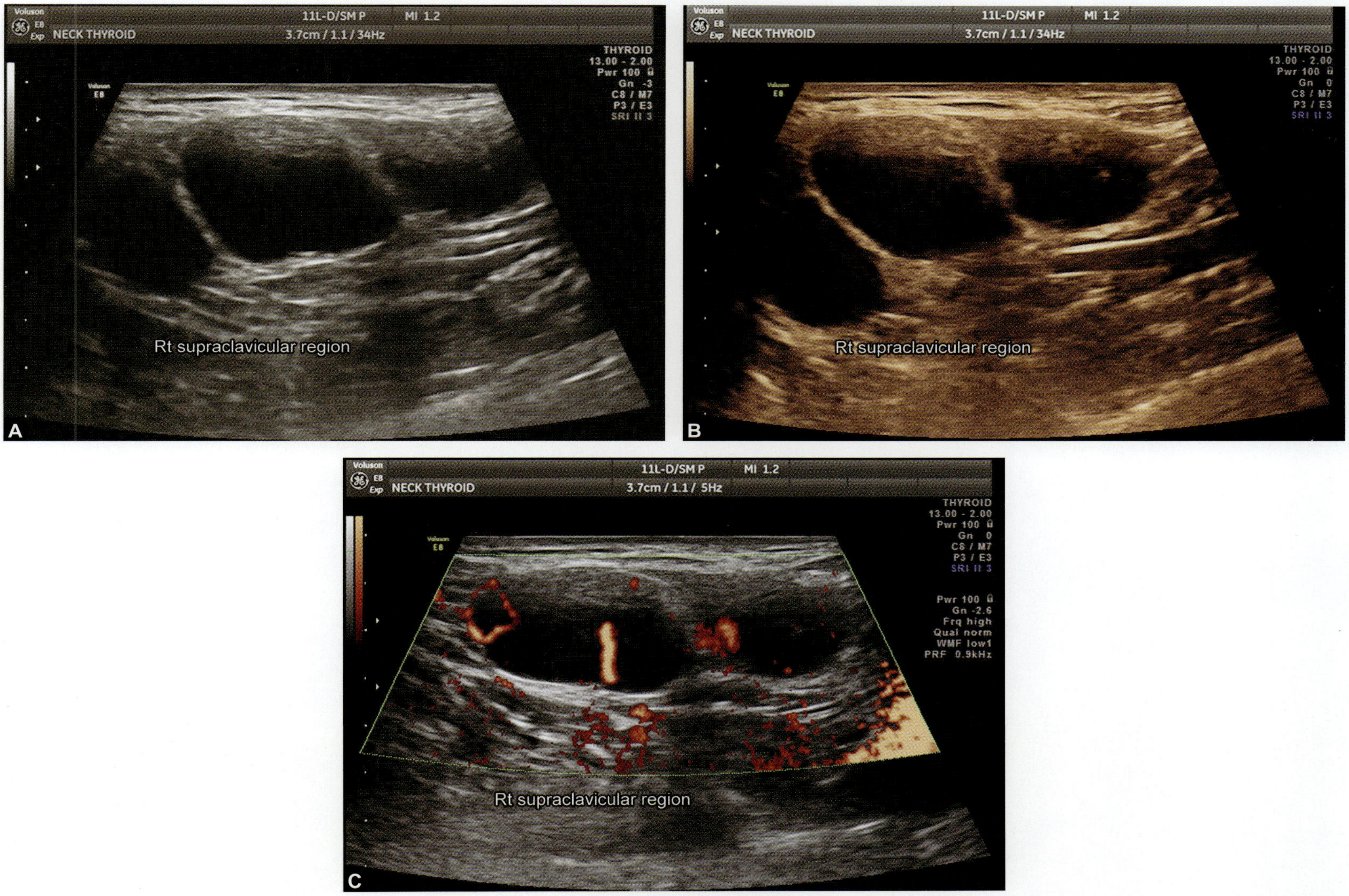

FIGURES 4.20A to C: Non-Hodgkin lymphoma. HRSG shows multiple enlarged nodal shadows in supraclavicular region. They are round in shape. Lymph node hilum is seen destroyed. No cystic degeneration is seen in them. On color flow imaging, vessels are seen feeding the mass from periphery to inside. FNAC confirms NHL.

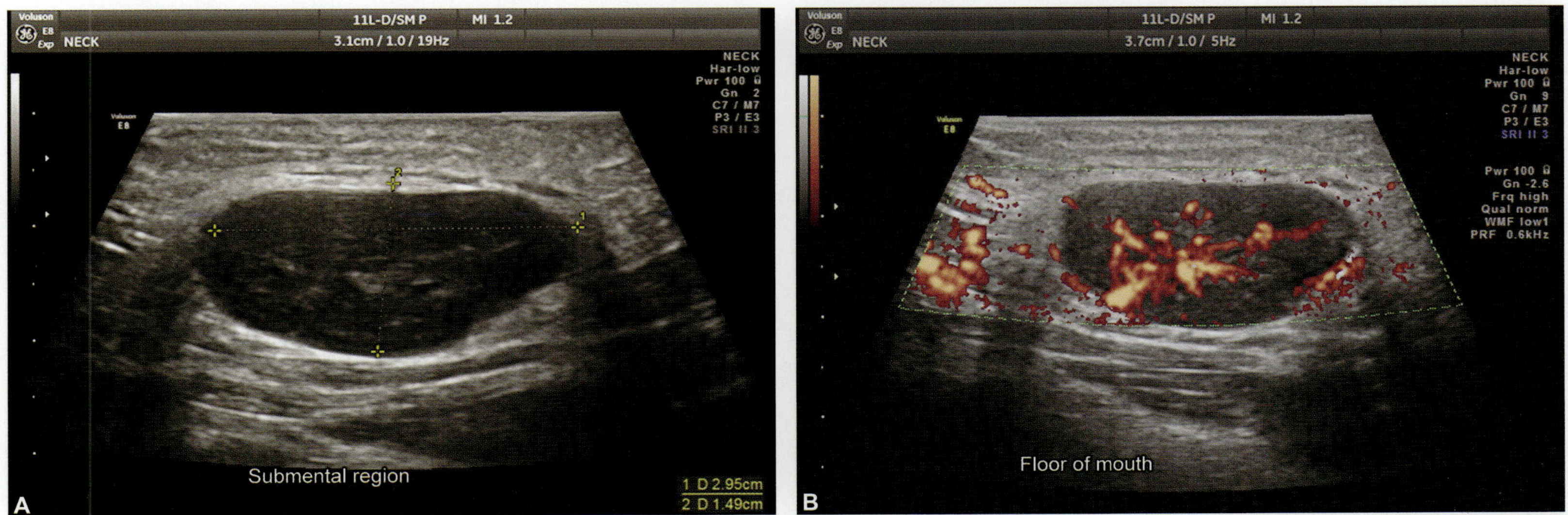

FIGURES 4.21A and B: A patient presented with soft tissue swelling in the submental region. HRSG shows a big well-defined hypoechoic nodal mass in the submental region. It is homogeneous and hypoechoic in texture. No calcification is seen into it. No cystic degeneration is seen. On color flow imaging, increased flow is seen into it.

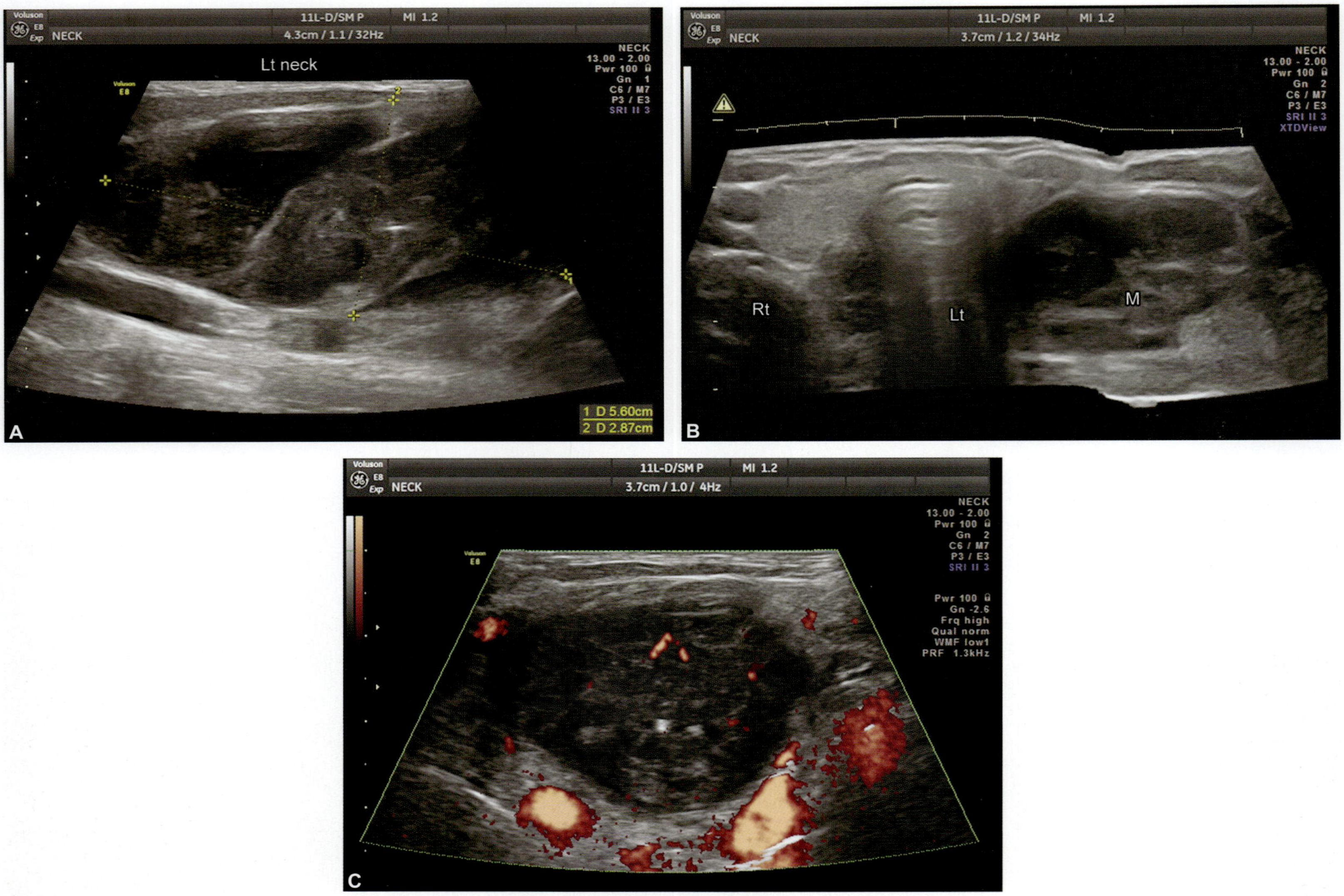

Figures 4.22A to C: Collar stud abscess. HRSG shows a big irregular low level echo complex mass in the left supraclavicular region. It is seen extending to the midcervical region. Low level echoes are seen into it. Thick echo collection is seen into it. But no cystic degeneration is seen. It is extending into the infraclavicular and retrosternal regions. On color flow imaging, moderate flow is seen in the mass. Enlarged nodal shadows are also seen into it in the posterior triangle.

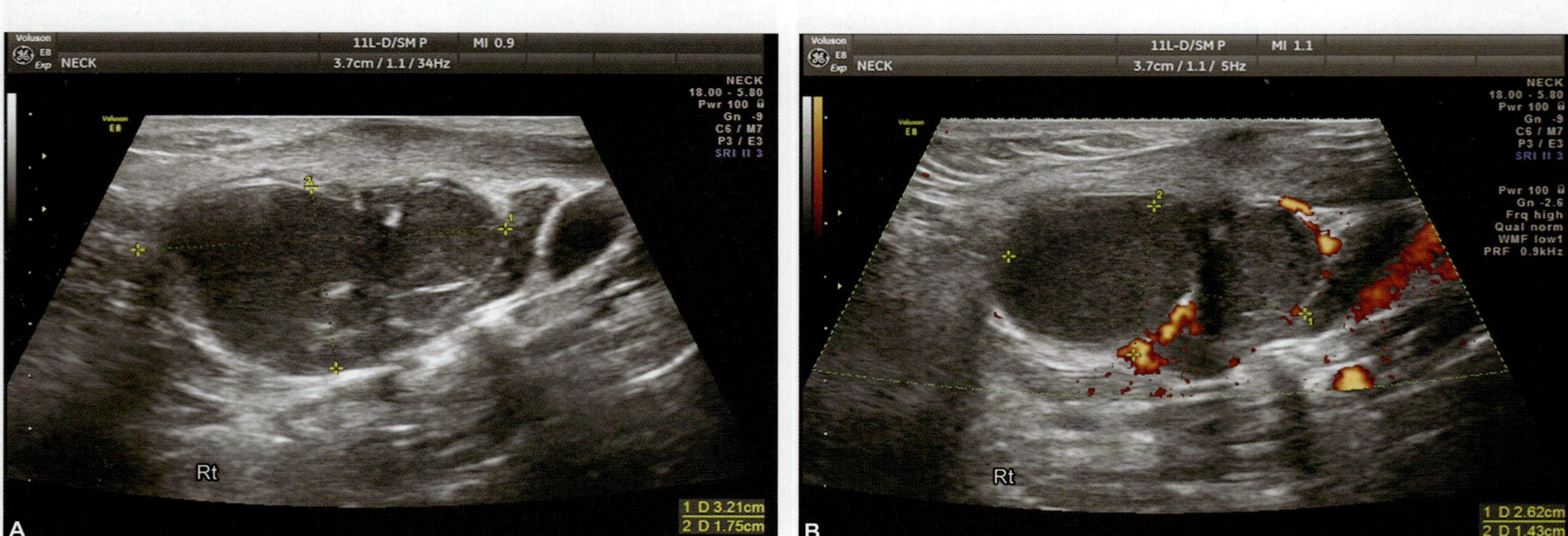

FIGURES 4.23A and B

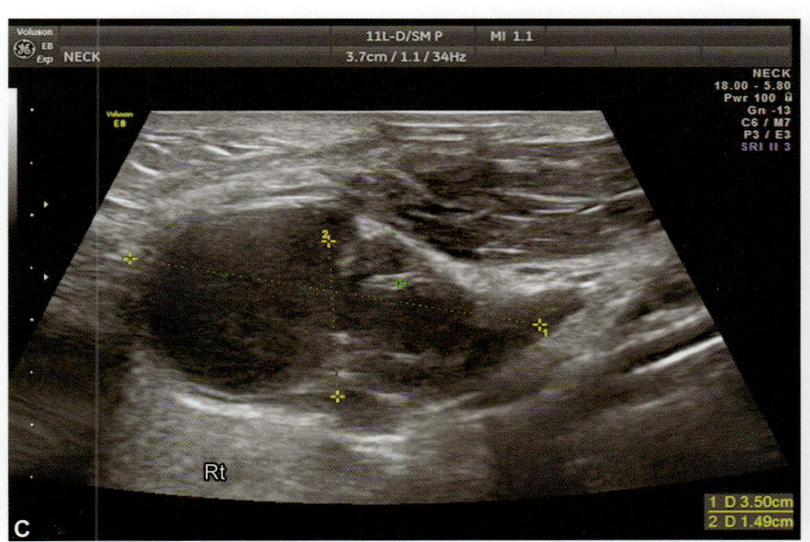

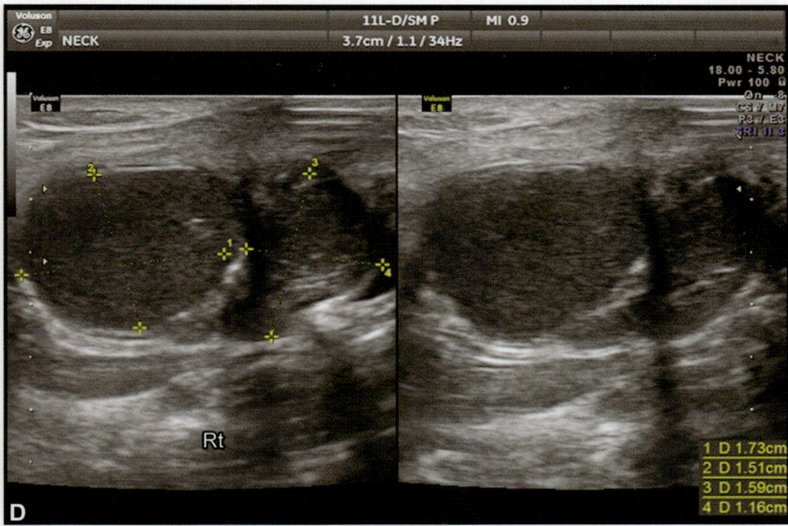

FIGURES 4.23C and D

FIGURES 4.23A to D: FUC of cold abscess. A known case of neck tuberculosis came in follow up. HRSG shows a pocket of thick collection seen in the right upper cervical region. Thick cheesy collection is seen in them. But no loculation is seen. Enlarged nodal shadows are also seen in right midcervical region. No necrosis is seen in them. Few enlarged nodes are also seen in the left mid cervical region. Enlarged nodes are also seen in left upper cervical region

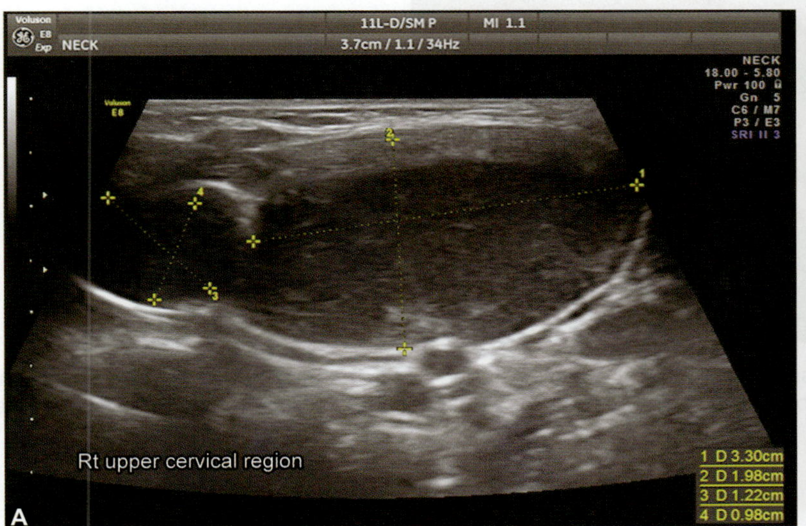

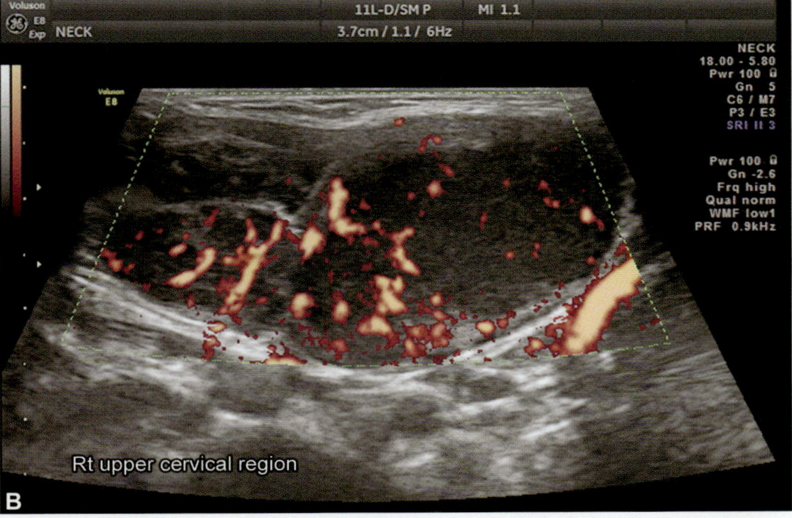

FIGURES 4.24A and B: A 5-year-old boy presented with soft tissue mass in the neck right upper cervical region. HRSG shows multiple nodal masses seen in right upper cervical regions. Big nodal mass is seen in right upper cervical region. Area of necrosis is seen into it. But no cystic degeneration is seen.

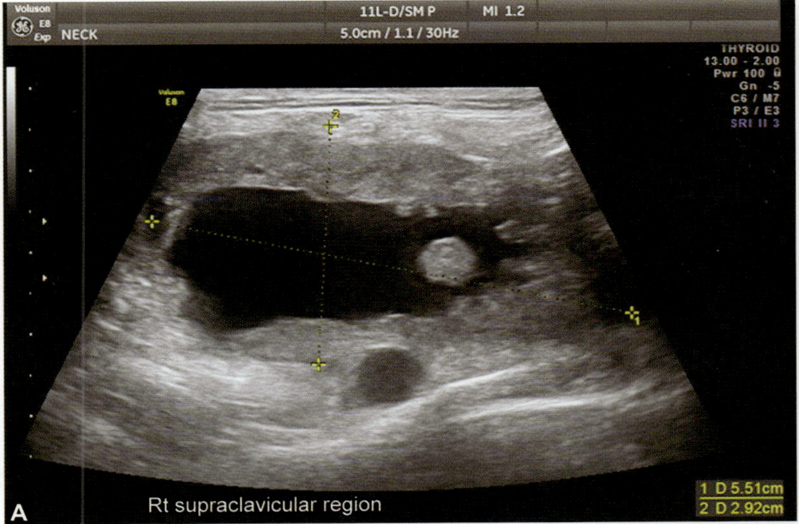

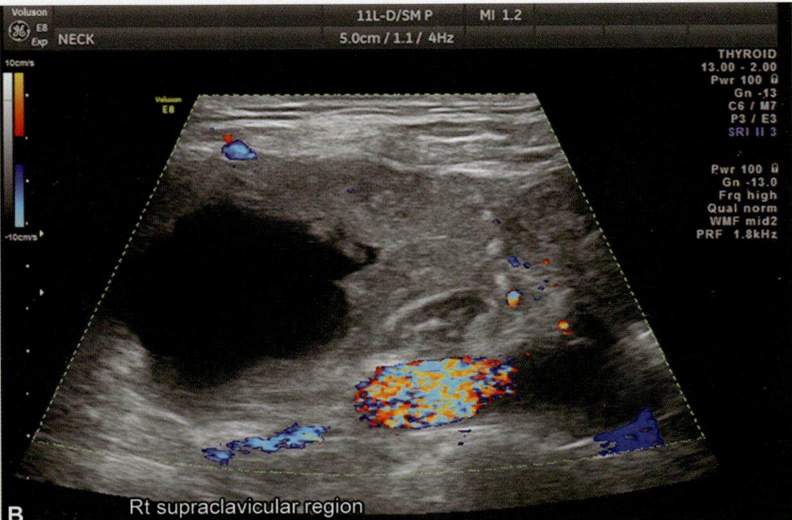

FIGURES 4.25A and B: FUC of neck tuberculosis. A known case of neck tuberculosis presented with fluid collection in right supraclavicular region. HRSG shows pocket of collection in right supraclavicular region. Few enlarged nodes are also seen in the supraclavicular region and midcervical region. No evidence of any necrosis is seen in them.

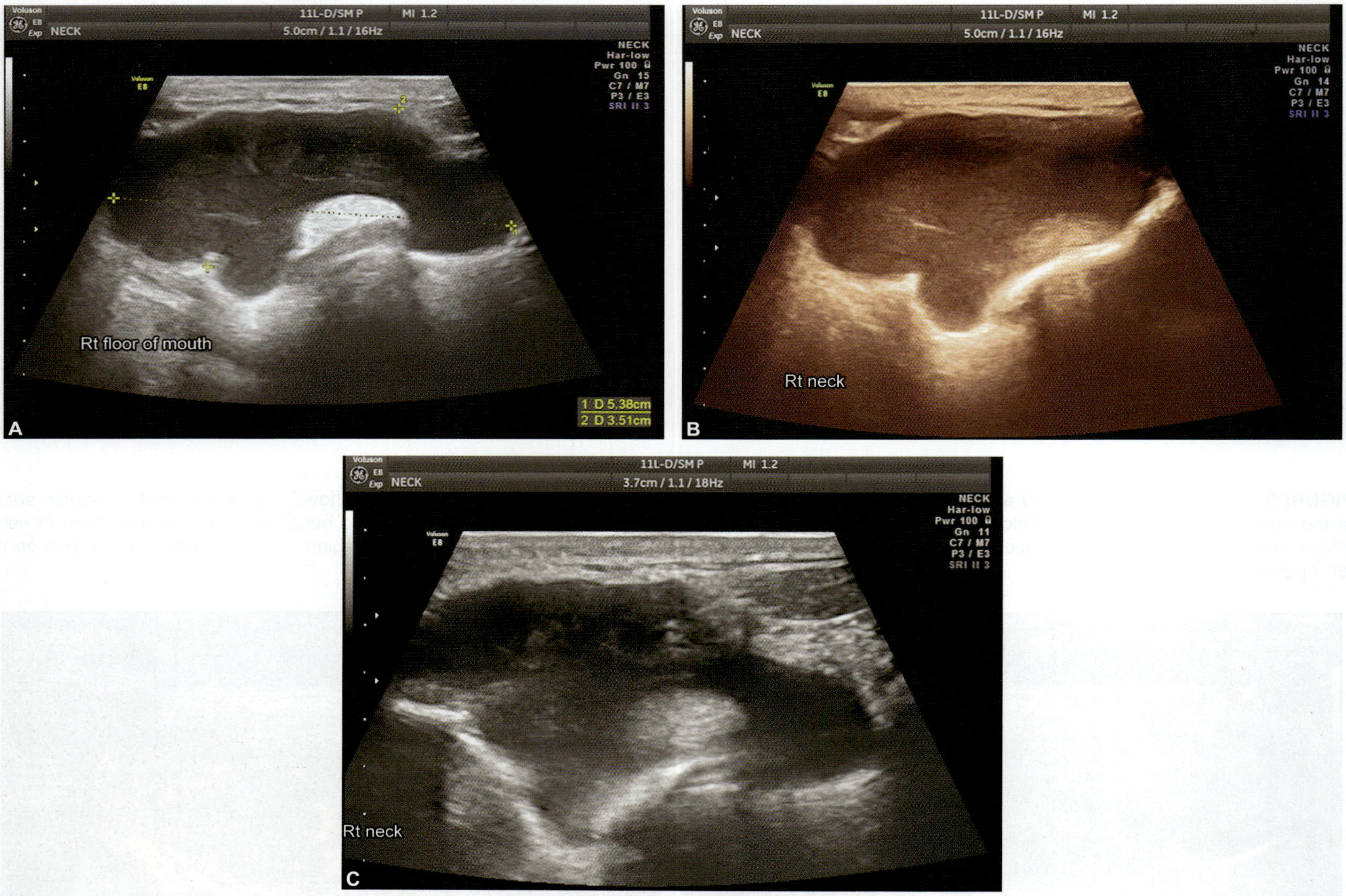

FIGURES 4.26A to C: Sublingual ranula. A patient presented with soft tissue swelling in the midline of the neck. It shows low level echo collection, which is seen extending down and going to floor of the mouth. Homogeneous echoes are seen in it. On aspiration clear fluid is seen in it suggestive of sublingual ranula.

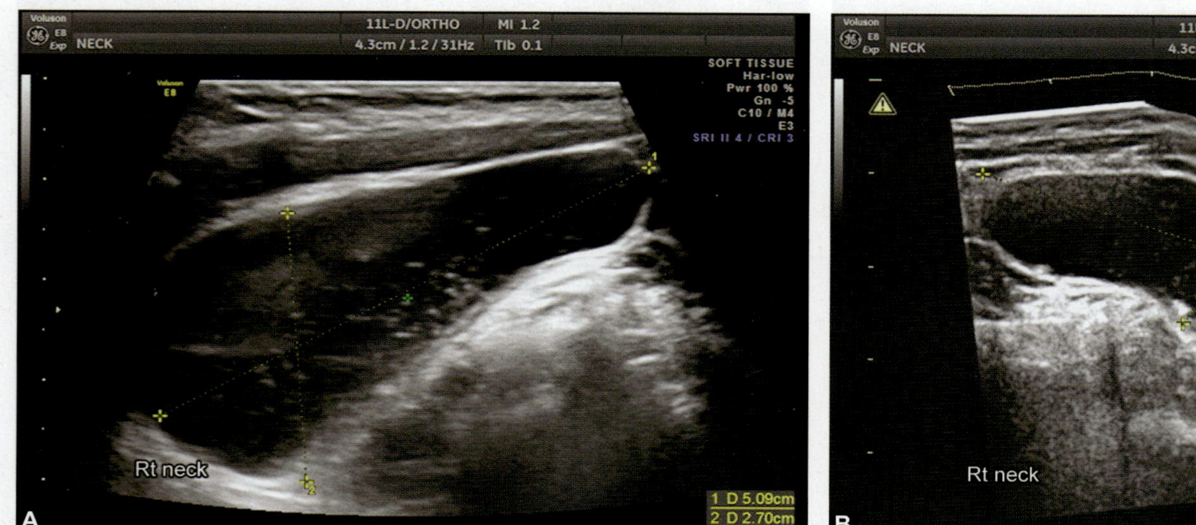

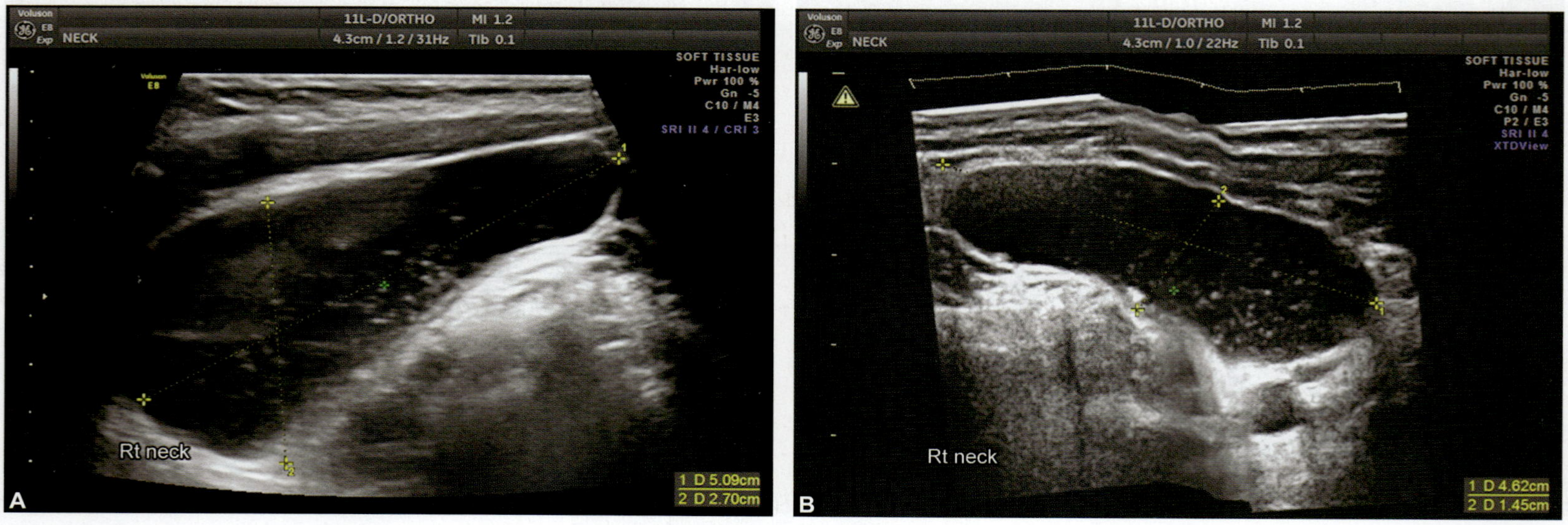

FIGURES 4.27A and B

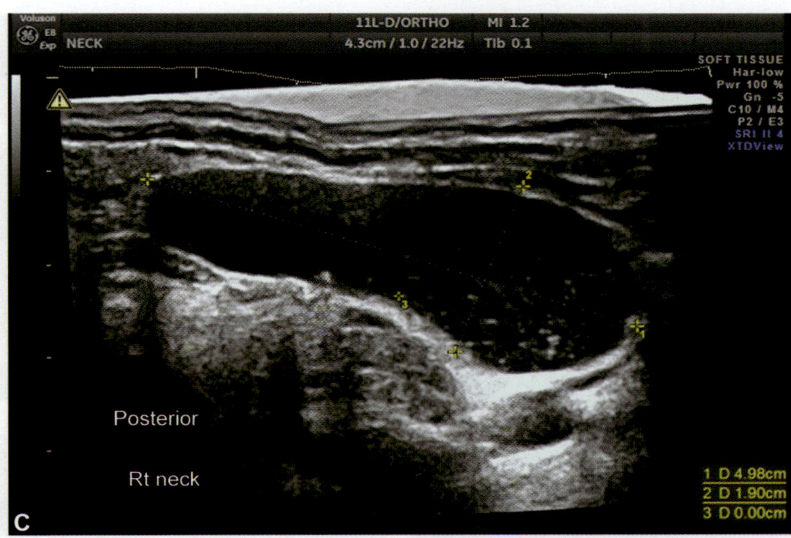

FIGURE 4.27C

FIGURES 4.27A to C: A patient presented with soft tissue swelling in the lateral side of right side of neck. HRSG shows a well-defined cystic mass in right side of the neck. It is extending from preauricular region going down to lower cervical region. Fine internal echoes are seen in the cyst with bright echogenic pattern. The cyst is separate from the neck vessels. On color flow imaging, no flow is seen in the cyst. It is separate from the thyroid gland. Few enlarged nodes are also seen in right upper cervical region. Findings are suggestive of brachial cleft cyst.

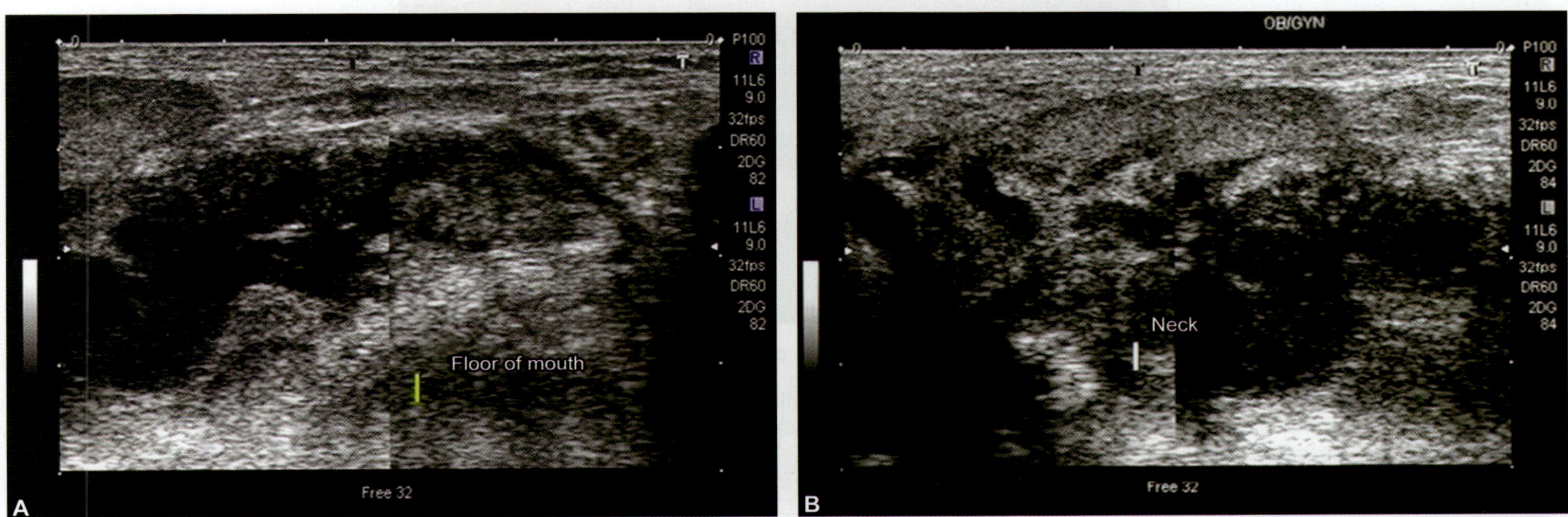

FIGURES 4.28A and B: Ludwig angina. A patient presented with diffuse soft tissue swelling in the neck with high fever. HRSG shows irregular ill-defined mixed echo complex mass in the neck. It is seen confined to subcutaneous tissue plane. Associated fat necrosis is also seen. Central area of necrosis is also seen. Perifocal edema is present. Normal anatomic relations are distorted. Findings are consistent with Ludwig angina.

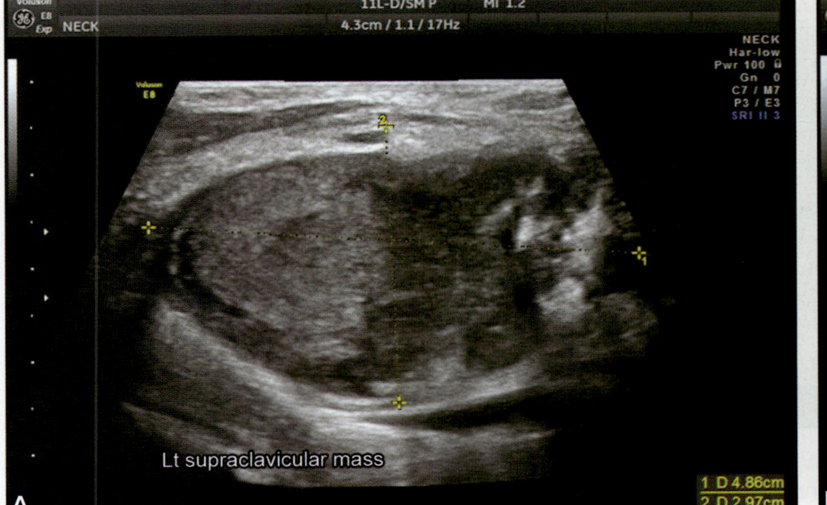

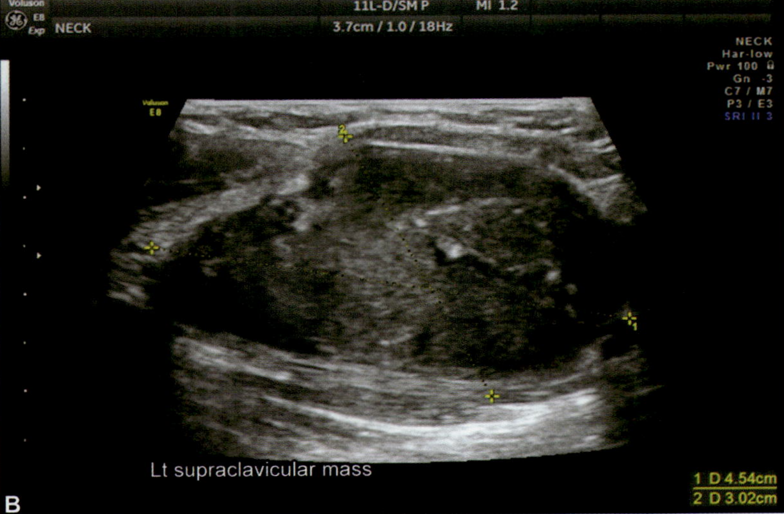

FIGURES 4.29A and B

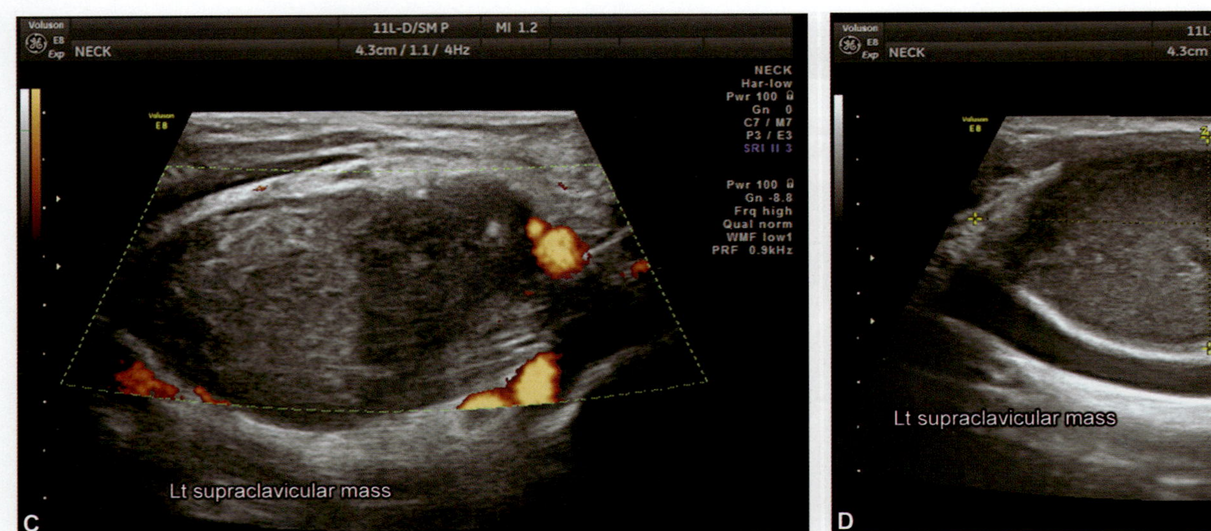

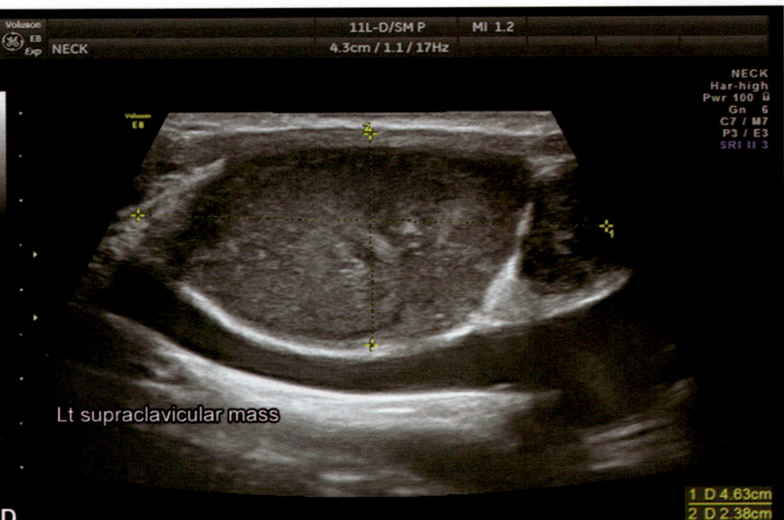

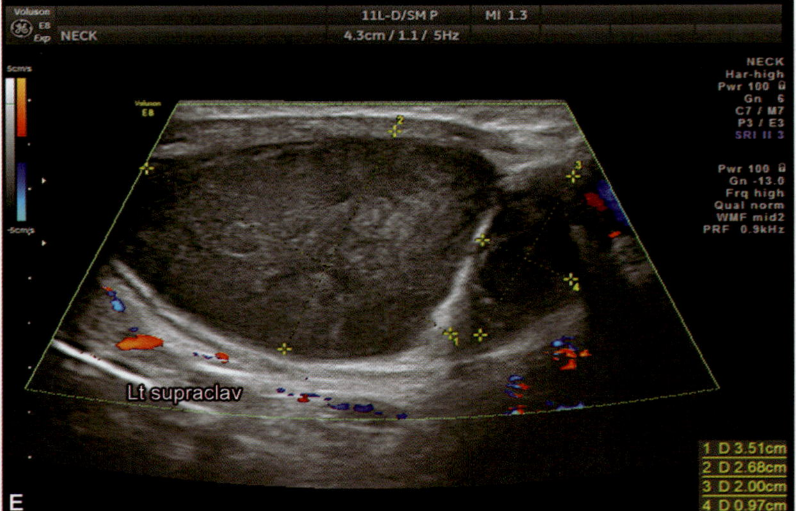

FIGURES 4.29C to E

FIGURES 4.29A to E: Supraclavicular abscess. A patient presented with soft tissue swelling in the neck. HRSG shows a big well encapsulated low level echo complex mass seen in the left supraclavicular region. Thick cheesy echoes are seen in it. But no cystic degeneration is seen. Few enlarged nodes are also seen on the left side of the neck.

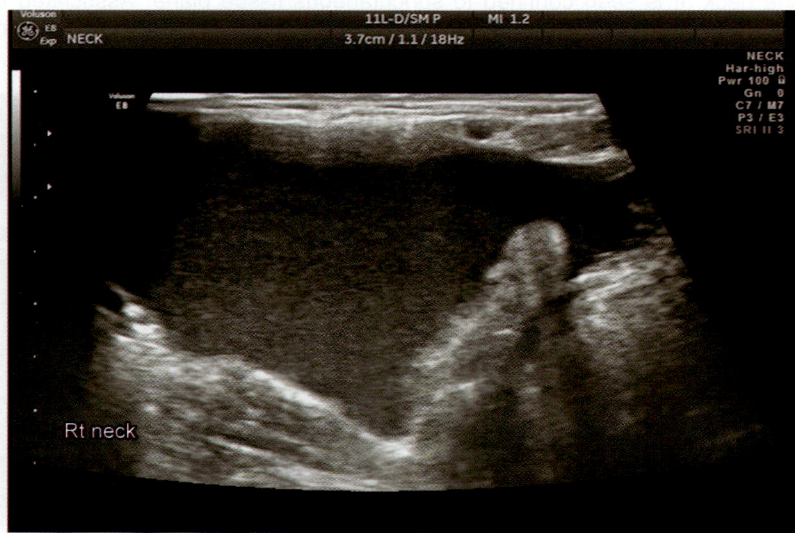

FIGURES 4.30: A young girl presented with soft tissue swelling in the right side of neck. HRSG shows a well-defined low level echo collection seen in right upper cervical region. It is seen superior to the submandibular gland. It is seen extending into the floor of the mouth. Low level echoes are seen into it. Thin septa is also seen into it. But no calcification is seen into it. It is separate from the submandibular and anteriomedial gland.

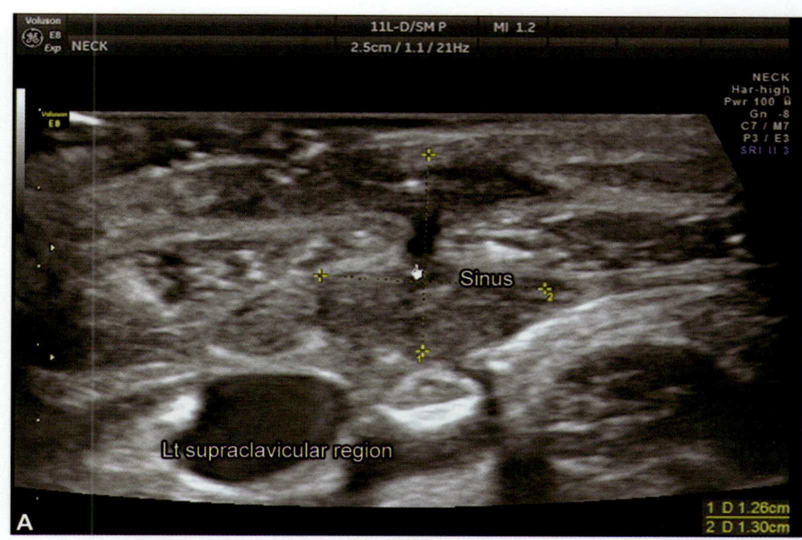

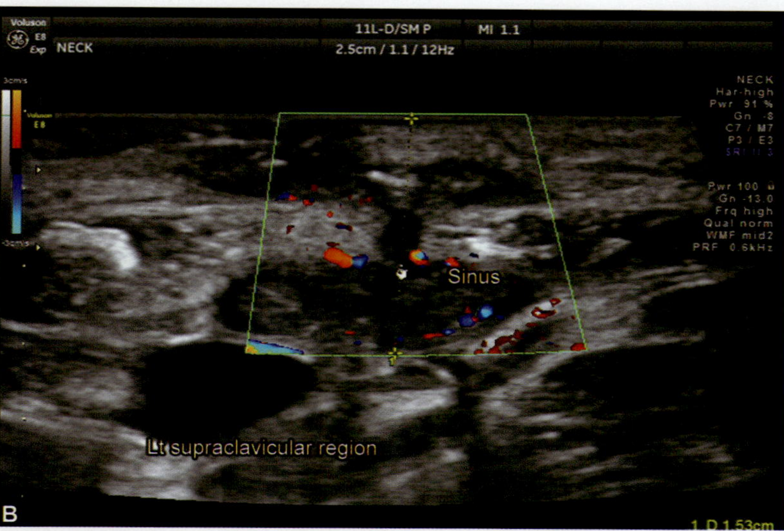

FIGURES 4.31A and B: HRSG shows a low level echo complex mass in the left supraclavicular region. A discharging sinus is also seen in the supraclavicular region. Enlarged nodal shadows are seen in the supraclavicular region. A low level echoes complex mass is seen in the retrosternal region. Cystic degeneration is seen into it suggestive of an abscess formation. The sinus is seen communicating with the abscess. It is 2 cm deep from the skin. Few enlarged nodes are also seen in the left upper cervical region. Enlarged nodal shadows are also seen in right side of the neck.

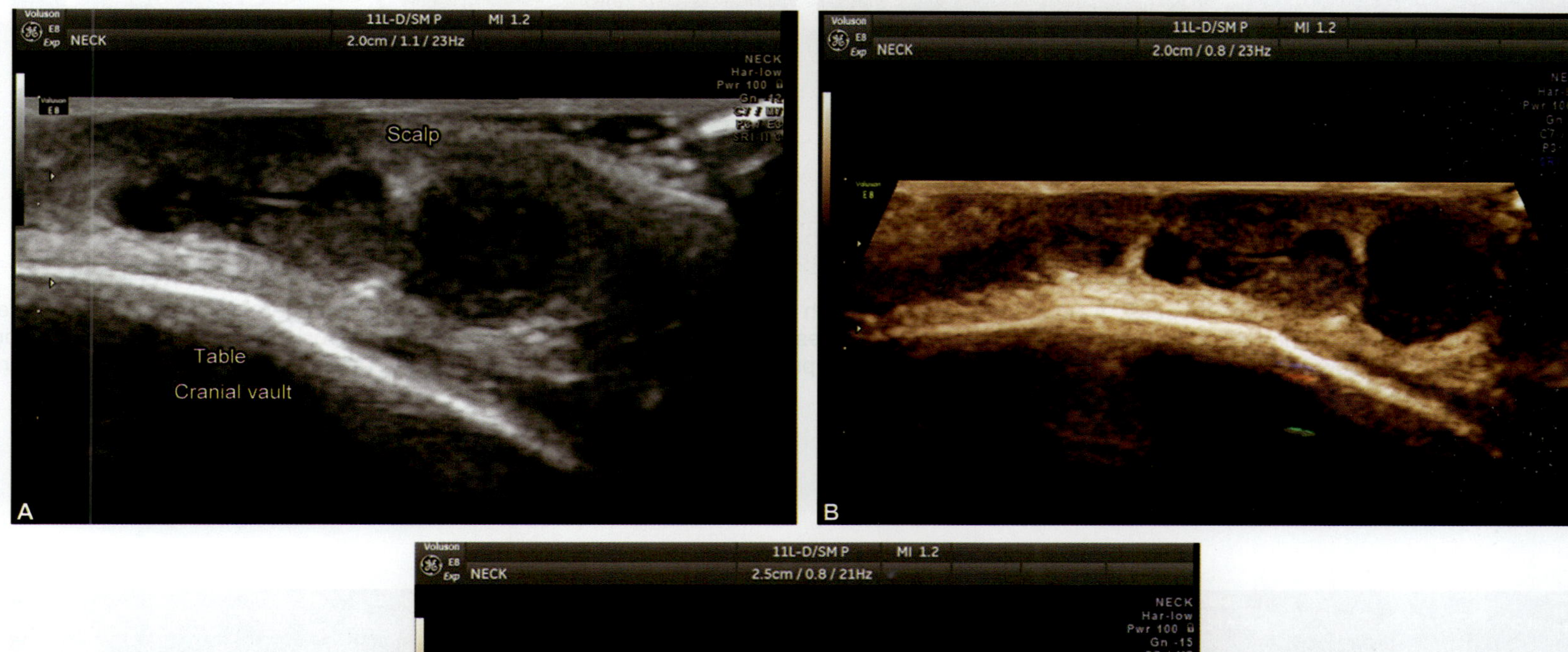

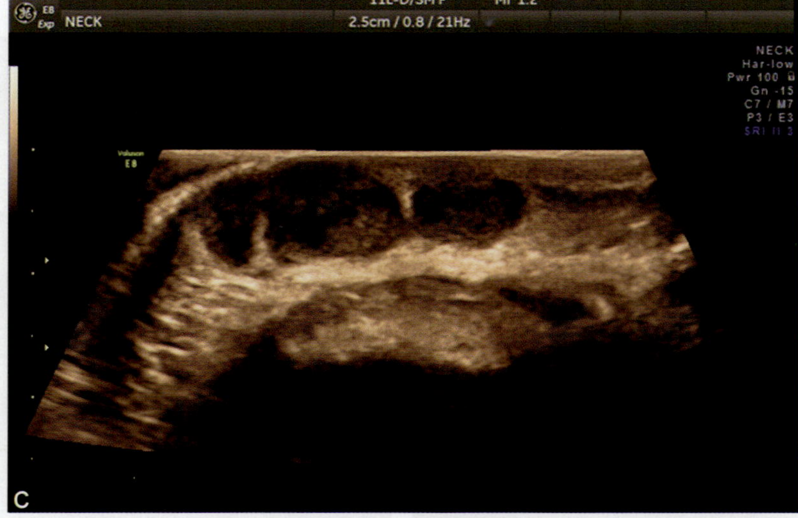

FIGURES 4.32A to C: A 3-month-old baby presented with soft tissue mass over the scalp and occiput. HRSG shows a multiloculated cystic low level echo complex mass in the scalp of the occiput. It is seen confined to the scalp. Low level echoes are seen in it. But no calcification is seen. On color flow imaging, few vessels are seen feeding it. On spectral Doppler tracing low arterial flow is seen in the mass. However, the mass is not seen invading the cranial vault. No intracranial extension is seen.

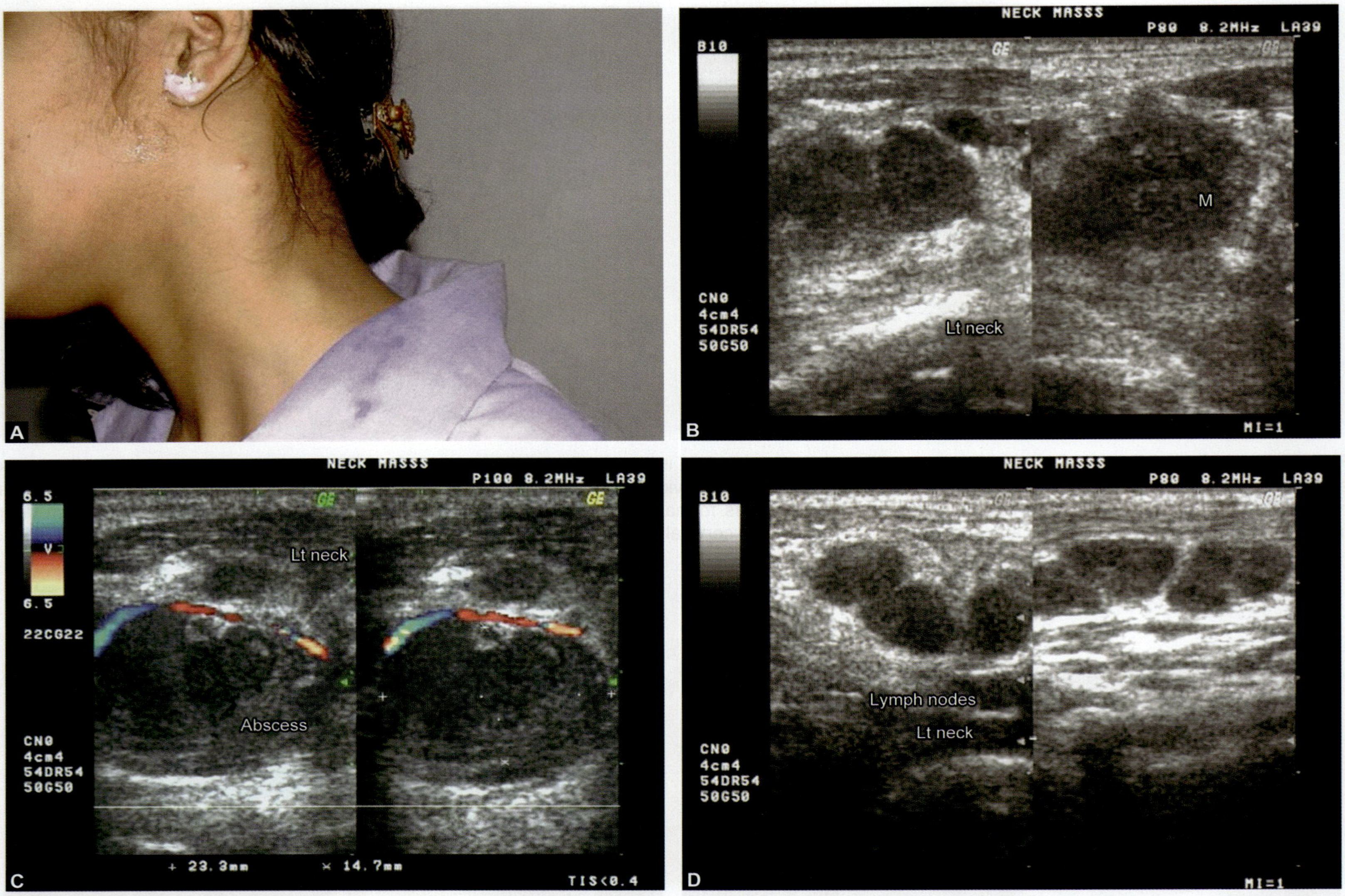

FIGURES 4.33A to D: Tubercular abscess. A young girl presented with soft tissue mass in left cervical area. No tenderness was present in the mass. HRSG shows well-defined thick wall low-level echo complex masses in right cervical area. Central area of necrosis is seen in them. On color Doppler imaging, poor flow is in the masses. However, capsular flow is present. Multiple enlarged lymph nodes are seen in upper cervical area in the same suggestive of tubercular lymphadenitis.

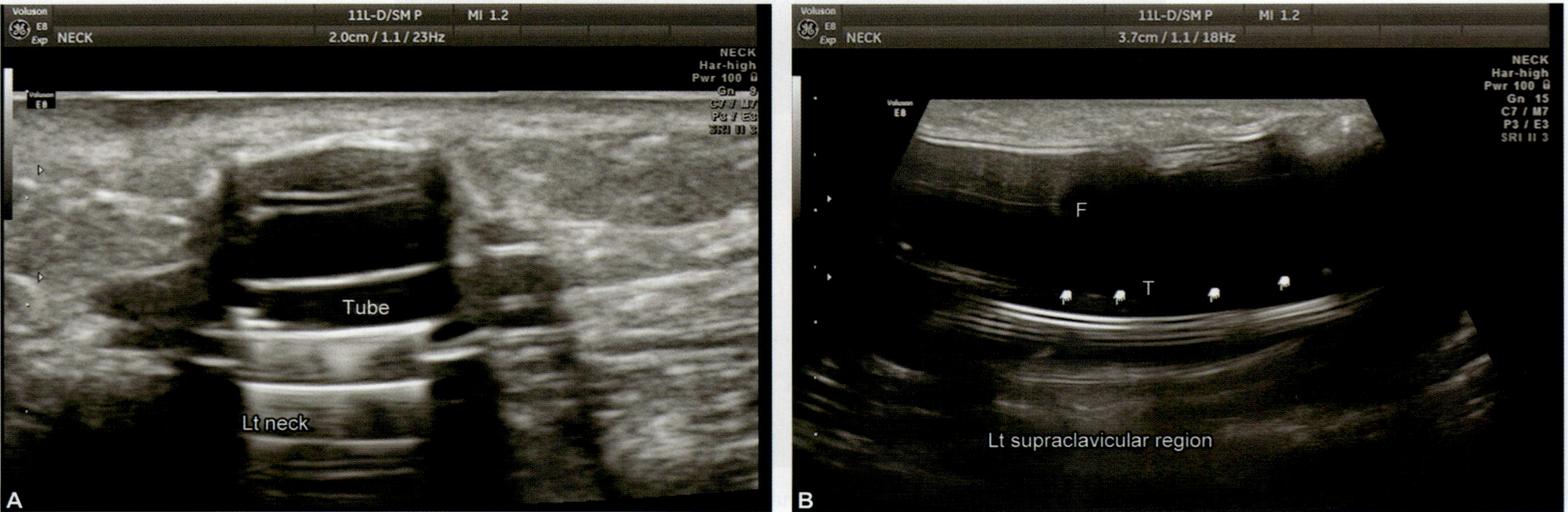

FIGURES 4.34A and B

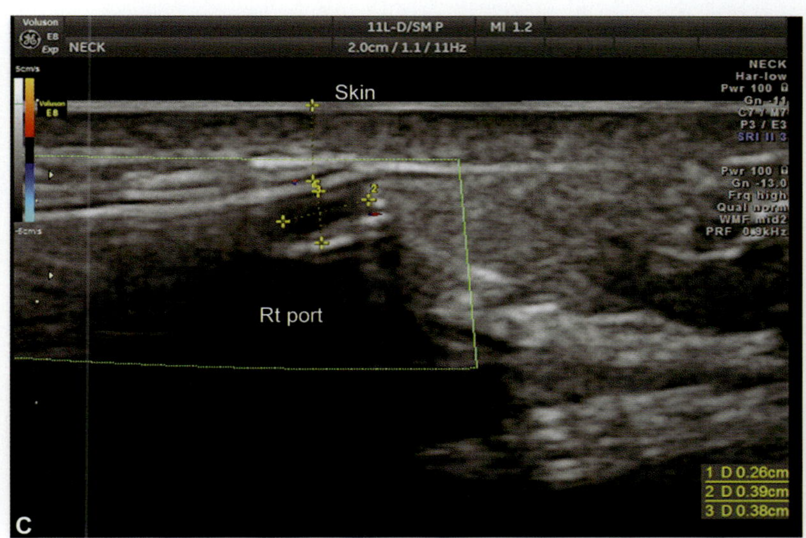

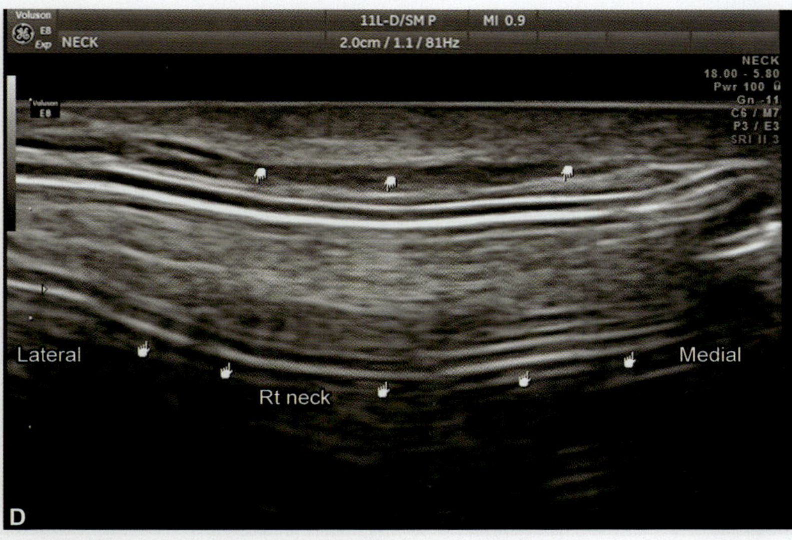

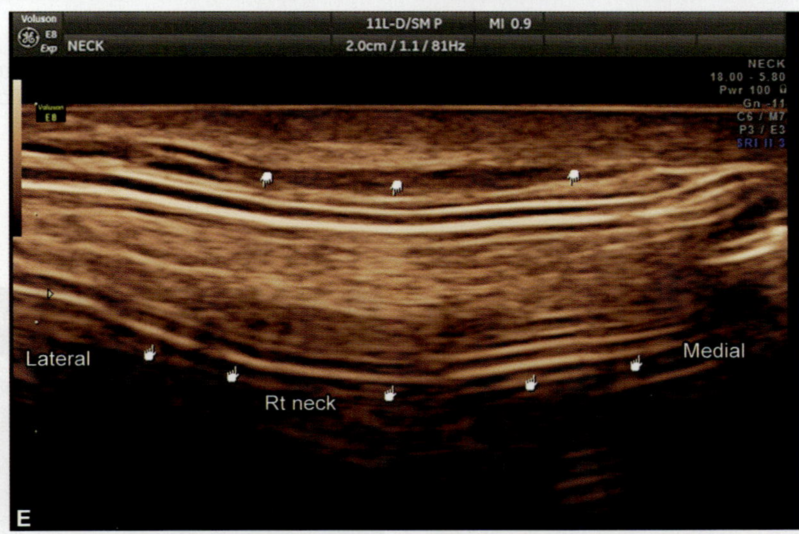

FIGURES 4.34C to E

FIGURES 4.34A to E: Tissue expander in neck. A patient of burn presented with tissue expander and its port in the right side of neck. HRSG shows a sonolucent ovoid shadow in the right side of the neck infraclavicular region lateral to the sternal notch about 2 cm away from the sternal notch. It is seen 3 mm deep from the skin surface. Echogenic tubular shadows are seen running parallel in the right supraclavicular region suggestive of tubes of the expander. The left side of the port is seen distended. A fluid-filled pocket is seen below the subcutaneous tissue suggestive of distended expander. The port is seen in position. It is 2 mm deep from the skin. The right port is 2.2 mm diameter and the left port is 5 mm in diameter.

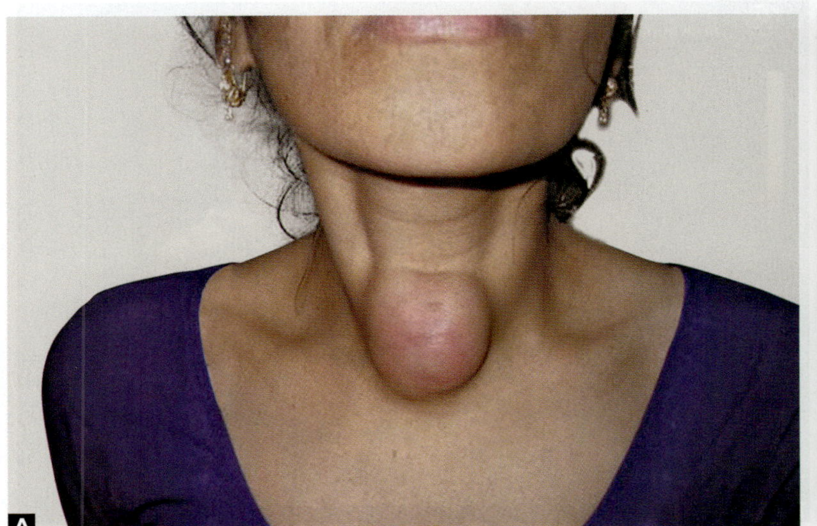

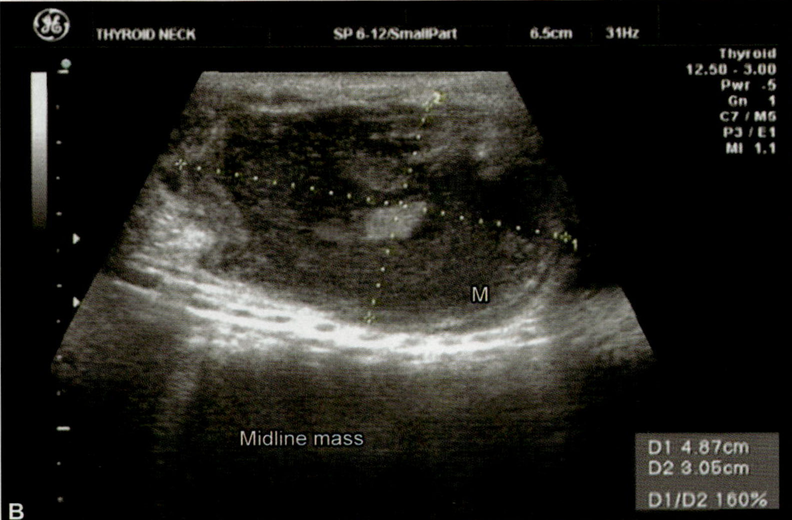

FIGURES 4.35A and B

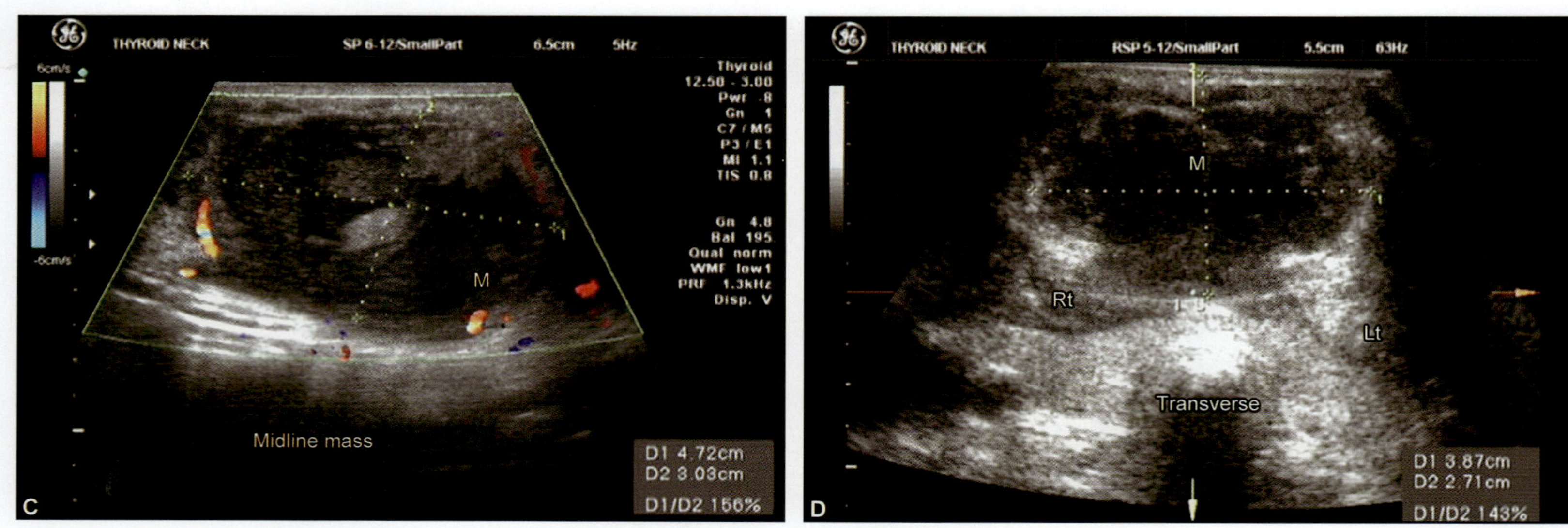

FIGURES 4.35C and D

FIGURES 4.35A to D: Pyogenic suprasternal abscess. A lady presented with well defined red and hot mass in the suprasternal notch. HRSG shows a thick walled, thick echo mass in the suprasternal area. Echogenic debris is also seen in it. On color flow imaging, low flow is seen. Aspiration showed a thick pyogenic abscess.

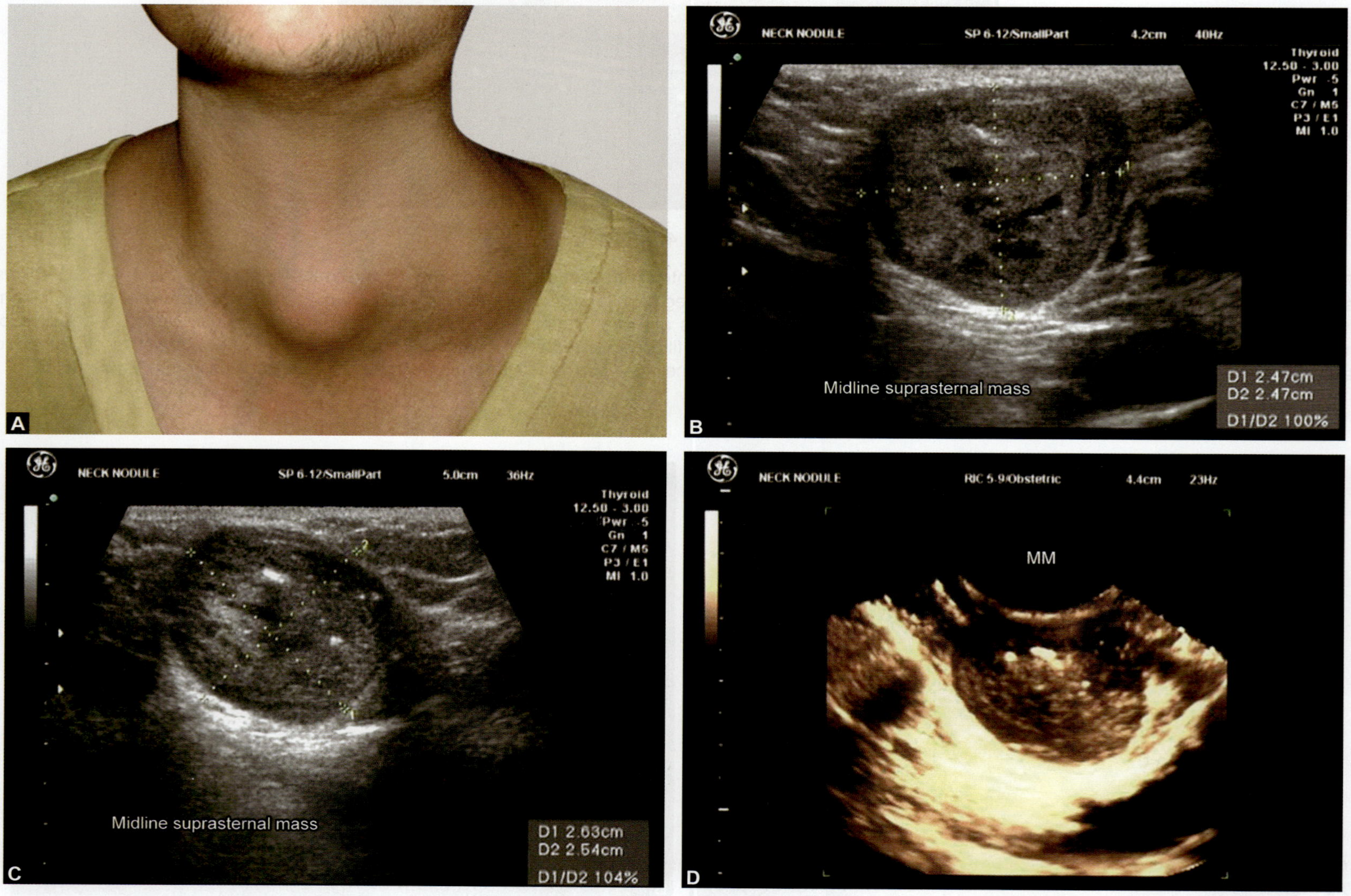

FIGURES 4.36A to D

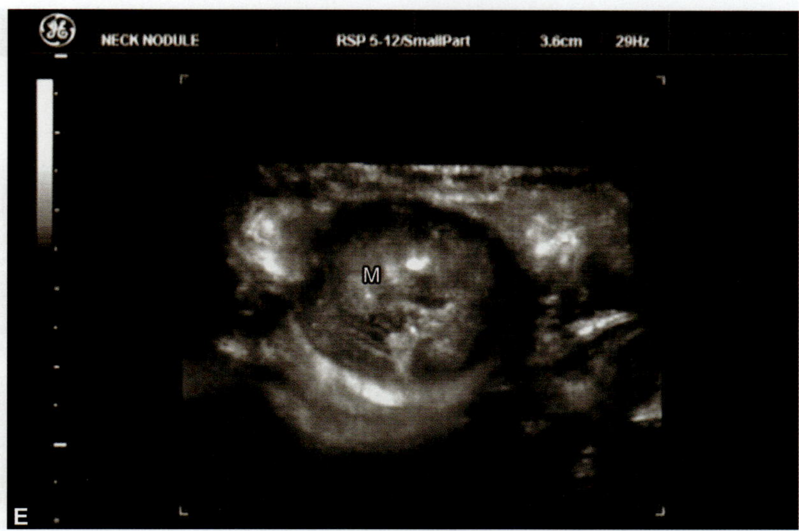

FIGURE 4.36E

FIGURES 4.36A to E: Localized pyogenic abscess (Antibioma). A young girl presented with cystic mass in the midline of the neck in suprasternal area. HRSG shows a thick jelly like mass in the suprasternal area. Few cystic areas are seen in it suggestive of degeneration. 3D imaging of the same patient shows the details of the mass. Biopsy confirmed an antibioma.

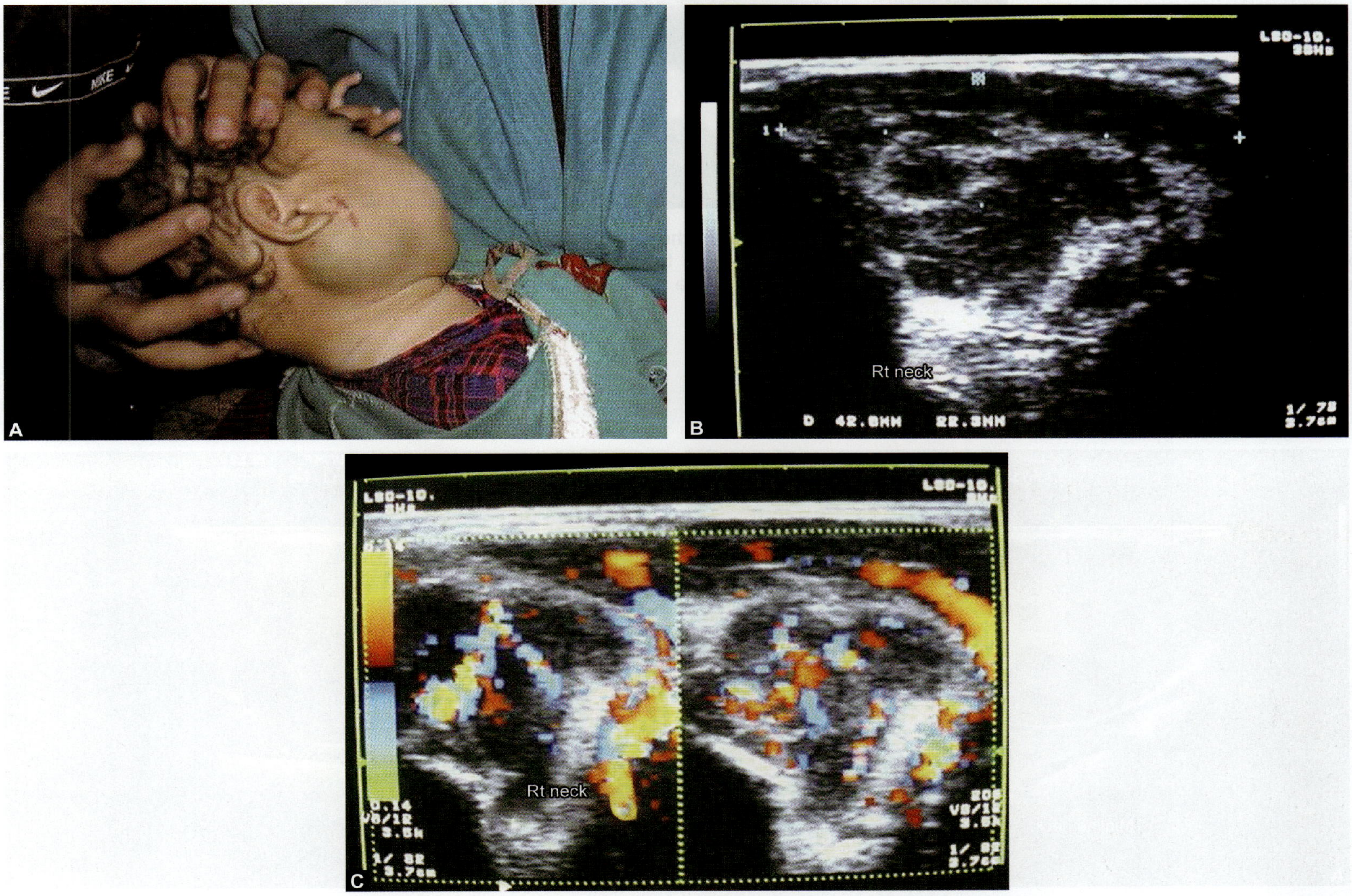

FIGURES 4.37A to C: Acute abscess in the right neck. A new born baby presented highly tender mass in right upper cervical and postauricular area. HRSG shows a low-level echo complex mass with irregular outlines and necrosis. Color Doppler imaging shows increased flow in the mass, suggestive of hyperemia. Findings are suggestive of an abscess.

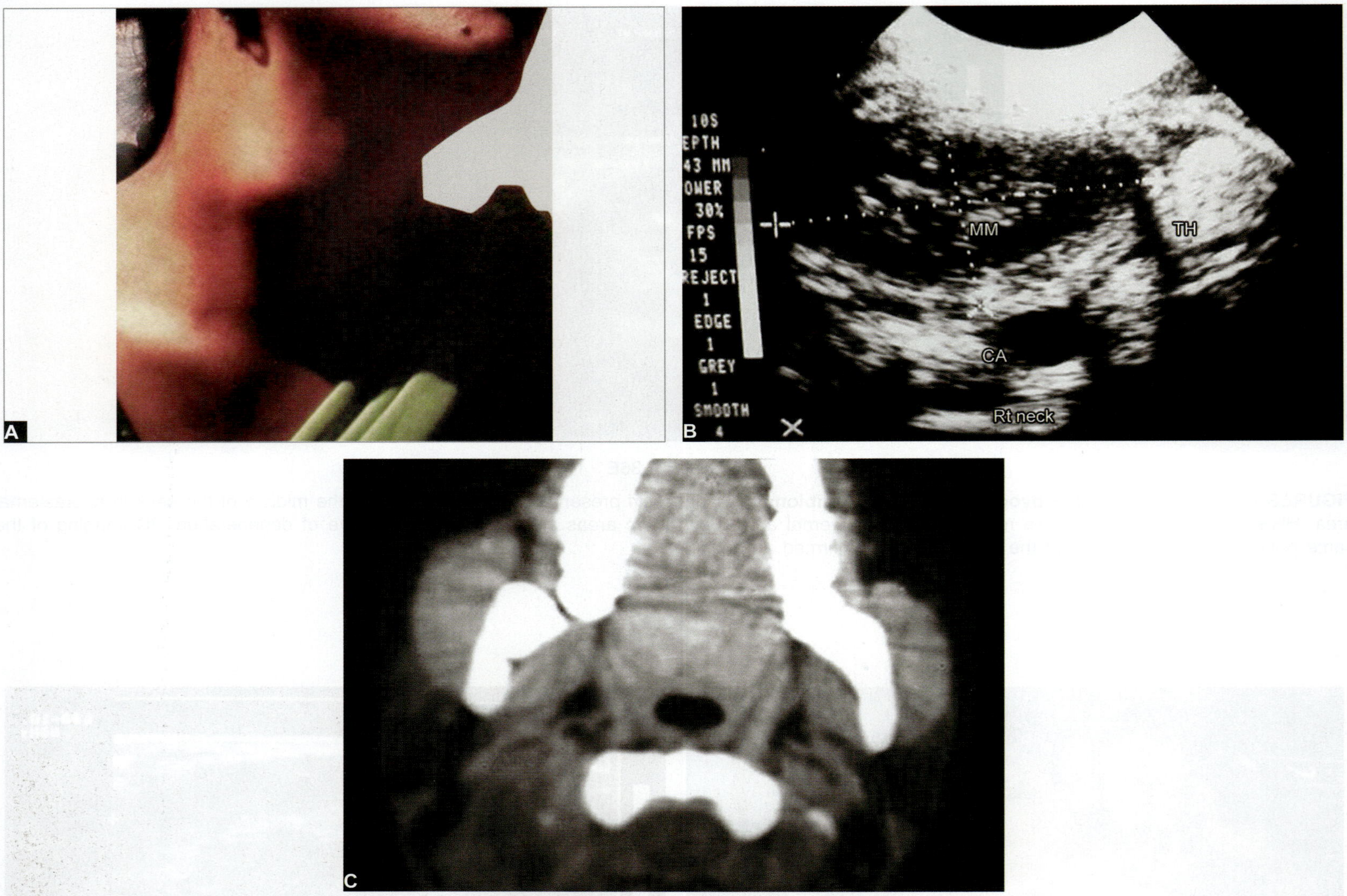

FIGURES 4.38A to C: Tubercular paravertebral abscess extending in the neck. A young lady presented with a nontender swelling in the right side of neck. HRSG shows a big thick-walled low-level echo complex mass in the midcervical area. Multiple internal echoes are seen in it suggestive of an abscess. CT scan of the same patient shows a hypodense mass in the paravertebral and paraphyrngeal area, known case of tubercular abscess.

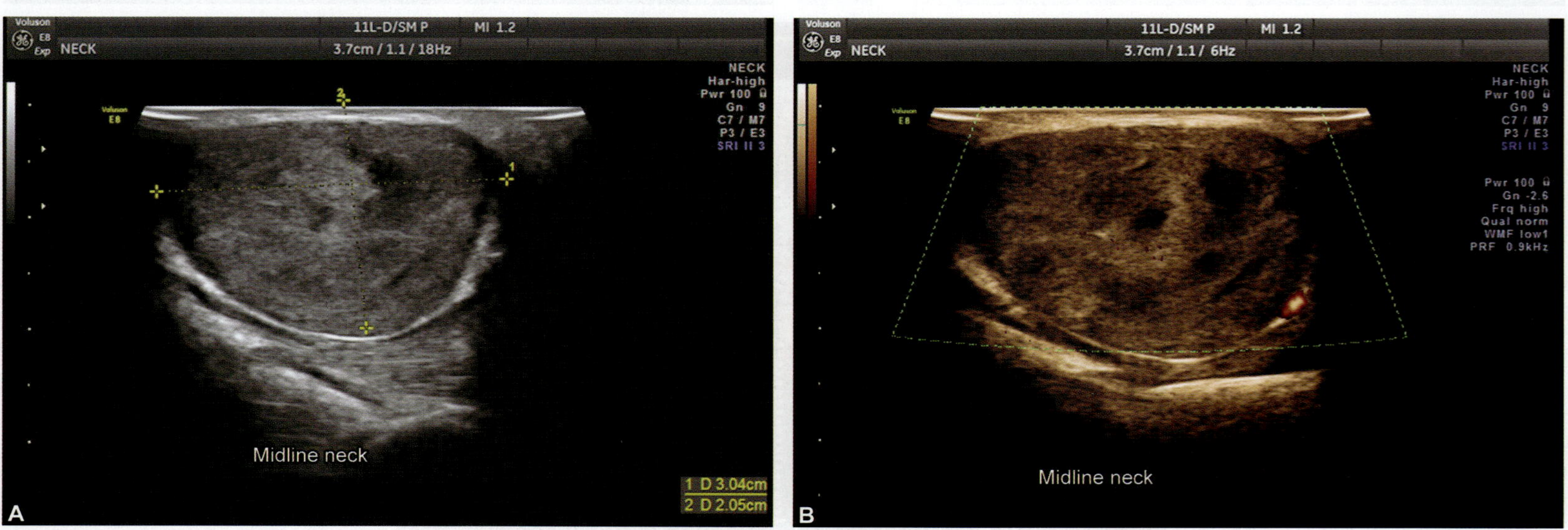

FIGURES 4.39A and B

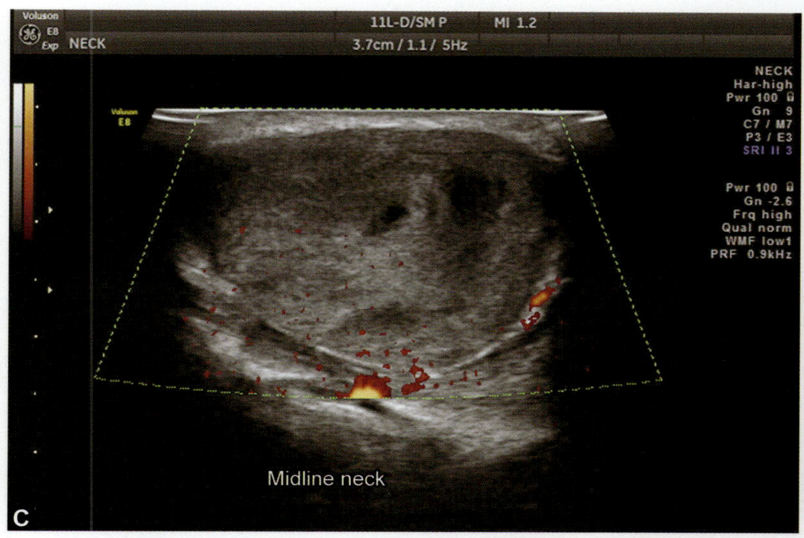

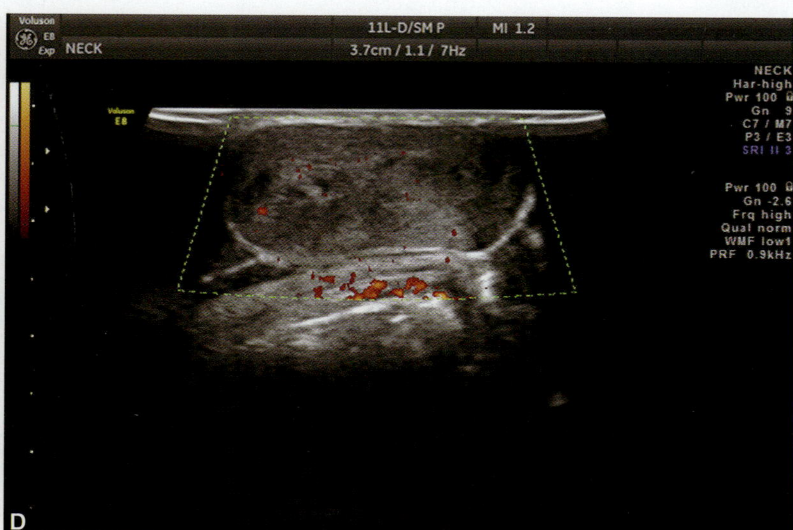

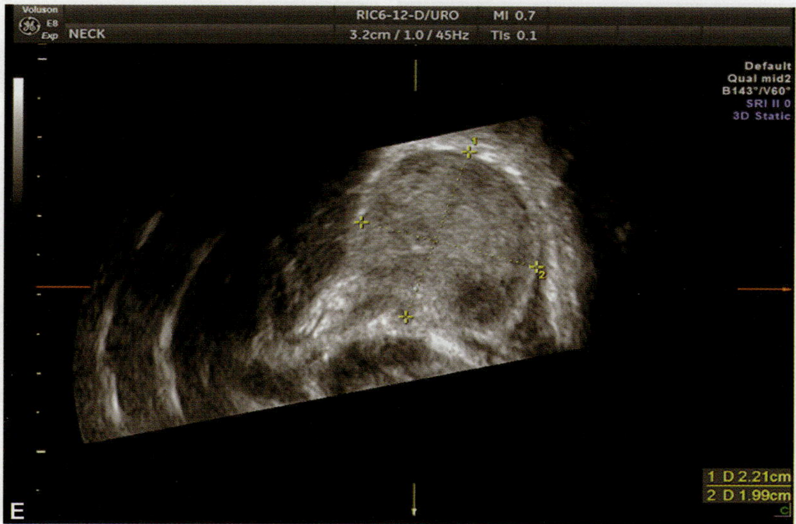

FIGURES 4.39C to E

FIGURES 4.39A to E: Infected thyroglossal duct cyst. A well-defined cyst seen in the midline. The cyst is seen anterior to the thyroid and it is separate from the thyroid. Homogeneous low level echoes are seen into it. But no evidence of any calcification is seen. No other focal mass is seen. On color flow imaging, no flow is seen in the cyst.

BENIGN NECK MASSES

Benign Tumors

The most common benign tumors found in neck are hemangiomas, fibromas, lipomas and tumors of nerves as neurofibromas. Sublingual dermoids are also seen as a congenital benign mass. The lymph node enlargement and lymph node masses are commonly found in the neck as primary lymph node disease or metastatic lymph node disease.

Hydatid Cyst

It is uncommon in the neck. However, it may be found in lower cervical and superior mediastinum. It appears to be a well defined sharply marginated cystic mass on HRSG. Echogenic septa and daughter cysts are also seen on ultrasound. Walls may be calcified and echogenic. On real time imaging, water lily sign is positive.

Nerve Tumors

The most common nerve tumors found in the neck are neurofibroma, ganglioneuroma and neurinomas. These are characteristically found along the nerve route, and associated atrophy of the muscle is found supplied by the involved nerve. The tumor is homogeneous in texture and well defined. They are hypoechoic in echogenicity. The margins are echogenic. Usually hyperplastic reactive lymph nodes are seen associated with the tumor. The tumor does not show any flow or little flow on color flow imaging. However, carotid body tumors chemodectomas are highly vascular. They are echogenic well-defined tumors, which are seen at the carotid artery bifurcation. The tumor may be seen adherent with the carotid sheath.

Nonspecific Lymphadenitis

There may be generalized enlargement of lymph nodes presenting as a mass in the neck. Ultrasonogram shows well-defined lobulated pattern of the mass. It shows homogeneous texture. No calcification or necrosis is seen in the mass. Pressure may be seen on the neck vessels due to large size of the mass. Fine needle aspiration cytology (FNAC) is the final investigation to confirm the diagnosis in these cases.

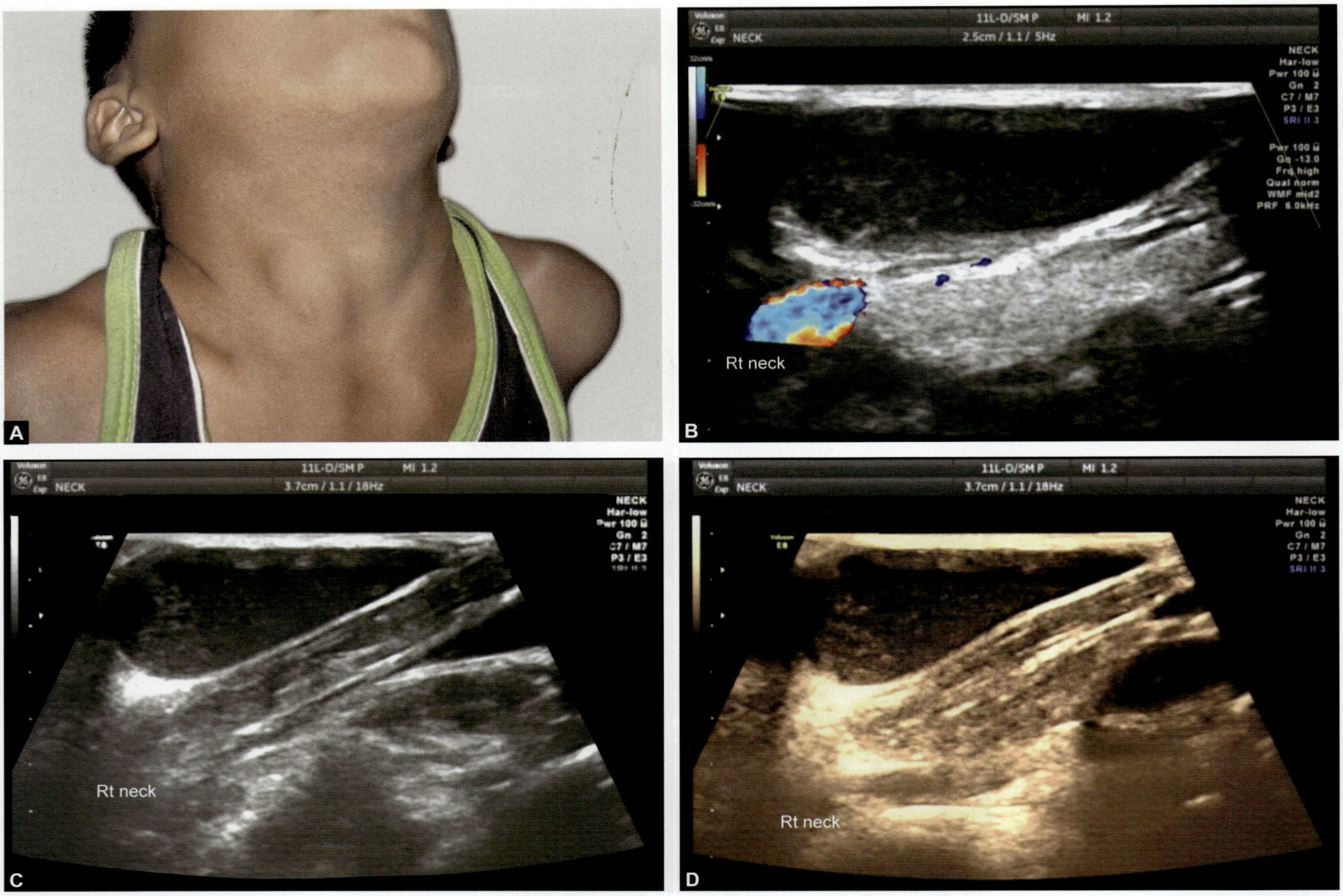

FIGURES 4.40A to D: Branchial cleft cyst. A young child presented with soft tissue swelling in the anteriolateral part of neck. HRSG shows a well-defined cyst in the neck. Homogeneous echoes are seen in it. No calcification or loculation is seen in the cyst. Findings are suggestive of branchial cleft cyst.

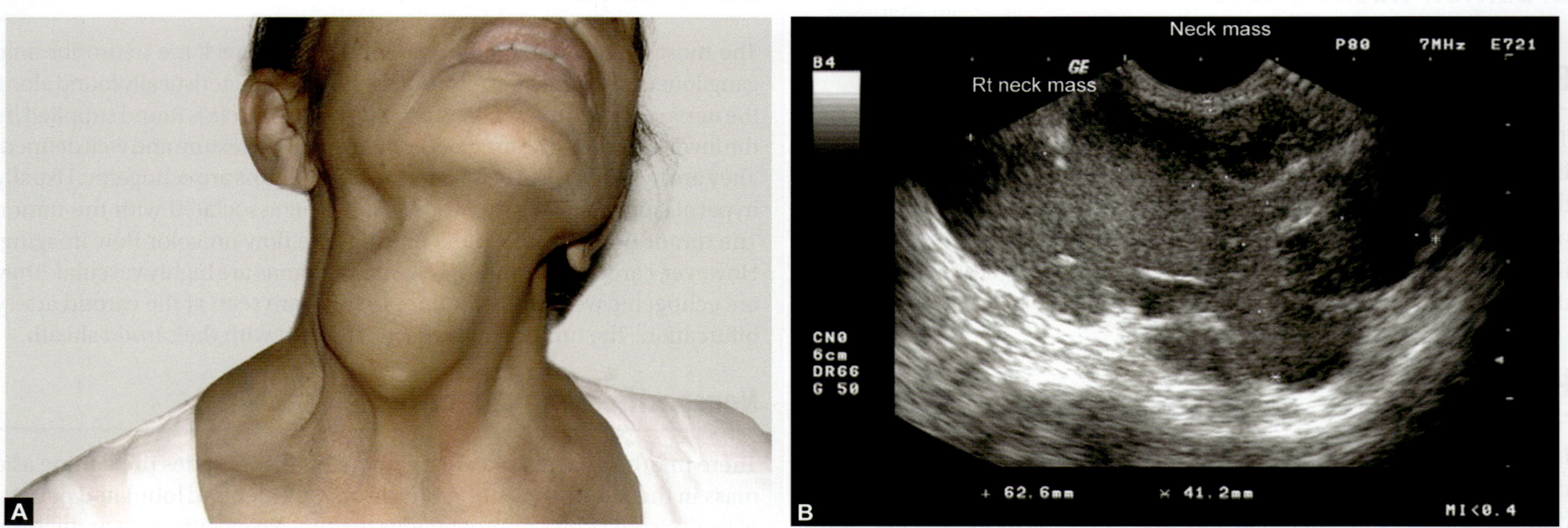

FIGURES 4.41A and B

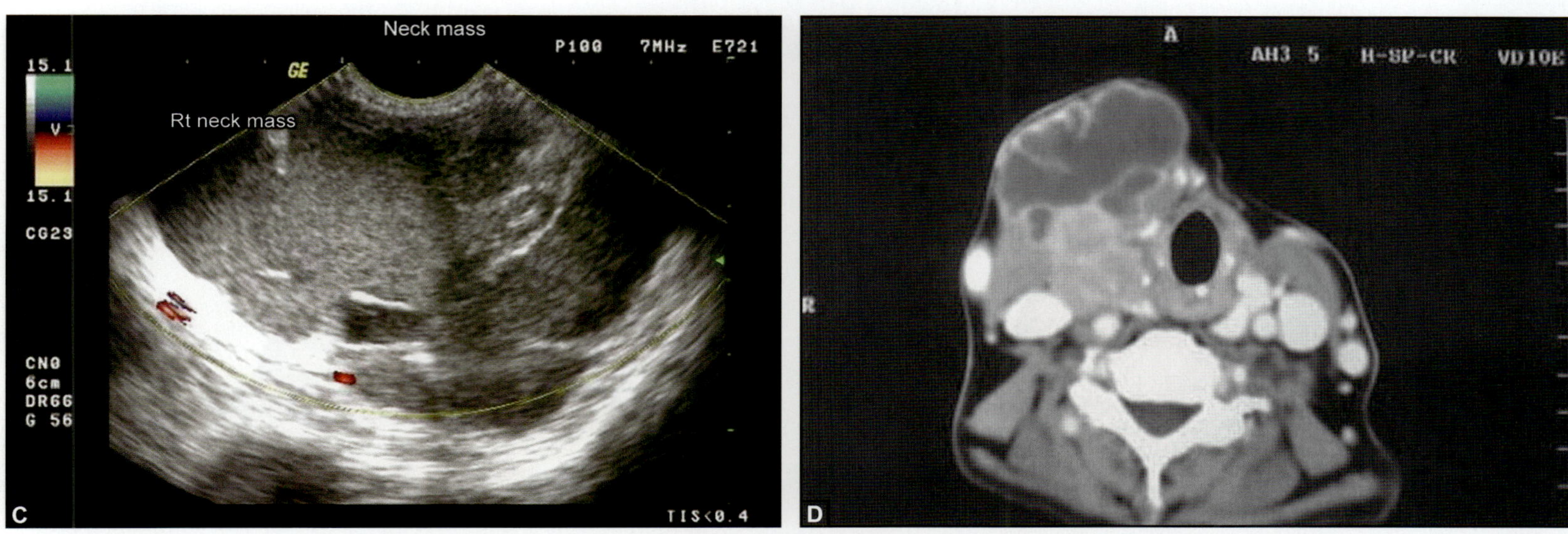

FIGURES 4.41C and D

FIGURES 4.41A to D: Infected branchial cyst. An old lady presented with a soft tissue mass in the neck. The mass is seen in the anterior triangle. HRSG shows a thick echo mass. No calcification is seen in it. No cystic degeneration is seen. Few echogenic septa are seen in the mass. CT of the same patient shows detail of the multiloculated cystic mass. FNAC confirmed branchial cyst.

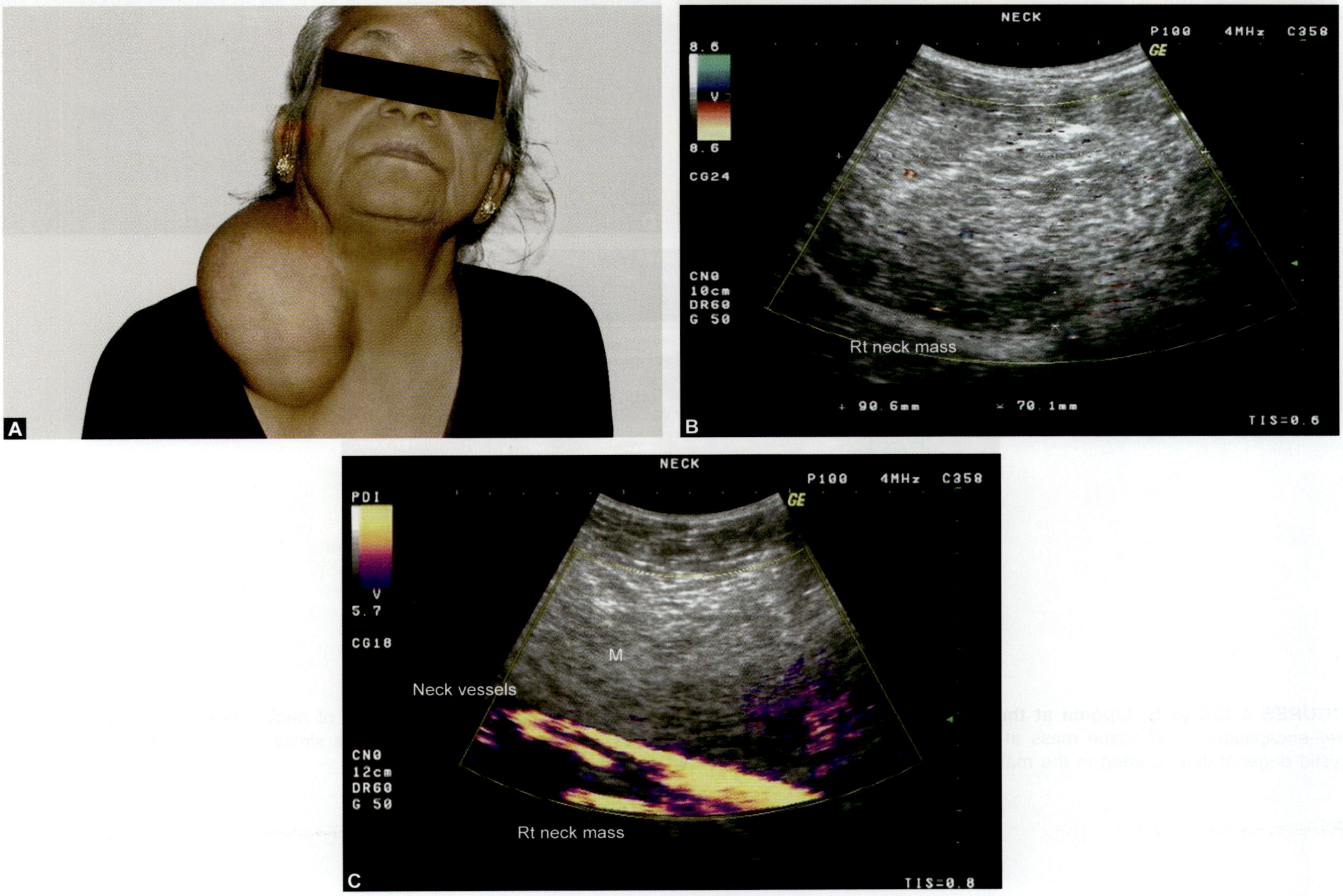

FIGURES 4.42A to C: An old lady presented with big soft tissue mass in the right side of the neck. The mass is coming out from anterior triangle of the neck. HRSG shows a big homogeneous soft tissue mass in the neck. The mass shows homogeneous echoes. No calcification is seen in the mass. No cystic degeneration is seen. The mass is not seen pressing over the neck vessels.

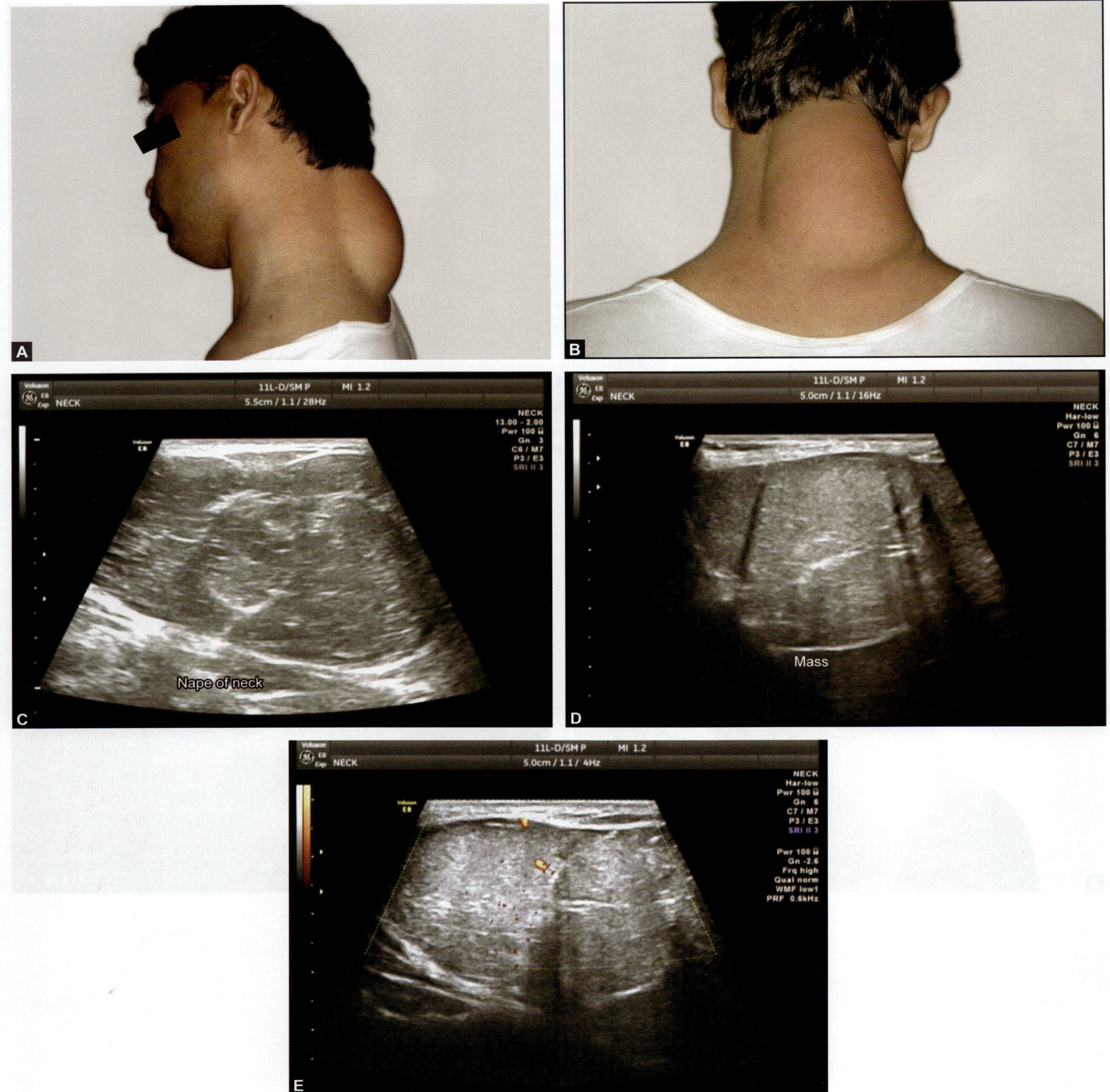

FIGURES 4.43A to E: Lipoma at the nape of neck. A patient presented with soft tissue mass at the nape of neck. HRSG shows a well-defined well-encapsulated soft tissue mass at the nape of the neck. It is homogeneous in texture. The echotexture is similar to the fat. No calcification or cystic degeneration is seen in the mass. On color flow imaging, poor flow is seen in it suggestive of lipoma.

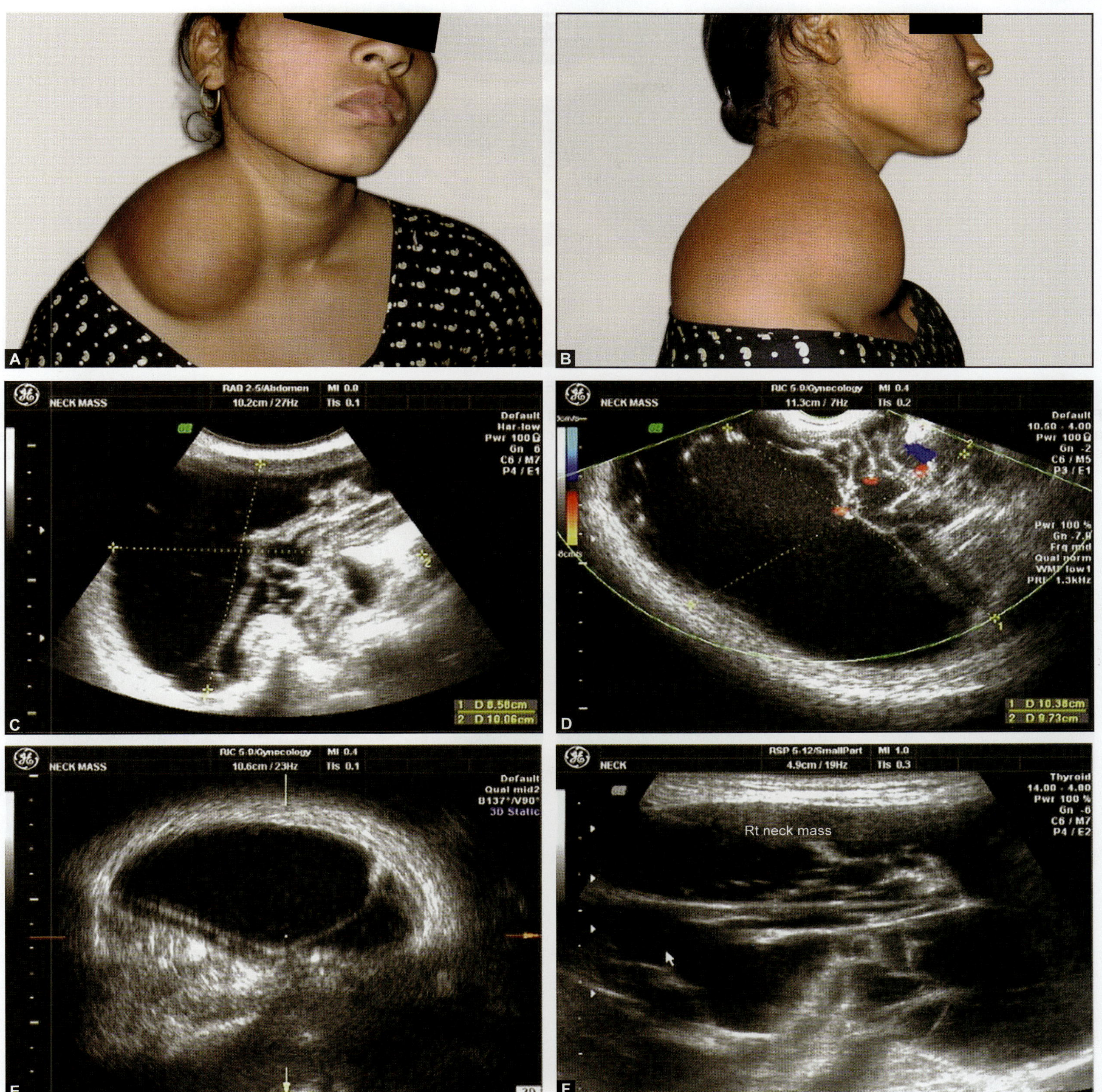

FIGURES 4.44A to F

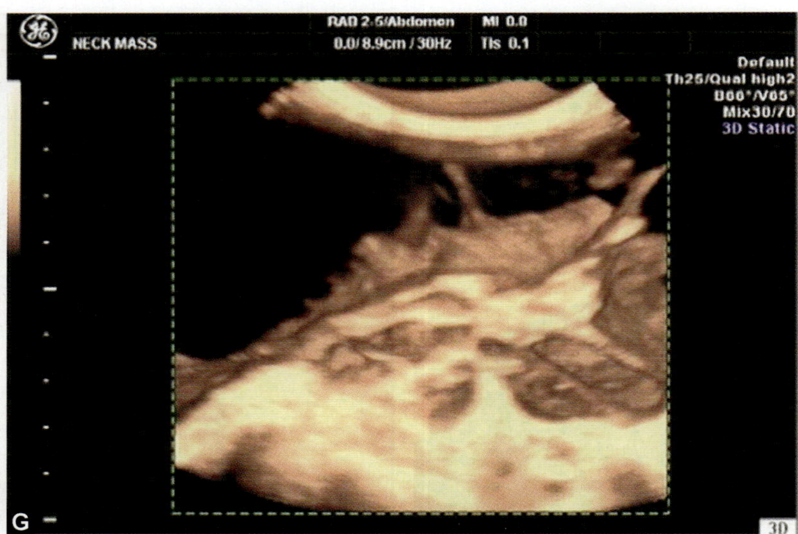

FIGURE 4.44G

FIGURES 4.44A to G: Cystic hygroma. A young lady presented with soft tissue cystic mass in the side of the neck. The mass is seen coming out anteriorly. HRSG shows a big multiloculated cystic mass in the neck. Thick echogenic septa are seen in it. On color flow imaging, few vessels are seen in the septa. 3D of the same of the same mass shows better details of the cyst. The septa stand out clearly. Biopsy confirmed cystic hygroma.

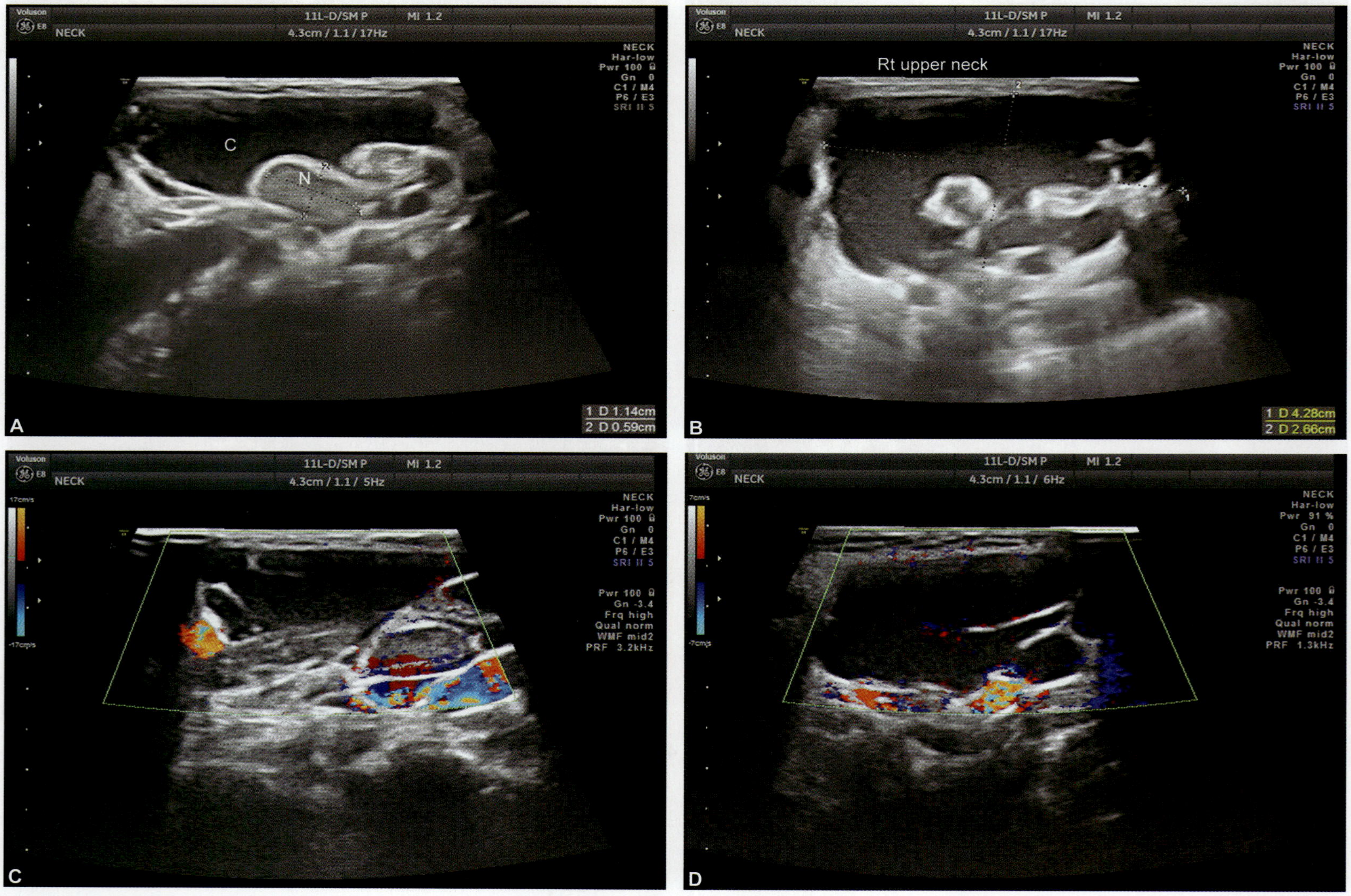

Figures 4.45A to D: Cystic hygroma. A 2.5-year-old boy presented with soft tissue mass in the right side of the neck. HRSG shows a multiloculated cystic mass in the neck. Thick septa are seen in the mass. Cheesy collection is also seen in the loculations. On color flow imaging, poor flow is seen in it. Findings are suggestive of cystic hygroma.

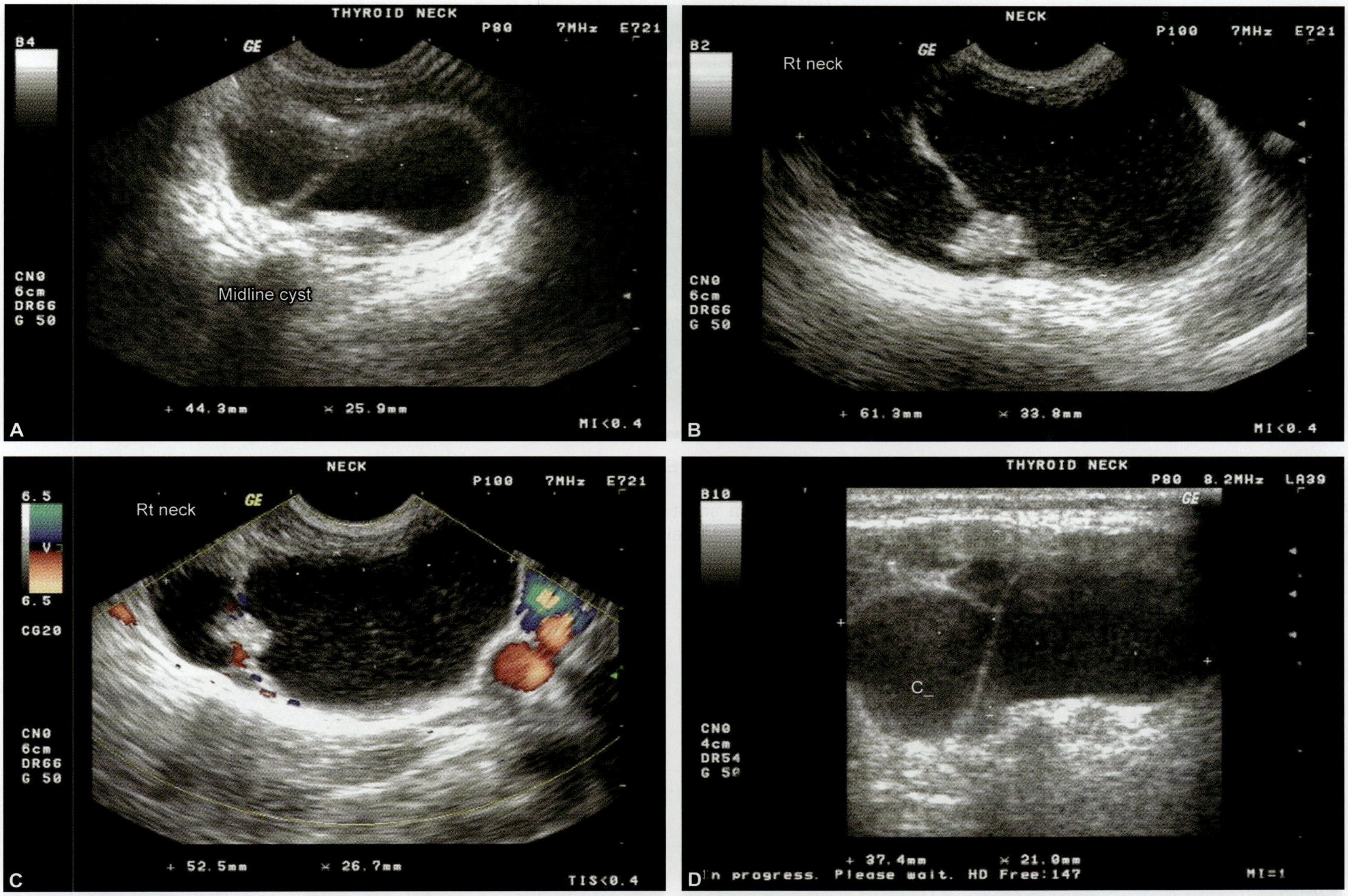

FIGURES 4.46A to D: Lymphatic cyst. A patient presented with a big cystic mass in the neck. HRSG shows big multiloculated cystic mass. Thick echogenic septum is seen in it. FNAC confirmed lymphatic cyst.

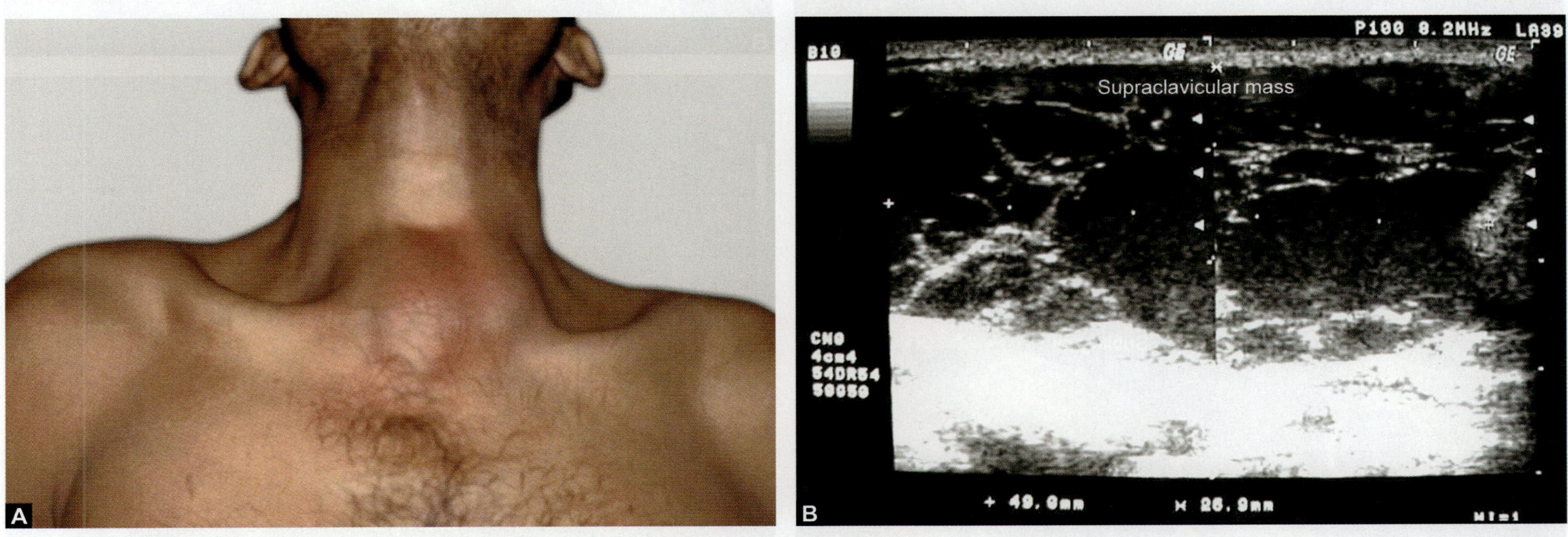

FIGURES 4.47A and B

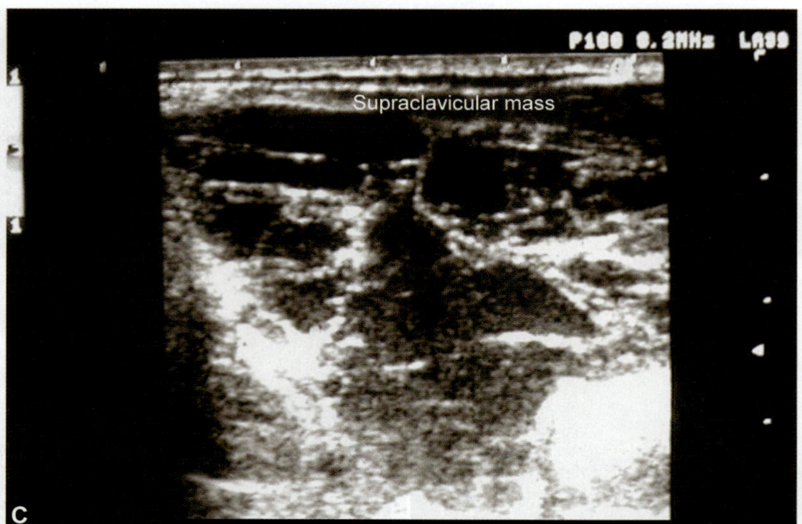

FIGURE 4.47C

FIGURES 4.47A to C: Lymphangioma. A patient presented with a soft tissue mass in the suprasternal area. HRSG shows a multiloculated cystic mass. Multiple thinned echogenic septa are seen in the mass. Few internal echoes are seen in the cyst, suggestive of debris. Color Doppler imaging shows poor flow in the mass. Biopsy of the mass was lymph angioma.

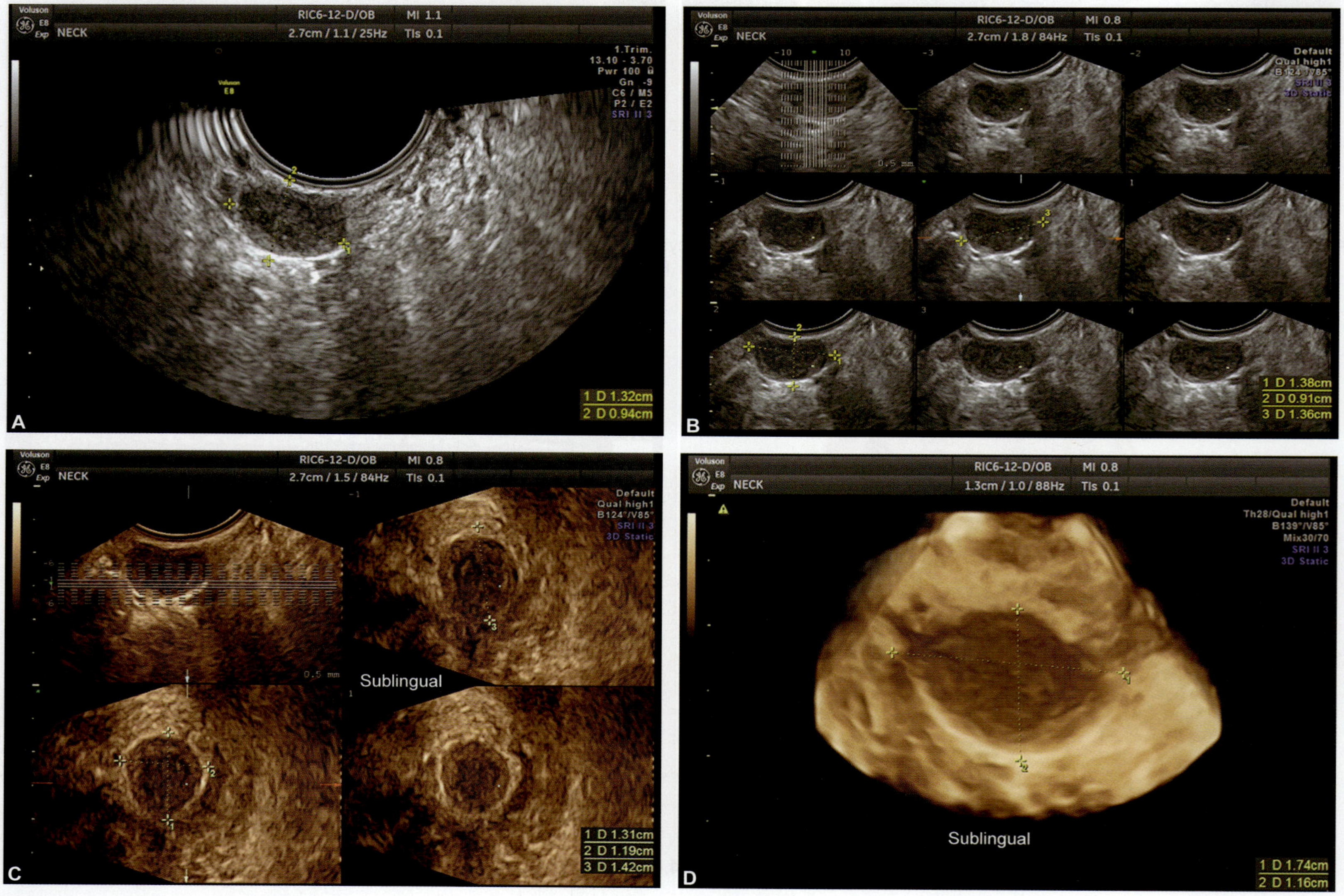

FIGURES 4.48A to D: Sublingual dermoid. A patient presented with soft tissue swelling in the sublingual region. HRSG shows a well-defined low-level echo complex mass in the sublingual region. It shows thick echoes. But no suggestion of any cystic degeneration is seen. Few echogenic nodules are seen in it. The three-dimensional and tomographic ultrasound imaging clearly show the content of the cyst. FNAC confirms sublingual dermoid.

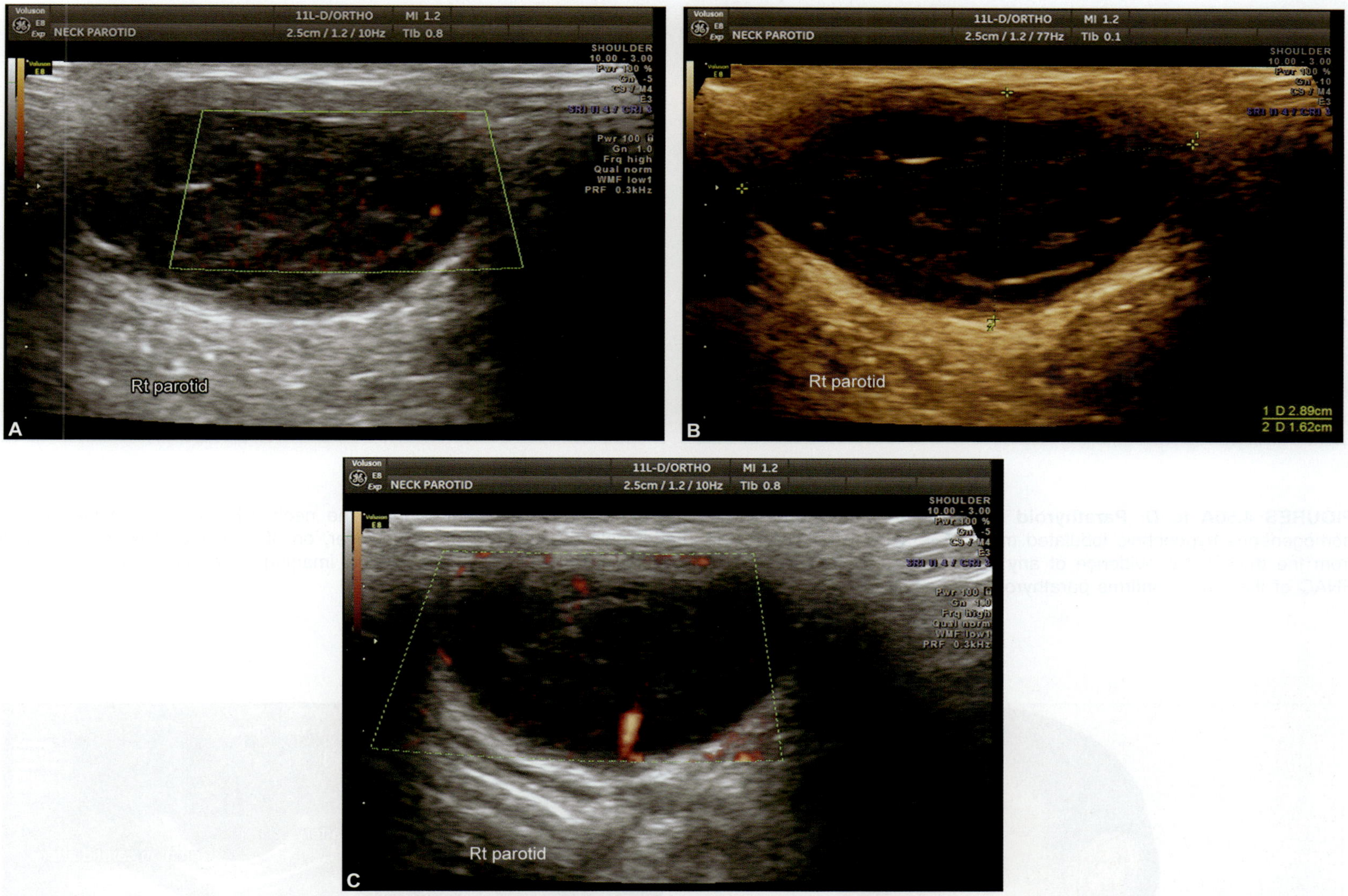

FIGURES 4.49A to C: A patient presented with preauricular swelling. HRSG shows a well-defined well-encapsulated mass seen in the preauricular region. It shows homogeneous echoes. No calcification is seen in it. It is separate from the parotid gland. The parotid gland is normal. Echotexture is homogeneous. No focal mass is seen in the parotid. The duct is not dilated. FNAC confirms organized abscess.

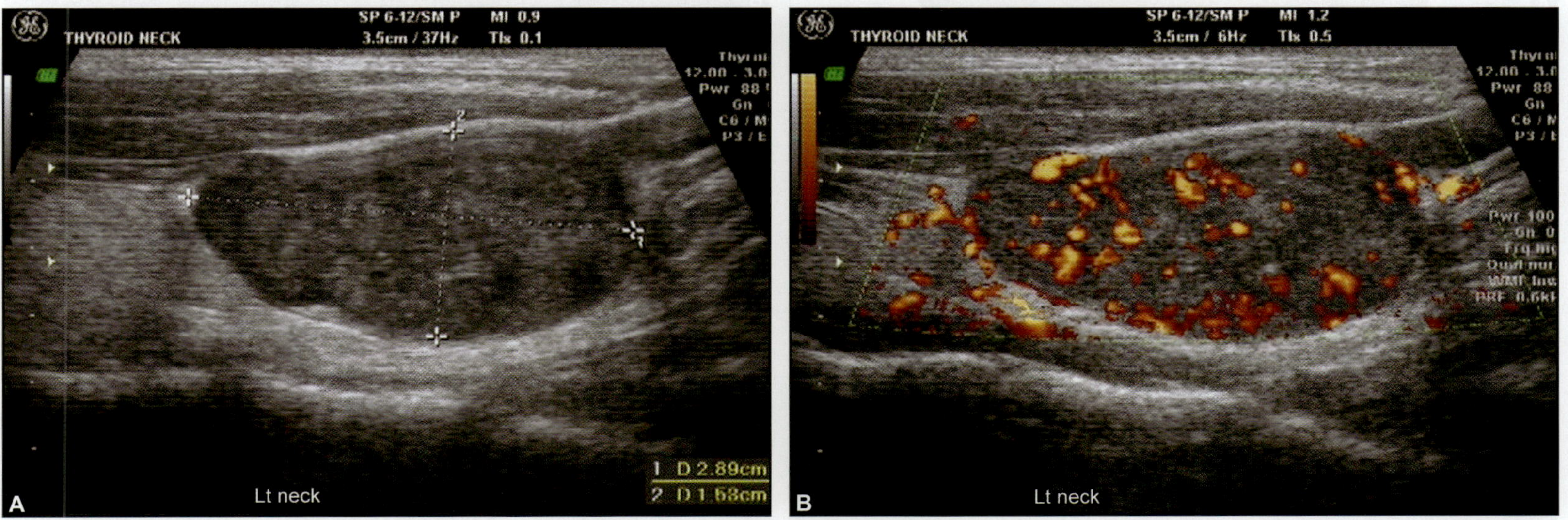

FIGURES 4.50A and B

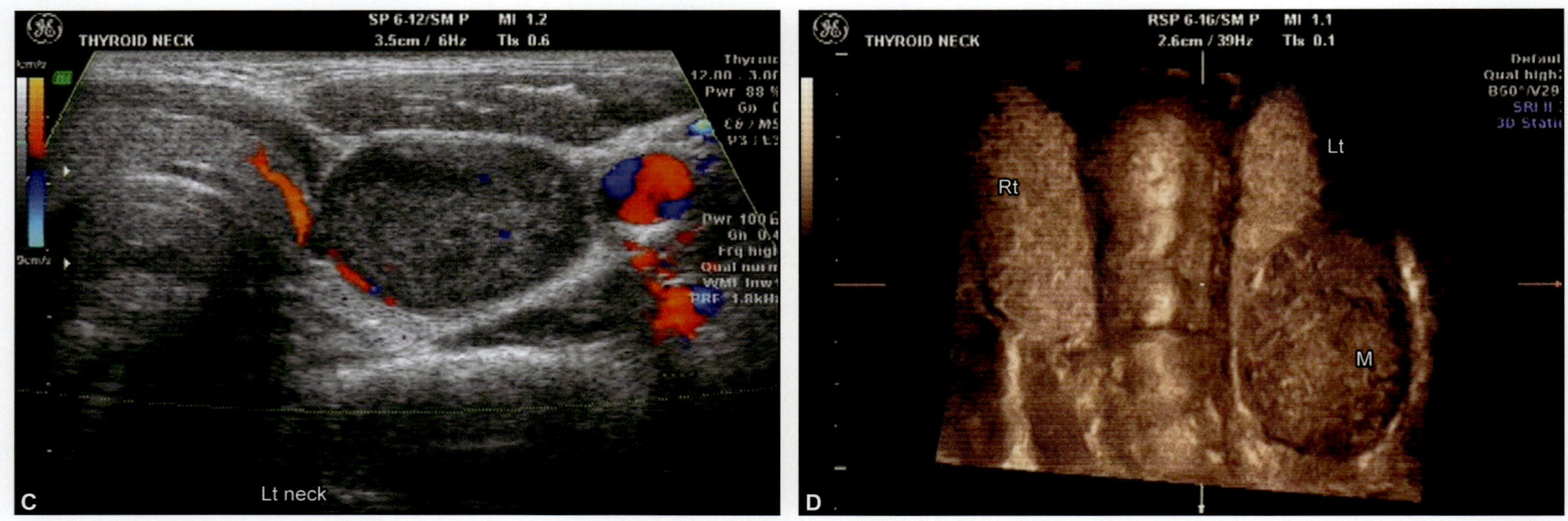

FIGURES 4.50C and D

FIGURES 4.50A to D: Parathyroid adenoma. A patient presented with soft tissue mass in left side of the neck. HRSG shows a well-defined homogeneous hypoechoic lobulated mass. It is seen in relation to the inferior pole of the left thyroid. However, on 3D imaging, it is seen separate from the thyroid. No evidence of any calcification or cystic degeneration is seen in the mass. On color flow imaging, moderate flow is seen in it. FNAC of the mass confirms parathyroid adenoma.

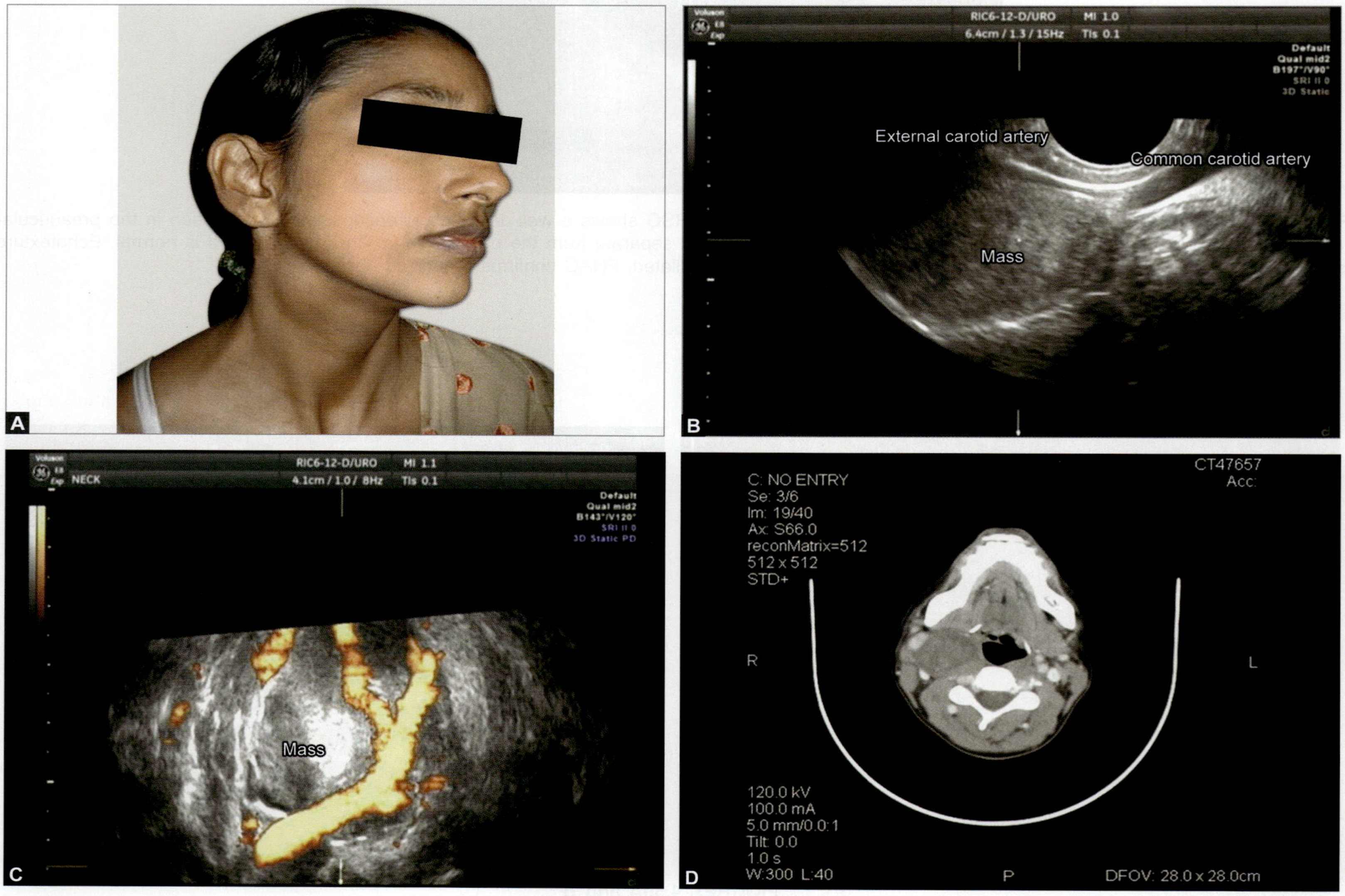

FIGURES 4.51A to D

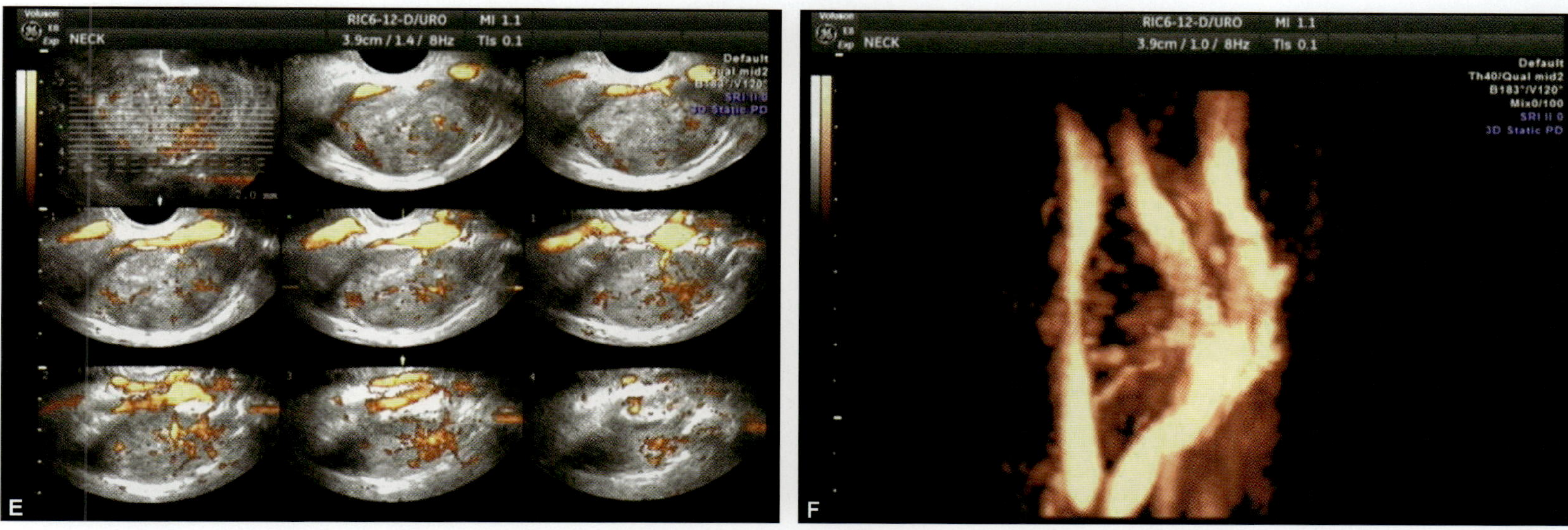

FIGURES 4.51E and F

FIGURES 4.51A to F: Carotid body tumor. A lady presented with soft tissue mass in the right upper cervical region. HRSG shows a well-defined lobulated soft tissue mass in the right upper neck. It is seen near the carotid artery bifurcation. It is homogeneous in texture. Pressure is seen on the external carotid artery. On 3D imaging, it is seen attached with carotid sheath. CT scan of the same patient confirms the ultrasound findings. FNAC of the mass confirms carotid body tumor.

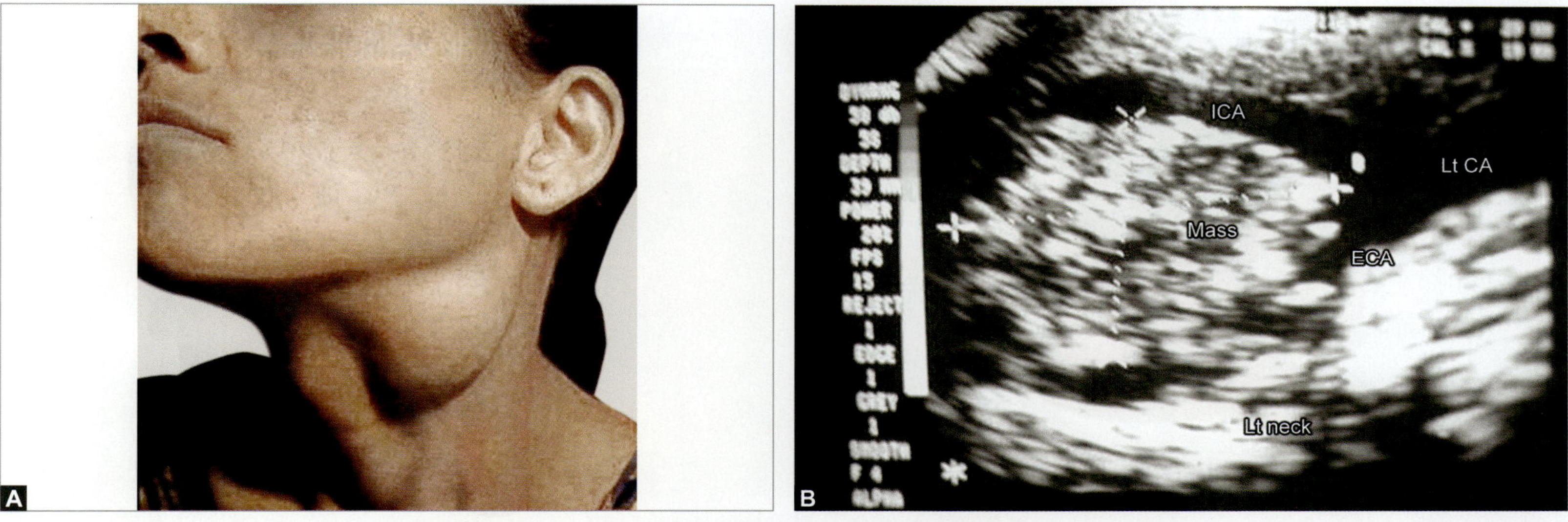

FIGURES 4.52A and B: Carotid body tumor. A young lady presented with a soft tissue mass in the left side of the neck in its upper part. It was nontender. HRSG shows a well-defined echogenic tumor mass seen in between the carotid bifurcation. The tumor is seen splaying in the internal and external carotid artery (ICA and ECA) and was adherent with carotid artery (CA) sheath. Biopsy shows carotid body tumor or chemodectomas.

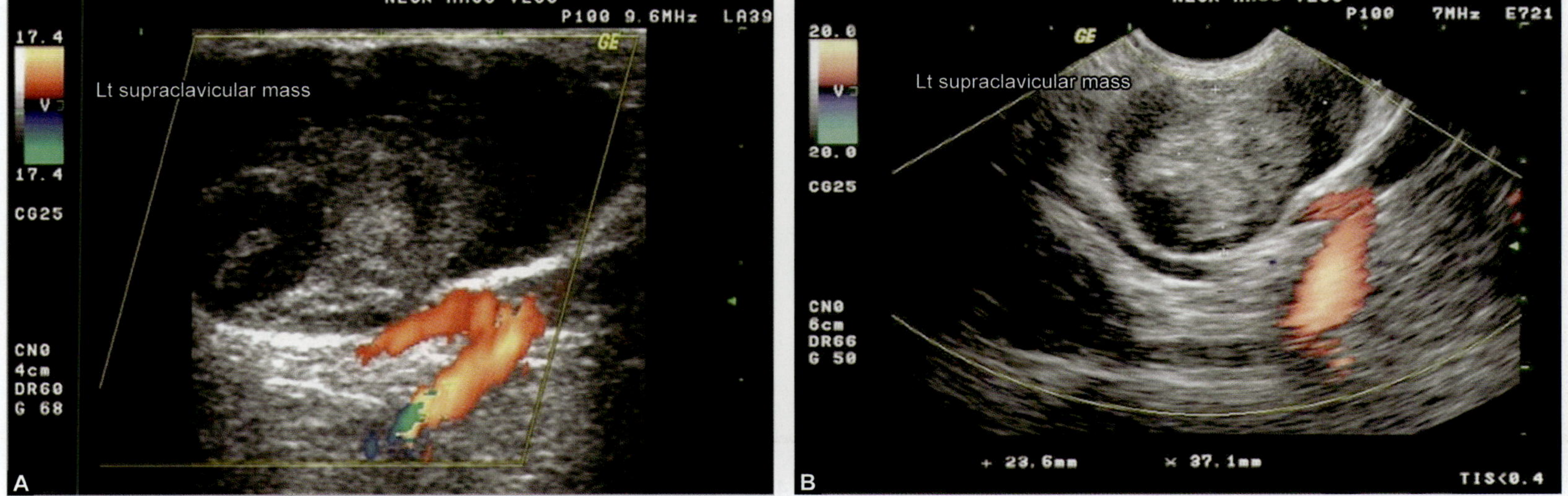

FIGURES 4.53A and B: Carotid body tumor (Potato tumor). A patient presented with soft tissue mass in the neck upper cervical region. The mass is seen in relation to the carotid vessels. It is homogeneous in texture. No necrosis is seen in it. No cystic degeneration is seen. However, it was not fixed with the carotid sheath. Biopsy confirmed carotid body tumor.

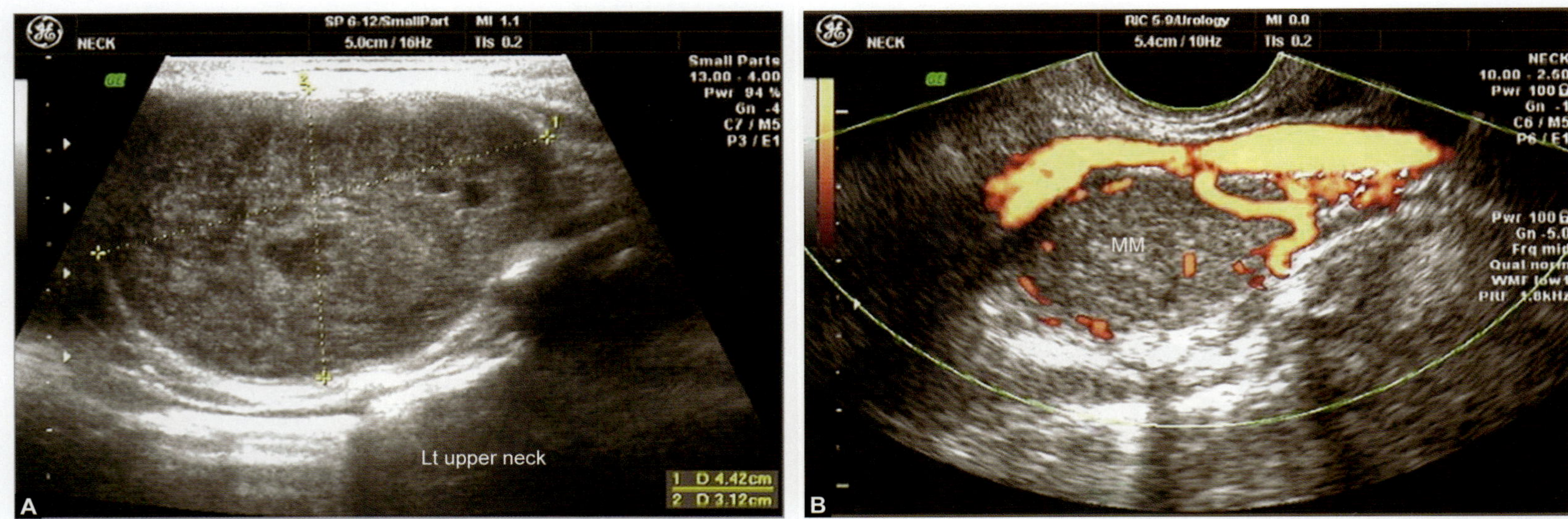

FIGURES 4.54A and B: Carotid body tumor. A patient presented with well-defined soft tissue mass in the neck. The mass is seen in relation to the carotid vessels. It is seen fixed with the carotid sheath. Color Doppler shows a feeding vessel in the mass. Biopsy confirmed carotid body tumor.

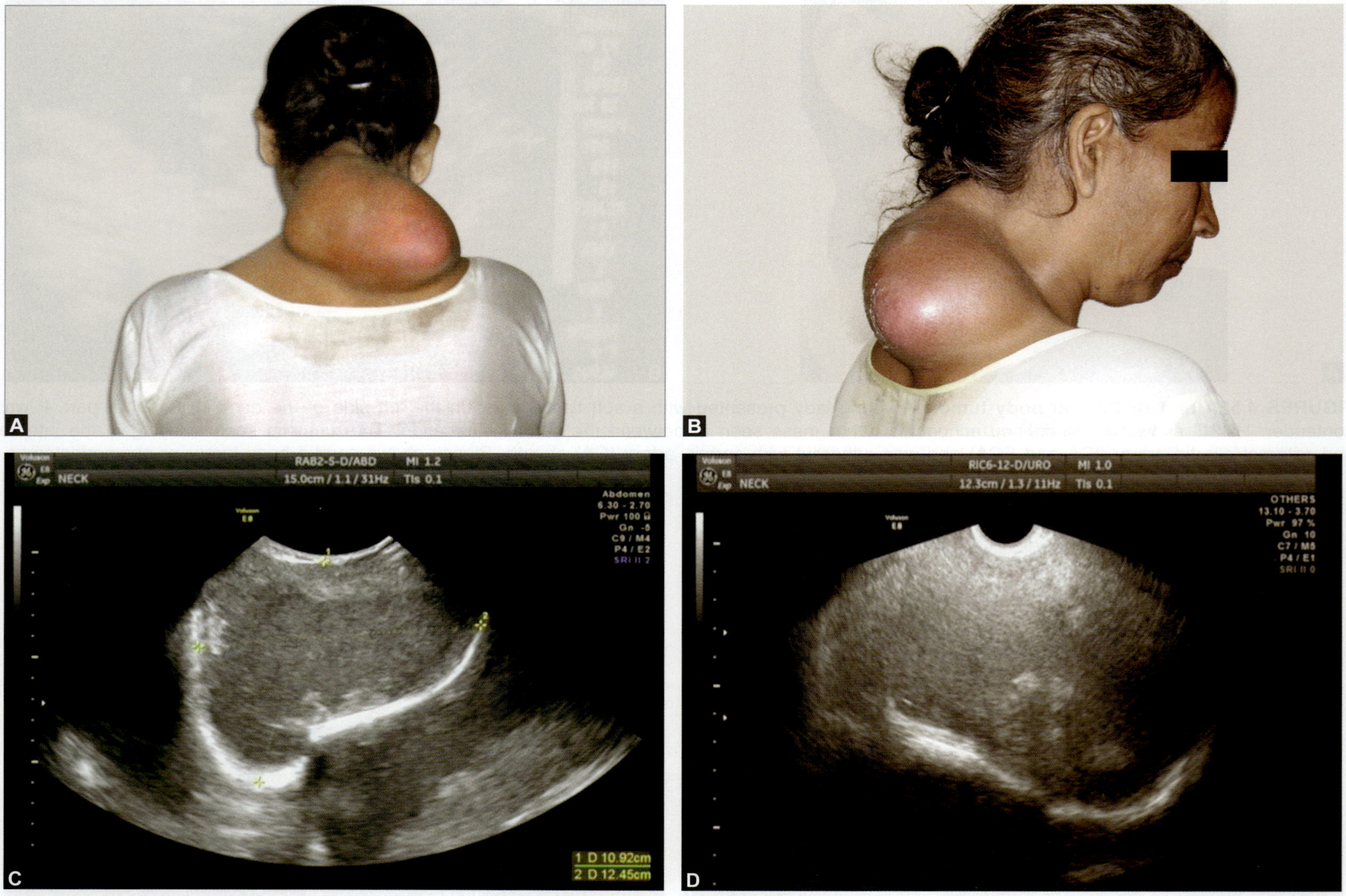

FIGURES 4.55A to D

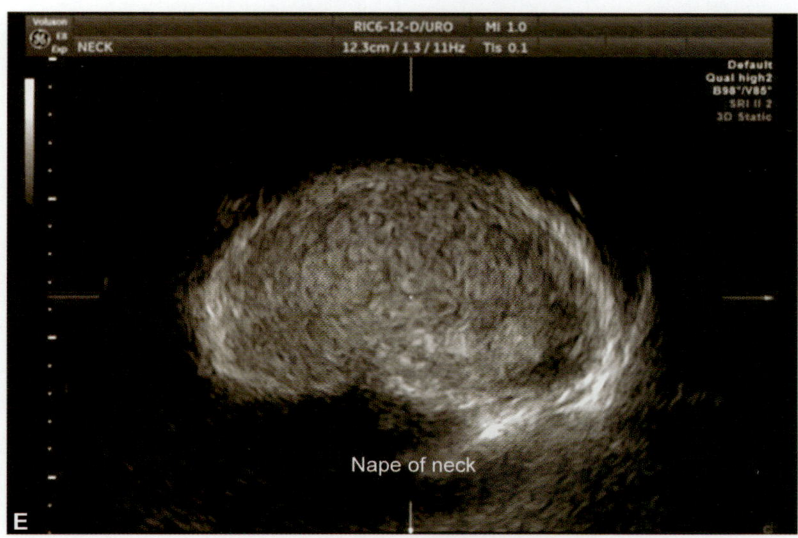

FIGURE 4.55E

FIGURES 4.55A to E: Huge sebaceous cyst. A patient presented with huge cystic mass at the base of the neck, which is tense on palpation. HRSG shows a big cystic mass at the nape of neck. Thick echoes are seen in the mass with homogeneous echo pattern. On 3D imaging, few echogenic nodules are also seen in it. On FNAC biopsy, it turned out to be sebaceous cyst.

NEUROGENIC TUMORS IN THE NECK

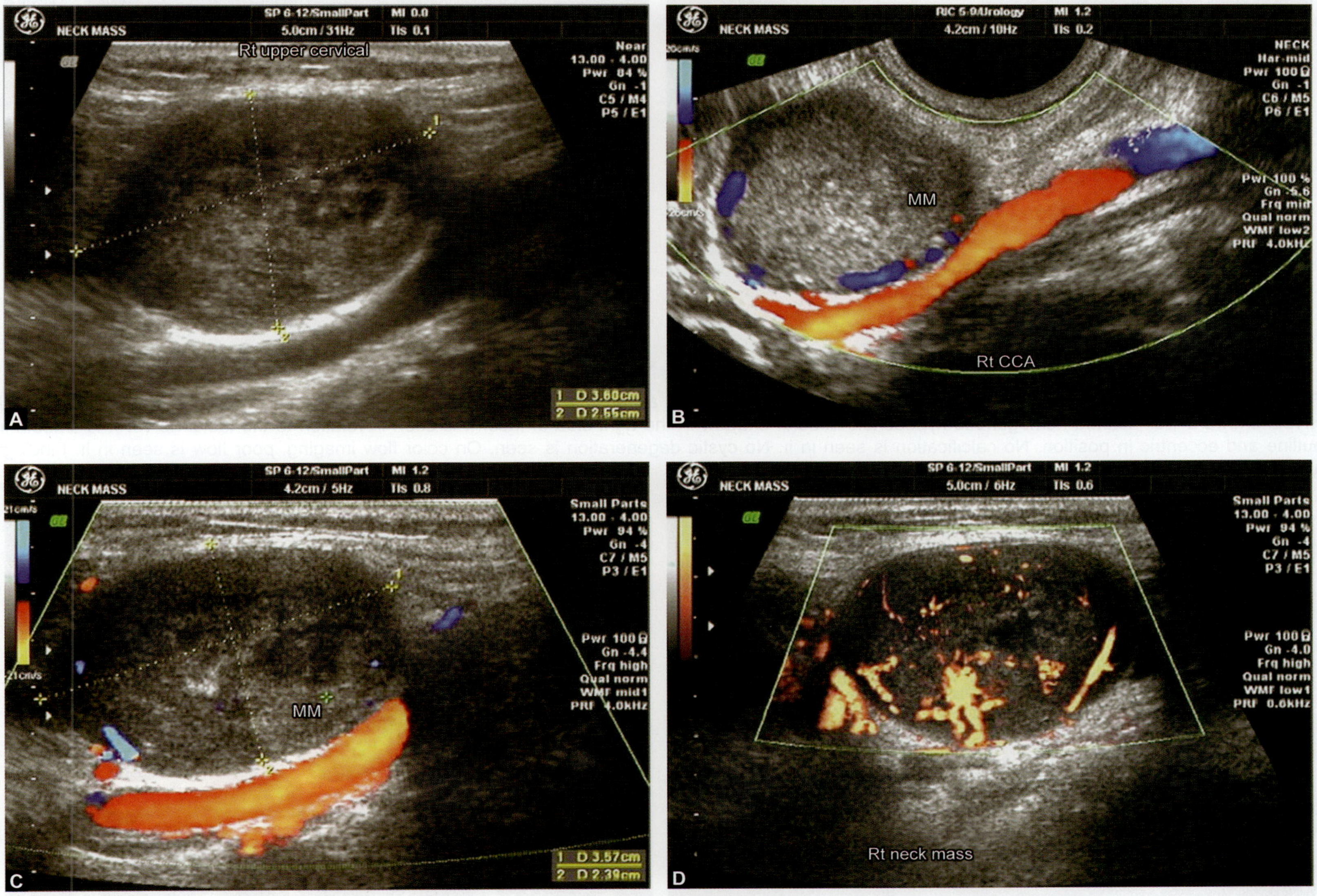

FIGURES 4.56A to D

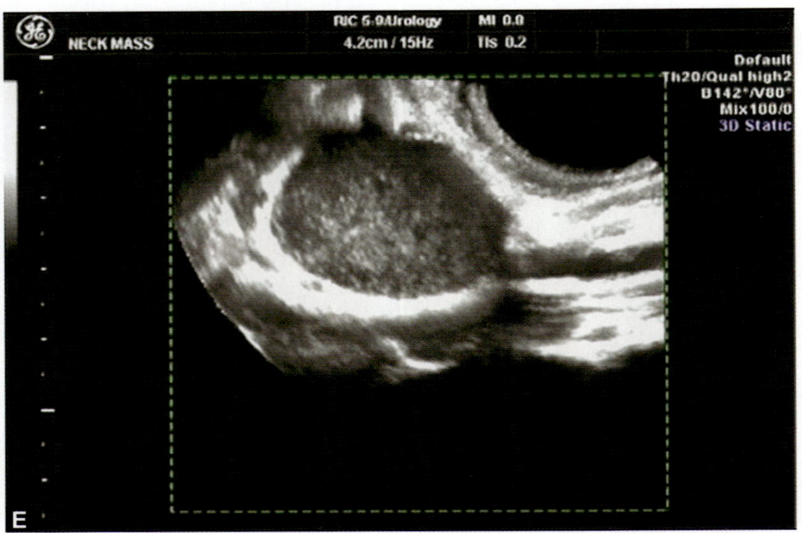

FIGURE 4.56E

FIGURES 4.56A to E: Schwann cell neuromas. An old lady presented with soft tissue mass in right side of the neck. The mass is homogeneous in texture with well-defined margins. No necrosis is seen in it. On color flow imaging, low flow is seen in the mass. It is separate from the neck vessels. 3D imaging of the mass shows finer details with relationship with the neck vessels. Biopsy shows Schwann cell neuromas.

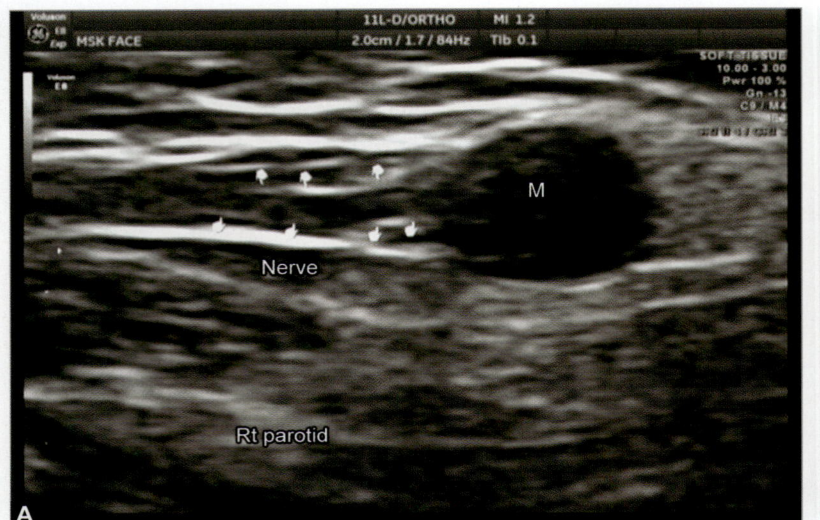

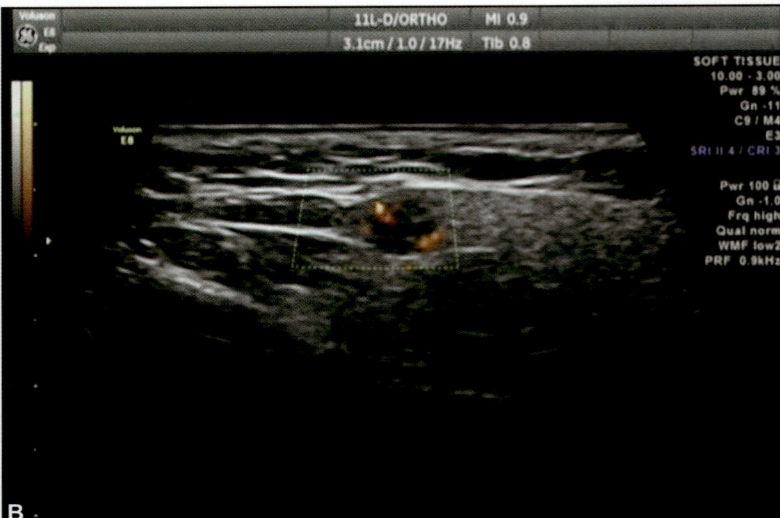

FIGURES 4.57A and B: Fascial nerve tumor. A patient presented with a palpable nodule in the right side of face in the region of parotid gland. HRSG shows a well-defined homogenous hypoechoic nodular shadow in the right side of face. It is seen in relation to the facial nerve. It is smooth in outline and eccentric in position. No calcification is seen in it. No cystic degeneration is seen. On color flow imaging, poor flow is seen in it. Findings are consistent with fascial nerve schwannoma.

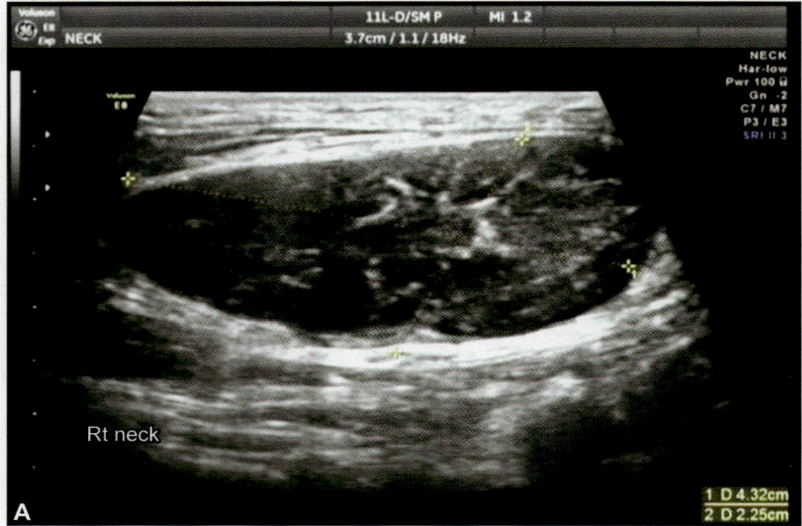

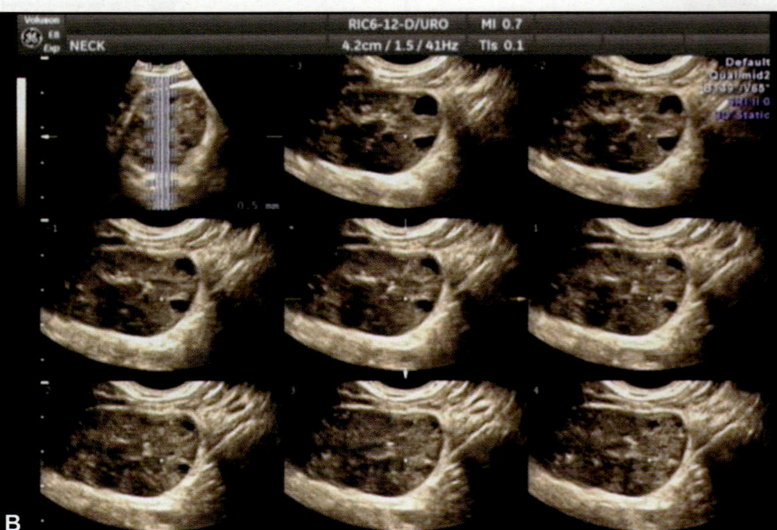

FIGURES 4.58A and B

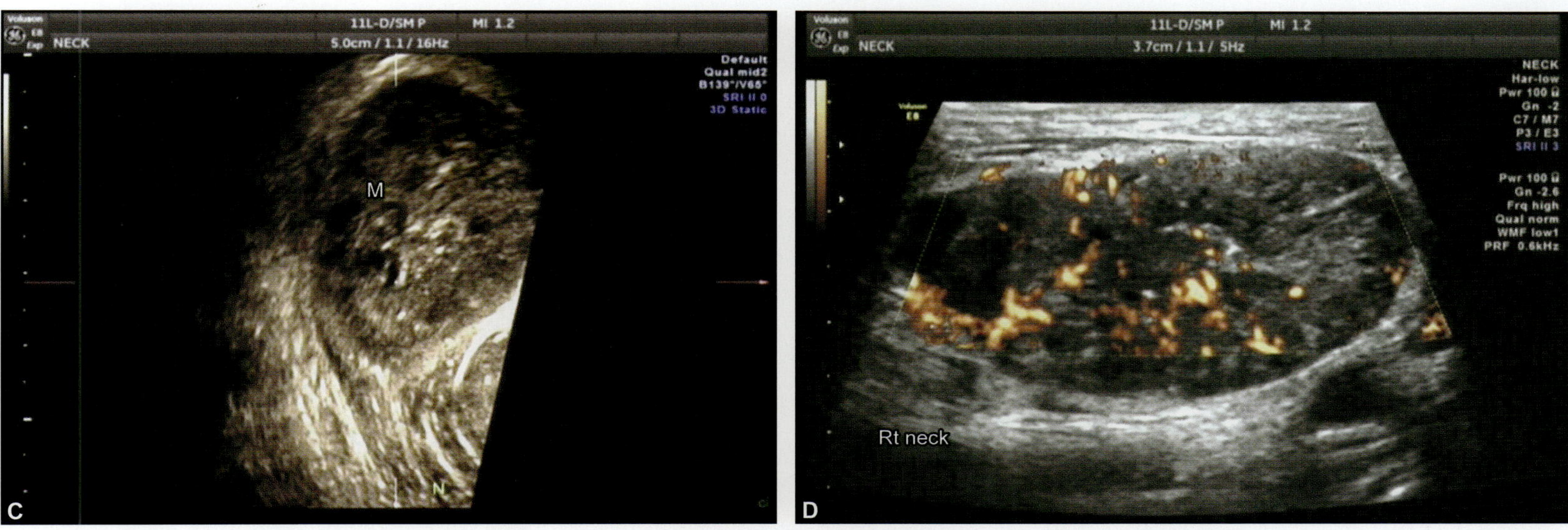

FIGURES 4.58C and D

Figures 4.58A to D: A patient presented with soft tissue mass in the right side of neck. HRSG shows a well-defined well-encapsulated fusiform soft tissue mass in the right side of the neck. It is seen in relation to vagus nerve. It is seen growing in one direction. On color flow imaging, few vessels are seen feeding it. Biopsy of the mass confirms vagus nerve schwannoma.

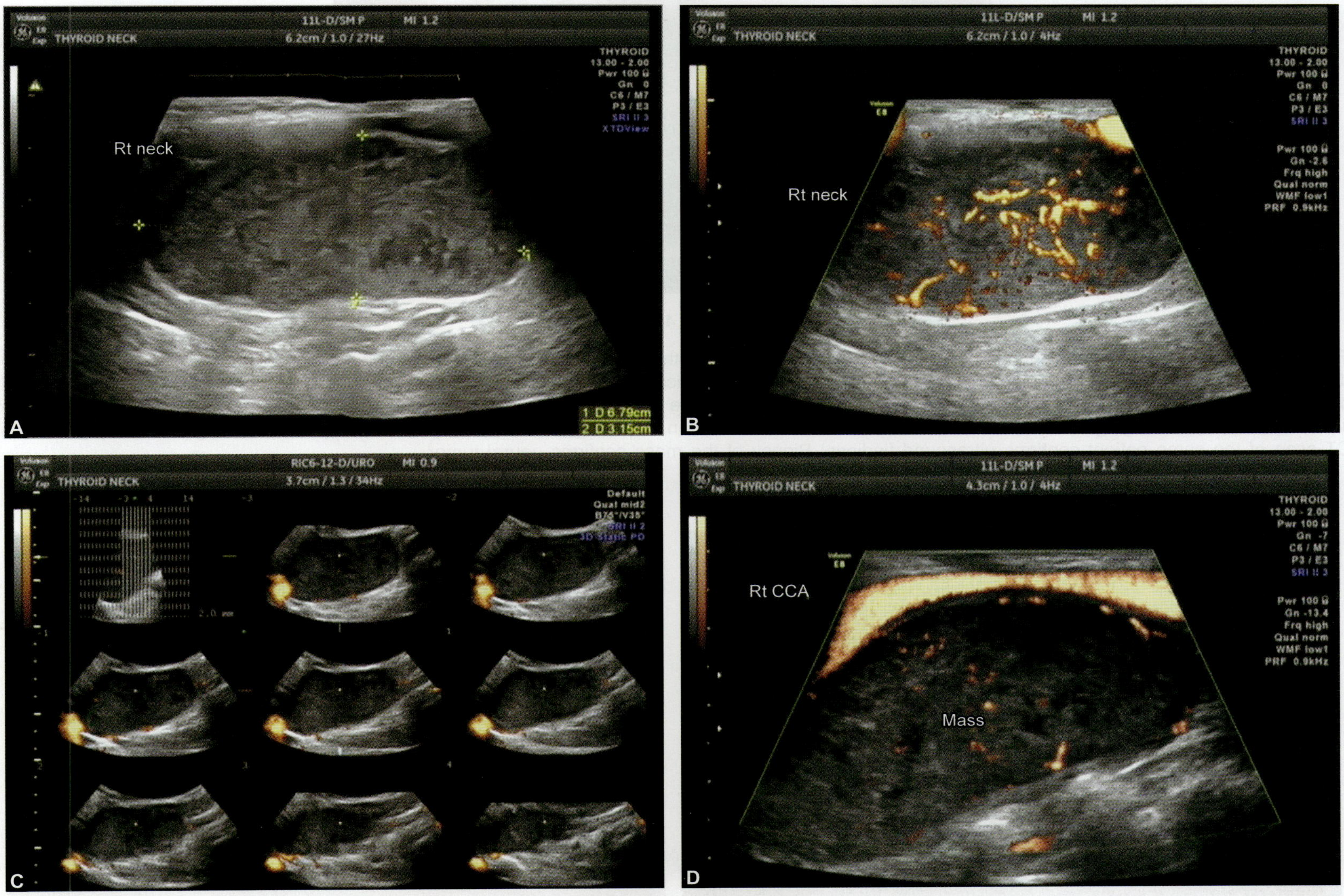

FIGURES 4.59A to D

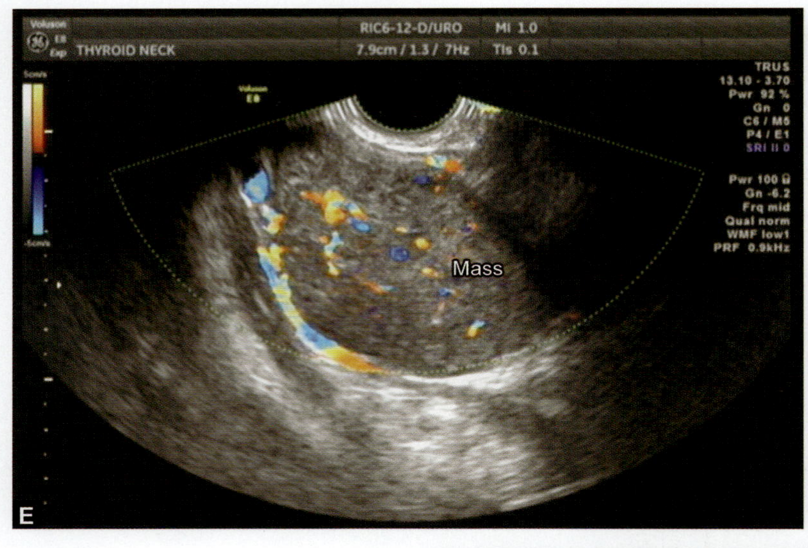

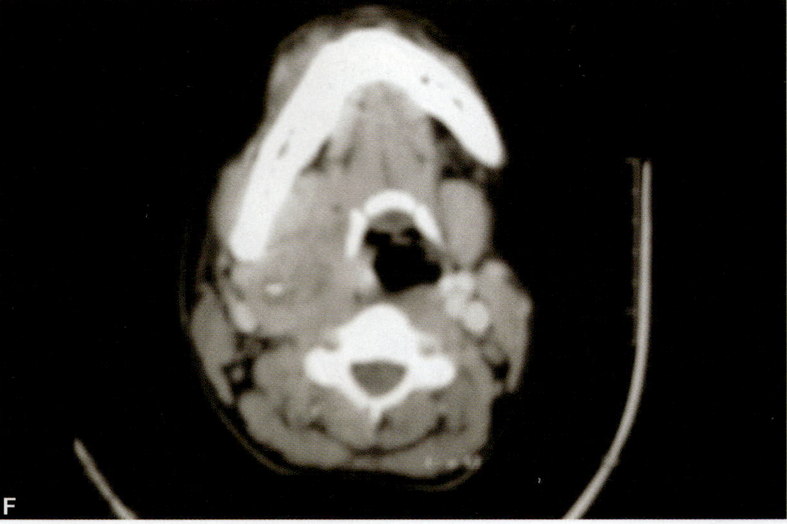

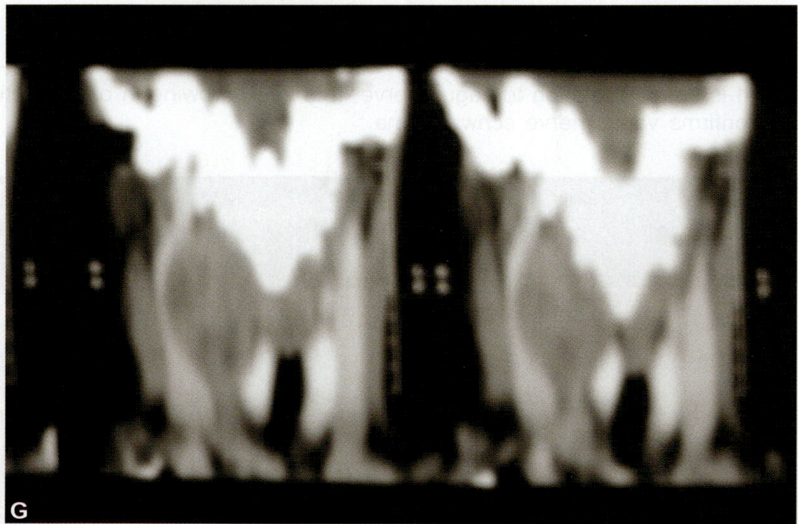

FIGURES 4.59E to G

FIGURES 4.59A to G: A patient presented with big soft tissue mass in the right side of neck. It is homogeneous in texture. HRSG shows a well-defined lobulated hypoechoic predominately solid mass in the upper cervical region pressing over the right lobe of the thyroid and displacing it with pressure on the neck vessels. The mass is well encapsulated. It is separate from the thyroid. No calcification seen in the mass. No cystic degeneration seen. On color flow imaging, moderate flow is seen in the mass. It is seen displacing the neck vessels anteriorly and pressing over the jugular vein. CT scan of the same patient confirms ultrasound findings. Biopsy of the mass confirms neural tumor.

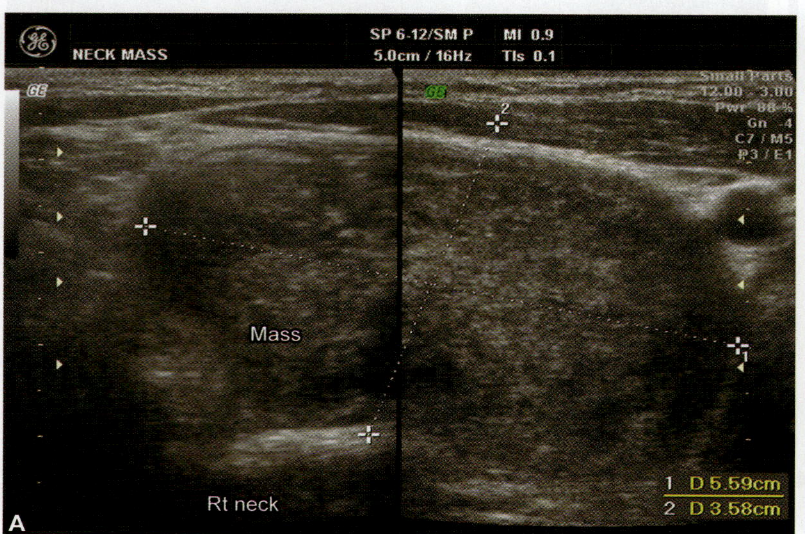

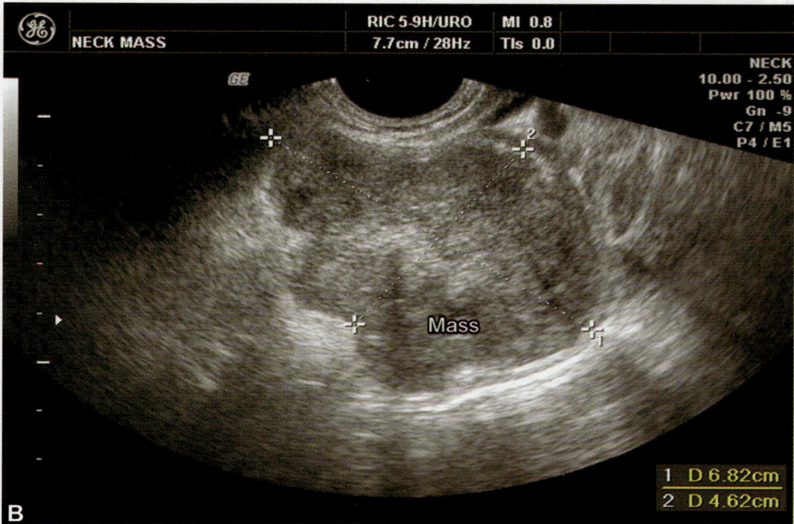

FIGURES 4.60A and B

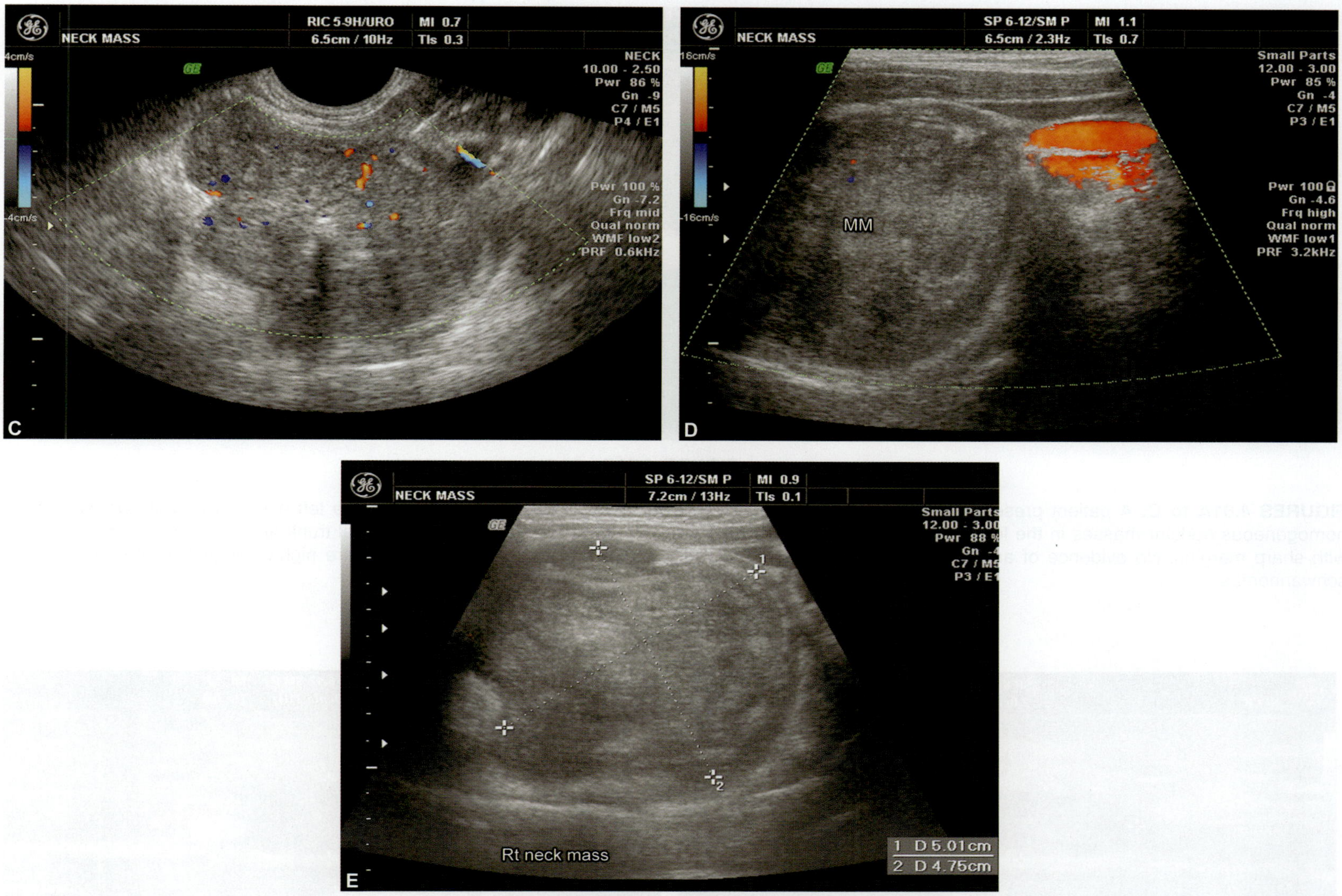

FIGURES 4.60C to E

Figures 4.60A to E: A patient presented with big soft tissue mass in right side of neck. HRSG shows a well-defined lobulated homogeneous soft tissue mass in the right side of neck in mid and upper cervical region. It is seen anterior to the neck vessels. The mass is seen lifting the right external carotid artery. But it appears to be separate from the carotid vessels. It is homogeneous in texture. On color flow imaging, low flow is seen in the mass. The mass is also separate from thyroid gland. No cystic degeneration is seen. Biopsy of the mass confirms nerve tumor.

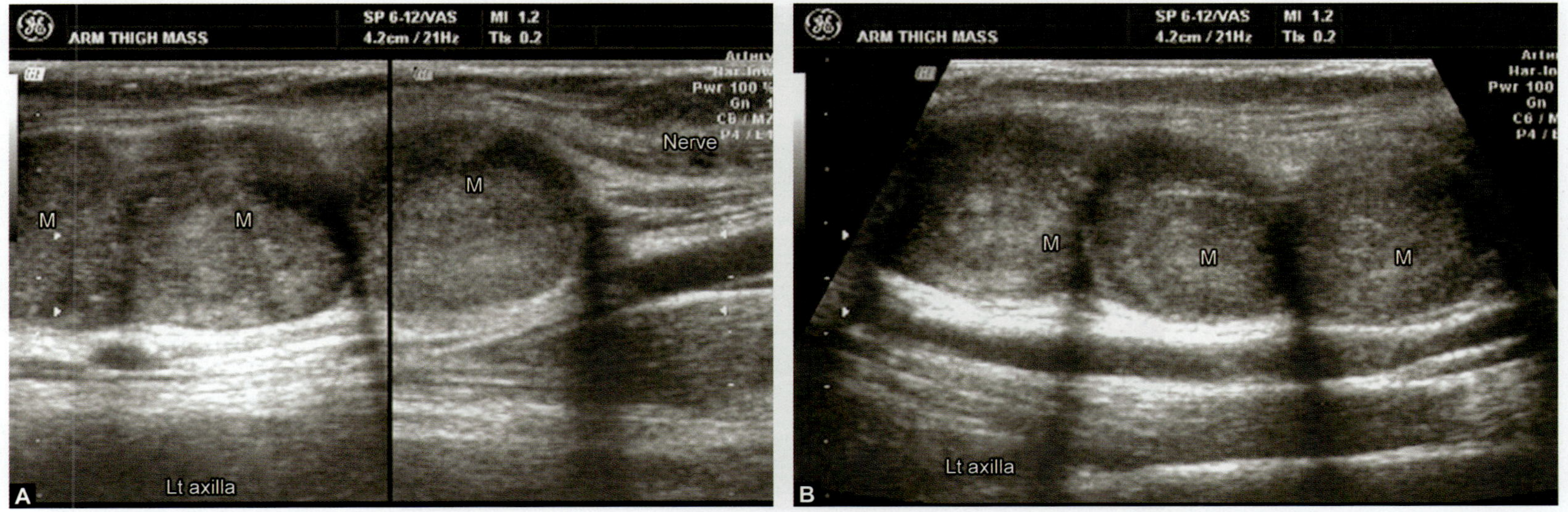

FIGURES 4.61A and B

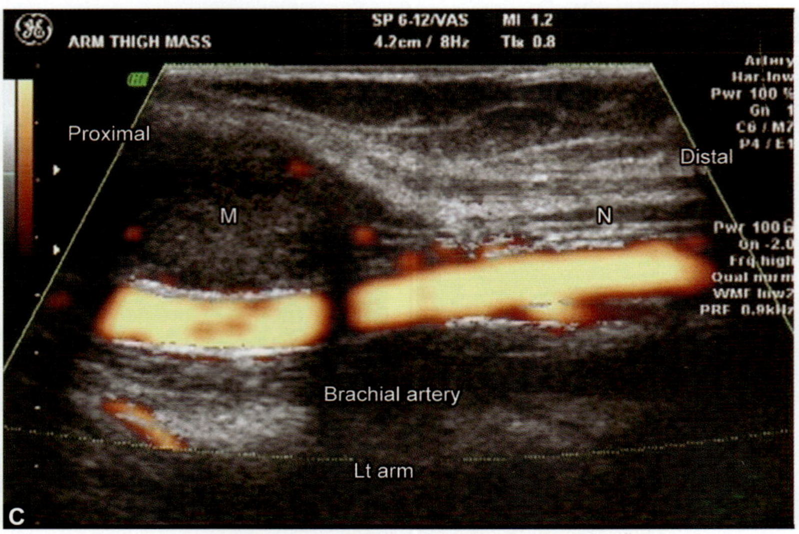

FIGURE 4.61C

FIGURES 4.61A to C: A patient presented with multiple masses in left lower neck, which are also seen in the left axilla. HRSG shows well-defined homogeneous nodular masses in the left infraclavicular region and left axilla. They are seen attached at brachial trunk and show bead like appearance with sharp margins. No evidence of any calcification or cystic degeneration is seen in them. HRSG findings are highly suggestive of brachial plexus schwannomas.

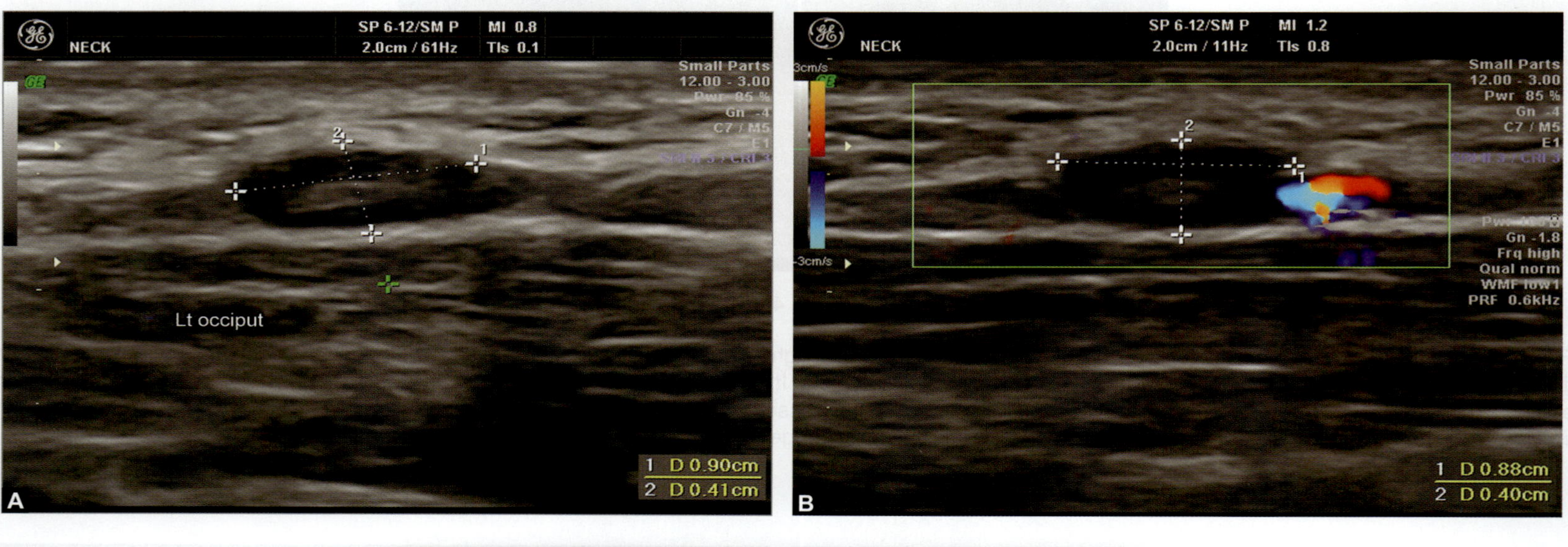

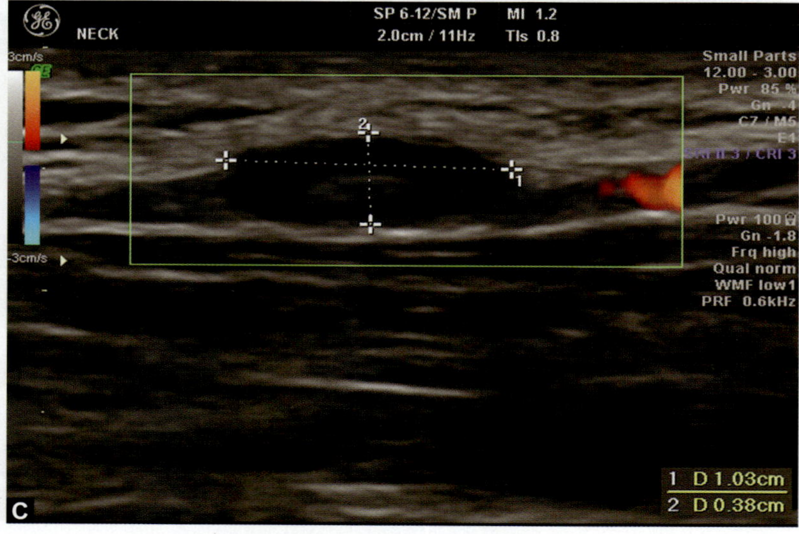

FIGURES 4.62A to C: Occiput neurofibroma. A patient presented with soft tissue nodular mass at the occiput. HRSG shows a well-defined hypoechoic fusiform nodular mass at occiput. It is seen in relation to the nerve and growing on either side of the nerve. It is smooth in outline. No calcification is seen in them. On color flow imaging, no flow is seen in it. Findings are suggestive of neurofibroma of the nerve.

PARASITIC INFESTATIONS

High resolution ultrasound is very useful and sensitive modality for evaluation of parasitic infestation like cysticercus, hydatid cyst and other worms in the body. Typical sonographic features are seen of different parasitic infestations in neck.

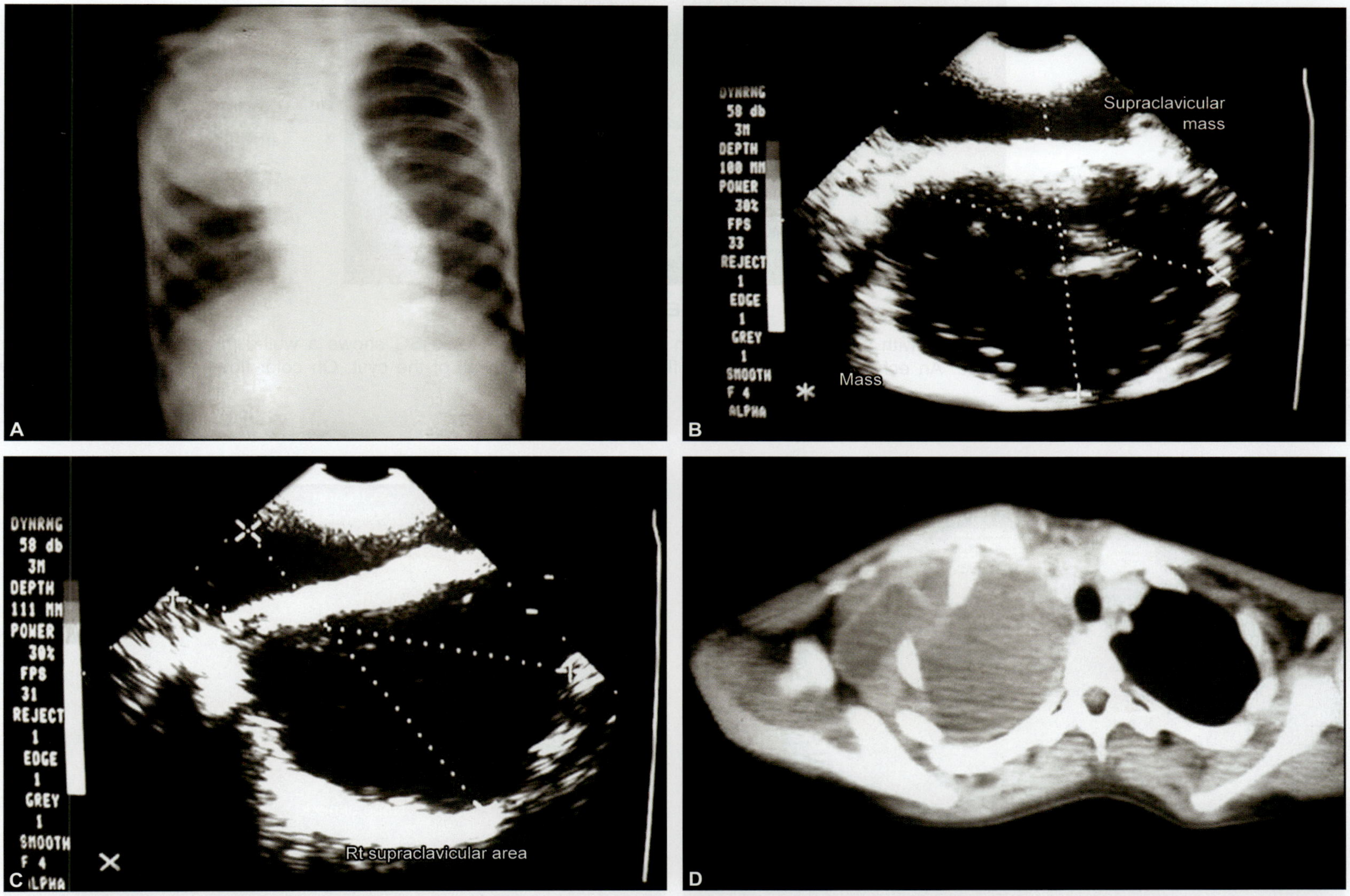

Figures 4.63A to D: Hydatid cyst in the neck. HRSG shows a thick-walled multiloculated cystic mass in right supraclavicular area. The septa are thickened and calcification is seen in them. Few internal echoes are seen in the cyst suggestive of hydatid cyst. CT scan of the same patient shows hypodense mass with homogeneous echoes. Biopsy confirms hydatid cyst.

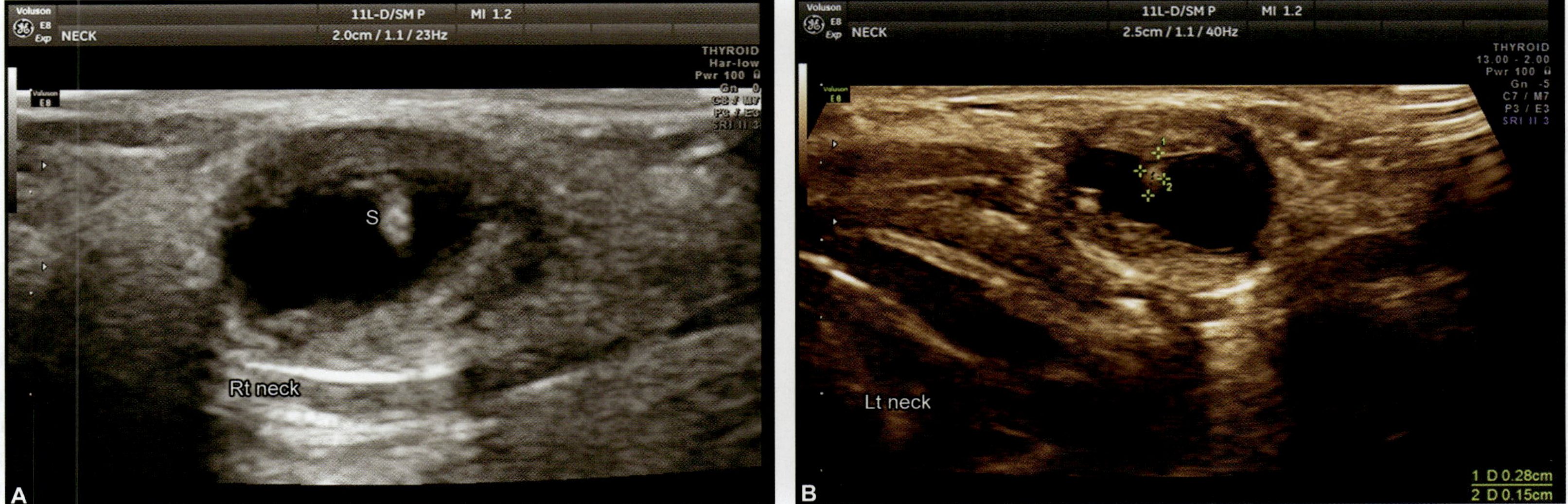

FIGURES 4.64A and B

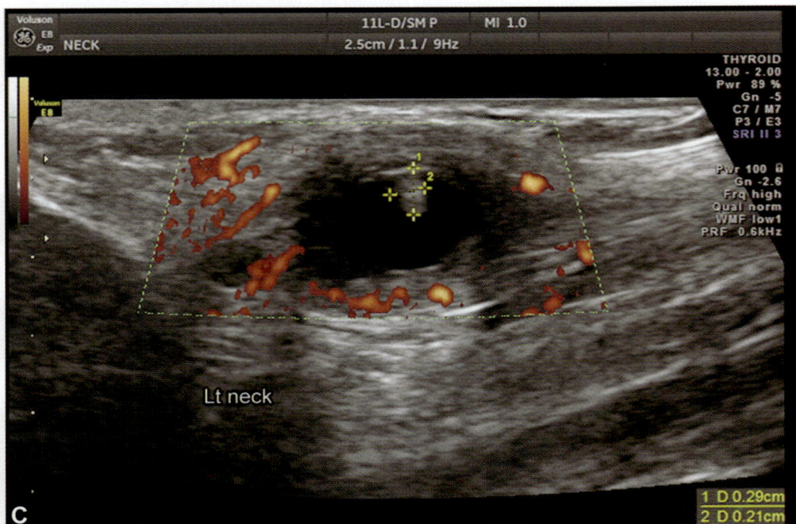

FIGURE 4.64C

FIGURES 4.64A to C: A young girl presented with soft tissue swelling in the right side of neck. HRSG shows a well-defined cystic shadow in the sternocleidomastoid muscle on the left side. An echogenic nidus is seen fixed with the inner wall of the cyst. On color flow imaging, moderate flow is seen in the cyst.

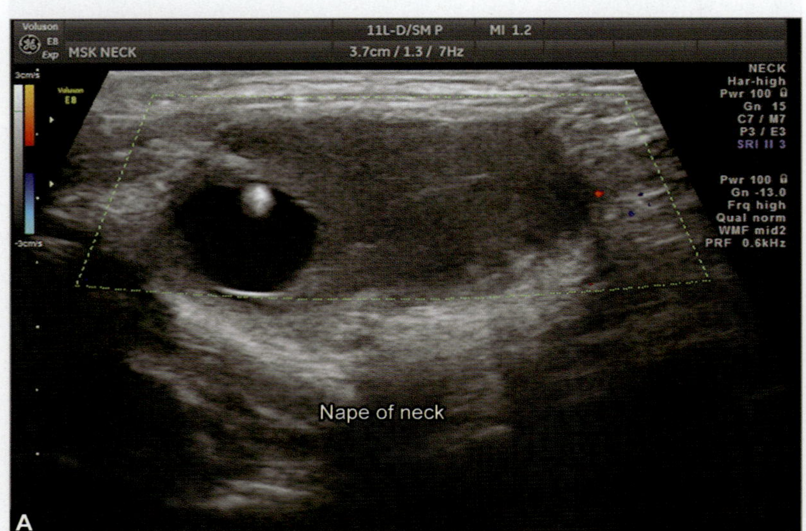

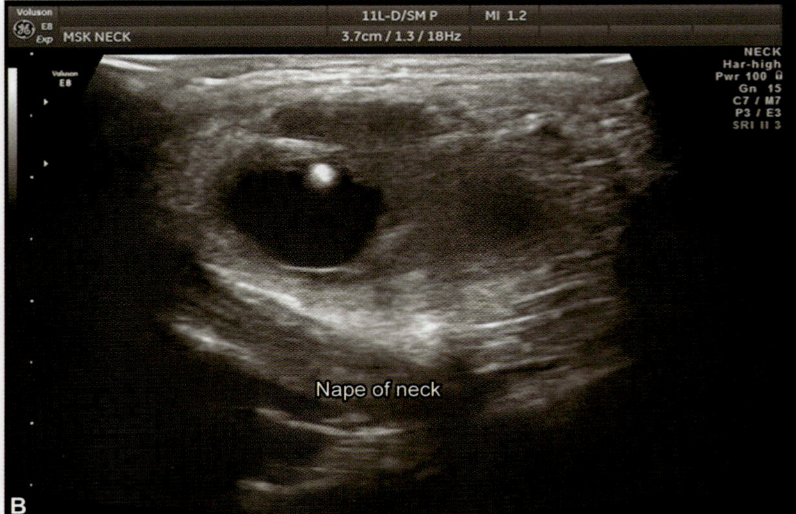

FIGURES 4.65A and B: An 8-year-old boy presented with soft tissue swelling at the nape of the neck. HRSG shows a well-defined cystic mass in the occipital muscle. The cyst shows echogenic nidus fixed with the inner wall of cyst. Associated muscle inflammation is also seen. Findings are suggestive of typical cysticercus cyst.

VASCULAR MASSES

HRSG is very sensitive and accurate in detecting vascular masses in the neck. Hemangiomas, cavernous venous malformations and artero venous malformations can be easily differentiated on HRSG. Color flow imaging is mandatory in deciding the nature of the mass.

Hemangiomas

These are soft, cystic and mobile mass present superficially or deep in the soft tissue planes. They may be pulsatile. Ultrasonogram shows low amplitude mass with jelly like consistency. Fine echogenic septa are seen in the mass. Echogenic hemorrhagic collection is seen when there is secondary Hemorrhage in the hemangioma. Color flow imaging is an added advantage in hemangioma.

Aneurysmal Dilatation

Aneurysmal dilatation of great vessels may bulge in the lower cervical region on either side or in the midline. It is highly pulsatile throbbing mass. It is seen as a well-defined mass with anechoic lumen. Ultrasonogram shows blood flow on Doppler color flow imaging can confirm the diagnosis. Walls may be calcified and thickened in long standing aneurysm. Echogenic thrombus may be seen in the aneurysm.

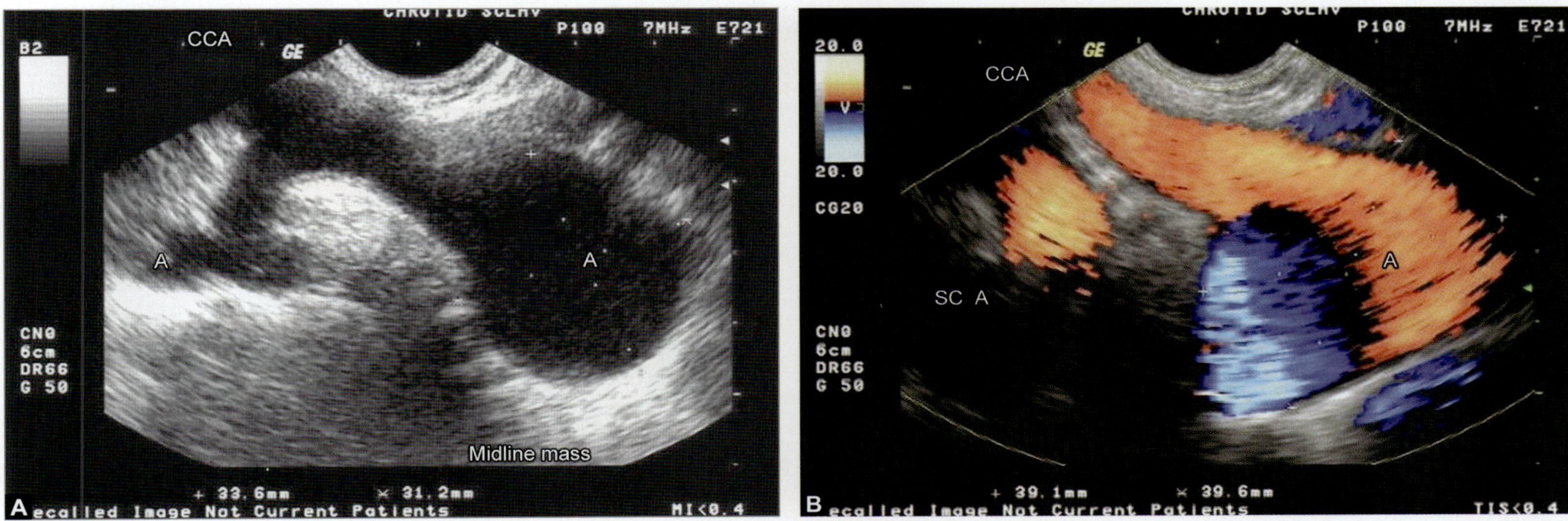

FIGURES 4.66A and B: Aneurysm of right carotid artery. A patient presented soft pulsatile swelling in the right supraclavicular area. Color Doppler imaging shows aneurysmal dilatation of proximal common carotid artery. The blood is seen flowing in the aneurysm in whirlpool fashion. No calcification is seen in the aneurysm.

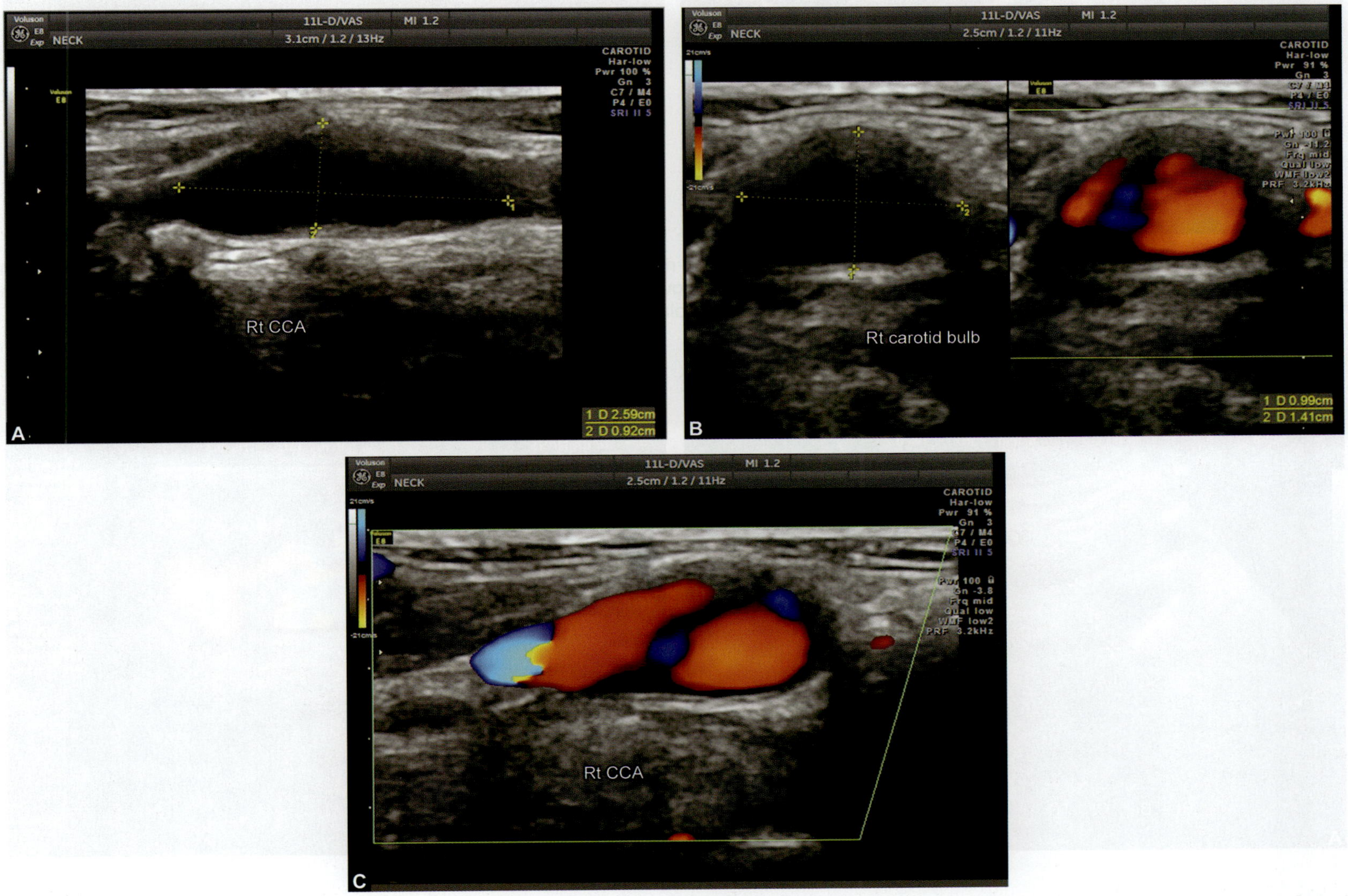

FIGURES 4.67A to C: Aneurysmal dilatation of right carotid bulb. A patient presented with pulsatile swelling in the right upper cervical region. HRSG shows aneurysmal dilatation of right carotid bulb. However, no calcification or plaque is seen in right carotid bulb.

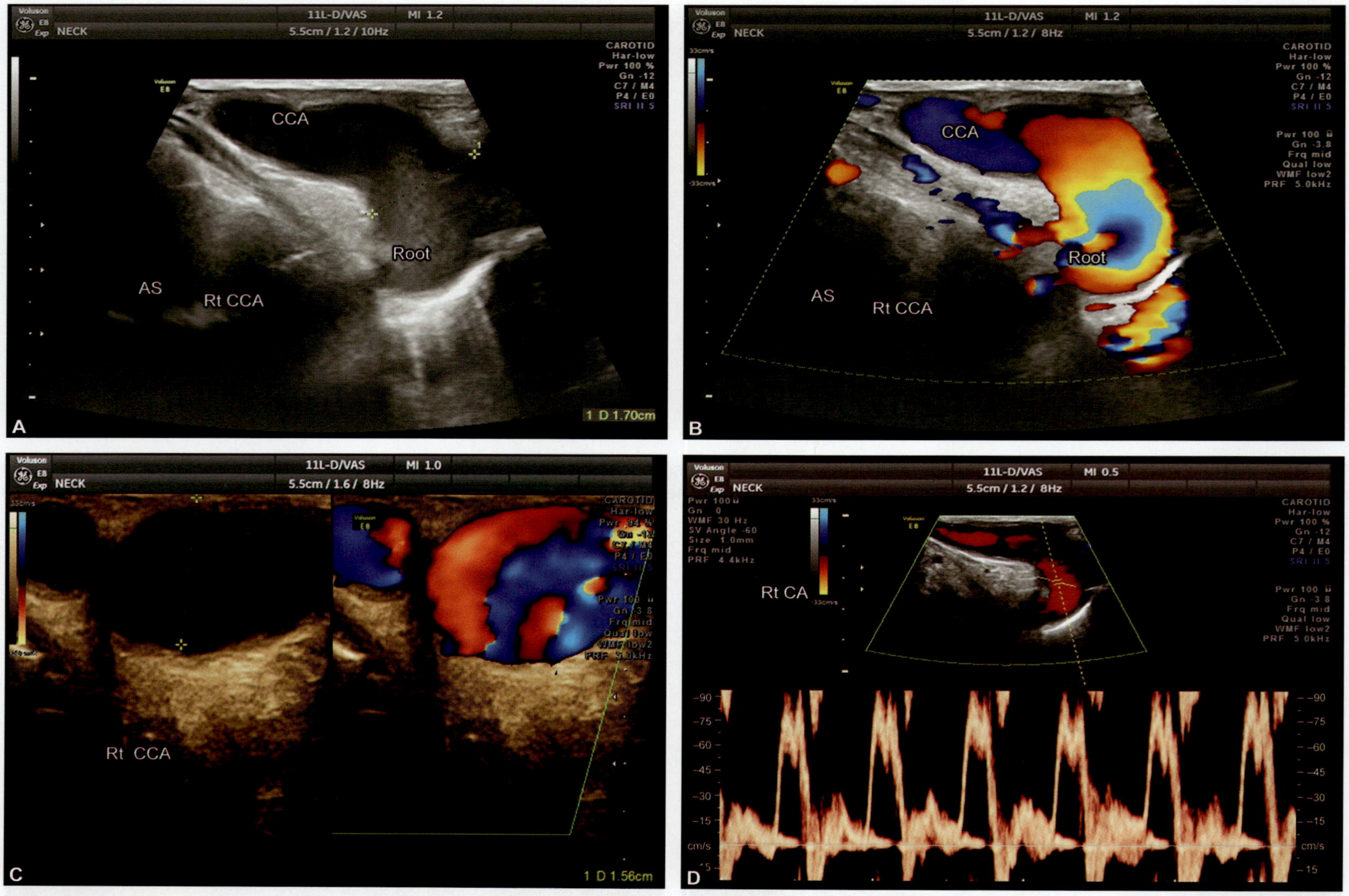

FIGURES 4.68A to D: A patient presented with pulsatile swelling in the right side of the neck. HRSG shows aneurysmal dilatation of root of right carotid artery. The root of right carotid is 16 mm in caliber. On color flow imaging, high flow is seen in the root. It is seen in whirlpool fashion. However, no thrombus is seen in the dilated aneurysm. On spectral Doppler tracing, high flow is seen in it.

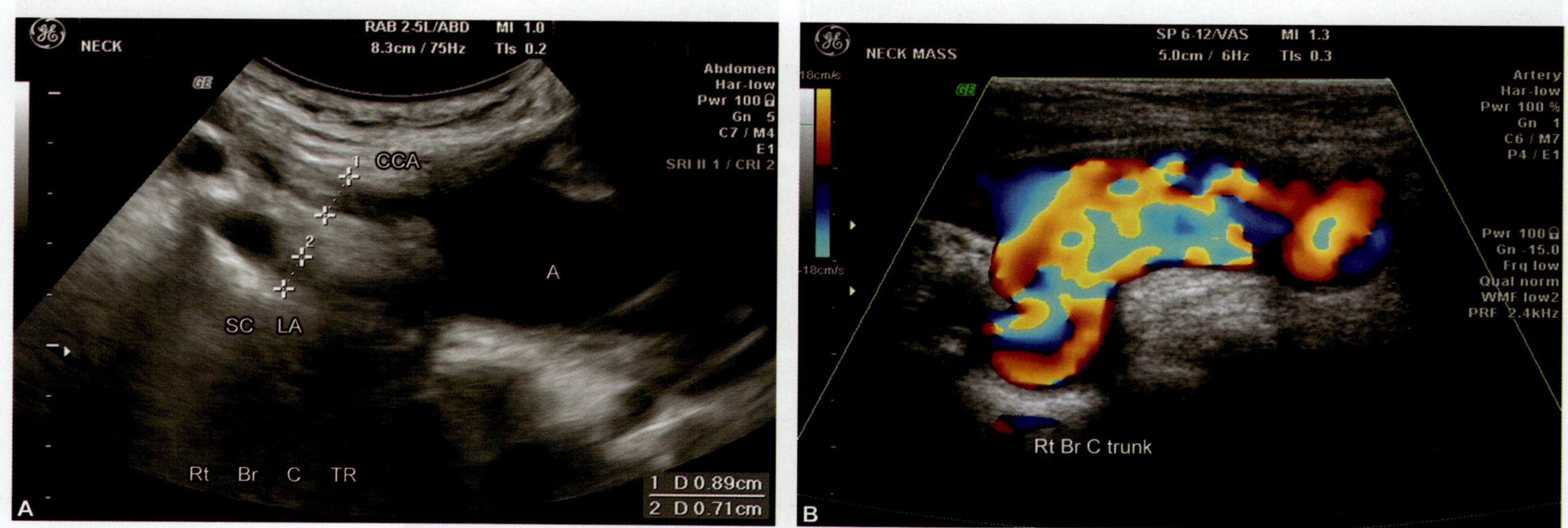

FIGURES 4.69A and B

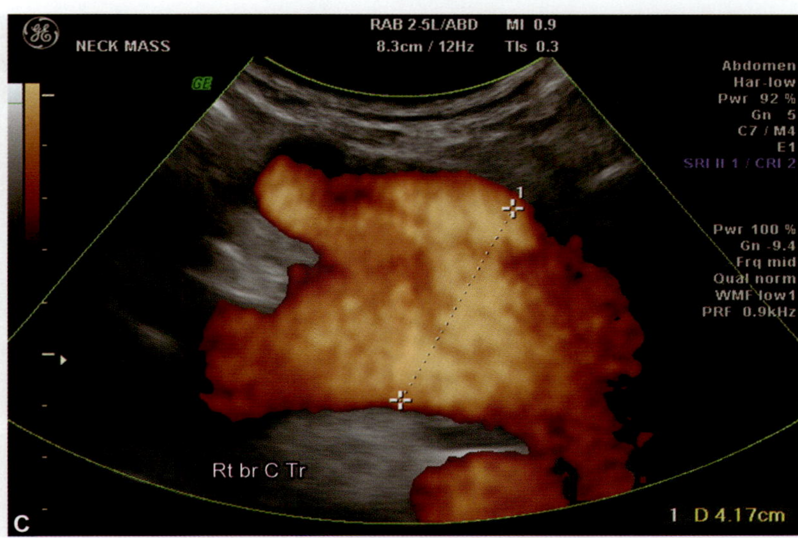

FIGURE 4.69C

FIGURES 4.69A to C: Aneurysm brachiocephalic trunk. A patient presented with soft tissue swelling in right lower neck. HRSG shows soft tissue mass in the right neck. The mass is cystic in nature. It is seen in relation to the right brachiocephalic trunk. It is pulsatile in nature. On color flow imaging, it shows blood flow in whirlpool fashion. On spectral Doppler tracing, bizarre blood flow is seen into it. Aneurysm dilatation of brachiocephalic trunk is seen. High flow pattern is also seen in right carotid and subclavian artery.

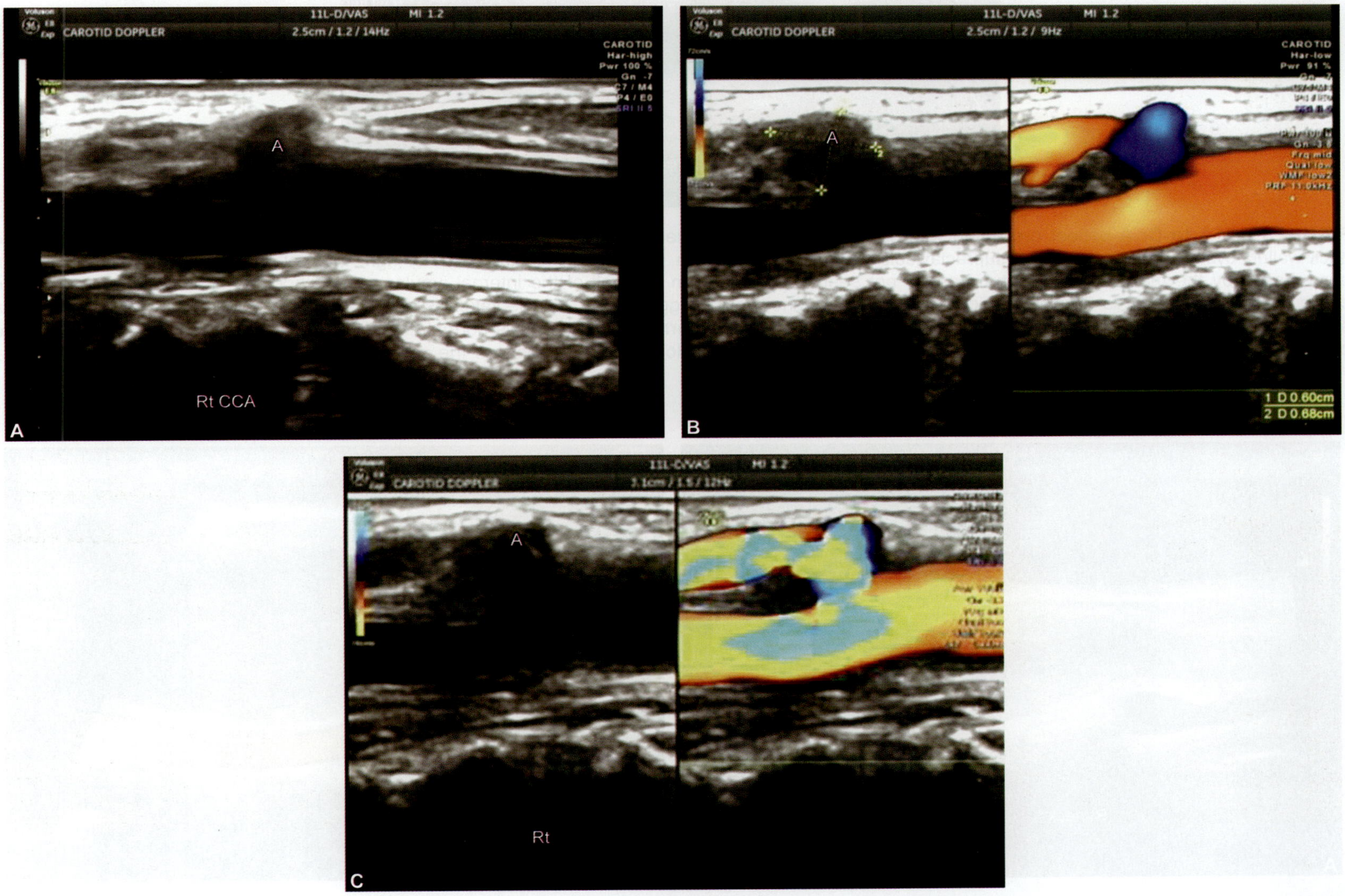

FIGURES 4.70A to C: Aneurysm of right CCA in distal part. A patient presented with small pulsatile swelling in right upper cervical region. HRSG shows a small aneurysm coming out from anterior wall of distal CCA before its bifurcation. On color flow imaging, blood is seen flowing in it. Aliasing is also seen in it. But no calcification is seen. Findings are suggestive of small aneurysm coming out from anterior wall of right CCA.

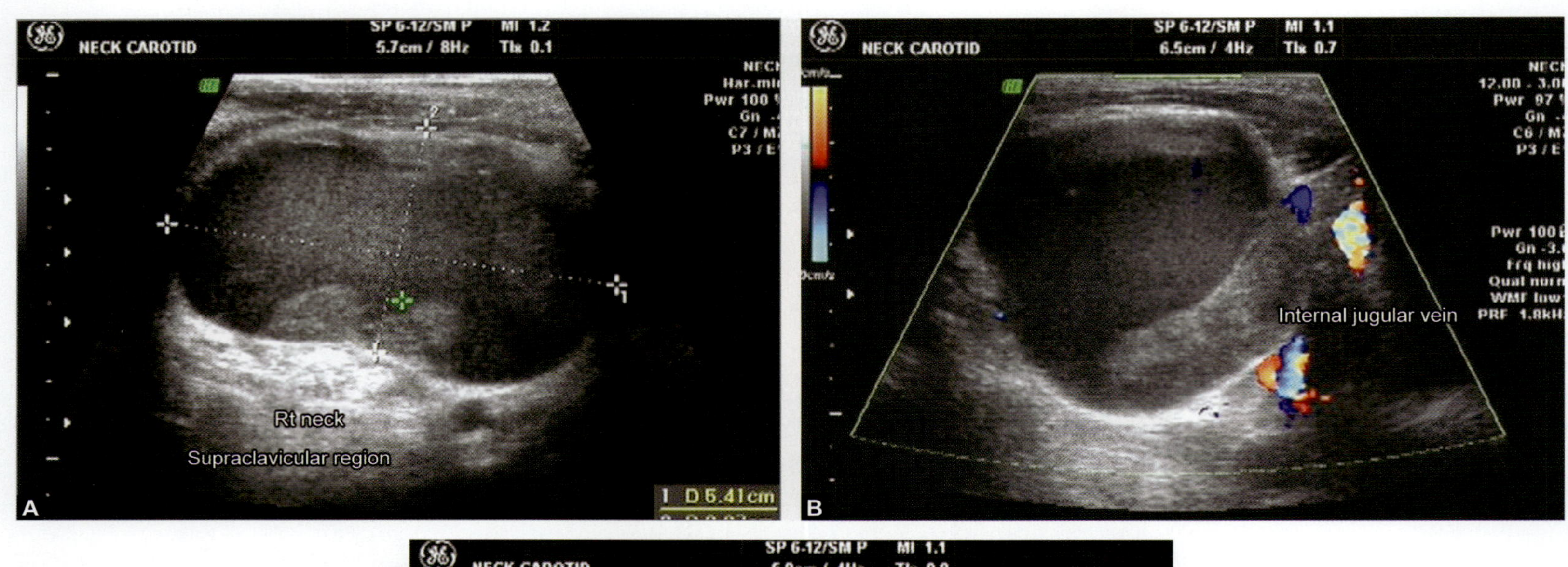

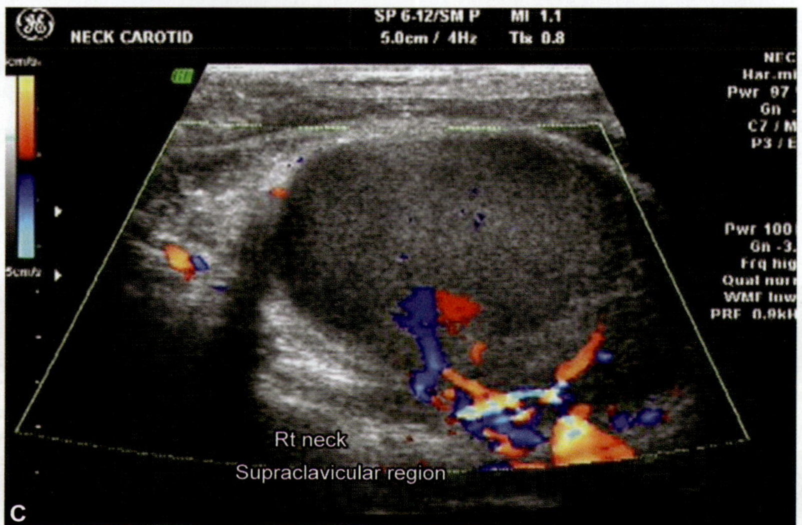

FIGURES 4.71A to C: A patient presented with soft tissue swelling in the right side of neck in supraclavicular region. HRSG shows a well-defined thick-walled cystic mass in the right supraclavicular region. It is seen in relation to the distal part of right internal jugular vein. The vein is seen compressed by the mass. However, the mass is not seen separated from the wall of the internal jugular vein. Echogenic debris is also seen in the cystic mass. However, it is filled with thick homogeneous echoes. No suggestion of any septation is seen into it. On color flow imaging, no flow is seen in the mass. However, capsular flow is seen into it. The proximal part of the vein shows normal flow. No evidence of any thrombus seen in the proximal part of the vein. It is also separate from the right carotid tree. No pressure is seen on the carotid artery.

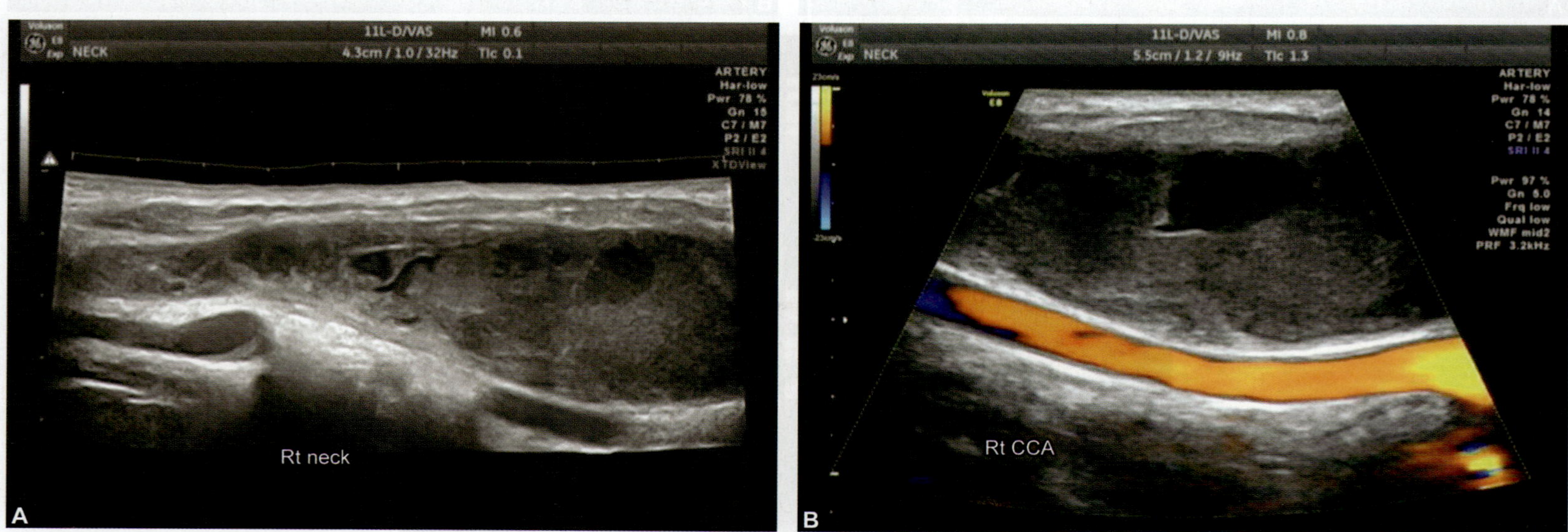

FIGURES 4.72A and B

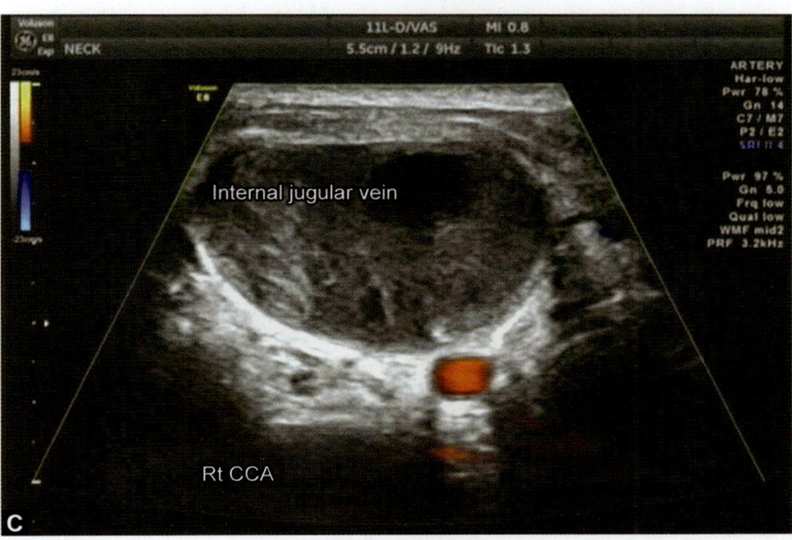

FIGURE 4.72C

FIGURES 4.72A to C: A patient presented with hard soft tissue swelling in the right side of the neck. HRSG shows big low-level echo complex mass in the right side of the neck. It is seen in relation to the internal jugular vein. The whole of the vein is distended. Thick echoes are seen into it. There is also evidence of fusiform dilation of the vein seen in its neck part suggestive of aneurysmal dilatation of the vein. Mixed echo complex shadows are seen filling it. On color flow imaging, no flow is seen in the vein suggestive of thrombosed vein with aneurysmal dilatation. The thrombus is seen extending right up to distal part of the vein, where it is seen merging with brachiocephalic trunk. Part of the vein is seen patent at brachiocephalic trunk.

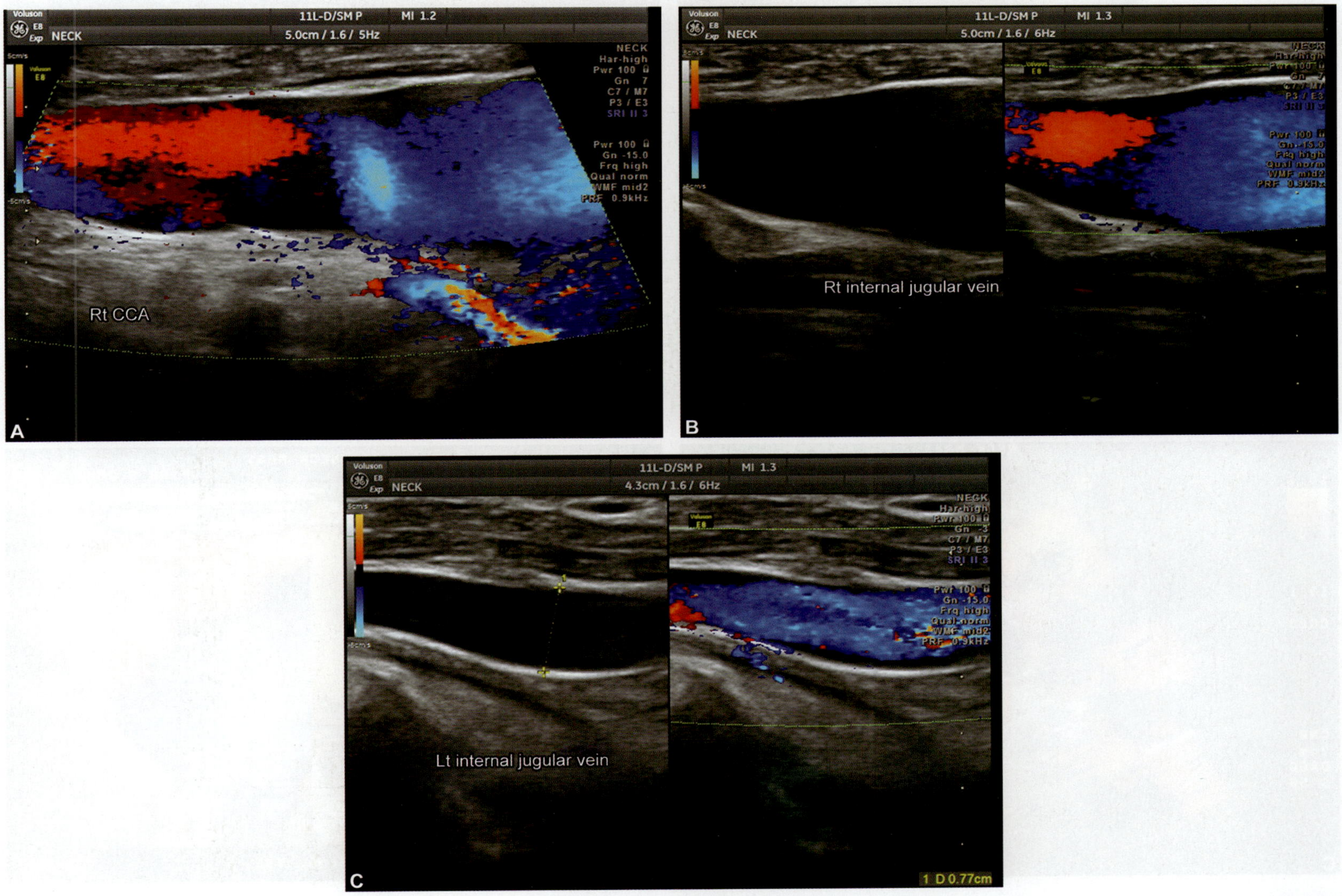

FIGURES 4.73A to C: Internal jugular vein ectasia. A patient presented with soft tissue swelling in right side of neck. The right internal jugular vein is dilated. It is 15 mm in caliber. However, no thrombus or calcification is seen. On color flow imaging, normal flow is seen in the vein. The left internal jugular vein is normal. It is 7.7 mm in caliber. Findings are suggestive of internal jugular vein ectasia.

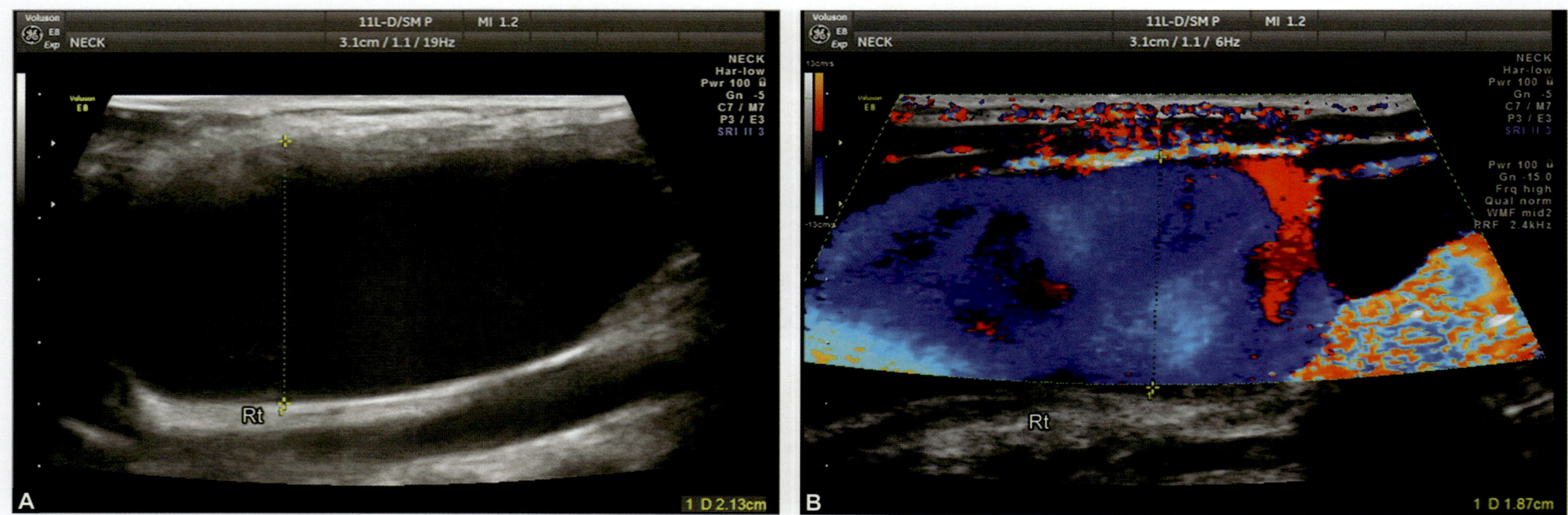

FIGURES 4.74A and B: Internal jugular vein ectasia. A 3-year-old child presented with soft tissue swelling in right side of neck, which becomes prominent while blowing the air. HRSG shows markedly dilated internal jugular vein, which is 2.1 mm in caliber. On blowing the air, it becomes engorged. No evidence of any thrombus or calcification is seen in it. Findings are suggestive of internal jugular vein ectasia.

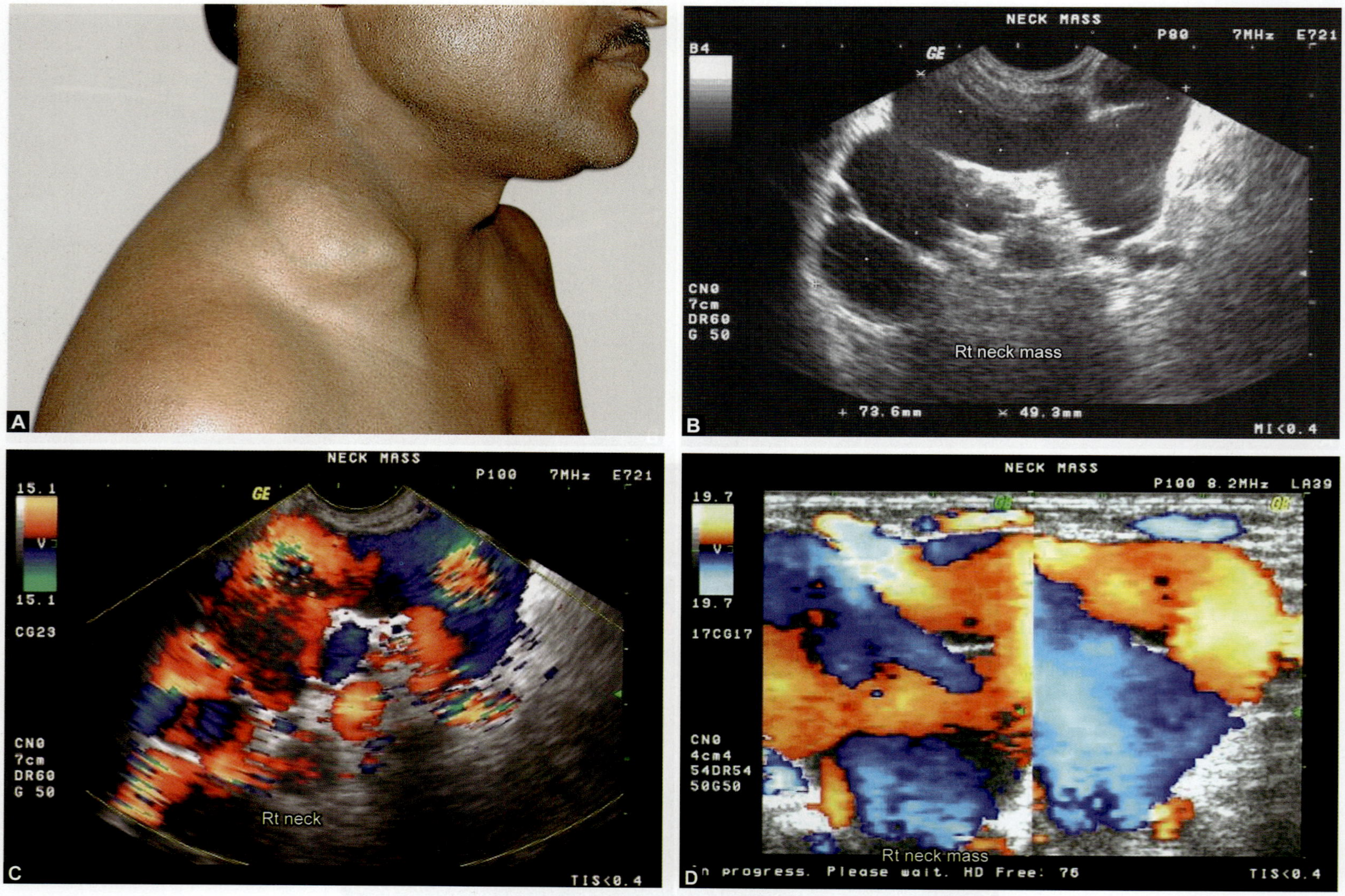

FIGURES 4.75A to D

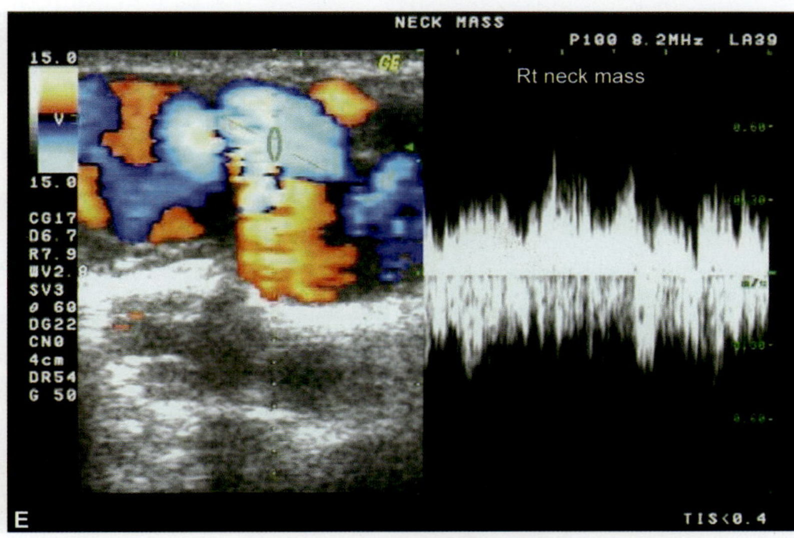

FIGURE 4.75E

FIGURES 4.75A to E: Localized anteriovenous malformation (AVM) of right supraclavicular region. A patient presented with cystic mass in the right supraclavicular region. HRSG shows multiple dilated vessels in the right supraclavicular region and upper cervical region. On color flow imaging, high flow is seen in the vessels. On spectral Doppler tracing, bizarre flow pattern is seen in it suggestive of AVM.

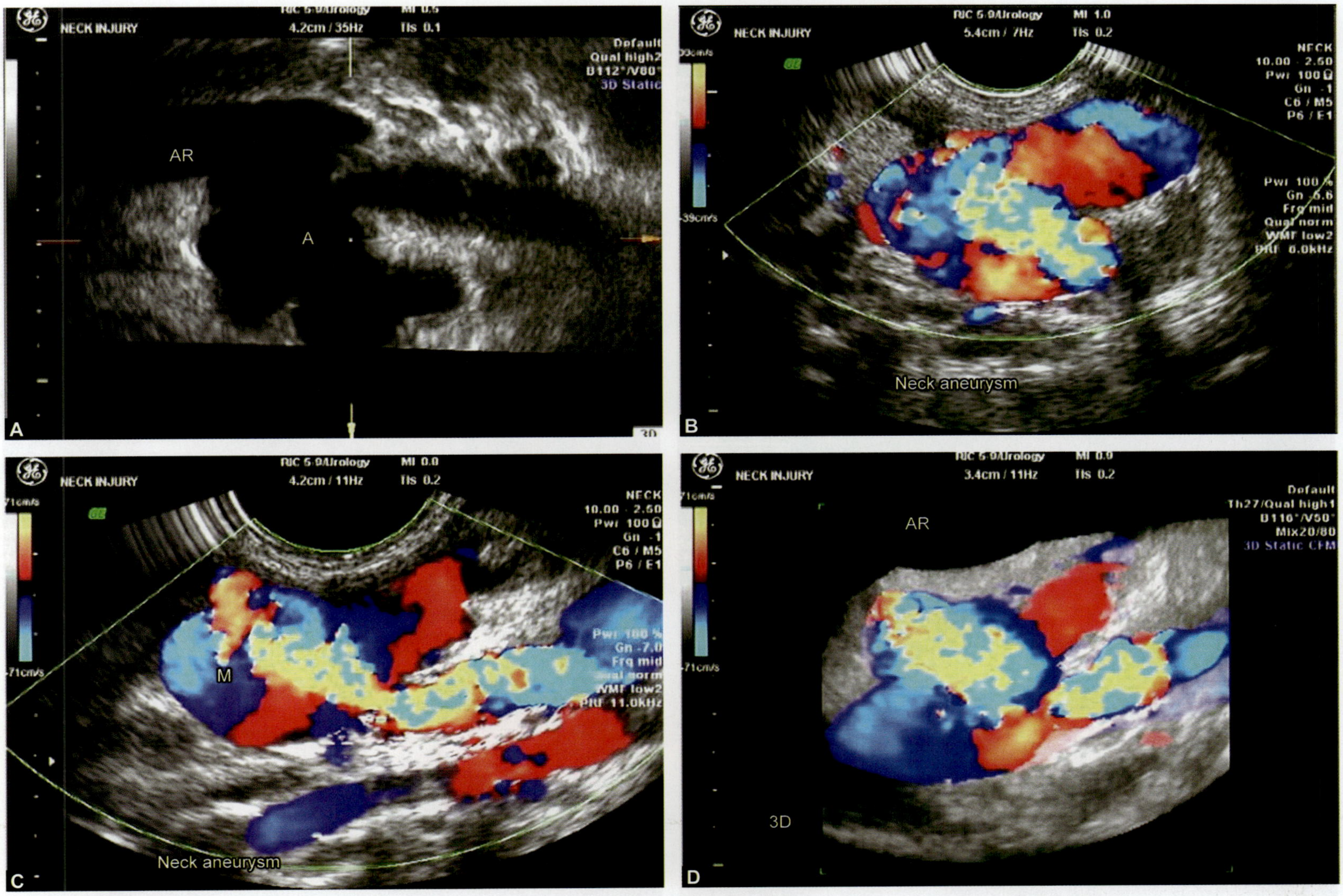

FIGURES 4.76A to D

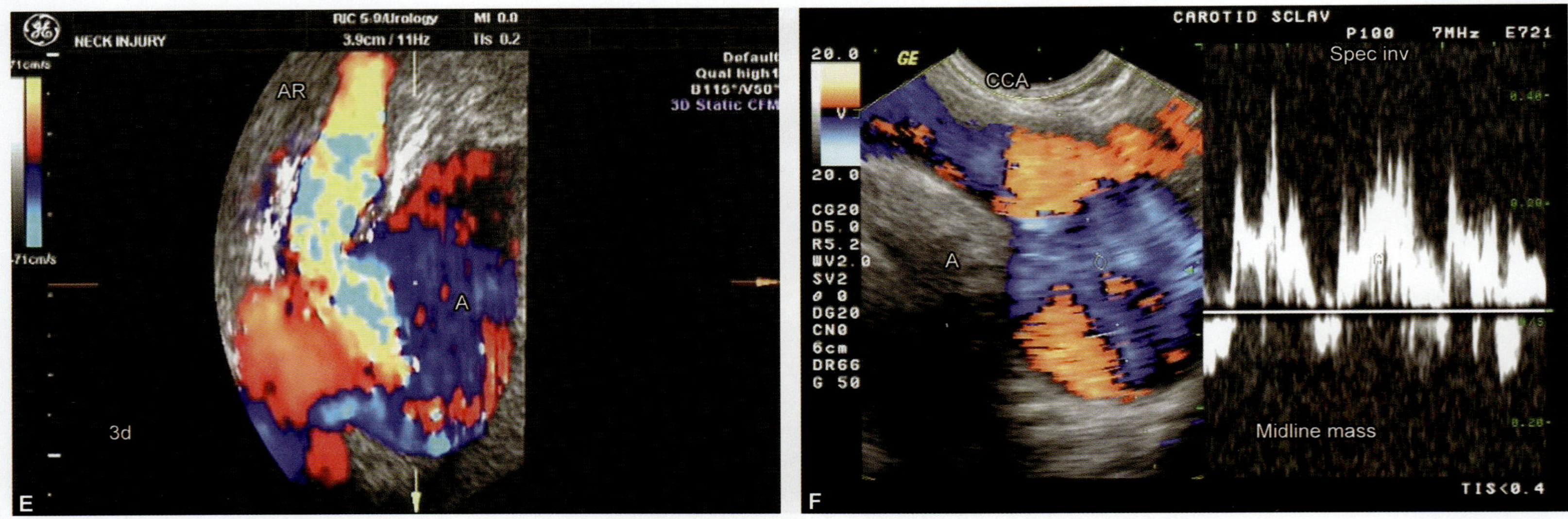

FIGURES 4.76E and F

FIGURES 4.76A to F: Three-dimensional (3D) traumatic aneurysm left brachiocephalic trunk. A young boy sustained sharp knife injury in the left side of the neck. No carotid artery pulsation seen on the left side. Soft tissue mass was seen in the neck. HRSG shows traumatic aneurysm of left brachiocephalic trunk. 3D imaging shows details of the aneurysm. 3D imaging of the aneurysm with color flow imaging shows filling of the aneurysm with the blood with bizarre fashion. The proximal brachiocephalic trunk is seen feeding the aneurysm.

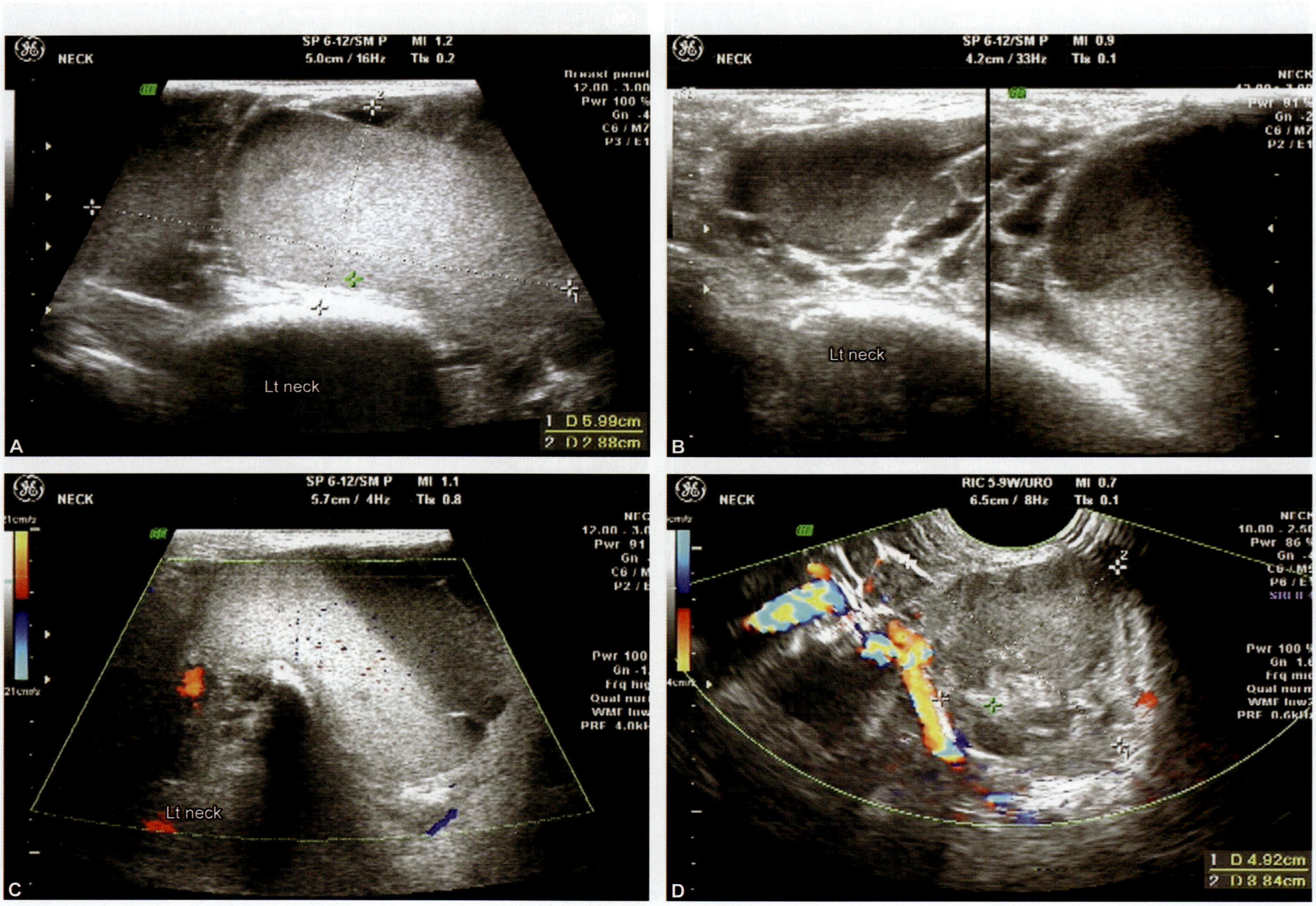

FIGURES 4.77A to D

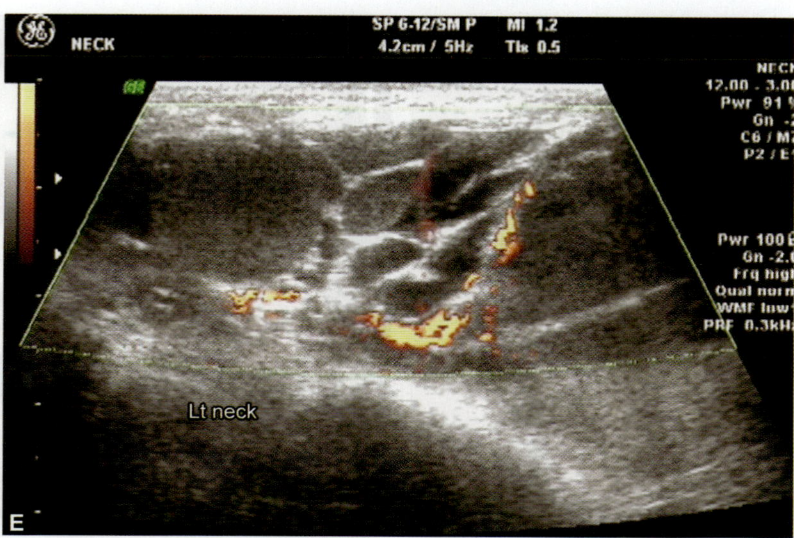

FIGURE 4.77E

FIGURES 4.77A to E: Lymphangioma. A 6-year-old child presented with soft tissue swelling in the left side of the neck. HRSG shows predominantly cystic mass in left side of neck. Thick collection is seen into it. No calcification is seen. It is seen in relation to left parotid gland. Normal glandular texture is lost. Normal anatomic relations are also distorted. On color flow imaging, capsular flow is seen into it. Multiple enlarged nodes are also seen in left upper cervical region. There is evidence of septa are seen in the mass. Multiple septations are seen into it. On color flow imaging, there is evidence of flow seen in the septa.

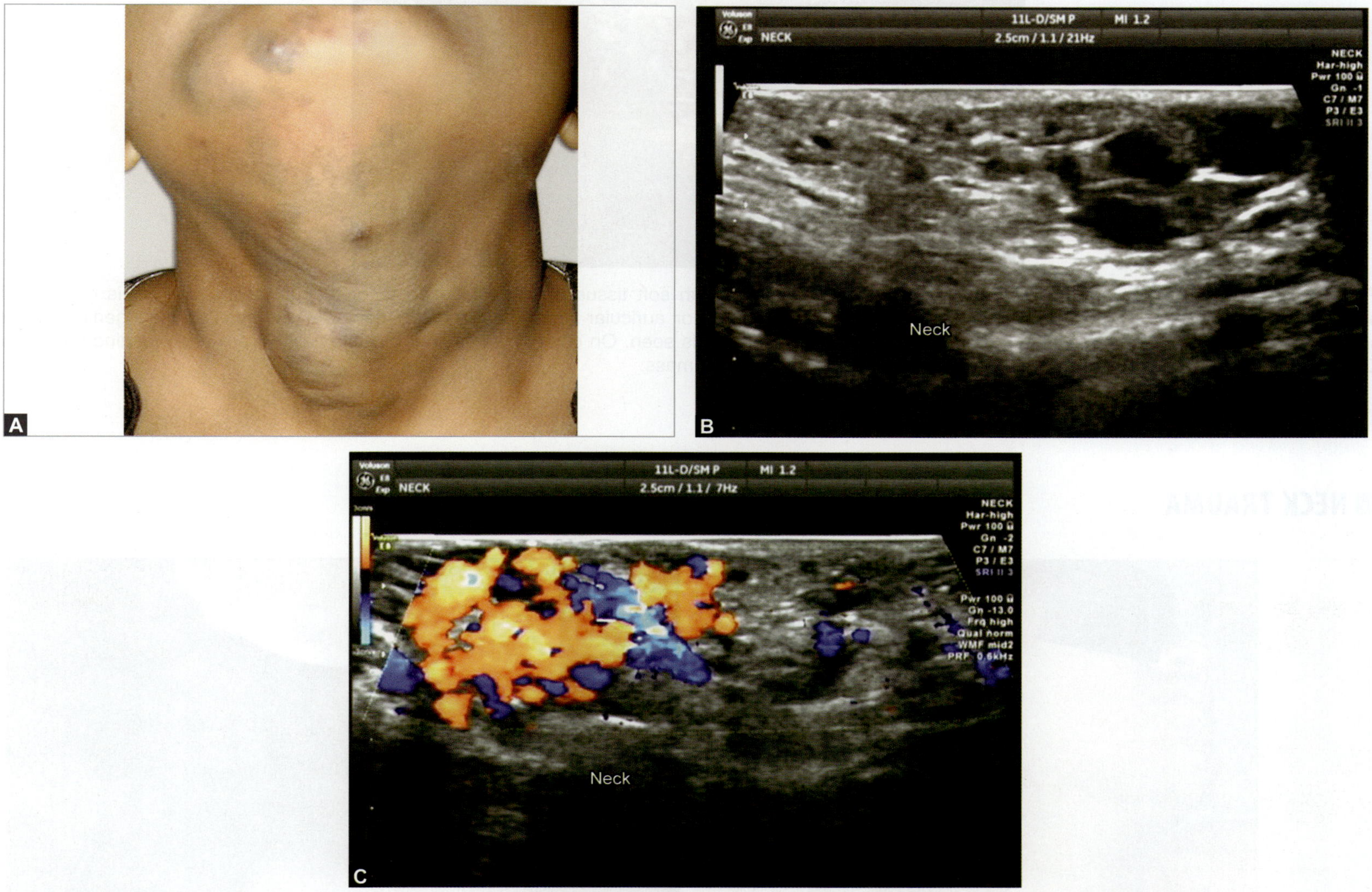

FIGURES 4.78A to C: A patient presented with diffuse soft tissue swelling in the anterior compartment of the neck. HRSG shows an irregular ill-defined inhomogeneous soft tissue mass in the midline of the neck. The mass is seen extending from upper part of the neck going up to the lower 1/3rd part of the neck. It is also seen extending to the lateral side of neck on either side. Part of the mass is seen extending to the floor of the mouth. The mass is seen confined in the superficial plane. It is not seen invading the deep muscles. It is separate from salivary gland on both sides. Multiple hypoechoic areas are seen into it. On color flow imaging, they appear to be dilated vessels. On spectral Doppler tracing, low venous flow is seen in them. Few large vessels are seen on the left side of the neck. The vessels are separate from the large vessels of the neck. No evidence of any echogenic foci are seen in the dilated vessels suggestive of phlebolith.

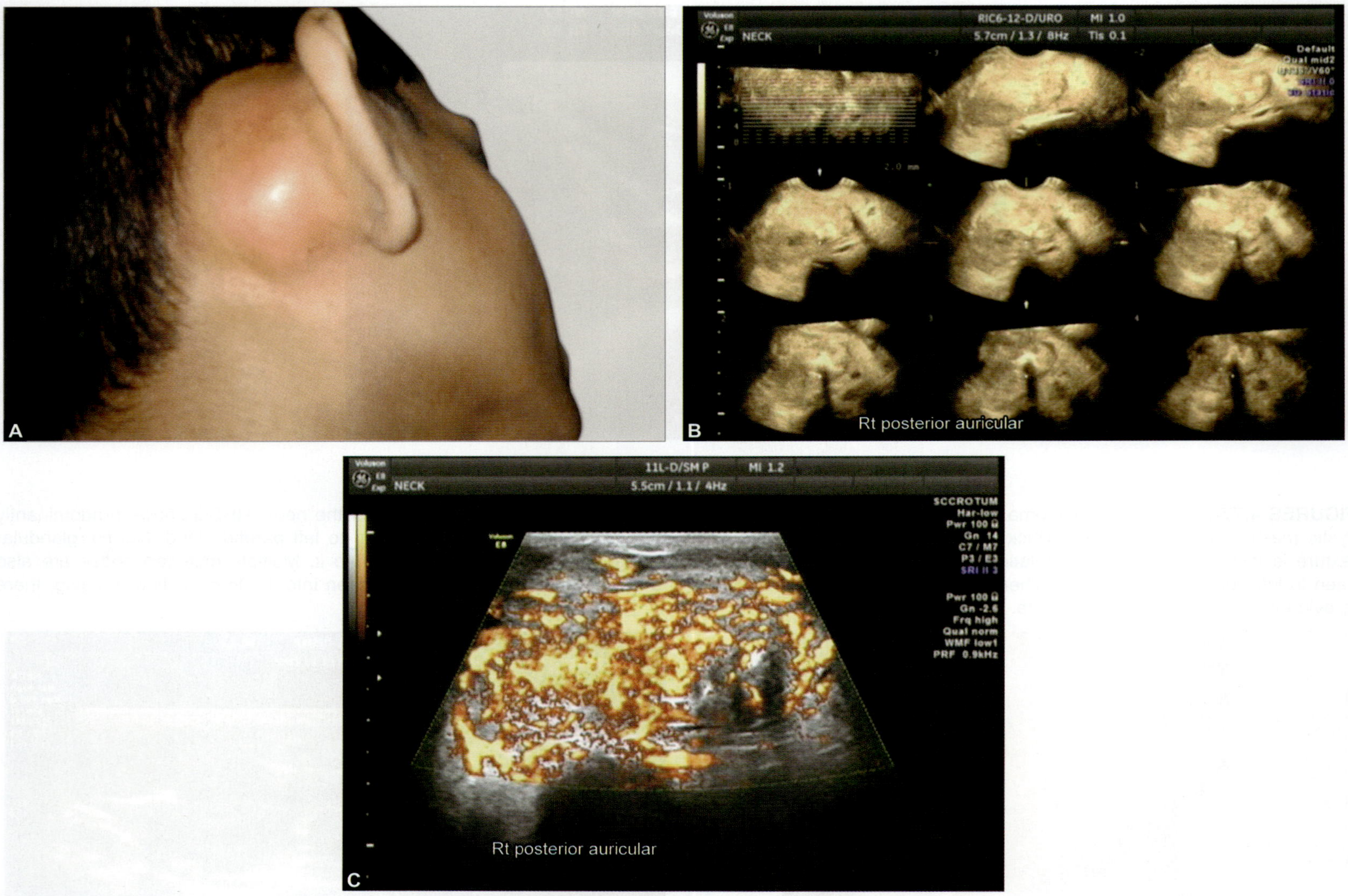

FIGURES 4.79A to C: Hemangiomatous mass. A patient presented with soft tissue welling in the posterior triangle of the neck. It is confined in posterior auricular region. HRSG shows a solid mass in the right posterior auricular region. It is homogeneous in texture. Few echogenic calcified specks are seen into it. But no cystic degeneration is seen. No loculation is seen. On color flow imaging, multiple vessels are seen feeding the mass. On spectral Doppler tracing, high arterial and venous flow is seen in the mass.

NECK TRAUMA

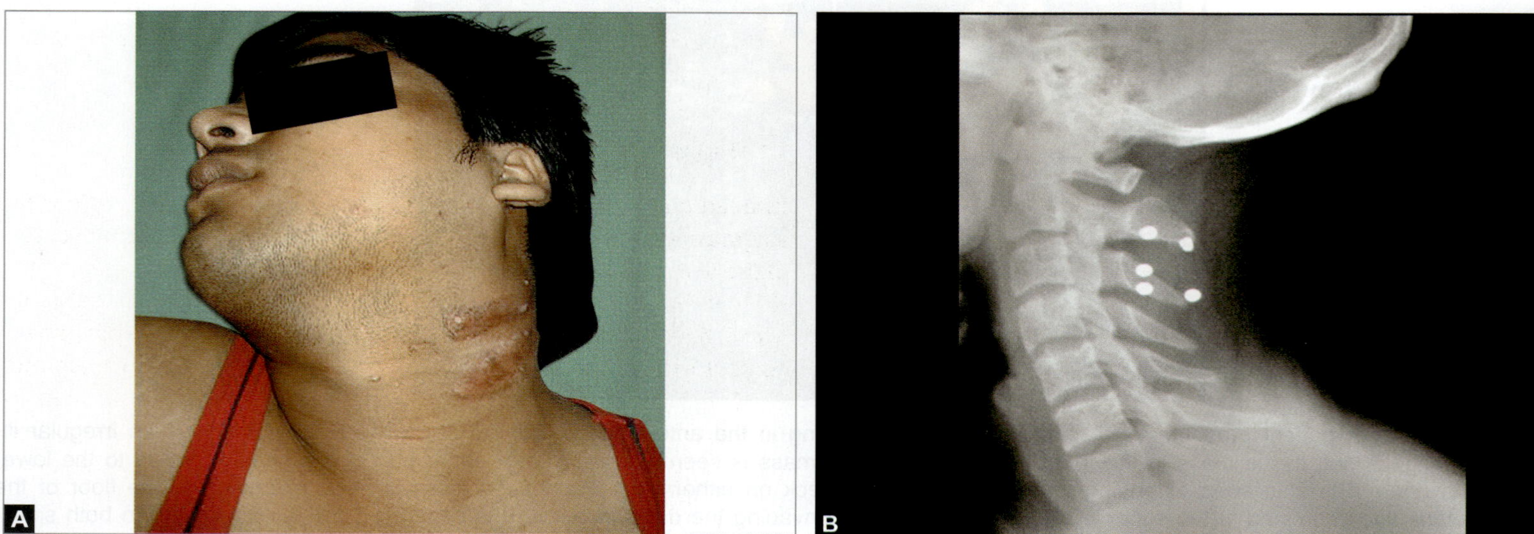

FIGURES 4.80A and B

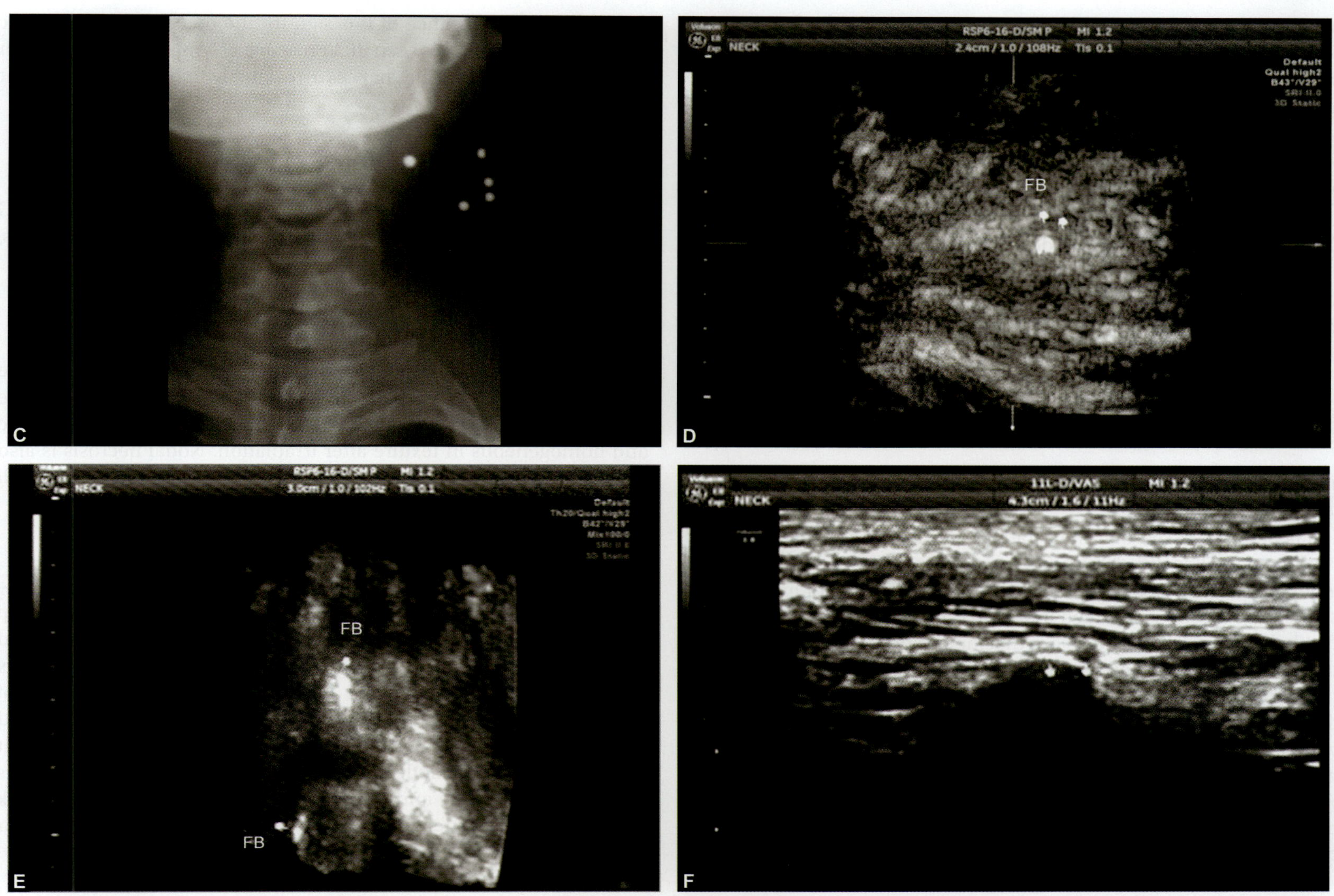

FIGURES 4.80C to F

FIGURES 4.80A to F: A patient presented with gunshot injury in the left side of neck. X-ray of cervical spine shows echogenic shadows with metallic density in the neck. They are seen in the paravertebral region. HRSG shows multiple echogenic shadows in the paravertebral region. But they are seen away from the spinal cord. The cord is seen intact. No intraspinal injury is seen. On ultrasound findings, the patient was not operated as he was not having any neurological deficit.

NECK MALIGNANT MASSES AND LYMPH NODES

Lymph Node Mass

Normally, lymph nodes of the neck are not resolved on ultrasonographic examination because the reflectivity of lymph nodes is similar to the subcutaneous fat. But when they are enlarged or involved in a disease process, they become hypoechoic and enlarged, therefore, they can be very well picked up on HRSG. Seven main chains of lymph nodes are present in the neck. They are as follows:

1. Internal jugular
2. Anterior jugular
3. Parotid chain
4. Submandibular chain
5. Anterior juxtavisceral
6. Retropharyngeal
7. Spinal accessory chain.

From clinical point of view, internal jugular, anterior jugular, parotid and submandibular chains are important. They are further grouped as superficial and deep chains. For convenience, they are further grouped as low cervical, midcervical and high cervical groups. Internal jugular, anterior jugular, parotid, submandibular, jugulodigastric and post-auricular chains are easily accessible on HRSG. However, other chains are not easily detected on HRSG, therefore, CT of MRI examination is required for their evaluation.

Clinical Assessment

In head and neck cancer, involvement of the neck nodes decides the staging of the disease, which is very important for further management of the disease. Clinical assessment of lymph node metastasis becomes difficult when the lymph nodes are small in size and nonpalpable. When they are less than 1 cm in size or when they are deeply present as posterior to sternocleidomastoid muscles they are nonpalpable. Clinical assessment is also difficult in post-surgical or post-irradiative neck due to extensive fibrosis or in a large head and neck cancer mass. Low accuracy of clinical assessment of disease in head and neck cancer is estimated up to 30%, which is very high in the group. Staging, management and treatment of disease become controversial. Therefore, different imaging modalities were tried to improve the results of clinical assessment like CT, MRI and HRSG. Among all of them, HRSG has been found to be highest sensitive. It can pick up nodes as small as 2 mm in size in superficial group.

The different parameters to distinguish reactive node from metastatic node are as follows:

Lymph Node Size

It is seen that normal lymph node has an axial diameter between 2 mm to 5 mm. In reactive enlargement of lymph node as in tonsil infections, the jugulodigastric nodes become enlarged. The size increases more than 2 cm in length and 1 cm in thickness. However, in metastatic lymph node enlargement, the size does not increase more than 2 cm and it remains under 1 cm in length and in thickness. But lymph node size and axial diameter has got limited value in the differential diagnosis of metastatic lymph node enlargement.

Lymph Node Shape

It has been observed that metastatic nodes have a tendency to be of round shape. Reactive lymph node enlargement appears to be more enlarged. Sakai et al. have defined the numerical index for lymph node shape. It is known as rounded index (RI). The longitudinal diameter is divided by axial diameter. It is seen that metastatic nodes have a RI of less than 1.5 cm, whereas reactive lymph nodes have RI of more than 2 cm.

Echo pattern—Normally, the lymph nodes are hypoechoic than the adjacent thyroid parenchyma. However, no specific echo pattern is reported for lymph node pathology. The metastatic nodes are less hypoechoic. When they are small, they have sharp margins. However, when they are large, they are heterogeneous in texture and show tumor necrosis. Microcalcification may be found in the metastatic nodes. Cystic changes are also found in them mainly in papillary carcinoma of thyroid.

Reactive nodes are homogeneous in texture. They have sharp margins and regular smooth shape. Macrocalcification is seen in them mainly on the granulomatous disease.

Lymph Node Hylum

In reactive lymph node enlargement, there is a highly reflective band seen in the central part of node or in lymph node sinus. It is seen running through the substance of node. It is considered to be a sign of nonmalignancy. Presence of lymph node hilum combined with RI index increases the significance of this sign for the detection of metastatic lymph node disease. It is seen that presence of lymph node hilum with RI index of more than 2, the chances of reactive lymph node enlargement are high.

Extranodal Tumor Extension

Extranodal tumor extension is a poor prognostic sign for patient. HRSG is very sensitive tool to assess extra-nodal tumor spread to muscles, jugular vein or carotid artery.

Post-radiotherapy Evaluation

Clinical assessment is difficult in post-irradiative neck due to extensive fibrosis. HRSG is very sensitive to detect presence of recurrence of disease in post-irradiative neck. Nodes become well-defined, hypoechoic and homogeneous in texture after irradiation. Nodal necrosis is also encountered. Recurrence of primary growth or disease can be very well assessed by HRSG.

Malignant Tumors

Malignant cervical tumors are very rare. They include lip sarcoma, malignant chemodectomas, malignant epithelioma and rhabdomyosarcoma. However, tumors of larynx and laryngopharynx when enlarged, they bulge as a mass in the neck. The extension of the growth can be assessed by HRSG. In carcinoma of larynx and laryngopharynx, associated lymph node enlargement and assessment of nonpalpable lymph node can be done on HRSG. Cervical lymphomas are also very common and big lobulated masses are seen in the neck with heterogeneous texture. Retrosternal extension of the mass can be assessed from the suprasternal notch. Echo texture, lymph node enlargement and vessel involvement can be assessed on HRSG.

HRSG is also a good tool to assess the treatment response and recurrence of growth in carcinoma of larynx or laryngopharynx. However, no specific sonographic feature is found in cervical malignancy. But the signs are suggestive of malignancy found elsewhere in body like irregular margins, heterogeneous texture, lobulated pattern and surrounding tissue invasion and infiltration and vessel involvements are the features that suggest the malignant nature of the mass. Biggest advantage of HRSG is to do the guided fine-needle aspiration biopsy of the tumor for histopathological examination to confirm the diagnosis.

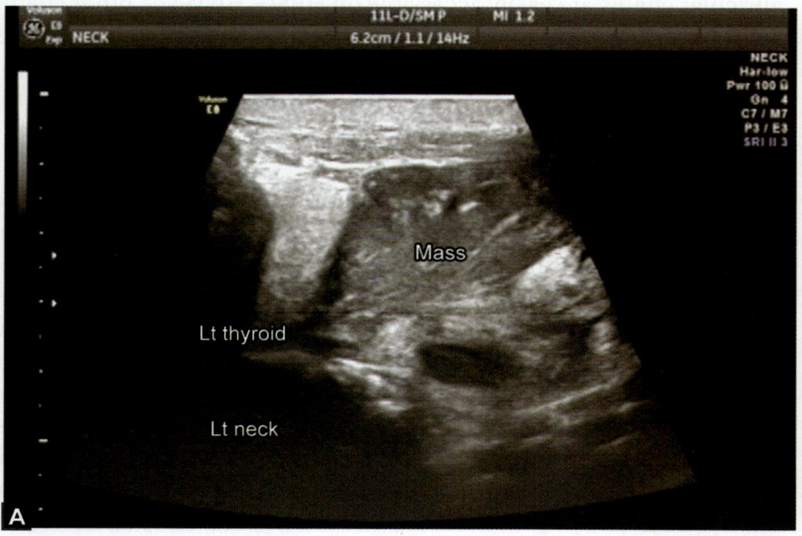

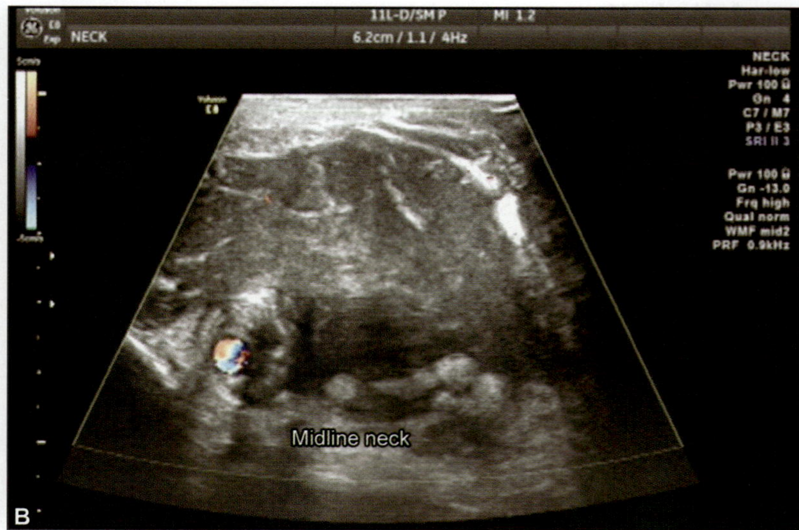

FIGURES 4.81A and B

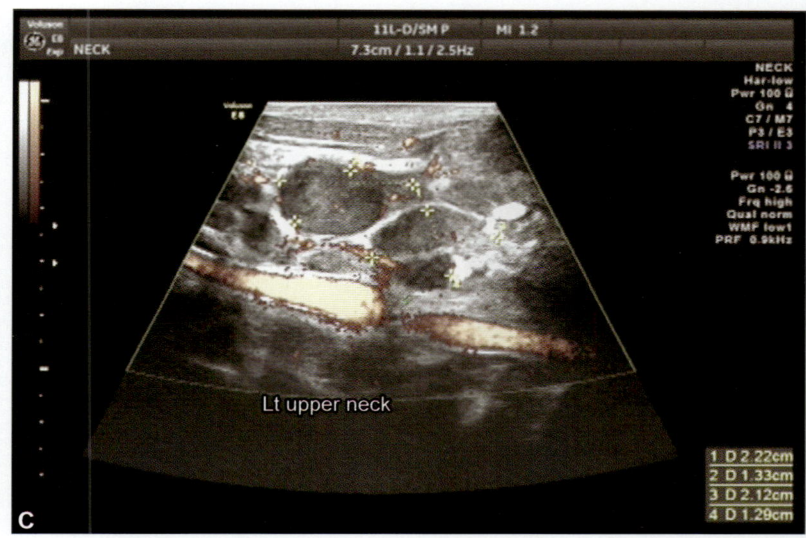

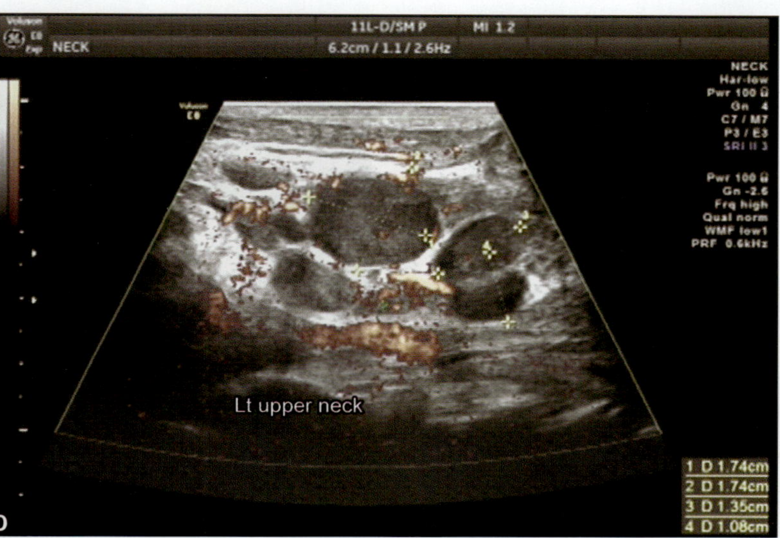

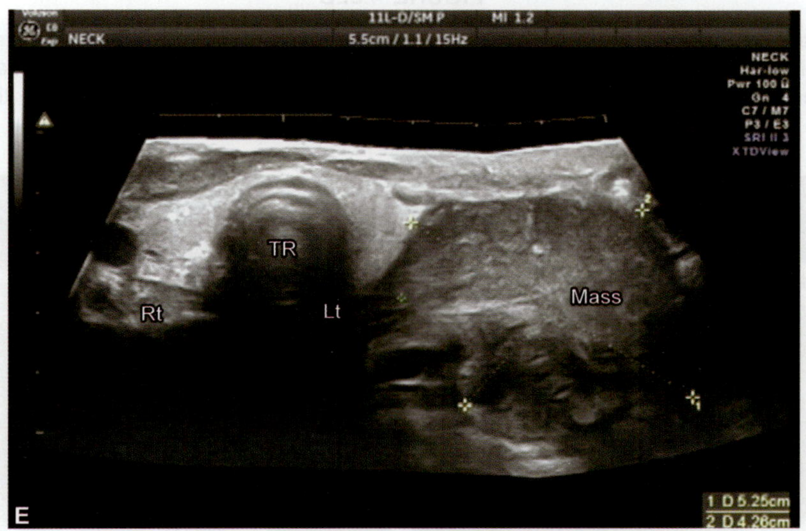

FIGURES 4.81C to E

FIGURES 4.81A to E: Lymphoma. A patient presented with soft tissue mass in left side of neck. There is evidence of big hypoechoic nodal mass in left side of neck. It is seen separate from thyroid. It is hypoehcoic in texture. Multiple enlarged nodes are sloe seen in left upper cervical region. The nodes are round in shape. Lymph node hilum is destroyed. On color flow imaging, peripheral flow is seen in the nodes. Findings are suggestive of lymphoproliferative disease. Biopsy of the mass confirms lymphoma.

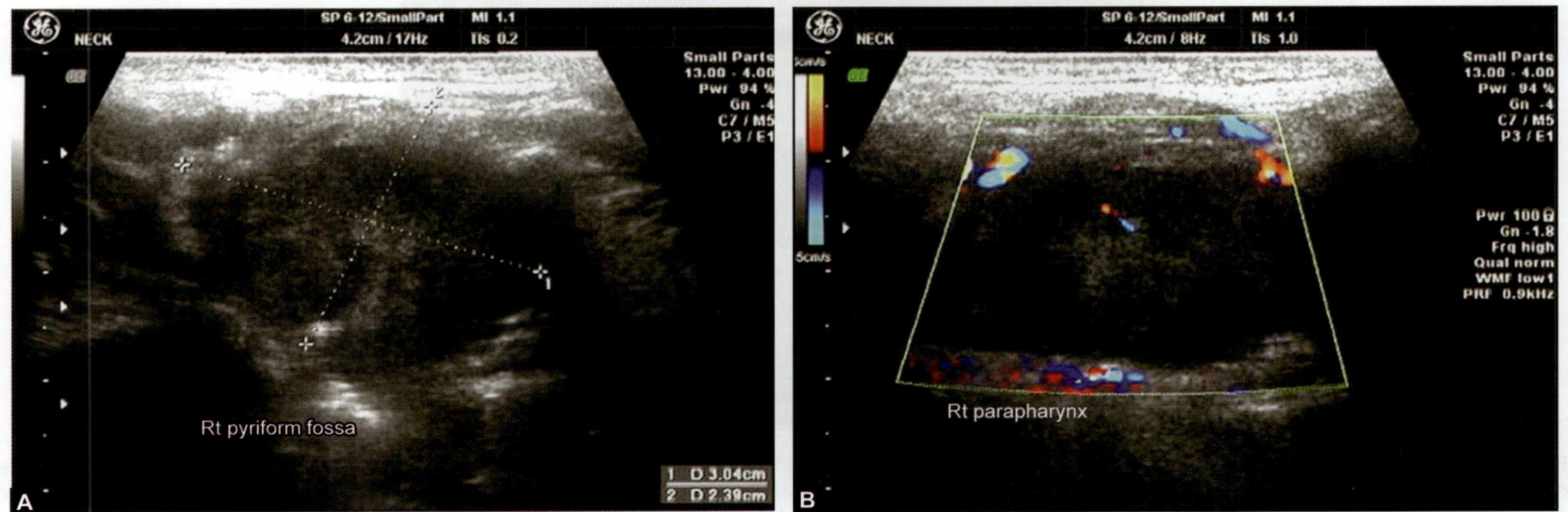

FIGURES 4.82A and B

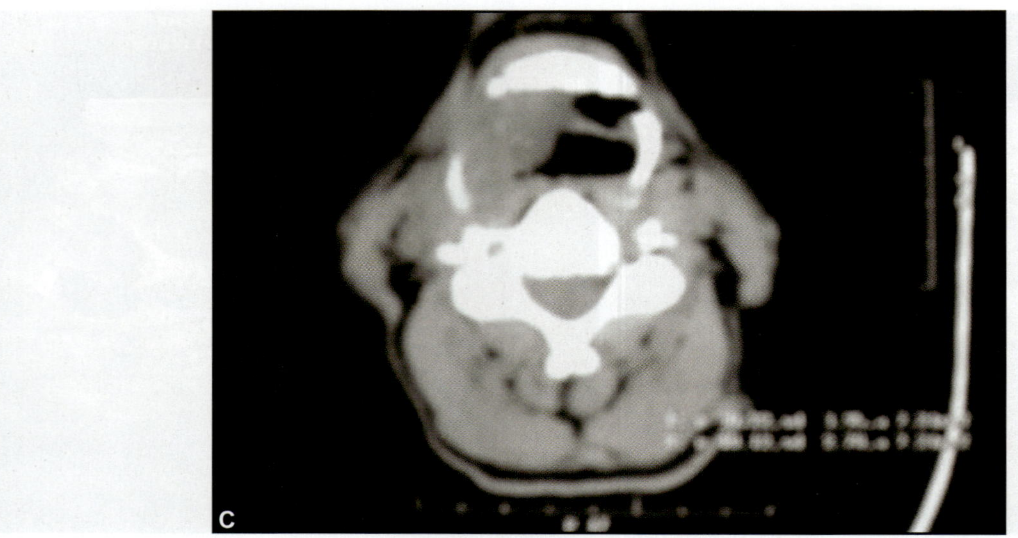

FIGURE 4.82C

FIGURES 4.82A to C: Parapharyngeal malignant mass. An old man presented with mass and fullness in the midline of the neck. HRSG shows a big heterogeneous hypoechoic mass in the paraphyrangeal space. Biopsy of the mass showed malignant squamous cell carcinoma. CT scan of the same patient confirmed the HRSG findings. The mass is seen invading right parapharyngeal space and also the pyriform fossa.

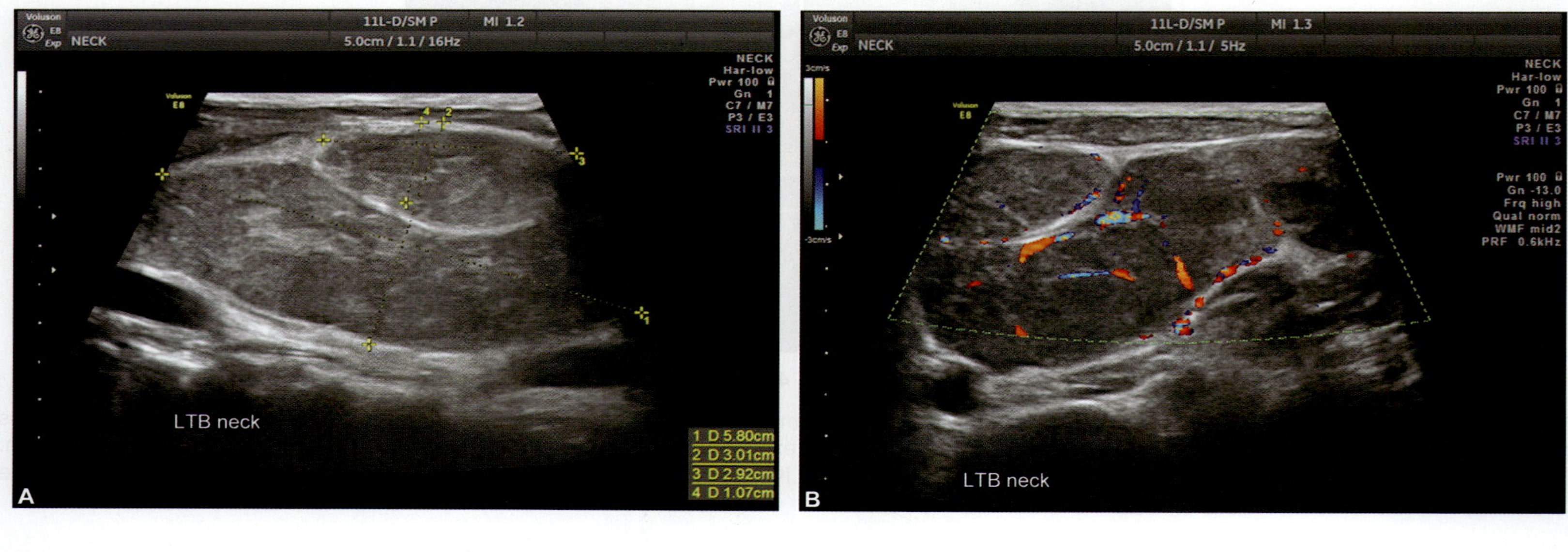

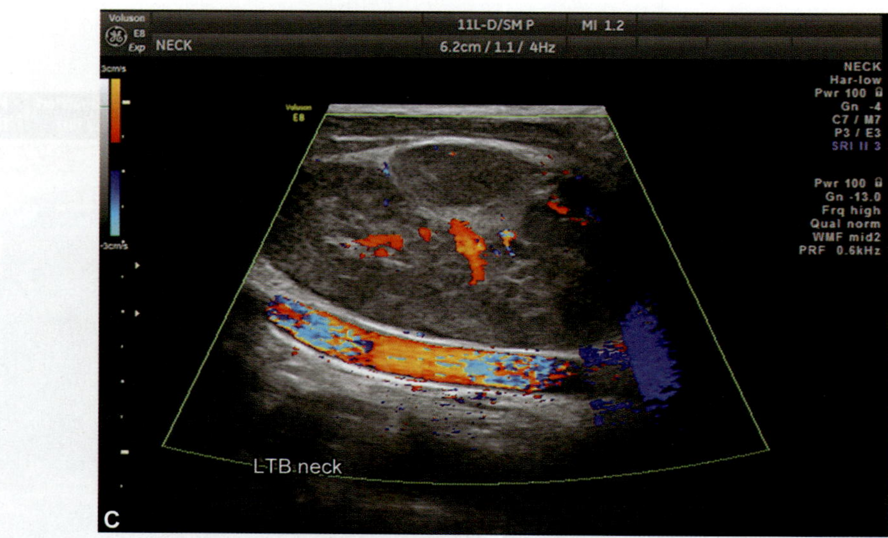

FIGURES 4.83A to C: A patient presented with nodular masses in left side of neck. HRSG shows multiple enlarged nodal shadows in the left side of the neck. They are hypoechoic in texture. They appear to be enlarged lymph nodes forming a mass. No necrosis is seen in them. No cystic degeneration is seen. Few enlarged nodes are also seen on the right side. But no necrosis is seen in them. On color flow imaging, low flow is seen in them.

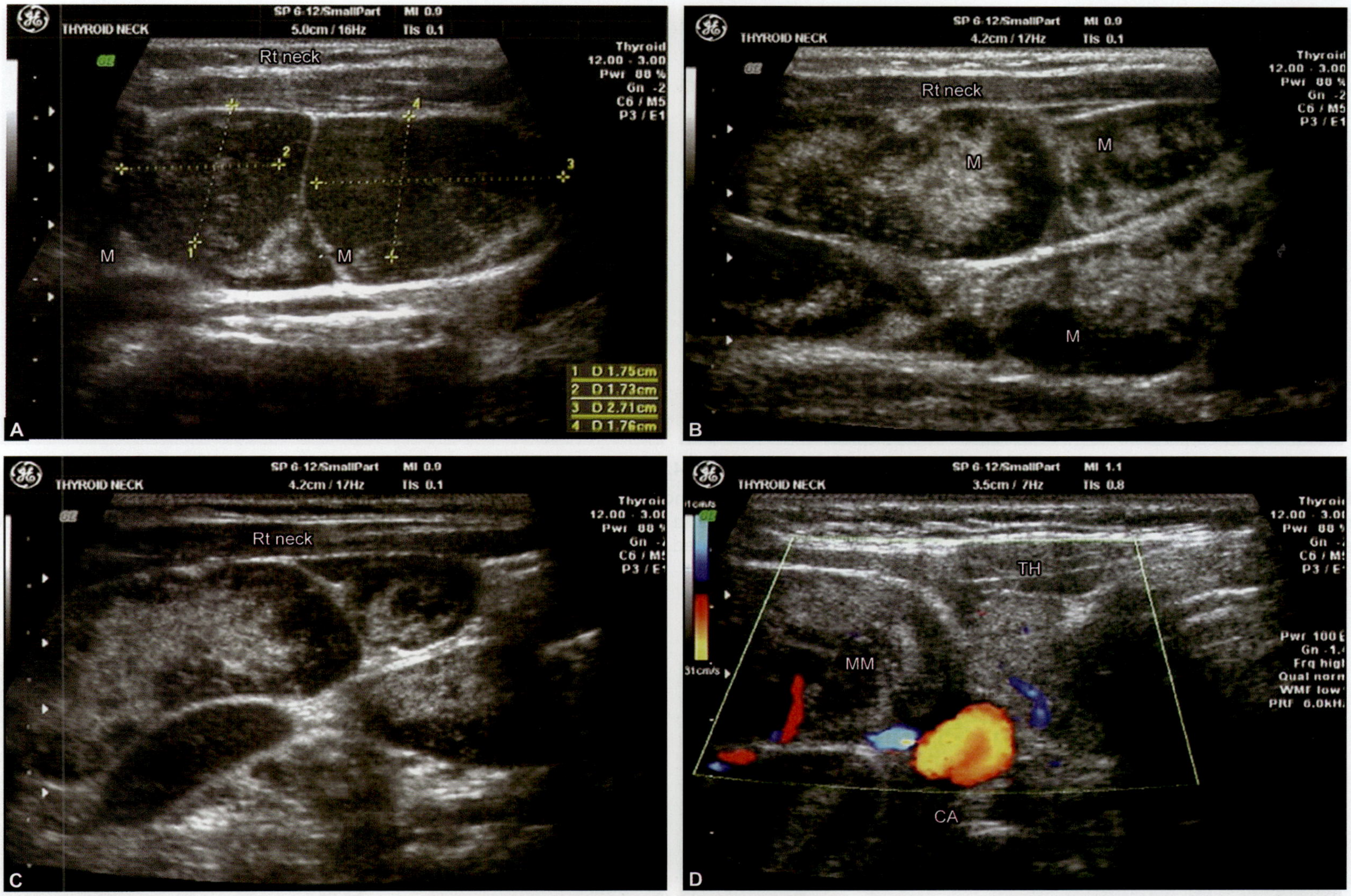

FIGURES 4.84A to D: Malignant enlarged lymph nodes in the neck. An old lady presented with multiple enlarged nodes in the right side of the neck. HRSG shows heterogeneous nodal enlargements. The nodes have lost the normal texture. The lymph node hilum is distorted. The ovoid shape of the node is lost. But no necrosis is seen in them. The color flow imaging shows the nodes are not invading the neck vessels. They are separate from the thyroid gland. Biopsy of the node shows metastatic nodal mass.

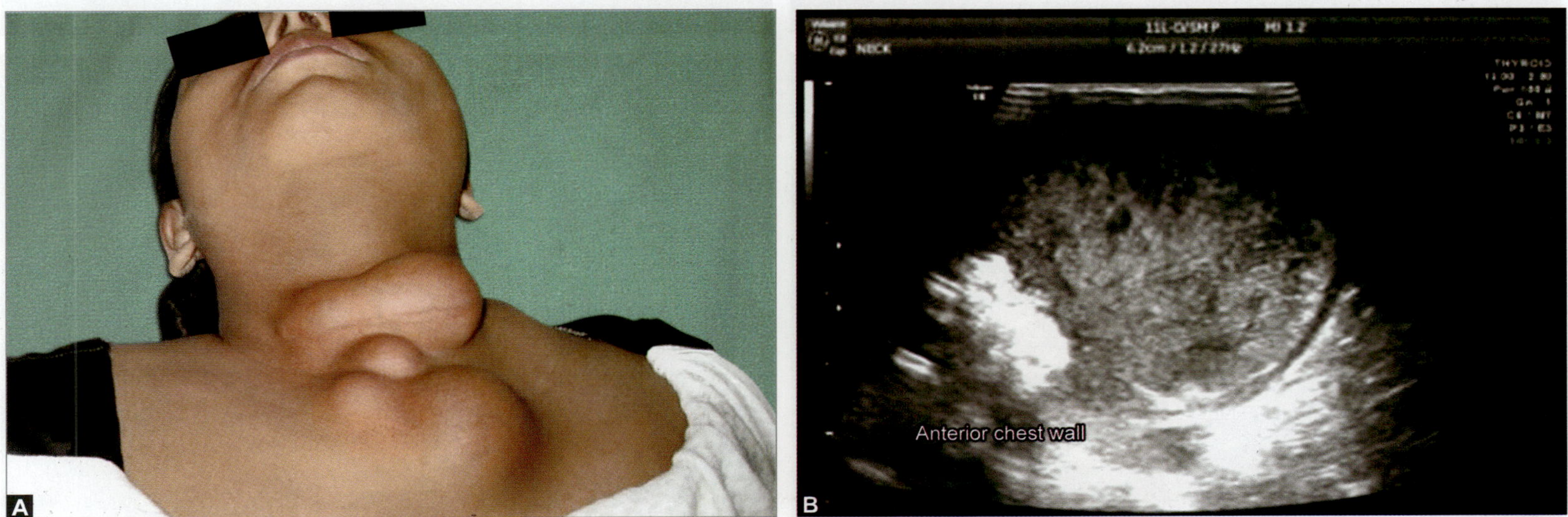

FIGURES 4.85A and B

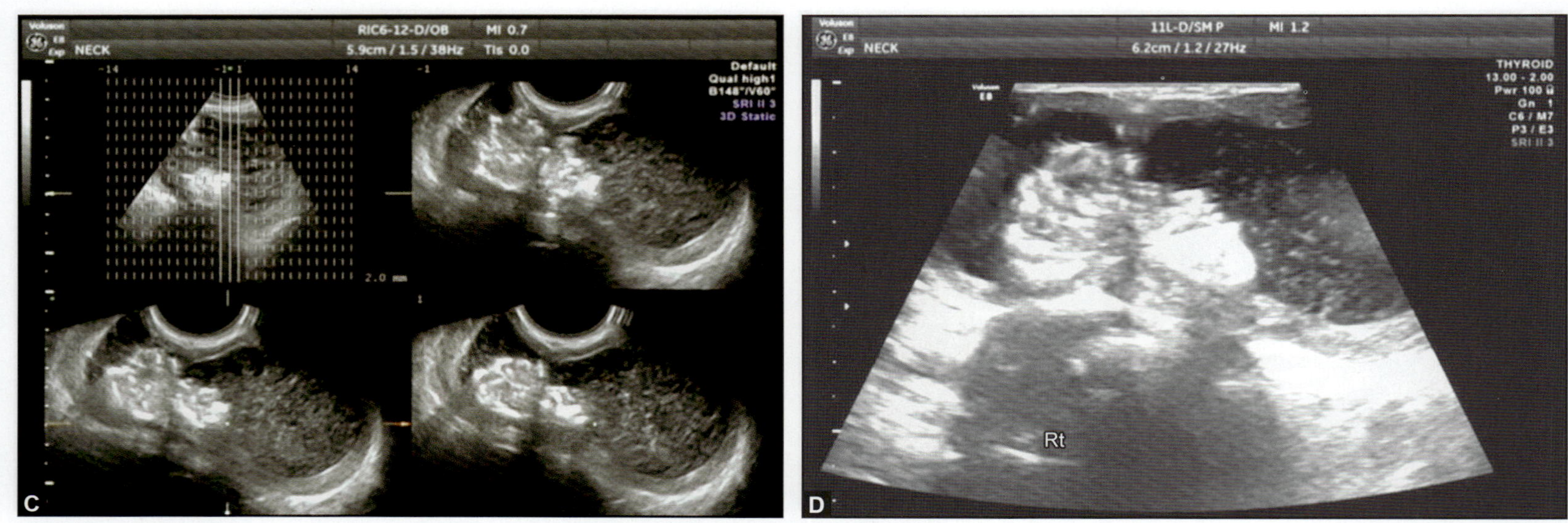

FIGURES 4.85C and D

FIGURES 4.85A to D: A young girl and known case of medullary carcinoma thyroid presented with multiple masses in the neck and suprasternal region. HRSG shows big low level echo complex masses in the neck and suprasternal region. Cystic degeneration is also seen in them. Soft tissue shadows are seen in the masses. Normal anatomic relations are distorted. Aspiration biopsy confirms recurrence of disease.

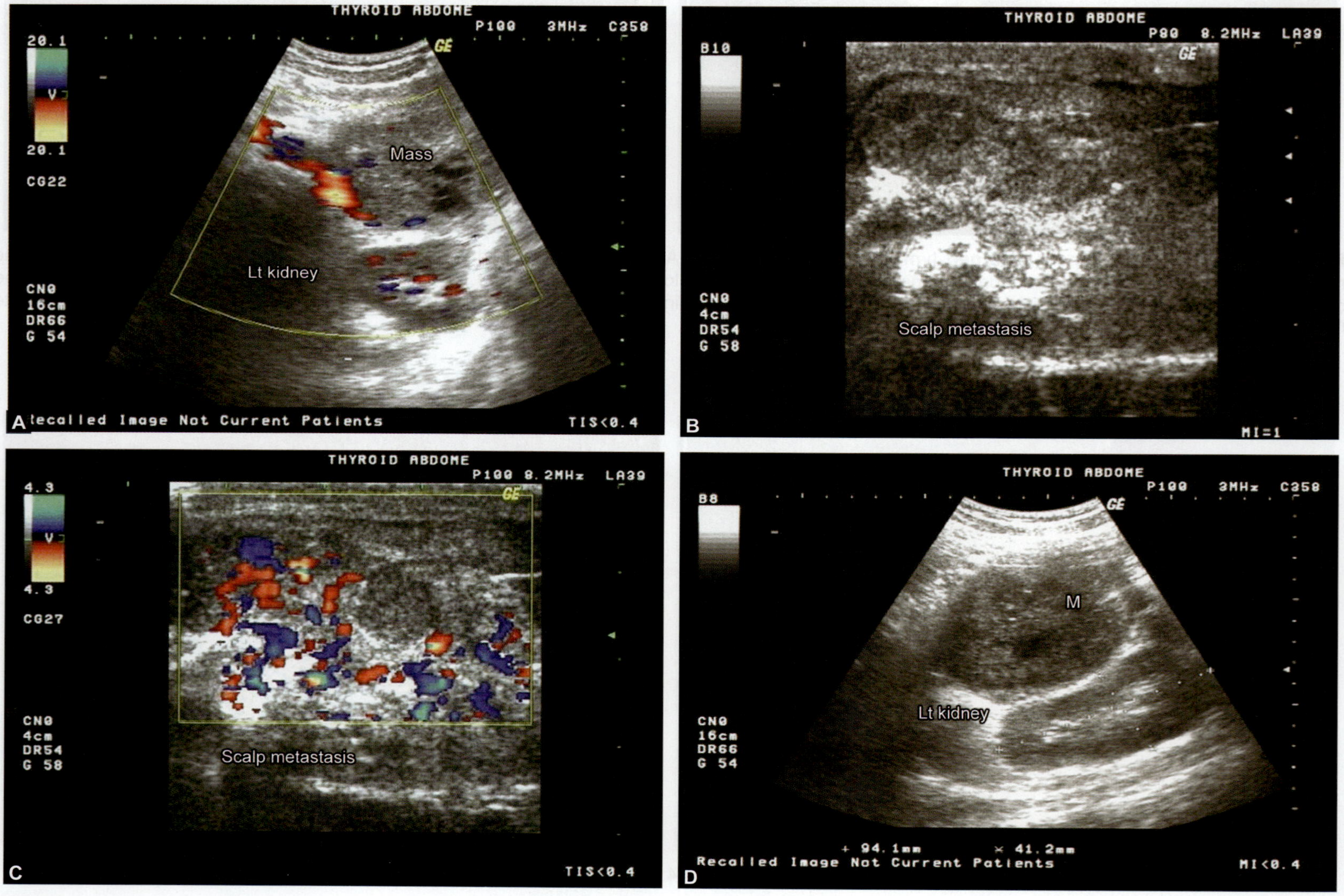

FIGURES 4.86A to D: Adrenal tumor metastasizing to scalp. HRSG shows a big irregular hypoechoic mass lesion in the left adrenal area. A well-defined hypoechoic mass is seen anterior to the left kidney. It has pushed the kidney down. However, renal outline is maintained. Biopsy of the mass shows adrenal tumor. HRSG of scalp of the same patient shows an irregular hypodense mass over the left scalp. It is irregular in outline with multiple hypodense areas. On color flow imaging, increased flow is seen in the mass. Biopsy of the mass shows metastatic deposits from the adrenal tumor.

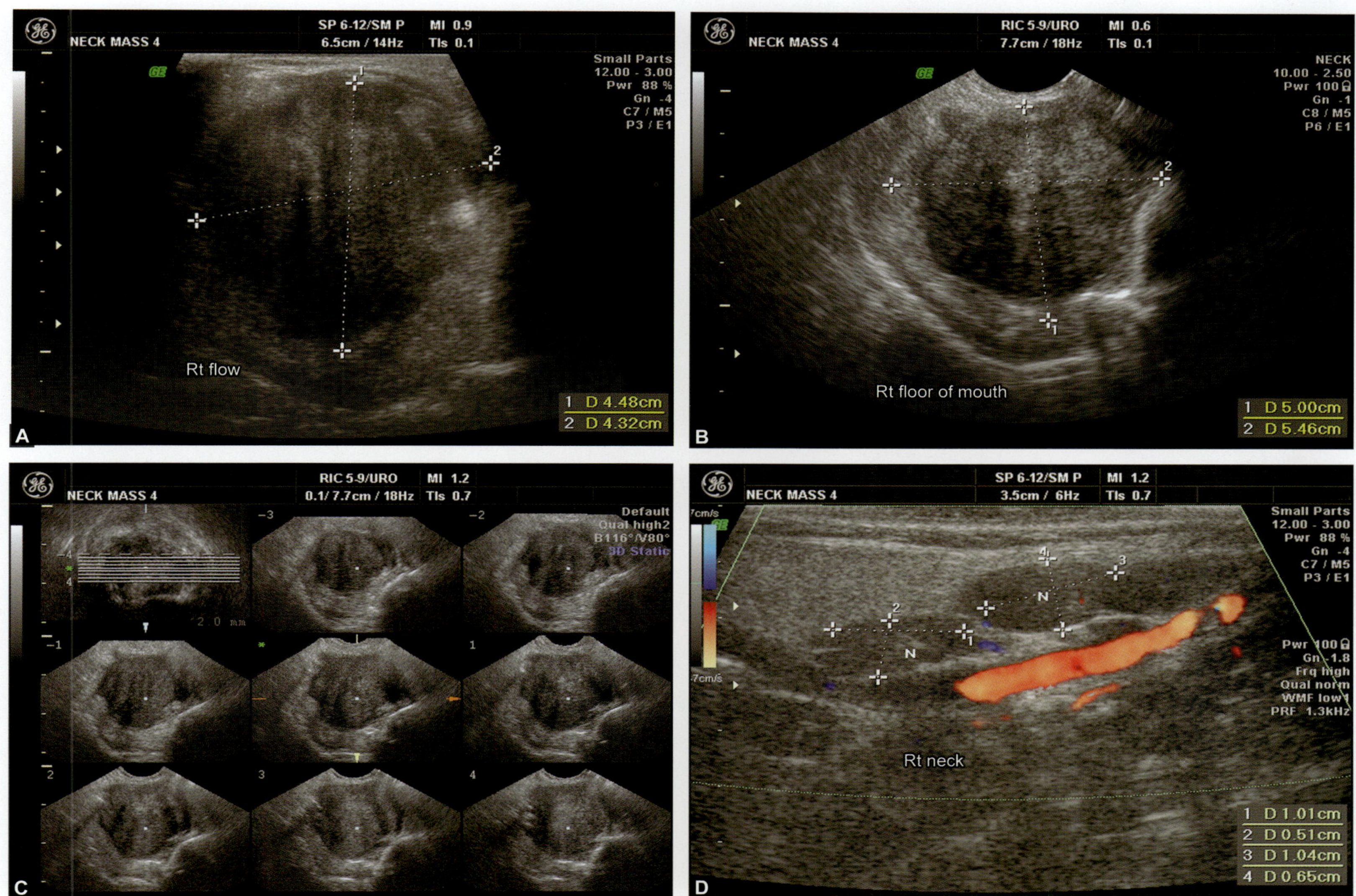

FIGURES 4.87A to D: A patient presented with soft tissue mass in the right side of the neck. HRSG shows a well-defined homogeneous hypoechoic mass on the right side of the mouth. It shows thick capsule. The mass shows homogeneous central area. Few calcified specks are seen in the mass. The mass is separate from the left submandibular gland. It appears to be separate from the tounge and also from right submandibular gland, right parotid gland. It is also separate from the thyroid. No necrosis is seen in the mass. On color flow imaging, no flow is seen in it. There is evidence of few enlarged nodes are seen in the right submental region. They appear to be homogeneous in texture.

CONCLUSION

HRSG is an important, rapid, noninvasive imaging technique to evaluate cervical lymph nodes in head and neck cancer patients. Most diseased nodes can be detected on HRSG. When sonographic criteria fail to differentiate between benign and metastatic nodes, USG-guided FNAC confirms the diagnosis. It is also very good tool to assess postsurgical or postirradiated neck for recurrence of disease. HRSG is an excellent modality for evaluating other neck masses including the salivary glands. It is first line of investigation in neck masses.

CHAPTER 5

Salivary Glands

PK Srivastava

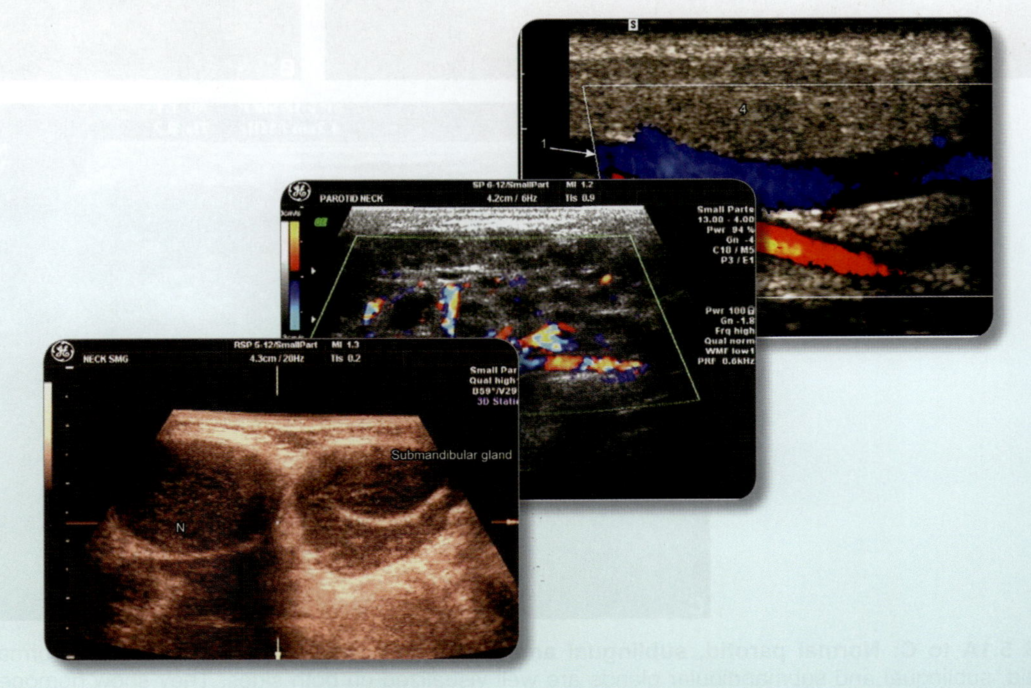

High-resolution ultrasonography is capable to image all the three major salivary glands, i.e. parotid, submandibular and sublingual glands. It can detect most of the lesions affecting them. A 7.5 or 10 MHz transducer is the ideal transducer to detect salivary glands. The gland can be imaged in multiple planes like axial, longitudinal or cross-section or oblique planes.

The parotid glands are the largest salivary glands. They lie over the ramus of mandible on each side. Each gland has got two lobes. One superficial lobe which rests over ramus of mandible and another deep lobe which is seen behind the ramus in between the mastoid and stern mastoid muscle and in front of the styloid process. The gland shows a homogeneous texture. It is more echogenic than the surrounding muscles. The margins of the gland are not well defined, and the retro-pharyngeal portions of the gland cannot be evaluated on HRSG. The parotid duct can be resolved on HRSG running in the substance of the gland longitudinally. However, the intraglandular portion of facial nerve is seen only in 30% of the cases. Small lymph nodes are commonly present in the gland, which can be seen as hypoechoic nodular shadow on HRSG. The submandibular gland is seen below the jaw and sublingual glands are seen in the floor of the mouth. They have got the similar echotexture to that of parotid gland. Sublingual glands are difficult to be resolved on HRSG. They can be seen as small triangular solid echogenic nodules in the floor of the mouth in axial scanning.

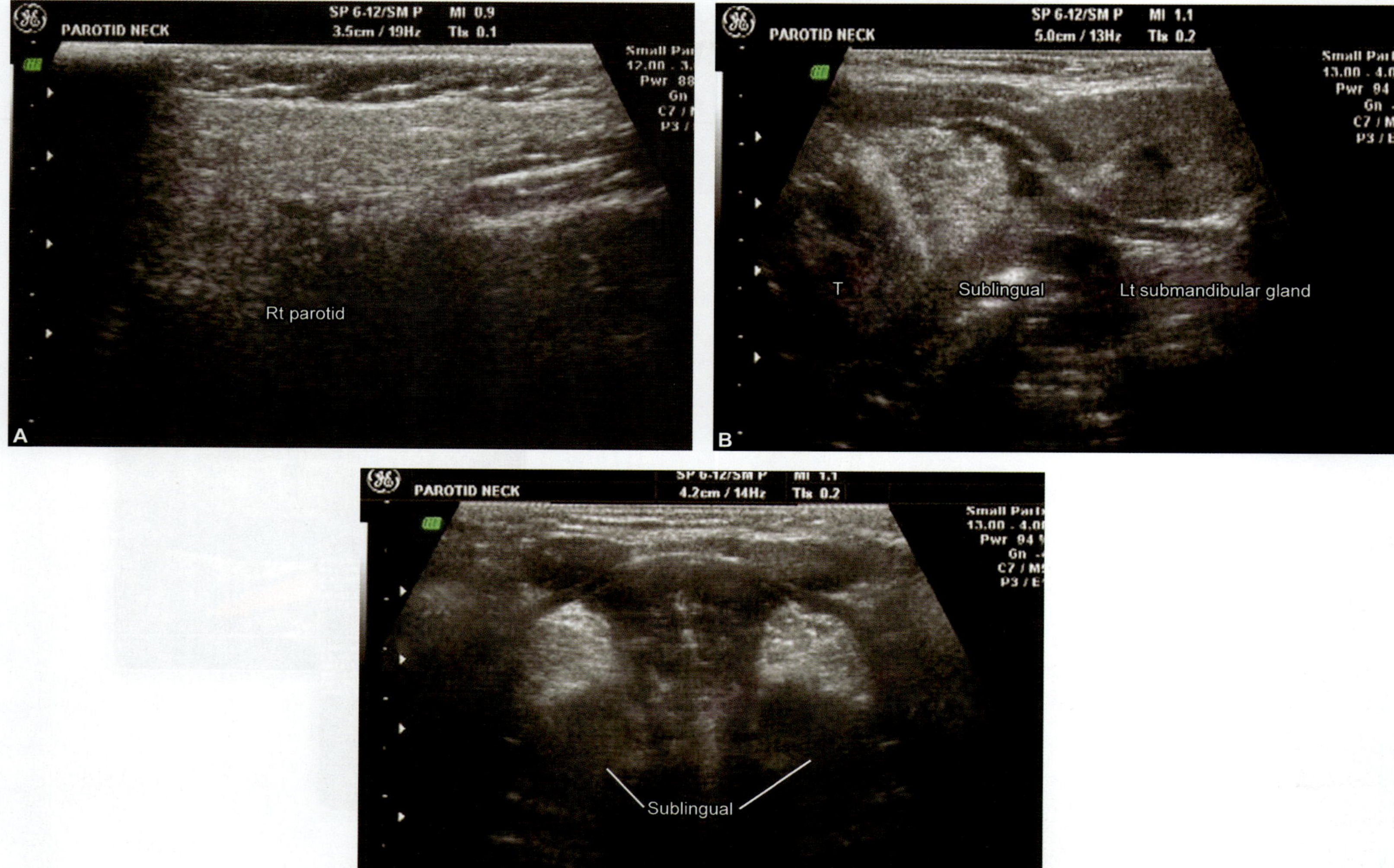

FIGURES 5.1A to C: Normal parotid, sublingual and submandibular glands. HRSG shows normal sonographic appearance of salivary glands. The parotid, sublingual and submandibular glands are well visualized on both sides. They show homogeneous texture with medium level echoes. Fine granular texture is seen in the gland. Few hypoechoic areas are seen in the gland may be because of vessels or dilated ductules.

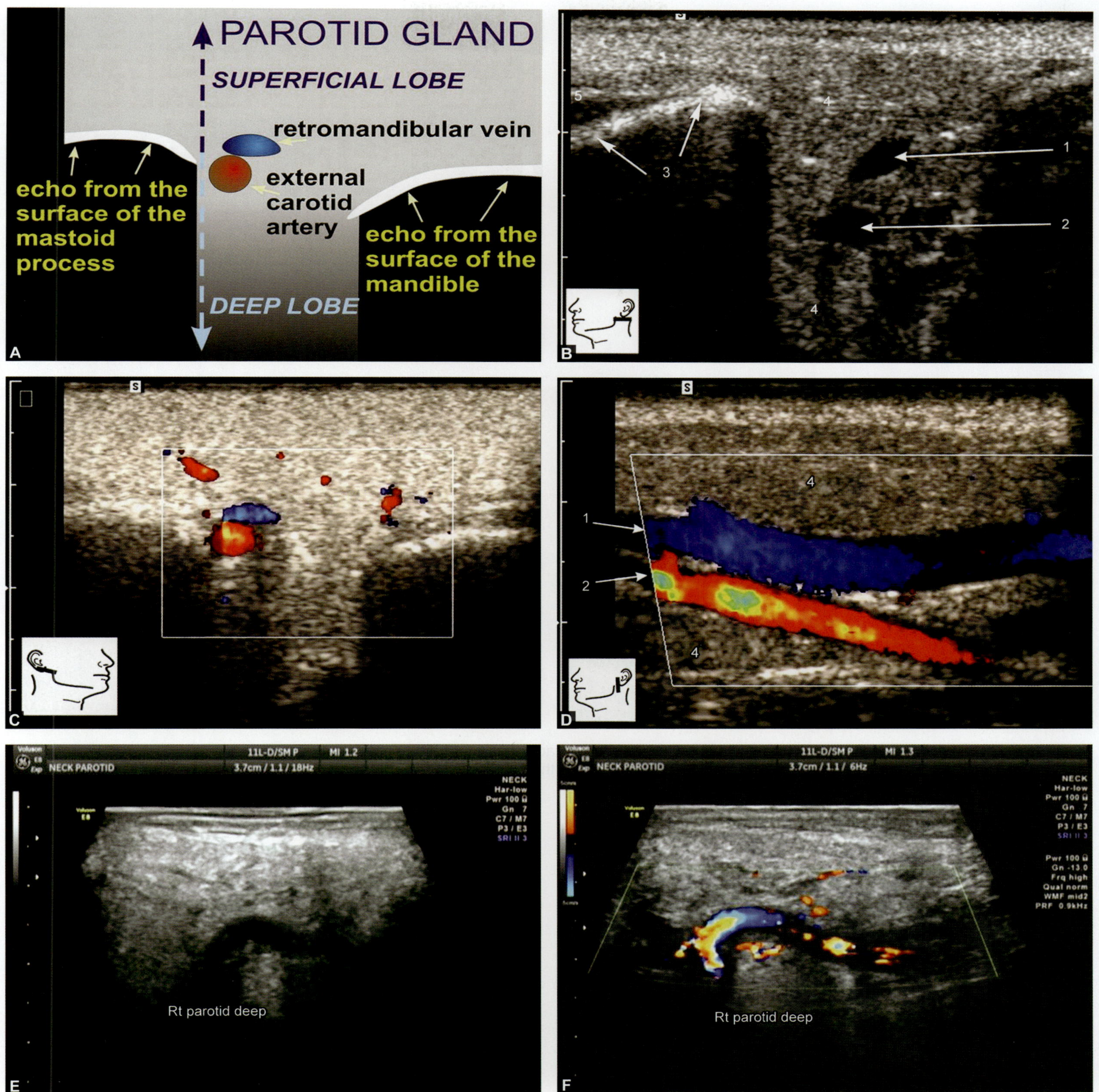

FIGURES 5.2A to F: Figure A shows normal diagrammatic representation of superficial lobe of parotid gland with its relation with mastoid process and ramus of mandible. Figures C and D show sonographic appearance of superficial lobe of parotid. 3: Mastoid process. 4: Gland, 1 and 2: Vessels. Figures E and F show deep lobe of parotid with vessels running through the gland.

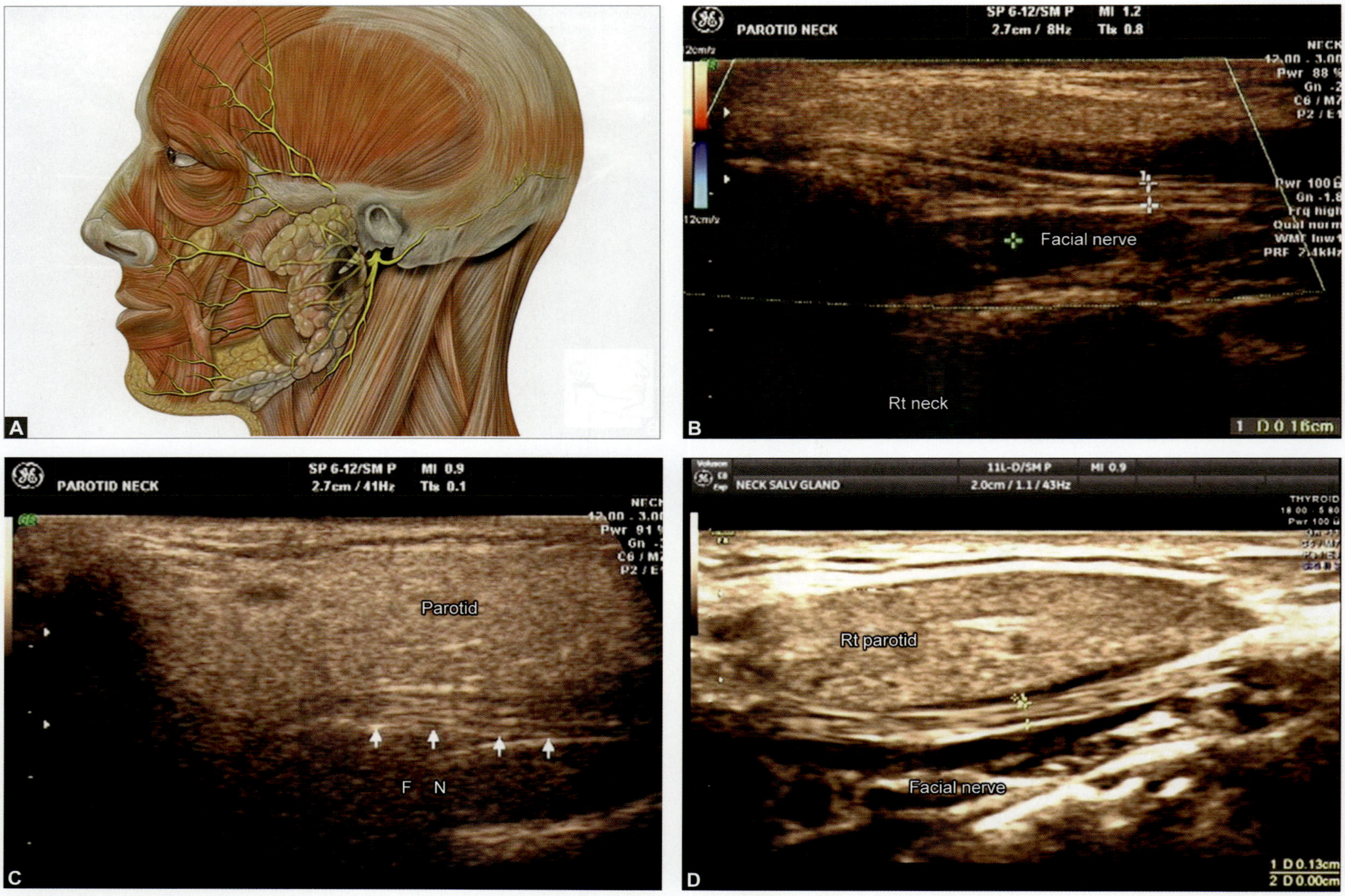

FIGURES 5.3A to D: Figure A shows diagrammatic representation of facial nerve and its relation with parotid gland. HRSG shows facial nerve running in relation to the parotid gland. Branches of the facial nerve are also seen beautifully in the gland.

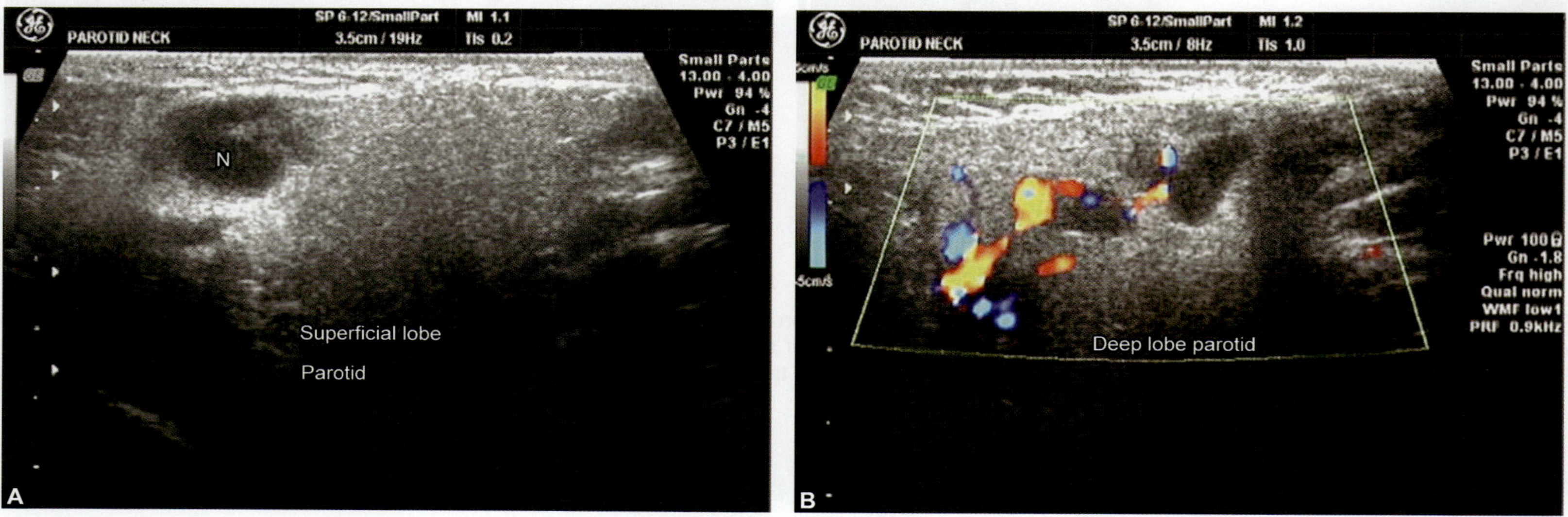

FIGURES 5.4A and B

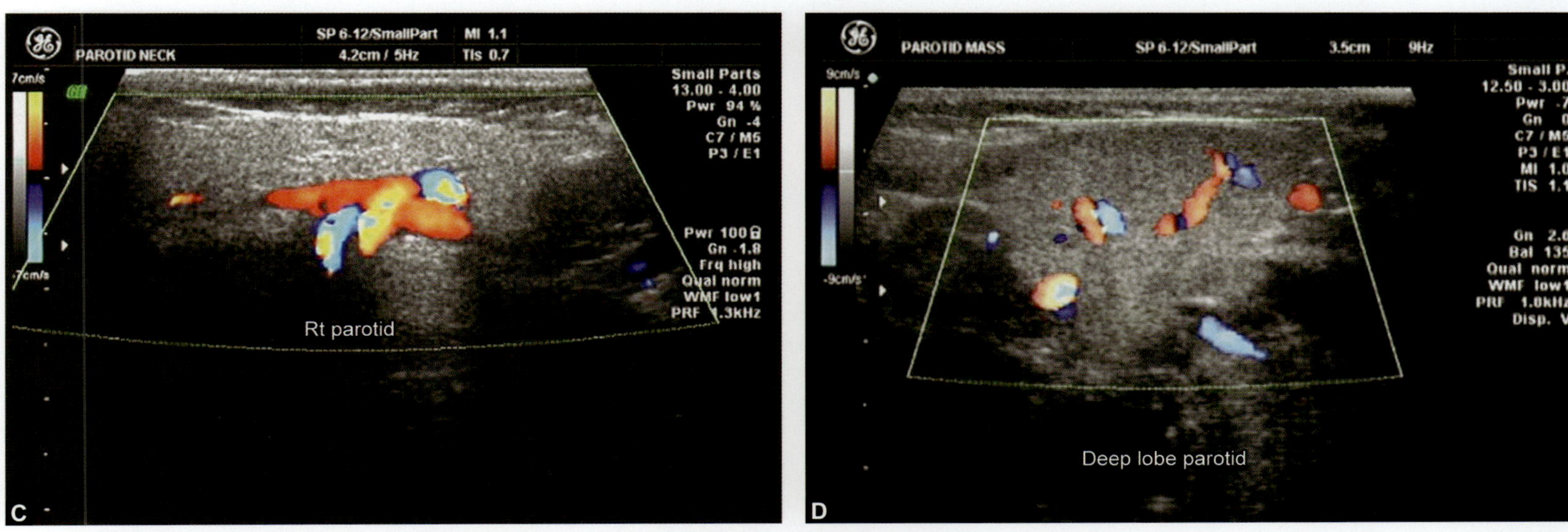

FIGURES 5.4C and D

FIGURES 5.4A to D: Normal parotid gland with sentinel node. HRSG shows normal parotid gland. A hypoechoic nodular shadow is seen in the outer lateral border of the gland, which is the sentinel node. The vessels are also seen running through the gland.

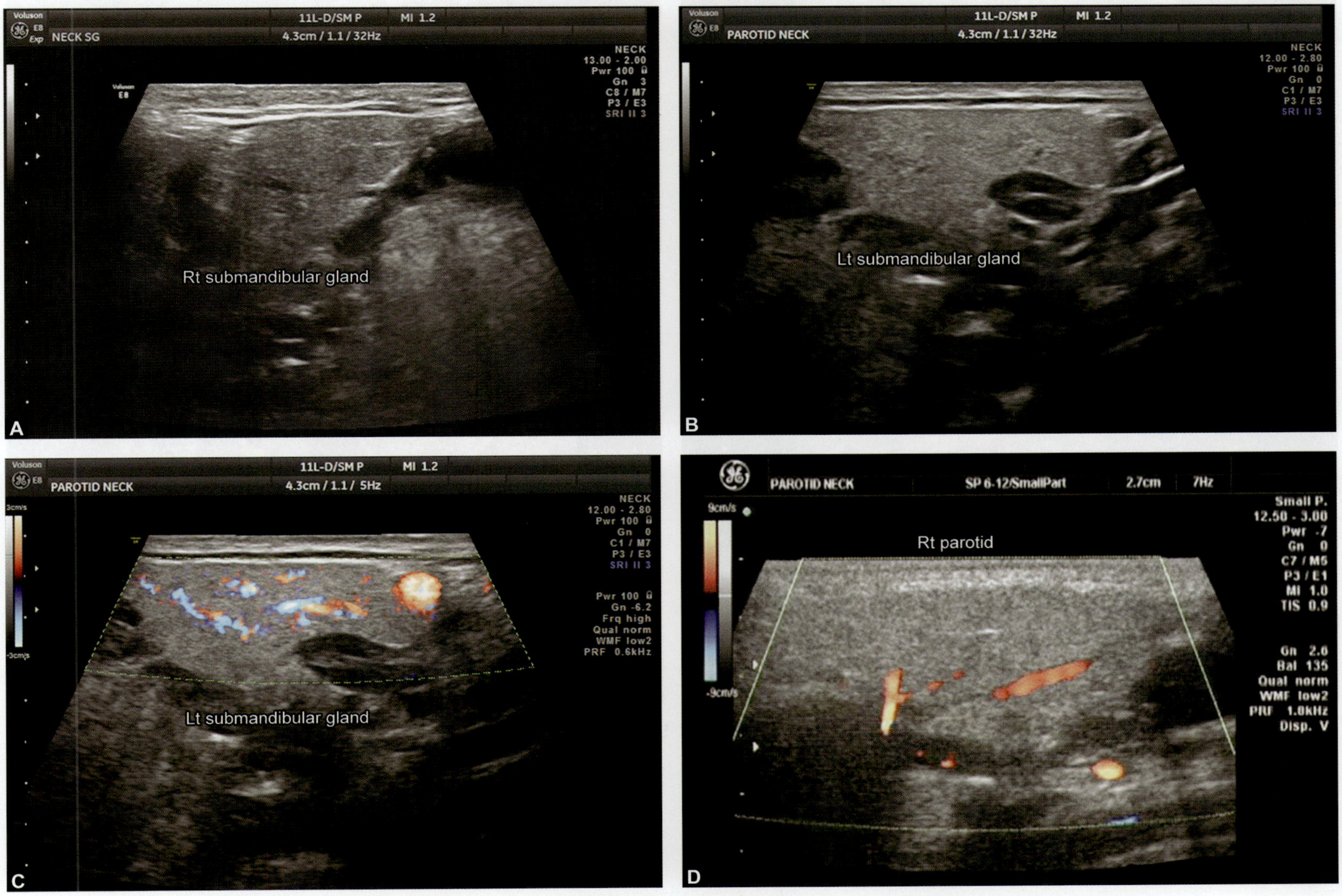

FIGURES 5.5A to D: Normal submandibular gland. HRSG shows normal submandibular gland in the submandibular gland fossa. Vessels are seen running through the gland.

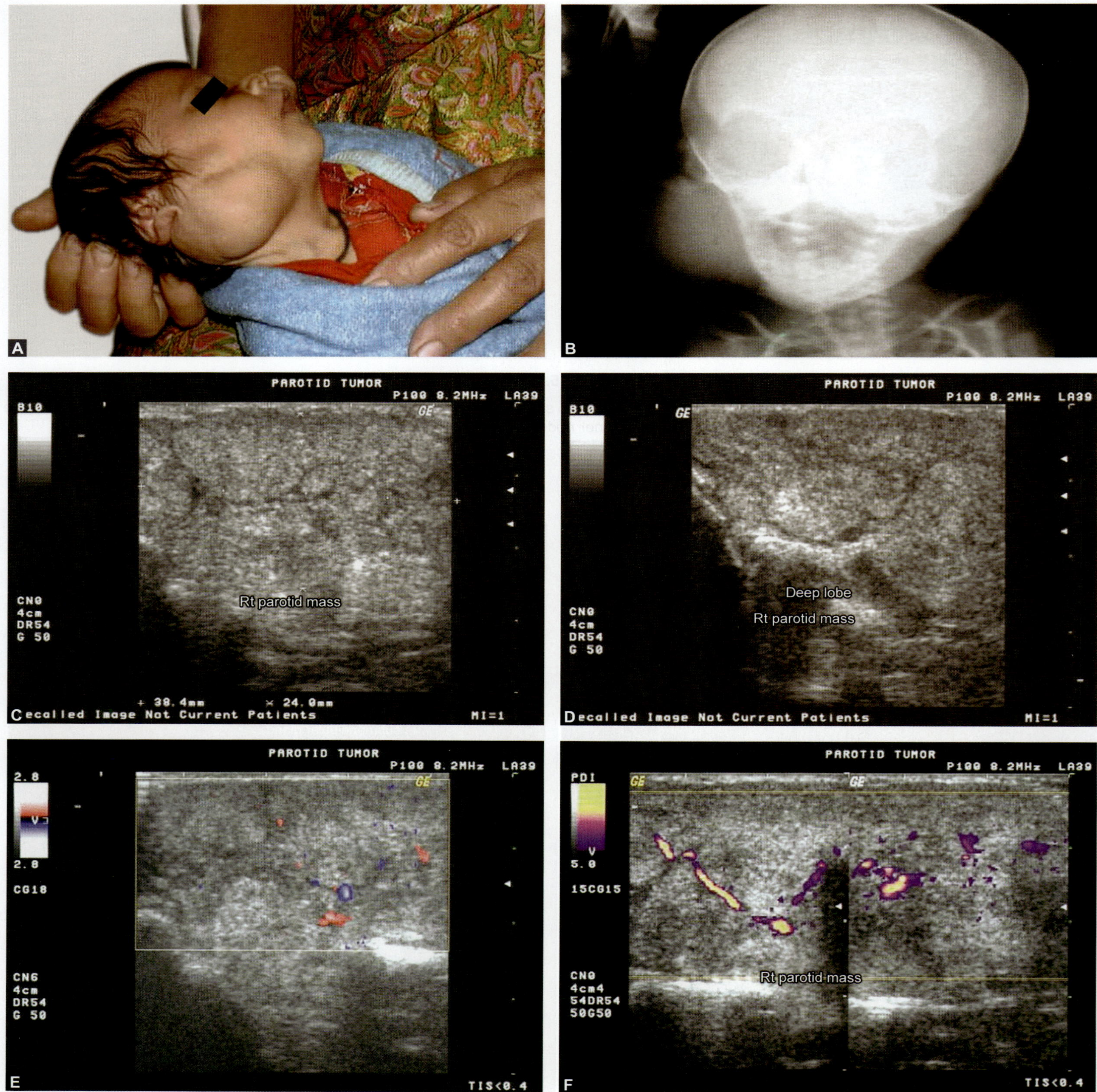

FIGURES 5.6A to F

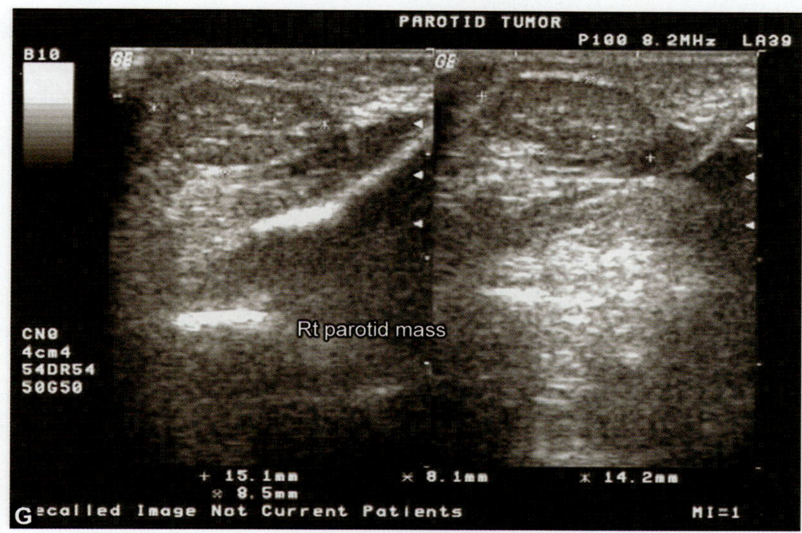

FIGURE 5.6G

FIGURES 5.6A to G: Plain X-ray of the head shows soft tissue mass over the right side of the neck. Skull bones are normal. HRSG shows a predominantly multilobulated solid mass in the right parotid region and upper cervical region. Few well-defined solid lobules are seen in the mass. No cystic degeneration is seen. HRSG shows the mass is going through the upper cervical area with multiple hypoechoic septa running in the mass. Color Doppler imaging shows little flow in the mass. Part of the normal glandular tissue is seen in the parotid mass.

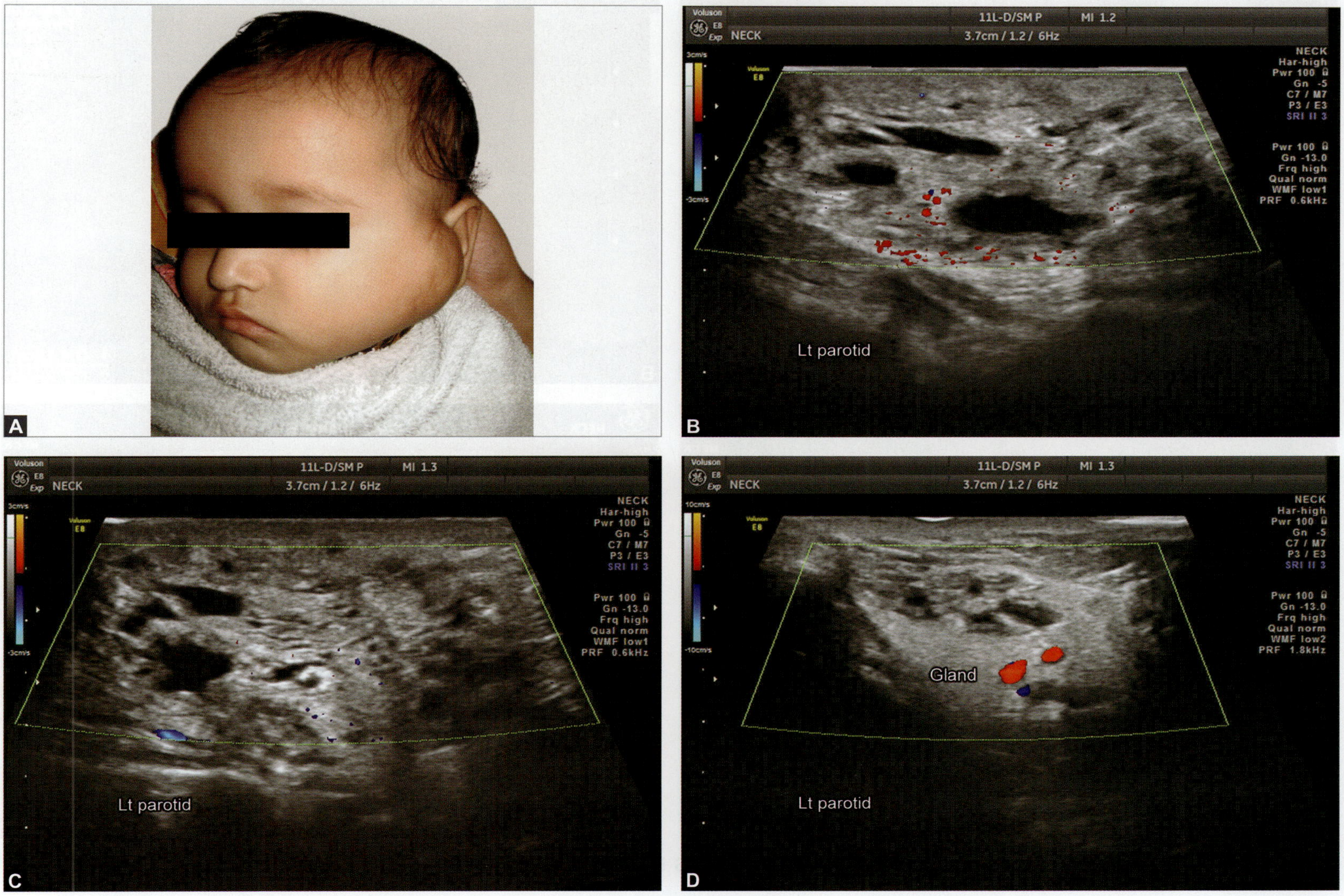

A

B

Lt parotid

C

Lt parotid

D

Gland

Lt parotid

FIGURES 5.7A to D

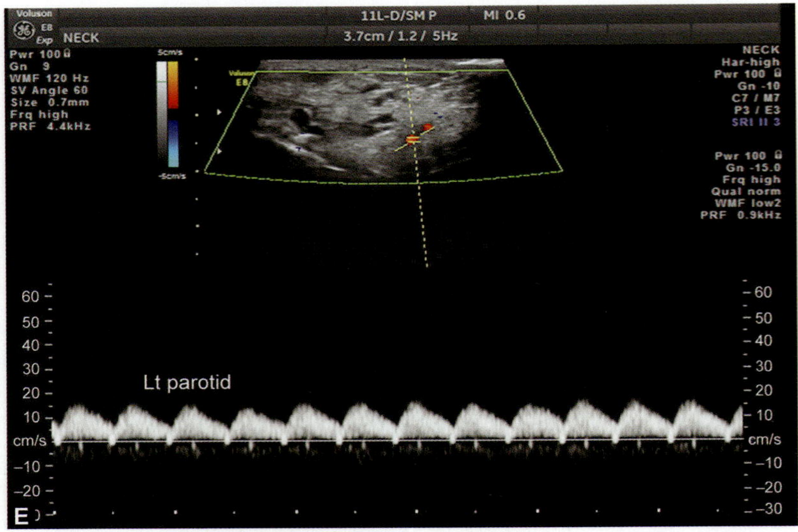

FIGURE 5.7E

FIGURES 5.7A to E: A 6-month-old baby presented with soft tissue swelling in left parotid gland. HRSG shows a multiloculated cystic mass in the left parotid gland. Low level echoes are seen in the cyst. On color flow imaging, few vessels are seen feeding the cyst wall. The FNAC from the mass confirms cystic hygroma.

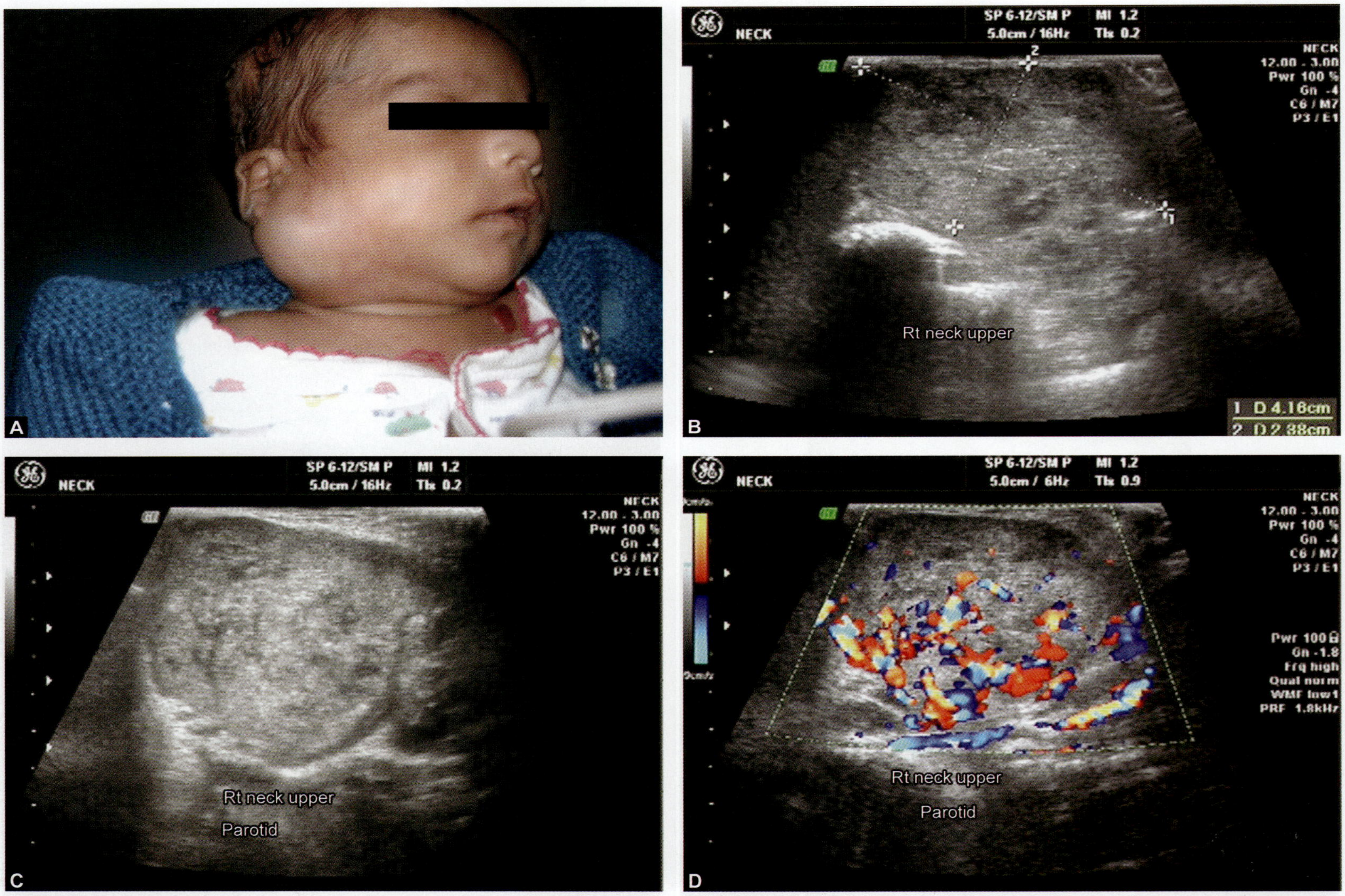

FIGURES 5.8A to D

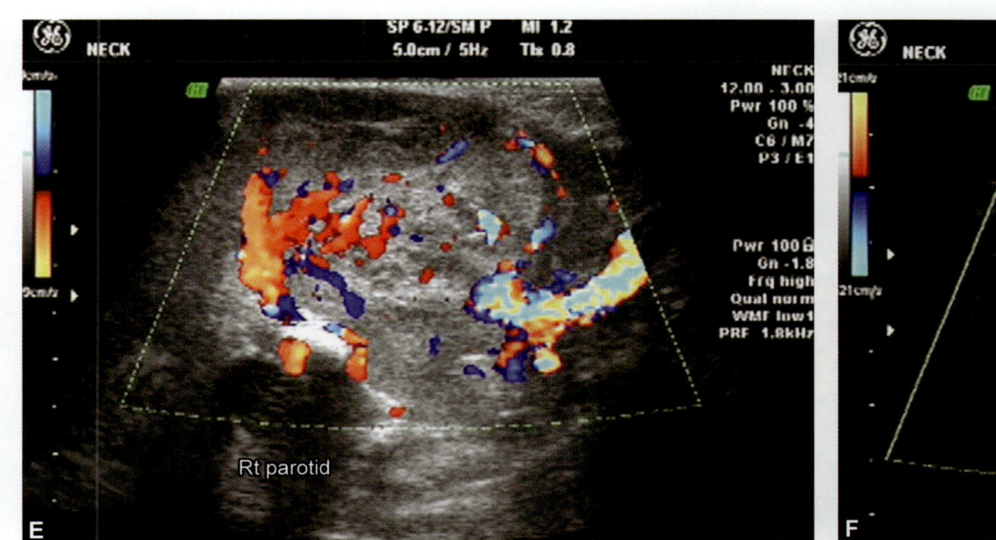

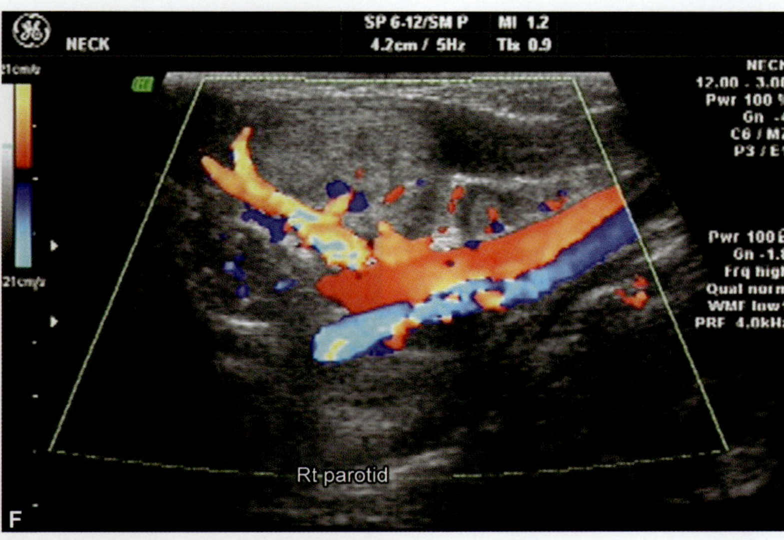

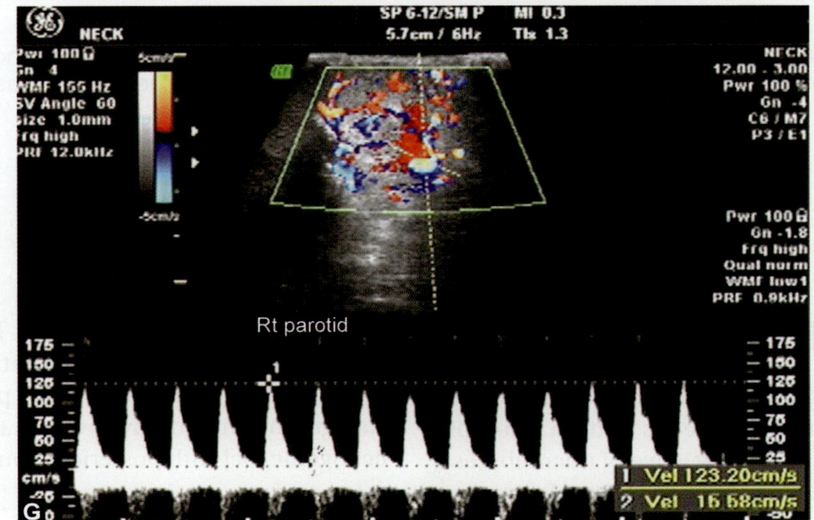

FIGURES 5.8E to G

FIGURES 5.8A to G: Angiolymphoma. A newborn baby presented with soft tissue mass in the right parotid gland. HRSG shows a predominantly solid mass in the right parotid gland. It shows hypoechoic areas. On color flow imaging, multiple vessels are seen feeding the mass. On spectral Doppler tracing, high flow is seen in the mass. FNAC of the mass confirms angiolymphoma.

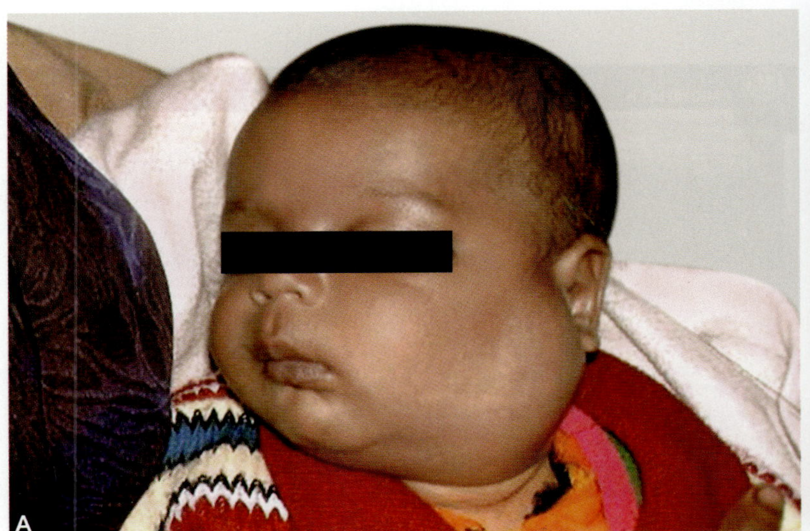

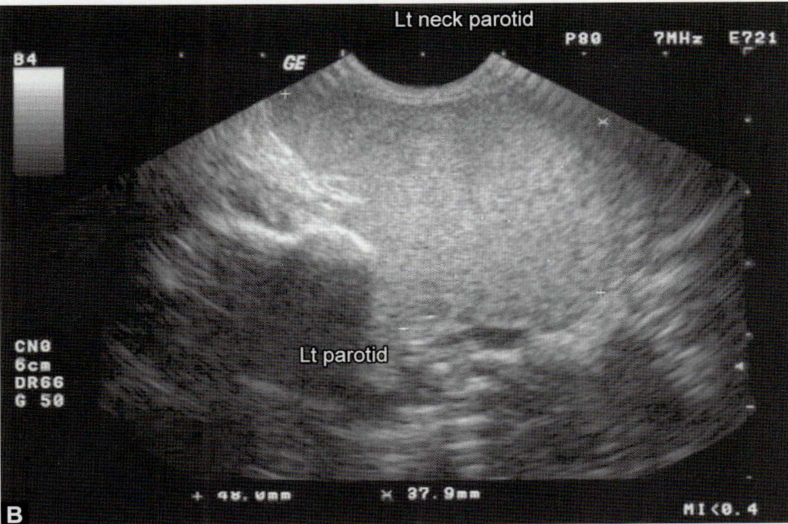

FIGURES 5.9A and B

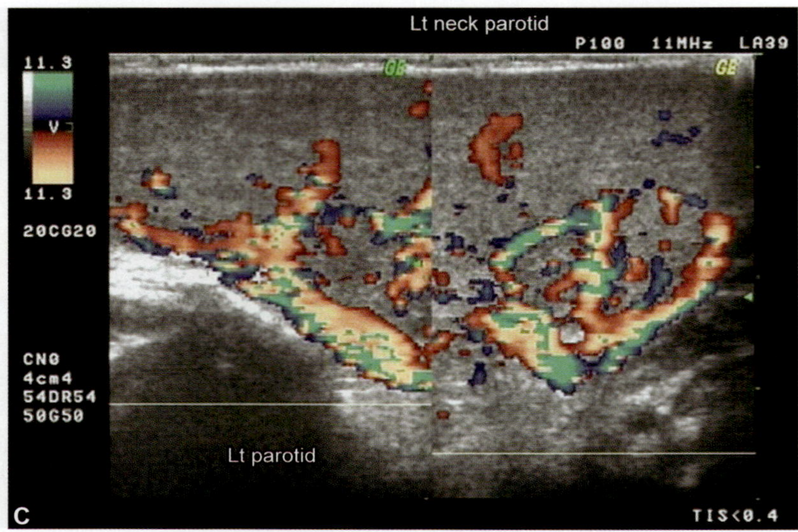

FIGURE 5.9C

FIGURES 5.9A to C: Angiolymphoma. A child was born with soft tissue mass over the parotid region. HRSG shows homogeneous soft tissue mass in the parotid region. Normal gland is not seen. **On color flow imaging,** multiple vessels are seen feeding the mass. Biopsy confirmed angiolymphoma.

ACUTE INFLAMMATION

In acute inflammation of parotid gland, it becomes enlarged and hypoechoic in texture and shows inhomogeneous pattern. Multiple hypoechoic pockets are seen in the gland suggestive of microabscess. Breaking down of glandular tissue may lead to large abscess formation.

It shows thick wall with low-level echo complex necrotic area. Ultrasonographic-guided aspiration of the pus can be done. Stone in the parotid duct can be easily picked up on HRSG. It is better than sialography and noninvasive in nature. The calculi are seen as a bright echogenic foci with posterior acoustic shadowing.

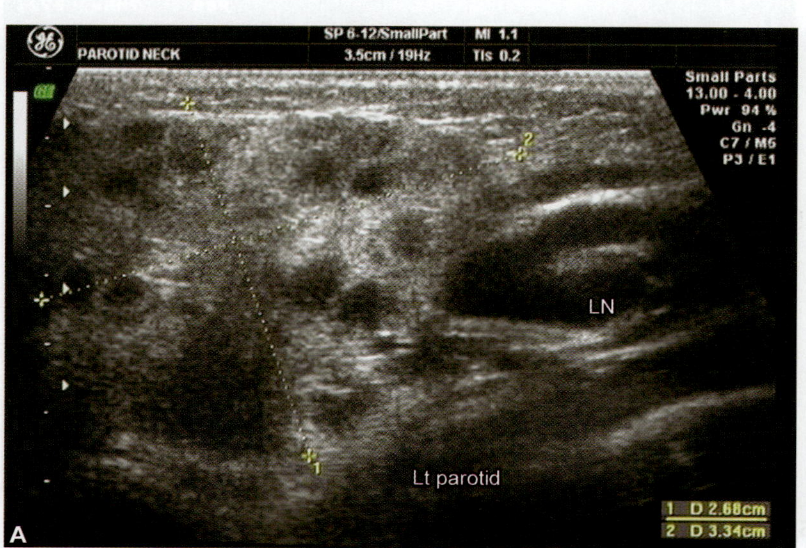

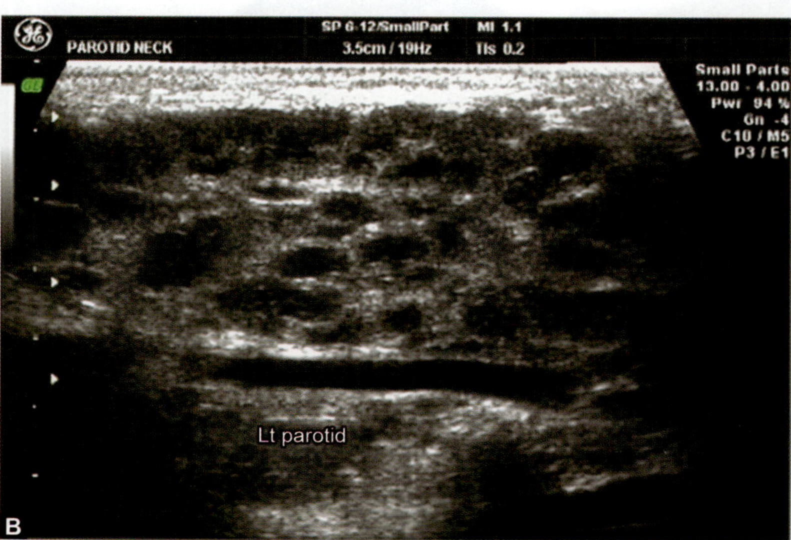

FIGURES 5.10A and B

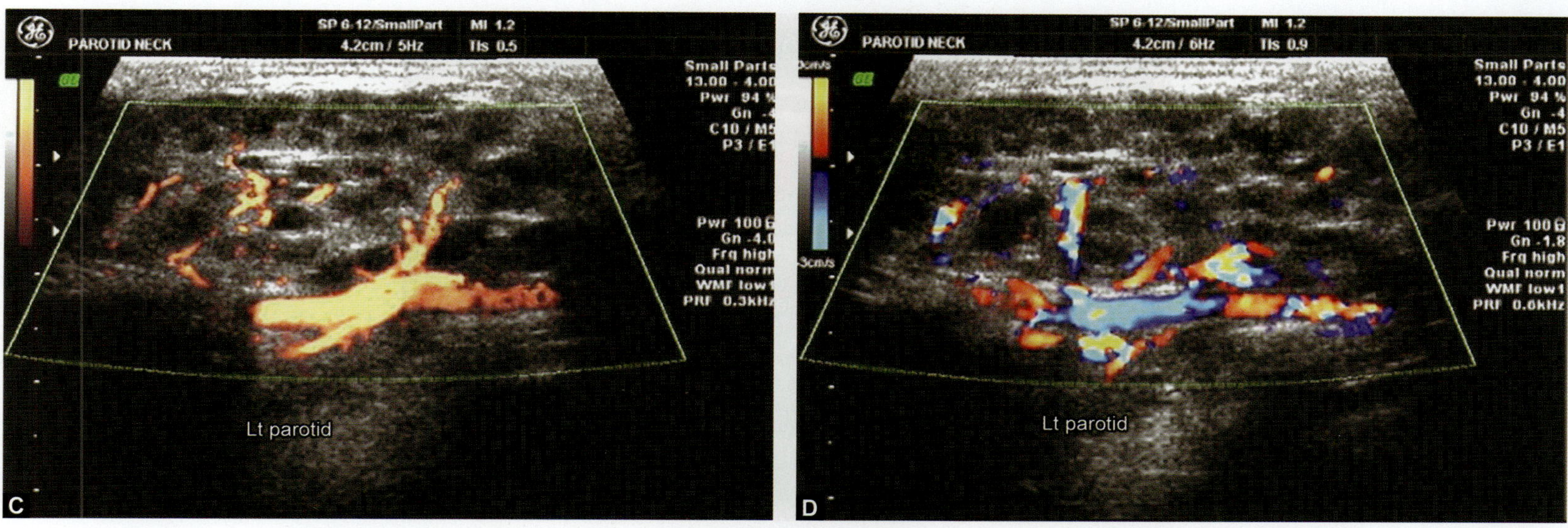

FIGURES 5.10C and D

FIGURES 5.10A to D: Acute inflammation in parotid gland. HRSG shows edematous hypoechoic enlargement of the left parotid gland. Margins are blurred in acute inflammation of the gland. Multiple hypoechoic foci are seen within the gland suggestive of small abscesses. HRSG shows heterogeneous enlargement of the left parotid gland with blurred outlines. Multiple small micro abscesses are seen in the gland. **On color Doppler imaging,** increased flow is in the gland suggestive of hyperemia.

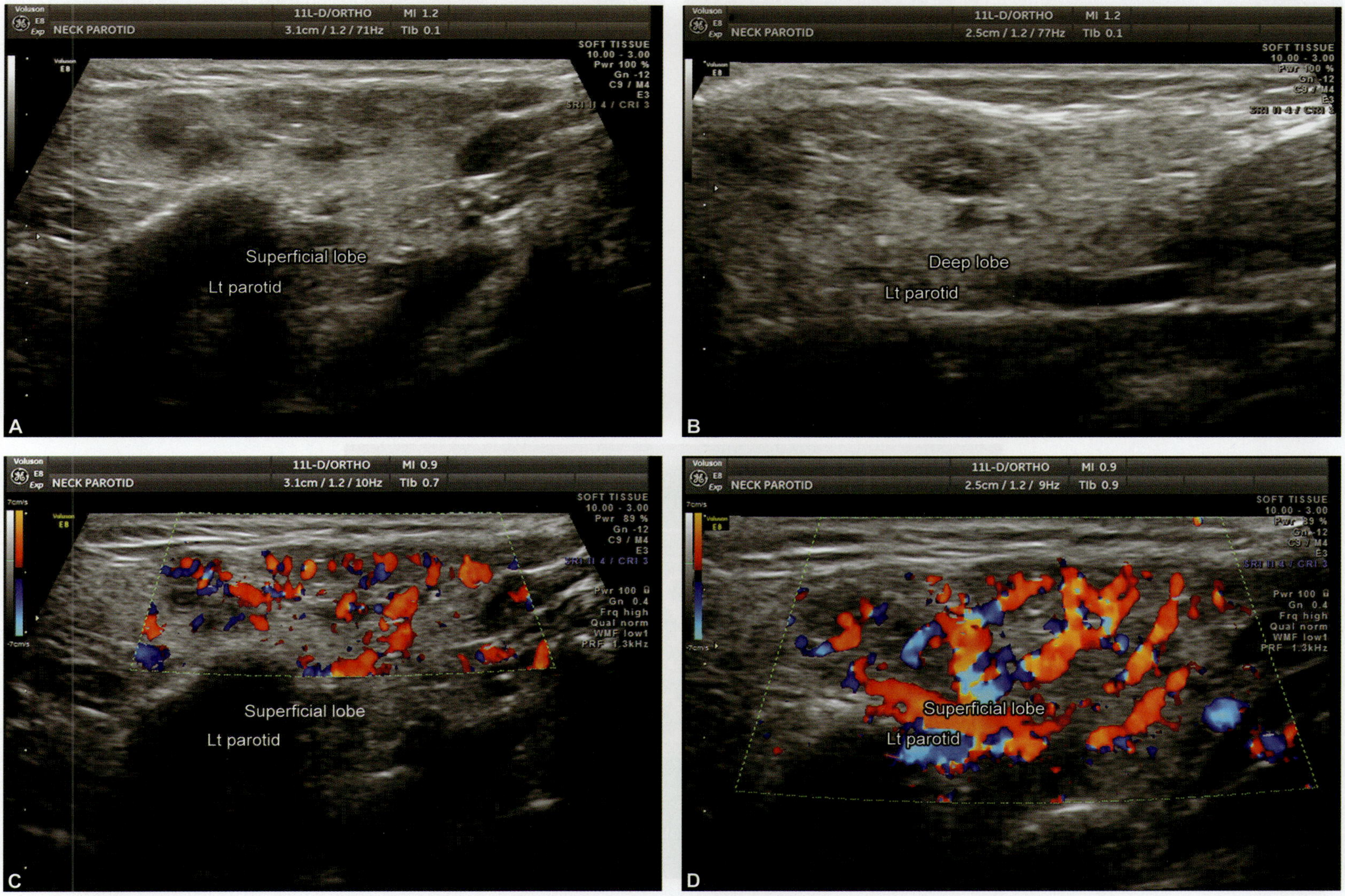

FIGURES 5.11A to D

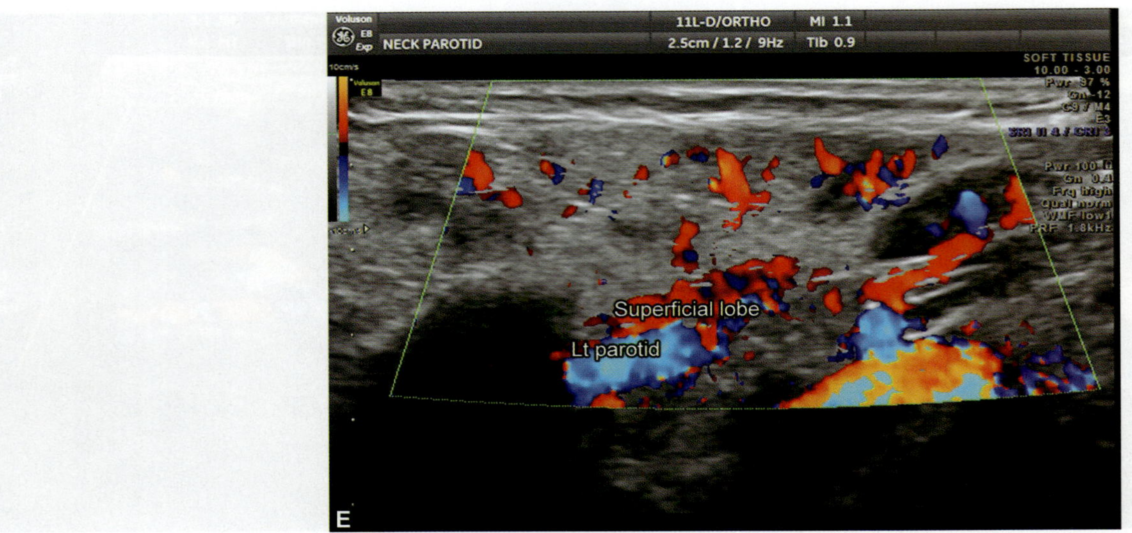

FIGURE 5.11E

FIGURES 5.11A to E: Acute inflammation of parotid gland. A 10-year-old girl presented with painful swelling in the left parotid gland. HRSG shows diffuse inflammation of superficial lobe of left parotid gland. The deep lobe is also seen hypoechoic and edematous. Small pockets are seen in the gland. On color flow imaging, multiple vessels are seen feeding the gland suggestive of acute inflammation of the gland.

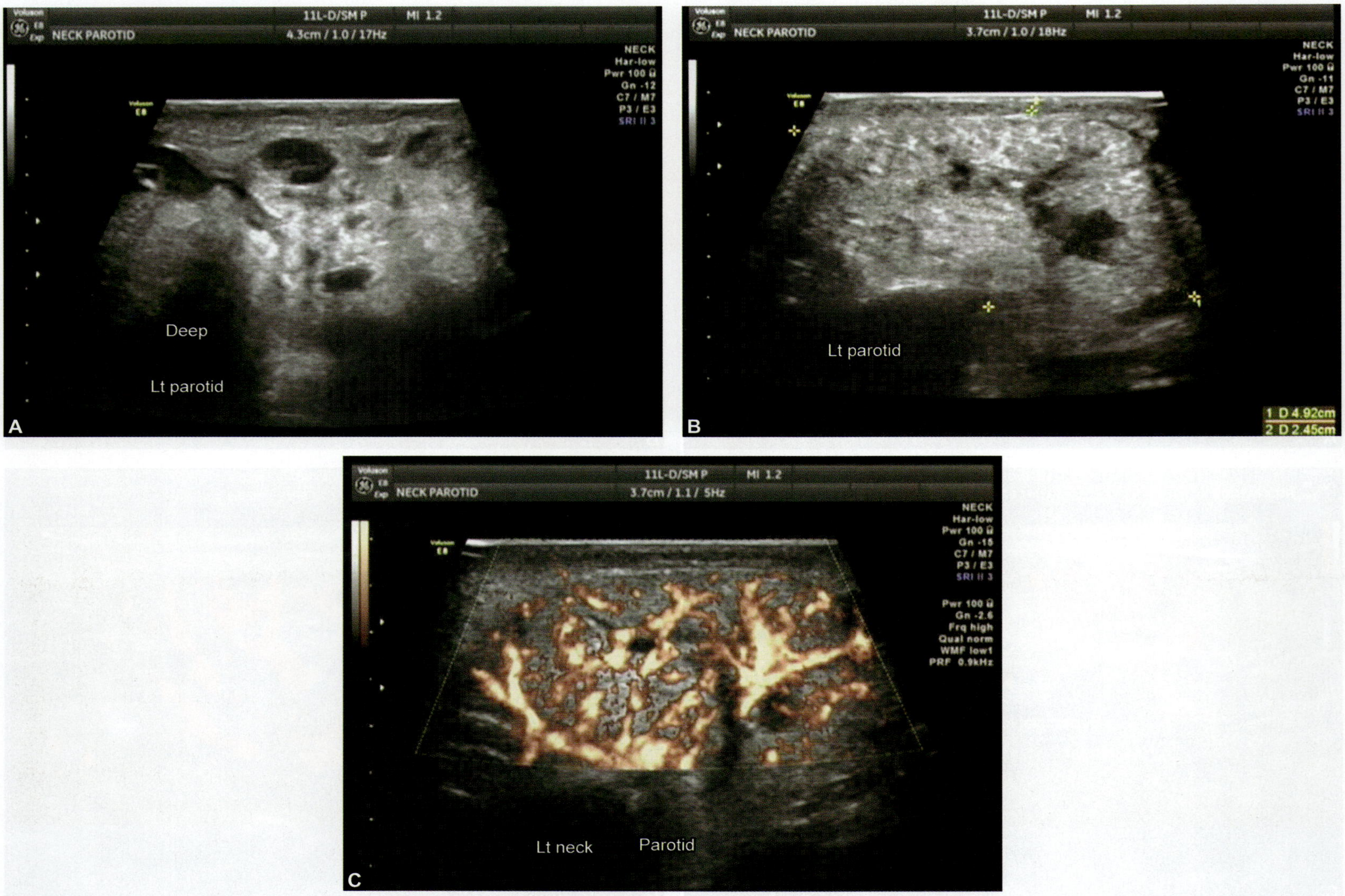

FIGURES 5.12A to C: Acute inflammation of deep lobe of parotid. A young girl presented with soft tissue swelling involving the deep lobe of gland. HRSG shows enlargement of the deep lobe. The gland is edematous. Hypoechoic areas are seen in the gland. Few hypoechoic pockets are seen suggestive of small abscess. On color flow imaging, increased flow is seen in the gland suggestive of acute suppurative parotitis.

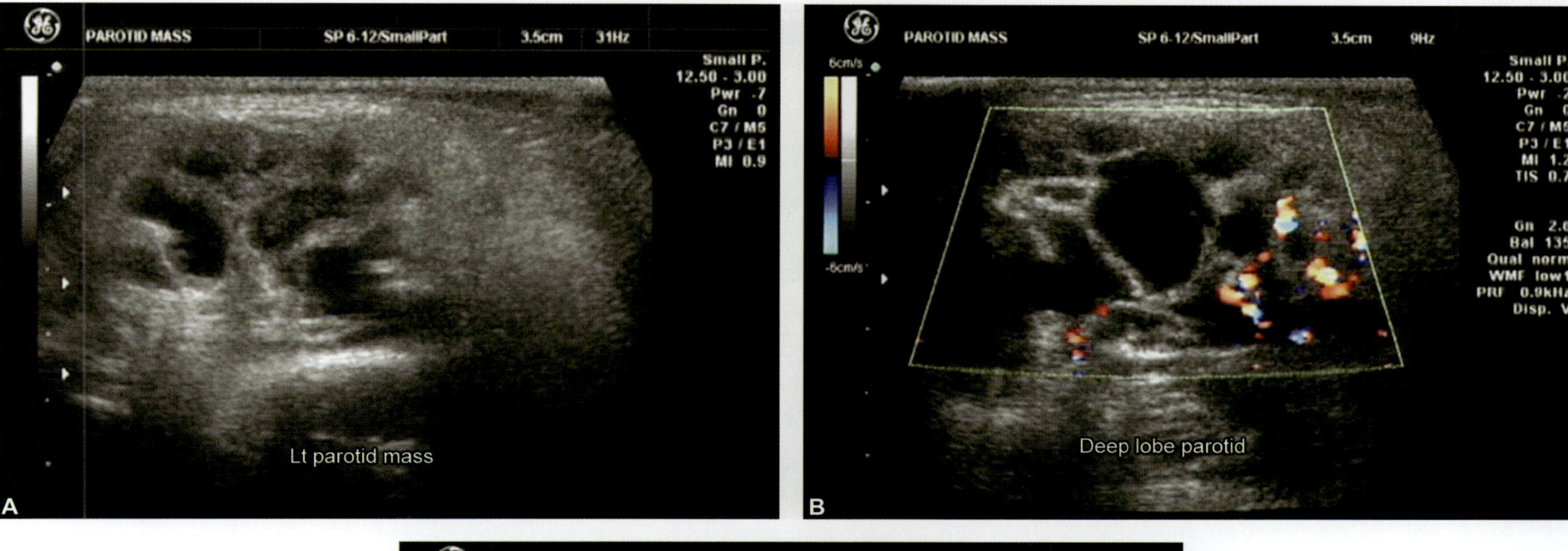

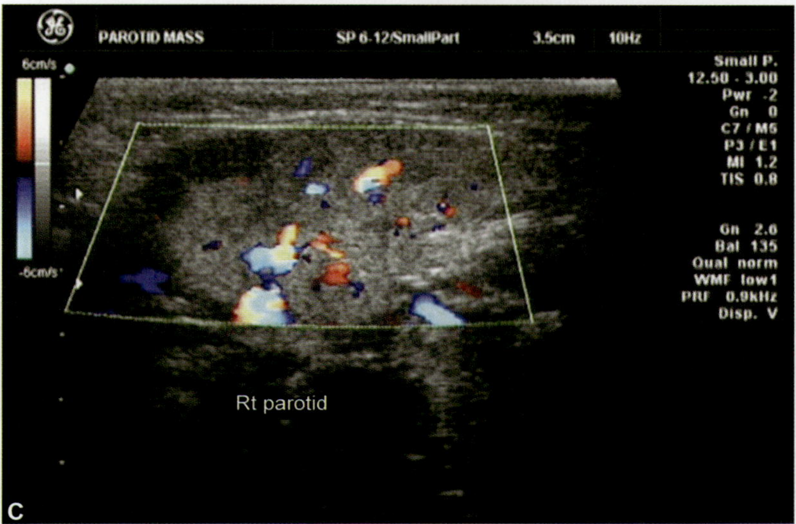

FIGURES 5.13A to C: Acute parotitis. A young child presented with acute swelling of the left parotid gland. HRSG shows edematous swelling enlarged parotid gland. Big abscess is seen in the gland. **On color flow imaging,** increased flow is seen in the gland left parotid is normal in appearance.

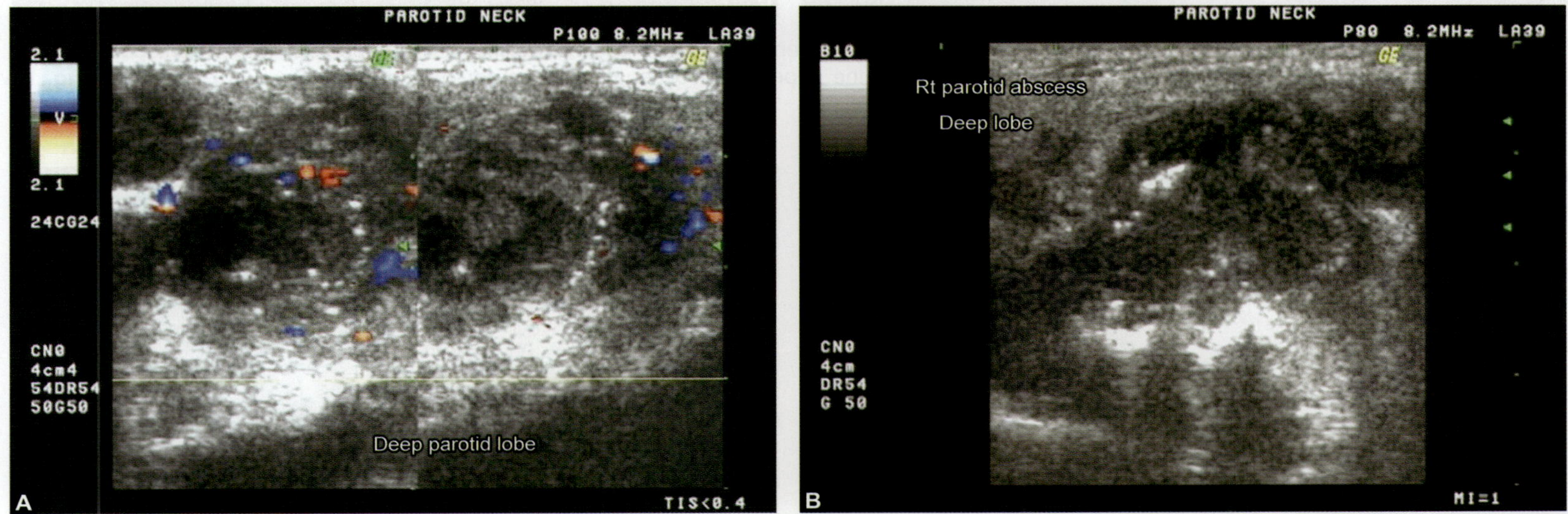

FIGURES 5.14A and B

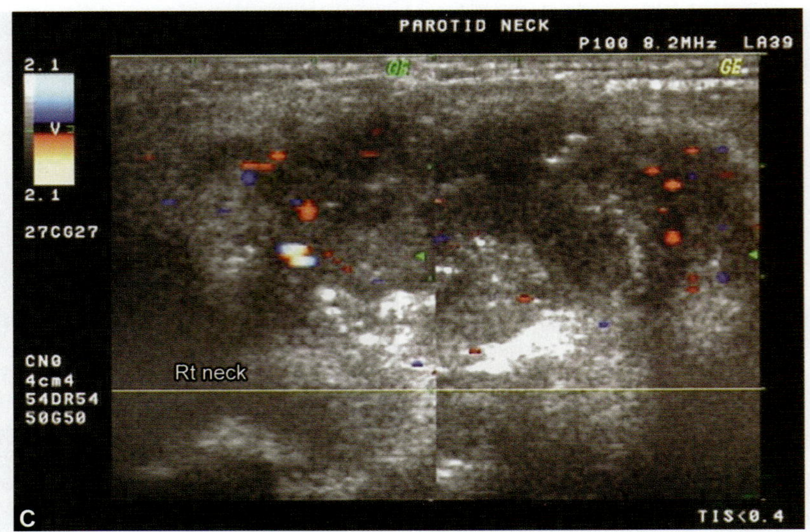

FIGURE 5.14C

FIGURES 5.14A to C: Acute narcotizing parotitis. A young girl presented with acutely painful swelling in right side of the neck with high fever. HRSG shows irregular hypoechoic enlarged deep lobe of parotid. Normal glandular texture is lost. It is grossly inhomogeneous. Multiple abscess are seen in the gland with necrosis suggestive of acute narcotizing parotitis. **On color flow imaging,** low flow is seen in the gland.

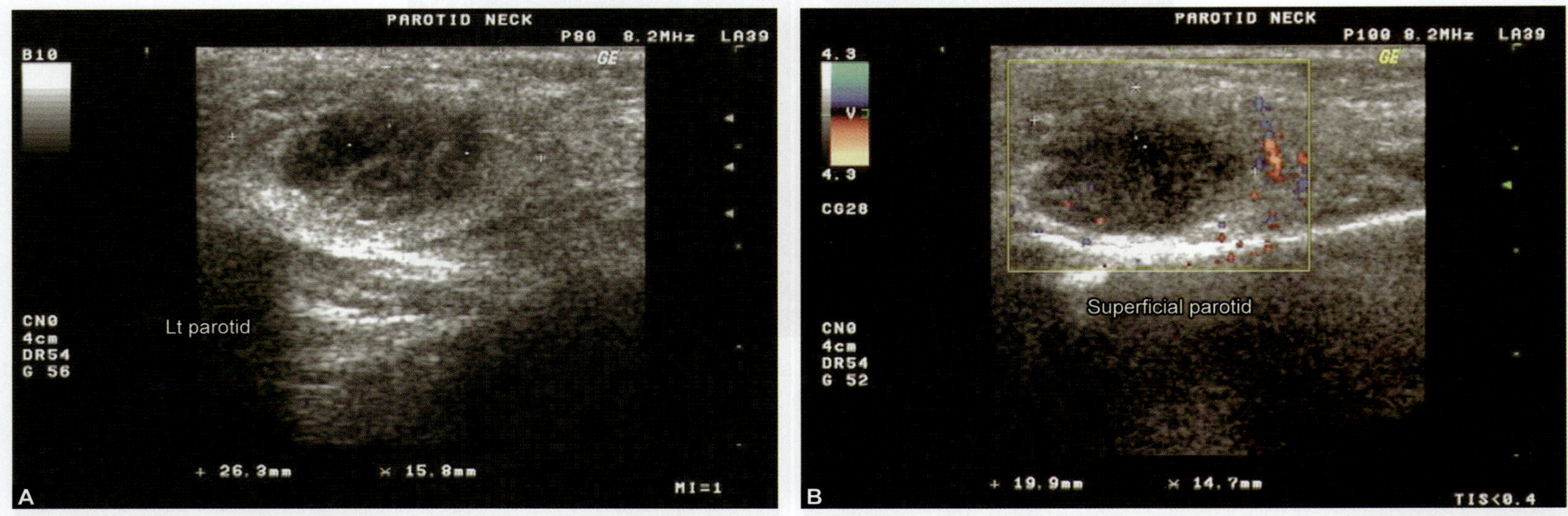

FIGURES 5.15A and B: Subacute parotid abscess. A young girl presented with soft tissue swelling in the superficial lobe of left parotid gland. HRSG shows a thick walled low level echo complex collection in the superficial lobe suggestive of chronic abscess. **On color flow imaging,** low flow is seen in it.

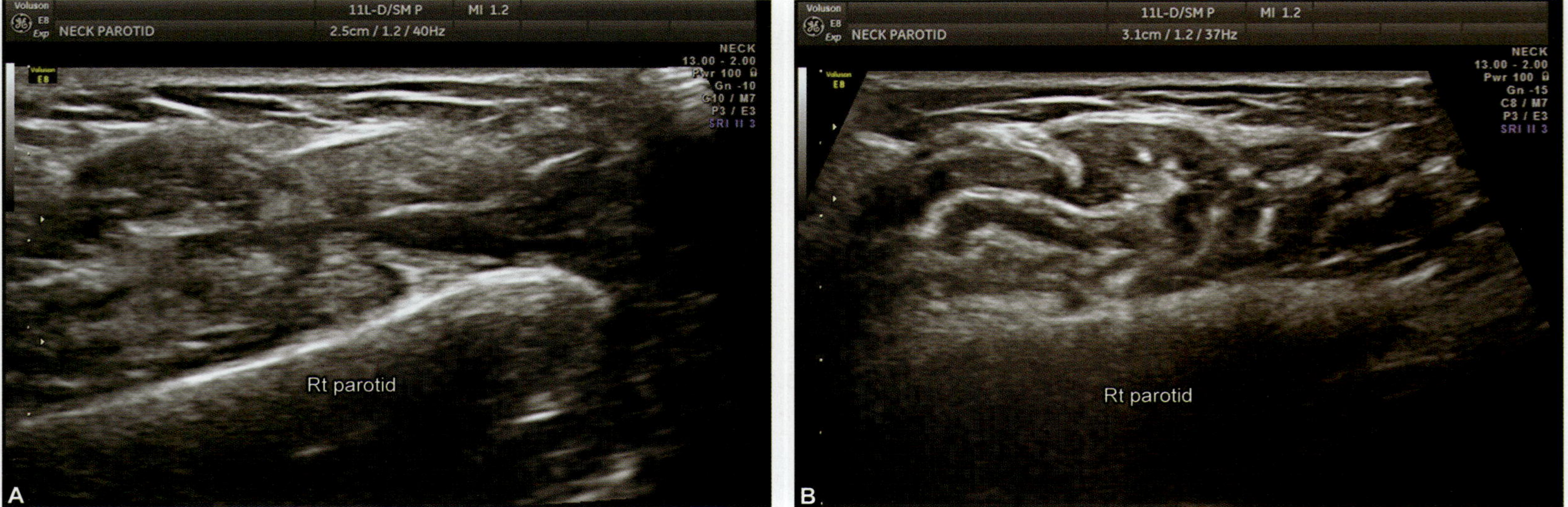

FIGURES 5.16A and B

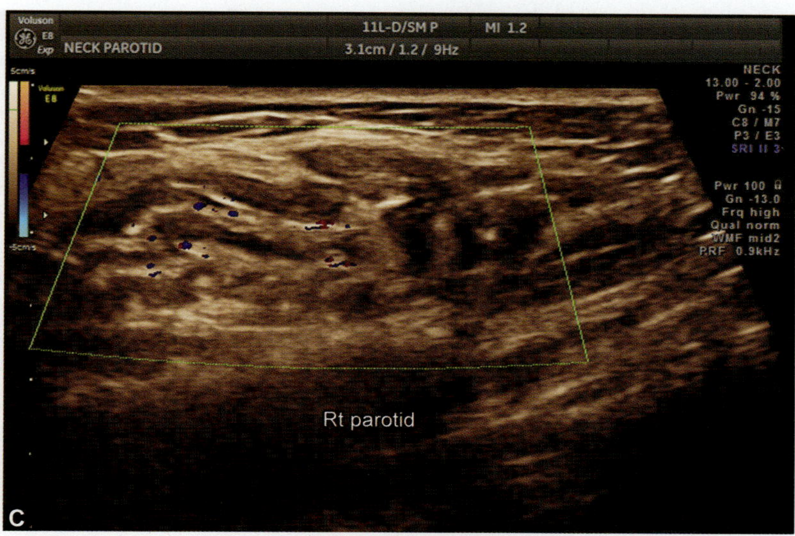

FIGURE 5.16C

FIGURES 5.16A to C: A patient presented with painful swelling in the right parotid gland. HRSG shows enlarged edematous parotid gland. The gland shows inhomogeneous texture. Multiple hypoechoic areas are seen in the gland. Perifocal edema is also present. The acni are also inflamed. Few echogenic foci are seen in the gland. However, no ductal dilatation is seen. The deep lobe of the gland is normal. Findings are suggestive of acute inflammation of right parotid gland involving superficial lobe.

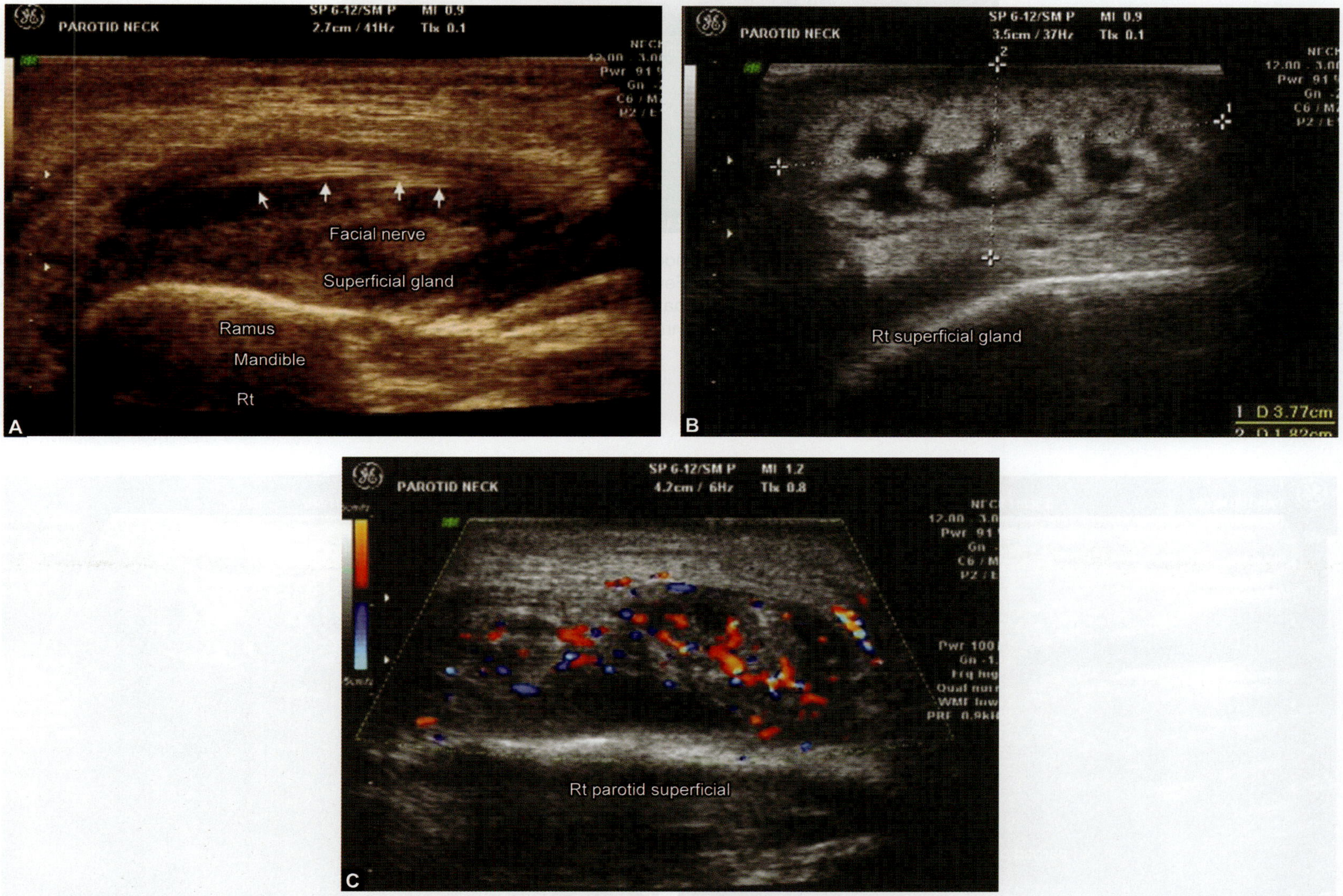

FIGURES 5.17A to C: Parotid abscess with pressure of facial nerve. A patient presented with soft tissue swelling over the right parotid region. HRSG shows marked edematous enlarged parotid gland. Multiple hypoechoic areas are seen in the parotid suggestive of multiple abscess. The abscess is seen pressing over the facial nerve and displacing it resulting into severe pain. **On color flow imaging,** increased flow is seen in the gland.

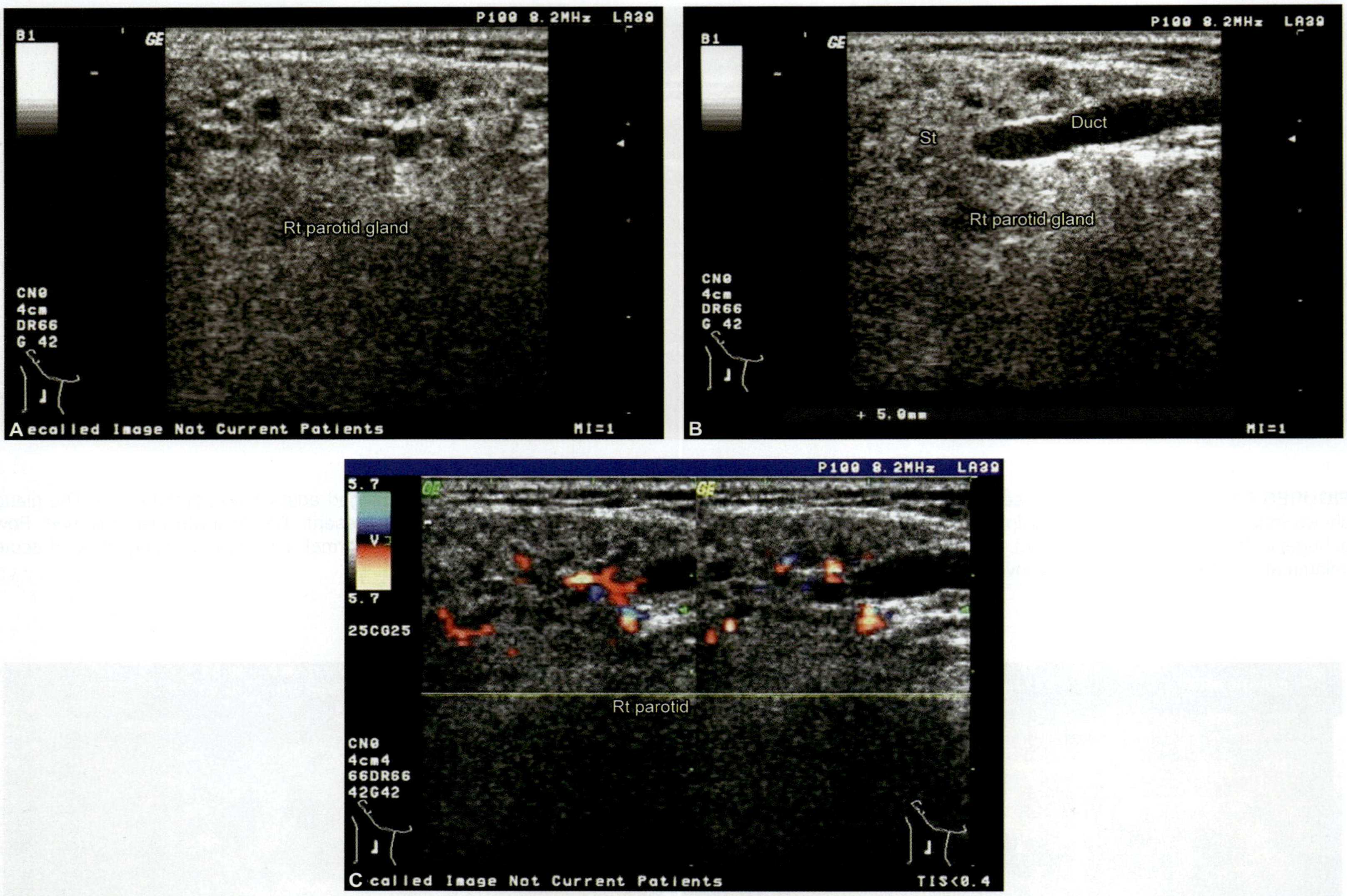

FIGURES 5.18A to C: Chronic recurrent sialectasia with lithiasis. A middle-aged women presented with chronic swelling of the right parotid gland. HRSG shows enlargement of the gland with multiple hypoechoic areas. Few fine calcified specks are seen in the substance of the gland suggestive of microlithiasis. But no abscess formation is seen. HRSG shows dilated parotid duct with blocking its mouth by an echogenic calculus. Color Doppler imaging shows little or poor flow in the gland suggestive of chronic inflammation.

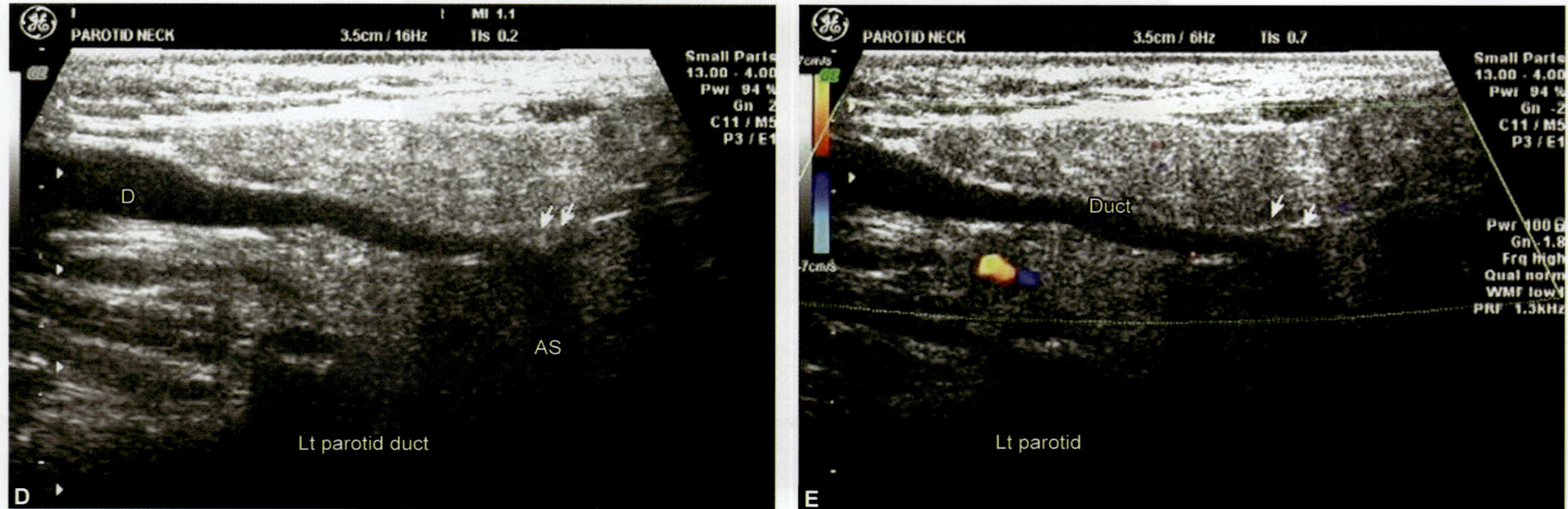

FIGURES 5.18D and E: Dilated parotid duct with impacted stone at the mouth of the duct. A patient presented with recreant painful swelling in the left parotid region. HRSG shows markedly dilated parotid duct. An echogenic shadow is seen impacted at the mouth of the duct. It is accompanied with acoustic shadowing suggestive of calculus.

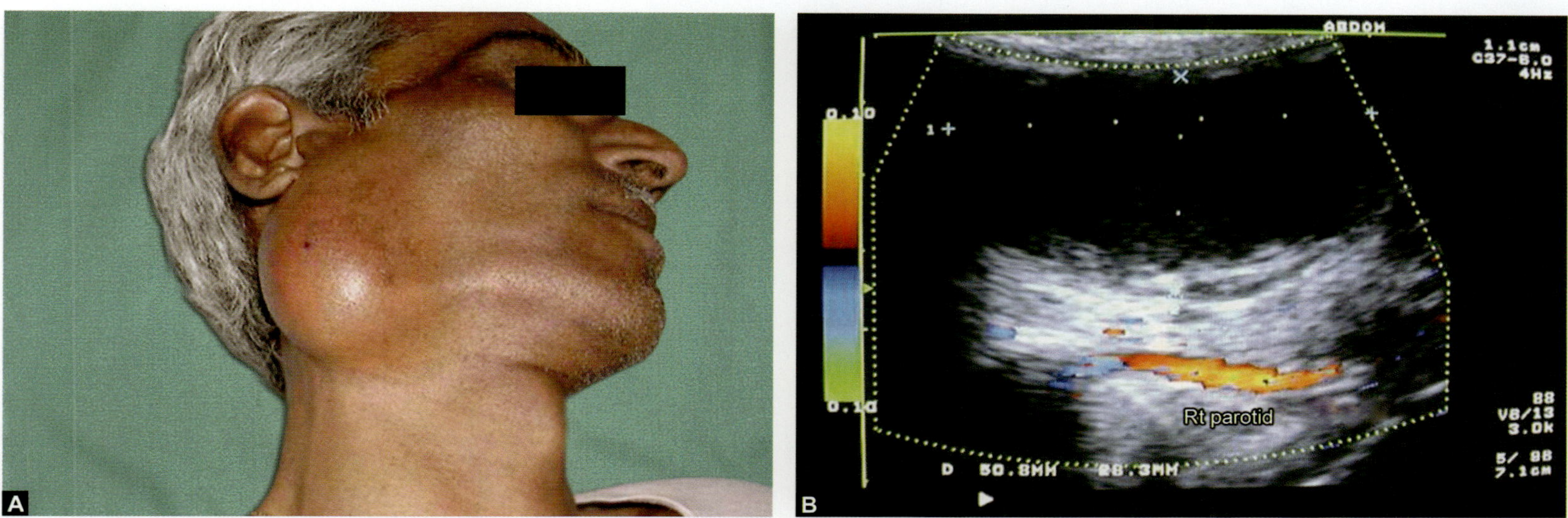

FIGURES 5.19A and B: Parotid abscess. A man presented with soft tissue tender mass over the right parotid area. HRSG shows a low-level echo complex mass in the parotid gland. Central area of necrosis is seen in it. Color flow imaging shows poor flow in the mass suggestive of parotid abscess.

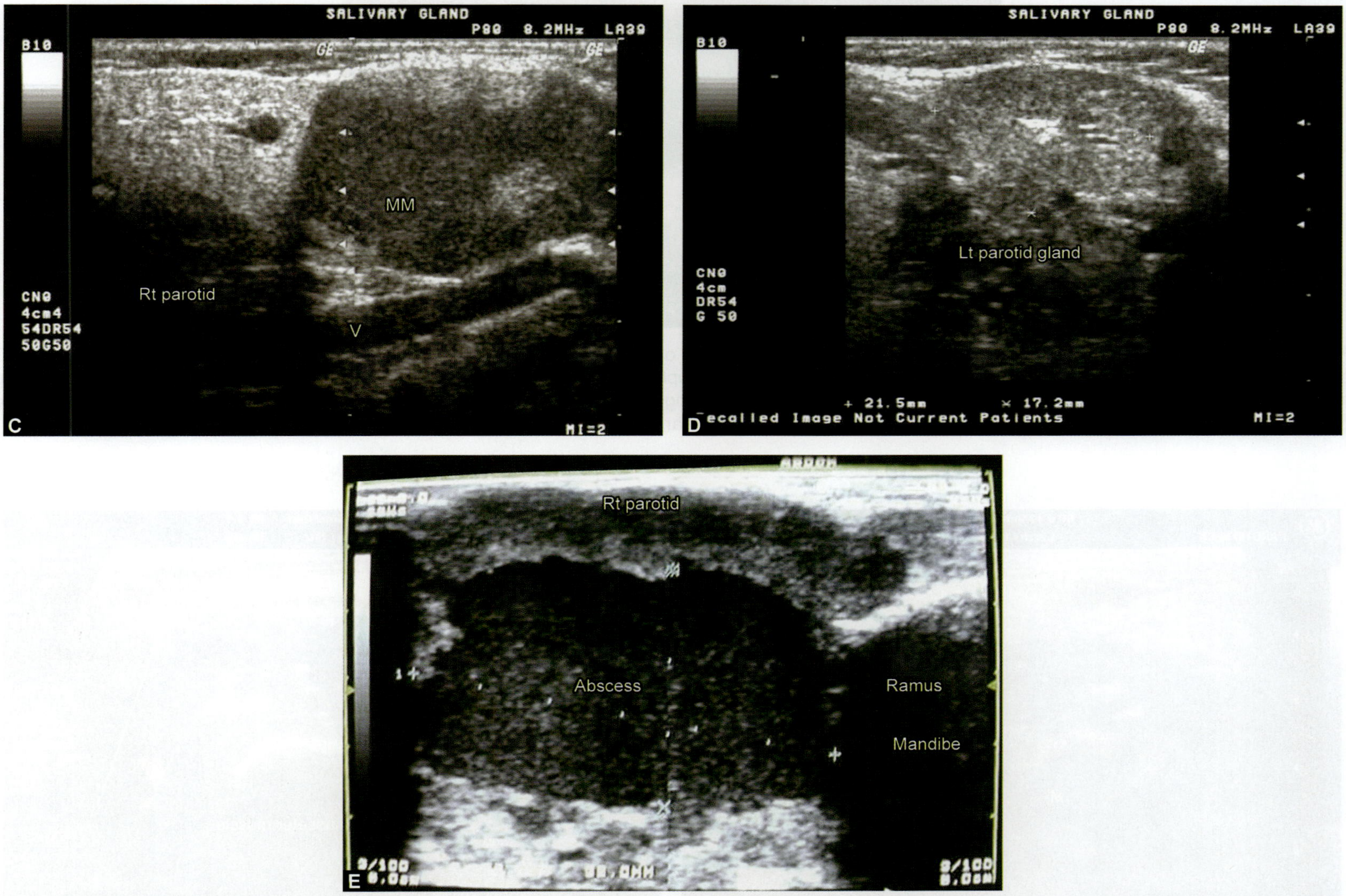

FIGURES 5.19C to E: Parotid abscess. A young girl presented with painful cystic mass. HRSG shows a well-defined echo complex mass in the parotid gland suggestive of an abscess. The left parotid gland is normal. HRSG of the same patient shows that the abscess is not pressing over the parotid duct. The duct is seen normaly. No evidence of any calculus is seen.

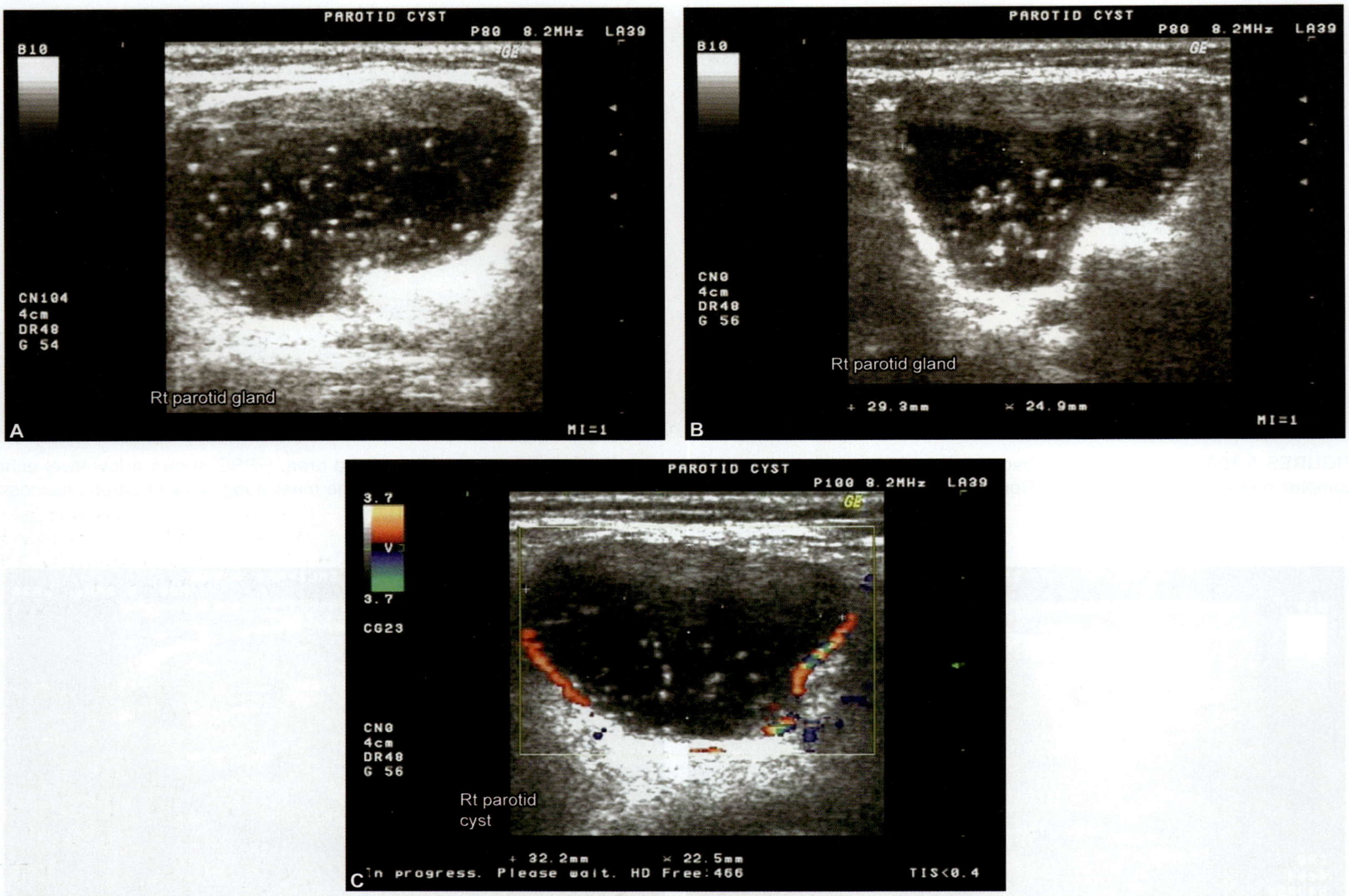

FIGURES 5.20A to C: Mucoid degeneration in the parotid gland. An old lady presented with a cystic swelling of the right parotid gland. HRSG shows a well-defined cystic mass in the parotid gland. The cyst has completely destroyed the normal glandular texture. However, it is having sharp margins. No septation or loculation is seen in the cyst. Multiple bright echogenic specks are seen floating in the cyst. Biopsy of the cyst shows mucoid degeneration. Color Doppler imaging of the cyst shows peripheral capsular enhancement of the cyst.

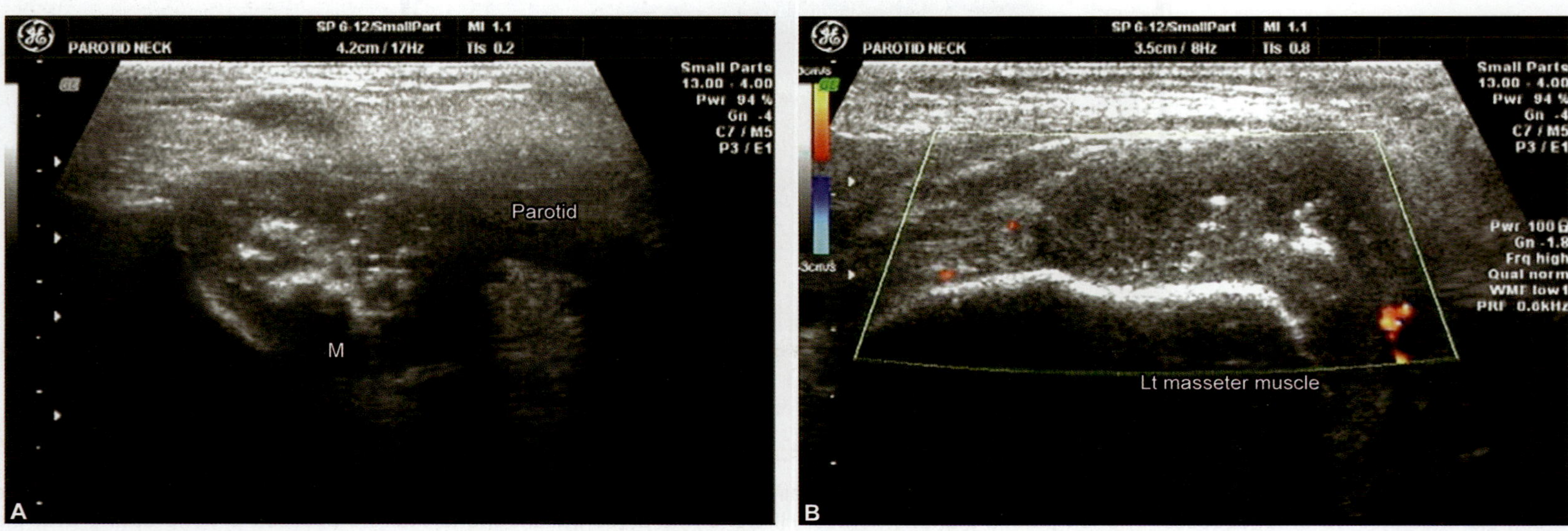

FIGURES 5.21A and B

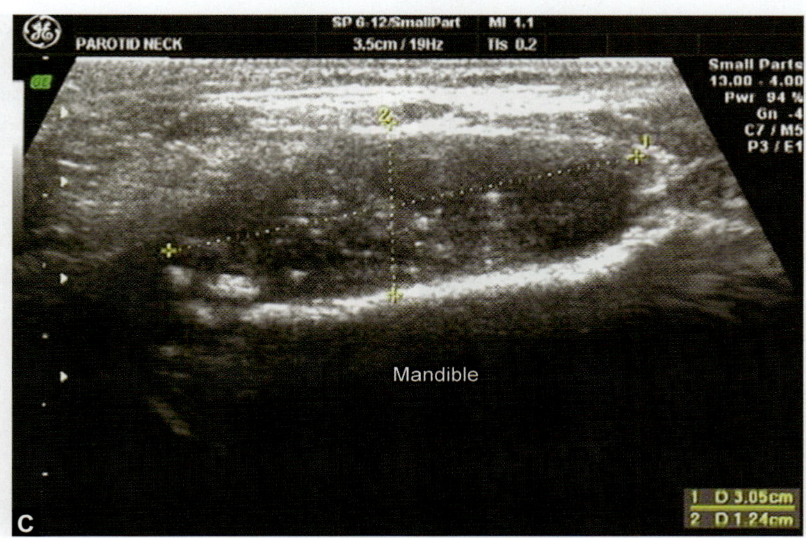

FIGURE 5.21C

FIGURES 5.21A to C: Tubercular abscess in the parotid. A young girl presented with chronic non-tender swelling involving the left parotid gland. HRSG shows mixed echo complex mass in the parotid echogenic specks are also seen in the mass. It is seen extending in the left masseter muscle. **On color flow imaging,** poor flow is seen in the abscess. Biopsy of the mass confirms chronic tubercular abscess.

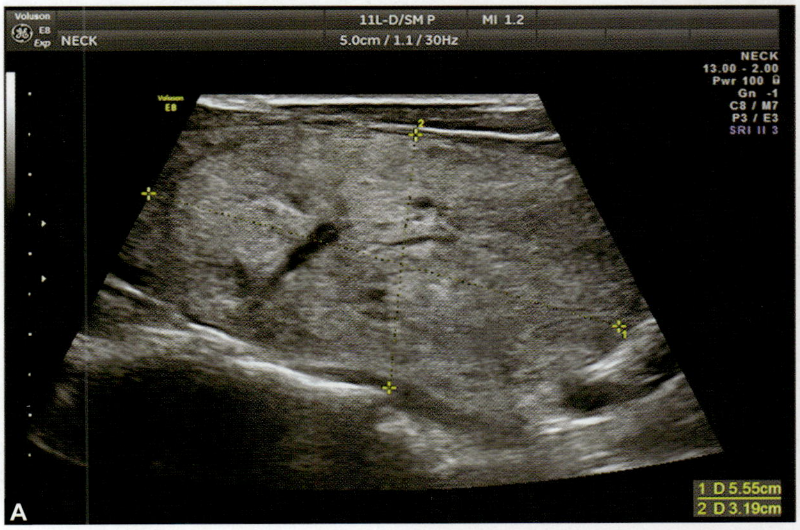

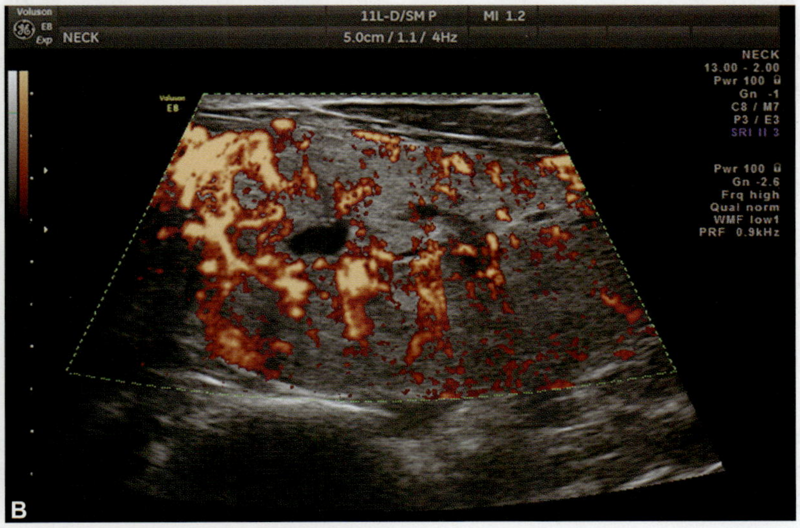

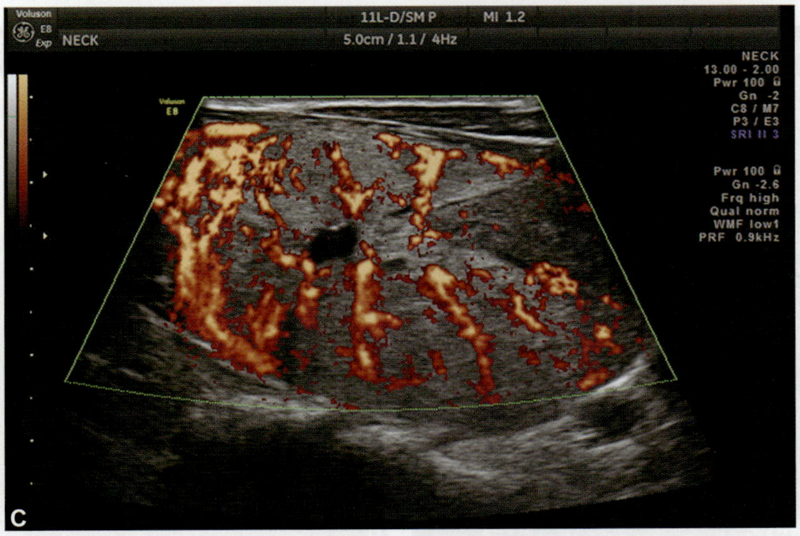

FIGURES 5.22A to C: Submandibular gland inflammation. A man presented with soft tissue swelling in the right submandibular gland fossa. HRSG shows diffuse enlargement of the submandibular gland. The gland is edematous and inhomogeneous in texture. Small abscesses are also seen in the gland. **On color flow imaging,** marked increased flow is seen in the gland suggestive of acute inflammation.

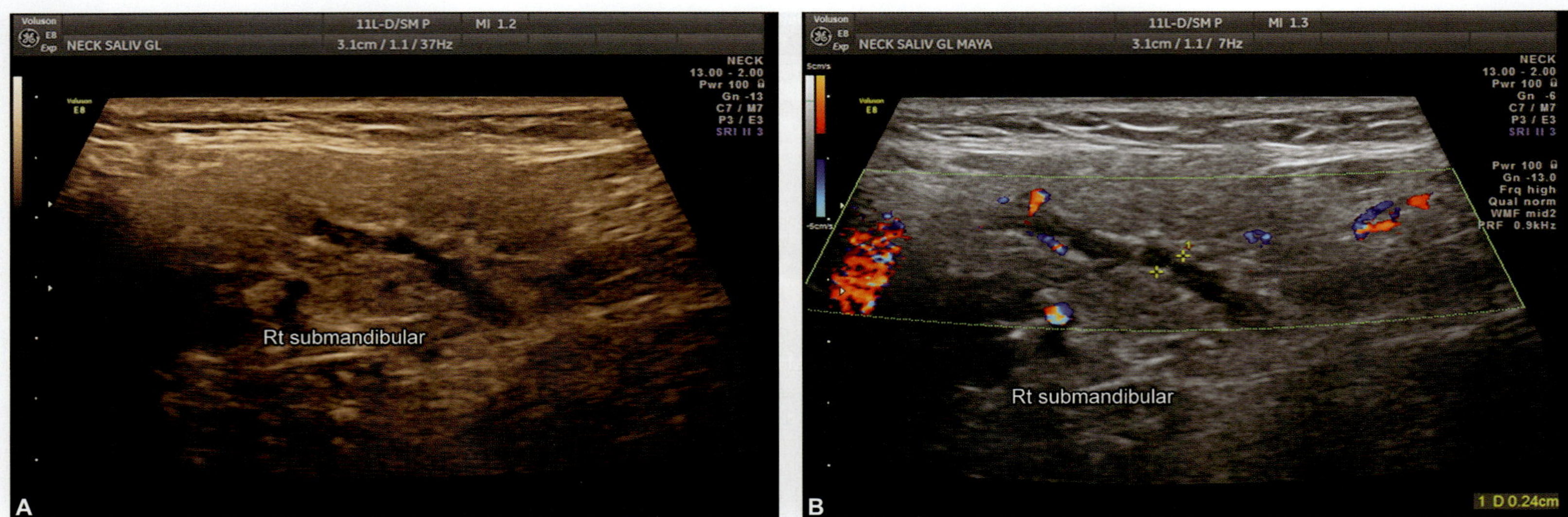

FIGURES 5.23A and B: Dilated SMG duct. A patient presented with swelling in the right SMG gland. HRSG shows swelling of the gland. The duct is seen dilated but no evidence of any calculus shadow is seen in the duct at the time of study. This may be because of transient blockage of the duct.

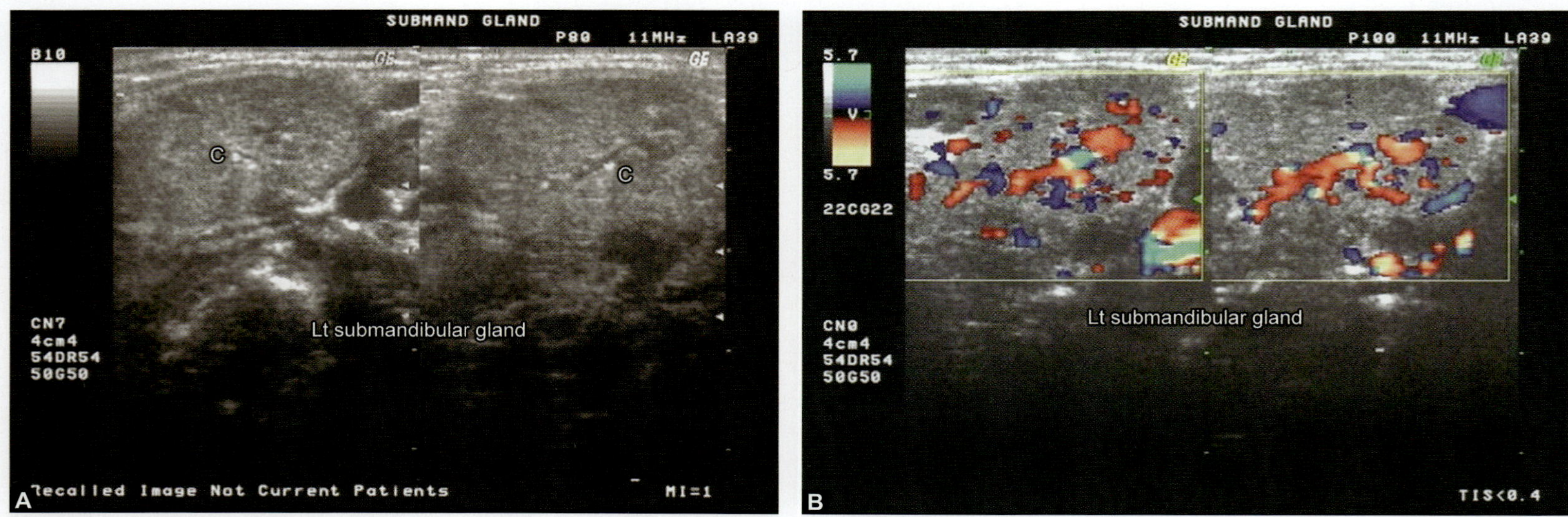

FIGURES 5.24A and B: Acute inflammation of the gland. A young girl presented with swelling in the left submandibular area. The gland is enlarged and increased in size. It is lobulated. However, the margins are maintained. The duct is dilated. Few calcified small calculi are also seen in the duct of the gland.

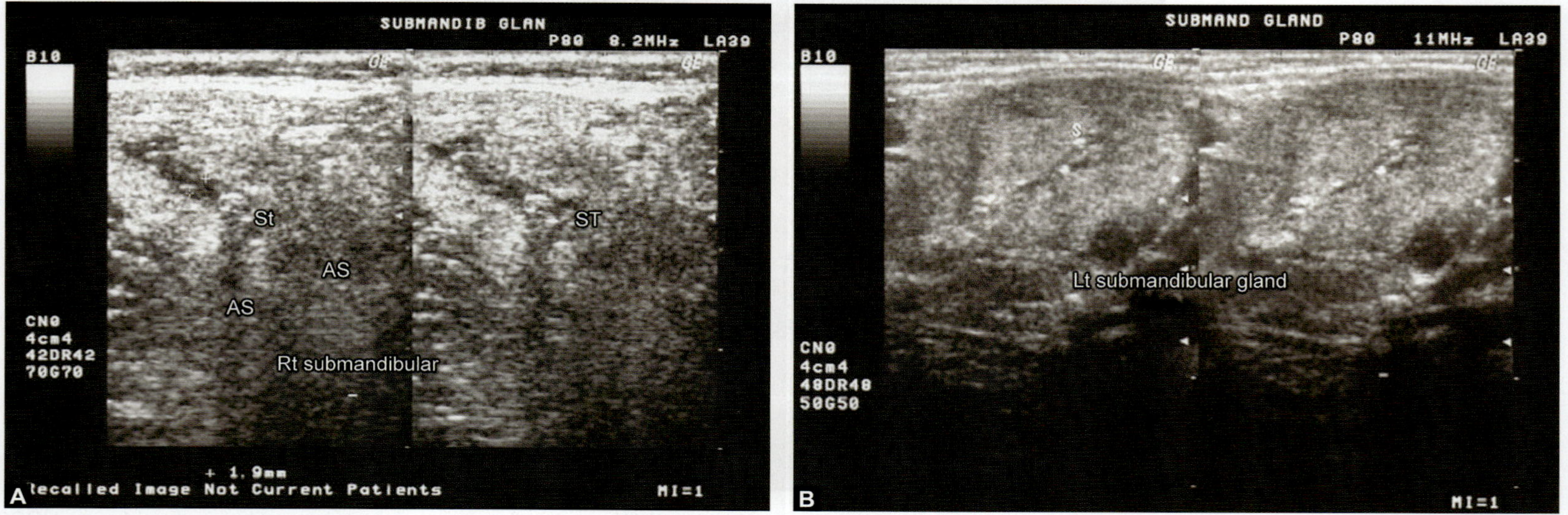

FIGURES 5.25A and B

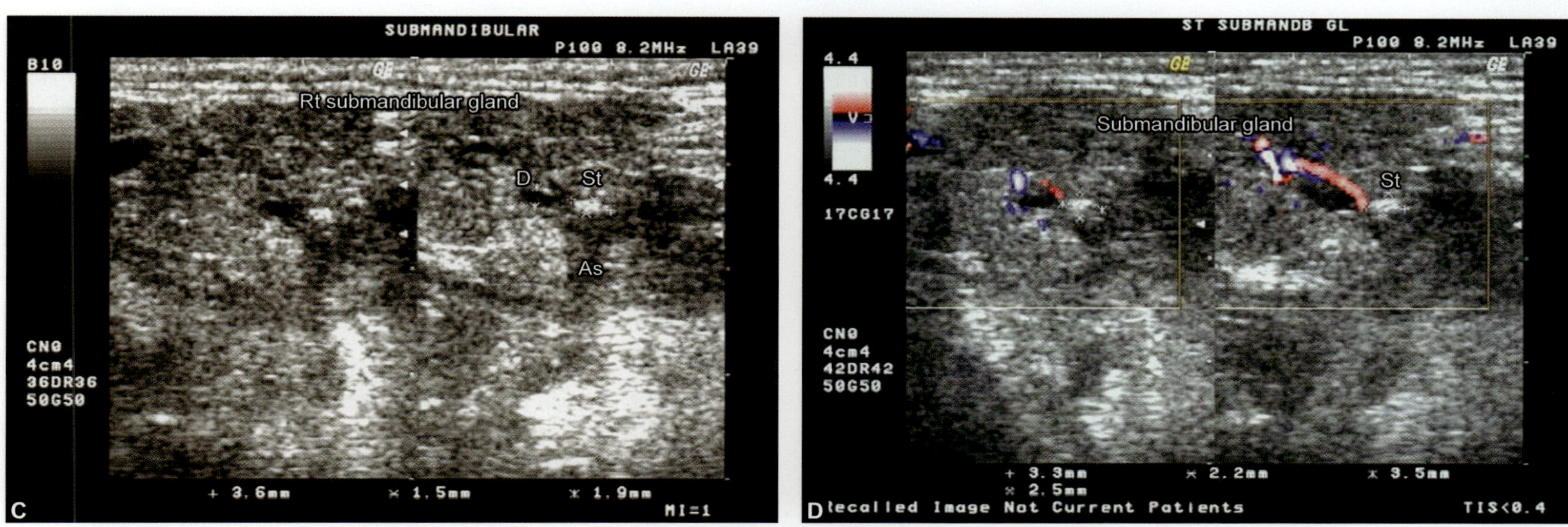

FIGURES 5.25C and D

FIGURES 5.25A to D: Chronic sialectasis with lithiasis. HRSG shows enlarged right submandibular gland. The lobules are increased in size. The main duct is dilated. Echogenic calcified foci are seen in the main duct suggestive of calculi. They are accompanied with acoustic shadowing. But no evidence of any cystic degeneration is seen. HRSG shows small abscess formation in the case of chronic recurrent sialectasis of the submandibular gland. On color Doppler imaging little flow is seen in the substance of the gland.

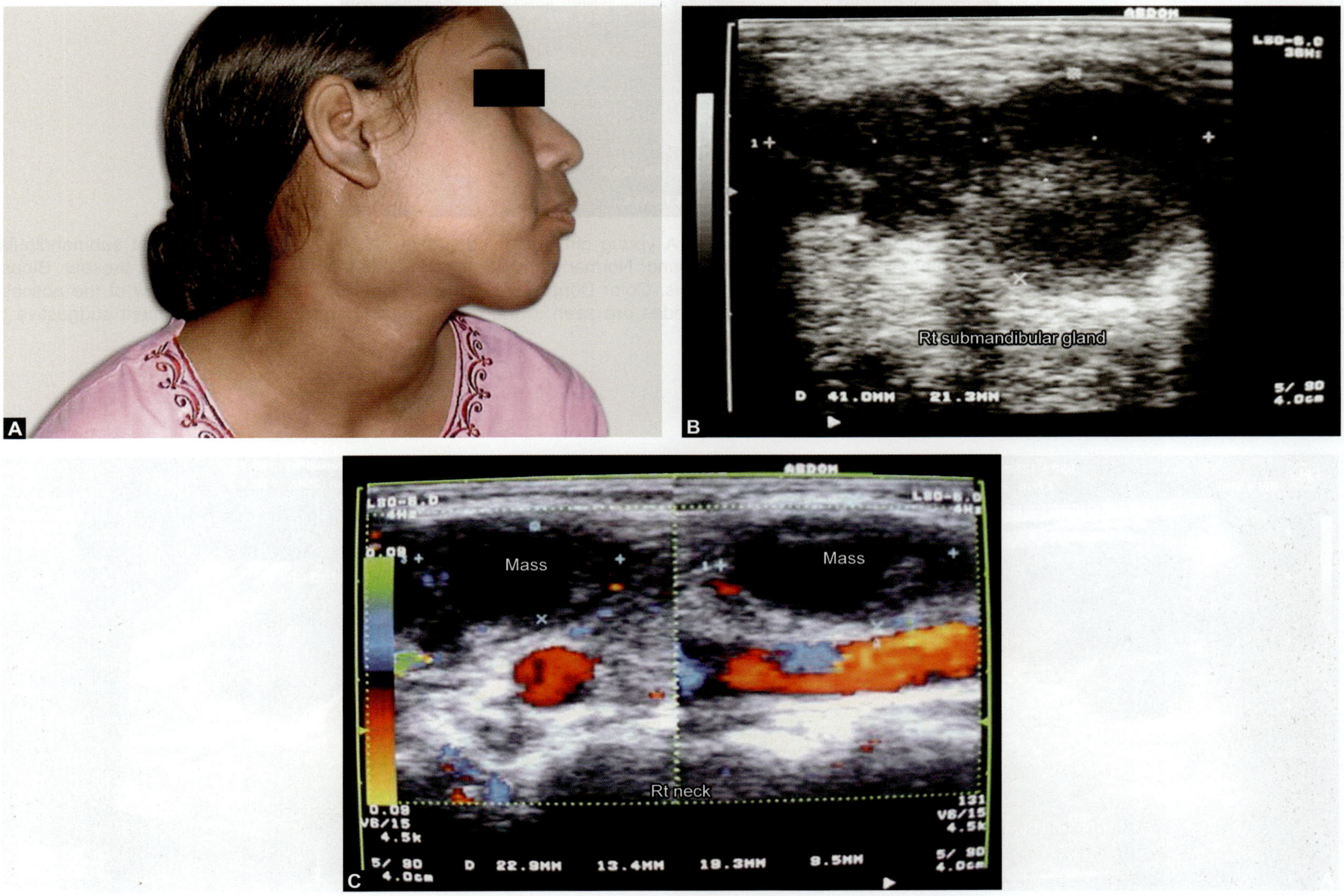

FIGURES 5.26A to C: Submandibular gland abscess—Pyogenic abscess. A young lady presented with a soft tissue mass in right submandibular area. HRSG shows a low-level echo complex mass with central area of necrosis. Echogenic debris is also seen in the mass. The mass was bilobed. Biopsy shows pyogenic abscess. Multiple enlarged lymph nodes are also seen in the upper cervical area suggestive of reactive lymph node enlargement.

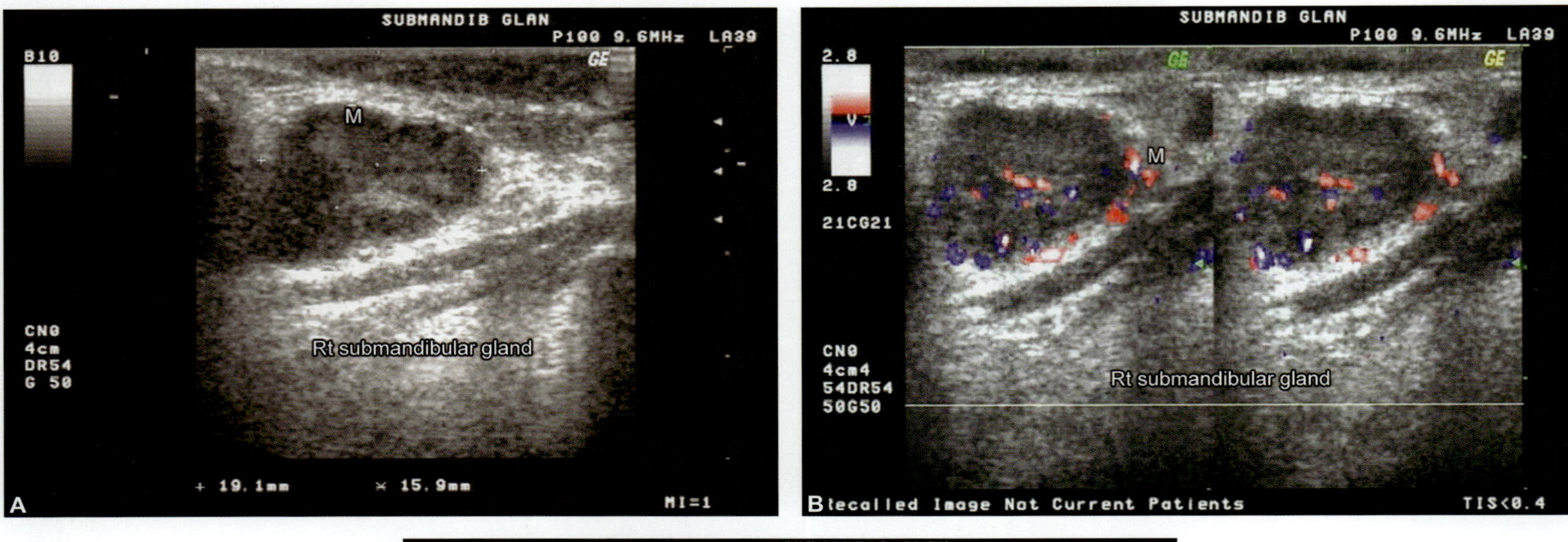

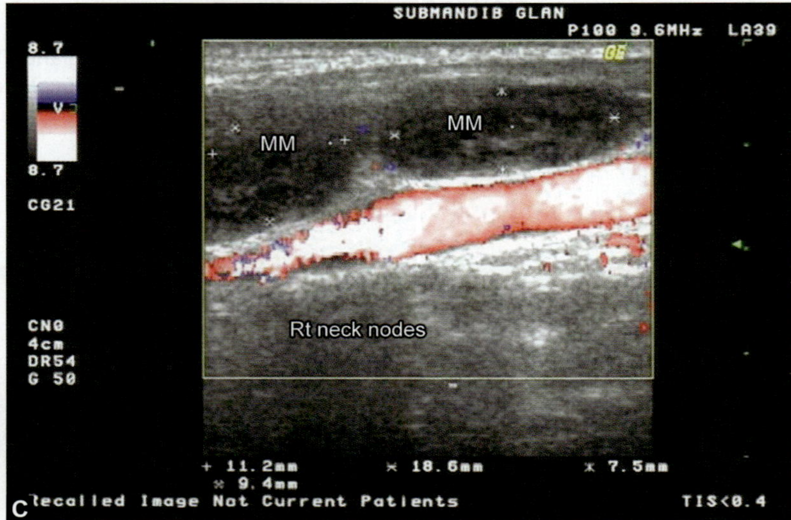

FIGURES 5.27A to C: Tubercular abscess in submandibular gland. A young girl presented with a soft cystic mass in the right submandibular area. HRSG shows low-level echo complex mass in the submandibular gland. Normal glandular texture is lost. No perifocal edema is present. Biopsy shows tubercular abscess. Patient was also having pulmonary tuberculosis. Color Doppler imaging the same patient shows little flow of the abscess cavity. However, capsular vascularity is seen. Multiple enlarged lymph nodes are seen in the upper cervical area in the same patient suggestive of tubercular lymphadenitis.

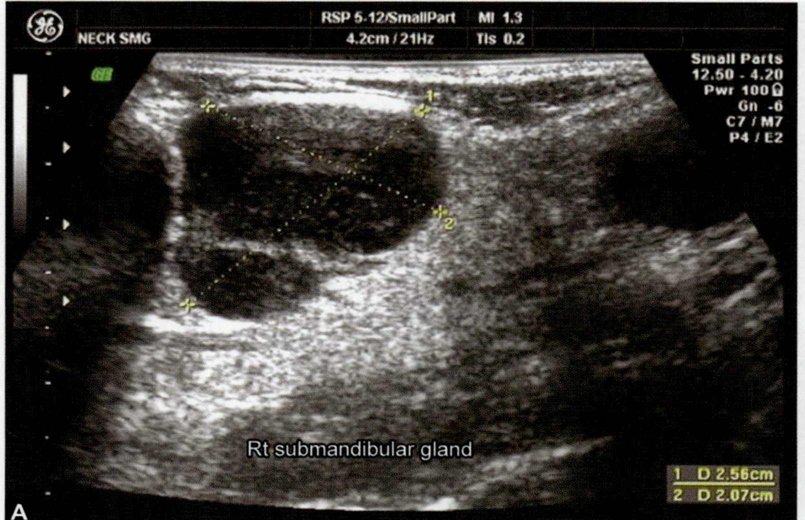

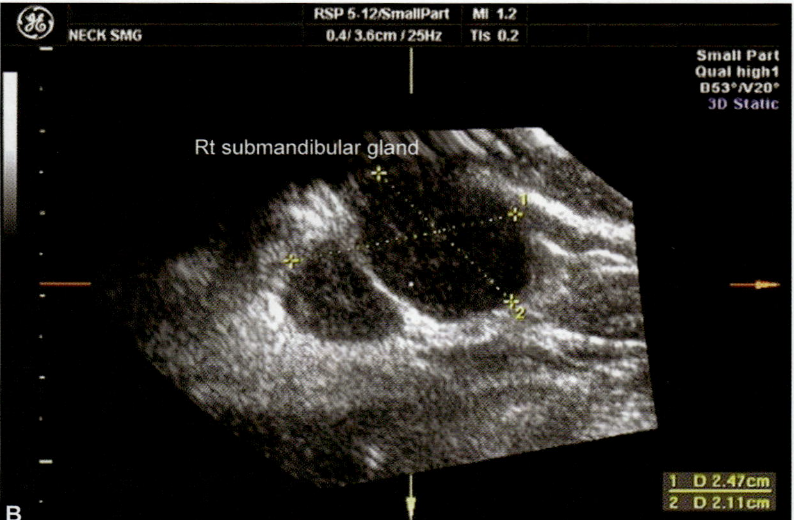

FIGURES 5.28A and B

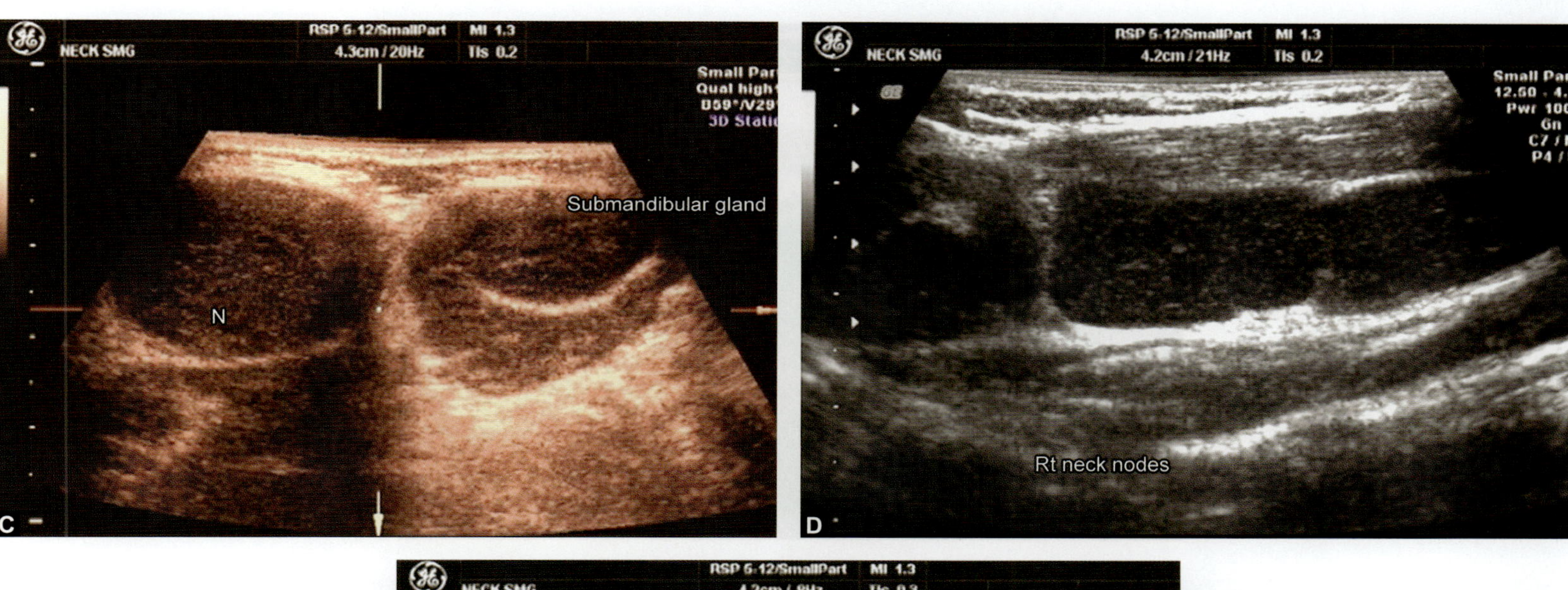

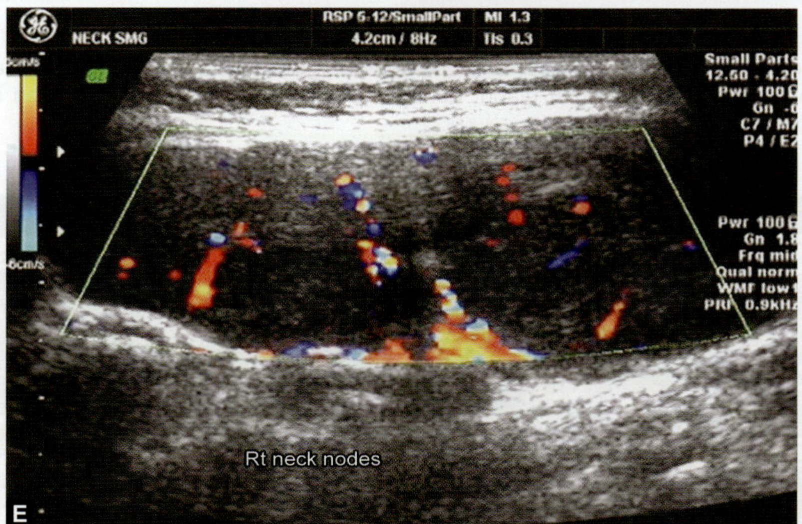

FIGURES 5.28C to E

FIGURES 5.28A to E: Submandibular gland tuberculosis. A young girl presented with swelling in the right submandibular gland. HRSG shows thick walled loculated cystic mass in the SMG. Echogenic septa is also seen in it. Thick collection is seen in the gland. 3D imaging of the gland shows details of the cystic cavity. Aspirate of the cyst came out to be thick pus suggestive of chronic infection. Multiple enlarged nodes are also seen in the right upper cervical and midcervical region. Increased flow is seen in them on color flow imaging. Biopsy confirmed tubercular abscess.

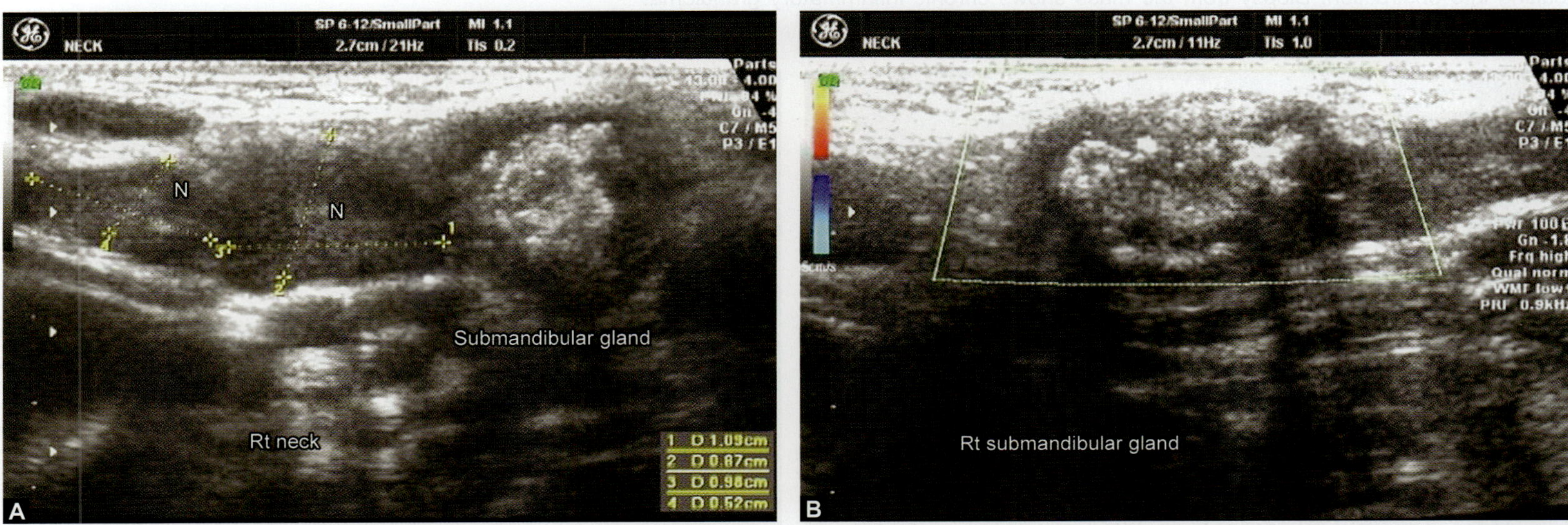

FIGURES 5.29A and B

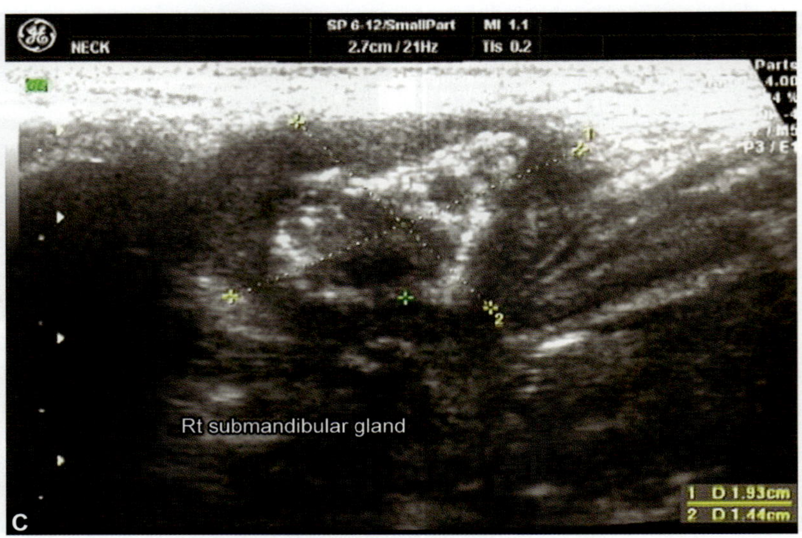

FIGURE 5.29C

FIGURES 5.29A to C: Chronic tubercular abscess. A young child presented with mass with non-tender mass in the right submandibular gland. HRSG shows thick echogenic collection in the submandibular gland. Echogenic calcified specks are also seen in it. Multiple enlarged nodes are also seen in the neck. Biopsy confirmed chronic tubercular abscess.

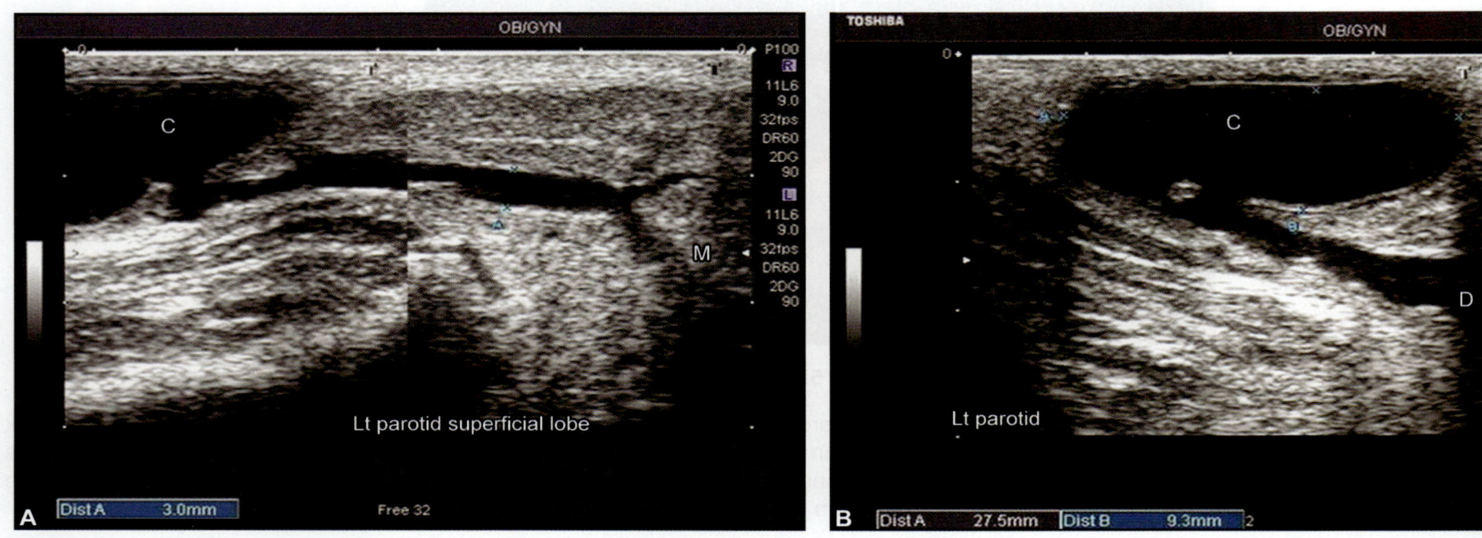

FIGURES 5.30A and B: Dilated duct with retention cyst. A young girl presented with soft tissue swelling in the left parotid gland. HRSG shows a well-defined cystic shadow in the left parotid gland. The parotid gland duct is also dilated. A soft tissue shadow is seen blocking the mouth of duct resulting into obstruction. Biopsy from the mass shows chronic inflammatory granuloma.

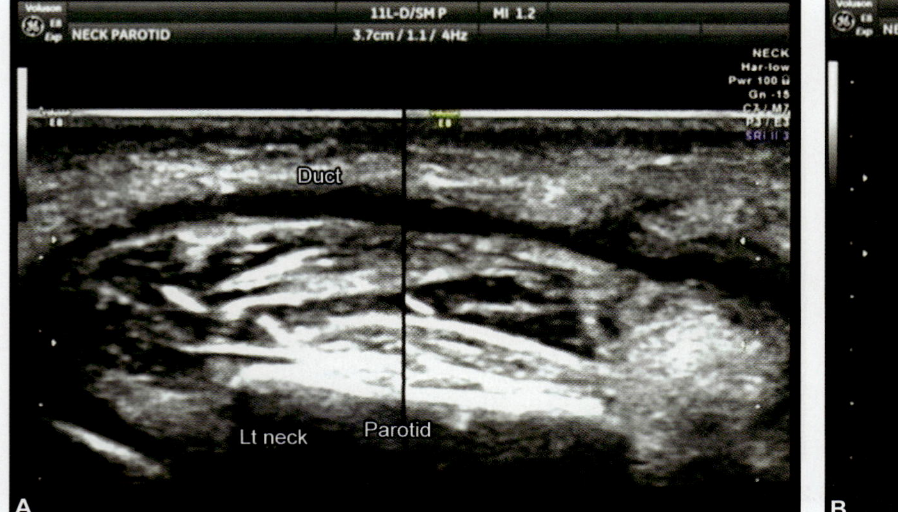

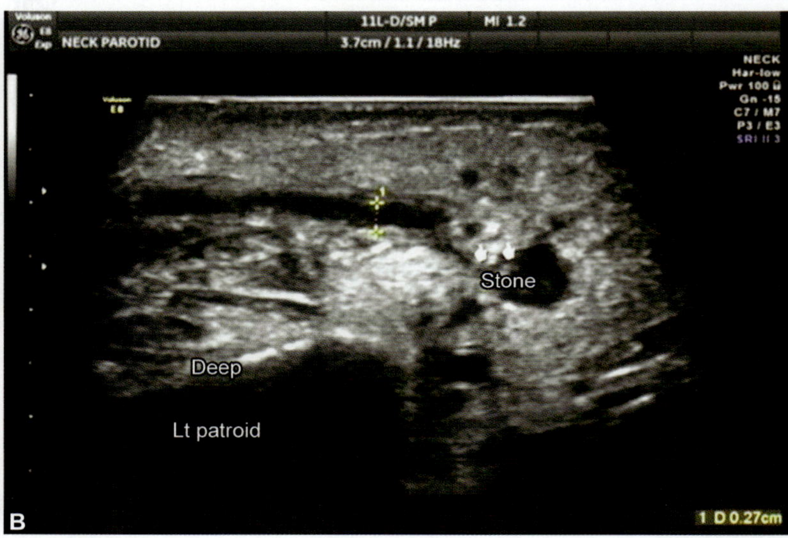

FIGURES 5.31A and B

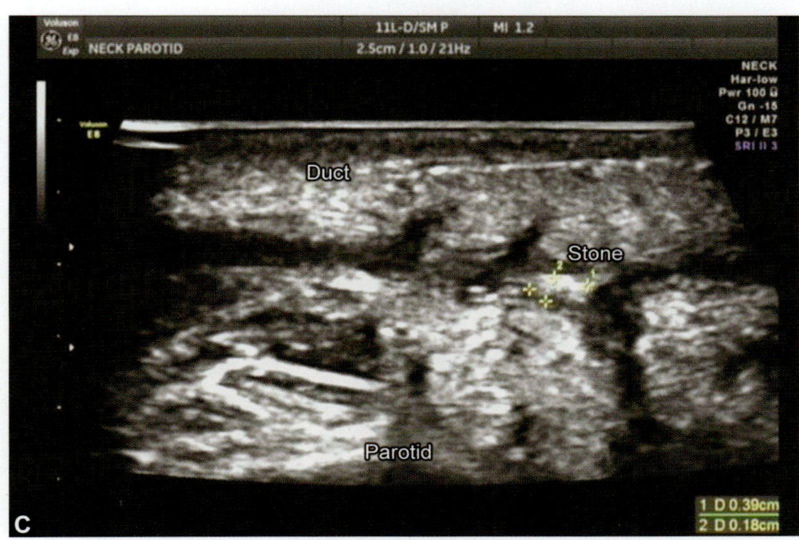

FIGURE 5.31C

FIGURES 5.31A to C: A 6-year-old girl presented with swelling of left parotid gland. HRSG shows diffuse enlargement of the gland. Inhomogeneous texture of the gland is seen. The parotid duct is also dilated. An echogenic shadow is seen in the distal part of duct suggestive of calculus. The ductal branches are also seen dilated suggestive of chronic inflammatory disease with stone formation.

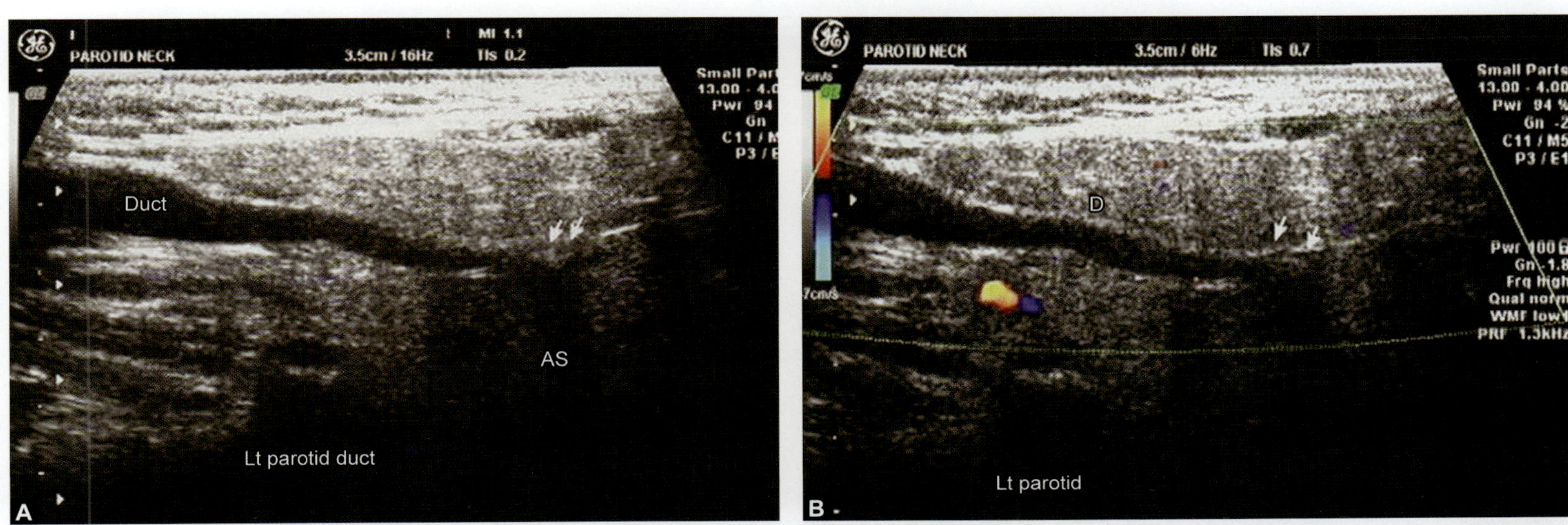

FIGURES 5.32A and B: Dilated parotid duct with impacted stone at the mouth of the duct. A patient presented with recurrent painful swelling in the left parotid region. HRSG shows markedly dilated parotid duct. An echogenic shadow is seen impacted at the mouth of the duct. It is accompanied with acoustic shadowing suggestive of calculus.

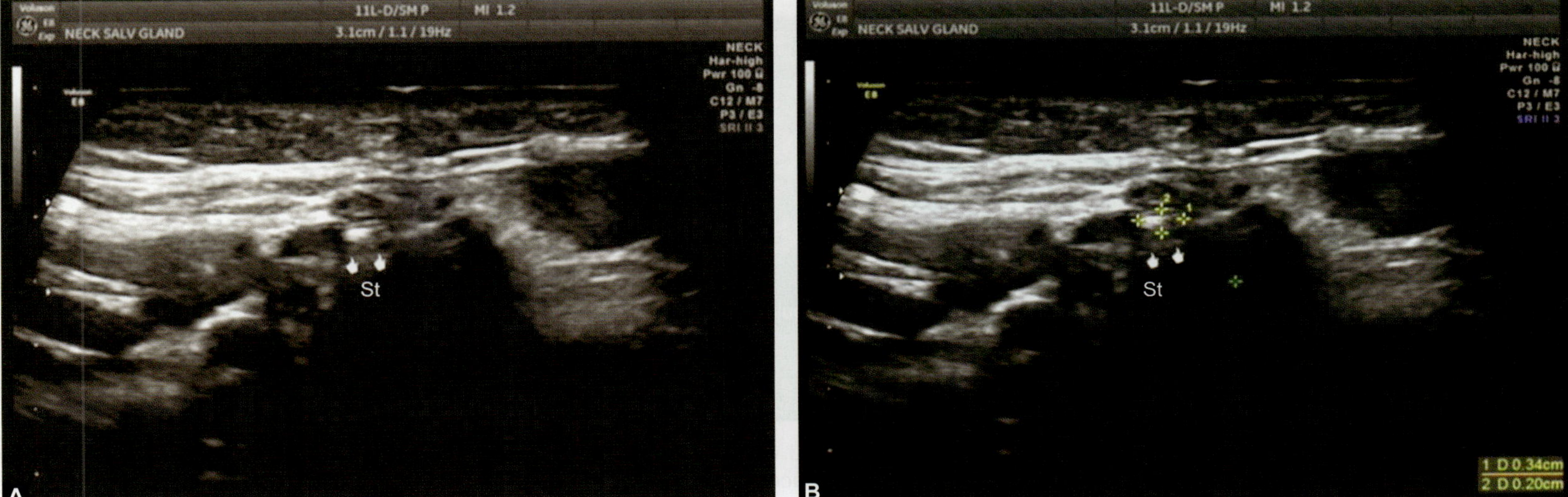

FIGURES 5.33A and B

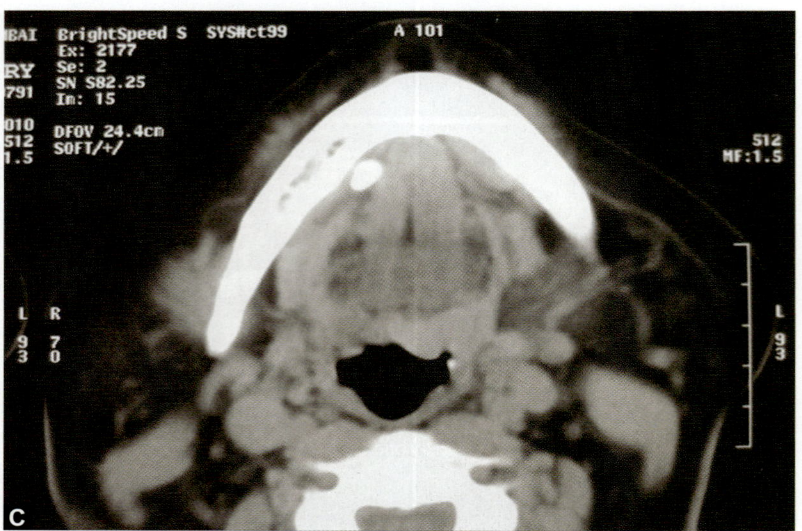

FIGURE 5.33C

FIGURES 5.33A to C: Submandibular gland calculus. A lady presented with soft tissue swelling in the right submandibular gland. HRSG shows inflamed edematous submandibular gland. The duct is also dilated. An echogenic shadow is seen at the mouth of duct suggestive of calculus. CT scan of the same patient clearly shows the calculus.

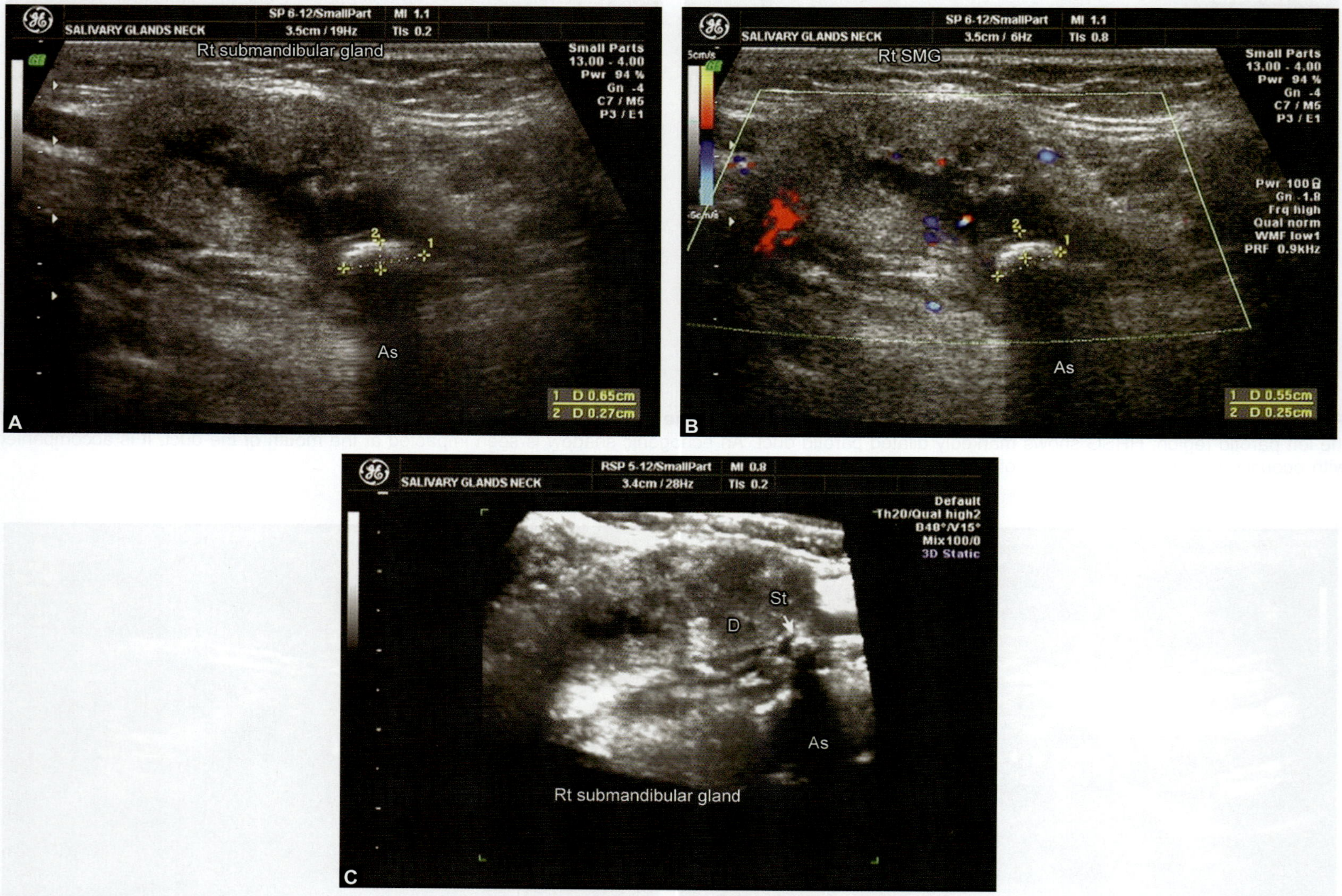

FIGURES 5.34A to C: Big submandibular calculus. A patient presented with a palpable nodular mass in right submandibular gland. HRSG shows a big echogenic shadow in the duct of the gland. It is accompanied with acoustic shadowing suggestive of a big calculus. The gland is also enlarged and hypoechoic in texture. The ductal branches are also dilated. 3D imaging of the gland shows details of the ductal dilatation with impacted stone at the mouth of the duct.

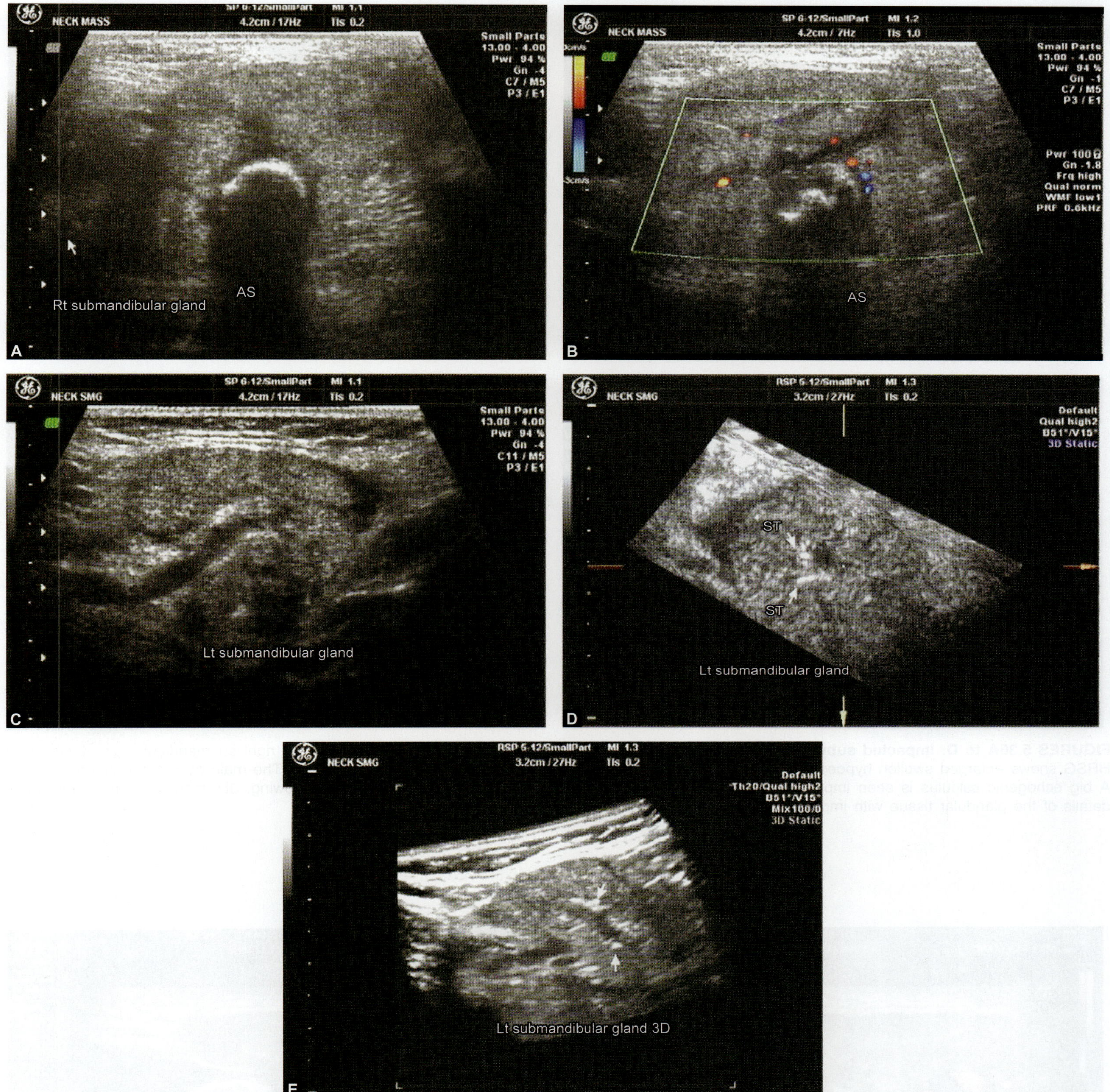

FIGURES 5.35A to E: Big submandibular calculus. A patient presented with recurrent pain and swelling in the right submandibular gland (SMG). HRSG shows a big calculus impacted in the duct of the gland. Small calculi are also seen in the ductal branches. The big calculus shows acoustic shadowing. 3D imaging of the gland shows small calculi impacted in the ductal branches.

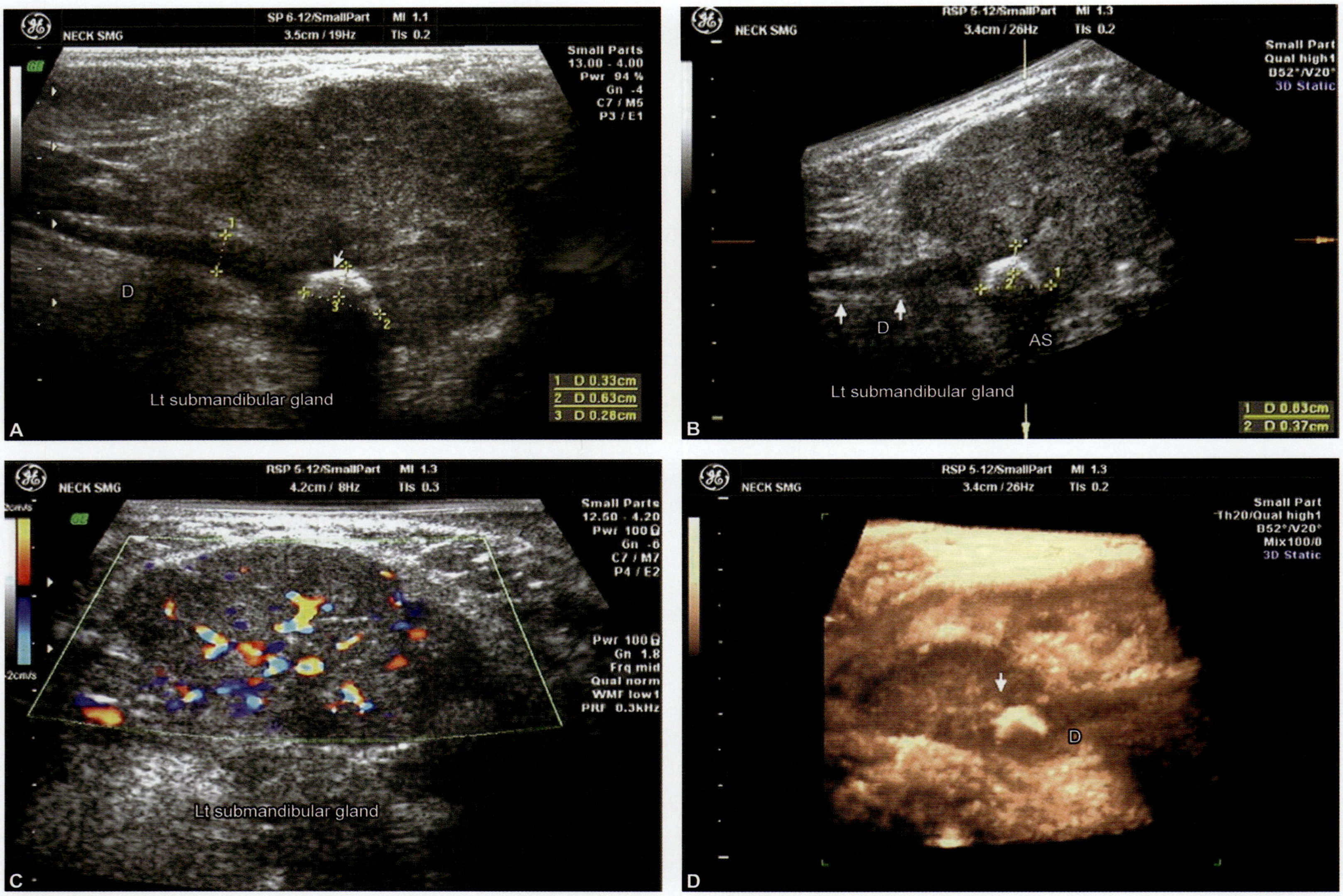

FIGURES 5.36A to D: Impacted submandibular gland calculus. A patient presented with painful swelling of right submandibular gland with fever. HRSG shows enlarged swollen hypoechoic gland. On color flow imaging, increased flow is seen in the gland. The main duct of the gland is dilated. A big echogenic calculus is seen impacted at the mouth of the duct. It is accompanied with acoustic shadowing. 3D imaging of the gland shows details of the glandular tissue with impacted stone in the mouth of the duct.

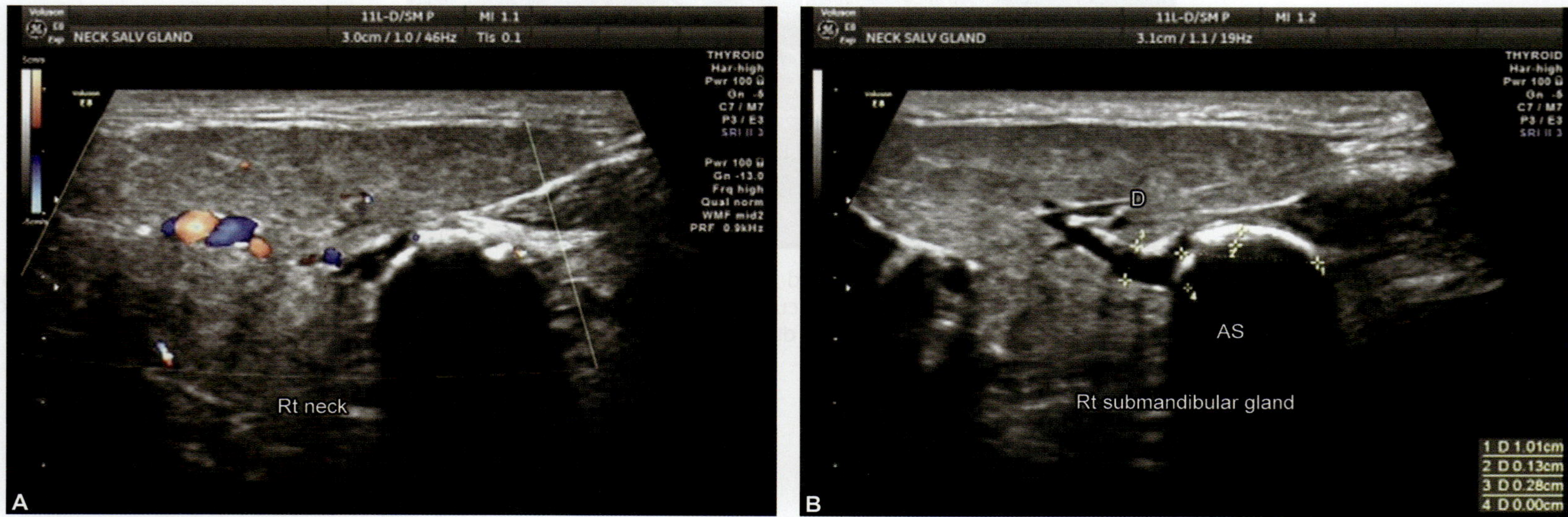

FIGURES 5.37A and B

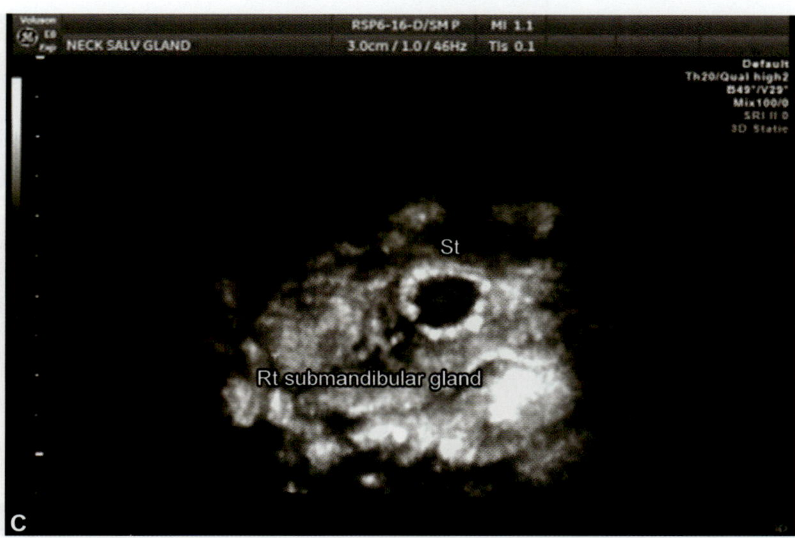

FIGURE 5.37C

FIGURES 5.37A to C: Big submandibular gland calculus. A patient presented with painful swelling in the right submandibular gland. HRSG shows a big impacted echogenic shadow in the duct of the gland. It is accompanied with acoustic shadowing. 3D ultrasound with TUI imaging shows the stone clearly and inflammation of the gland.

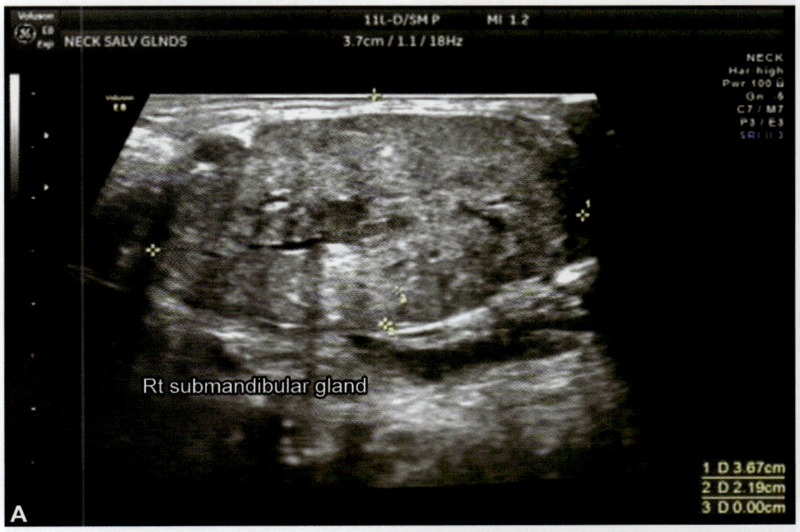

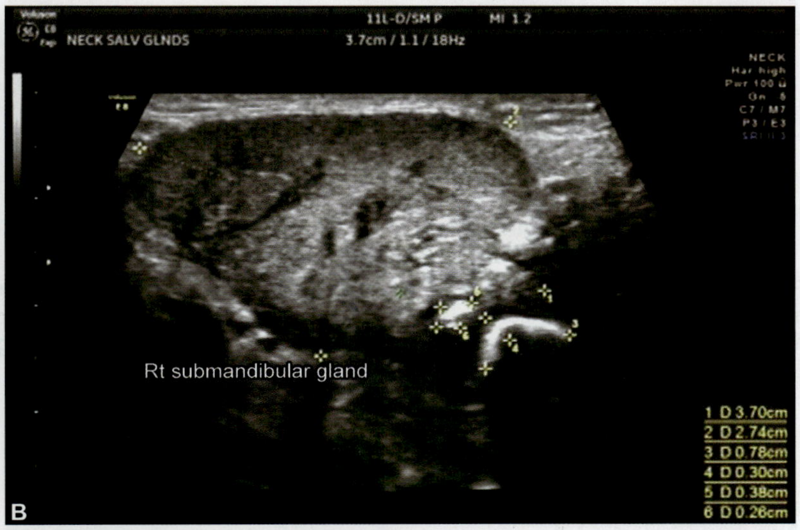

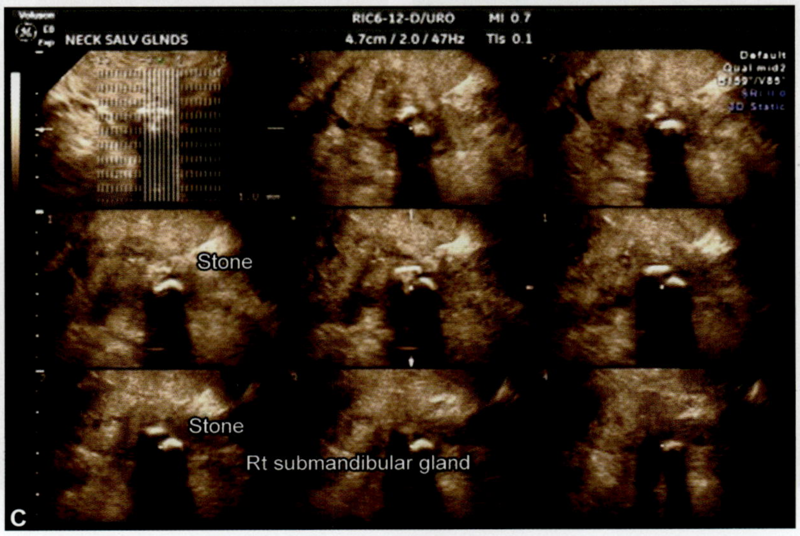

FIGURES 5.38A to C: Right submandibular gland calculi. A lady presented with soft tissue swelling in right submandibular gland. HRSG shows diffuse enlargement of the gland. Multiple small echogenic foci are seen in the gland. Two big echogenic shadows are seen impacted in the duct, which are accompanied with acoustic shadowing. 3D imaging of the gland shows the calculi impacted in the duct.

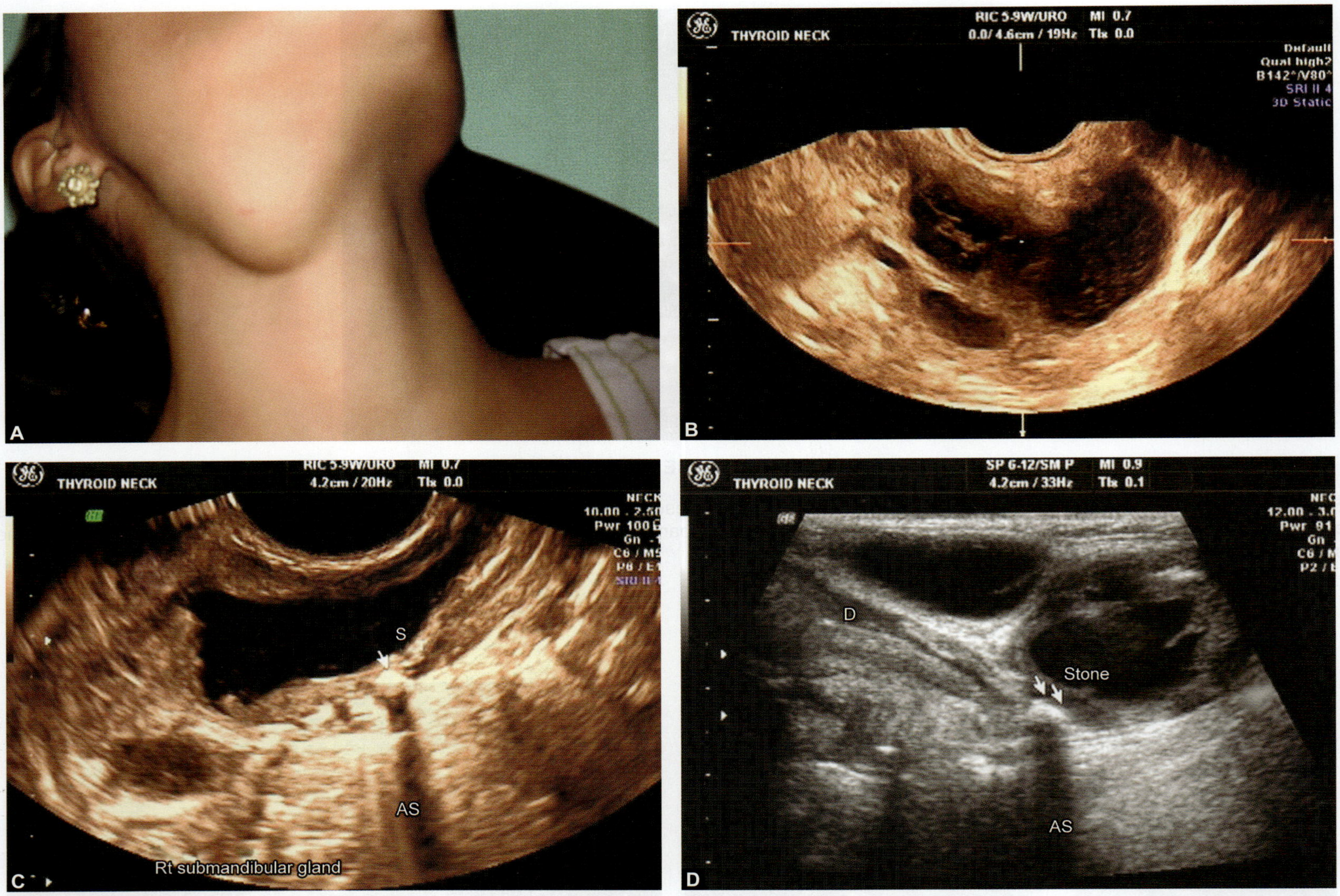

FIGURES 5.39A to D: A young lady presented with soft tissue swelling in right submandibular gland fossa. HRSG shows a low level echo complex mass in submandibular gland. The gland duct is also dilated. On 3D imaging, multiple calculi are seen in the duct, which are accompanied with acoustic shadowing. Low level echoes are also seen in the collection suggestive of chronic abscess formation.

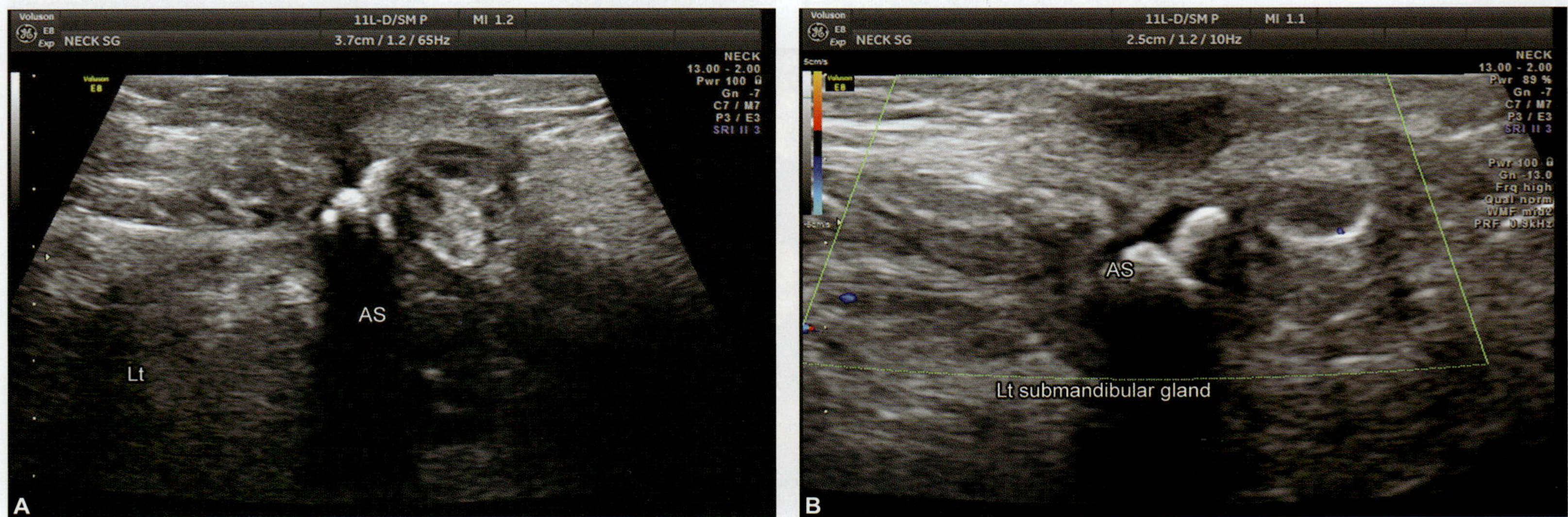

FIGURES 5.40A and B

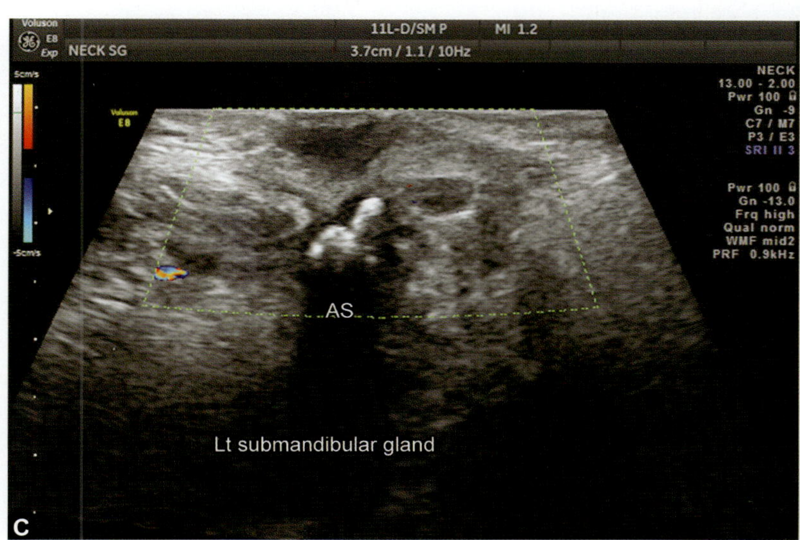

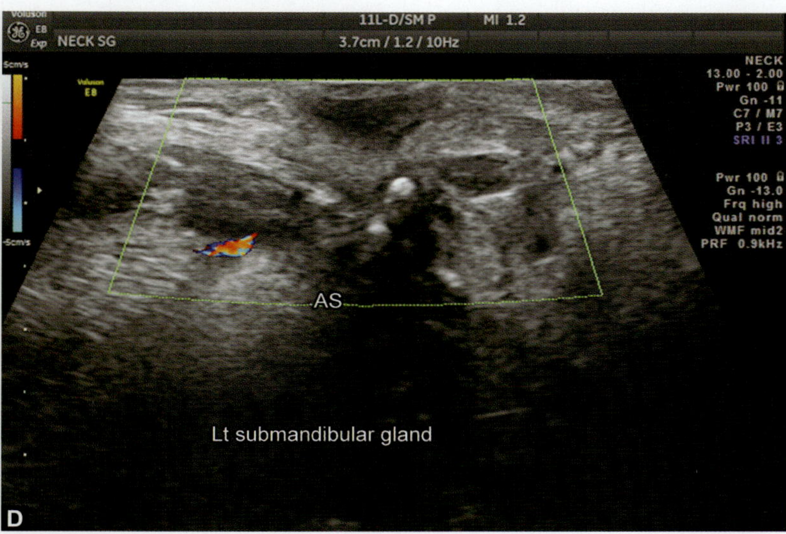

FIGURES 5.40C and D

FIGURES 5.40A to D: Chronic submandibular gland inflammation with multiple calculi. An old lady presented with a hard swelling in the left submandibular gland fossa. HRSG shows irregular ill-defined inhomogeneous heterogeneous texture of the submandibular gland. Dense echogenic foci are seen in the substance of gland, which are accompanied with dense acoustic shadowing. Normal glandular texture is lost. Biopsy from gland shows chronic inflammatory disease.

SALIVARY GLAND MASSES

Salivary gland masses can be easily picked up on HRSG. The aims of ultrasonographic imaging in a palpable mass in salivary gland is to confirm the presence of the mass, to differentiate between intra and extra glandular mass, and the nature of the mass whether it is solid or cystic. Detection of parotid mass is very accurate and its sensitivity is 100% as it can detect subclinical nodules, although identification of nature of mass is more difficult and FNAC can confirm the diagnosis.

Pleomorphic adenomas, mixed parotid gland tumor are more common and they remain silent for many years. By and large, all the benign tumors of parotid gland are echo poor and homogeneous in texture. They are sharply demarcated. Malignant tumors are grossly heterogeneous and irregular in outline. Irregular pockets of collection are seen in the tumor suggestive of hemorrhage. Associated lymph node enlargement around the lesion is suggestive of malignancy. However, HRSG guided biopsy is ultimate to confirm the diagnosis. HRSG is also helpful in staging of the disease for proper treatment and management.

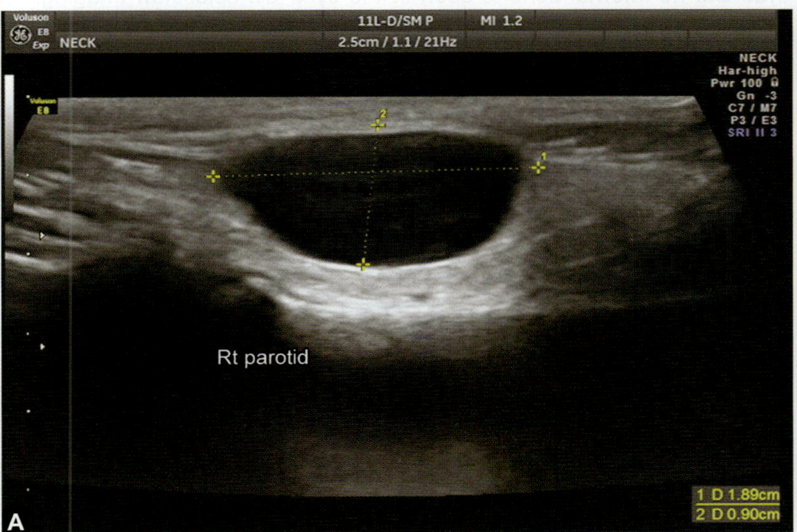

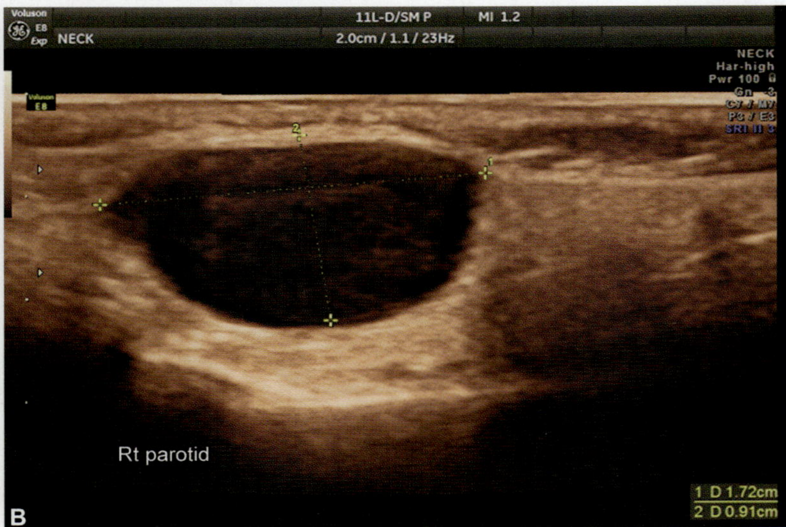

FIGURES 5.41A and B

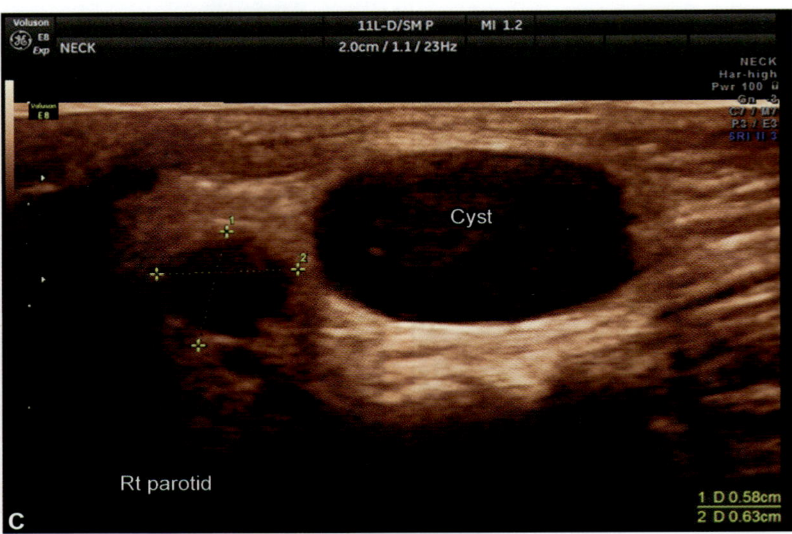

FIGURE 5.41C

FIGURES 5.41A to C: Simple parotid cyst. A young boy presented with soft tissue swelling in right parotid gland. HRSG shows a well-defined cystic shadow in the parotid gland. The cyst shows clear fluid. Post-cystic enhancement is also seen posterior to the cyst. A nodal shadow is also seen near the cyst suggestive of enlarged sentinel node.

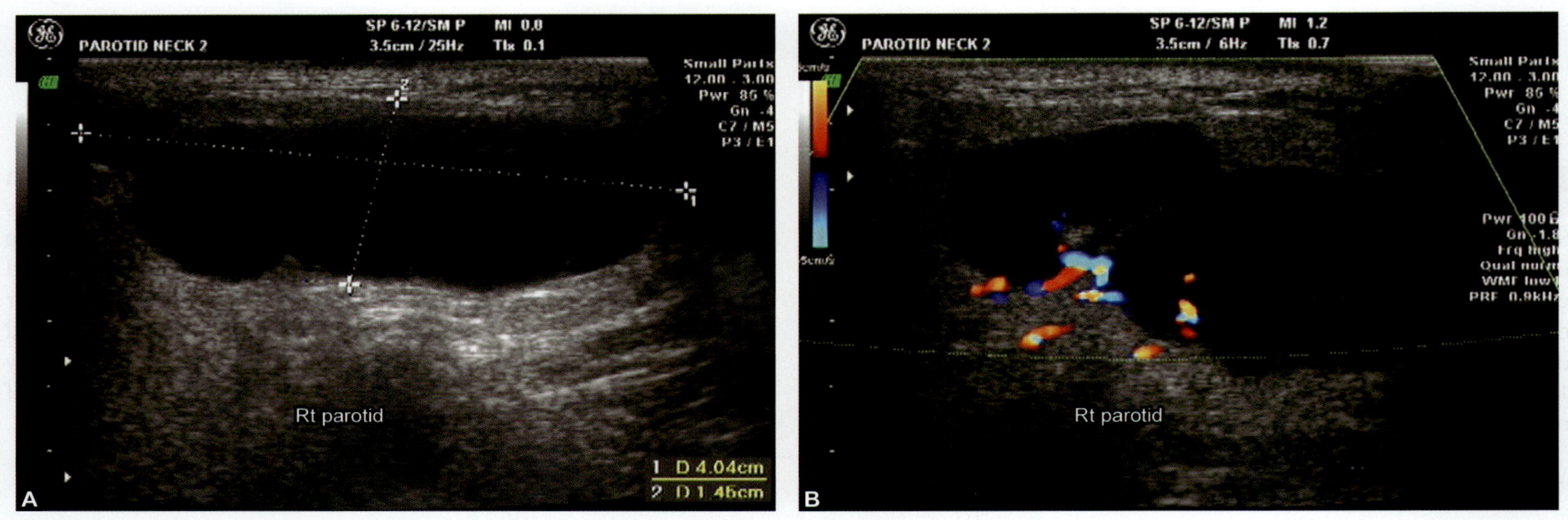

FIGURES 5.42A and B: Big cystic swelling in parotid gland. A patient presented with soft tissue swelling in right parotid gland. HRSG shows a big cystic mass in the parotid gland. A small thin septa is also seen in the cyst. But no internal echo is seen in the cyst. On color flow imaging, few vessels are seen feeding the septa of the cyst.

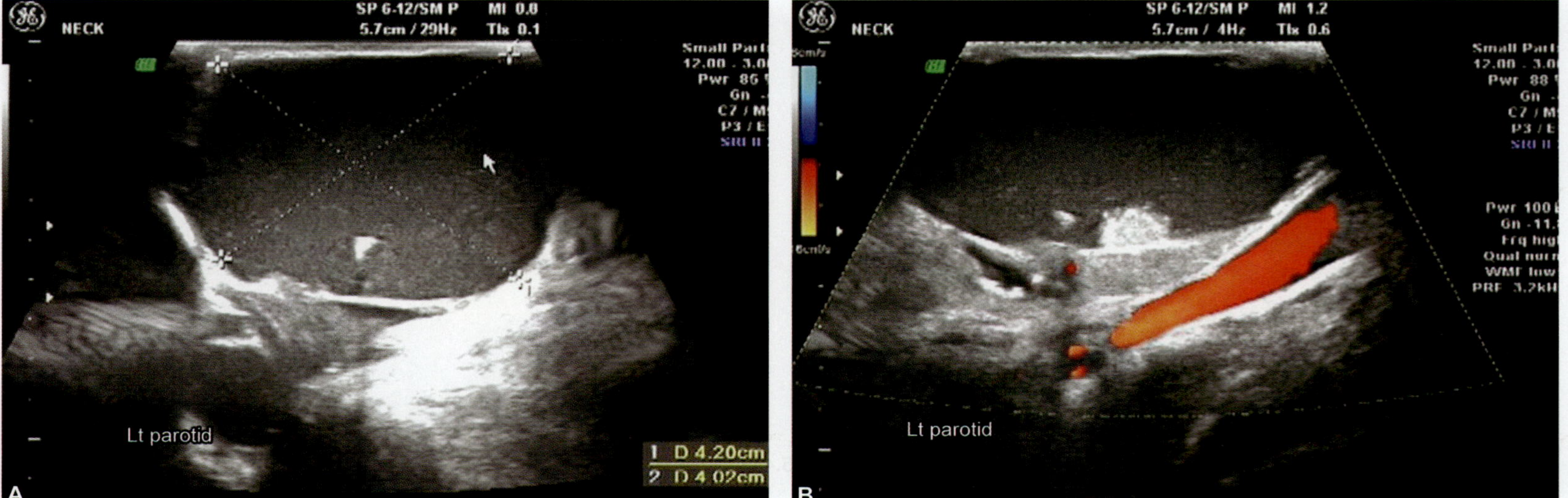

FIGURES 5.43A and B

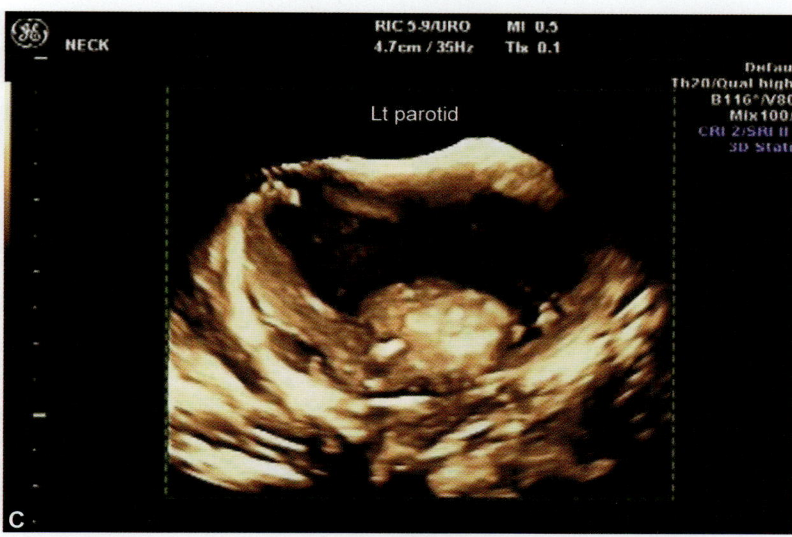

FIGURE 5.43C

FIGURES 5.43A to C: Big retention cyst in the left parotid gland. A patient presented with soft tissue cystic mass in left parotid gland. HRSG shows a big cystic shadow in left parotid gland. Homogeneous echoes are seen in it. However, a small echogenic nodule is also seen in the cyst. 3D imaging shows the nodule very clearly. USG guided FNAC shows benign nature of the nodule.

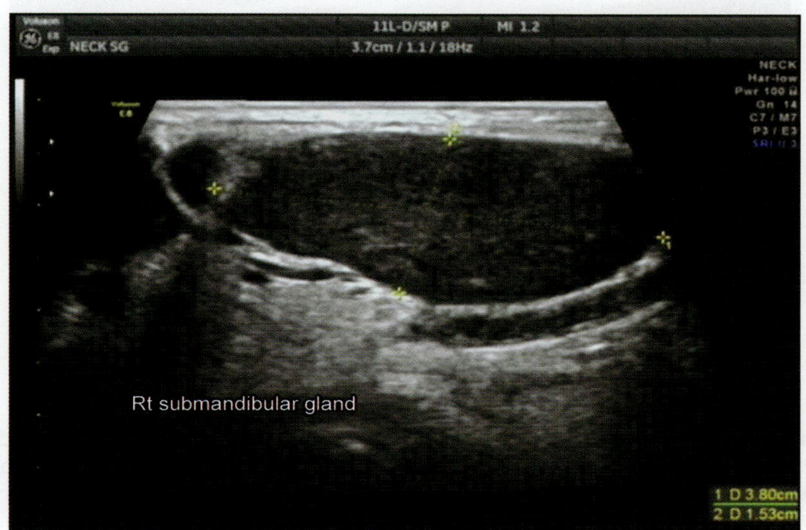

FIGURE 5.44: Submandibular gland cyst. A patient presented with soft tissue swelling in the right submandibular gland. HRSG shows a well-defined cystic mass in the right submandibular gland. Thick echoes are seen in the cyst. But no septation is seen.

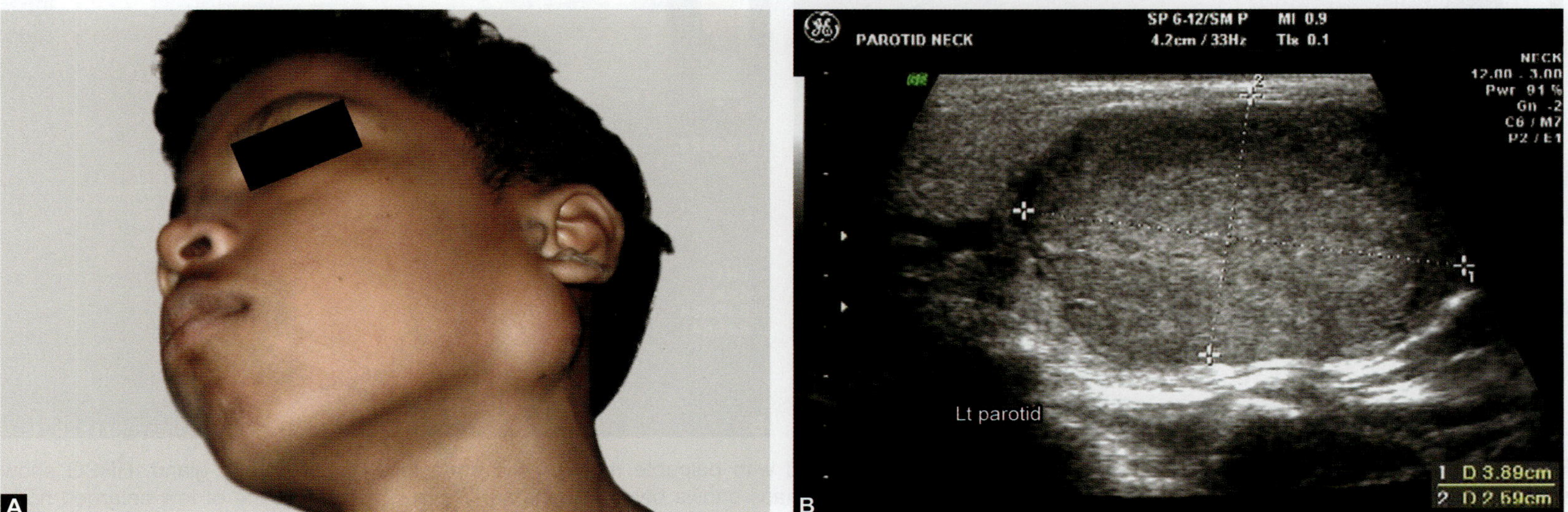

FIGURES 5.45A and B

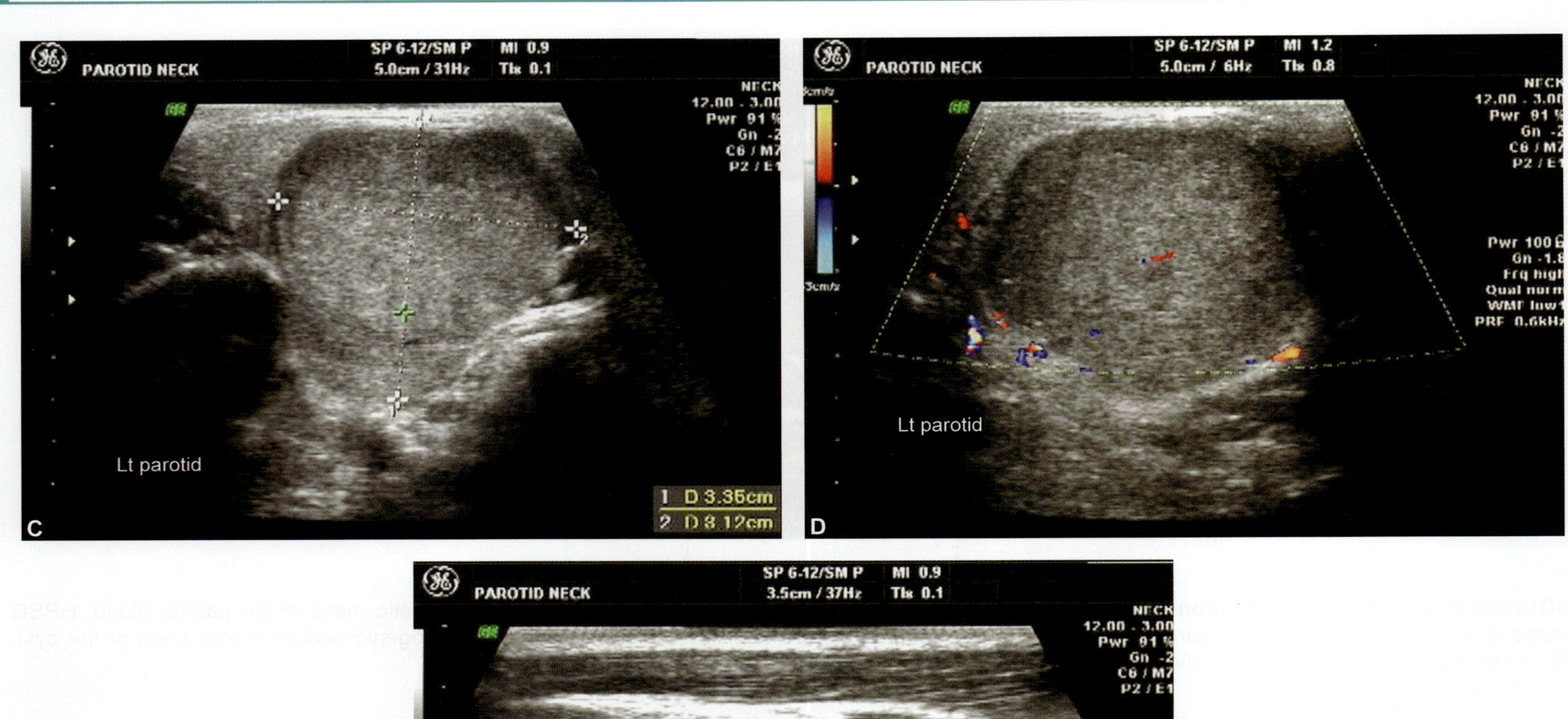

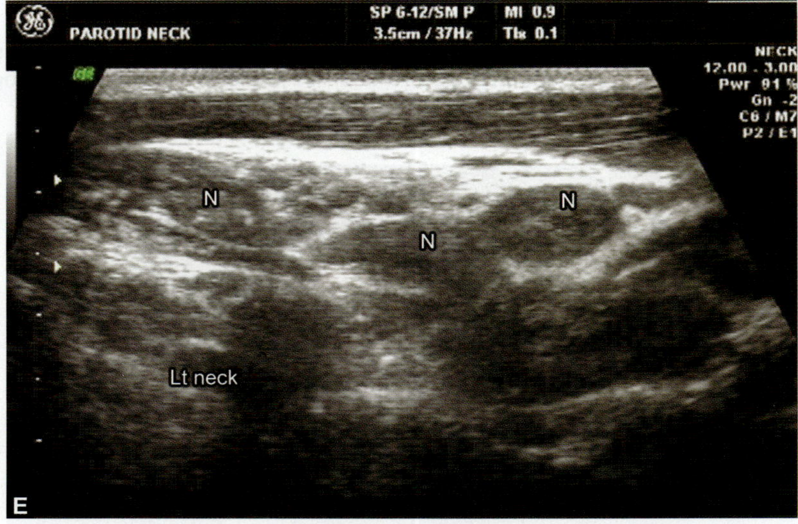

FIGURES 5.45C to E

FIGURES 5.45A to E: Adenoma parotid. A young boy presented with soft tissue mass in the left parotid gland. HRSG shows a well-defined homogeneous soft tissue mass in left parotid gland. No calcification is seen in the mass. No cystic degeneration is seen. On color flow imaging, few vessels are seen feeding the mass. Few enlarged nodes are also seen in left upper cervical region. FNAC of the mass confirms pleomorphic adenoma.

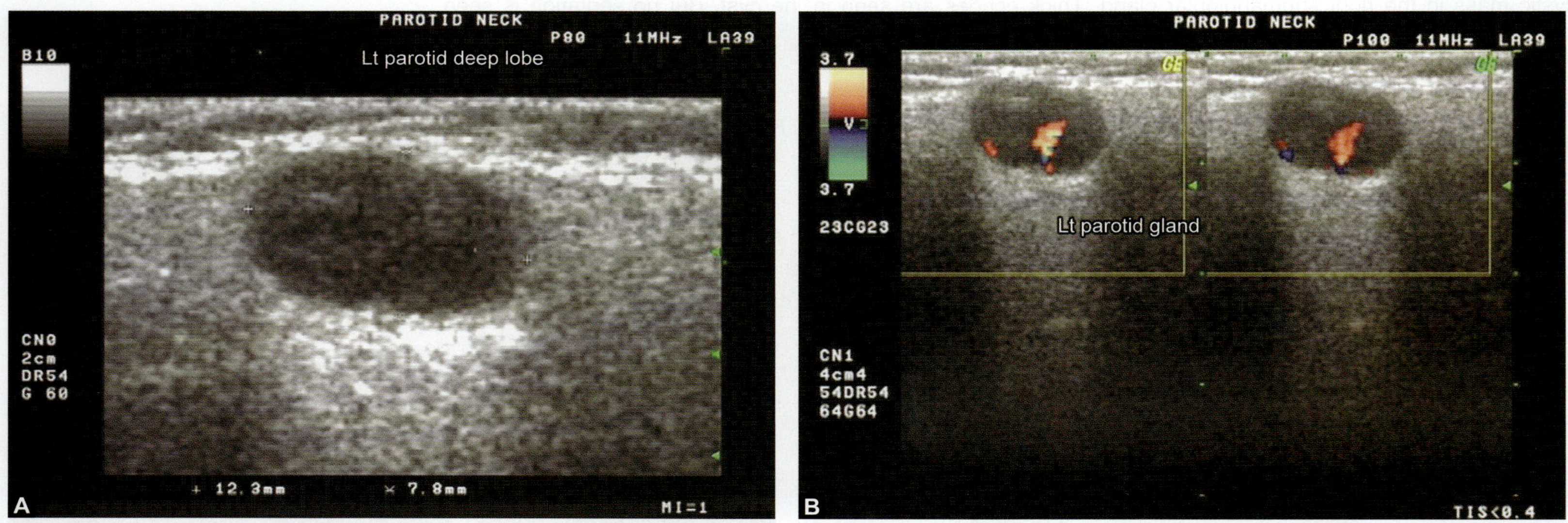

FIGURES 5.46A and B: Benign adenoma parotid. A patient presented with palpable mass in the deep lobe of left parotid gland. HRSG shows well-defined homogeneous hypoechoic mass in the gland. Biopsy of the mass shows benign adenoma. There is also evidence of few enlarged nodes seen in the upper cervical region. On color flow imaging normal flow is seen in them.

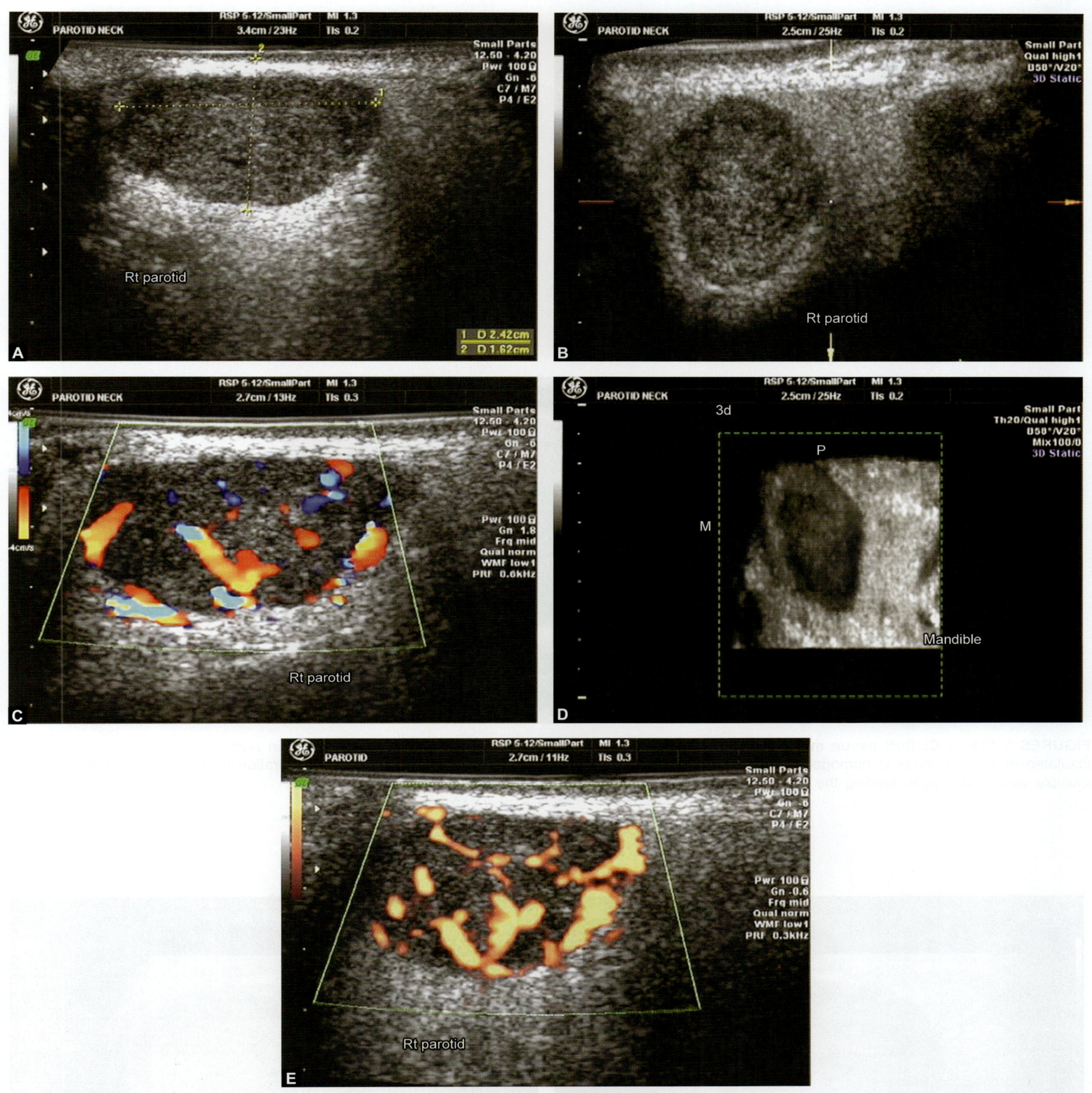

FIGURES 5.47A to E: A lady presented with soft mass in the right parotid gland. HRSG of the gland shows well-defined homogeneous mass. It shows sharp margins. No necrosis or calcification is seen in it. 3D of the same mass shows better details of the mass. Color flow imaging of the mass shows increased flow in the mass. Biopsy of the mass proves benign pleomorphic adenoma.

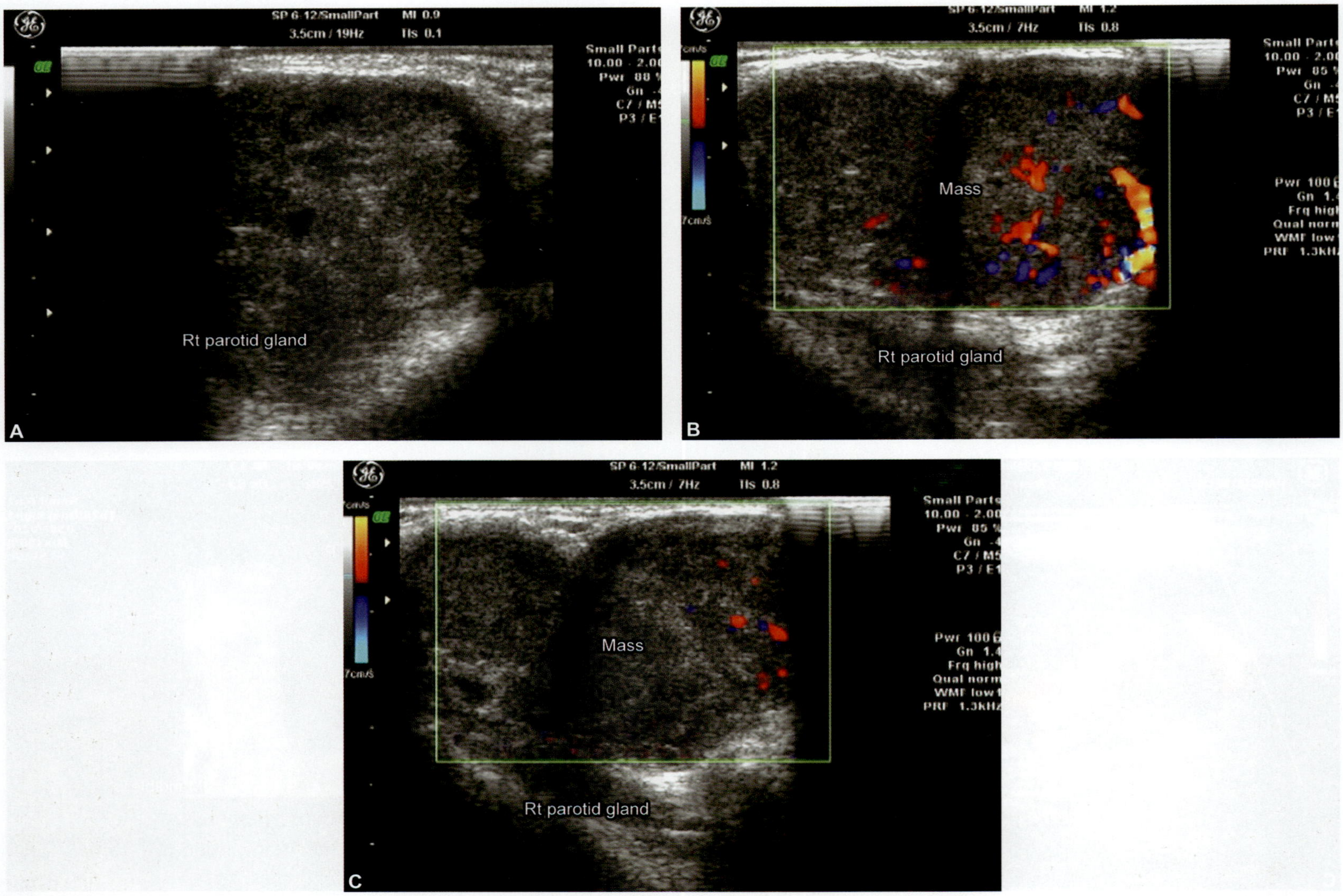

FIGURES 5.48A to C: Soft tissue mass in right parotid gland. A patient presented with soft tissue mass in right parotid gland. HRSG shows a lobulated mass. The mass is homogeneous in texture. No calcification is seen in the mass. No cystic degeneration is seen. On color flow imaging, multiple vessels are seen feeding the mass. Biopsy of the mass confirms pleomorphic adenoma.

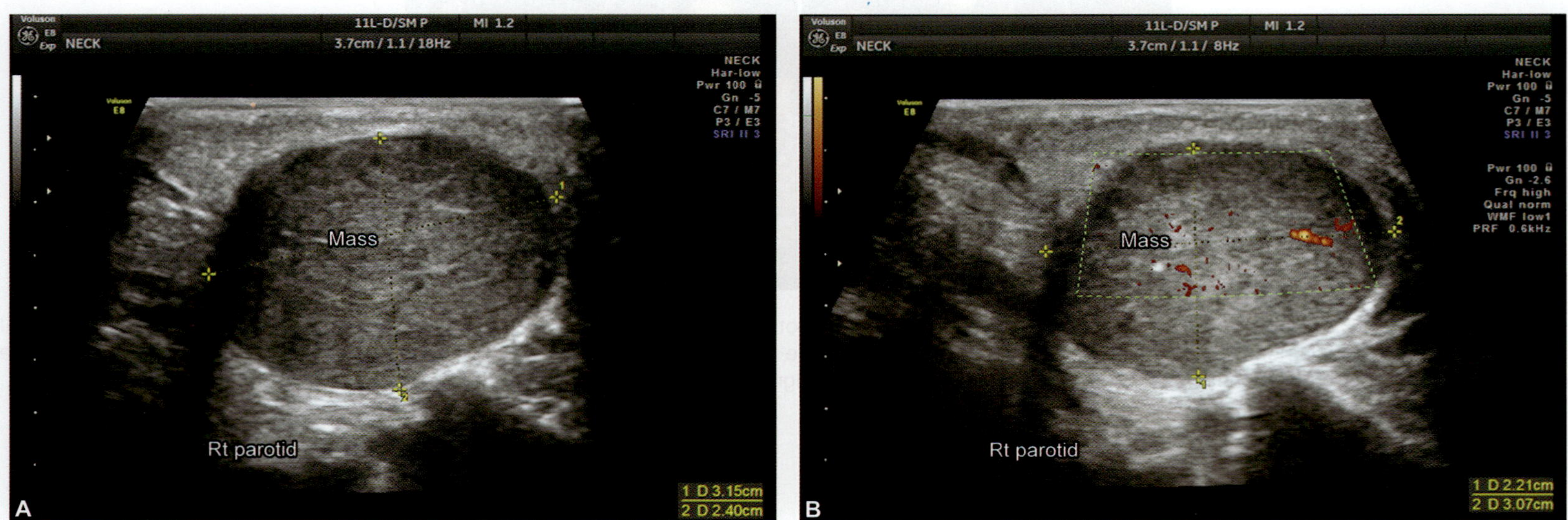

FIGURES 5.49A and B

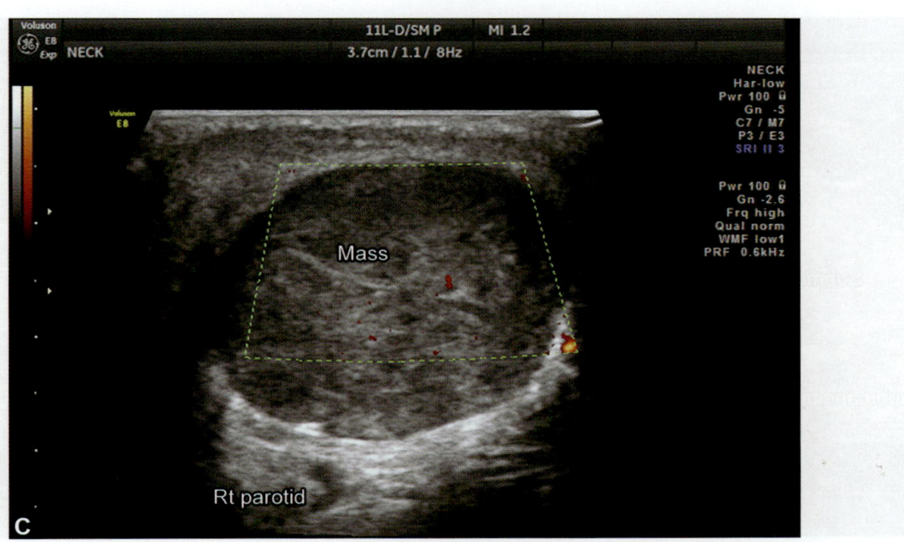

FIGURE 5.49C

FIGURES 5.49A to C: A patient presented with soft tissue mass in the right parotid gland. HRSG shows a well-defined homogeneous soft tissue mass in the gland. No necrosis is seen in the mass. On color flow imaging, poor flow is seen in the mass. FNAC of the mass confirms slow growing adenoma.

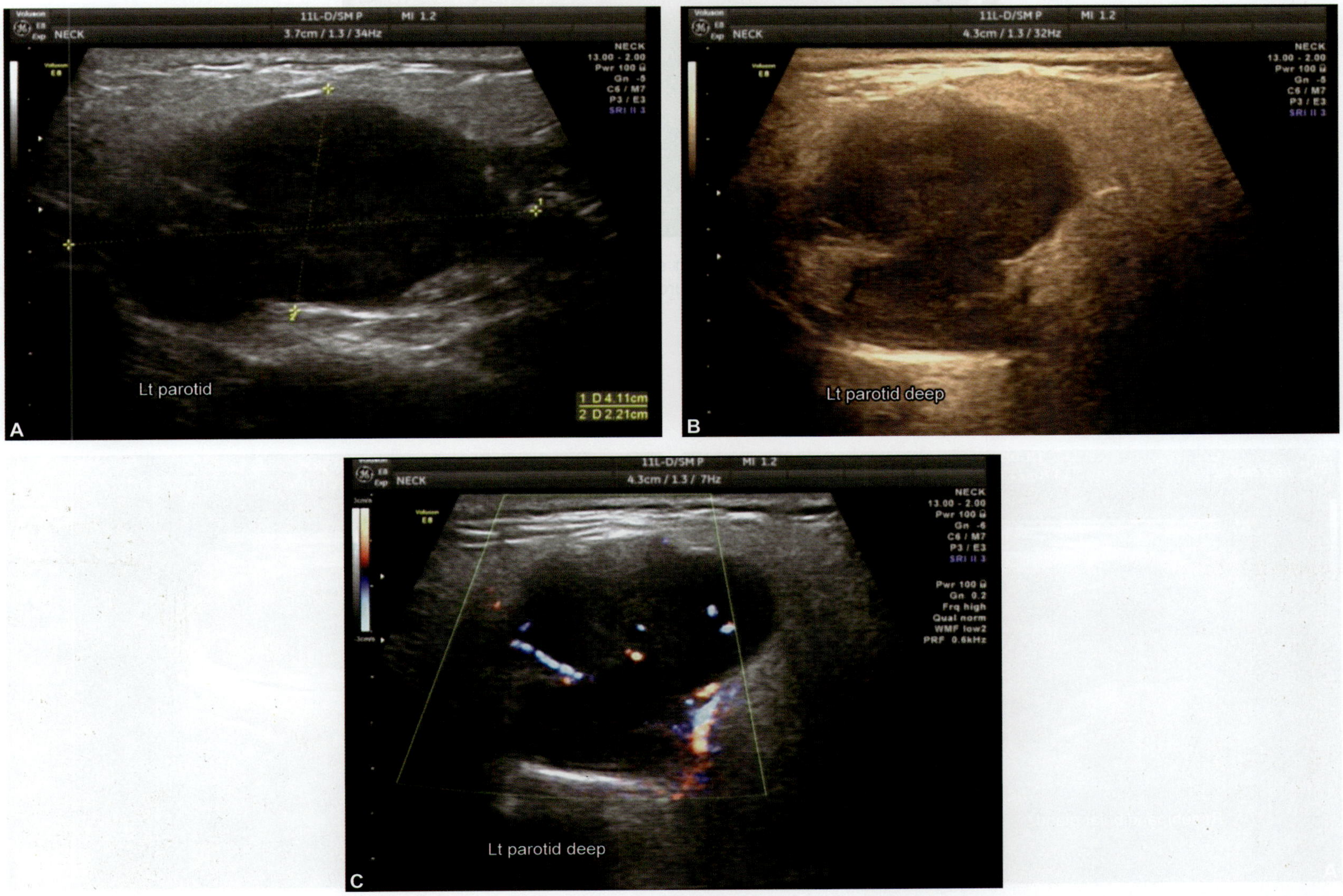

FIGURES 5.50A to C: A 12-year-old child presented with soft tissue mass in left parotid gland. The mass is seen involving superficial and deep lobe. It is homogeneous in texture. No calcification is seen in the mass. No cystic degeneration is seen. On color flow imaging, few vessels are seen feeding the mass. FNAC of the mass confirms benign mass.

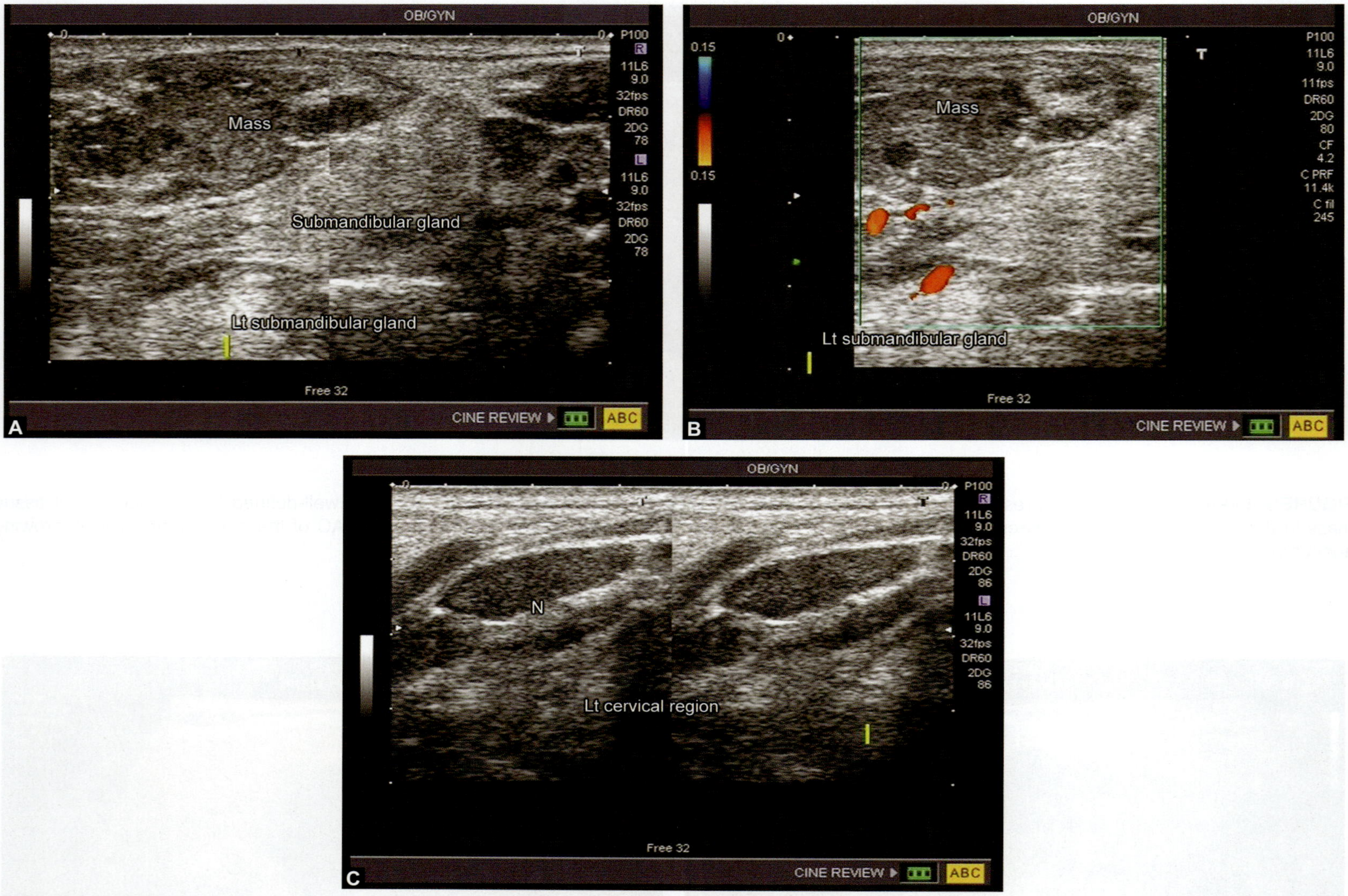

FIGURES 5.51A to C: A patient presented with soft tissue swelling in left submandibular gland. HRSG shows a well-defined homogeneous mass in left submandibular gland. The mass is well-defined homogeneous in texture. Multiple enlarged nodes are also seen in left upper cervical region. On color flow imaging, low flow is seen in the mass.

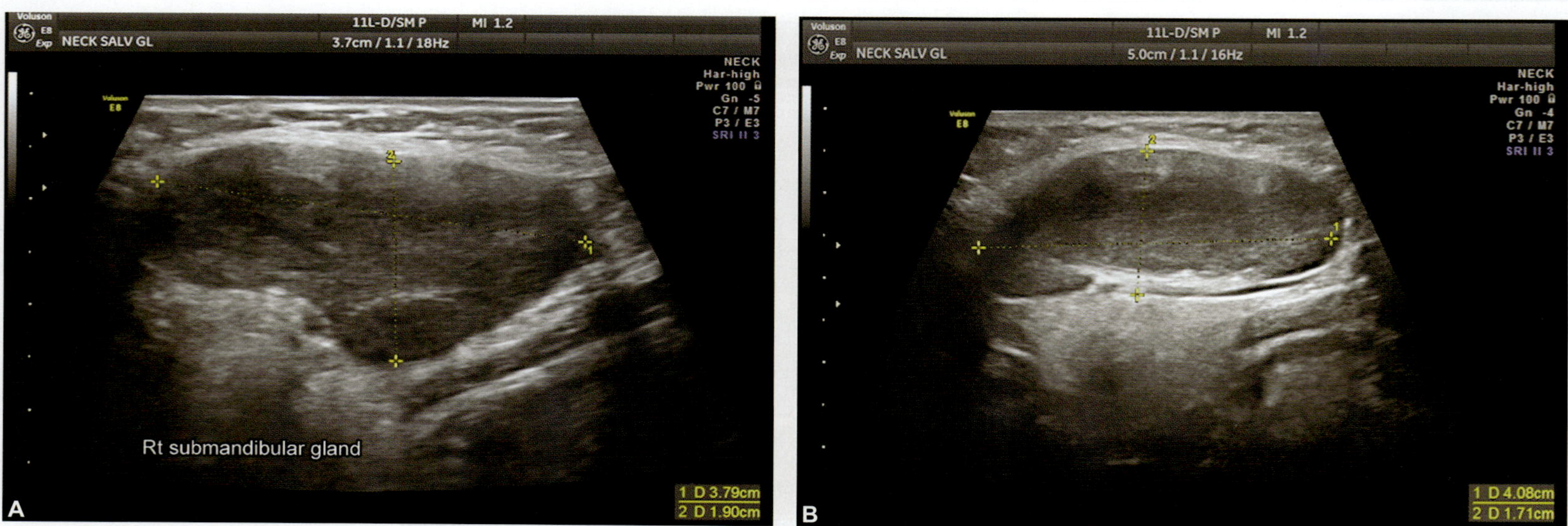

FIGURES 5.52A and B

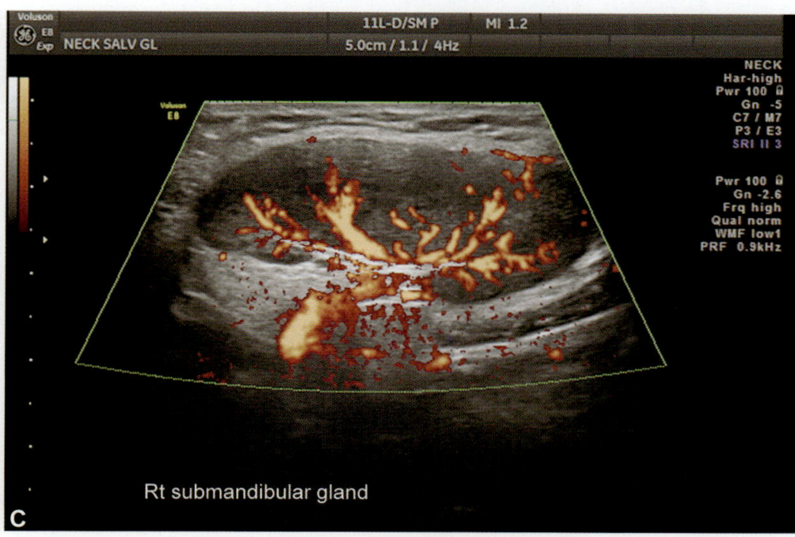

FIGURE 5.52C

FIGURES 5.52A to C: A young girl presented with soft tissue swelling in right submandibular gland which is firm on palpation. HRSG shows a well-encapsulated soft tissue mass in right submandbular gland. The mass is smooth in outline. No calcification is seen in the mass. No cystic degeneration is seen. On color flow imaging, multiple dilated vessels are seen in the mass. Enlarged lymph nodes are seen in the right submandibular gland. On color flow imaging, increased flow is seen in the gland suggestive of reactive nodal enlargement.

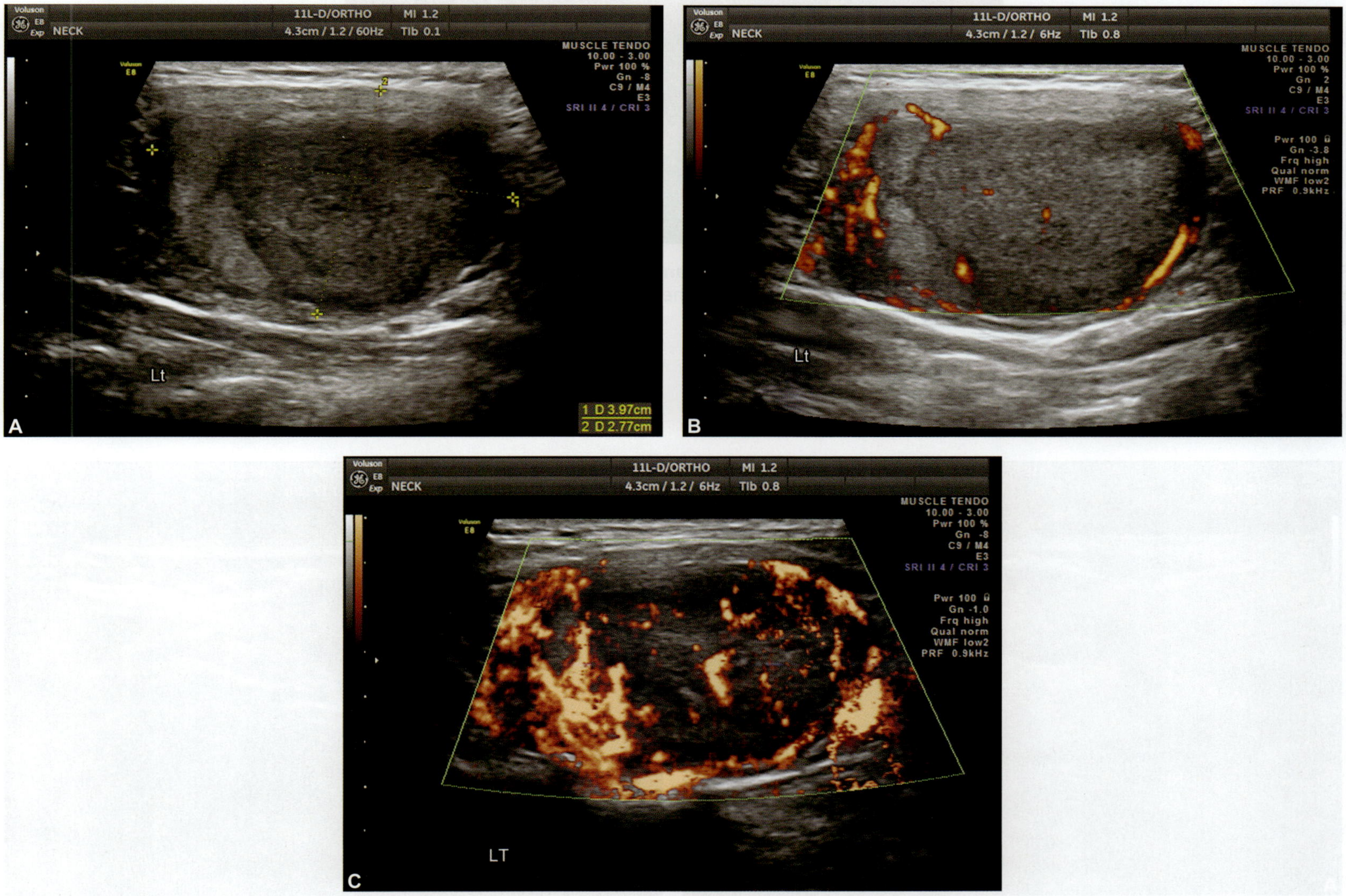

FIGURES 5.53A to C: A lady presented with soft tissue mass in the left submandibular gland. HRSG shows a complex echo mass in the left submandibular gland. It shows homogeneous texture. On color flow imaging, increased flow is seen in it. No calcification or cystic necrosis is seen in the mass. FNAC of the mass confirms pleomorphic adenoma.

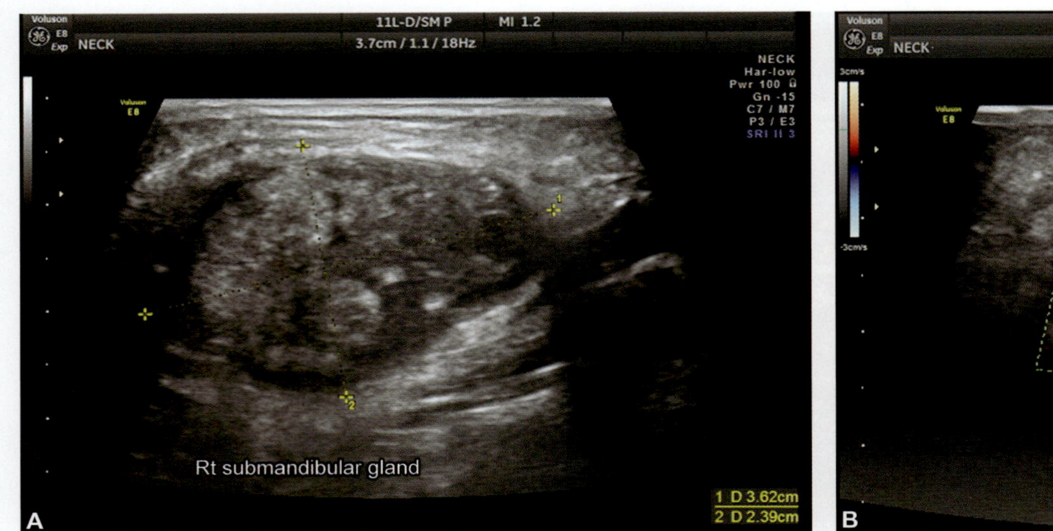

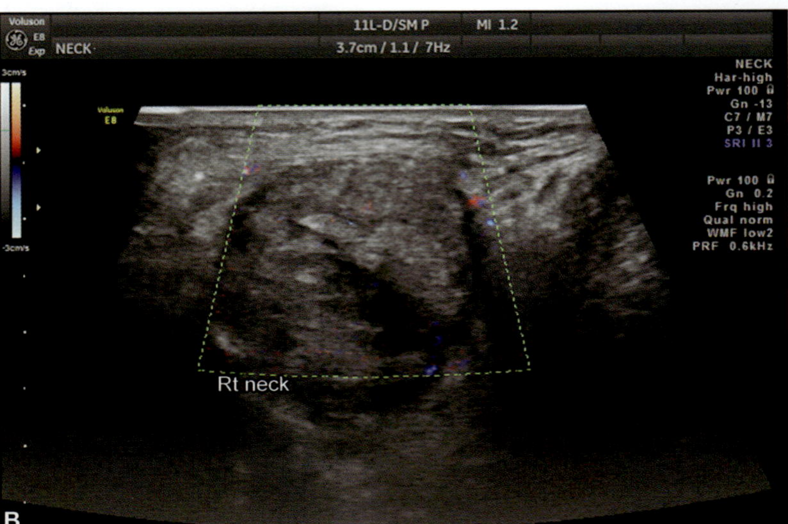

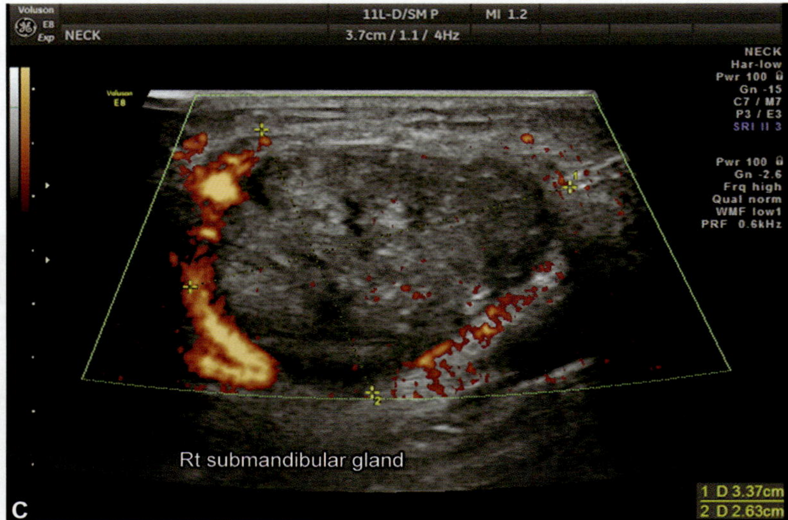

FIGURES 5.54A to C: Complex mass in the right submandibular gland. A patient presented with mass in the right submandibular fossa. The mass shows heterogeneous texture. Multiple echogenic foci are seen in the mass. Low level echoes are also seen in it. On color flow imaging, poor flow is seen in it. Biopsy of the mass confirm chronic abscess.

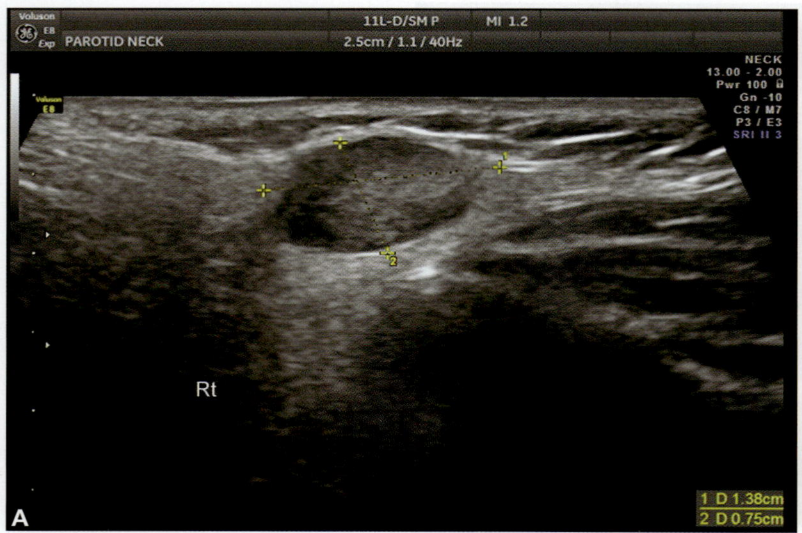

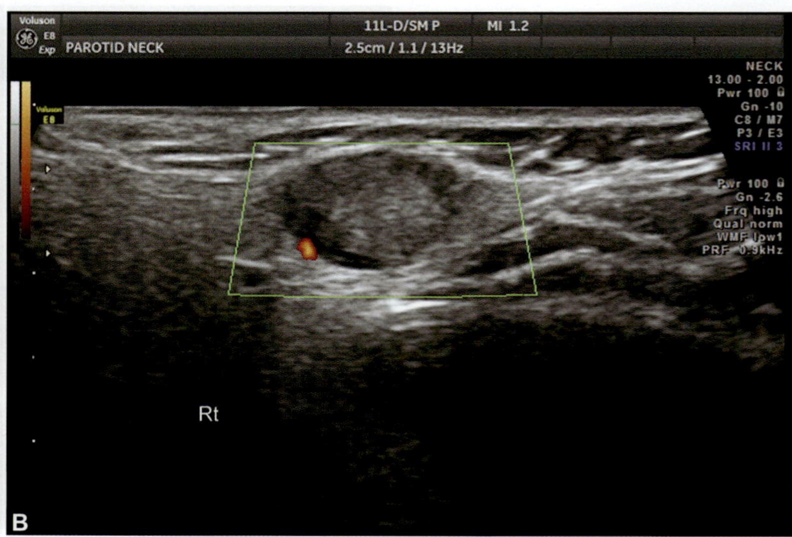

FIGURES 5.55A and B

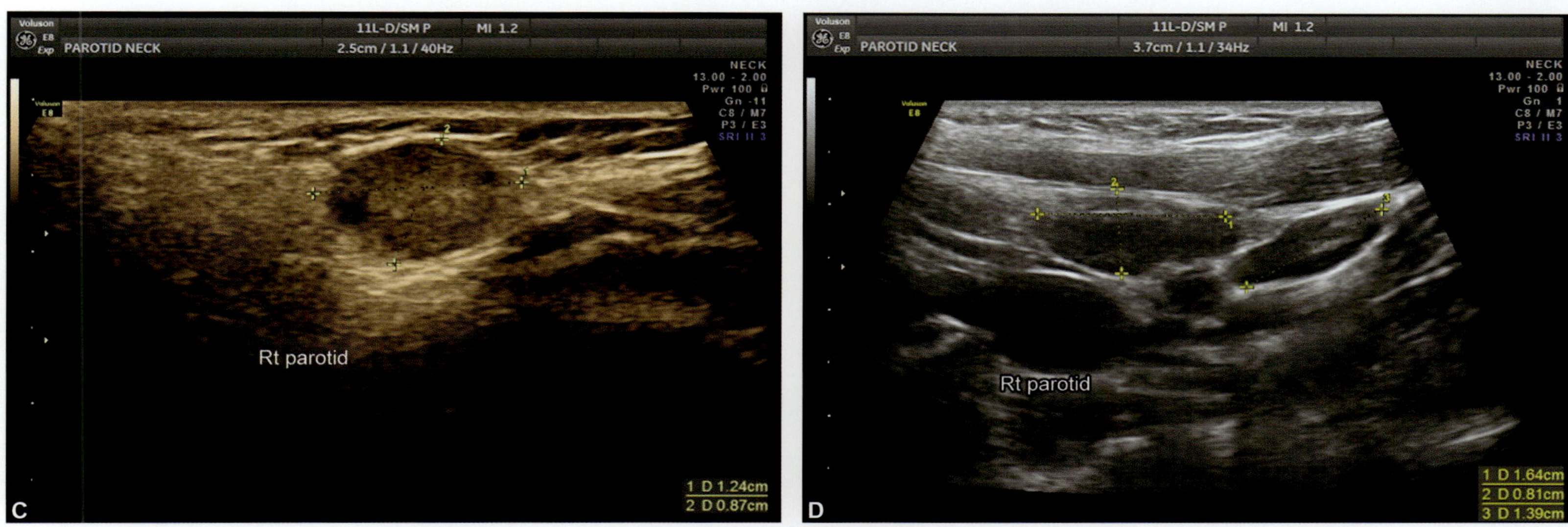

FIGURES 5.55C and D

FIGURES 5.55A to D: A patient presented with nodular shadow in the right parotid gland. HRSG shows a well-defined mass in the right parotid gland. It shows homogeneous texture and it is well-encapsulated. No calcification is seen in it. No cystic degeneration is seen. On color flow imaging, low flow is seen in it. Multiple enlarged nodes are also seen in the right upper cervical region. FNAC from the mass confirms benign adenoma. The lymph nodes are reactive nodal enlargement.

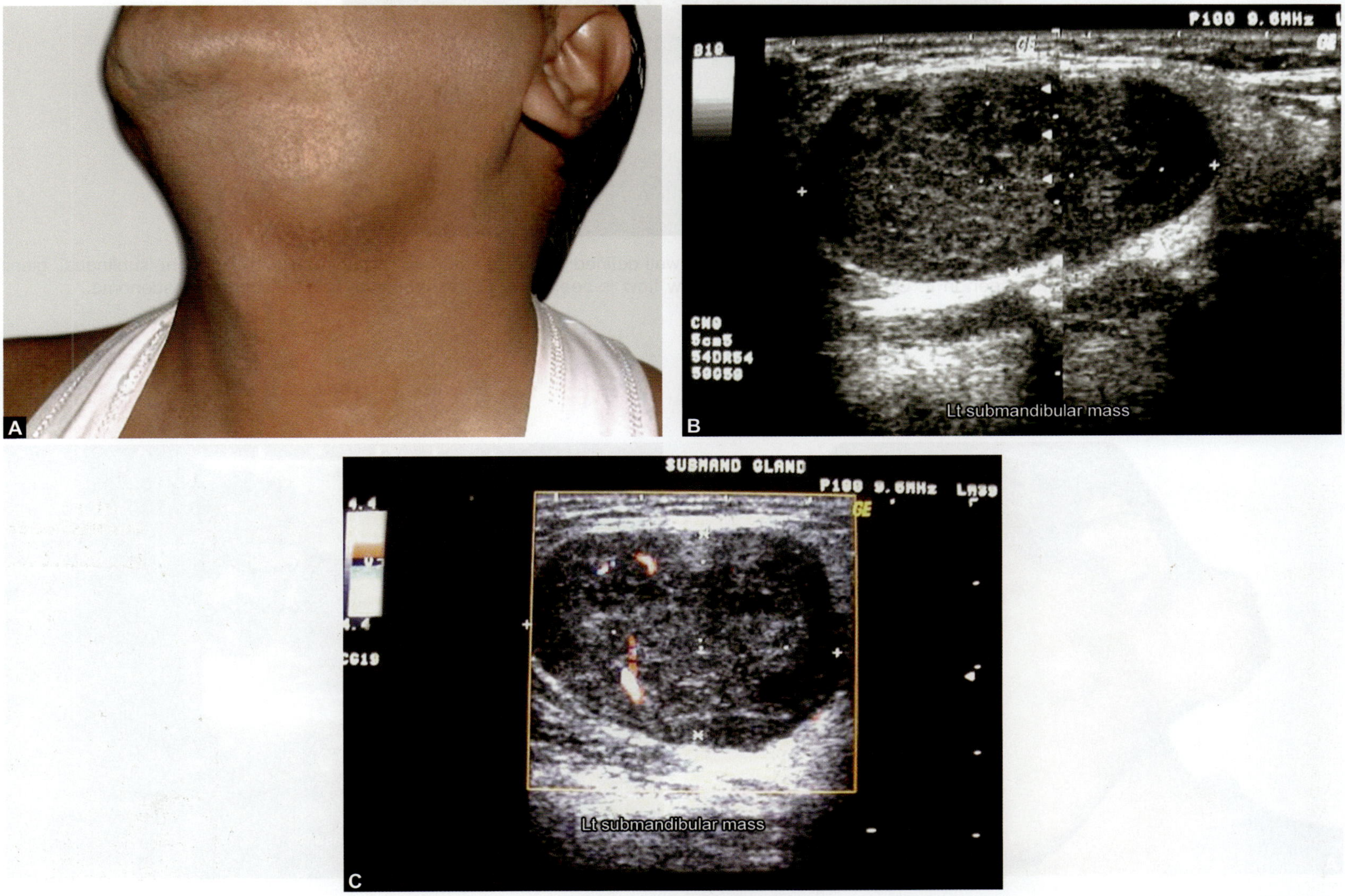

FIGURES 5.56A to C: Submandibular gland pleomorphic adenoma. A patient presented with a soft tissue mass swelling over the left submandibular area. HRSG shows a well-encapsulated hypodense mass in the submandibular area. The mass shows medium level echoes. No cystic degeneration is seen in the mass. No perifocal edema is present. Color Doppler imaging of the mass shows poor flow. Biopsy of the mass shows pleomorphic adenoma.

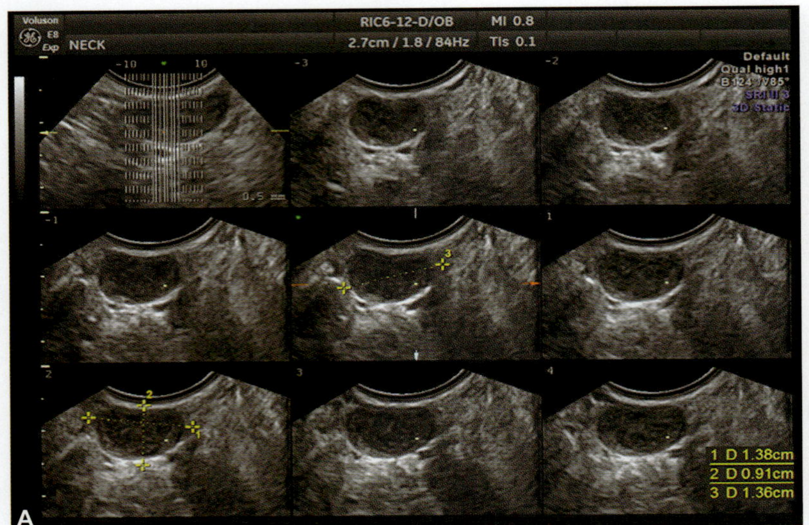

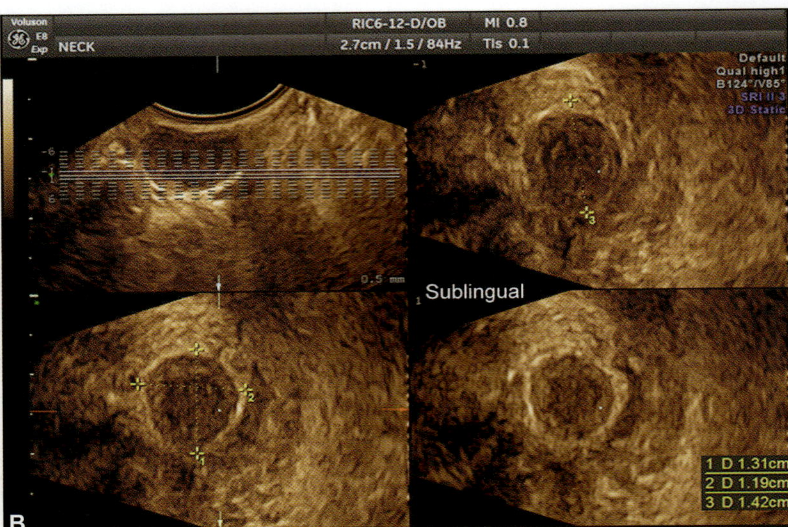

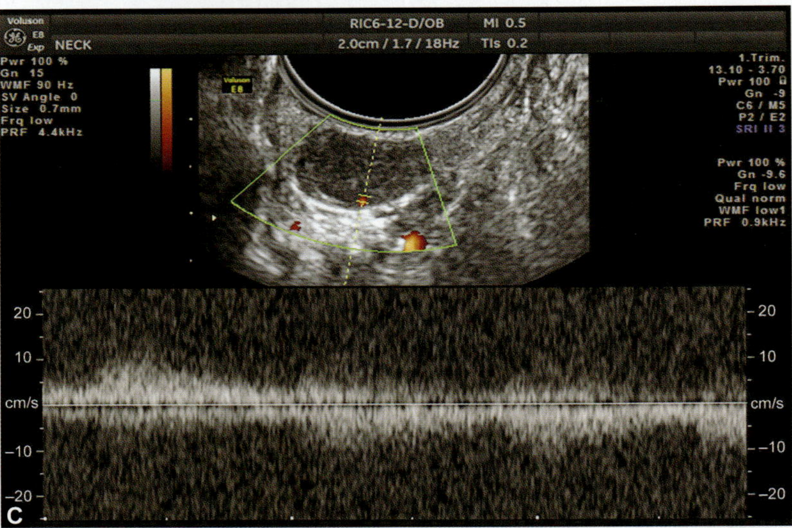

FIGURES 5.57A to C: Sublingual gland adenoma. HRSG shows a well-defined encapsulated soft tissue mass in the right sublingual gland. Homogeneous echoes are seen in it. On color flow imaging, low flow is seen in it. Biopsy confirms benign sublingual adenoma.

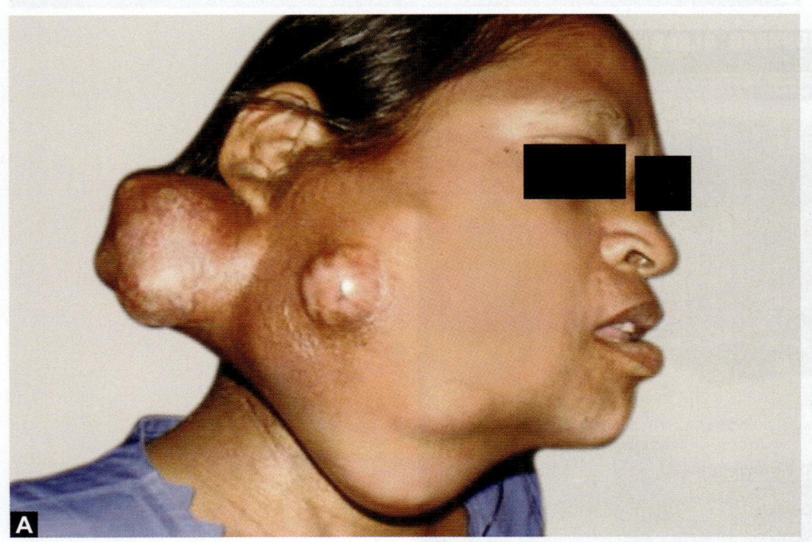

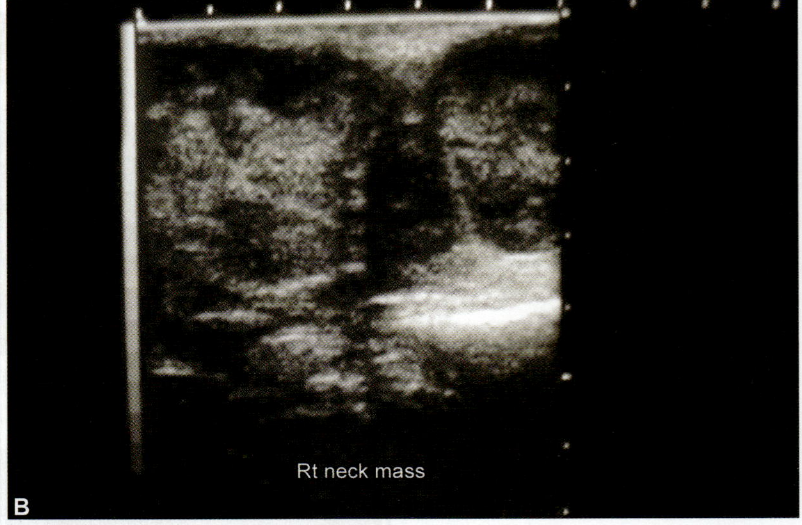

FIGURES 5.58A and B

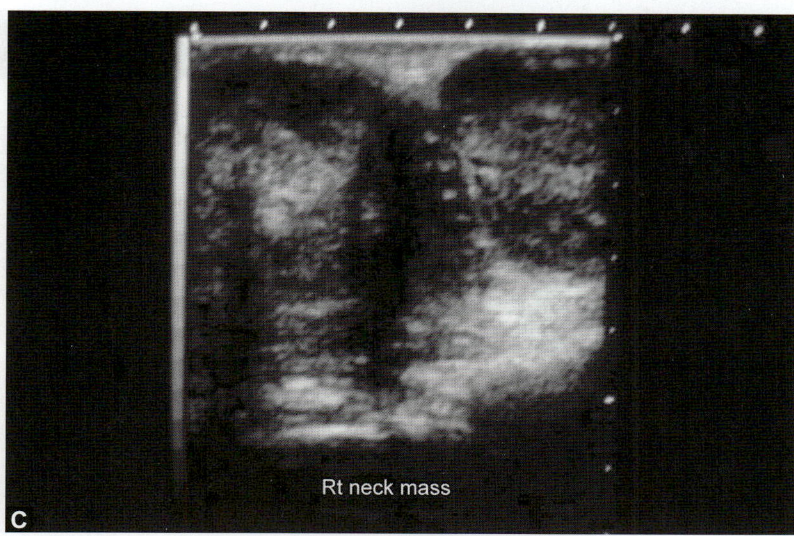

FIGURE 5.58C

FIGURES 5.58A to C: A lady presented with big lobulated nodular masses involving the right parotid gland. HRSG shows multilobulated soft tissue mass involving the whole of parotid gland. No necrosis is seen in them. No cystic degeneration is seen. Biopsy showed pleomorphic adenoma.

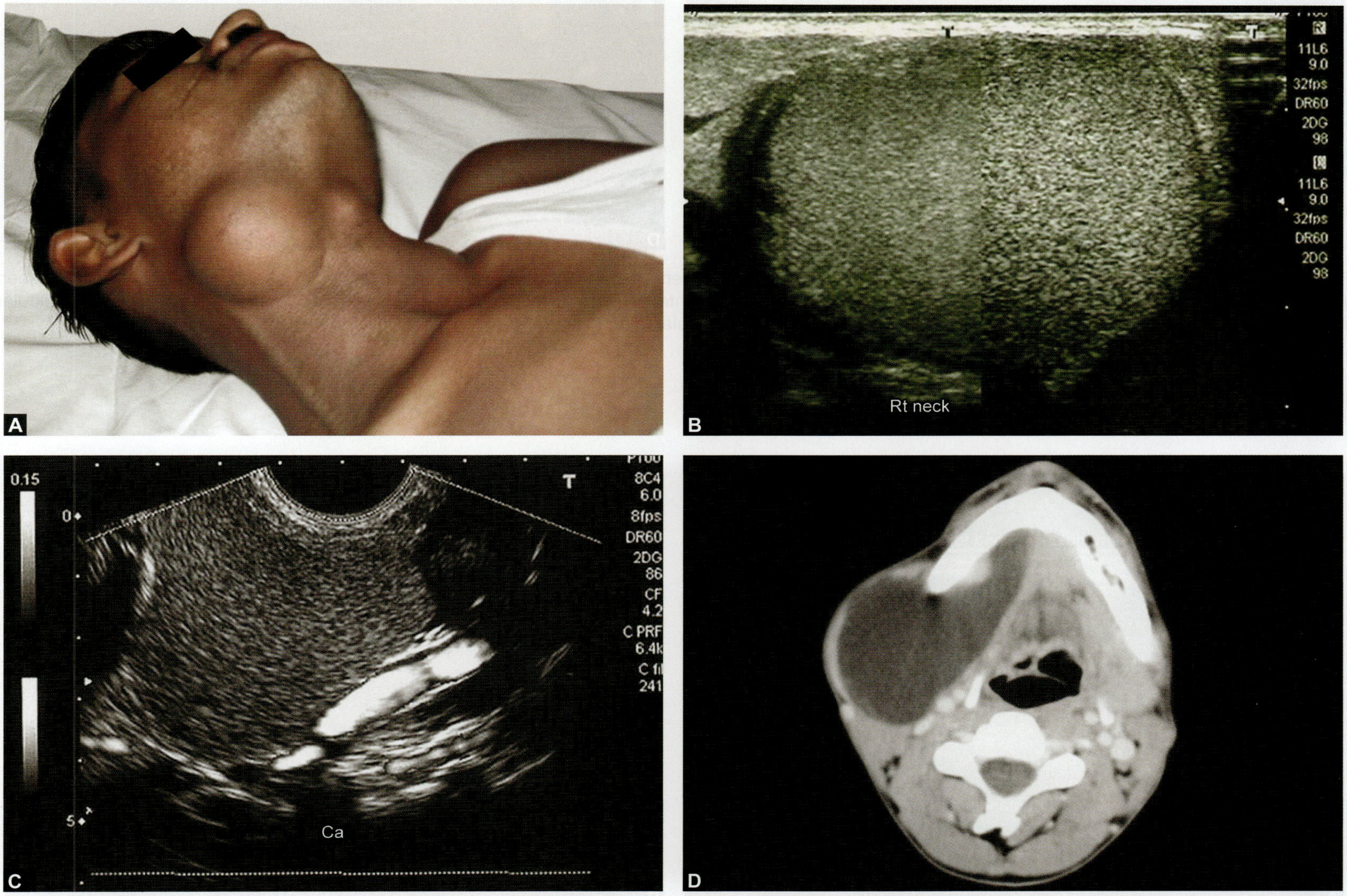

FIGURES 5.59A to D: Submandibular gland ranula. A patient presented with soft cystic swelling in the right submandibular gland fossa. HRSG shows a big cystic mass in the submandibular gland fossa. The cyst shows tongue-like projection. Homogeneous echoes are seen in it suggestive of thick collection. CT scan also shows the cystic mass with a tongue-like projection suggestive of SMG ranula.

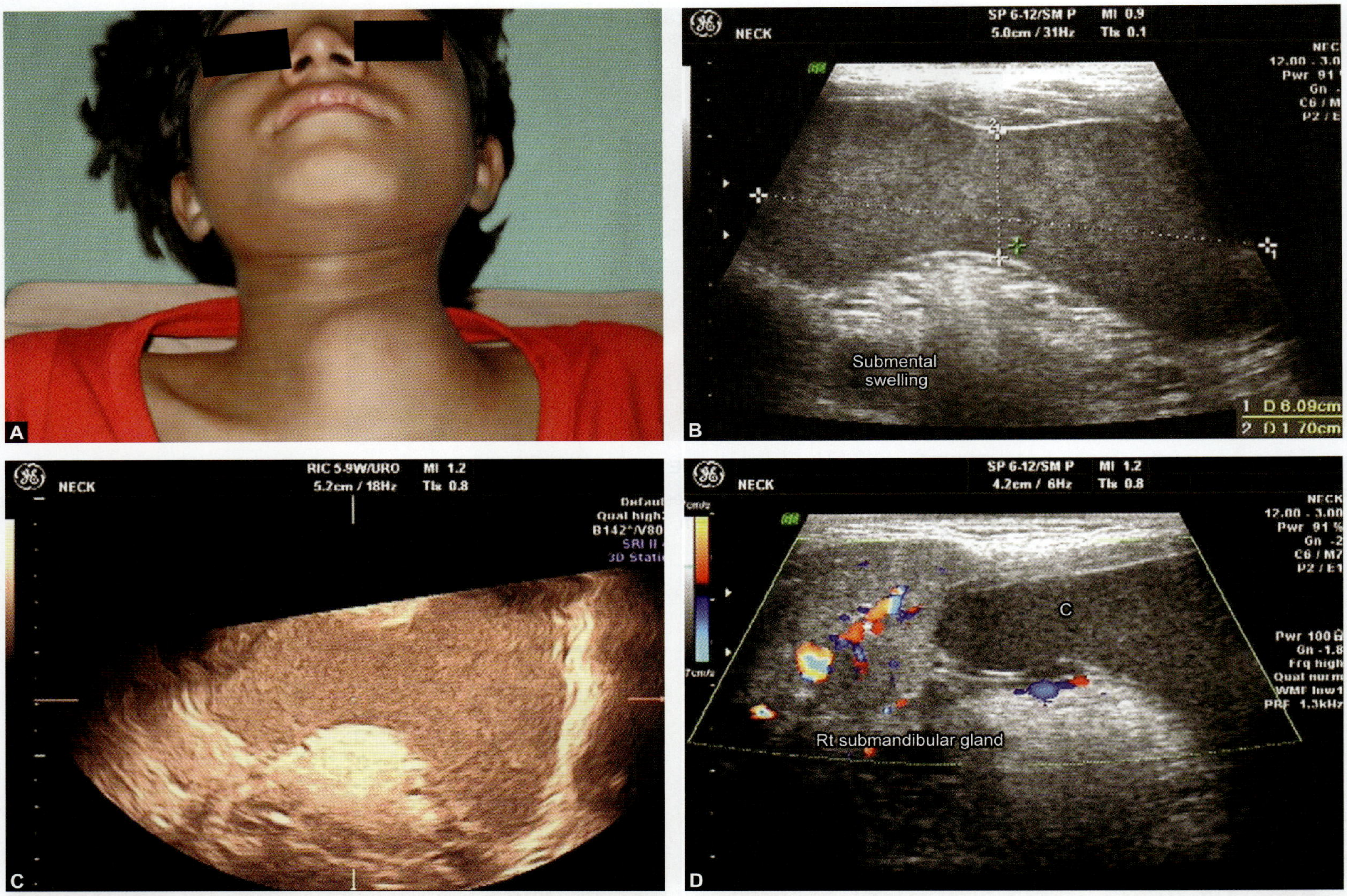

FIGURES 5.60A to D: Submandibular gland ranula. A young girl presented with soft tissue swelling in the right submandibular fossa. It is seen going down and coming to the midline. The swelling is seen in the submental region and going down anteriorly. It is seen in relation to submandibular gland. Homogeneous echoes are seen in it suggestive of big submandibular gland ranula.

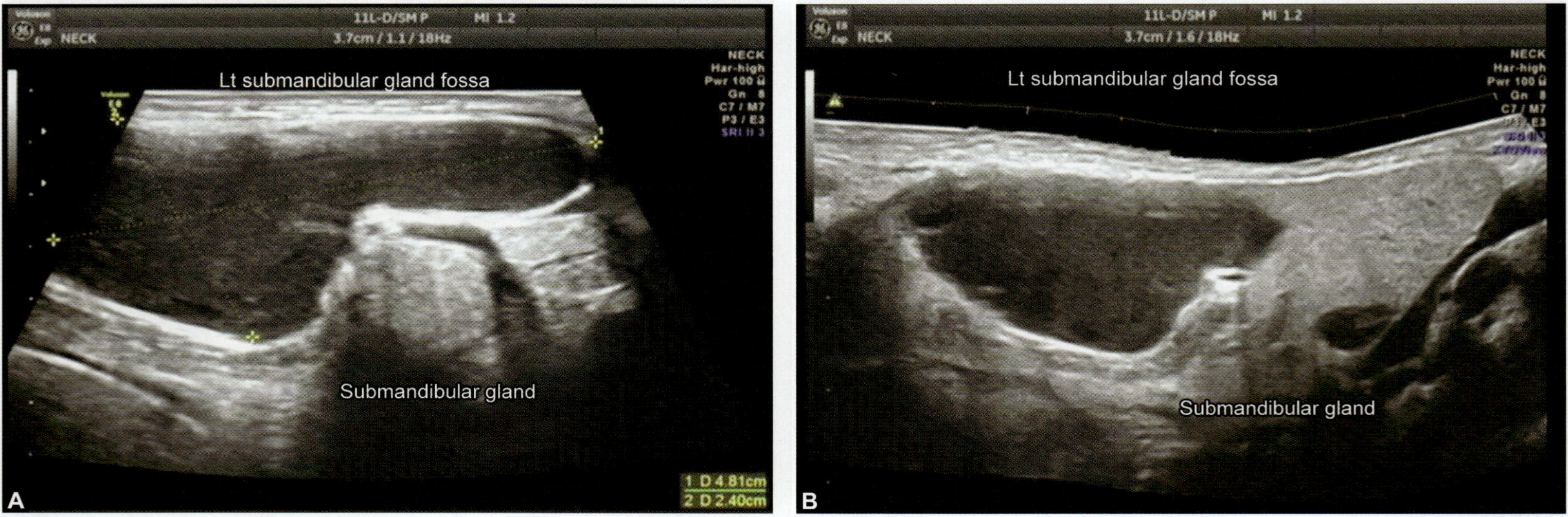

FIGURES 5.61A and B

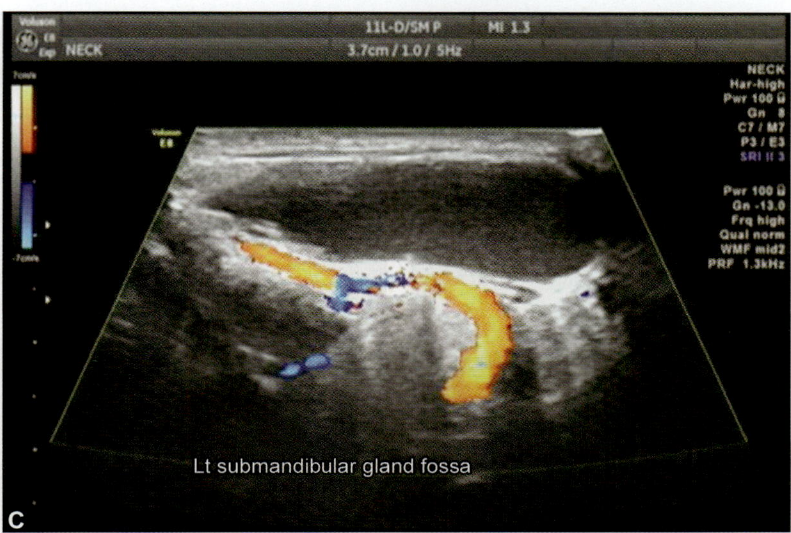

FIGURE 5.61C

FIGURES 5.61A to C: Submandibular gland (SMG) ranula. A big cystic mass is seen in the left submandibular gland fossa. It is seen in relation to left submandibular gland. Homogeneous echoes are seen in it with thick echo collection suggestive of left SMG ranula.

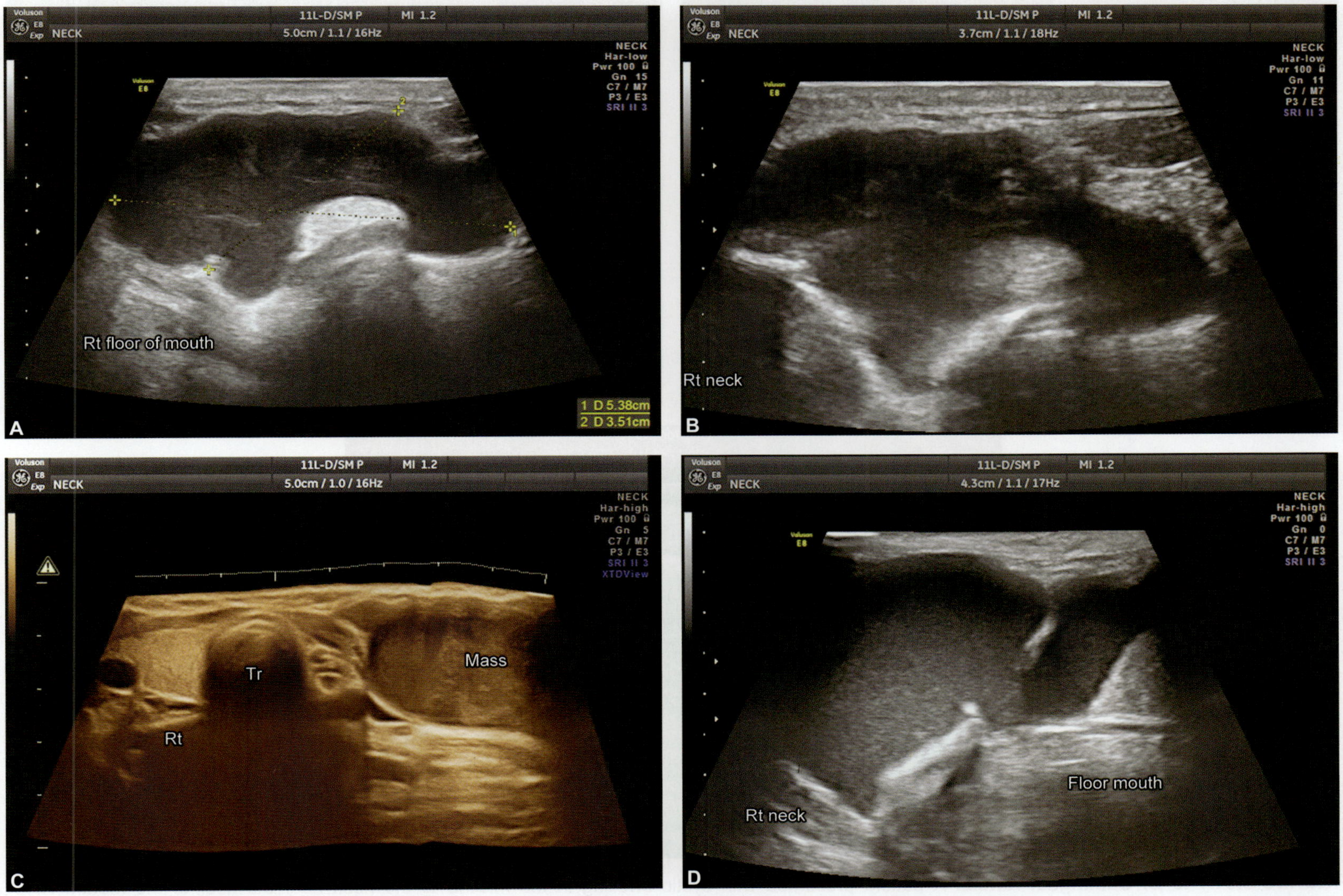

FIGURES 5.62A to D: Sublingual ranula. A patient presented with soft tissue swelling in the midline of the neck. It shows low level echo collection, which is seen extending down and going to floor of the mouth. Homogeneous echoes are seen in it. On aspiration clear fluid is seen in it suggestive of sublingual ranula.

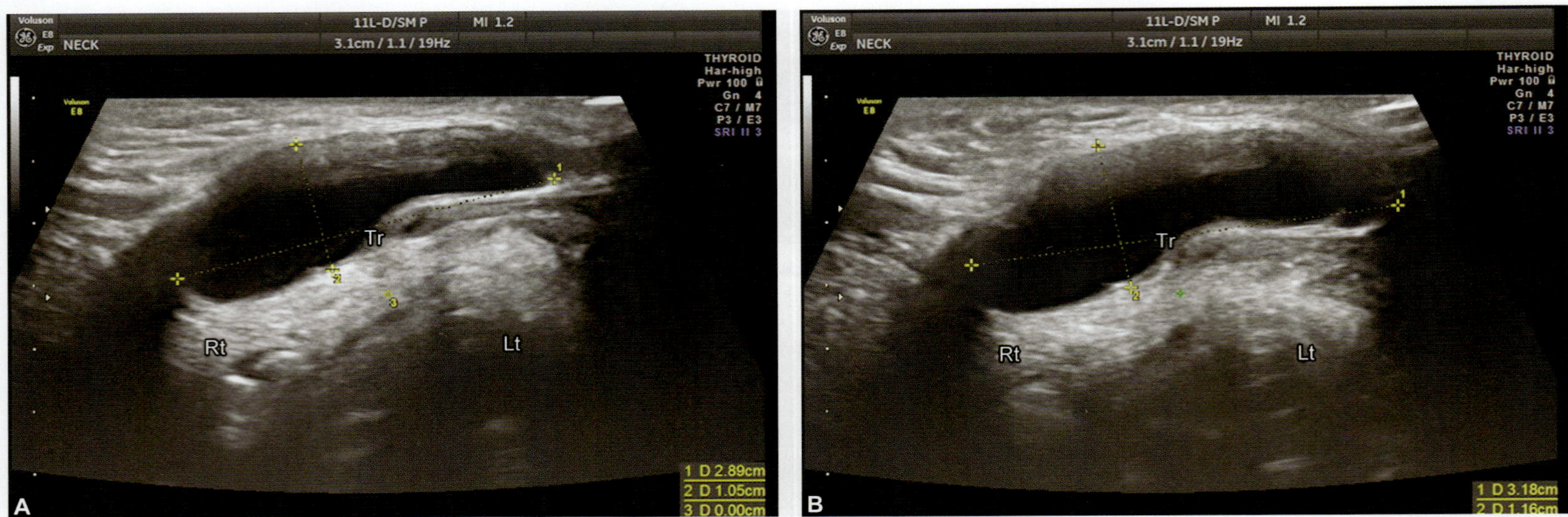

FIGURES 5.63A and B: Sublingual ranula. A 16-year-old girl presented with cystic swelling in the floor of the mouth. HRSG shows a pocket of collection in relation to sublingual gland. Low level echoes are seen in it suggestive of sublingual ranula.

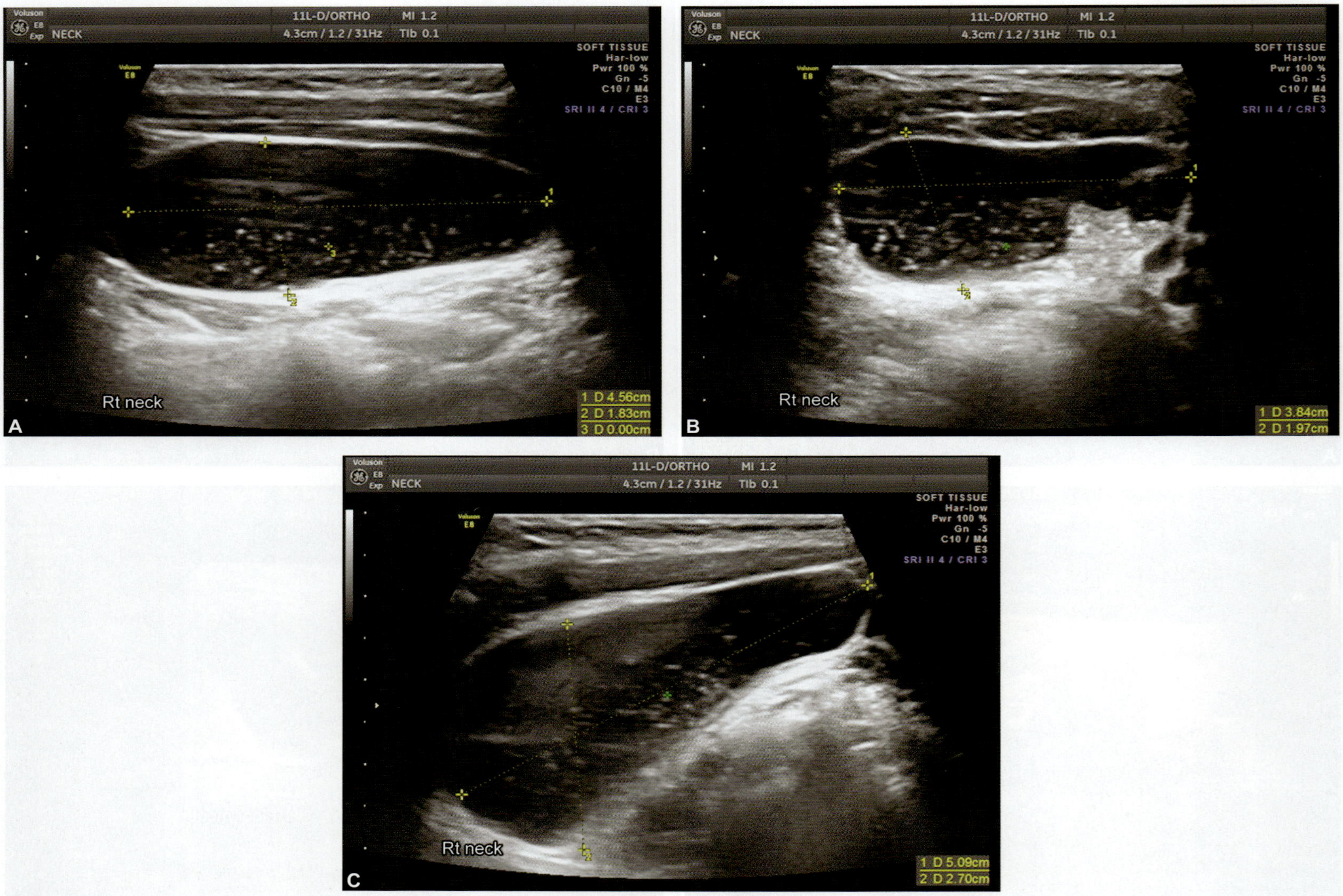

FIGURES 5.64A to C: Sublingual ranula. A patient presented with cystic swelling in the midline of the neck near the floor of the mouth. HRSG shows a cystic swelling with a tongue-like projection in it. Homogeneous low level echoes are seen in it. No septation is seen in it. Aspiration biopsy confirms sublingual ranula.

VASCULAR MASSES IN THE SALIVARY GLAND

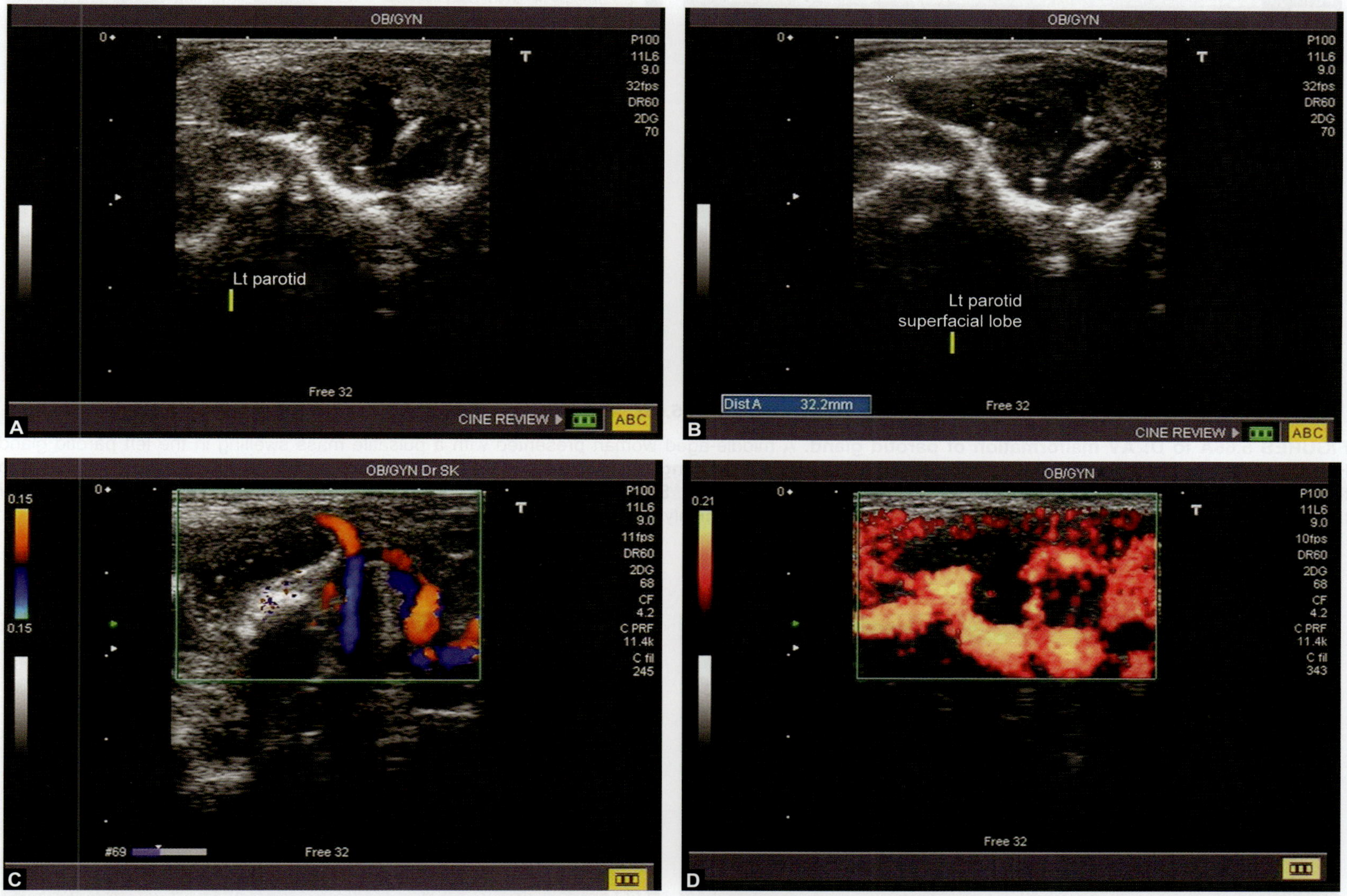

FIGURES 5.65A to D: A patient presented with a soft tissue mass in the left parotid gland involving the superficial lobe. HRSG shows a low level echo complex mass in the gland. On color flow imaging, multiple vessels are seen feeding the mass suggestive of hemangiomatous mass.

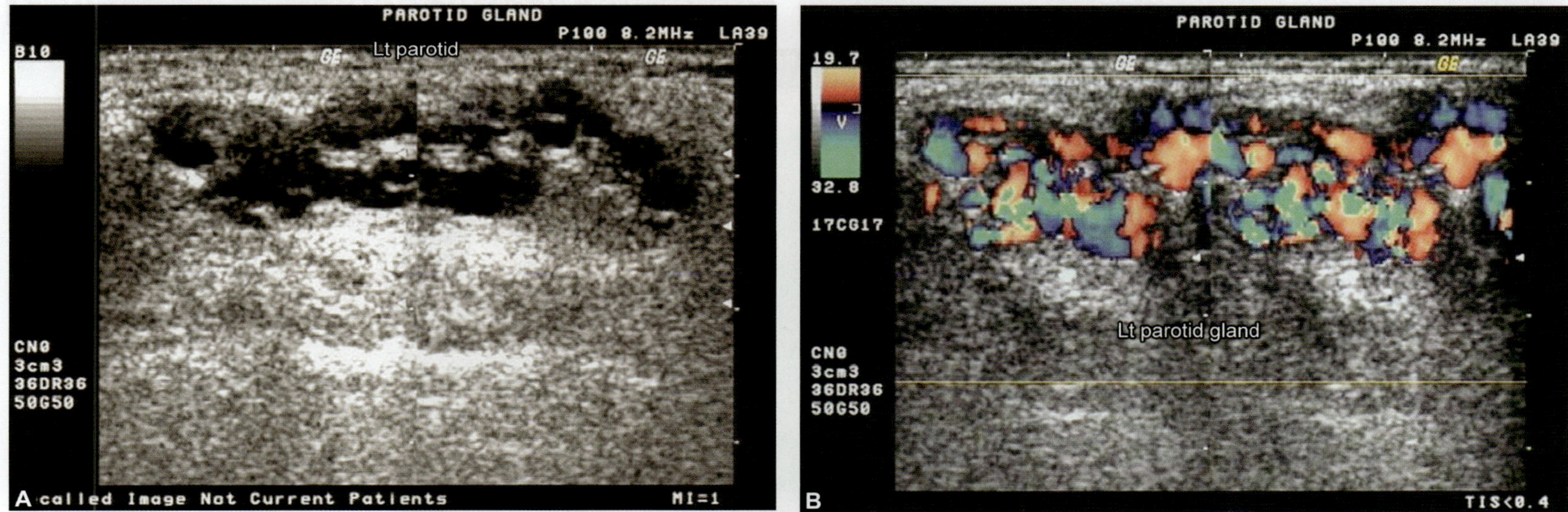

FIGURES 5.66A and B

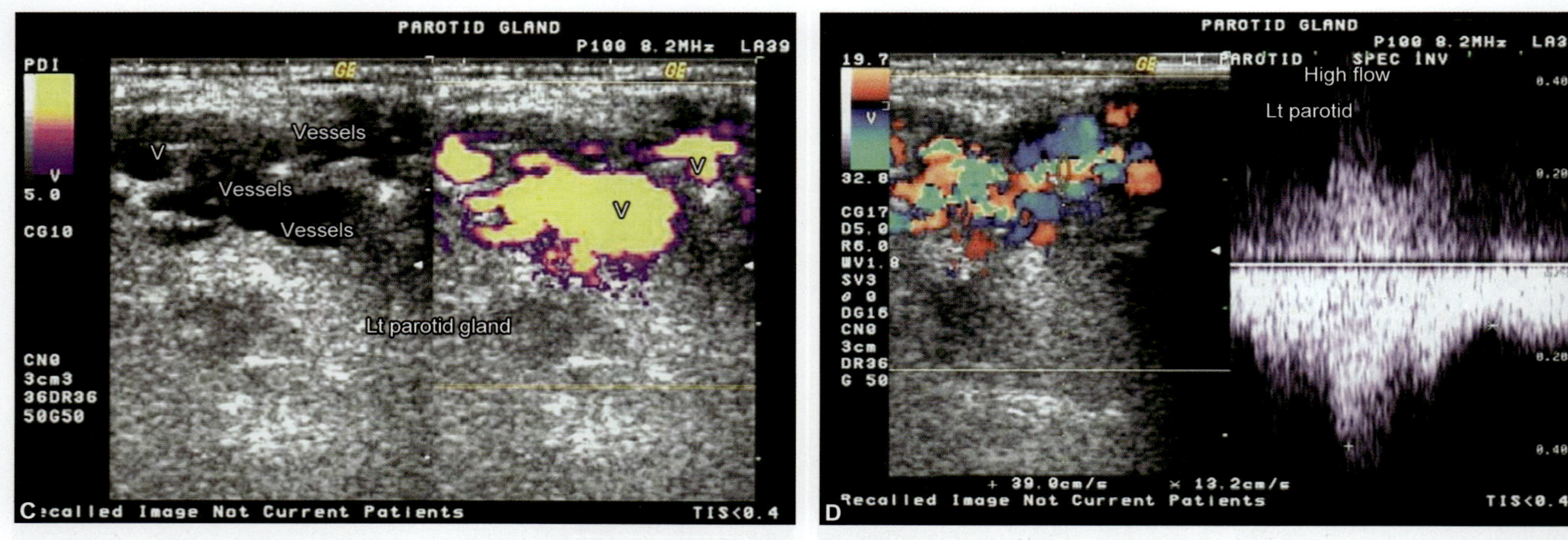

FIGURES 5.66C and D

FIGURES 5.66A to D: AV malformation of parotid gland. A middle-aged woman presented with a pulsatile mass swelling in the left parotid gland. HRSG shows multiple dilated vessels in the gland. **Color Doppler imaging** of the same patient shows high blood flow in the vessels filling whole of the gland. Power Doppler imaging shows irregular filling of the sinusoides. **Spectral Doppler imaging** shows high flow in the vessels running through the gland with arterial and venous flow pattern. Doppler findings are highly suggestive of AV malformation in the parotid gland.

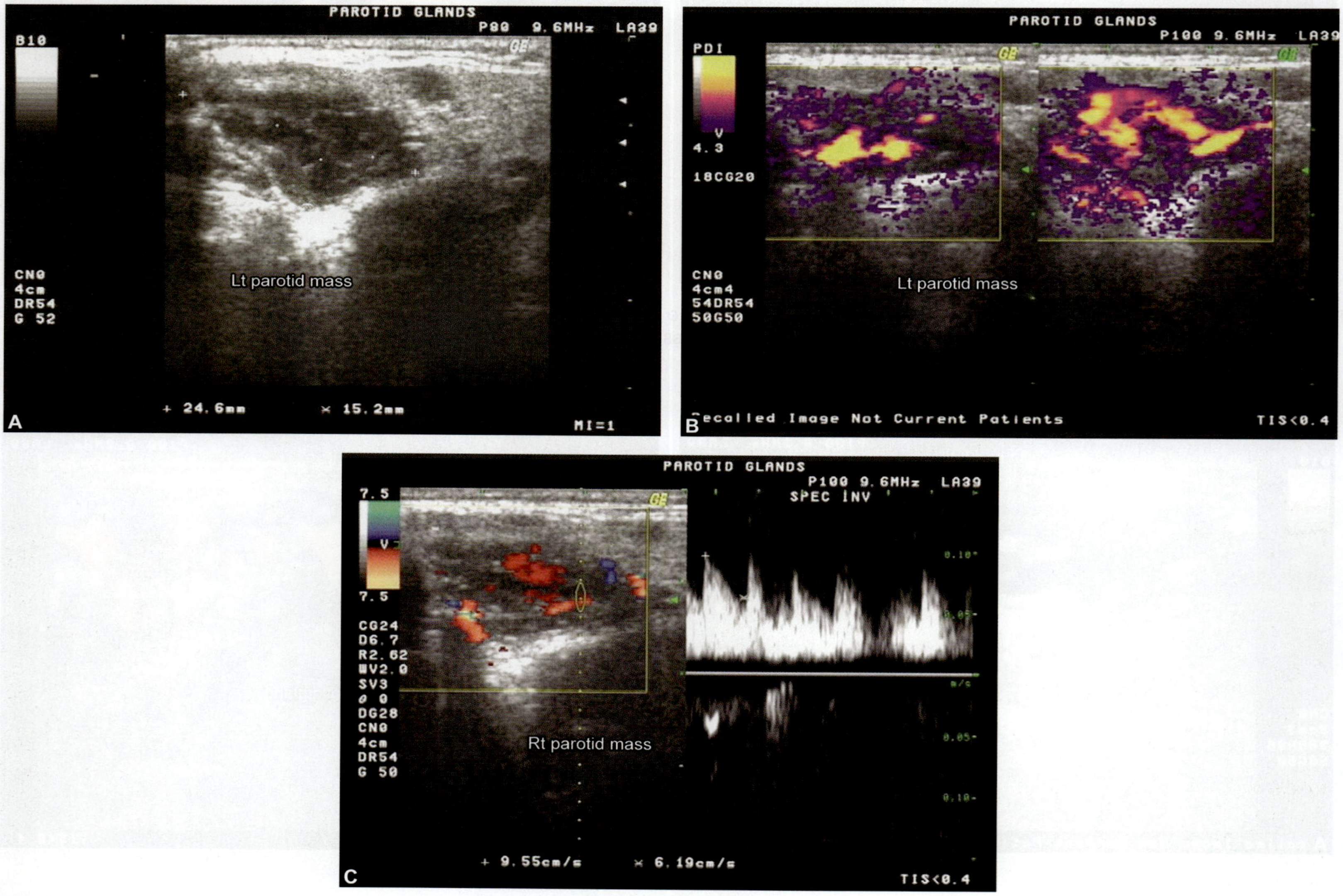

FIGURES 5.67A to C: Cavernous venous malformation in the parotid gland. A young boy presented with a cystic mass in the left parotid gland. HRSG shows multiple dilated vessels in the gland. Normal glandular texture is lost. Power Doppler imaging shows low flow in the blood vessels suggestive of venous flow. Spectral Doppler flow-imaging shows pulsatile venous flow in the mass. Biopsy shows cavernous venous malformation.

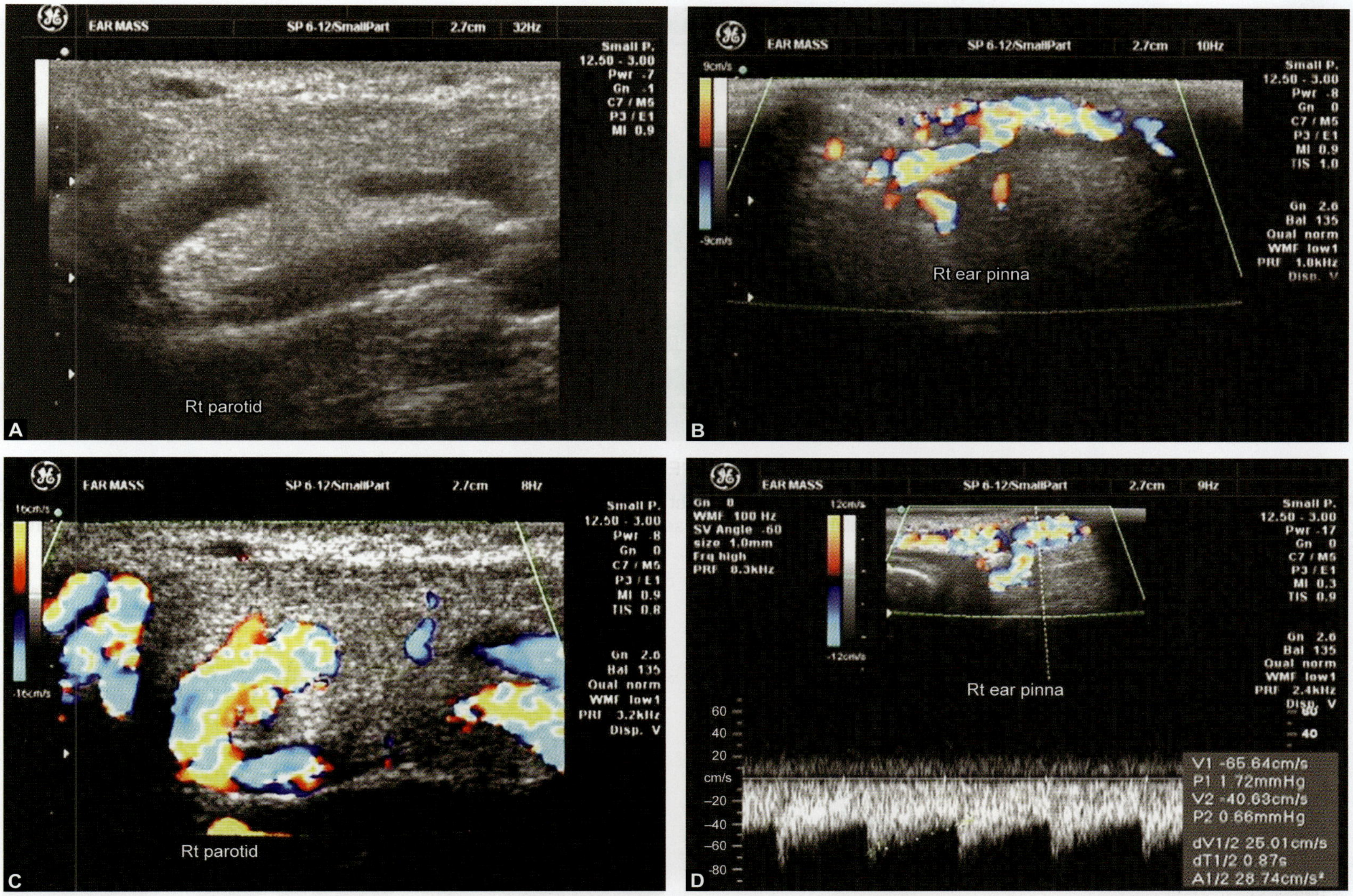

FIGURES 5.68A to D: Parotid AVM. A patient presented with swelling over the right parotid region and also thickened pinna of the right ear. HRSG shows smooth enlargement of right parotid gland. Multiple dilated vessels are seen in the gland. **Color Doppler imaging** shows dilated vessels in the parotid gland. The vessels are also seen feeding pinna of the ear. **On spectral Doppler tracing** increased flow seen in the vessels confirmed the finding of AVM.

MALIGNANT SALIVARY GLAND MASSES

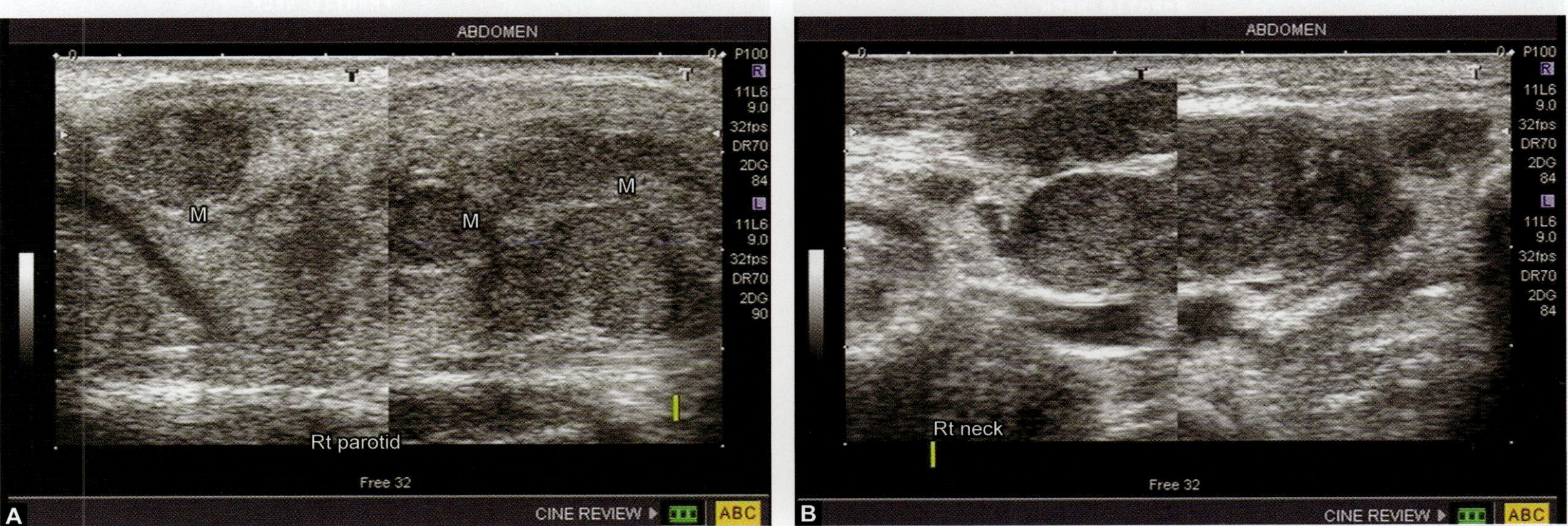

FIGURES 5.69A and B

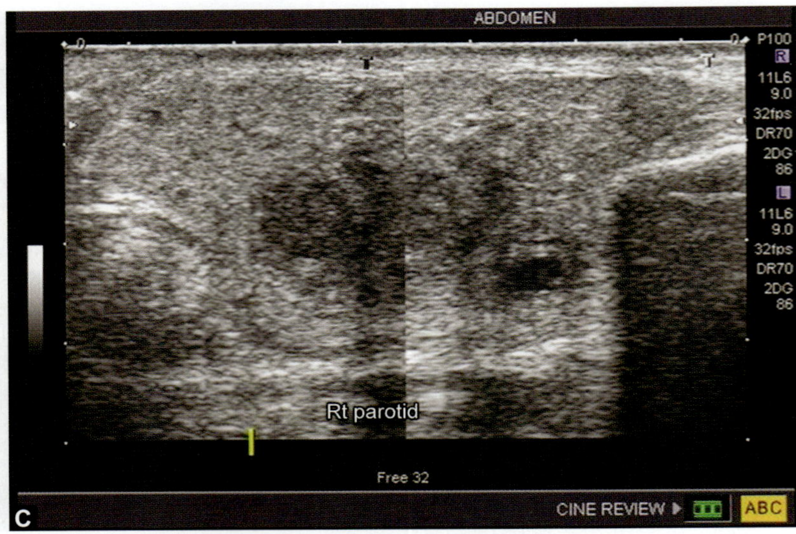

FIGURE 5.69C

FIGURES 5.69A to C: A patient presented with hard swelling in the right parotid region. HRSG shows a heterogeneous mass in the right parotid gland. Normal glandular texture is lost. Multiple irregular ill-defined masses are seen in the gland, which are solid in nature. FNAC of the mass confirms malignant tumor.

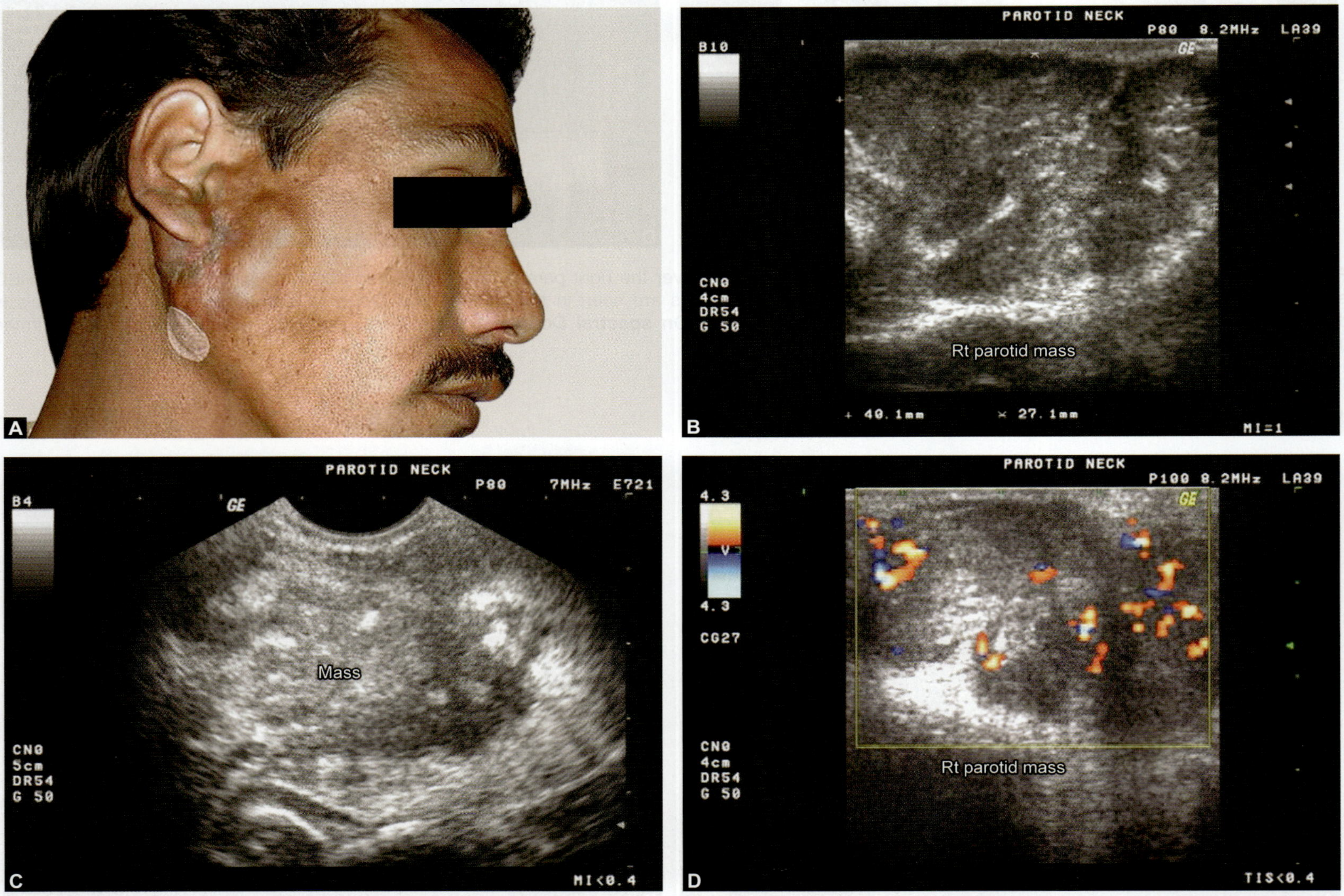

FIGURES 5.70A to D: Adenocarcinoma of parotid. A patient presented with irregular soft tissue mass over the right parotid area. HRSG shows a big irregular heterogeneous mass invading the parotid gland. The mass is seen invading the deep lobe of parotid. The capsule of the gland was also broken of the gland. Biopsy confirmed invasive adenocarcinoma.

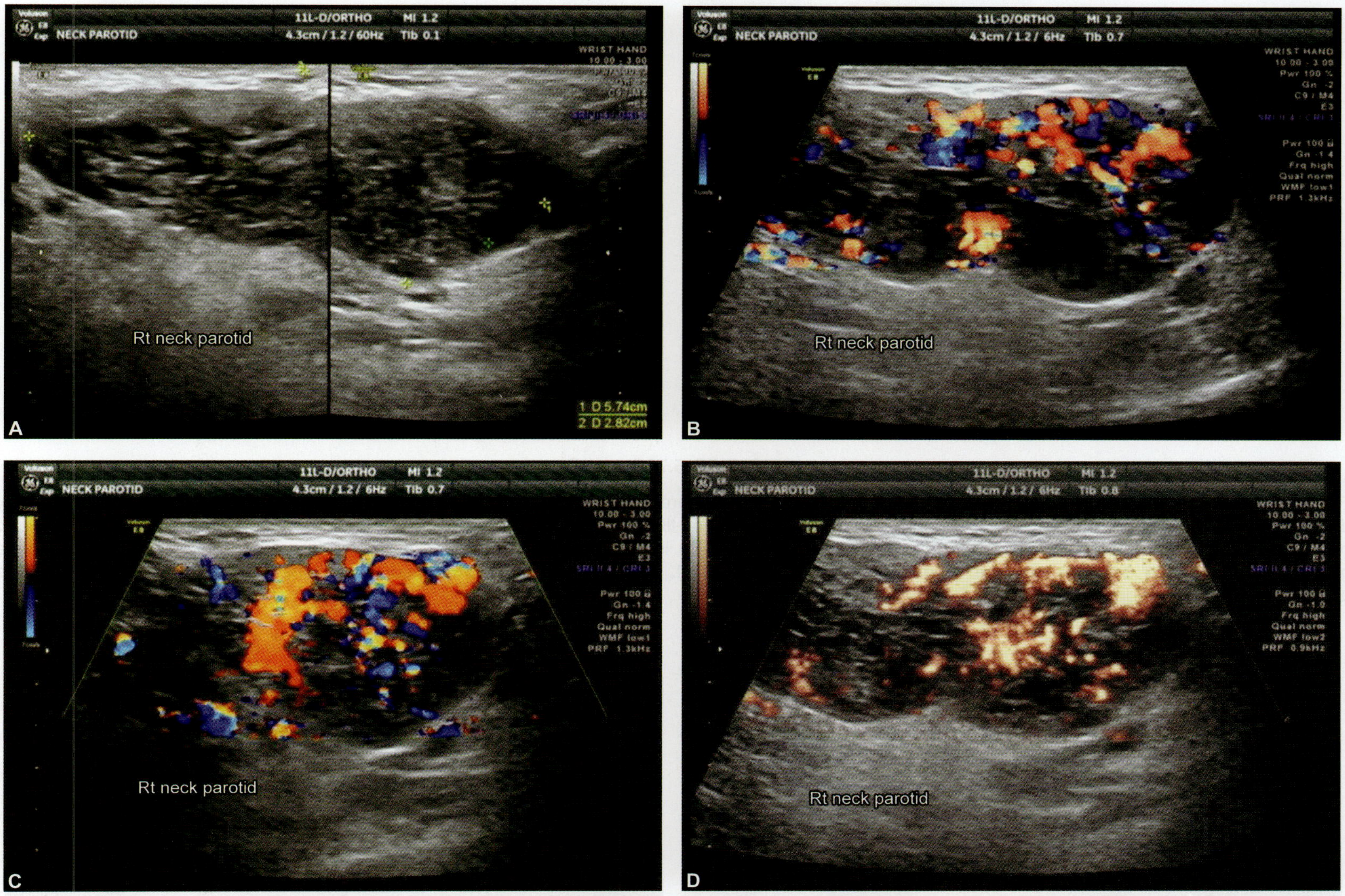

FIGURES 5.71A to D: Parotid CA. A patient presented with a diffuse soft tissue mass in right parotid gland. HRSG shows a big irregular heterogeneous mass in the parotid gland. Normal glandular texture is lost. Capsule of the mass is seen broken. On color flow imaging, increased flow is seen in the mass. Biopsy of the mass confirmed adenocarcinoma of parotid.

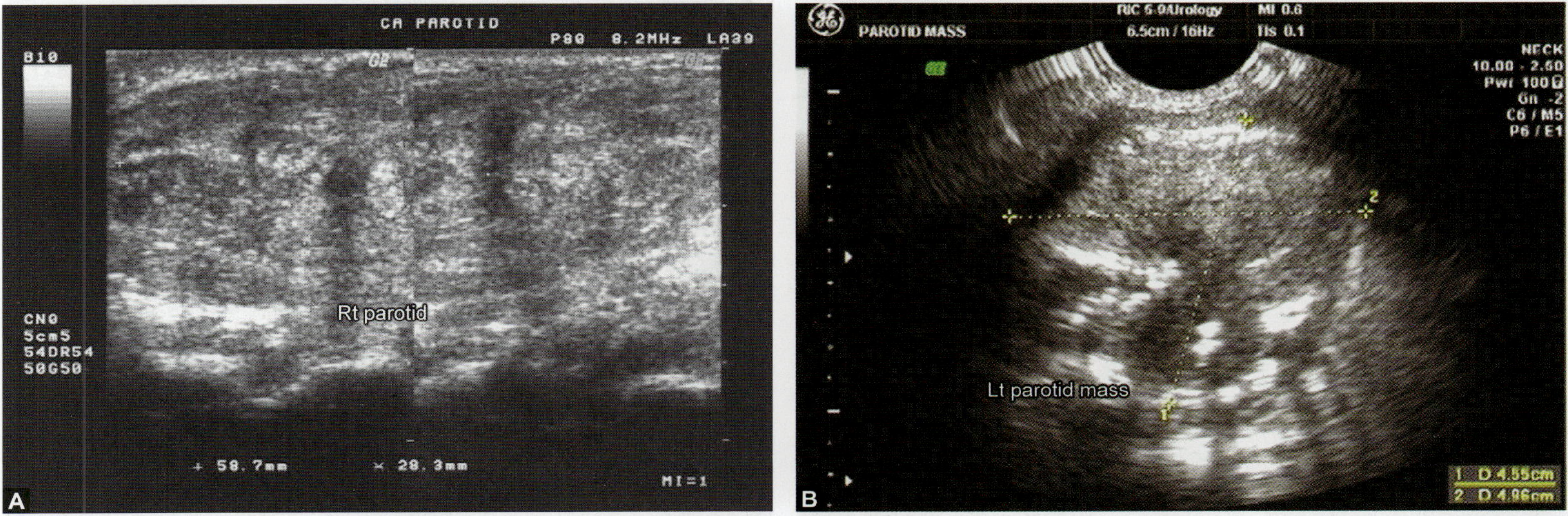

FIGURES 5.72A and B

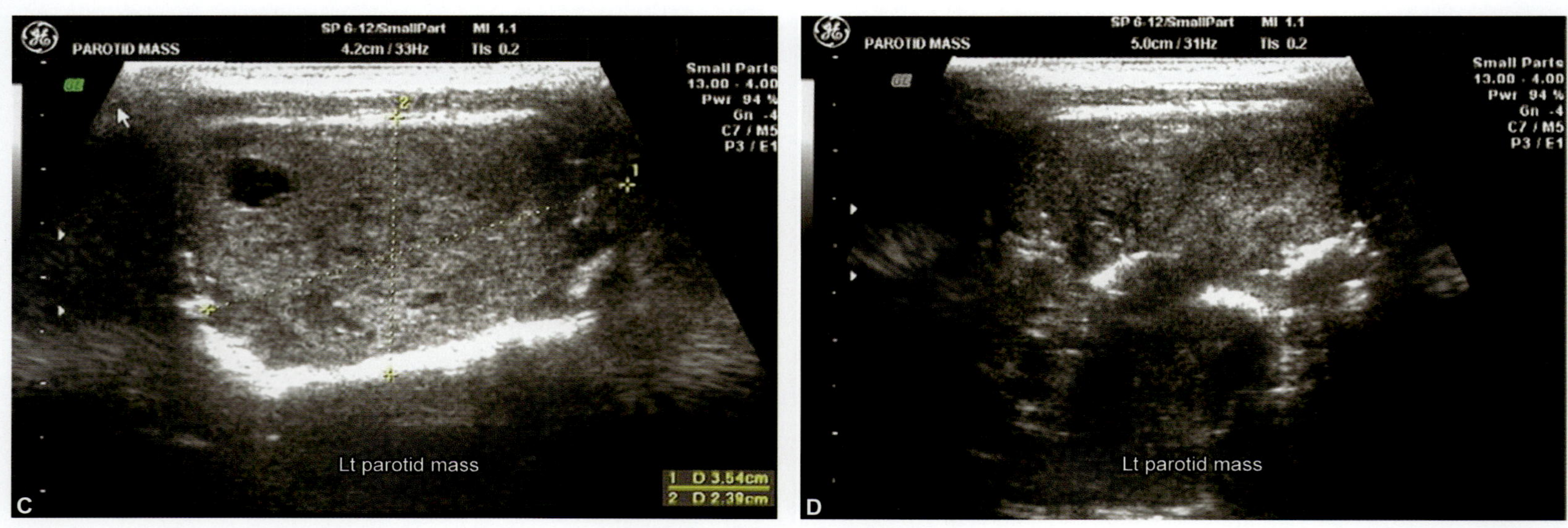

FIGURES 5.72C and D

FIGURES 5.72A to D: Malignant adenocarcinoma parotid. A patient presented with a big mass in the right parotid gland. The mass has totally destroyed. The capsule is broken and it is seen invading the adjacent tissue planes. Biopsy confirmed invasive adenocarcinoma. A young child presented with a big soft tissue mass in the left parotid region. The mass is coming out from the parotid gland. It is seen broken the capsule of the gland and invading the adjacent structure. Normal glandular texture is lost. Echogenic calcification is also seen in the mass. Biopsy showed invasive adenocarcinoma.

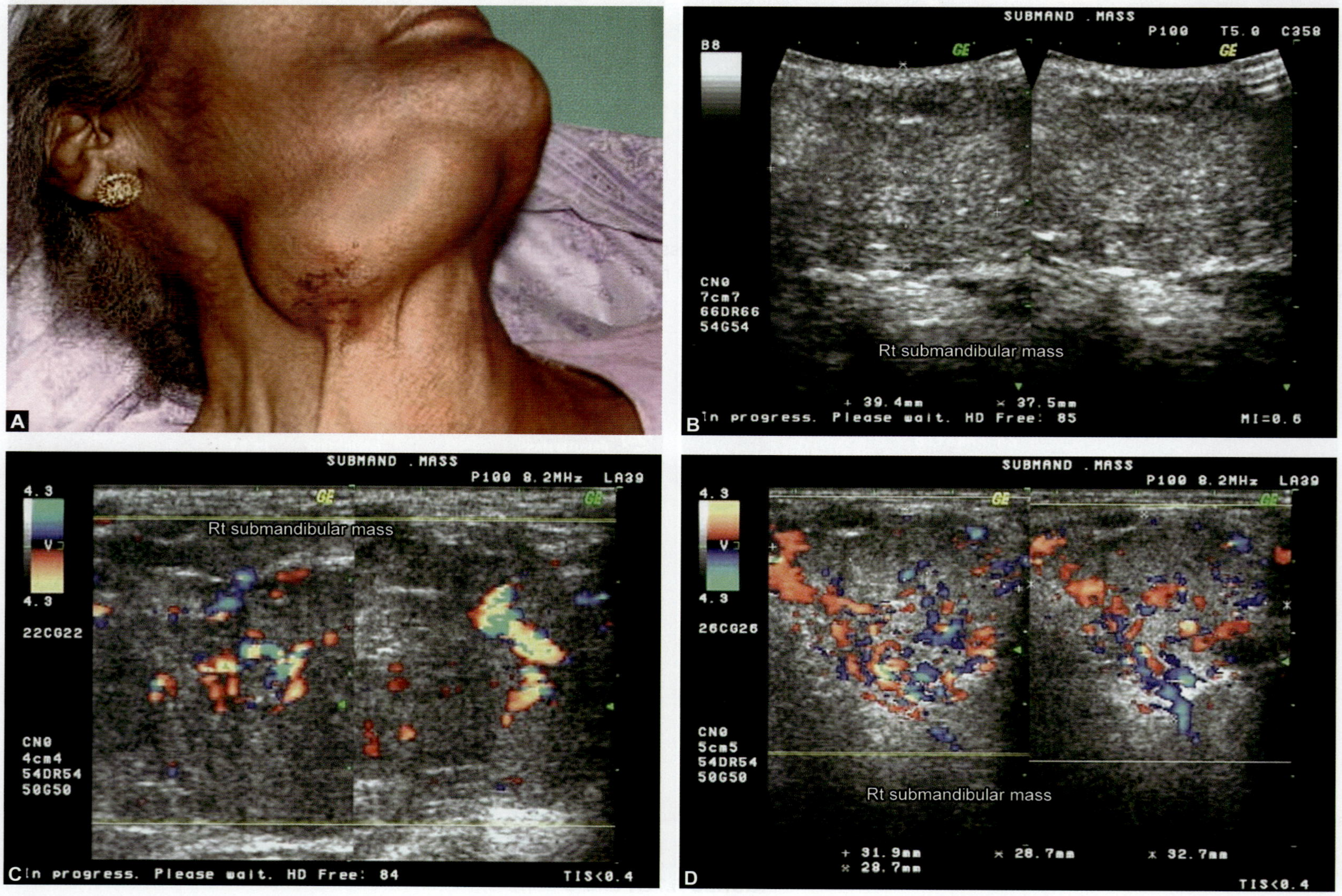

FIGURES 5.73A to D: Malignant mass in the neck. Old lady presented with a solid mass in the right submandibular region. HRSG shows a big irregular heterogeneous solid mass invading the right parotid gland. No necrosis is seen in it. No cystic degeneration is seen. Color Doppler of the mass shows increased vascularity in the mass. However, the flow pattern is bizarre. Biopsy of the mass shows carcinoma.

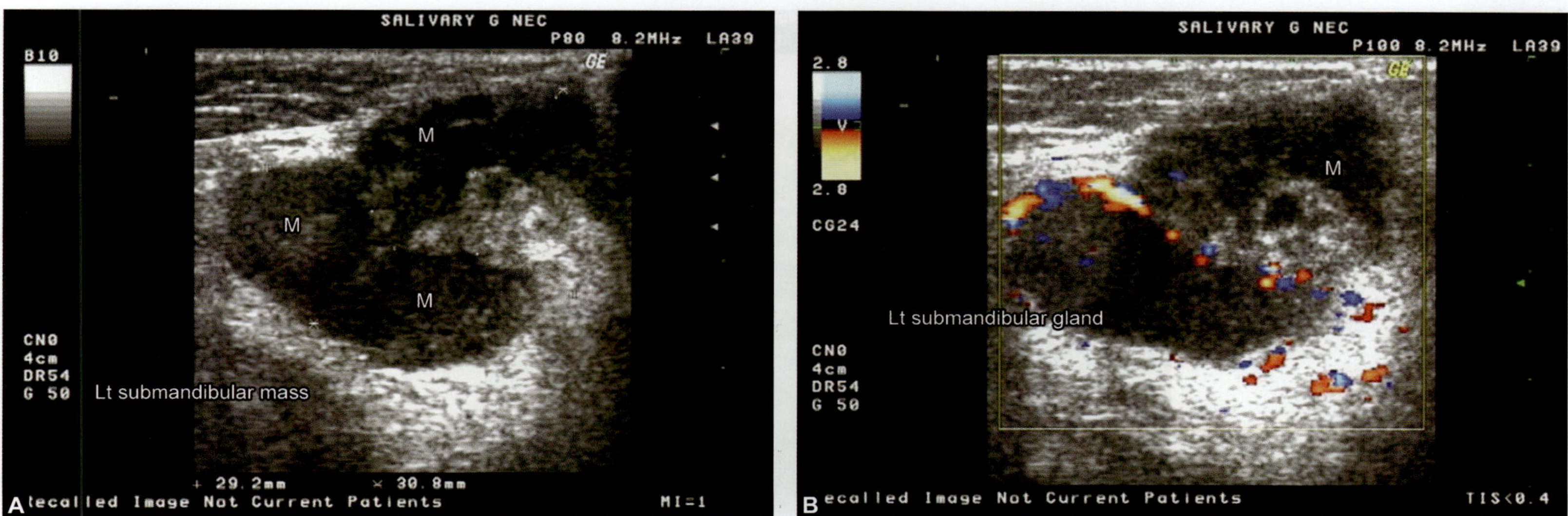

FIGURES 5.74A and B: Malignant mass in the submandibular gland. A middle-aged man presented with heterogeneous mass in the left submandibular gland. Normal glandular texture is lost. The capsule is broken. The mass is seen invading the soft tissue planes. Biopsy confirmed invasive adenocarcinoma.

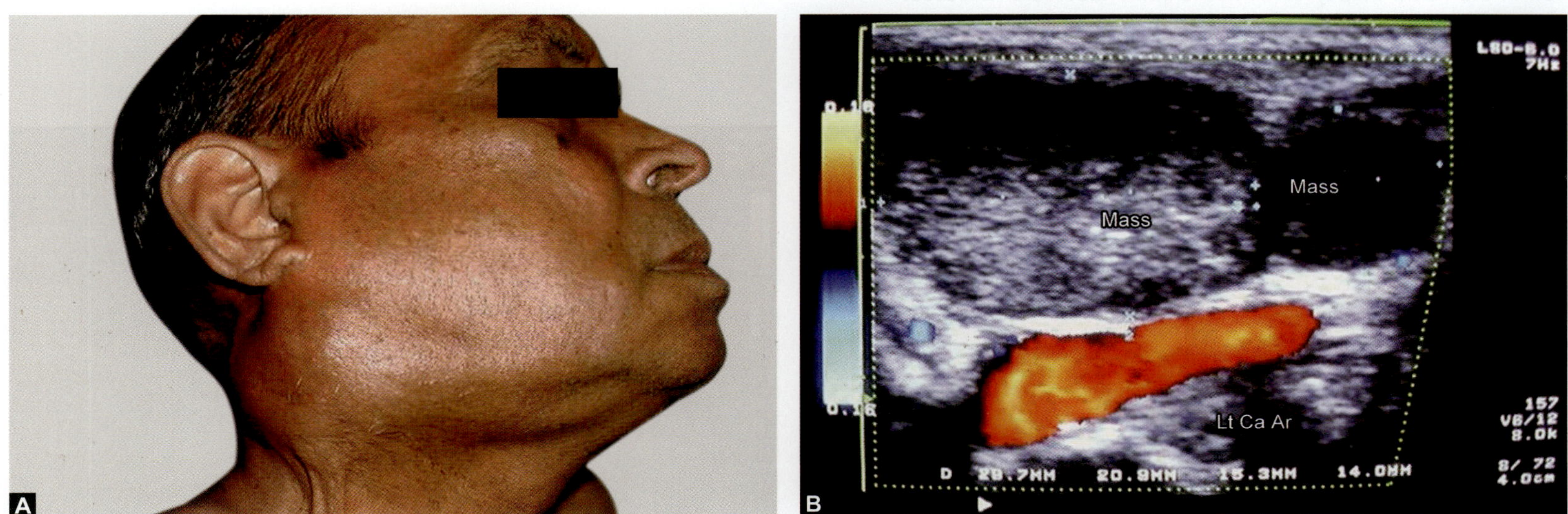

FIGURES 5.75A and B: Malignant cyst. An old man presented with a solid cystic mass over the right submandibular area. HRSG shows complex mass in submandibular gland. Biopsy of the mass confirmed adenocarcinoma.

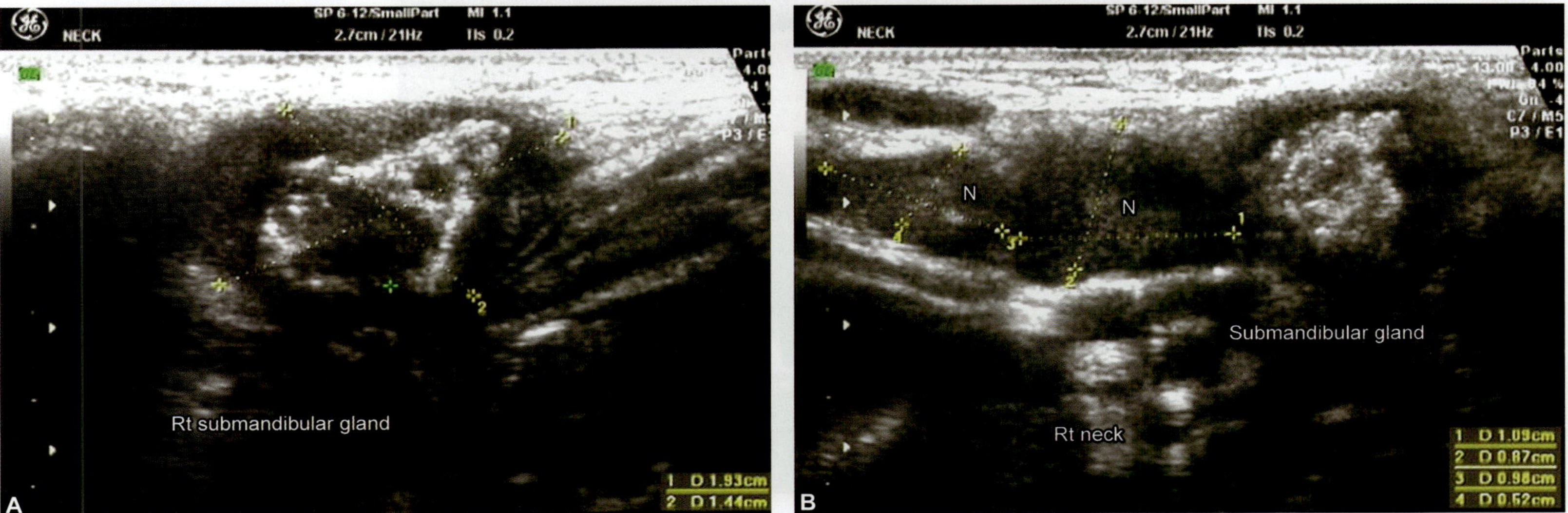

FIGURES 5.76A and B

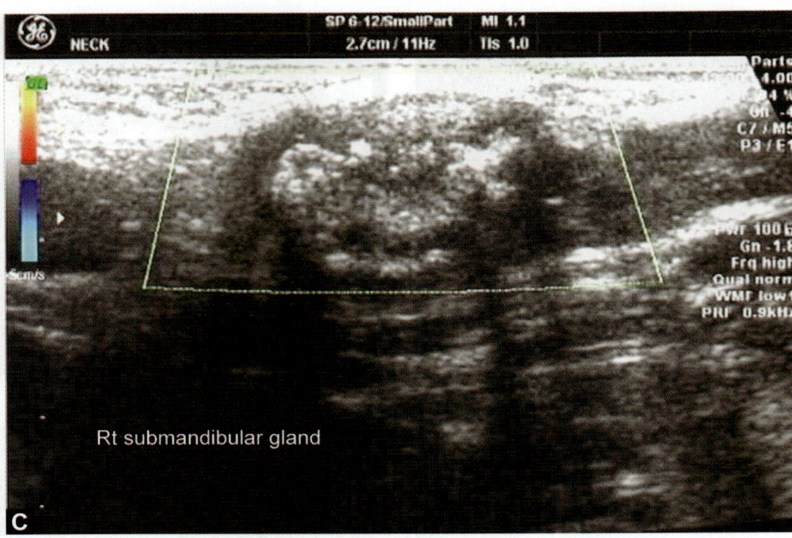

FIGURE 5.76C

FIGURES 5.76A to C: Chronic tubercular abscess. A young child presented with mass with non-tender mass in the right submandibular gland. HRSG shows thick echogenic collection in the submandibular gland. Echogenic calcified specks are also seen in it. Multiple enlarged nodes are also seen in the neck. Biopsy confirmed chronic tubercular abscess.

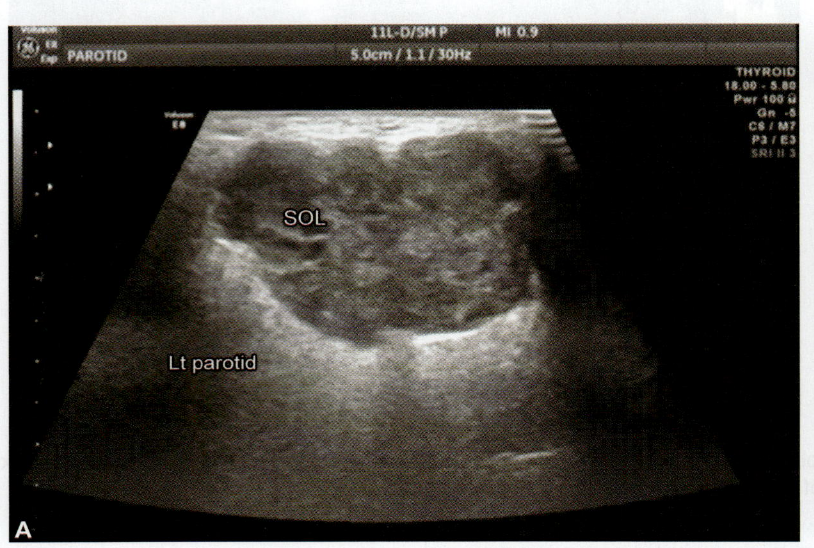

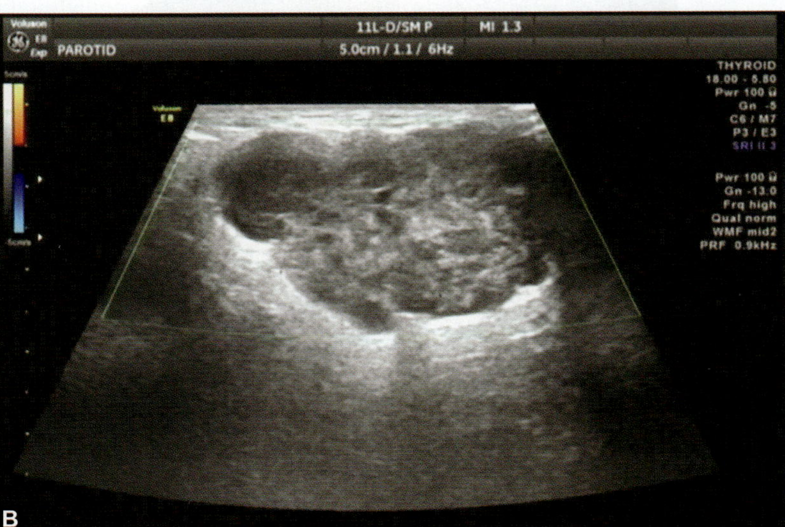

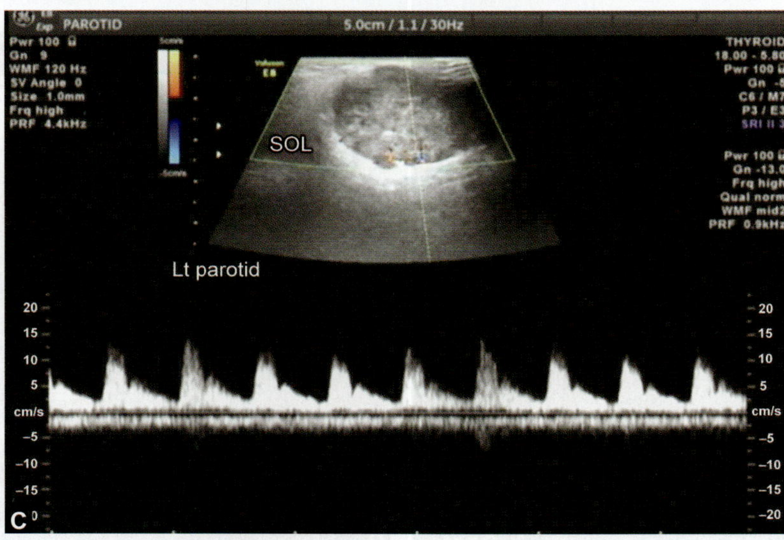

FIGURES 5.77A to C: Heterogeneous mass in left parotid gland. A big irregular ill-defined soft tissue mass in the left parotid gland. The mass is predominantly solid. It shows irregular margins. On color flow imaging, moderate flow is seen in the mass. Biopsy of the mass confirms malignant mass.

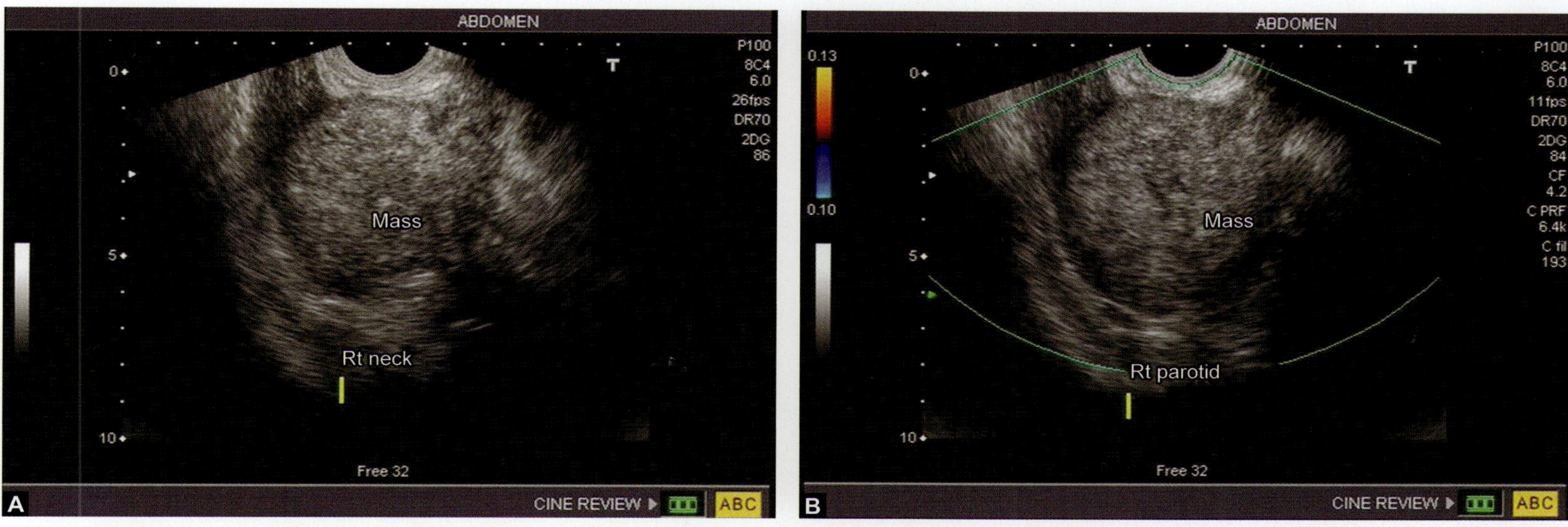

FIGURES 5.78A and B: Parotid mass. A patient presented with heterogeneous mass in the parotid gland. It is predominantly solid. Margins are irregular. On color flow imaging, it shows poor flow. FNAC of the mass confirm malignancy.

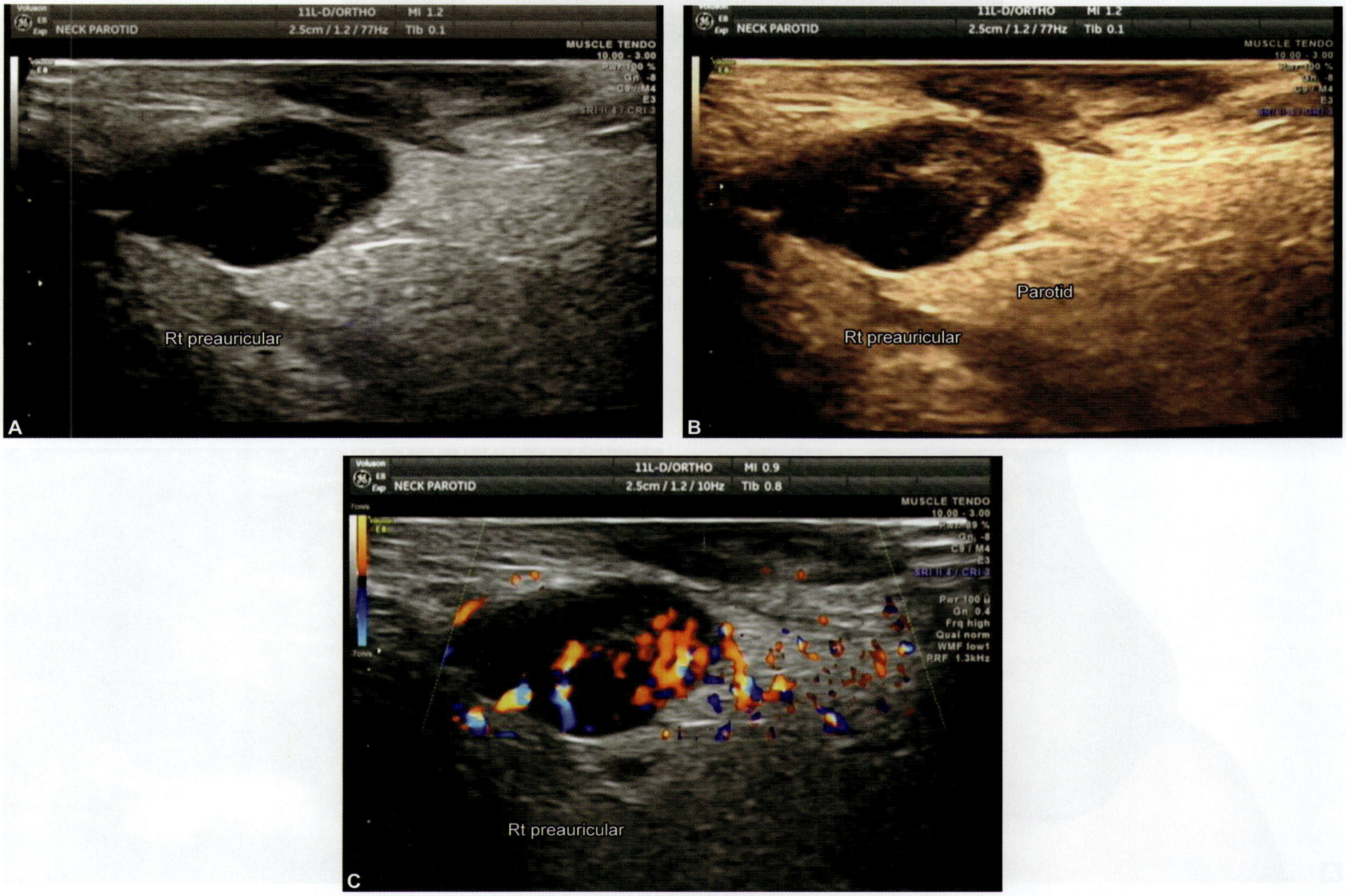

FIGURES 5.79A to C: Metastatic deposit in the parotid gland. A known case of melanoma presented with soft nodular shadow in the preauricular region on right side. HRSG shows a hypoechoic low level echo complex mass, which is seen extending in the parotid gland. On color flow imaging, it shows moderate flow. FNAC of the mass confirms metastatic deposits of sublingual gland.

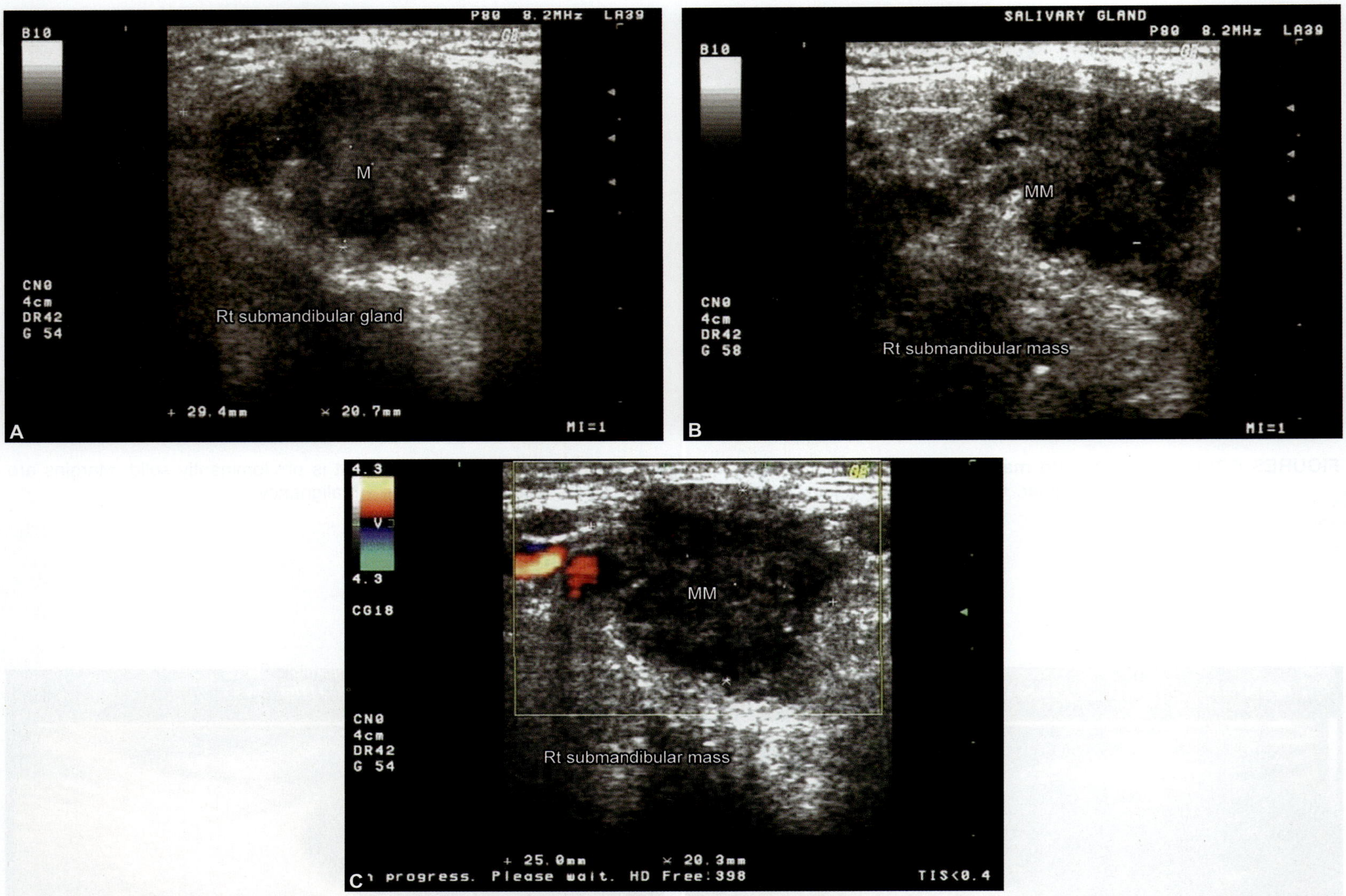

FIGURES 5.80A to C: Malignant mass at the submandibular gland. HRSG shows an irregular heterogeneous mass in the right submandibular area. Margins are irregular. Capsule is broken. Color Doppler imaging shows poor flow in the mass. There is also suggestion of finger like projection seen coming out from the mass invading the fascial planes. No cystic degeneration is seen in the mass. Biopsy of the mass shows malignant epidermoid carcinoma.

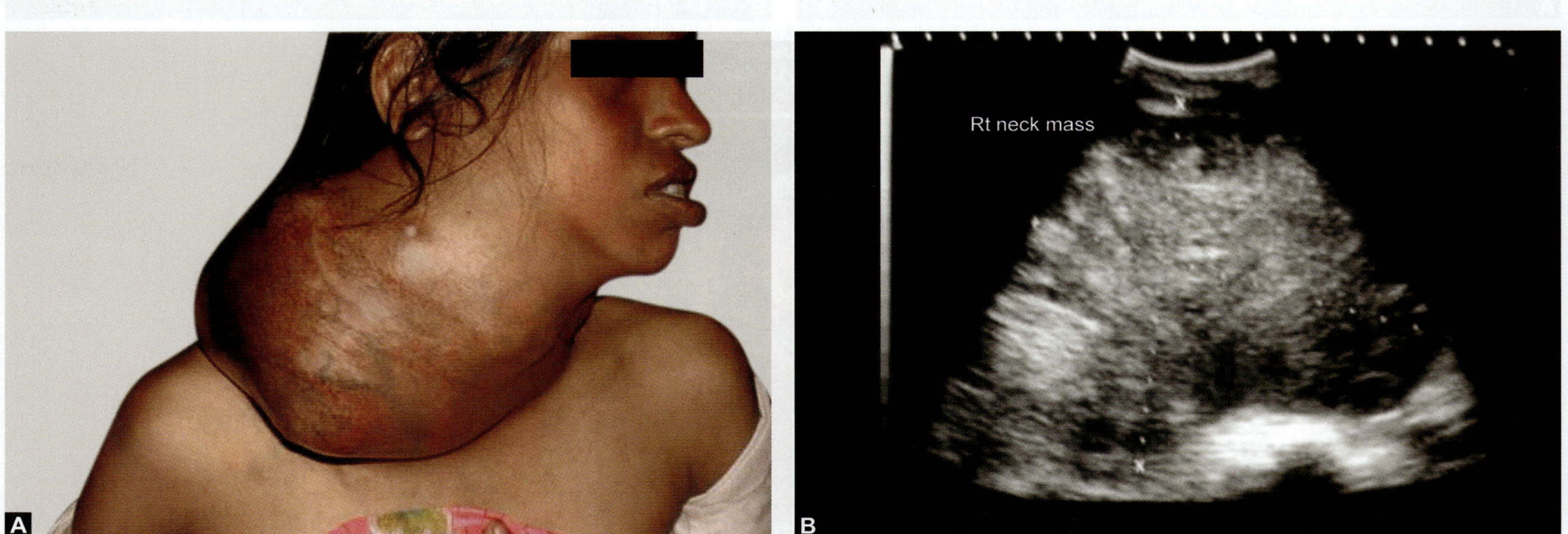

FIGURES 5.81A and B

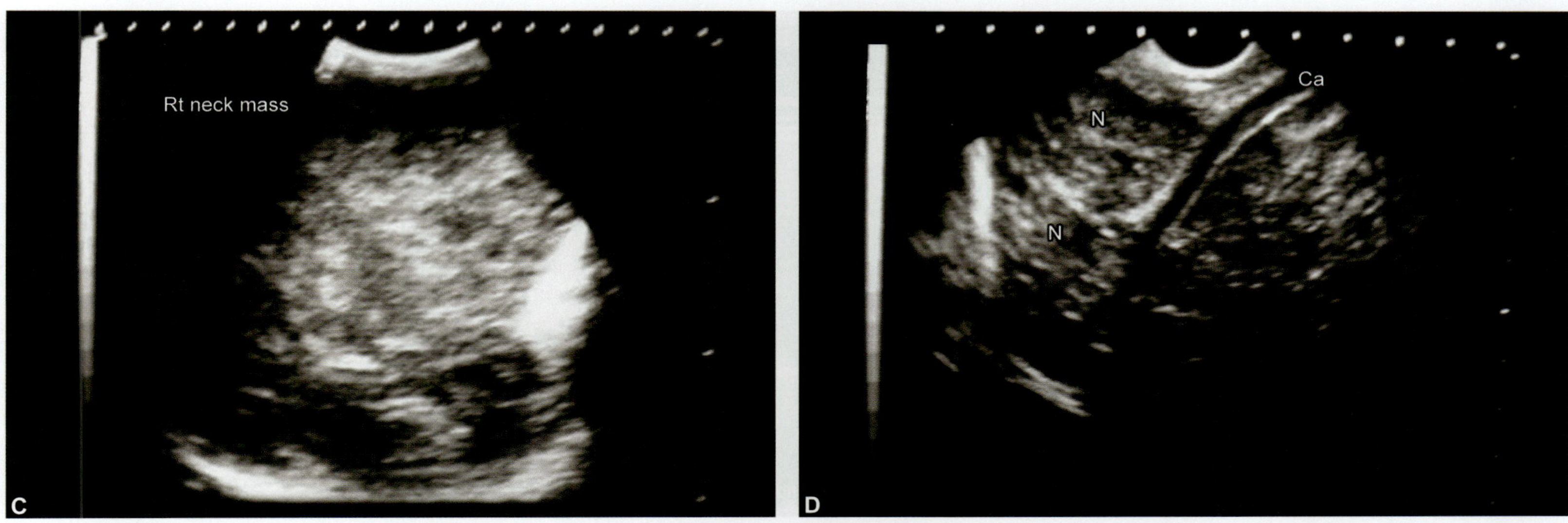

FIGURES 5.81C and D

FIGURES 5.81A to D: Spindle cell carcinoma of the neck. A lady presented with big mass in the neck region. HRSG shows a big heterogeneous mass invading the neck. Normal anatomy is destroyed. Biopsy of the mass shows spindle cell carcinoma. However, the mass is not seen invading the neck vessels. Though it is seen pressing over the neck vessels. However, they are not invaded by the mass.

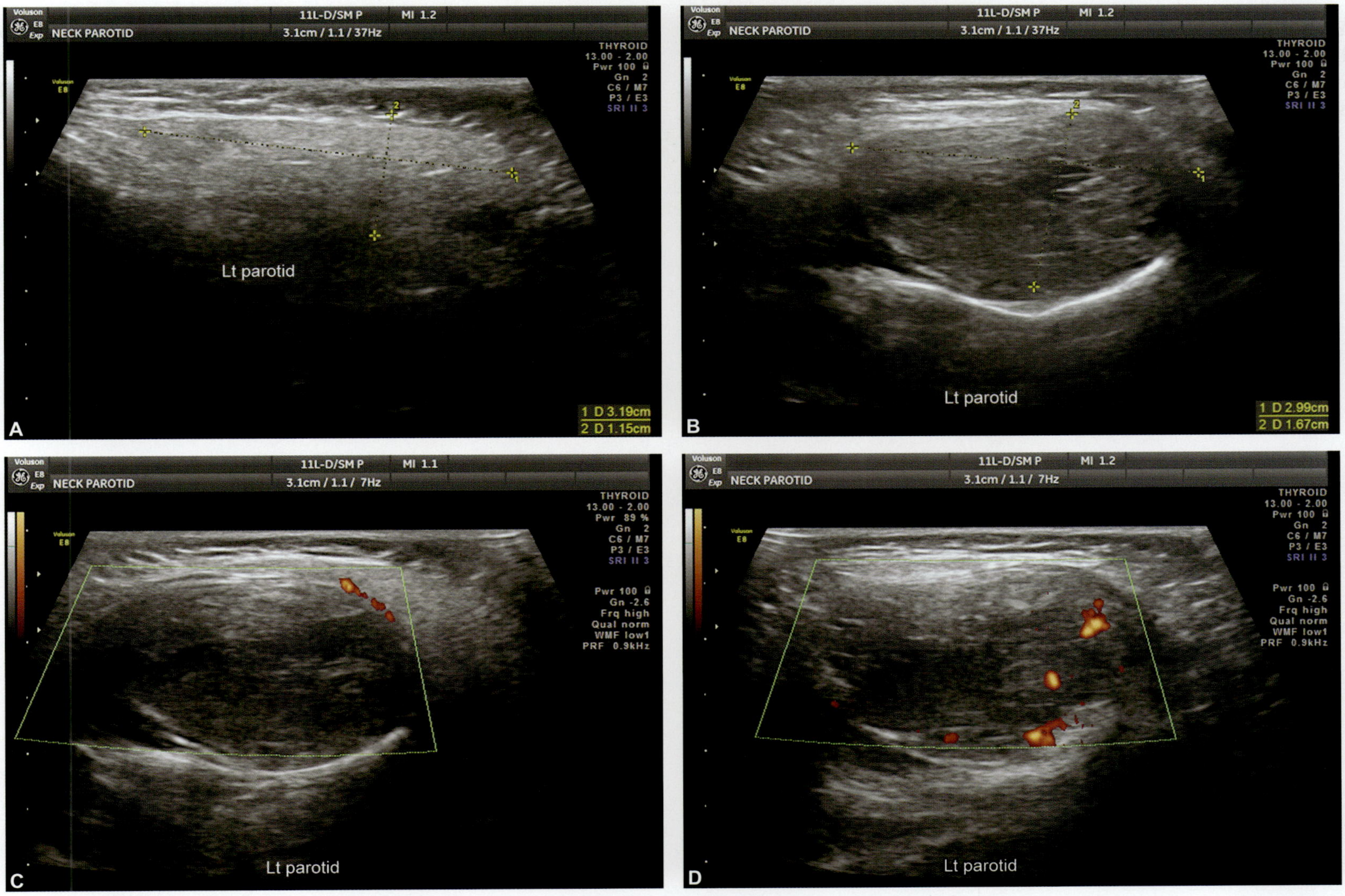

FIGURES 5.82A to D

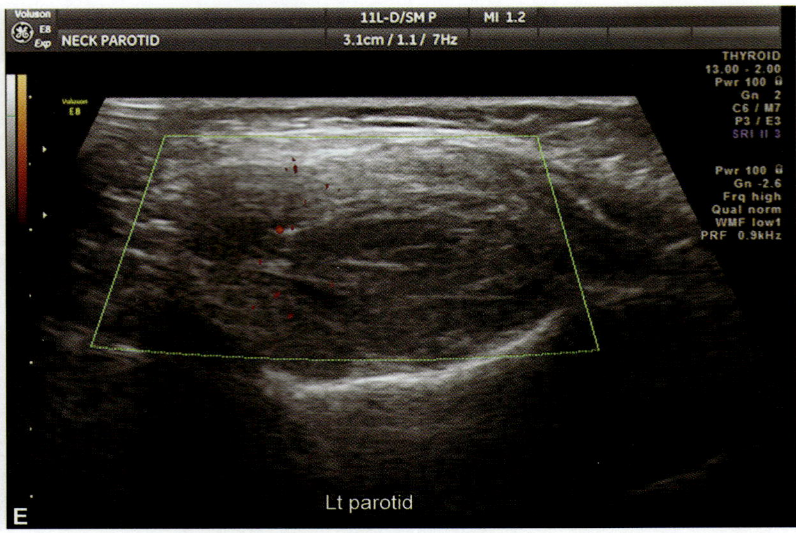

FIGURE 5.82E

FIGURES 5.82A to E: A young girl presented with soft tissue swelling in the left side of neck in the parotid region. HRSG shows an irregular ill-defined mass in the left cheek. The mass is separate from the parotid gland. It is seen coming out from the masseter muscle. It is heterogeneous in texture. On color flow imaging, poor flow is seen in the mass. On biopsy is turn out to be muscle tumor. The parotid gland is normal.

CONCLUSION

High-resolution sonography (HRSG) is an important, rapid, noninvasive imaging technique to evaluate cervical lymph nodes in head and neck cancer patients. Most diseased nodes can be detected on HRSG. When sonographic criteria fail to differentiate between benign and metastatic nodes, USG-guided FNAC confirms the diagnosis. It is also very good tool to assess post-surgical or post-irradiated neck for recurrence of disease. HRSG is an excellent modality for evaluating other neck masses including the salivary glands. It is first line of investigation in neck masses.

CHAPTER 6

Neurosonography of Neonatal Brain

PK Srivastava

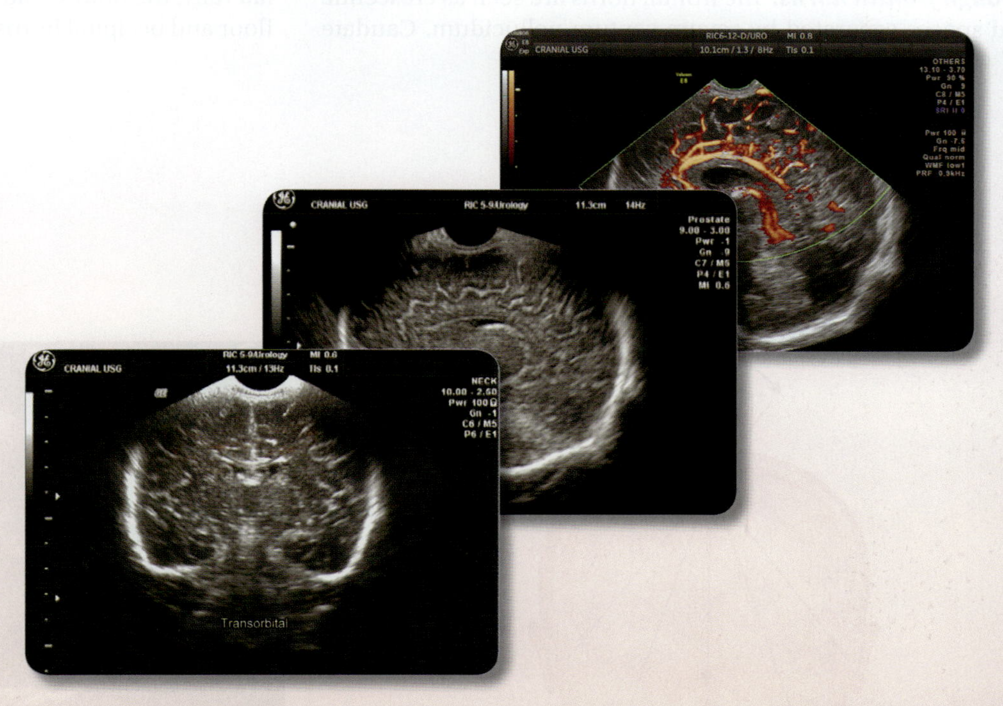

INTRODUCTION

With the advent of high-resolution sonography and lately addition of color Doppler have paved the way for detailed evaluation of neonatal brain. The fact that it can be taken to the bedside makes it an ideal imaging tool in the evaluation of critically ill premature newborn babies.

TECHNIQUE AND INSTRUMENTATION

To obtain undisturbed images, mild sedation is helpful. The newborn suspected to have suffered anoxia/birth injury is seen in the main department. The pre-term baby is examined at bedside with portable machine having high resolution probe without disturbing the life-support. The anterior fontanelle is used as acoustic window and multiple coronals, sagittal and parasagittal scans are taken using 5.0/7.5 MHz sector transducers. Positioning the transducer just above the external auditory meatus does axial scanning. By this technique, we get excellent view of lateral ventricles. The technique is used for measurement of lateral ventricular ratio (LVR) in the diagnosis of hydrocephalus.

NORMAL ANATOMY

Coronal Scans

Placing the probe transversely in anterior fontanelle and sweeping the probe from front to back obtain the imaging in coronal plane. It gives excellent details of ventricular system and adjoining brain parenchyma as described by Shuman et al.

Plane through frontal horns: The frontal horns are seen as crescentic fluid-filled spaces separated by cavum septum pellucidum. Caudate nucleus occupies the lateral concavity of the frontal horns. Corpus callosum, which forms the roof of lateral ventricles is seen as concave hypoechoic band.

Plane through thalamus: With the slight shift of probe posteriorly from the plane of frontal horns, section through thalami is obtained. In this plane, the lateral ventricles are seen as arcuate fluid-filled structures, thalami appear as hypoechoic structures separated by silt-like third ventricle. The echogenic choroid plexus is seen prominently occupying the body of lateral ventricles.

Plane through quadrigeminal cistern: The cerebellum and quadrigeminal cistern appear as an echogenic tree. Body of lateral ventricle is seen superiorly, and temporal horn is seen inferiorly. The tentorium cerebelli appear as thick echogenic band on either side of cerebellum. The middle cerebral artery can be recognized pulsating on real-time in echogenic Sylvain fissure laterally.

Plane through trigone of lateral ventricle: The choroid plexus occupies most of the lateral ventricle. The parietal lobe is seen superiorly. The tentorium forms the inverted V posteriorly.

Sagittal Scans

The sagittal scans are obtained by placing the probe parallel to the anterior fontanelle. The first plane obtained is in the midline. The cavum septum pellucidum is seen as comma-shaped structure just above the third ventricle, corpus callosum is seen as hypoechoic band running just above, whereas fourth ventricle and echogenic cerebellar vermis are appreciated posterior to cavum septum pellucidum. By slight angulations laterally, one visualizes caudate nucleus, shallow lateral ventricle and cerebellar hemispheres posteriorly. By further angulations laterally, the body of lateral ventricle with choroid plexus resting on its floor and occipital horns can be appreciated.

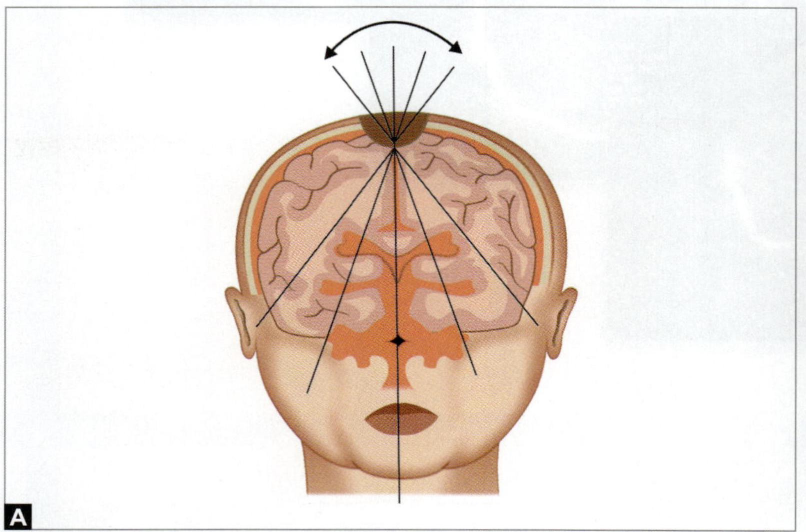

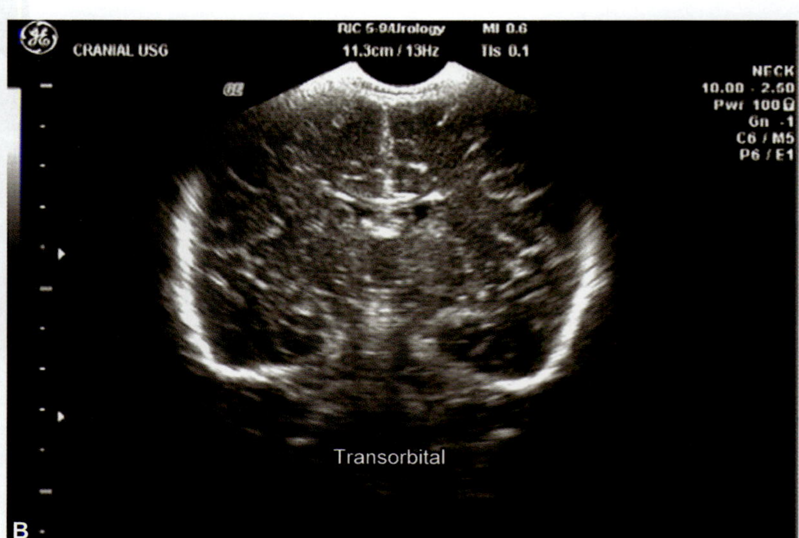

FIGURES 6.1A and B: Line diagram shows scanning plane through anterior fontanelle, in coronal and transorbital planes. Normal brain anatomy-Transorbital view—the coronal plane shows normal brain anatomy. Anterior horn, third ventricle and both thalami are seen in the trans-orbital views. *Courtesy:* Textbook of Diagnostic Ultrasound by Rumack.

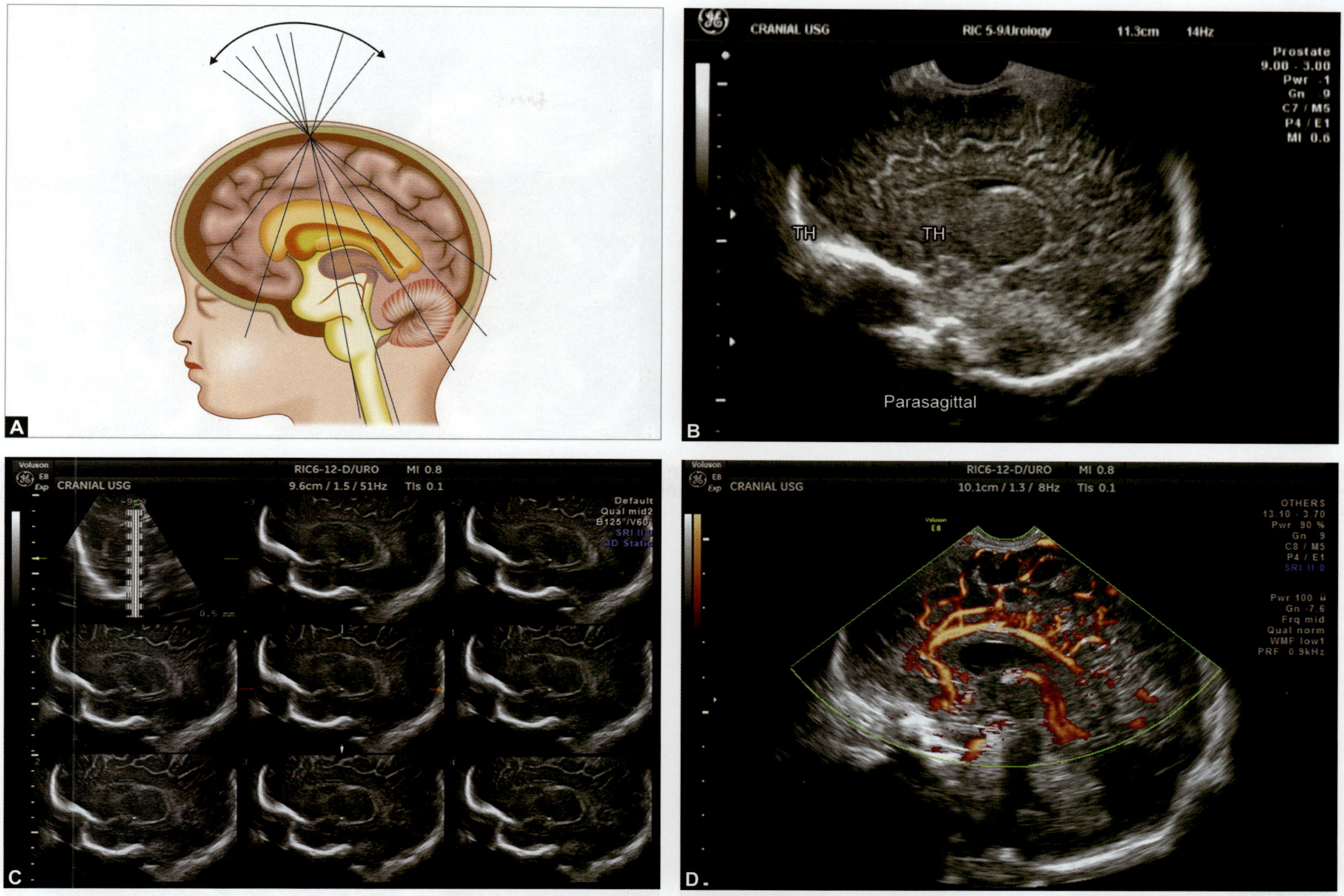

FIGURES 6.2A to D: Line diagram-parasagittal view. The line diagram shows scanning planes in parasagittal axis. Rocking movement of transducer can scan whole of the brain in parasagittal view. Normal parasagittal plane- HRSG shows normal infant brain anatomy in parasagittal planes. Cavum septum pellucidum is seen a small collapsed fluid-filled shadow. The thalamus is seen well-defined rounded body. Collapsed fourth ventricle is seen as a streak. Normal salci and gyri are seen. The tomographic ultrasound imaging (TUI) shows detailed anatomy of the brain. The thalamus is clearly defined. On color flow imaging, pericallosal artery and its branches are clearly seen.

Courtesy: Textbook of Diagnostic Ultrasound by Rumack.

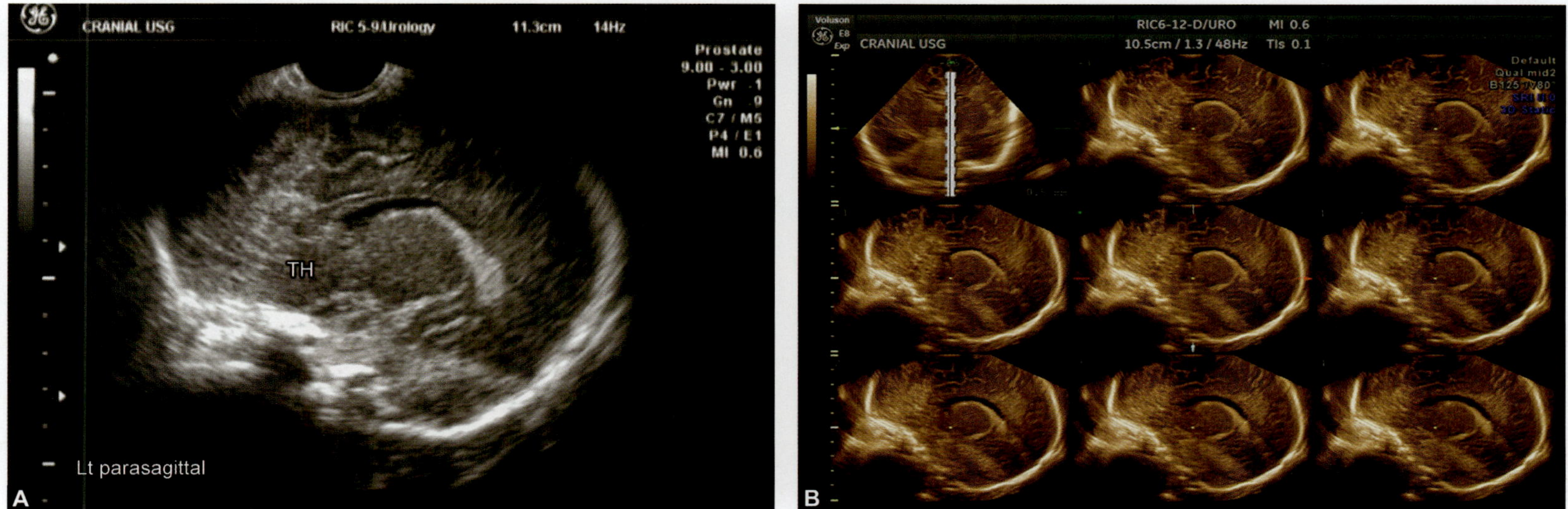

FIGURES 6.3A and B: Normal parasagittal view. HRSG shows normal infant brain in parasagittal planes. Body of the third ventricle is seen and echogenic choroid plexus is seen filling the body at the atrium. Head of the caudate nucleus is also seen adjacent to the thalamus. The tomographic ultrasound imaging (TUI) shows different sections of the brain in sagittal plane.

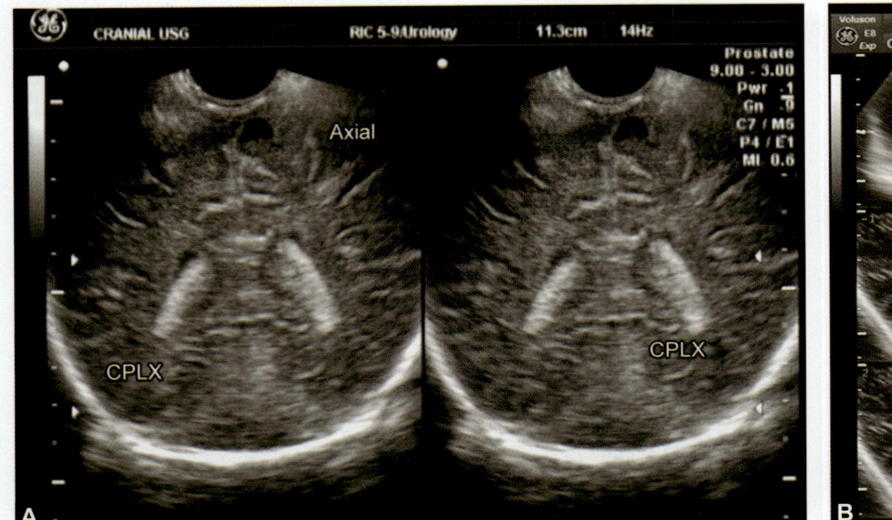

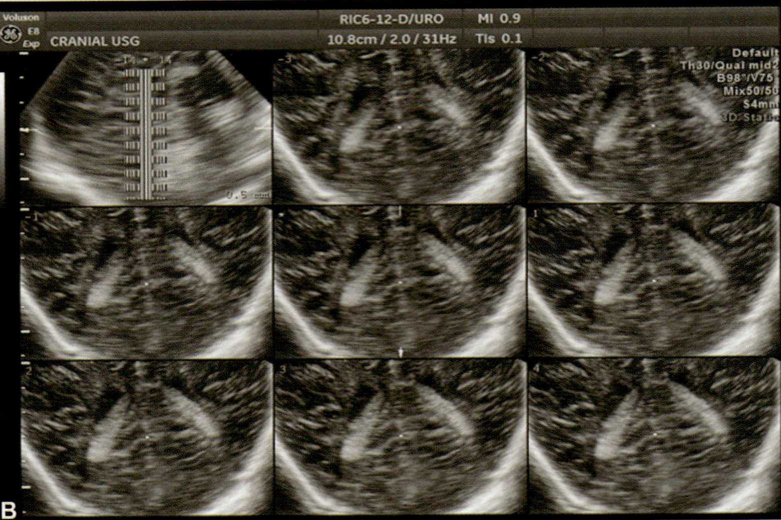

FIGURES 6.4A and B: Normal axial view. HRSG shows normal axial view of the brain parenchyma. Body of the lateral ventricles is seen. Echogenic choroid plexus fill the lateral ventricles. Parietal lobes show normal sulci and gyri. The tomographic ultrasound imaging (TUI) shows detailed anatomy of the choroid plexus and normal brain parenchyma.

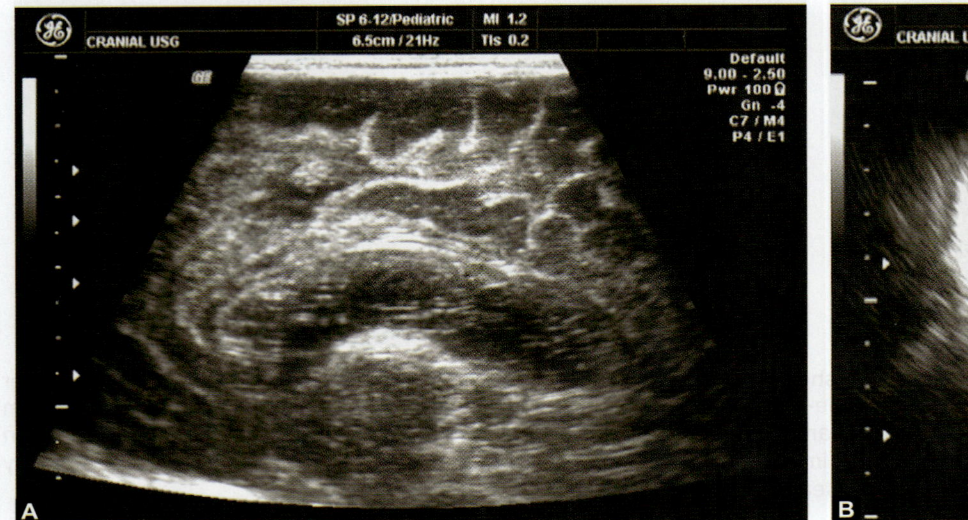

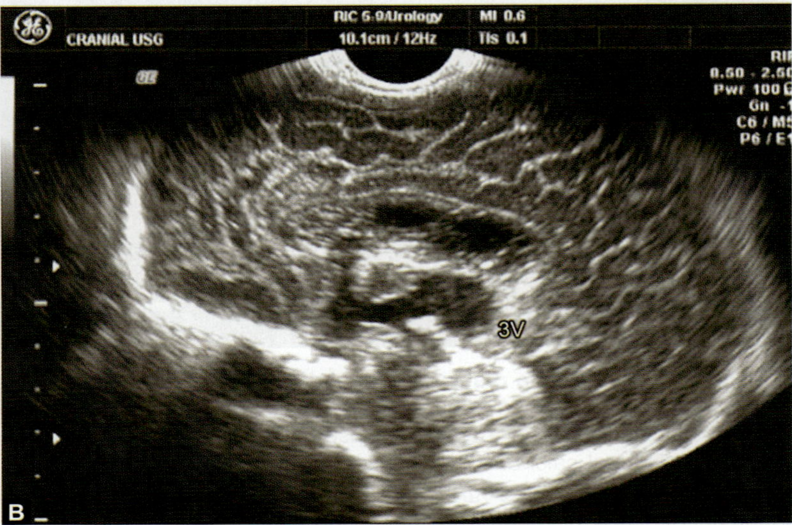

FIGURES 6.5A and B: Normal sulci and gyri on high resolution. High resolution ultrasound shows the details of the sulci and gyri of the brain parenchyma. The sulci and gyri stand out clearly on HRSG.

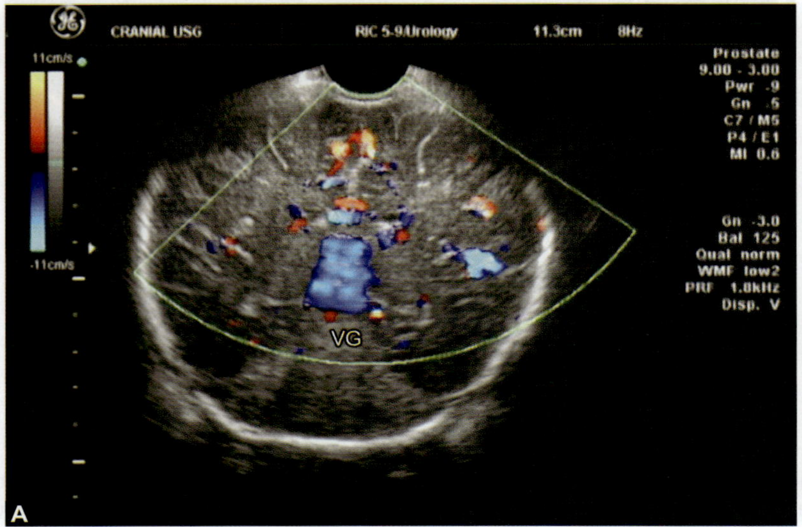

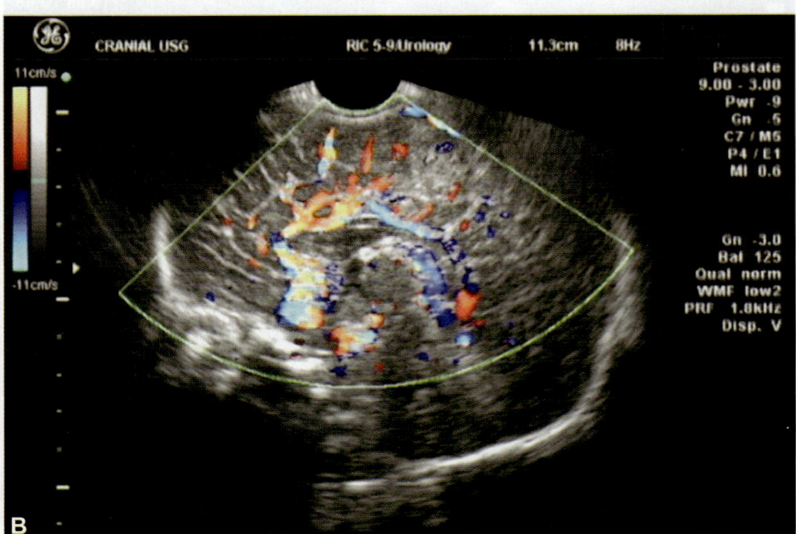

FIGURES 6.6A and B

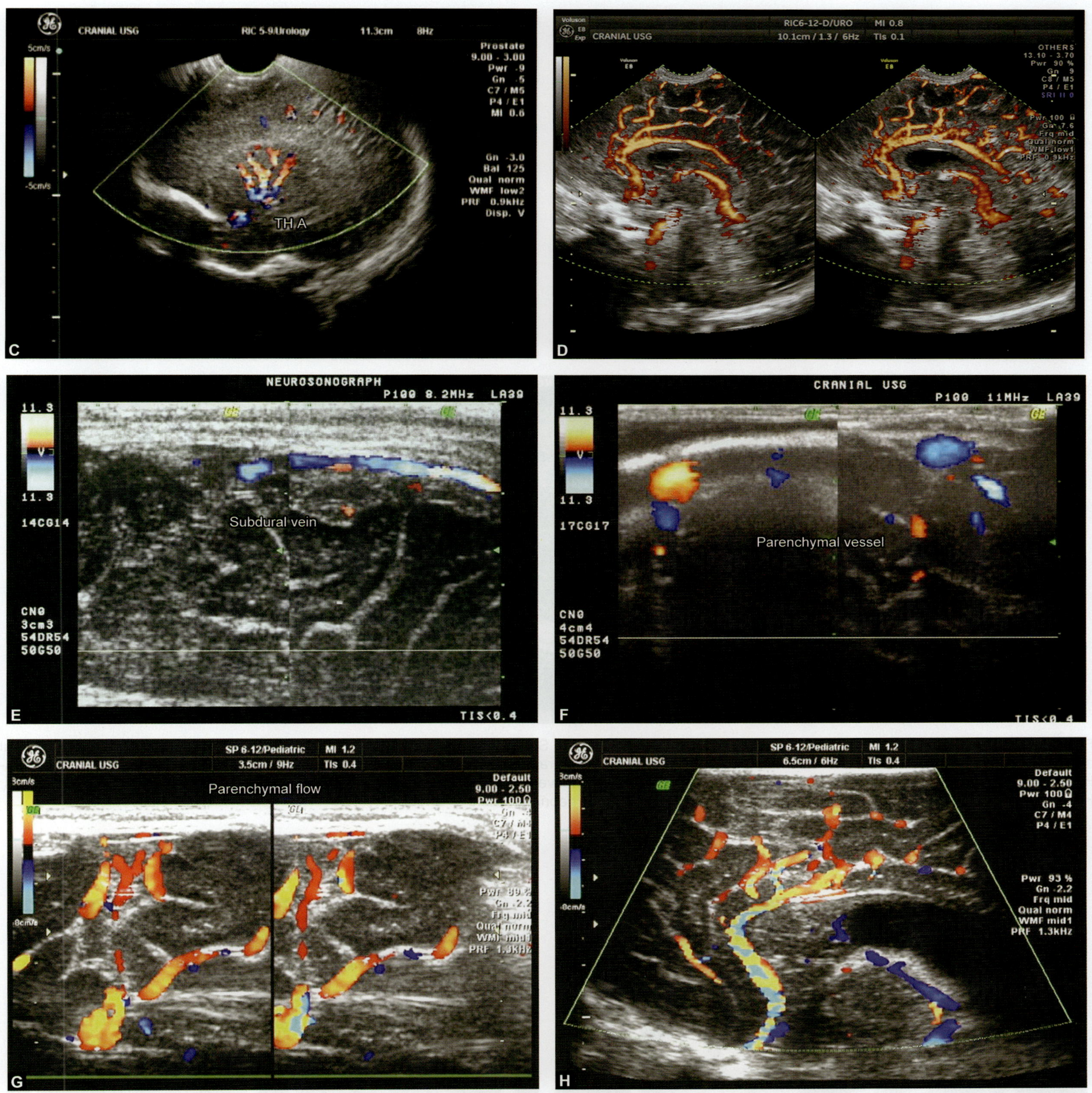

FIGURES 6.6C to H

FIGURES 6.6A to H: Normal brain parenchymal flow. Color flow imaging shows normal parenchymal flow in the brain parenchyma. The vein of Galen is seen as the dominant vessel. Normal thalamic and internal capsular flow: Color Doppler imaging shows normal internal capsular and thalamic flow supplied by lenticulo striate arteries, branches of middle cerebral artery.

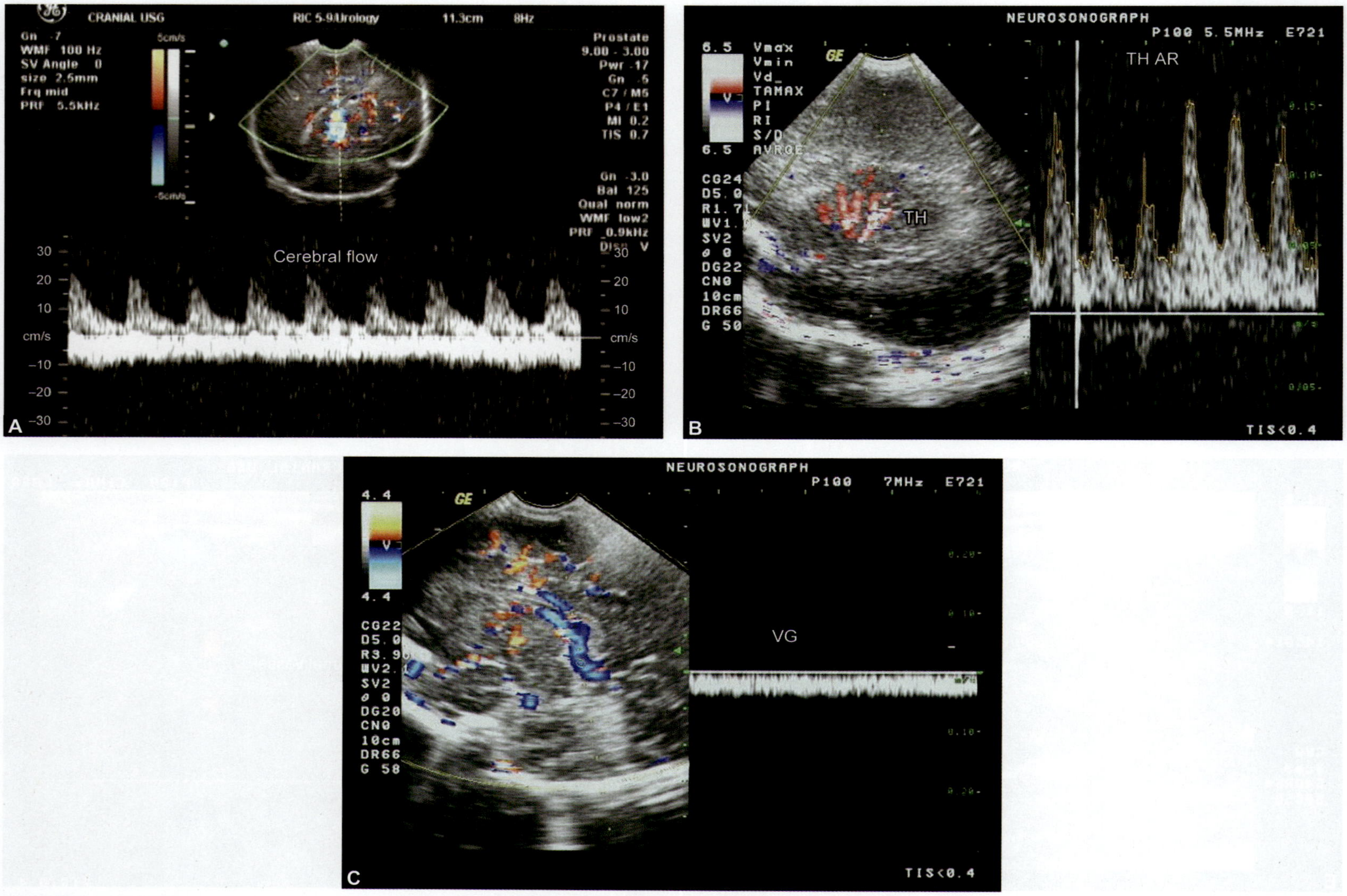

FIGURES 6.7A to C: Spectral Doppler flow in the cerebral arteries. Spectral Doppler tracing flow shows arterial flow pattern the intracerebral arteries. Spectral Doppler flow in vein of Galen (VG). Spectral Doppler tracing flow shows monophasic flow pattern of vein of Galen. Dural Sinus-HRSG shows normal dural sinus running in the superior surface of the vein. Color Doppler imaging shows normal venous flow in the dural sinus. High resolution color flow imaging shows normal parenchymal flow in neonatal brain.

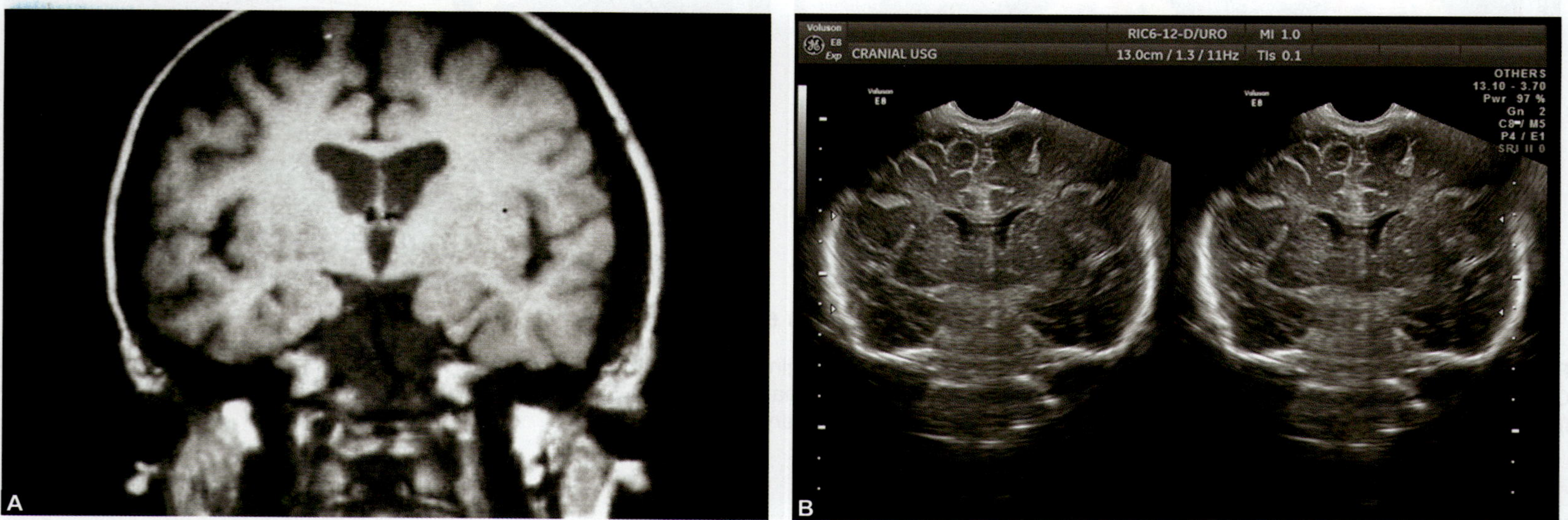

FIGURES 6.8A and B: MRI of the normal brain. MRI of the normal brain shows normal brain anatomy which is comparable to the normal sonographic anatomy of the brain. Normal sonographic image of infant brain: HRSG shows normal image of brain parenchyma in coronal plane. The image is comparable to the MRI of the same patient.

CONGENITAL ANOMALIES

Congenital malformations are quite common and with the availability of high-resolution sonography most of the disorders can be diagnosed prenatally. Brain malformations are classified based on the various stages of development of the brain. De Myer had suggested the classification in early seventies, which had been modified by Harwood-Nash and Rumack and Johnson, accordingly the brain malformations can be classified as follows:

Disorders of Organogenesis

Disorders of neural tube closure: Chairi malformation, Dandy-Walker malformation, agenesis of the corpus callosum, lipoma of the corpus callosum, teratoma disorders of diverticulation, septo-optic dysplasia, holoprosencephaly, aventricular cerebrum.

Disorders of proliferation: Microcephaly.

Disorders of sulcation and migration: Lissencephaly, schizencephaly, heterotopias, destructive lesions, disorders of organization, disorders of myelination

Disorders of histogenesis: Phakomatosis (tuberous sclerosis, neurofibromatosis), neoplasia, vascular lesions.

Among the malformations, disorders of neural tube closure are frequently encountered in our day-to-day practice and need further attention.

Chiari Malformation

Chairi malformations have been classified into Chiari I to IV, however, Chiari II is most frequently seen, and its early recognition becomes important, as invariably it is associated with meningomyelocele.

The salient sonographic features are as follows:
- Bat wing appearance of frontal horns due to anterior and inferior pointing
- Cavum septum pellucidum completely or partially absent
- Enlarged third ventricle
- Enlargement of mass intermedia
- Non-visualization of fourth ventricle.

The above changes can be explained on account of downward herniation of cerebellar tonsils into upper spinal canal.

Dandy-Walker Malformation

The salient sonographic features are as follows:
- Large posterior fossa cyst community with fourth ventricle
- Hypoplastic cerebellar hemispheres
- Associated hydrocephalus.

Associated with other anomalies in 68% cases, i.e. agenesis of corpus callosum, encephalocele, aqueductal stenosis.

Dandy-Walker variant

- Small posterior fossa cyst
- Mild hydrocephalus.

Differential diagnosis of Dandy-Walker malformation
- Arachnoid cyst—no communication with fourth ventricle
- Large cysterna magna—no hydrocephalus.

Agenesis of Corpus Callosum

Agenesis of corpus callosum may present as complete agenesis, partial agenesis or hypoplasia, 80% of the cases are associated with other anomalies such as Dandy-Walker, Chiari malformation and midline cysts.

The salient sonographic features are as follows:
- Distorted sulci/gyri anatomy
- Superior extension of third ventricle
- Parallel lateral ventricles
- Absent cavum septum pellucidum
- Absent cingulate gyrus.

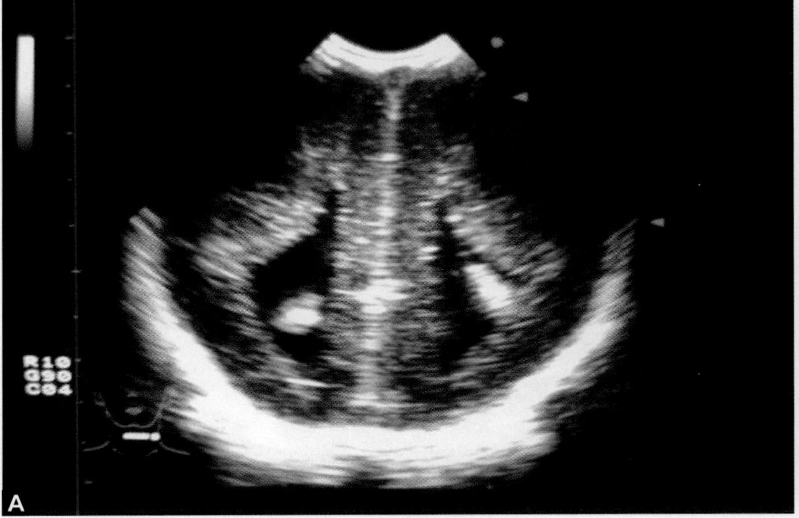

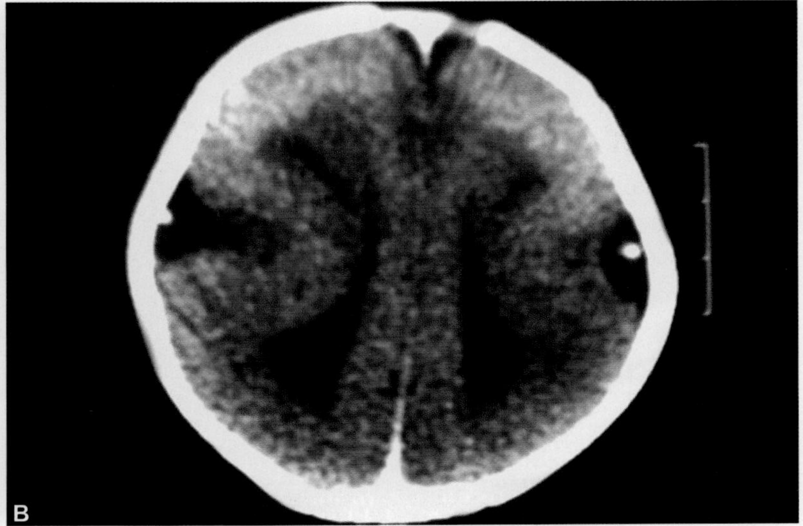

FIGURES 6.9A and B: Agenesis of corpus callosum. HRSG shows parallel placed lateral ventricles suggestive of agenesis of corpus callosum. The ventricles are seen widely separated. The sulci and the gyri are seen running in radial fashion. Typical sonographic findings are agenesis of corpus callosum. CT scan of the same patient also shows parallel lateral ventricles. Thus, confirms the sonographic findings.

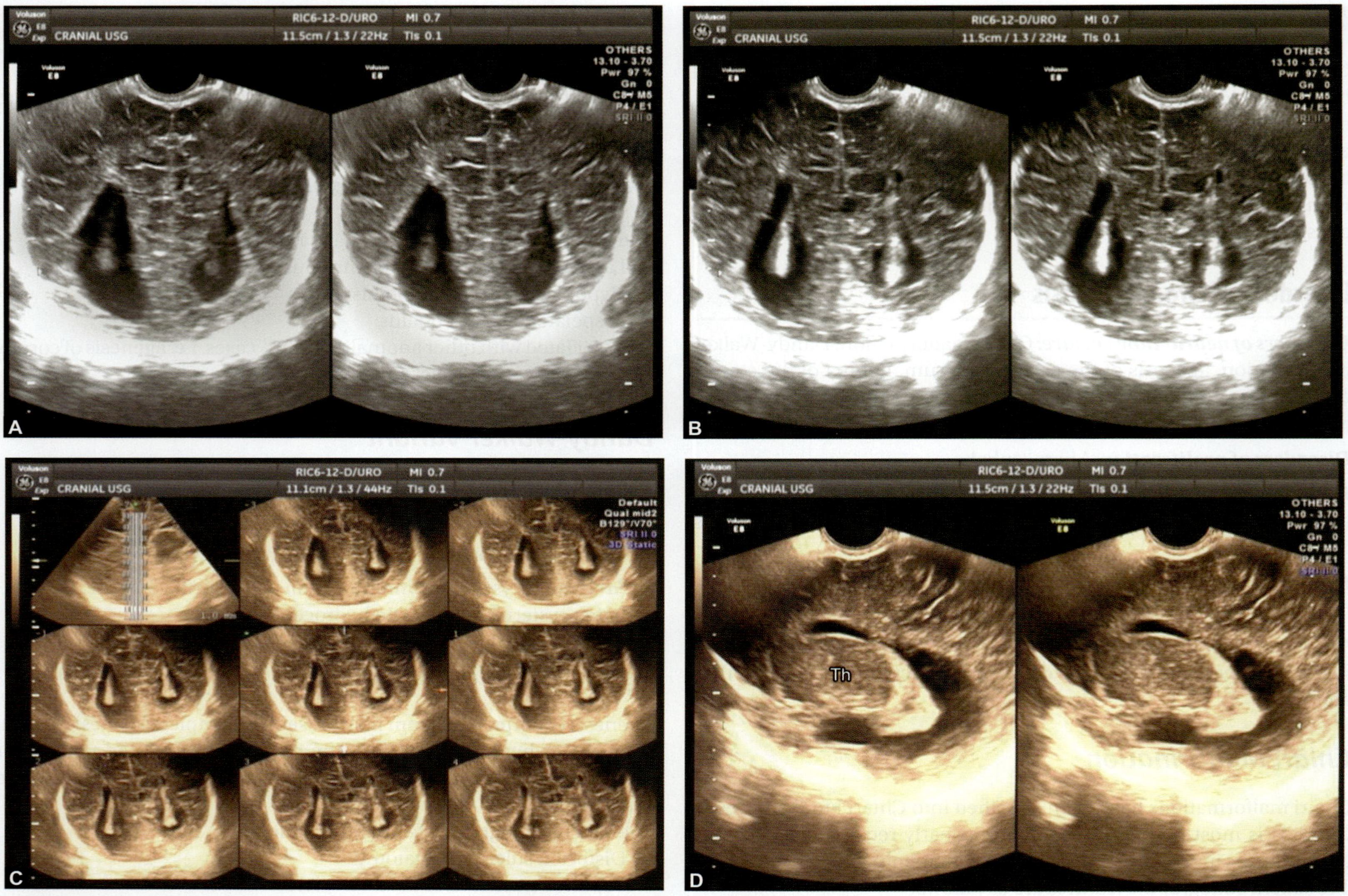

FIGURES 6.10A to D: Agenesis of corpus callosum. HRSG shows agenesis of corpus callosum. The lateral ventricles are seen parallely placed. The TUI imaging shows choroid plexus seen filling the lateral ventricles in parasagittal vein. The choroid plexus is seen extending upto anterior part of lateral ventricle. Typical sign of agenesis of corpus callosum.

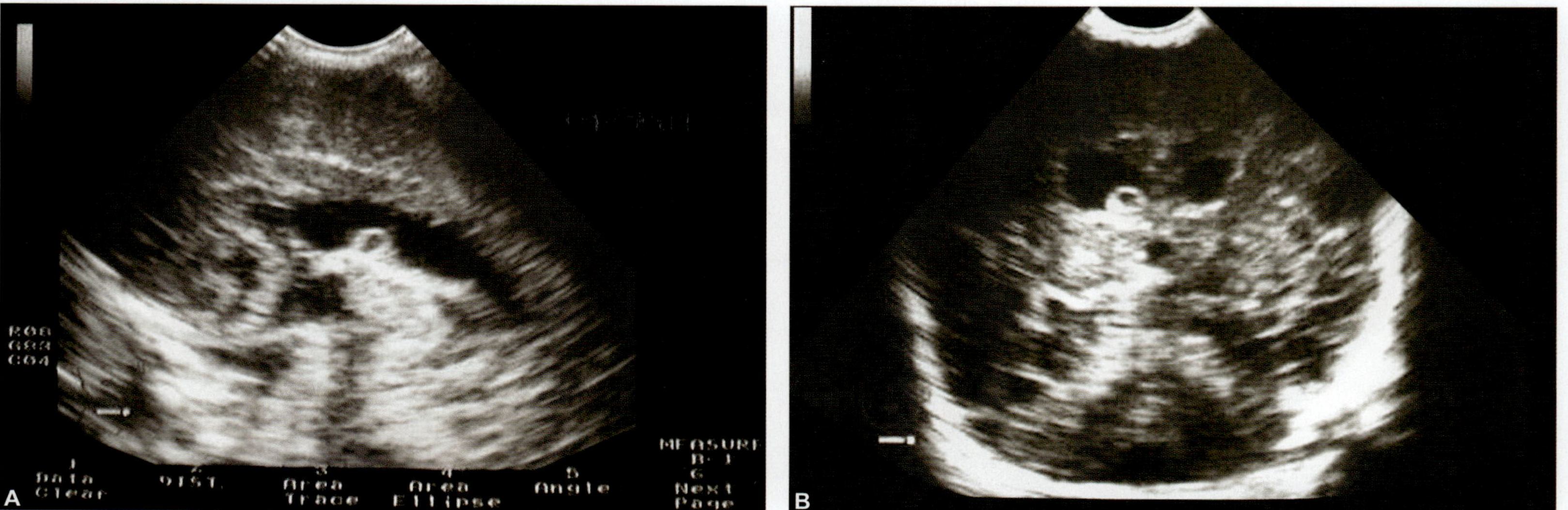

FIGURES 6.11A and B: Choroid plexus cyst. An infant child presented with fullness of the fontanelle. HRSG shows mild dilatation of the ventricles. A well-defined thin walled cyst is seen attached with the choroid plexus suggestive of choroid plexus cyst.

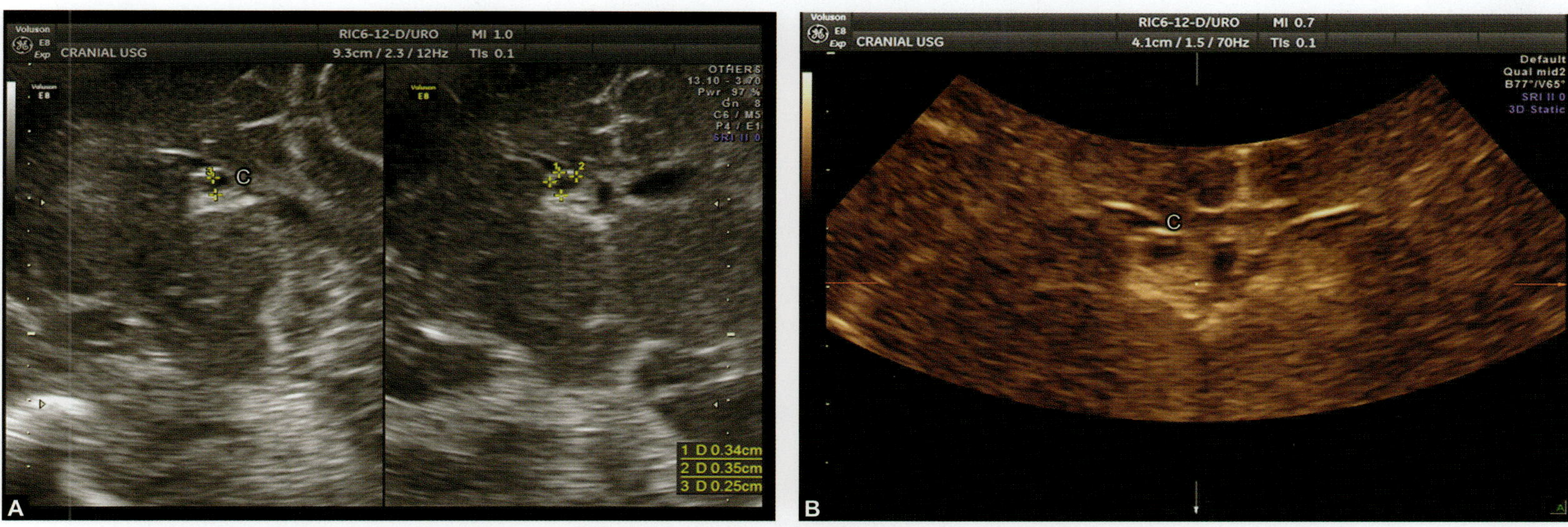

FIGURES 6.12A and B: Small choroid plexus cyst. HRSG shows a small choroid plexus cyst in the left ventricle. HRSG shows the cyst wall very clearly.

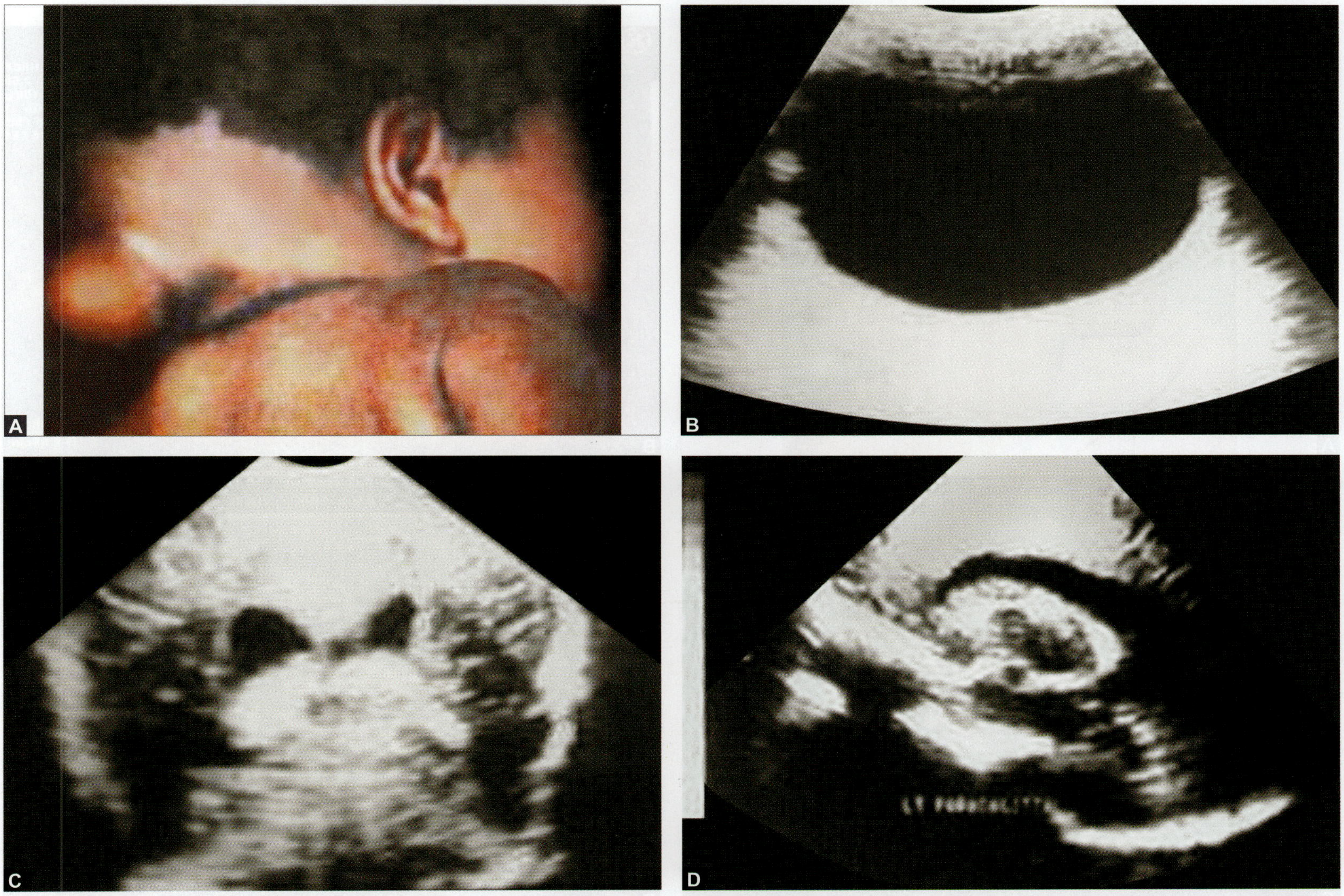

FIGURES 6.13A to D: Occipital meningocele. A young boy presented with a cystic mass in the occiput. HRSG shows thin-walled cyst in the mass. No brain herniation is seen in the cyst. No septation, calcification or any membranous shadow is seen in the cyst. HRSG shows mild pressure on the outflow tract involving the fourth ventricle by the cyst. Fullness of the lateral ventricles is seen due to the pressure by the cyst.

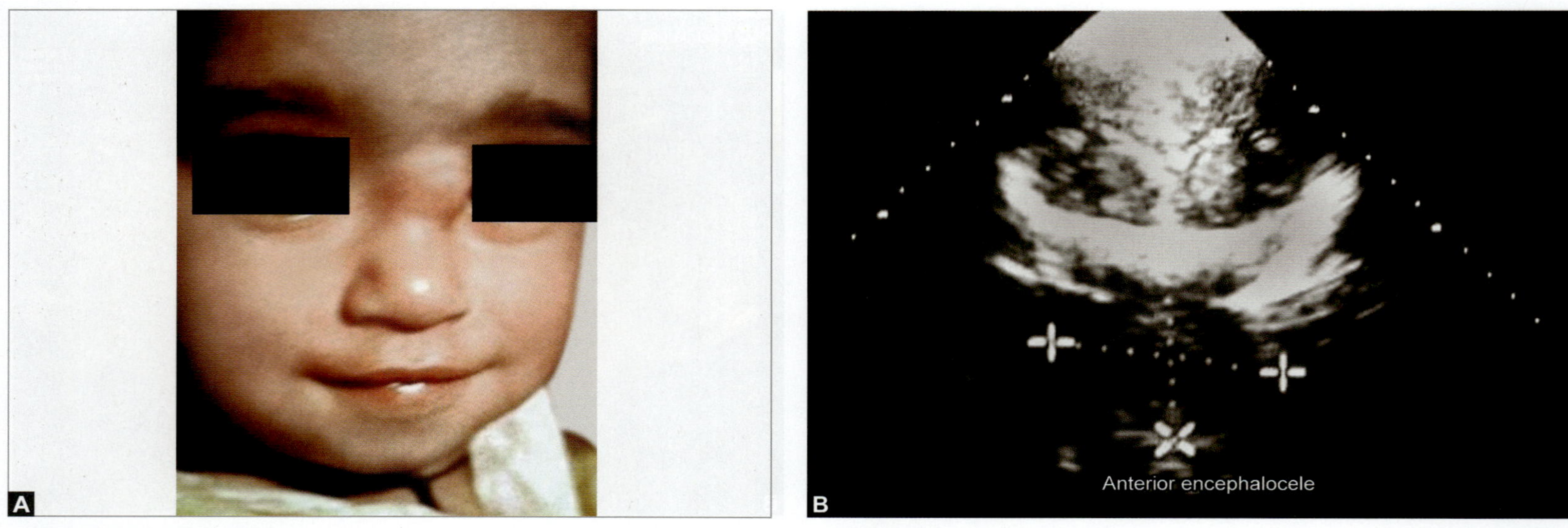

FIGURES 6.14A and B: Anterior meningocele. A young boy presented with a cystic mass over the nasion. A well-defined thick walled cystic mass is seen in the mass. Homogeneous low-level collection is seen in it. No septation or loculation is seen suggestive of anterior meningocele.

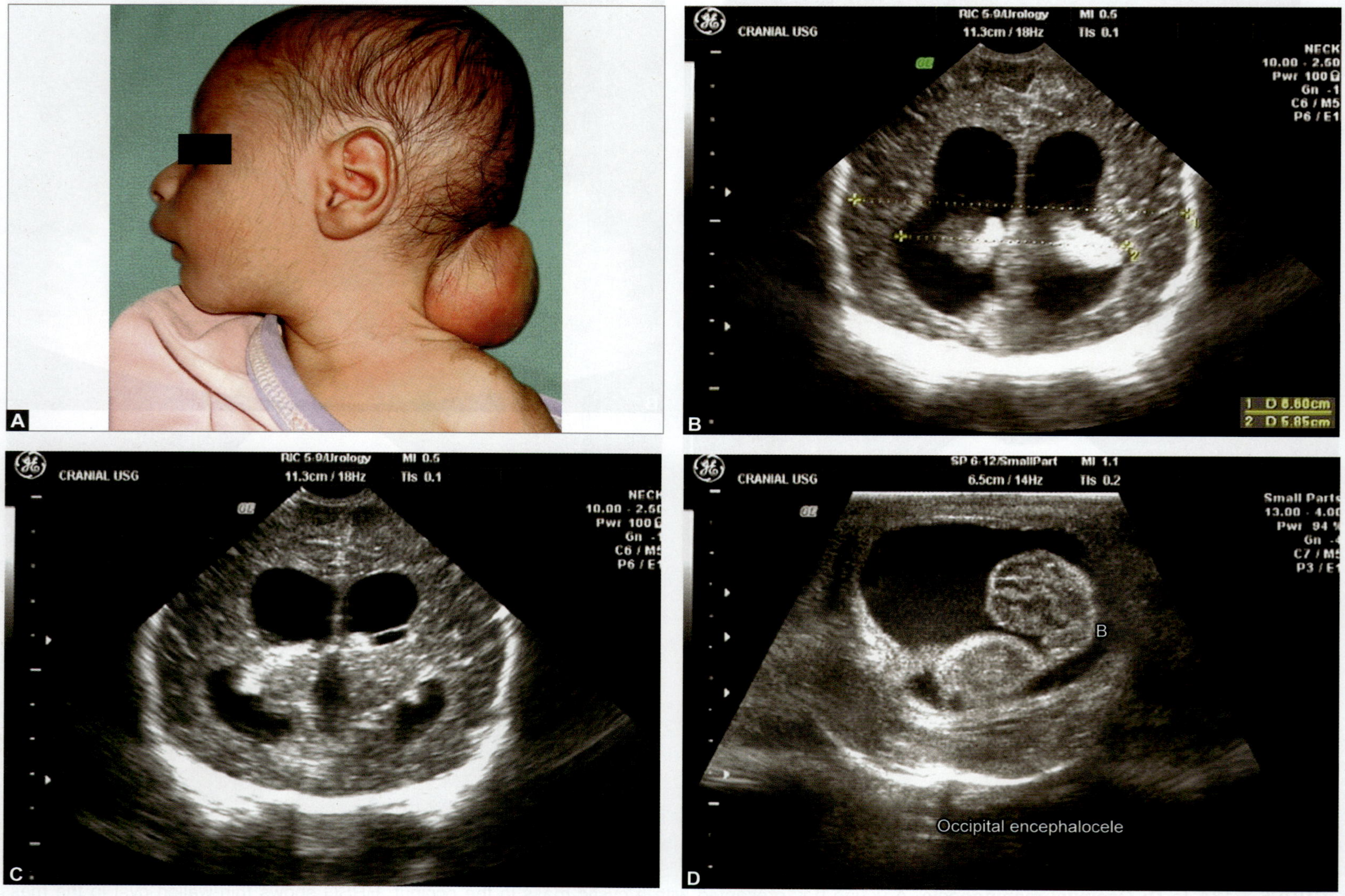

FIGURES 6.15A to D

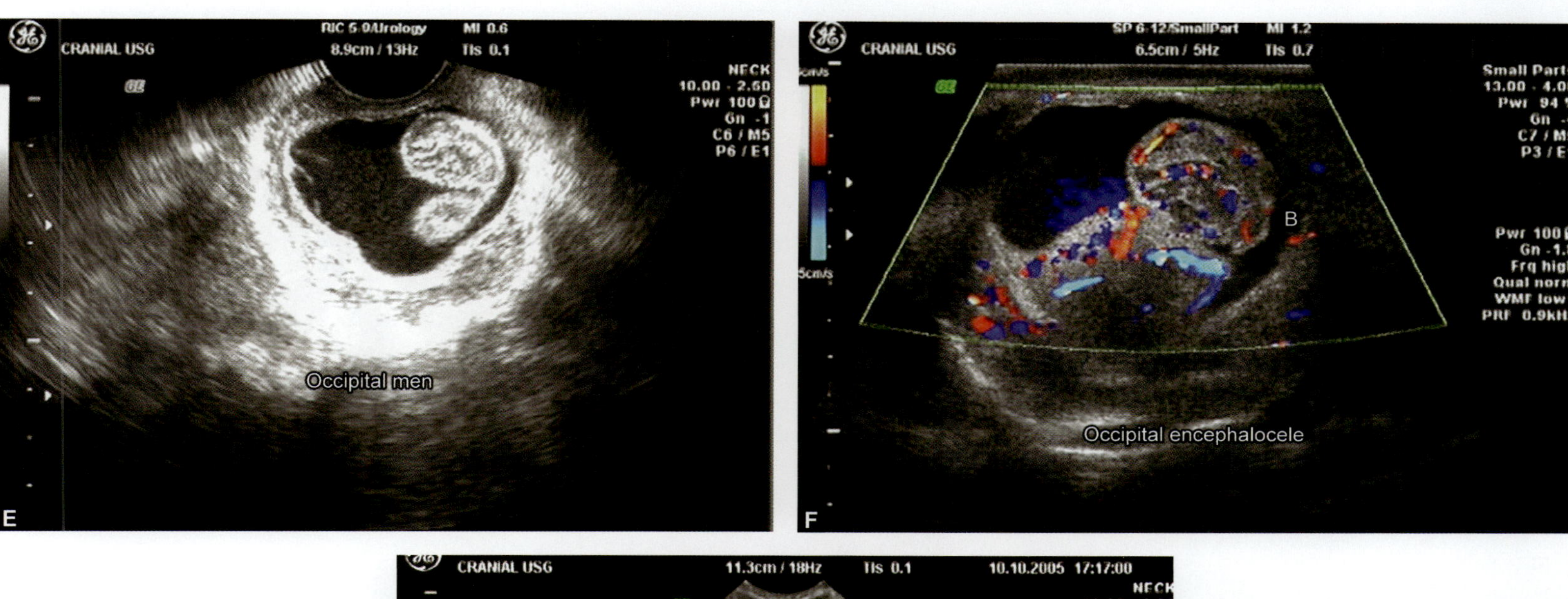

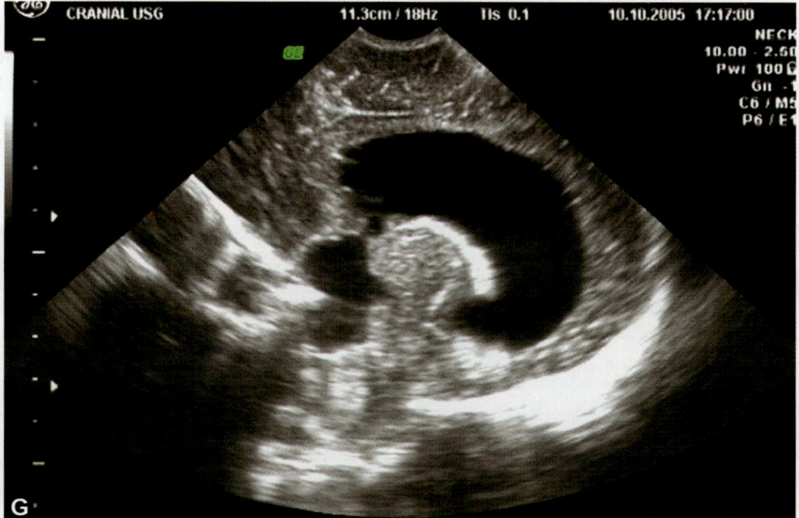

FIGURES 6.15E to G

FIGURES 6.15A to G: Occipital encephalocele. An infant is born with soft tissue swelling over the occiput. Cranial ultrasound shows dilated ventricles. Cephalo ventricular ratio is altered. But no pressure is seen on brain parenchyma. High-resolution ultrasound of the occipital cystic mass shows herniation of the brain tissue in the cyst suggestive of encephalocele, and part of the cerebellum is seen in the cyst. On color flow imaging vessels are seen in the brain tissue. 3D imaging of the same patient shows defect in the occiput. The brain is seen herniating through the defect in the cyst.

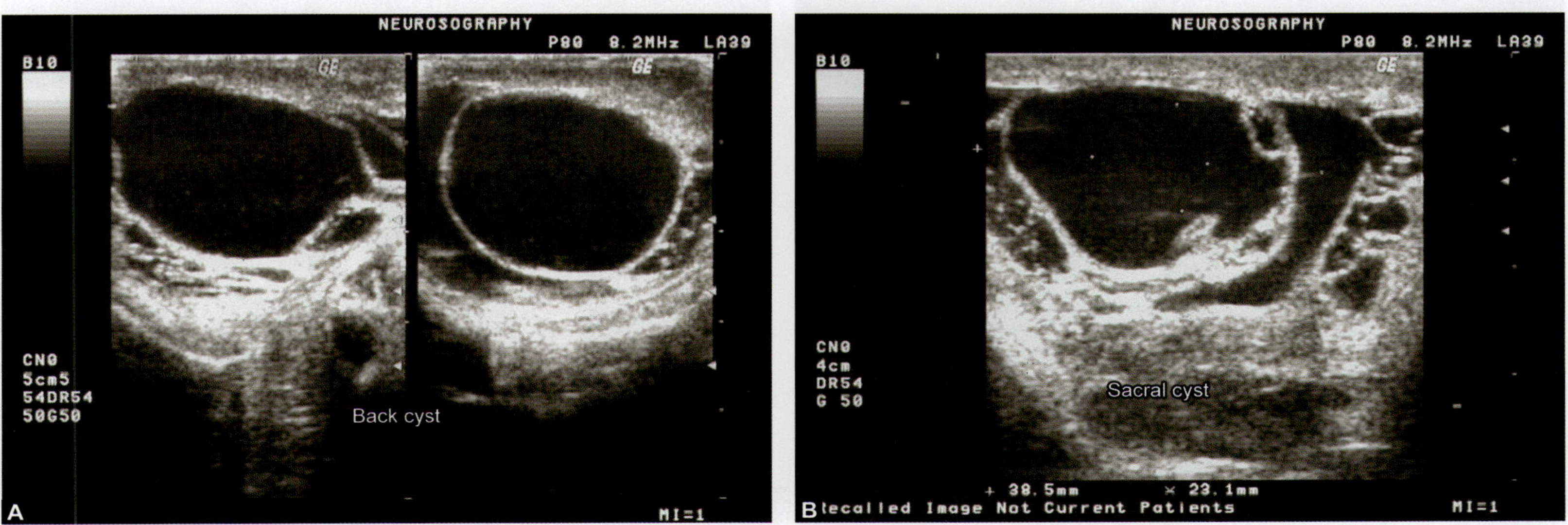

FIGURES 6.16A and B

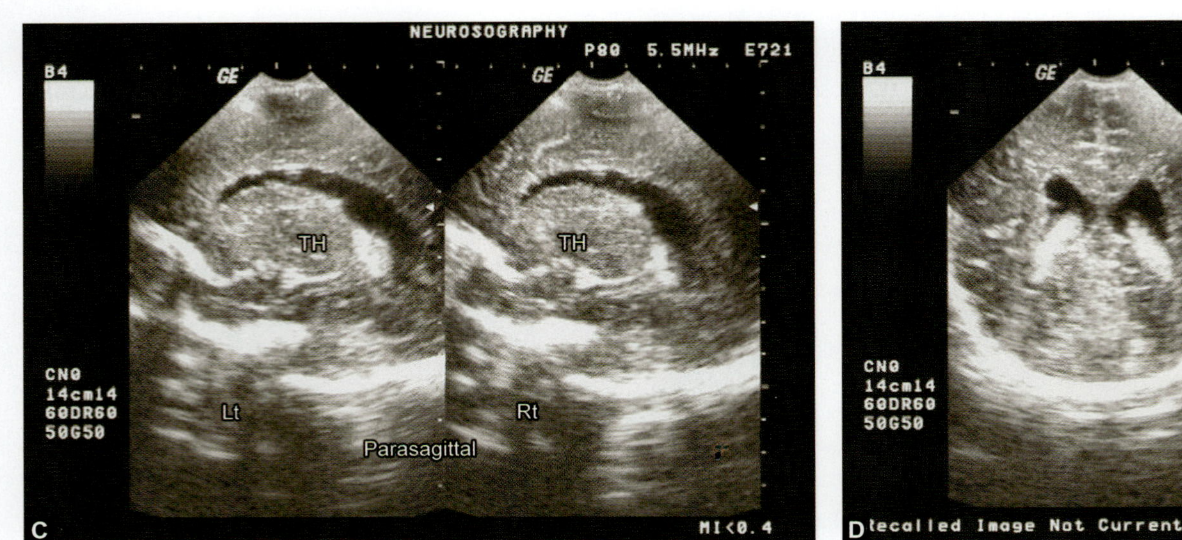

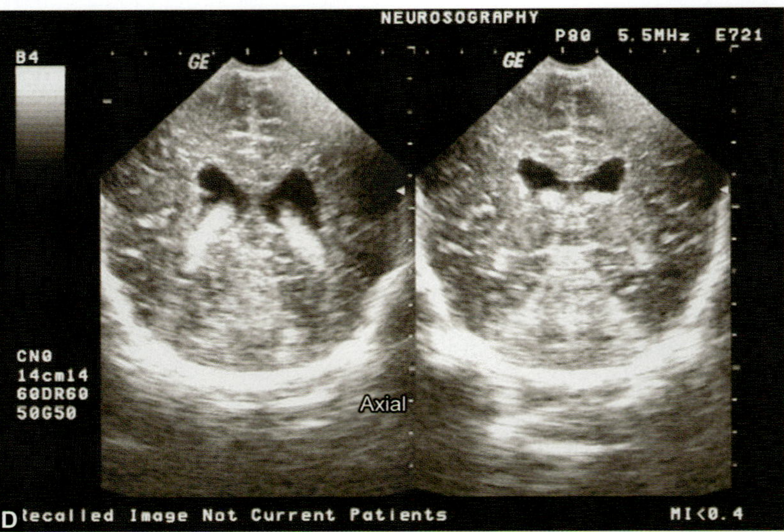

FIGURES 6.16C and D

FIGURES 6.16A to D: Sacral meningocele. HRSG shows a cystic mass in the sacral region in an infant. Echogenic septa are seen in the cyst. But no soft tissue shadow is seen suggestive of a meningocele. Cranial ultrasound of the same patient shows mild fullness of ventricular system involving the lateral ventricles due to the pressure by the sacral cyst. But no periventricular leak is seen.

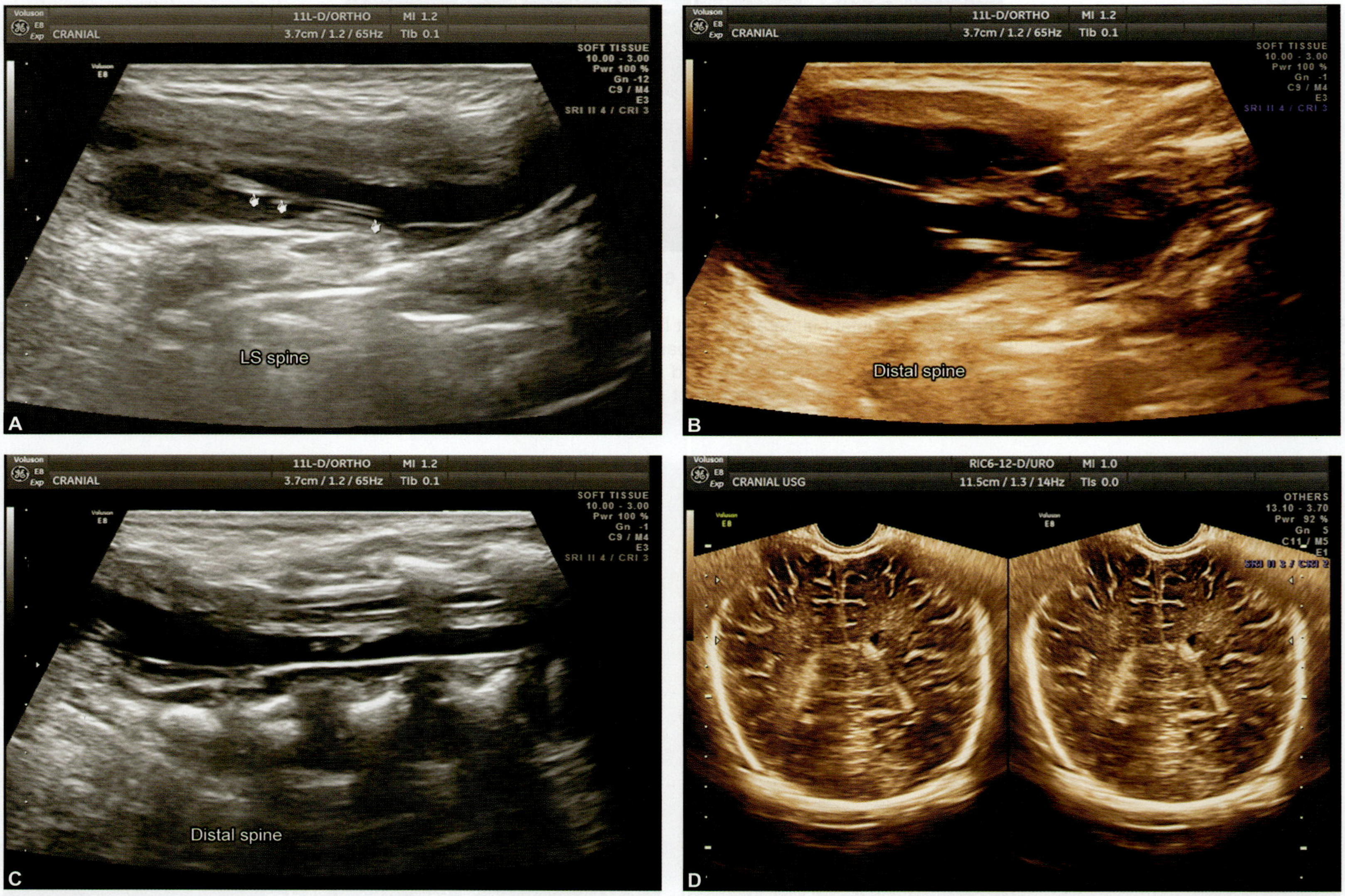

FIGURES 6.17A to D: Sacral meningocele. A patient presented with lumbosacral meningocele. HRSG shows a cystic shadow in the lower lumbar region. Thin strands are seen in it. A thin septum is also seen in the meningocele. The nerve routes are also seen passing through the meningocele. The cranial ultrasound of the same patient does not show dilated ventricles because of the back pressure. The ventricles are normal and brain parenchyma shows normal texture.

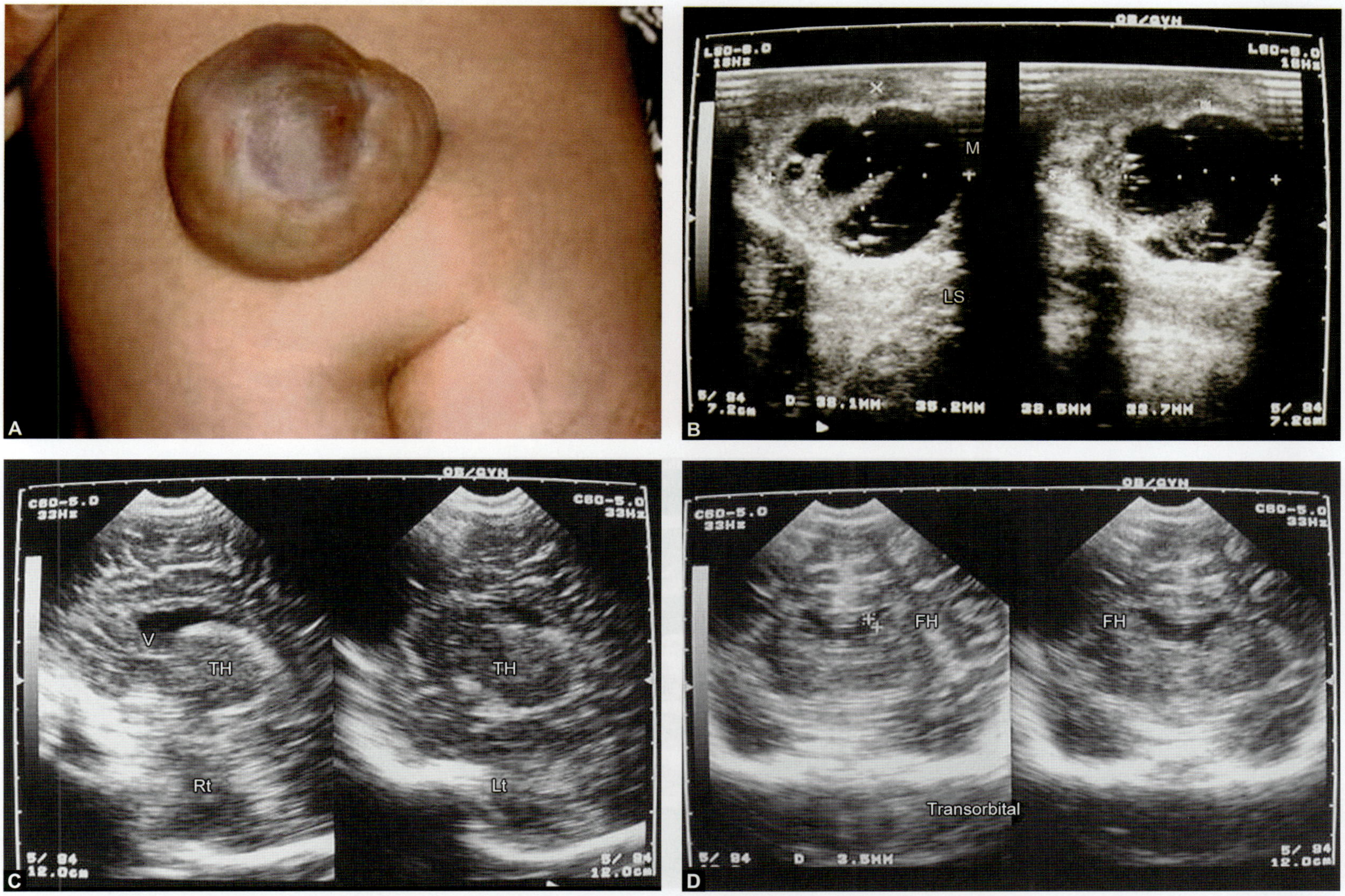

FIGURES 6.18A to D: Sacral meningocele. An infant was born with a soft tissue mass over the sacral area. HRSG shows multi loculated cystic mass with multiple echogenic septa suggestive of sacral meningocele. No membranous herniation is seen in it. Cranial ultrasound of the same patient shows normal ventricular system. No back pressure is seen on the ventricles by the meningocele.

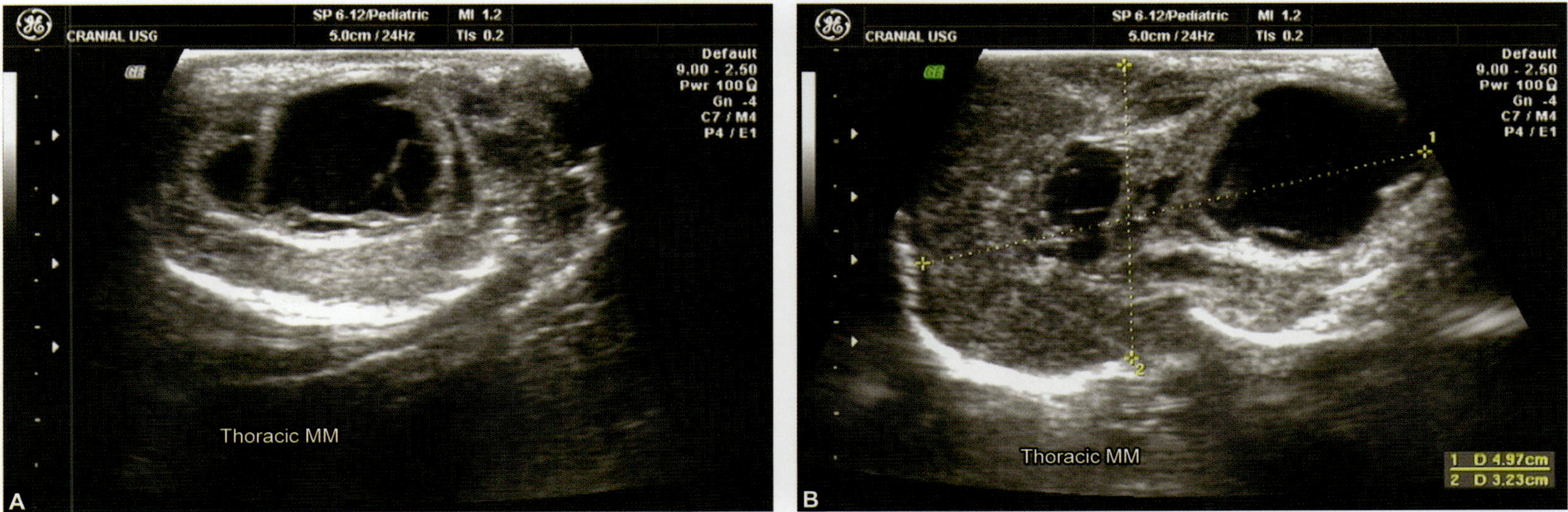

FIGURES 6.19A and B

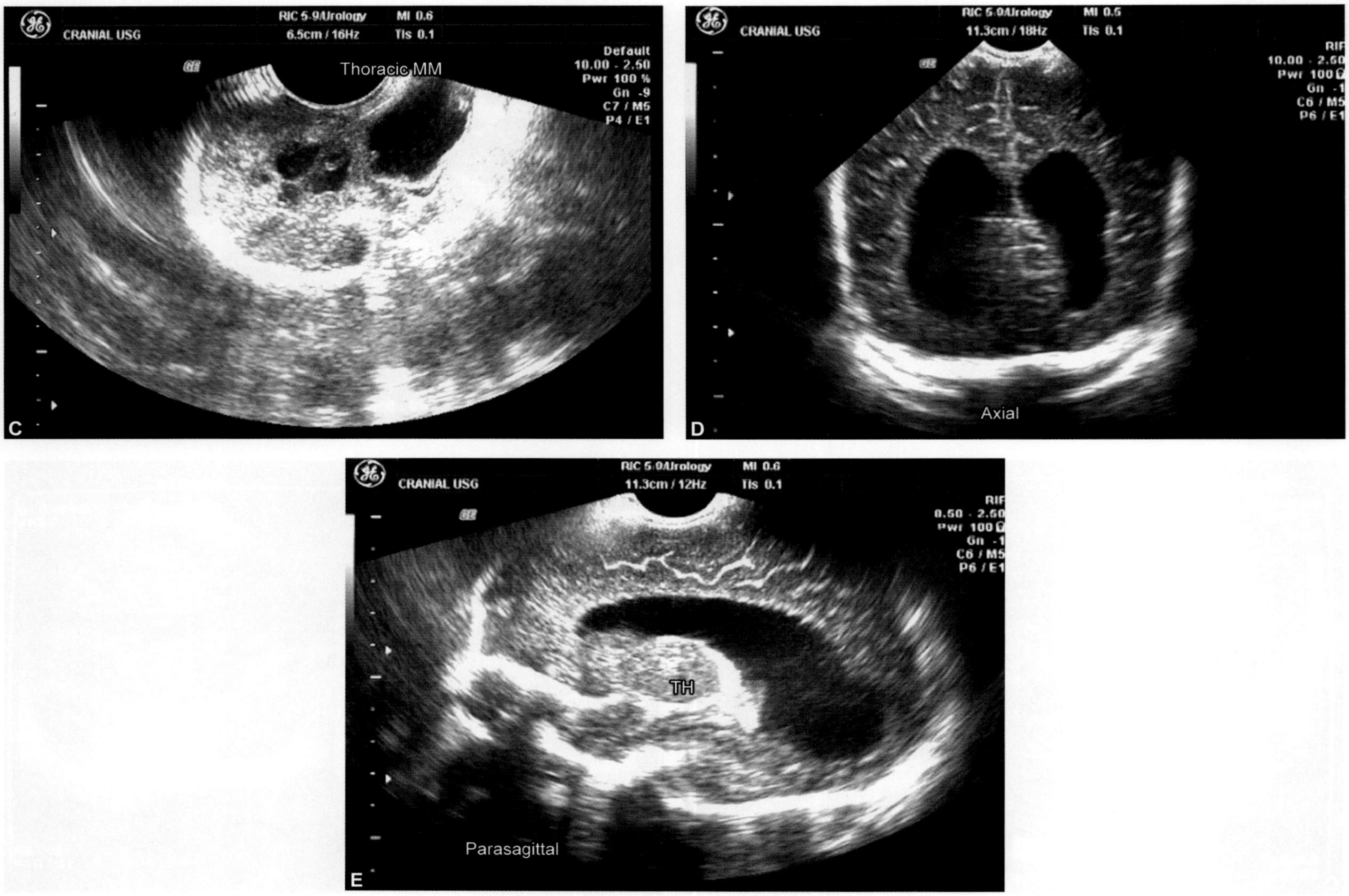

FIGURES 6.19C to E

FIGURES 6.19A to E: Thoracic meningomyelocele. A child was born with big thoracic meningomyelocele. HRSG shows a multi loculated thick walled cystic mass. The mass shows herniation of the membranes. The cranial ultrasound of the same patient shows dilated ventricles due to obstructive pathology.

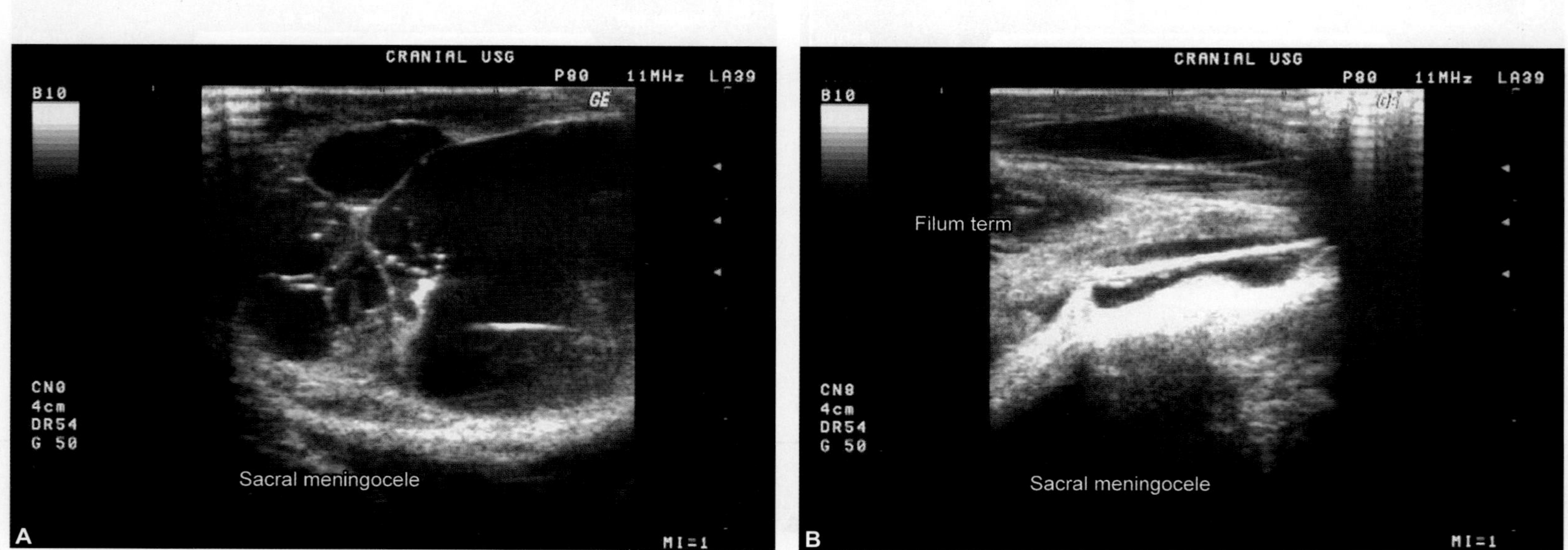

FIGURES 6.20A and B

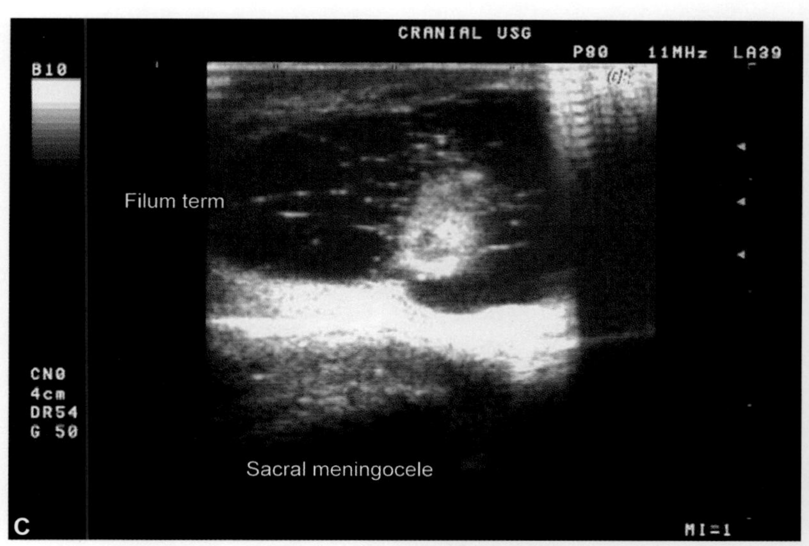

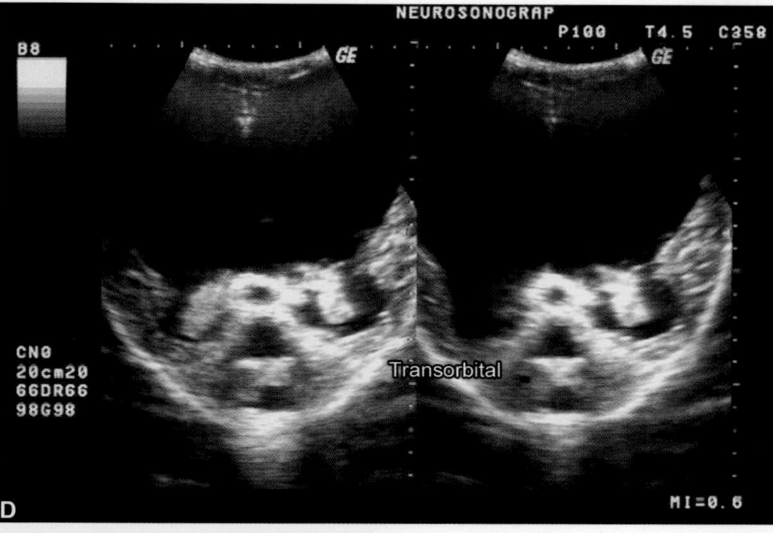

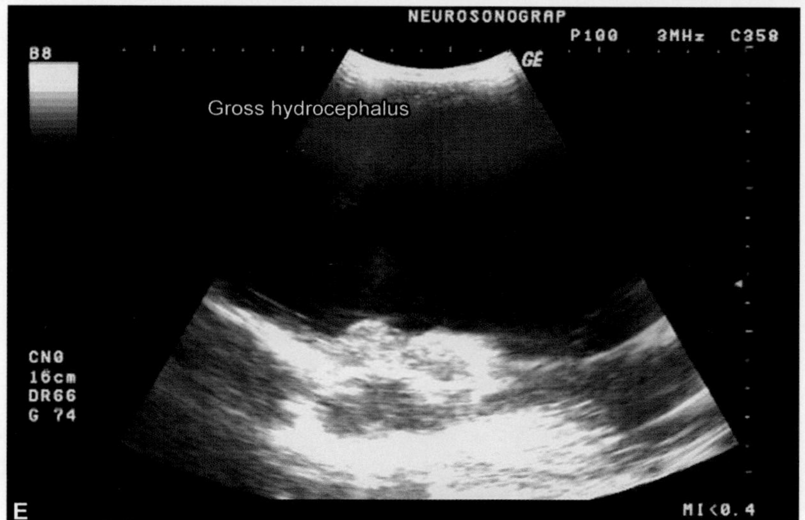

FIGURES 6.20C to E

FIGURES 6.20A to E: Lumbosacral meningomyelocele. An infant is born with a big cystic mass in the lumbosacral region. HRSG shows a complex cystic mass in the LS region. Multiple membranes are seen in it suggestive of meningomyelocele. The filum terminal is seen floating in the cyst. The fibril pattern of filum terminal is well appreciated on HRSG. Cranial ultrasound of the same patient shows gross hydrocephalous. The dilated ventricles press over brain parenchyma with thinning of parenchyma

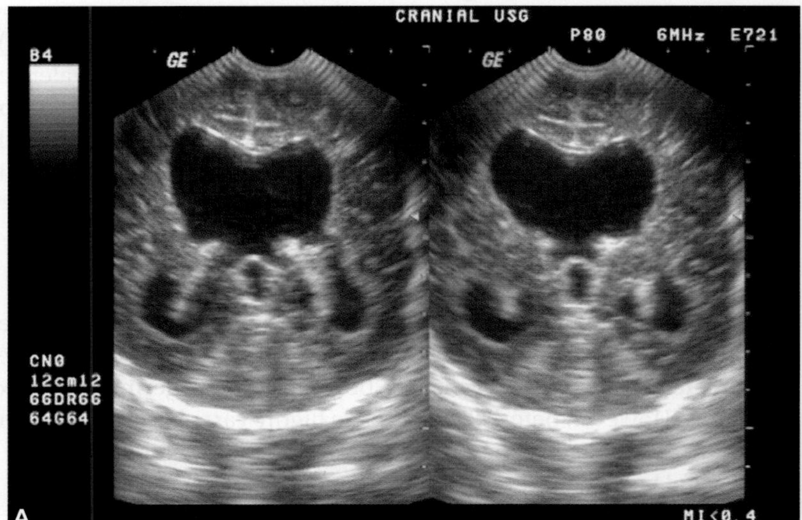

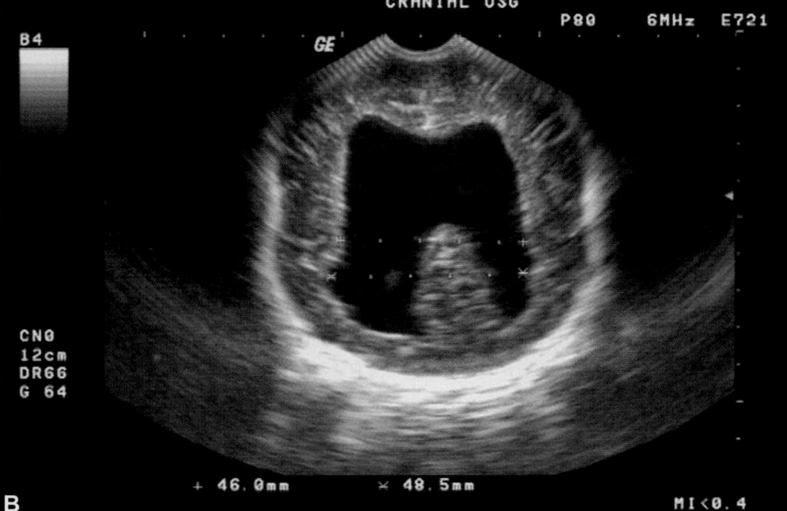

FIGURES 6.21A and B: Septooptic dysplasia with lobar holoprosencephaly. HRSG shows flattening of the frontal horns with evidence of absence of septum pellucidum. The anterior horns are fused and squared shaped. However, the occipital horn is separate.

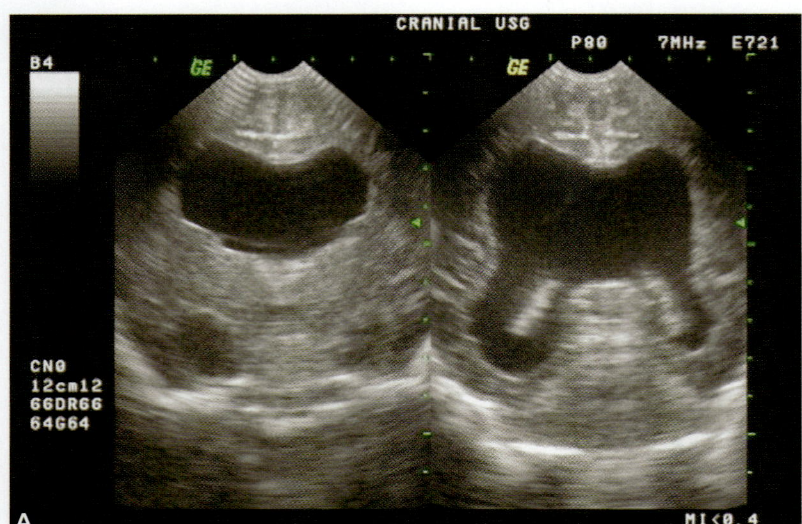

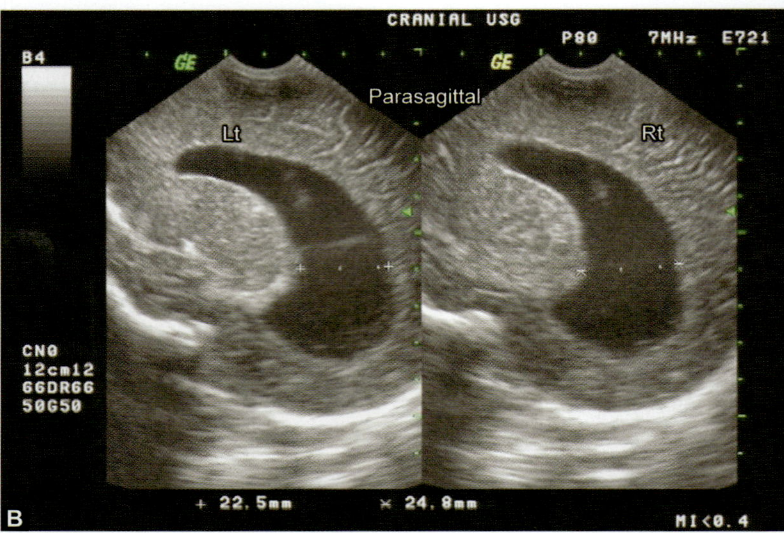

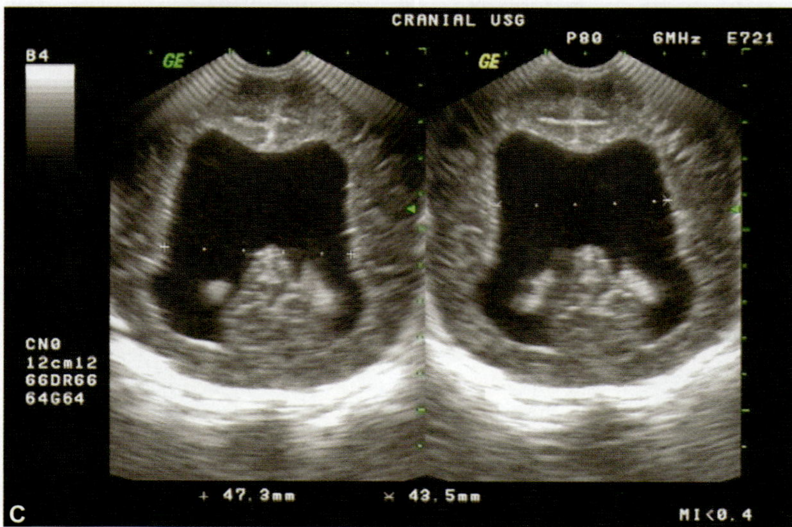

FIGURES 6.22A to C: Lobar holoprosencephaly. HRSG shows details of the holoprosencephaly. The frontal horns are fused. However, the occipital horns are separated. The ventricles are dilated.

HYDROCEPHALUS

Hydrocephalus is the most common sequelae of hemorrhage in pre-term infants leading to obstruction at the level of third of fourth ventricle. The other possible cause may be interference in absorption of CSF due to inflammatory ependymitis or basilar arachnoiditis due to hemorrhage/ infection. Rarely, over production of CSF from choroid plexus papilloma may be responsible for production of hydrocephalus (non-obstructive).

Ultrasonographic Diagnosis of Hydrocephalus

Various qualitative and quantitative methods have been described for diagnosis of hydrocephalus. The lateral ventricular ratio (LVR) method described by Rumack and Jhonson has been commonly used. The measurements are made from midline echo to the inner surface of lateral ventricle and from midline to inner table of skull on axial ultrasonography. The normal LVR is up to 35%, LVR of 35–40% is considered mild hydrocephalus, LVR of 41–50% is considered moderate, and LVR of more than 50% is severe hydrocephalus. In fetus, the ventricular measurement at the level of atrium is found to be more accurate, wherein less than 10 mm is considered to be normal. However, with sonographer gaining experience, the ventricular dilatation can be appreciated on routine coronal and sagittal scans without any critical measurements.

Ventricular dilatation can be documented weeks before clinical signs of hydrocephalus are noticed. Serial sonograms on weekly intervals are recommended to look for progress of hydrocephalus.

Intracranial Hemorrhage

Intracranial hemorrhage (ICH) and periventricular leukomalacia (PVL) are the most common CNS problems in premature infants. Prevalence of ICH in infants born at less than 32 weeks of gestation or with birth weight less than 1500 g is 30–55%. All such infants should be screened routinely on days 4–7 after birth. Infants with ICH should be followed weekly to detect early hydrocephalus.

Pathophysiology

The germinal matrix, which contains rich vascular stroma is a fragile structure present in the region of caudothalamic groove in the inferiolateral wall of lateral ventricle, beyond 32 weeks germinal matrix involutes. However, before 32 weeks it is highly vascular and fragile in the event of increased cerebral blood flow and raised blood pressure. Papile et al have nicely graded the extent of hemorrhage as follows:

Grade I Subependymal hemorrhage related to germinal matrix.
Grade II Intraventricular extension without hydrocephalus.
Grade III IVH + Hydrocephalus.
Grade IV IVH + Parenchymal extension

Ultrasonography is the most effective method for detection and follow-up of various grades of hemorrhage, mostly newborns are affected within 7 days, hence, first sonographic evaluation is recommended after 7 days of birth.

Subependymal Hemorrhage (SEH)

SEH is seen as an area of increased echogenecity in the inferolateral wall of lateral ventricle, acute hemorrhage is hyper echogenic and is similar in echogeneicity to choroid plexus. In few cases, the SEH liquefy centrally resulting in cyst formation, which may persist for months.

Intraventricular Hemorrhage (IVH)

The hemorrhage may rupture through ependymal lining into the ventricles. Sonography reveals an echogenic clot filling and expending the pathways of CSF and may reach up to basal cisterns. At times it is difficult to diagnosis IVH if it is not associated with hydrocephalus, clot commonly adheres to the choroid plexus and is indistinguishable from it. However, with due course of time, the clot becomes hypoechoic in the center due to liquefaction, the clot contracts and gradually decreases in size.

Intraparenchymal Hemorrhage (IPH)

The SEH may extend into surrounding parenchyma. The intraparenchymal hemorrhage is commonly seen (approximately in 8%) in the fetus born with birth-weight of less than 1500 g. Though it is commonly believed that intraparenchymal hemorrhage is extension of SEH, however, few studies have revealed that in neonates, the intraparenchymal hemorrhage may be manifestation of secondary hemorrhage within an area of periventricular infarction. It shows all the features of hemorrhage seen elsewhere in the body being echogenic in the beginning and leading to formation of porencephalic cyst as the clot resorbs.

Periventricular Leukomalacia (PVL)

PVL develops as a consequence of ischemia in the periventricle white matter leading to gliosis or cystic changes depending upon the severity.

Sonographically, PVL appears as focal areas of increased echogenicity in periventricular region. The involvement is bilateral and symmetrical. In several cases, it appears as periventricular cystic formation, however, since sensitivity of ultrasonography is 30% only. In cases of strong clinical suspicion with negative sonography, MRI is indicated.

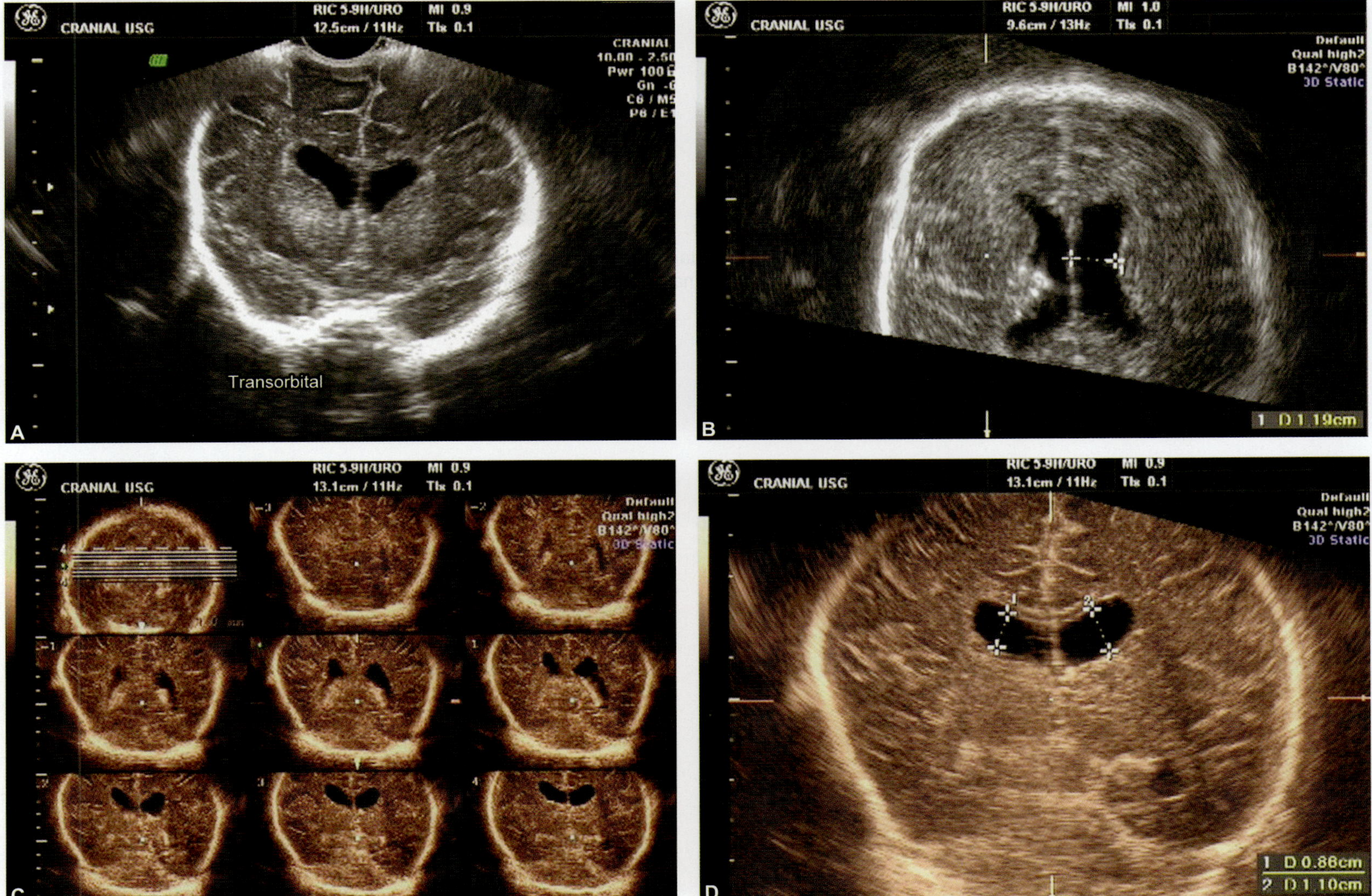

FIGURES 6.23A to D: Mildly dilated frontal horn and lateral ventricles. A 10-day-old child presented with mild fullness of anterior fontanels. HRSG shows mild fullness of frontal horn. The lateral ventricles also show mild dilatation. They are 12 mm in size, which is just above the normal limit (Normal < 10 mm). However, no periventricular leak is seen. No pressure is seen on brain parenchyma. The TUI imaging shows all sections of ventricles clearly.

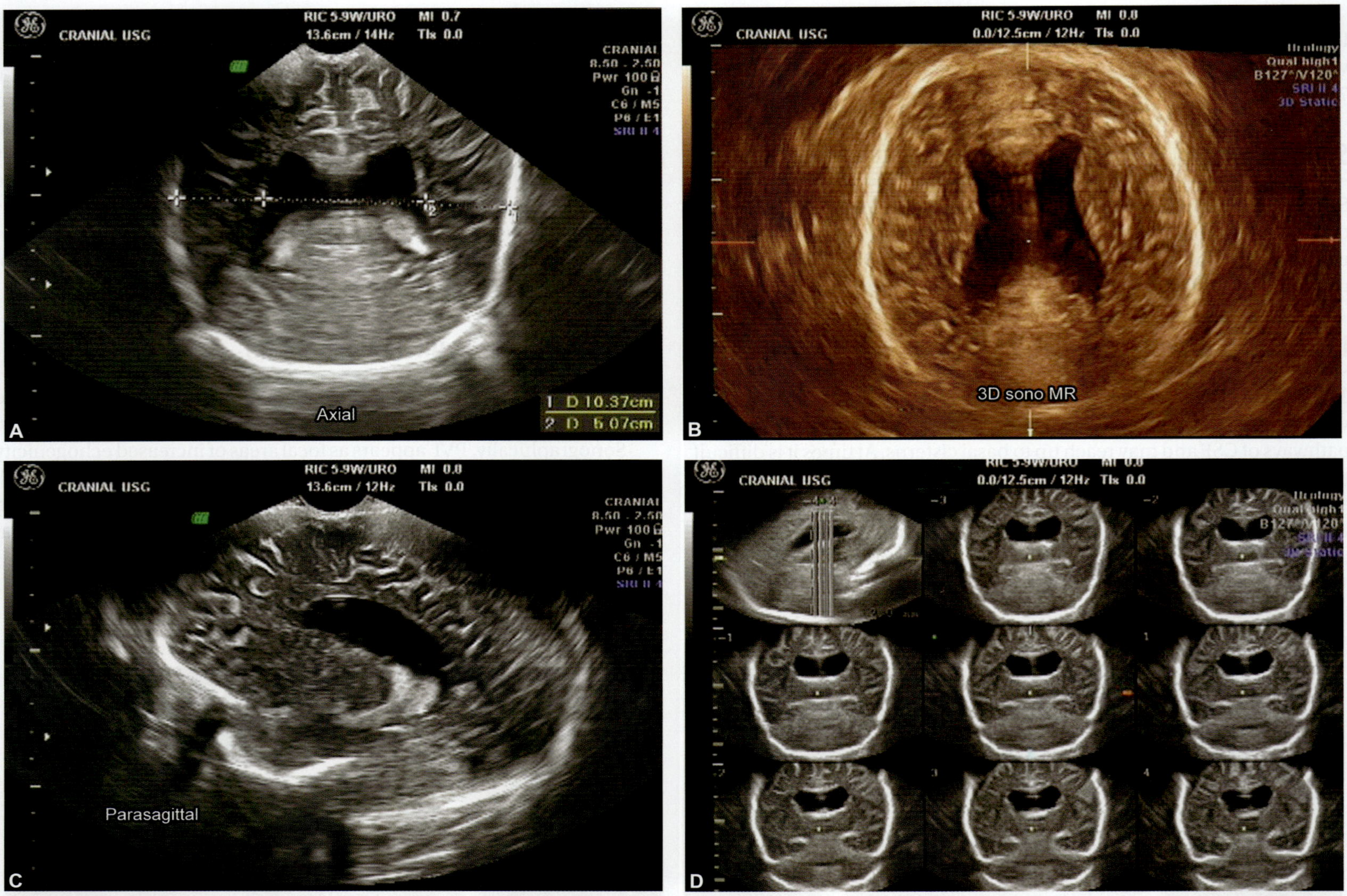

FIGURES 6.24A to D: A baby presented with fullness of anterior fontanel. HRSG shows dilated frontal horn and lateral ventricles. However, cephalo-ventricular ratio is maintained (normal < .5). But no periventricular leak is seen.

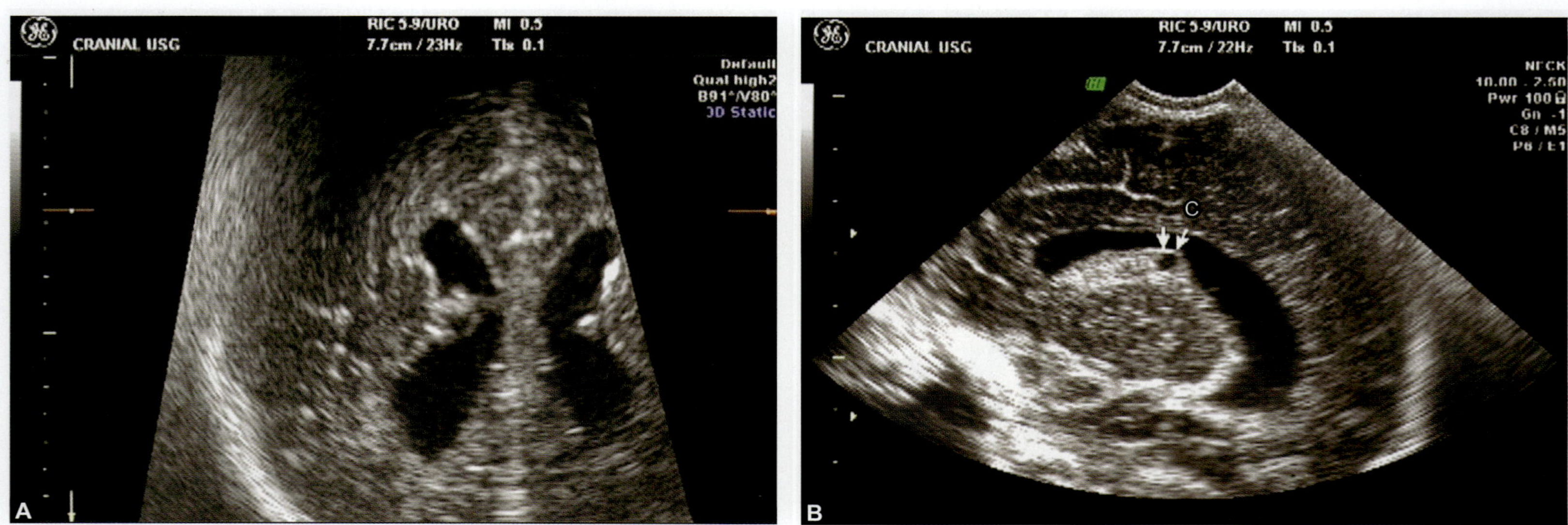

FIGURES 6.25A and B

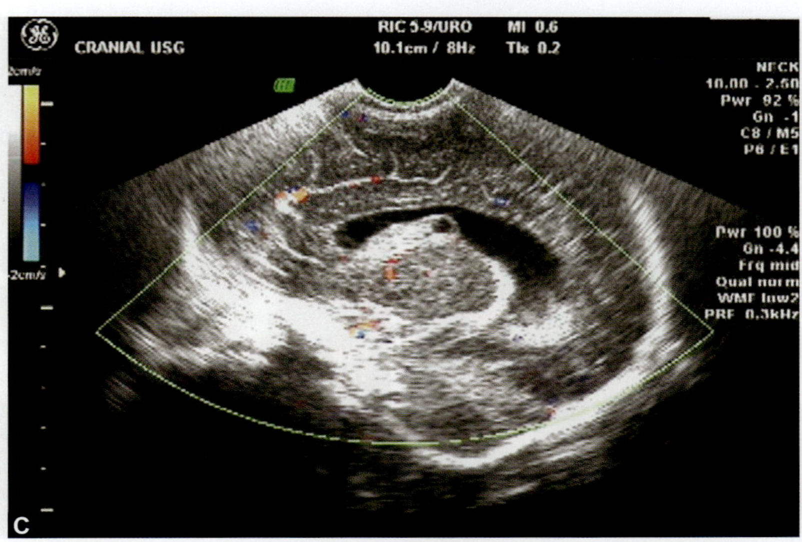

FIGURE 6.25C

FIGURES 6.25A to C: Small choroid plexus cyst in dilated ventricles. An 11-day-old baby presented with fullness of anterior fontanelle. HRSG shows mild fullness of lateral ventricle. A small cyst is seen in the choroid plexus on left side, which is seen clearly on ultrasound.

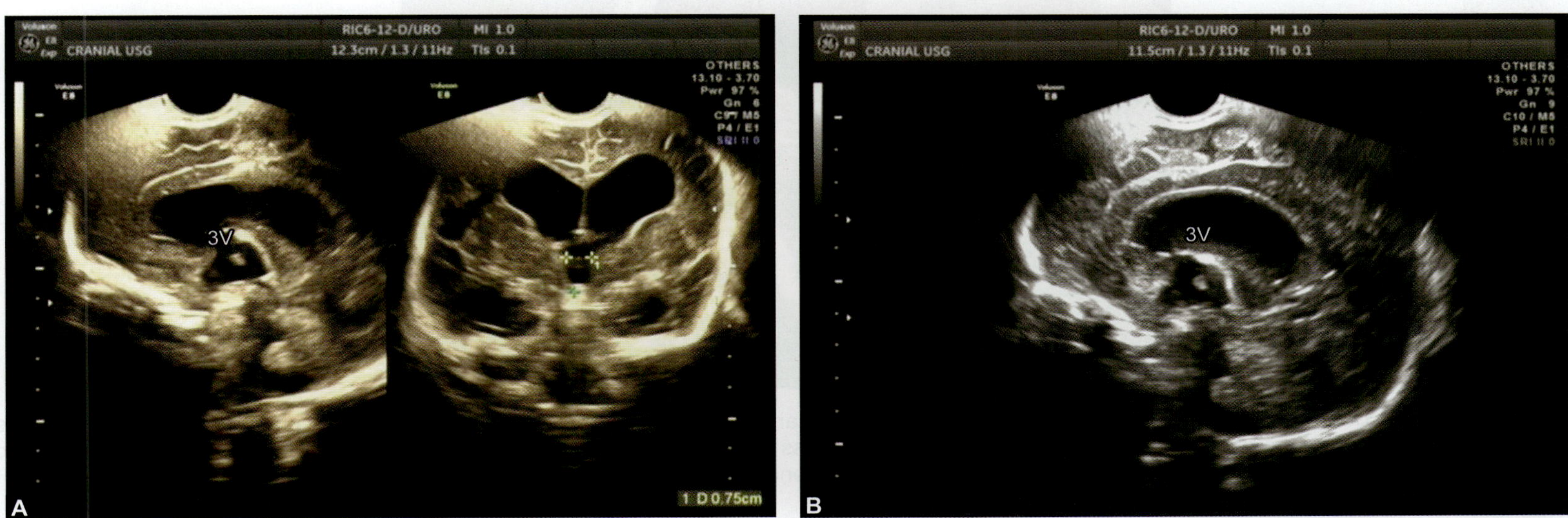

FIGURES 6.26A and B: Dilated lateral 3rd ventricle. A patient presented with tense anterior fontanel. HRSG shows dilated lateral ventricles. The 3rd ventricle is also dilated. It is 7.5 mm in size (normal < 3 mm). But no periventricular leak is seen. Findings are suggestive of aqueduct stenosis.

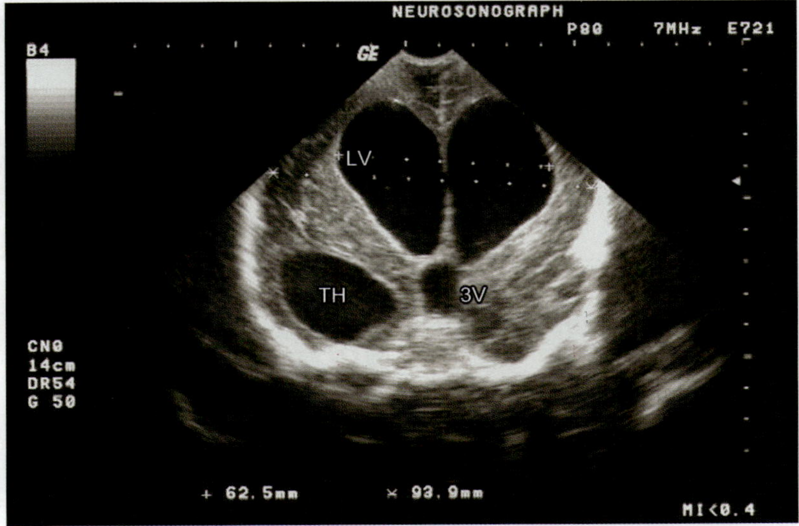

FIGURE 6.27: Gross hydrocephalus. Neurosonography shows grossly dilated ventricles involving all the four ventricles with marked pressure on the brain parenchyma.

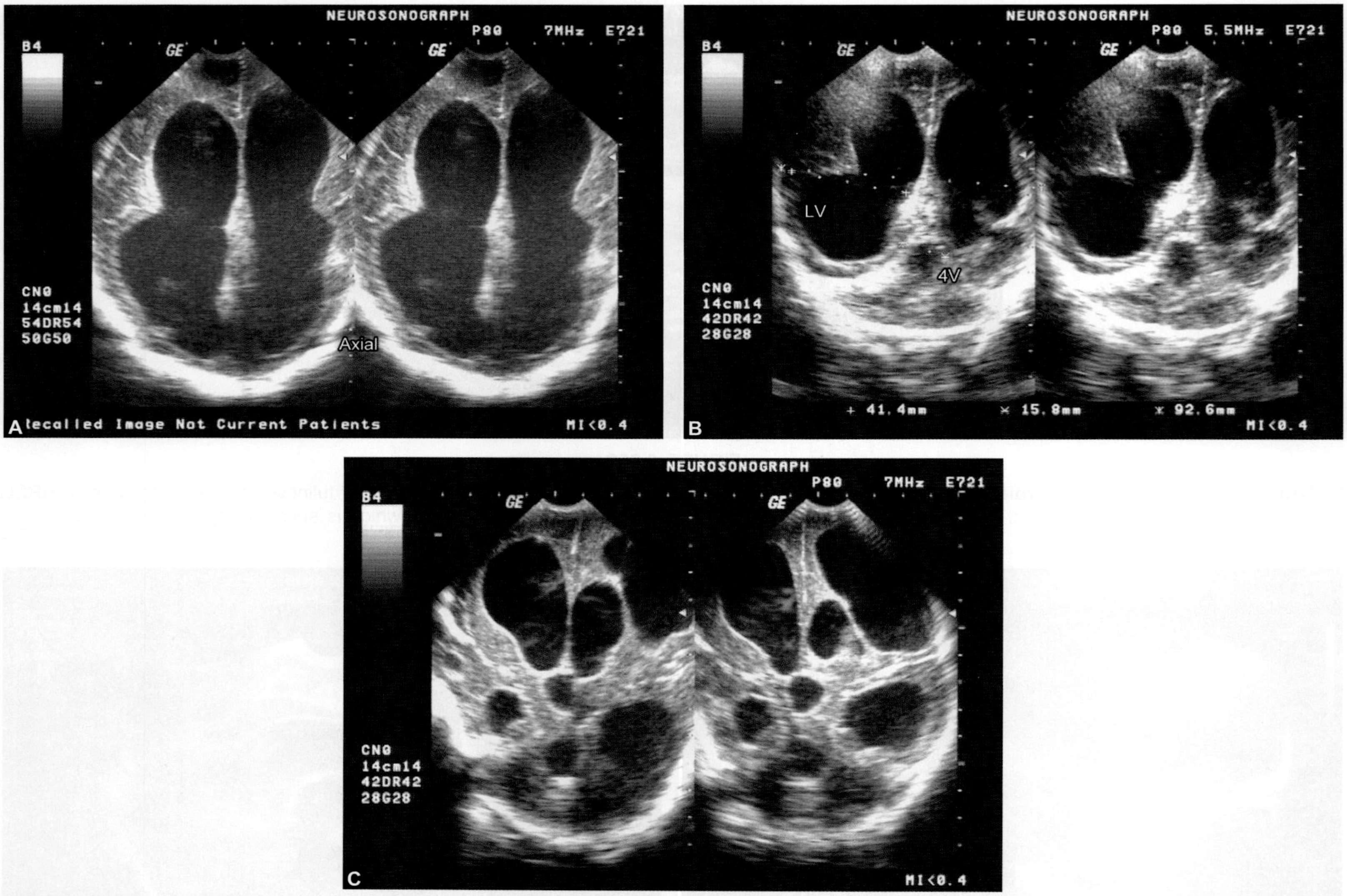

FIGURES 6.28A to C: Gross hydrocephalus. The lateral ventricles are markedly dilated. Forth ventricle is also dilated in brain parenchyma suggestive of gross hydrocephalus. Axial and the parasagittal planes also show gross dilatation of all the four ventricles. The occipital horn, temporal horn and forth ventricles are grossly dilated. Marked pressure is seen in brain parenchyma.

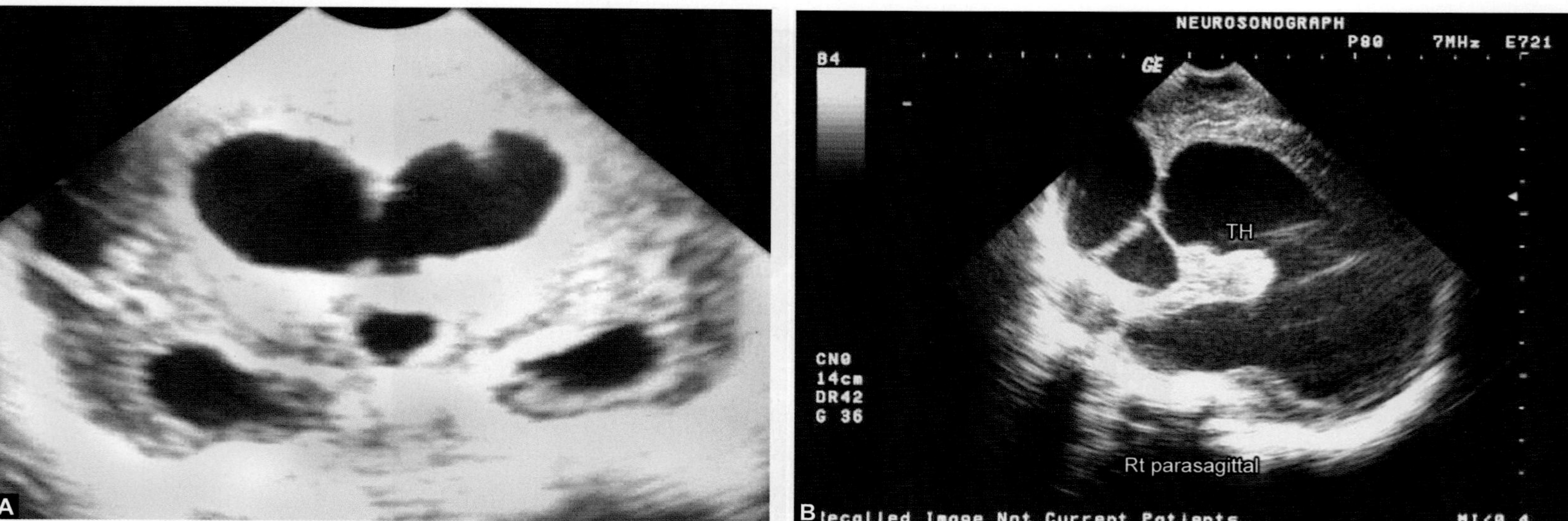

FIGURES 6.29A and B: Obstructed hydrocephalus. HRSG shows dilated ventricles involving all the four ventricles in a case of obstructed hydrocephalus due to basal arachnoiditis due to brain infection.

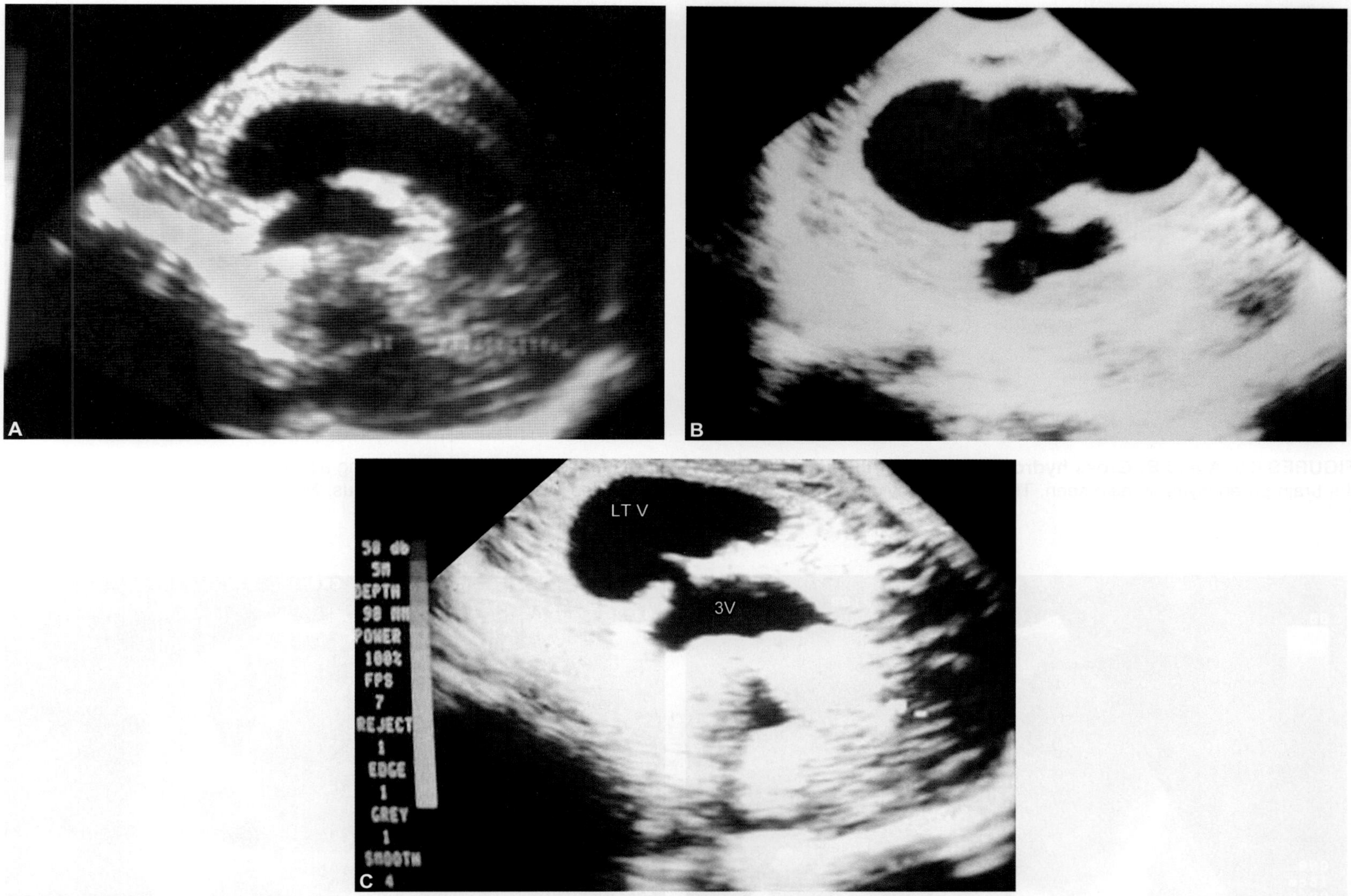

FIGURES 6.30A to C: Aqueduct stenosis. HRSG shows obstructed hydrocephalus due to aqueduct stenosis. The third ventricle and lateral ventricles are grossly dilated. Fourth ventricle is not dilated. The aqueduct of Sylvius is seen obstructed resulting into dilated third ventricle, lateral ventricle. The foramen of Monro is seen distended.

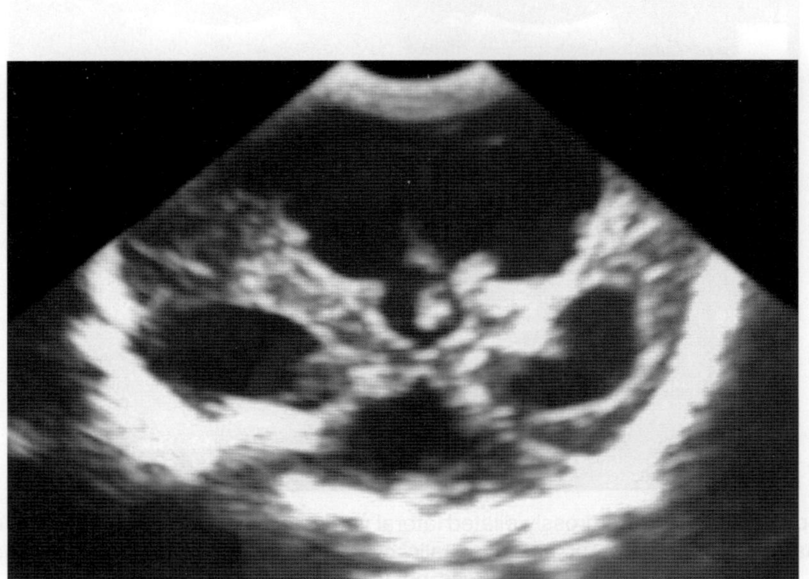

FIGURE 6.31: Dandy-Walker cyst. HRSG shows a big cystic mass in the fourth ventricle with a Dandy-Walker cyst. It has obstructed the outflow tract resulting into obstructed hydrocephalus.

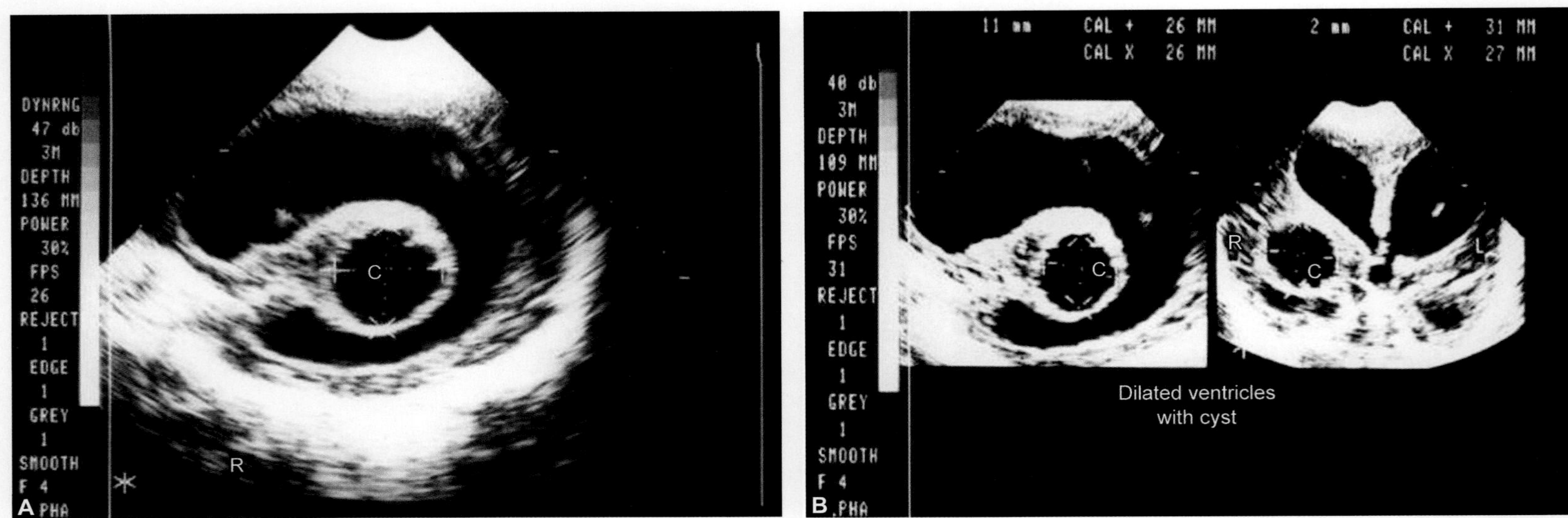

FIGURES 6.32A and B: Gross hydrocephalus with thalamic cyst. HRSG shows gross hydrocephalus involving all the ventricles. Pressure thinning of the brain parenchyma is also seen. There is also evidence of a well-defined thin walled cyst seen in the thalamus. No internal echo is seen in the cyst.

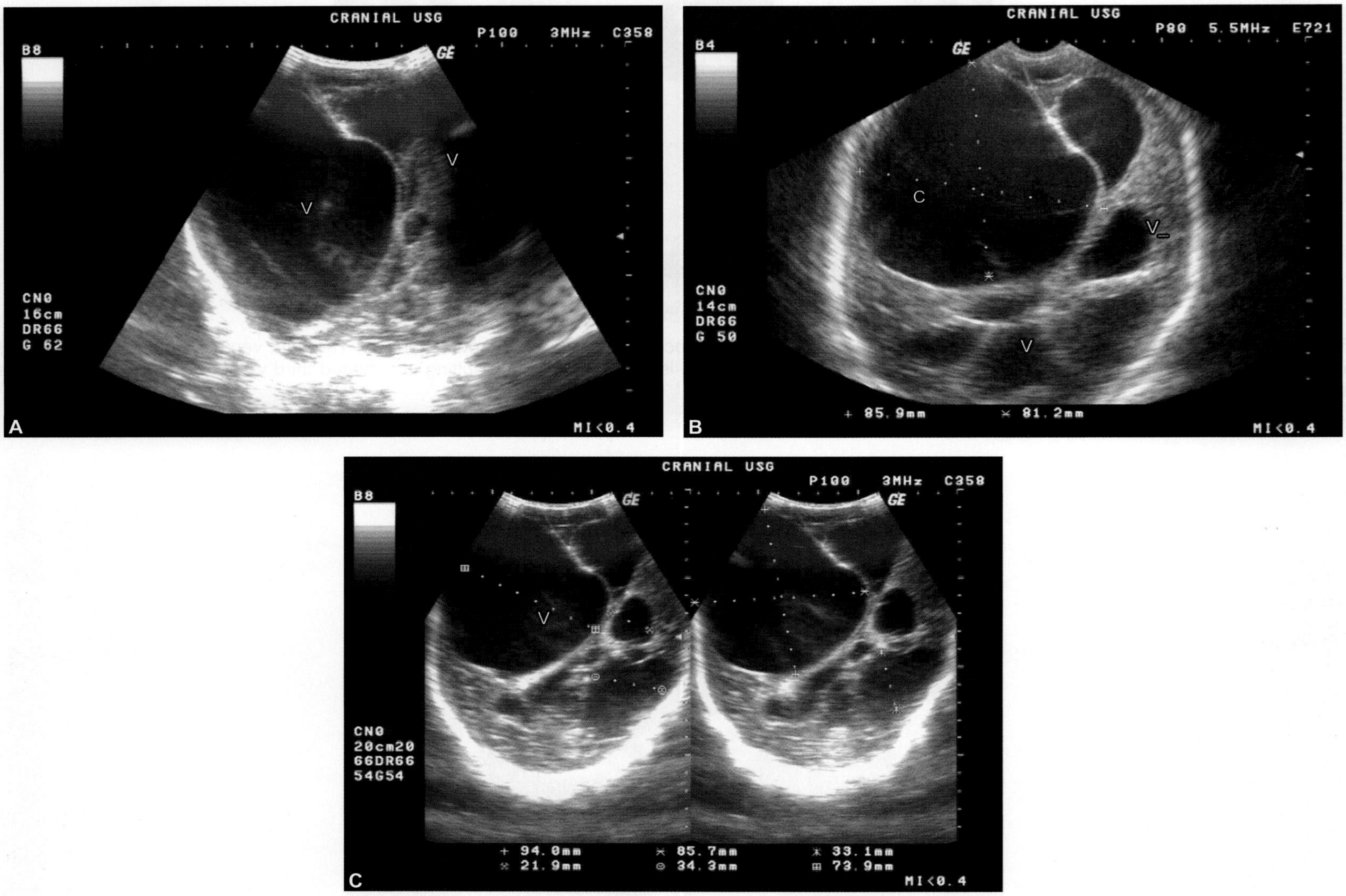

FIGURES 6.33A to C: Porencephalic cyst. HRSG shows grossly dilated lateral ventricle in parasagittal plane. The dilated ventricle is seen communicating with a cystic mass in the high parietal area suggestive of porencephalic cyst. The cyst is seen pressing and displacing the right ventricle to the opposite. It is seen pressing over the outflow tract resulting in to gross obstructed hydrocephalus.

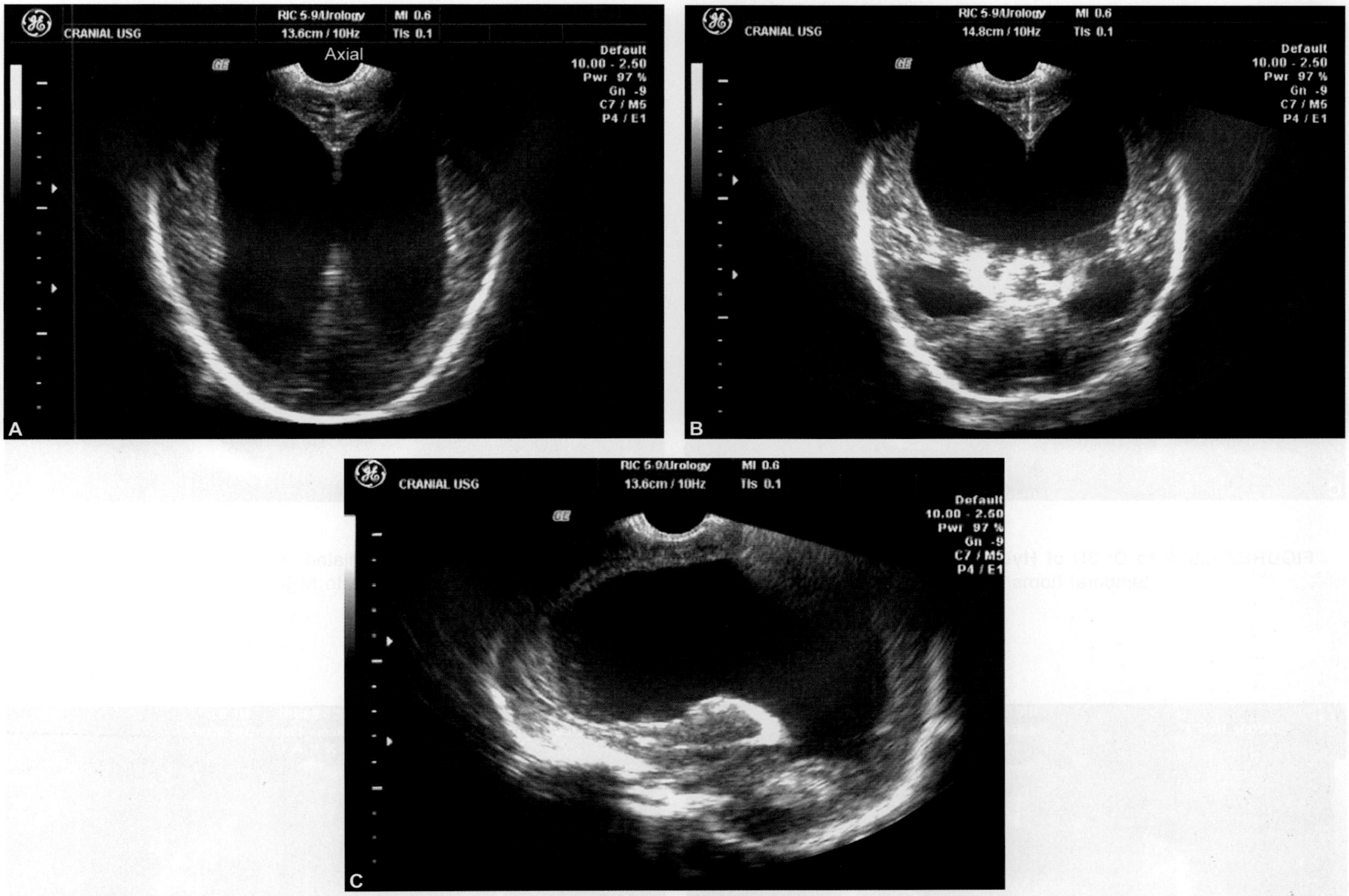

FIGURES 6.34A to C: Gross hydrocephalus. HRSG shows gross dilatation of the ventricles. All the ventricles are dilated. Brain parenchyma is seen compressed by the fluid pressure. Third ventricle is also well seen on HRSG.

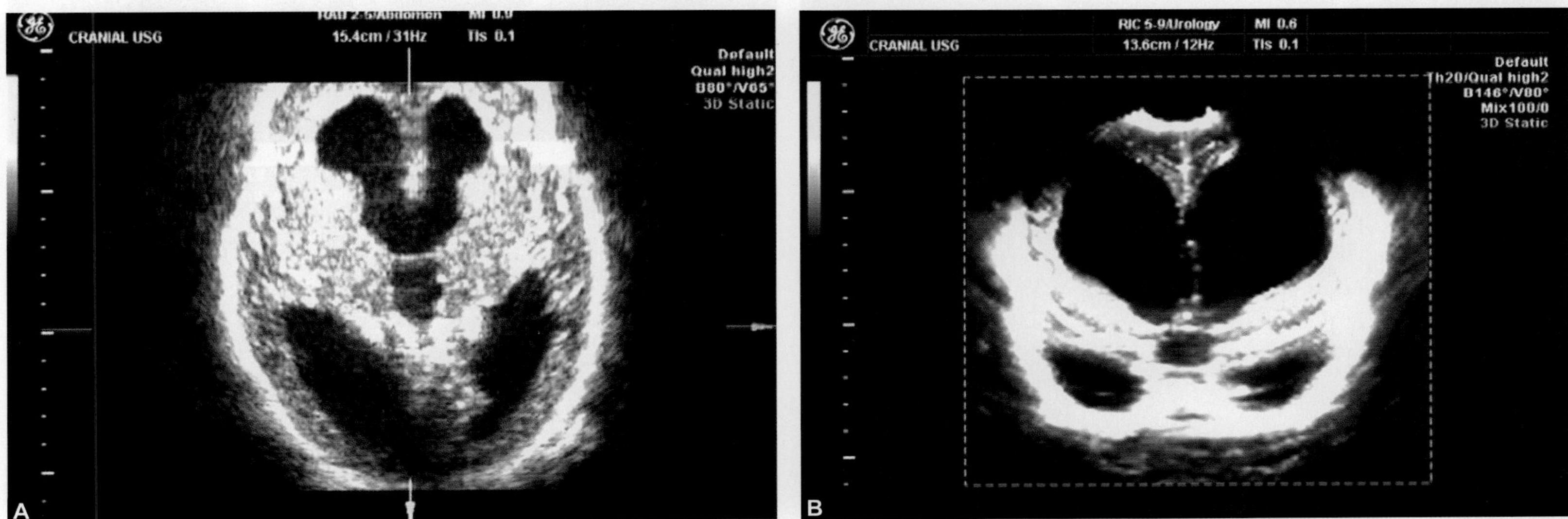

FIGURES 6.35A and B

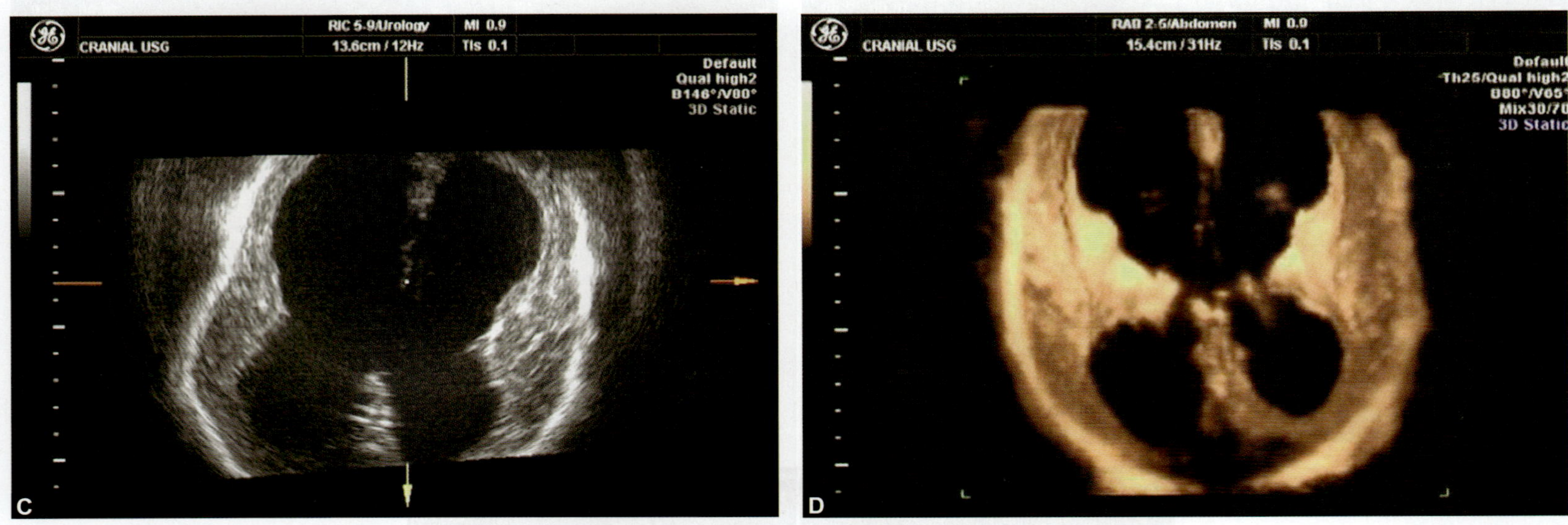

FIGURES 6.35C and D

FIGURES 6.35A to D: 3D of Hydrocephalus. 3D ultrasound of the same patient shows the details of dilated ventricles. The frontal horns, temporal horns and occipital horns are well visualized. 3D images are well comparable to MRI images.

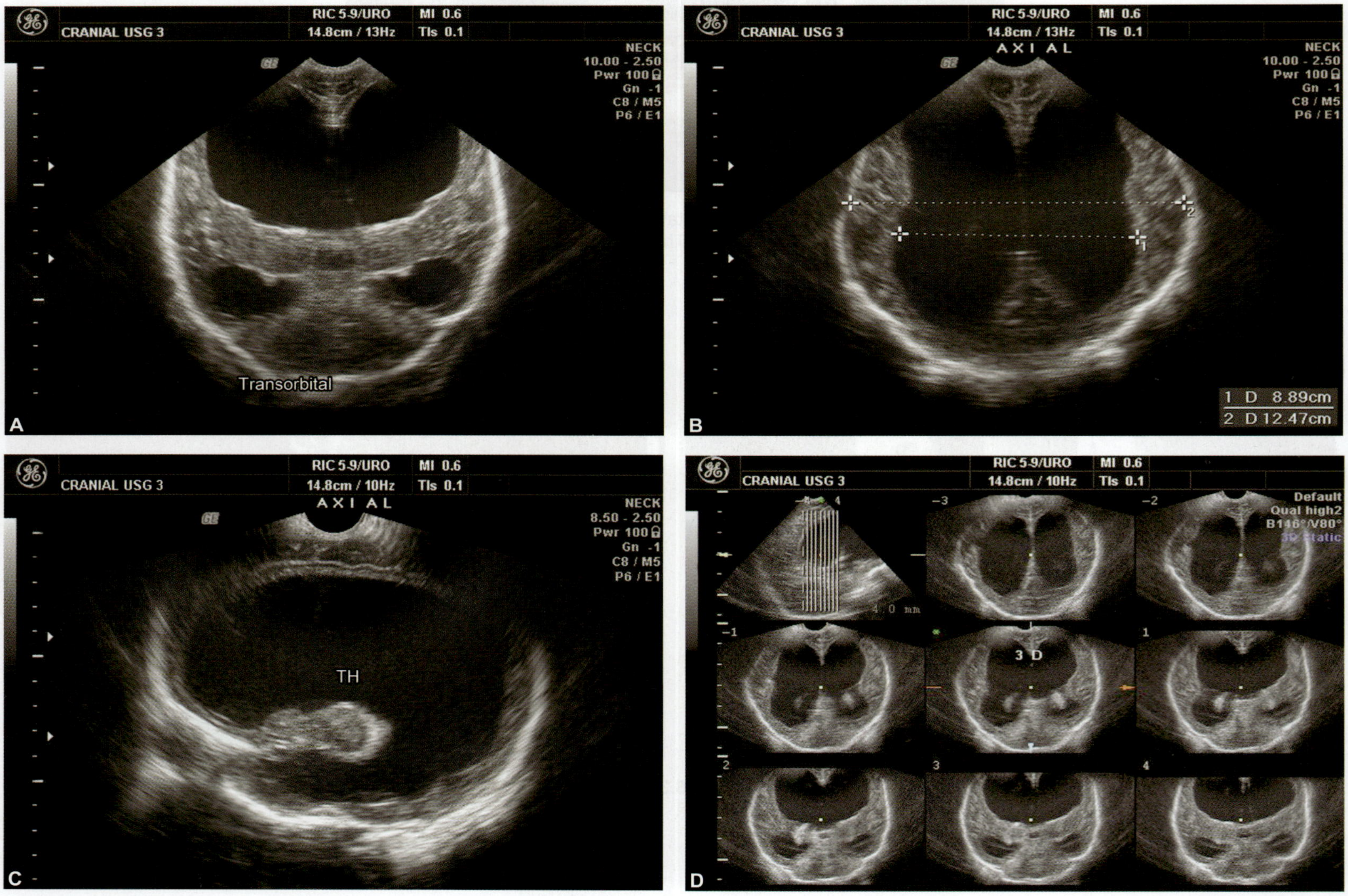

FIGURES 6.36A to D: Gross hydrocephalus with thinning of brain parenchyma. HRSG shows markedly dilated ventricles. All the four ventricles are dilated. Periventricular leak is seen. Pressure is seen on brain parenchyma resulting into thinning of brain parenchyma.

INTRAVENTRICULAR HEMORRHAGE

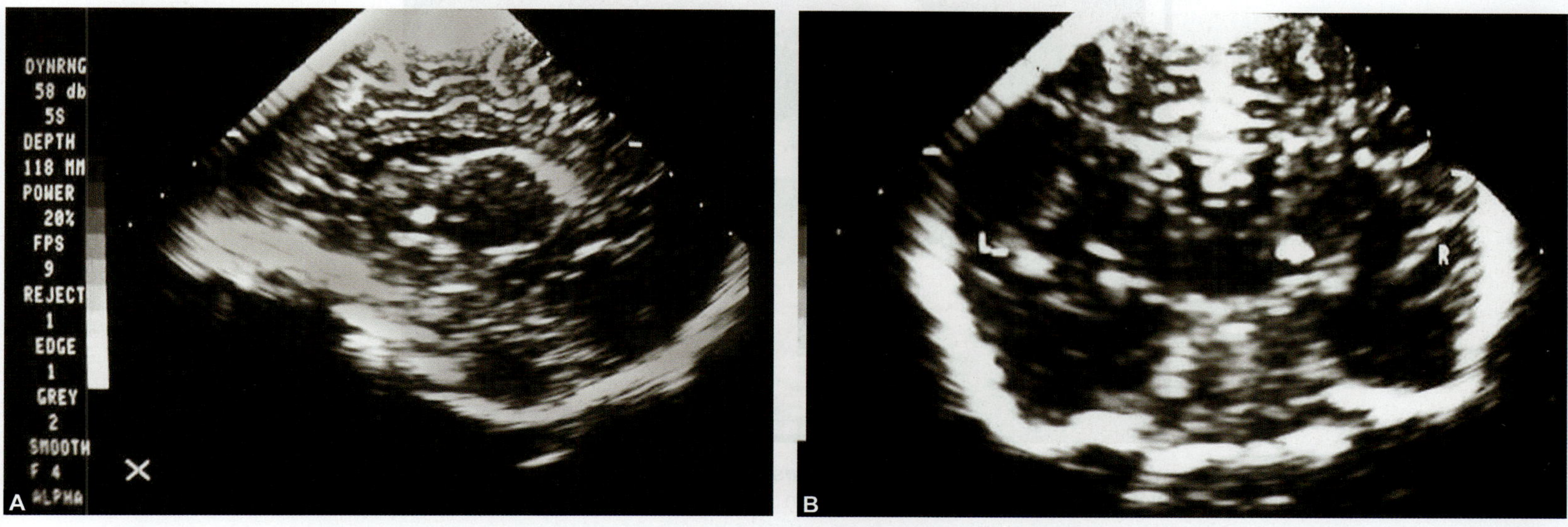

FIGURES 6.37A and B: HRSG shows a small echogenic focus in the epindymal region in parasagittal axis. The coronal plane shows the bleed in the floor of frontal horn suggestive of subependymal bleed.

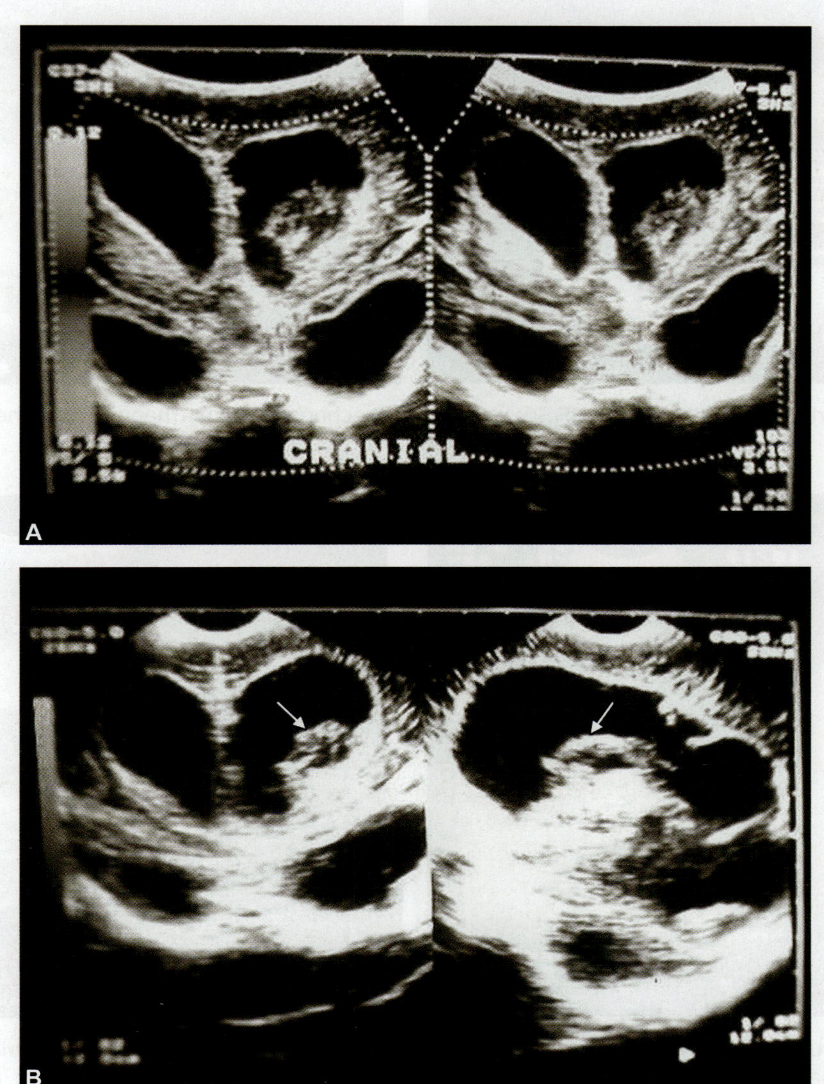

FIGURES 6.38A and B: Intraventricular hemorrhage. HRSG shows an echogenic clot in the frontal horn of the ventricle. The ventricle wall is irregular. Echogenic thin strands are seen in the ventricles. On color flow imaging increased flow is seen in the ventricular wall suggestive of ventriculitis.

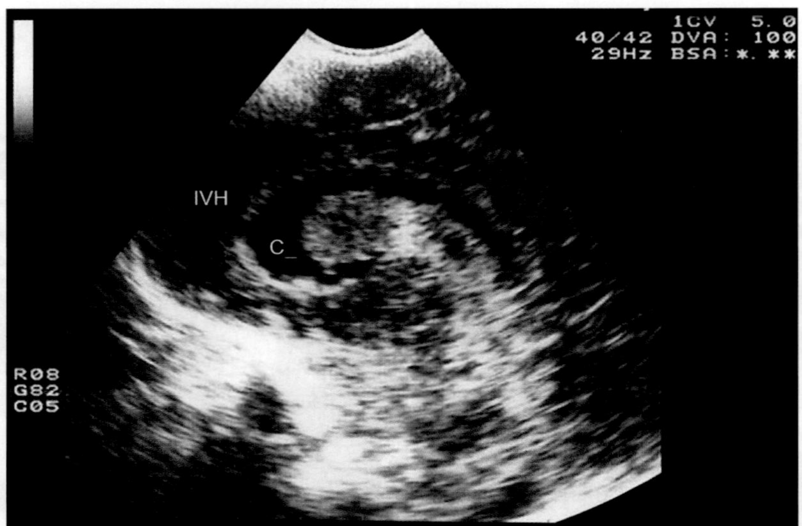

FIGURES 6.39: Intraventricular hemorrhage. HRSG shows a big echogenic haemorrhagic clot in the lateral ventricle. The clot is seen obstructing the foramen resulting into obstructed hydrocephalus.

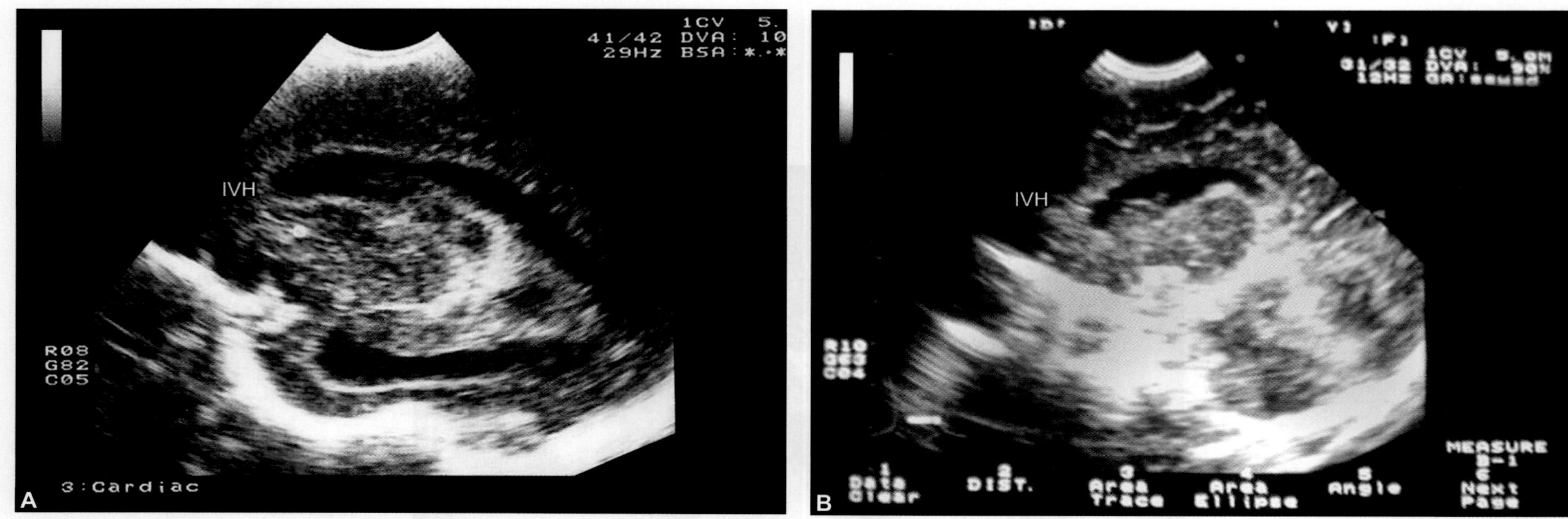

FIGURES 6.40A and B: Intraventricular hemorrhage. HRSG shows a big echogenic hemorrhagic clot in the lateral ventricle. The clot is seen obstructing the foramen resulting into obstructed hydrocephalus.

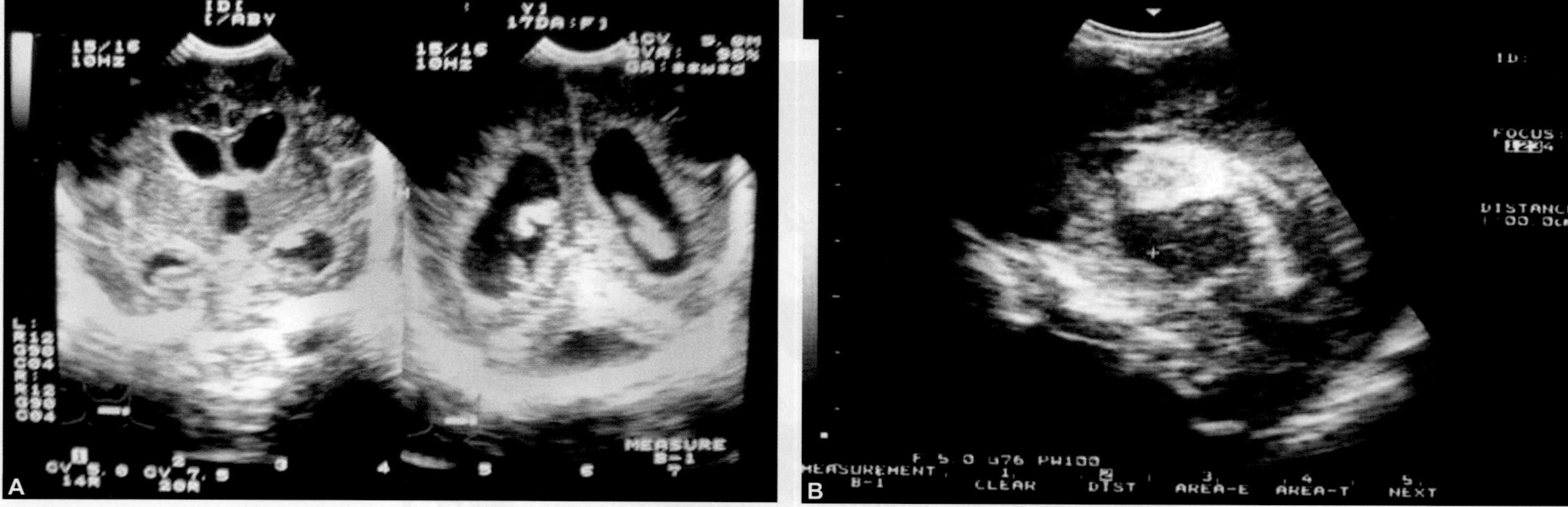

FIGURES 6.41A and B: Intraventricular hemorrhage. HRSG shows echogenic-floating clot in the lateral ventricle associated hydrocephalus is also seen. Dense intraventricular hemorrhage—HRSG shows dense echogenic hemorrhagic collection filling whole of the lateral ventricle. Chalky white collection is seen in the hemorrhage.

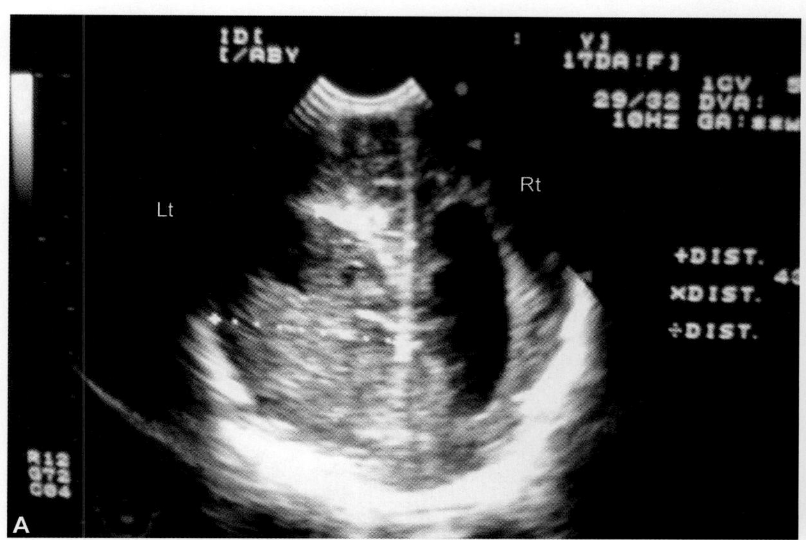

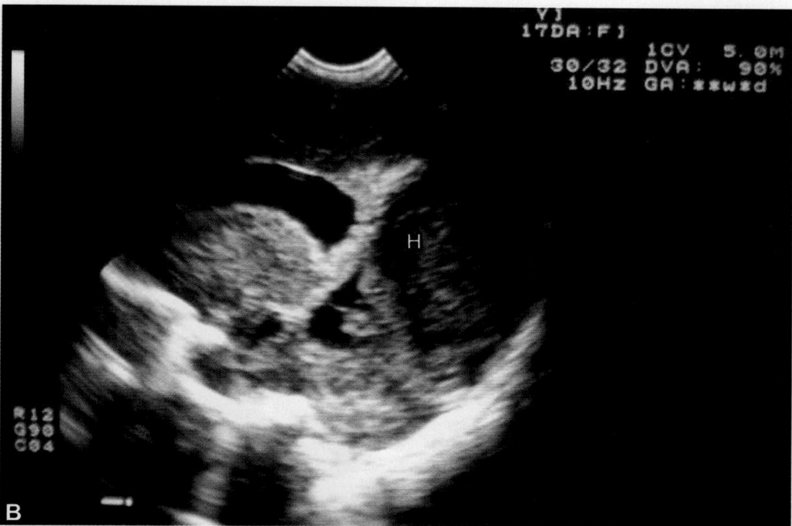

FIGURES 6.42A and B: Cerebral hemorrhage. A patient presented with semi unconscious state with low GC. HRSG shows a big cerebral hemorrhage involving the left cerebral cortex. The hemorrhage is seen causing mass effect and midline shift. Obstructed hydrocephalus is also seen.

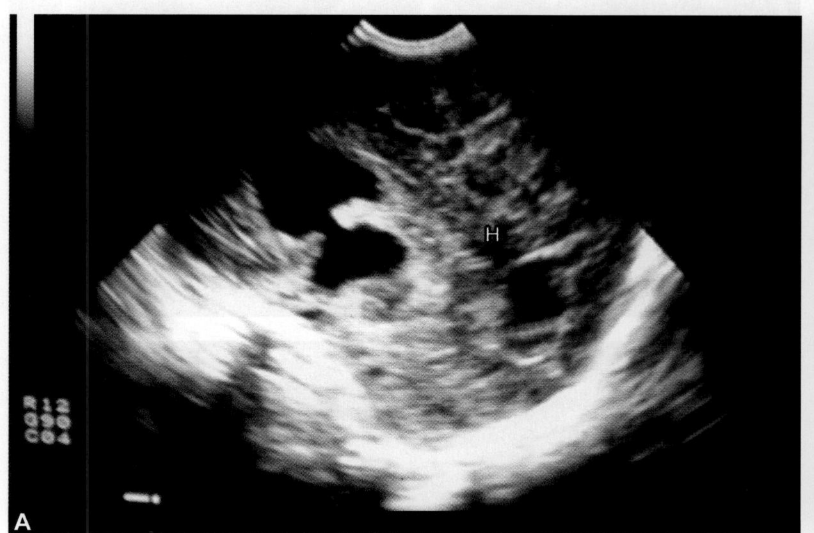

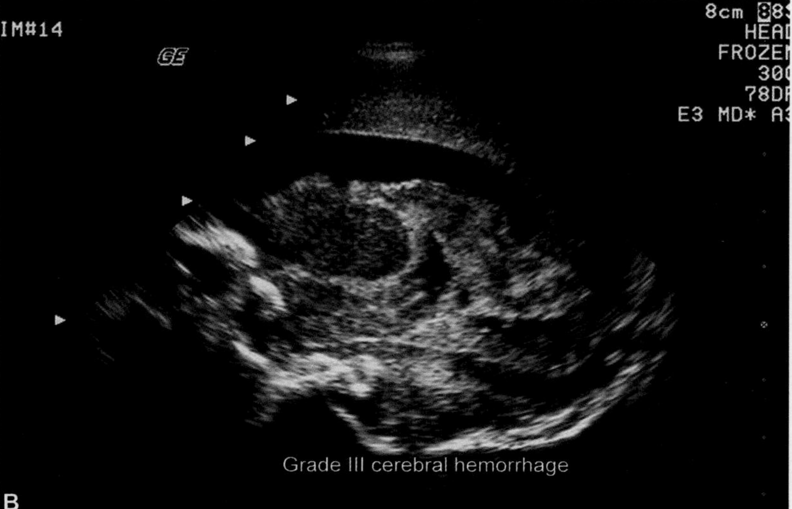

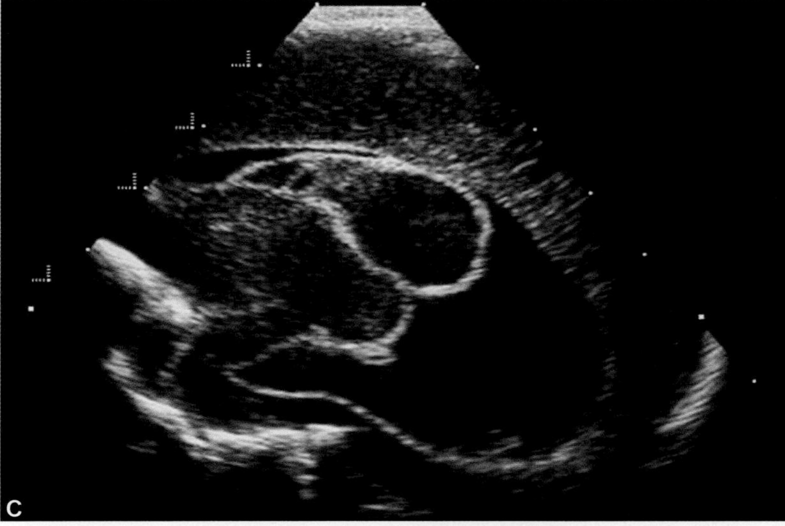

FIGURES 6.43A to C: Intraventricular hemorrhage. HRSG shows a big echogenic hemorrhagic clot in the ventricle. However, the hemorrhage is seen confined to the ventricular cavity suggestive of grade III hemorrhage. Retracting hemorrhagic clot: HRSG shows retracting clot filling the ventricular cavity.

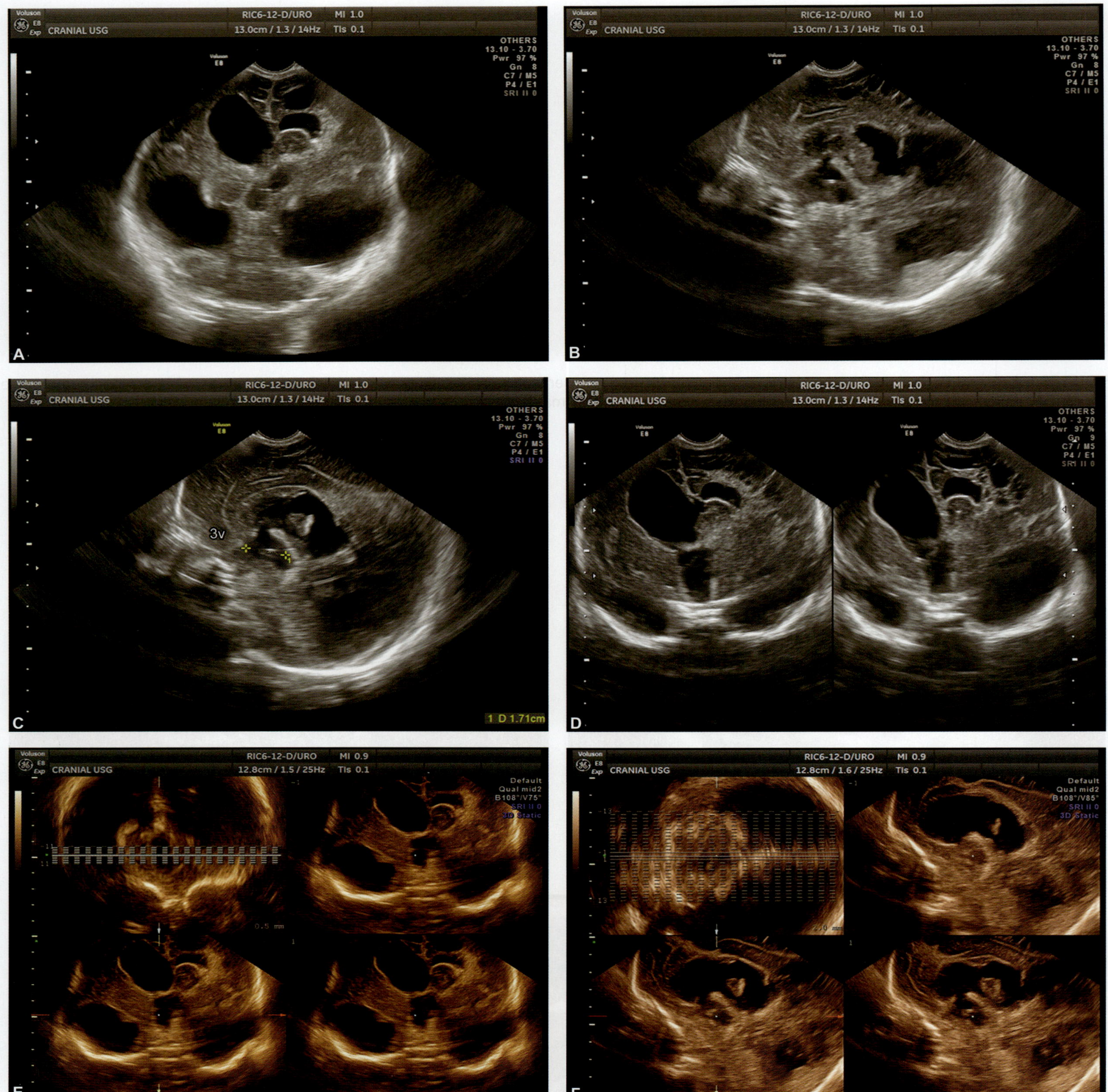

FIGURES 6.44A to F: A 14-day-old baby presented with low GC with fever. HRSG shows dilated ventricles. Echogenic shadows are seen filling the right frontal horn and right ventricle suggestive of intraventricular hemorrhage. Echogenic clot is also seen in the ventricle. The clotted blood is seen obstructing the 3rd ventricle resulting into obstructed hydrocephalous. The TUI imaging shows the echogenic clot obstructing the 3rd ventricle.

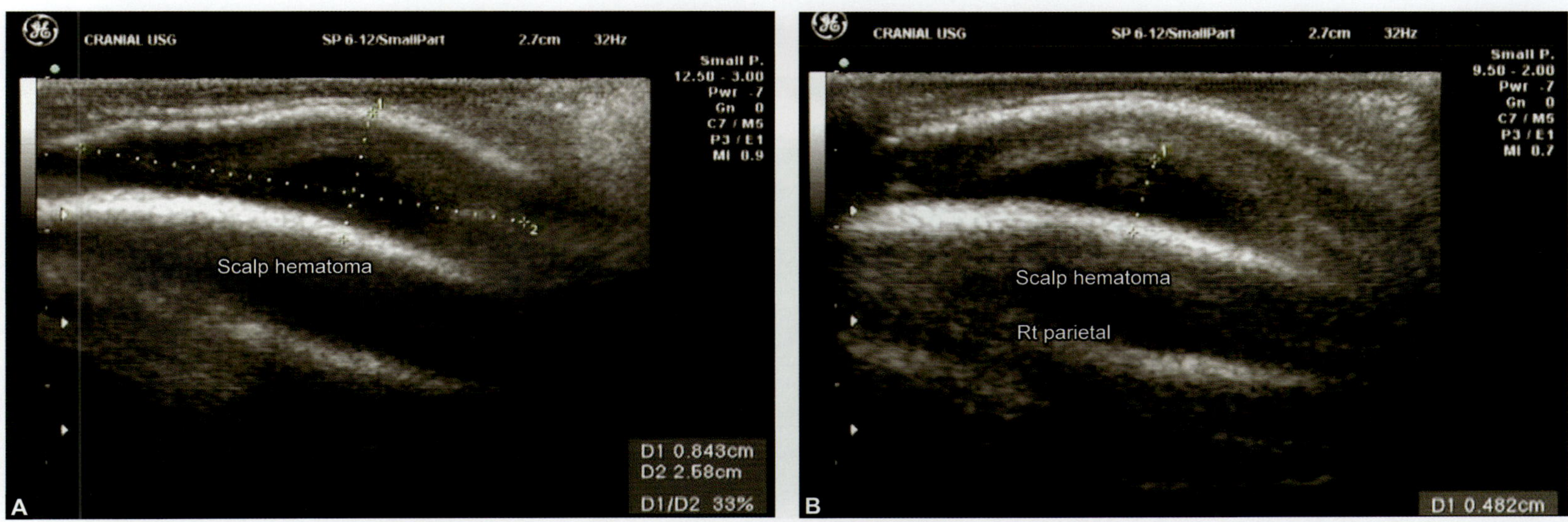

FIGURES 6.45A and B: Scalp hematoma. A patient presented a soft tissue swelling over the parietal scalp after a fall injury. HRSG shows big low-level collection in the scalp layer suggestive of scalp hematoma. However, the bones appear to be intact.

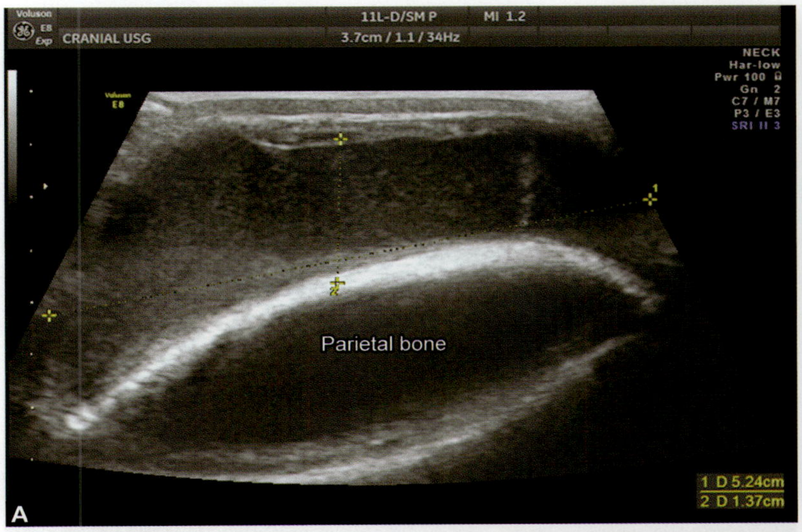

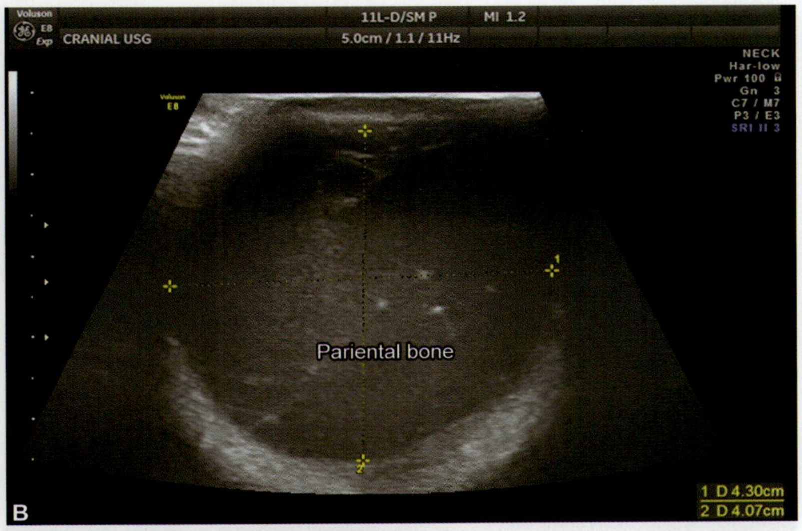

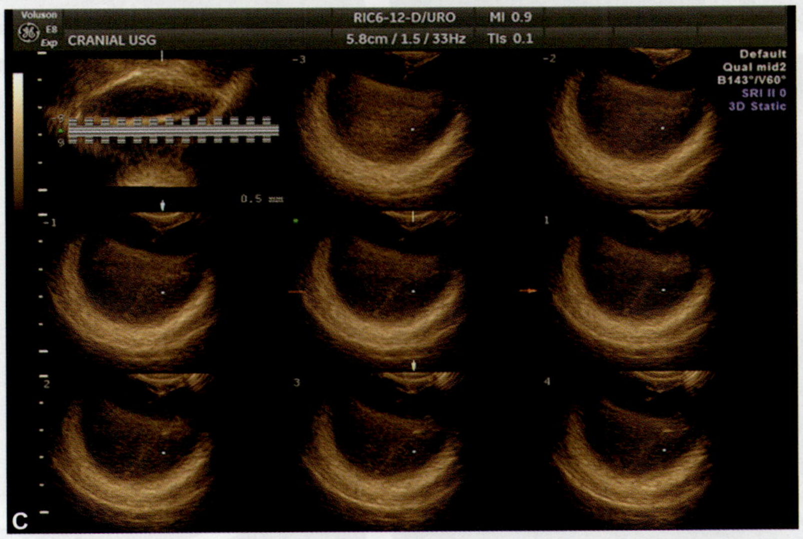

FIGURES 6.46A to C: Huge parietal bone hematoma. A 15-day-old baby sustained head injury and presented with a big soft tissue swelling. HRSG shows a big loculated pocket of collection in the parietal bone. Thick echoes are seen in the collection. No septation is seen in it. The skull table is clearly seen. No evidence of any fracture of skull table is seen.

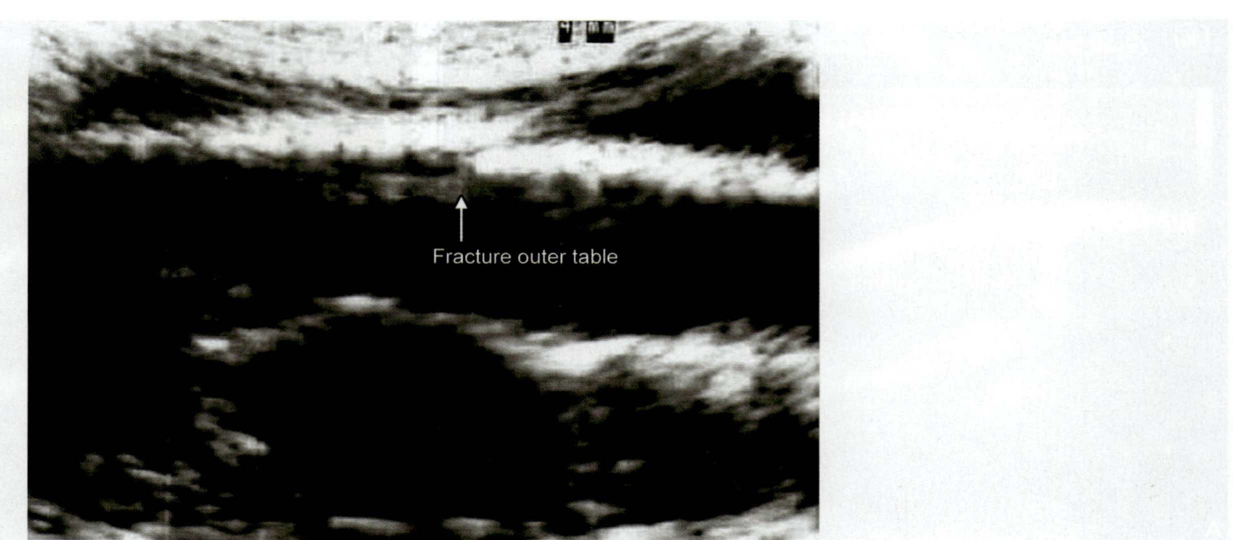

FIGURE 6.47: Parietal bone fracture. A baby sustained injury to the head after had a fall and presented with soft swelling over the scalp. HRSG shows fracture of the outer table of the parietal bone. The bony fragments are seen well in apposition on HRSG.

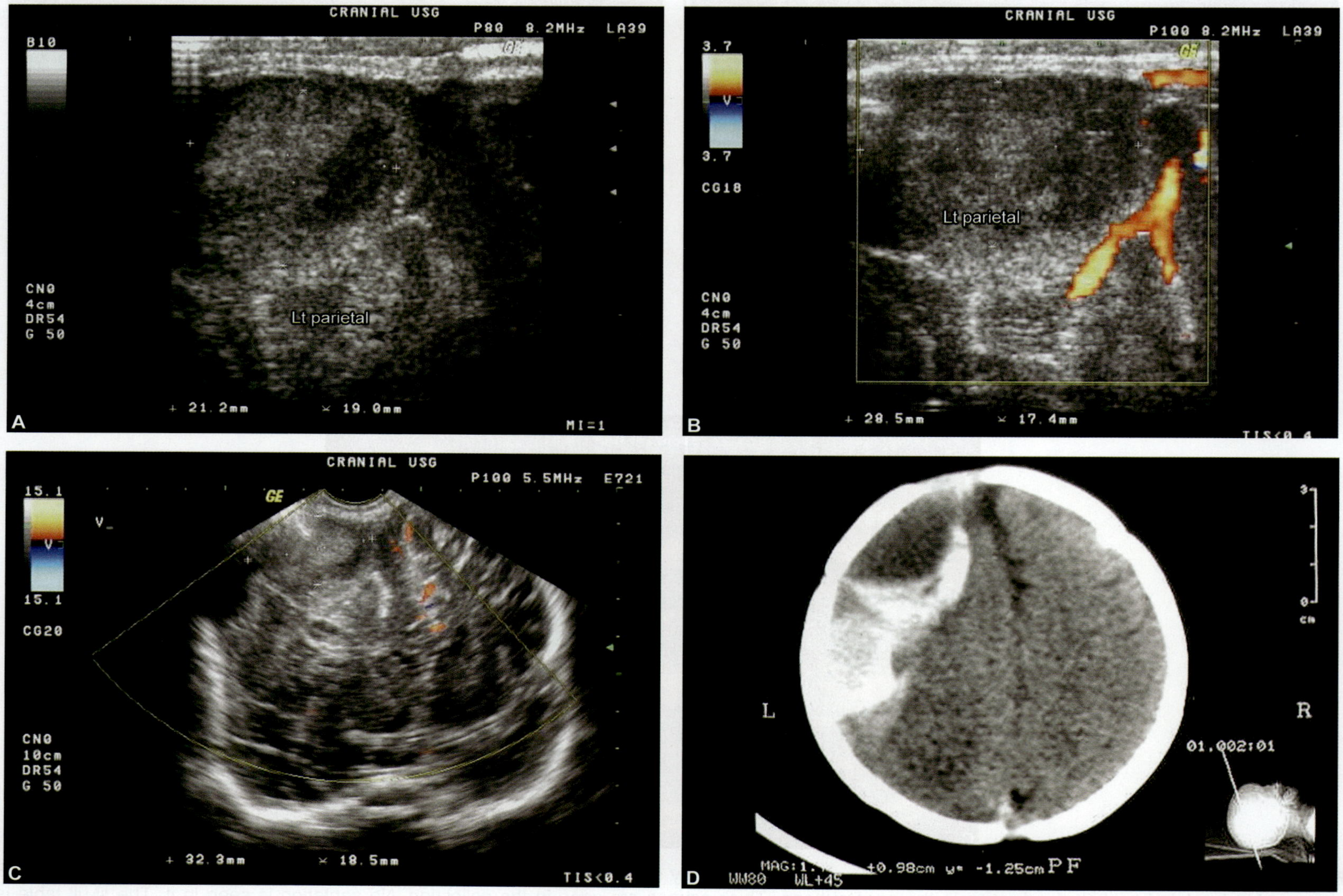

FIGURES 6.48A to D: Big parietal hematoma. A patient presented in unconscious state after had a fall. HRSG shows big parietal hematoma with associated subdural hematoma. It is seen pressing and displacing the contralateral brain. On color Doppler imaging, the hematoma is seen pressing and displacing the vessels. CT scan of the same patient shows the hematoma with mass effects and confirms the sonographic findings.

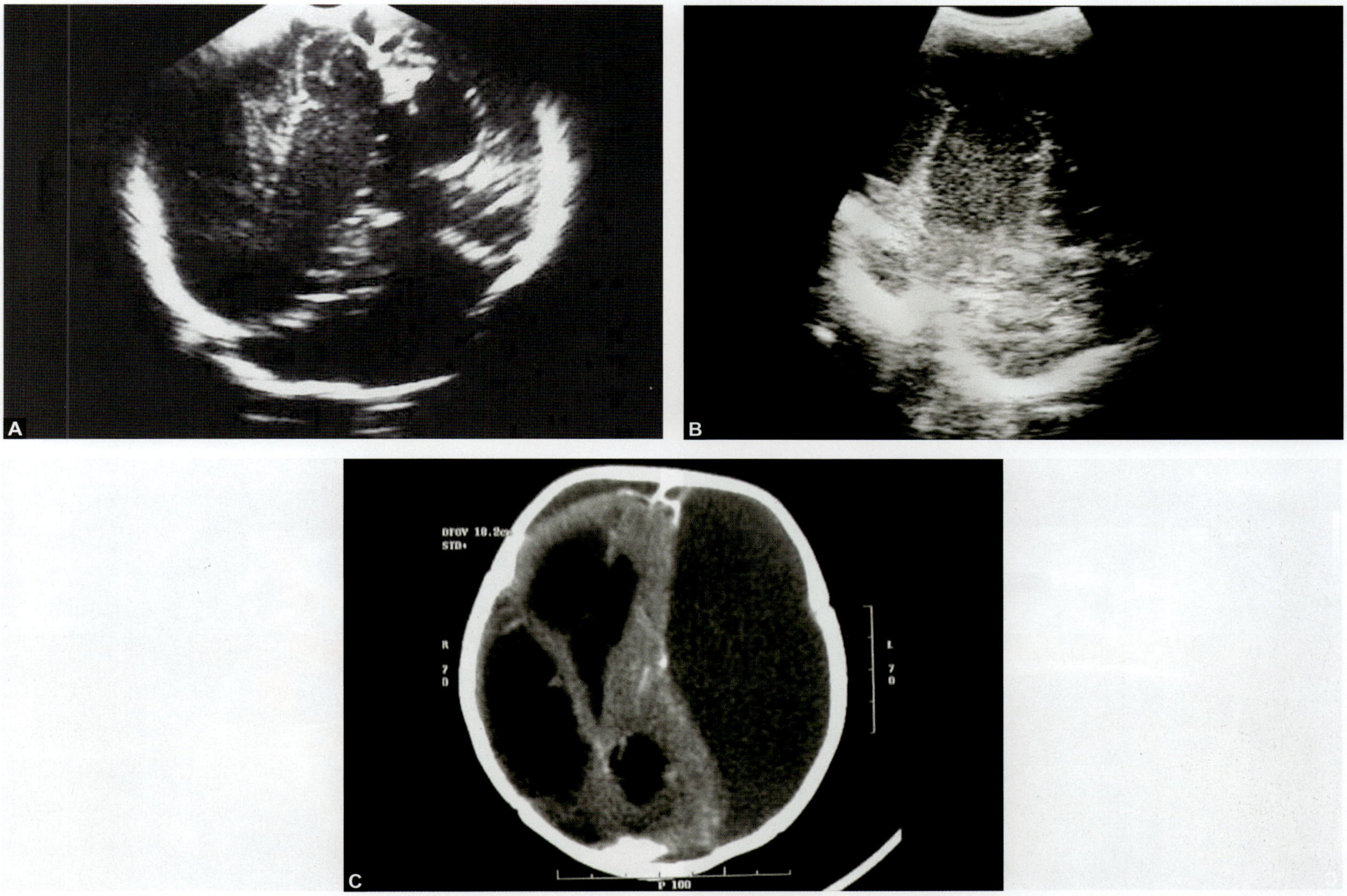

FIGURES 6.49A to C: Chronic subdural hematoma. A patient presented in unconscious state. HRSG shows a big low level echo collection in the subdural space. It is seen pressing and displacing the brain parenchyma. Marked thinning of the brain parenchyma is seen. Aspiration of the fluid confirmed chronic subdural hematoma. CT scan of the same patient shows details of the subdural hematoma. The hematoma is seen completely displacing the brain parenchyma with marked thinning.

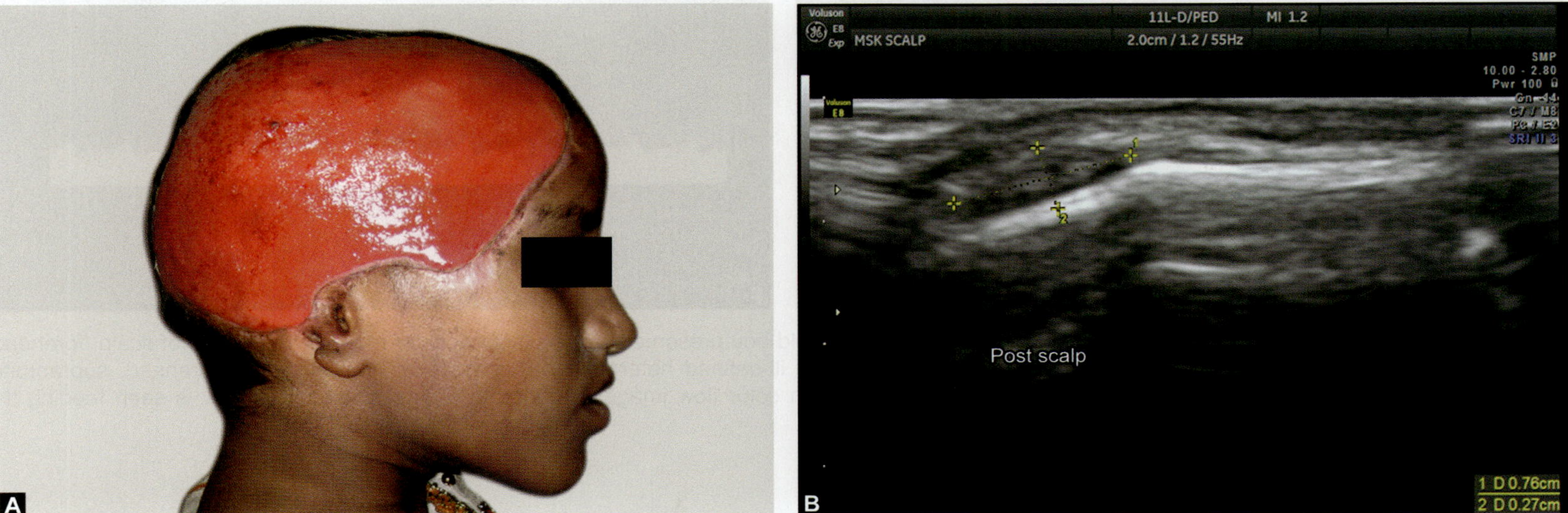

FIGURES 6.50A and B: Scalp hematoma. A young girl presented with scalp injury. The scalp has been ripped off. HRSG shows intact scalp bone. No fracture is seen in the bone. Small hematoma is seen above the skull table.

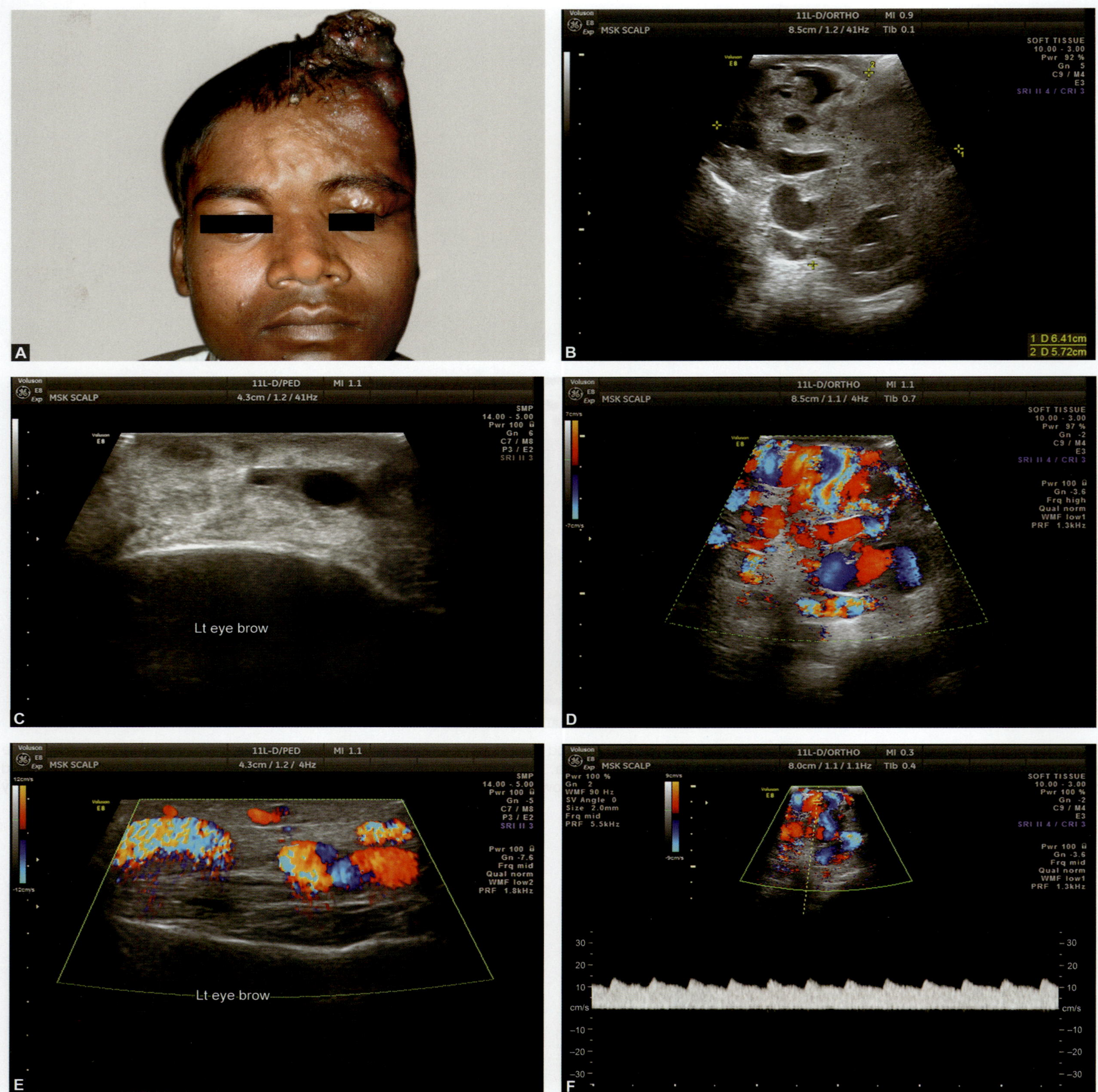

FIGURES 6.51A to F: Scalp and forehead vascular mass. An 18-year-old boy presented with multiple nodular masses in left side of scalp, forehead, left supra orbital region and left upper lid. HRSG shows a big irregular ill-defined heterogeneous mass involving left scalp, forehead, supraorbital region and left upper lid. Multiple vessels are seen feeding the mass. On color flow imaging, moderate arterial and venous flow is seen feeding the mass. The vessels are seen invading the skull table.

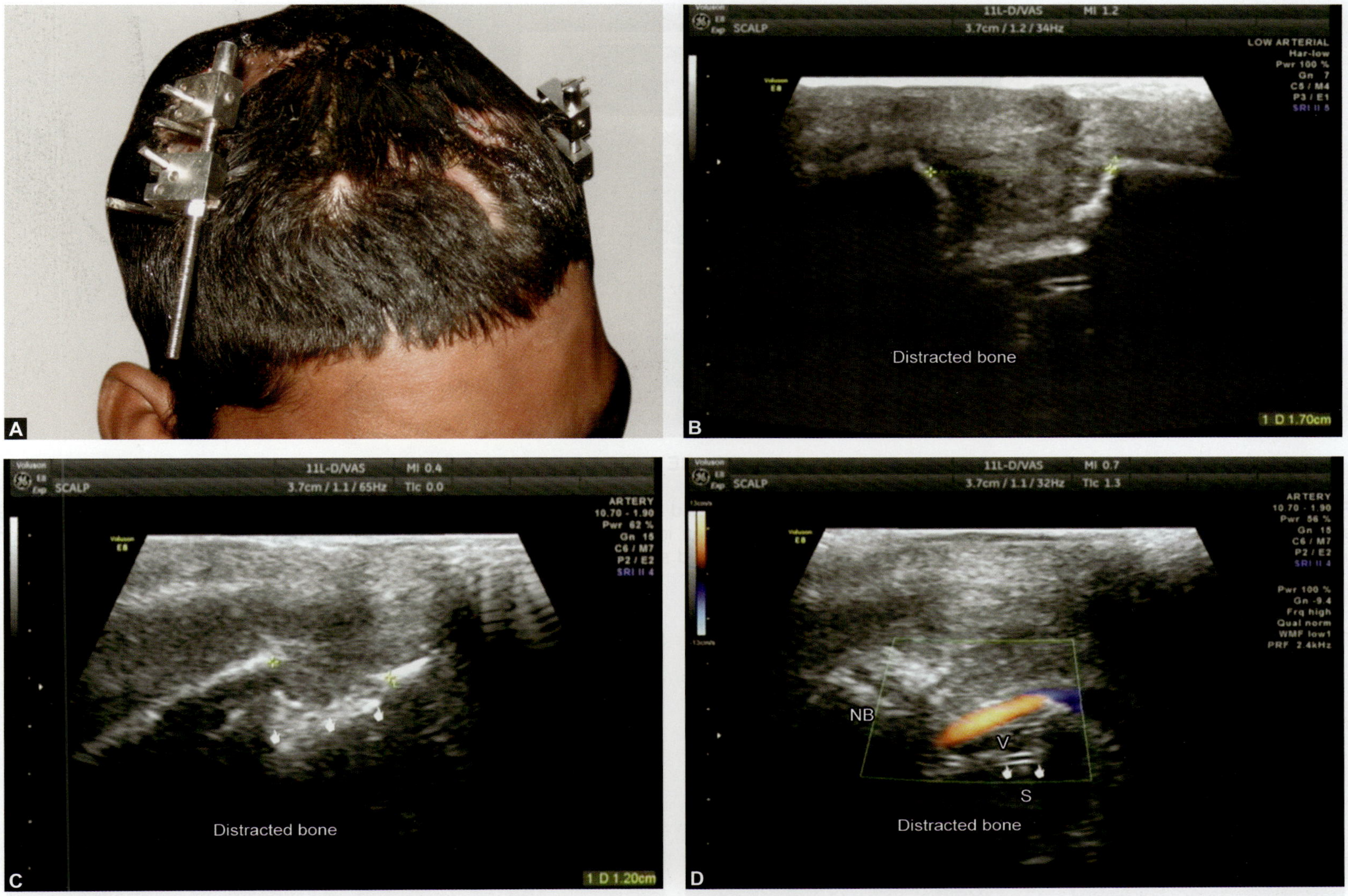

FIGURES 6.52A to D: Scalp injury with fracture of the bone. A patient presented with trauma to the skull. HRSG shows fracture of the bone. On distraction operation new bone formation is seen between the fractured segment. Callus formation is seen. New vessels are also seen feeding it suggestive of neo angiogenesis. HRSG is a very good modality for evaluation of new bone formation and neo angiogenesis.

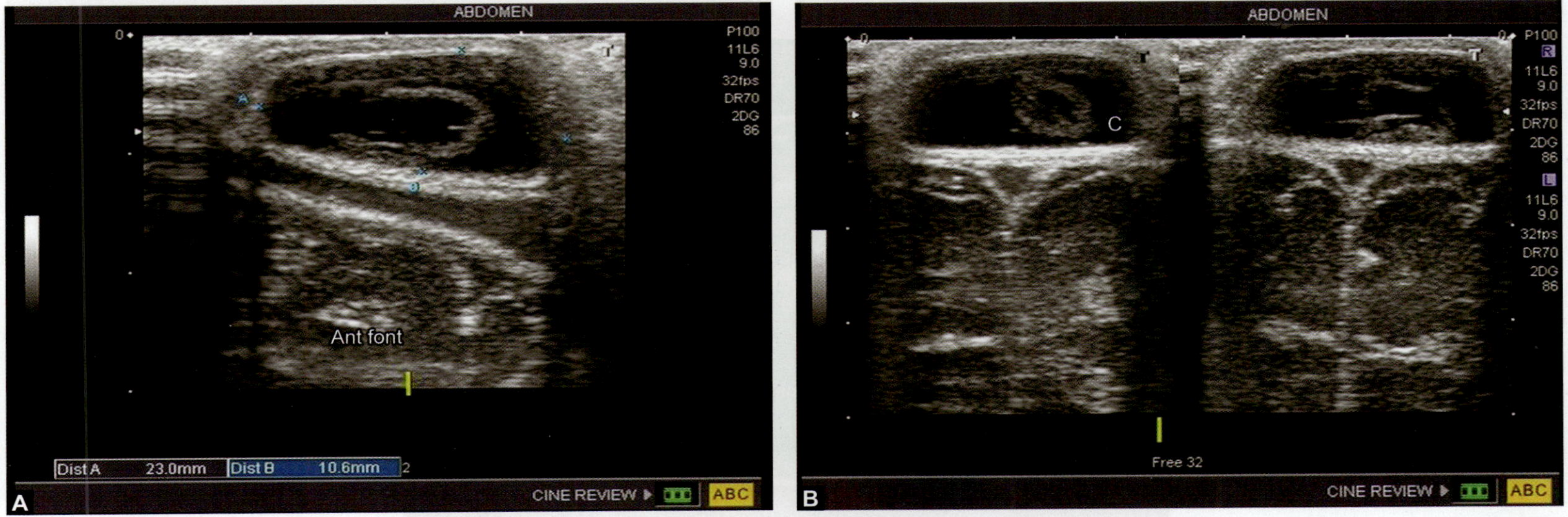

FIGURES 6.53A and B

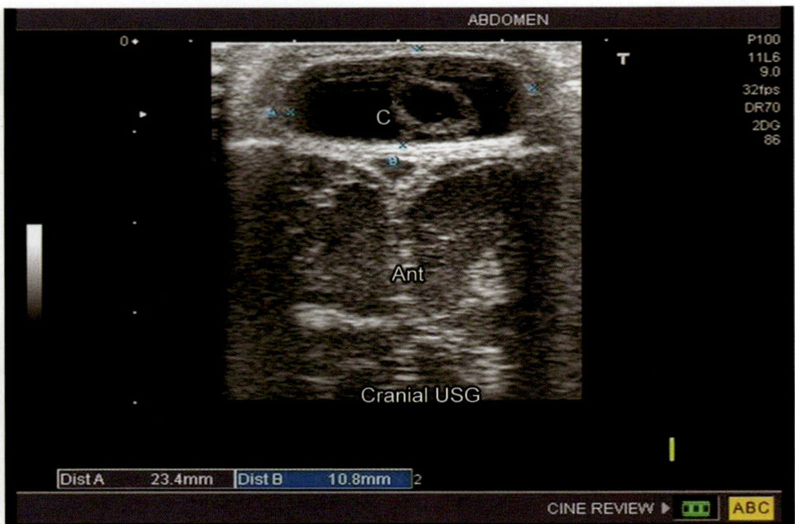

FIGURE 6.53C

FIGURES 6.53A to C: Organized hematoma in the scalp. A 2-month-old child presented with soft tissue swelling over the anterior fontanel. HRSG shows a complex echo mass in the scalp. Echogenic shadows are seen in it. On color flow imaging, no flow is seen in it. The skull table is seen intact. On aspiration, clotted blood was seen in it suggestive of organized skull hematoma.

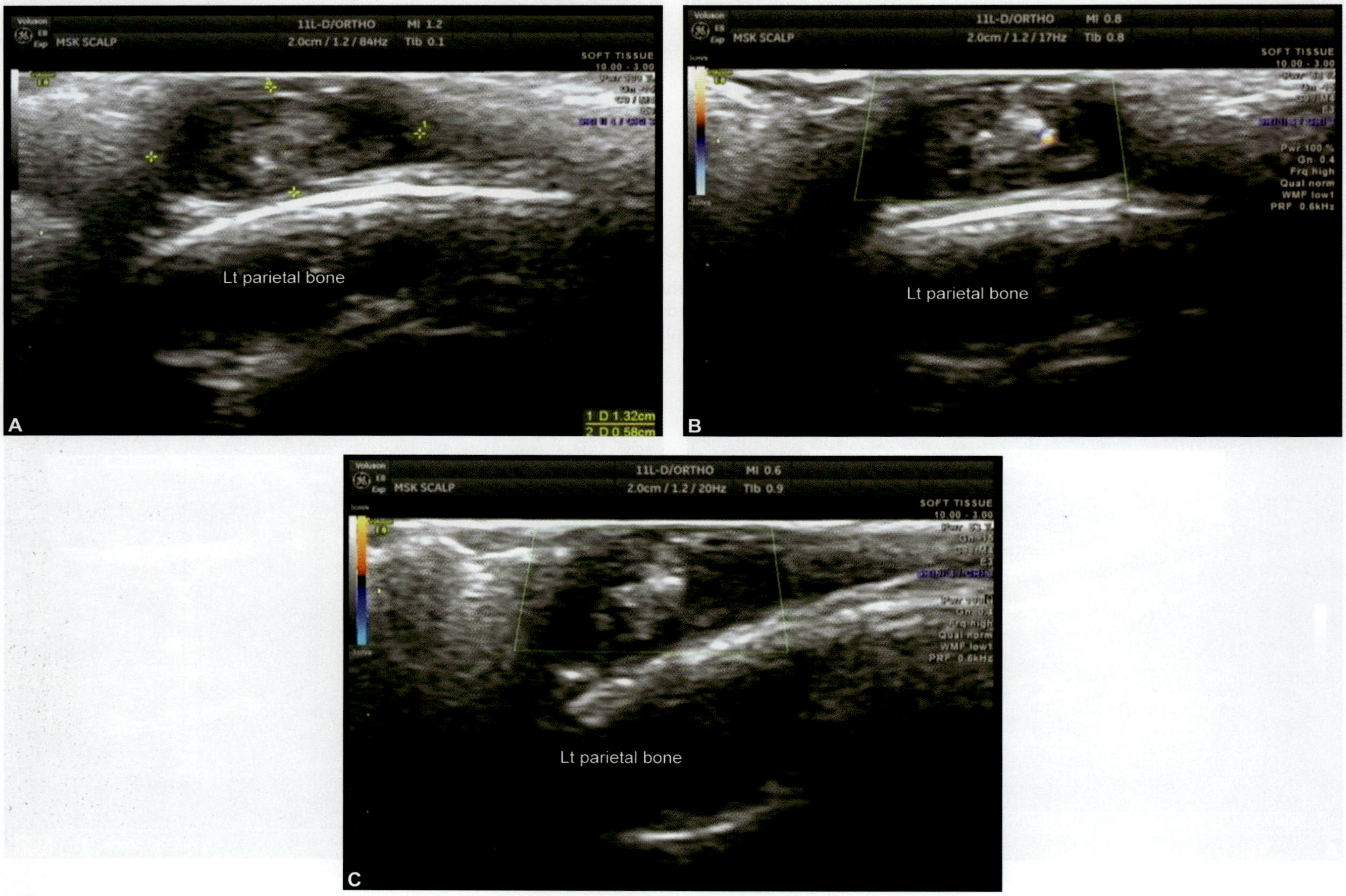

FIGURES 6.54A to C: A lady presented with soft tissue masses over the scalp. HRSG shows multiple well-defined heterogeneous soft tissue masses in the scalp. No cystic degeneration is seen. No calcification is seen. They are confined to the scalp. No evidence of any skull table invasion is seen. On color flow imaging, no flow is seen. Findings are consistent with skull warts.

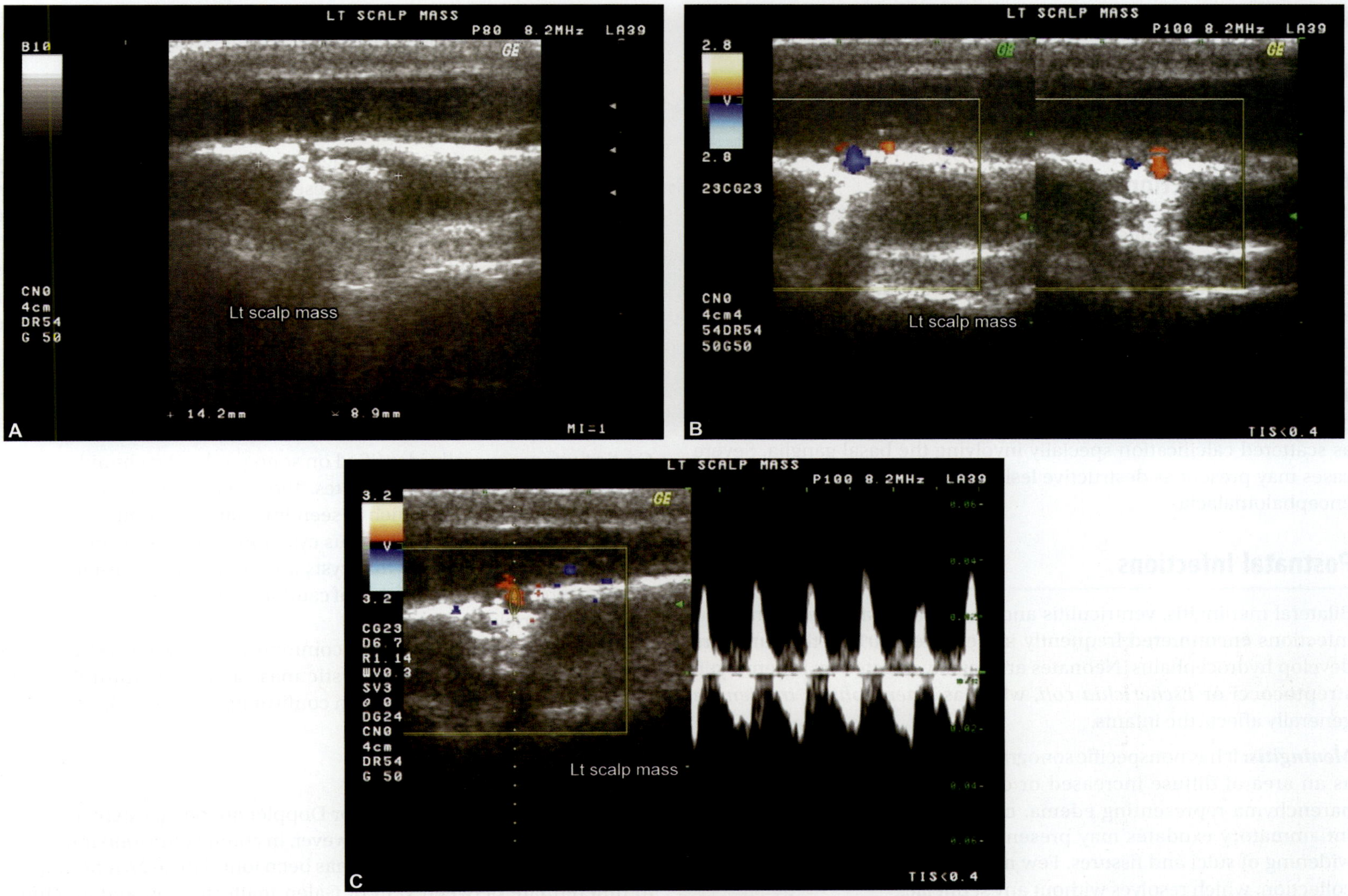

FIGURES 6.55A to C: Scalp mass. A patient presented with soft tissue mass over the scalp. HRSG shows soft tissue mass over the scalp. Bony erosion is also seen, on color flow imaging increased flow is seen in it. Biopsy showed metastatic deposit.

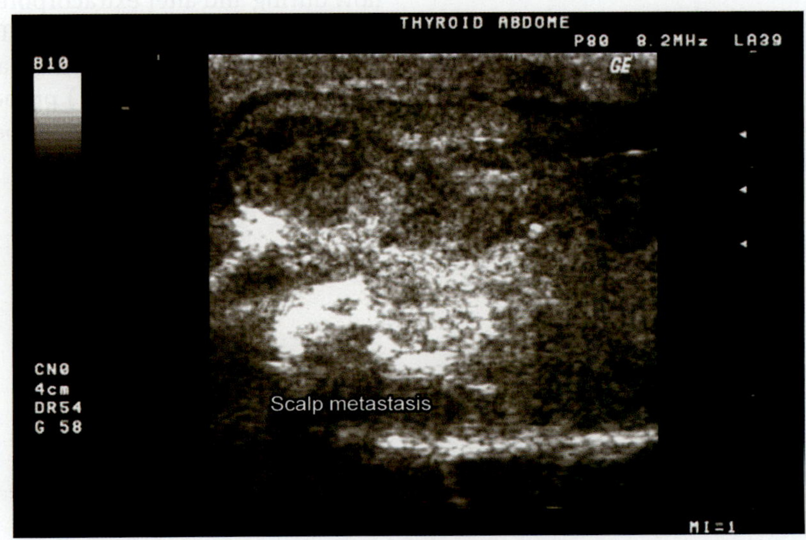

FIGURE 6.56: Scalp metastasis. A patient of CA thyroid presented with soft tissue mass over the scalp. HRSG shows an irregular ill defined mass over the scalp. It is seen invading the skull table. Margins are ill defined. Biopsy of the mass confirms scalp metastasis.

INTRACRANIAL INFECTIONS

The intracranial infections can be divided into:

i. Antenatal acquired.
ii. Postnatal acquired.

Antenatal Infections

Most common infections acquired in utero are due to *Cytomegalovirus*, herpes simplex, rubella or *Toxoplasma*. *Cytomegalovirus (CMV)* typically presents with periventricular calcification. The typical features are present at or immediately after birth. Though initially they may be small enough not to cause shadowing their persistence after 1 to 2 weeks of birth differentiates them from subependymal hemorrhage. Toxoplasmosis is the second most common infection. Unlike periventricular distribution is seen in CMV, toxoplasmosis presents as scattered calcification specially involving the basal ganglia. Severe cases may present as destructive lesions presenting as multiple cystic encephalomalacia.

Postnatal Infections

Bilateral meningitis, ventriculitis and encephalitis are common brain infections encountered frequently in neonates. 30% of the survivors develop hydrocephalus. Neonates are usually affected by β-hemolytic streptococci or *Escherichia coli*, whereas *Haemophilus influenzae* generally affects the infants.

Meningitis: It has nonspecific sonographic appearances. It may present as an area of diffuse increased or decreased echogenicity of brain parenchyma representing edema, cerebritis, or evolving infarction. Inflammatory exudates may present as increased echogenicity and widening of sulci and fissures. Few may present with extra/axial fluid collection, which resolves without any sequelae.

Ventriculitis: It is a serious complication and presents with characteristic sonographic findings. The findings include floating debris in ventricles with septation and ventricular dilatation. The development of Intraventricular septa poses a great problem in effective shunting.

Multiple cystic encephalomalacia (MCE): It is a serious complication of bacterial meningitis with poor outcome. Ultrasonography shows multiple bilateral cystic lesions involving the brain parenchyma with or without ventriculomegaly. Early detection helps in malignant and family counseling.

Abscess and infarctions: These are commonly seen in neonates with poor resistance. Focal areas of increased echogenicity represent vasculitis, cerebritis or infarction. Abscess presents as an area of cavitations with thickened wall with or without debris.

INTRACRANIAL MASSES

The brain tumors in the neonatal age group are uncommon and mostly are congenital. Most tumors are present as hydrocephalus, which can easily be picked up by ultrasonography. Ultrasonography is found to be excellent screening modality, however, for detailed delineation contrast. CT of MRI is preferred method of imaging. In many cases, these tumors may present as hemorrhage, and one should be aware about their presentations. The commonly occurring tumors in this age group are astrocytomas choroid plexus papilloma and ependymoma.

Cystic Tumors

Cystic tumors are easily identified on sonography. Arachnoid cysts are frequently encountered in neonates. The other common cystic lesions are porencephalic cyst, which is seen invariable in continuation with ventricular system. Choroid plexus cyst presents as cystic mass within choroid plexus. Subependymal cysts are formed as a consequence of SEH and are found in the region of caudothalamic groove involving the lining of ventricles.

Galenic venous malformation commonly describes as vein of Galen aneurysm is seen as midline cystic mass above the third ventricle. Doppler ultrasonography helps in confirming the diagnosis.

Color Doppler USG

Though duplex Doppler and color Doppler are being extensively used in various clinical conditions, however, in cranial ultrasonography, it is still struggling to find its place. It has been found to be extremely useful to differentiate between vein of Galen malformation and arachnoid cyst. It has also been used to detect patency of intracerebral vessels. Sagittal sinus thrombosis has been accurately diagnosed using color Doppler technique.

In severe respiratory disease where extracorporeal membrane oxygenation is increasingly being used, color Doppler has been found to be useful to study the collaterals vessel pathways that maintain blood flow during and after extracorporeal membrane oxygenation.

Lately transcranial Doppler (TCD) has been used in diagnosis of increased intracranial pressure leading to vascular spasm. TCD utilizes high frequency (2.25 MHz) probe. In near future with development of technology, it may prove to be an effective tool for evaluation of intracerebral circulation.

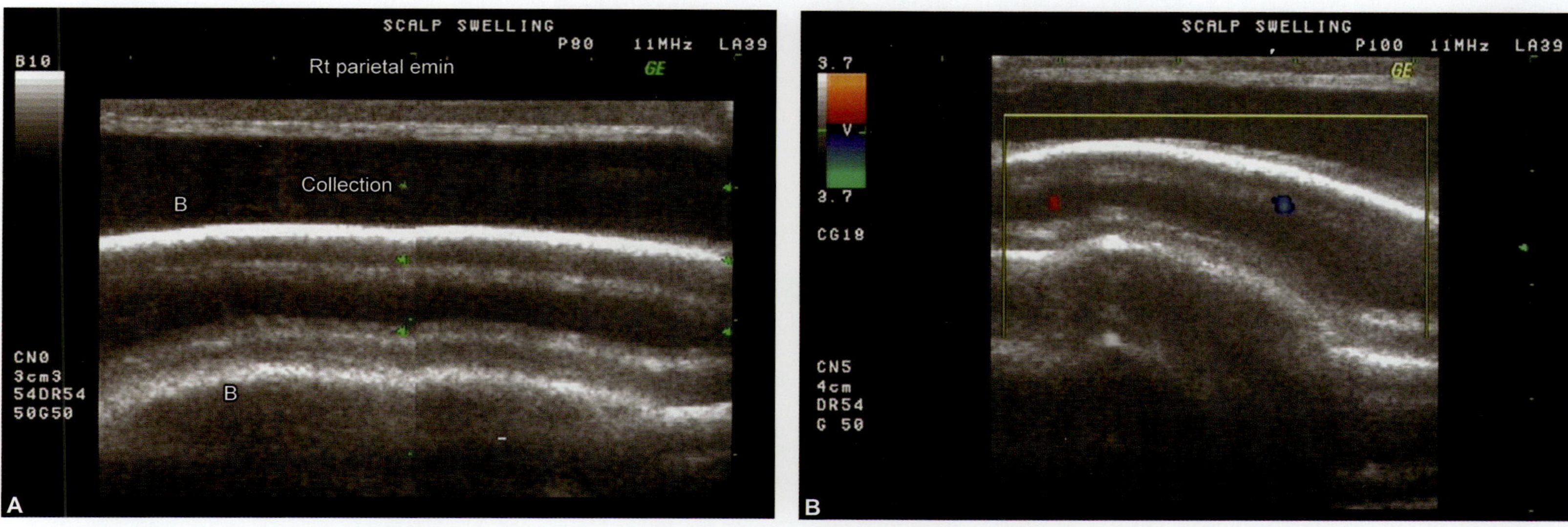

FIGURES 6.57A and B: Scalp infection. A child presented with tender hot swelling over the parietal region. HRSG shows low-level echo collection in the scalp. However, the collection was limited only to the scalp layer. No subdural collection was seen. Aspiration confirmed pyogenic collection.

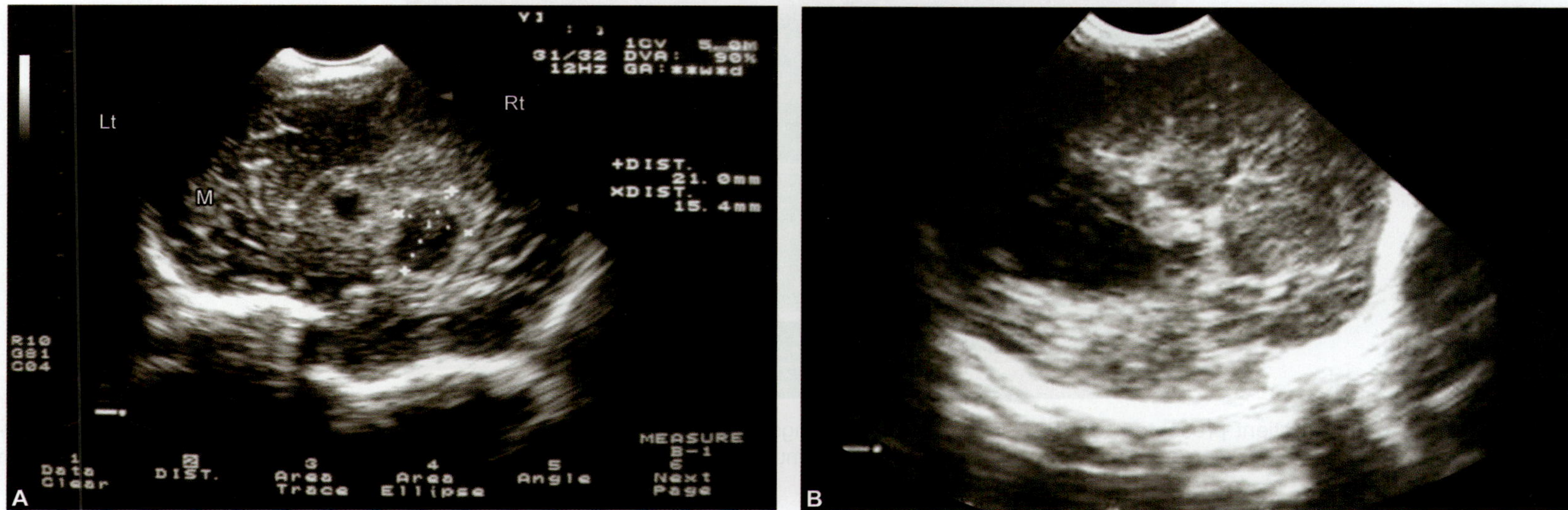

FIGURES 6.58A and B: Brain abscess. A patient presented with high fever. HRSG shows irregular low-level echo complex mass in the right parietal lobe suggestive of brain abscess. HRSG shows irregular hypoechoic low-level echo complex mass in the left parietal lobe. The mass is seen involving the thalamic region.

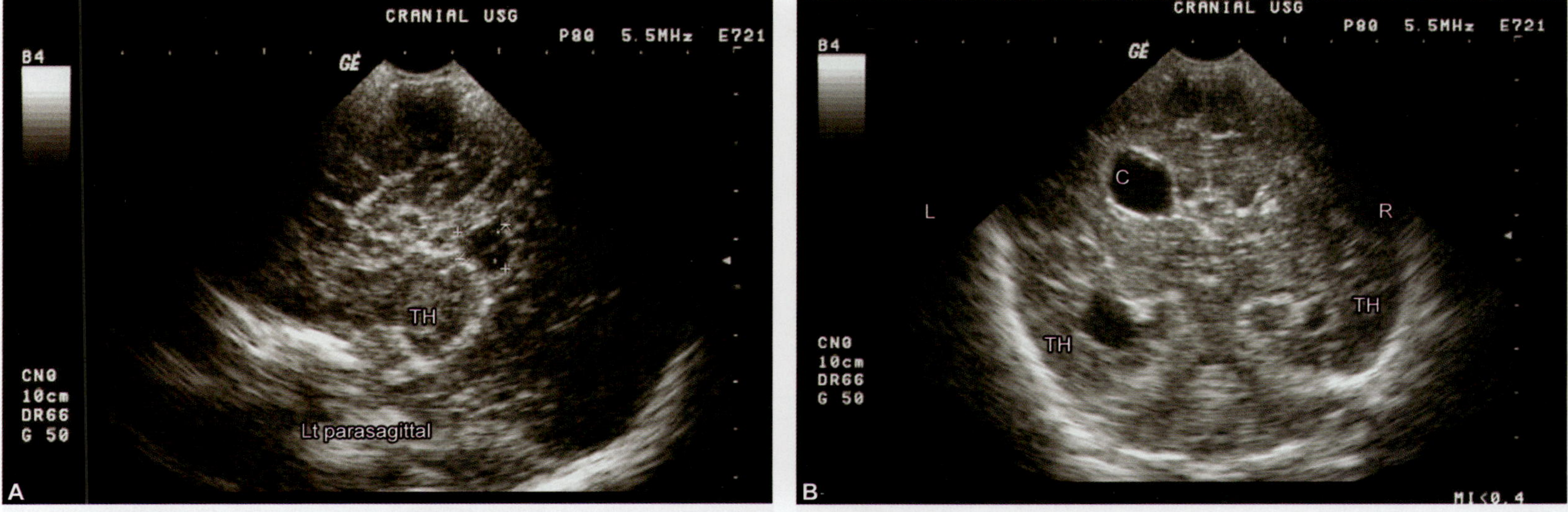

FIGURES 6.59A and B: Brain abscess with parietal cyst. A patient presented with high fever with fullness of the ventricles. HRSG shows low-level echo complex mass in the parathalamic region suggestive of an abscess. There is also evidence of well-defined thin walled cyst seen in the left parietal lobe.

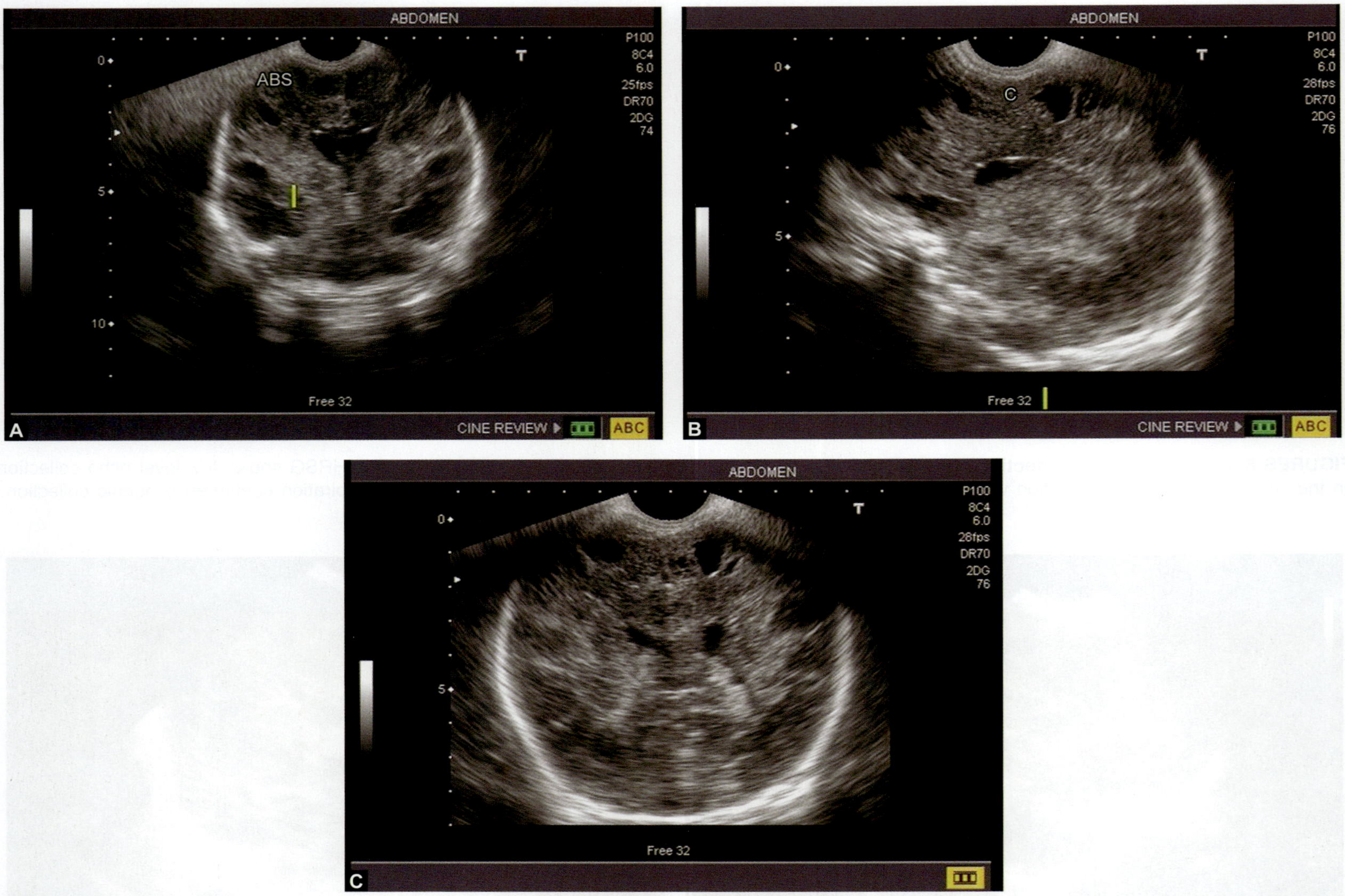

FIGURES 6.60A to C: A patient presented with high fever. The LP findings suggestive of septic meningitis. HRSG of the brain shows multiple low-level echo complex masses involving both cerebral cortex suggestive of multiple abscess. The left parietal lobe also shows gliosis. Associated brain edema is also seen.

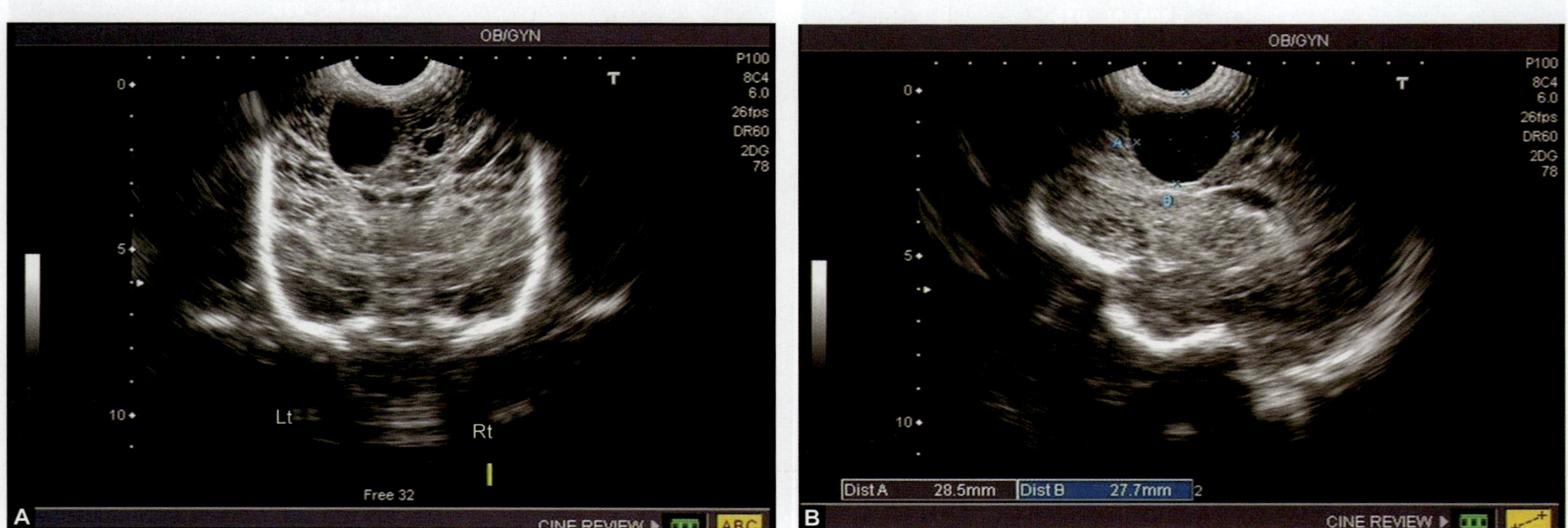

FIGURES 6.61A and B

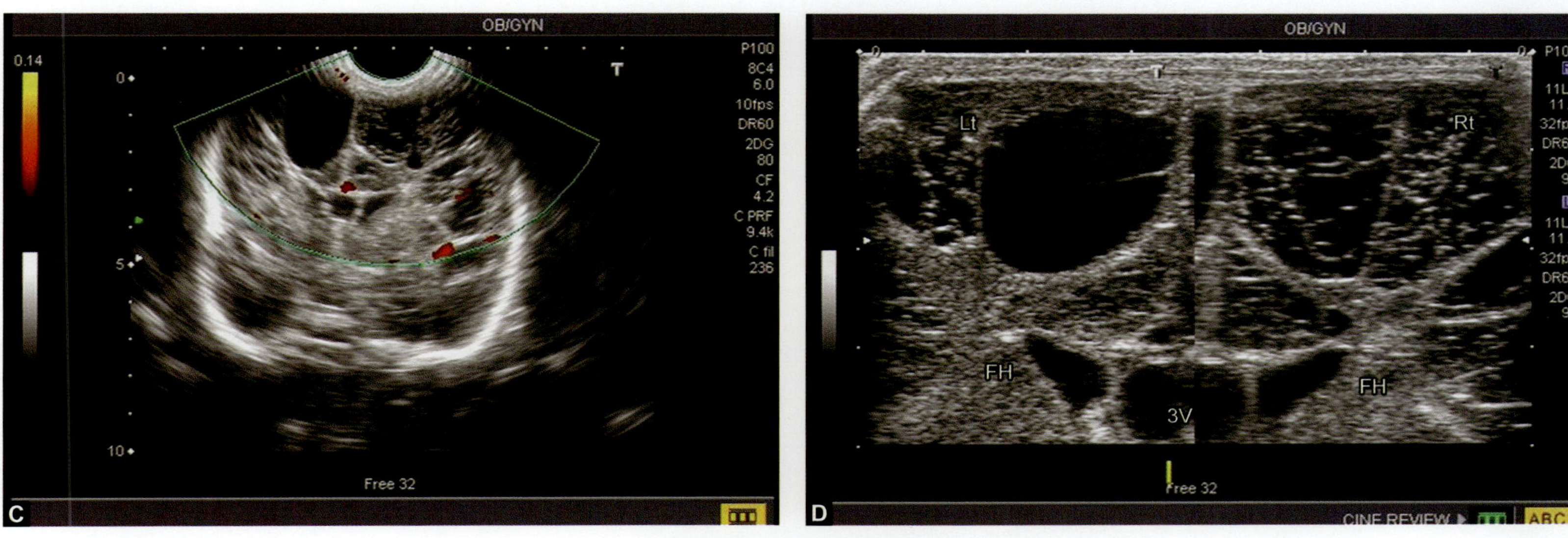

FIGURES 6.61C and D

FIGURES 6.61A to D: Big brain abscess with gliosis with hydrocephalus. A small baby presented with tense anterior fontanel with low general condition. HRSG shows a big irregular ill-defined mass in right parietal lobe. Thick echoes are seen in it suggestive of big abscess. The left parietal lobe shows a cystic mass due to gliosis. The adjacent brain parenchyma shows the abscess cavity with debris. Pressure is seen on ventricles resulting into obstructed hydrocephalus.

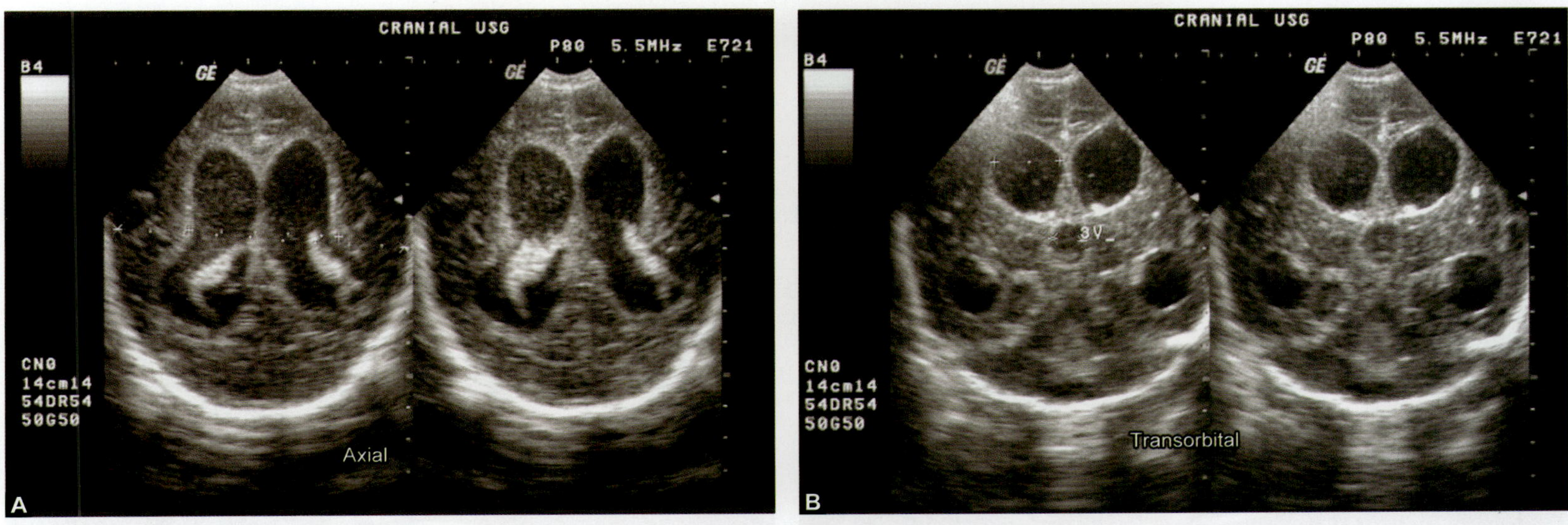

FIGURES 6.62A and B: Ventriculitis with hydrocephalus. A child presented with high fever and fullness of the fontanelle. HRSG shows dilated ventricles. Echogenic collection is seen in the ventricles. The walls of the ventricles are echogenic. Sonographic findings are suggestive of ventriculitis. Spinal fluid examination confirmed the pyogenic meningitis.

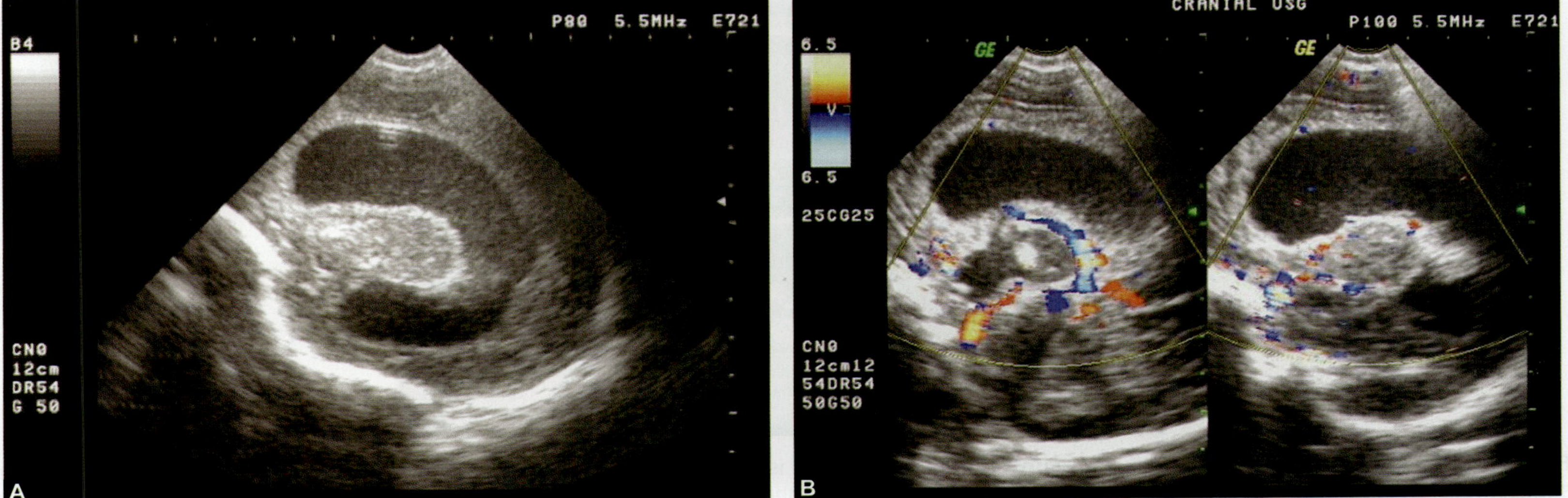

FIGURES 6.63A and B: Ventriculitis with hydrocephalus. Echogenic collection is seen filling the lateral ventricles. On color flow imaging, high flow is seen in periventricular vessels.

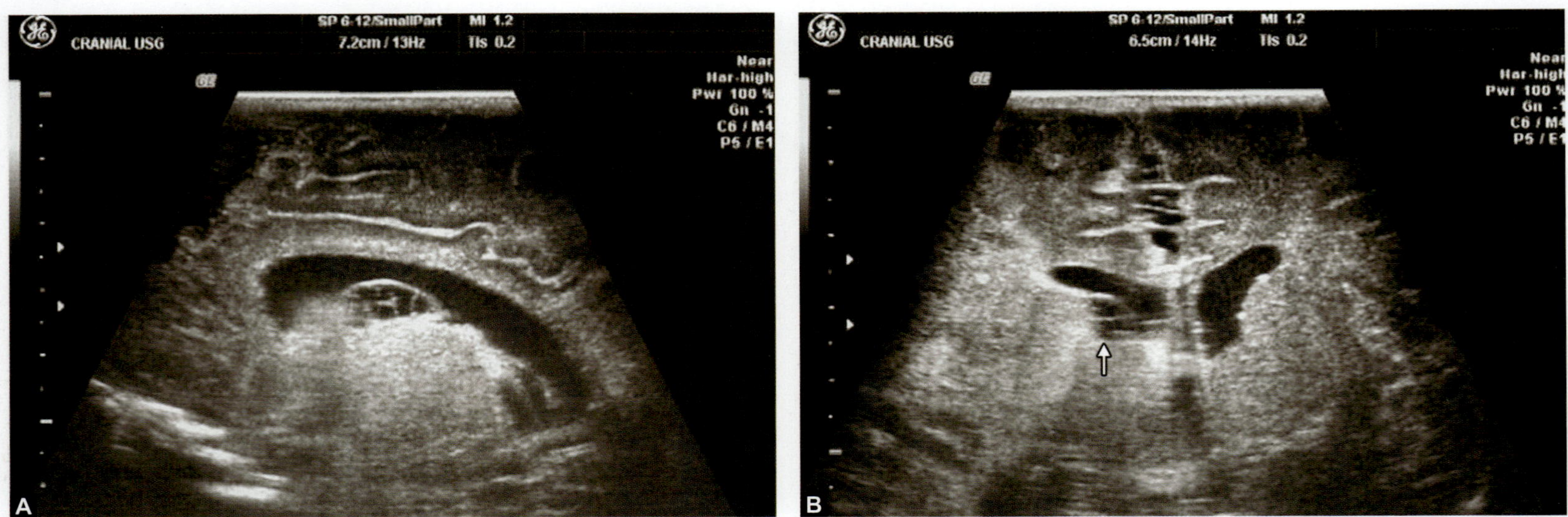

FIGURES 6.64A and B: Pyogenic ventriculitis. Shows dilated ventricles. Echogenic collection is seen in the ventricles. Fine echogenic strands are seen running in the ventricles suggestive of protein bands in a case of pyogenic meningitis.

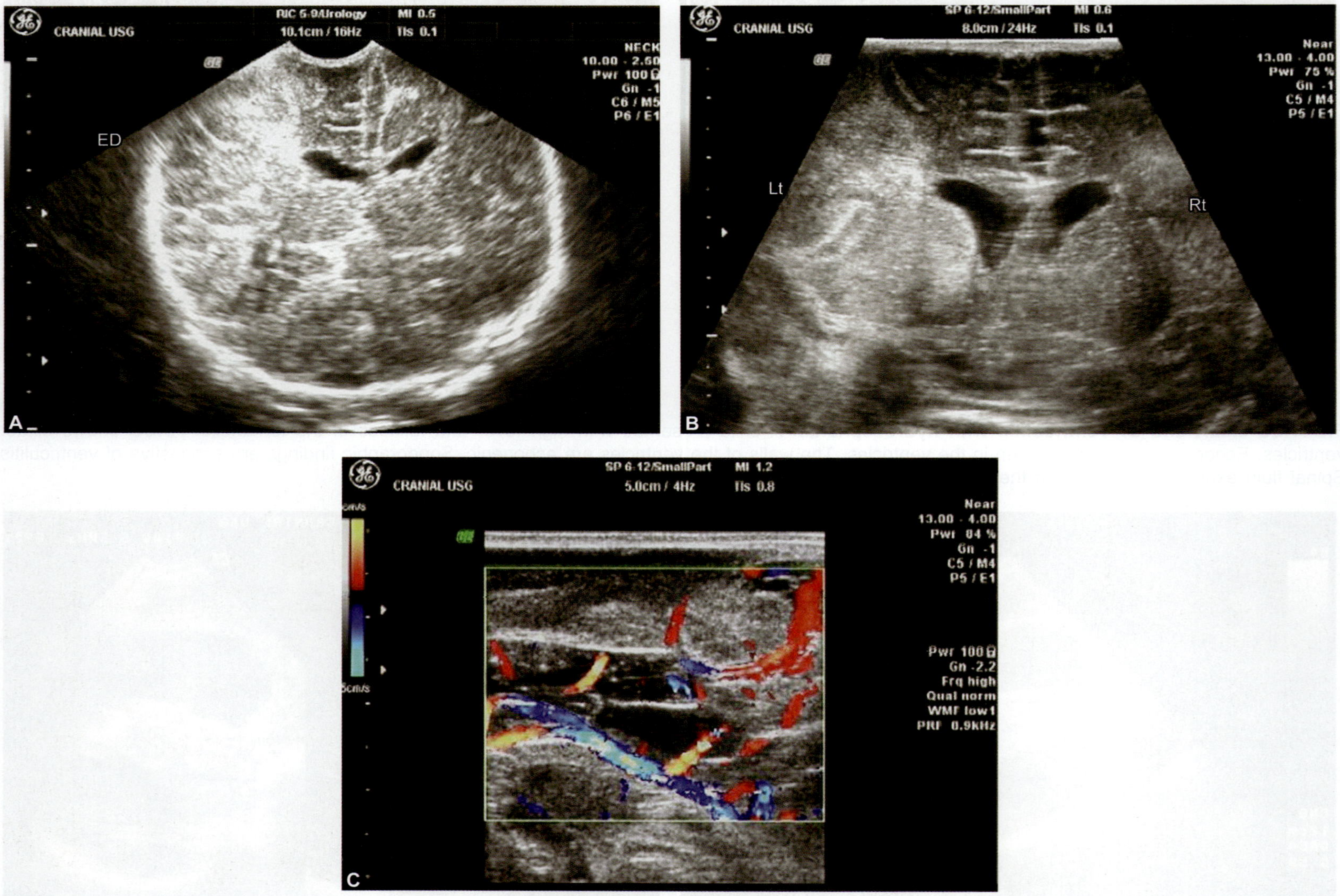

FIGURES 6.65A to C: Pyogenic ventriculitis with brain edema. There is also evidence of echogenic brain parenchyma seen in the same patient suggestive of associated brain edema. The sulci and gyri are effaced by the brain edema. On color flow imaging, increased flow is seen in the brain parenchyma due to hyperemia.

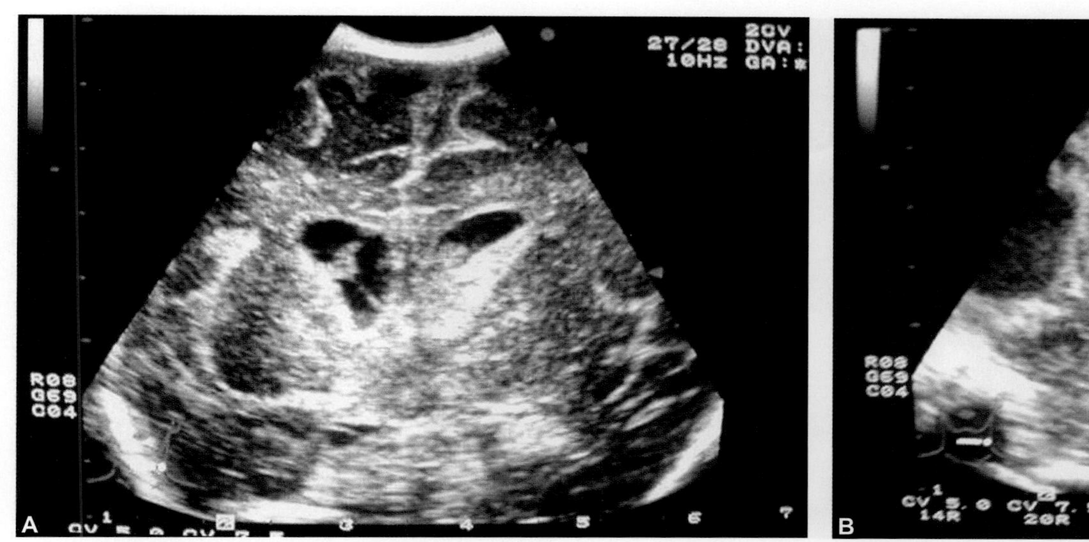

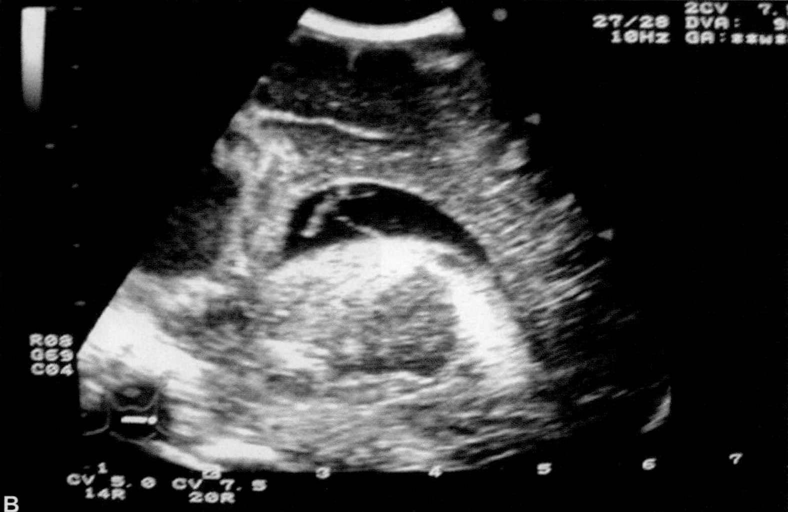

FIGURES 6.66A and B: Meningitis with ventriculitis. A patient presented with high fever with fullness of the ventricles. HRSG shows mild dilatation of the ventricles. Ventricular walls are echogenic. Fine echogenic strands are seen floating in the ventricles suggestive of ventriculitis with meningitis.

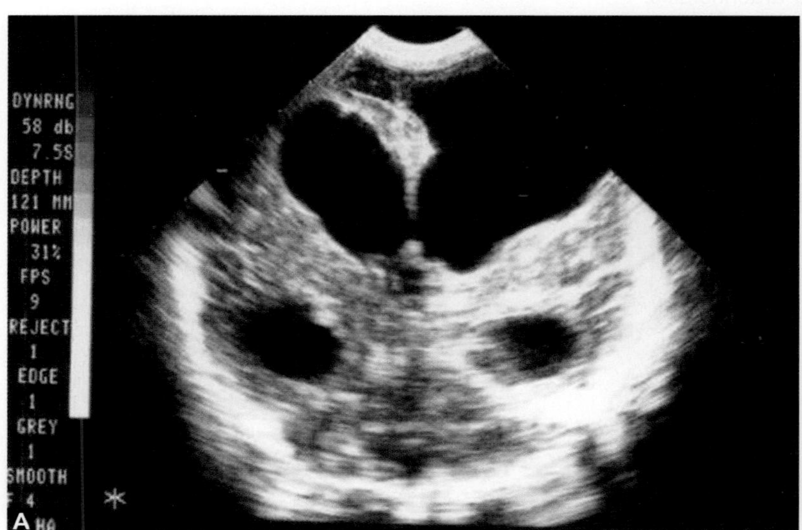

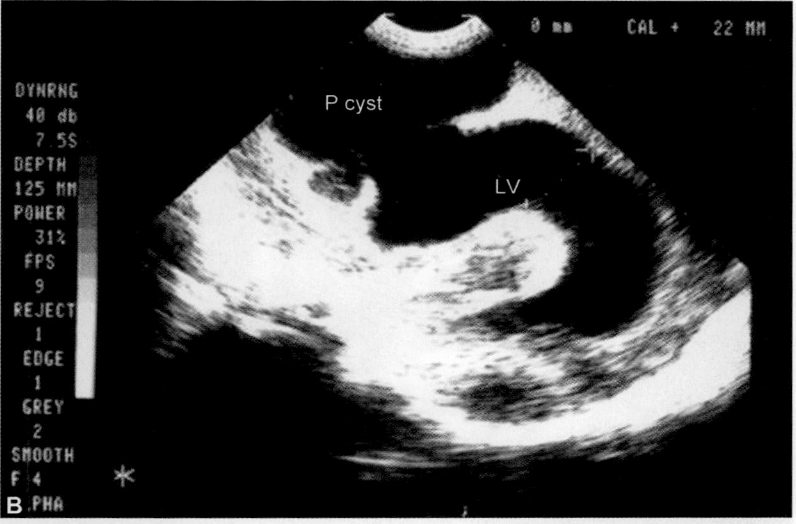

FIGURES 6.67A and B: Porencephalic cyst. HRSG shows well-defined cystic mass communicating with lateral ventricle on the left side suggestive of a big porencephalic cyst. The contraletral frontal horn and temporal horns are also dilated.

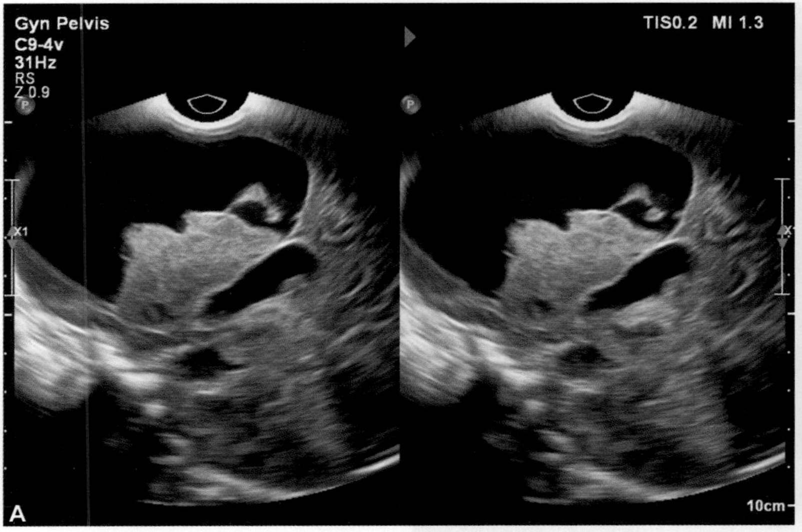

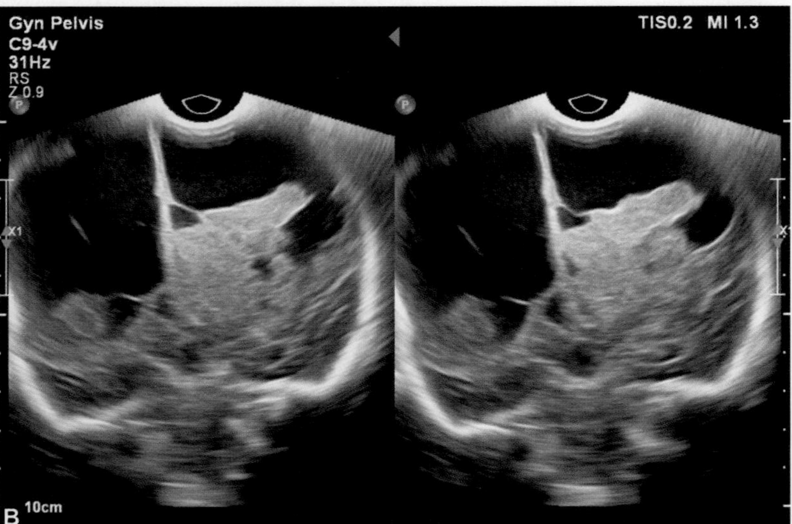

FIGURES 6.68A and B

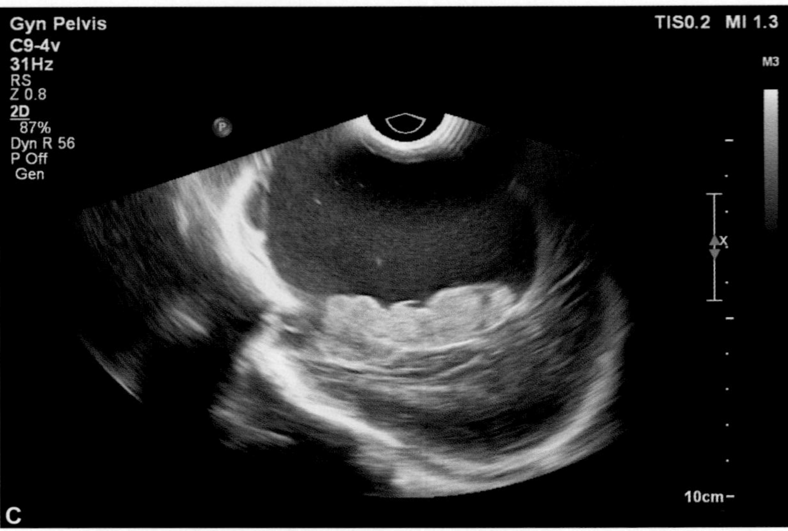

FIGURE 6.68C

FIGURES 6.68A to C: Ventriculitis with hydrocephalus. A patient of pyogenic meningitis presented with high fever with fullness of fontanelle. HRSG shows dilated ventricles. Echogenic cerebral fluid is seen filling the ventricles. Fine echogenic strands are seen in the ventricles. The ventricular walls are also irregular in outline. Obstructed hydrocephalus is seen due to basal arachnoiditis.

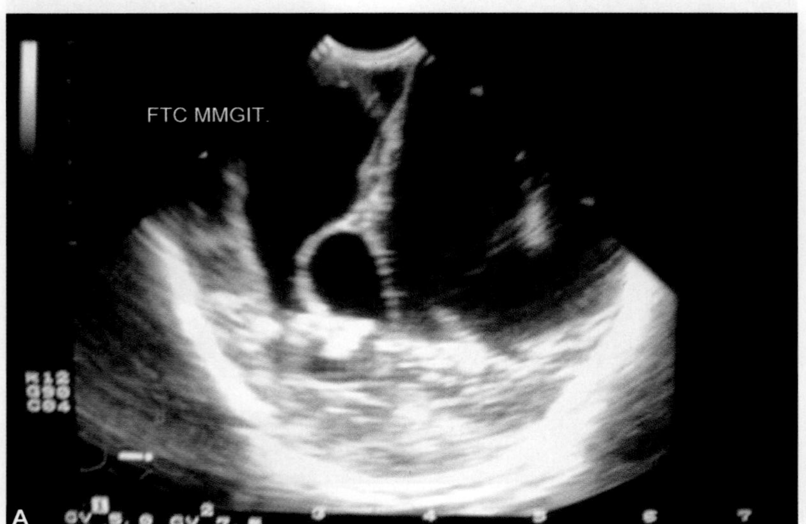

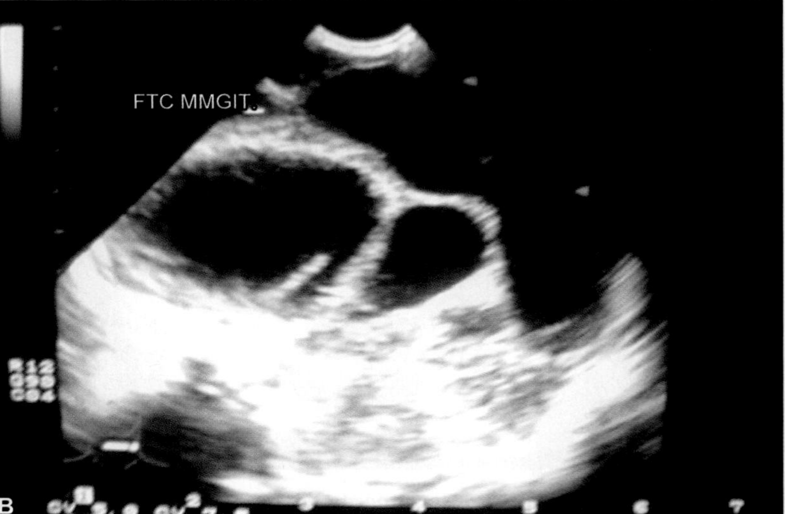

FIGURES 6.69A and B: Post meningitis hydrocephalus with gliosis. A patient presented with gross hydrocephalus after meningitis. HRSG shows distorted brain anatomy. Marked fluid collection is seen in the ventricles. Brain parenchyma is thinned out. Echogenic strands are also seen in the ventricles. Ultrasound is very good for evaluation of sequelae of cranial infections.

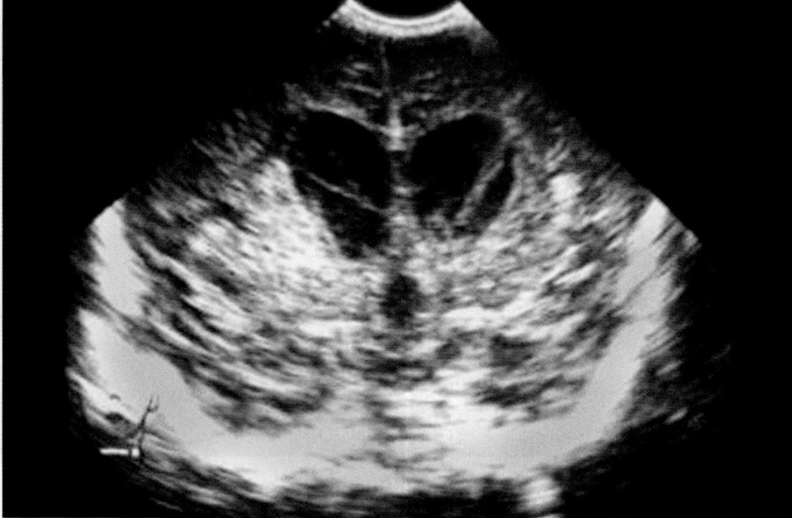

FIGURE 6.70: Ventriculitis with hydrocephalus. HRSG shows dilated frontal horns. Echogenic collection is seen in the ventricles. Fine echogenic strands are seen running in the ventricles.

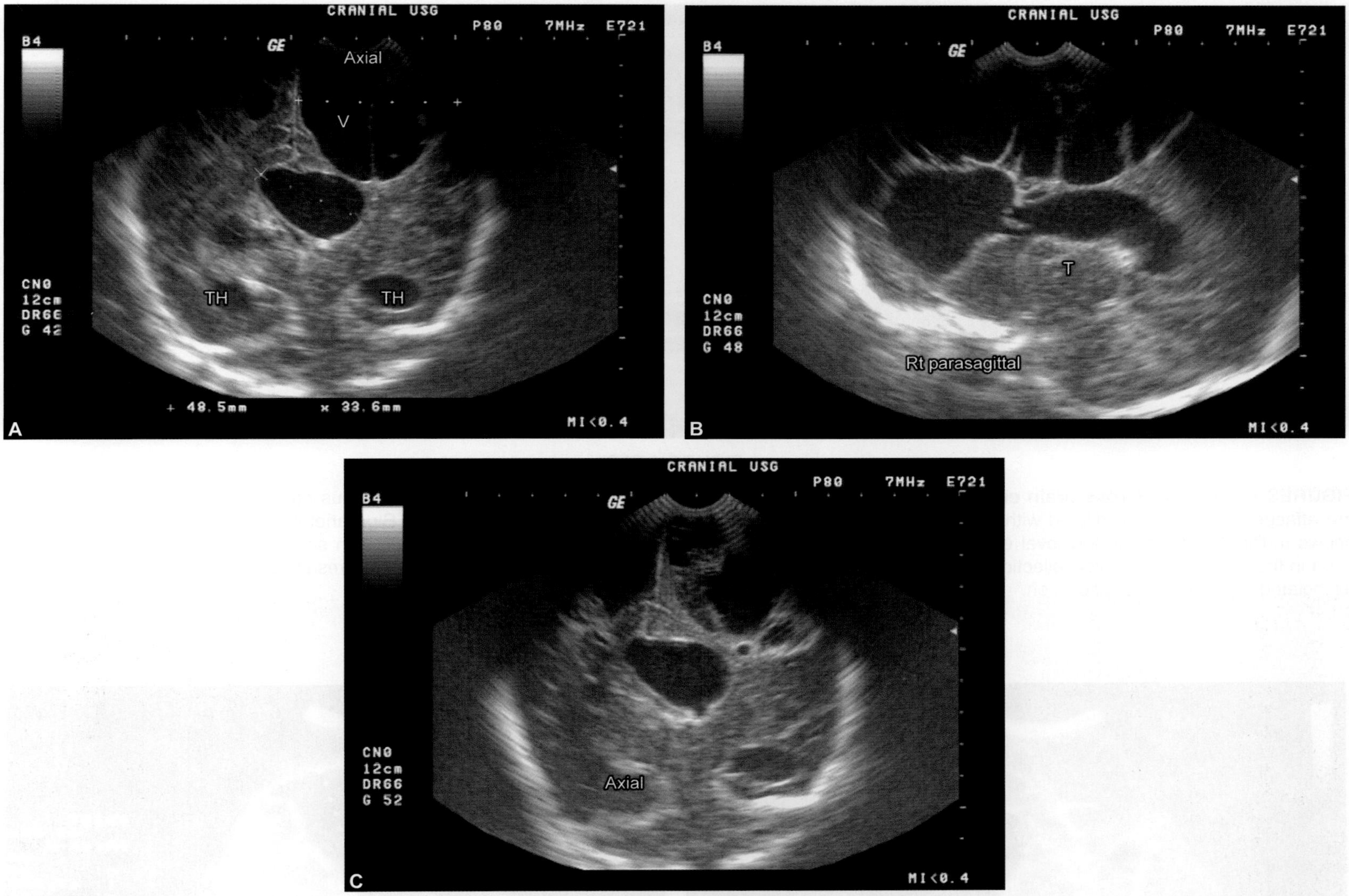

FIGURES 6.71A to C: Post meningitis porencephalic cyst with hydrocephalus. A patient presented with progressively increasing hydrocephalus after meningitis. HRSG shows marked dilatation of the ventricles. A big cyst is seen communicating with the right frontal horn suggestive of porencephalic cyst. Echogenic strands are seen floating in the cyst suggestive of pyogenic exudative collection.

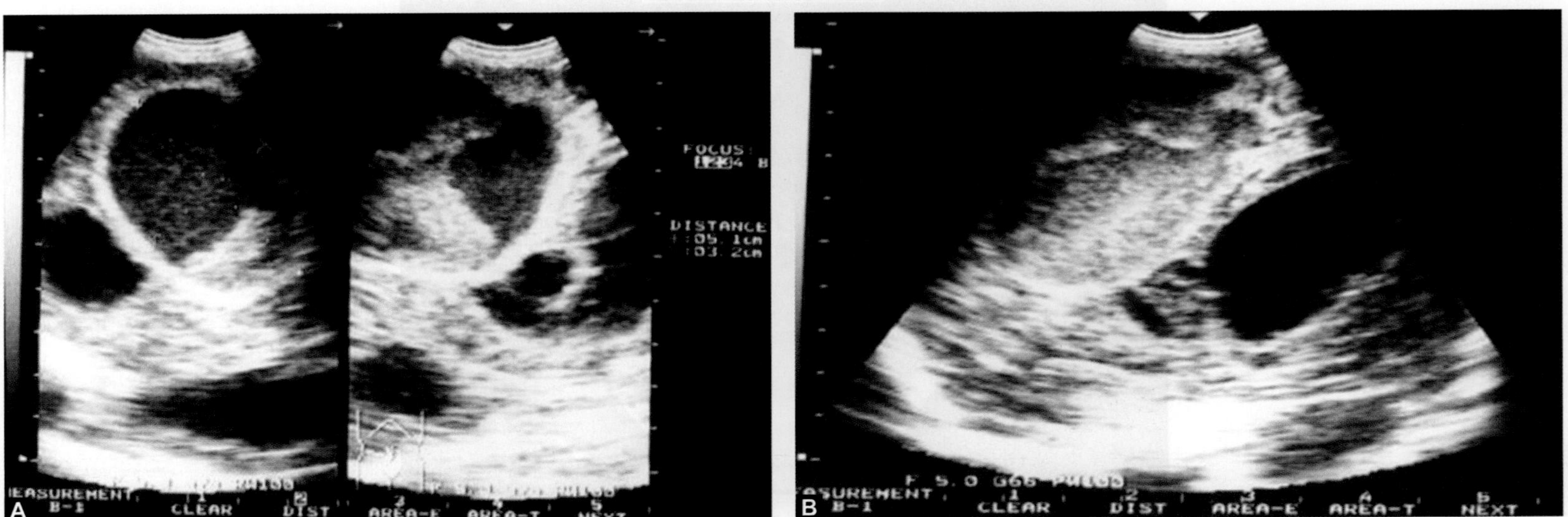

FIGURES 6.72A and B

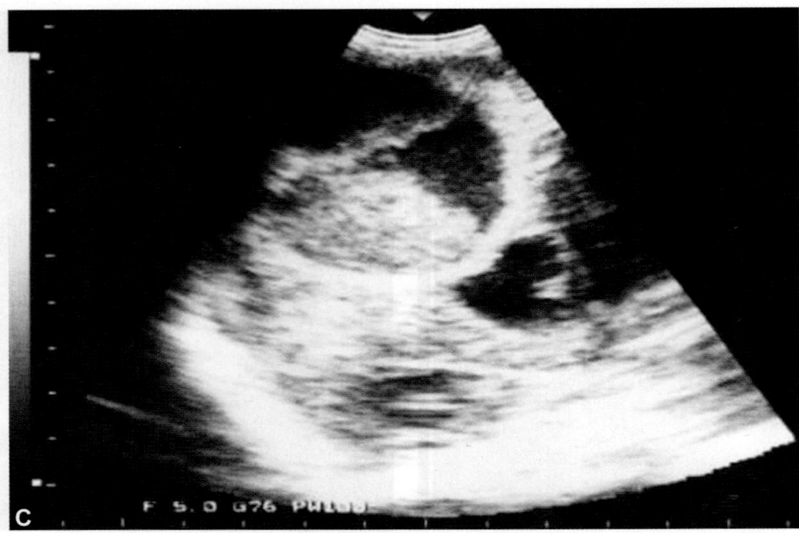

FIGURE 6.72C

FIGURES 6.72A to C: Gross brain edema with ventriculitis. HRSG shows gross brain edema. The edematous parenchyma is wide. Sulci and gyri are effaced. Ventricles are dilated with echogenic collection. Fibersbands are also seen in the ventricles. Big parietal lobe abscess: Neurosonography shows multiple thick walled low-level echo complex masses in the fronto parietal area in a child presented with septicemia. Echogenic debris is also seen in the abscess. Low-level collection is seen filling the abscess cavity. It is seen pressing over the ventricles resulting into obstructed hydrocephalus associated mass effect is also seen.

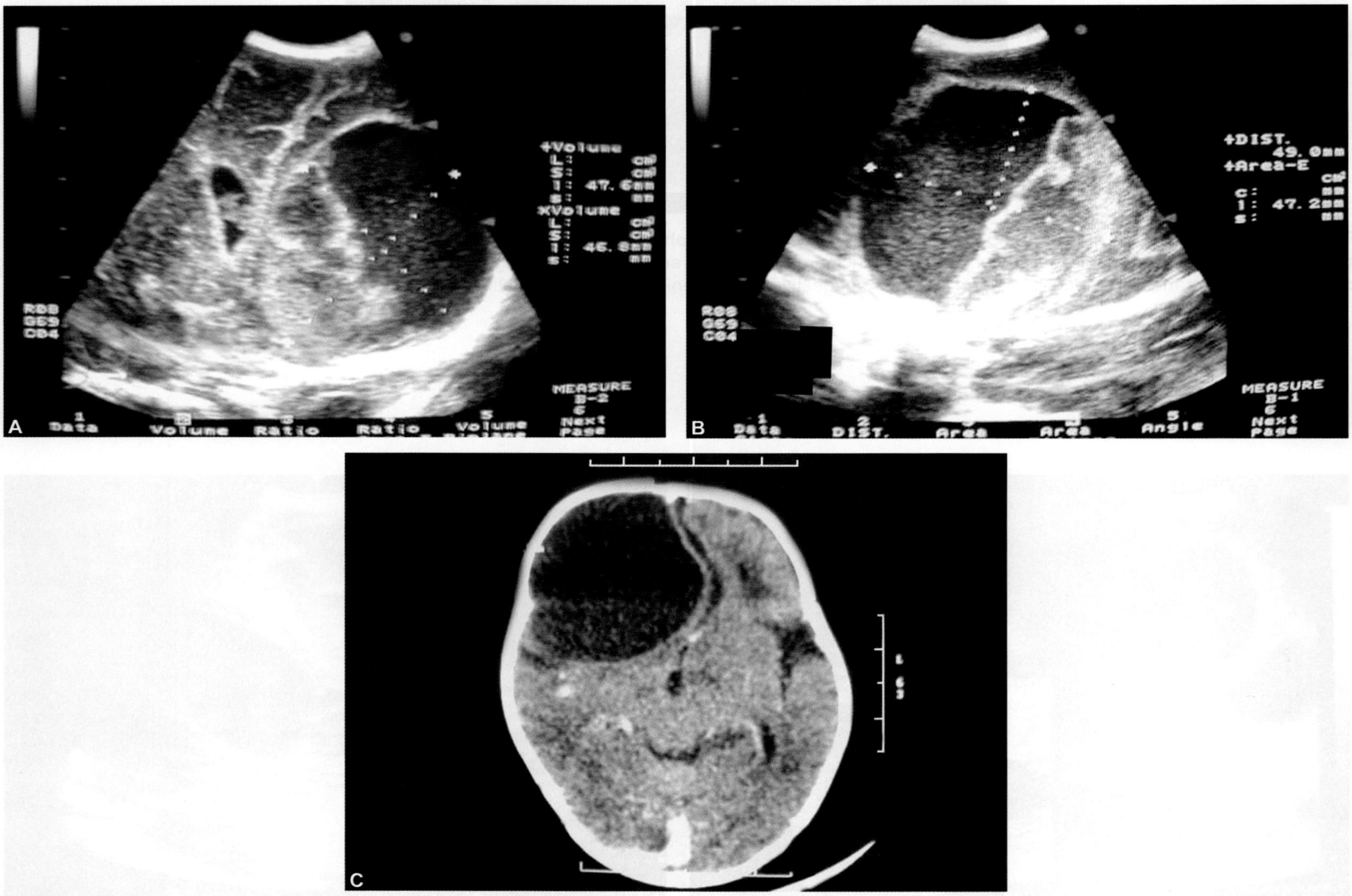

FIGURES 6.73A to C: Big parietal abscess. HRSG shows a big thick walled cystic mass in the right frontal parietal region. Echogenic collection is seen in the abscess. Layering sign is positive. Marked perifocal edema is present with mass effect suggestive of big brain abscess. CT scan of the same patient shows big abscess in the right frontal parietal region with mass effect.

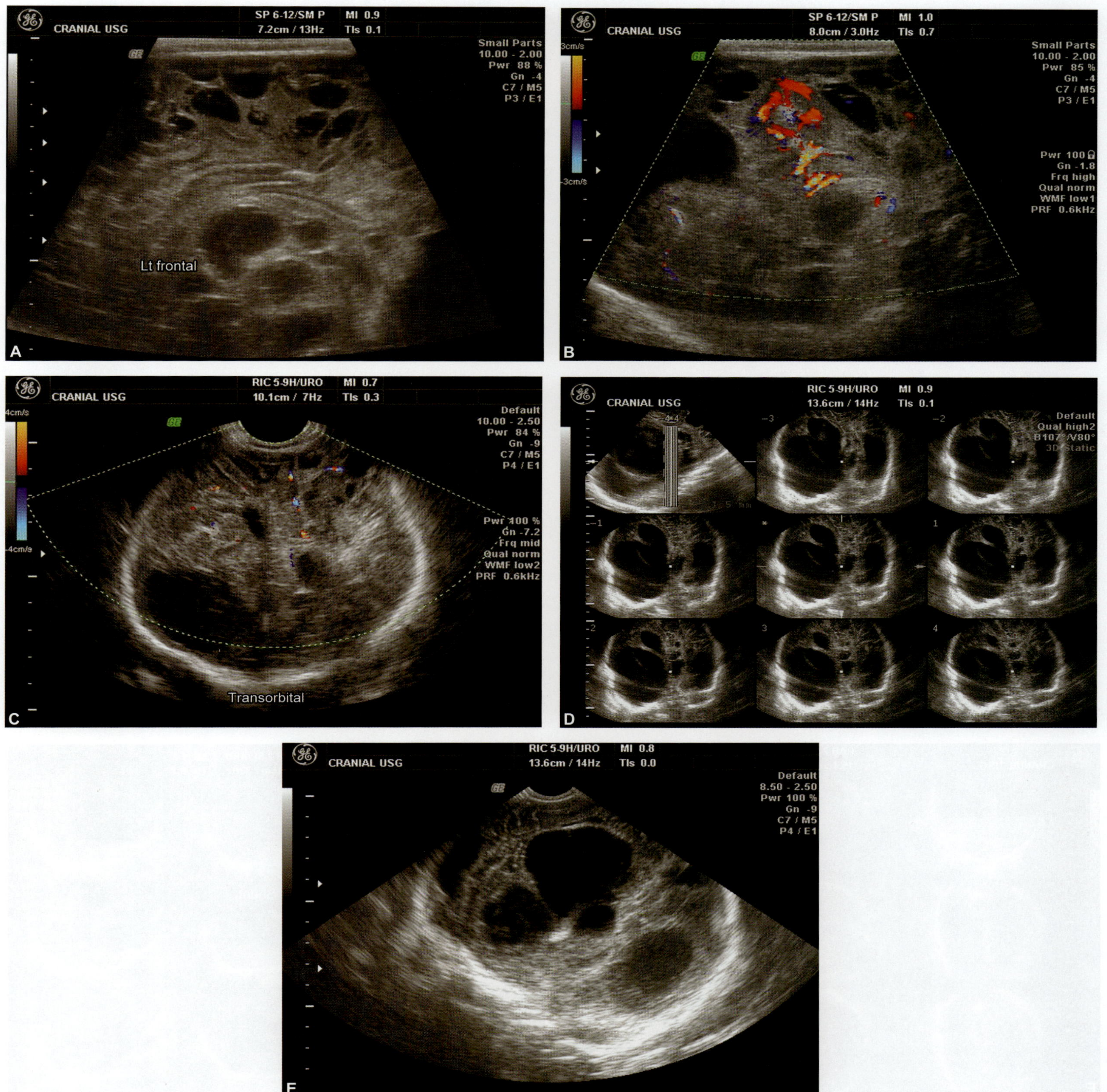

FIGURES 6.74A to E: Multiple brain abscess with gliosis. A 4-month-old baby presented with high fever with septicemia and tense anterior fontanel. HRSG shows multiple irregular ill defined low level echo complex masses in both parietal lobe, frontal lobe. A big low-level attenuating mass is seen in left temporal lobe. Echogenic debris is seen in them suggestive of multiple abscesses. The TUI imaging clearly shows multiple brain abscesses. Associated gliosis is also seen with pressure on the right side of the brain.

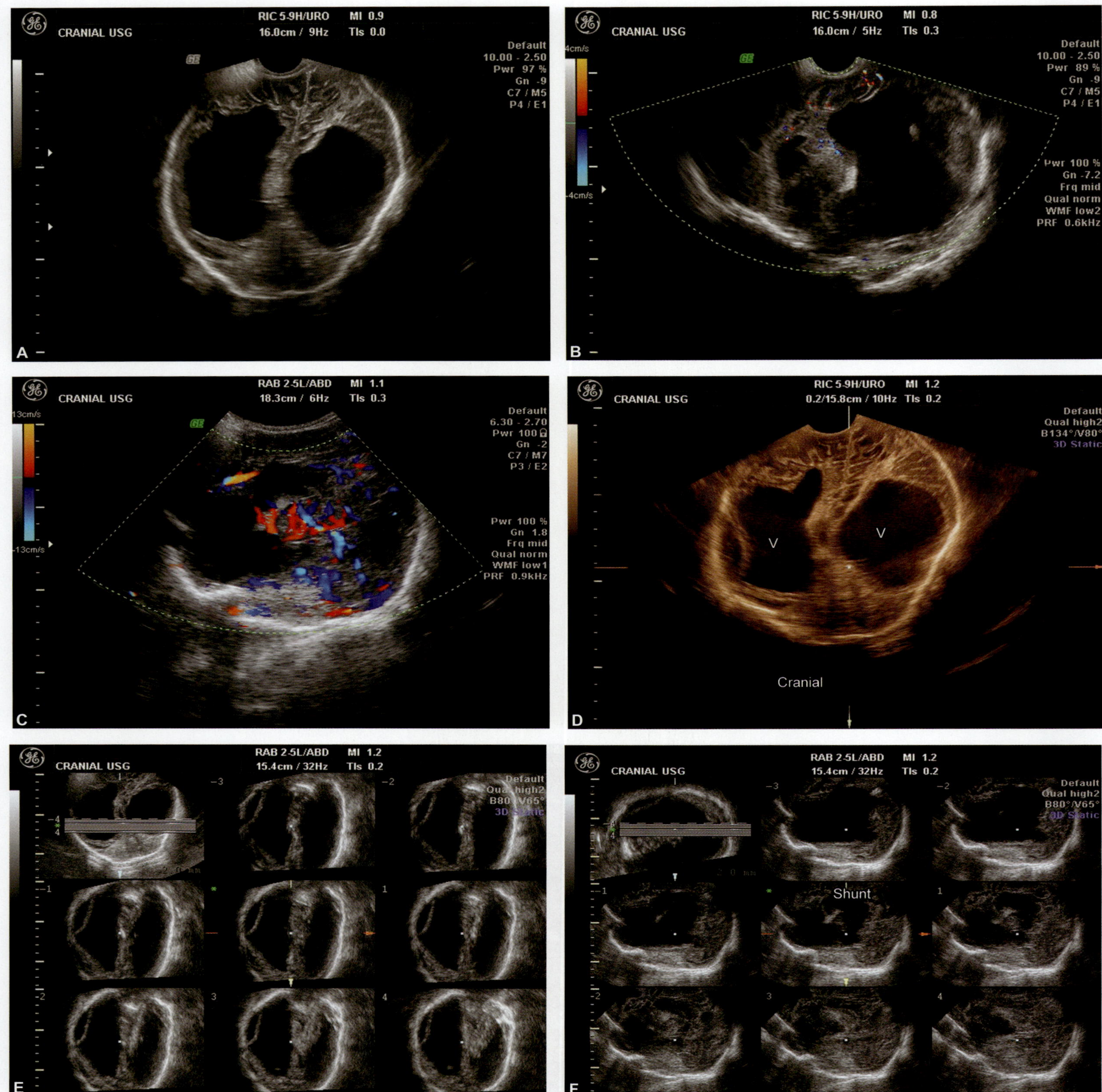

FIGURES 6.75A to F: Multiple brain abscess with gliosis with hydrocephalus. The same patient came in follow-up after two months. HRSG shows gliotic cysts in both cerebral cortex. The big one on the left side due to necrosis. The ventricles are also dilated. Echogenic strands are seen in dilated ventricles suggestive of ventriculitis. Thinning of brain parenchyma is also seen. The baby underwent shunt operation and an echogenic shunt is seen in the dilated ventricle suggestive of blockage of the shunt.

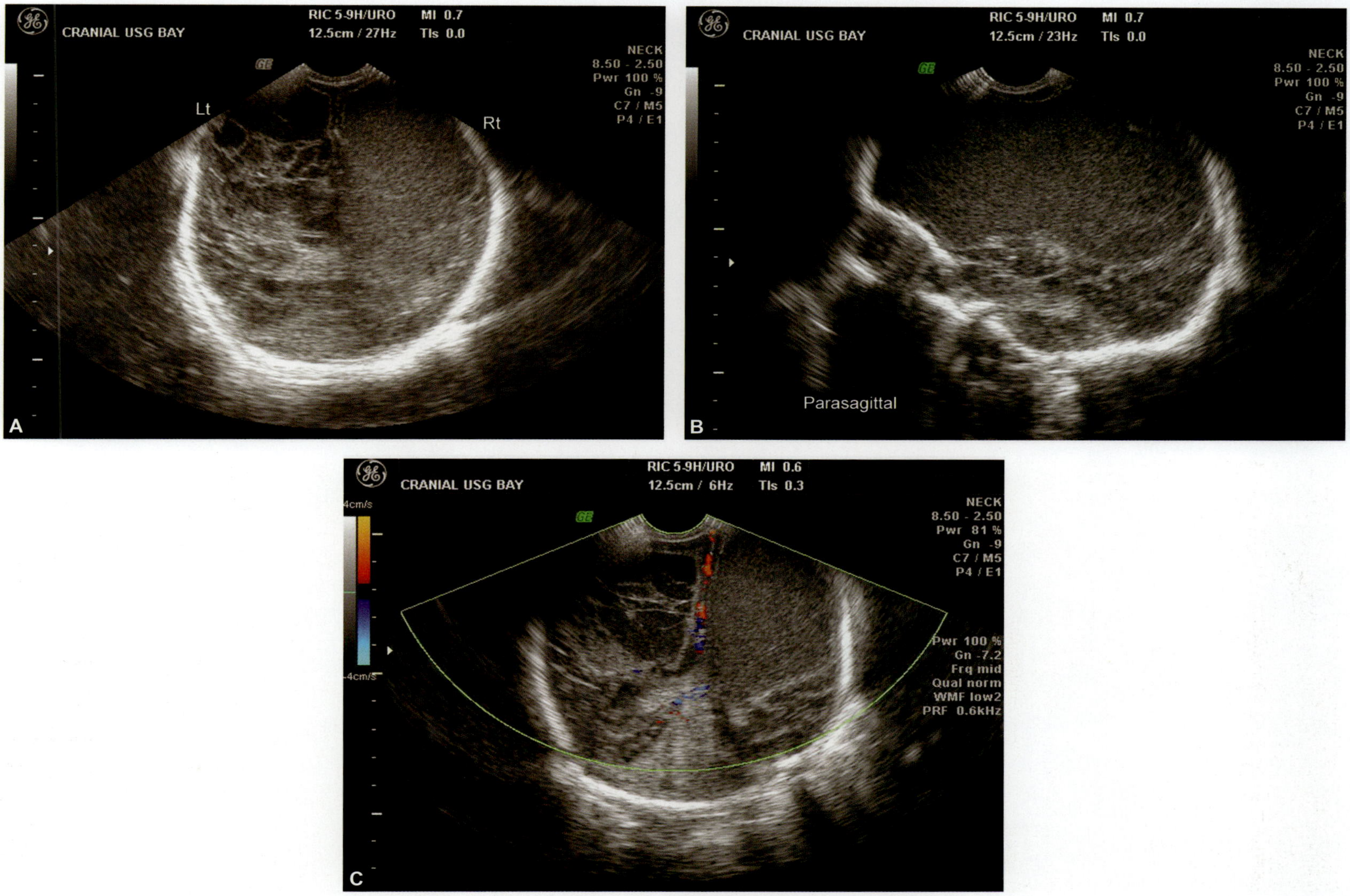

FIGURES 6.76A to C: Huge brain abscess with thinning of the brain parenchyma with gliosis. A 10-month-old baby presented with tense collection in the brain. The left side of the cortex shows heterogeneous low-level echo collection with multiple septations. The right side of the cortex shows thick echo collection suggestive of pyogenic collection. Thinning of the brain parenchyma is seen. Normal anatomic relations are distorted.

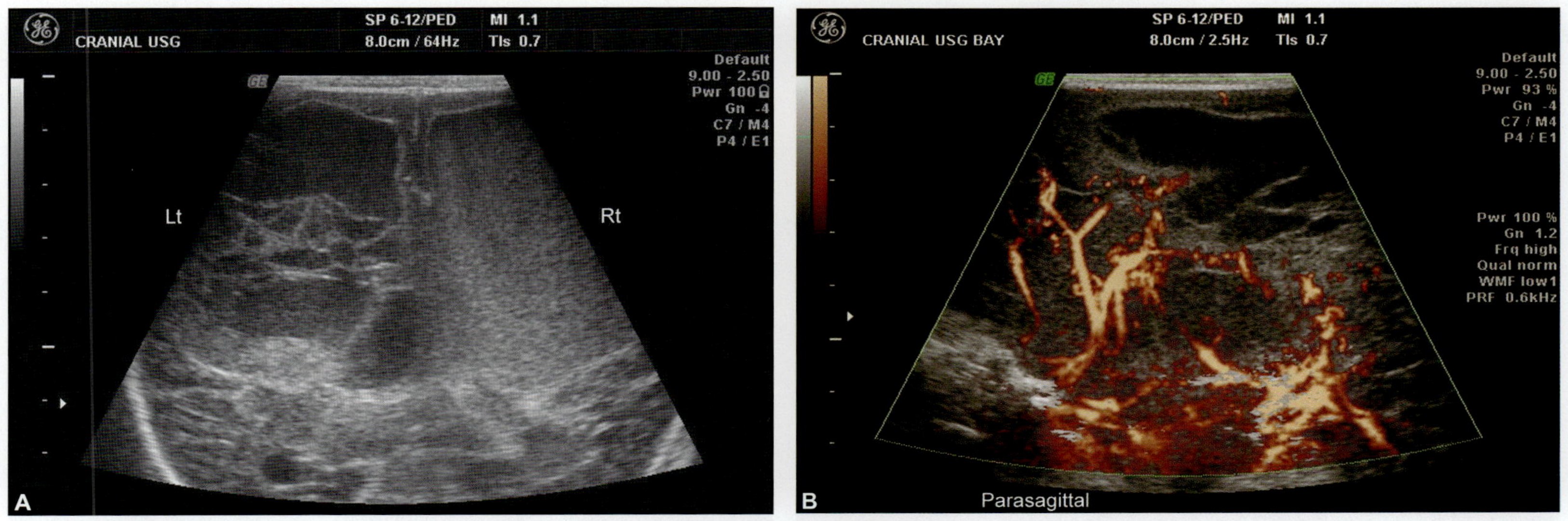

FIGURES 6.77A and B

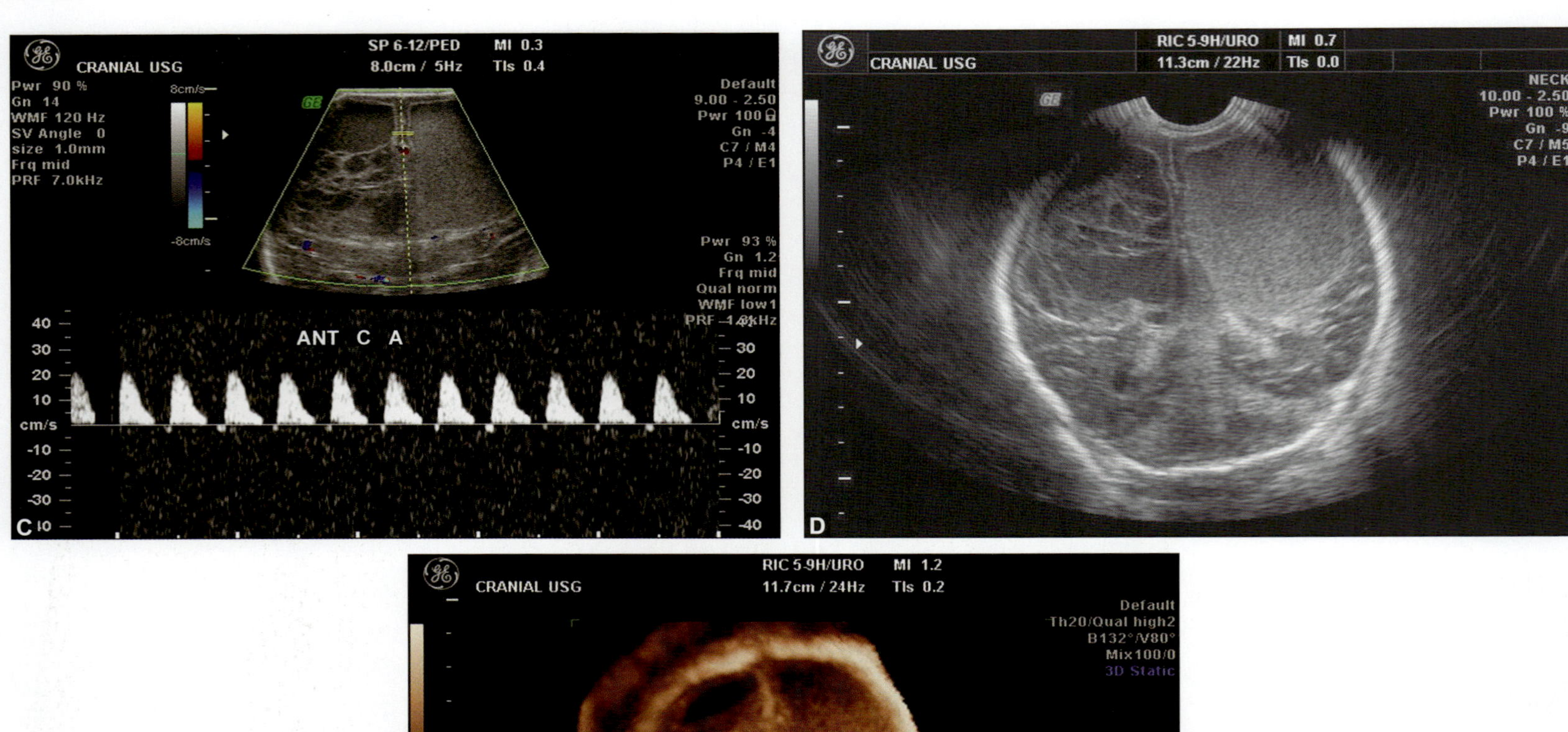

FIGURES 6.77C to E

FIGURES 6.77A to E: On color flow imaging, crowding of the vessels is seen. On spectral Doppler tracing, high resistance flow is seen in the cranial arteries because of the pressure on artery. The 3D ultrasound of the skull shows big abscess in left cortex and pyogenic collection in right side of cortex.

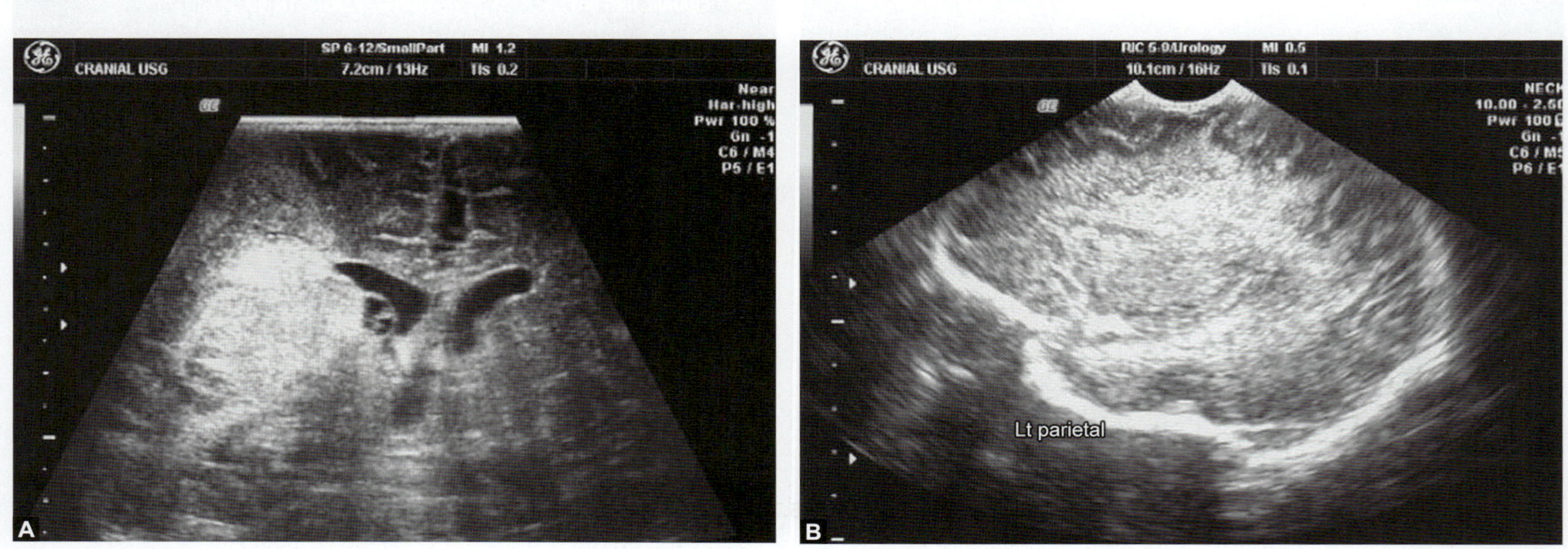

FIGURES 6.78A and B: Gross brain edema with ventriculitis. HRSG shows gross brain edema. The edematous parenchyma is wide. Sulci and gyri are effaced. Ventricles are dilated with echogenic collection. Fiber bands are also seen in the ventricles.

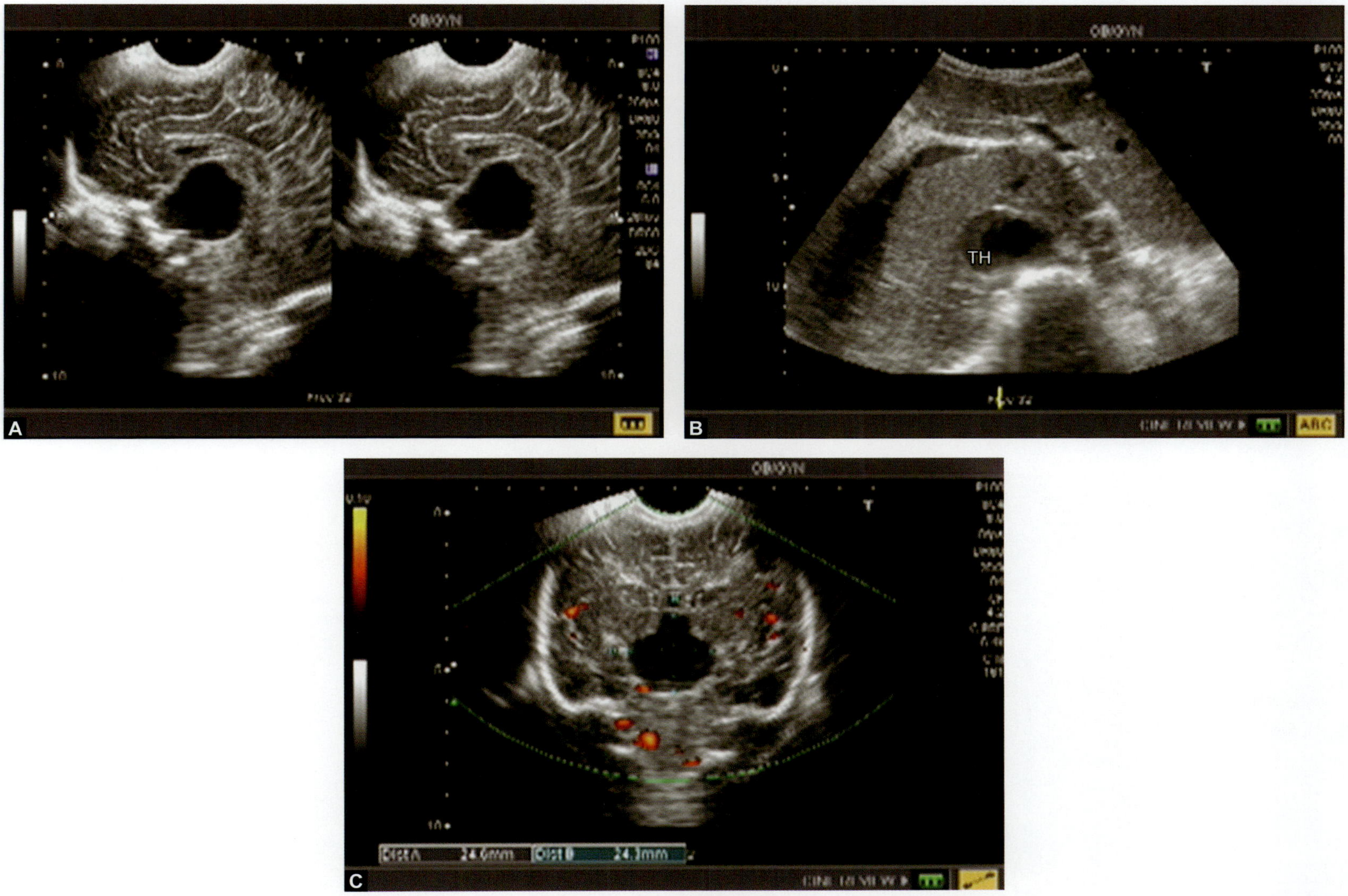

FIGURES 6.79A to C: Brain abscess with thalamic gliosis. A patient presented with low GC. HRSG shows a cystic mass in the region of thalamus suggestive of cystic degeneration of the thalamus. Associated perifocal edema is also present.

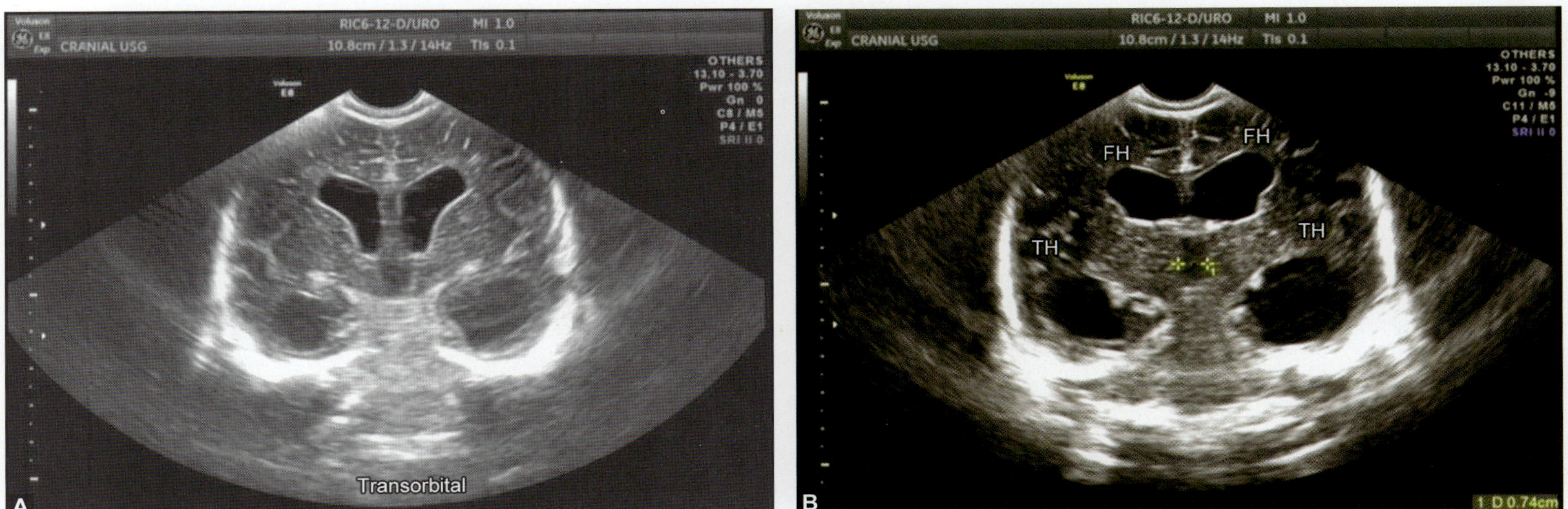

FIGURES 6.80A and B

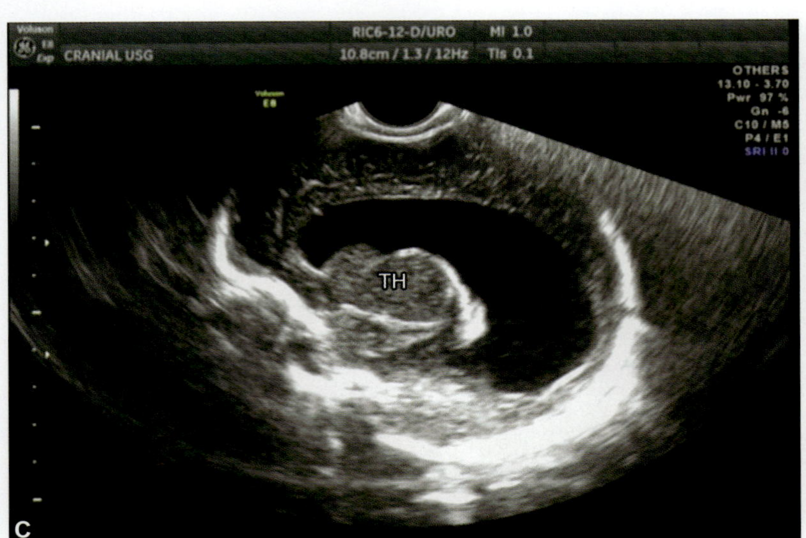

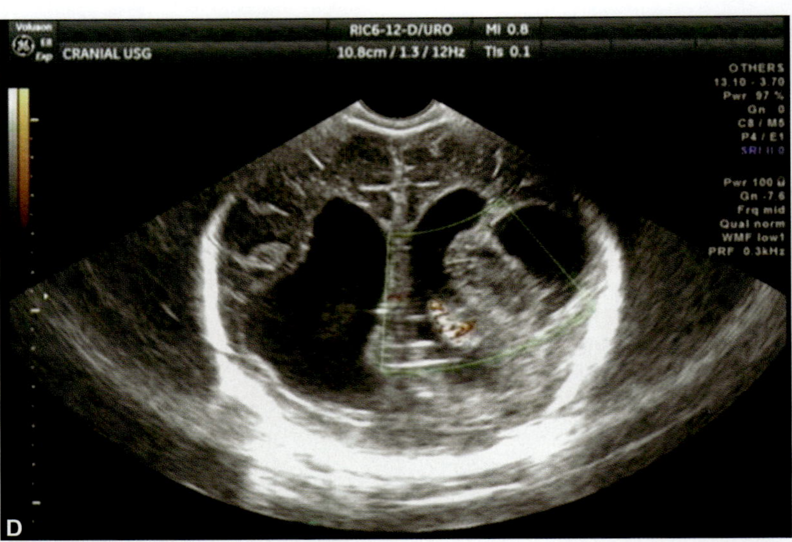

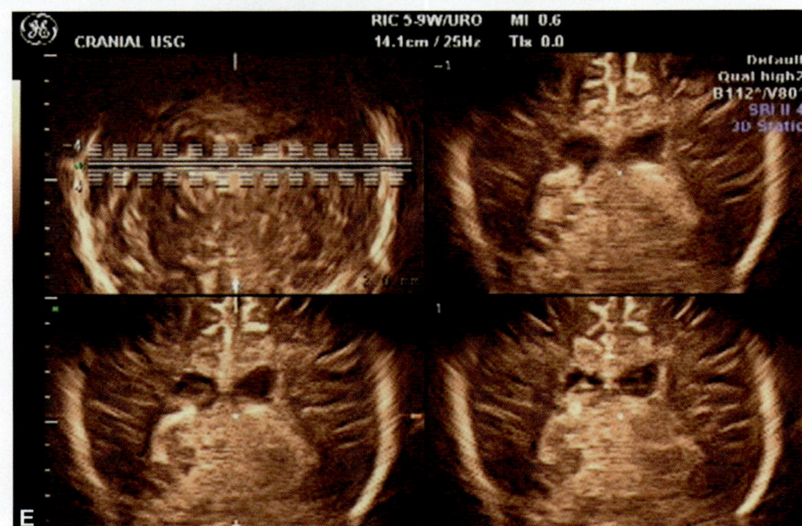

FIGURES 6.80C to E

FIGURES 6.80A to E: A patient presented with hydrocephalus involving three ventricles. The 4th ventricle was not dilated. HRSG shows an irregular ill defined echogenic mass coming out from the right ventricle. It is seen crossing the midline and obstructing the ventricles. It is highly echogenic. Few calcified foci are seen in it. The findings are suggestive of teratomatus mass.

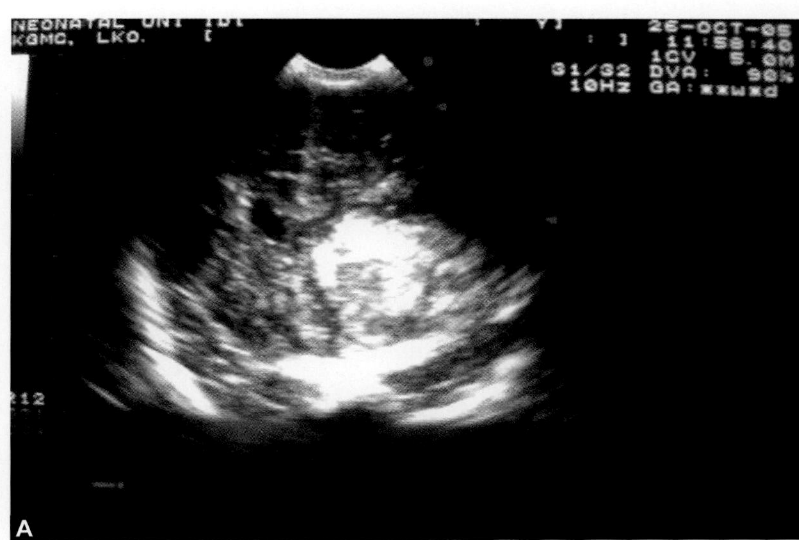

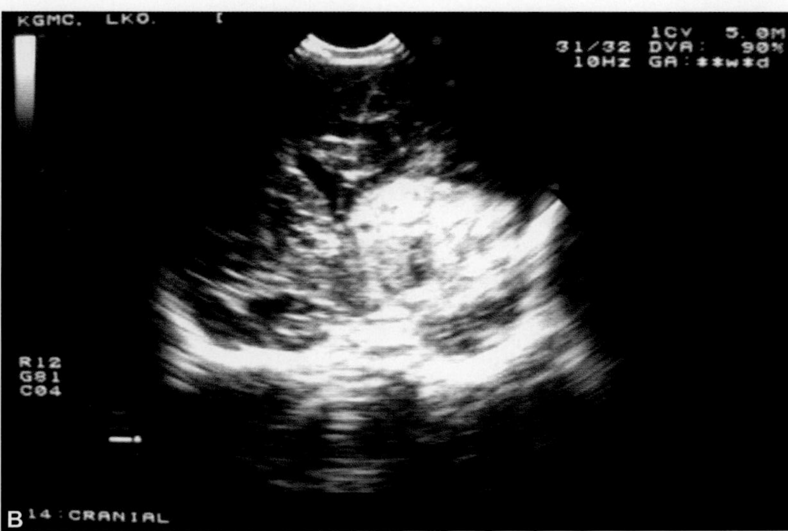

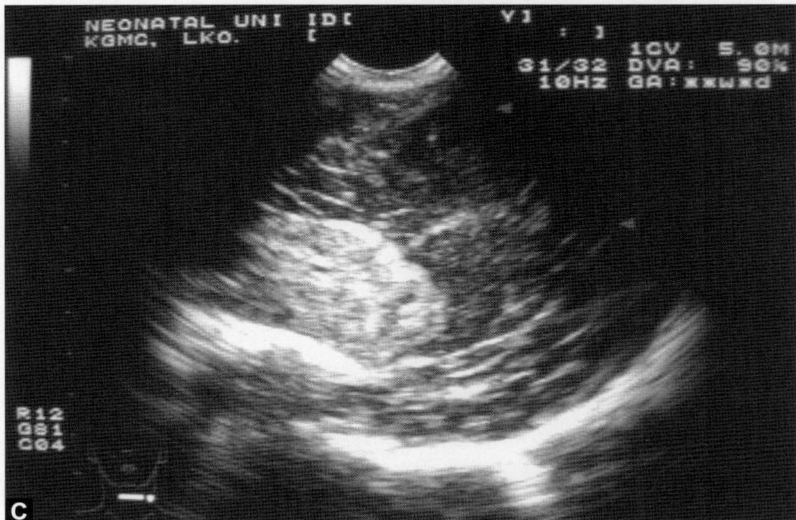

FIGURES 6.81A to C: Intracranial tumor glioma. A two-month-old child presented with fall and subsequent coma. HRSG shows a big irregular highly echogenic mass in the right parietal lobe. The mass is seen pressing over the right lateral ventricle with mass effect. The mass is seen pressing over the ventricles. Obliteration of the ventricle is seen. Contralateral shift is also seen. Biopsy of the mass confirmed glioma.

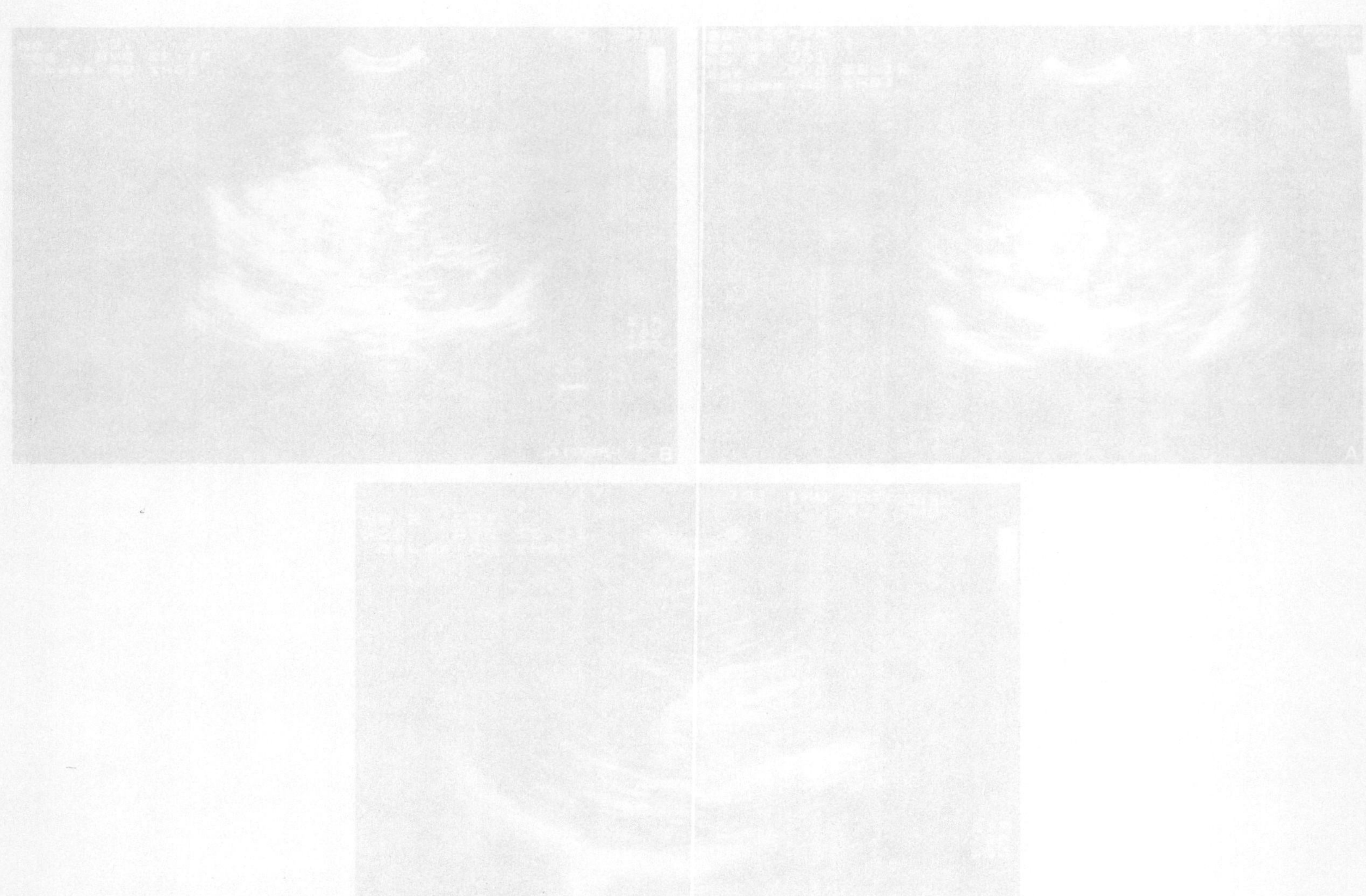

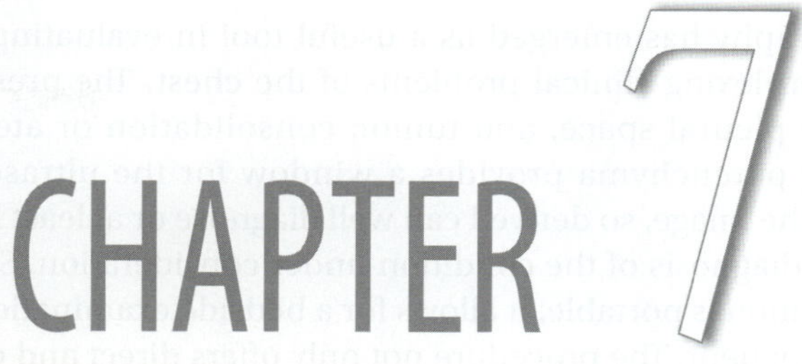

Peripheral Chest

PK Srivastava

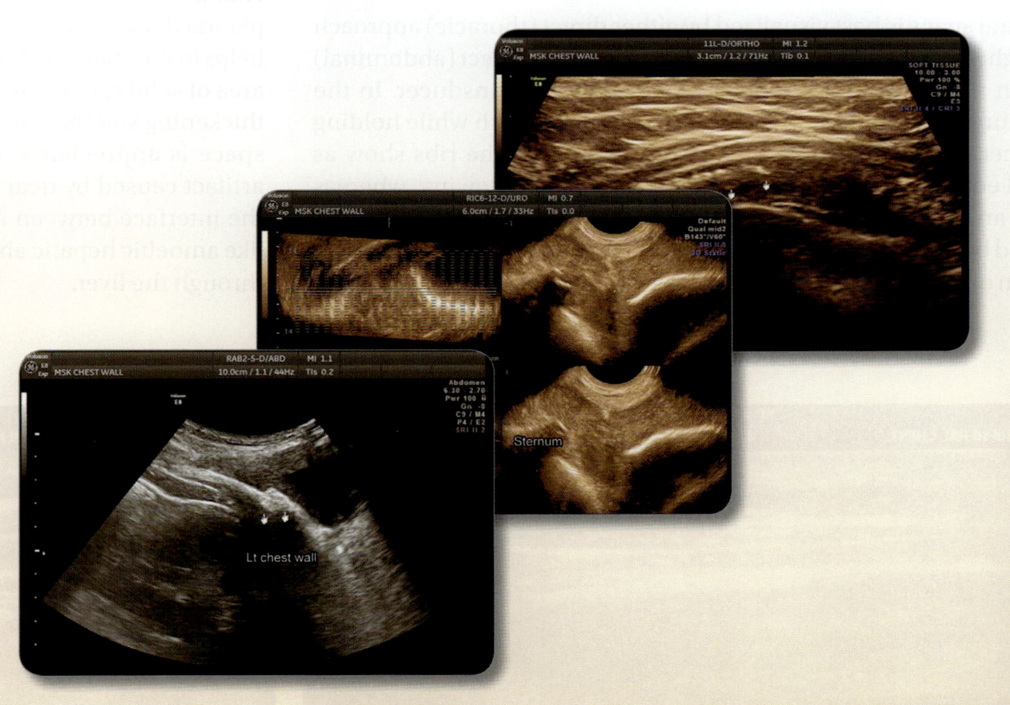

INTRODUCTION

Ultrasonography has emerged as a useful tool in evaluating a wide range of perplexing clinical problems of the chest. The presence of fluid in the pleural space, and tumor, consolidation or atelectasis in the lung parenchyma provides a window for the ultrasound to penetrate. The image, so derived can well diagnose or at least limit the differential diagnosis of the condition under consideration. Since the instrumentation is portable, it allows for a bedside examination of the critically ill patient. The procedure not only offers direct and constant visualization of pleural, parenchyma or mediastinal abnormalities, but can also facilitate and guide the safe and accurate placement of needles for diagnostic or therapeutic aspiration of pleural, parenchyma and mediastinal abnormalities, and the role and methodology of ultrasonographic-aided invasive interventions in the diagnosis and treatment.

PERIPHERAL CHEST

HRSG is excellent modality for evaluation of peripheral chest, masses like abscess formation, hematoma, parasitic cyst in the chest wall, vascular masses like hemangioma, cavernous venous malformation, Arteriovenous malformation, metastatic tumors or deposits and early rib infections like osteomyelitis and bony tumors of the rib. HRSG can tell local involvement of the chest wall or distant involvement of other organ in the same sitting. Congenital anomalies like cystic hygromas can be very well evaluated on HRSG.

PLEURAL SPACE

The pleural space is best visualized by either direct (thoracic) approach using high frequency (5 Mhz) linear transducer or indirect (abdominal) approach using lower frequency (3.5 Mhz) sector transducer. In the normal lung an examination through thoracic approach while holding transducer perpendicular to the intercostal spaces, the ribs show as rounded echogenicities with prominent acoustic shadowing, whereas parietal and visceral pleura are seen as thin bright echogenic lines separated by a dark line of normal pleural fluid. The air filled lung causes reflection of the sound beam producing a pattern of bright echoes which diminish with increasing distance from a transducer—an indicator of the air filled lung. In the abdominal (indirect) approach the normal air filled lung above the bright echogenic diaphragm is an indicator of absence of pleural fluid. A static scan encompassing large region of interest involving lower thorax and upper abdomen showing normal appearances.

A pleural effusion on ultrasonography is recognized as an area of echolucency separating the parietal and visceral pleura. With the abdominal approach, the presence of hypoechoic fluid above the diaphragm, the absence of the mirror image reflection of the liver or spleen above the diaphragm or visualizations of lung through the window created by fluid collection, are the findings that indicate the presence of a pleural effusion. As opposed to the criteria for fluid masses in the abdomen, posterior echo accentuation does not serve as an indicator of fluid in the chest because of air around the lesion. Lymphoma and leukemic involvement may show as anechoic lesion like fluid, hence warranting an optical gray scale setting using varying frequency transducers. On the contrary the complex pleural fluid show up as echogenic, making it difficult to differentiate from solid tissue. However, the ultrasonographic examination is often able to detect prominent septation of pleural spaces, which is usually missed on chest radiography or CT examination. Discrimination of pleural fluid to be transudates or exudates is usually not possible on ultrasonographic appearance alone and requires a diagnostic thoracocentesis. However, the ultrasonography can determine the appropriate site and approach for aspiration of fluid from the pleural space.

This modality also offers the means to characterize the focal pleural lesions, which may be a loculated effusion, thickened fibrous pleura of a solid pleural tumor. Presence of fluid in a lesion is suggested by moving septation or floating echogenic shadows in the lesions and change in shape with respiration. Linear plaque like calcification of pleural thickening of punctate internal calcification of the tumor further helps in the characterization of lesion. Ultrasonography can also identify area of solid tumor within the pleural effusion or a focal area of pleural thickening suitable for guided needle biopsy. Presence of air in pleural space is appreciated as bright echo with prominent reverberation artifact caused by near complete reflection of the ultrasound beam at the interface between air and tissue. The juxta diaphragmatic lesions like amoebic hepatic abscess with thoracic complications are well seen through the liver.

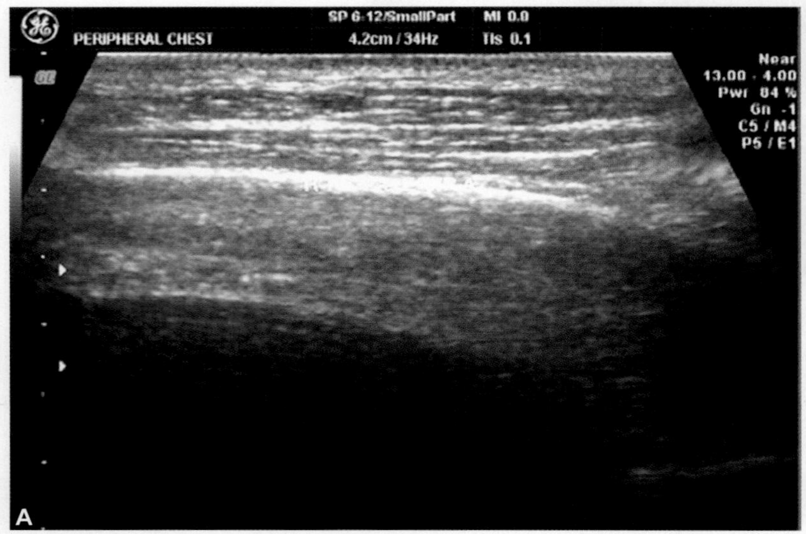

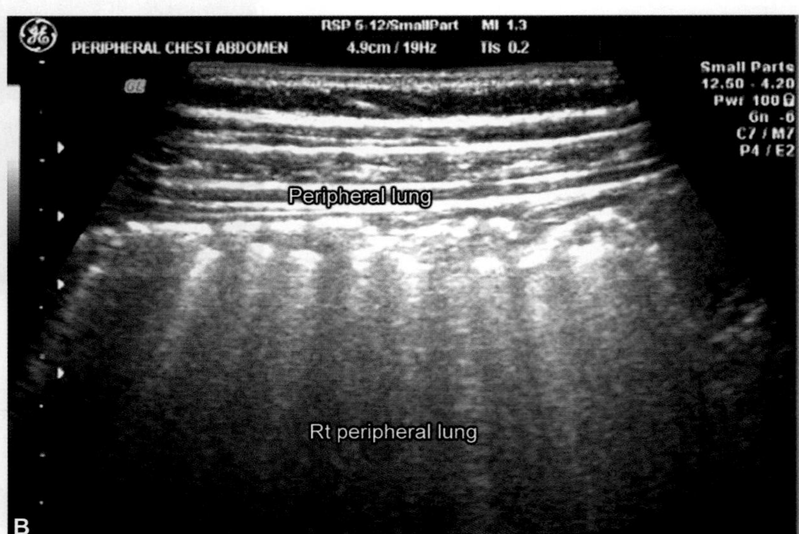

FIGURES 7.1A and B

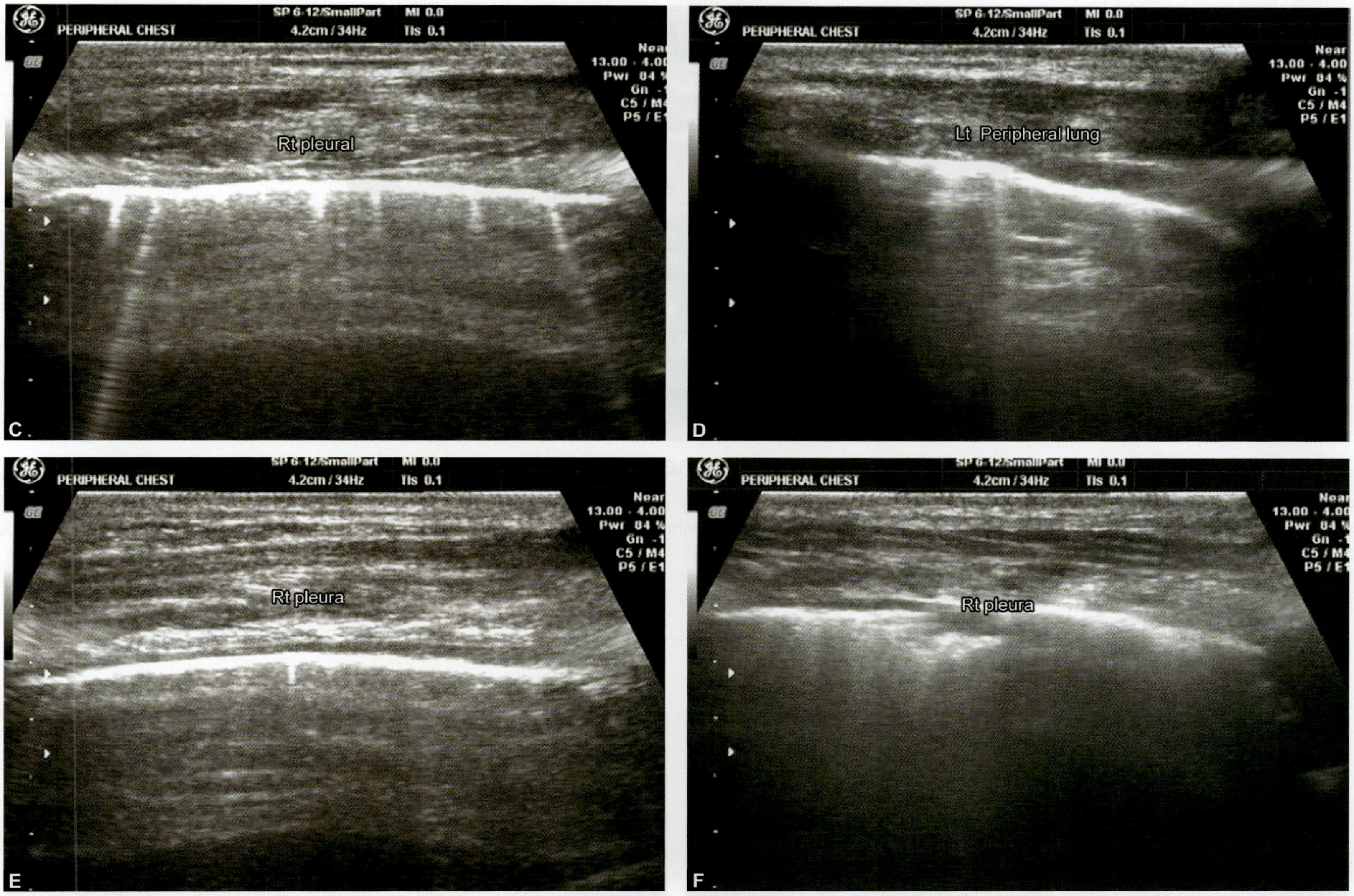

FIGURES 7.1C to F

FIGURES 7.1A to F: HRSG shows bright echogenic line representing the pleura. Parietal and visceral layers are not separated in normal conditions. The peripheral lung is seen bright soft tissue interface on high-resolution ultrasound. On HRSG pleural shadow shows artifacts due to interposing ribs. Rib shadow casting the acoustic shadowing. HRSG shows bright interface of the peripheral lung. Bright echogenic shadows are seen in the peripheral lung with comet tail artifacts due to air filled lung. Subcutaneous tissue is well visualized. The echogenic strip of bright echoes shows the pleural layer. Reverberation artifacts are seen posterior to the pleural shadow.

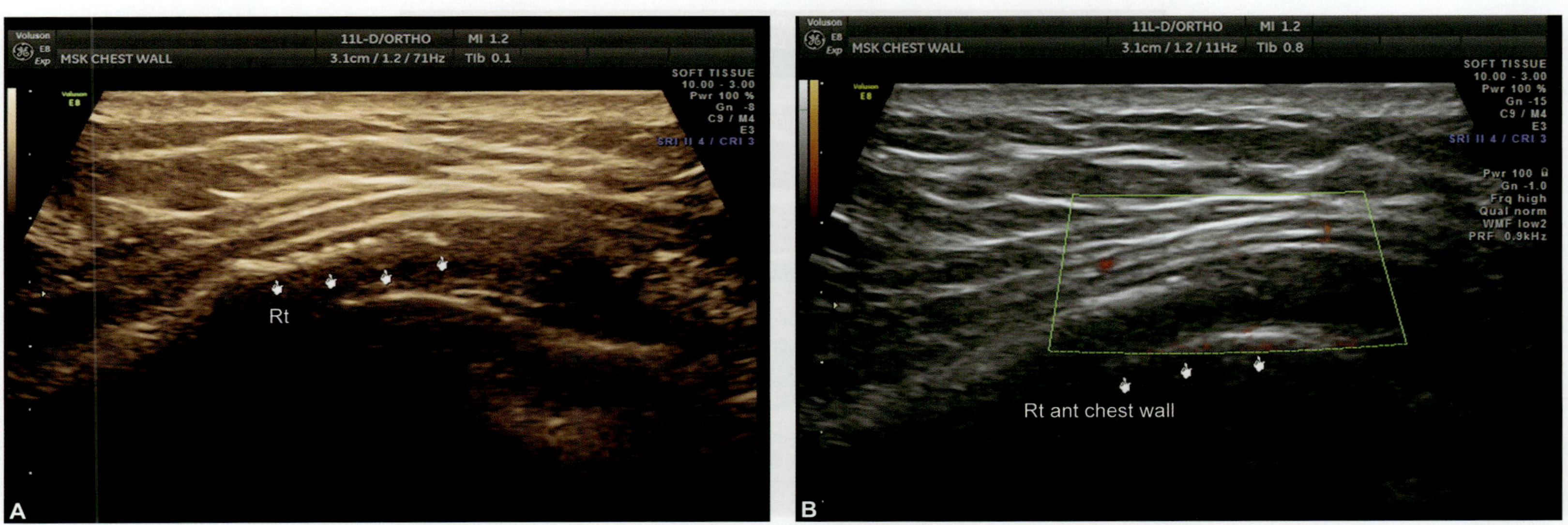

FIGURES 7.2A and B

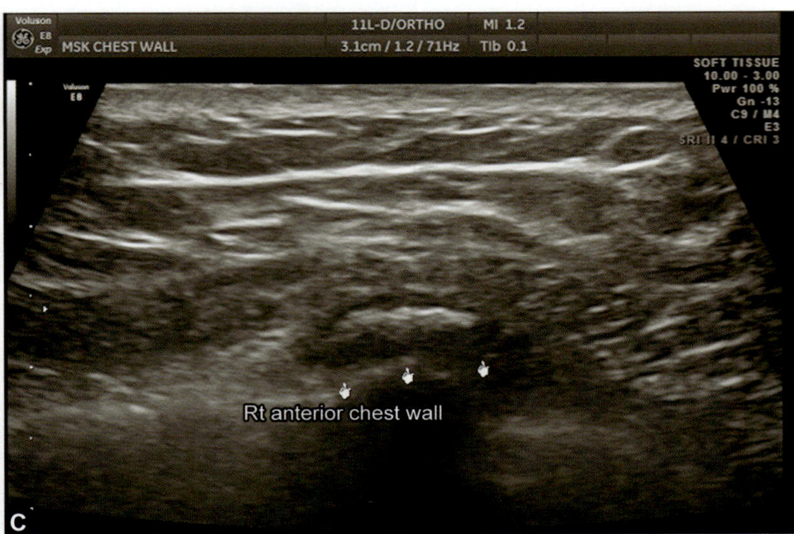

FIGURE 7.2C

FIGURES 7.2A to C: A patient presented with soft tissue swelling over the right anterior chest wall. HRSG shows an echogenic linear calcified shadow in the intercostal muscle. It is accompanied with acoustic shadowing. No perifocal edema is seen in it. Findings are suggestive of amorphous calcification in the chest wall muscle.

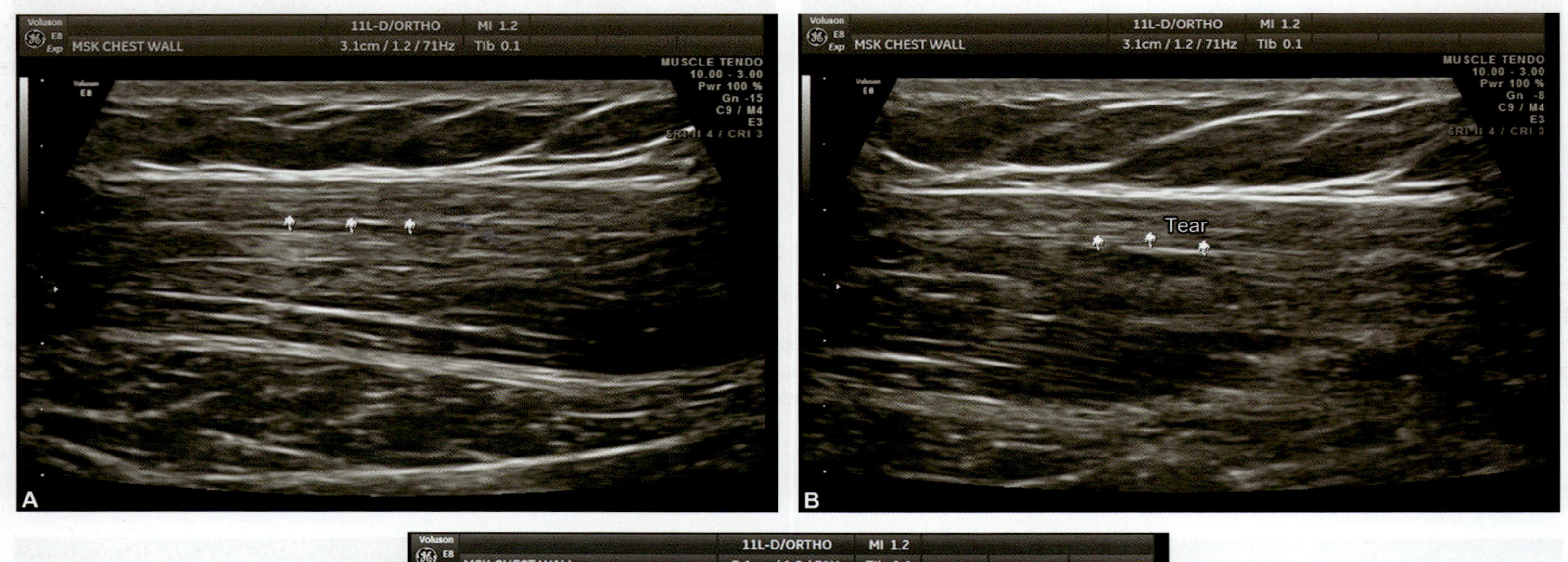

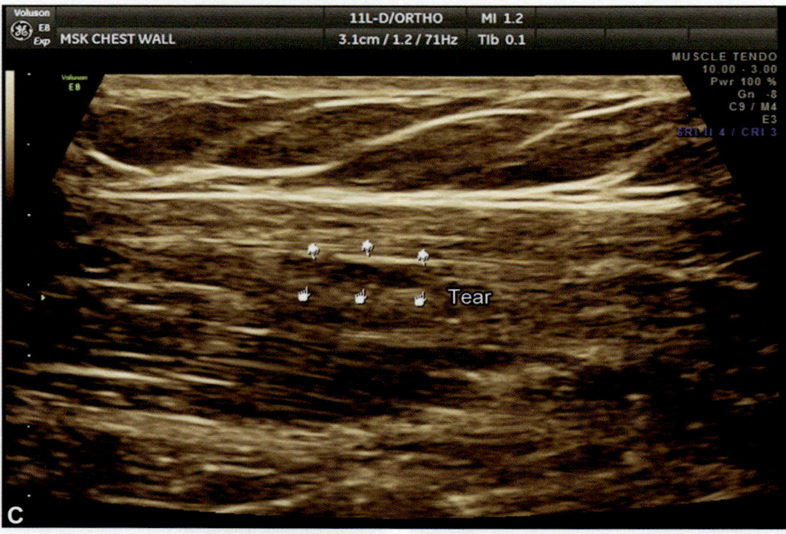

FIGURES 7.3A to C: Intercostal muscle tear. A patient presented with pain in the left intercostal region. HRSG shows a hypoechoic cleft in the intercostal muscle suggestive of intercostal muscle tear.

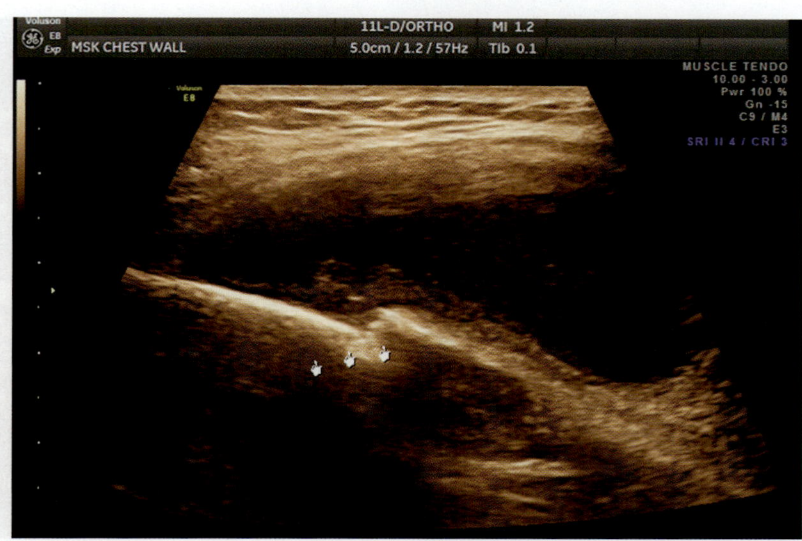

FIGURE 7.4: Rib fracture with hematoma formation. A patient sustained anterior chest wall trauma on left side. HRSG show fracture of the rib. The fractured segments are seen in apposition.

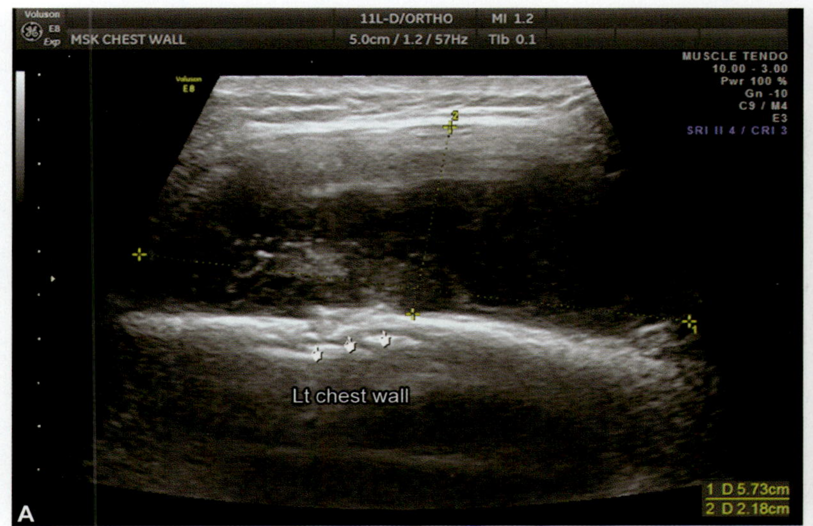

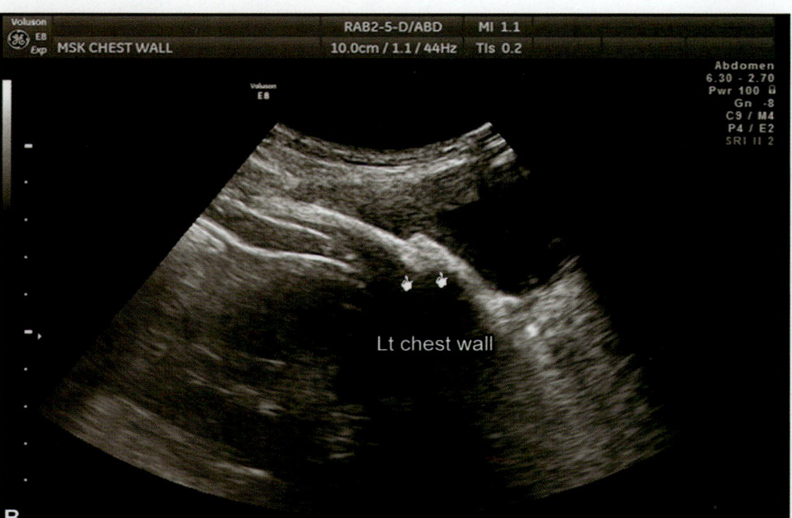

FIGURES 7.5A and B: There is also evidence of low level echo collection seen anterior to fractured rib. Thick echoes are seen in it suggestive of hematoma formation.

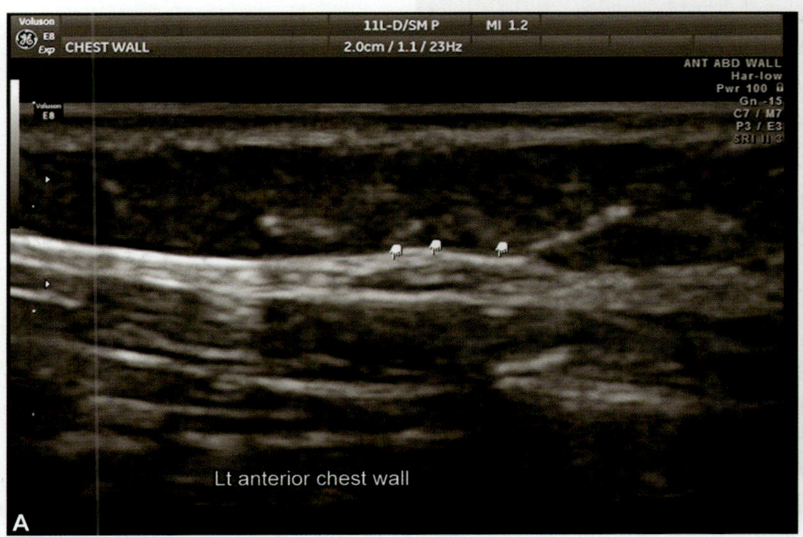

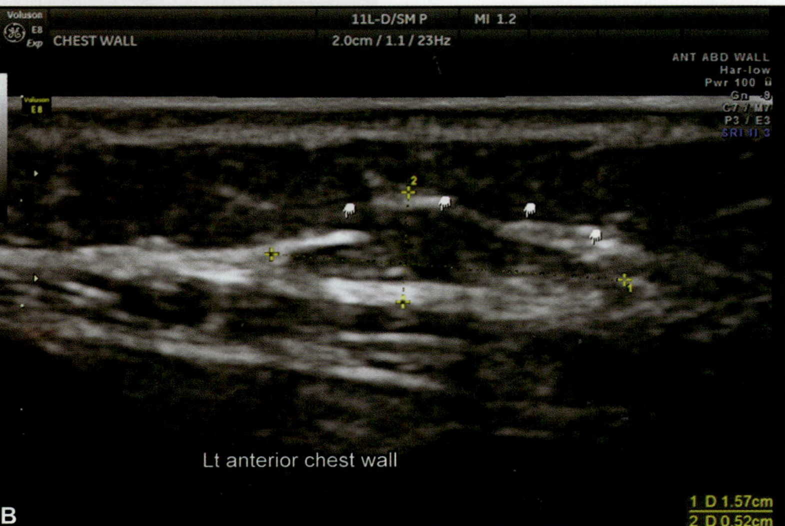

FIGURES 7.6A and B

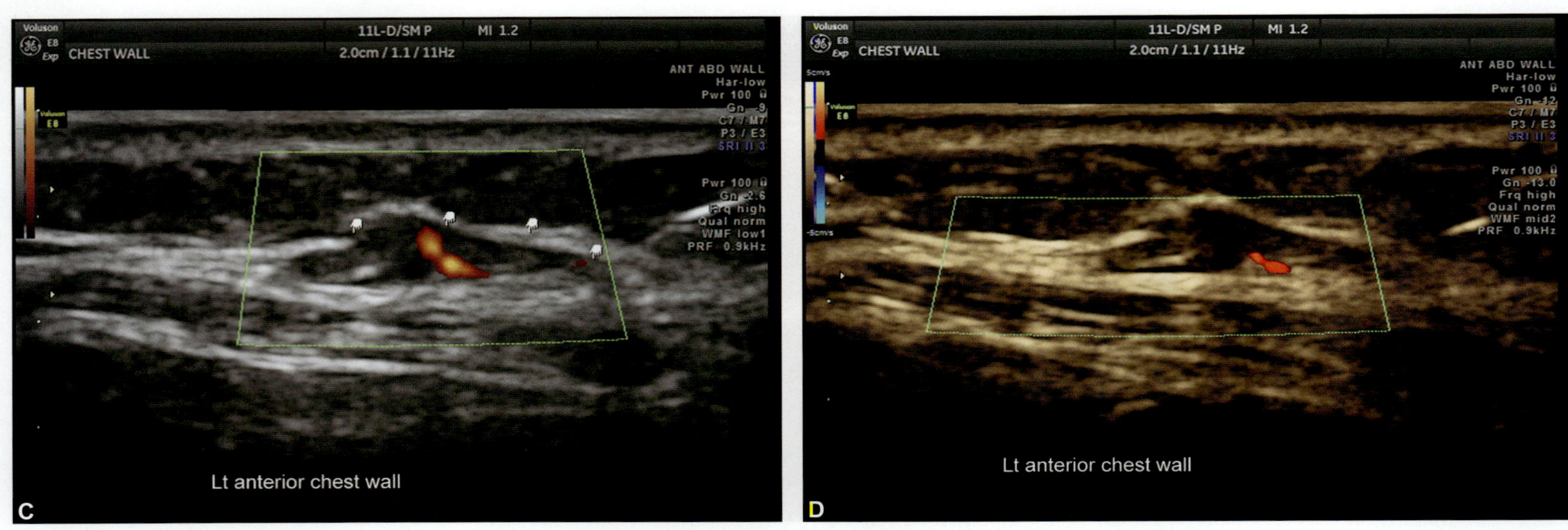

FIGURES 7.6C and D

FIGURES 7.6A to D: HRSG shows an irregular ill defined hypoechoic soft tissue shadow in relation to the superior border of the 8th rib. The rib shows thinning with evidence of erosion of the bony surface. The lesion is expansile in nature. Few vessels are seen feeding it. Biopsy of the mass shows chronic granulomatous disease suggestive of tuberculosis.

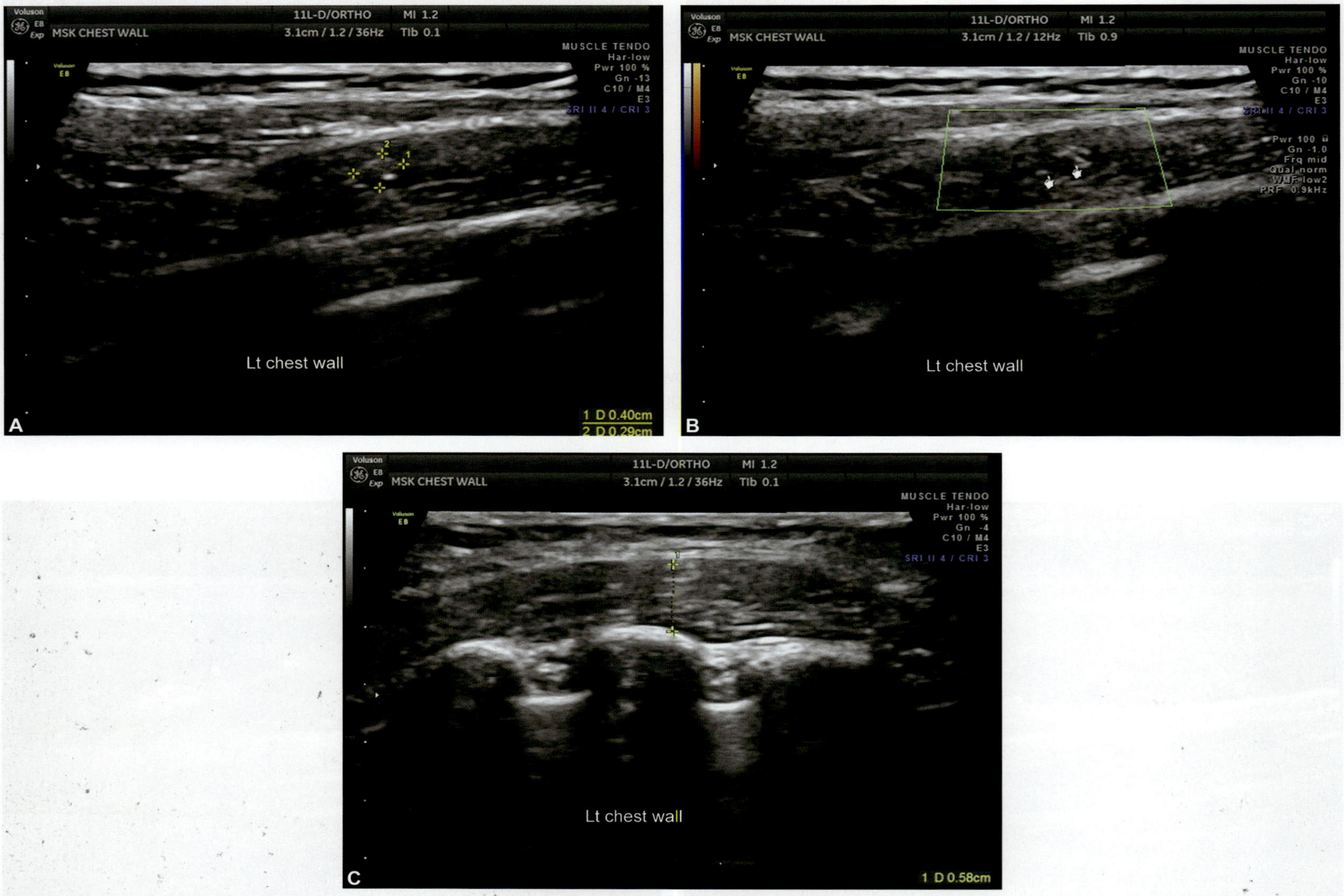

FIGURES 7.7A to C: A young girl presented with soft tissue trauma to left anterior chest wall with painful nodular shadow. HRSG shows an irregular ill-defined nodular mass in the intercostal muscle. Echogenic foci are seen in the mass. But no perifocal edema is seen. Findings are suggestive of old muscle tear with calcification in the process of healing.

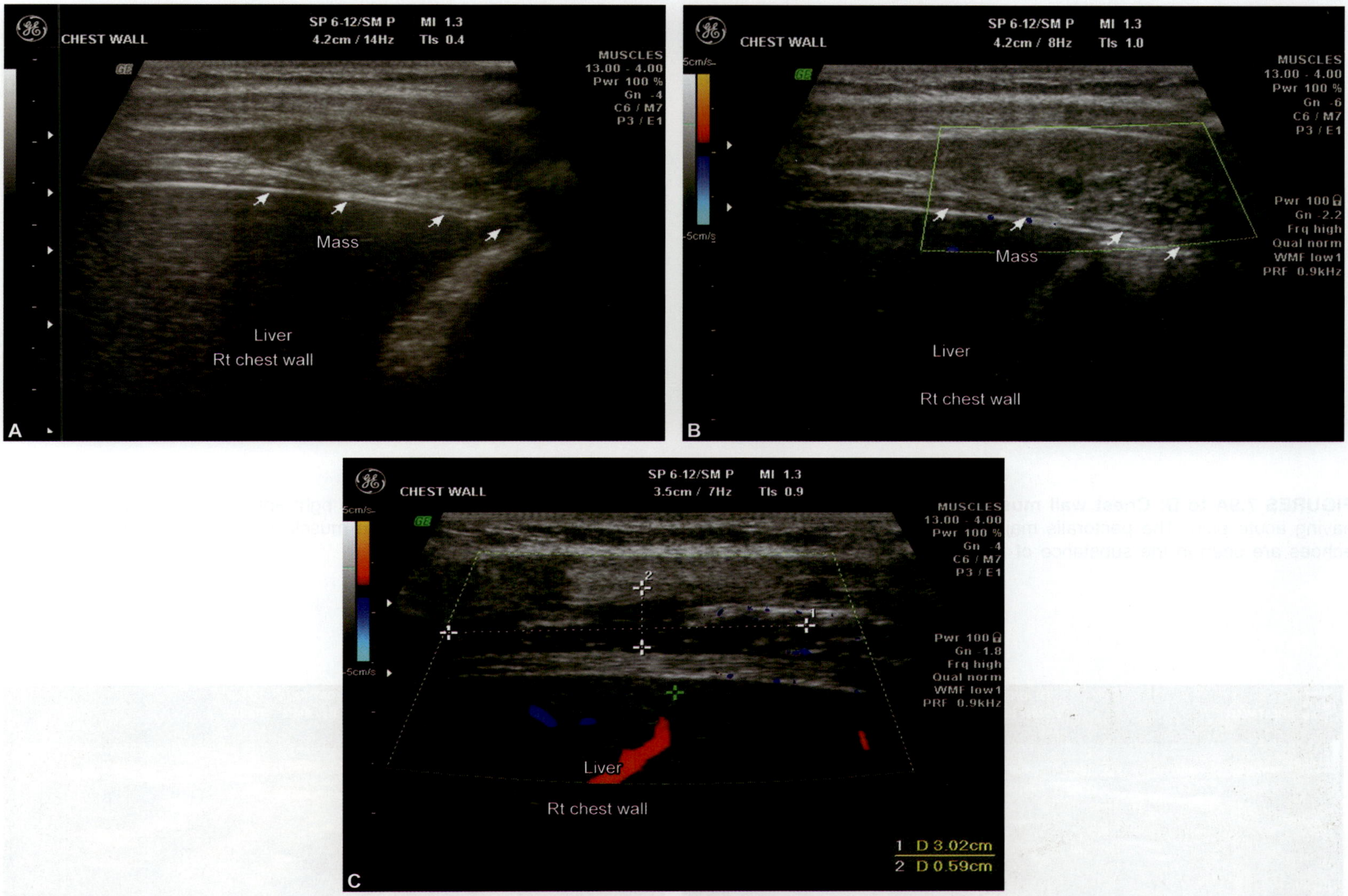

FIGURES 7.8A to C: Chest wall abscess. A young boy presented with soft tissue swelling over the right anterior chest wall. HRSG shows low level echo complex mass in the anterior chest wall. Thick wall is seen around it with central area of necrosis. Associated perifocal edema was presented suggestive of chest wall abscess.

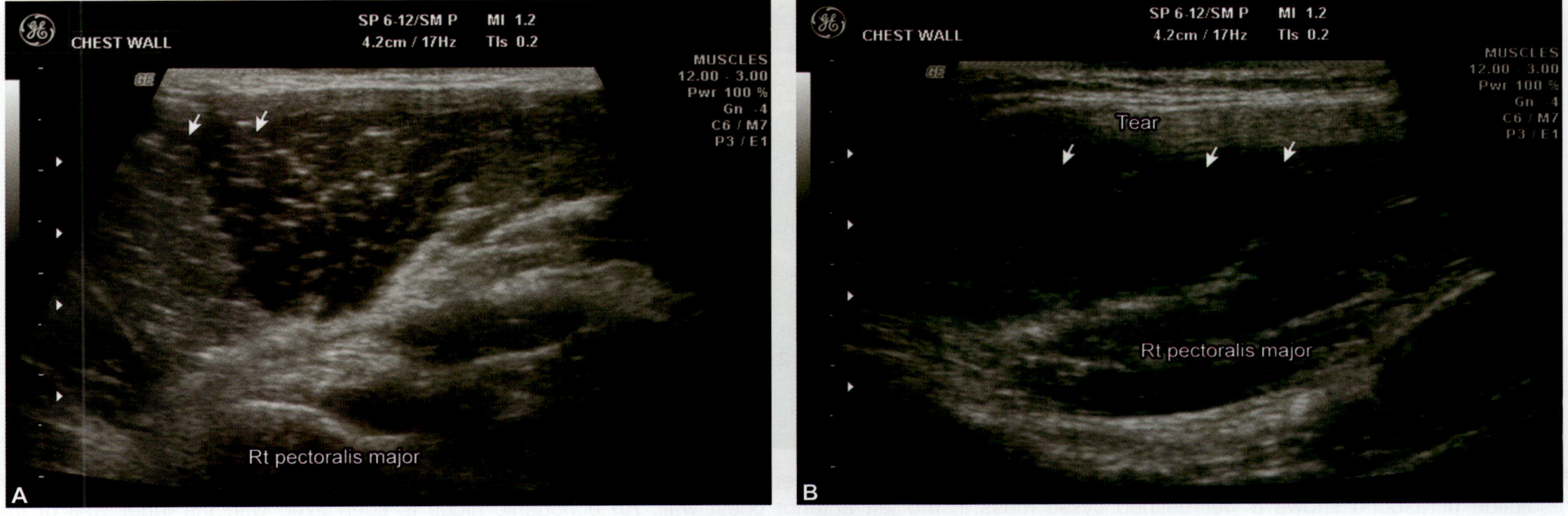

FIGURES 7.9A and B

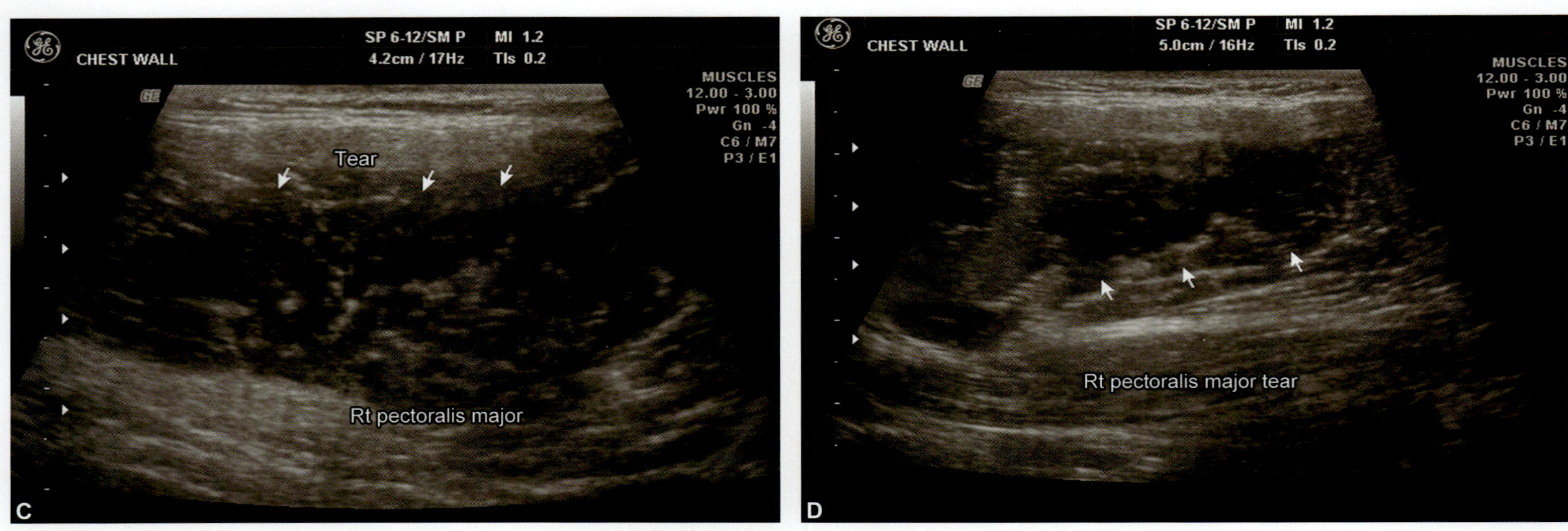

FIGURES 7.9C and D

FIGURES 7.9A to D: Chest wall muscle tear. A 20-year-old man presented with soft tissue swelling over the right anterior chest wall. He was also having acute pain. The pectoralis major muscle is markedly edematous and inhomogeneous in texture. The muscle fibers are seen torn. Low level echoes are seen in the substance of muscle suggestive of big muscle tear with hematoma formation.

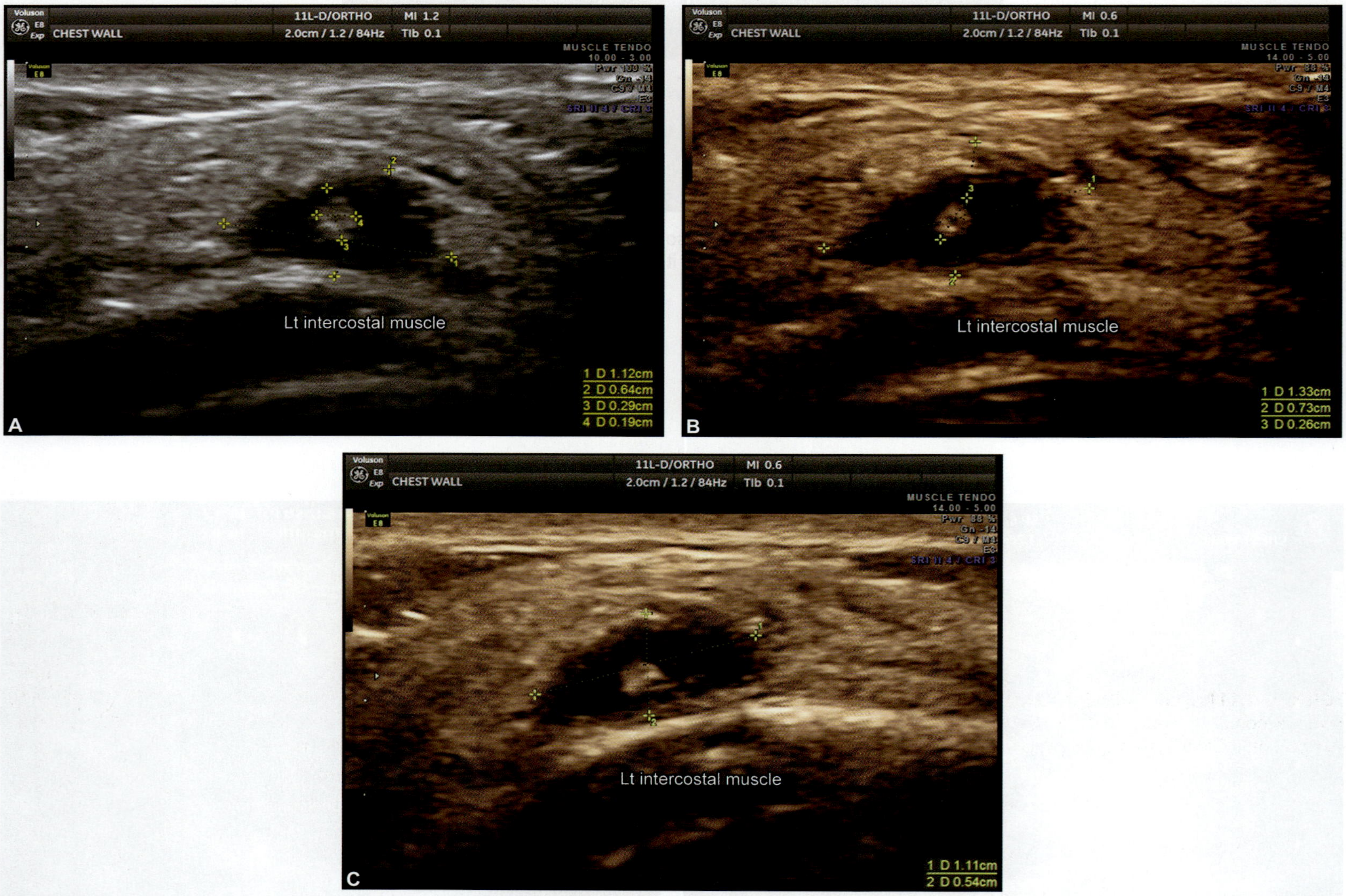

FIGURES 7.10A to C: Cysticercus cyst in intercostal muscle. A patient presented with soft tissue swelling in the left anterior chest wall. High resolution ultrasound shows a well-defined cystic mass in the left anterior chest wall. An echogenic nidus is seen fixed with the inner wall of the cyst suggestive of cysticercus cyst.

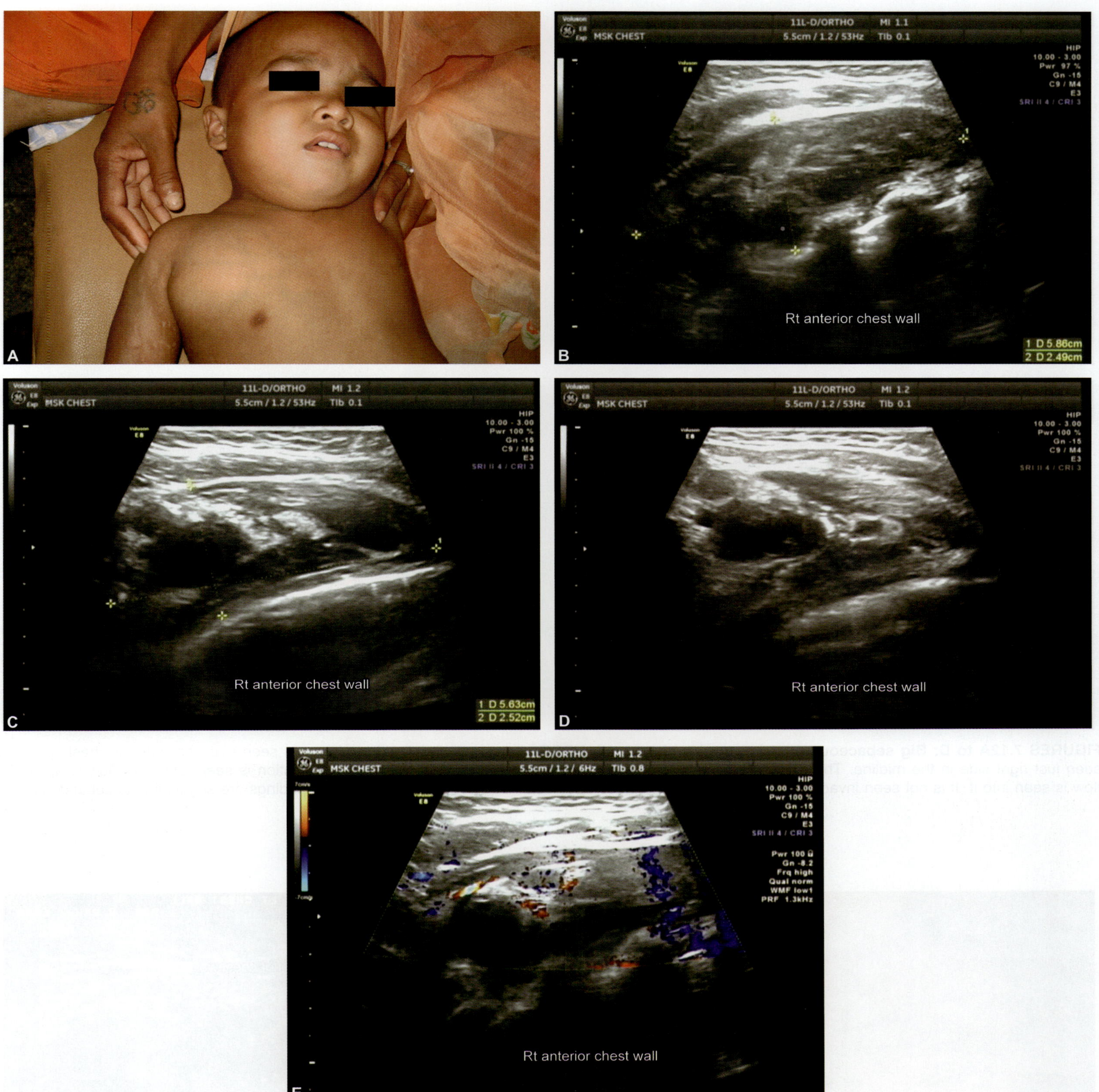

FIGURES 7.11A to E: Anterior chest wall abscess. A 1.5-year-old baby presented with soft tissue swelling over the right anterior chest wall. HRSG shows a complex echo mass in the anterior chest wall. It shows heterogeneous texture. Central area of necrosis is seen in it. Perifocal edema is also present. On color flow imaging, poor flow is seen in it. Findings are suggestive of chest wall abscess.

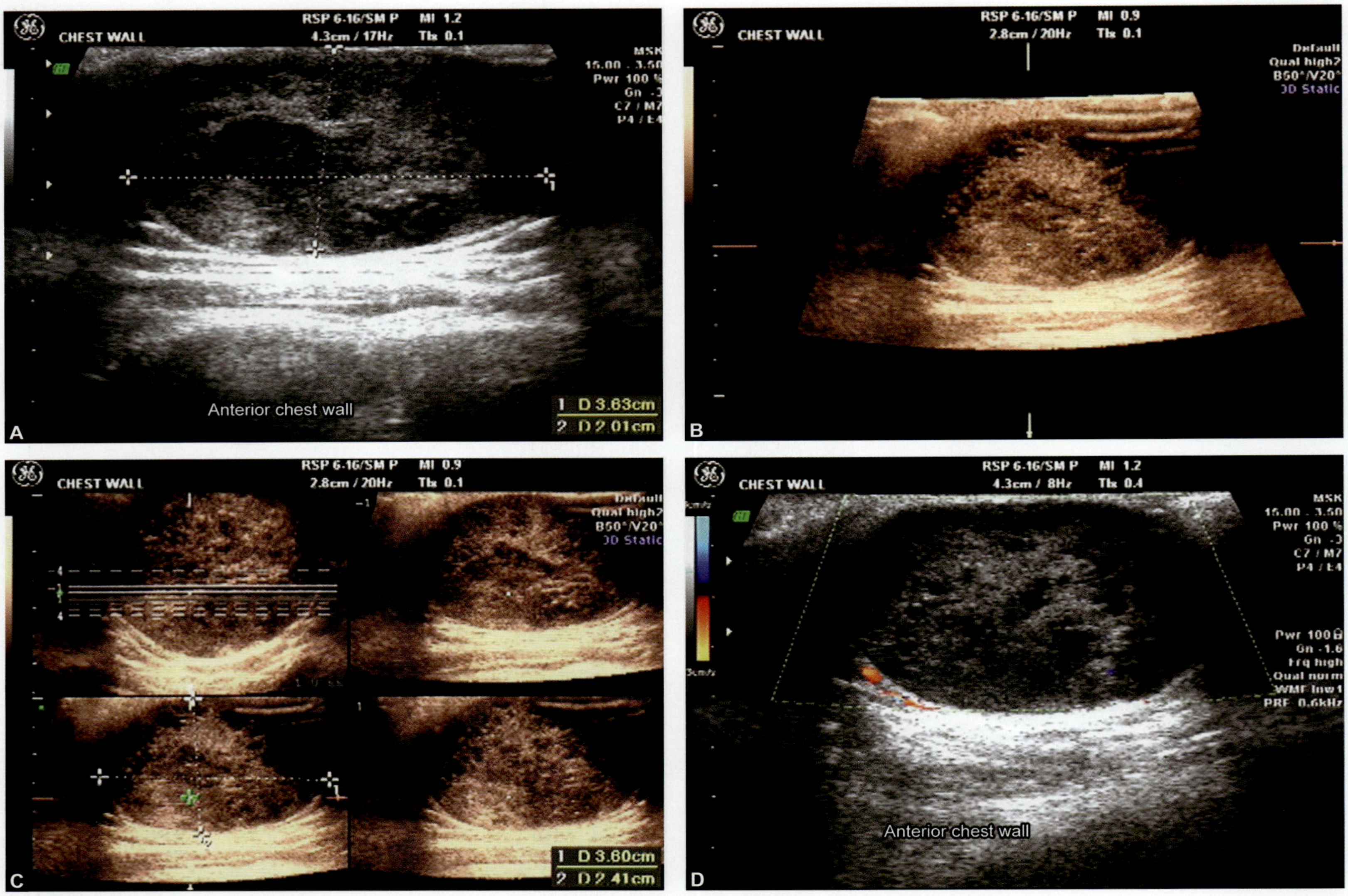

FIGURES 7.12A to D: Big sebaceous cyst in anterior chest wall. HRSG shows a well-defined cystic mass seen over the anterior chest wall. It is seen just right side in the midline. Thick jelly like echoes is seen into it. But no septation is seen. No calcification is seen. On color flow imaging, no flow is seen into it. It is not seen invading the chest wall muscle. It is seen confined to subcutaneous plane. Findings are suggestive of sebaceous cyst.

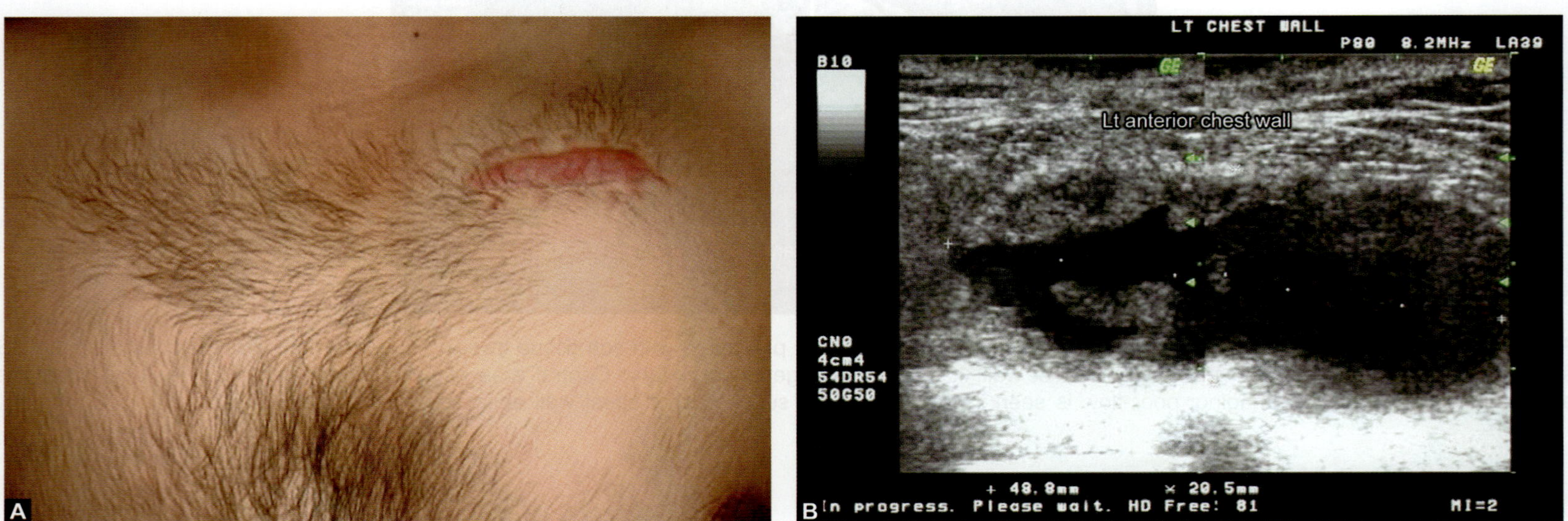

FIGURES 7.13A and B

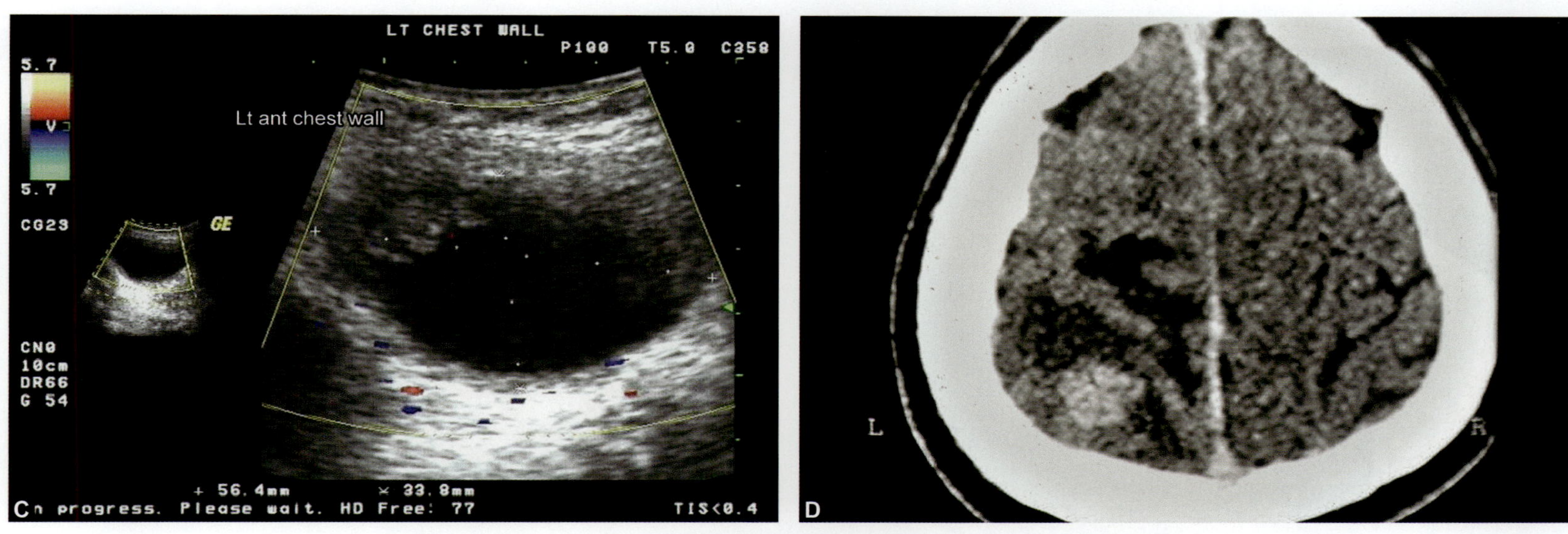

FIGURES 7.13C and D

FIGURES 7.13A to D: Tubercular abscess anterior chest wall muscle. A young boy presented with soft tissue swelling over the left anterior chest wall. HRSG shows low-level echo collection in the muscle. Thick echogenic wall is seen around it. Debris is also seen. No perifocal edema is present indicating a cold abscess. Cranial CT of the same patient shows a hyperdense focus in the left parietal lobe with perifocal edema suggestive of tuberculoma.

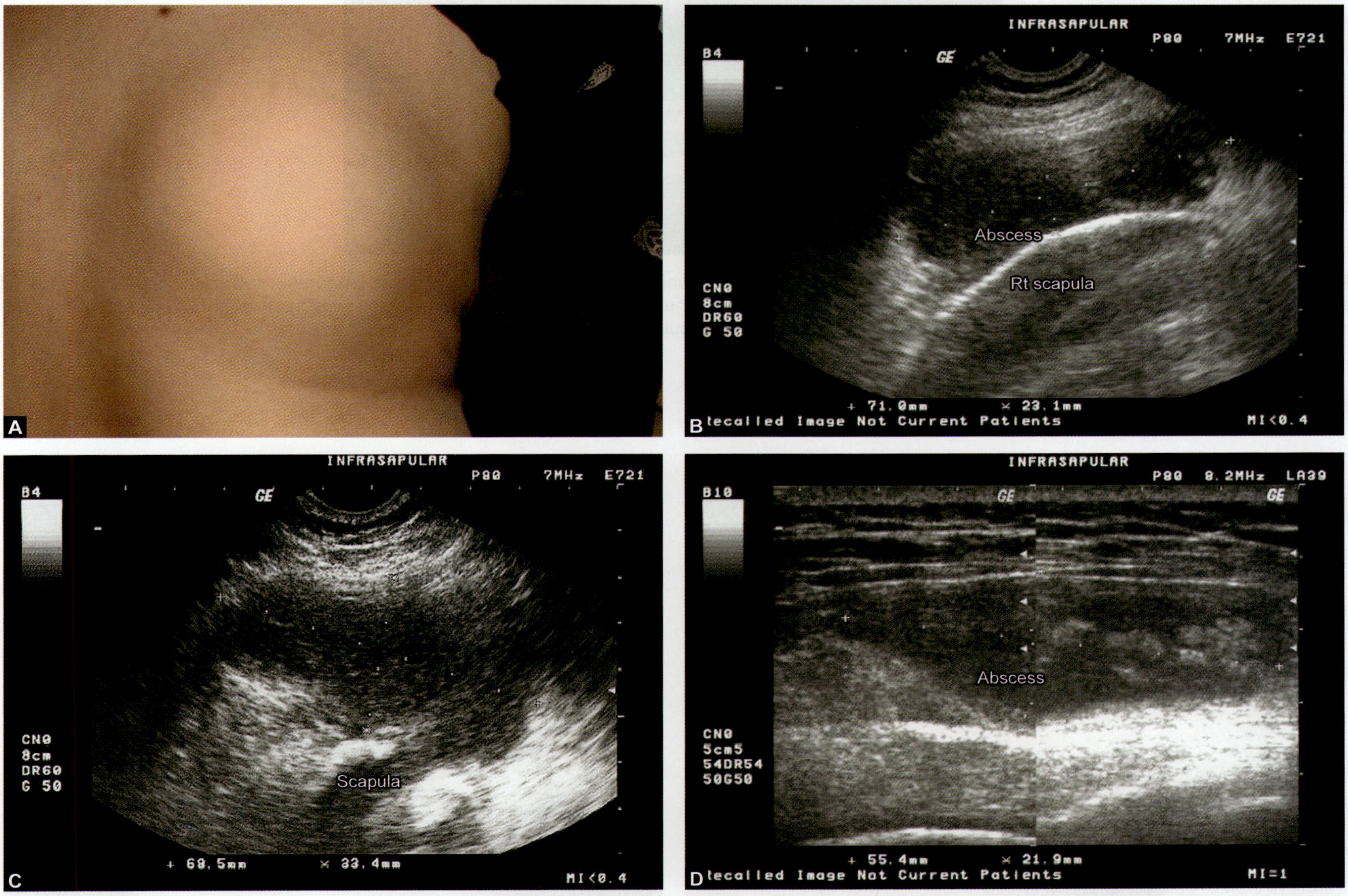

FIGURES 7.14A to D: Tubercular abscess over the right scapular region. A young girl presented with soft tissue non-tender mass lesion over the right Infrascapular region over the posterolateral chest wall. HRSG shows a low level echo complex mass over the infrascapular region. No perifocal edema is present. The inferior border of the scapula shows bony destruction. The collection turns out to be chronic inflammatory abscess suggestive of tubercular abscess. The abscess is also seen extending in to the right paraspinal muscles. Central area of necrosis is seen in it. But no perifocal edema is present.

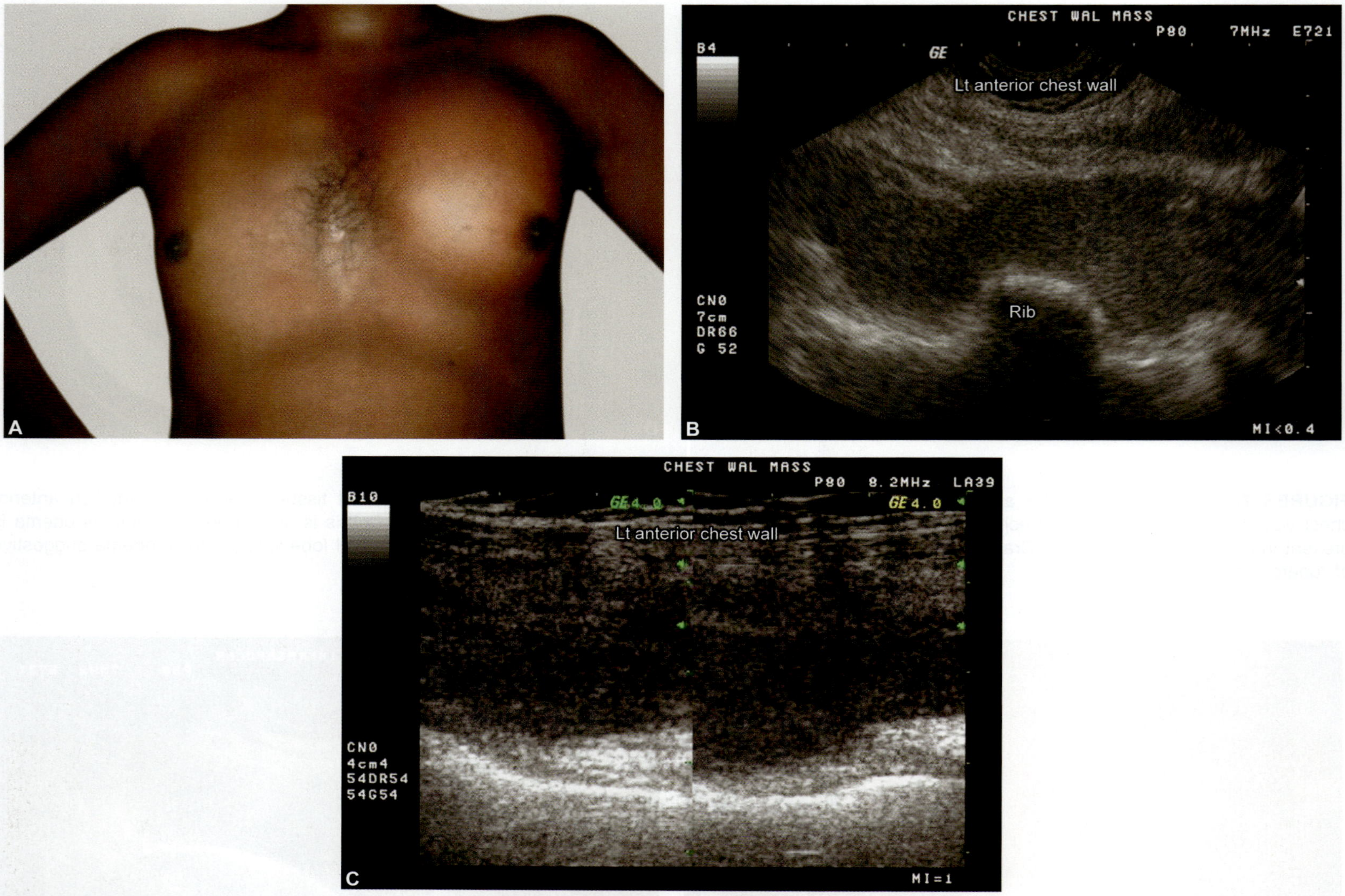

FIGURES 7.15A to C: Tubercular abscess anterior chest wall. A young man presented with painless non-tender soft tissue mass over the left anterior chest wall. HRSG shows thick low-level echo cystic mass over the anterior chest wall. Thick collection is seen in it. However, the collection is not seen eroding the rib or the bony cage. Aspiration confirmed tubercular abscess.

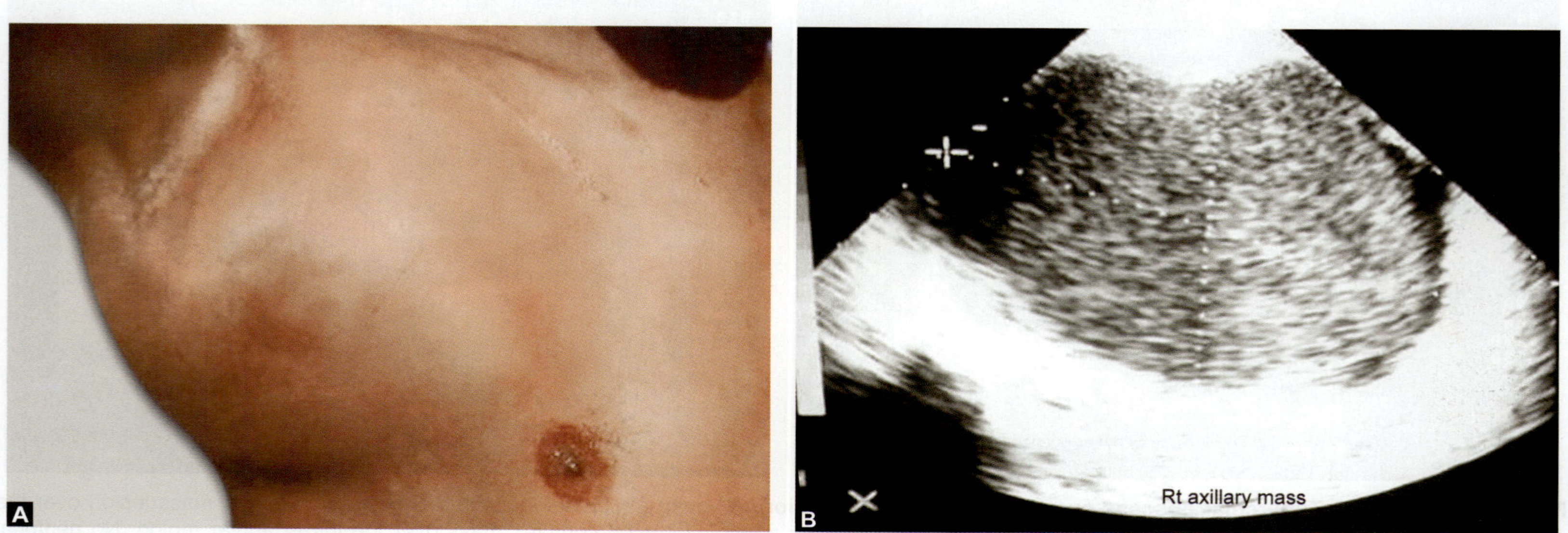

FIGURES 7.16A and B: Pyogenic abscess. A young man presented with a big tender over the right anterior chest wall and extending to the axilla. HRSG shows a low level echo complex mass. Homogeneous collection is seen in it. Layering sign is positive. Perifocal edema is present. No septation or loculation is seen in the mass suggestive of a big pyogenic abscess.

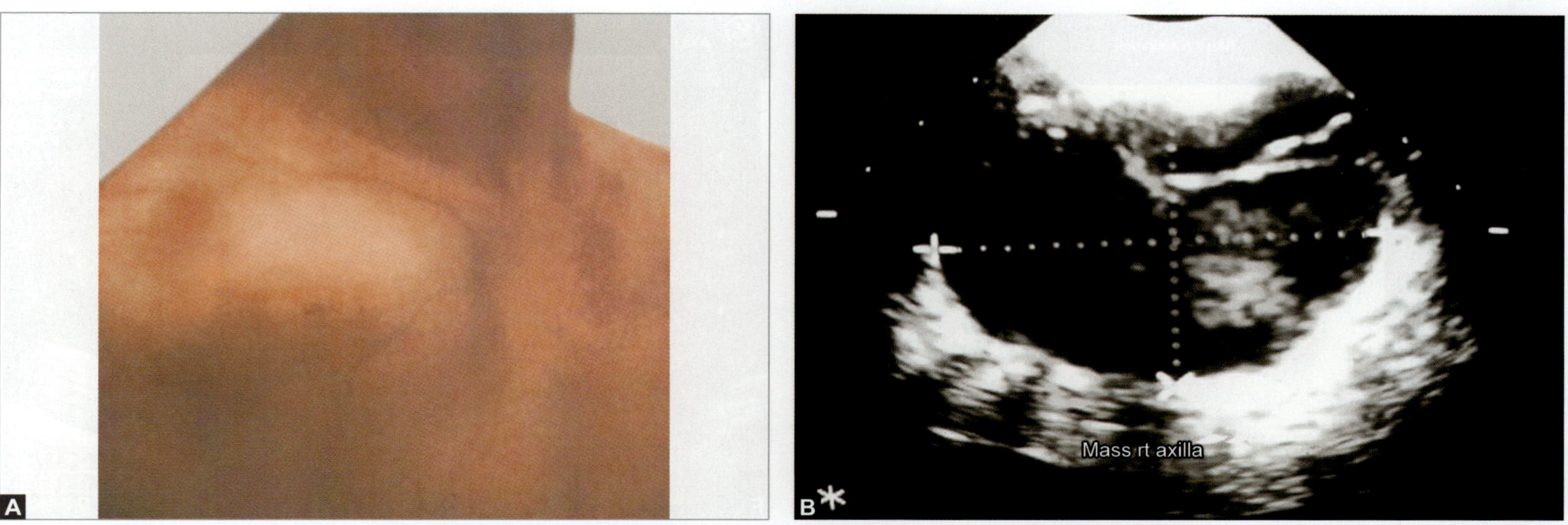

FIGURES 7.17A and B: Hydatid cyst in the infraclavicular region. A young man presented with a soft tissue mass over the right infraclavicular region. HRSG shows a well-defined cystic mass. Echogenic membrane is seen floating in the cyst suggestive of hydatid cyst. Low-level echo collection is also seen in it

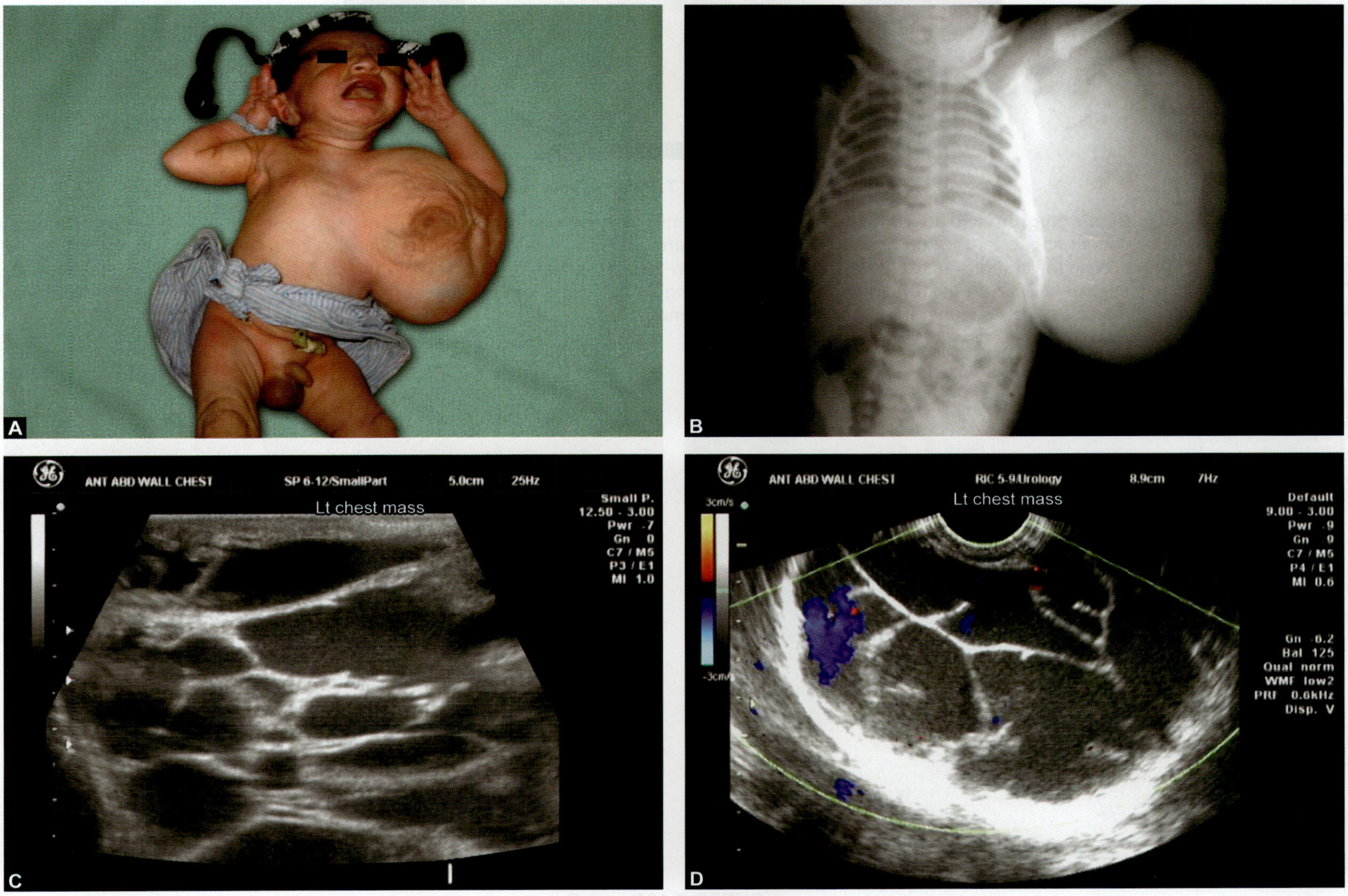

FIGURES 7.18A to D

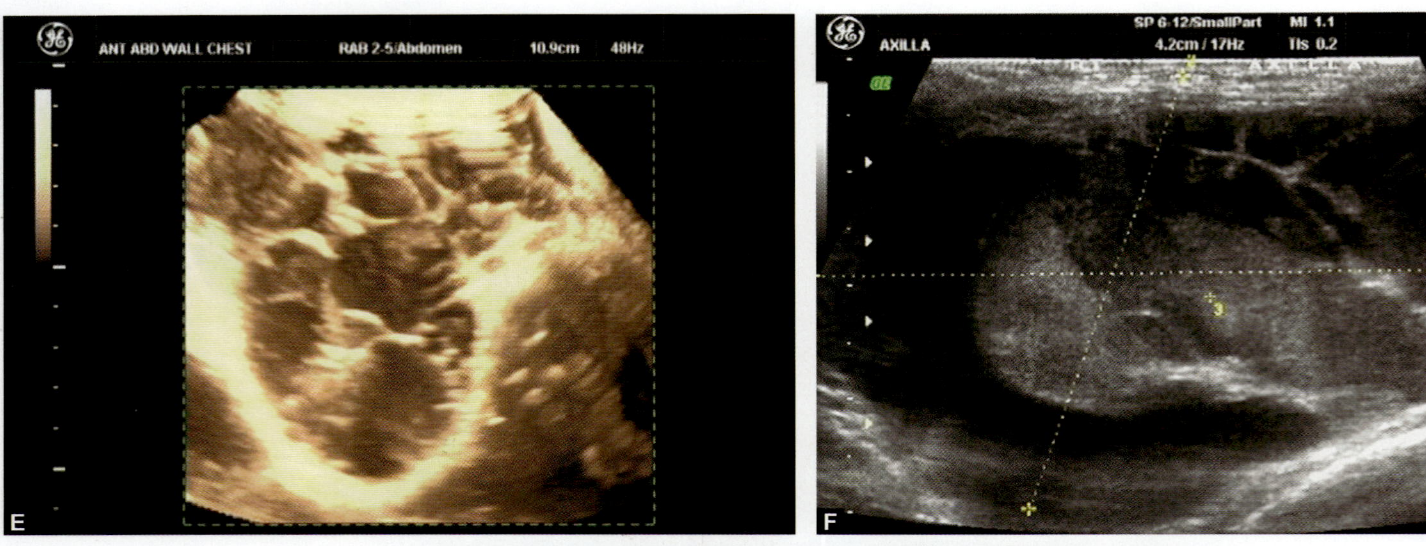

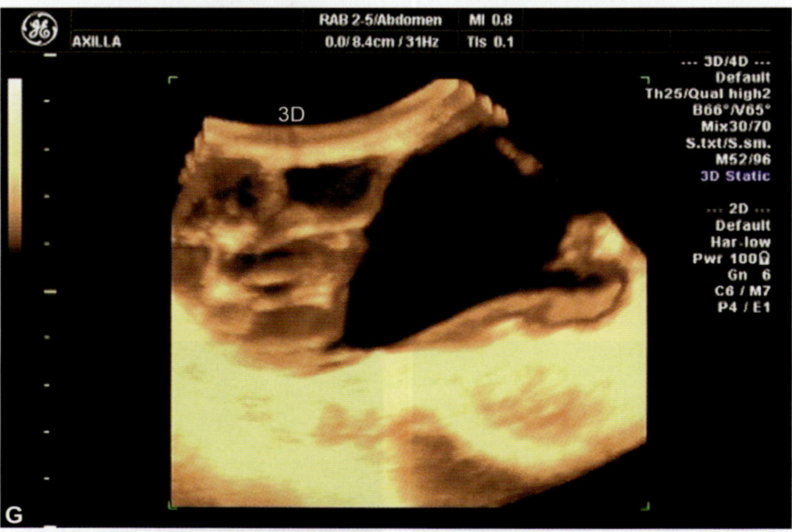

FIGURES 7.18E to G

FIGURES 7.18A to G: Cystic hygroma fixed with the chest wall. A child is born with big soft tissue mass hanging from the left anterior chest wall. X-ray of the same patient shows soft tissue shadow over the left thorax. HRSG of the same patient multiseptate cystic mass fixed with the left anterior chest wall. Bright echogenic septa are seen in the cyst. Thick low-level collection is also seen in the cyst suggestive of big cystic hygroma. On color flow imaging, no flow is seen in the cystic hygroma. 3D imaging of the same patient shows details of the cystic hygroma. It is not seen fixed with the chest wall muscles. The peripheral lung appears to be normal.

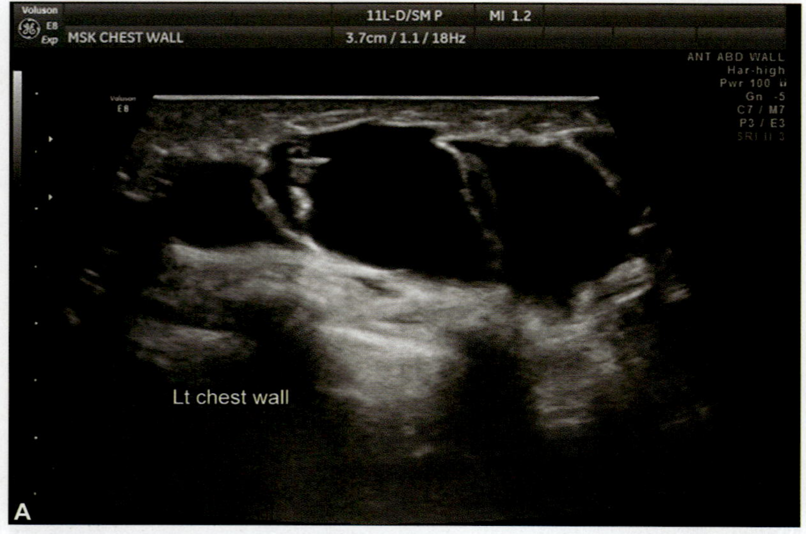

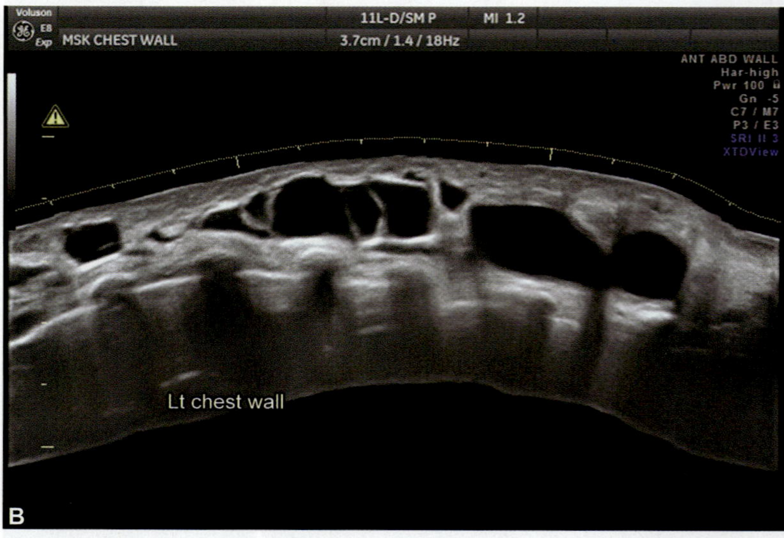

FIGURES 7.19A and B

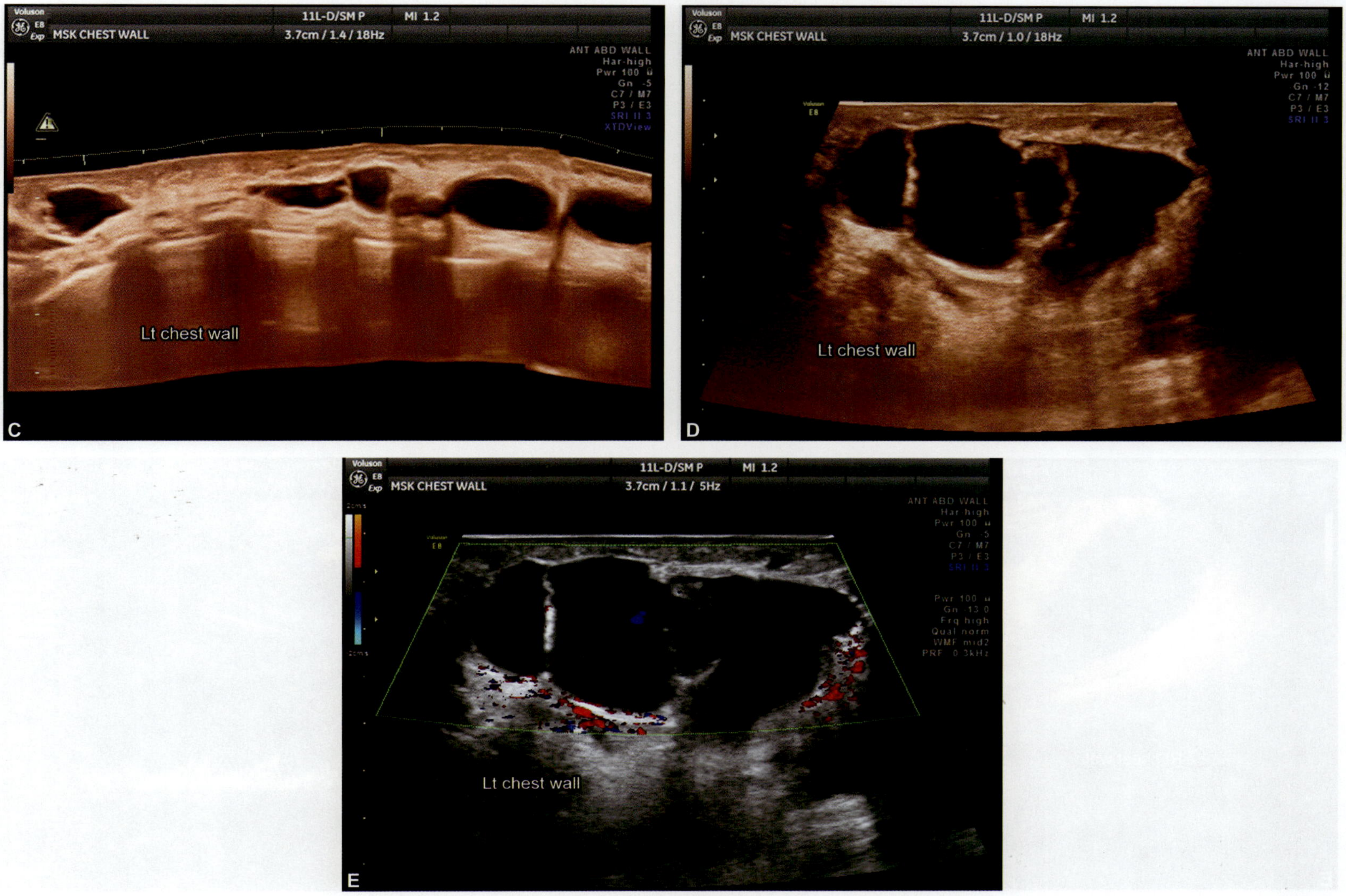

FIGURES 7.19C to E

FIGURES 7.19A to E: Chest wall cystic hygroma. HRSG shows a big soft tissue mass is seen on the left anterior chest wall. The mass is seen extending from left Infrascapular region going down up to lower limit of the paralumbar region. It shows multiple well-defined cystic masses. It is multiloculated. Thin-walled septa is seen in the mass. But no calcification is seen. On color flow imaging, low flow are seen in the septa. No other focal mass lesion is seen. The mass is superficial in nature. It is not seen invading the chest wall muscles. Findings are suggestive of cystic hygroma.

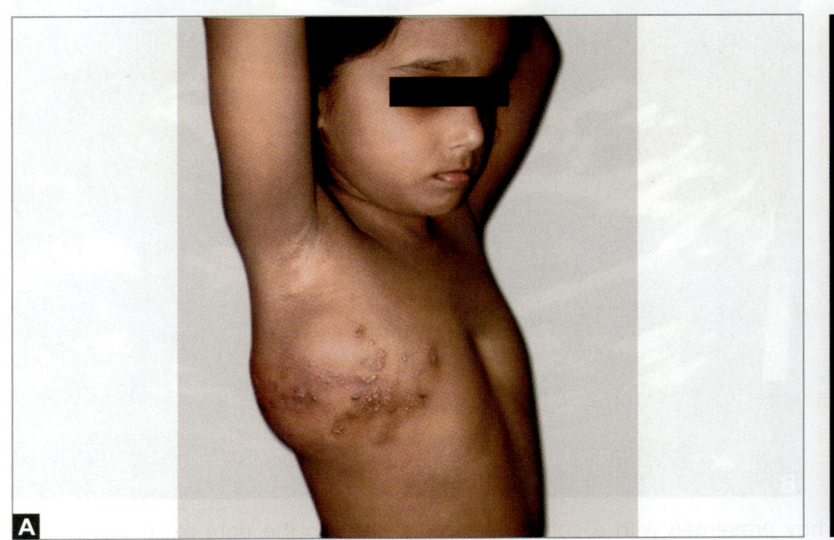

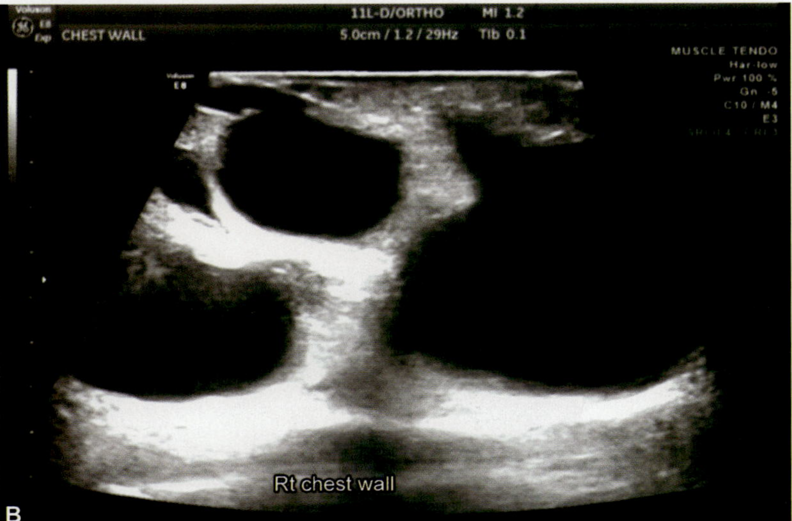

FIGURES 7.20A and B

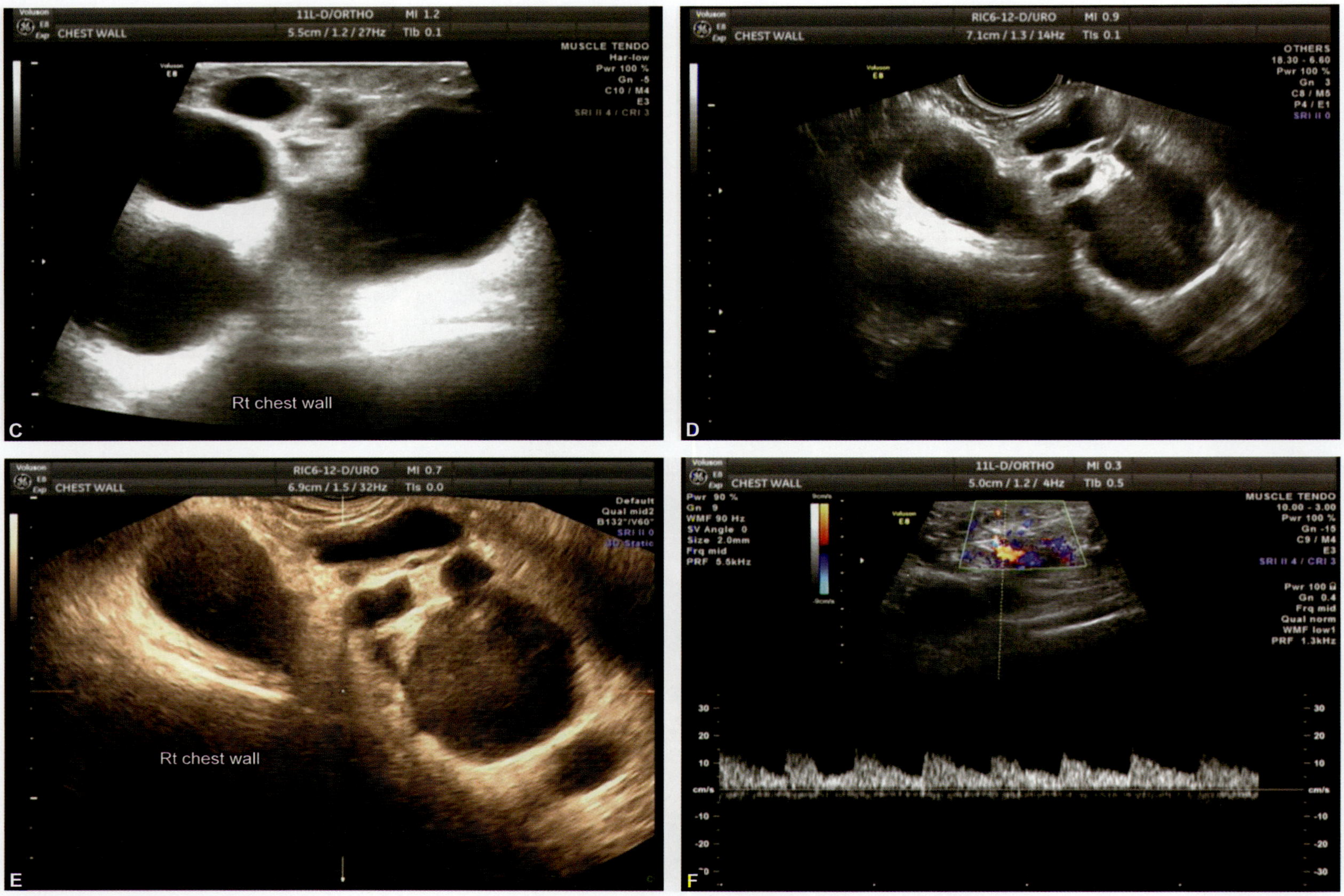

FIGURES 7.20C to F

FIGURES 7.20A to F: Lymphangioma. A young girl presented with a big soft tissue mass involving right anteralateral chest wall. It is soft in consistency. HRSG shows a multiloculated cystic mass in the anterolateral chest wall. Thick septa are seen in the mass. Cheesy collection is also seen in the cyst. No calcification is seen in them. On color flow imaging, low arterial flow is seen in the septa. Findings are suggestive of lymphangioma.

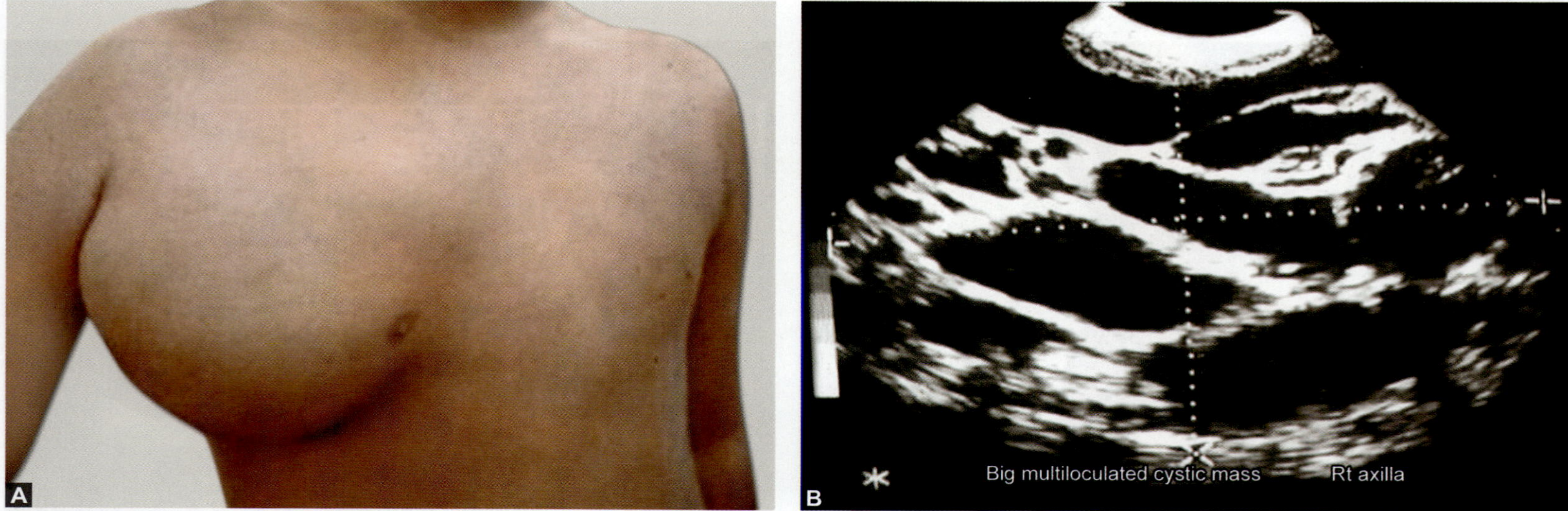

FIGURES 7.21A and B: Cystic hygroma anterior chest wall. A young boy presented with a soft tissue cystic mass in the right axilla and anterior chest wall. HRSG shows a multiseptate multiloculated soft tissue mass. The septa are well defined. Locullae are anechoic. However, few locullae show internal echoes, typical finding of cystic hygroma.

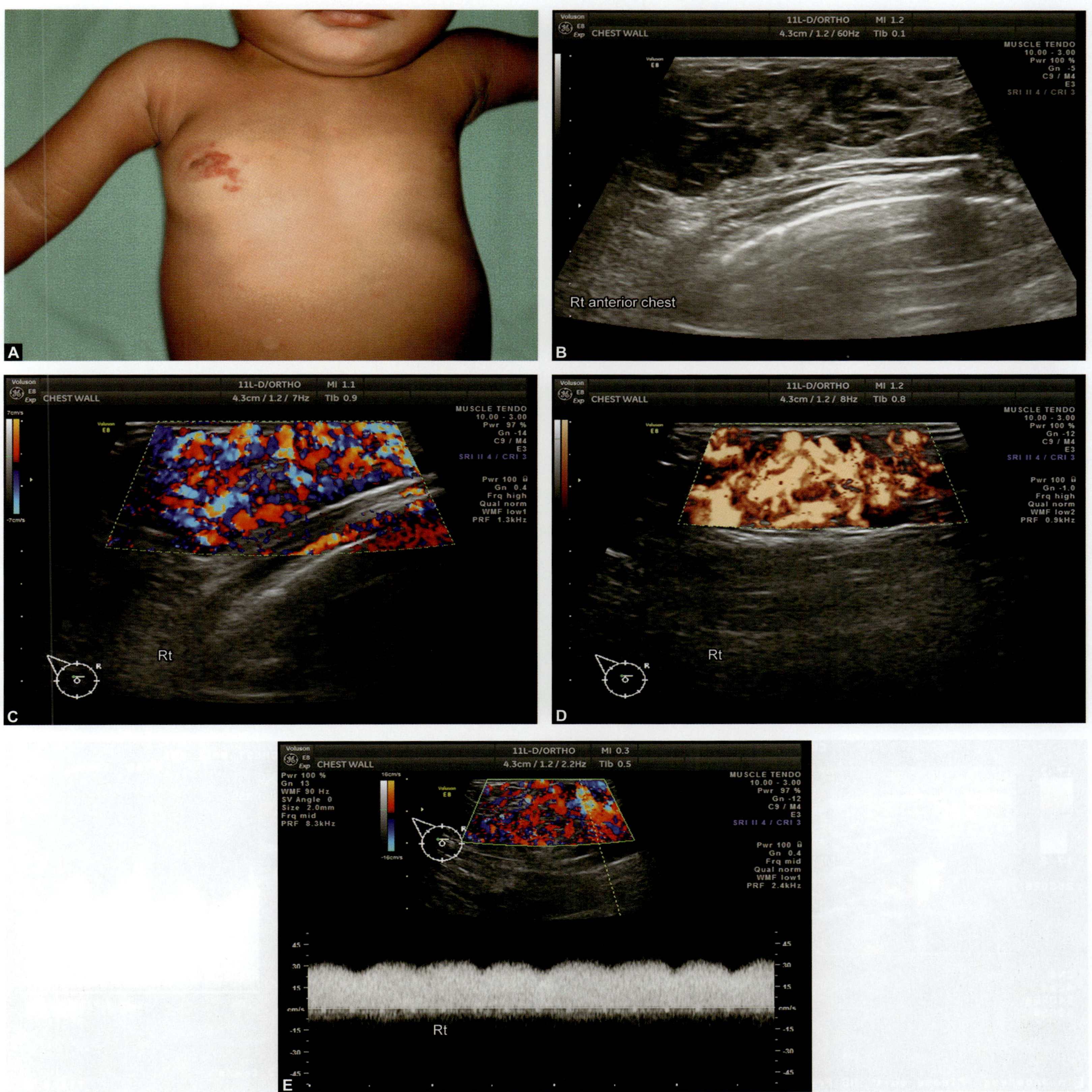

FIGURES 7.22A to E: Hemangiomatous mass in right anterior chest wall. A 1-year-old baby presented with a soft tissue mass involving right anterior chest wall in the region of areola and periareolar region. HRSG shows a low level echo complex mass n the subcutaneous tissue plane. Multiple vessels are seen in the mass. On color flow imaging, moderate arterial flow is seen in them. However, the vessels are not seen invading the chest wall. Findings are suggestive of highly vascular hemangiomatous mass.

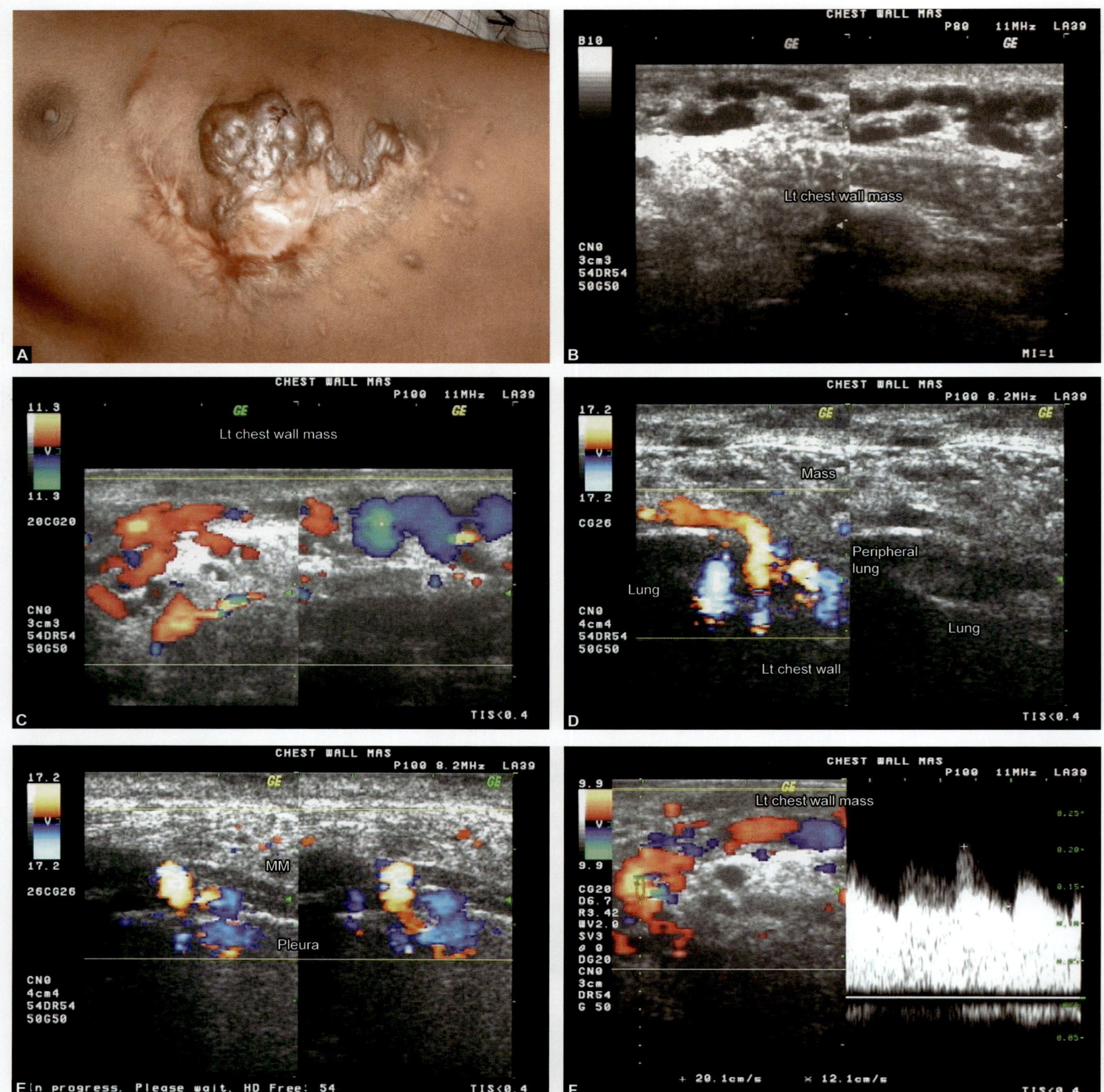

FIGURES 7.23A to F: Vascular mass over the anterior chest wall. A young man presented with a vascular mass over the left anterior chest wall. Multiple dilated vessels are seen in the mass. HRSG shows multiple dilated channels in the mass suggestive of vessels. On color flow imaging, low blood flow is seen in the vessels. HRSG shows the vessels are seen invading the chest wall and also perforated the pleura. They are seen going to the peripheral lung. Therefore, it is suggestive of deeper invasion of the vascular mass. On spectral Doppler tracing, the mass shows arterial flow with prolonged diastolic flow. Venous flow was also seen in the vessels suggestive of AV fistula in the mass.

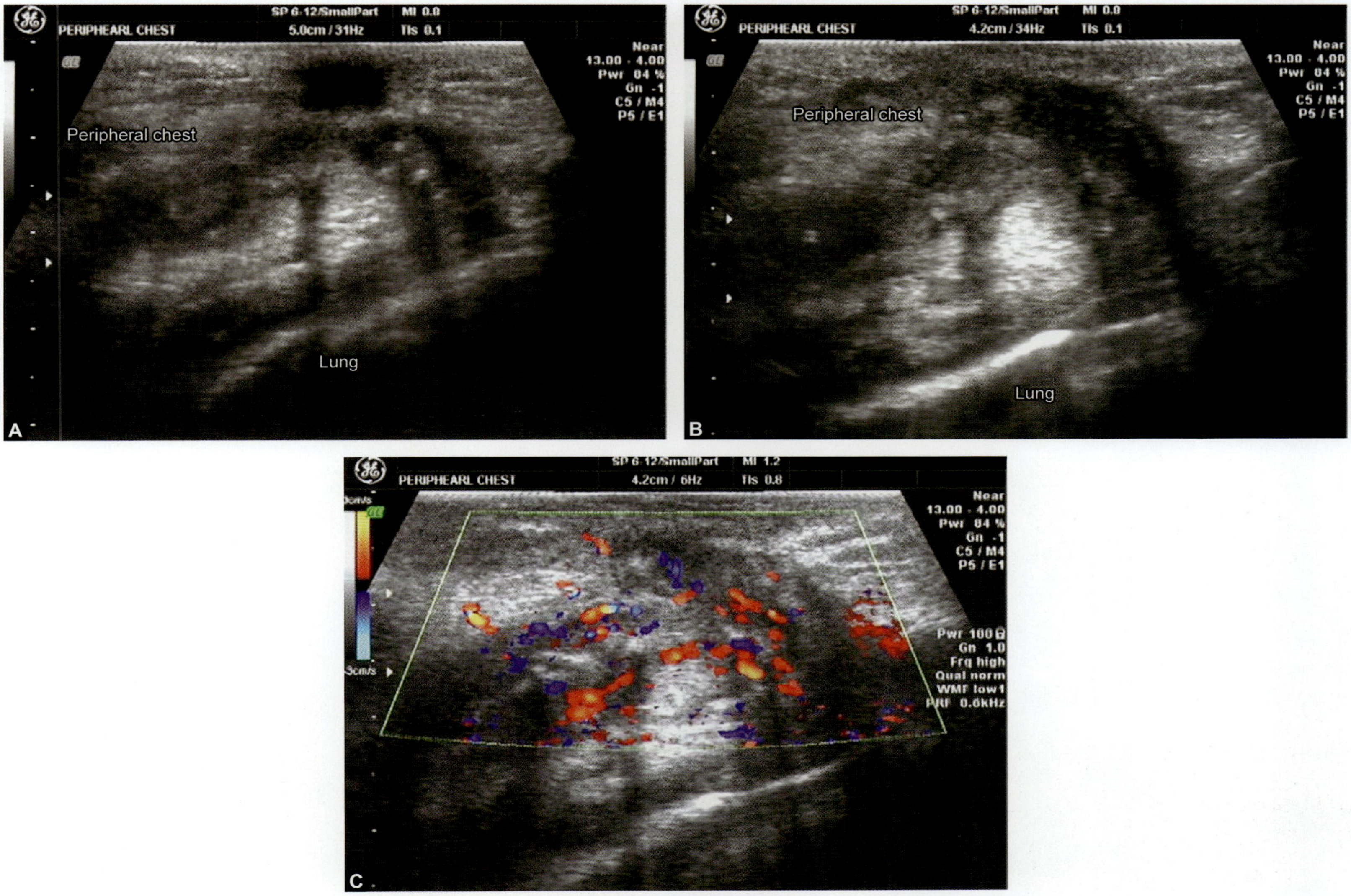

FIGURES 7.24A to C: FTC operated hydatid cyst peripheral chest. A patient operated for hydatid cyst peripheral chest presented with pain and swelling over the scar line. HRSG shows irregular hypoechoic areas over the scar tissue suggestive of granulomatous tissue with secondary infection. On color flow imaging, increased flow is seen around the scar suggestive of secondary infection.

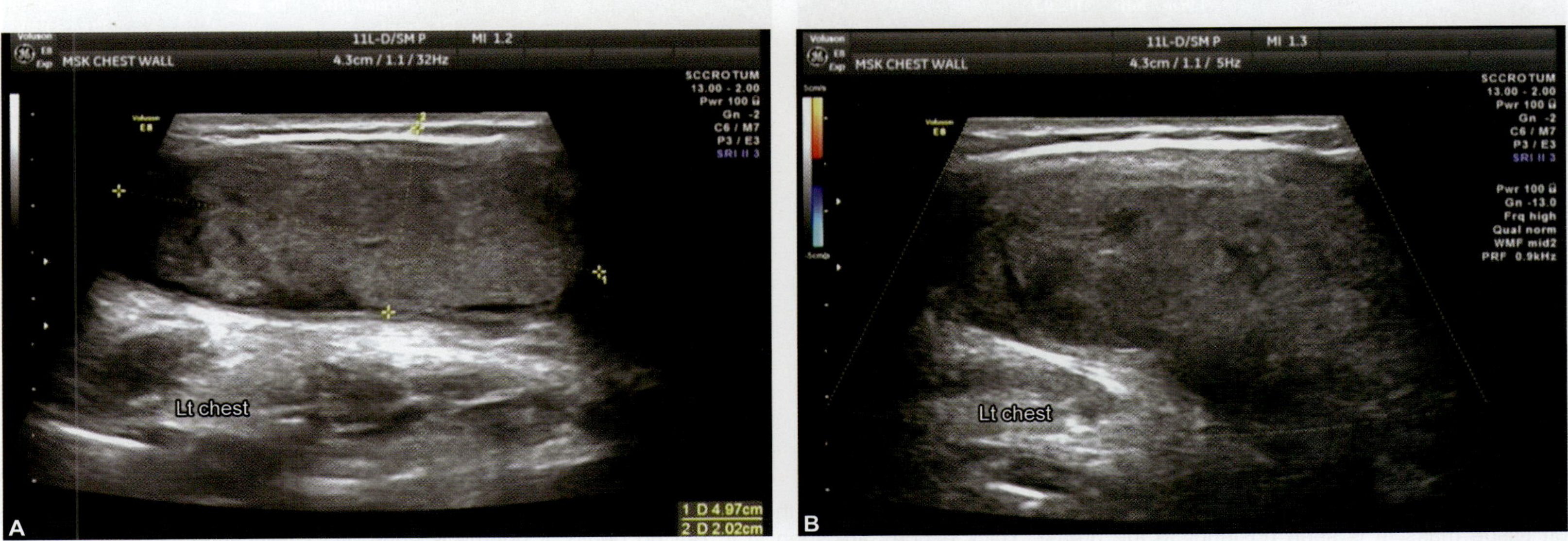

FIGURES 7.25A and B

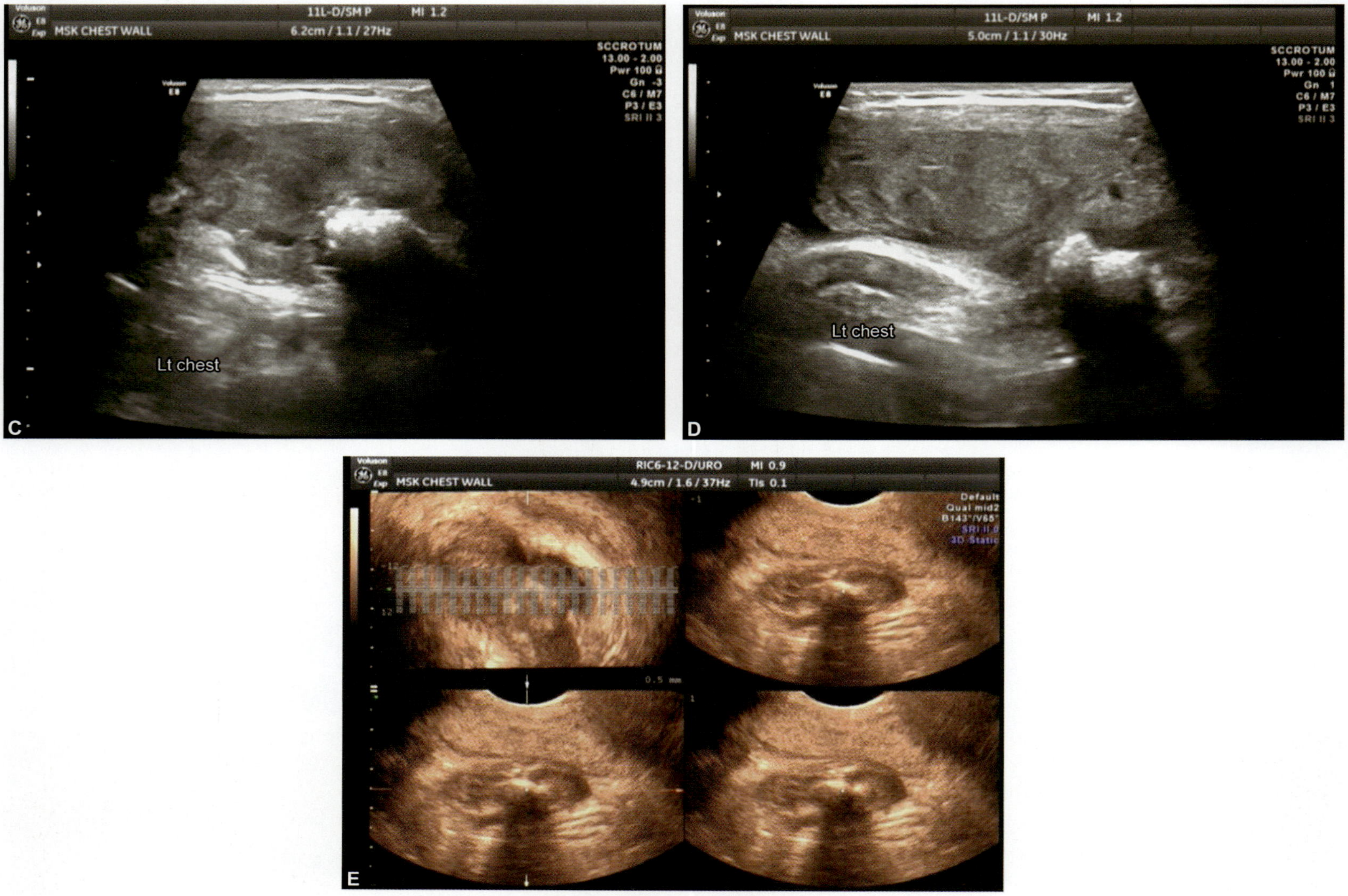

Lt chest

C

Lt chest

D

E

FIGURES 7.25C to E

FIGURES 7.25A to E: A patient presented with soft tissue mass over the left chest wall. HRSG shows an irregular thick-walled soft tissue mass over the left subcostal region. Thick echoes are seen in it. Thick cheesy collection is seen in it. No septation is seen in it. No loculation is seen. There is evidence of associated erosion also seen. But no evidence of any extension of the mass is seen in the pleural cavity or subdiaphragmatic space. Findings are suggestive of caries rib with cold abscess.

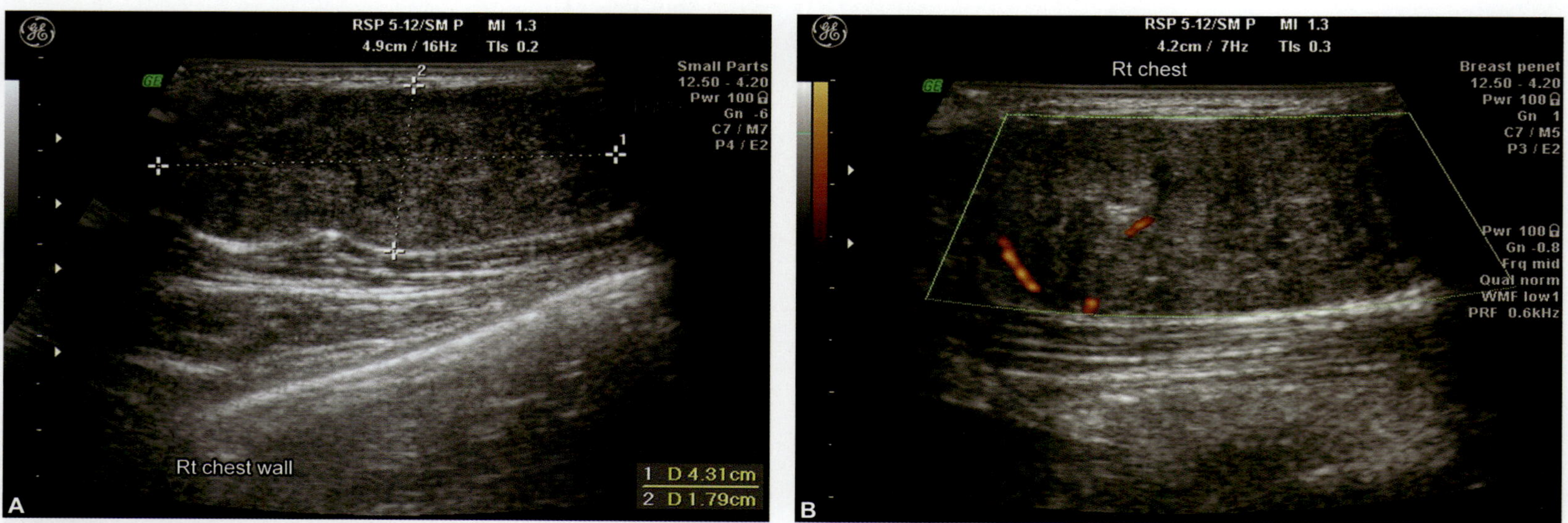

FIGURES 7.26A and B: A young girl presented with soft tissue mass in the right chest wall. HRSG shows a well encapsulated homogeneous echo soft tissue mass. It is seen posterior to the breast. Thick echoes are seen in it. But no perifocal edema is seen. No calcification is seen. On color flow imaging, poor flow is seen in it. Biopsy of the mass confirms organized abscess, which turned out to be a cold abscess.

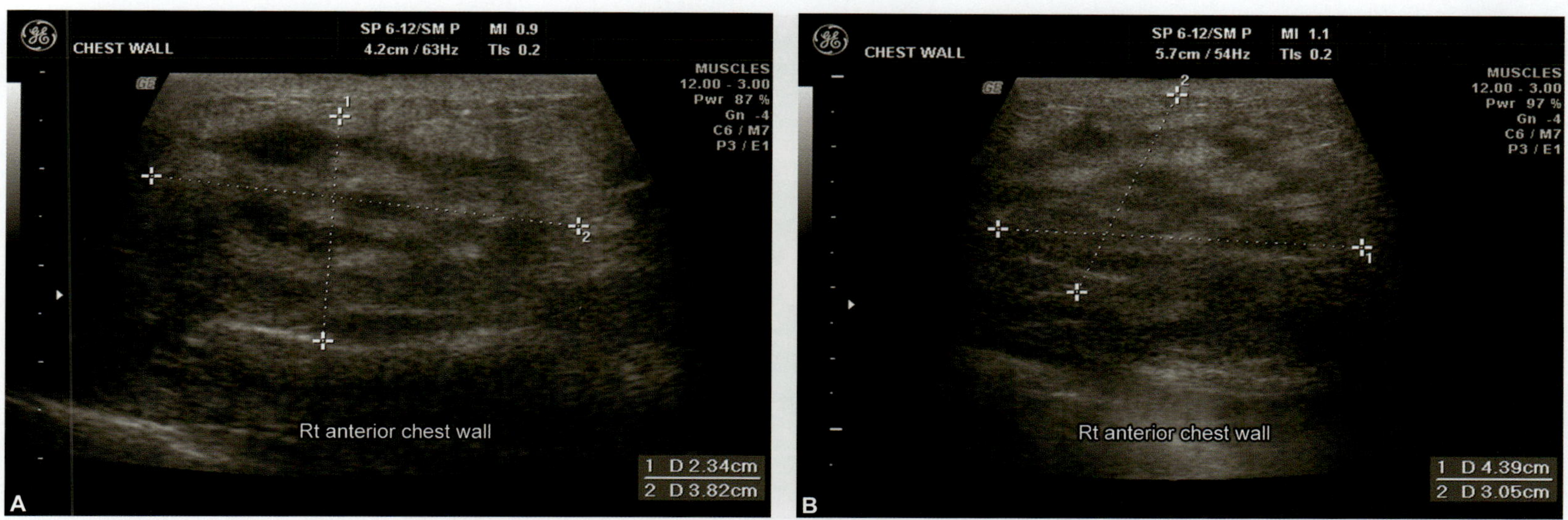

FIGURES 7.27A and B: HRSG shows an irregular ill-defined low level echo complex mass in anterior chest wall. It shows central area of necrosis. Perifocal edema is also present. But no cystic degeneration is seen. However, subcutaneous soft tissue edema is present suggestive of pyogenic abscess.

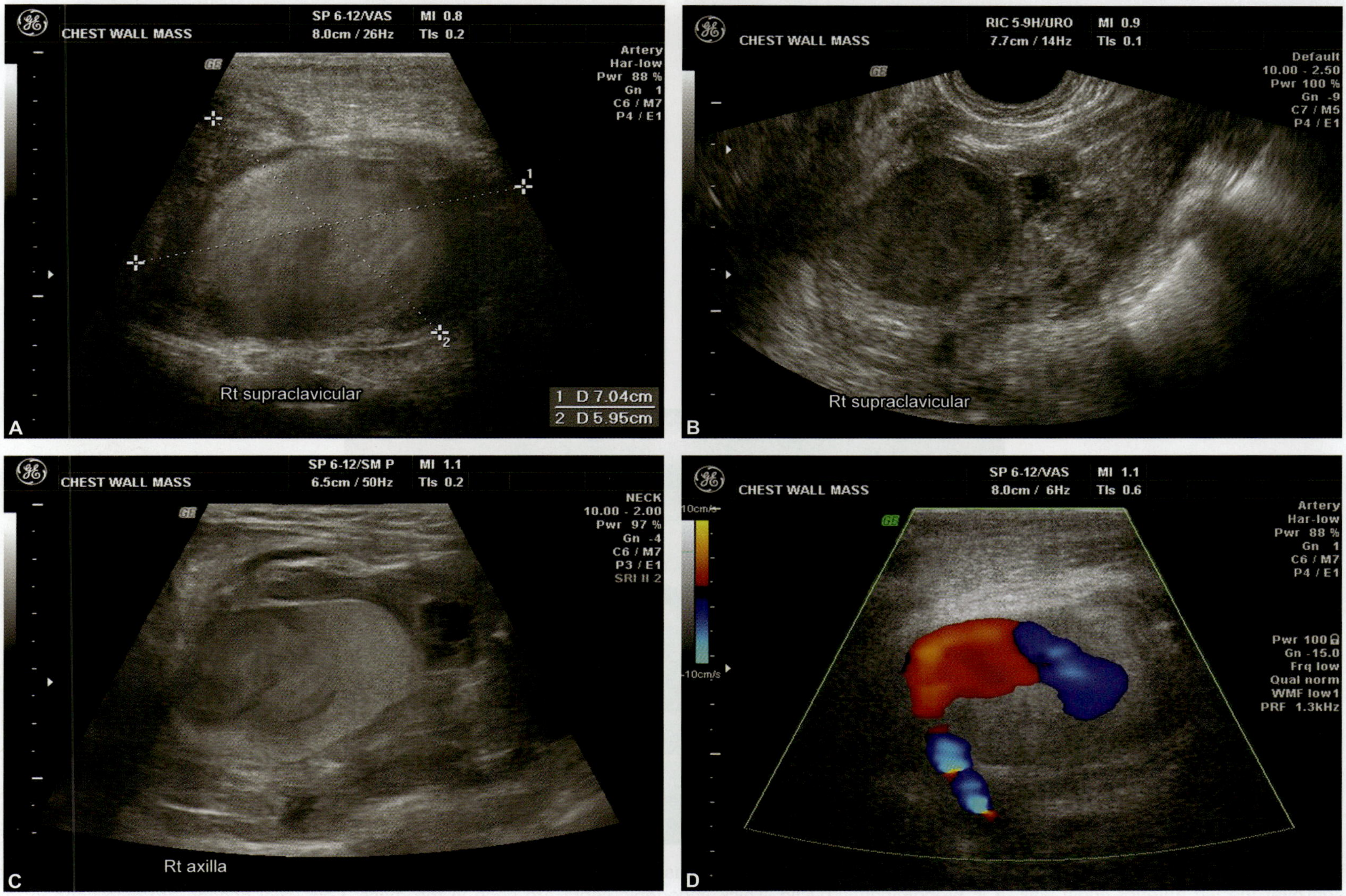

FIGURES 7.28A to D

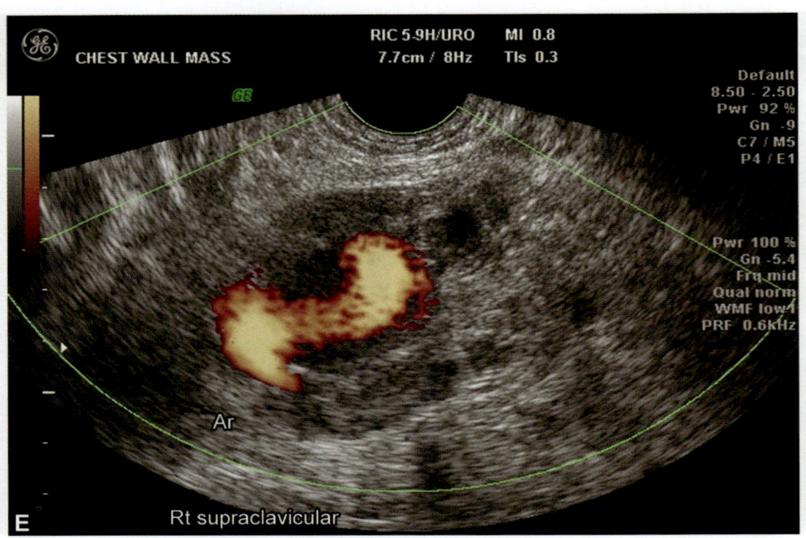

FIGURE 7.28E

FIGURES 7.28A to E: Bleeding aneurysm. A patient presented with a pulsatile swelling in right axilla, which is seen extending to the lateral chest wall. HRSG shows a big low level echo complex mass on anterior side of chest and medial side of right axilla. The mass shows thick echoes. It shows whirlpool movements. On color flow imaging, blood is seen moving in the mass. It is seen in relation to the proximal axillary artery suggestive of bleeding aneurysm. On spectral Doppler tracing, bizarre flow is seen in the aneurysm. No evidence of any calcification or thrombus is seen in the aneurysm.

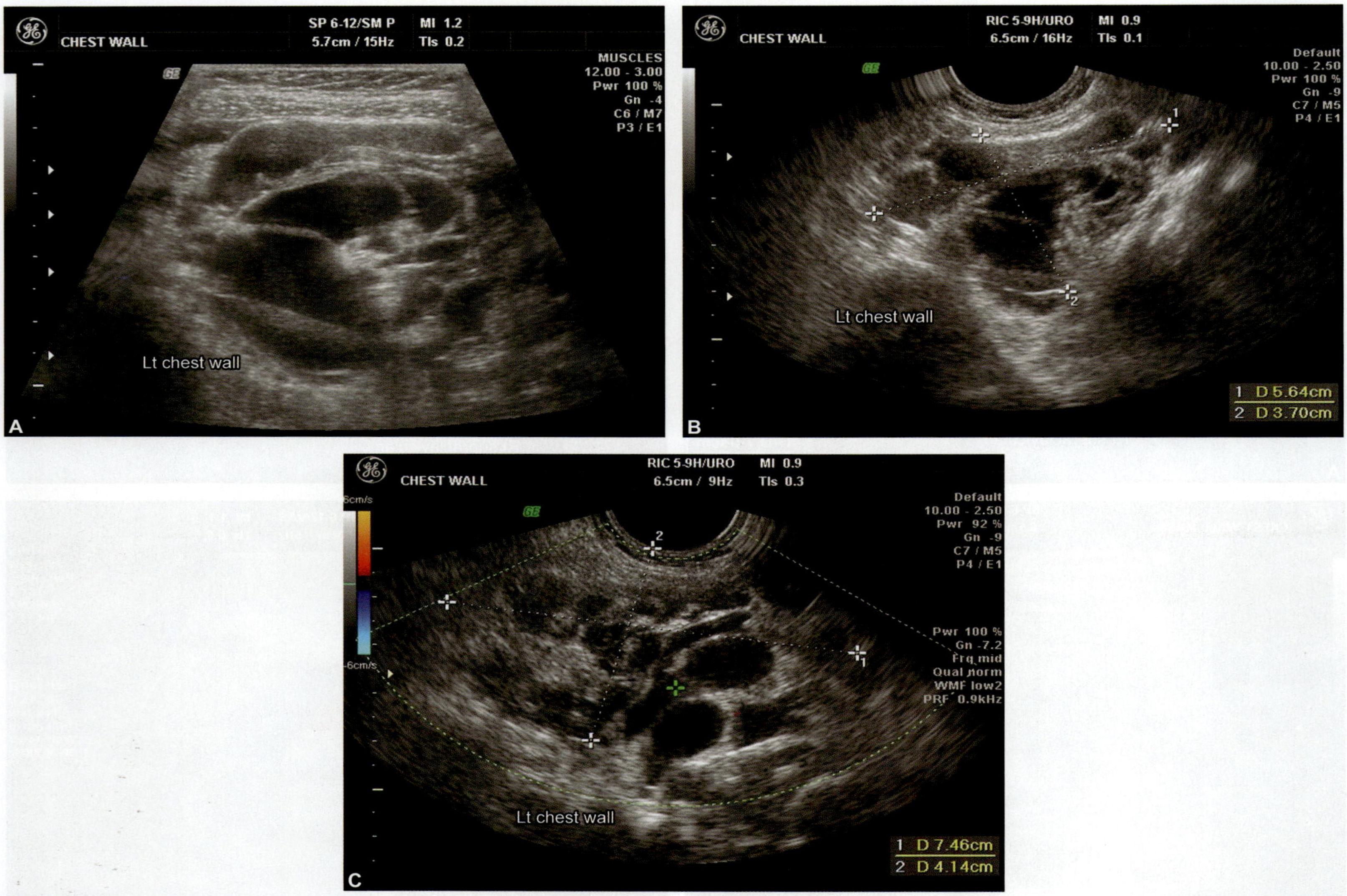

FIGURES 7.29A to C: A 5-month-old baby presented with soft tissue mass over the left chest wall. HRSG shows a low level echo complex mass seen over the left anterior chest wall. It is predominantly cystic. Thick echogenic septa are seen in the mass. Low level echoes are also seen in the cyst. On color flow imaging, no flow is seen in the cyst. However, low arterial flow is seen in the septa. Findings are suggestive of lymphangioma.

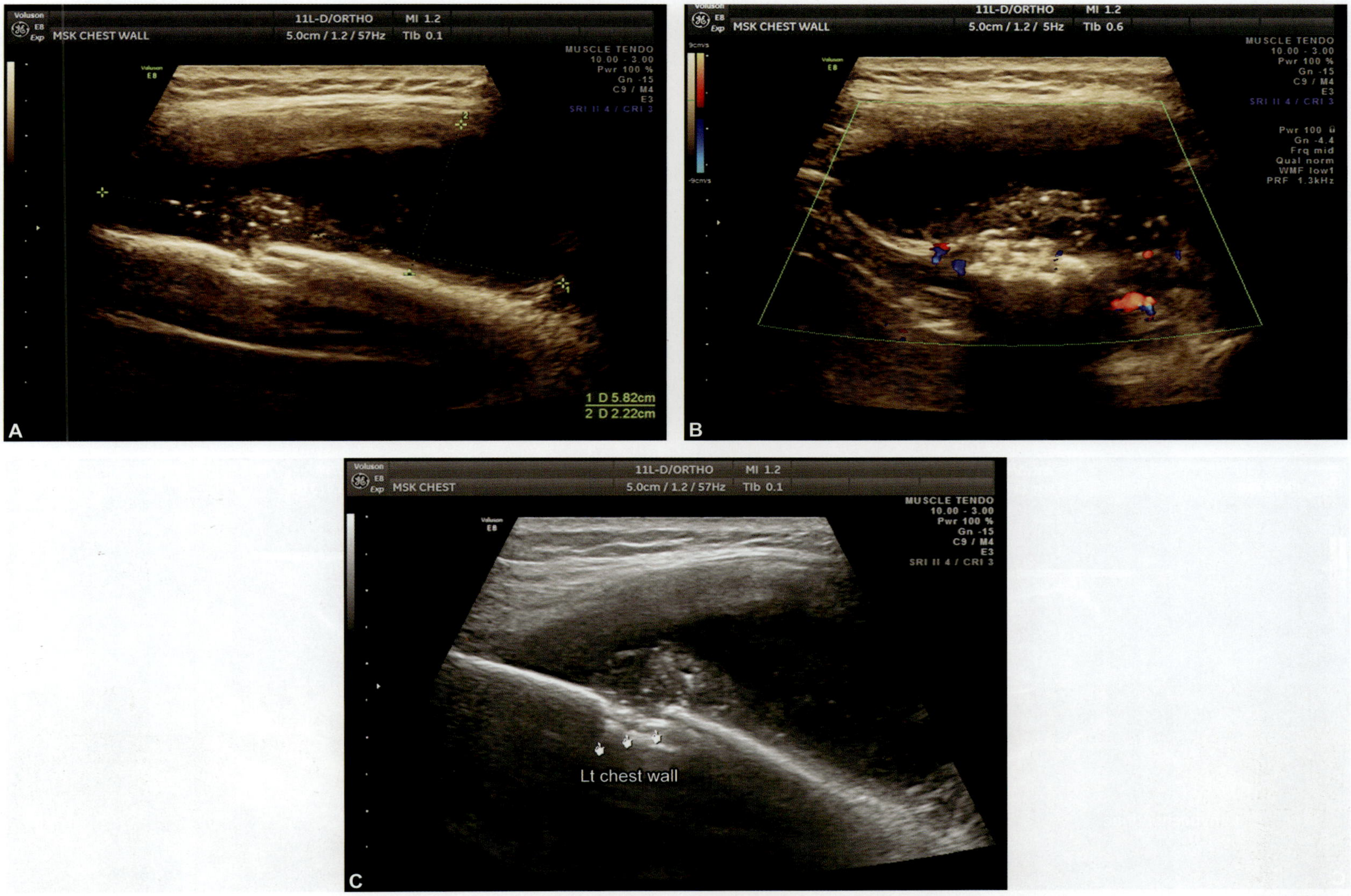

FIGURES 7.30A to C: Tubercular abscess with rib erosion. HRSG shows an irregular thick walled low level echo complex mass over the left side of the left chest wall in the infrascapular region. Thick collection is seen into it. Low level echoes are also seen into it. Echogenic debris is also seen into it. On color flow imaging, no flow is seen into it. Fracture of the rib is seen. However, the fractured segments are seen in close approximation. Associated erosion of the rib is also seen.

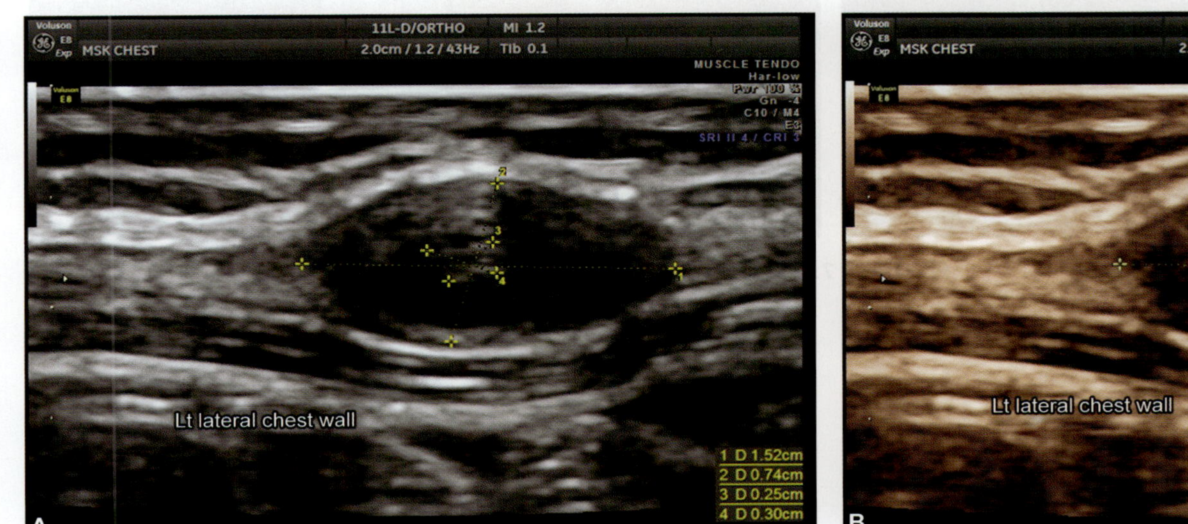

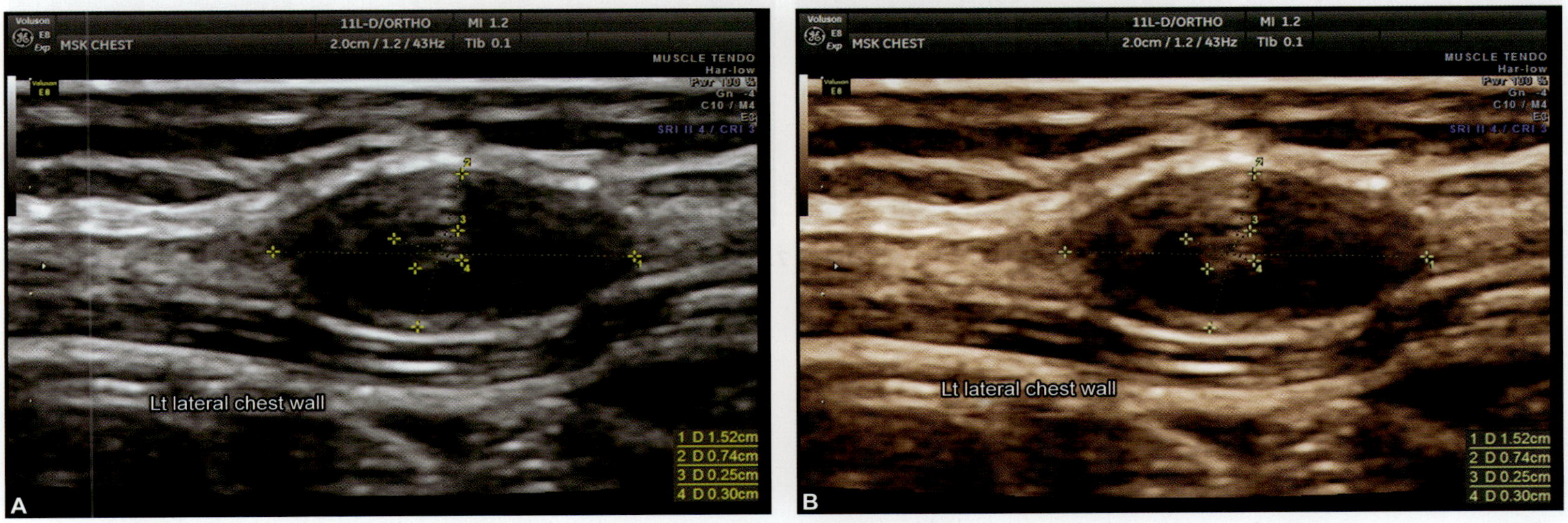

FIGURES 7.31A and B: A patient presented with soft tissue swelling in left lateral chest wall. HRSG shows a complex cystic mass in the intercostal muscle. An echogenic nidus is seen in the inner wall of cyst suggestive of cysticercus cyst.

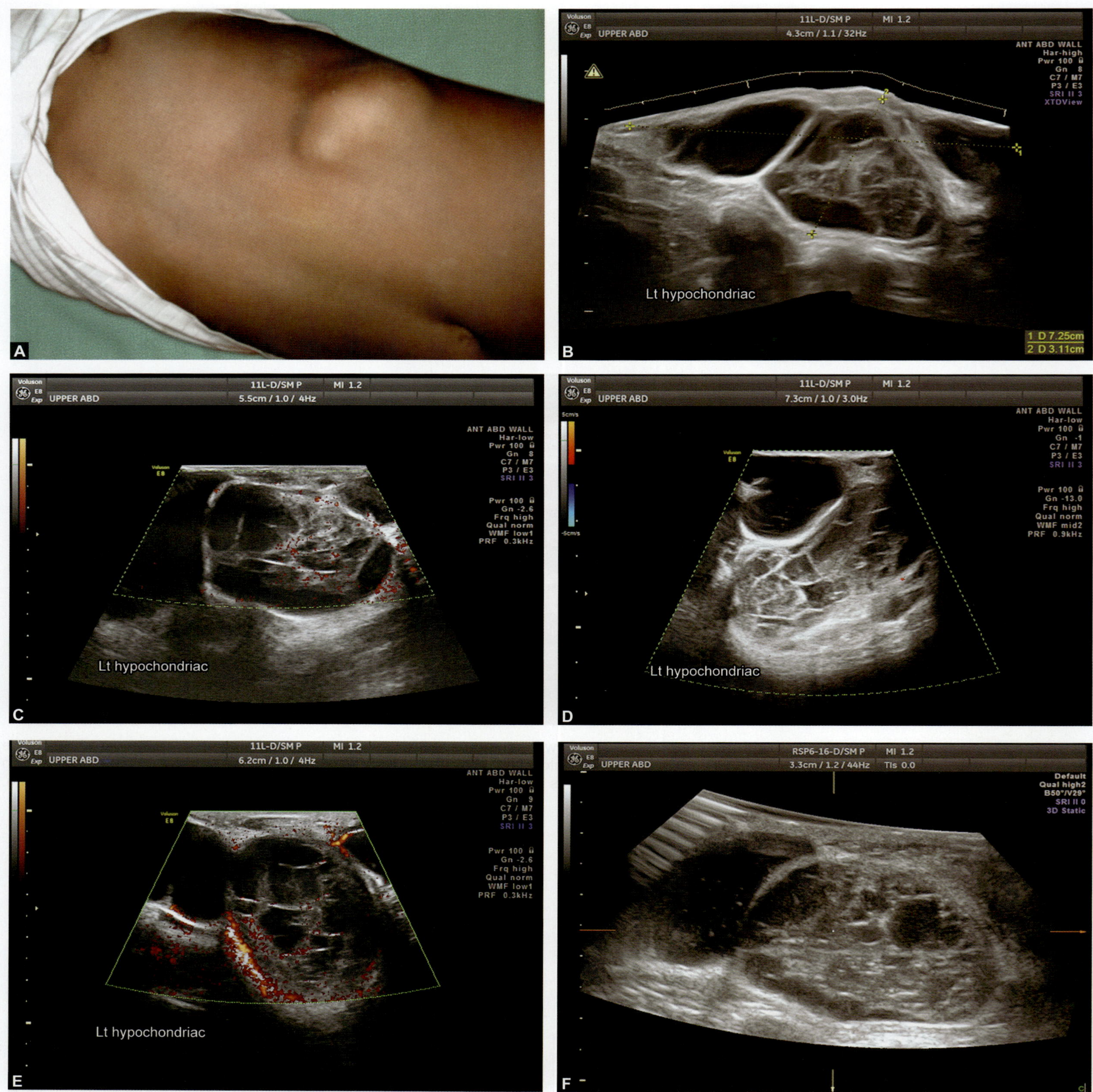

FIGURES 7.32A to F

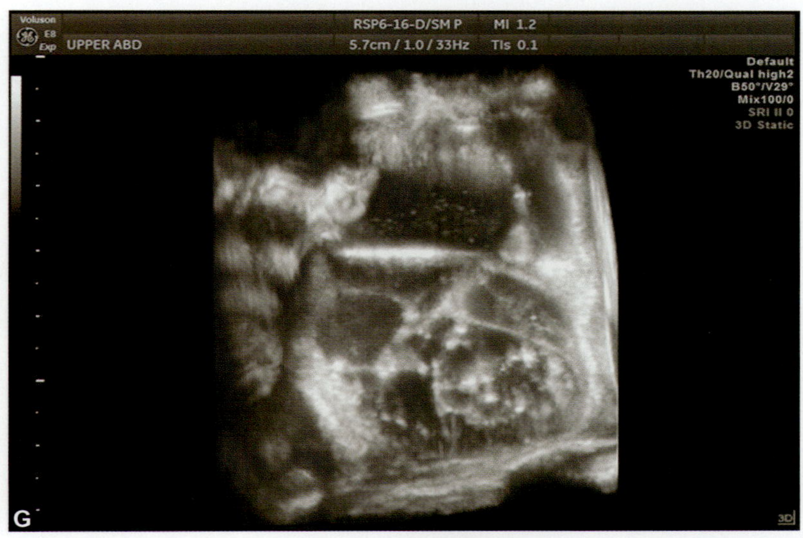

FIGURE 7.32G

FIGURES 7.32A to G: A patient presented with soft tissue mass over the left subcostal region, which is seen going down. HRSG shows a well encapsulated multiloculated predominantly cystic mass seen in the left subcostal region. It is seen in the subcutaneous tissue plane. Multiple echogenic septa are seen in it. Thick cheesy shadows are also seen in it. But no evidence of any calcification is seen. No intra cystic soft tissue mass is seen. On color flow imaging, low flow is seen in the septa. But no evidence of any intracystic flow is seen. The mass is not seen invading the deeper tissue. Findings are suggestive of lymphangioma.

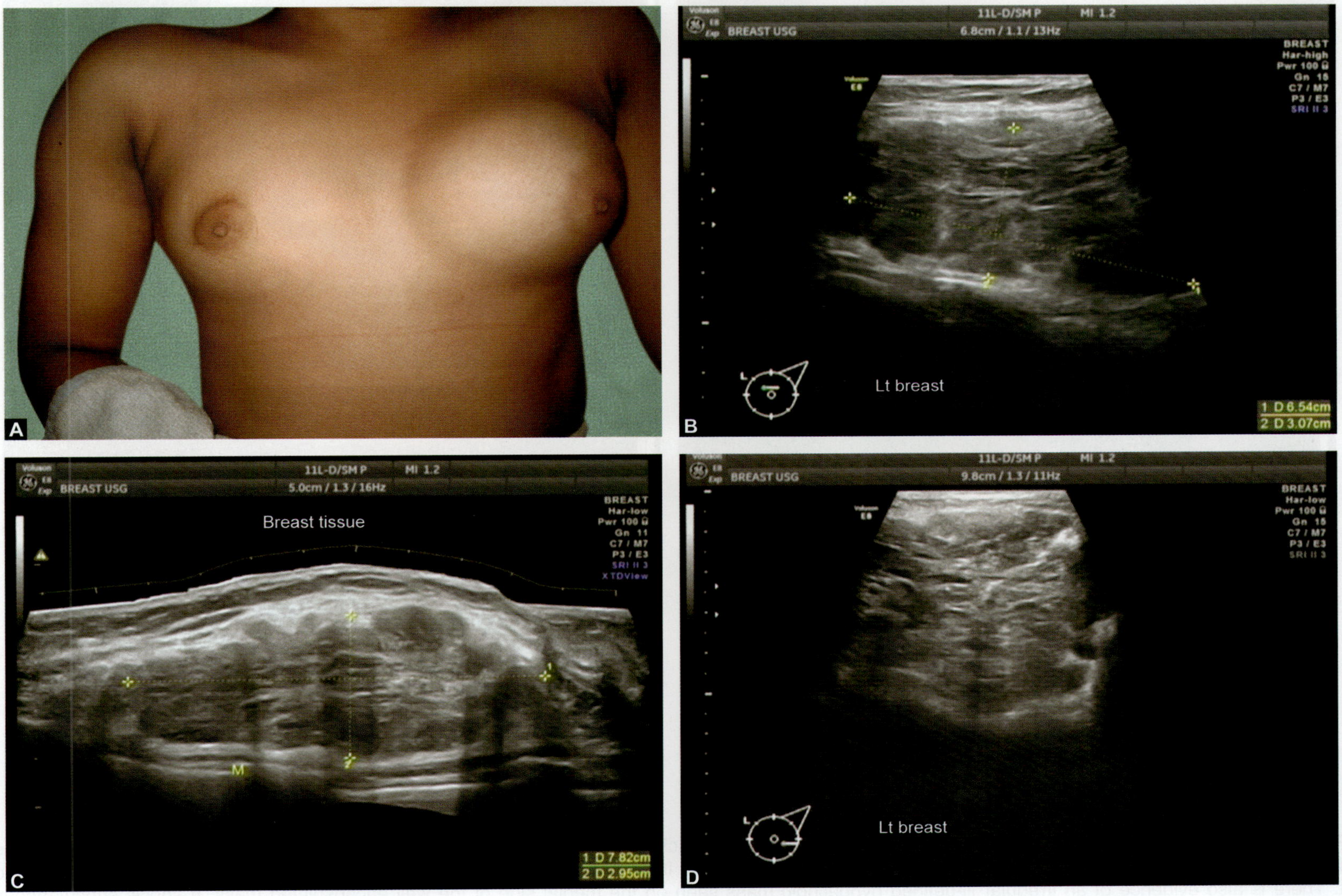

FIGURES 7.33A to D

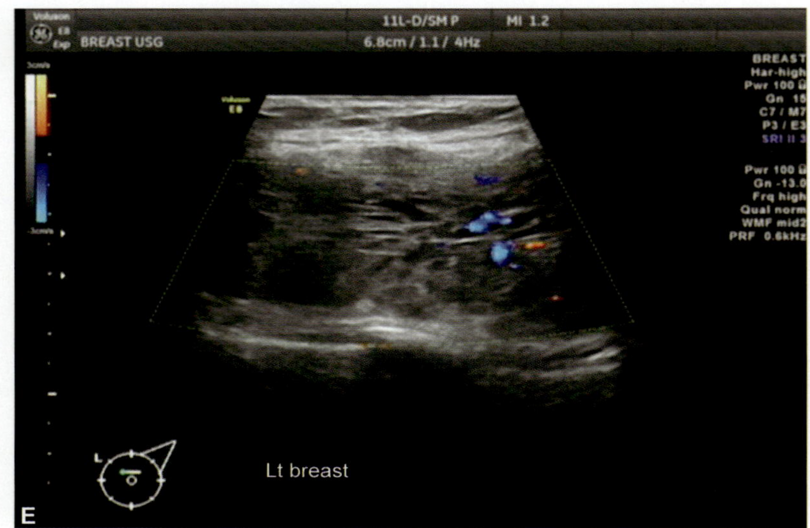

FIGURE 7.33E

FIGURES 7.33A to E: A young girl presented with markedly increased left breast. HRSG shows a big lobulated predominantly solid soft tissue mass is seen in the left breast. The mass is seen posterior to the breast tissue. It is solid in nature. No calcification is seen. No cystic degeneration is seen in the mass. Normal anatomic relations are distorted. Normal breast tissue is seen pushed up by the mass. On color flow imaging, poor flow is seen in the mass. Biopsy of the mass confirms muscle tumor.

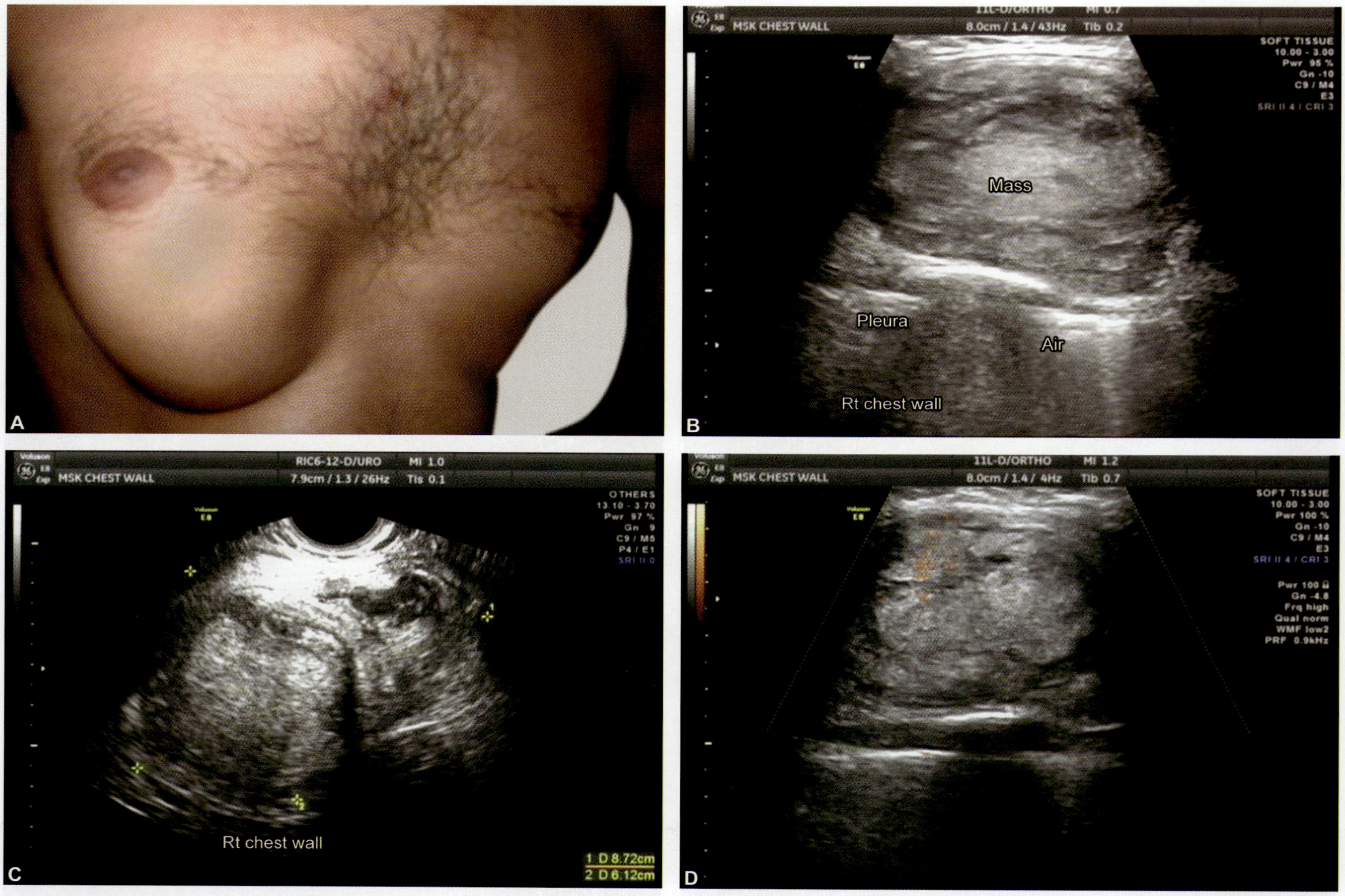

FIGURES 7.34A to D: A patient presented with soft tissue mass in right chest wall. HRSG shows a thick walled well encapsulated soft tissue mass seen over the right anterior chest wall. Thick echo collection is seen into it. But no calcification is seen. On color flow imaging, no flow is seen into it. There is also evidence of an irregular ill-defined hypoechoic mass seen on the medial side of the well encapsulated mass. It shows subcutaneous collection. But no cystic degeneration is seen. Findings are suggestive of cold abscess.

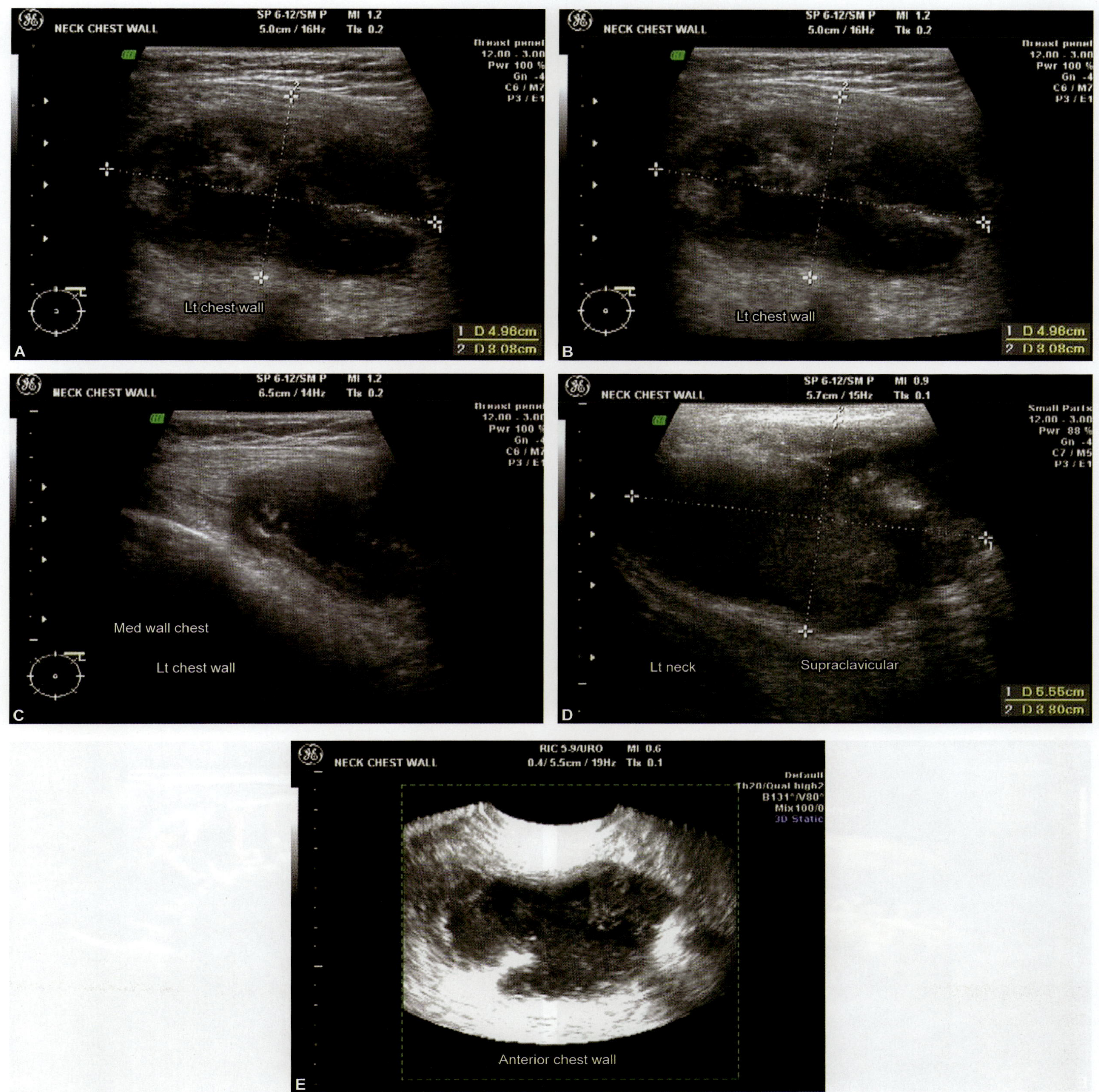

FIGURES 7.35A to E: 3D imaging of the same patient shows pocket of thick collection in anterior chest wall.

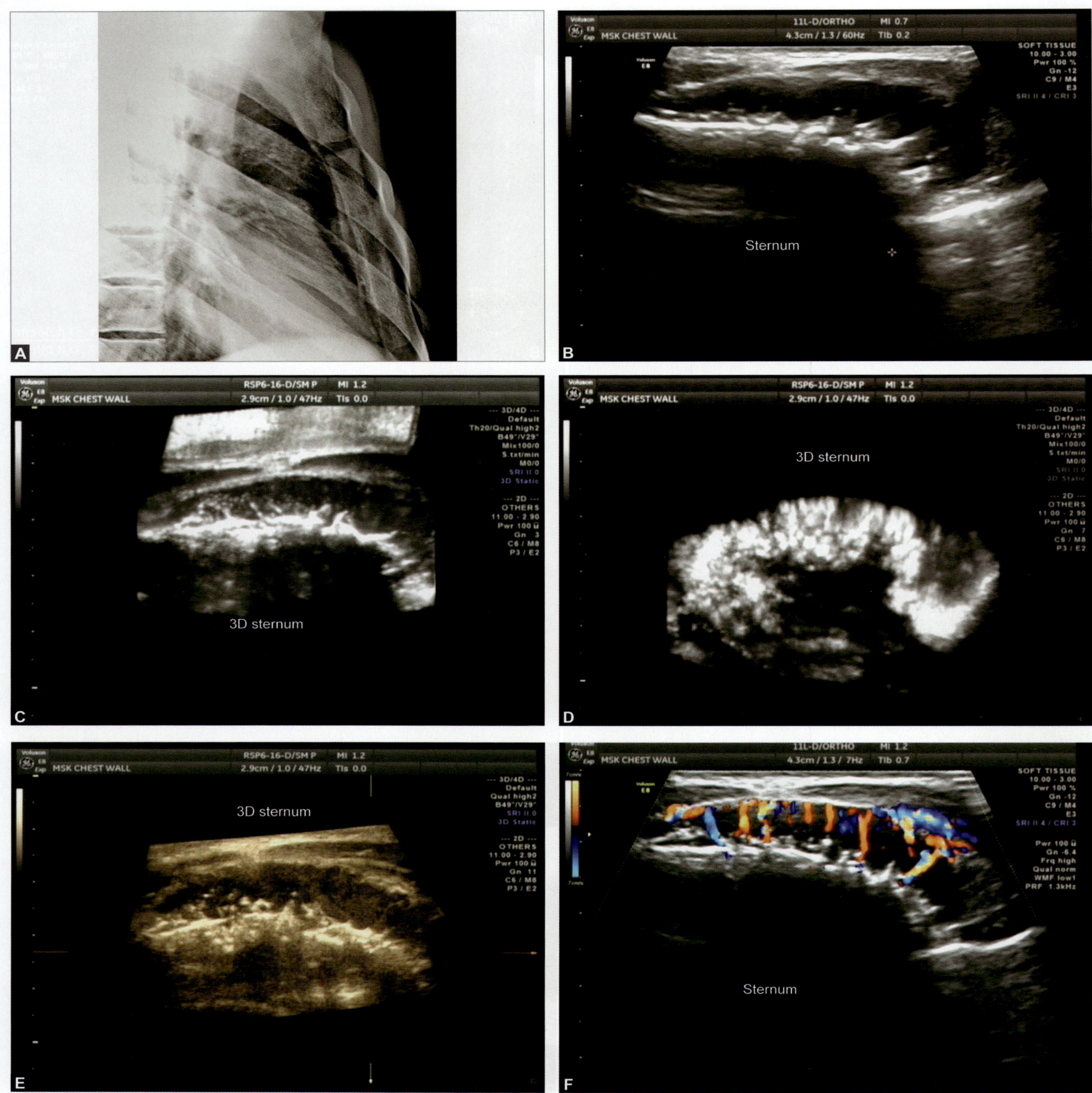

FIGURES 7.36A to F

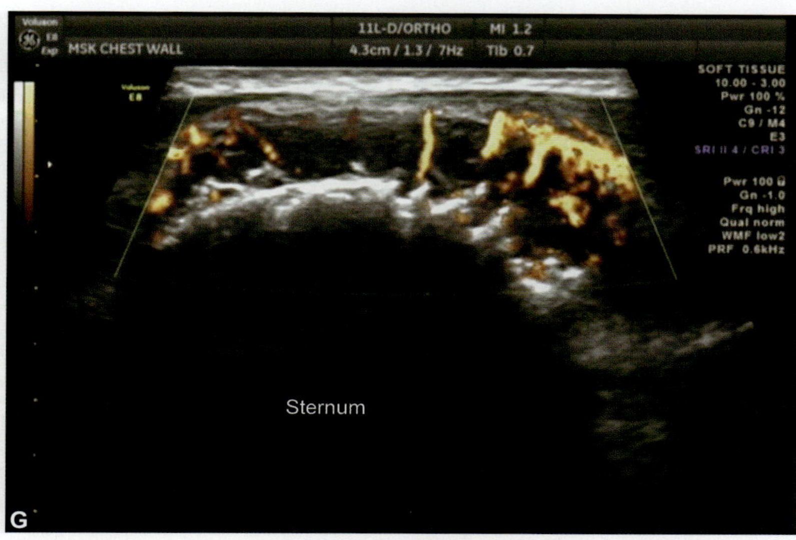

FIGURE 7.36G

FIGURES 7.36A to G: Ewings sarcoma sternum. A patient presented with soft tissue swelling over the sternum. The plain X-ray shows an ill-defined soft tissue swelling. HRSG shows a soft tissue mass coming out from the sternum. The sternal margins are irregular in outline. Breitling of the margin is seen. Multiple echogenic specks are also seen in the mass. 3D imaging shows the mass invading the sternum. On color flow imaging, multiple vessels are seen feeding the mass. Biopsy of the mass confirms ewing's sarcoma.

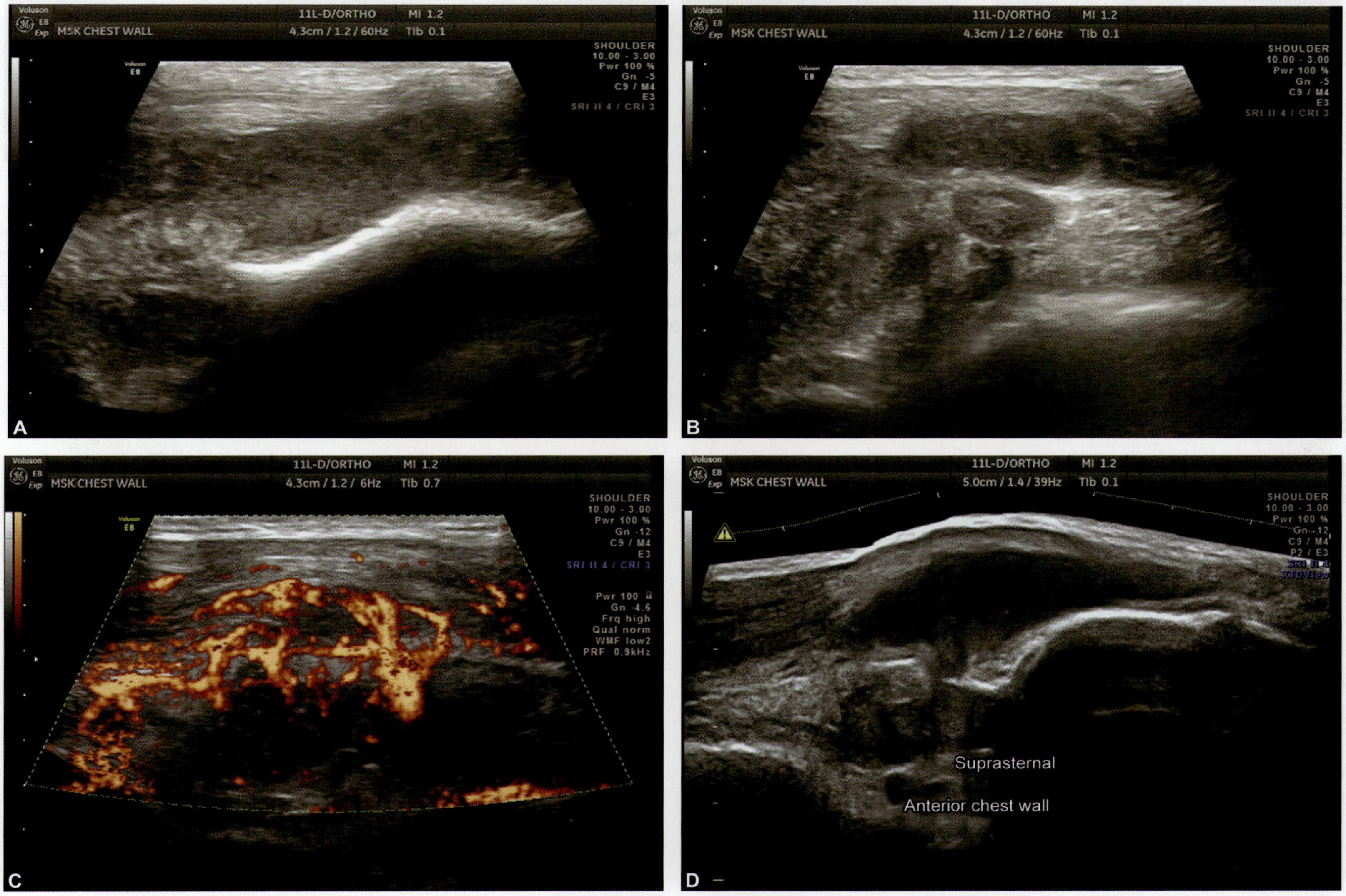

FIGURES 7.37A to D

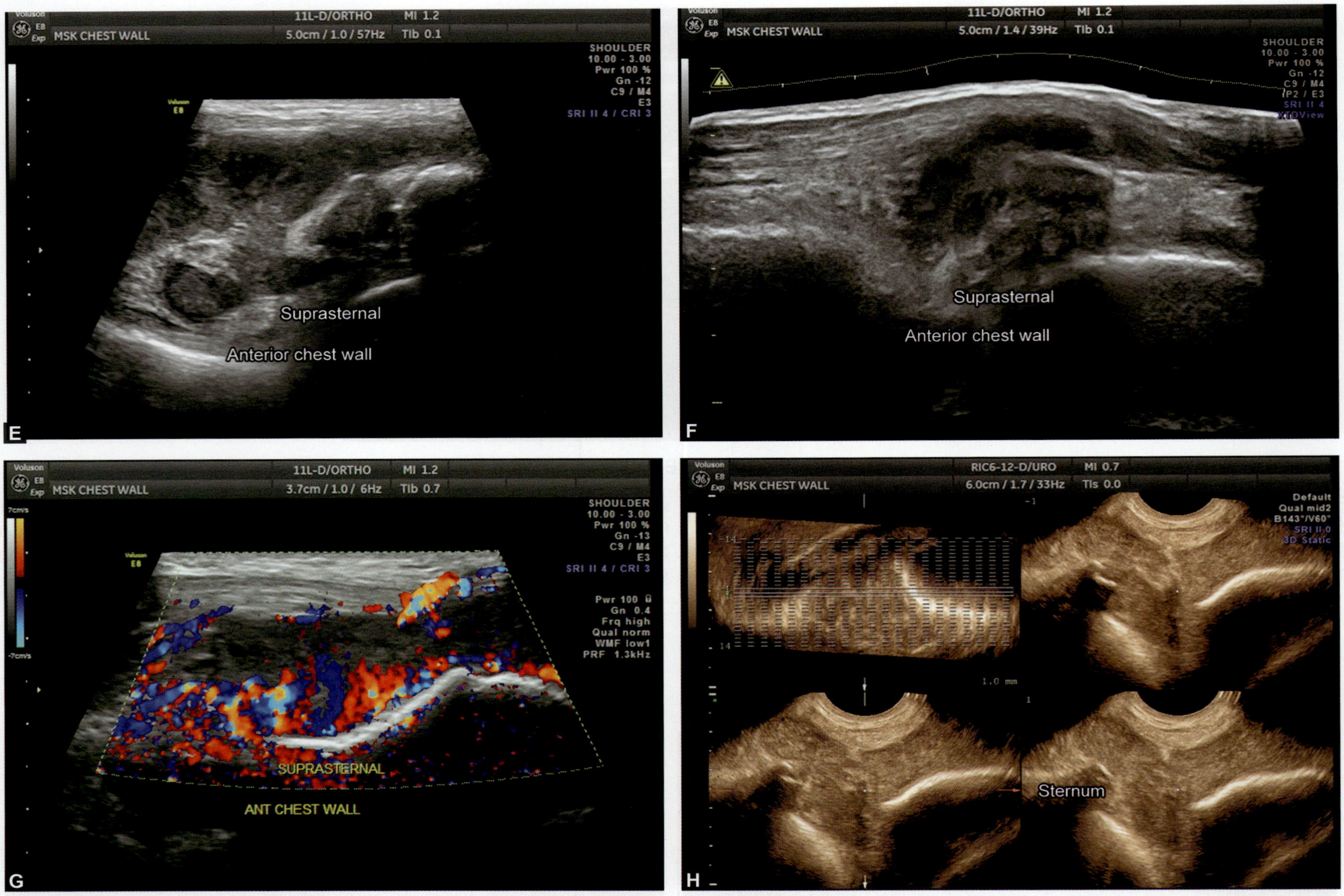

FIGURES 7.37E to H

FIGURES 7.37A to H: A patient presented with soft tissue mass over the anterior chest wall. HRSG shows an irregular ill-defined low level echo complex mass in anterior chest wall anterior to the sternum. Thick echoes are seen in it. It shows soft tissue shadows with jelly like consistency suggestive of granulomatous tissue. Erosion of the sternum is also seen and it is seen extending posterior to the sternum. On color flow imaging, high flow is seen in it. But no sinus formation is seen. Multiple enlarged nodes are also seen in the right supraclavicular region. Few enlarged nodes are also seen in the left supraclavicular region. No necrosis is seen in them. Findings are suggestive of tubercular abscess with bony erosion.

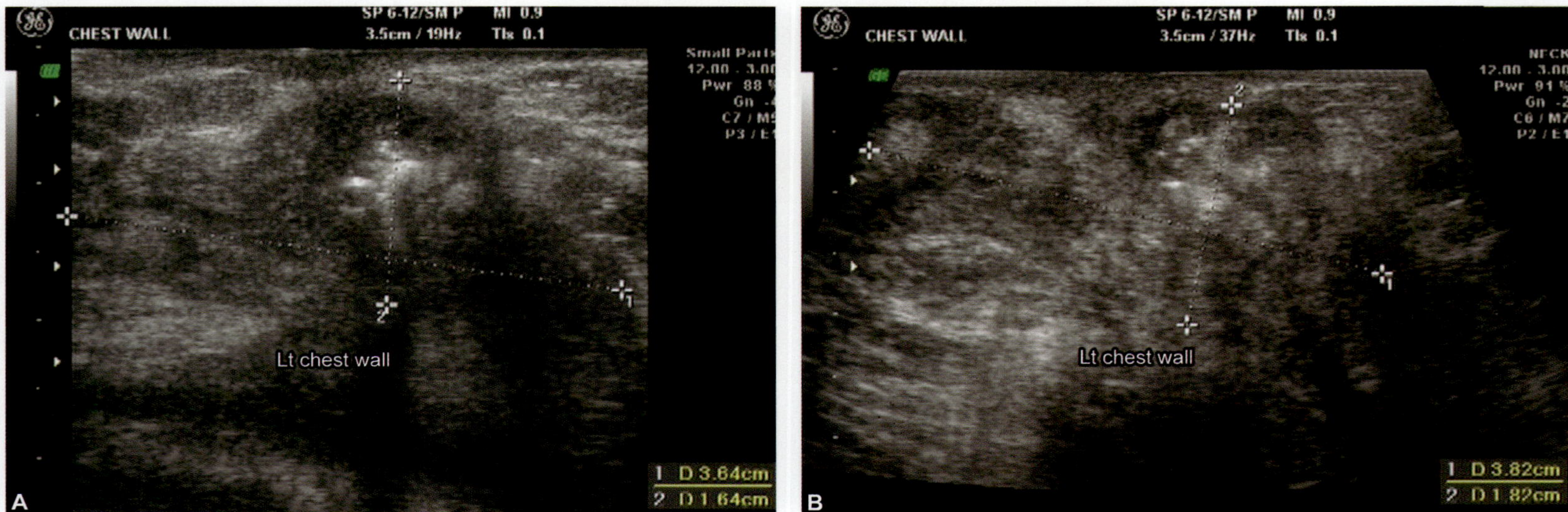

FIGURES 7.38A and B

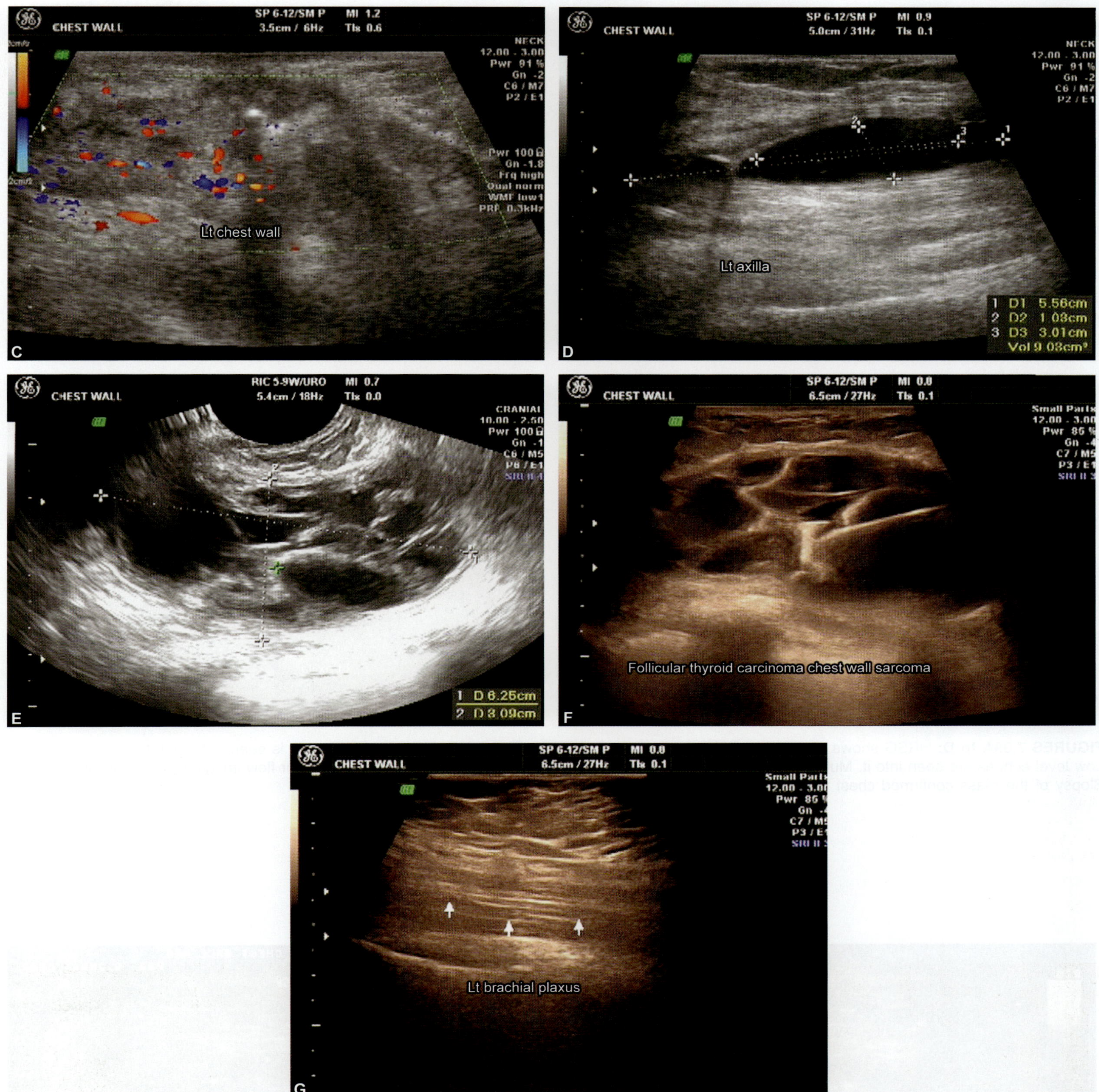

FIGURES 7.38C to G

FIGURES 7.38A to G: A patient presented with soft tissue swelling over the chest wall. (A to E) HRSG shows a heterogeneous mass involving the chest wall muscles. It is ill defined. Echogenic specks are seen in the mass. On color flow imaging, low vascularity is seen in the mass. Enlarged nodal shadows are also seen in left axilla. Biopsy of the mass confirms soft tissue sarcoma; (F to G) The same patient presented with soft tissue swelling after operation of the mass. HRSG shows multiloculated collection in the anterior chest wall. Thick septa are seen in the collection due to postsurgical complications. The brachial plexus cord is well visualized. However, no pressure is seen on the cord.

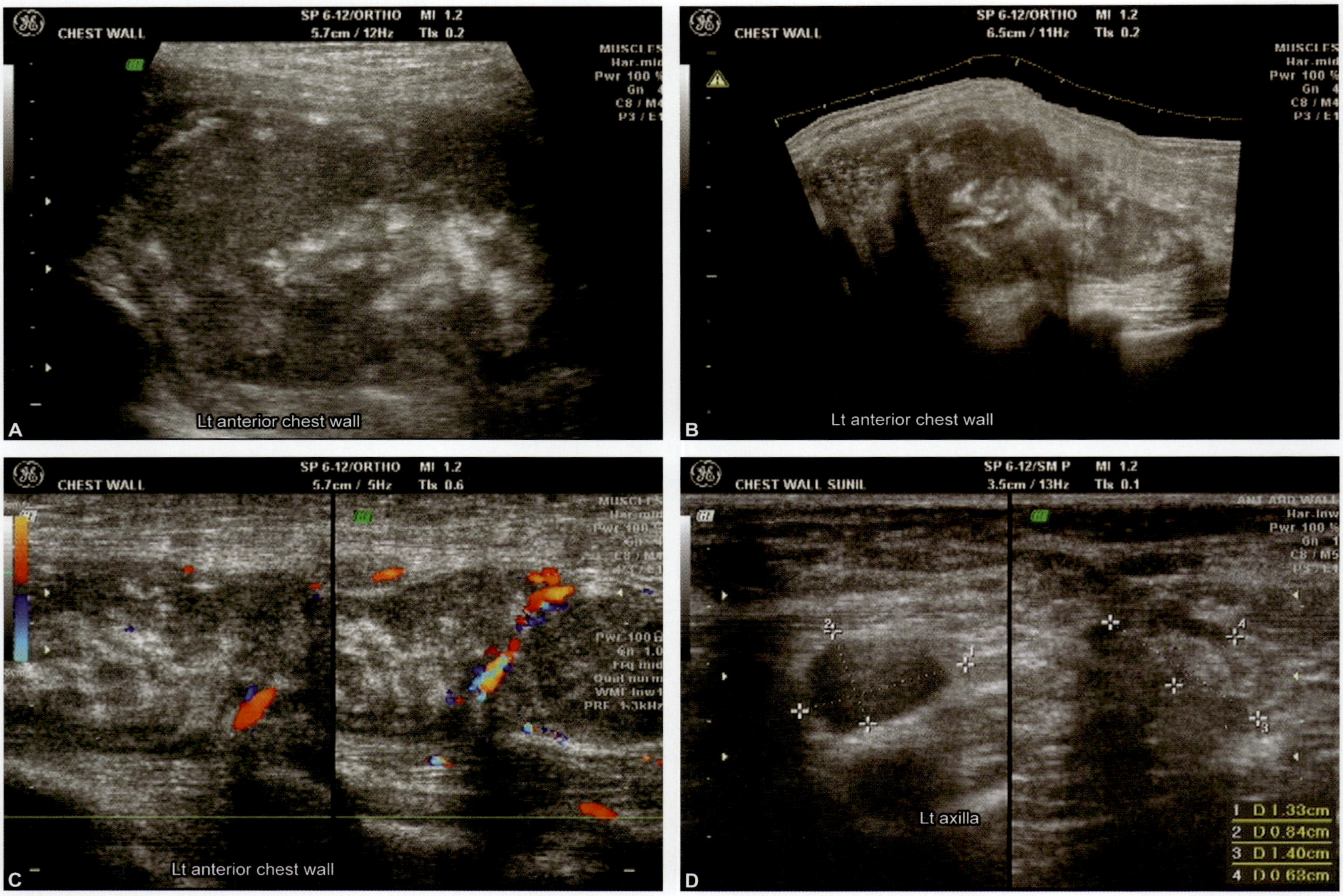

FIGURES 7.39A to D: HRSG shows a big low level echo complex mass seen in the left anterior chest wall. It is seen in the pectoralis major muscle. Low level echoes are seen into it. Multiple echogenic foci are also seen. But no cystic necrosis is seen. On color flow imaging, small vessels collection. Biopsy of the mass confirmed chest wall sarcoma.

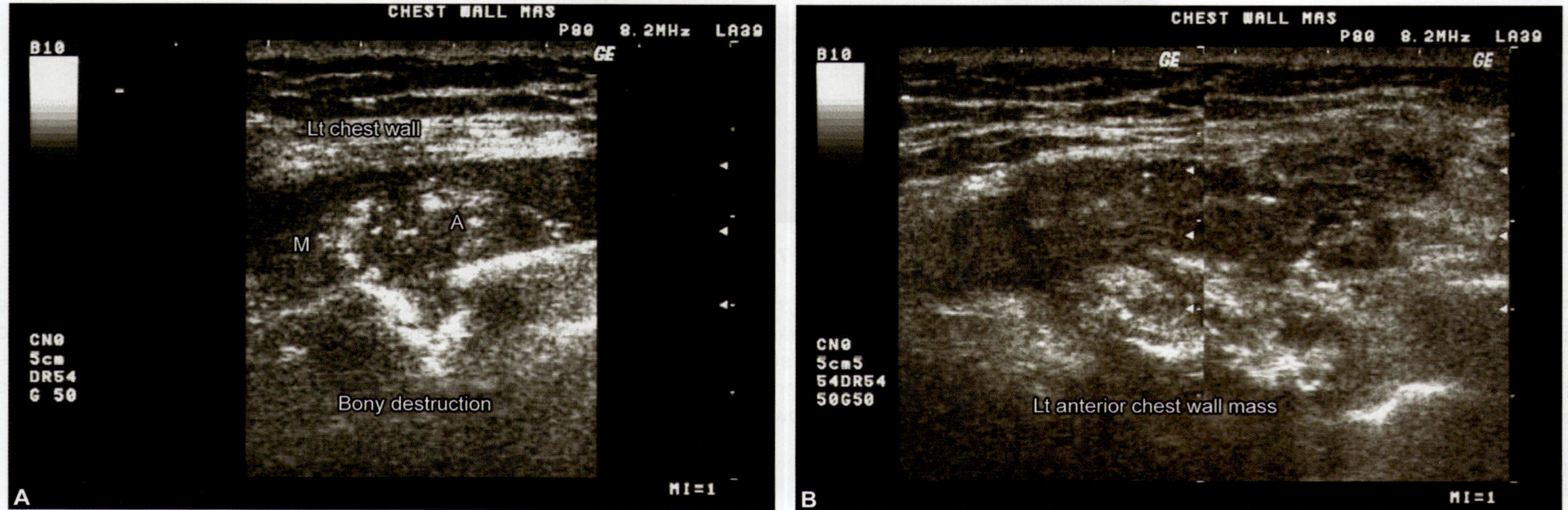

FIGURES 7.40A and B: Tumor mass invading chest wall and the rib. HRSG shows an irregular heterogeneous mass invading the rib of the left chest wall and the mass has destroyed the rib. It is also seen invading the muscles of the chest wall. Biopsy confirmed invasive chondrosarcoma.

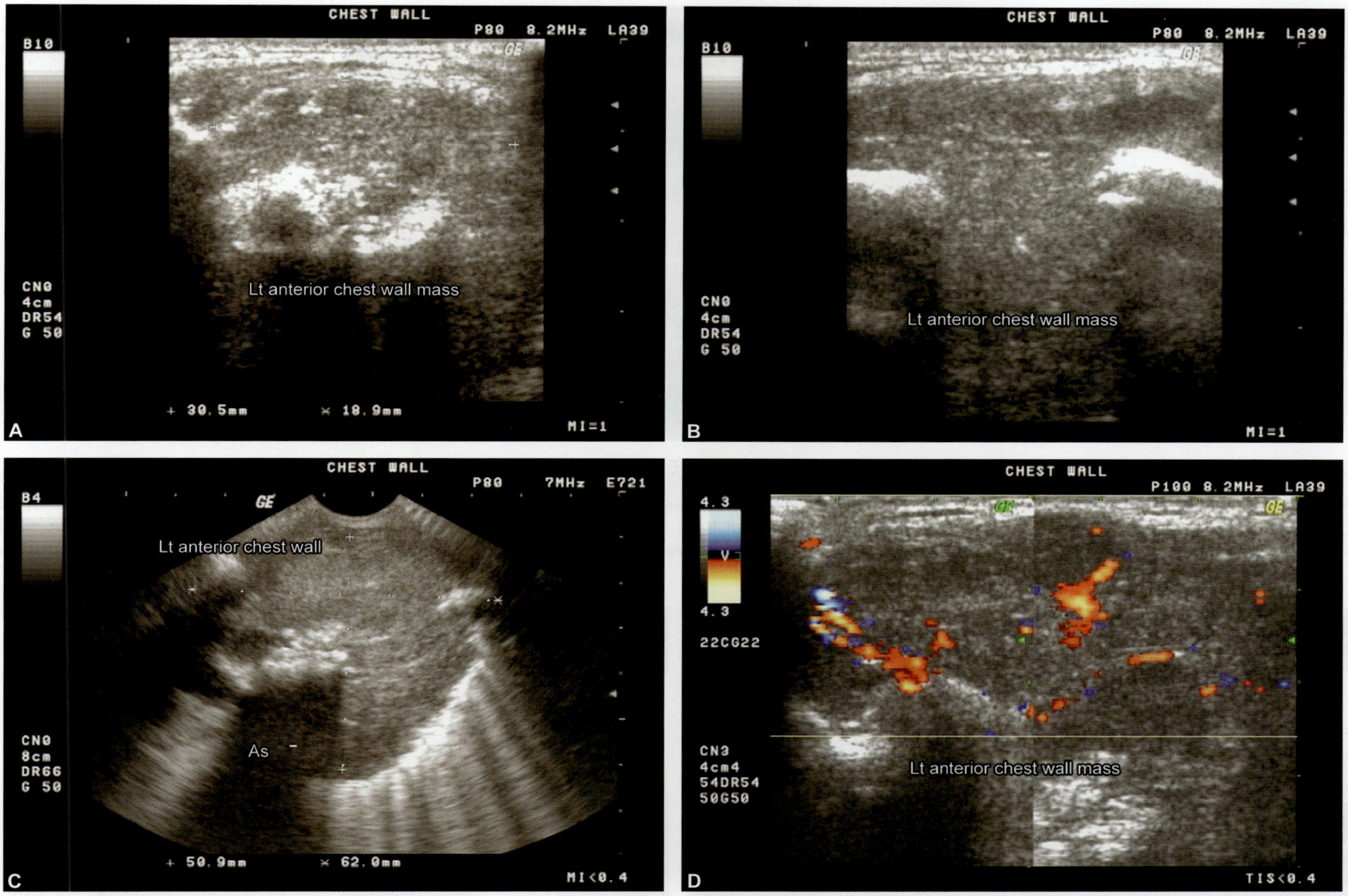

FIGURES 7.41A to D: Big heterogeneous malignant mass invading the chest wall and pleura and peripheral lung. A patient presented with big heterogeneous soft tissue mass fixed with the chest wall. The mass is seen invading the peripheral chest. It is also seen going down deep and invading the rib cage with the bony destruction. Pleural invasion with invasion of peripheral lung is also seen. On color flow imaging, low flow seen in the mass. Biopsy of the mass shows malignant rhabdomyosarcoma.

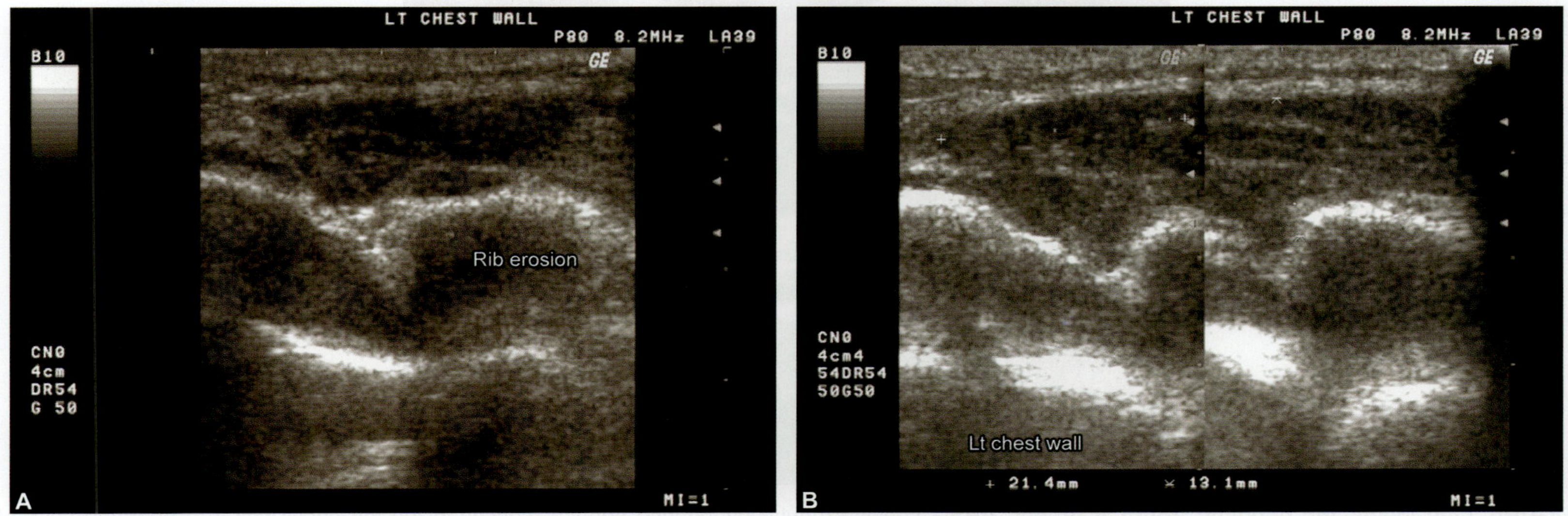

FIGURES 7.42A and B

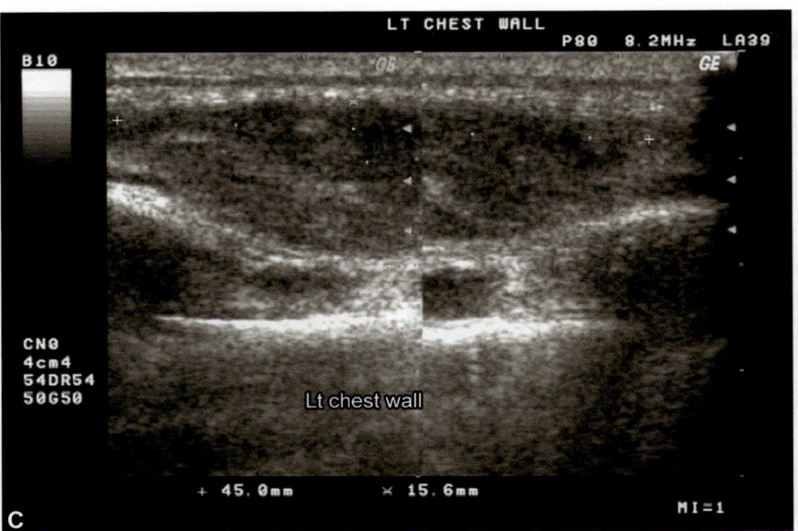

FIGURE 7.42C

FIGURES 7.42A to C: Rib tumor invading the chest wall. A patient presented with persistent soft tissue mass over the chest wall, which was hard. On clinical examination, HRSG shows a soft tissue mass coming out from the rib. It is seen invading the chest wall muscle. Rib erosion is also seen suggestive of malignant tumor. High-resolution ultrasound shows soft tissue component of the tumor. Biopsy of the tumor confirmed chondrosarcoma.

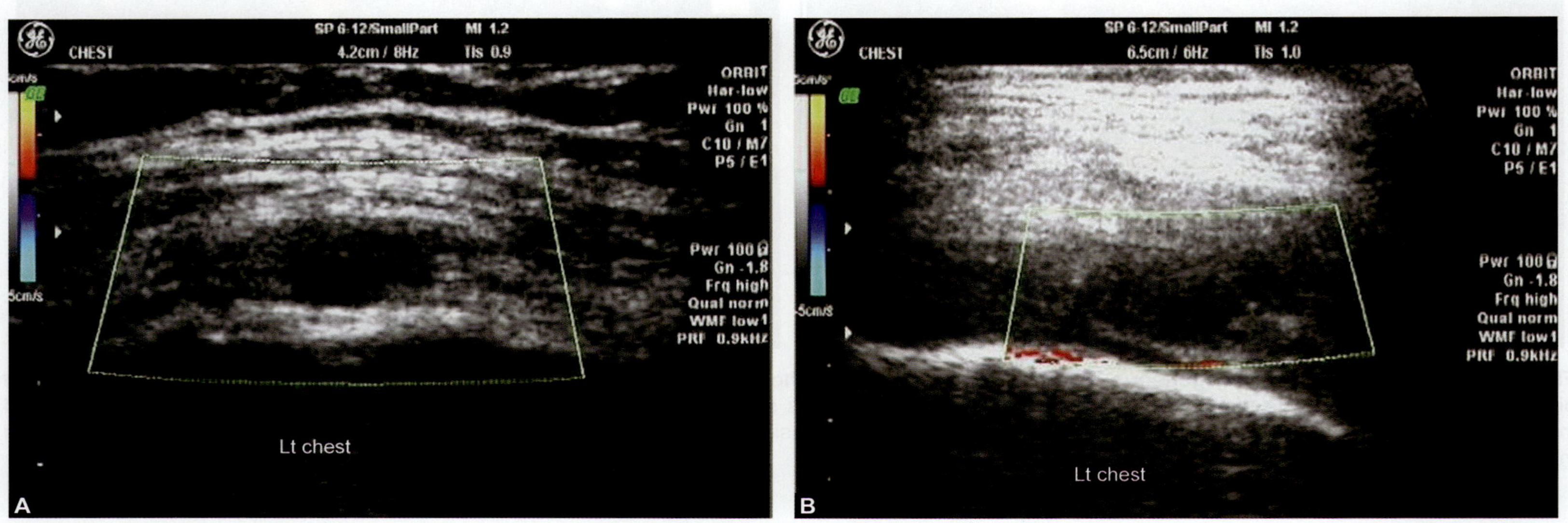

FIGURES 7.43A and B: Metastatic deposit. A patient of CA breast presented with soft tissue mass over the chest wall. HRSG shows a hypoechoic irregular mass over the chest wall suggestive of metastatic deposit.

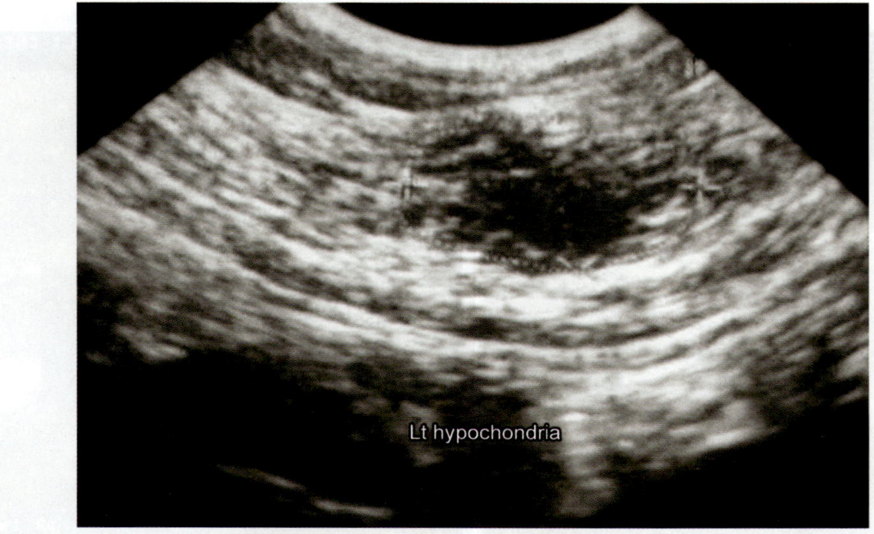

FIGURE 7.44: Metastatic deposits from CA breast. HRSG shows irregular hypodense nodular masses in the left chest wall in a operated case of CA breast. They are well-defined smooth in outline suggestive of enlarged lymph nodes. Irregular hypoechoic mass is also seen in the chest wall. Biopsy of the mass shows metastatic deposits.

Indications for High-resolution Sonography

- Simple pleural effusion
- Encysted pleural effusion
- Lamellar pleural effusion
- Pleural calcification
- Empyema
- Hemothorax
- Pleural thickening
- Pleural tumors
- Primary tumors are rare
- Benign tumors
- Mesothelioma, fibroma
- Lymphoma
- Metastatic tumors—Most common cause is carcinoma bronchus.

Large collection of the fluid in the pleural space may cause hemothorax resulting into collapse of the lung toward hilum. It results into inversion of diaphragm. It can be best evaluated on real time. HRSG shows paradoxical movements on real time imaging.

Mesothelioma is benign tumor. They are poorly echogenic or hypoechoic homogeneous in texture. The most common cause is due to prolonged exposure to asbestos. Homogeneous nodular pleural thickening is seen on HRSG.

LUNG PARENCHYMA

Ultrasonographic examination of the lung parenchyma to determine the nature of lesion is possible only when the barrier of air in lung periphery is broken by collapse of lung or filling in by fluid and inflammatory cells (in consolidation). Consolidated lung is hypoechoic as compared to aerated lung, liver or spleen. Air within bronchi surrounded by consolidated lung produces highly reflective linear branching echoes that can be recognized as sonographic air bronchogram. Aerated alveoli surrounded by consolidated lung produce highly reflective globular echoes that can be recognized as sonographic air alveolograms. In the consolidated lung, fluid-filled bronchi or pulmonary vessels can be seen as anechoic tubular branching structures. Differentiation between the two can be recognized as observing pulsation in vessels or using Doppler. The identification of sonographic air bronchogram, air alveologram, fluid bronchogram and/or pulmonary vasculature helps to differentiate consolidated lung from parenchyma masses and pleural lesions. Besides ultrasonographic examination is useful to differentiate pneumonia alone from pneumonia with pleural effusion of empyema. Atelectatic lung appears as wedge-shaped density moving synchronously with respiration through the pleural fluid and have crowded fluid or air filled bronchi within the collapsed portion of the lung.

Lung abscesses have thick irregular walls with echogenic debris and air within the internal fluid and area are often associated with surrounded area of consolidations. An empyema is confined within the pleural space and tends to have smooth walls of uniform thickness. It also compresses and displaces the surrounding lung parenchyma. The radiographic dilemma of differentiating lung abscess from empyema is resolved to large extent by ultrasonography. With the real time sonography, a lung abscess during inspiration, demonstrates expansion of its entire circumference, whereas in case of empyema only the visceral pleural surface show motion. Hydatid cyst has characteristics appearance on daughter cysts, lifting up of membrane or sonographic water lily sign. They may have associated hepatic involvement or some other pathology.

Lung tumors, both peripheral and central, depending on size and relation to chest wall can usually be visualized by ultrasonography. They usually have well-defined outlines and stand out in presence of surrounding air filled lung, consolidation or collapse. Although most of the lesions that are smaller than 5 cm are hypoechoic compared to aerated lung. The increased echogenicity of larger lesions may be caused by internal echolucency with hyperechoic walls while calcification is seen as echogenic speck with or without posterior shadow. For centrally located lung tumors associated consolidation or collapse is required as a window to permit visualization. Tumors that are surrounded by consolidation lung appear as hyperechoic masses within the hypoechoic fluid filled lung. Ultrasonography can help in diagnosing invasion of the chest wall by using lung tumor. Besides this modality permit us to identify various pathologies present in case of opaque hemithorax.

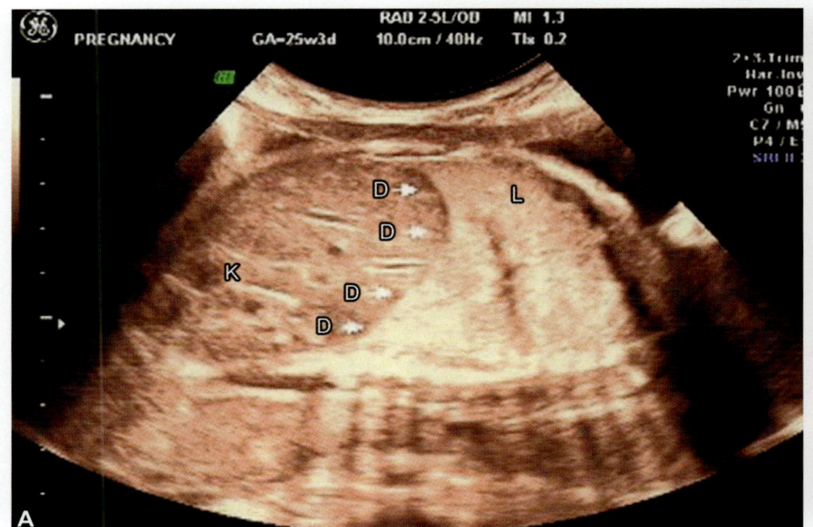

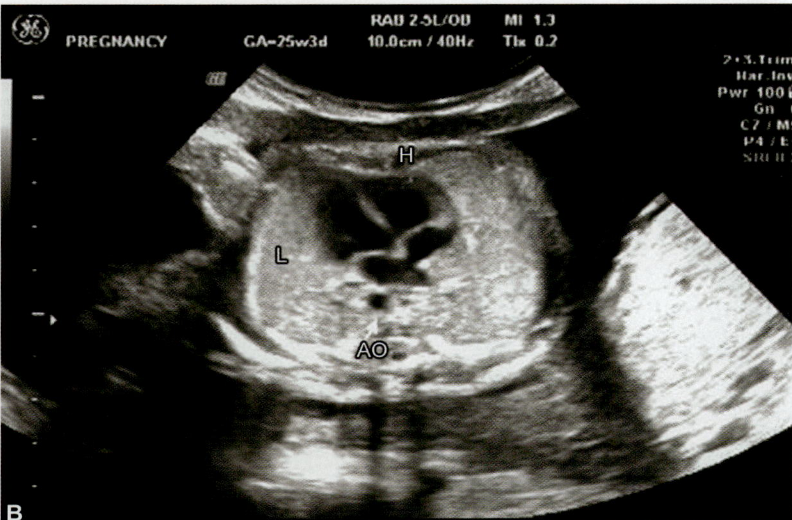

FIGURES 7.45A and B

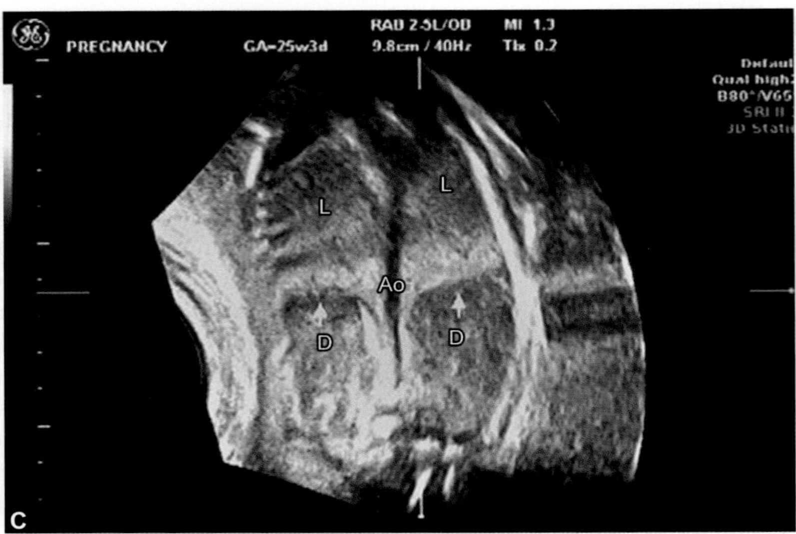

FIGURE 7.45C

FIGURES 7.45A to C: Fetal lung. HRSG is very good modality for evaluation of fetal lung. The lung is seen as echogenic soft tissue shadows in the thorax encasing the fetal heart. The dome of diaphragm is seen as a hypoechoic curvy linear bands. Separating the thorax and the abdomen. Figure 7.45B shows 3D coronal image of fetal lung.

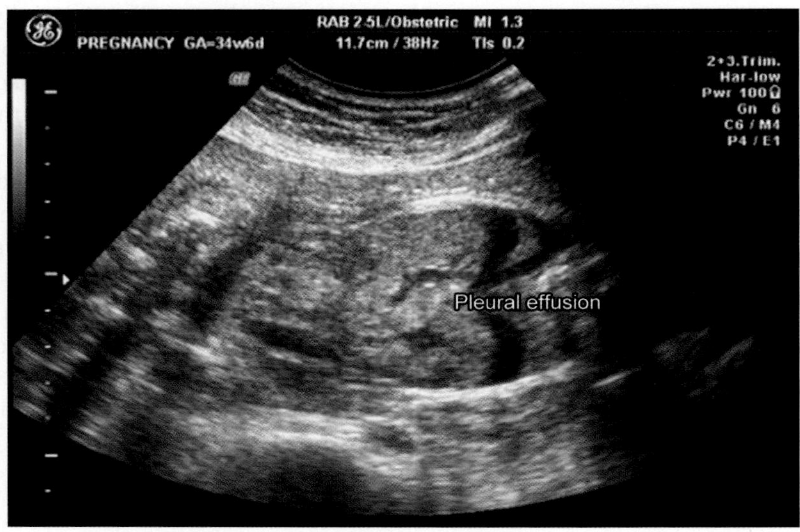

FIGURE 7.46: Bilateral small pleural effusion in fetus. HRSG shows pleural effusion in both thoracic cavity in the fetal lung.

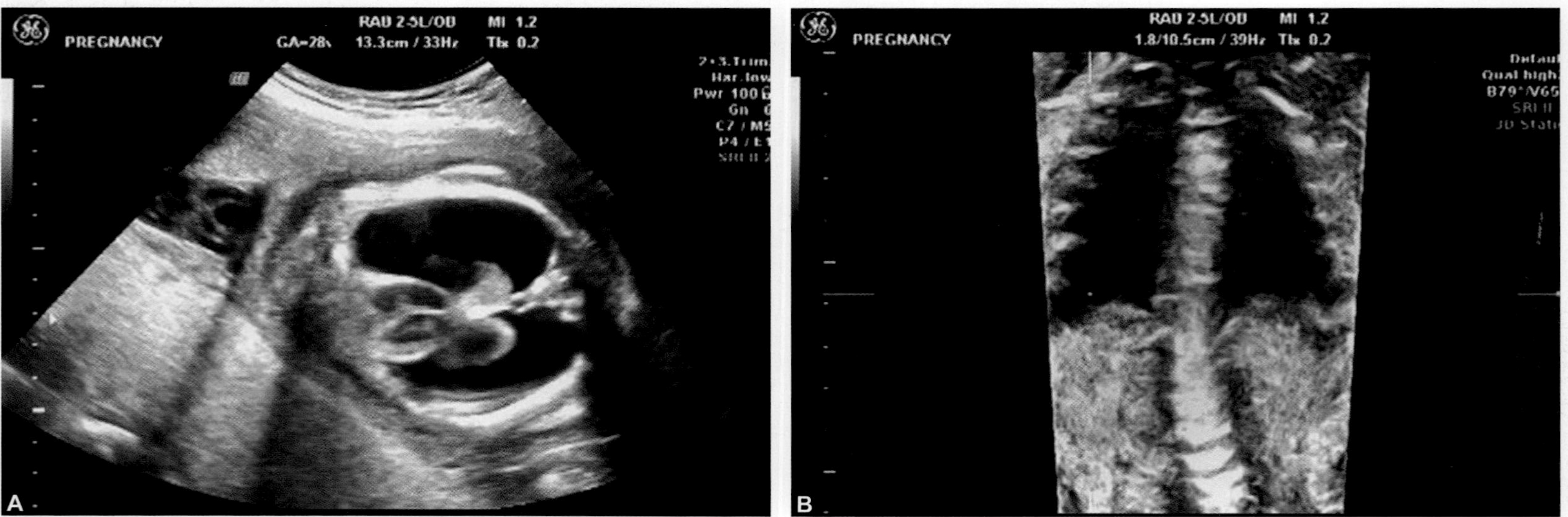

FIGURES 7.47A and B

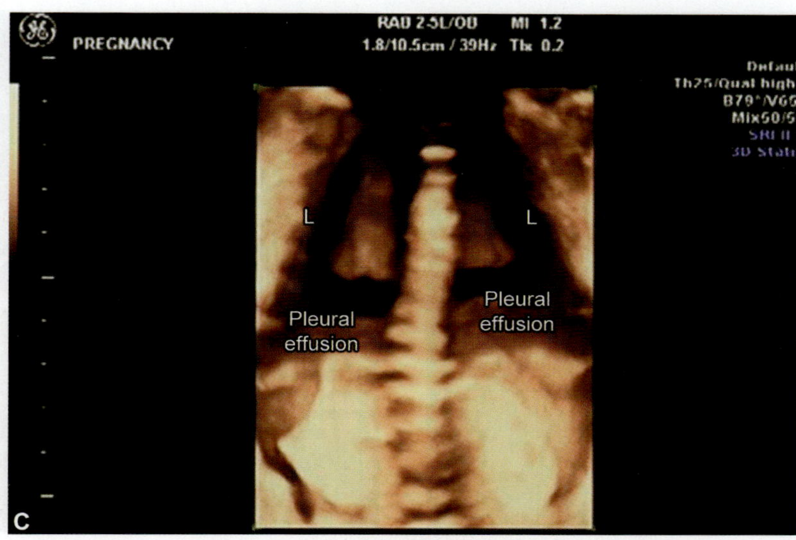

FIGURE 7.47C

FIGURES 7.47A to C: Bilateral pleural effusion with 3D imaging (SONO MR). HRSG shows gross amount of fluid collection in both pleural cavity of the fetus. The heart is seen compressed. 3D coronal imaging of fetal thorax shows collapsed lung with bilateral pleural effusion.

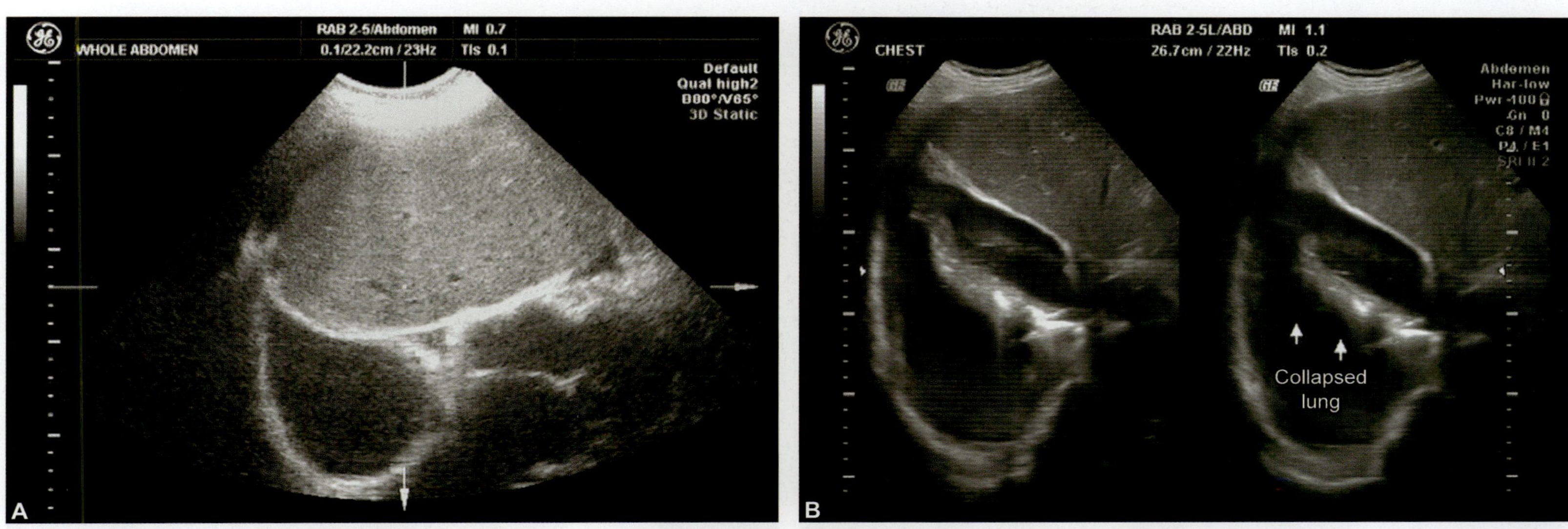

FIGURES 7.48A and B: Simple pleural effusion with ascites. HRSG shows small amount of fluid collection in the right pleural cavity. Fluid is also seen in the peritoneal cavity. **Massive pleural effusion with collapsed lung.** HRSG shows gross amount fluid collection in the right pleural cavity. The associated collapsed of the lung shows air entrapment as echogenic shadows.

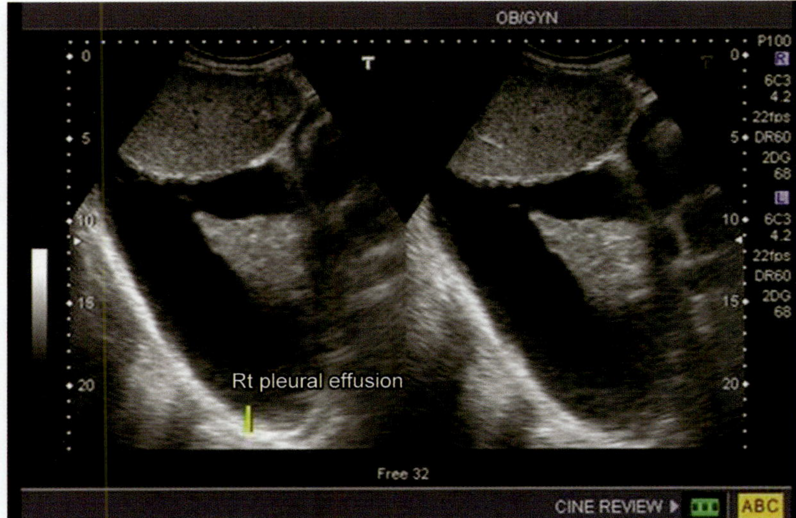

FIGURE 7.49: Collapsed lung with pleural effusion. HRSG shows gross amount of fluid collection in the right pleural cavity. Associated collapse of the lung is also seen as a triangular soft tissue shadow.

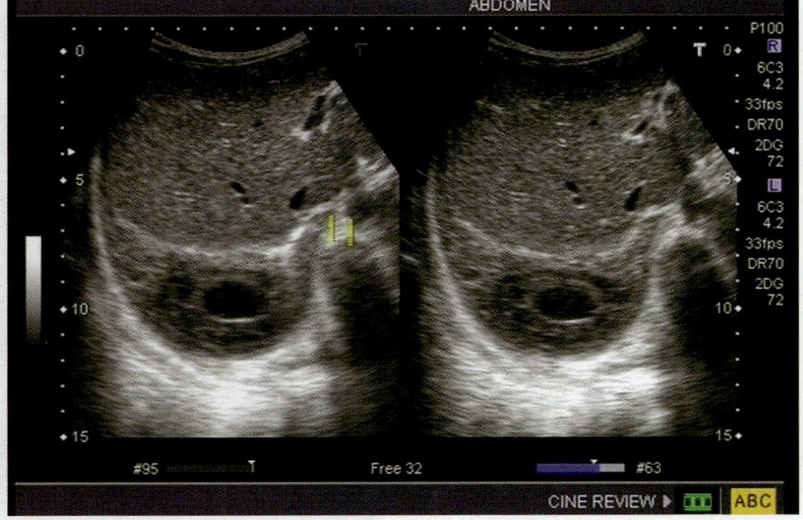

FIGURE 7.50: Pyothorax. HRSG shows thick echo collection in the right pleural cavity. Thick cheesy shadows are seen in the pleural cavity. A small pocket of fluid collection is seen in the centre. On aspiration thick pus was taken out suggestive of pyothorax.

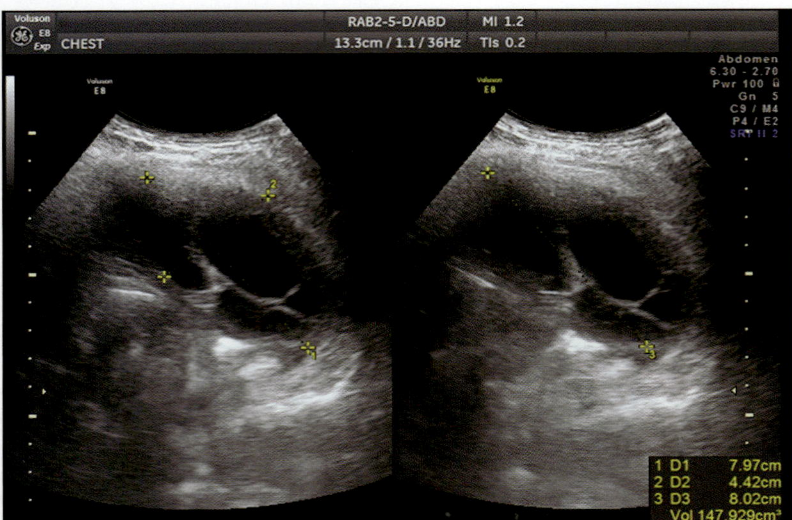

FIGURE 7.51: Loculated pleural effusion. A patient presented with fluid collection in the left pleural cavity. HRSG shows pocket of thick collection in the left pleural cavity. Multiple echogenic bands are seen in the collection suggestive of loculated collection.

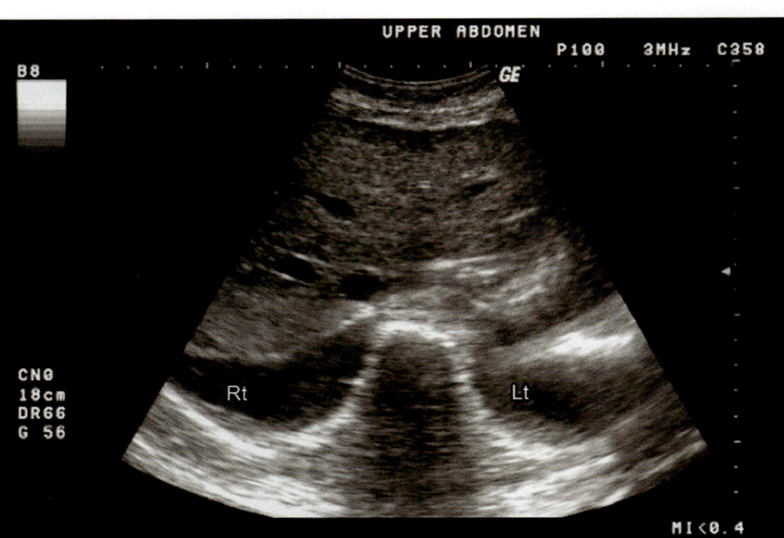

FIGURE 7.52: Bilateral pleural effusion. A patient presented with breathlessness. HRSG shows bilateral pleural effusion. Left lung is collapsed and it is seen floating in the left pleural effusion as an echogenic shadow.

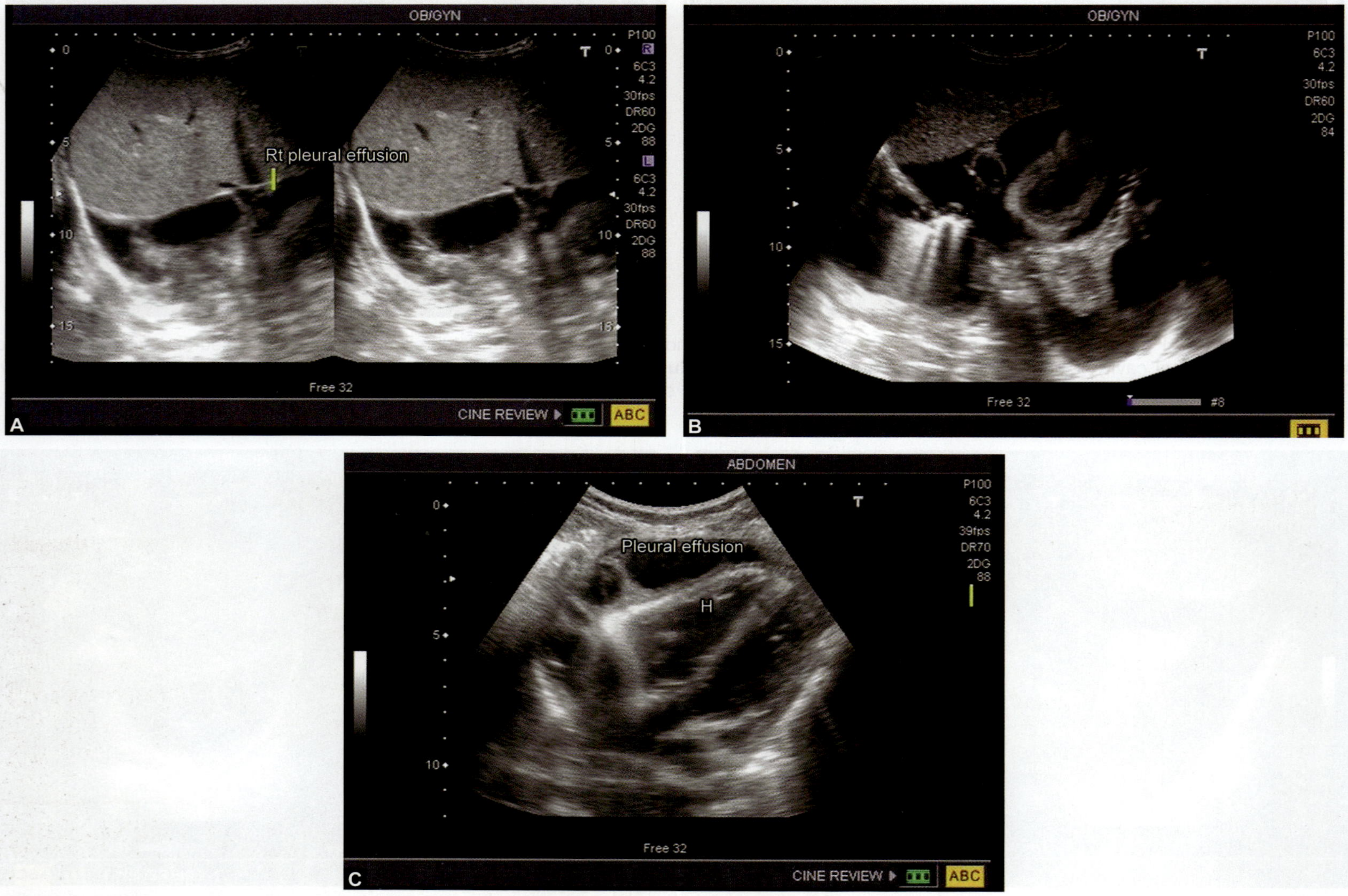

FIGURES 7.53A to C: Pleural effusion with associated pericardial effusion. A patient presented with dyspnea. HRSG shows right-sided pleural effusion. Associated segmental collapse of the lung is also seen. There is also evidence of gross pericardial effusion seen. The liver was also enlarged and hepatic veins were congested due to gross cardiac dysfunction.

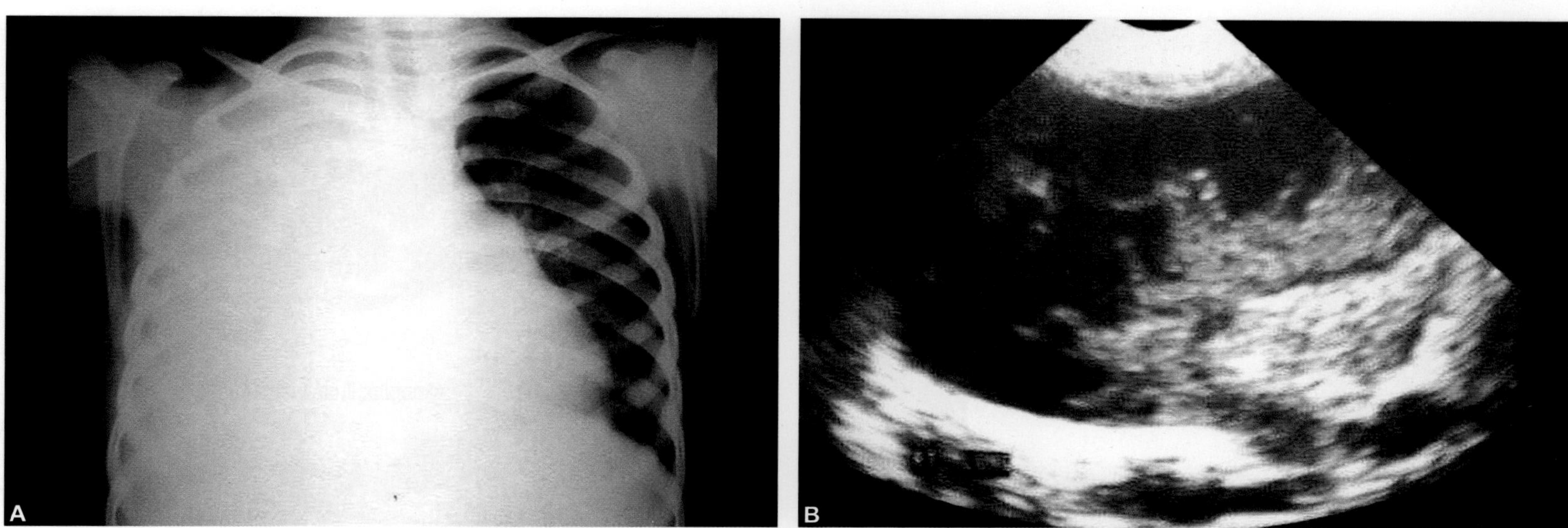

FIGURES 7.54A and B: Massive pleural effusion. Plane X-ray chest of the patient shows right-sided hemithorax with radiodense opacities filling whole of the right thorax of a young child. HRSG shows massive fluid collection in the right pleural cavity. The lung is seen collapsed and floating in the fluid collection. Multiple fibrous bands are seen in the collection. Echogenic debris is also seen in the collection.

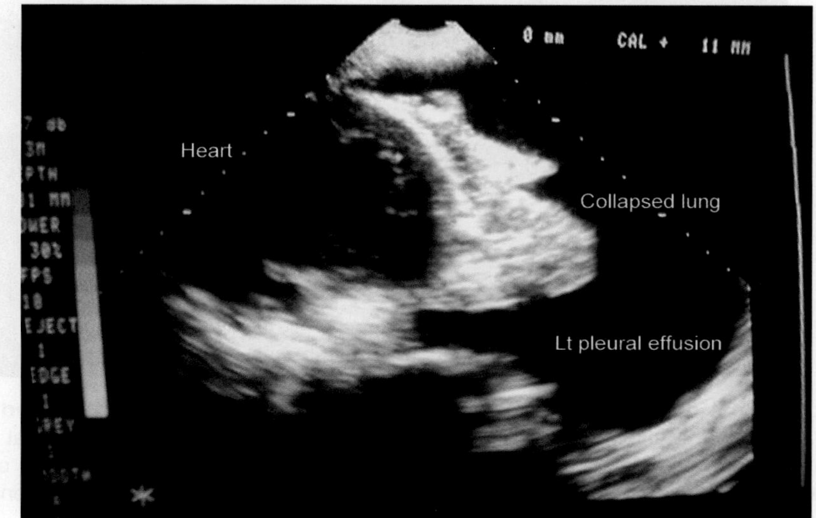

FIGURE 7.55: Massive pleural effusion. HRSG shows gross amount of fluid collection in the left pleural cavity. The lung is collapsed and compressed by the pressure of the fluid. Heart is also seen shifted to the right side.

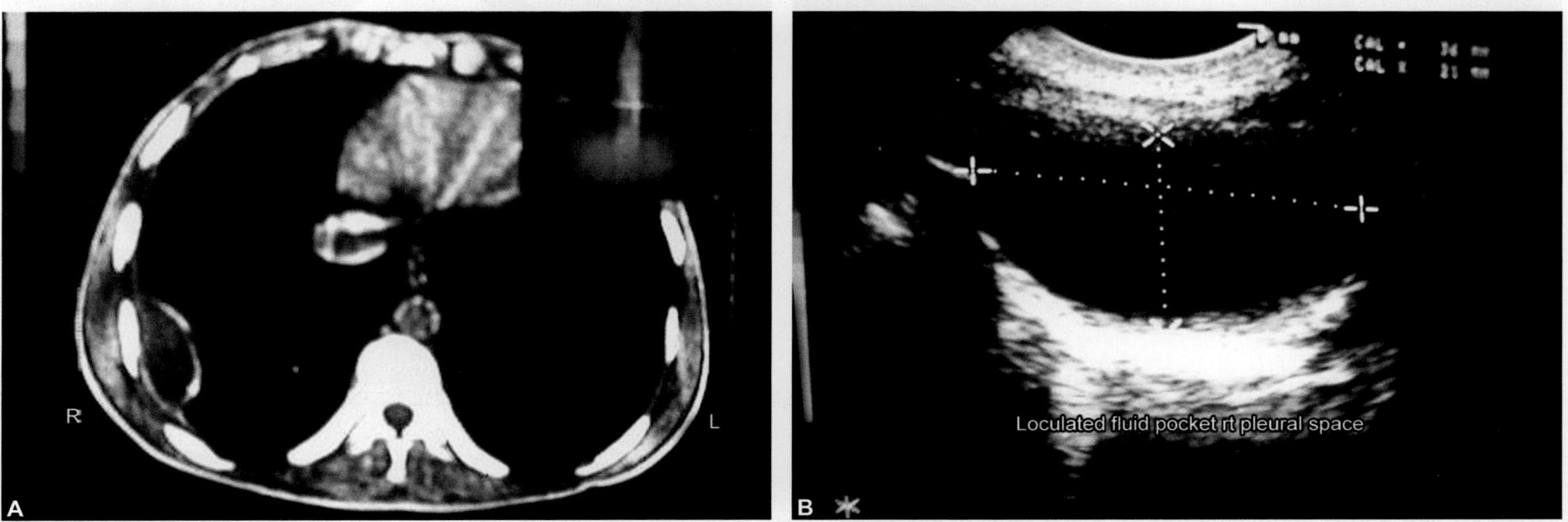

FIGURES 7.56A and B: Loculated anterior pleural effusion. CT scan of the patient shows a hypodense shadow in the anterior part of the right lung. HRSG of the same patient shows encysted fluid collection in the anterior part of the right lung.

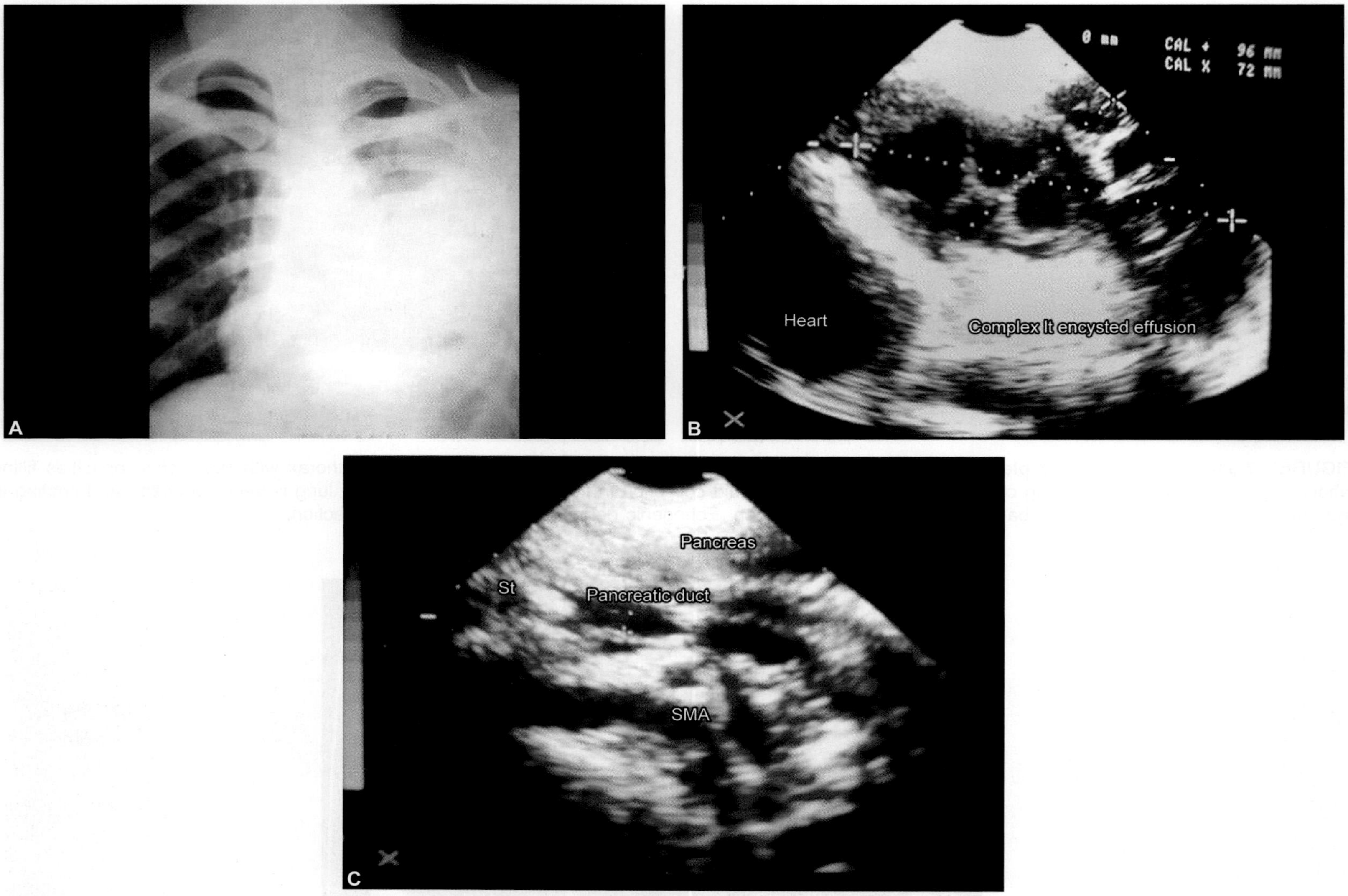

FIGURES 7.57A to C: Plane X-ray of chest of the patient shows left-sided radioopacity with obliterated CP angle. HRSG of the same patient shows multiloculated left-sided pleural effusion. Multiple echogenic septa are seen in the collection. Abdominal sonography of the same patient shows chronic calcific pancreatitis with dilated pancreatic duct. Multiple calculi are seen in the pancreatic duct. Tail of the pancreas is enlarged hypoechoic irregular in outline. The pancreatitis is the cause of recurrent left-sided pleural effusion in the same patient. Pancreatitis involving the tail of the pancreas is known to cause reactive pleural effusion on the left side.

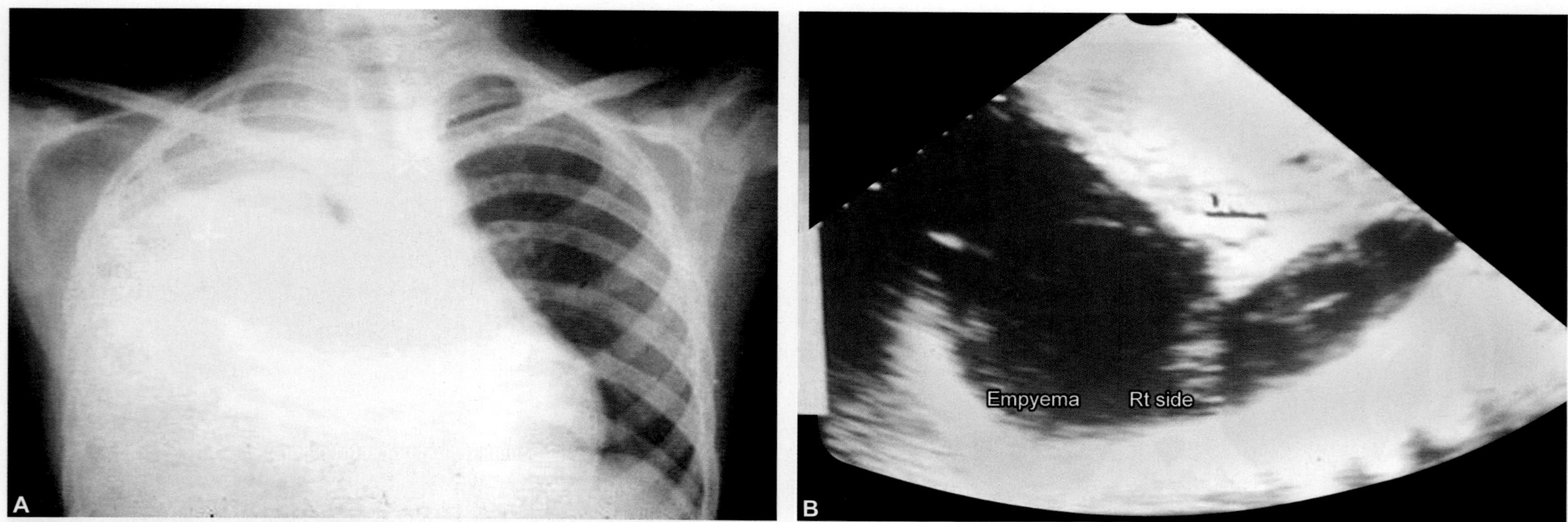

FIGURES 7.58A and B: Empyema thorax. Plane X-ray of the patient shows right-sided hemithorax suggestive of radiodense opaque shadow is seen filling the right pleural cavity and opacify the thorax. HRSG of the same patient shows big thick low level echo collection filling the pleural cavity. The lung is seen collapsed and sharp borders of the collapsed lung are seen. On aspiration of the fluid pyogenic collection was seen coming out from the fluid.

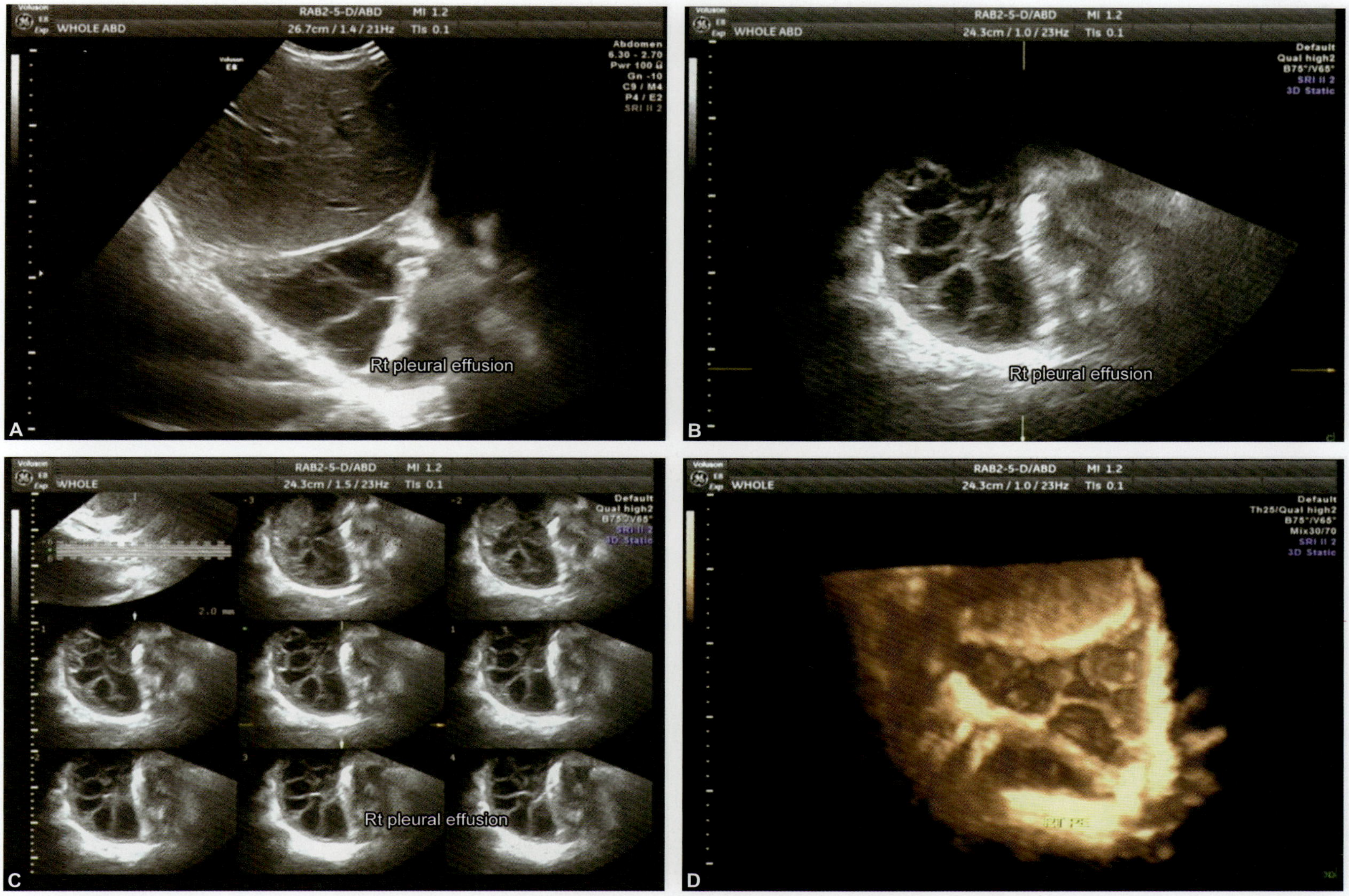

FIGURES 7.59A to D: A patient presented with high fever with dyspnea. HRSG shows a multiloculated pocket of thick collection in right pleural cavity. 3D ultrasound with TUI shows multiple echogenic septa in the collection forming multiple loculations. On aspiration thick pus was aspirated.

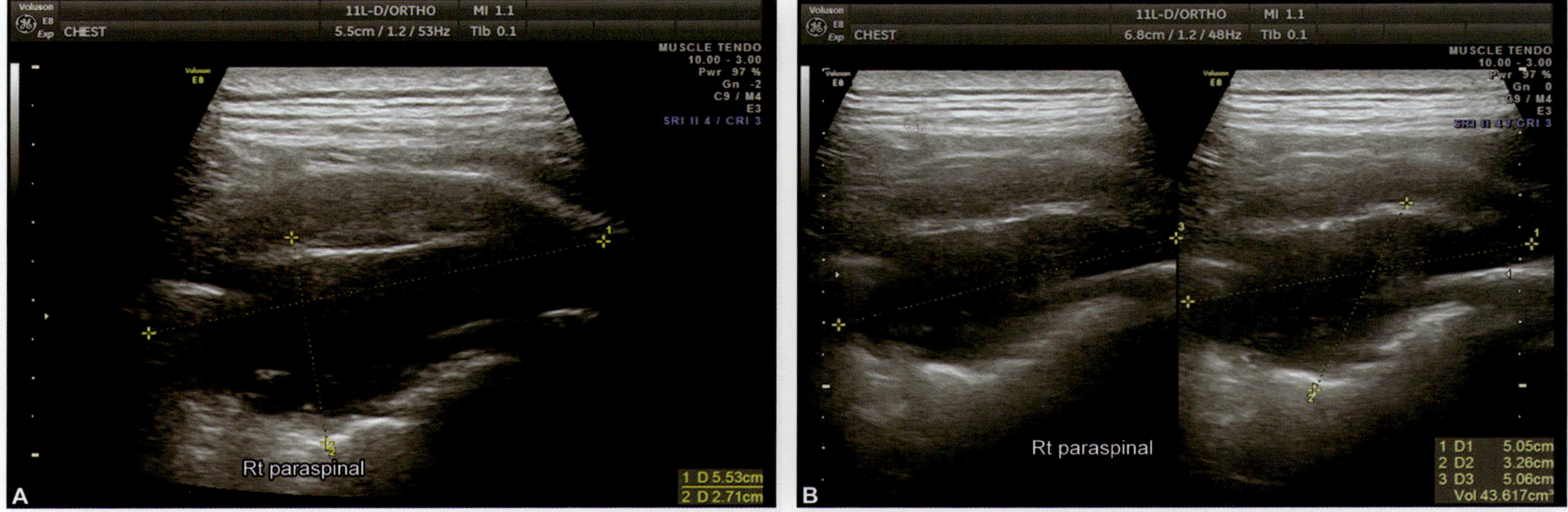

FIGURES 7.60A and B

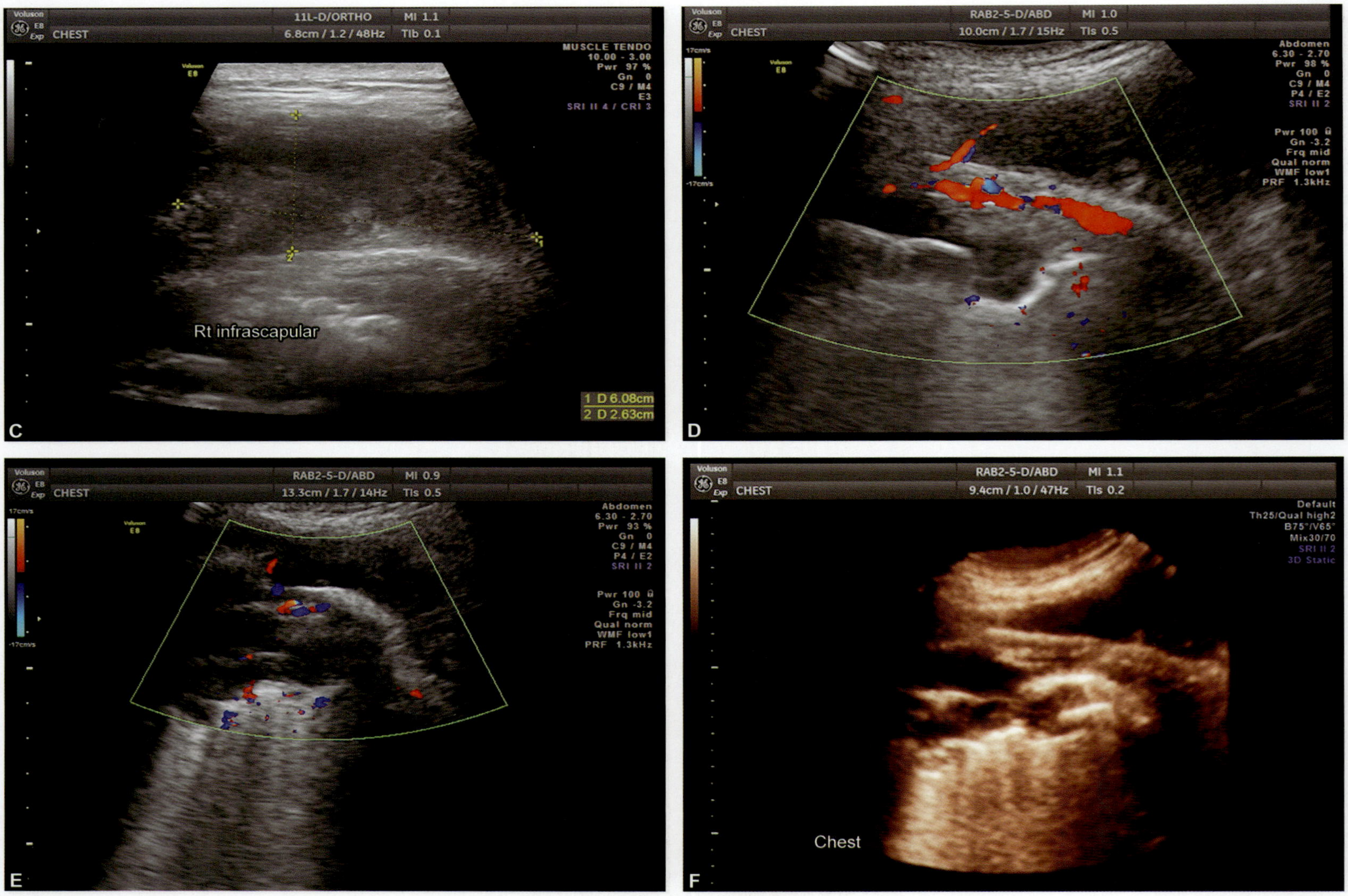

FIGURES 7.60C to F

FIGURES 7.60A to F: A patient presented with high fever not responding to treatment. HRSG shows pocket of thick collection in the right infrascapular region. Thick echoes are seen in it. There is also evidence of a small communication seen from the collection to the right pleural cavity. Thick cheesy pocket of collection is seen in it. On color flow imaging, few vessels are seen feeding it. Low arterial flow is seen in it suggestive of granulomatous collection. Small collection is seen also seen in right pleural cavity. Findings are suggestive of chronic infective pyogenic collection.

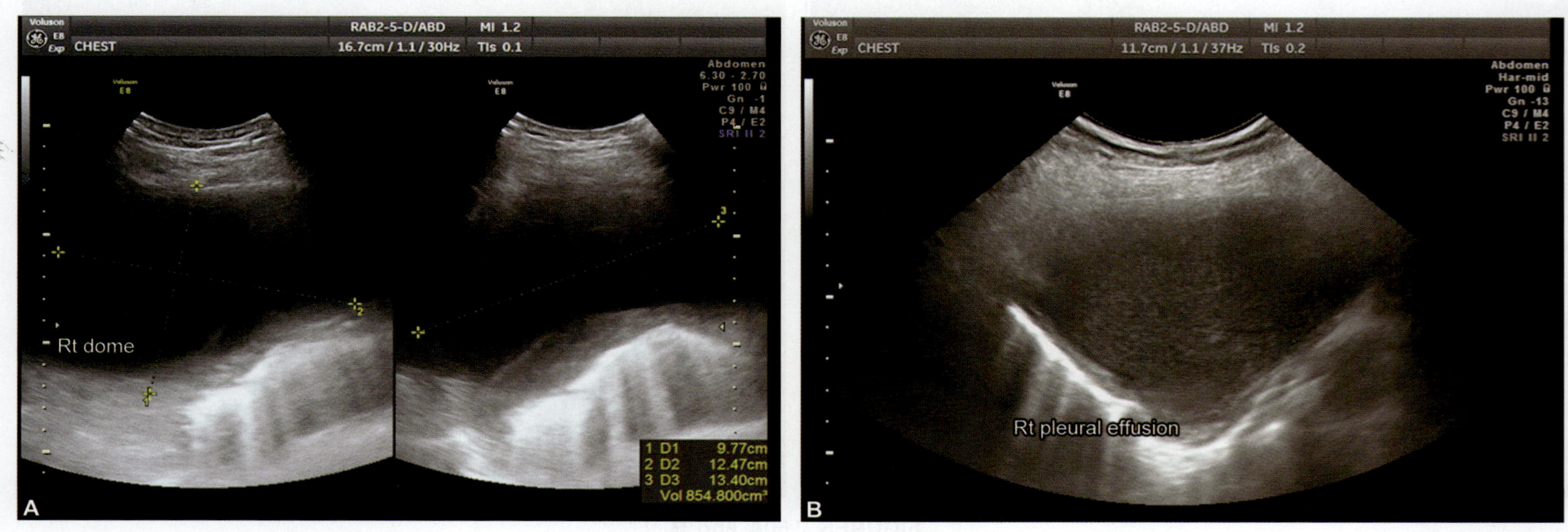

FIGURES 7.61A and B: Massive pleural effusion. HRSG shows large amount of fluid collection in the right pleural cavity. The lung is seen collapsed and compressed.

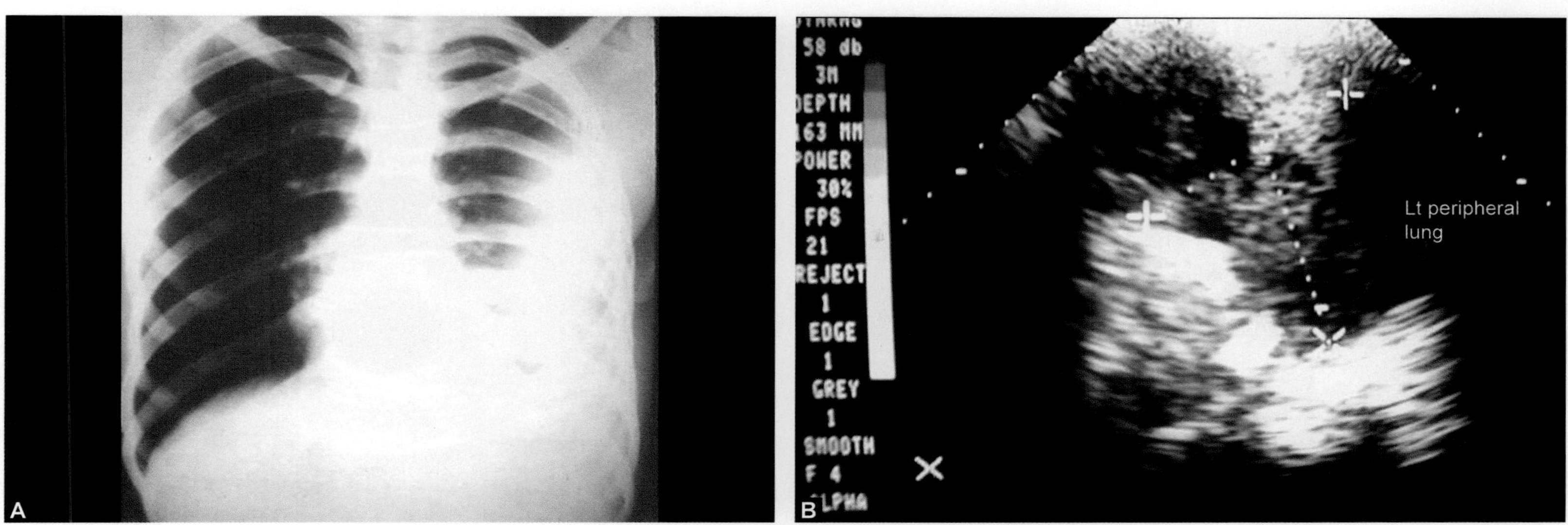

FIGURES 7.62A and B: Peripheral lung mass. Plane X-ray of the cyst shows a radiodense opacity in the left thorax with obliterated costophrenic angle. HRSG of the same patient shows a soft tissue mass in the left mid zone and lower zone. The mass shows irregular margin. Irregular hypoechoic areas are also seen in it suggestive of an abscess. USG-guided biopsy of the mass shows bronchogenic carcinoma.

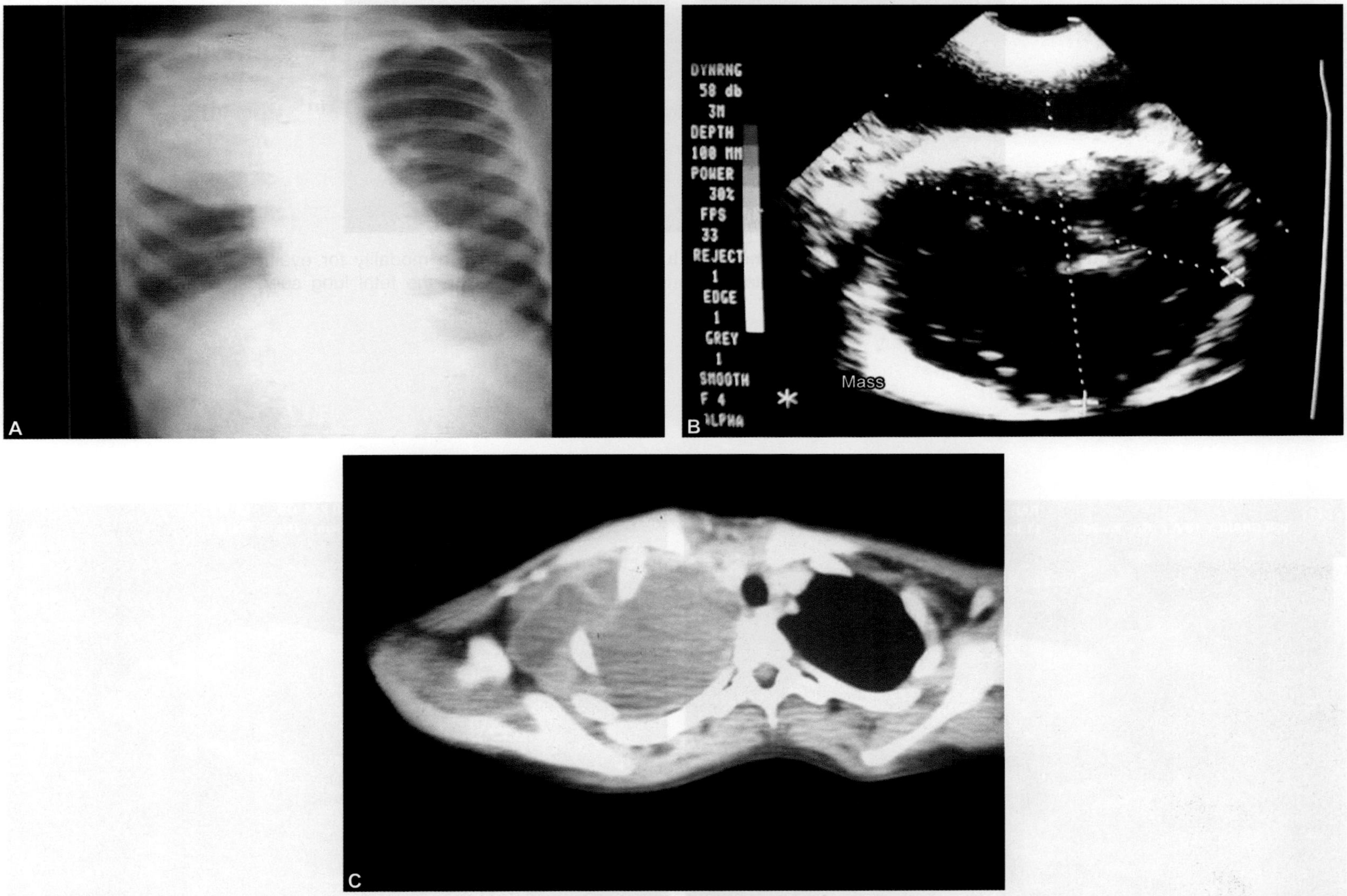

FIGURES 7.63A to C: Hydatid cyst of the lung. X-ray of the young girl shows a well-defined homogeneous mass in the right upper zone. The mass shows sharp margins. HRSG of the same patient shows a multiloculated cystic mass in the right supraclavicular and infraclavicular area going to the upper part of the right thorax. Echogenic calcification is also seen in the mass. CT scan of the same patient shows homogeneous soft tissue mass with thick septa. Biopsy of the mass shows hydatid cyst.

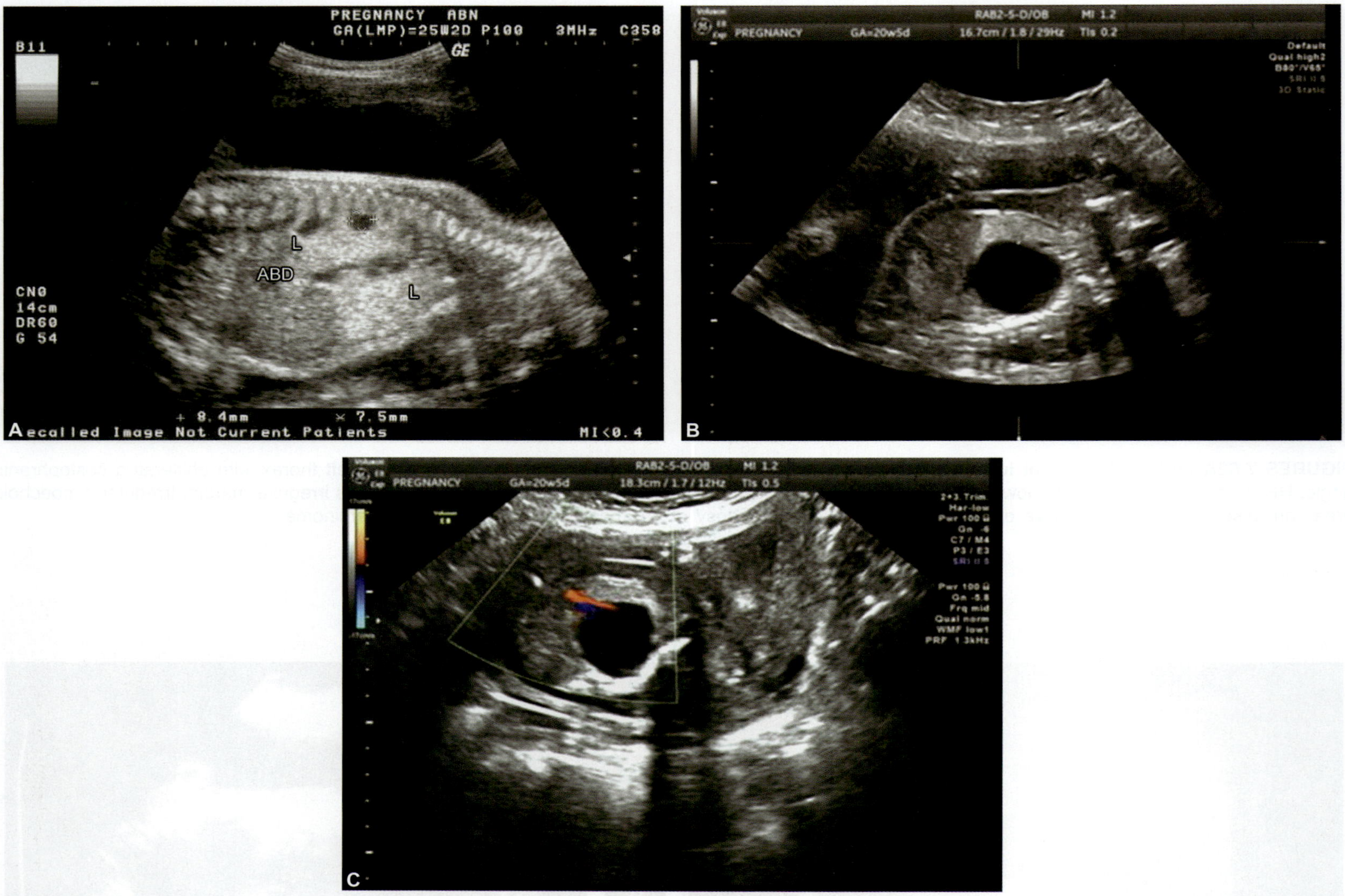

FIGURES 7.64A to C: Cystic adenomatoid malformation in the fetal lung. HRSG is very good modality for evaluation of cystic masses in the lung in fetus. Figure 7.64A shows multiple small cysts in the fetal left lung. A big cyst is seen in the fetal lung suggestive of cystic adenomatoid malformation of lung.

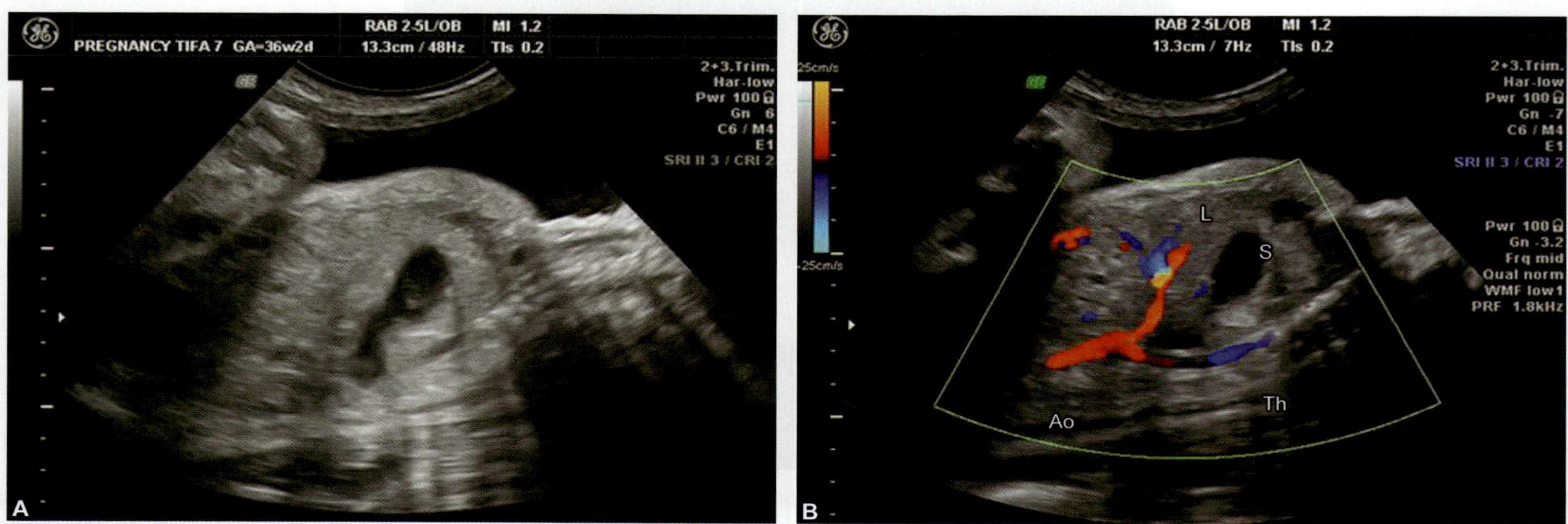

FIGURES 7.65A and B: Diaphragmatic hernia in fetal thorax. HRSG shows a cystic mass seen herniating in the fetal thorax. It is seen displacing the fetal heart suggestive of stomach herniating in the fetal thorax.

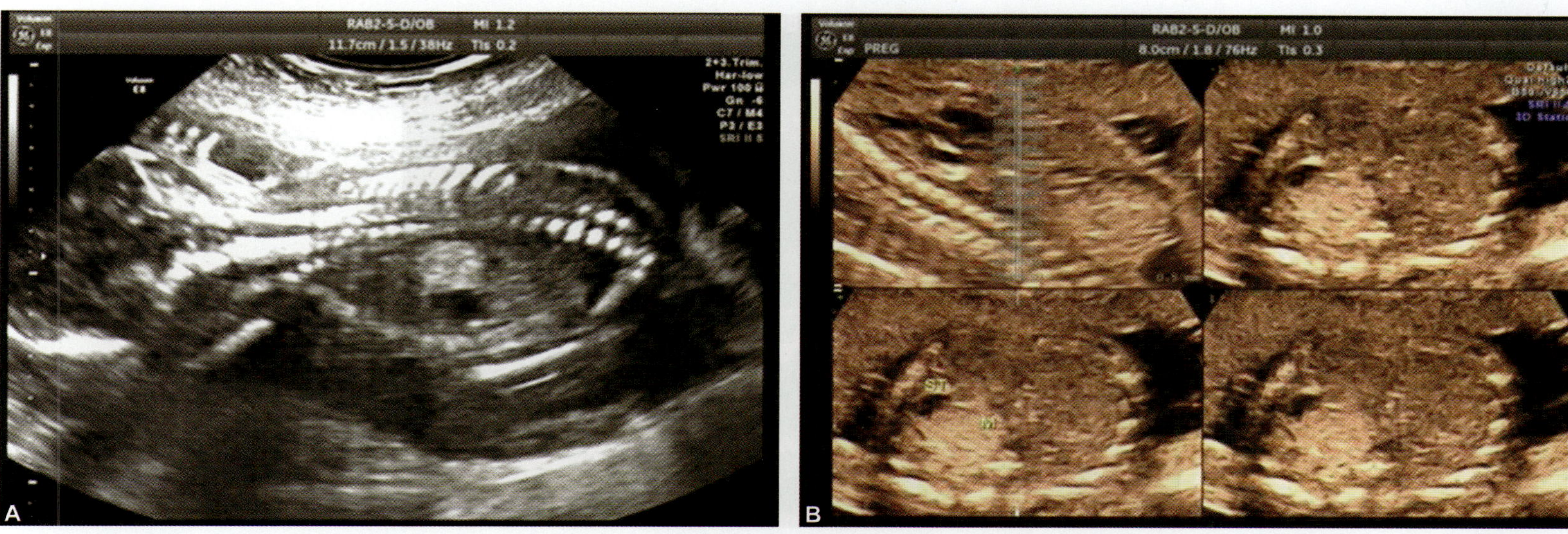

FIGURES 7.66A and B: Extralobar sequestration. Fetus shows a highly echogenic soft tissue shadow below the diaphragm in the fetus. It is seen above the stomach. It is typical finding of extralobar sequestration in the lung.

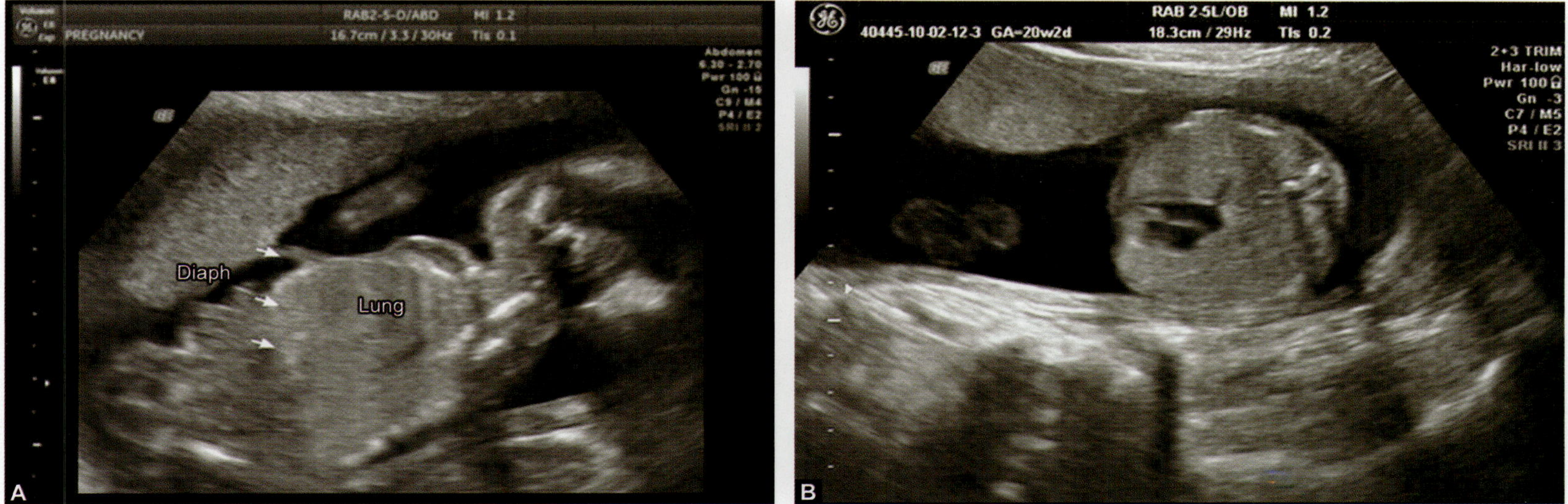

FIGURES 7.67A and B: Chronic high airway obstruction. HRSG shows markedly enlarged fetal lungs, which are seen going down in the fetal abdomen and occupying almost 2/3rd of the fetal abdomen. The heart is sandwiched between the markedly enlarged lungs suggestive of chronic high airway obstruction due to tracheal atresia.

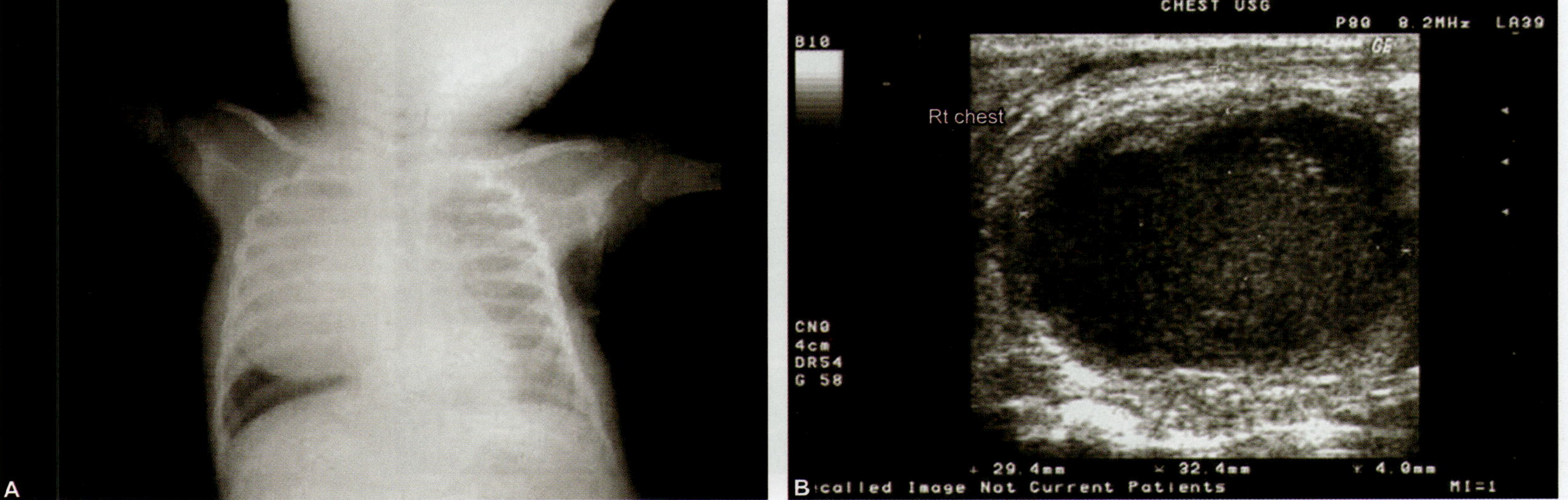

FIGURES 7.68A and B

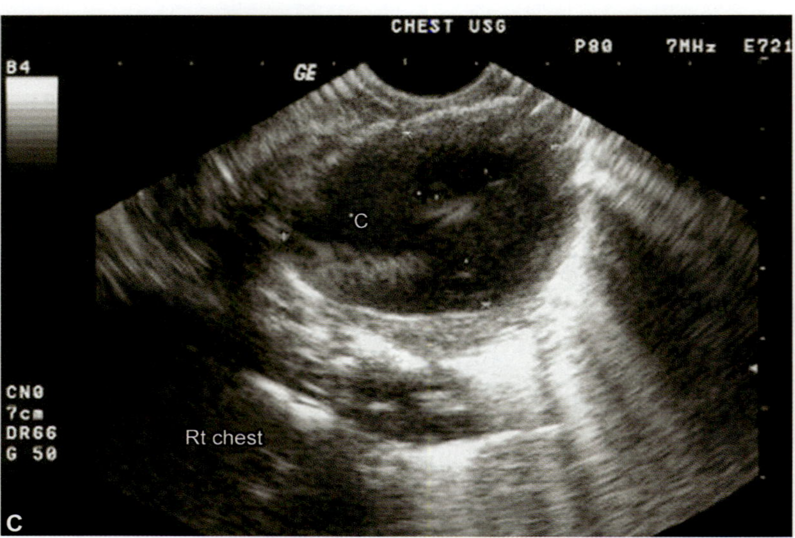

FIGURE 7.68C

FIGURES 7.68A to C: Cystic adenomatoid malformation of lung. A newborn child presented with dyspnea. X-ray chest shows well define homogeneous opacity in the right lung. HRSG of the same patient shows well-defined cyst in the right lung. No septation is seen in it.

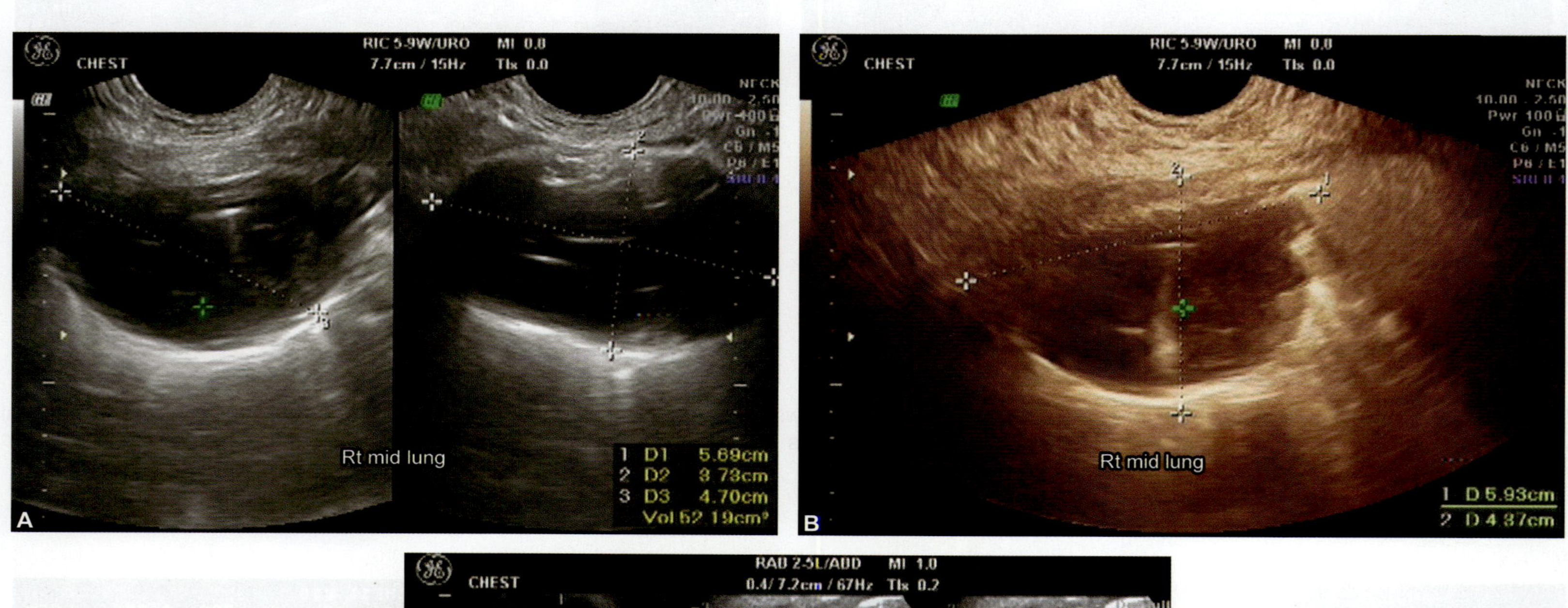

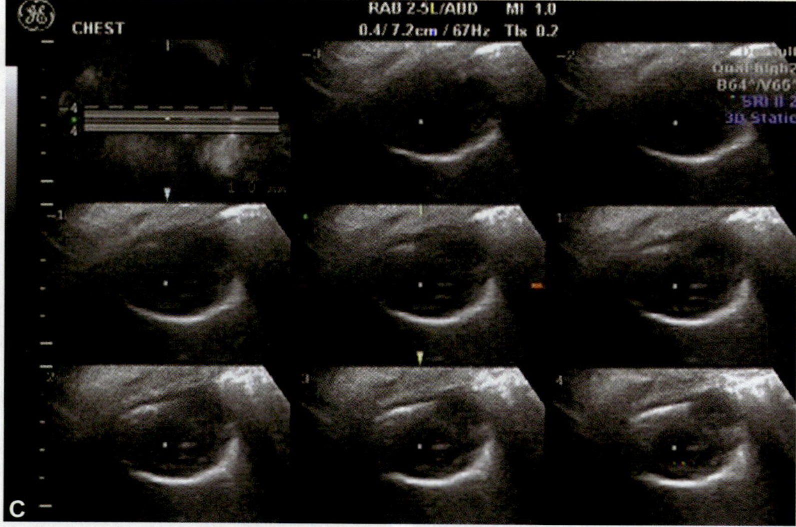

FIGURES 7.69A to C: A patient presented with soft tissue shadow in the right lung on X-ray. HRSG shows well defined pocket of fluid collection in the mid part of the right peripheral lung. It shows echogenic walls fluid collection is seen into it. Multiple internal echoes are seen into it. But no evidence of any calcification is seen. No membrane is seen floating in the collection suggestive of encysted pleural effusion.

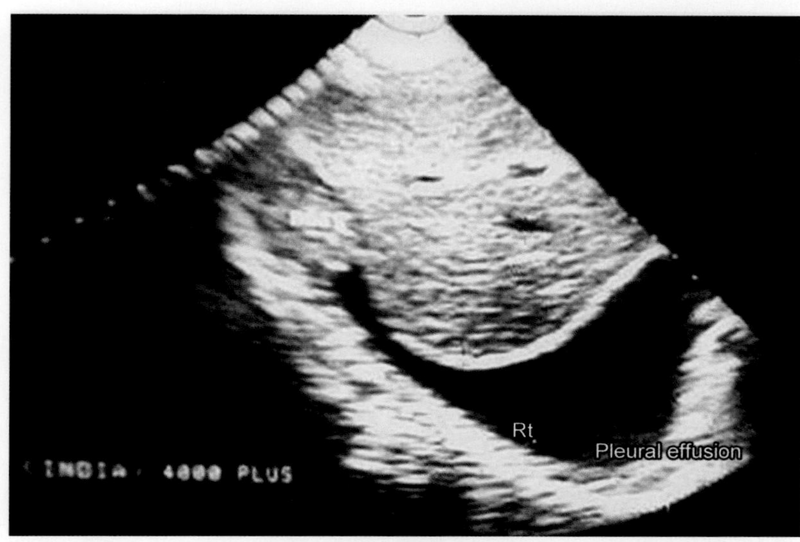

FIGURE 7.70: Mesothelioma of pleura. HRSG shows a well-defined homogeneous hyperechoic nodular mass coming out from the pleura on the right side on the anterior recess. No calcification is seen in the mass. No cystic degeneration is seen. Associated pleural effusion is also seen. Biopsy of the mass shows mesothelioma.

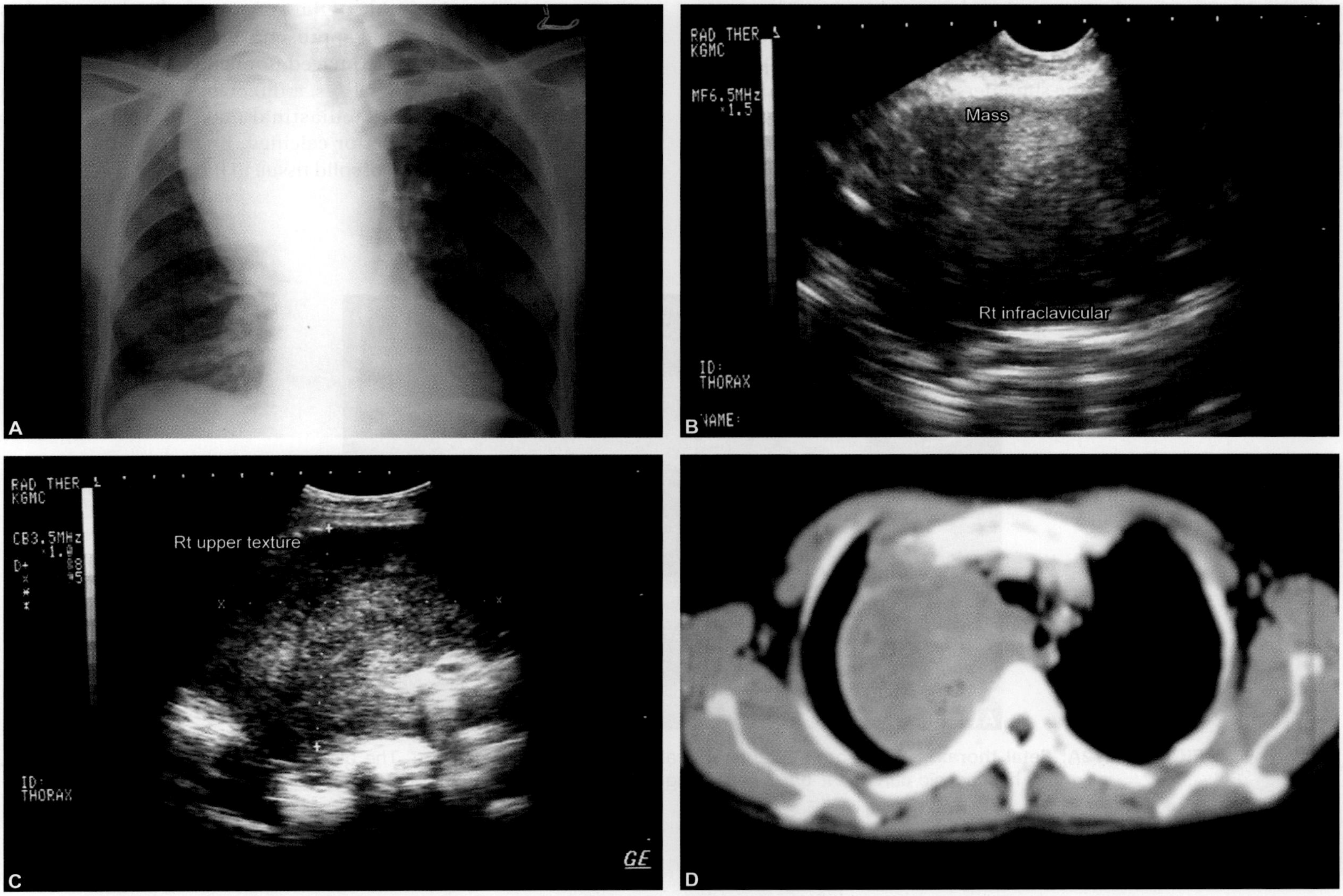

FIGURES 7.71A to D

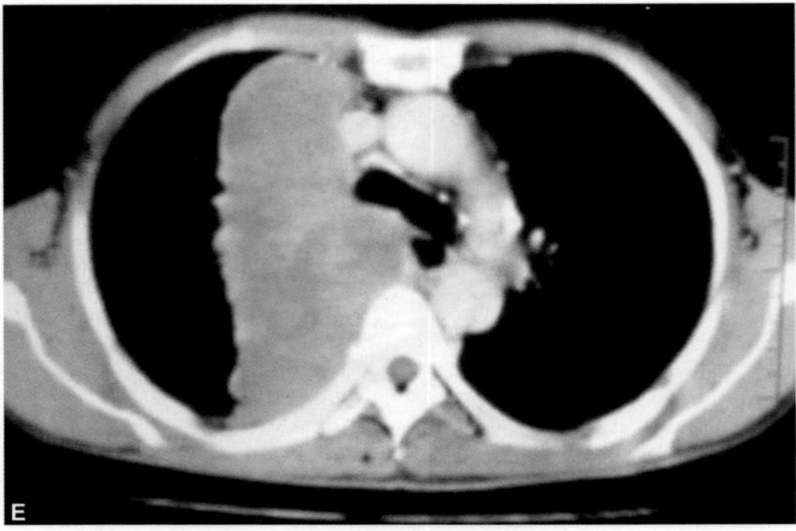

FIGURE 7.71E

FIGURES 7.71A to E: A patient presented with short breath. X-ray chest shows big opacity in the right thorax. HRSG shows big soft tissue mass in the right peripheral lung and also seen in upper and mid lobe region. It is homogeneous in texture. No calcification is seen in it. NO cystic degeneration is seen. CT scan of the same patient confirmed the biopsy of the mass showed bronchogenic carcinoma.

MEDIASTINUM

Although shadowing bone and the reflective lung surrounds mediastinum, most of its area can still be effectively examined with careful attention to technique and patient positioning. The upper mediastinum is accessible to sonographic examination by the use of a suprasternal approach. Patients are examined in a supine position with a pillow place beneath the shoulders and the neck extended. The transducer is placed at the base of the neck and angled caudally behind the manubrium. Visualization is done in oblique sagittal and coronal planes. Parasternal scanning of the mediastinum is aided by placing the patient in the appropriate lateral decubitus position. The ascending aorta, anterior mediastinum and subcarinal region is best imaged from a right parasternal approach with patient in a left lateral position. The pulmonary trunk and left side of the anterior mediastinum are best imaged with a left parasternal approach with patient in right lateral position. Posterior masses are imaged from a posterior paravertebral approach. Further for large masses, a direct look through intercostal space can be undertaken. Mediastinal masses can be precisely characteristic cystic, vascular or calcified. By sonographic Doppler imaging precise localization of solid tissue in tumor achieved.

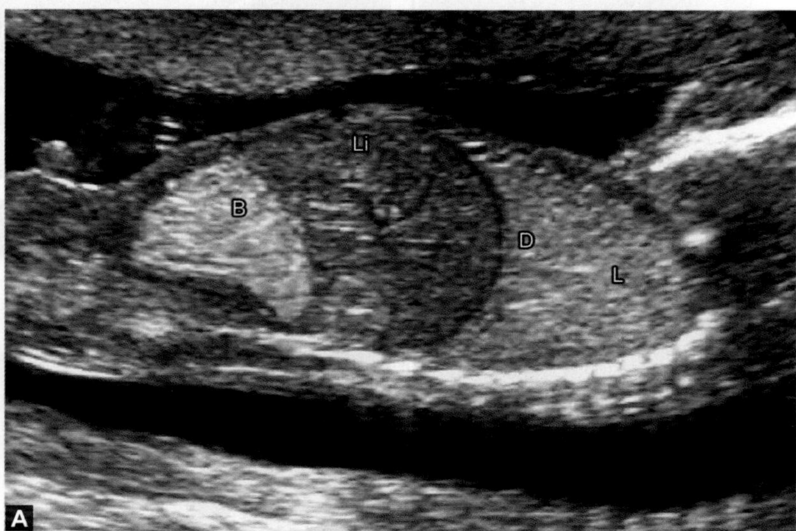

FIGURE 7.72A: Fetal thorax. HRSG shows fetal thorax, abdomen and the diaphragm. The diaphragm is seen as a hypoechoic curvilinear band separating the abdominal cavity and the thorax.

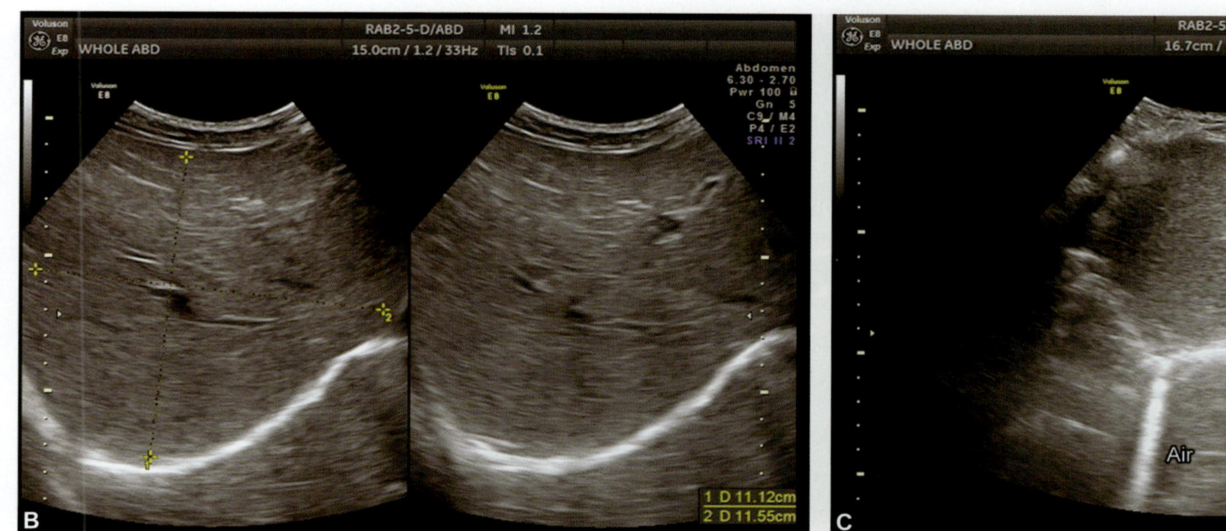

FIGURES 7.72B and C: Normal diaphragm. HRSG shows normal diaphragm as an echogenic curvilinear band, which is seen below the liver. It is smooth in outline and shows movement on dynamic scanning. Figure 7.72B shows strong reverberation artifacts due to air.

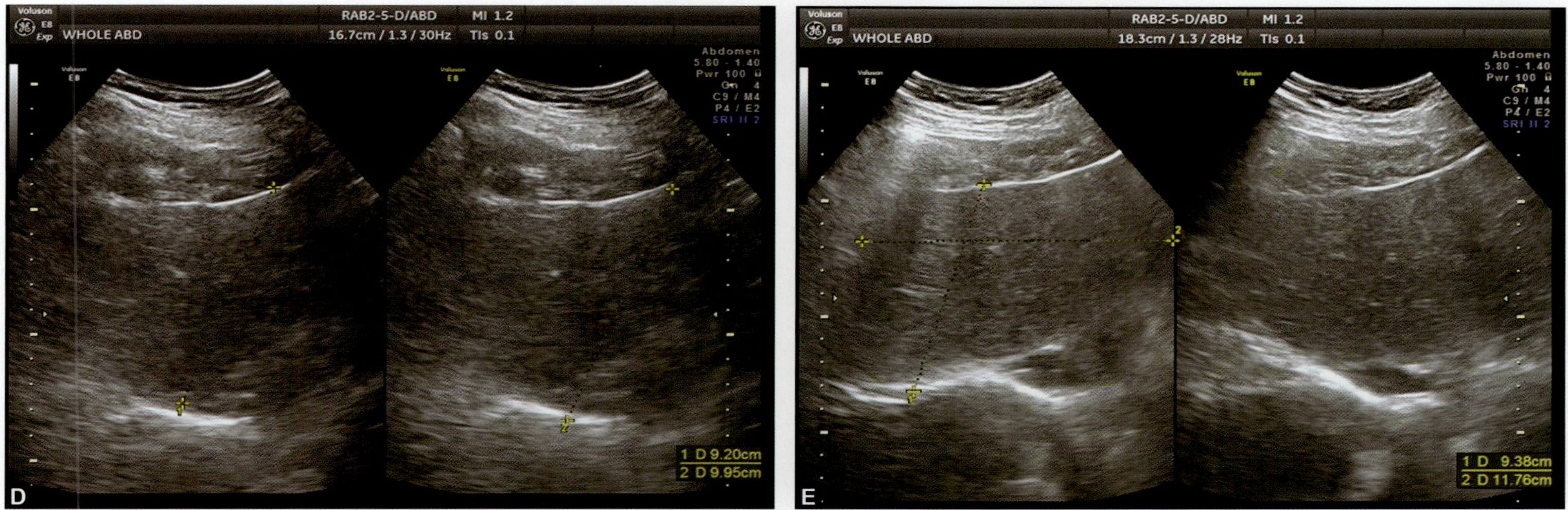

FIGURES 7.72D and E: Chilaiditi syndrome. HRSG shows interposition of bowel loops between the liver and dome of diaphragm, which is the typical feature of Chilaiditi syndrome. The bowel loops are seen filled with air.

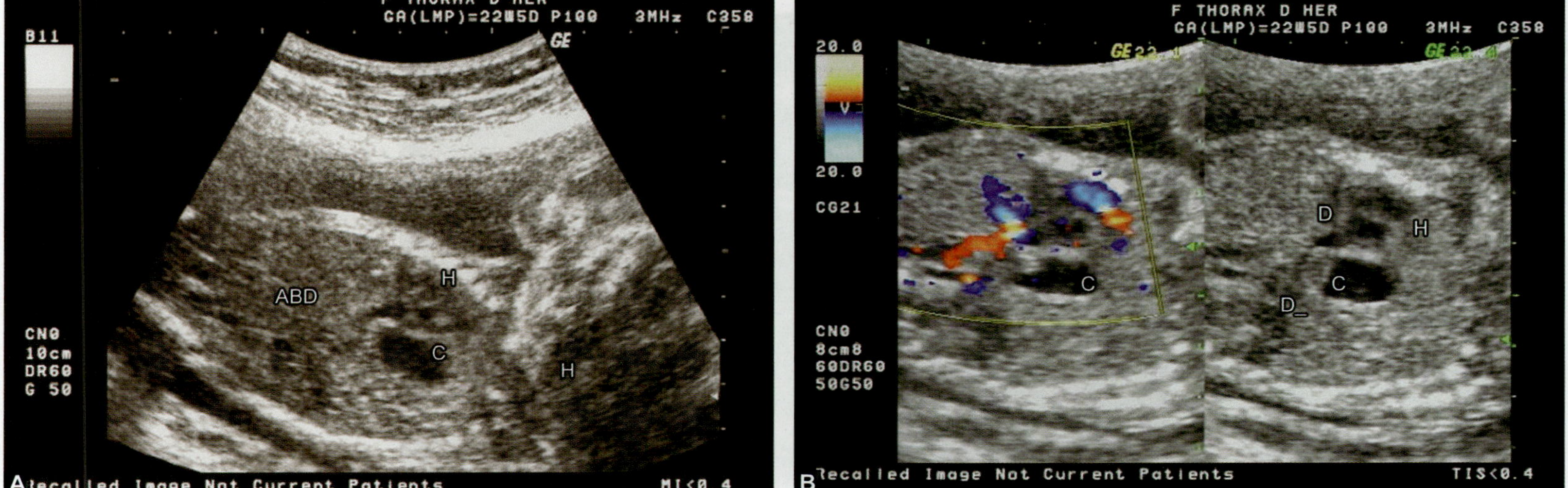

FIGURES 7.73A and B: Diaphragmatic hernia. HRSG shows a fetal thorax having a cystic mass in the thorax suggestive of herniated stomach in the fetal thorax. Color Doppler imaging of the patient shows shifting of the heart to the right side. Herniated stomach is seen as a non-vascular cystic structure.

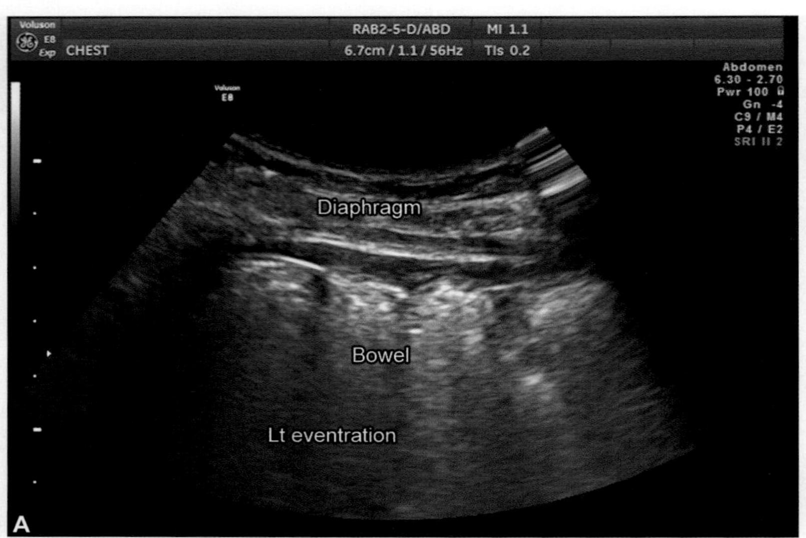

FIGURES 7.74A: Eventration of diaphragm. HRSG shows eventration of diaphragm on the left side. The normal dome-shaped appearance of the diaphragm is lost and it is seen flattened and pulled up. The bowel loops are seen below the diaphragm.

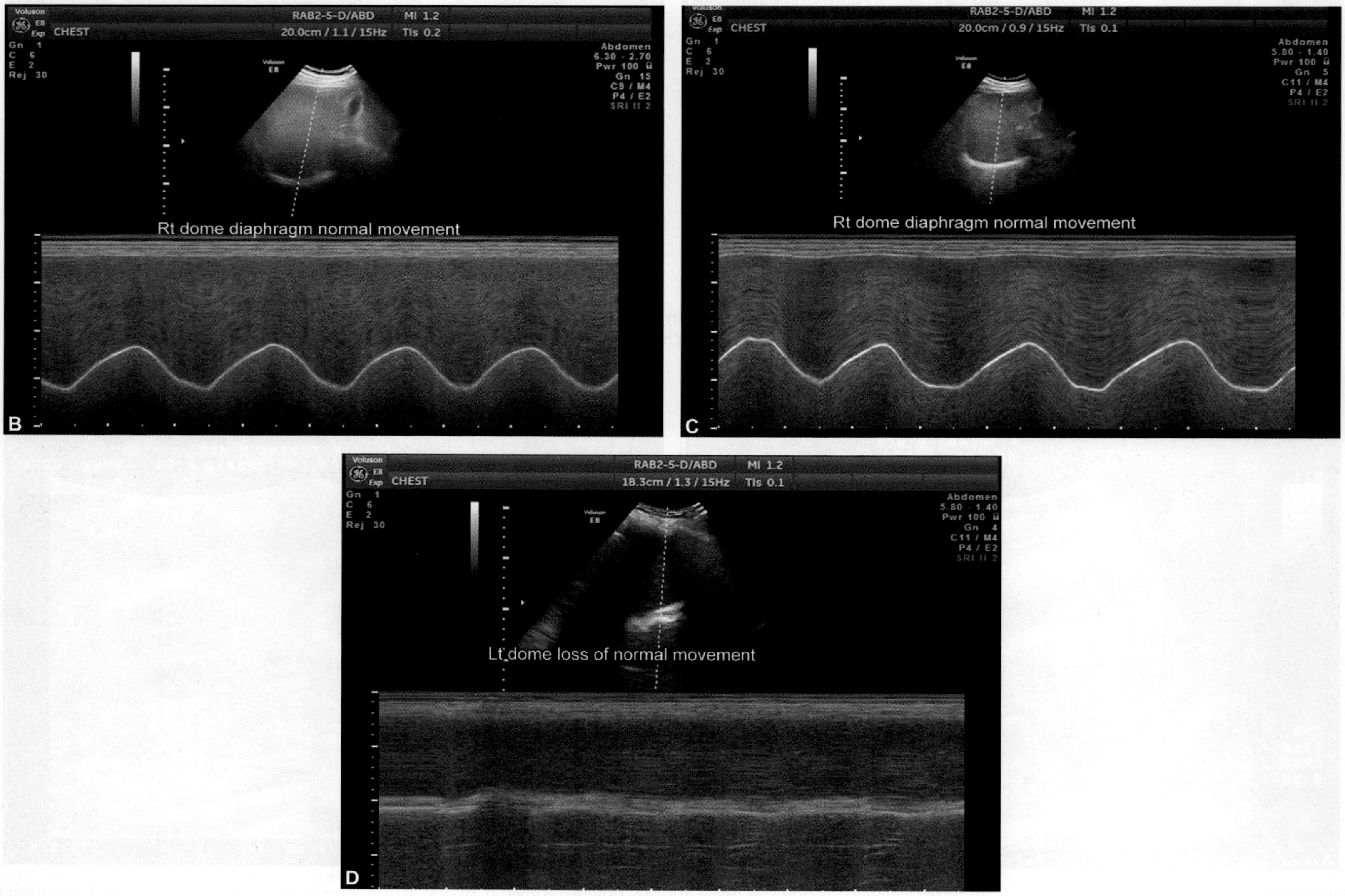

FIGURES 7.74B to D: Normal dynamic movements of diaphragm on M-mode. The normal dynamic movement of diaphragm is seen on M-mode as wavy lines. However, in eventration of diaphragm this normal movement of diaphragm is lost, which is easily appreciated on M-mode.

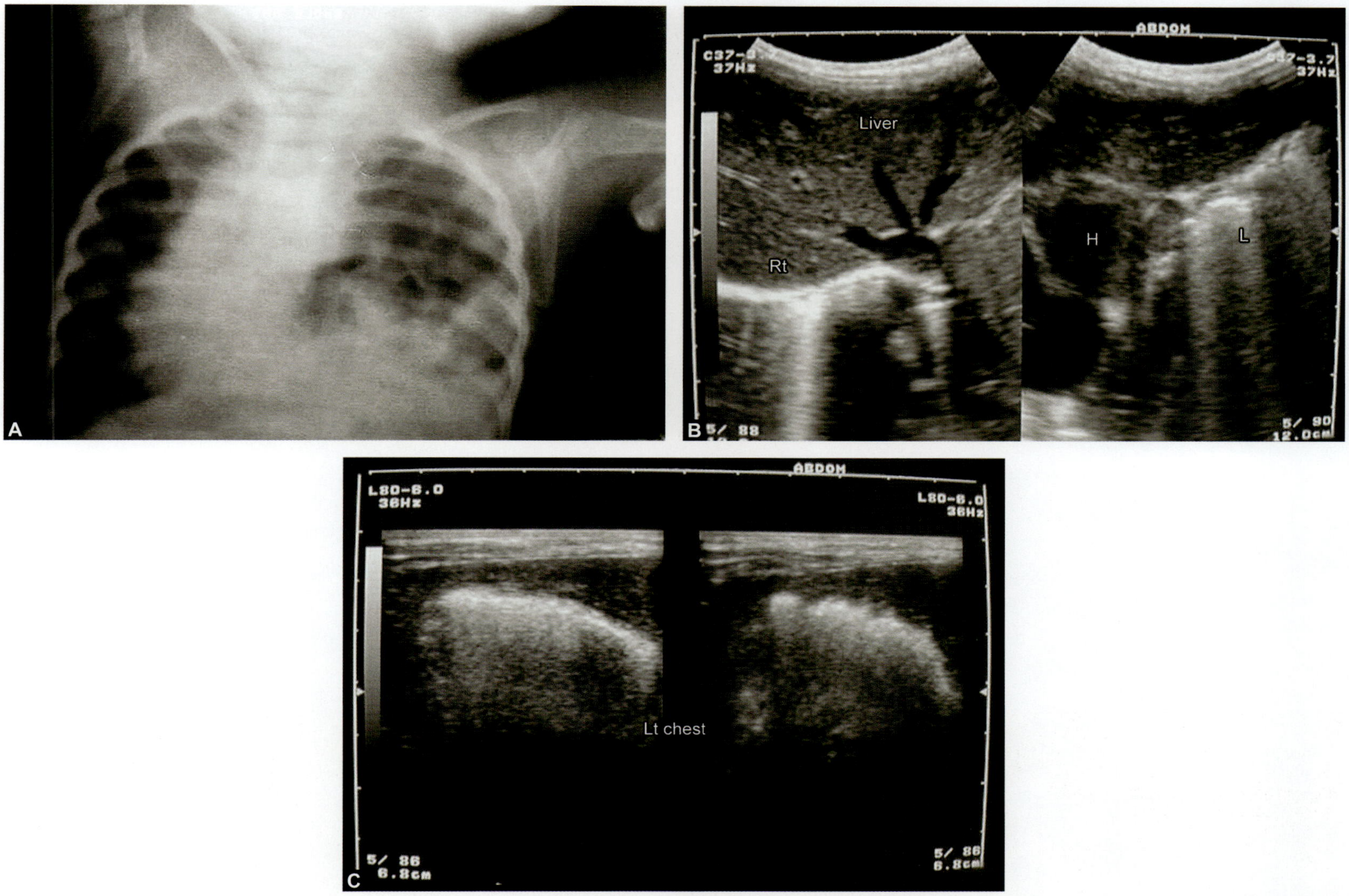

FIGURES 7.75A to C: Diaphragmatic hernia. X-ray of a child shows a loculated cystic mass in the left thorax. The heart is seen shifted in the right thorax. HRSG shows a herniated bowel loop in the thorax. The bowel loop is filled with air and seen as an echogenic shadow in the thorax. Heart is also seen pushed to the right side.

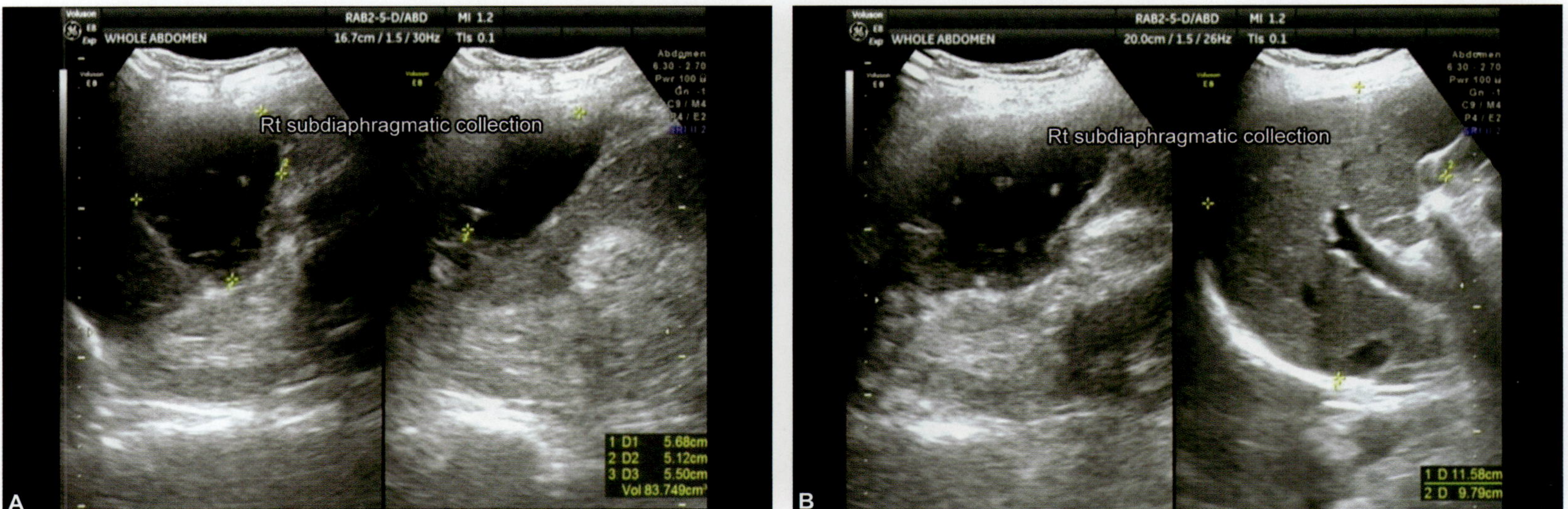

FIGURES 7.76A and B: Subdiaphragmatic collection. HRSG shows subdiaphragmatic collection. Thick low level collection is seen in the subdiaphragmatic space.

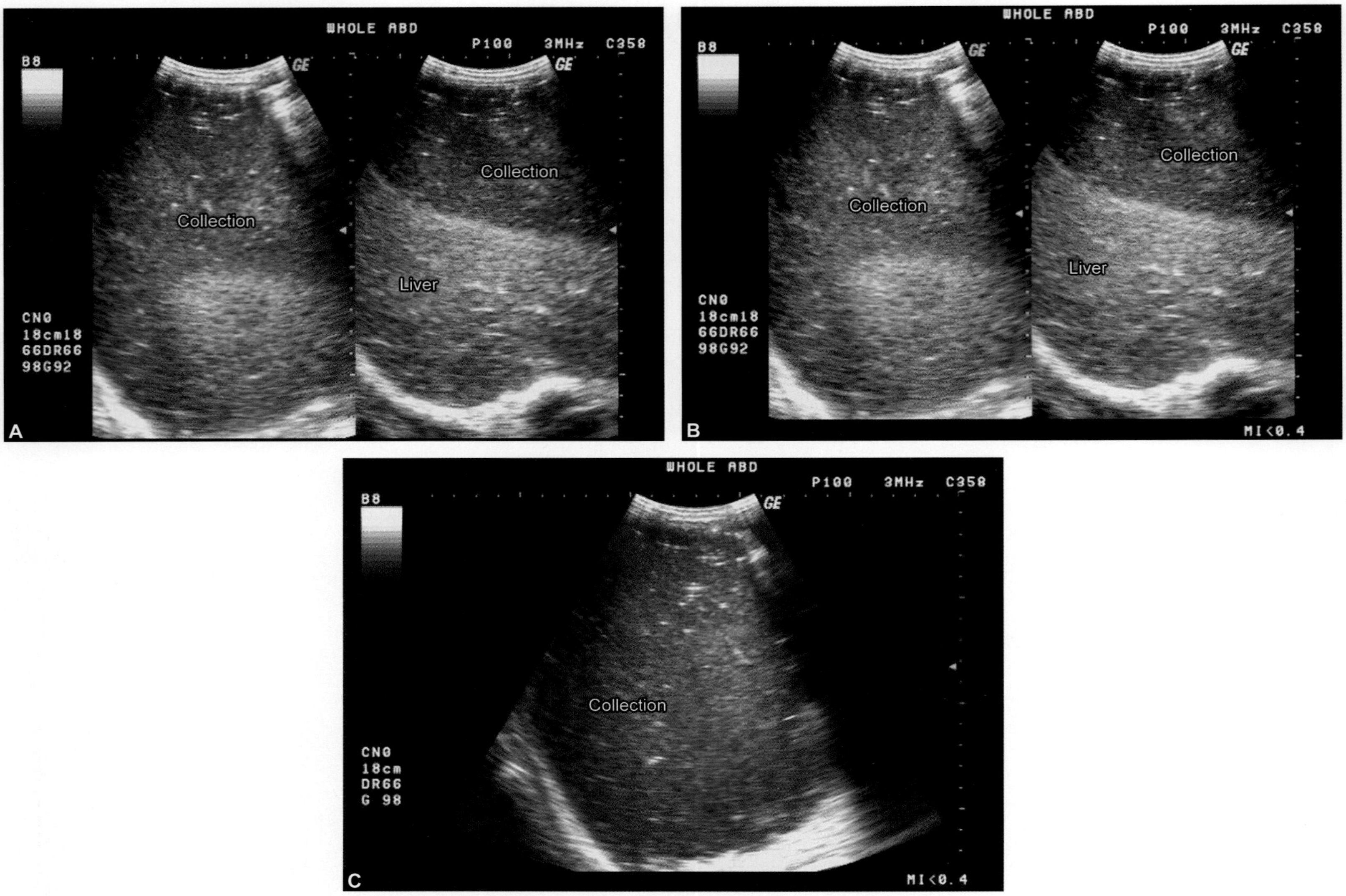

FIGURES 7.77A to C: Big subdiaphragmatic abscess. A patient presented with high fever with dyspnea. HRSG shows big collection in the right subdiaphragmatic space. Thick echoes are seen in it. Aspiration of the collection came out to be pyogenic collection.

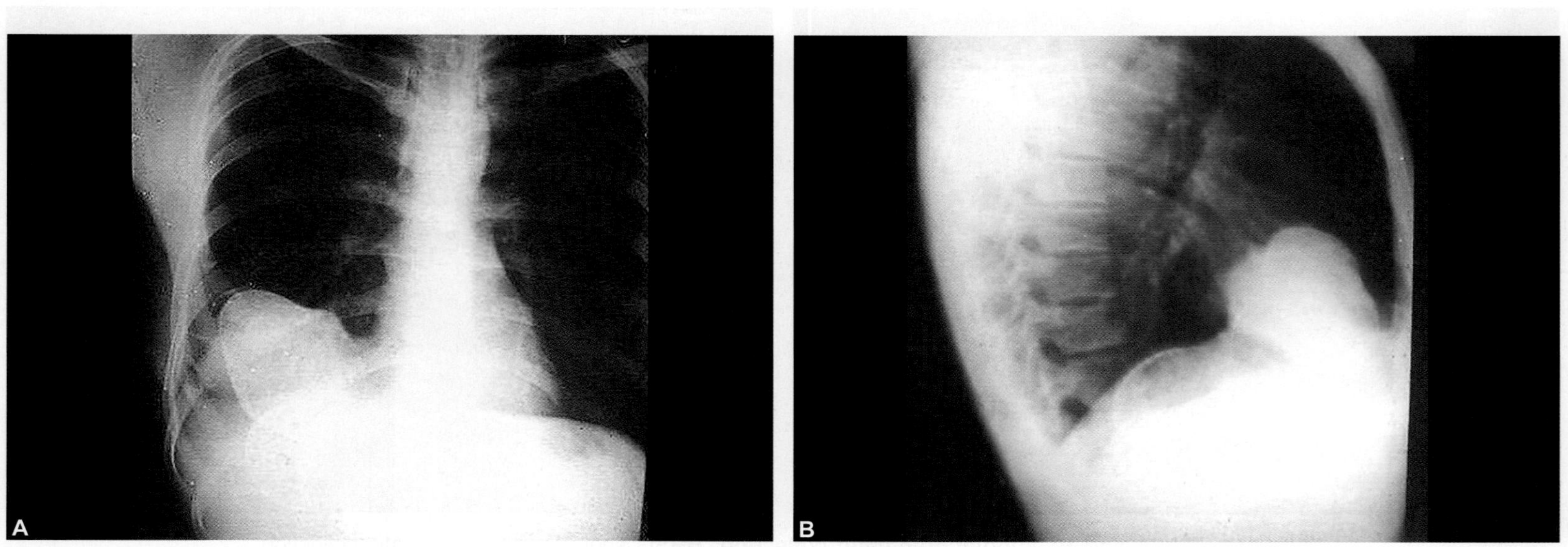

FIGURES 7.78A and B

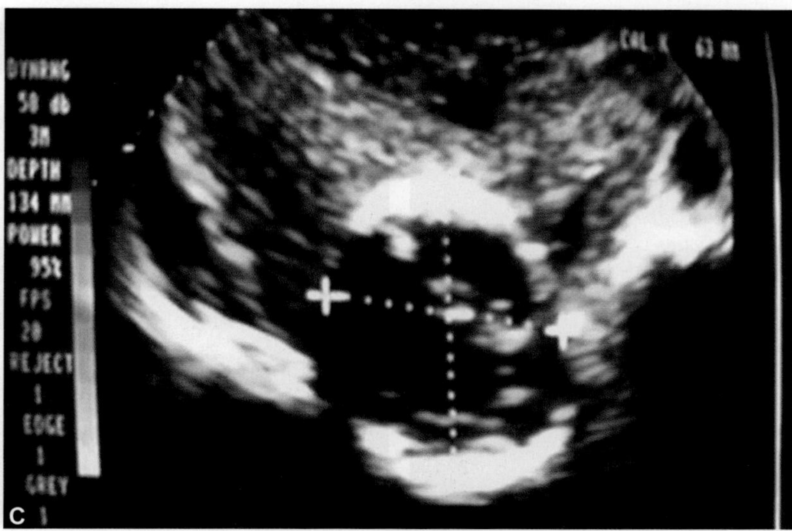

FIGURE 7.78C

FIGURES 7.78A to C: Hydatid cyst in the subdiaphragmatic area. Plane X-ray chest AP lateral view shows a well-defined radiodense shadow in the right subdiaphragmatic space. It is having sharp margins with wavy outline. Diaphragm lifting is also seen. HRSG shows a thick-walled cystic mass in the subdiaphragmatic space. Echogenic calcification is seen in the mass. Calcified specks are also seen in it suggestive of hydatid cyst. Small associated pleural fluid is also seen in the right pleural cavity.

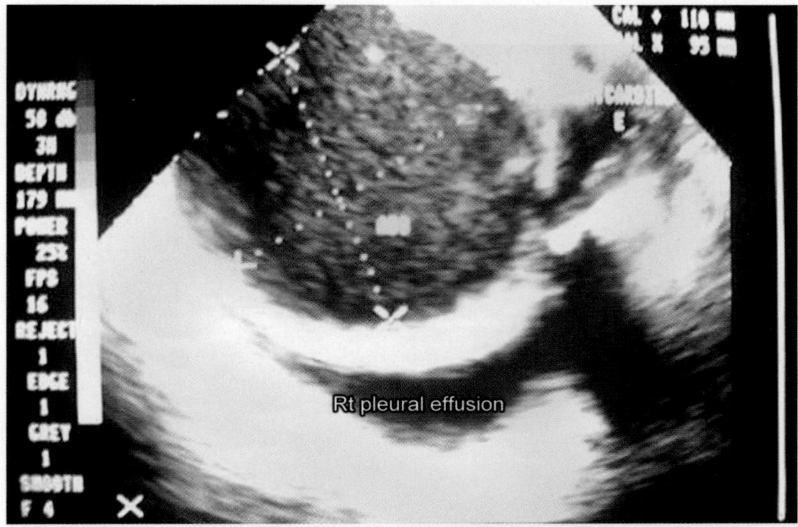

FIGURE 7.78D: Metastatic invasion of diaphragm. HRSG shows destruction of right dome of diaphragm by multinodular heterogeneous mass in right lobe of the liver. The diaphragmatic sleeve is destroyed and eaten up by the mass in a case of acute lymphatic leukemia. The liver shows the leukemic infiltrate in the liver parenchyma.

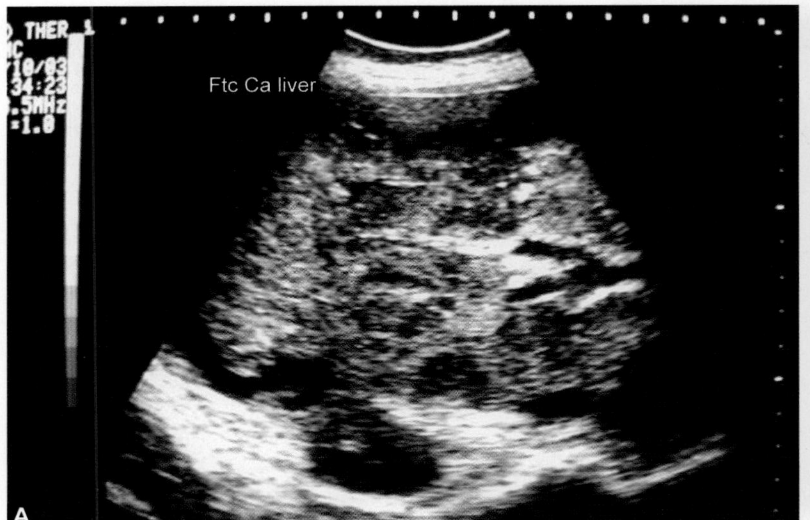

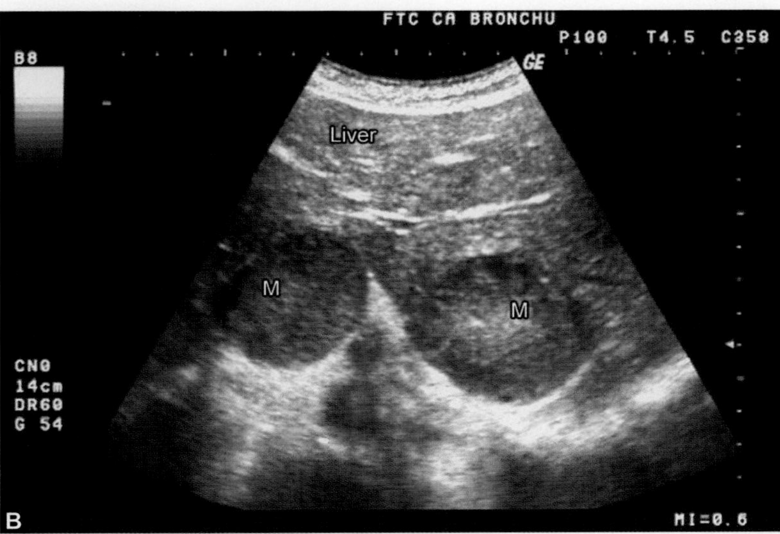

FIGURES 7.79A and B

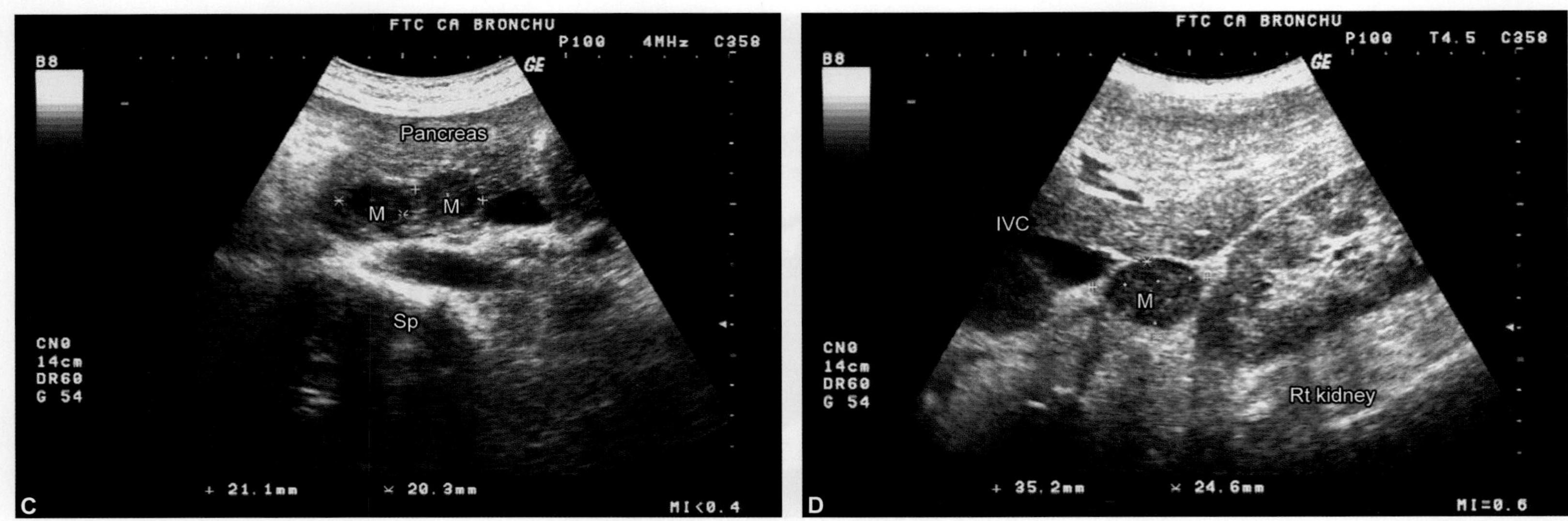

FIGURES 7.79C and D

FIGURES 7.79A to D: Metastatic deposits are also seen in both lobes of the liver in the same patient. Hypoechoic nodular masses are seen in the pancreas in the same patient of CA bronchus. Biopsy of the masses shows metastasis of adeno carcinoma. HRSG also shows right adrenal metastasis in the same patient of CA bronchus.

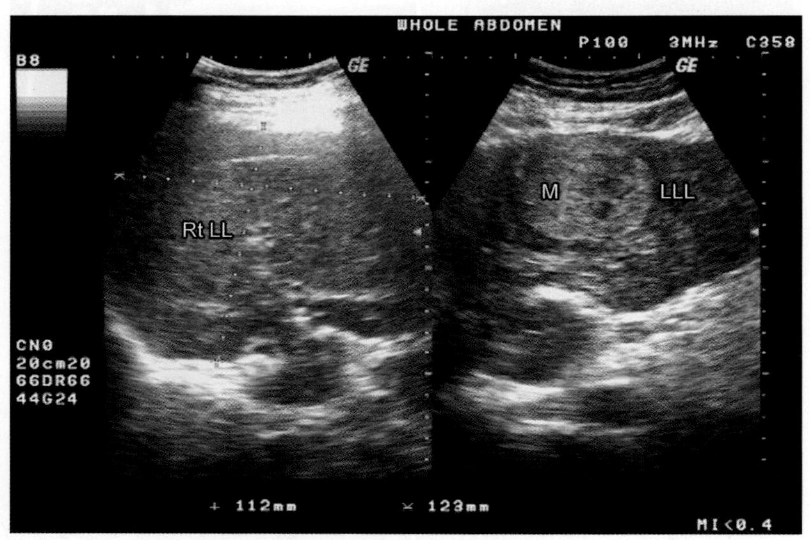

FIGURE 7.80: Metastatic mass in the right dome of the diaphragm. HRSG shows a hypoechoic mass invading the right lobe of the liver posterior segment in a case of carcinoma bronchus breast. The mass is also seen invading the right dome of the diaphragm.

CHAPTER 8

Breast

PK Srivastava

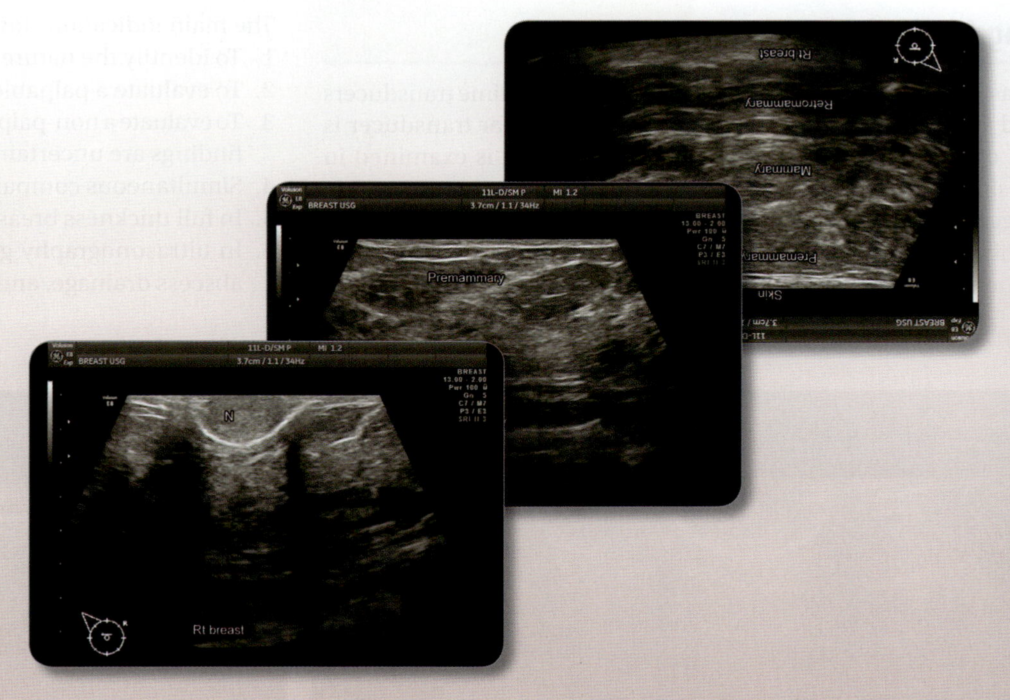

INTRODUCTION

The breast or mammary glands are modified sweat glands. They are exocrine organs. Their main function is the secretion of milk during pregnancy (lactation). Breast being superficial organ is ideal for HRSG evaluation. The other techniques like CT scanning, MRI or mammography has got limitations. Sonomammography due to its versatility has become a choice of investigation for breast imaging. Though X-ray mammography is still preferred for mass screening program for detection of breast cancer, but with use of sonomammography the nature of lesion, its surrounding tissue invasion and lymph node enlargement can be better evaluated.

Normal Anatomy

Breast is superficially placed anterior to pectoralis major, serratus anterior and external oblique muscles and the sixth rib. It is bounded medially by sternum and laterally by the margins of axilla. Second or third ribs and inferior border form the superior border by the seventh costal cartilage.

The size of normal breast varies depending on the age, functional state of the breast and amount of fibroadipose tissue in the breast. There is increase in the size in puberty due to stimulation by estrogen hormone and decrease in the size after menopause due to decrease in hormonal stimulation. The breast has got three layers.

1. ***Subcutaneous layer:*** It contains skin and subcutaneous fat.
2. ***Mammary layer:*** It contains glandular tissues, ducts and connective tissue.
3. ***Retromammary layer:*** It contains retromammary fat, muscle and deep connective tissue.

Scanning Method

Since breast is superficially placed, high-resolution real-time transducers of 7.5 and 10 MHz are the requisite transducers. Linear transducer is preferred over sector and convex probes. The patient is examined in sitting position. It allows a full thickness study of breast tissue.

The biggest advantage of breast ultrasonographic imaging is to assess the mobility of the breast tissue and any other lesion in the breast. Use of high frequency transducers as 10 MHz can give additional information about cancer nidus or microcalcification and reactive halo around the nidus. Doppler ultrasonography can give better information about benign or malignant mass in the breast.

Normal Sonoappearance of Breast

Normal ultrasonographic appearance of breast depends on many factors like age of patient, size of breast and functional state of the breast. Breast tissue is seen in three distinct layers. Most anterior is skin and subcutaneous fat. It appears to be a highly reflective layer on HRSG. The middle layer contains the glandular tissue, which is seen sandwiched between subcutaneous layer and retromammary layer. Rounded fat lobules are seen distributed between the glandular layers. They are uniformly reflective in young breast. The ducts are seen as tubular structures running towards the nipple or areola. The maximum normal caliber of ducts is 3 mm. In postmenopausal woman, glandular tissue decreases in amount and fatty tissue predominates and it becomes less echogenic. The ducts are also not seen in this breast. The young breasts are denser due to high percentage of glandular tissue. Dense breast is difficult to be seen on X-ray mammography. Therefore, sonomammography is better investigation to evaluate young breast. Nipple and areola attenuate the sound beam. This casts the shadowing, which is seen as a hypoechoic band posterior to nipple and areola. Glandular tissue predominates during pregnancy and ducts are dilated and radiating towards nipple from all directions. They can be seen well on HRSG. The axilla contains fibrofatty layer. It is having mixed echo texture. Normal lymph nodes are not identified on HRSG. However, when they are enlarged they can be easily picked up on HRSG.

Indications of Sonomammography

The main indications for breast sonography are as follows:

1. To identify the nature of palpable mass in the breast.
2. To evaluate a palpable mass in young females.
3. To evaluate a non-palpable mass in breast where X-ray mammography findings are uncertain.
4. Simultaneous comparison of both breasts.
5. In full thickness breast tissue study.
6. In ultrasonography guided breast procedures like cyst punctures, abscess drainage, and fine-needle aspiration cytology (FNAC), etc.

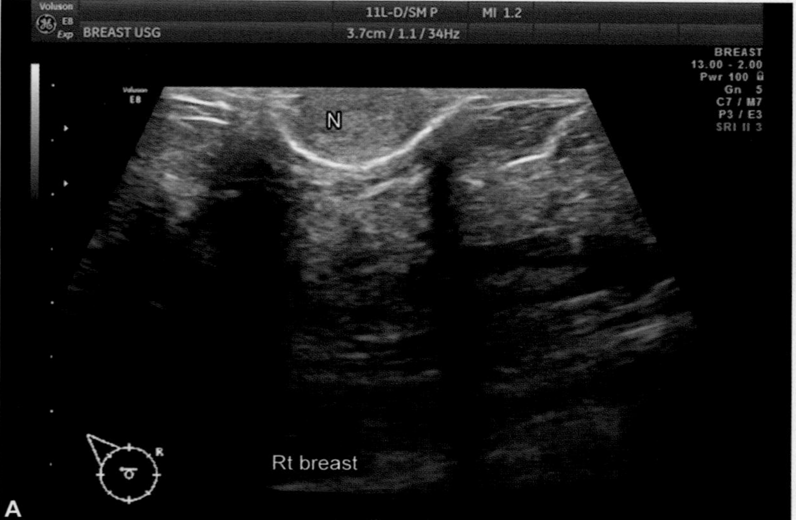

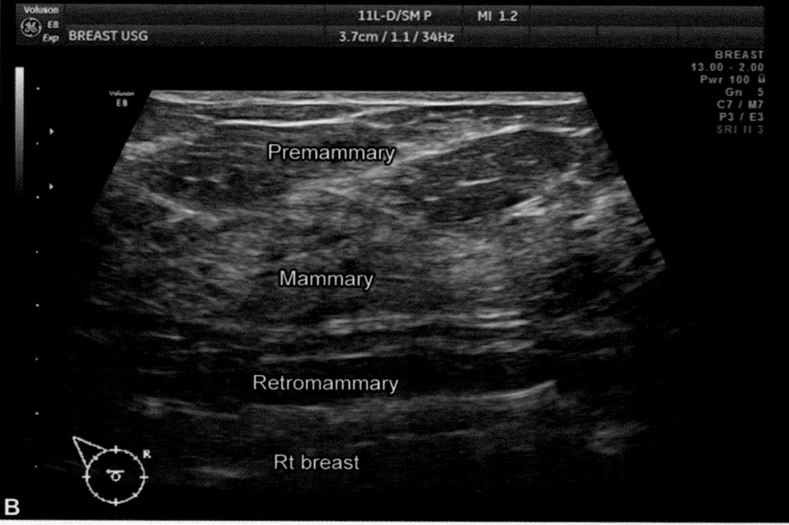

FIGURES 8.1A and B

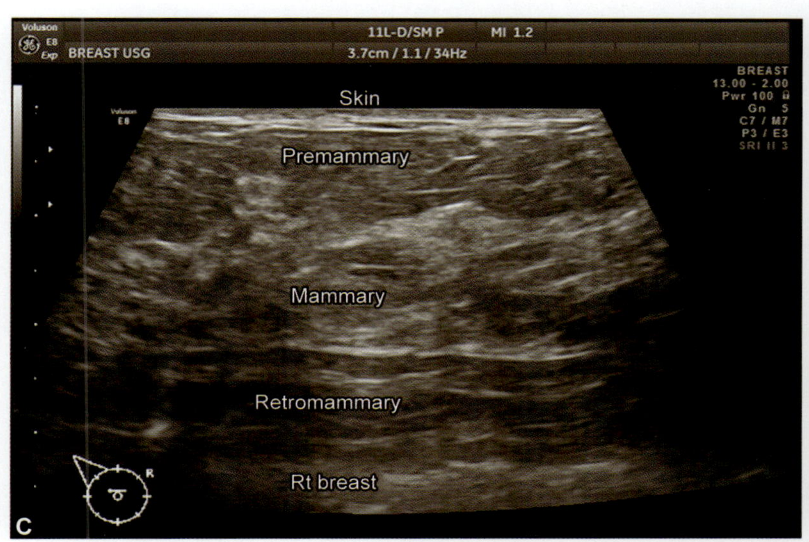

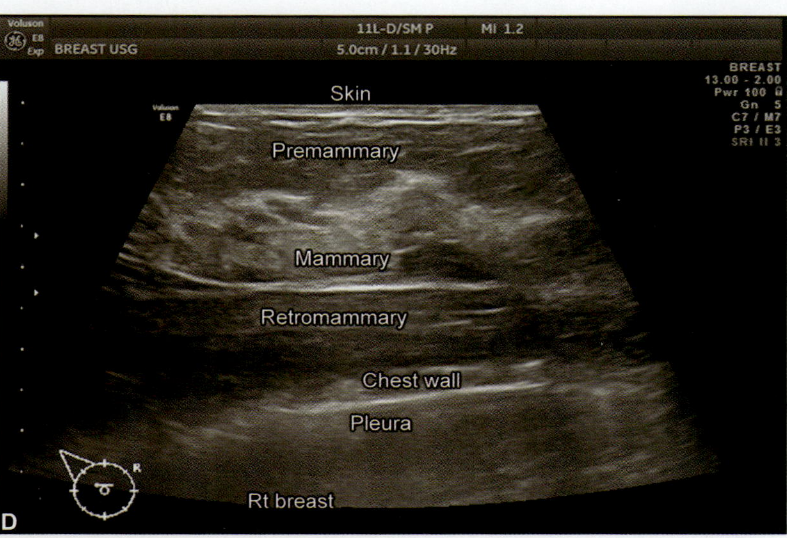

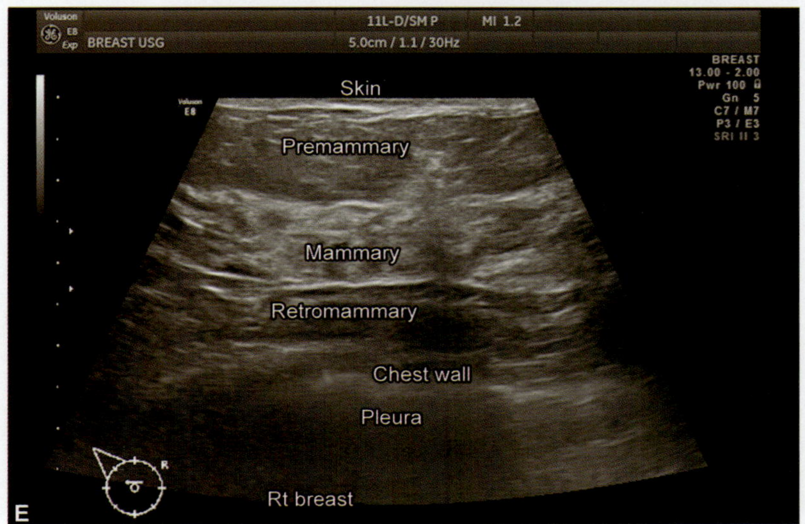

FIGURES 8.1C to E

FIGURES 8.1A to E: Normal breast. HRSG shows the normal breast appearance. Echogenic line is skin. Hypoechoic layer posterior to the skin is subcutaneous fat. A hypoechoic layer after the subcutaneous fat is premammary layer. The mammary layer shows main glandular components of the breast. Multiple fibro glandular lobules are seen dispersed in the glandular tissue. The retromammary layer is seen posterior to the mammary chest wall and a hyper reflective layer is seen after the chest wall is the pleura. HRSG shows normal breast. The skin, subcutaneous fat, mammary layer and retromammary layers are well-visualized. HRSG shows few ducts seen running to the areola. Normal duct diameter should not exceed 3 mm. HRSG shows nipple areola complex. Nipple is seen as a hypoechoic well-defined oval shadow. Echogenic border of the nipple is seen. Normal nipple cast shadowing.

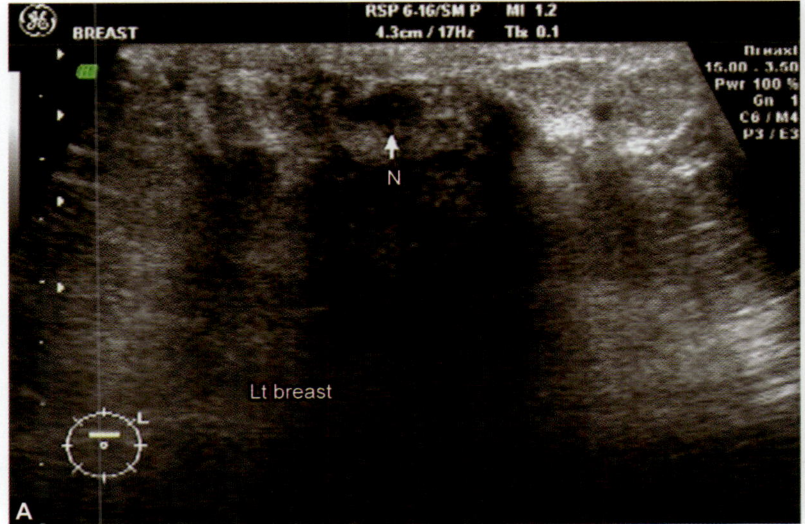

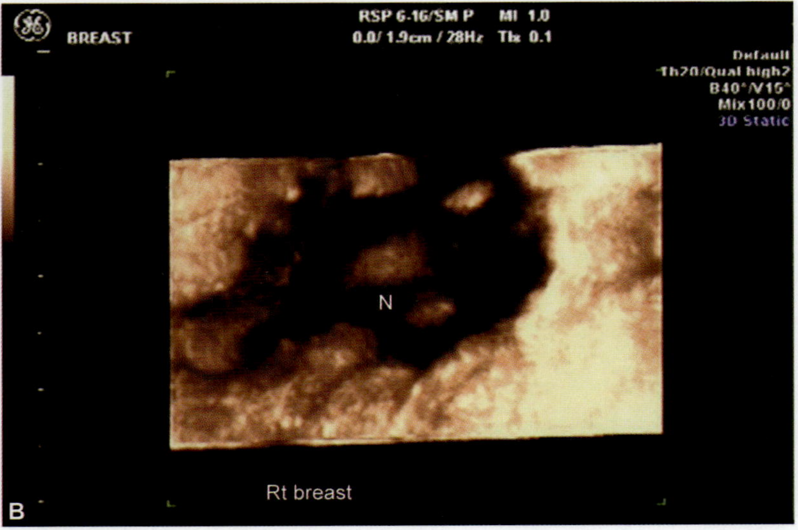

FIGURES 8.2A and B

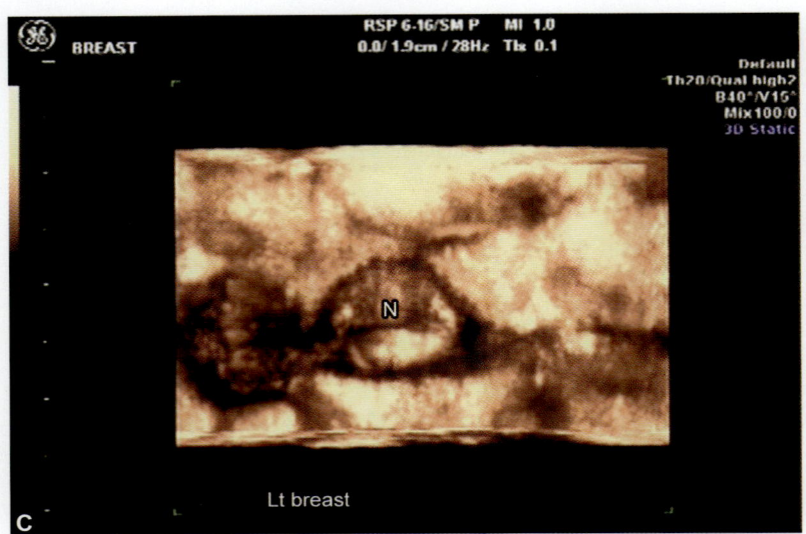

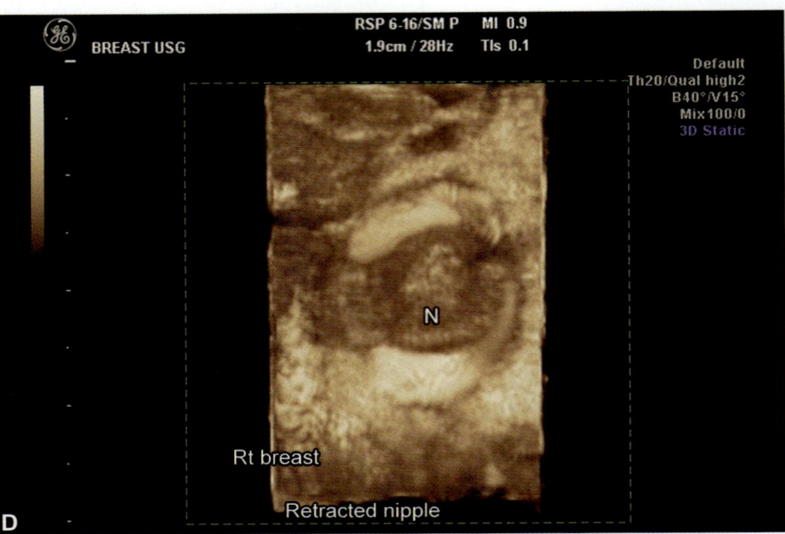

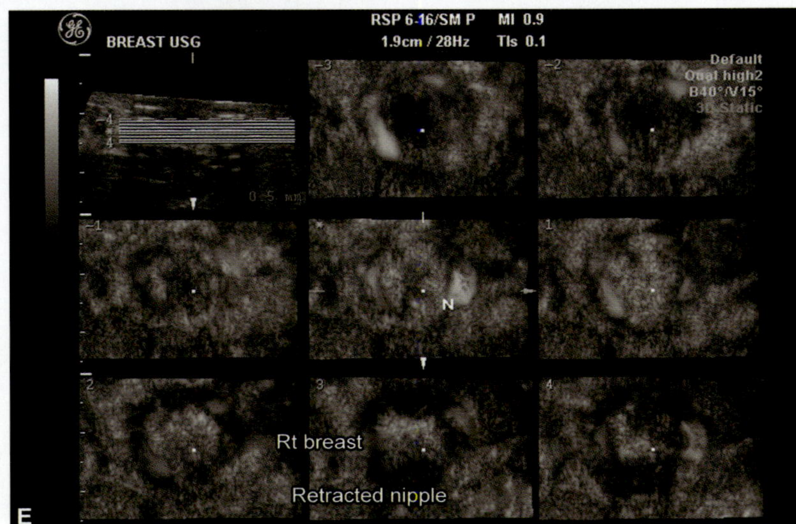

FIGURES 8.2C to E

FIGURES 8.2A to E: Retracted nipple. HRSG shows retracted nipple, which is not clearly seen on 2D ultrasound. The 3D ultrasound shows the retracted nipple very clearly. No suggestion of any focal mass is seen in the region of nipple areola complex.

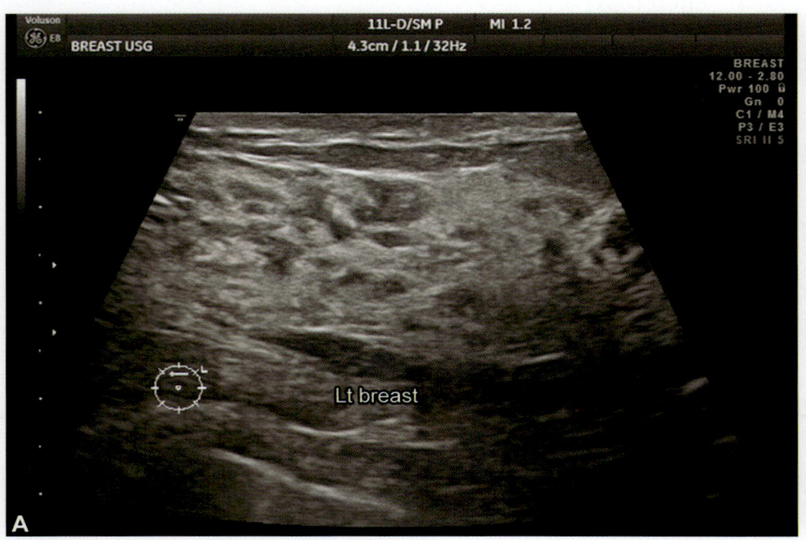

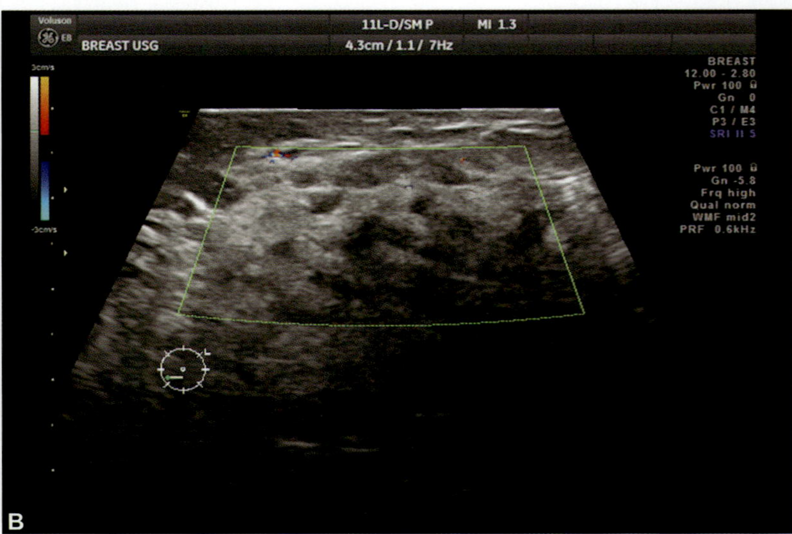

FIGURES 8.3A and B

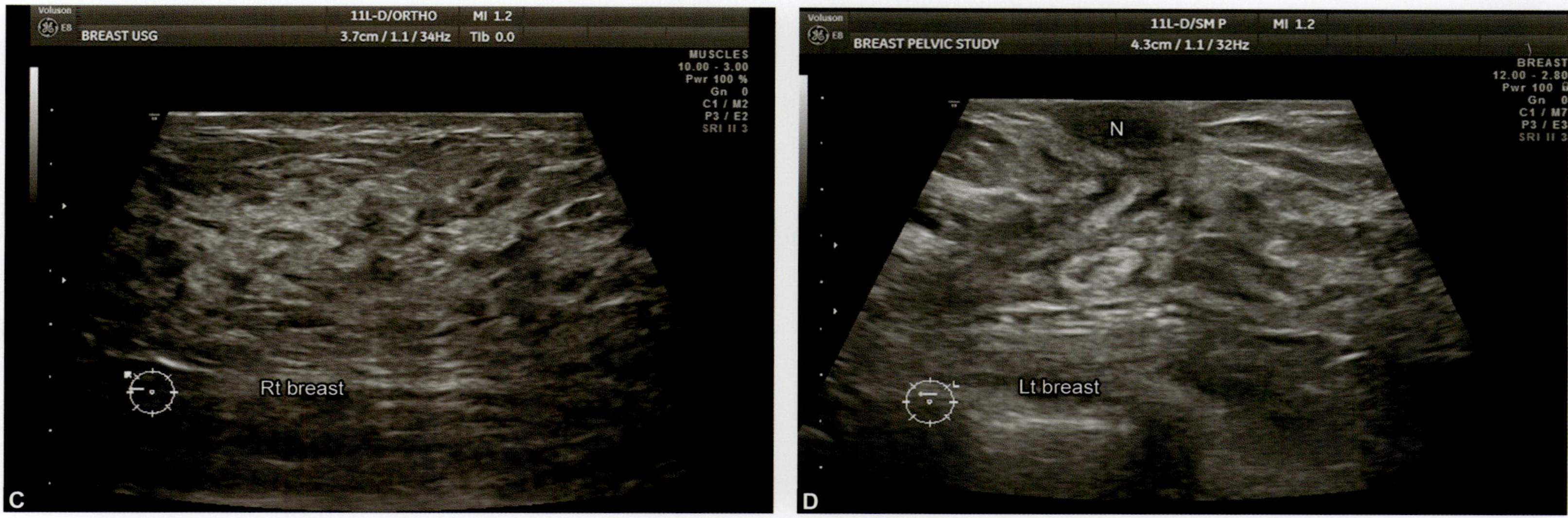

FIGURES 8.3C and D

FIGURES 8.3A to D: Normal ducts. HRSG shows multiple dilated ducts cut in the cross section in both the breast. They are seen running to areola. Normal caliber of the duct is less than 2 mm.

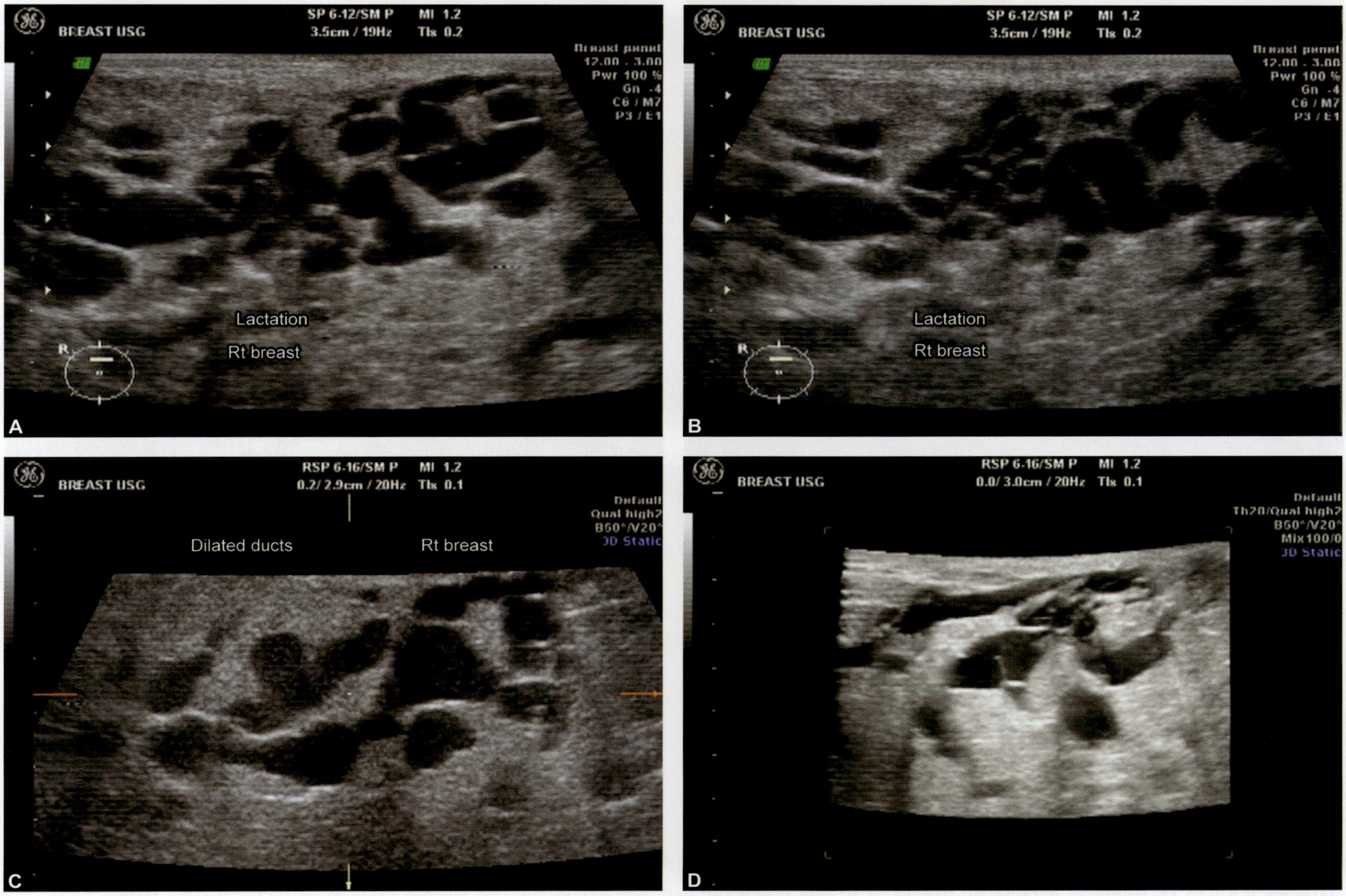

FIGURES 8.4A to D

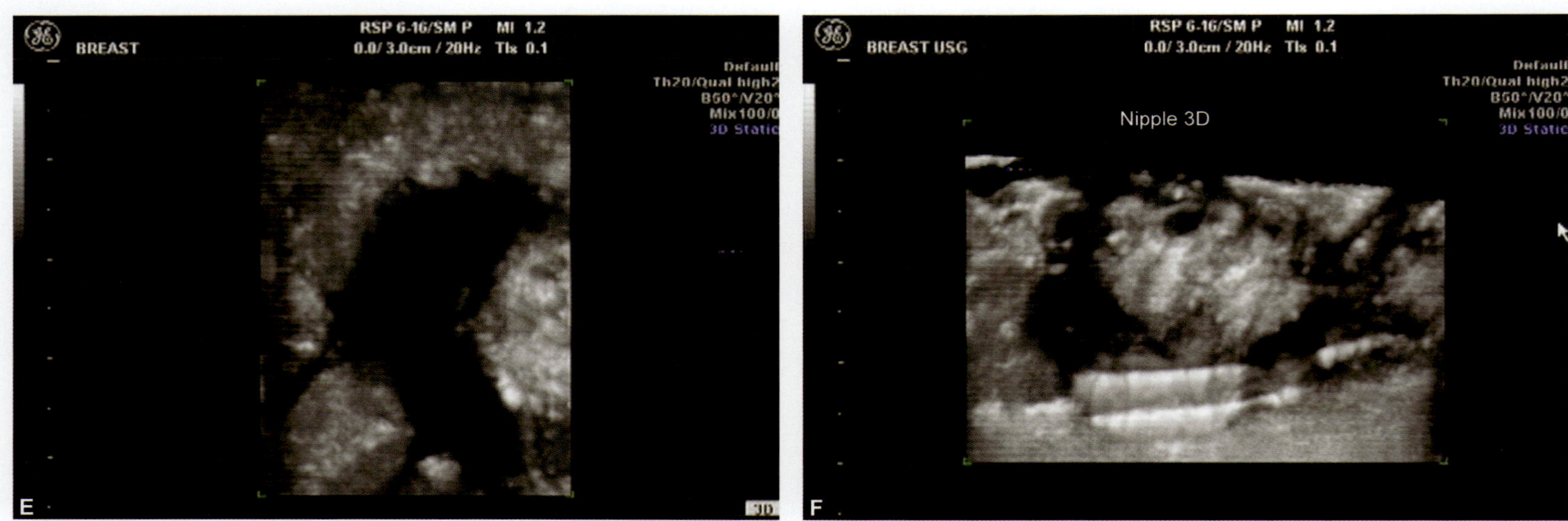

FIGURES 8.4E and F

FIGURES 8.4A to F: Dilated ducts in lactating woman. HRSG shows multiple dilated ducts in a lactating woman. They are running to areola from all the directions in spider leg pattern. On 3D imaging, the ducts are seen clearly. On volume contrast imaging, opening of the duct is seen at the mouth of the nipple.

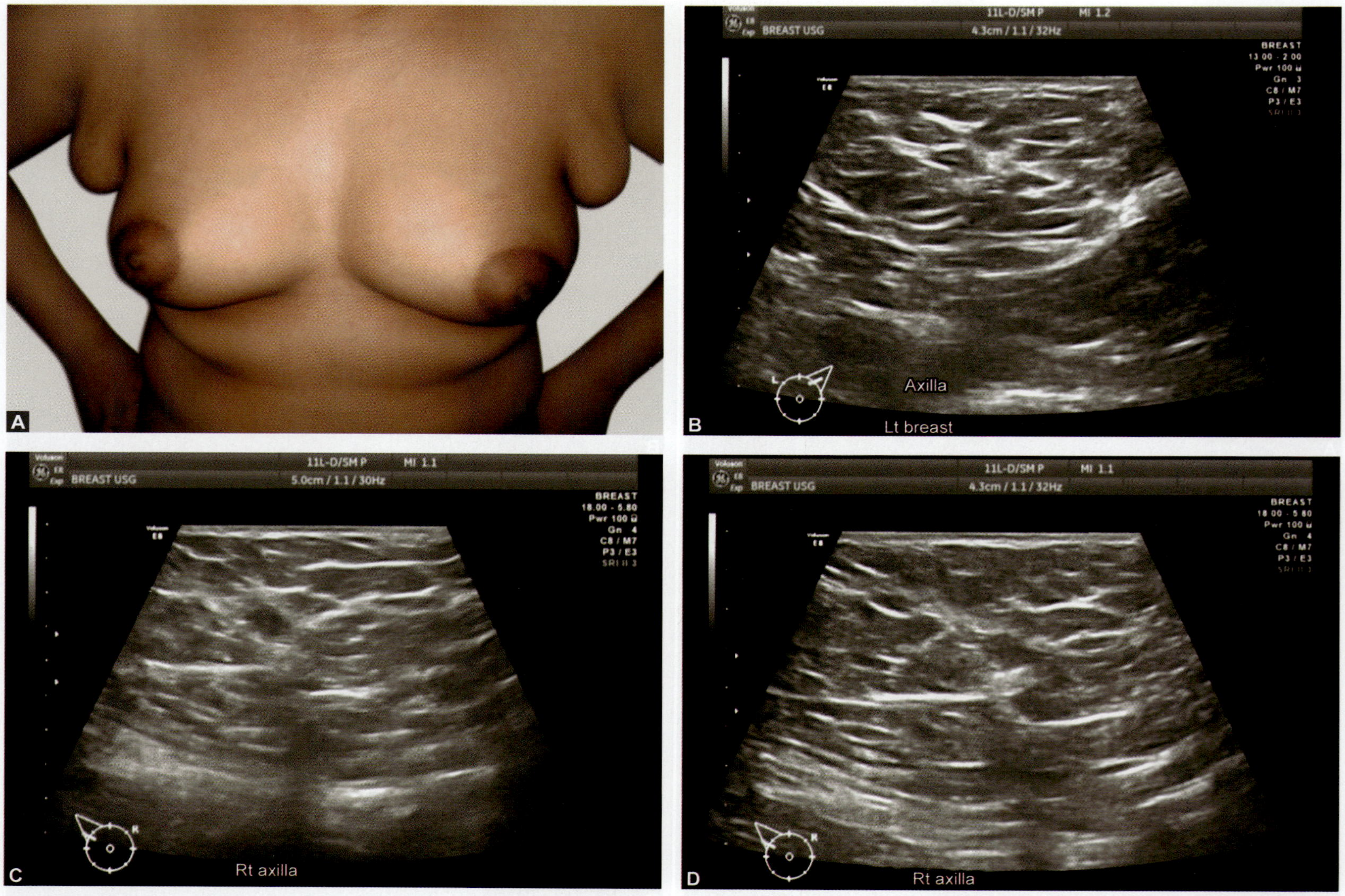

FIGURES 8.5A to D: Bilateral accessory breast. A patient presented with soft tissue swelling in both axilla in 25-year-old lady. HRSG shows soft tissue shadows in the tail of the breast on both sides. They are seen extending to both axilla. The soft tissue texture is similar to the breast tissue echotexture suggestive of bilateral accessory breast.

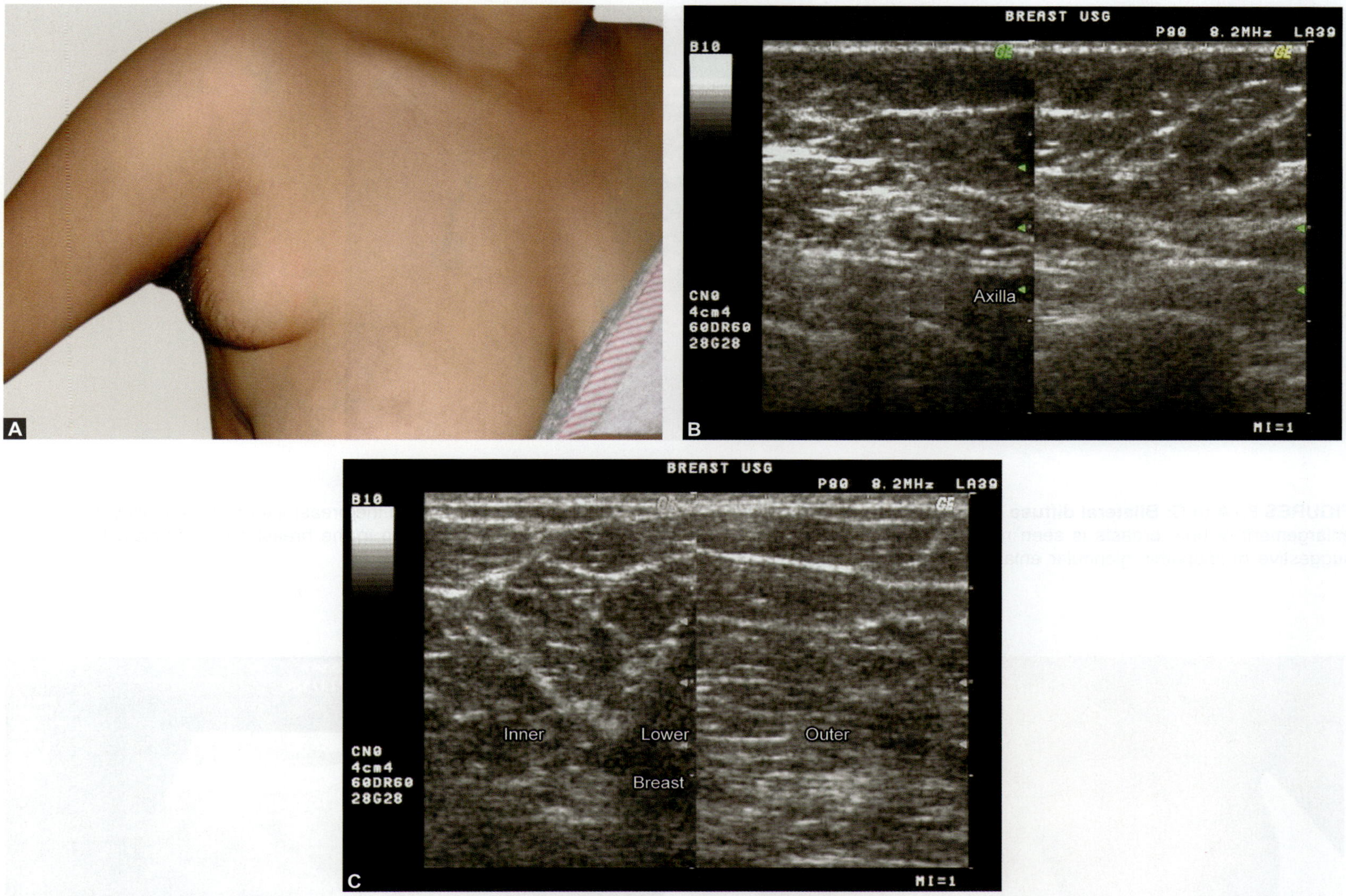

FIGURES 8.6A to C: Accessory breast. A patient presented with a soft tissue shadow in the right axilla. HRSG shows the soft tissue shadow in the right axilla is having echotexture similar to the breast suggestive of accessory breast. The normal breast tissue is seen in the upper inner and outer quadrant of the breast, which is similar to the soft tissue texture seen in right axilla.

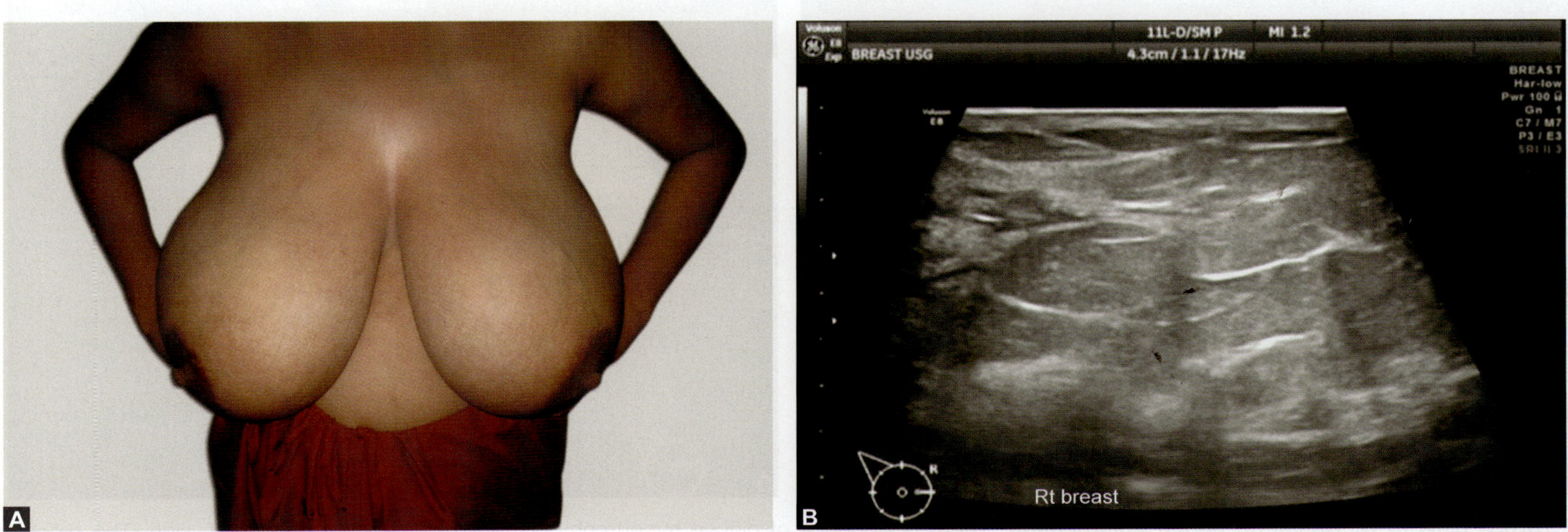

FIGURES 8.7A and B

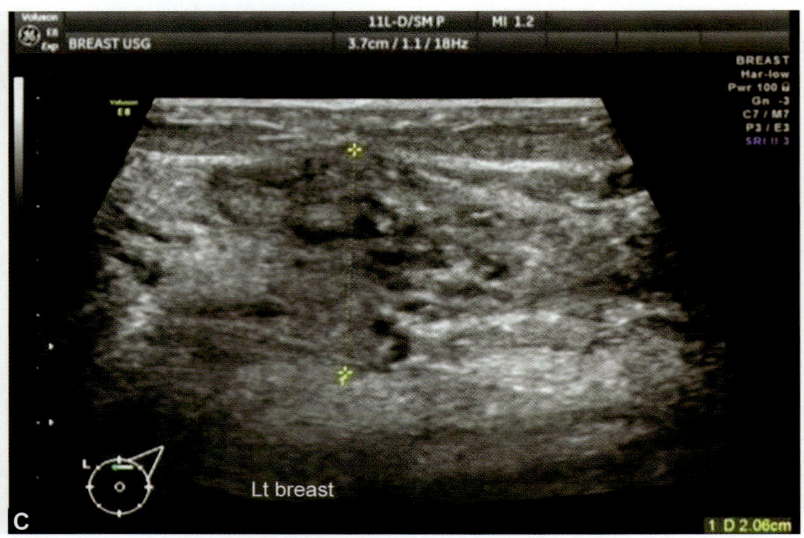

FIGURE 8.7C

FIGURES 8.7A to C: Bilateral diffuse breast hypertrophy. A patient presented diffuse enlargement of both the breast after first pregnancy. Progressive enlargement of both breasts is seen resulting into massive glandular enlargement. No focal mass is seen in the breast on either side. Findings are suggestive of idiopathic glandular enlargement on both sides.

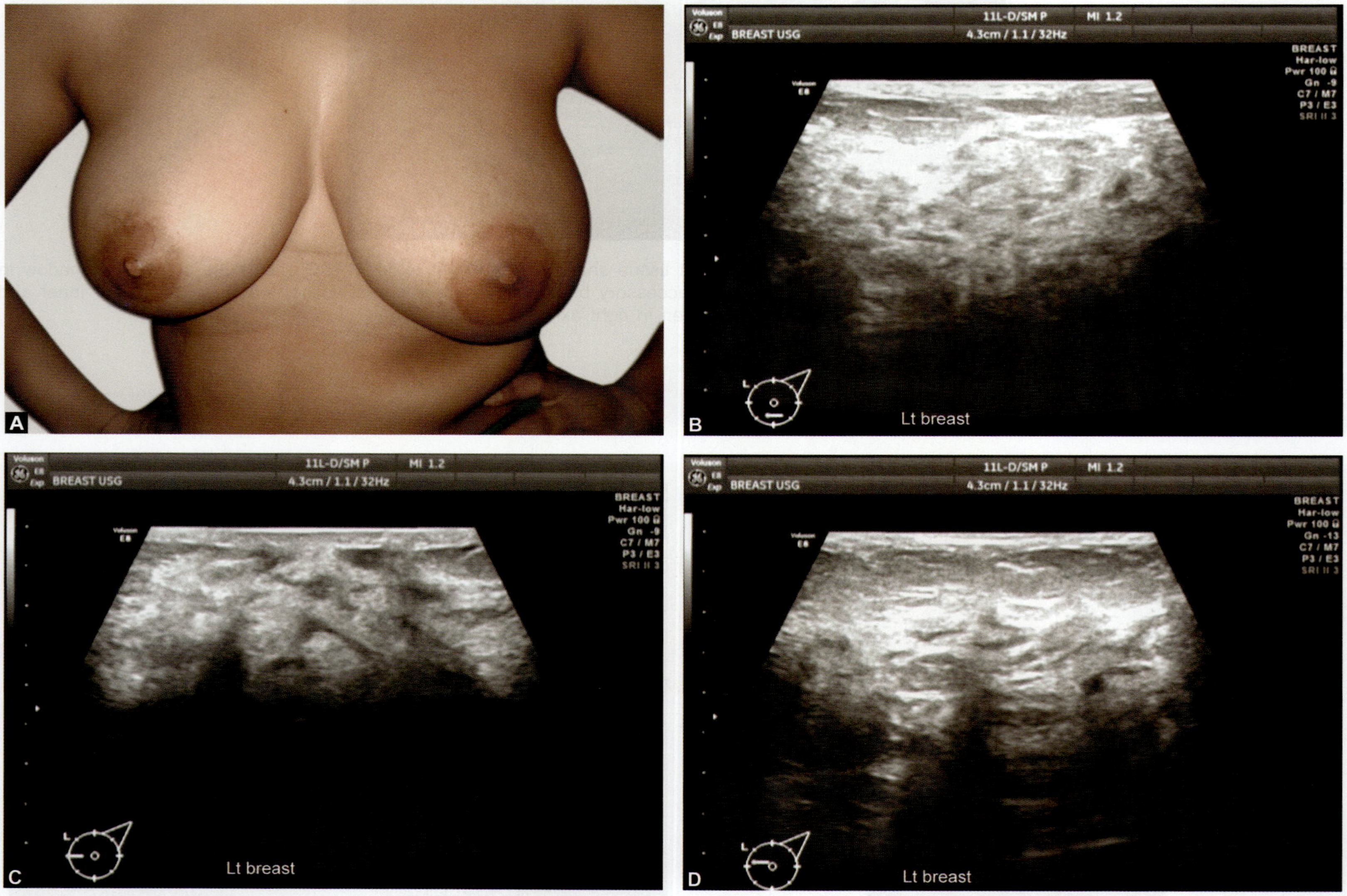

FIGURES 8.8A to D: Unilateral breast enlargement. There is evidence of diffuse hypertrophy of breast tissue seen on the left side. The granular tissue appears to be increased in size. Premammary and mammary and retromammary zones are normal on left side. No evidence of any focal mass is seen in them. The areola and periareolar area are free.

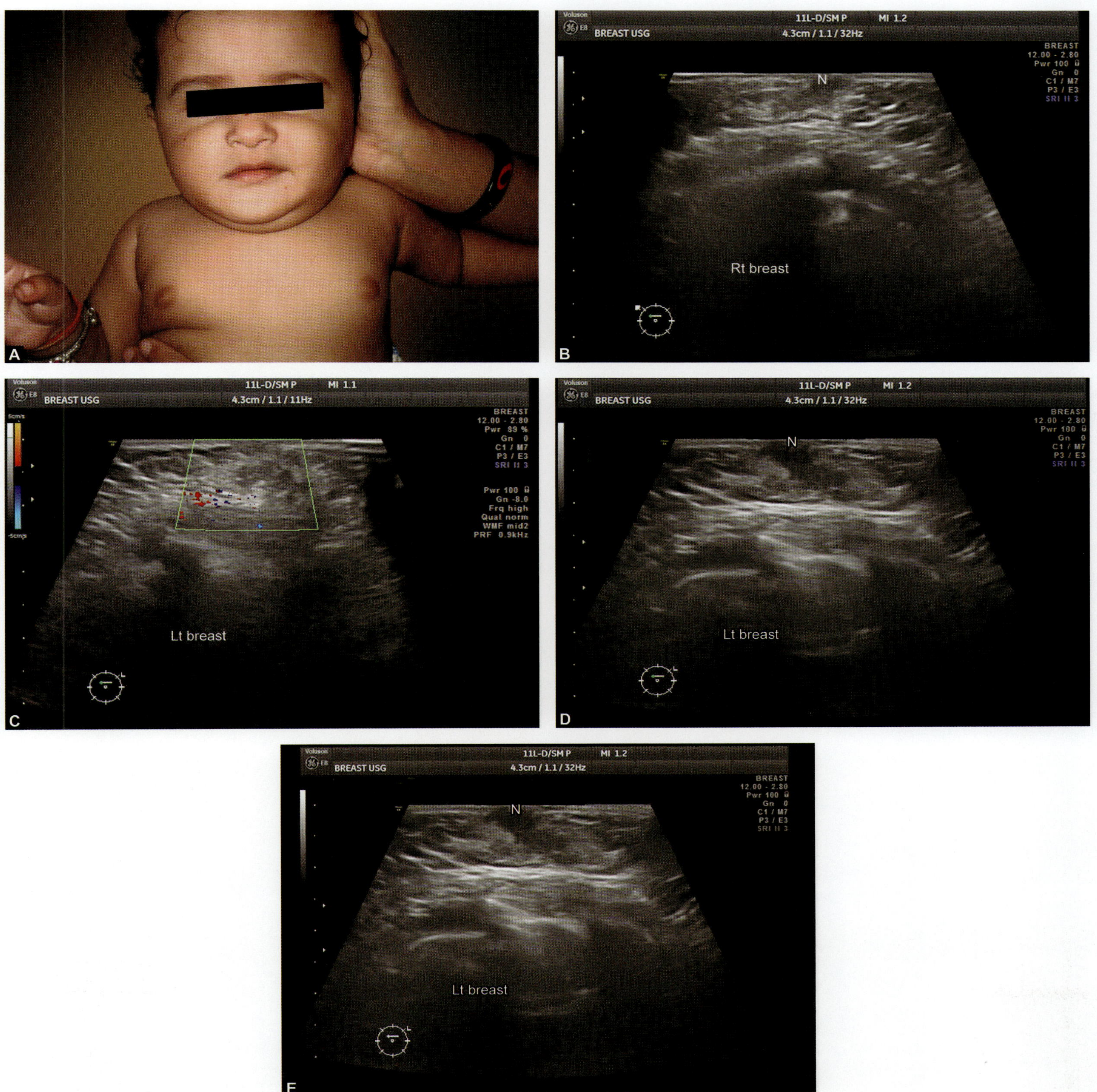

FIGURES 8.9A to E: Unilateral hypertrophy of the breast. A 5-month-old baby presented with unilateral hypertrophy of right breast. HRSG shows diffuse enlargement of breast tissue. But no focal mass is seen in the breast. No calcification is seen suggestive of unilateral hypertrophy.

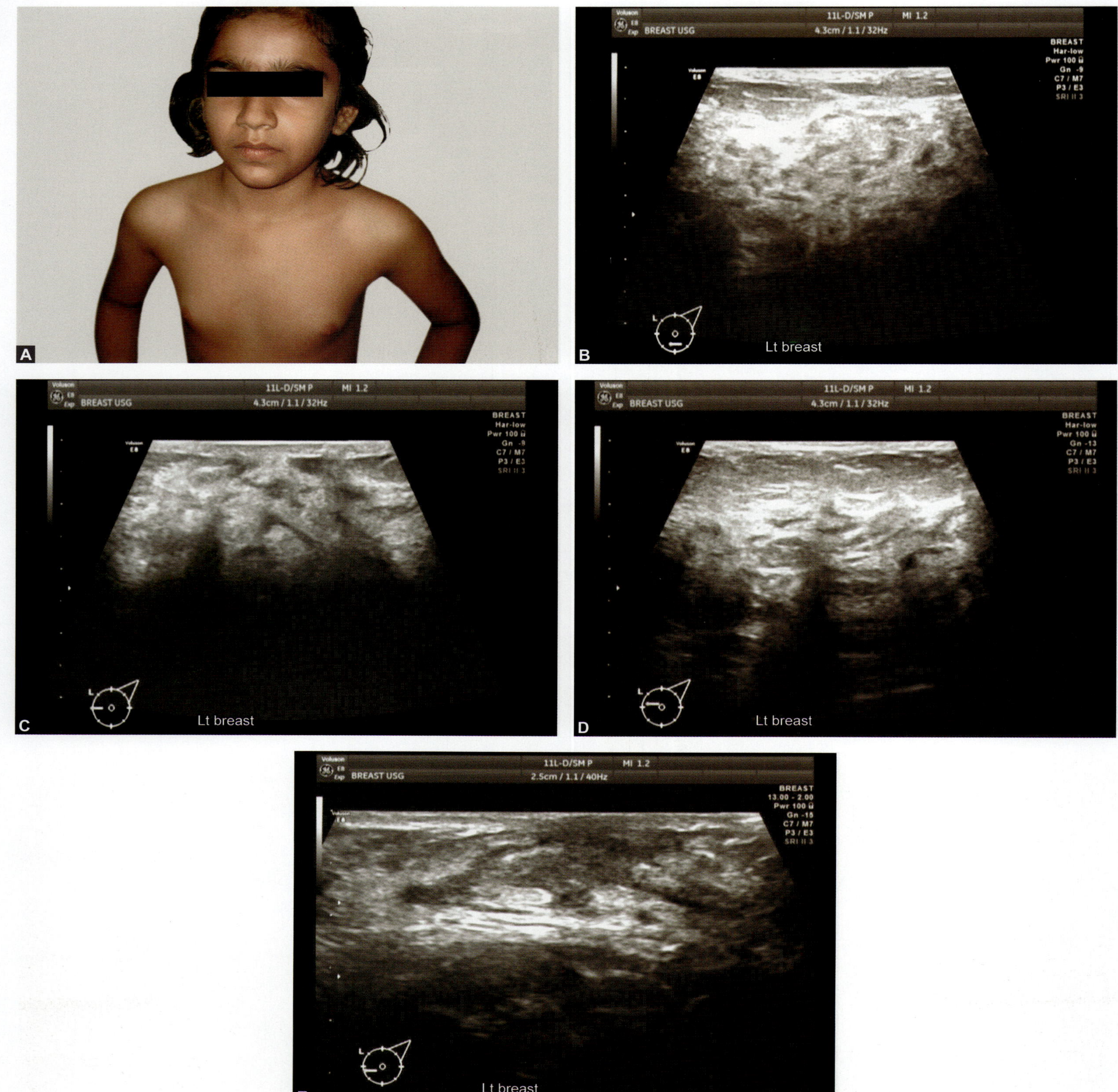

FIGURES 8.10A to E: A young girl presented with left breast enlargement. HRSG shows diffuse enlargement of glandular tissue in the left breast. No evidence of any focal mass is seen in the left breast. Areola and periareolar regions are free. The right breast is normal. Findings are suggestive of diffuse glandular enlargement in the left breast suggestive of unilateral breast enlargement.

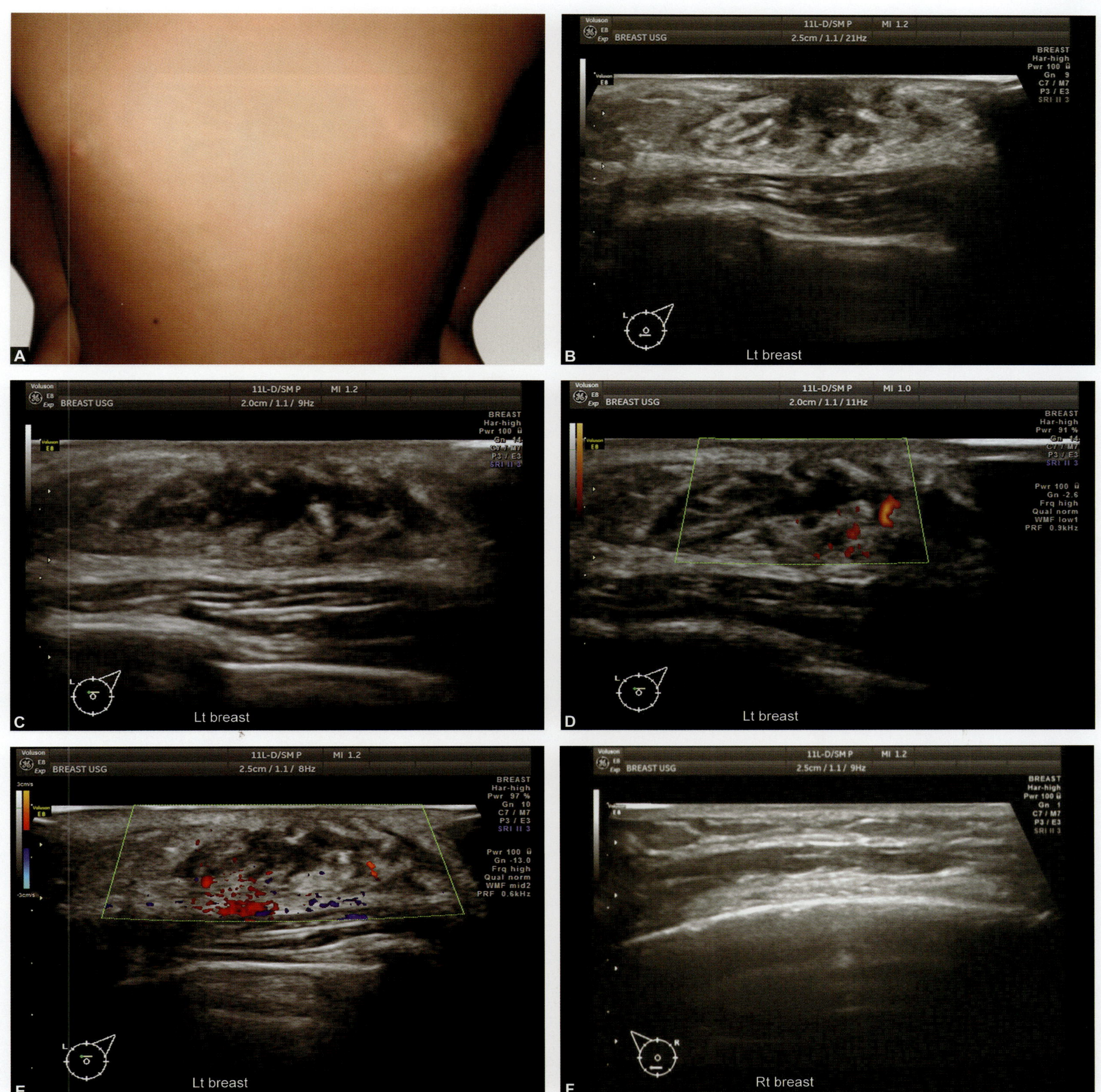

FIGURES 8.11A to F: Unilateral breast enlargement. An 8-year-old girl presented with left side breast enlargement. HRSG shows diffuse glandular tissue enlargement of left breast. No focal mass is seen in the breast. No calcification is seen. The right breast is normal. Unilateral breast enlargement in young girl is first sign of precocious puberty.

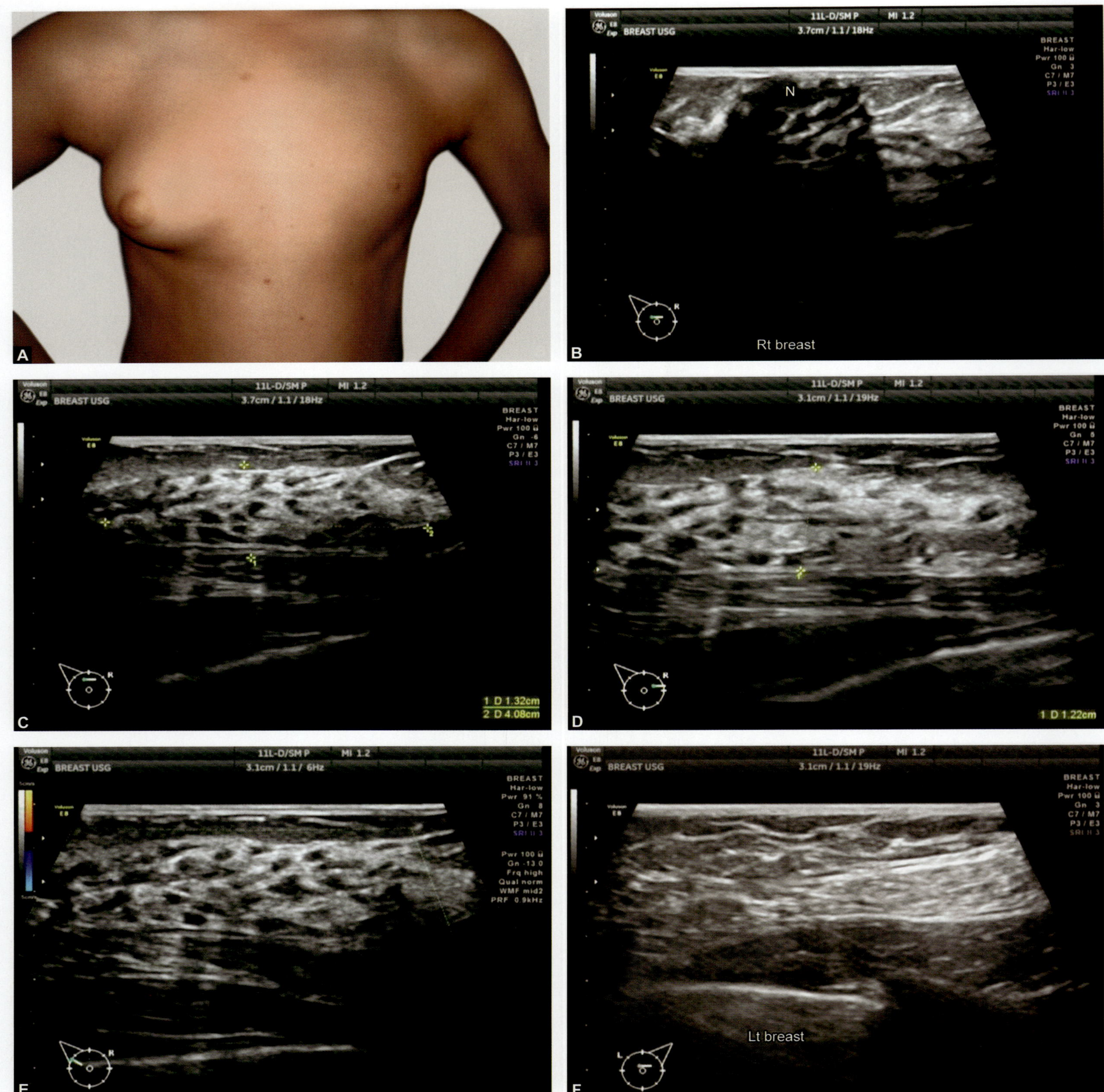

FIGURES 8.12A to F: Unilateral gynecomastia. A 12-year-old boy presented with marked enlargement of right breast. HRSG shows diffuse glandular enlargement in the right breast. No evidence of any focal mass is seen in the breast tissue. No calcification is seen. Left side of breast is normal. Findings are suggestive of unilateral gynecomastia.

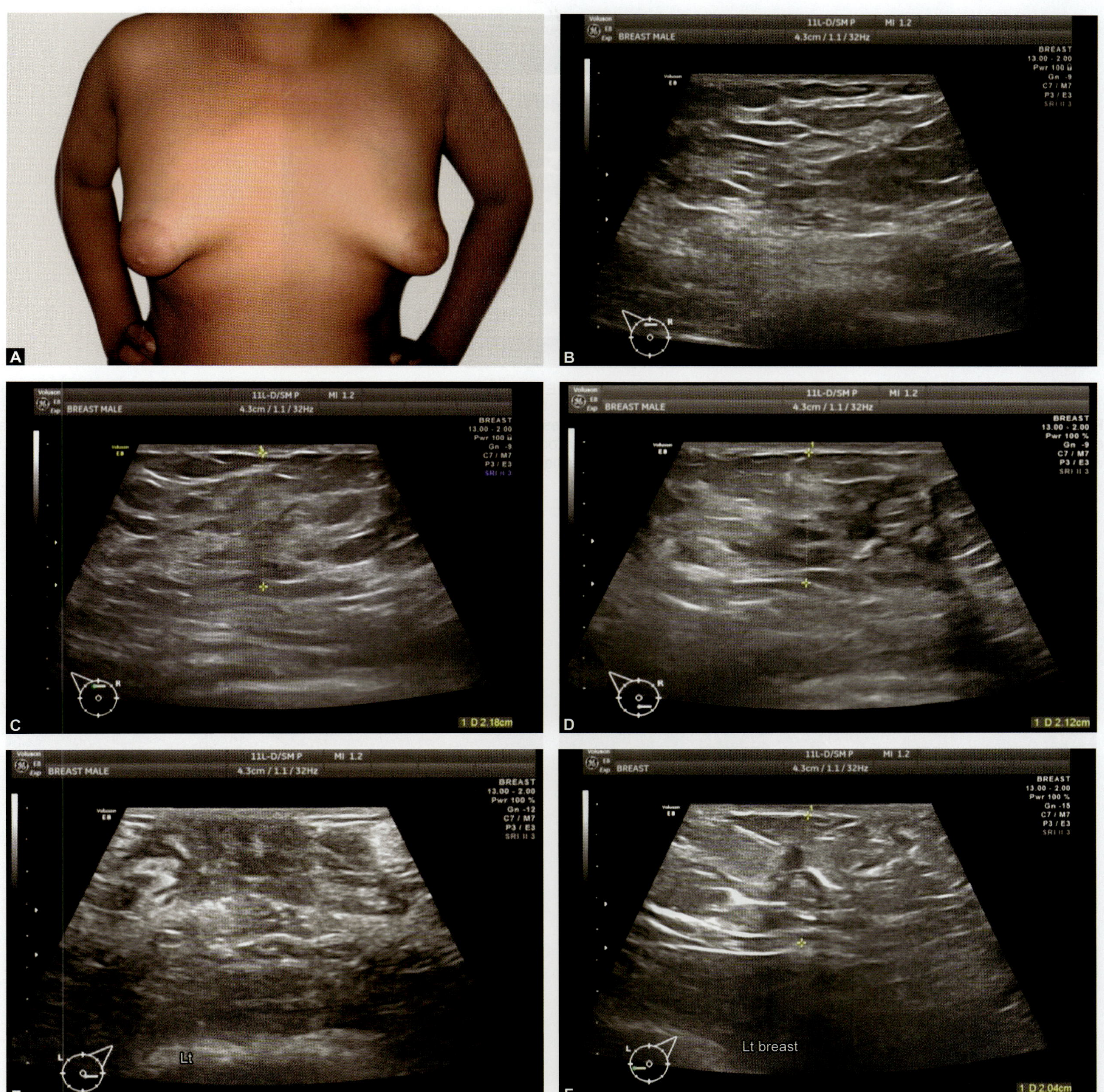

FIGURES 8.13A to F

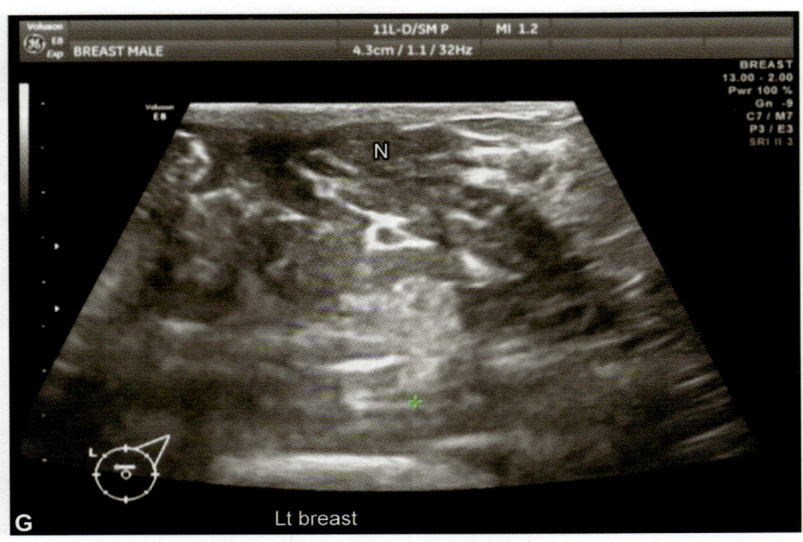

FIGURE 8.13G

FIGURES 8.13A to G: Bilateral gynecomastia. A 14-year-old boy presented with bilateral enlargement of both breasts. HRSG shows diffuse enlargement of glandular tissue in both the breasts. No evidence of any focal mass lesion is seen on either side. No calcification is seen. The chest wall muscles are normal. Findings are suggestive of bilateral gynecomastia.

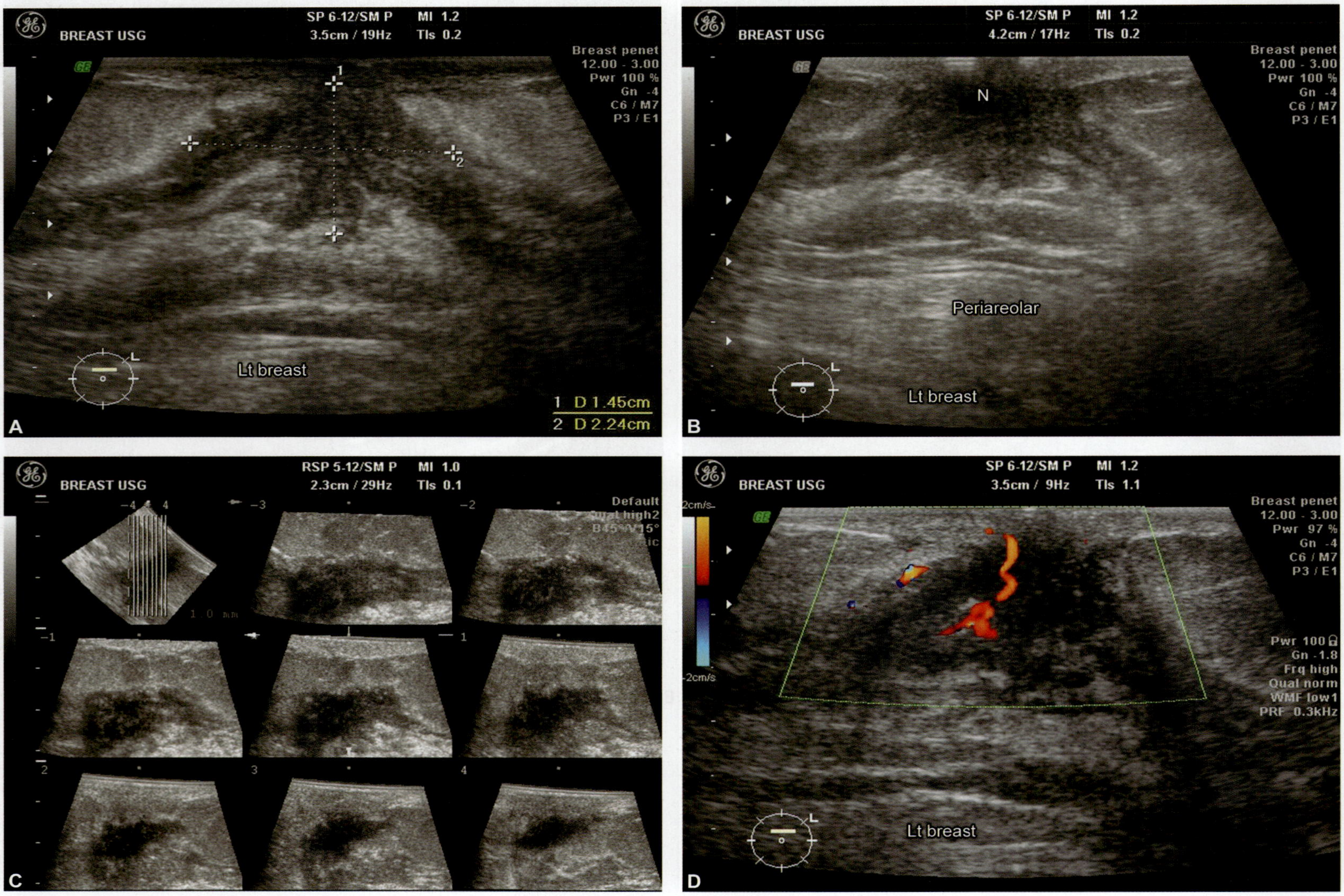

FIGURES 8.14A to D

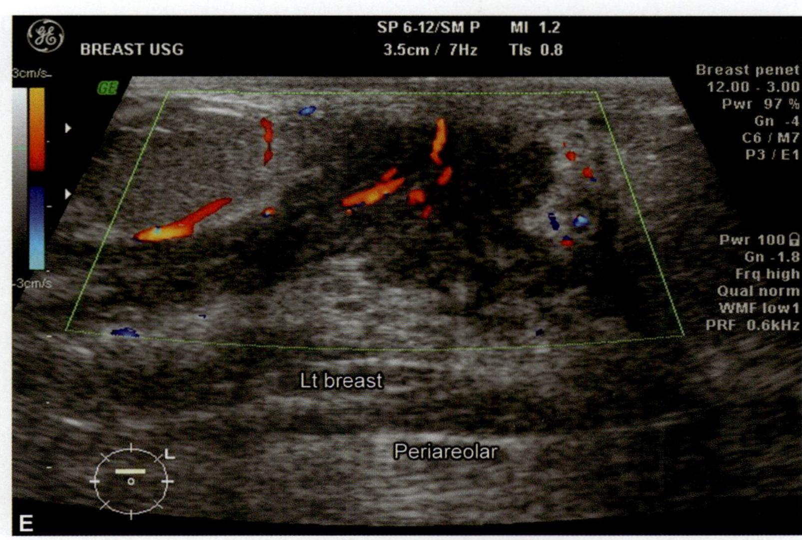

FIGURE 8.14E

FIGURES 8.14A to E: Proliferative gynecomastia. A patient presented with diffuse painful enlargement of left breast. HRSG shows irregular ill-defined inhomogeneous hypoechoic mass in the left breast. It is seen confined to the glandular tissue. No suggestion of any focal mass is seen in it. On color flow imaging, increased flow is seen in the inflamed breast tissue. Findings are suggestive of proliferative gynecomastia.

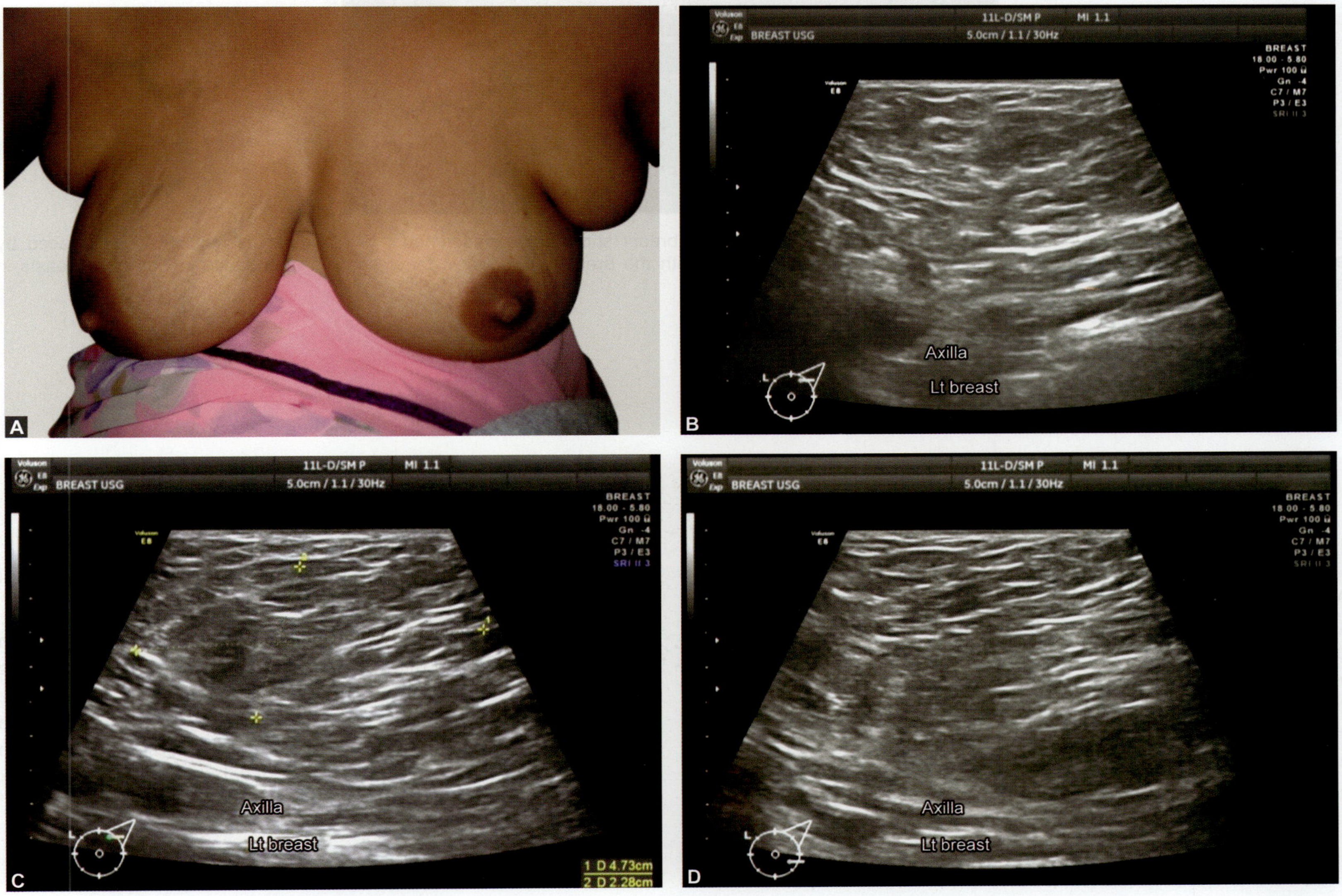

FIGURES 8.15A to D: Pad of fat in axilla. A patient presented with soft tissue masses in the region of tail of both breast. HRSG shows well-defined homogeneous echogenic masses on either side. They show echotexture similar to fat. No calcification is seen in them. No cystic degeneration is seen. Findings are suggestive of pad of fat on either side.

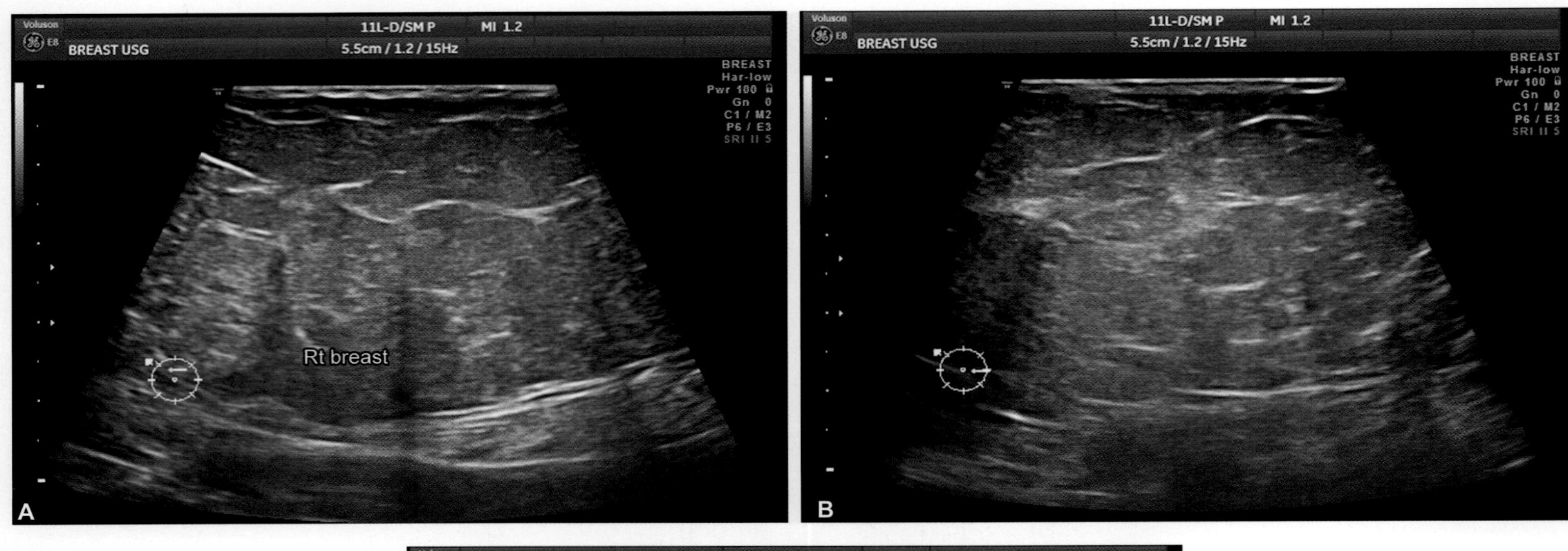

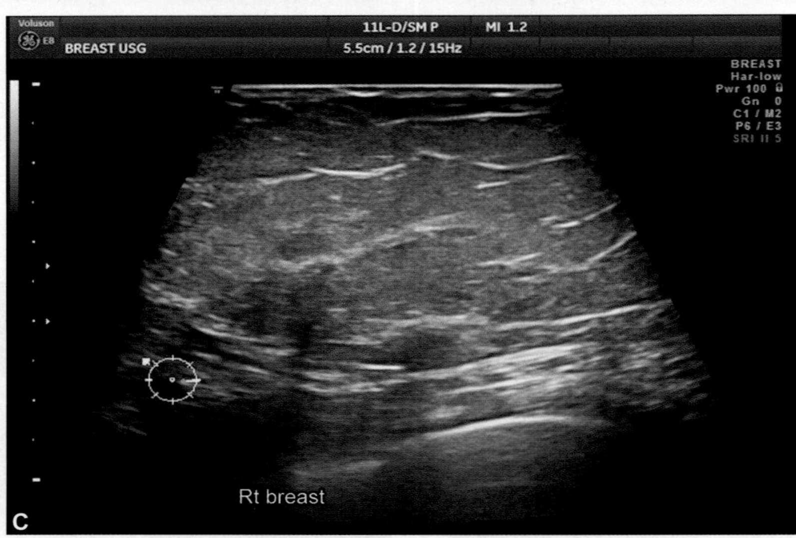

FIGURES 8.16A to C: Postmenopausal breast. The postmenopausal breast show decreased amount of glandular tissue, which is replaced by echogenic fat. HRSG shows decreased amount of glandular tissue in both the breasts. Echogenic fat is seen in abundance in both the breasts in postmenopausal lady.

Inflammatory Breast Masses

A breast abscess may result due to infected galactocele or due to secondary infection in the cyst. It appears to be a thick walled, echo poor low level echo complex mass. It shows heterogeneous texture with areas of attenuation and debris. The diagnosis of breast abscess can be confirmed by aspiration of the pus from it under USG guidance. However, a breast abscess can mimic a narcotizing tumor or fat necrosis.

Fat necrosis: It is difficult condition to be diagnosed on USG. As it causes sound beam attenuation and due to fibrosis, aspiration biopsy is also not very fruitful. Therefore, at times open biopsy is required. It resembles as carcinoma and it become difficult to exclude breast carcinoma.

Tuberculosis of the breast: Tuberculosis of the breast is uncommon condition. However, the disease can attack the breast from surrounding tubercular focus as in sternum, rib, chest wall or systemic focus elsewhere in body. A patient presents with soft tissue swelling in the breast, which is most of the time, is not painful. HRSG shows low-level echo collection with multiple internal echoes suggestive of debris. Liquefaction is rare. Inflammatory nodes are seen in axilla.

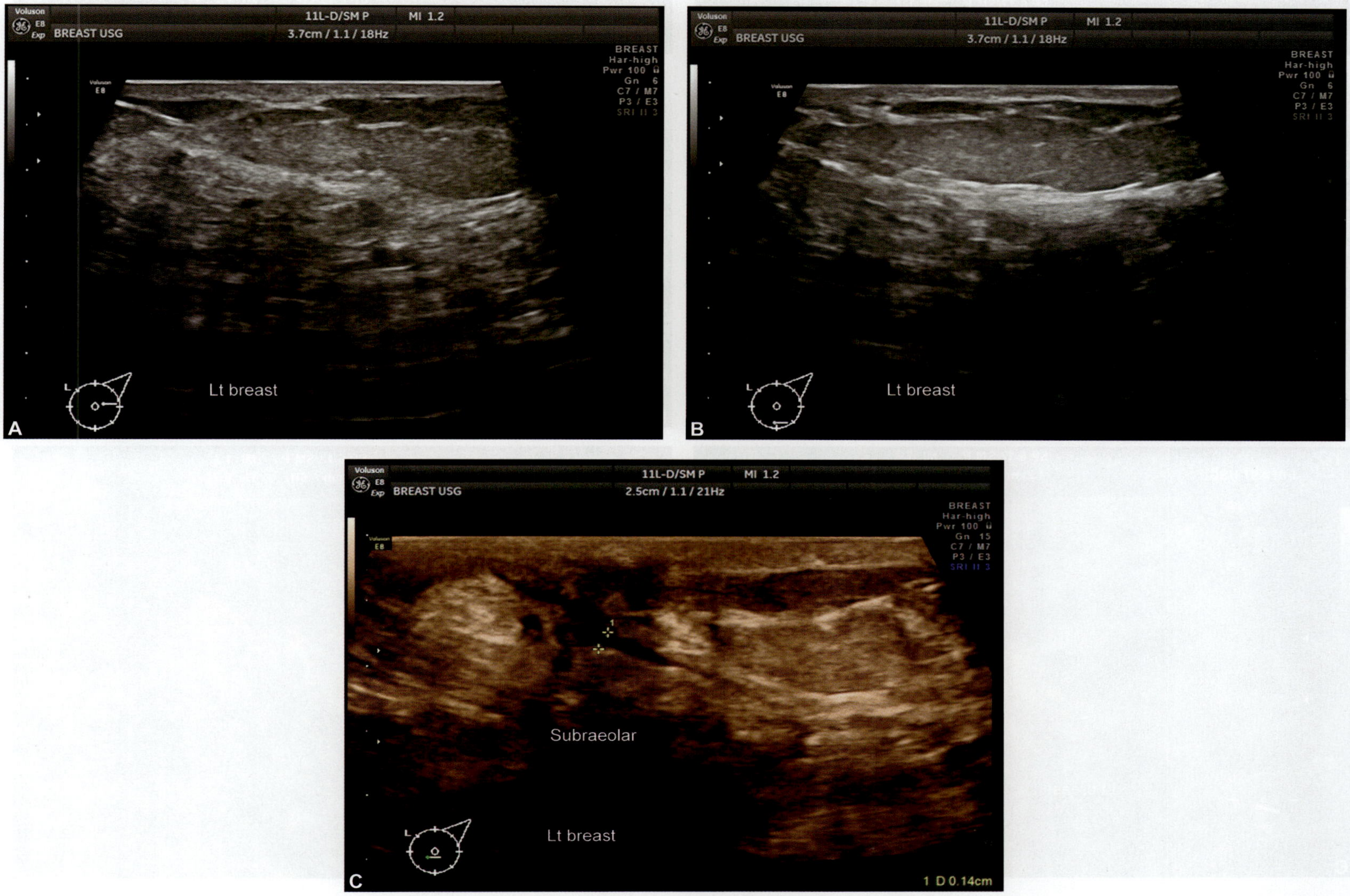

FIGURES 8.17A to C: Acute mastitis. A patient presented with acute pain in the left breast. HRSG shows irregular low level echo complex mass in the premammary zone. Homogeneous echoes are seen in it. But no cystic necrosis is seen. Findings are suggestive of acute mastitis involving premammary zone.

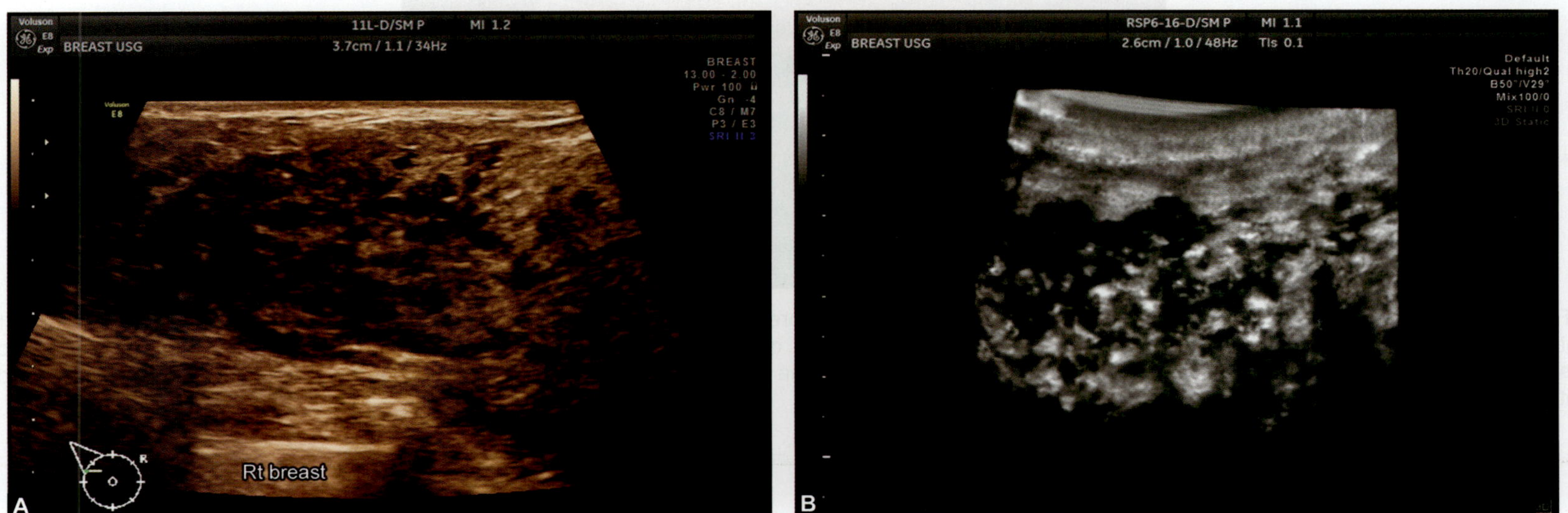

FIGURES 8.18A and B: Acute mastitis. An 18-year-old girl presented with acute pain in the right breast. HRSG shows diffuse edema of the right breast. Multiple hypoechoic areas are seen in the breast, which are discrete in distribution. The 3D imaging shows inflamed breast tissue. Associated fat inflammation is also seen suggestive of acute mastitis.

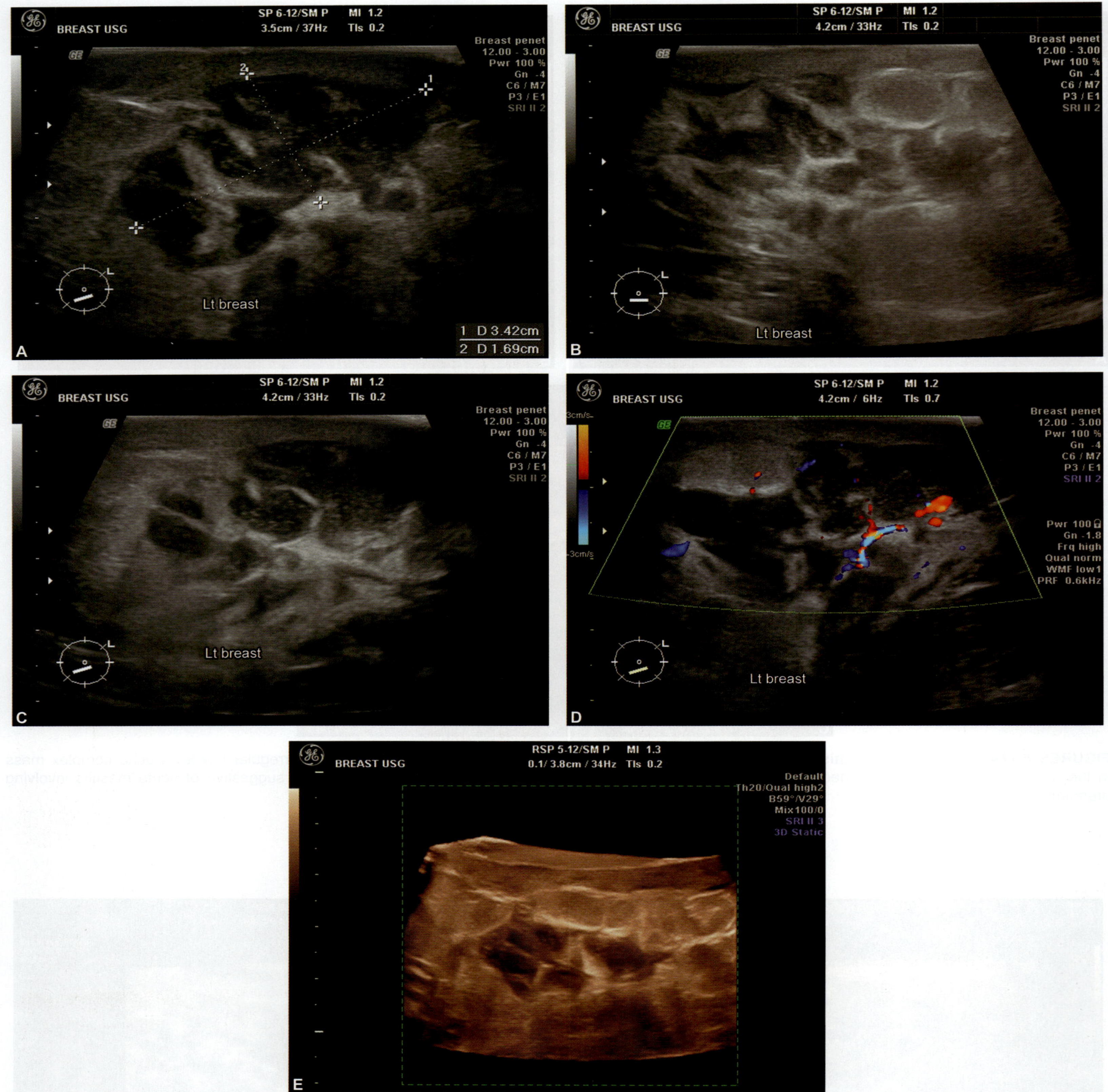

FIGURES 8.19A to E: Breast abscess formation. A 20-year-old lady presented with painful lump in the left breast. HRSG shows a big irregular ill-defined low level echo complex mass in the left breast in lower outer quadrant. Thick echoes are seen in the mass. Echogenic septa are also seen in it. Associated fat necrosis is also seen. Marked soft tissue edema is seen around it. On color flow imaging, peripheral flow is seen around it. Findings are suggestive of acute abscess formation.

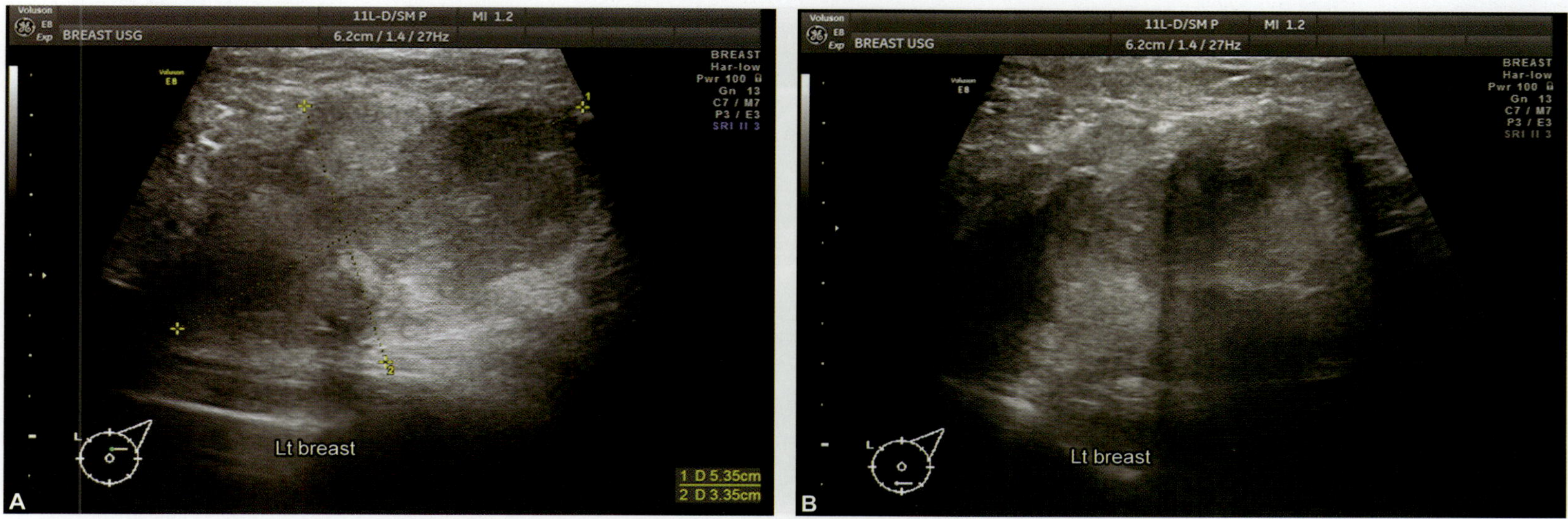

FIGURES 8.20A and B: Big breast abscess. A patient presented with big painful lump in left breast. HRSG shows a big low level echo complex mass in left breast. Central area of necrosis is seen in it. Associated perifocal edema is also present suggestive of breast abscess.

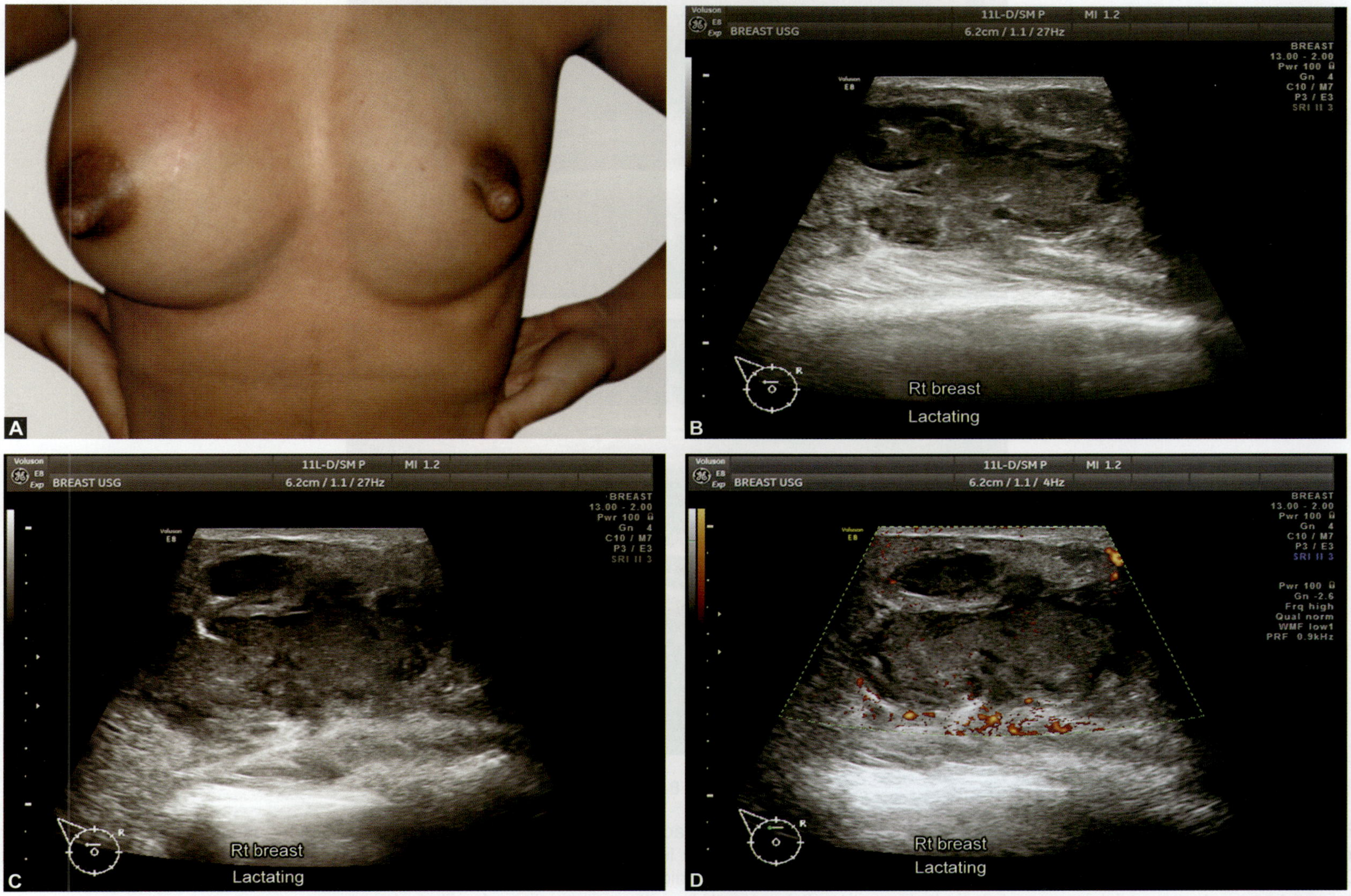

FIGURES 8.21A to D

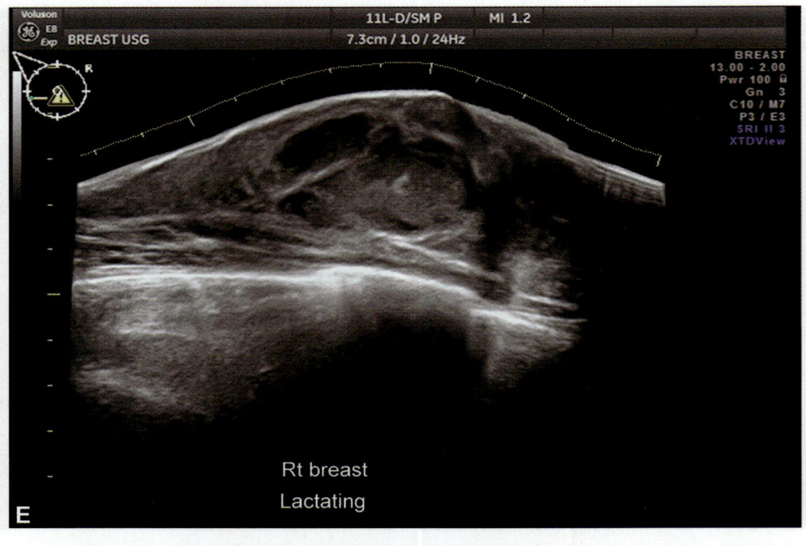

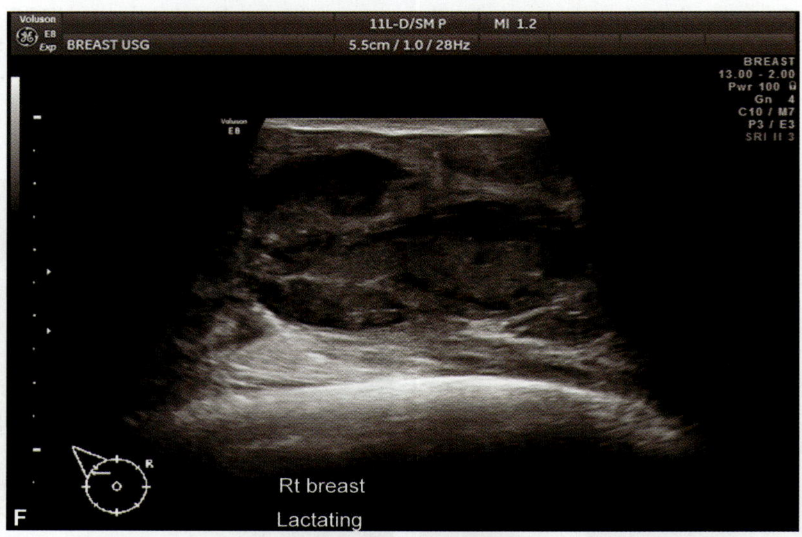

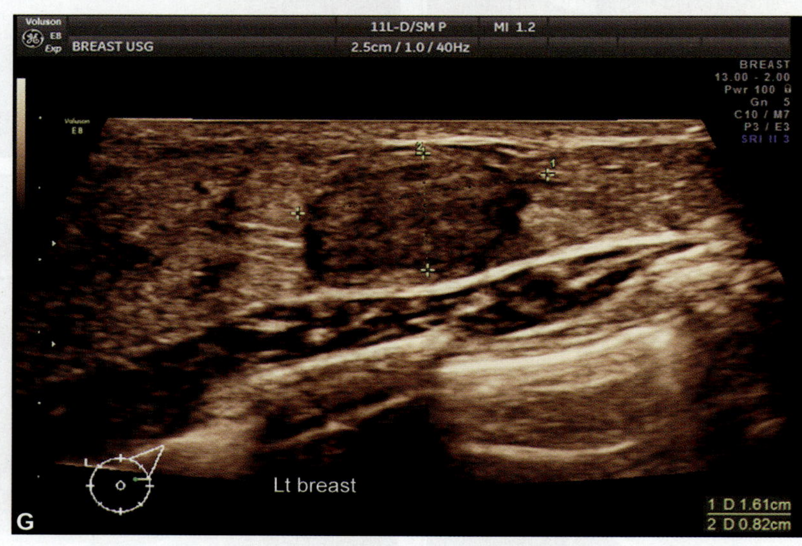

FIGURES 8.21E to G

FIGURES 8.21A to G: Big breast abscess. A 28-year-old lady having lactation presented with diffuse painful enlargement of the right breast with red hot skin in the upper part of breast. HRSG shows a big irregular low level echo complex mass in the right breast. Thick echoes are seen in it. Central area of necrosis is seen. Perifocal edema is present. Few echogenic septa are seen it suggestive of a big abscess. Left breast shows a well-defined homogeneous nodular mass at 3 o' clock position. It is smooth in outline suggestive of a fibroadenoma.

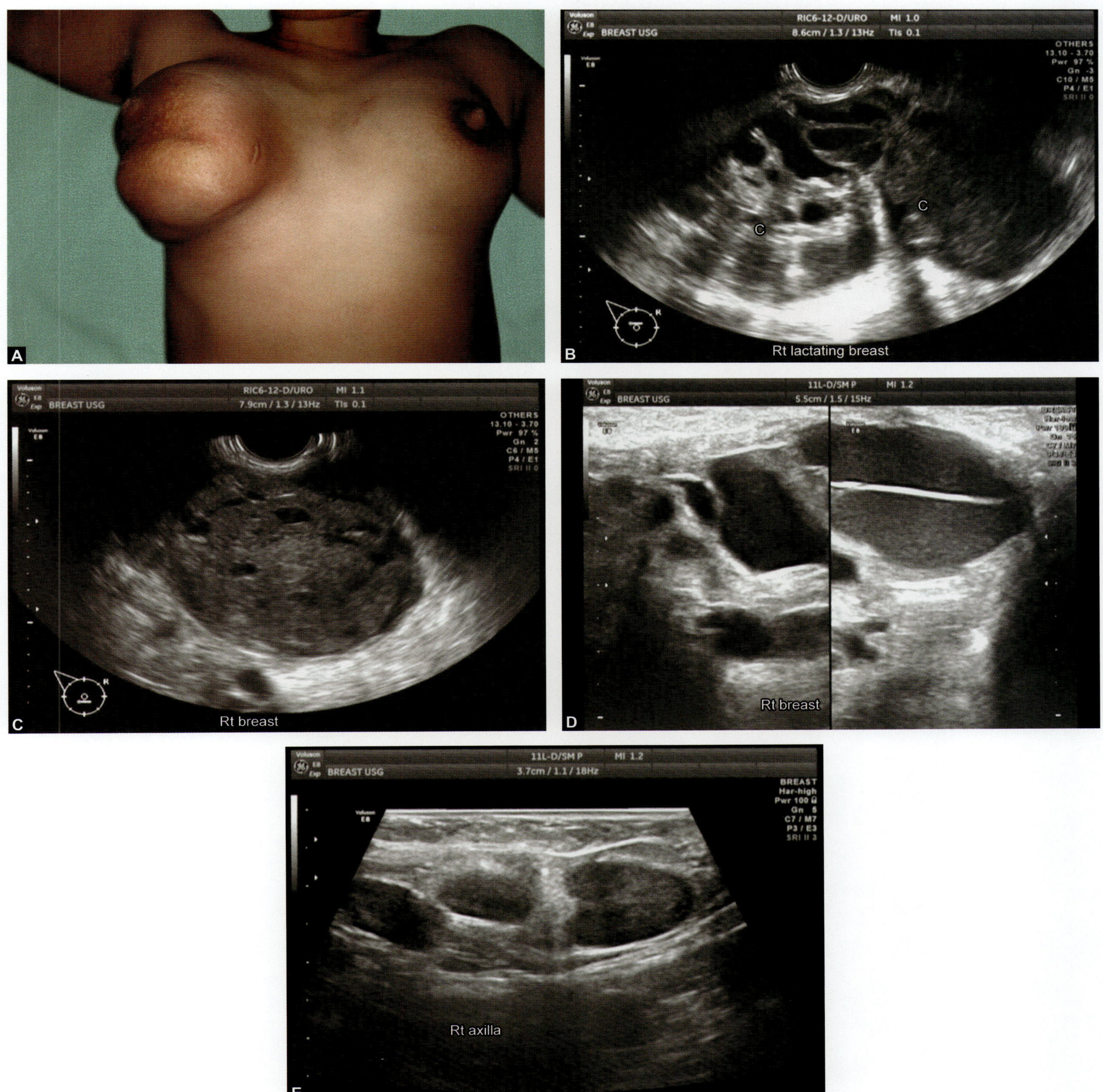

FIGURES 8.22A to E: Lactating breast abscess. A 24-year-old lactating mother presented with big painful enlargement of right breast. HRSG shows a big irregular low level echo complex mass involving whole of the right breast. Thick echoes are seen in it. Echogenic septa are also seen. Low level debris is seen in the mass. Normal anatomy is distorted. Multiple enlarged nodes are also seen in right axilla suggestive of reactive nodal enlargement. Findings are suggestive of big lactating breast abscess with inflammatory nodal enlargement in right axilla.

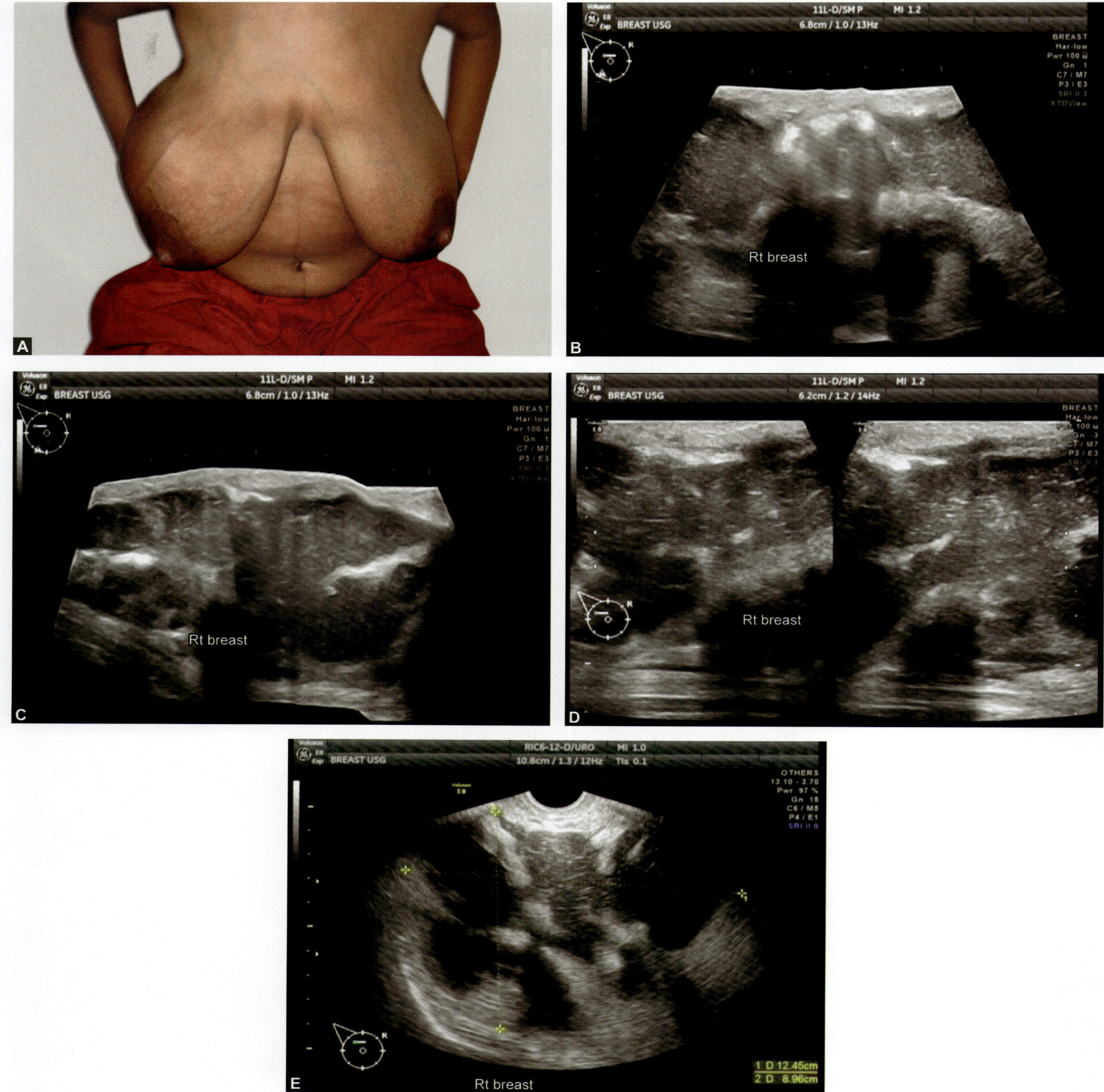

FIGURES 8.23A to E: Galactocele right breast. The right breast is enlarged. HRSG shows a big pocket of collection seen in the right breast in the upper outer quadrant. Multiple echoes are seen in the collection. Thick septa are also seen. The collection shows floating echoes. Turbidity is also seen in the collection. Multiple enlarged nodes are also seen in the right axilla. The nodes show echogenic hylum suggestive of reactive nodal enlargement. Findings are suggestive of big galactocele in right breast.

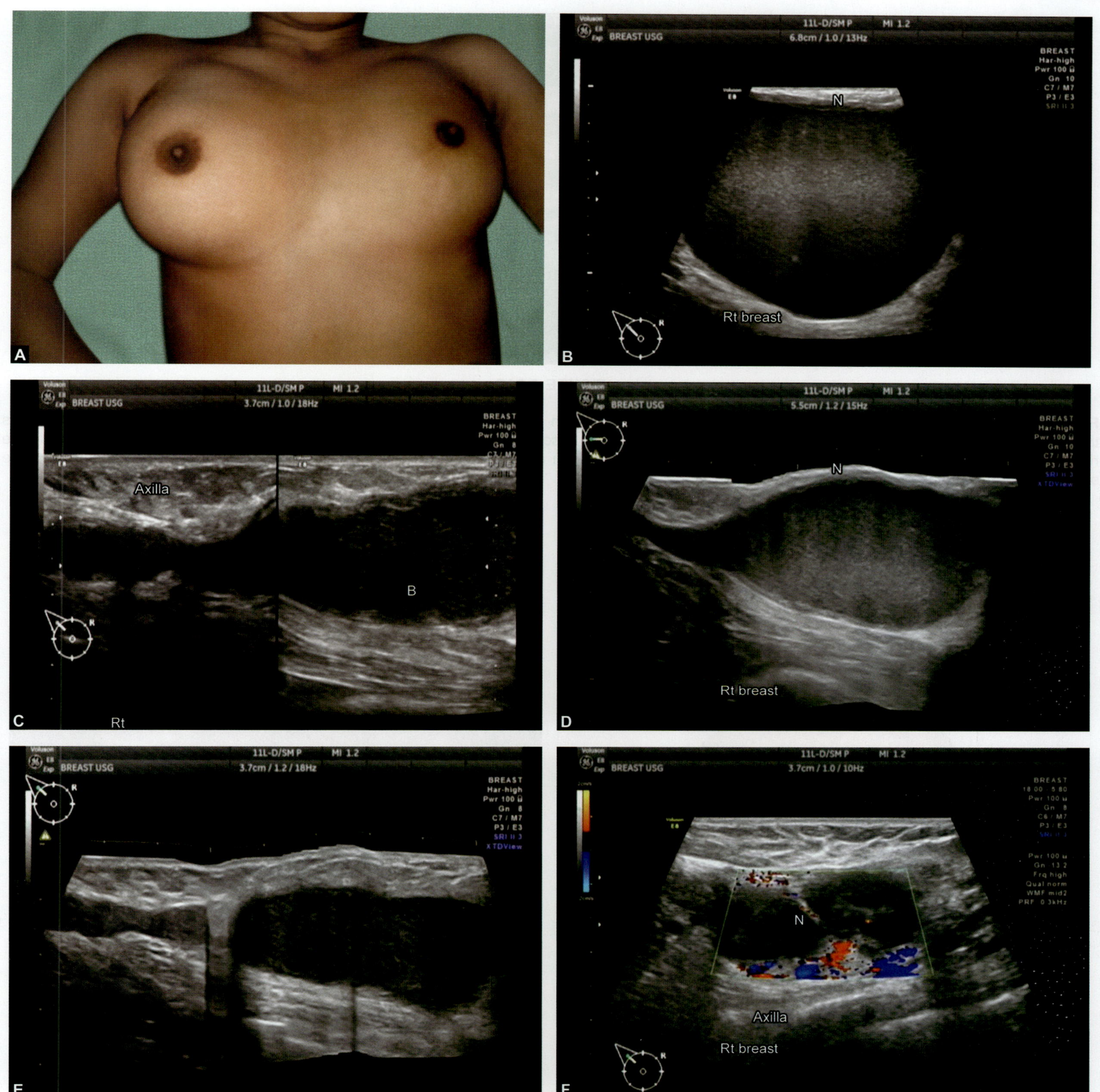

FIGURES 8.24A to F

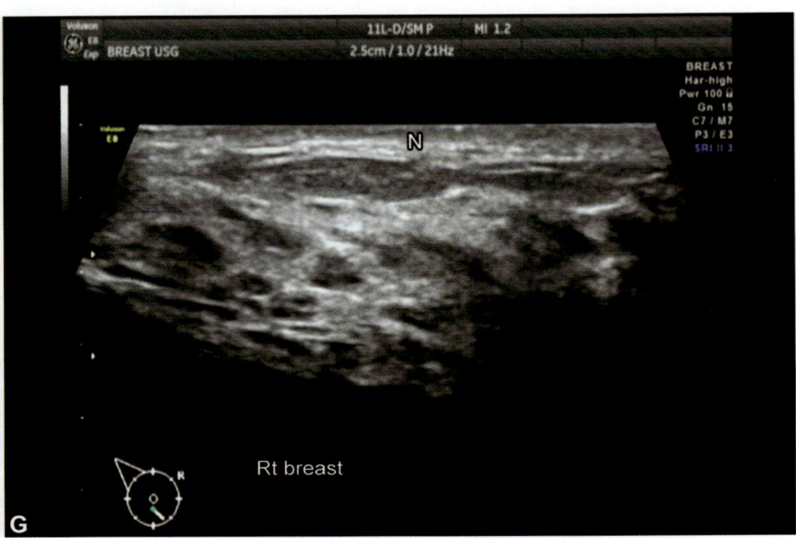

FIGURE 8.24G

FIGURES 8.24A to G: Breast tuberculosis. A young girl presented with diffuse enlargement of right breast with a semi-hard lump. HRSG shows thick low level echo collection in the right breast. A tract of collection is seen going to the right axilla. Multiple enlarged nodes are also seen in the right axilla. They are hypoechoic. No septation seen in the collection. On color flow imaging, no flow is seen in the collection pocket. Findings are suggestive of tubercular abscess in the right breast.

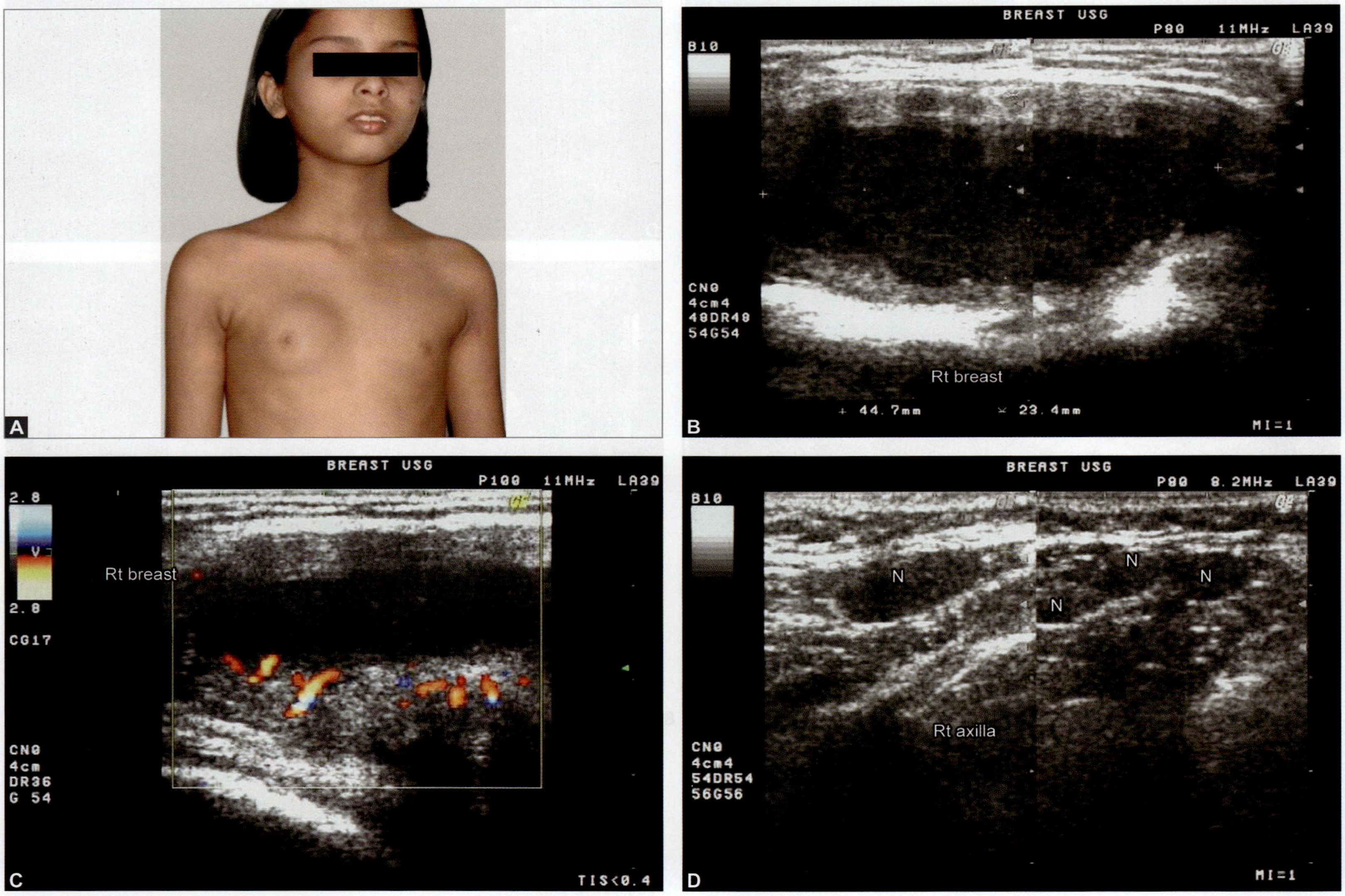

FIGURES 8.25A to D: Tubercular abscess. A young girl presented with slowly growing mass in the right breast. It was non-tender. Patient presented with low-grade fever. HRSG shows a thick low-level echo complex mass in the breast. Walls are thickened. On color flow imaging, peripheral wall flow is seen in it. Aspiration of the abscess confirmed tubercular abscess. Multiple enlarged nodes are also seen in the right axilla. Nodal biopsy also confirmed tubercular abscess.

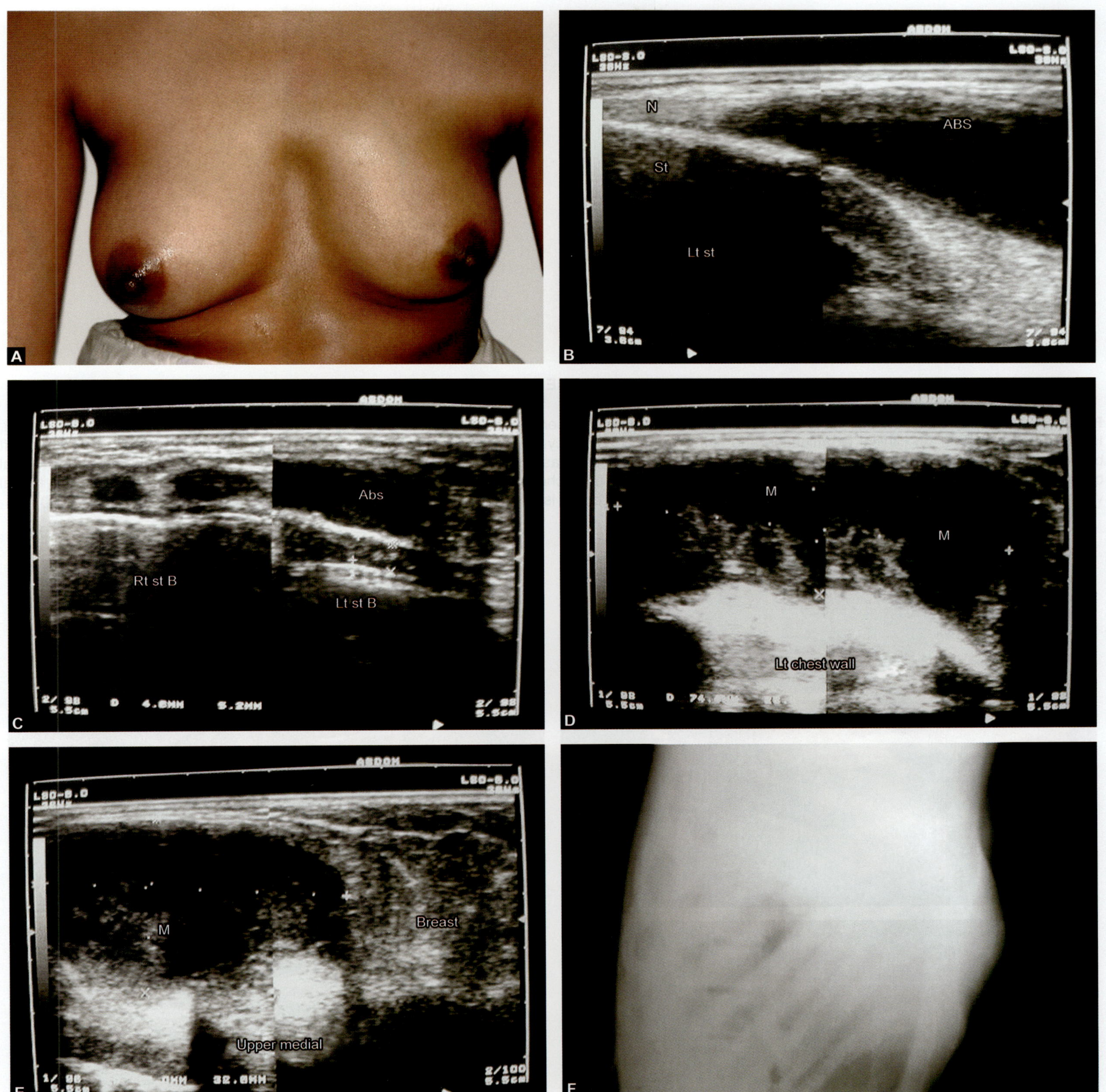

FIGURES 8.26A to F

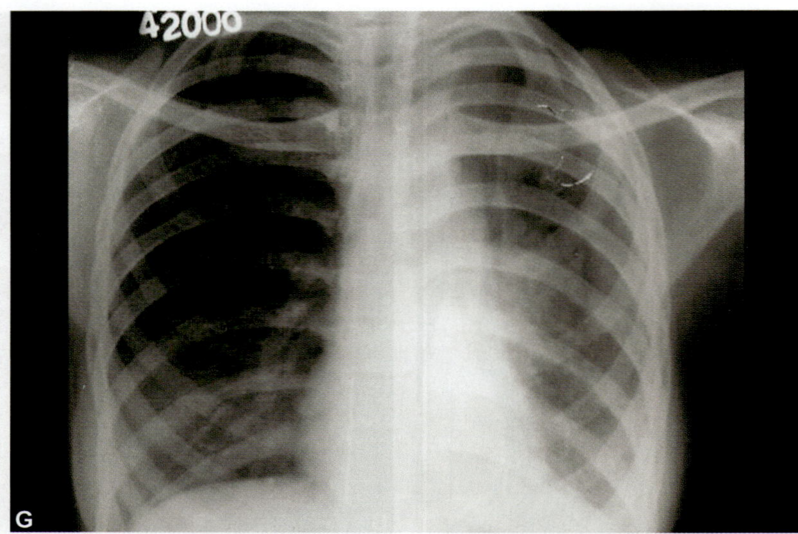

FIGURE 8.26G

FIGURES 8.26A to G: Tubercular abscess left breast. A young girl presented with soft tissue swelling over the upper medial quadrant of left breast. It was not very tender on clinical examination and semihard in consistency. HRSG shows low-level echo complex collection coming out from the left border of sternum and going to the upper medial quadrant to the left breast. HRSG shows thick low-level echo collection involving the upper medial quadrant of the left breast suggestive of an abscess. On aspiration thick cheesy material was taken out suggestive of tubercular abscess. P/A, lateral view shows tubercular infiltration involving the left lung. Soft tissue bulge is seen over the sternum on plain X-ray.

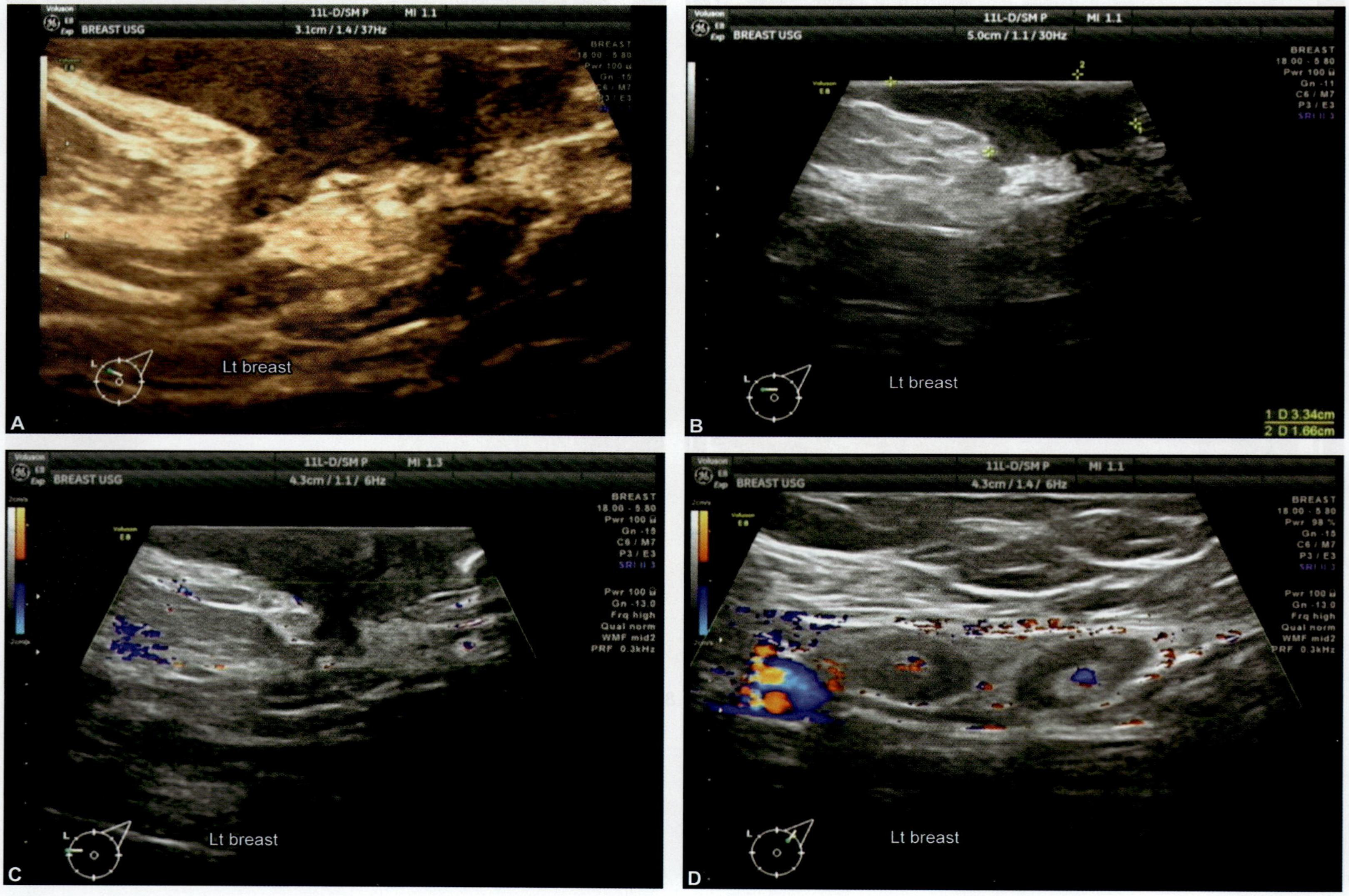

FIGURES 8.27A to D: Tubercular abscess. HRSG shows an irregular ill-defined pocket of collection in the breast in the upper inner quadrant. Thick echoes are seen in the collection. A sinus is seen to the periareolar region from the pocket of collection. But no septation is seen. No calcification seen. On color flow imaging, no flow is seen in the collection. There evidence of multiple enlarged nodes seen in the left axilla. Lymph node hilum is seen intact.

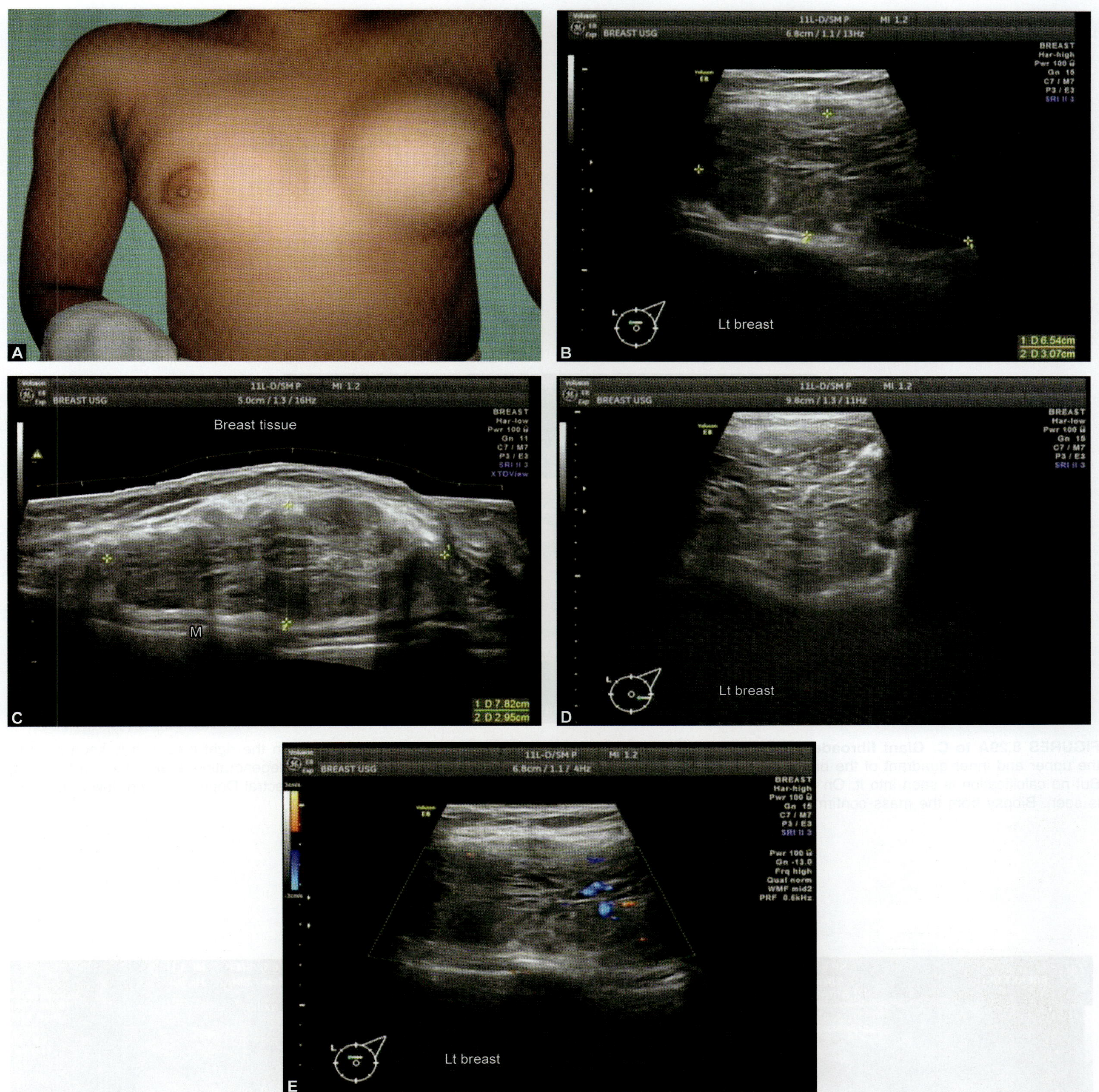

FIGURES 8.28A to E: A young girl presented with markedly increased left breast. HRSG shows a big lobulated predominantly solid soft tissue mass is seen in the left breast. The mass is seen posterior to the breast tissue. It is solid in nature. No calcification is seen. No cystic degeneration is seen in the mass. Normal anatomic relations are distorted. Normal breast tissue is seen pushed up by the mass. On color flow imaging, poor flow is seen in the mass. Biopsy of the mass confirms muscle tumor.

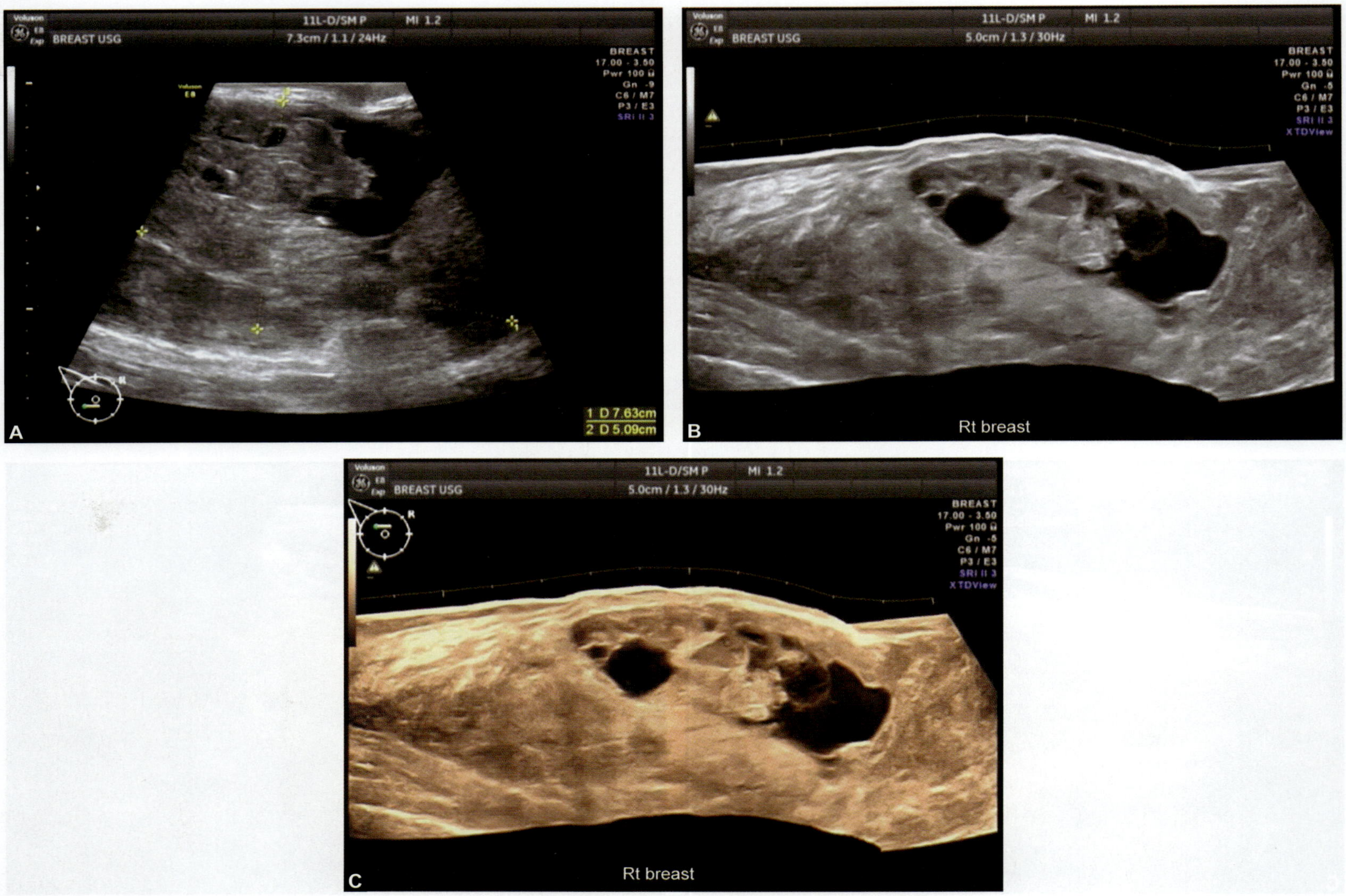

FIGURES 8.29A to C: Giant fibroadenoma with necrosis. HRSG shows a huge predominantly solid mass in the right breast. It is seen involving the upper and inner quadrant of the breast and also seen extending to the outer quadrant. But area of cystic degeneration is also seen in the mass. But no calcification is seen into it. On color flow imaging, few small vessels are seen feeding the mass. On spectral Doppler tracing, low arterial flow is seen. Biopsy from the mass confirms giant fibroadenoma with necrosis.

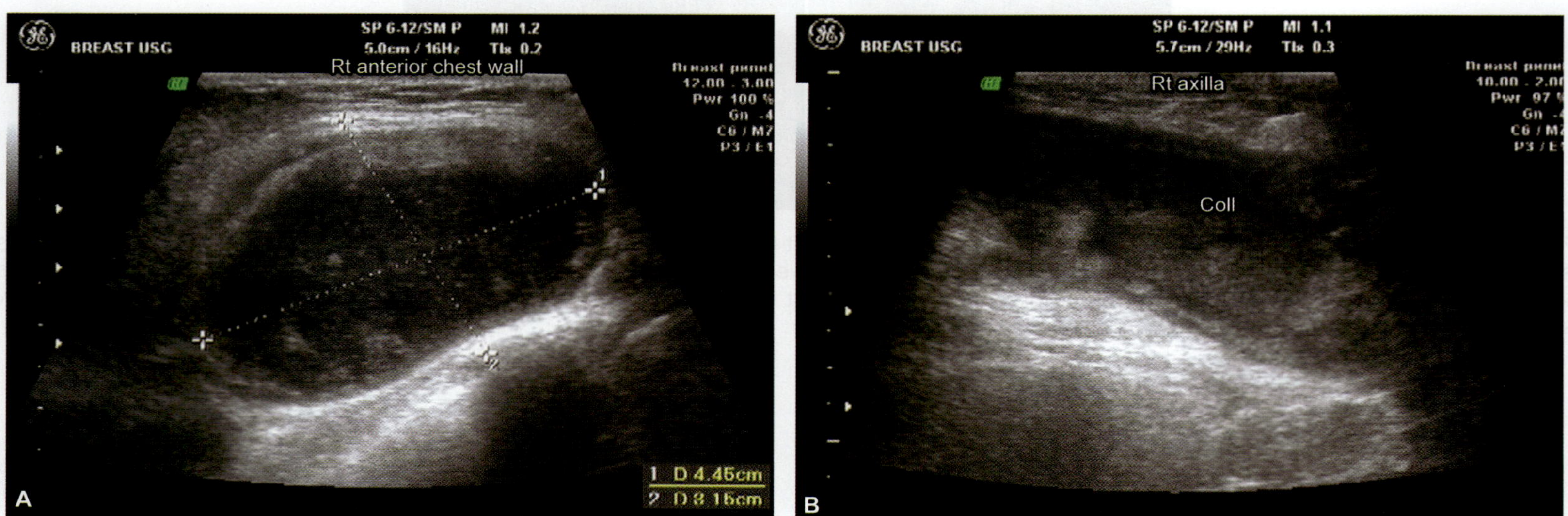

FIGURES 8.30A and B

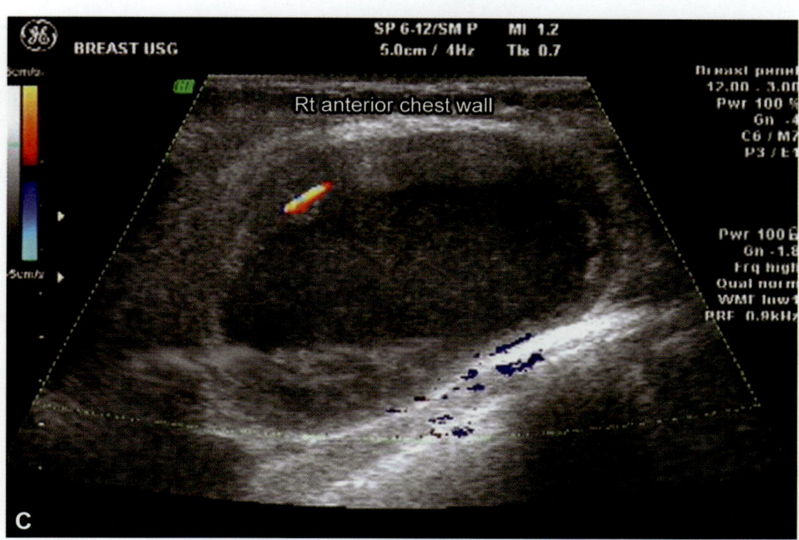

FIGURE 8.30C

FIGURES 8.30A to C: HRSG shows a big thick-walled cystic mass in the anterior chest wall. Multiple internal echoes are seen into it. But no calcification is seen. No septation seen. The mass is not seen invading the chest wall muscle. There is also evidence of thick low-level collection seen in the right axilla. It is seen going in the axillary recess. Thick echoes are seen into it. Aspiration biopsy confirmed organized abscess.

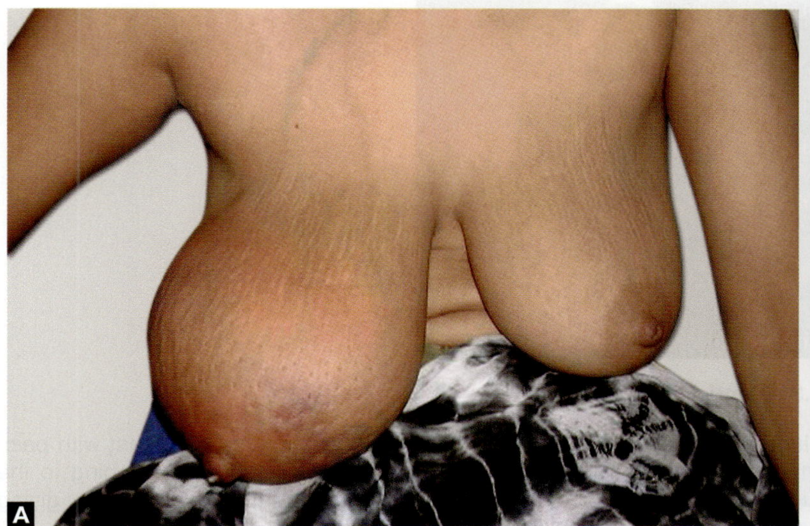

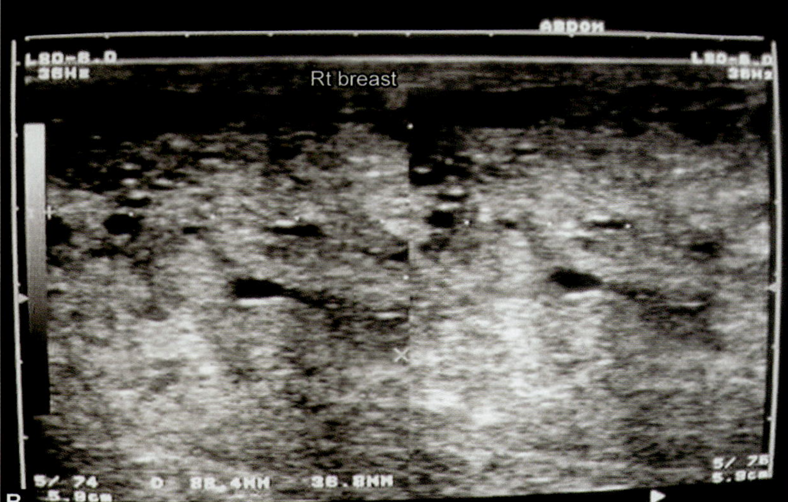

FIGURES 8.31A and B: Filarial breast. A patient presented with markedly enlarged tender, hot, inflamed right breast with acute mastalgia. The breast is almost doubles in size of the left breast. HRSG shows diffuse enlargement of the breast, involving whole of the breast. The ducts were dilated and engorged. Marked soft tissue edema is present. But no focal mass lesion is seen. The patient was having positive history of filaria infestation and it was acute filarial involvement of right breast. HRSG shows grossly edematous right breast with multiple dilated tubules in the same patient.

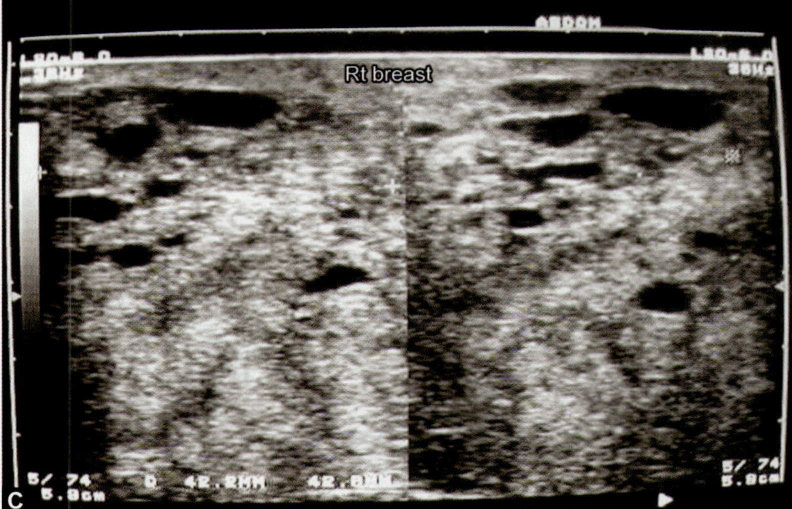

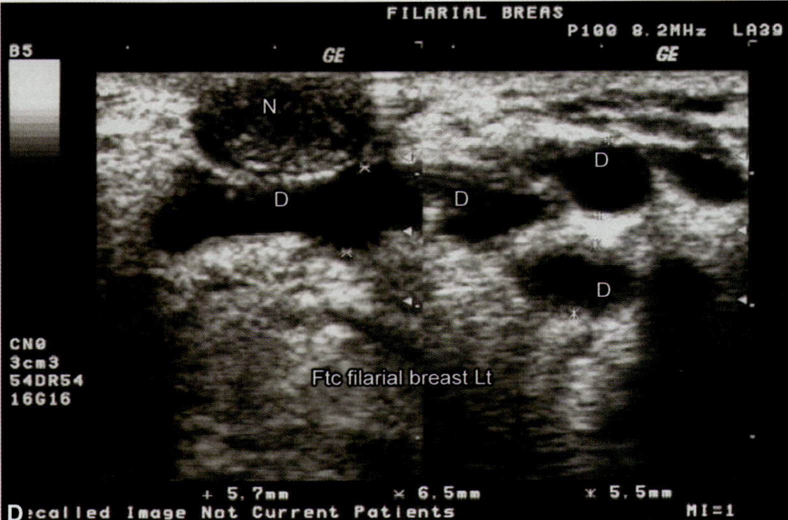

FIGURES 8.31C and D

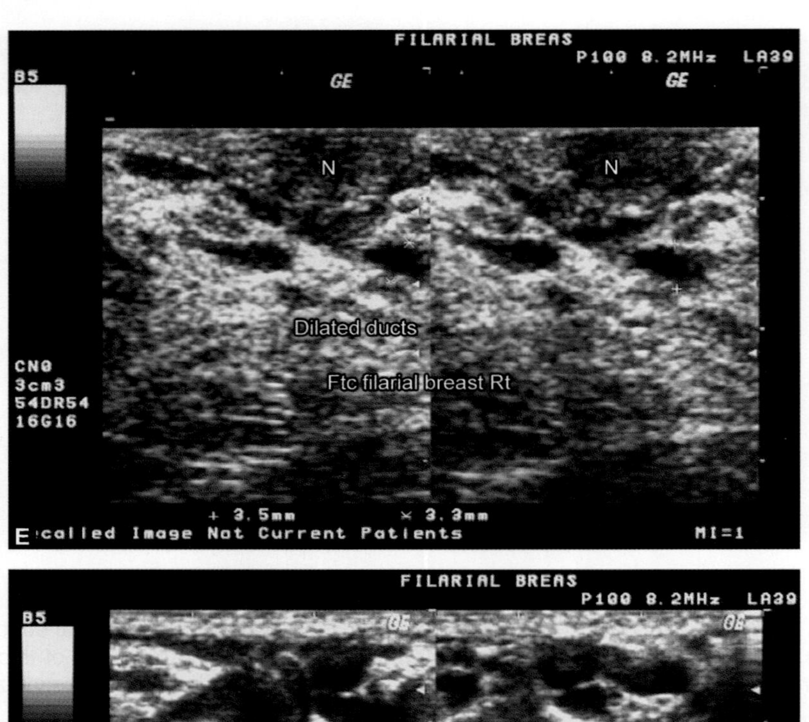

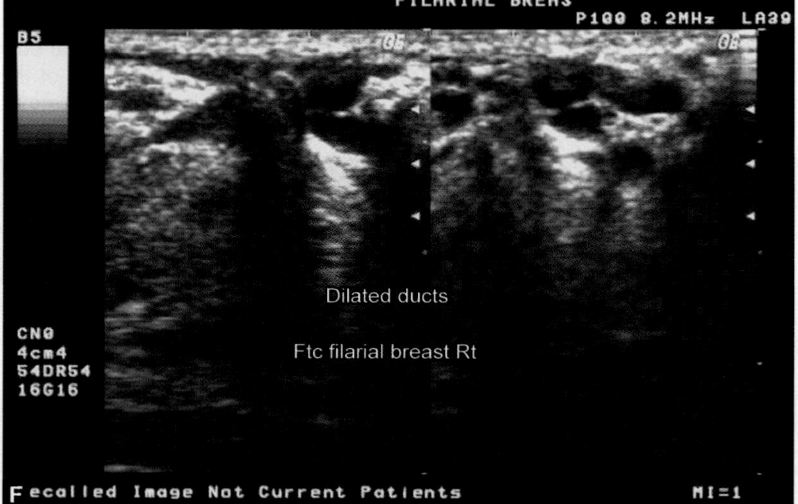

FIGURES 8.31E and F

FIGURES 8.31C to F: Bilateral filarial breast. A known case of bilateral filarial breast infestation presented with enlarged engorged breast with pain. HRSG shows markedly dilated tubules. They are running to the areola. The ducts are engorged. Rt breast also shows dilated ducts running to the tubules. Gross dilatation of the ducts is seen involving both the breast suggestive of filarial ductal dilatation with engorgement. Patient was giving history of white milk like fluid coming out from the both breasts in large quantity suggestive of chyle.

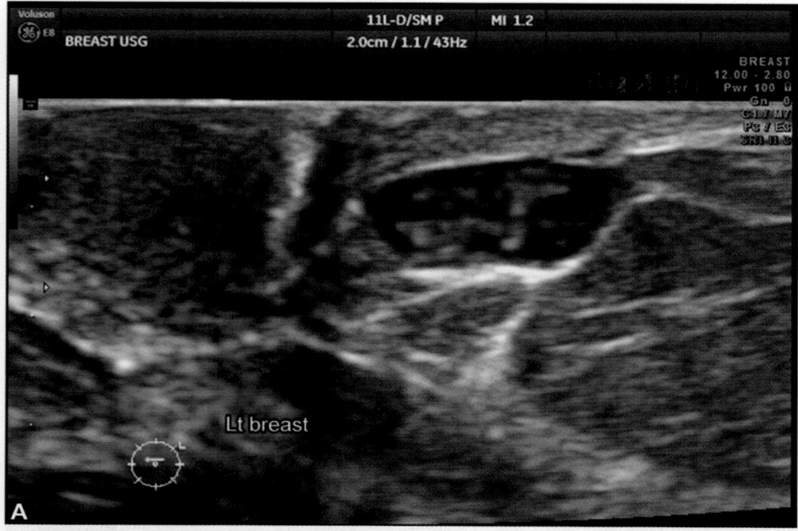

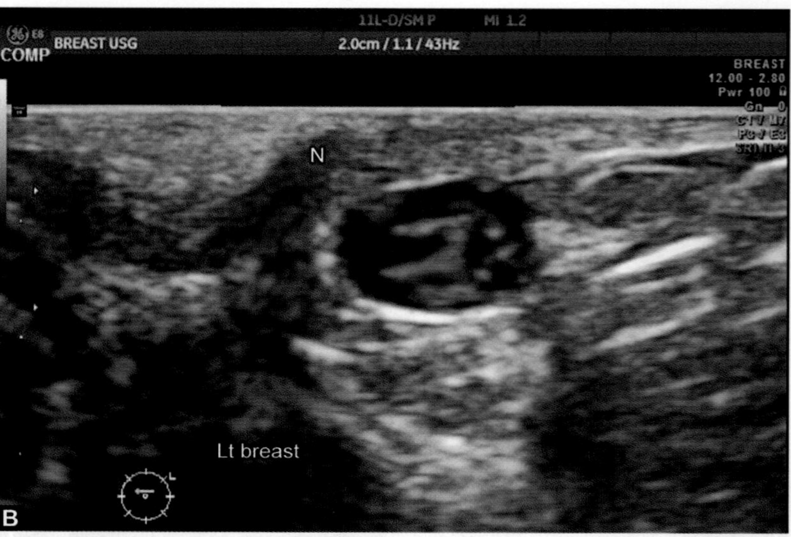

FIGURES 8.32A and B: Filarial mass in the right breast. A patient presented with soft tissue mass in left breast. HRSG shows a low level echo complex mass in right breast. Multiple echogenic shadows are seen in the mass, which show dancing movements on real time imaging suggestive of filarial with microfilaria.

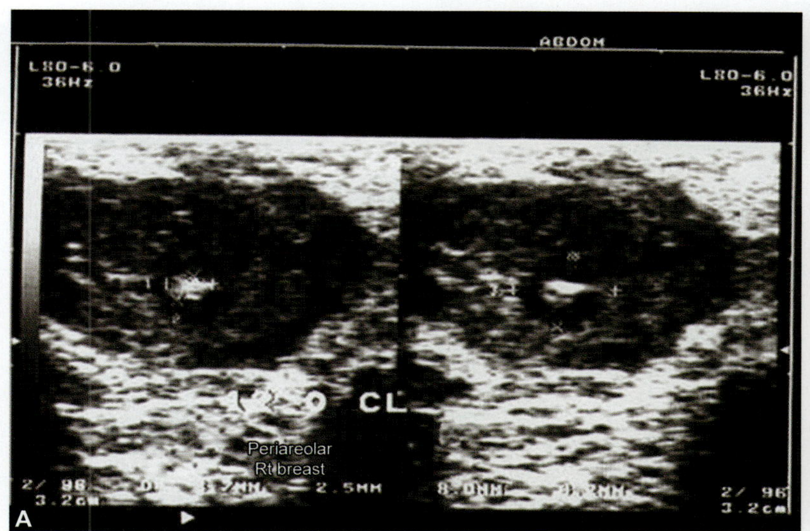

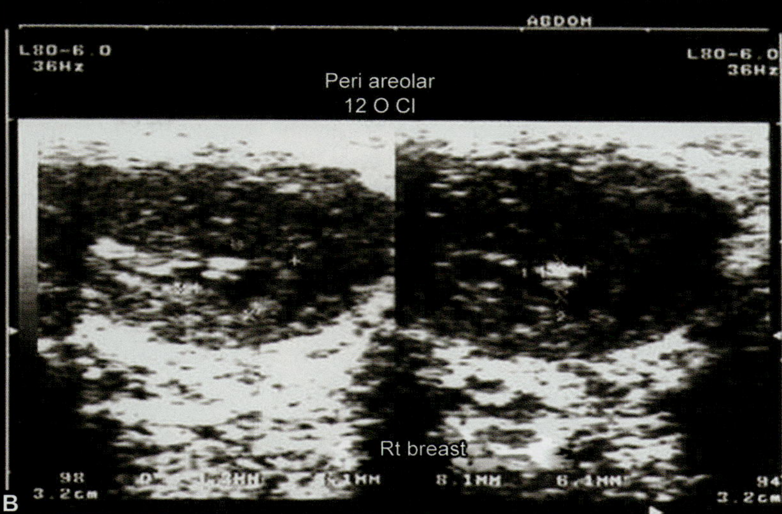

FIGURES 8.33A and B: Cysticercus cyst in the breast. HRSG shows a homogeneous mass shadow in the breast in a patient presented with a lump. A well-defined cyst is seen in the mass. An echogenic nidus is seen fixed with the inner wall of the cyst suggestive of scolex. This is a typical sonographic appearance of cysticercus cyst. It is an unusual finding and not commonly seen in breast. On color Doppler imaging, low flow is seen in the cyst suggestive of hyperemia.

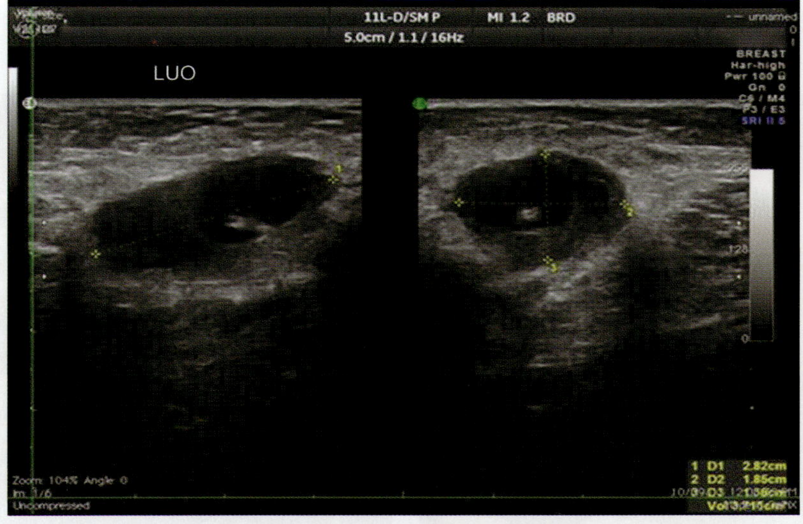

FIGURE 8.34: Cysticercus cyst in breast. A patient presented with soft tissue nodular mass in the left breast. HRSG shows a thick walled cystic mass in the left breast. An echogenic nidus is seen fixed with the inner wall of cyst suggestive of cysticercus cyst. Findings are typical of cysticercus cyst. (*Image Courtesy:* Dr Rahul Sachdev, BR Diagnostics, New Delhi)

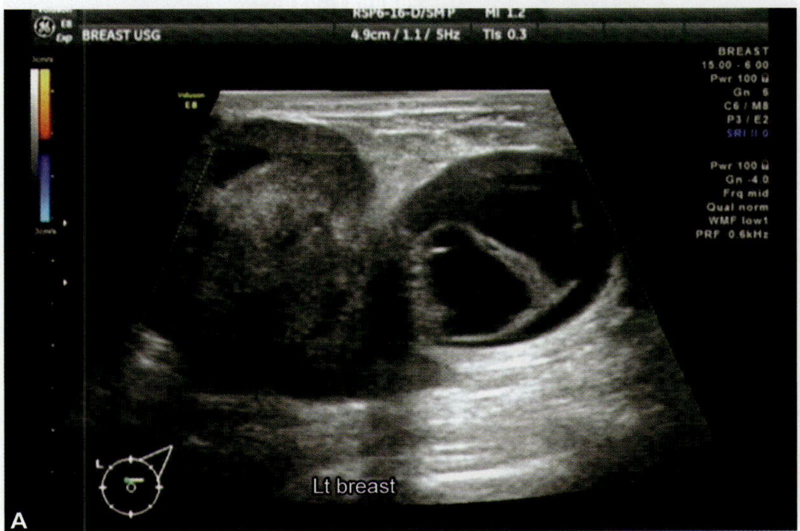

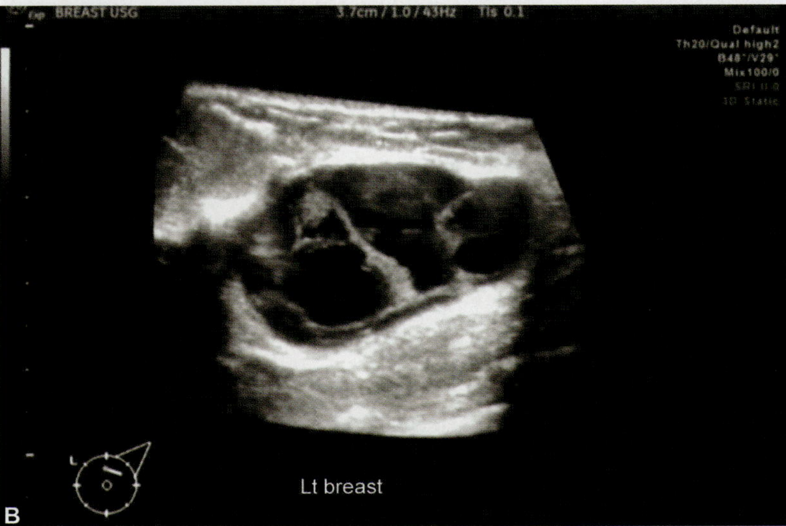

FIGURES 8.35A and B

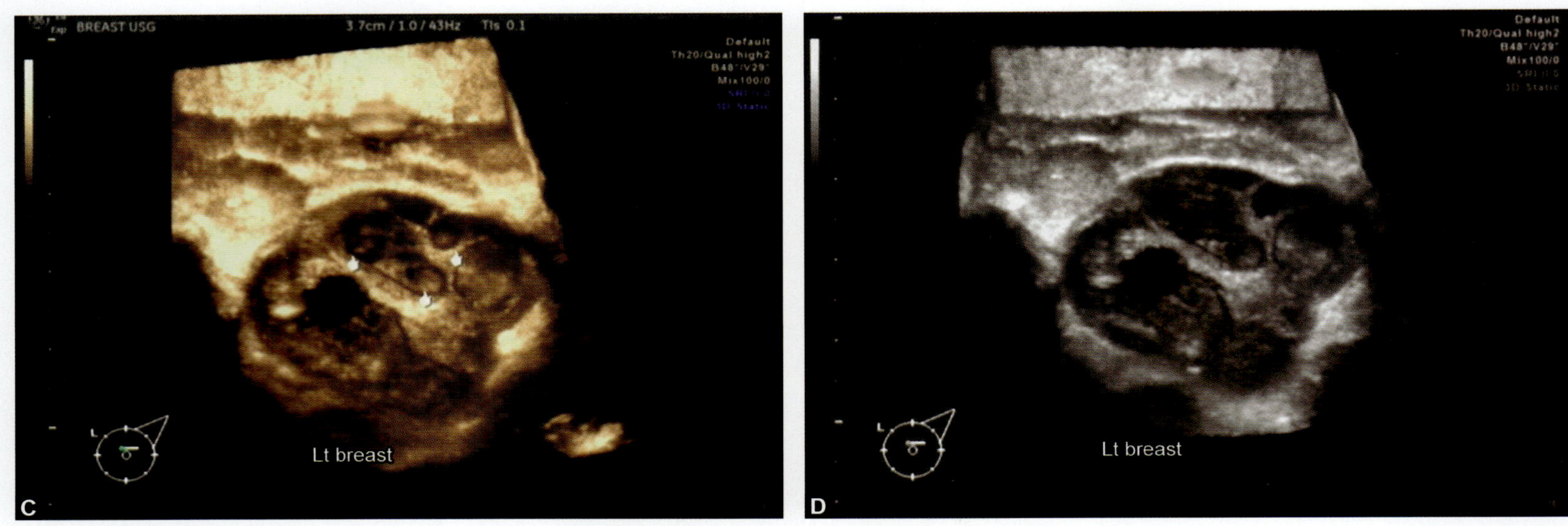

FIGURES 8.35C and D

FIGURES 8.35A to D: Hydatid cyst in breast with fibroadenoma. A 16-year-old girl presented with lump in left breast in upper and middle part. HRSG shows a big multiloculated cystic mass in the left breast. Thick echogenic septa are seen in it. Multiple daughter cysts are seen in the big cyst. On 3D imaging, the daughter cysts stand out clearly typical of hydatid cyst. Another lobulated mass is seen near the cystic mass, which is smooth in outline and homogeneous in texture. No calcification or cystic degeneration is seen in it. Findings are suggestive of a big fibroadenoma with hydatid cyst in left breast.

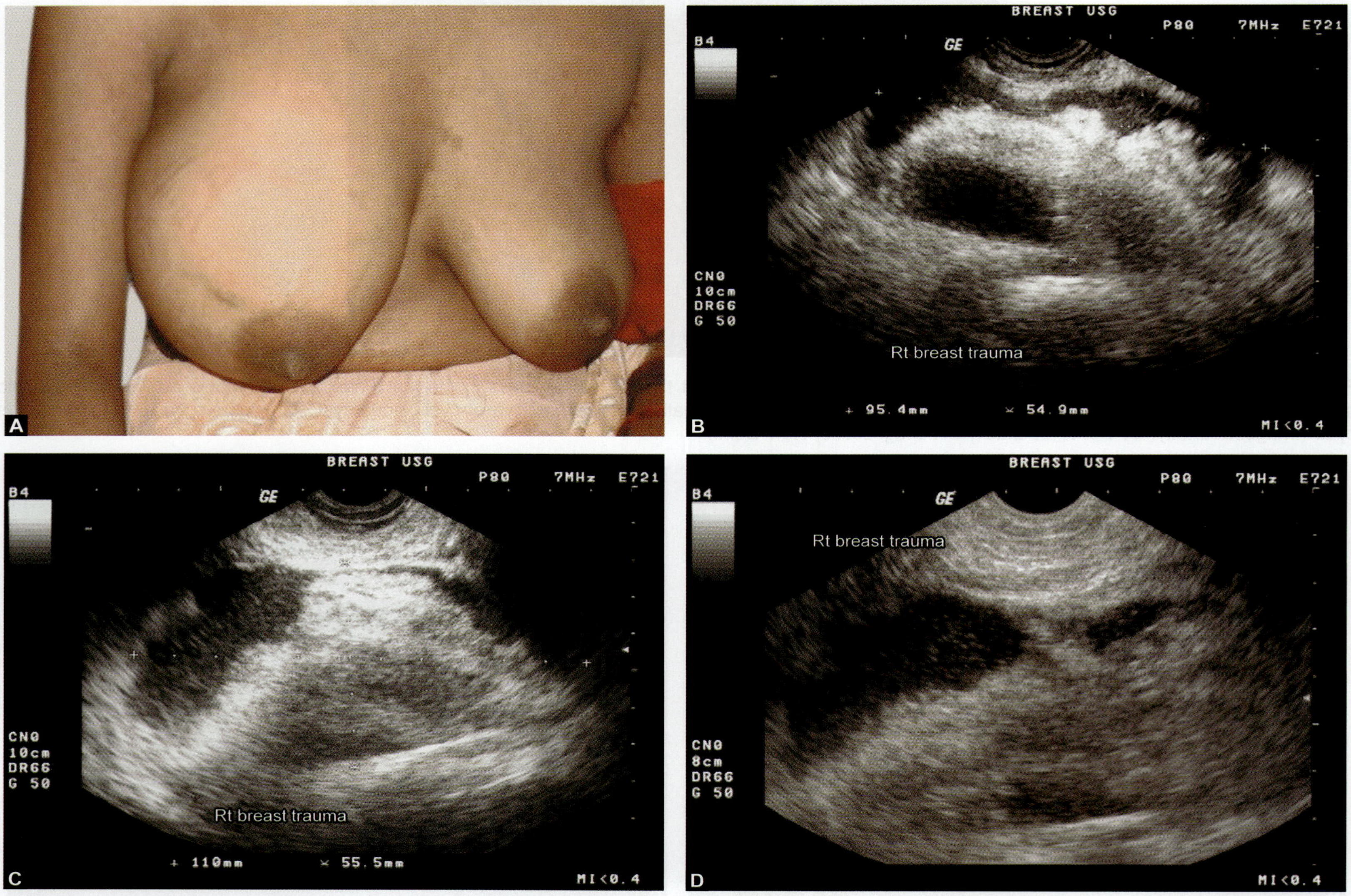

FIGURES 8.36A to D

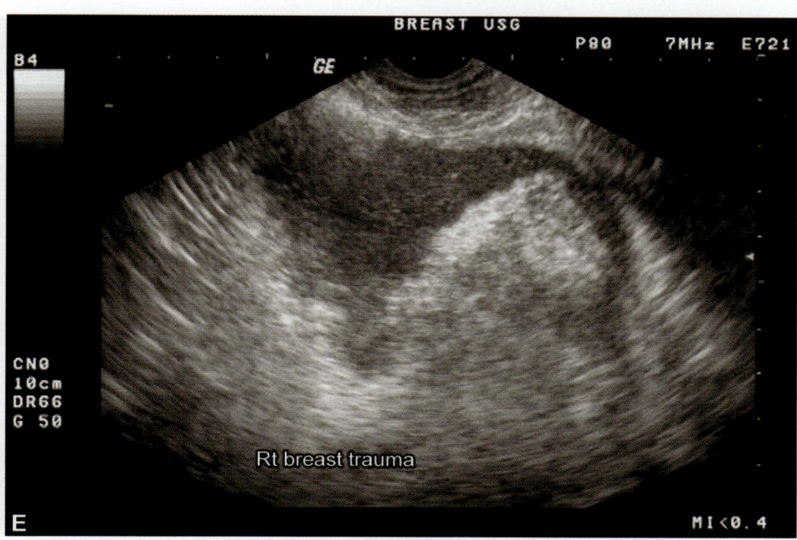

FIGURE 8.36E

FIGURES 8.36A to E: Ruptured breast. A patient presented with acute swelling of the breast after sustaining blunt trauma to the breast. HRSG shows rupture of the breast capsule with hematoma formation. The floating echogenic shadows are suggestive of fresh blood. The collected blood is seen gravitating on the dependant part. The ruptured breast tissue is seen floating in the hemorrhagic collection.

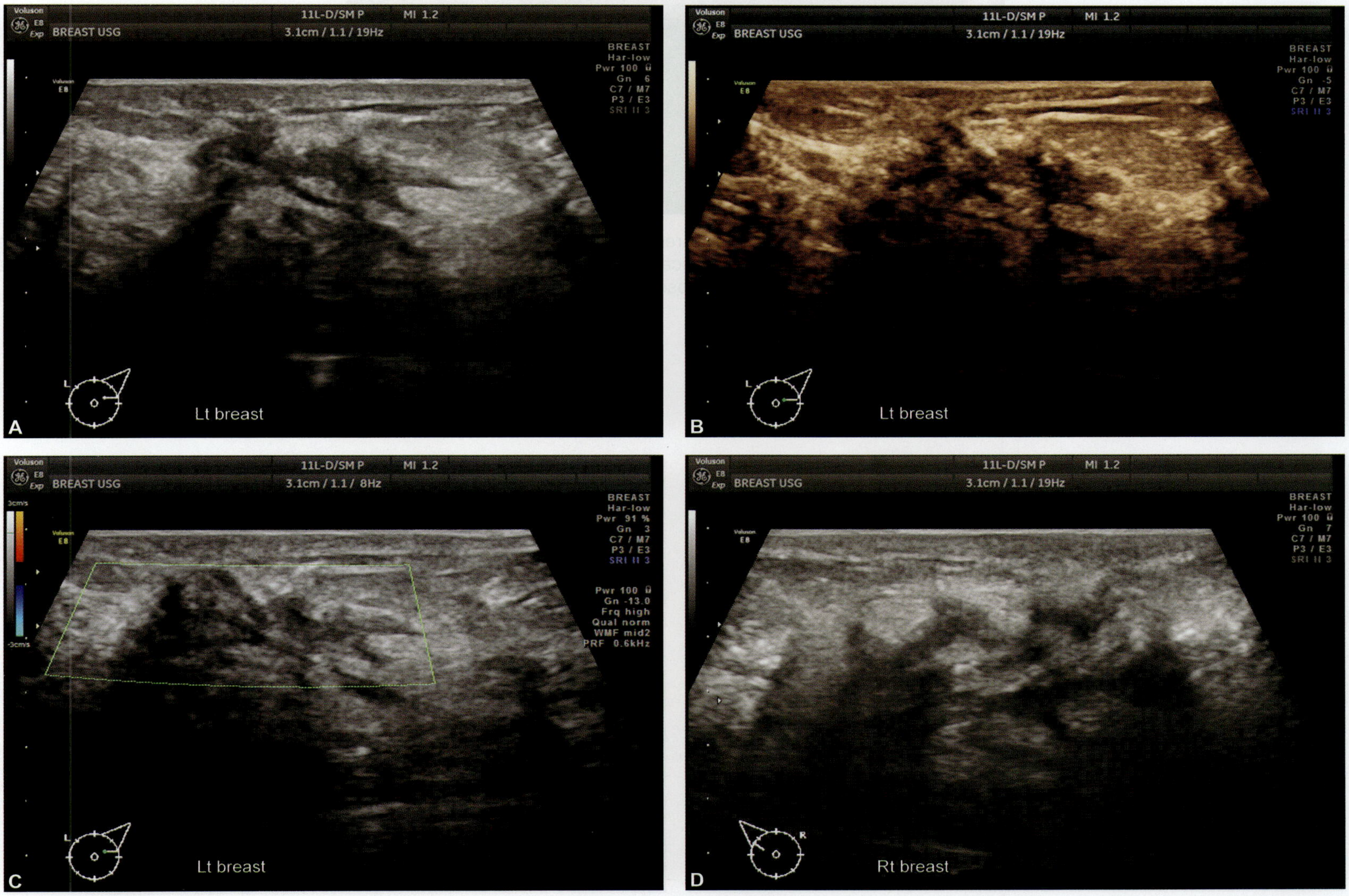

FIGURES 8.37A to D: Fat necrosis. A patient presented with ill-defined painful swelling in the left breast. HRSG shows irregular ill-defined low level echo complex shadow in the periareolar region in the mammary zone. But no focal mass is seen. Associated soft tissue edema is also seen. FNAC from the mass shows fat necrosis.

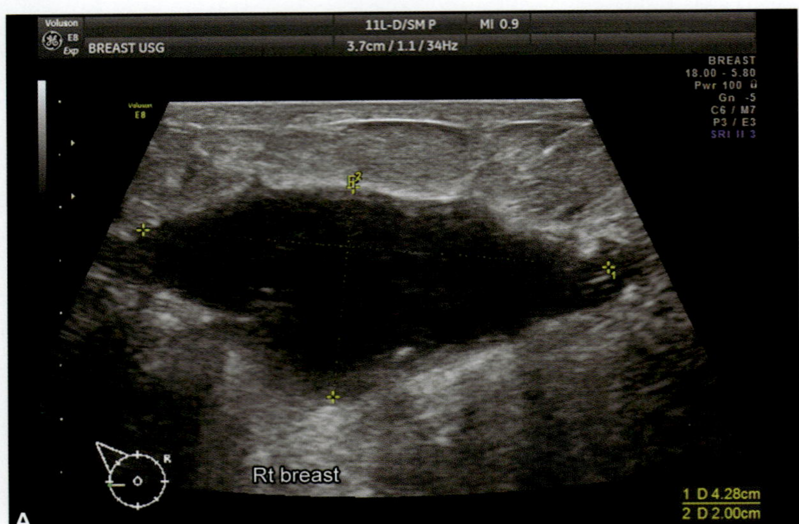

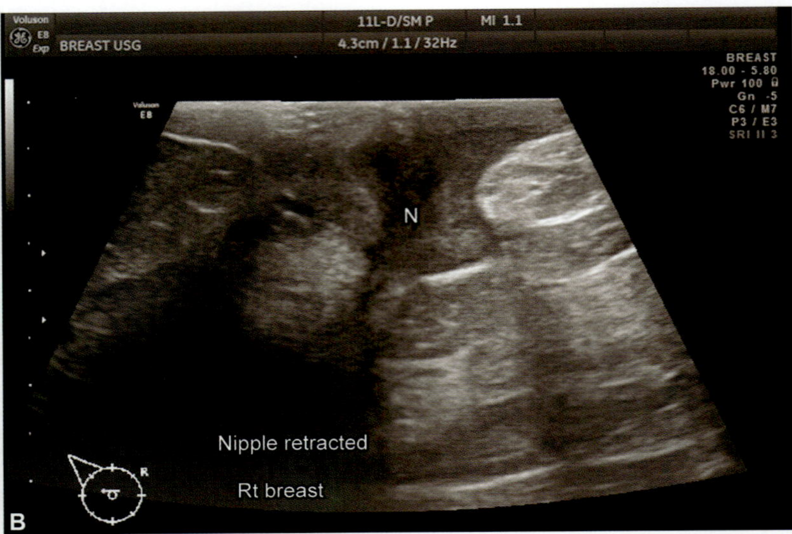

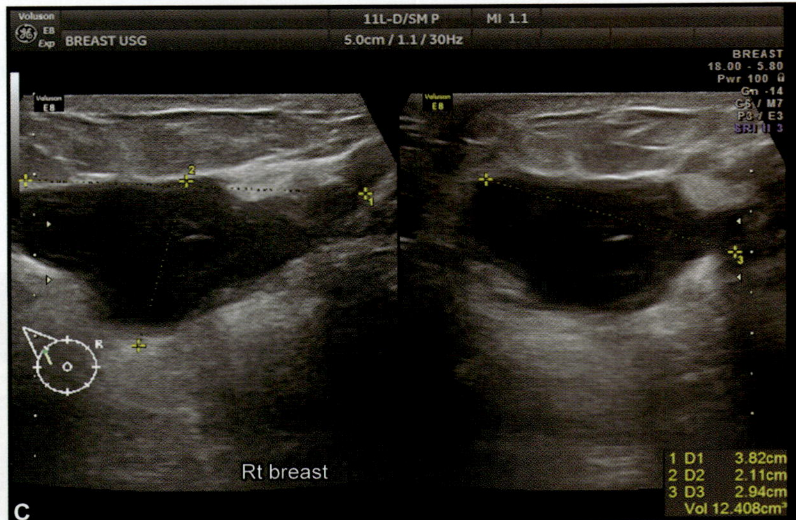

FIGURES 8.38A to C: Fat necrosis with abscess formation. A patient presented with painful lump in right breast at 8 o'clock position. HRSG shows an irregular ill-defined low level echo complex mass in right breast. Perifocal edema is also present. The nipple is seen retracted. The subcutaneous soft tissue fat is seen inflamed. FNAC from the mass confirms chronic abscess with fat necrosis.

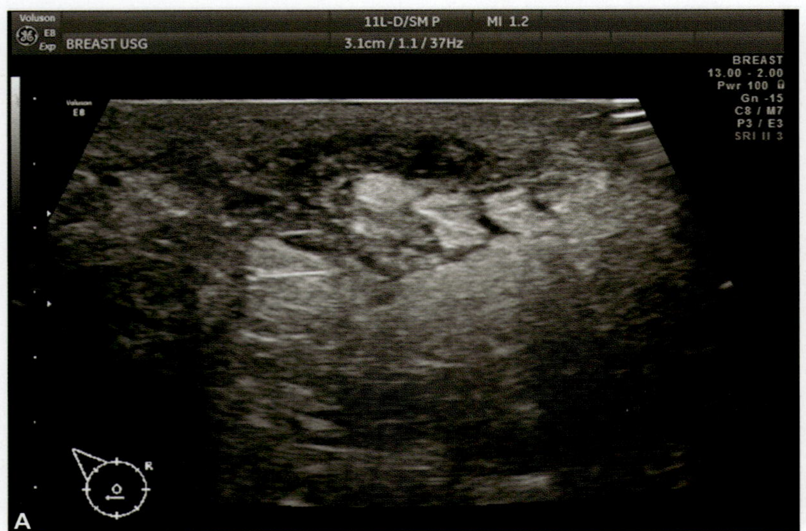

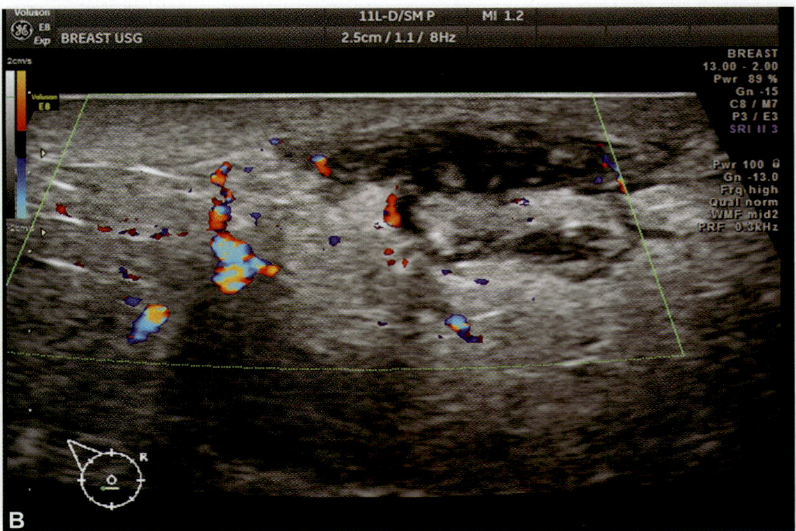

FIGURES 8.39A and B

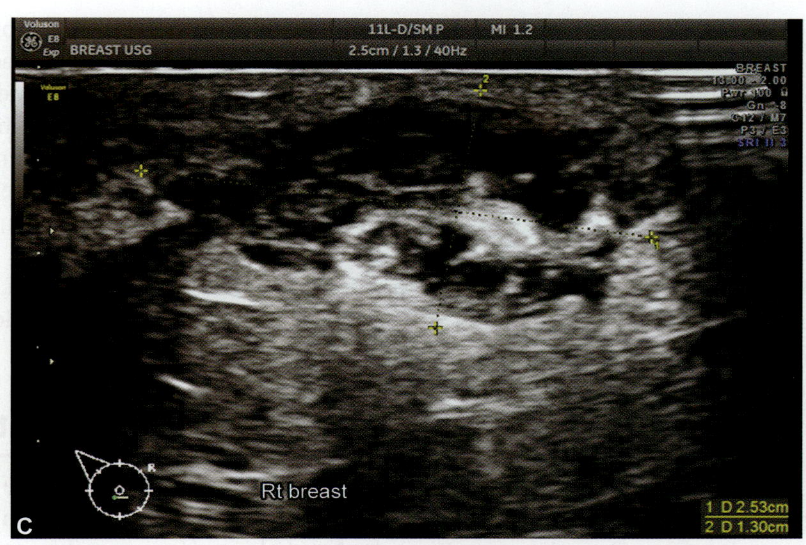

FIGURE 8.39C

FIGURES 8.39A to C: Fat necrosis with abscess formation. A patient presented with painful lump in right breast at 6 o'clock position. HRSG shows irregular ill-defined soft tissue mass in the right breast. Area of necrosis is seen in it. FNAC confirms fat necrosis with abscess formation.

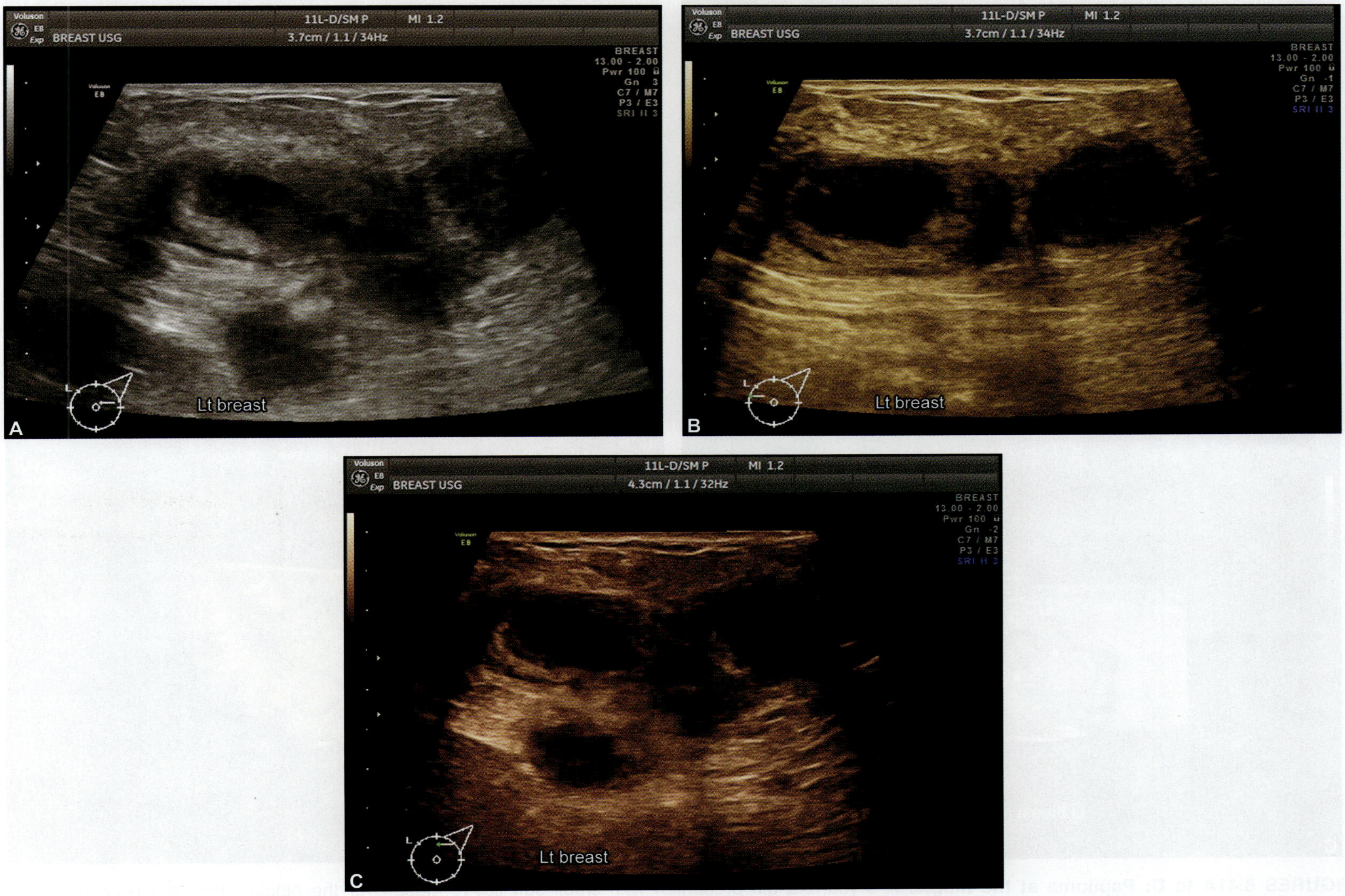

FIGURES 8.40A to C: Loculated breast abscesses. A 22-year-old girl presented with painful lumps in the left breast. HRSG shows thick loculated pocket of collection. Central area of necrosis is seen in them. Associated perifocal edema is also present. Findings are suggestive of loculated breast abscesses.

BENIGN BREAST MASSES

The benign breast masses are grouped as follows:

- Fibroadenoma
- Adenomata and papillomata
- Breast cyst
- Hematoma.

Fibroadenoma

Fibroadenomas are well-defined, lobulated solid, encapsulated masses present anywhere in the breast. They are homogeneous in texture. They are highly mobile and clinically termed as "breast mouse" due to their frequent changing position. When they are present near to skin, they are sharply marginated on HRSG. The capsule is echogenic. The mass is incompressible. No retrotumoral effect or shadowing is seen in fibroadenoma. At times there may be many fibroadenomas in one breast and they are more common in young breast. Presence of fibroadenoma in both breasts is also common. Macrocalcification is seen in few fibroadenomas. It may cast acoustic shadowing. At times areas of cystic necrosis are also seen in the tumors. Usually the fibroadenoma is small to medium size. But giant fibroadenoma is also reported. They are irregular in outline and heterogeneous in texture. Margins are ill-defined. It becomes difficult to differentiate it from a malignant breast lump. The overlap in ultrasound image of fibroadenoma and malignant breast lump is well-established. Therefore, other features of fibroadenoma like mobility of mass, its compressibility, homogeneous texture and its tendency to lie along are important. The long axis of adenoma is more than the transverse axis and known as **LAP** (Longitudinal / Anteroposterior) **ratio.** It should be more than 1.4 in fibroadenoma. However, wherever there is any doubt about the diagnosis, a biopsy is must to establish the diagnosis.

Adenomata and Papillomata

Adenomata and papillomata are the other benign masses. They are difficult to be differentiated from fibroadenoma on ultrasonographic features alone. However, they tend to appear near Periareolar area and usually surrounded by a rim of fluid. Hamartomas are usually sharply marginated and well demarcated. An internal structure is heterogeneous with calcification. Lipoma is well-defined echo poor mass with homogeneous texture.

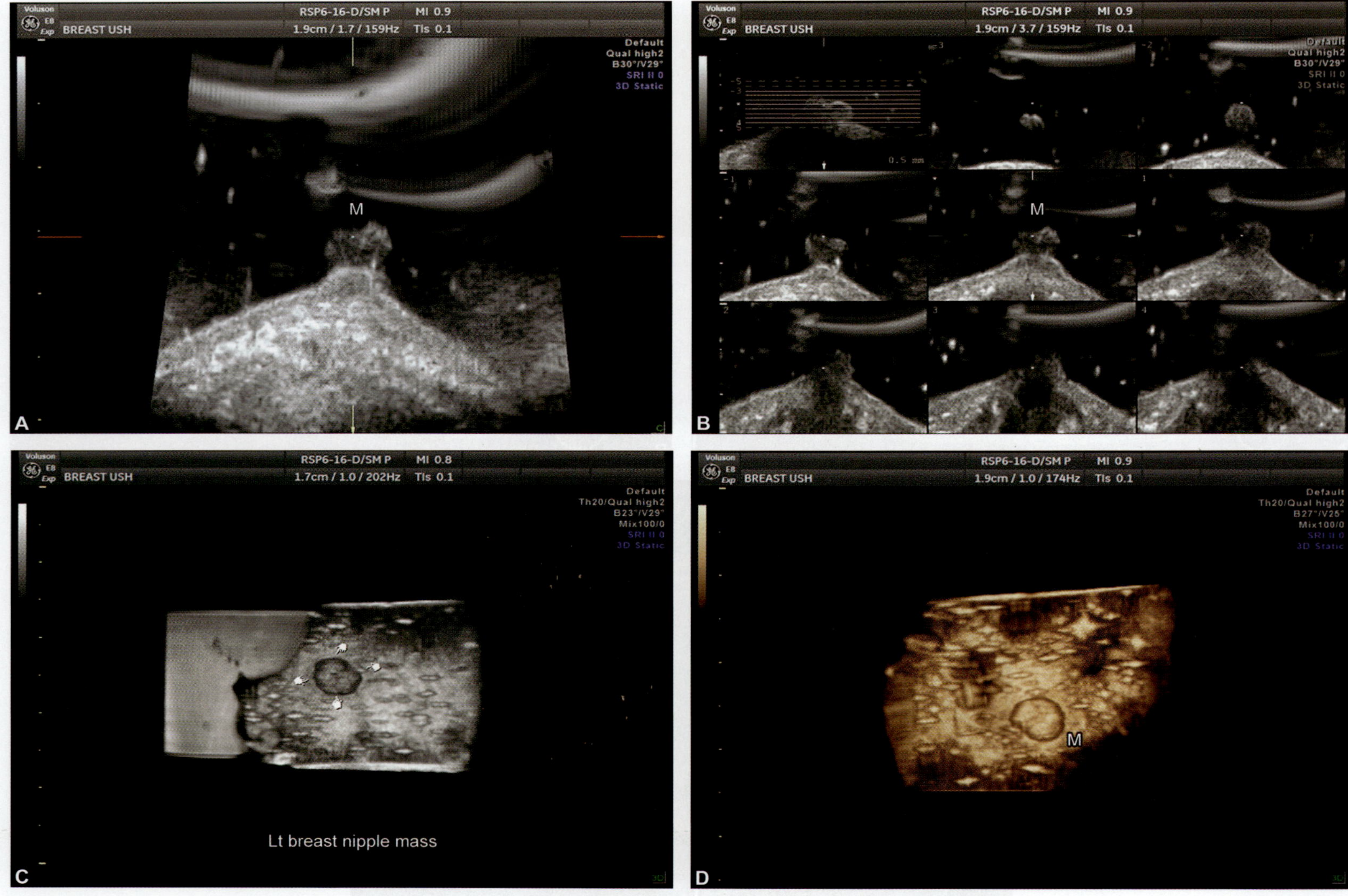

FIGURES 8.41A to D: Papiloma at the nipple. A 9-year-old girl presented with small soft tissue mass over the nipple. High resolution ultrasound with 3D imaging shows a well-defined soft tissue mass just sitting above the nipple. It is separate from the nipple. The TUI and 3D imaging clearly shows the mass and the nipple separately. On excision biopsy, small papilloma is confirmed.

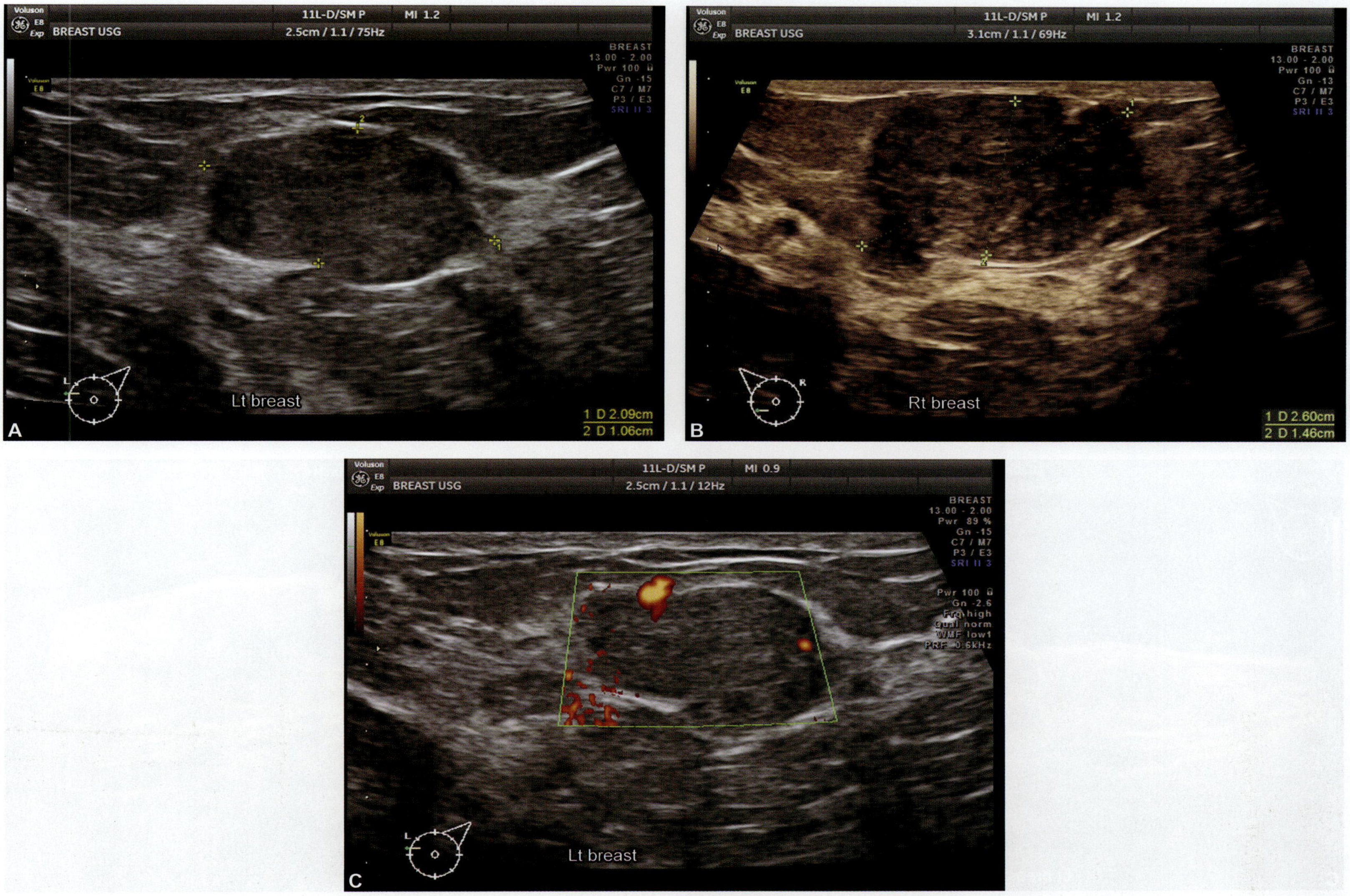

FIGURES 8.42A to C: Fibroadenoma in the breast. A young girl presented with soft tissue mass at 10 o'clock position in left breast. HRSG shows a well-defined lobulated cystic mass in the left breast at 10' O clock position. It is smooth in outline. Another mass is seen at 12 o' clock position. They grow in transverse direction and homogeneous in texture. No calcification is seen in them. No cystic degeneration is seen. Findings are suggestive of fibroadenomas.

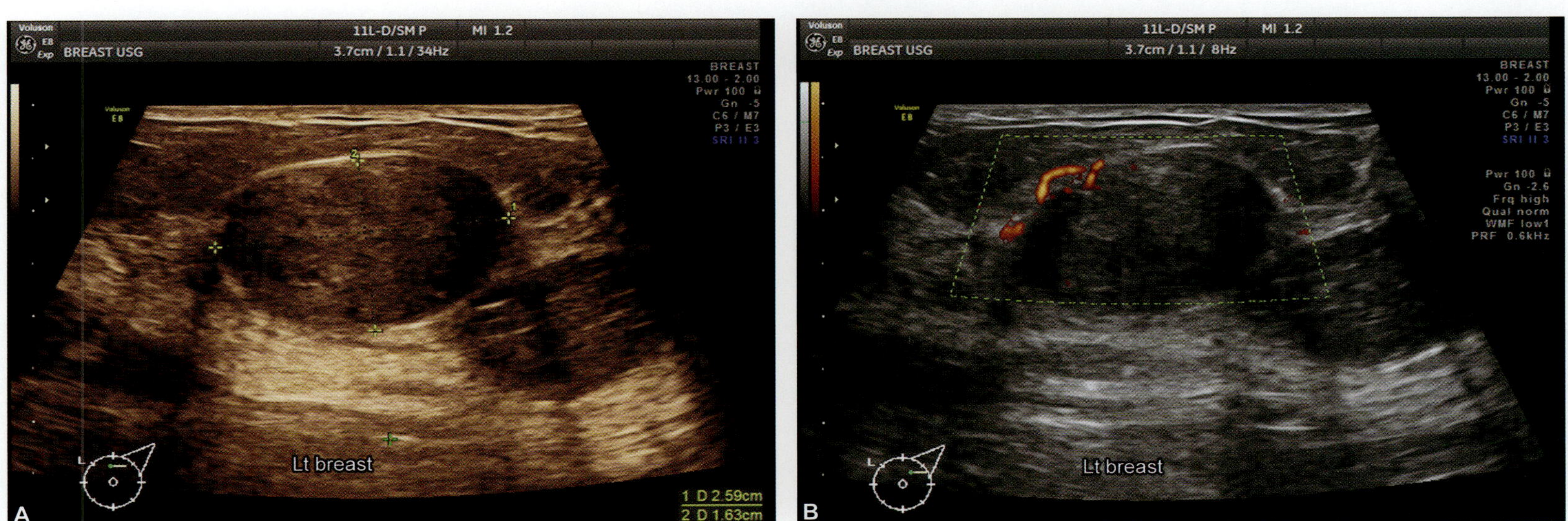

FIGURES 8.43A and B: Fibroadenoma in left breast. A young girl presented with lobulated soft tissue mass in the left breast in upper outer quadrant. HRSG shows two well-defined lobulated masses in left breast at 12 and 1 o'clock position. They are smooth in outline. No calcification or cystic degeneration is seen. They tend to grow in transverse direction. On color flow imaging, it shows peripheral vascularity. Findings are consistent with fibroadenomas.

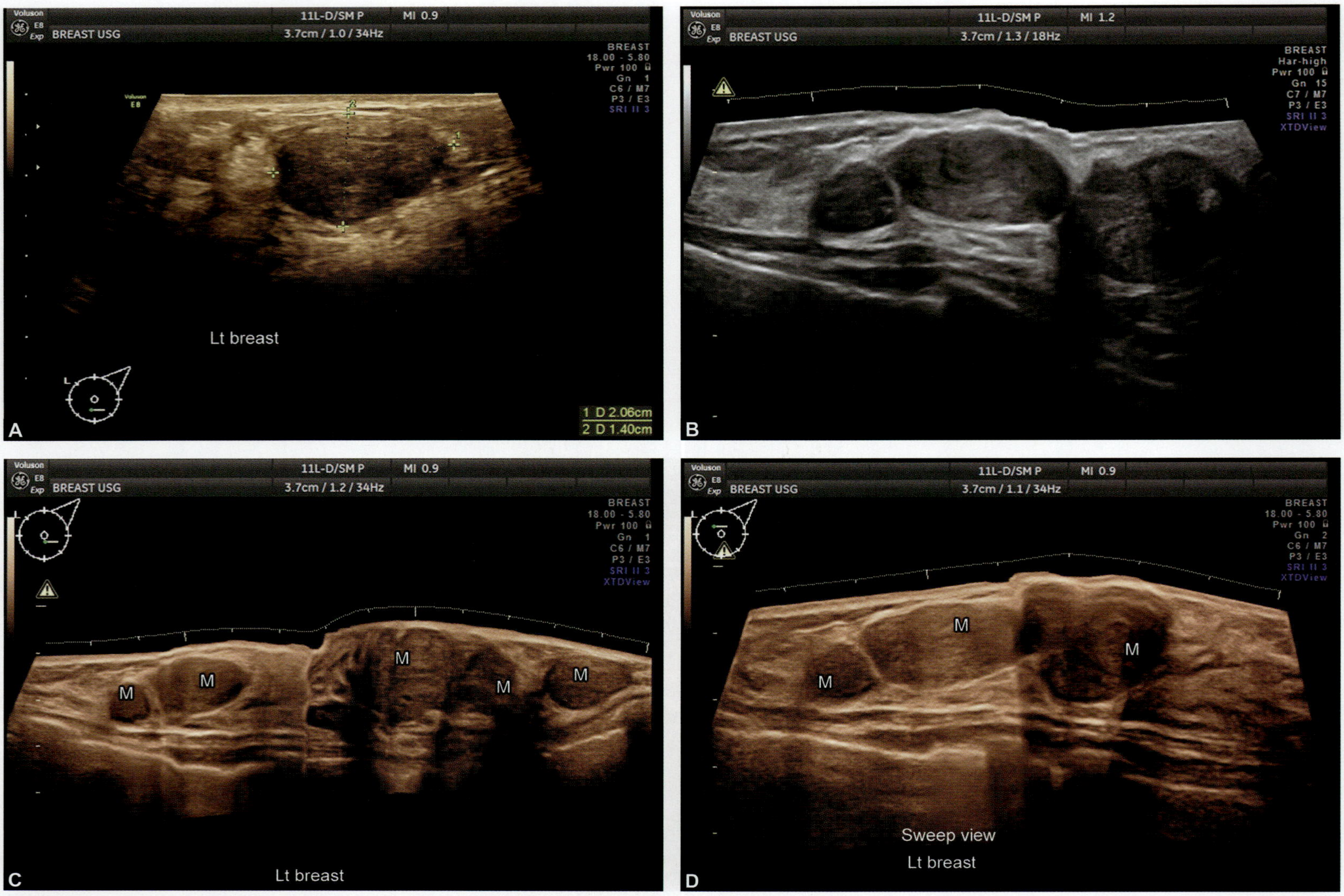

FIGURES 8.44A to D: **Multiple fibroadenomas.** A 22-year-old girl presented with nodular masses in the left breast. HRSG shows multiple well-defined lobulated masses in the left breast. The extended field of view shows all the masses beautifully. They are smooth in outline. No calcification or cystic degeneration is seen. Findings are consistent with multiple fibroadenomas.

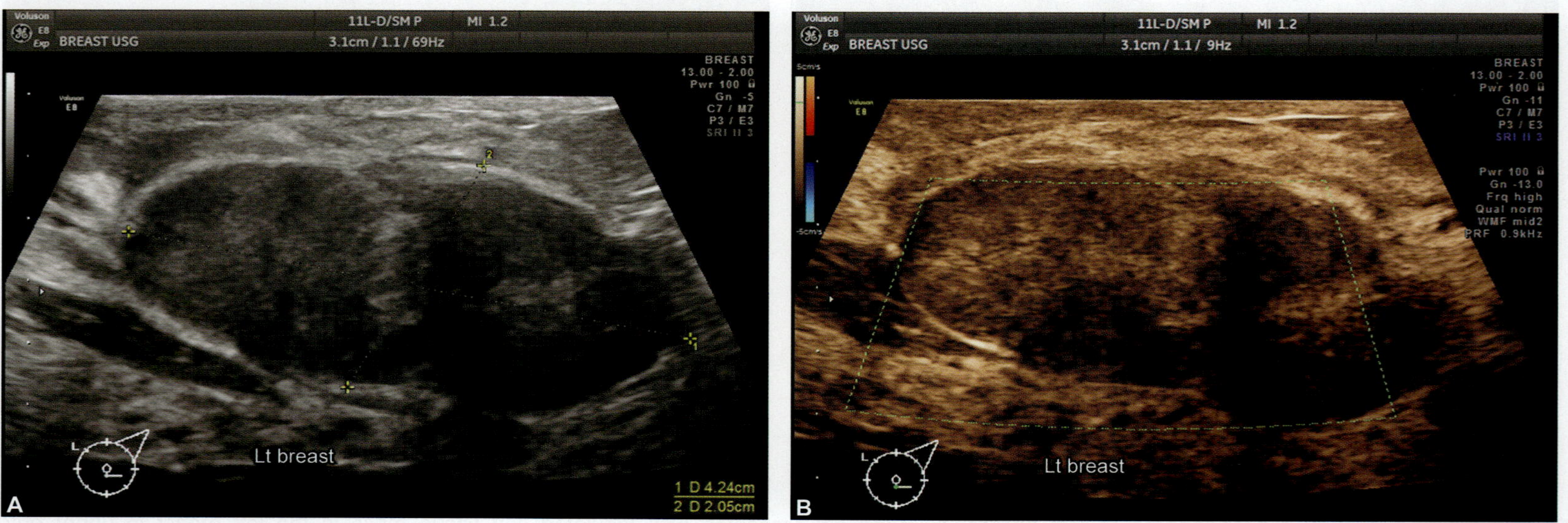

FIGURES 8.45A and B: Big fibroadenoma. HRSG shows a big lobulated soft tissue mass in the left breast at 4 and 5 o'clock position. It is well-encapsulated and smooth in outline. No calcification or cystic degeneration is seen in it. Findings are suggestive of big fibroadenoma.

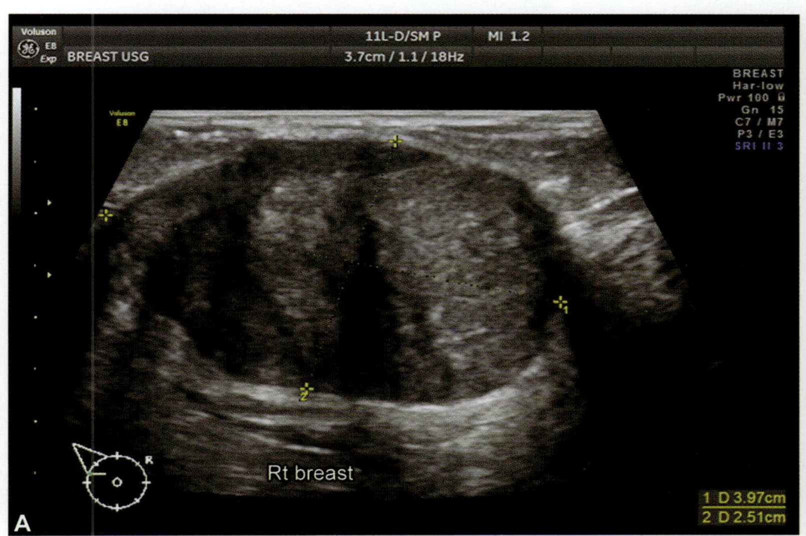

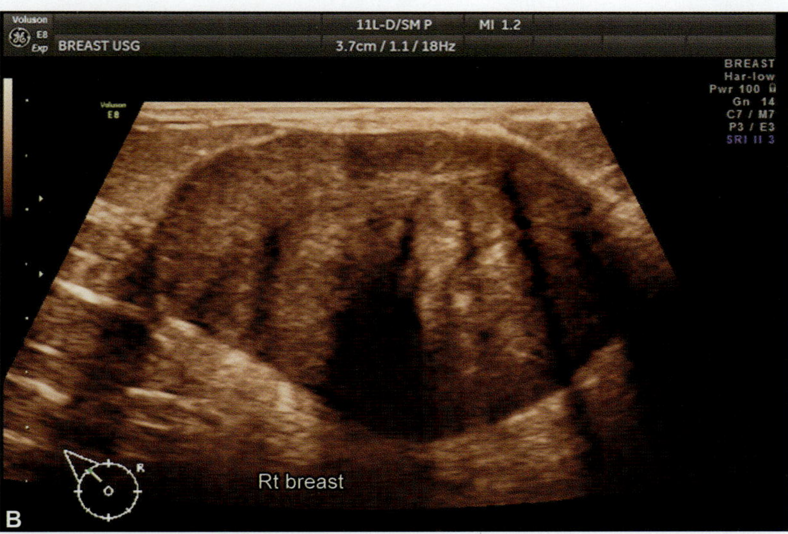

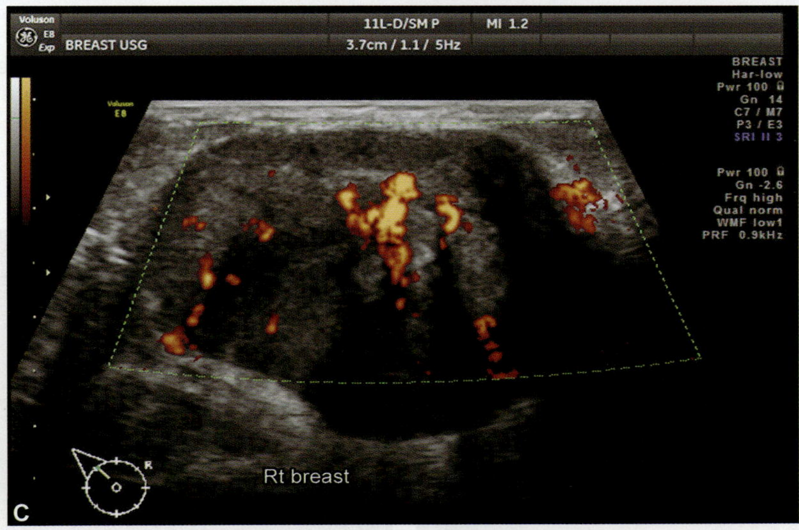

FIGURES 8.46A to C: Big fibroadenoma with macrocalcification. HRSG shows a big lobulated mass in right breast at 10 and 11 o'clock position. Echogenic foci are seen in it, which are accompanied with acoustic shadowing suggestive of macrocalcification. But no necrosis is seen in the mass. On color flow imaging, few vessels are seen feeding the mass suggestive of fibroadenomas with macrocalcification.

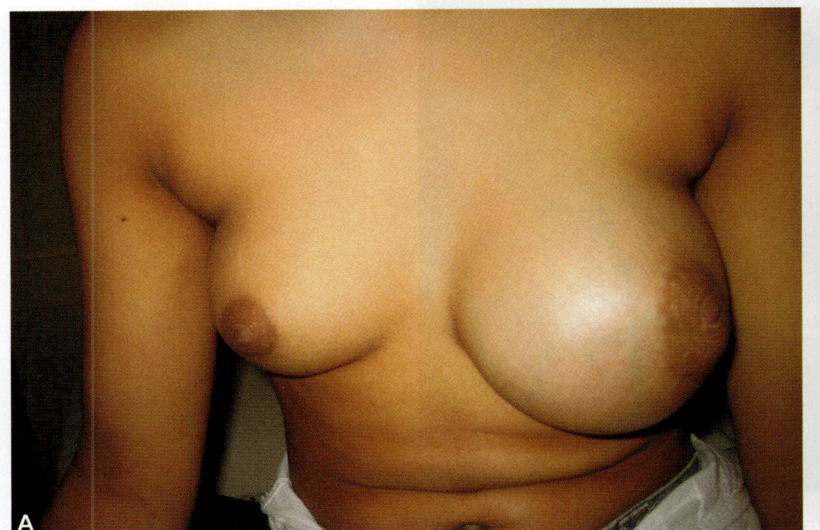

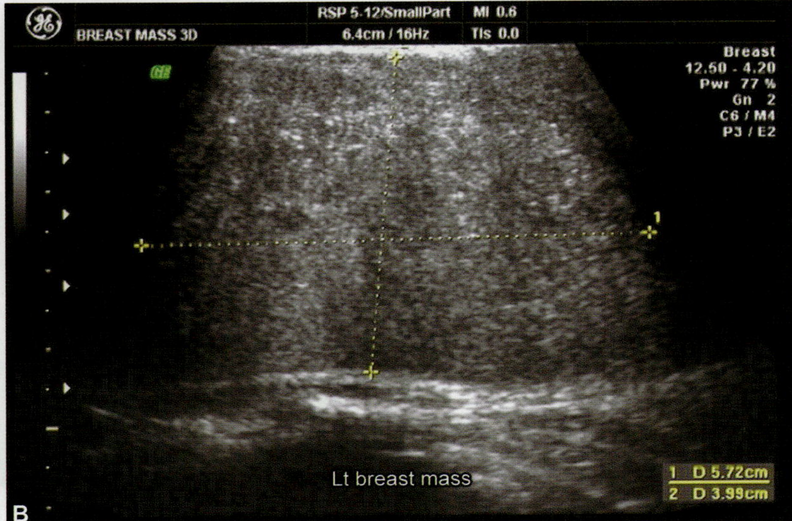

FIGURES 8.47A and B

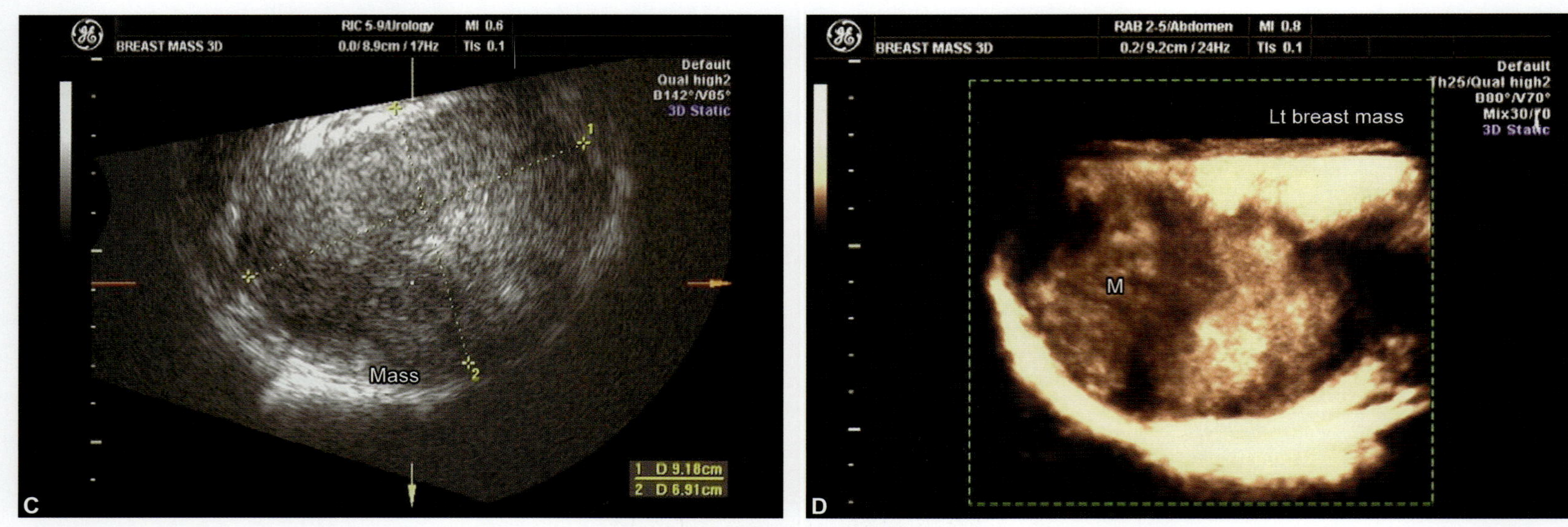

FIGURES 8.47C and D

FIGURES 8.47A to D: Big fibroadenoma breast. A young girl presented with big soft tissue mass in the left breast. Diffuse enlargement of the breast is seen. HRSG shows a well-defined encapsulated soft tissue mass in the left breast. The mass shows sharp margins with homogeneous texture. No calcification or cystic necrosis is seen in the mass suggestive of huge fibroadenoma. 3D imaging of the mass shows the details of the mass. Depth of the mass is well-appreciated on 3D imaging.

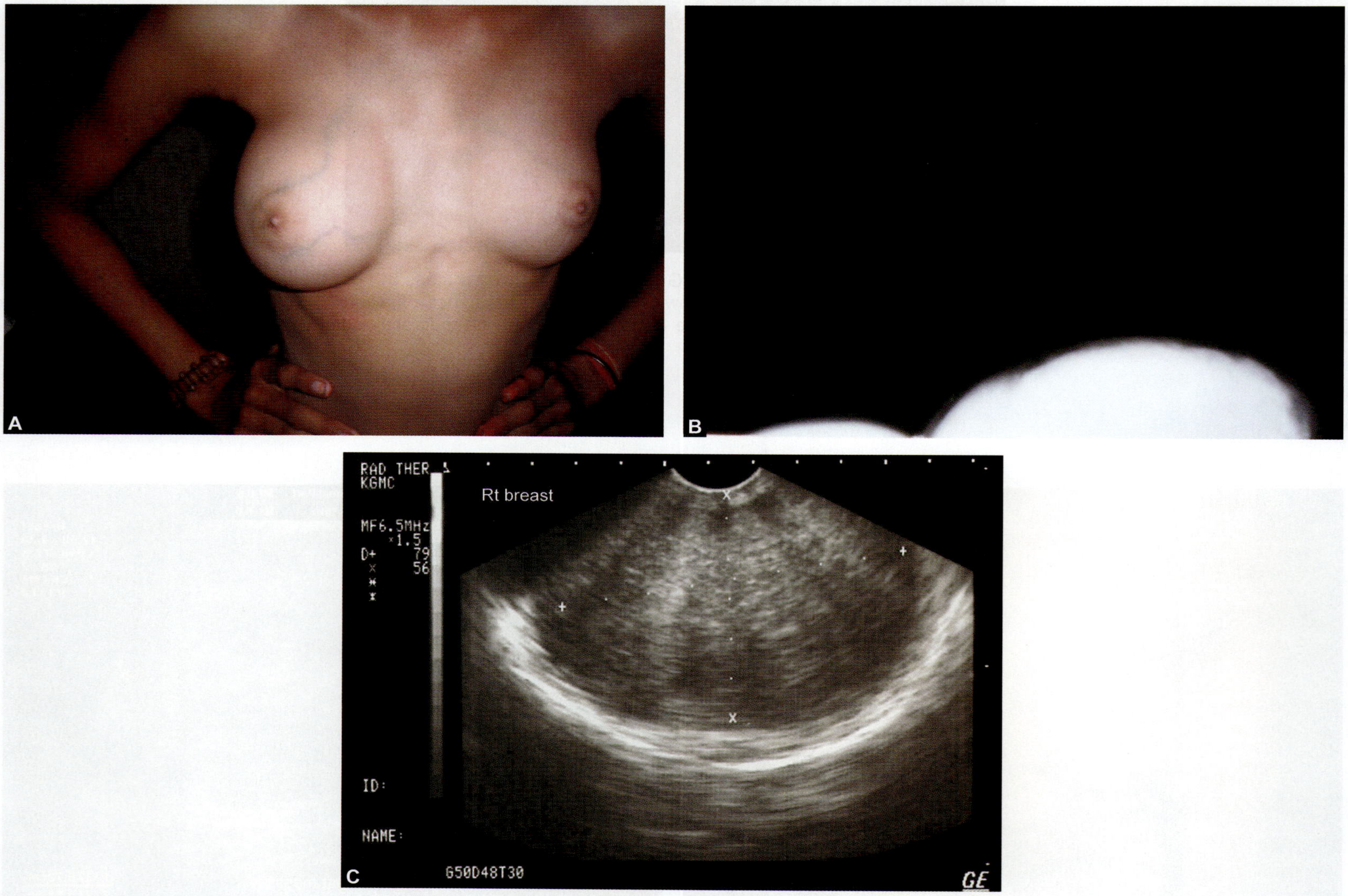

FIGURES 8.48A to C: Big fibroadenoma breast. A young girl presented with big mass in the right breast. The mass was non-tender. X-ray mammogram shows radiodense opacity in the right breast. No mass details are seen on X-ray mammogram. HRSG shows big homogeneous lobulated soft tissue mass in the right breast. The mass is well-encapsulated. Normal breast tissue is seen outside of the mass in the right upper outer quadrant. Biopsy confirms a big fibroadenoma.

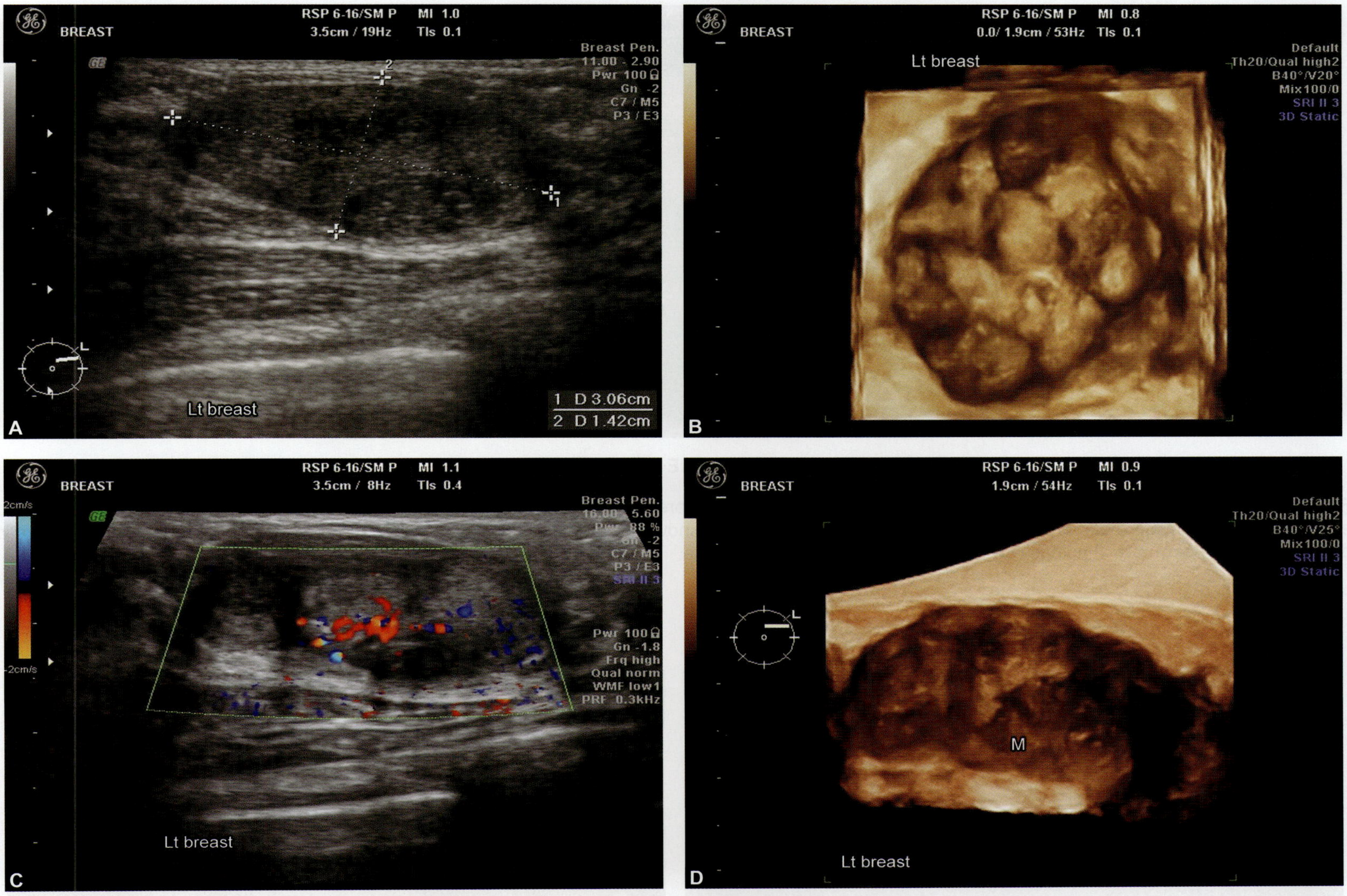

FIGURES 8.49A to D: A young girl presented with soft tissue mass in the left breast. HRSG shows well-defined hypoechoic ovoid shadow seen in the left breast at 2 and 3 o'clock position. Few hypoechoic areas are seen into it. But no evidence of any cystic degeneration is seen. Macronodules are seen in the left breast mass. Macrocalcification is also seen. On color flow imaging, moderate flow is seen into it. Another soft tissue shadow is seen at 11 o'clock position. It measures 8 x 5 mm in size. It is hypoechoic in texture. No calcification is seen into it. On 3D imaging, the texture of the mass is clearly seen and multiple lobulations in the mass. Left axilla is free. No other focal mass is seen on the left side.

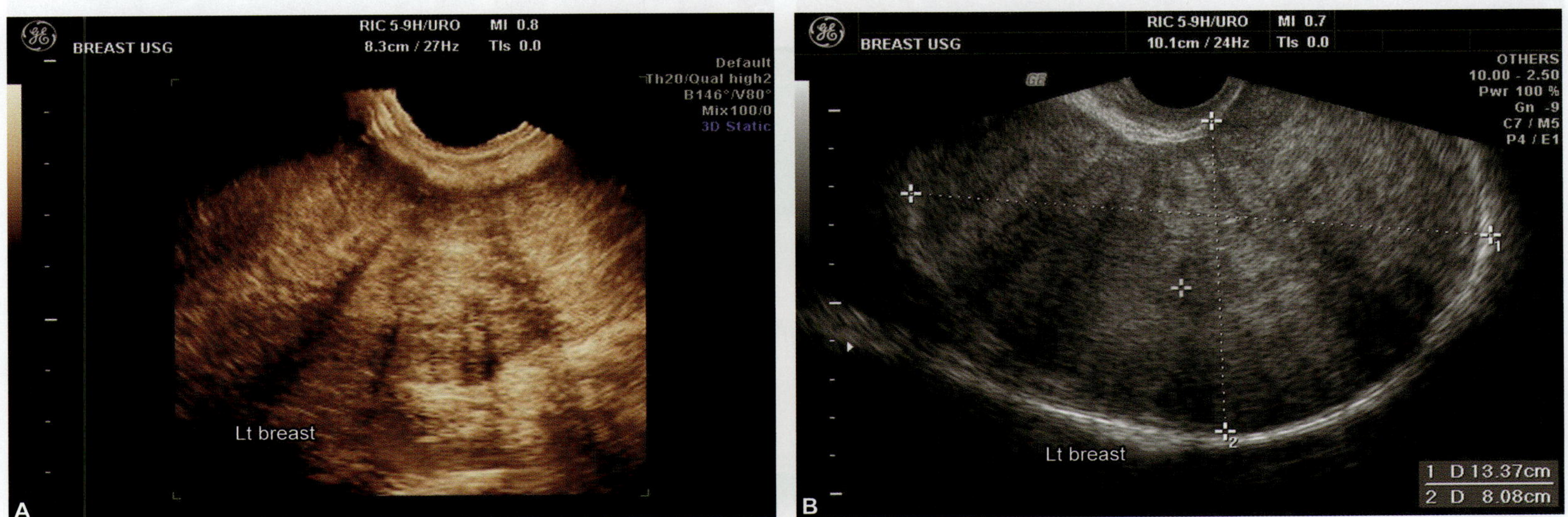

FIGURES 8.50A and B

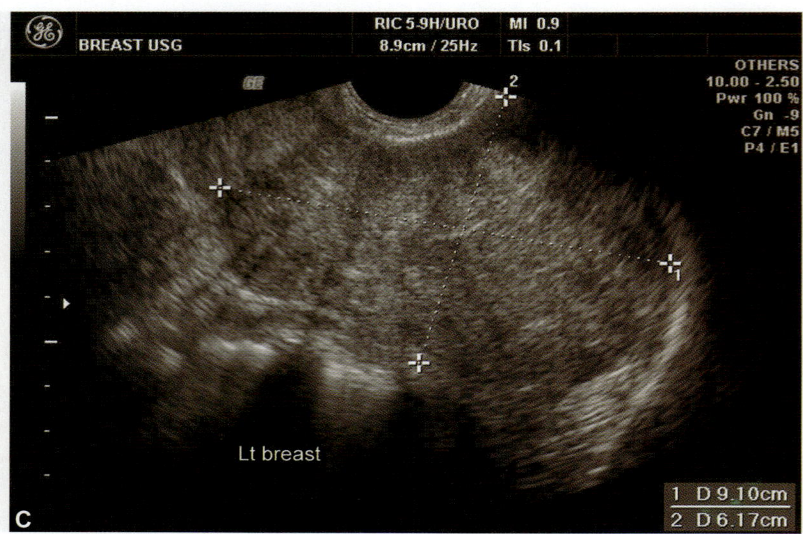

FIGURE 8.50C

FIGURES 8.50A to C: Giant fibroadenoma. A young 19-year-old girl presented with huge mass in the left breast. HRSG shows a well-defined encapsulated soft tissue mass involving the left breast. The 3D imaging shows the entire mass. It is homogeneous in texture. No calcification or cystic degeneration is seen in it. Findings are suggestive of giant fibroadenoma.

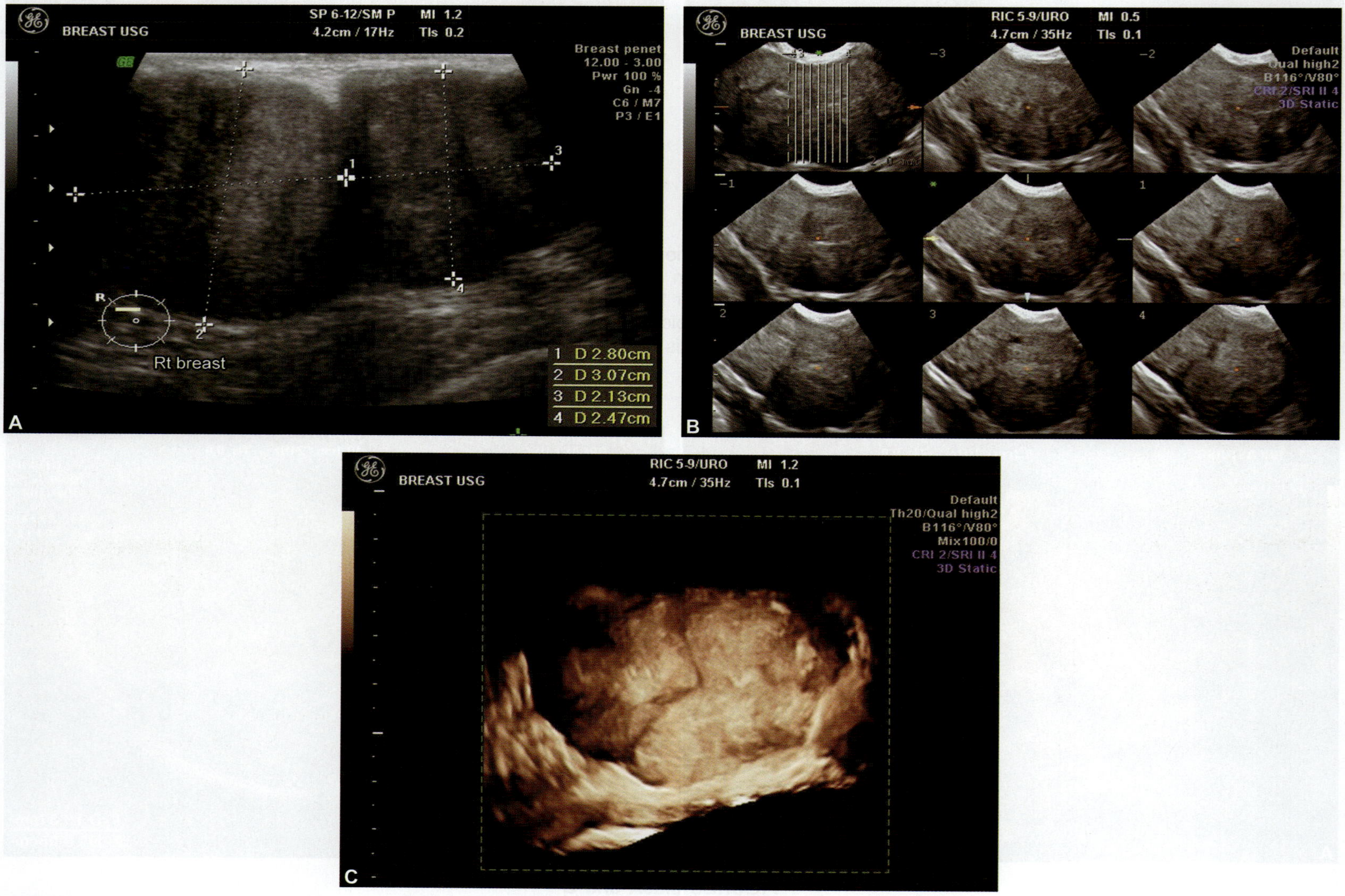

FIGURES 8.51A to C: Giant lobulated fibroadenoma. HRSG shows a huge lobulated mass in right breast in an 18-year-old girl. Multiple lobules are seen in the mass. The mass is homogeneous in texture. No necrosis is seen in it. The 3D imaging shows multiple lobules seen in the mass. Biopsy of the mass confirms giant lobulated fibroadenoma.

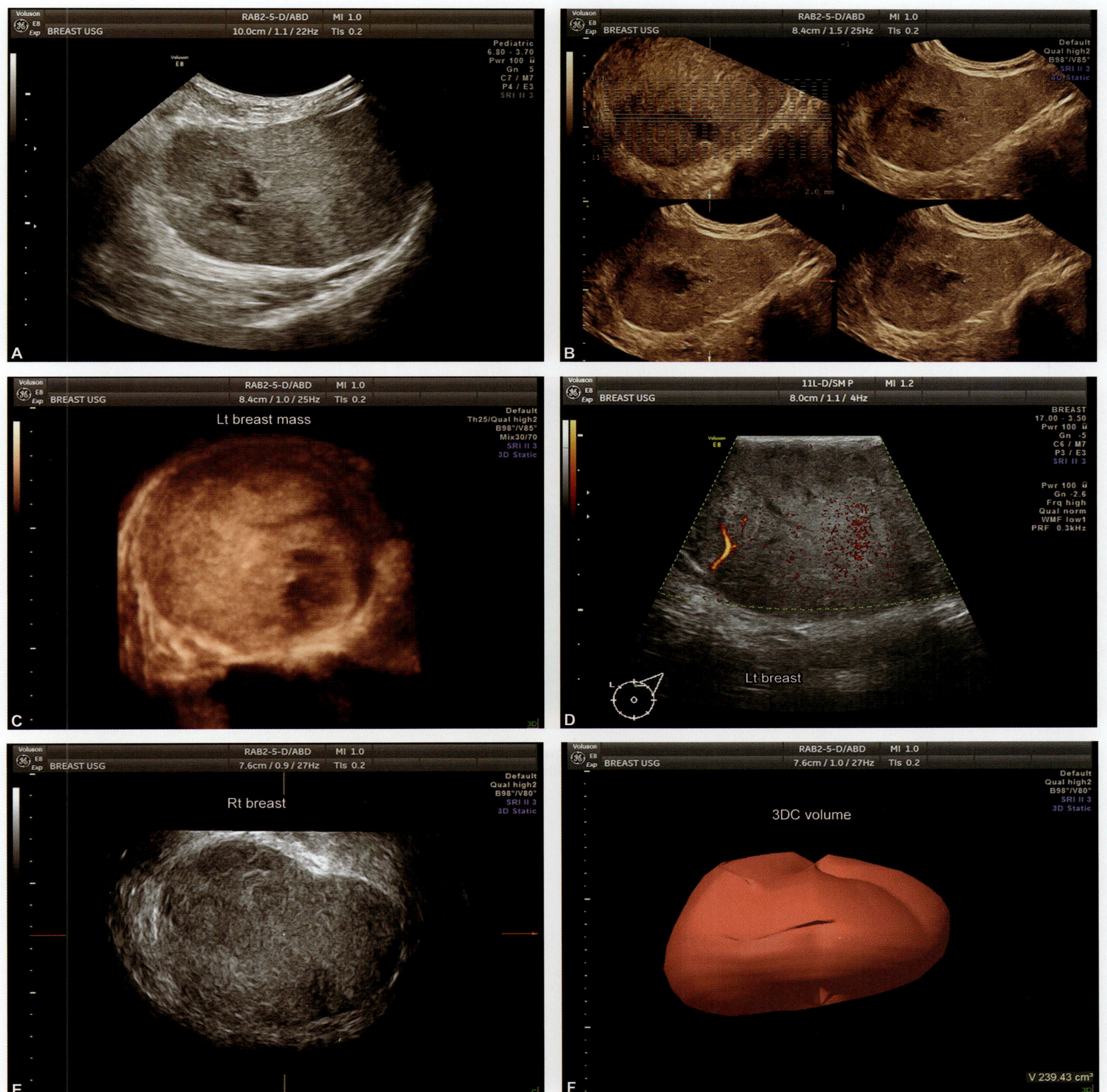

FIGURES 8.52A to F: Huge fibroadenoma. A 17-year-old girl presented with lumps in both the breast. HRSG shows big masses in both the breasts. However, the left breast mass is bigger than the right breast mass. The 3D imaging shows the entire mass. Small area of necrosis is also seen in the mass. 3D volume imaging shows the VOCAL image of the mass. Biopsy of the mass confirms fibroadenomas in both the breasts.

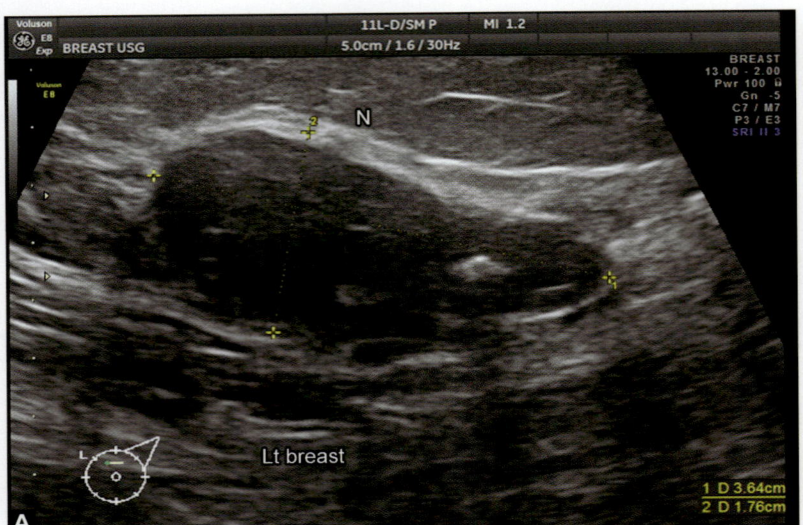

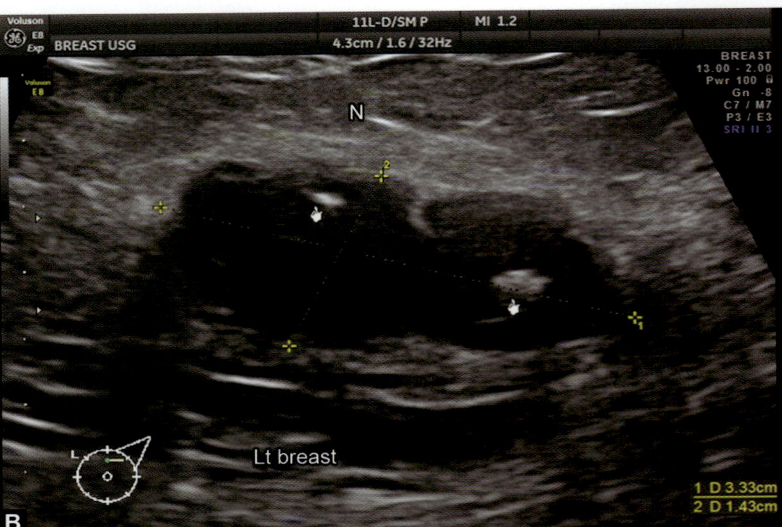

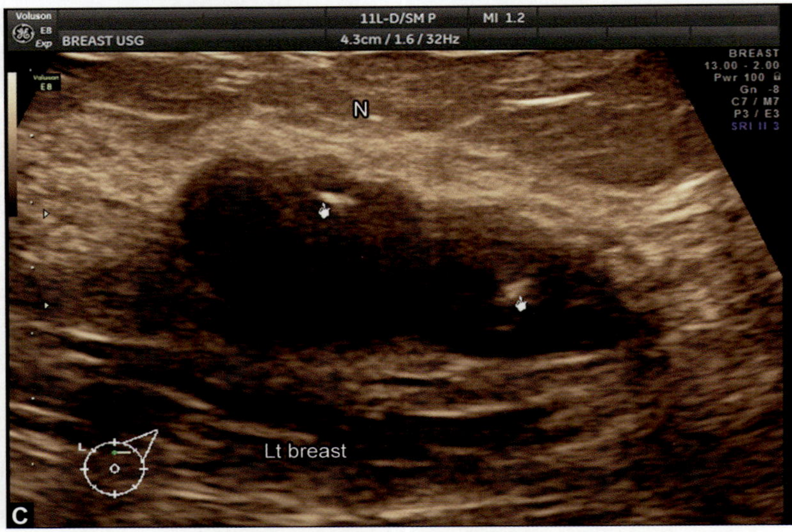

FIGURES 8.53A to C: Macrocalcification in fibroadenoma. HRSG shows a big mass in left breast at 12 and 10 o'clock position. Big echogenic foci are seen in the mass, which are accompanied with acoustic shadowing suggestive of macrocalcification.

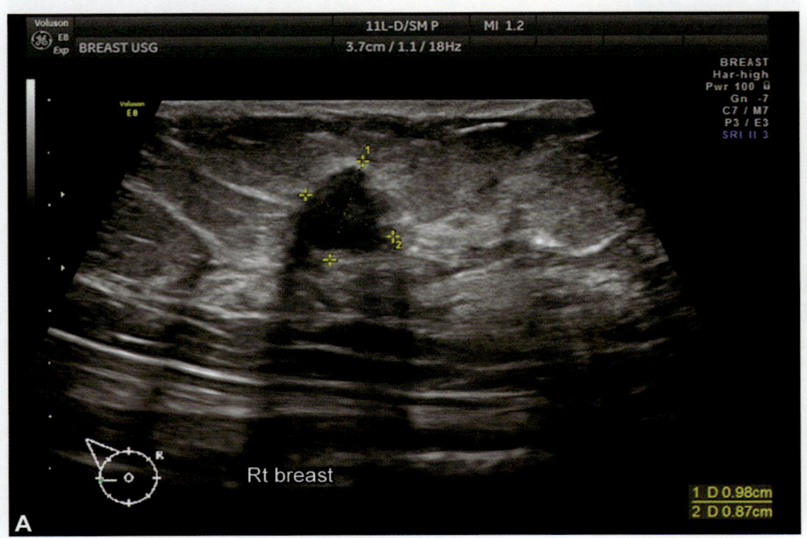

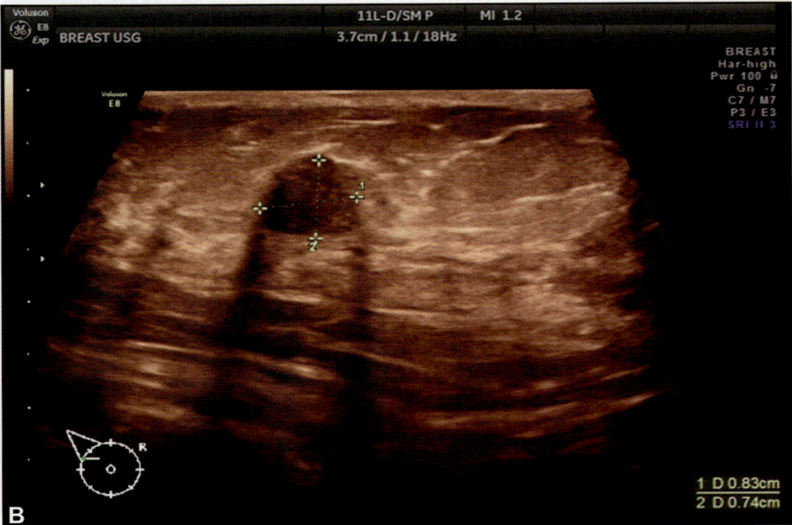

FIGURES 8.54A and B: Dense peripheral calcification in small fibroadenoma. HRSG shows a well-defined lobulated mass in right breast at 11 o'clock position. Dense rim calcification is seen in the mass, which is accompanied with acoustic shadowing.

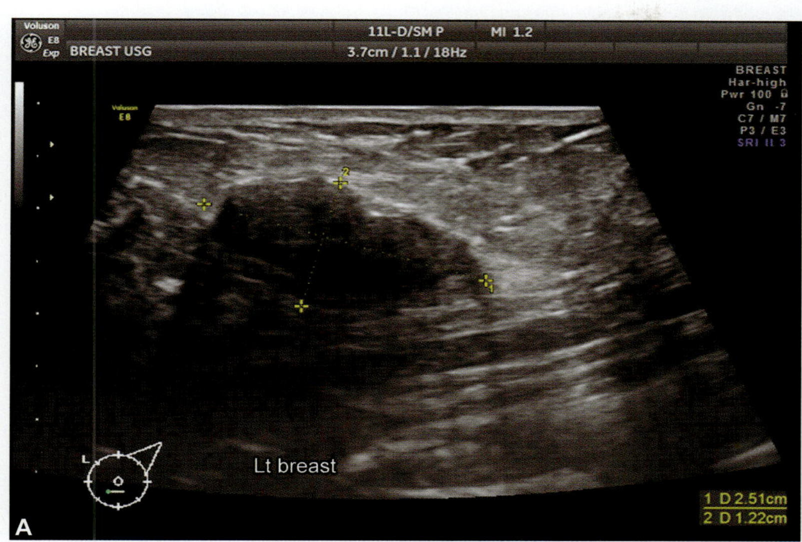

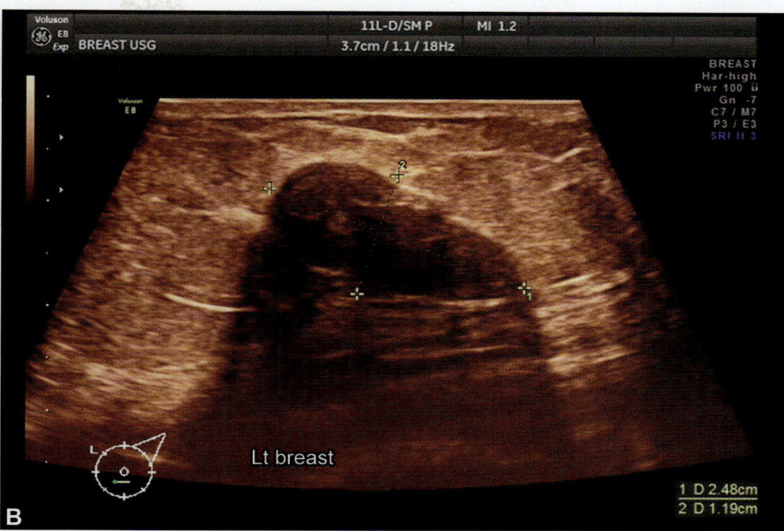

FIGURES 8.55A and B: Dense capsular calcification in fibroadenoma. A patient presented with lump in the left breast at 6 o'clock position. HRSG shows lobulated soft tissue mass in the left breast at 5 and 6 o'clock position periareolar region. Capsular calcification is seen into it. But no cystic degeneration is seen. On color flow imaging, no flow is seen into it. No other focal mass is seen. The left axilla is free.

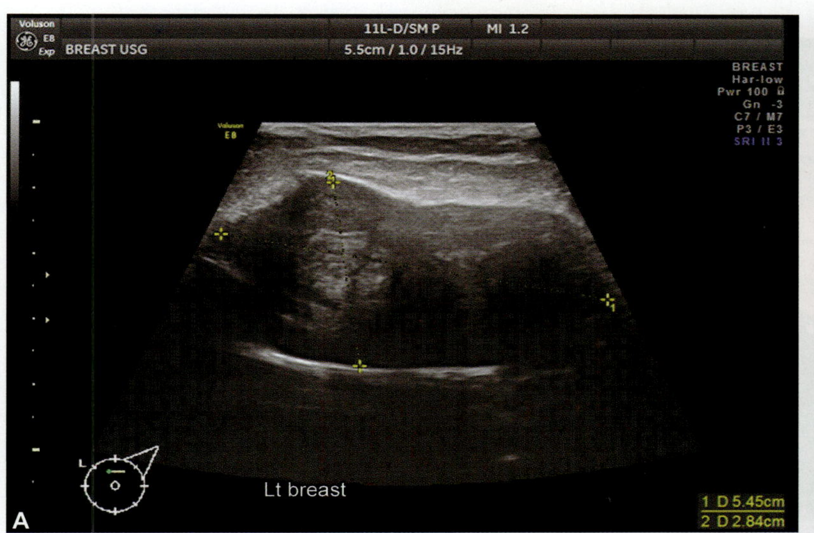

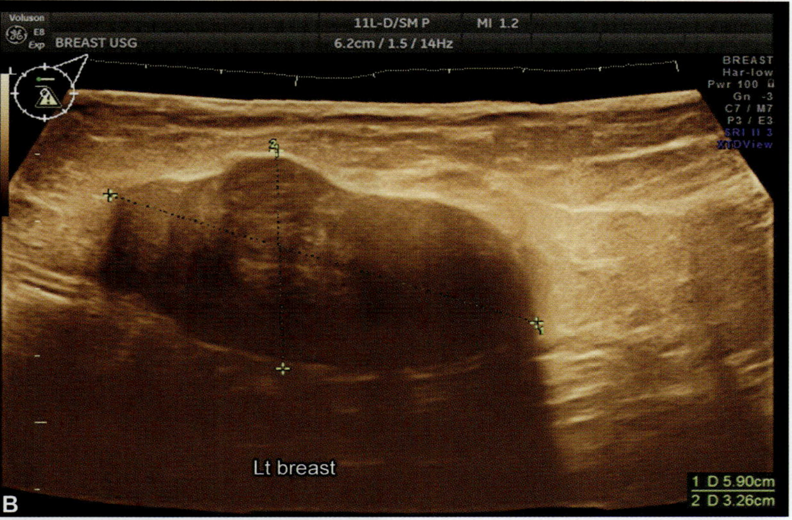

FIGURES 8.56A and B: Capsular calcification in fibroadenoma. A patient presented with hard lump in left breast at 12 o'clock position. HRSG shows a well-defined well-encapsulated hypoechoic mass. It measures 55 x 28 mm in size. Dense capsular calcification is seen in the mass, which is accompanied with acoustic shadowing. But no cystic degeneration is seen in the mass. Findings are suggestive of big fibroadenoma with capsular calcification.

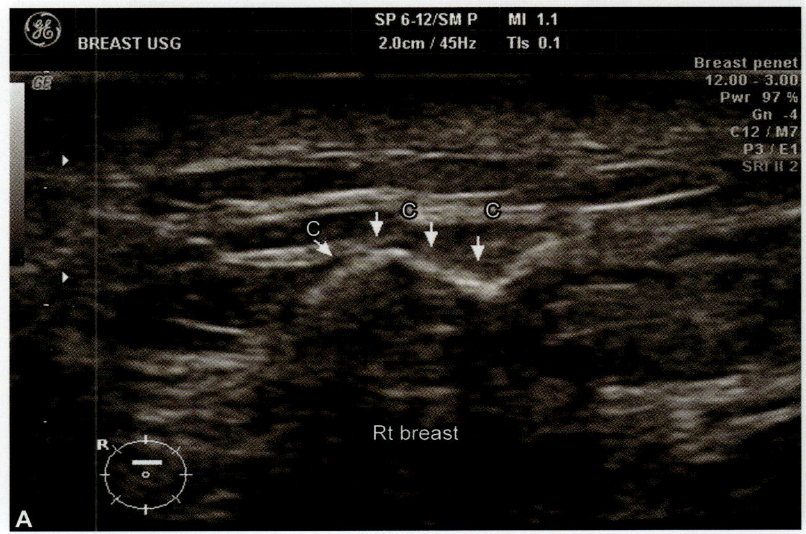

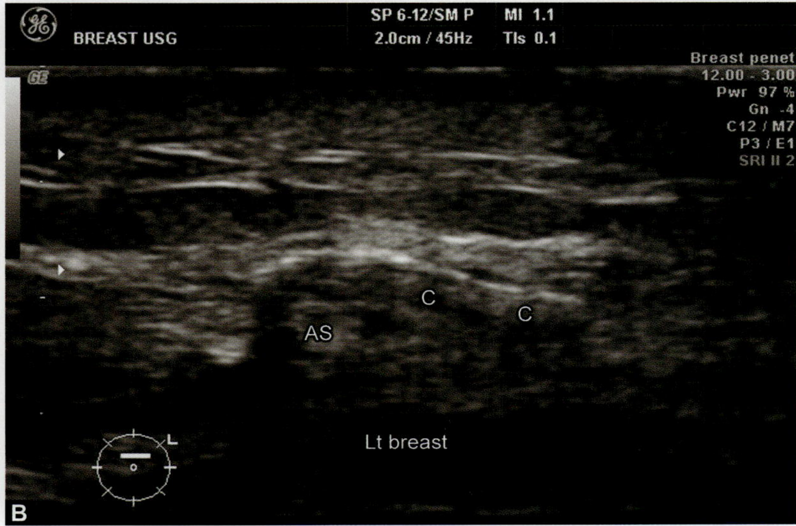

FIGURES 8.57A and B

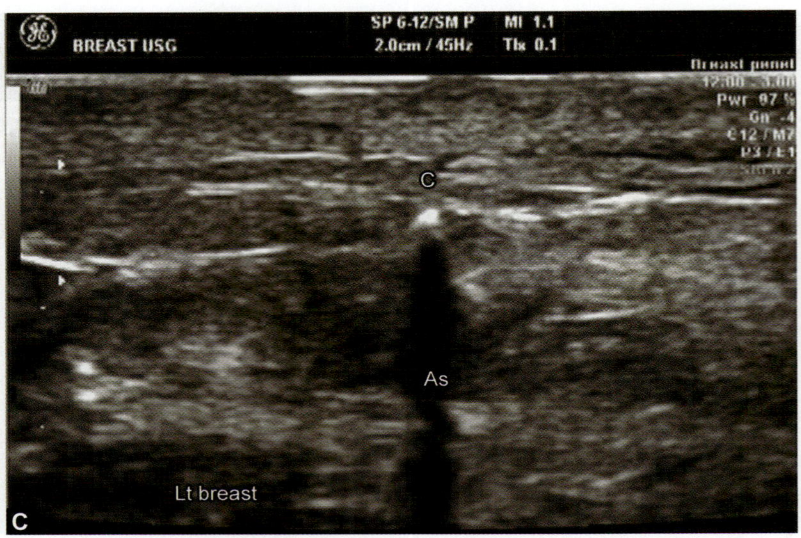

FIGURE 8.57C

FIGURES 8.57A to C: Linear cord-like calcification in the breast. A patient presented with nodularity in the right breast. HRSG shows a linear cord like calcification at 12 o'clock position periareolar region, which is accompanied with acoustic shadowing. But no focal mass is seen in the breast.

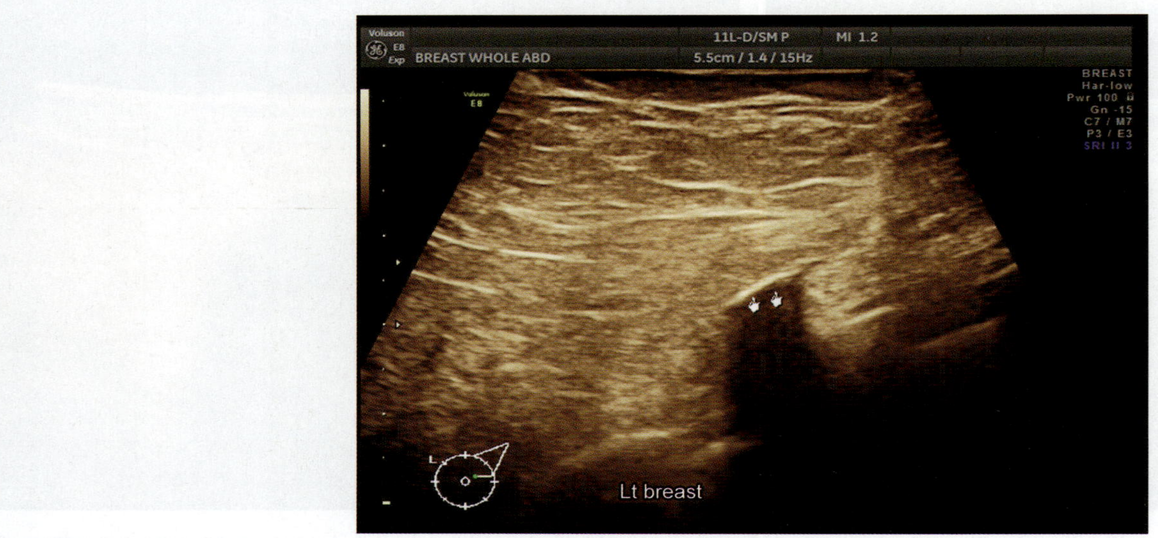

FIGURE 8.58: Dense linear calcification in the breast. HRSG shows dense echogenic linear shadow in the left breast between 2 o'clock and 3 o'clock position. It is accompanied with dense acoustic shadowing. No other focal mass lesion is seen. Findings are suggestive of dense linear calcification.

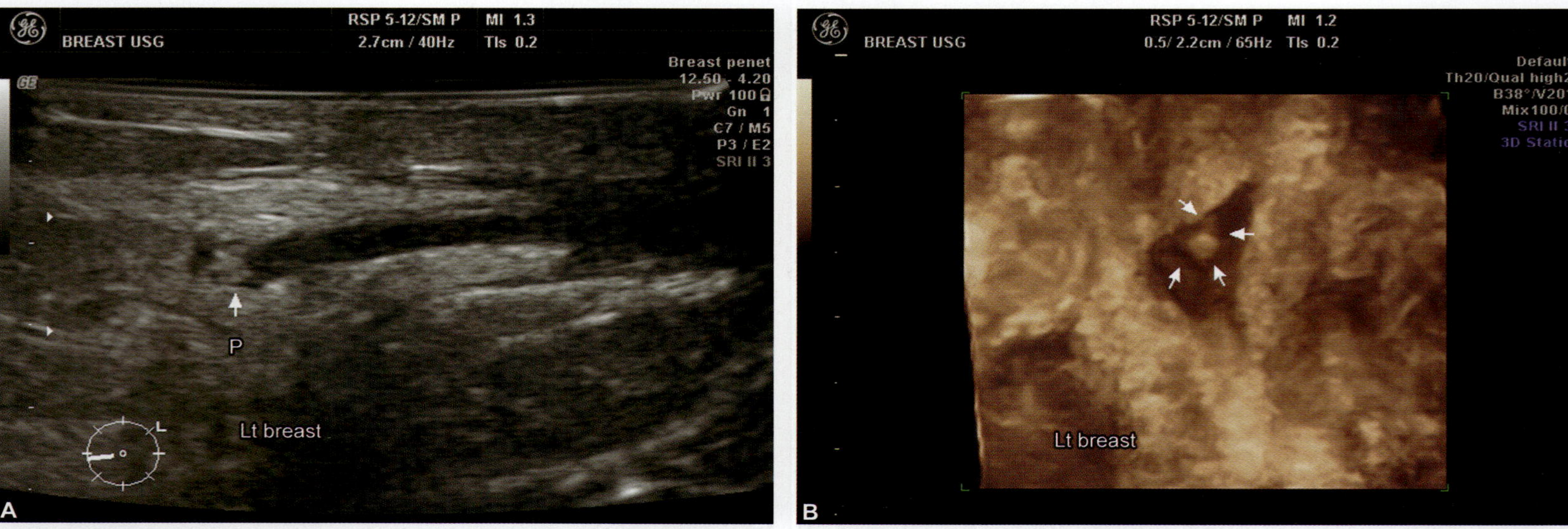

FIGURES 8.59A and B: Small ductal papilloma. A patient presented with discharge from the nipple. HRSG shows a dilated duct at 9 o'clock position. A small soft tissue shadow is seen at the proximal part of duct. On 3D imaging, it is clearly seen in the duct. It is smooth in outline. No calcification is seen in it. FNAC confirms small intraductal papilloma.

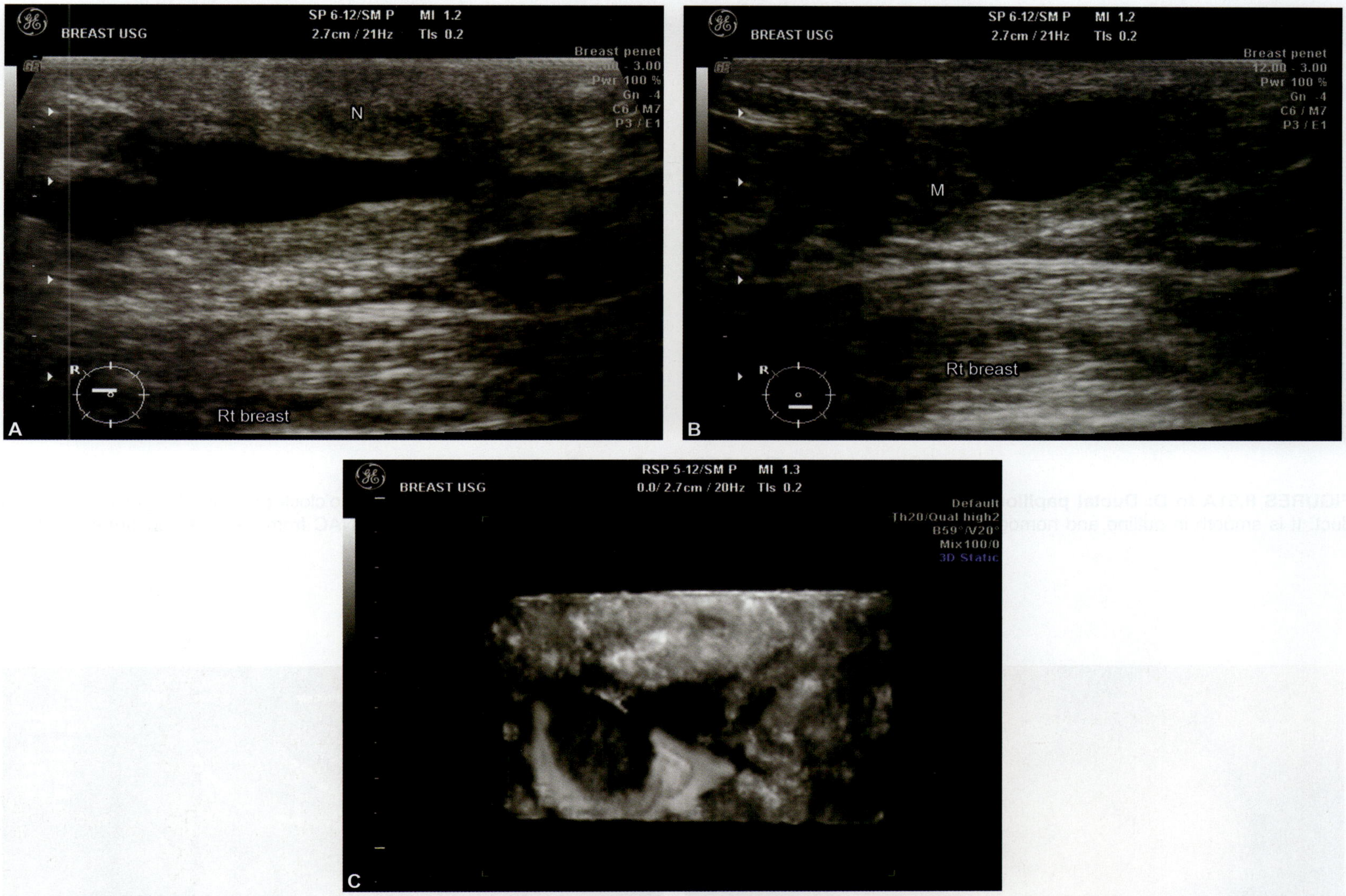

FIGURES 8.60A to C: Ductal papilloma. A patient presented with discharge from the nipple. HRSG shows a dilated duct at 9 o'clock position. It is seen going to areola. A soft tissue mass is seen in the duct. It is homogeneous in texture and smooth in outline. No calcification is seen in the mass. 3D volume contrast imaging shows the mass confined to the duct. FNAC from the mass confirms papilloma.

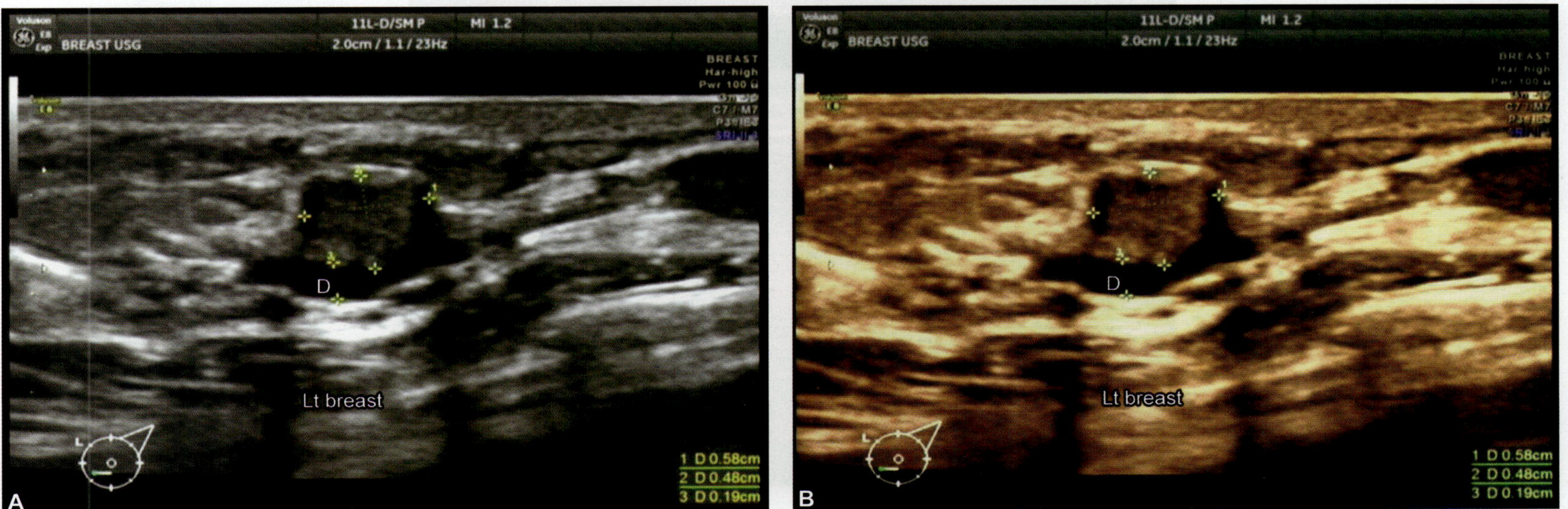

FIGURES 8.61A and B

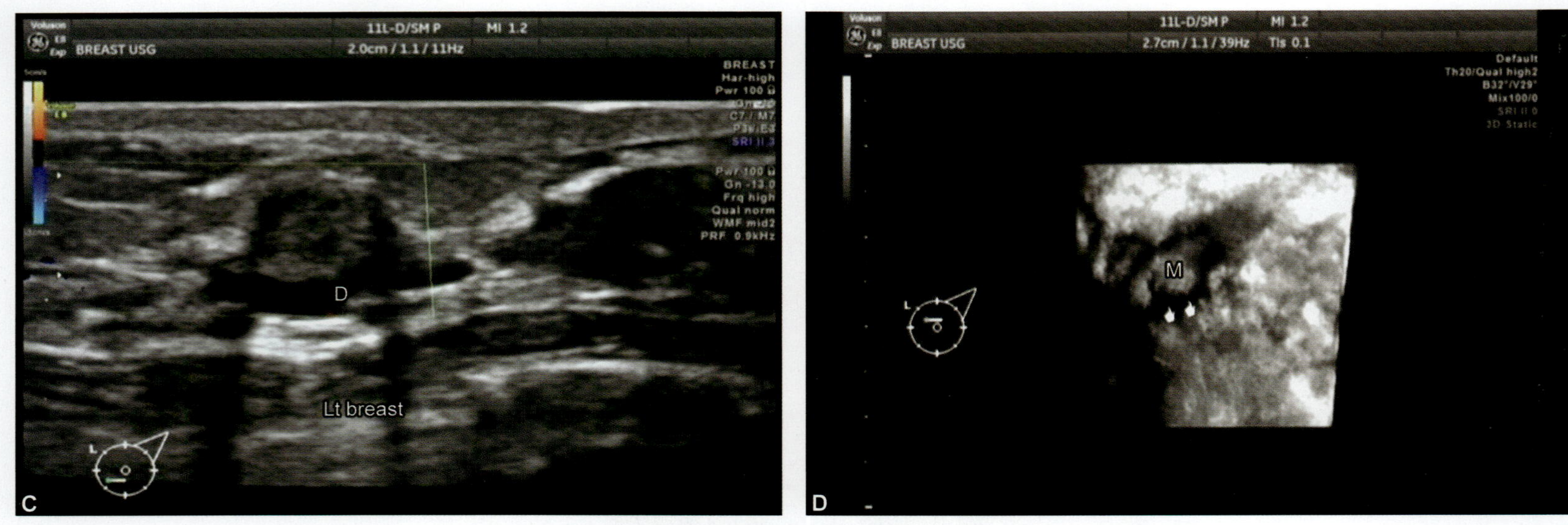

FIGURES 8.61C and D

FIGURES 8.61A to D: Ductal papilloma. HRSG shows a well-defined soft tissue mass in the left breast at 7 o'clock position. It is seen in a dilated duct. It is smooth in outline and homogeneous in texture. 3D imaging shows the mass confined to the duct. FNAC from the mass confirms papilloma.

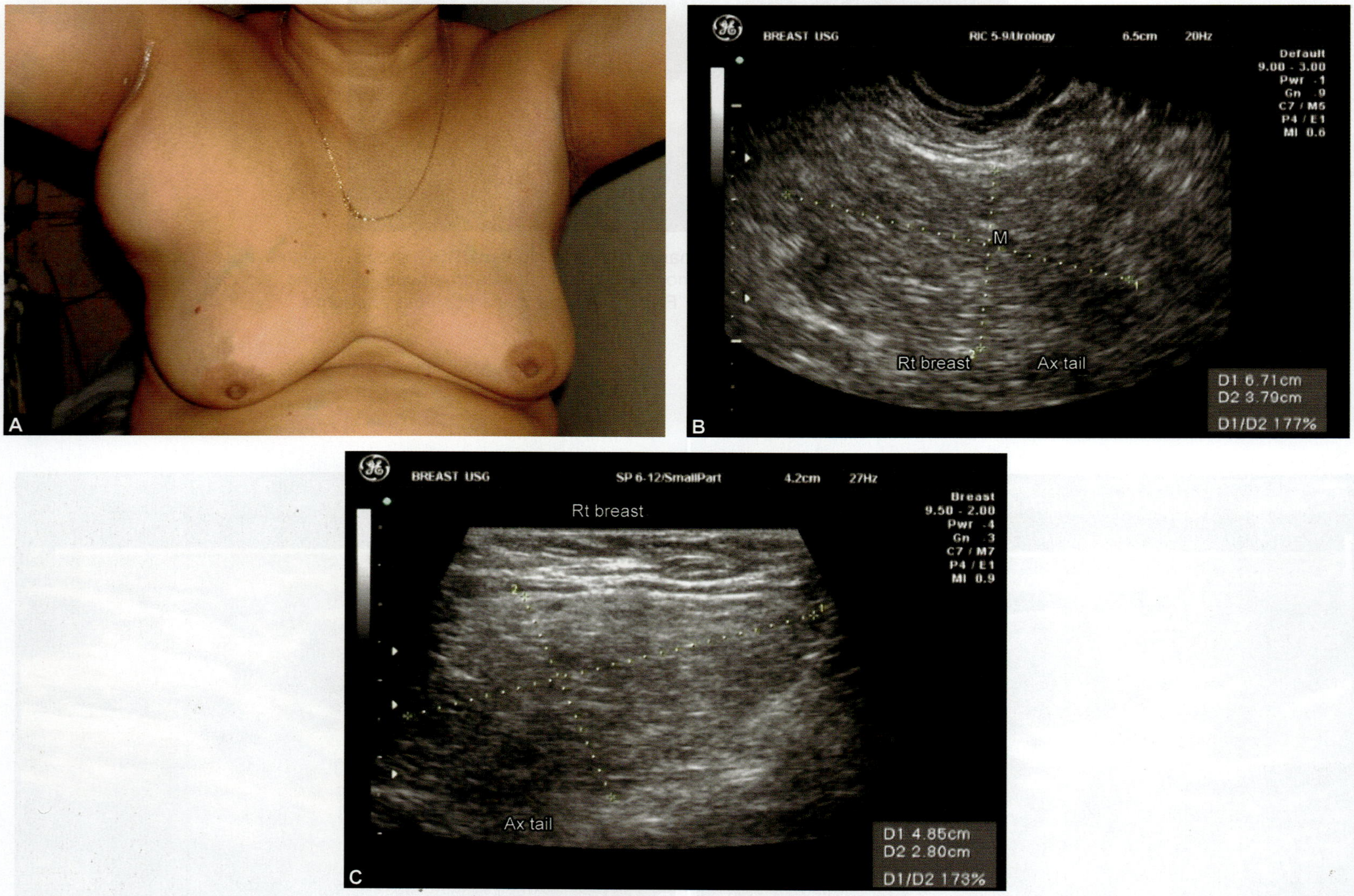

FIGURES 8.62A to C: Lipoma breast. A patient presented with soft tissue mass in the right axilla and also reaching up to right upper outer quadrant. HRSG shows well-defined homogenous mass in the breast. The mass shows medium level echoes. No calcification is seen in it. Biopsy of the mass shows lipoma of the breast.

MALIGNANT BREAST LESIONS

Breast carcinoma is one of the most common malignancies in women. The incidence of carcinoma of breast is on increase, and early detection offers better treatment and survival rate. Although X-ray mammography is still choice of investigation for mass screening program for detection of carcinoma breast, yet ultrasonography contributes significantly in making the diagnosis and disease infiltration in the local tissue. Ultrasonographic feature of typical breast carcinomas are as follows: -

1. Echo poor or hypoechoic texture of the mass.
2. Irregular border and outlines.
3. Posterior acoustic shadowing.
4. Heterogeneous texture.
5. Surrounding reflective zone (halo).

The sonographic criteria's for breast malignancy described by Stavros and his colleagues are as follows:

A. Spiculation
B. Taller than wide (Larger AP than transverse dimensions)
C. Angular margins
D. Markedly hypoechoic (composed to fat)
E. Shadowing
F. Calcifications
G. Duct extension
H. Branch pattern
I. Microlobulation

Individual criteria for benign lesions (smooth and well-circumscribed) are:

A. Absence of any malignant findings
B. Markedly hyperechoic (compared to fat)
C. 3 or fewer gentle lobulations
D. Thin, echogenic capsule.

MALIGNANT MASSES—FINDINGS

Spiculation

This consists of alternating hypoechoic and relatively hyperechoic straight lines radiating out perpendicularly from the surface of the nodule.

Taller than Wide

It indicates that a part or the entire solid nodule is greater in its AP dimension than it is in either the craniocaudal or transverse dimensions. This suggests growth across the tissue planes.

Angular Margins

Angular margins refer to the contour of the junction between the hypoechoic or Isoechoic solid nodule and the surrounding tissues. These may be acute, obtuse or nearly 90°. This finding has the highest sensitivity of any of the individual findings approaching 75%.

Markedly Hypoechoic

The central part of the majority of nodules is very hypoechoic. This suggests malignant change, but the converse is not true.

Shadowing

Some breast malignancies attenuate the sound beam and cause acoustic shadowing.

Calcification

Sonography is not as sensitive as mammography to detect punctate calcification. However, when detected are highly suggestive of malignancy.

Branch Pattern

A malignant breast nodule may have projections from the surface of the nodule extending in radial fashion within a duct toward the nipple and/or within duct away from the nipple. These findings suggest the extension of the nodule into or along the ductal system.

Microlobulation

Presence of small lobulations on the surface of a solid breast nodule is worrisome for malignancy. Microlobulations are often associated with angular margins.

Other additional features like skin thickening, disturbed trabeculae pattern, distorted tissue planes and microcalcification are also encountered on HRSG. But typical combination of nidus, halo and posterior shadowing is found in 40 to 50% of the breast cancers. The tumors nidus is echo poor and ill-defined in outlines. It is heterogeneous in texture. It may be uniform when it is small or under 1 cm in size. However, in large mass, it becomes grossly heterogeneous with distorted and disrupted normal echo pattern.

Posterior acoustic shadowing: It is caused due to the fibrosis caused by the tumor. It is seen on 40 to 60% of cases. However, it is also seen in fat necrosis, post-surgical or re-nonspecific findings.

Irregular borders: These are also one of the features of carcinoma of breast. Thus, it is also an unreliable sign and may be found in many benign conditions such as fibroadenoma, abscess, hematomas and fat necrosis.

Skin thickening and edema: Localized thickening of skin and skin edema are the features of inflammation in breast cancer. It also occurs in radiation therapy. HRSG can reveal the thickening skin. The thickened dermis becomes more echogenic than the normal pattern due to tumor infiltration, fibrosis or edema. Engorged lymphatics and interstitial fluid collection can be noticed on HRSG. Asymmetrical ductal dilatation is the feature of intraductal carcinoma. However, it may be seen in few benign conditions as intraductal papilloma.

Microcalcifications: These are the most important X-ray mammographic markers for non-palpable breast cancers, especially intraductal carcinomas. Occasionally with HRSG, microcalcification can be picked up specially when it is present within the mass. They are seen as tiny echogenic specks in the breast parenchyma and can be seen with high-gain setting. The size of microcalcification detected on X-ray mammogram and soft tissue abnormalities picked up on HRSG are the good indicators for breast carcinoma. However, detection of microcalcification on currently available ultrasonographic scanners is an unreliable parameter for confirmation of breast cancer. Therefore, other associated features should be looked for the final diagnosis.

Size of tumor: When carcinoma is diffuse, it disrupts the normal breast tissue pattern. It is replaced by a poorly reflective mass, which does not cause shadowing. It becomes difficult to distinguish it from the benign mass, and FNAC is required to establish the diagnosis.

HRSG can detect non-palpable nodes in axilla and also metastatic deposits in the liver in the same sitting, thus, helps in the staging of disease.

Ultrasound-guided Biopsy

Localization of breast lump for biopsy can be easily done with ultrasonographic imaging. Free-hand technique is the best to do USG guided FNAC. The lump is identified on USG and making a mark on the skin does localization. The depth of lesion can be found out on HRSG. Needle tip is guided into substance of the mass under USG and guided biopsy is done. It is simple, rapid and non-invasive technique for doing biopsy of the breast mass.

BIRADS Nomenclature and Categories

American College of Radiology (ACR) has developed standard reporting patterns for mammographic imaging of breast lesions. It is known as Breast, Imaging, Reporting and Data System (BIRADS). It is useful to classify the breast lesion under BIRADS risk categories for every mammogram. Though BIRADS is developed for mammogram, but same principles can be applied for sonomammograms. Since, most sonomammograms are targeted after clinical or mammographic suspicion of breast lesion, therefore, BIRADS is very useful in sonomammograms. As per the ACR the different categories of BIRADS are as follows:

BIRADS Category	Description	Risk of malignancy (%)	Management
1	Suspicious clinical presentation with doubtful X-ray mammogram normal sonomammogram	0	Clinical follow-up
2	Benign breast lesions on ultrasound like cysts, ductal ectasia, reactive lymph node enlargement, Benign solid breast masses-lipomas, fibroadenomas	0	Clinical follow-up Periodic screening
3	Probably benign lesions-Chances of malignancy <2 Complex cysts, intraductal papilloma, subset of fibro-adenomas	<2	Patient choice for follow-up and biopsy
4	Large group of breast lesions with suspicion of malignancy. This group is divided into two subcategories:	3–49	Biopsy
	• Mildly suspicious of breast malignancy	2–<50	Additional imaging—MRI
	• Moderately suspicious	50–89	Biopsy
5	Malignant masses	90 or >90	Biopsy

Advantages of Sonomammography over X-ray Mammography

Sonomammography has got distinctive advantages over X-ray mammography. They are as follows:

1. Sensitivity of sonomammography in carcinoma breast is high up to 95%.
2. Better differentiation between solid and cystic masses. It is superior to X-ray in radiologically dense breast as in young females, and breast density below 35 years of age is usually a limitation in X-ray mammography.
3. Ultrasound-guided tumor biopsy can be done from the tumor substance.
4. In mastalgia X-ray mammography is contraindicated.
5. In pregnancy sonomammography is preferred.
6. In massive breast lesions.
7. In severe physically disability.

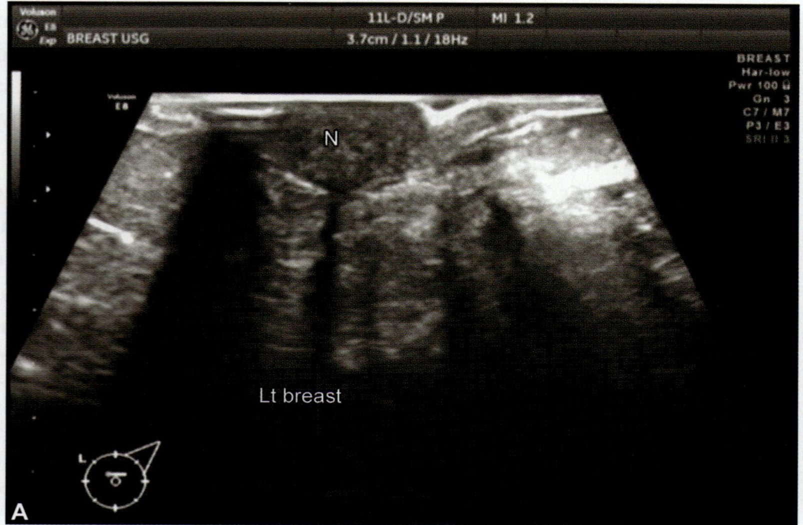

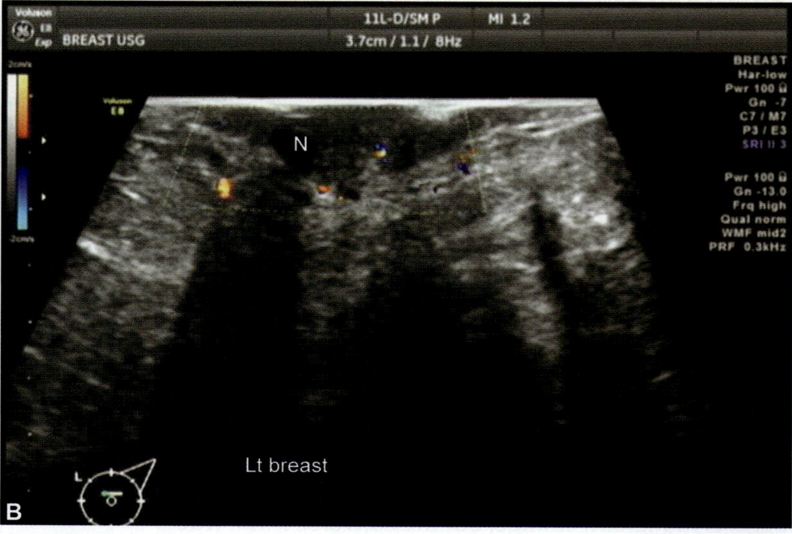

FIGURES 8.63A and B

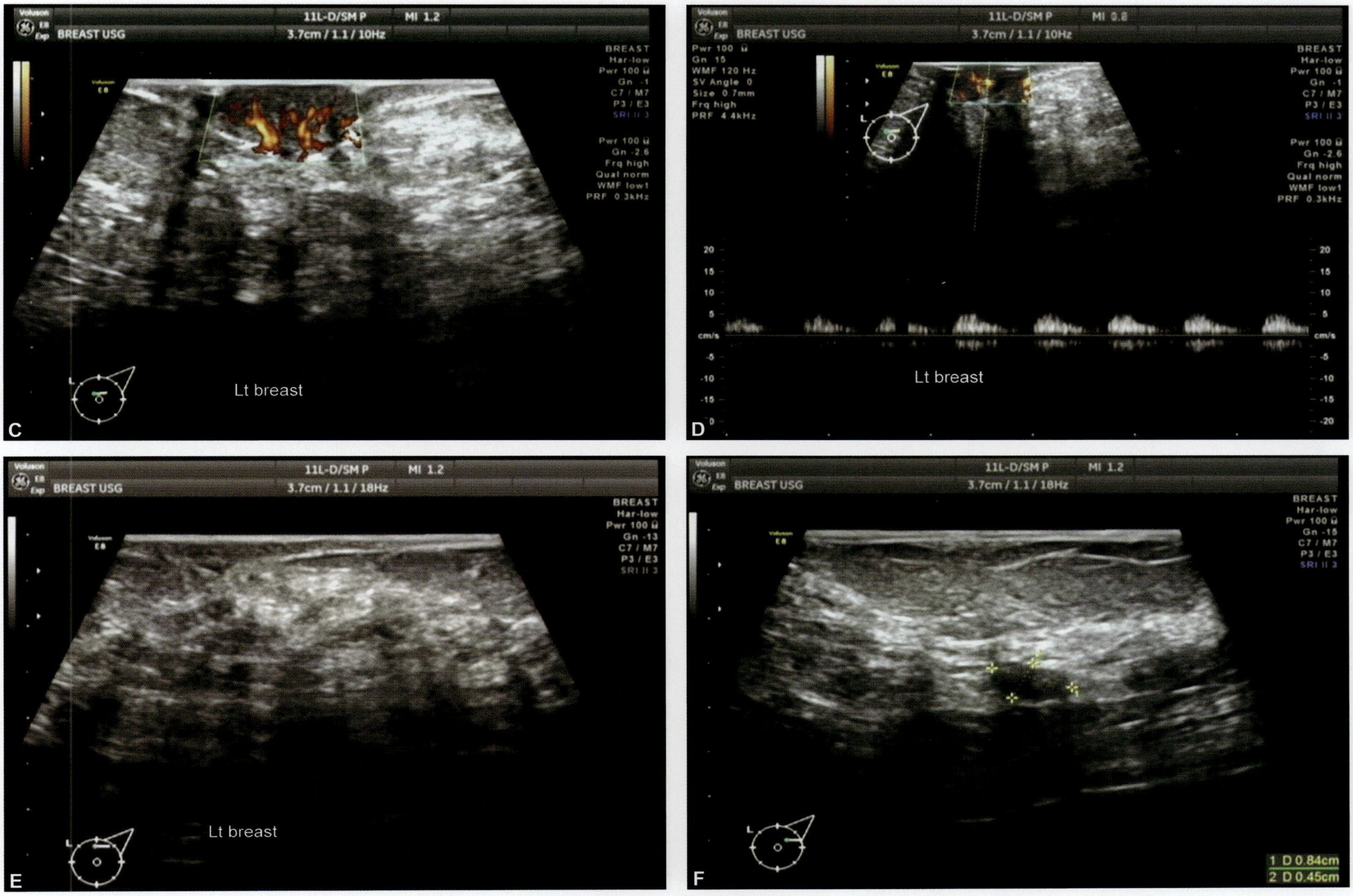

FIGURES 8.63C to F

FIGURES 8.63A to F: Paget's disease. A patient presented with redness of the nipple and areola with flaky and crusty skin over the nipple. HRSG shows inhomogeneous texture of the nipple. Hypoechoic areas are seen in the nipple. **On color flow imaging**, multiple vessels are seen feeding the areola and the nipple. On spectral Doppler tracing, low arterial flow is seen. There is also evidence of few enlarged lymph nodes seen in the left axilla, which are round in shape. The lymph node hylum is lost. The cytological examination confirms Paget's disease with malignant lymph nodes in the left axilla.

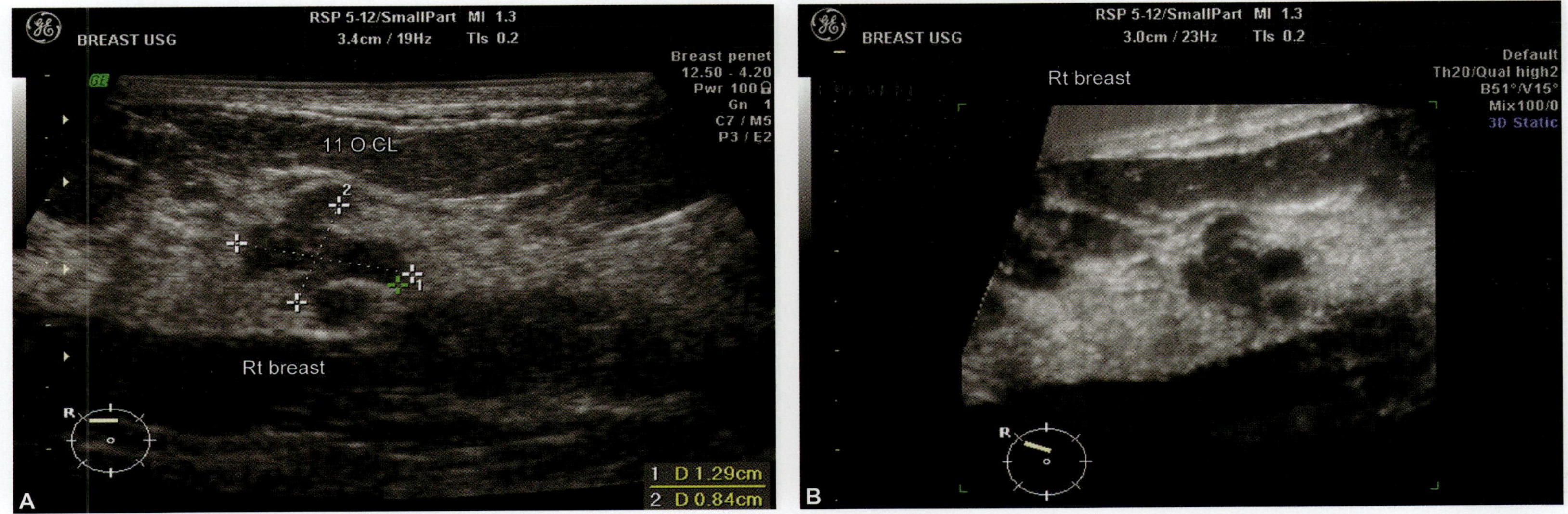

FIGURES 8.64A and B: A 40-year-patient presented with irregular nodularity in the upper part of the right breast. HRSG shows an irregular ill-defined soft tissue mass in the mammary zone. It shows multiple lobulations. However, it is confined to the mammary zone. 3D volume contrast imaging shows multiple lobulations in the mass. Biopsy confirms malignancy.

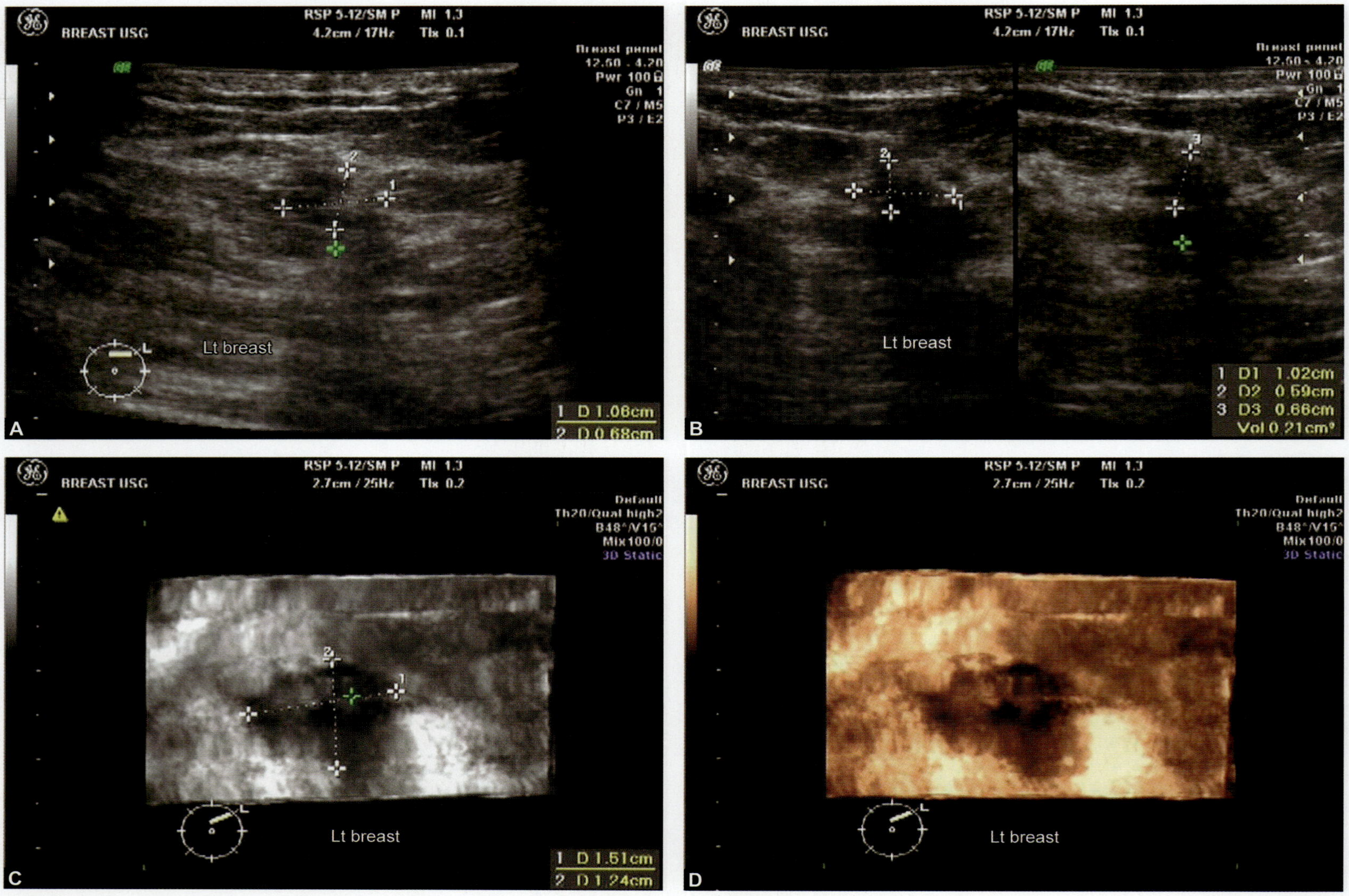

FIGURES 8.65A to D: A lady presented with irregular ill-defined nodule in the left breast. HRSG shows an irregular mass at 1 o'clock position in the left breast. It is confined to the mammary zone. 3D ultrasound shows the mass is taller than wide. Multiple microlobulations are seen in it. Biopsy of the mass confirms malignancy.

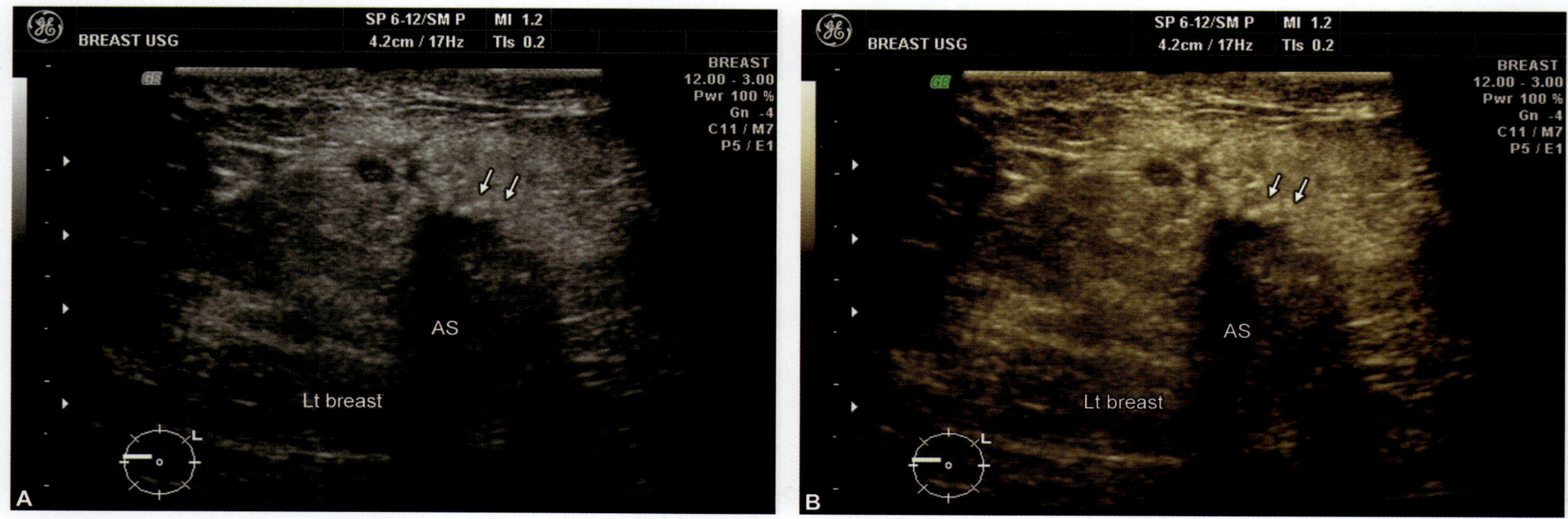

FIGURES 8.66A and B

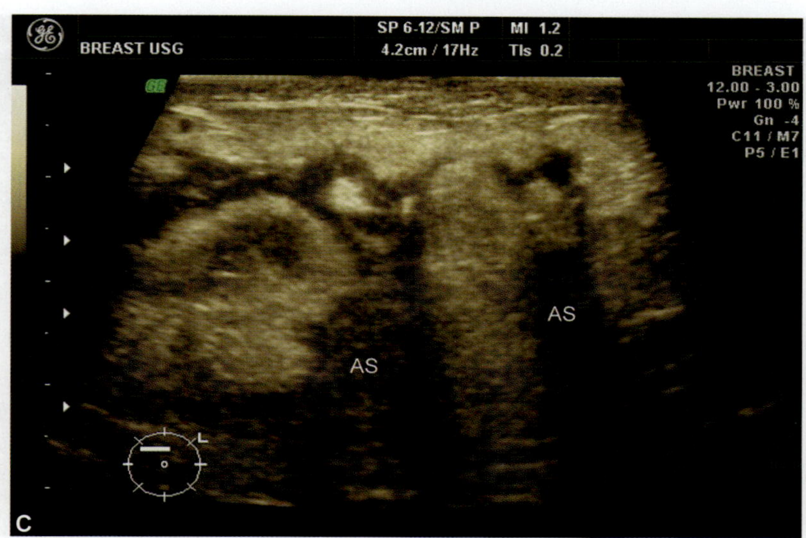

FIGURE 8.66C

FIGURES 8.66A to C: A lady presented with irregular nodular mass in the left breast. HRSG shows heterogeneous nodular masses in the left breast in upper inner quadrant. HRSG shows irregular nodular masses at 9 and 11 o'clock position. Echogenic specks are seen in them, which are accompanied with acoustic shadowing. The tumor nidus is small. Findings are suggestive of multifocal malignant masses. Biopsy confirms multifocal intraductal CA.

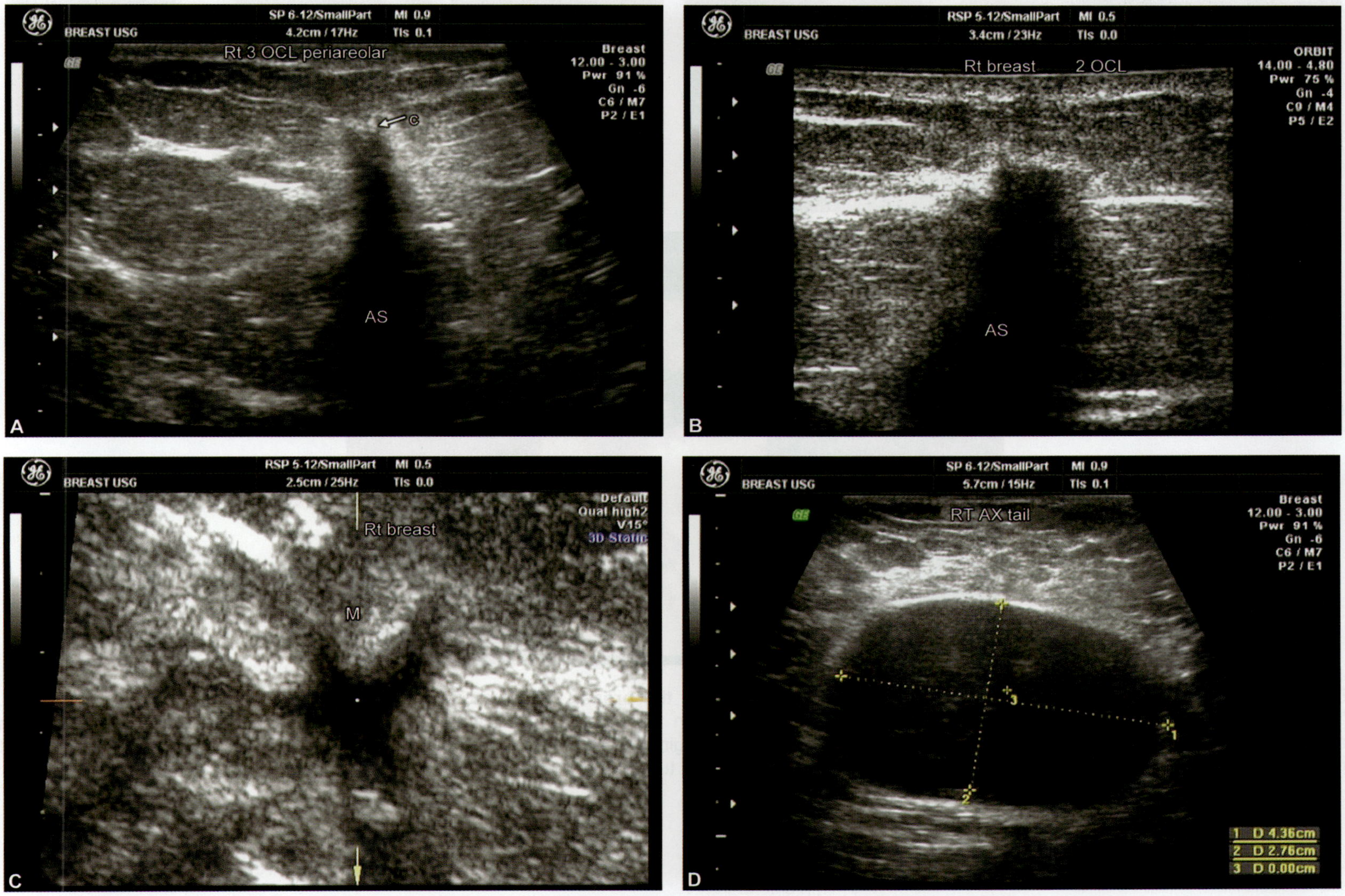

FIGURES 8.67A to D: 3D imaging of the same patient shows calcified focus in the tumor, which was responsible for dense acoustic shadowing. **3D imaging** of the tumor shows tumor nidus. Branching pattern of the mass is well-appreciated on 3D imaging. The calcified shadow is also seen clearly in the tumor. Enlarged node is seen in the axilla. The node is round in shape with hylum distorted suggestive of malignant node in the same patient.

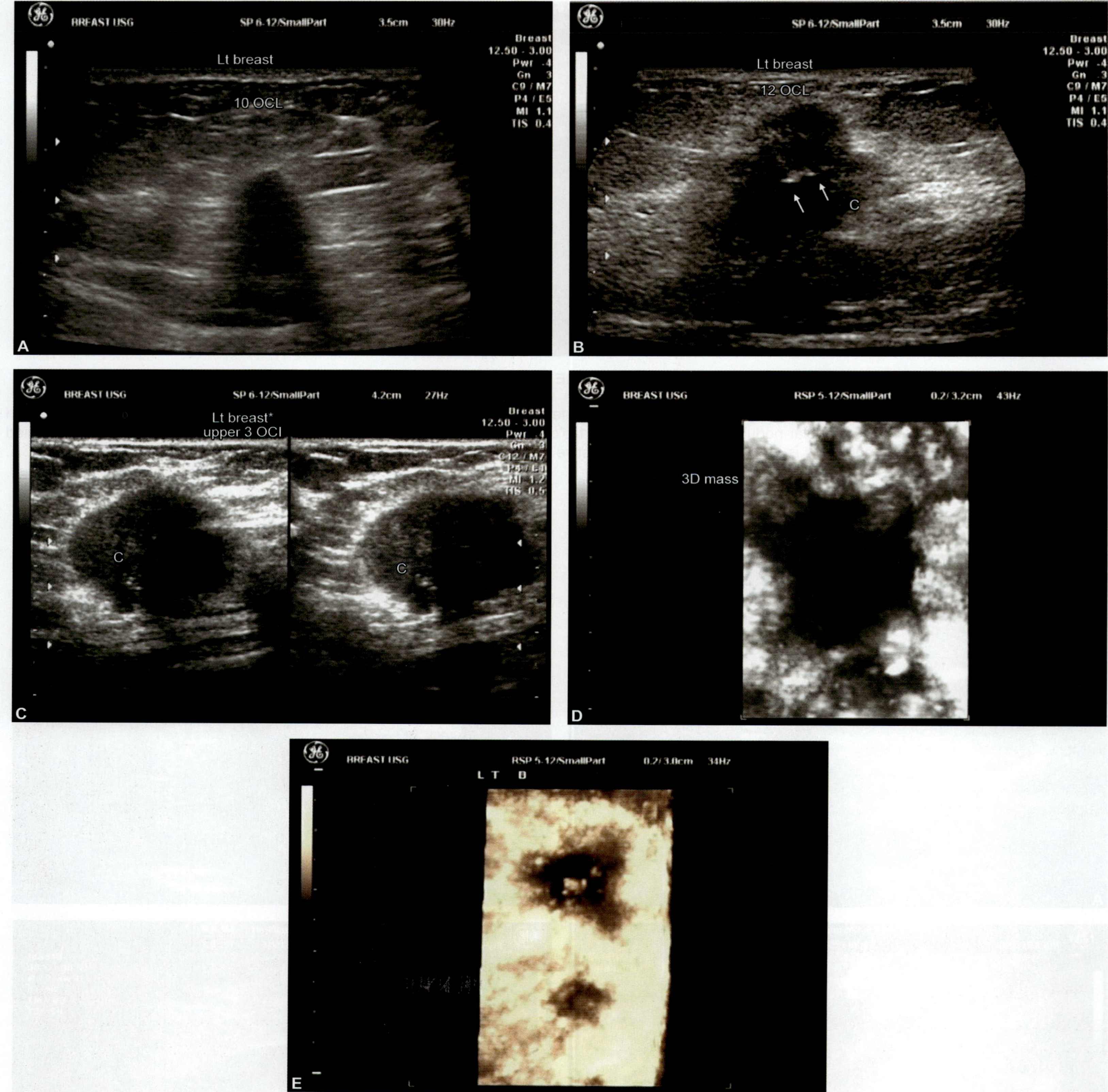

FIGURES 8.68A to E: Heterogeneous mass with microcalcification in the breast. HRSG shows an irregular heterogeneous mass in the breast. The mass shows dense acoustic shadowing. Microcalcification is seen in the mass. The calcified specks are highlighted with image compression technique. They are seen bright echogenic specks in the mass. 3D imaging of the mass shows star appearance with branching pattern typical of malignant nature of the mass. Microcalcification is seen embedded in the tumor bed.

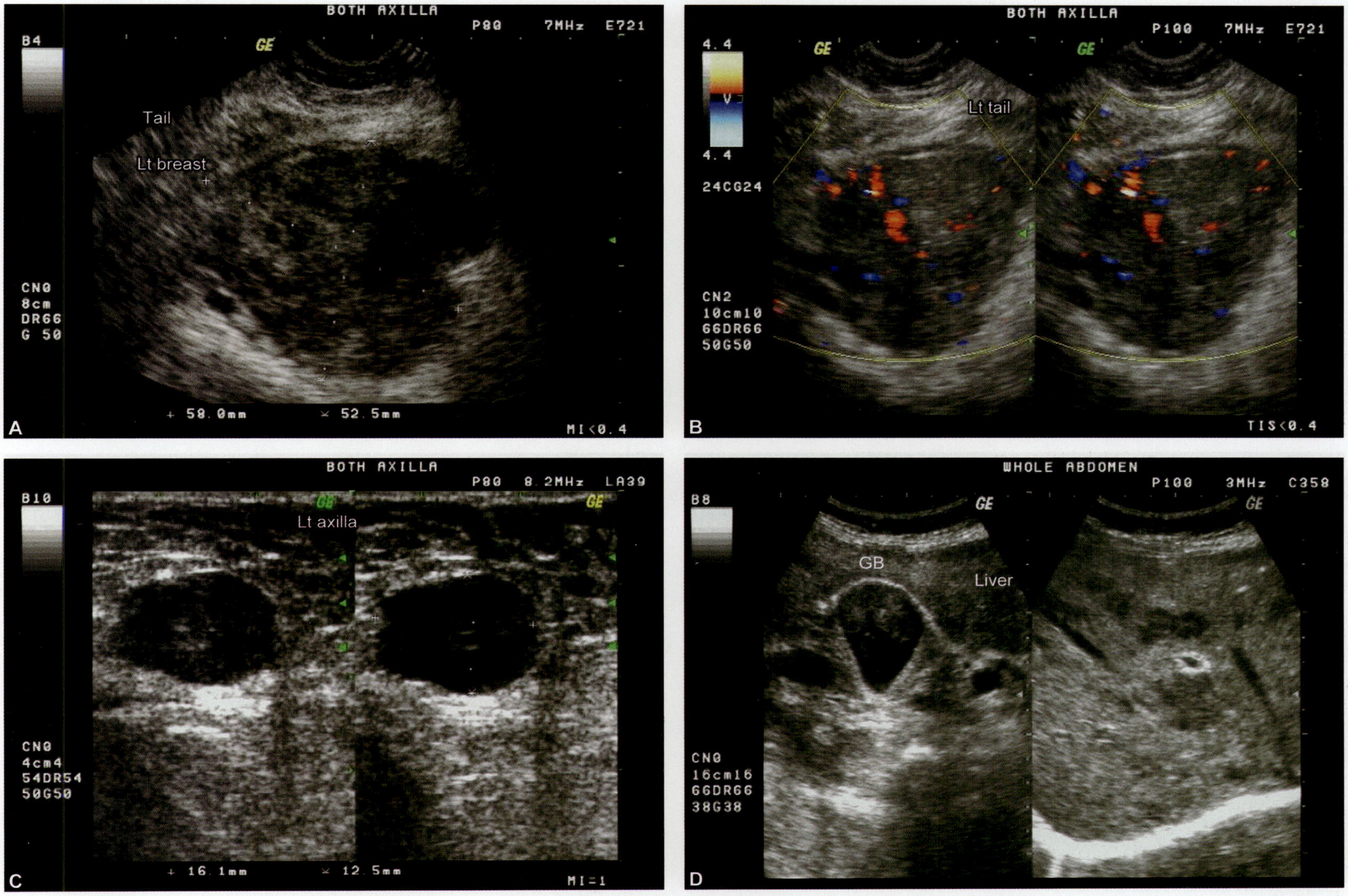

FIGURES 8.69A to D: Big heterogeneous mass with retromammary invasion. A patient presented with big mass in the breast. HRSG shows big heterogeneous mass in the breast. The mass is seen invading the retromammary layer. It is also seen invading the auxiliary tail. **On color flow imaging** multiple vessels are seen feeding the mass. HRSG shows enlarged nodes in the axilla with malignant changes in the nodes. They are round in shape. Lymph node hylum is destroyed. The liver also shows multiple irregular hypoechoic masses suggestive of metastatic deposits.

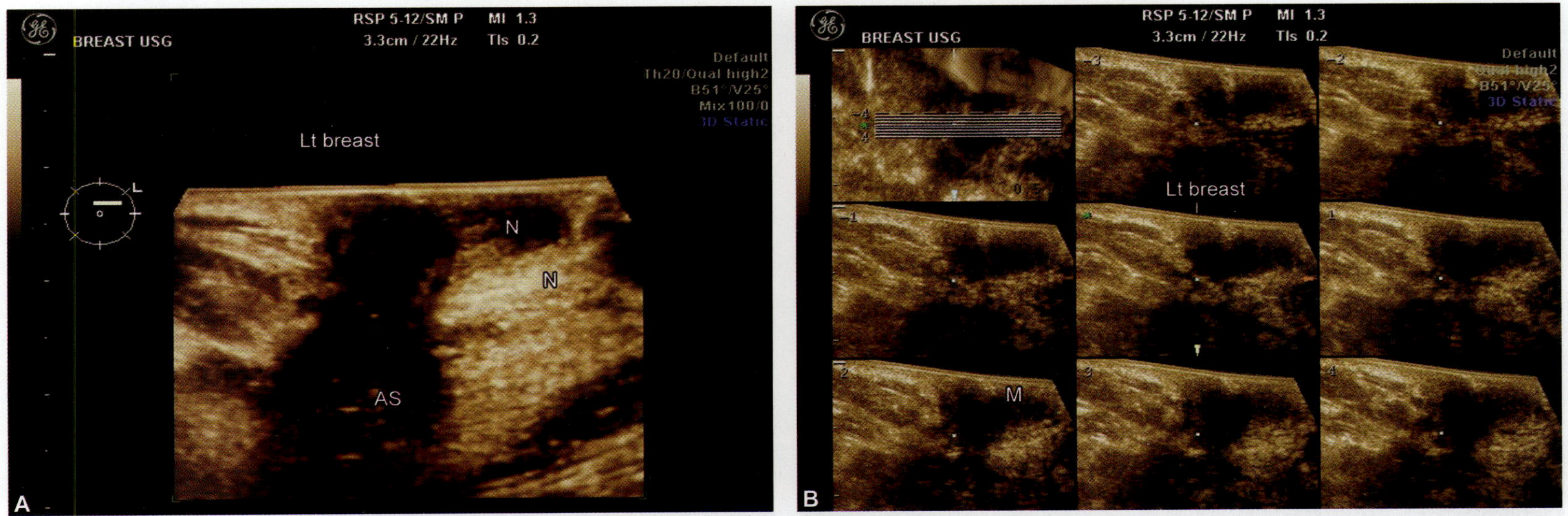

FIGURES 8.70A and B

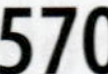

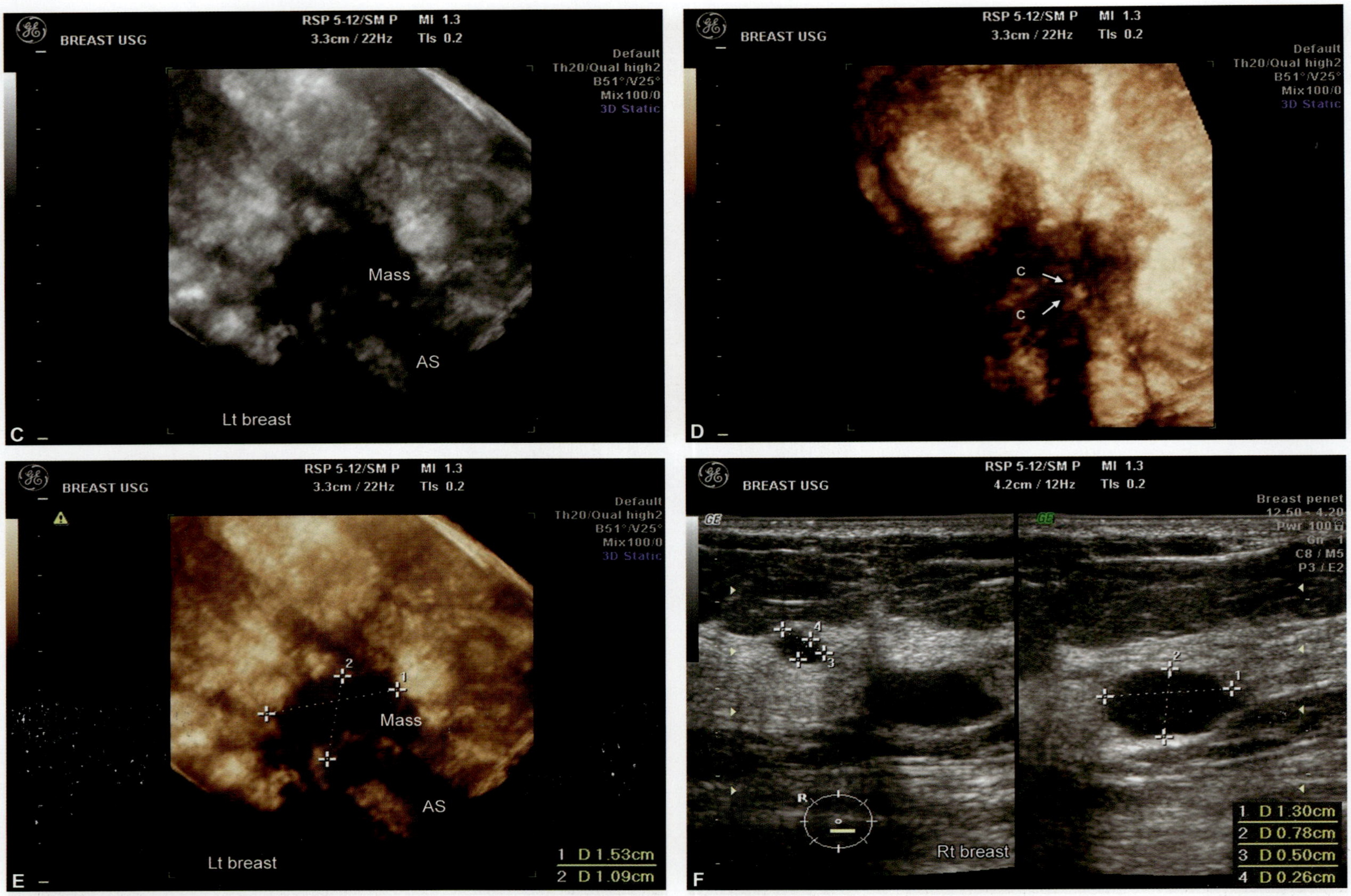

FIGURES 8.70C to F

FIGURES 8.70A to F: A patient presented with heterogeneous mass in the left breast. HRSG shows a big irregular heterogeneous mass at 12 and 1 o'clock position. The mass is taller than wide. On 3D ultrasound with tomographic imaging, the tumor nidus is seen. Echogenic specks are seen in the tumor nidus suggestive of microcalcification. It is accompanied with strong shadowing. Multiple lobulations are also seen in the mass. Enlarged lymph nodes are also seen in the axilla. Findings are suggestive of malignant mass with microcalcification. The right breast also shows small nodular masses, which are smooth in outline. No calcification is seen in them suggestive of small fibroadenomas.

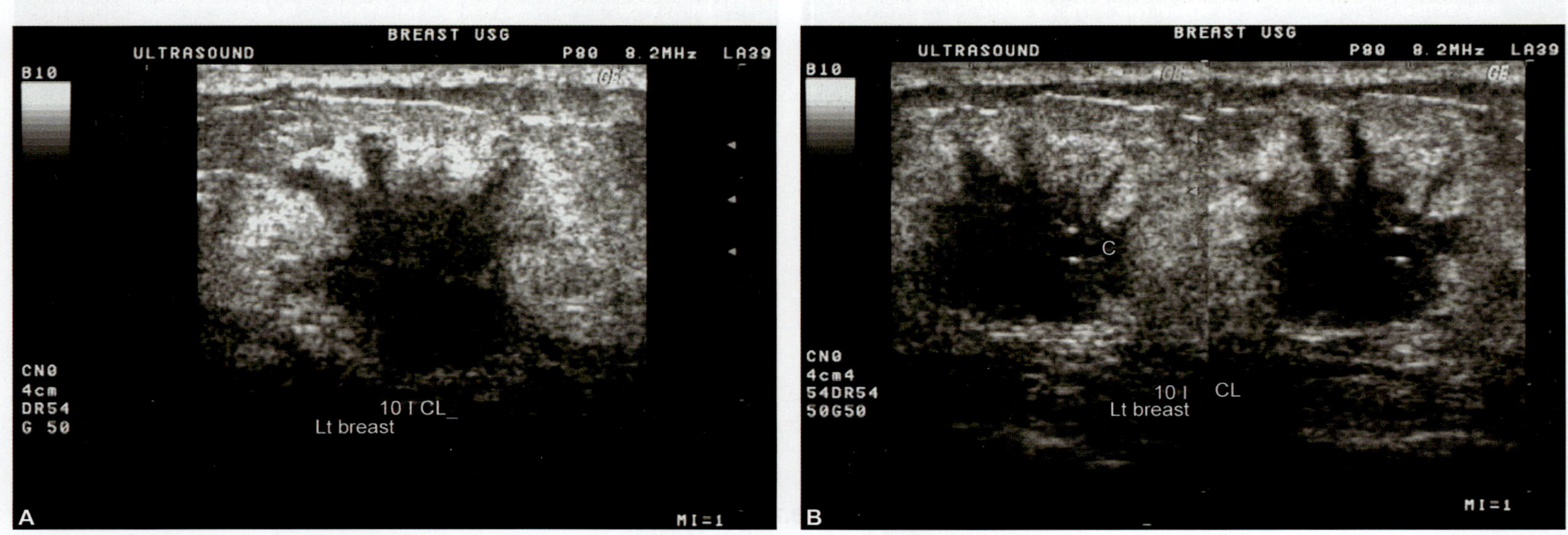

FIGURES 8.71A and B

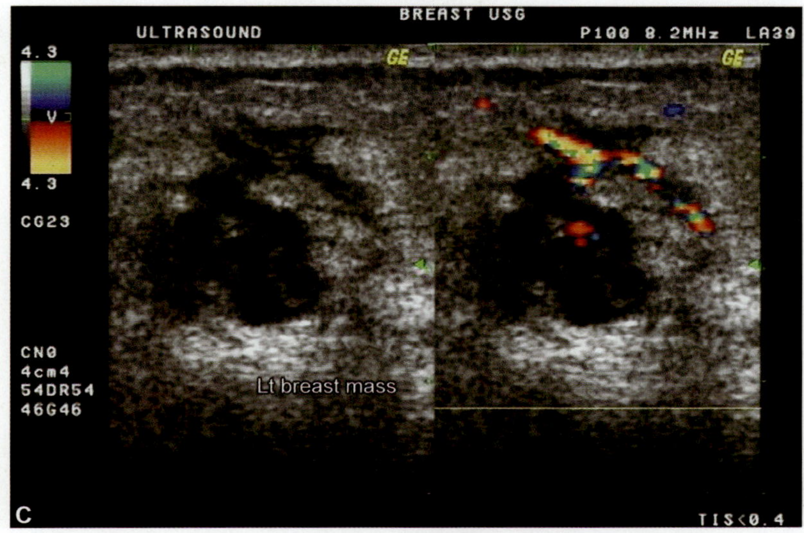

FIGURE 8.71C

FIGURES 8.71A to C: Heterogeneous mass with spiculated pattern. HRSG shows irregular heterogeneous mass in the breast. Fine spicules are seen coming out from the mass with "*Sunray Appearance*", typical of the malignant nature of the mass. Echogenic microcalcification is also seen in the mass. **On color flow imaging,** a big vessel is seen feeding the tumor. High flow is seen in the vessels on spectral Doppler tracing.

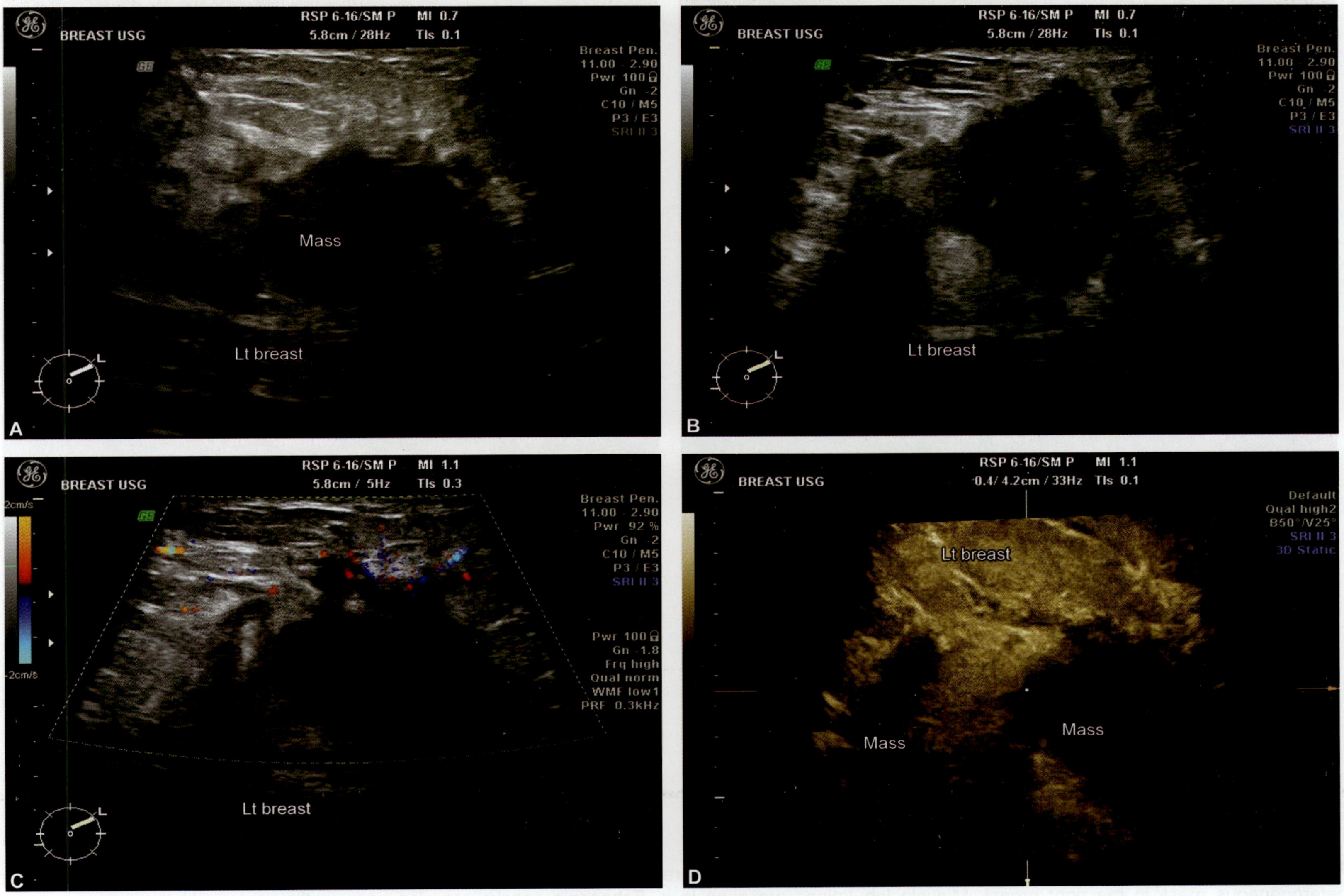

FIGURES 8.72A to D

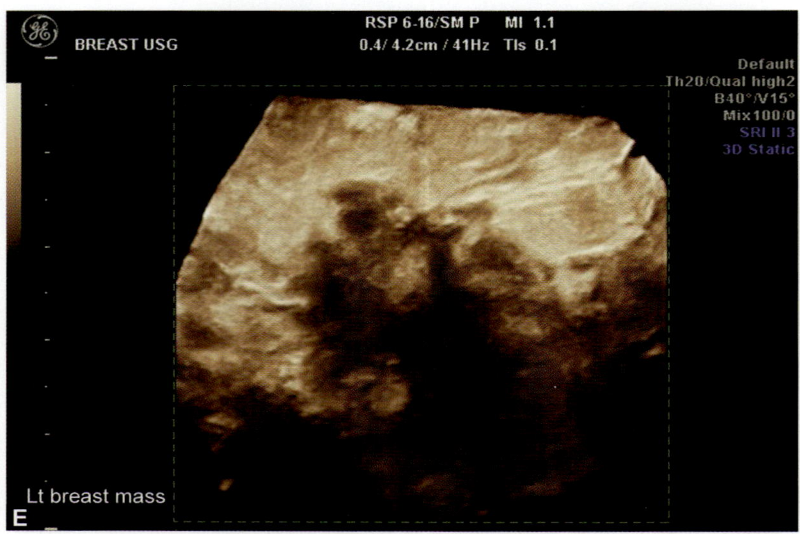

FIGURE 8.72E

FIGURES 8.72A to E: A patient presented with hard lump in the left breast. HRSG shows irregular heterogeneous mass in the left breast measuring 30 x 35 x 33 mm and volume of the mass is 17 cm^3. The mass is seen involving upper and outer quadrant. It shows echogenic calcifications suggestive of microcalcifications. Multiple heterogeneous foci are seen in the mass suggestive of multicentric mass. It is seen involving mammary zone. No retromammary invasion seen at the time of study. Findings are suggestive of big multicentric heterogeneous mass in the left breast suggestive of malignant mass. Intraductal carcinoma.

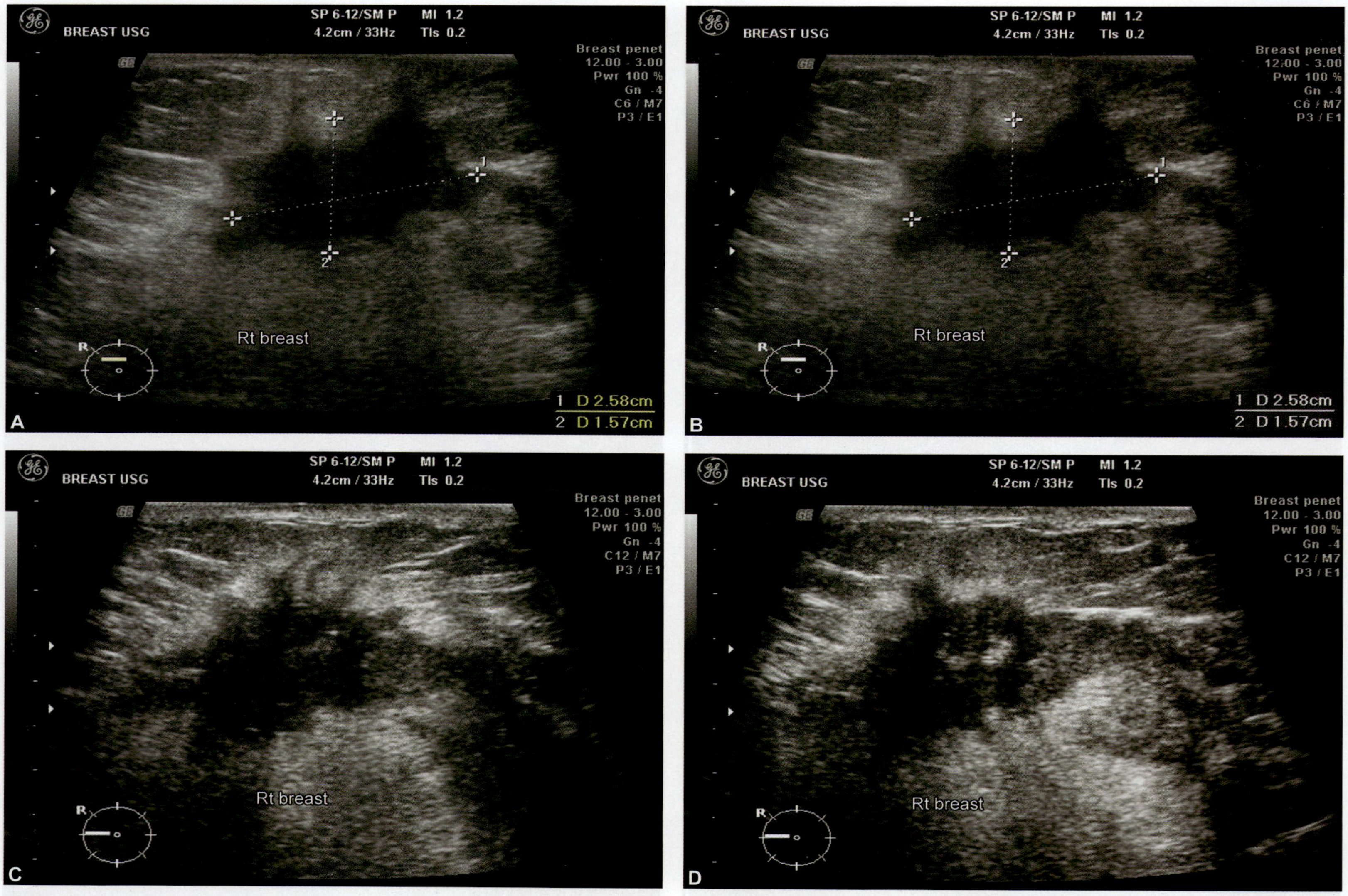

FIGURES 8.73A to D: A patient presented with hard lump in the right breast at 9 and 10 o' clock position. HRSG shows a big irregular ill-defined heterogeneous mass in the right breast. Multiple lobulations are seen in it. Echogenic specks are also seen in the mass, which are accompanied with acoustic shadowing. Margins of the mass show *sunray appearance*. The mass is seen invading the retromammary layer. Biopsy of the mass confirms malignant carcinoma.

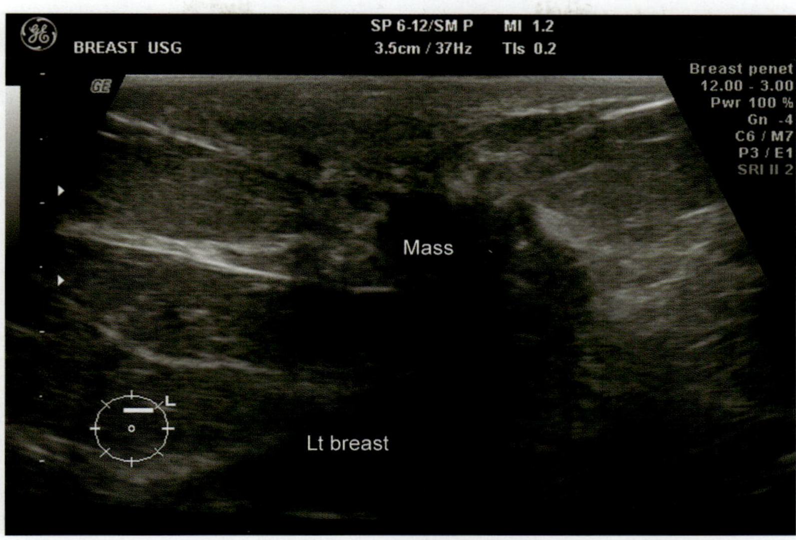

FIGURE 8.74: A 65-year-old lady presented with mass in the left breast. HRSG shows a big heterogeneous soft tissue mass in the left breast in the mammary zone. Echogenic specks are seen in the mass, which are accompanied with acoustic shadowing. Enlarged lymph nodes are also seen in the axilla suggestive of malignant mass.

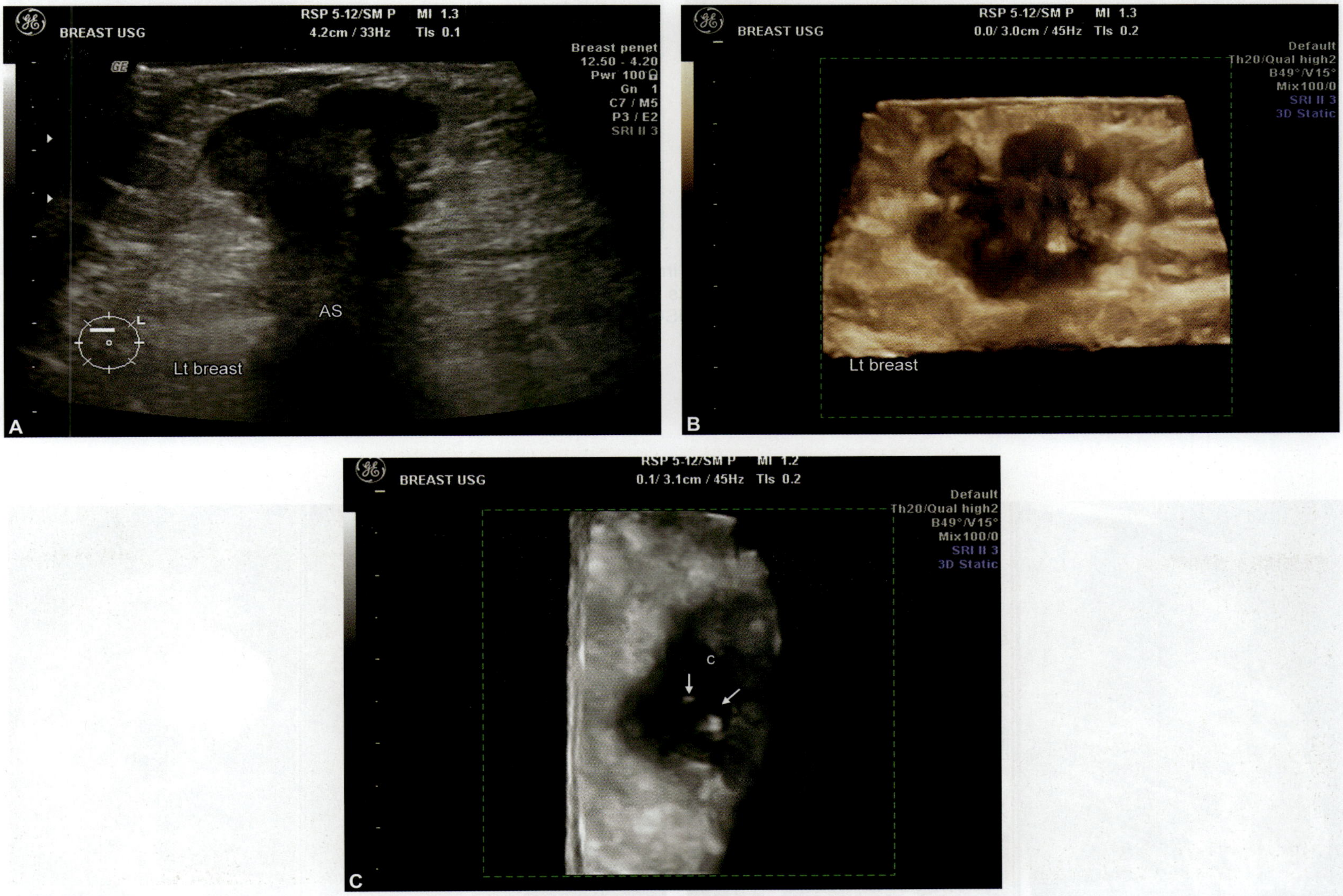

FIGURES 8.75A to C: A patient presented with hard lump in the left breast at 11 o'clock position. HRSG shows big irregular ill-defined mass at 11 o'clock position. On 3D imaging multiple lobulations are seen in the mass. Echogenic specks are also seen in the mass suggestive of microcalcification. Findings are suggestive of malignant mass.

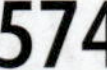

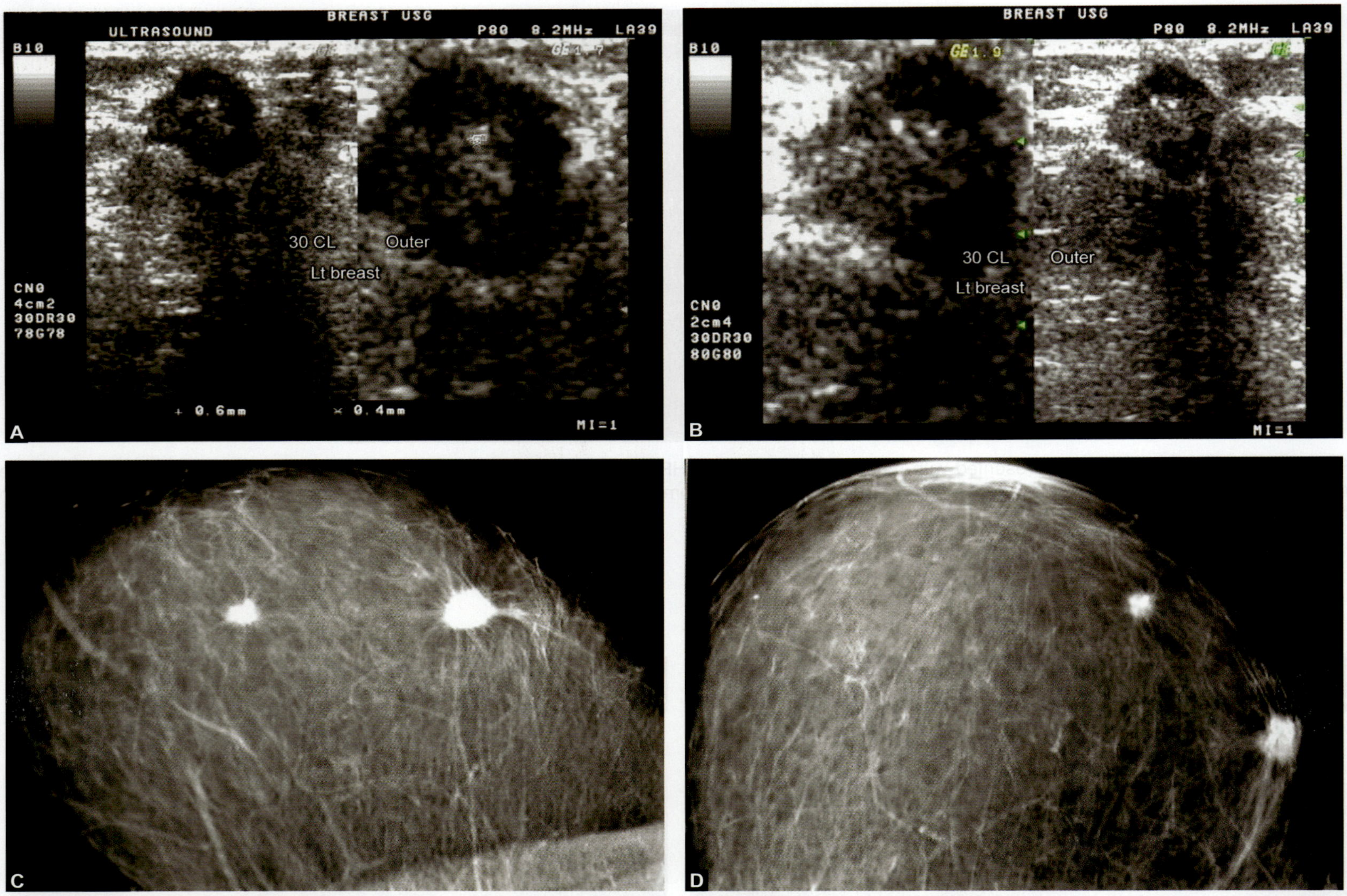

FIGURES 8.76A to D: Multifocal malignant breast tumor. HRSG shows irregular heterogeneous masses in the left breast. The masses show microlobulations coming out from the margins. Small echogenic calcified specks are also seen in the masses suggestive of microcalcification. The digital mammography of the same patient shows the masses as described on USG and confirmed the USG findings.

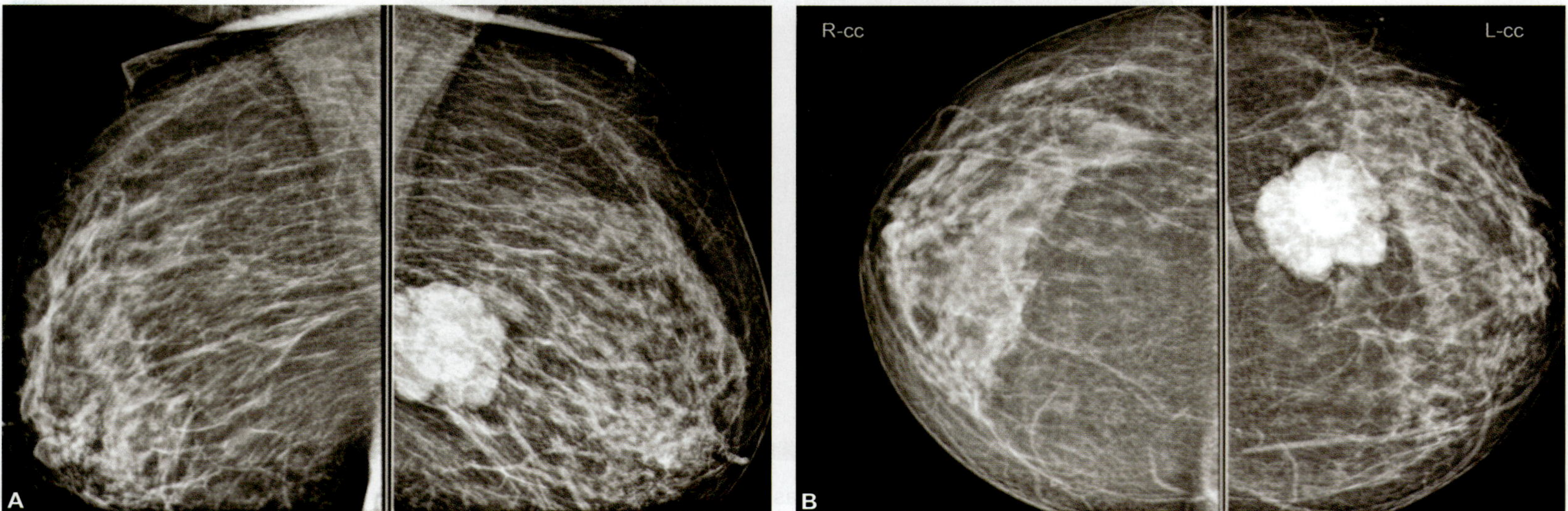

FIGURES 8.77A and B

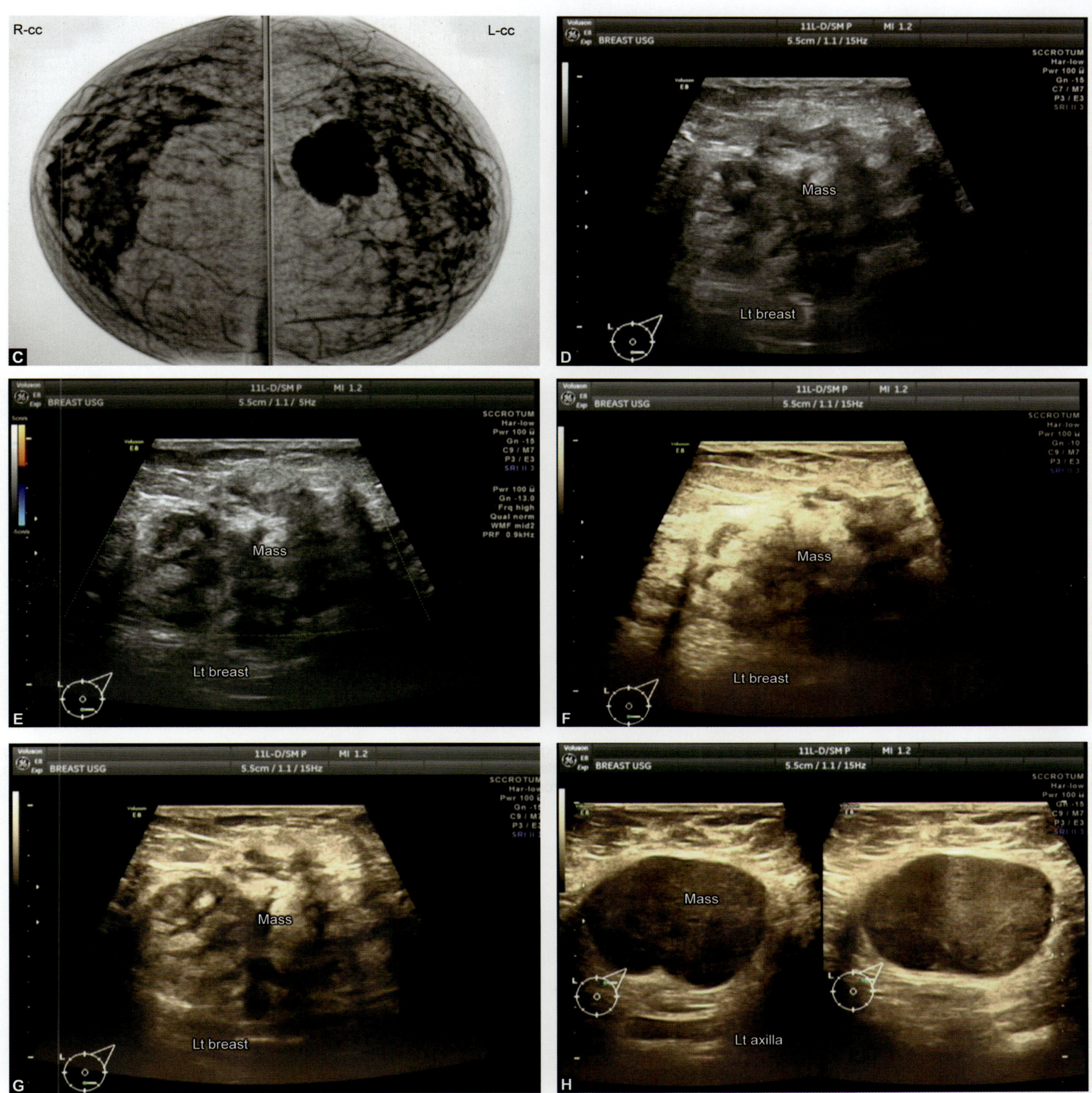

FIGURES 8.77C to H

FIGURES 8.77A to H: A patient presented with big mass in the left breast at 4 and 5 o'clock position. The breast mammogram shows heterogeneous mass in the left breast. HRSG shows big irregular heterogeneous soft tissue mass in the left breast. The mass shows lobulated margins. It is irregular in outline. It is seen invading the mammary and retromammary layers. Microcalcification is also seen in the mass. But no cystic degeneration is seen. It is not seen fixed with chest wall. Big hypoechoic nodal mass seen in the left axilla suggestive of enlarged lymph node. Lymph node hylum is destroyed. Normal texture is lost. Findings are suggestive of big irregular heterogeneous mass in the left breast in the lower quadrant invading the mammary and retromammary layers with enlarged lymph node in the left axilla with normal right breast study. Biopsy of the mass confirms BIRADS-5 malignancy.

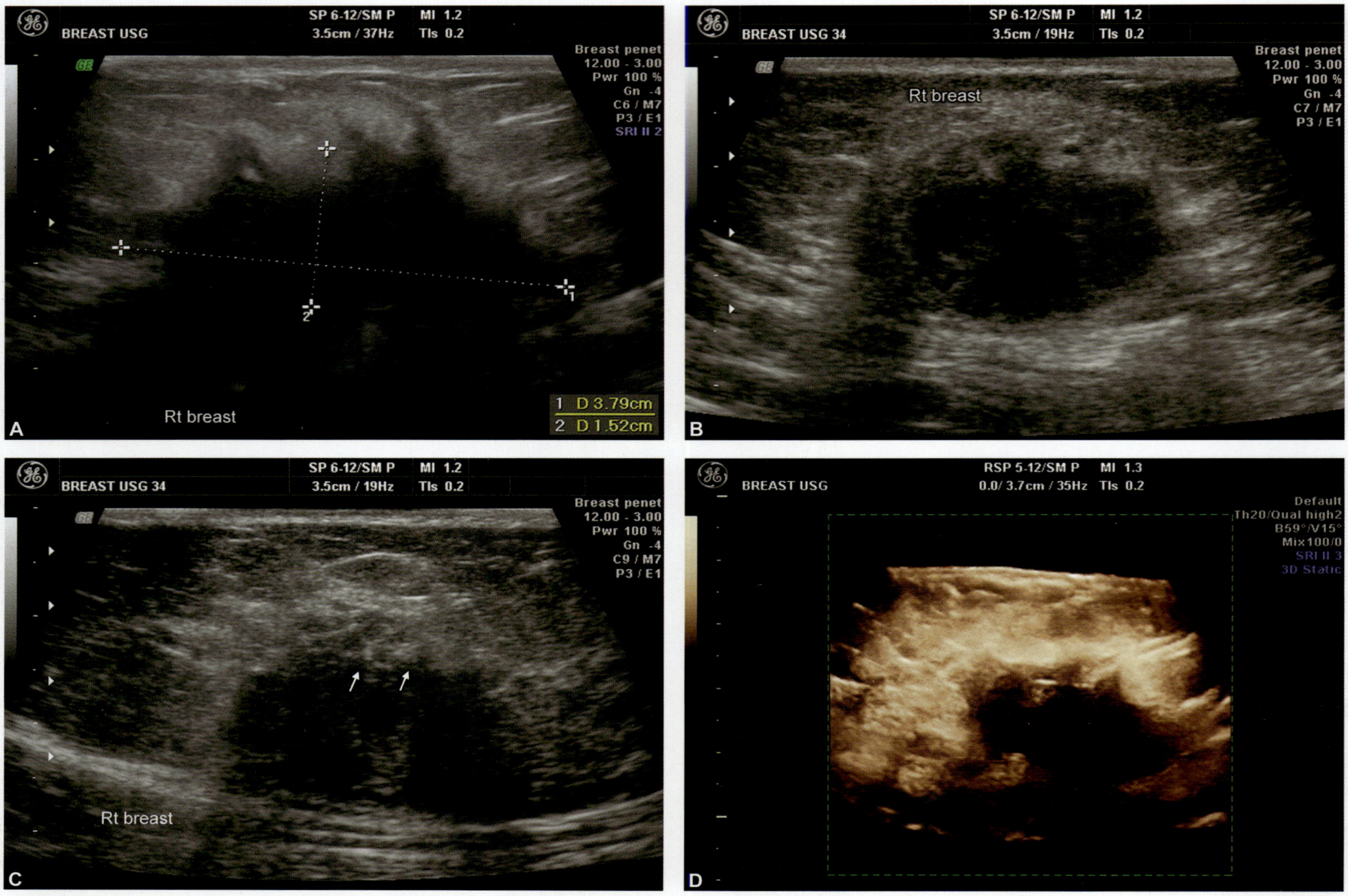

FIGURES 8.78A to D: HRSG shows a big heterogeneous mass in the right breast. The mass measures 40 x 15 mm in size. It is heterogeneous in texture. Multiple spiculation are seen in the mass. Echogenic foci are also seen in the mass suggestive of microcalcification. Tumor nidus is seen with acoustic shadowing. The mass is seen invading the retromammary zone. But chest wall muscles are not invaded by the mass.

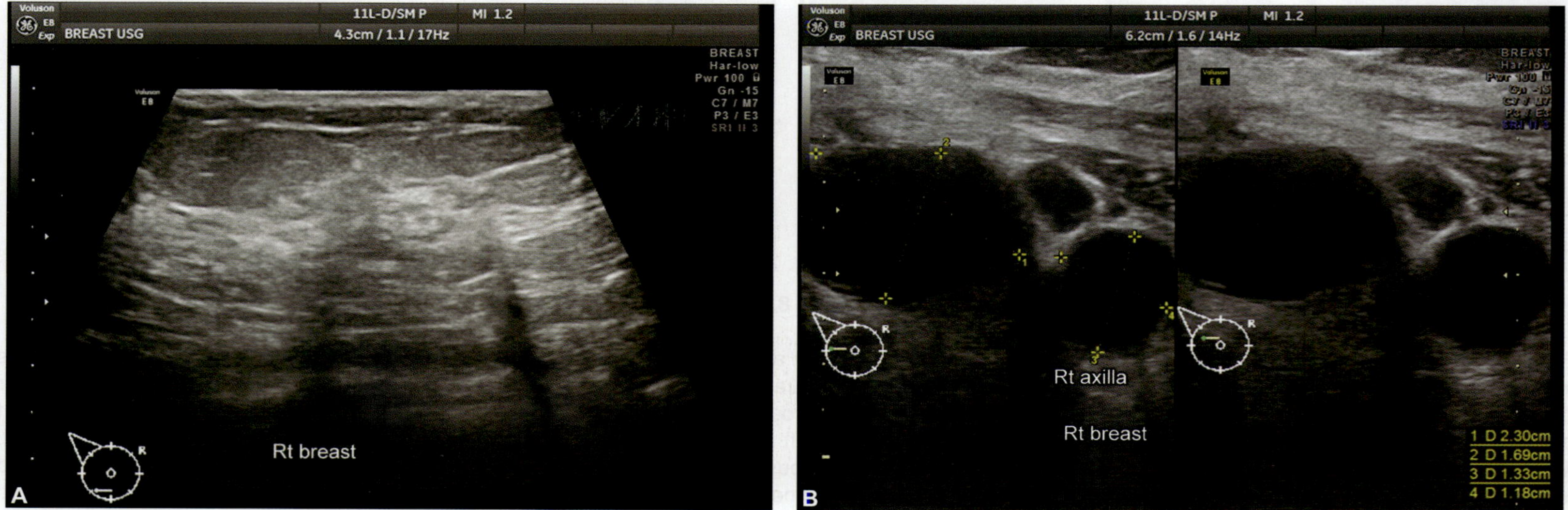

FIGURES 8.79A and B: A patient presented with hard lump in the right breast. HRSG shows an ill-defined soft tissue mass in the mammary zone at 6 and 7 o'clock position. Echogenic specks are seen in the mass. Multiple hypoechoic nodular masses are also seen in the right axilla suggestive of enlarged lymph nodes. Lymph node hylum is seen destroyed. Findings are suggestive of highly malignant mass in the breast.

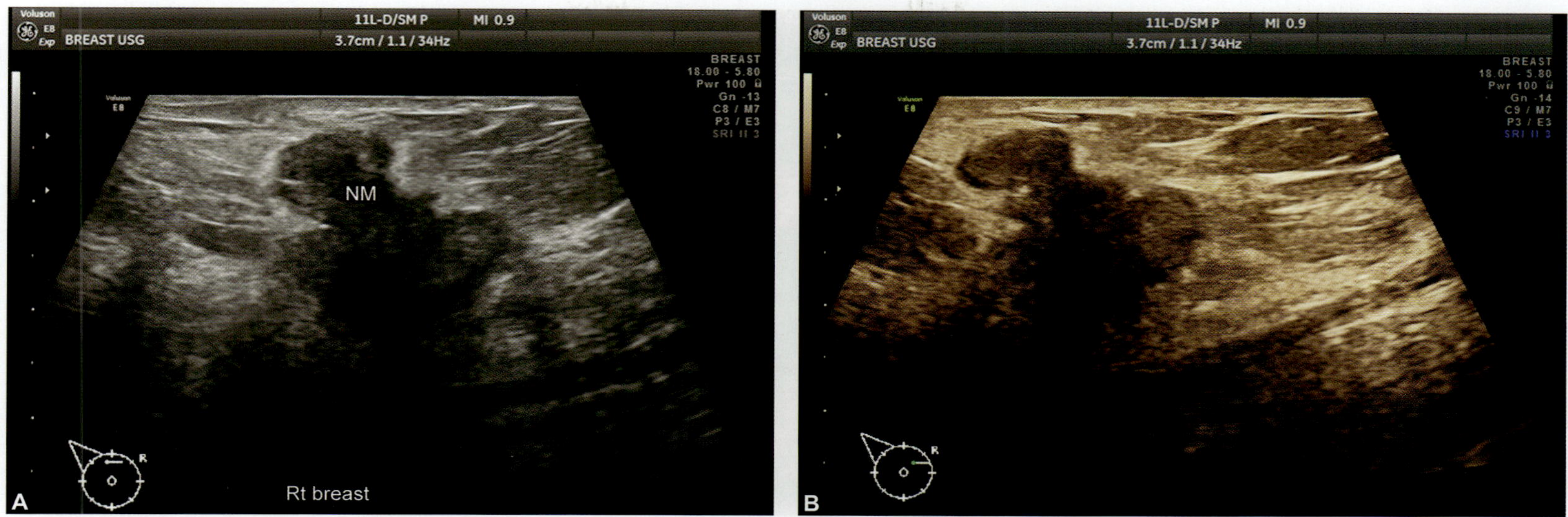

FIGURES 8.80A and B: A patient presented with a lump in the right breast. HRSG shows a big irregular mass in the right breast. It is taller than wide. Multiple lobulations are seen in the mass. Echogenic calcification is also seen in it suggestive of malignant mass.

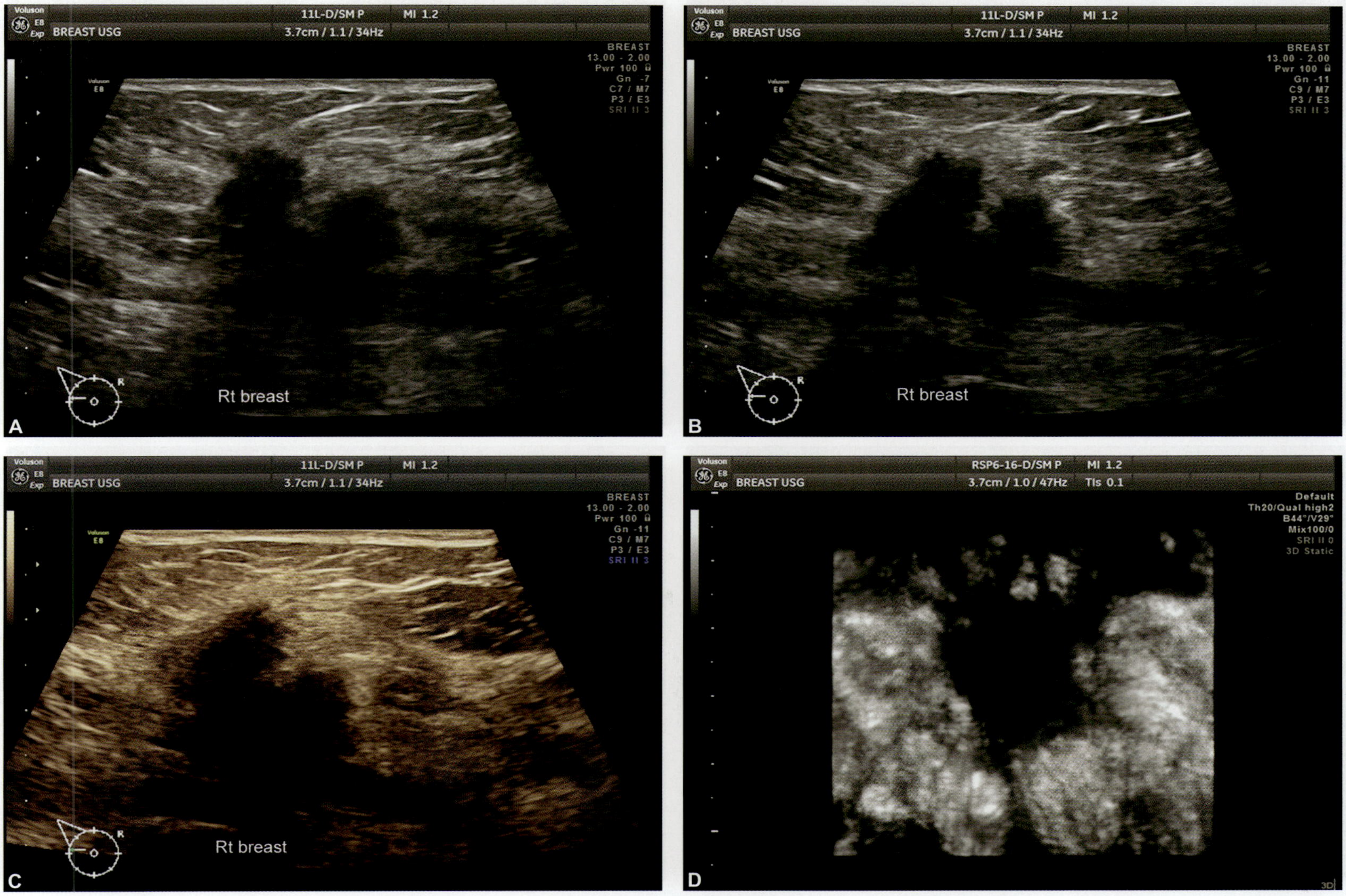

FIGURES 8.81A to D

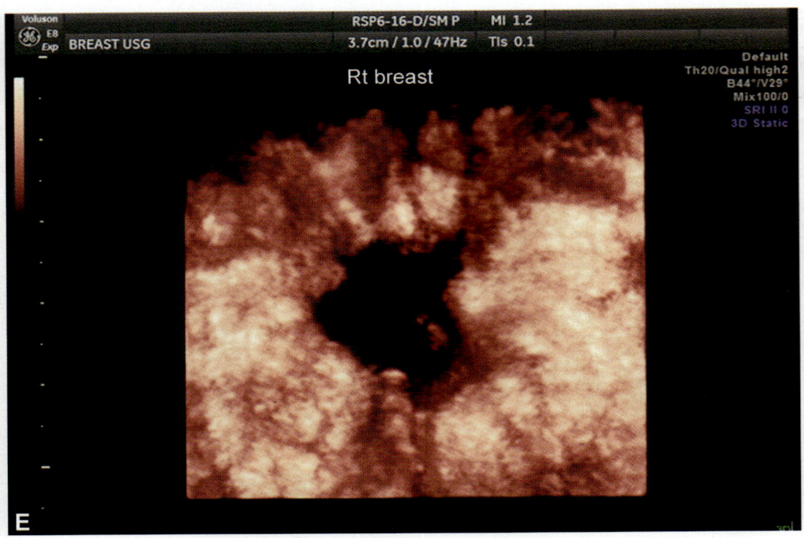

FIGURE 8.81E

FIGURES 8.81A to E: Intraductal carcinoma. A patient presented with a small nodular lump in the right breast at 9 o'clock position. HRSG shows a highly heterogeneous mass in the right breast. It is seen confined to the mammary zone. Small tumor nidus is seen in it. Echogenic calcified specks are also seen in it, which are accompanied with acoustic shadowing. On 3D imaging, multiple speculations are seen in the mass. However, no lymph node enlargement is seen. Biopsy of the mass confirms intraductal carcinoma.

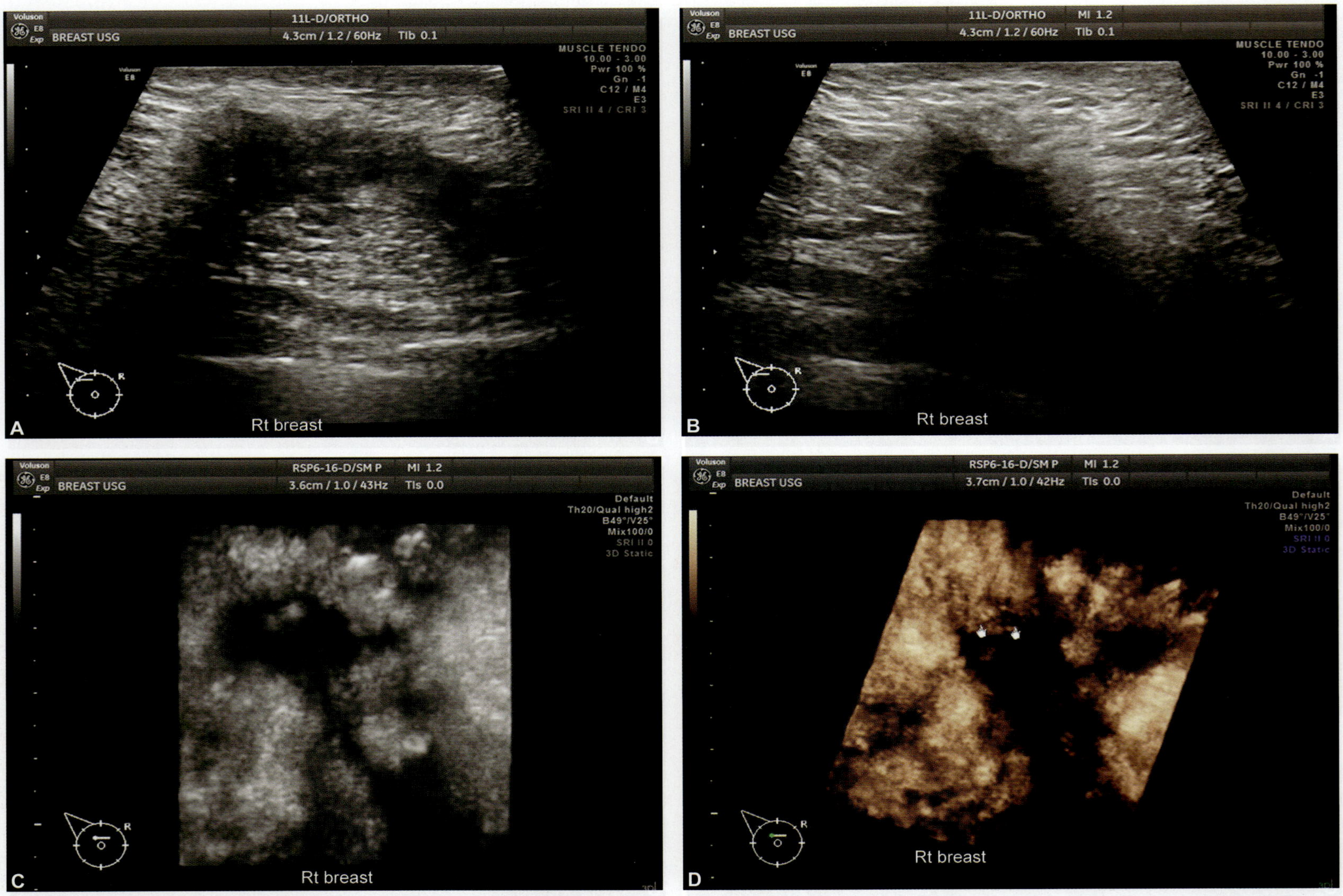

FIGURES 8.82A to D: Intraductal carcinoma. A patient presented with a solid lump in the right breast at 1 o'clock position. HRSG shows a big irregular soft tissue mass in the right breast. Echogenic microcalcification is also seen in the mass. Small tumor nidus is also seen in the mass, which is seen clearly on 3D imaging. It shows strong acoustic shadowing. Multiple lobulations are seen in the mass. Biopsy of the mass confirms intraductal carcinoma.

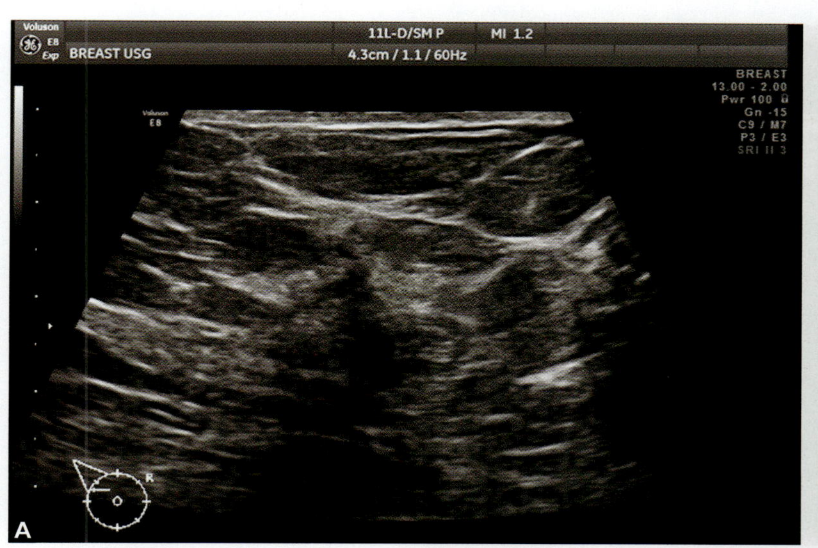

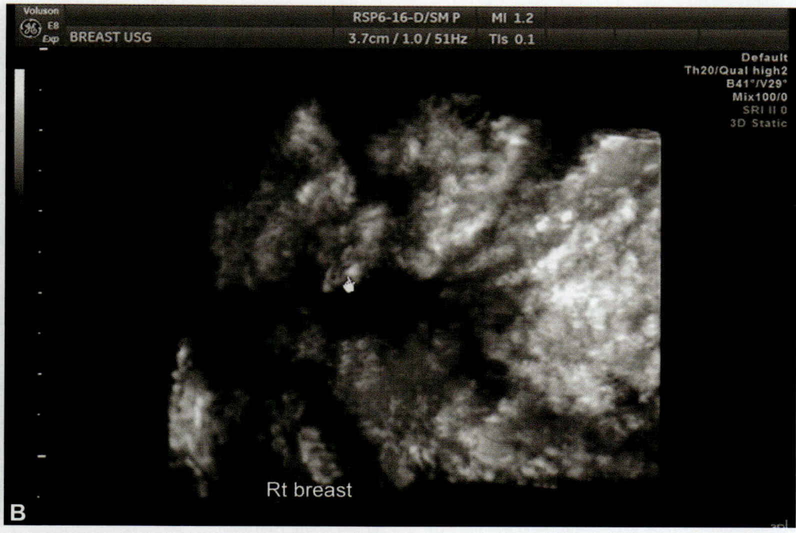

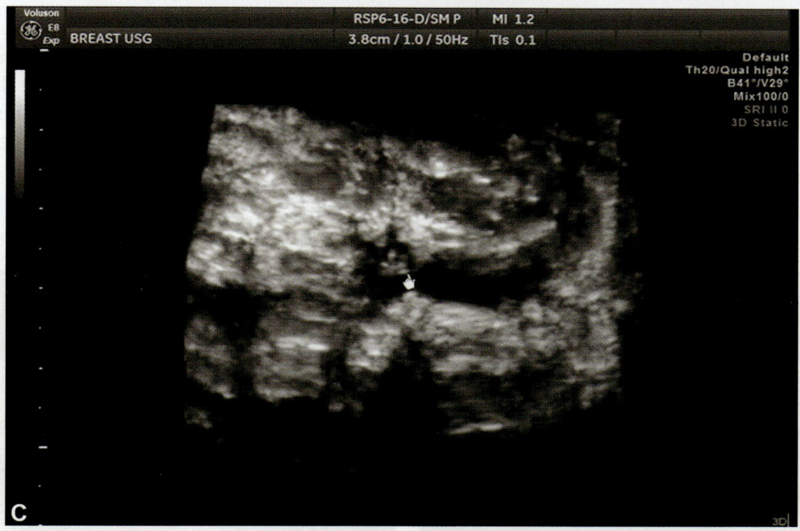

FIGURES 8.83A to C: A patient presented with small nodular shadow in right breast. HRSG shows a small irregular ill-defined mass in the right breast. 3D imaging shows microcalcification. Multiple speculations are also seen in the mass. The tumor nidus is seen in the mass. Biopsy of the mass confirms carcinoma breast.

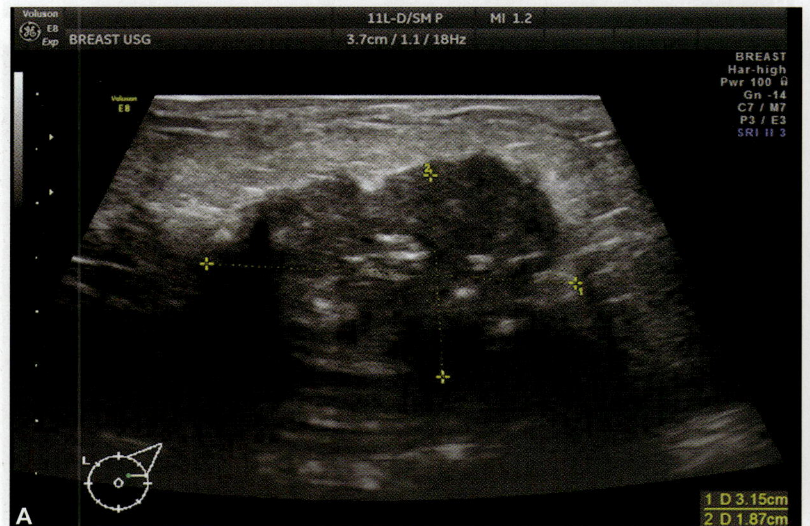

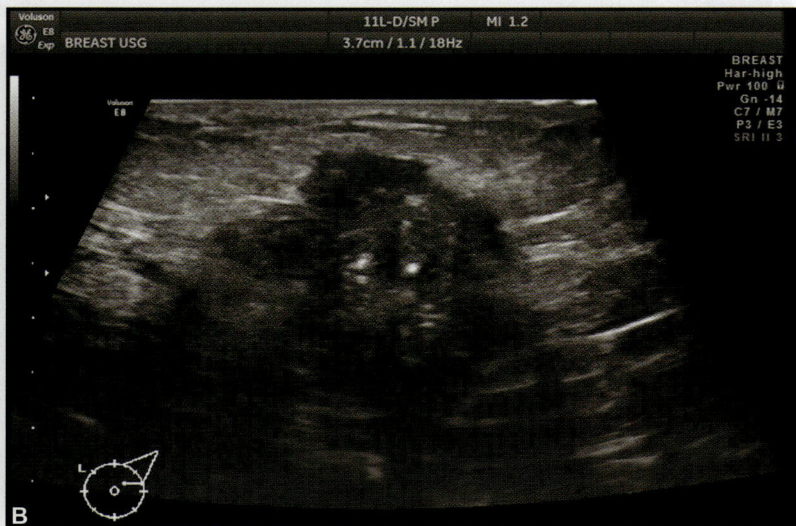

FIGURES 8.84A and B

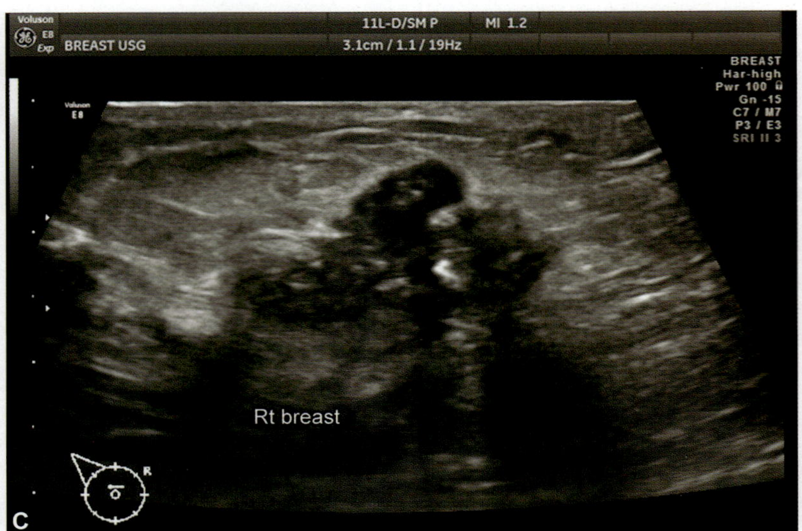

FIGURE 8.84C

FIGURES 8.84A to C: Carcinoma breast invading the chest wall. A patient presented with hard lump in the left breast. On clinical examination it appears to be fixed with the chest wall. HRSG shows a big irregular ill-defined heterogeneous mass in the left breast. Multiple echogenic specks are seen in the mass suggestive of microcalcification. Multiple lobulations are also seen in the mass. The mass is seen invading the retromammary zone and also the chest wall muscles. Biopsy of the mass confirms highly invasive intraductal carcinoma breast.

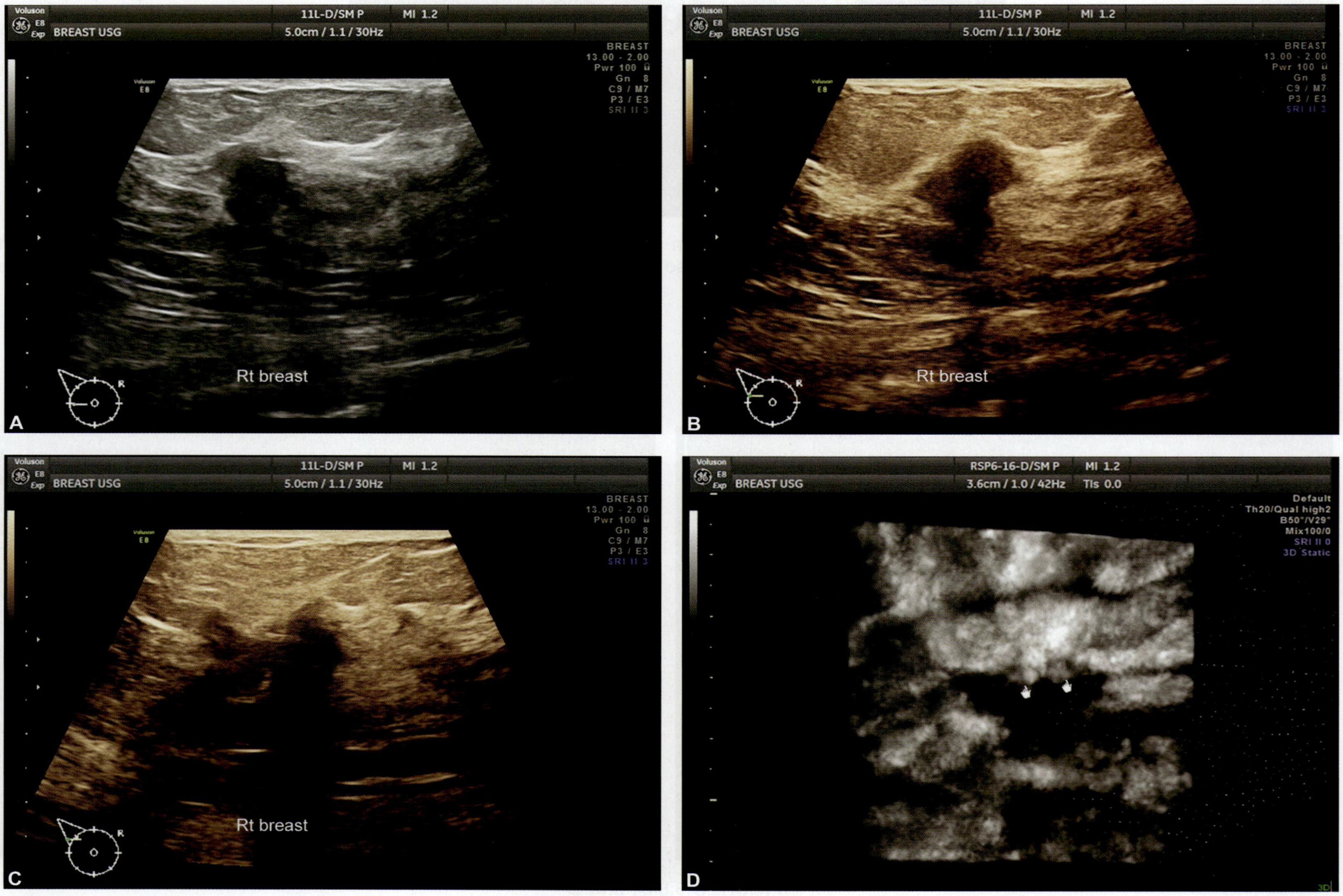

FIGURES 8.85A to D

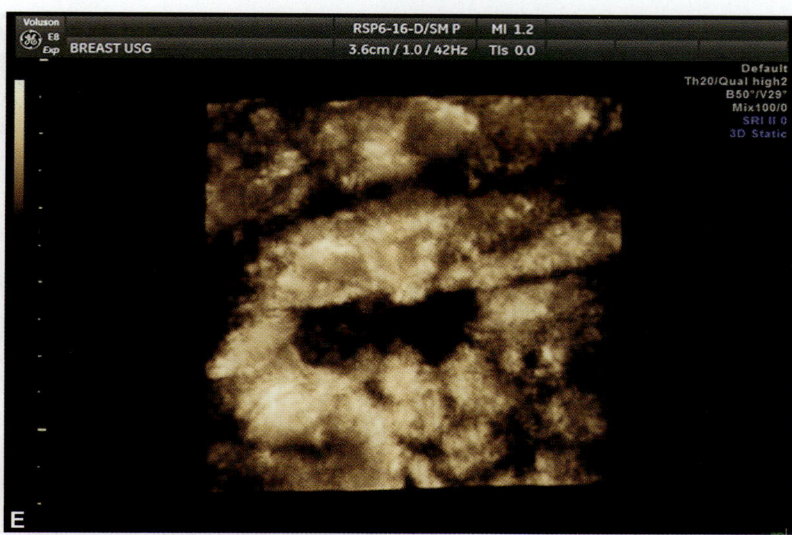

FIGURE 8.85E

FIGURES 8.85A to E: Nonpalpable breast carcinoma. A patient presented with irregularity in the right breast at 9 and 10 o'clock position. But no lump was palpable. HRSG shows an irregular heterogeneous mass in the right breast at 9 and 10 o'clock position. It is 4 cm away from areola. Echogenic foci are seen in it. Two tumor nidus are seen in the mass, which are accompanied with acoustic shadowing. The mass is confined to the mammary zone. No lymph node enlargement is seen in axilla.

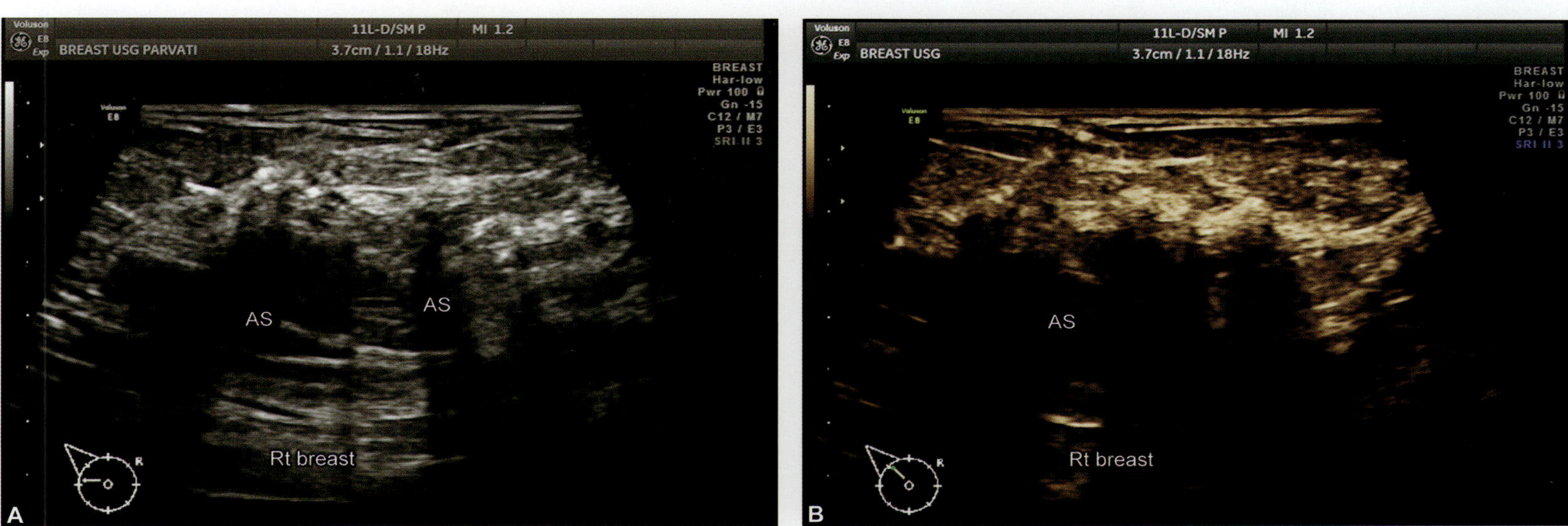

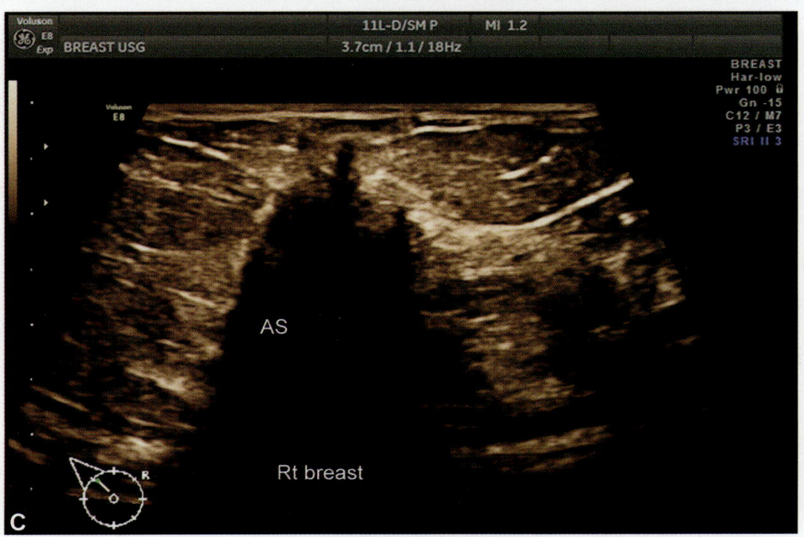

FIGURES 8.86A to C: Malignant mass in the breast. A patient presented with a hard lump in the right breast at 9 o'clock position. HRSG shows a big ill-defined irregular dirty looking mass in the right breast. Multiple echogenic specks are seen in the mass. Multiple tumor nidus are seen in the mass, which are accompanied with acoustic shadowing. Biopsy of the mass confirms invasive breast carcinoma.

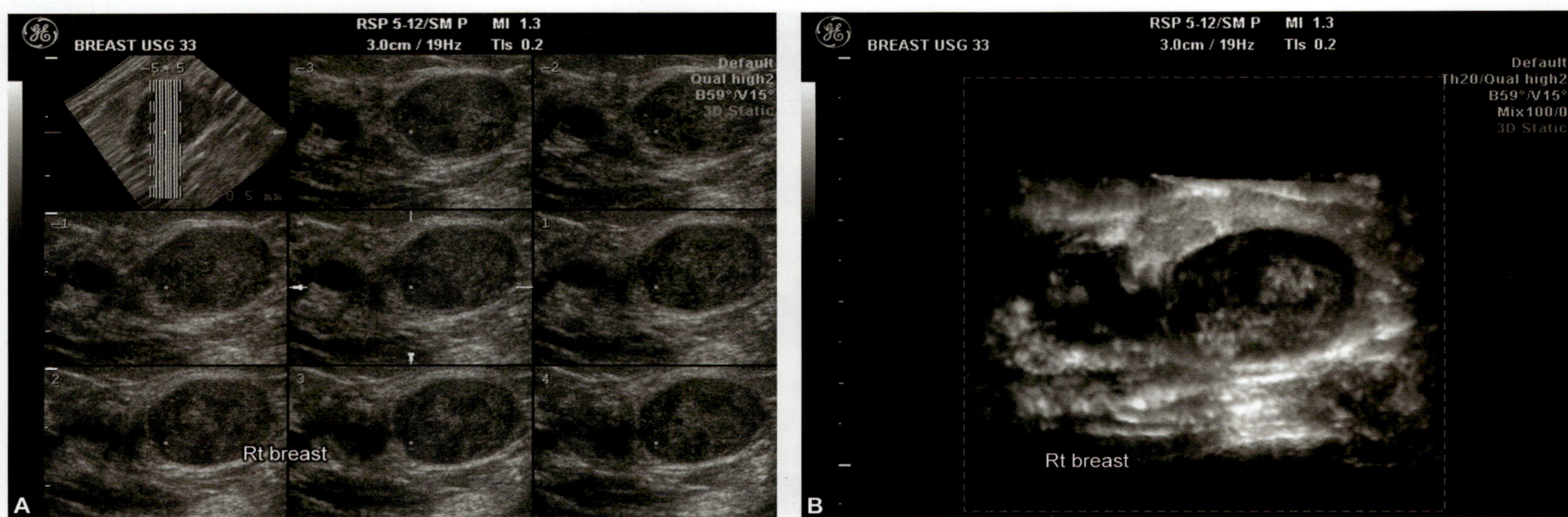

FIGURES 8.87A and B: CA breast confined to the mammary zone. A patient presented with a soft tissue mass in the right breast. The 2D imaging shows a well-defined soft tissue mass in the mammary zone at 7 o'clock position. However, on 3D volume contrast imaging heterogeneous texture of the mass is clearly seen. A small tumor nidus is seen in the mass. Biopsy of the mass confirms malignancy.

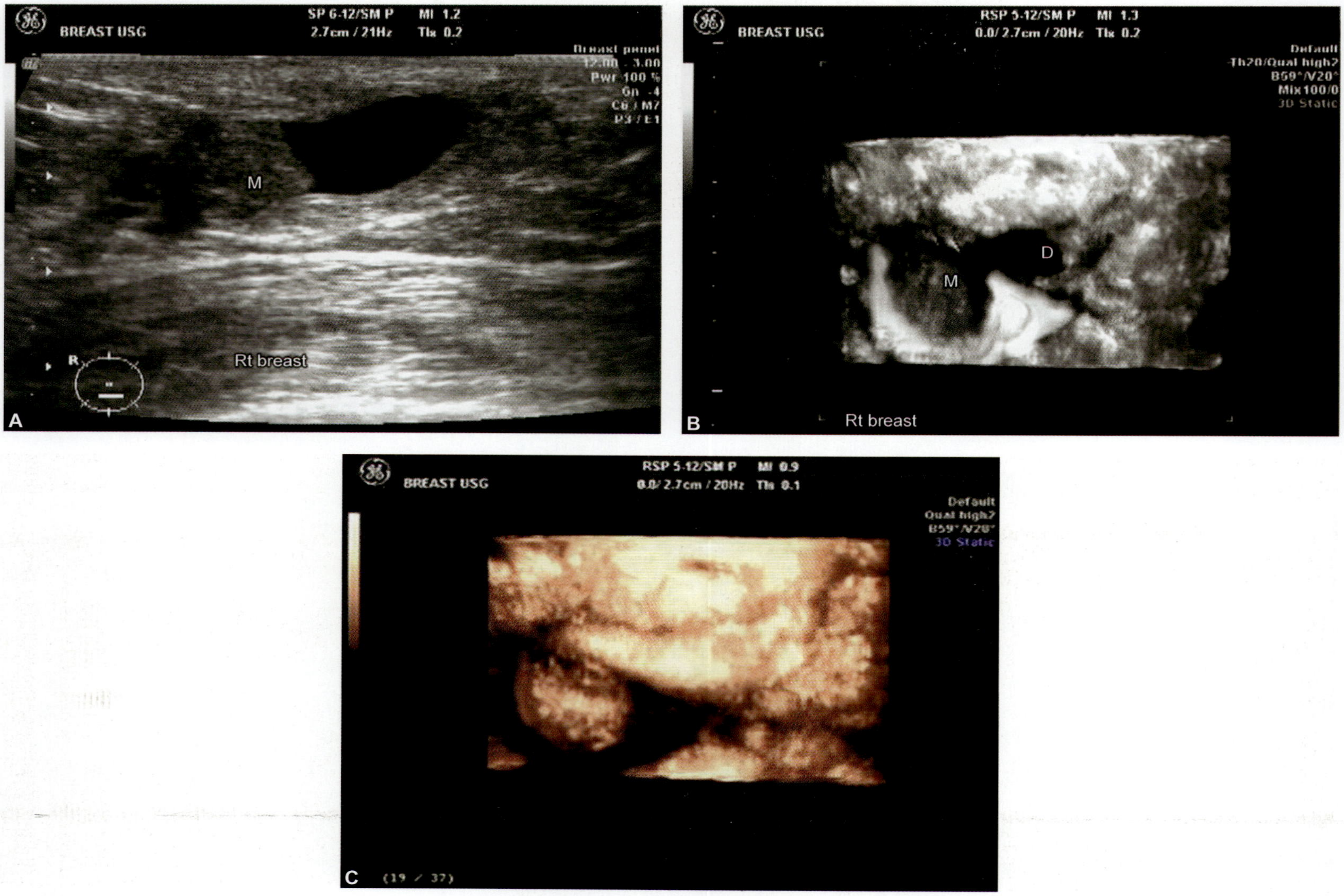

FIGURES 8.88A to C: Ductal carcinoma. A lady presented with bleeding from the nipple in right breast. HRSG shows dilated duct at 6 o'clock position. A soft tissue mass is seen in the duct. On 3D imaging the mass is seen invading the duct wall. Biopsy of the mass confirms intraductal CA.

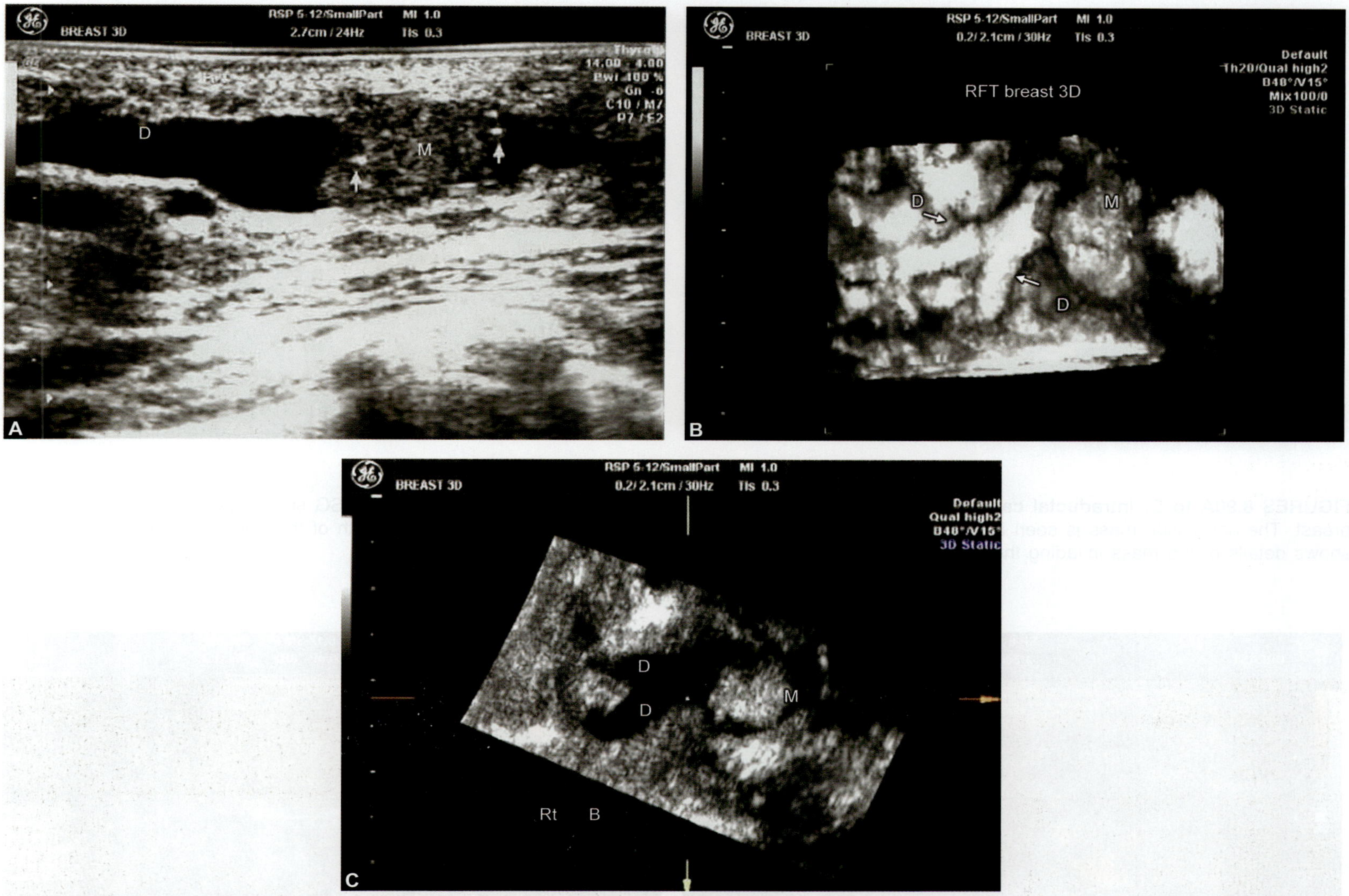

FIGURES 8.89A to C: Intraductal carcinoma. A patient presented with blood from the nipple with a palpable lump in periareolar area. HRSG shows dilated ducts in the periareolar area. A big soft issue mass is seen in one of the ducts. The duct is markedly dilated. Microcalcification is also seen in the mass. Biopsy confirmed intraductal carcinoma. 3D imaging of the same patient shows dilated ducts. The mass is seen blocking mouth of two ducts. It is clearly delineated on 3D imaging.

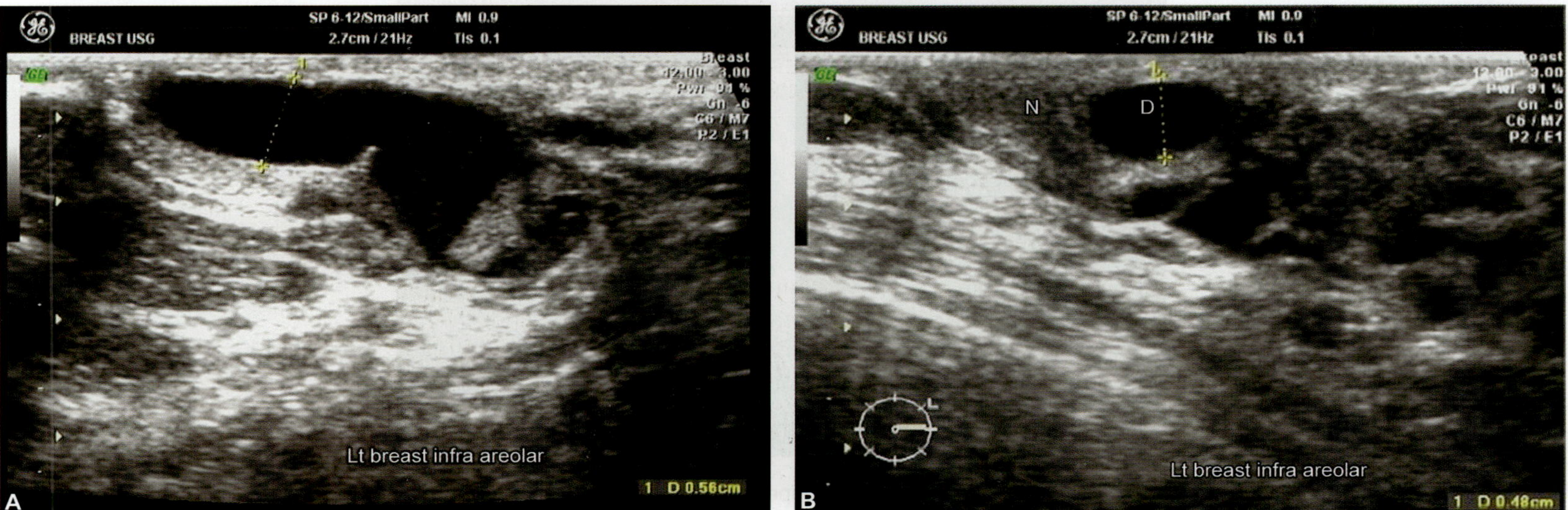

FIGURES 8.90A and B

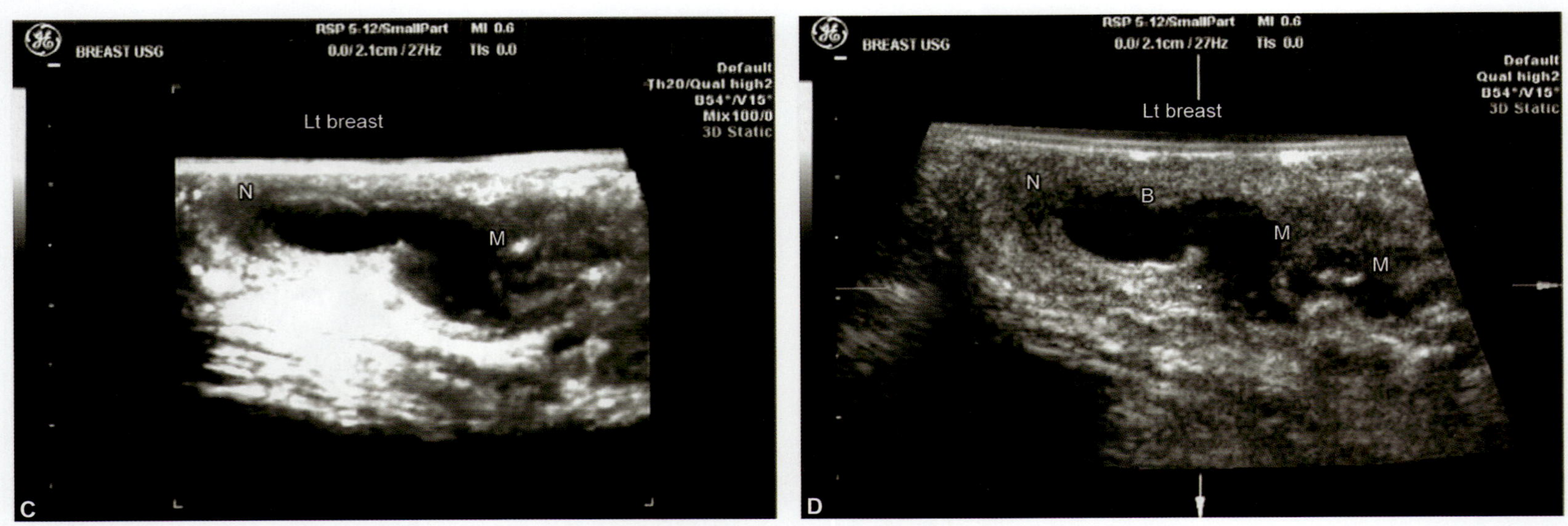

FIGURES 8.90C and D

FIGURES 8.90A to D: Intraductal carcinoma. A patient presented with blood discharge from the nipple. HRSG shows grossly dilated ducts in the breast. The soft tissue mass is seen in the duct. The mass is seen invading the duct and blocking the mouth of the duct. 3D imaging of the mass shows details of the mass invading the duct.

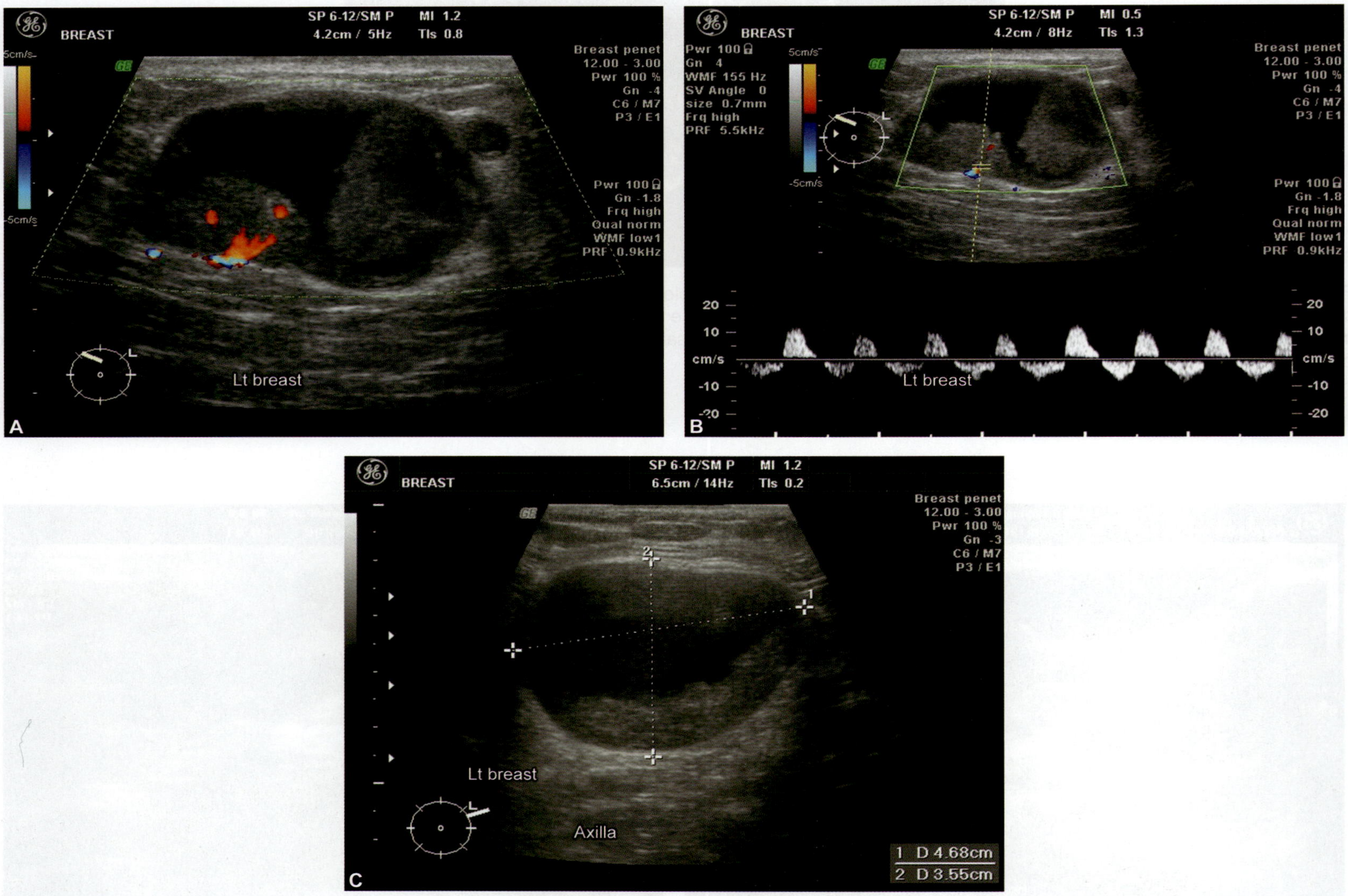

FIGURES 8.91A to C: A patient presented with lump in the left breast upper and inner quadrant. HRSG shows a heterogeneous mass in the breast, which measures 45 x 25 mm in size. Cystic necrosis is seen in the mass. But no calcification is seen. **On color flow imaging**, few vessels are seen feeding the mass. There is also evidence of another dilated duct seen in periareolar area. It runs from 11 o'colock position to areola measuring 5 mm in caliber. Soft tissue mass is seen in the duct. Few hypoechoic masses are seen at 2 o'clock position in the left breast. A big cystic mass is seen in the left axilla. The mass measures 45 x 35 mm in size. Central area of necrosis is seen in it. Biopsy confirms necrotizing carcinoma breast.

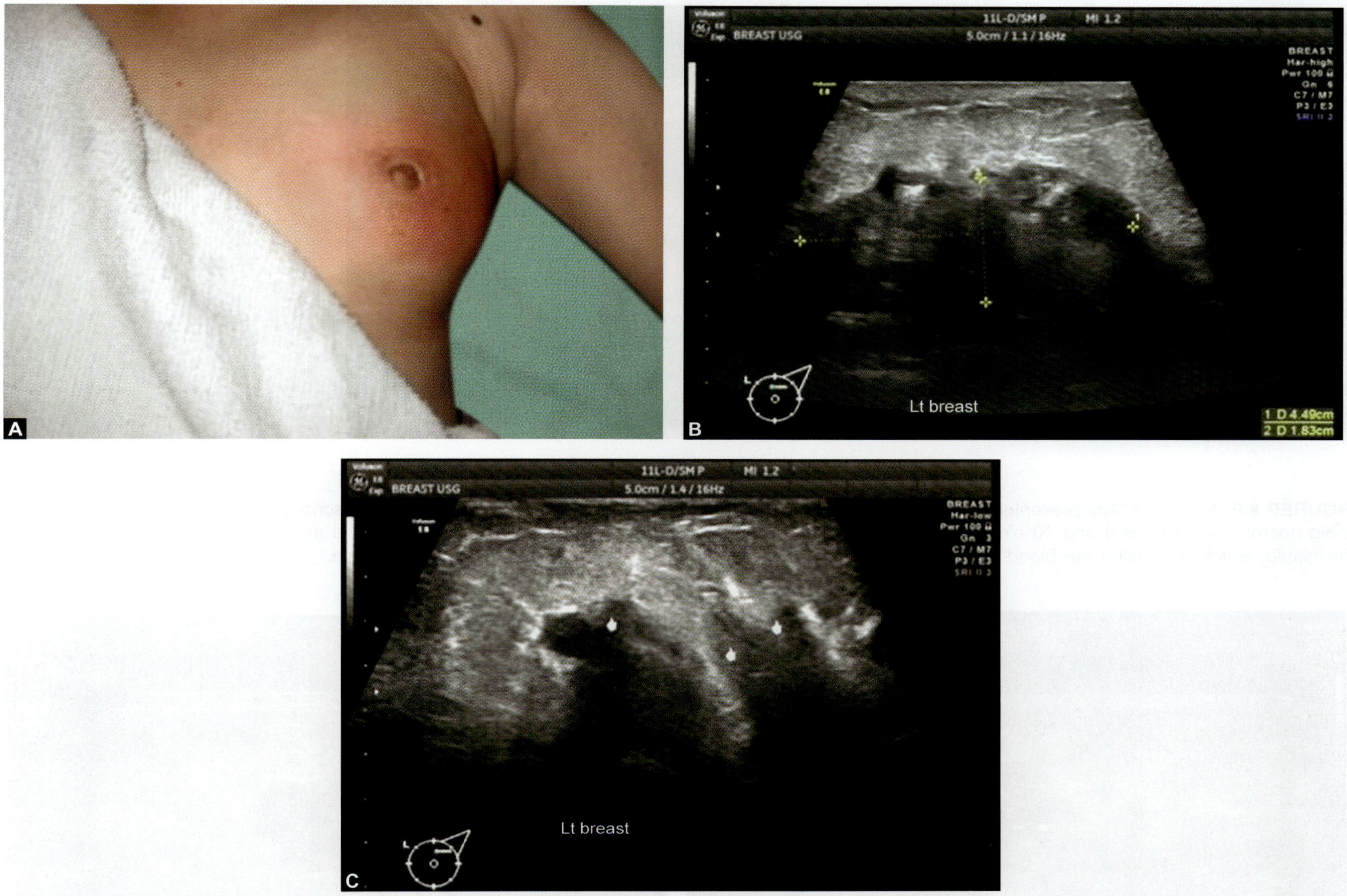

FIGURES 8.92A to C: Inflammatory carcinoma breast. A patient presented with red hot left breast. HRSG shows big irregular ill-defined heterogeneous mass in the left breast. Margins are shaggy. Hypoechoic areas are seen in the mass. Echogenic calcified specks are also seen in the mass suggestive of microcalcification. Multiple focal tumor nidus are seen in the mass, which are accompanied with acoustic shadowing. Biopsy of the mass confirms inflammatory intraductal carcinoma.

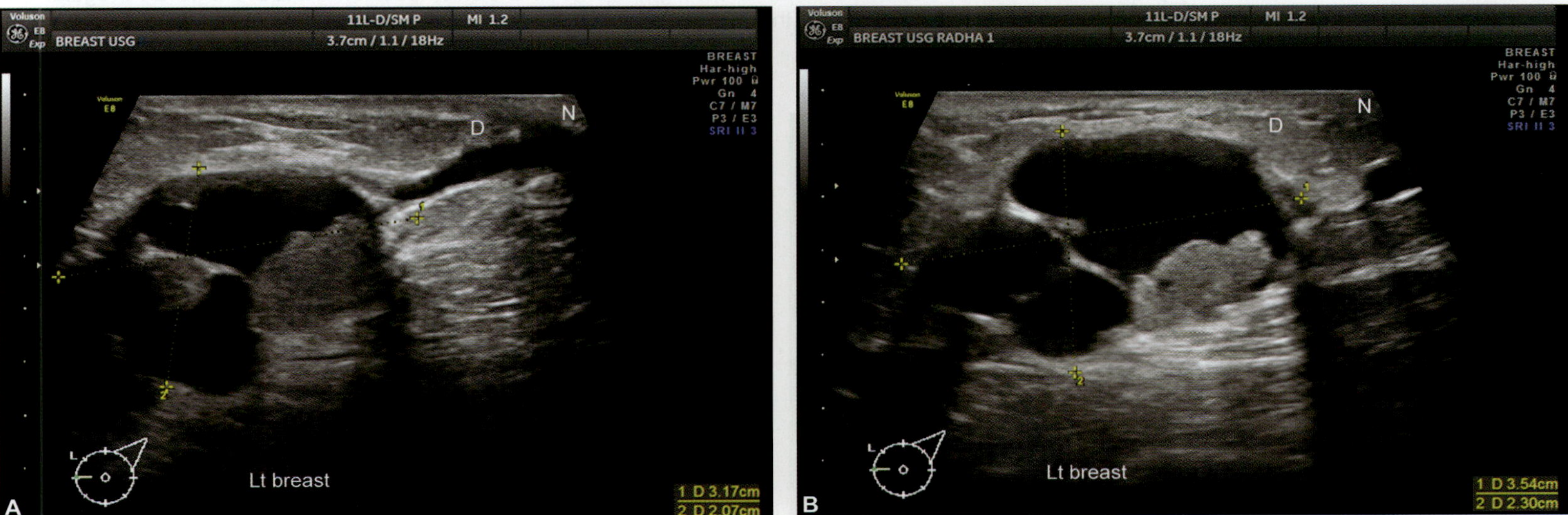

FIGURES 8.93A and B

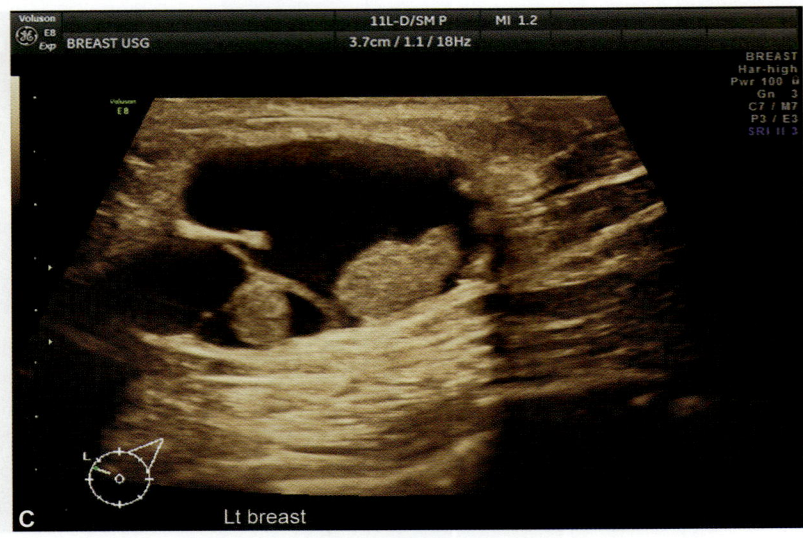

FIGURE 8.93C

FIGURES 8.93A to C: A lady presented with mass in the left breast at 9 o'clock position. She also had blood discharge from the nipple. HRSG shows a big necrotizing mass at 9 and 10 o'clock position. Soft tissue masses are seen in the mass. A dilated duct is also seen running from the mass to the nipple, which is causing the blood discharge. Biopsy of the mass confirms necrotizing intraductal carcinoma.

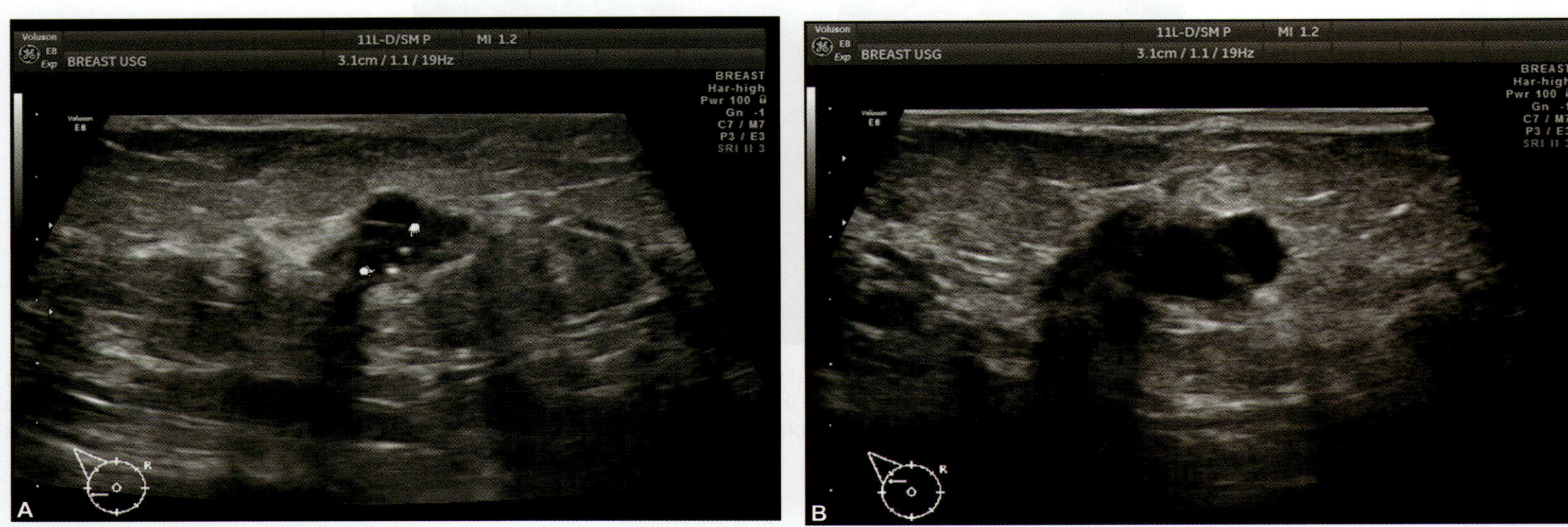

FIGURES 8.94A and B: An old lady presented with small nodular shadow in the right breast at 8 o'clock position. HRSG shows an irregular mass confined to the mammary zone. Echogenic microcalcification is seen in the mass. Small tumor nidus is also seen in it, which is accompanied with acoustic shadowing. Biopsy of the mass confirms intraductal carcinoma.

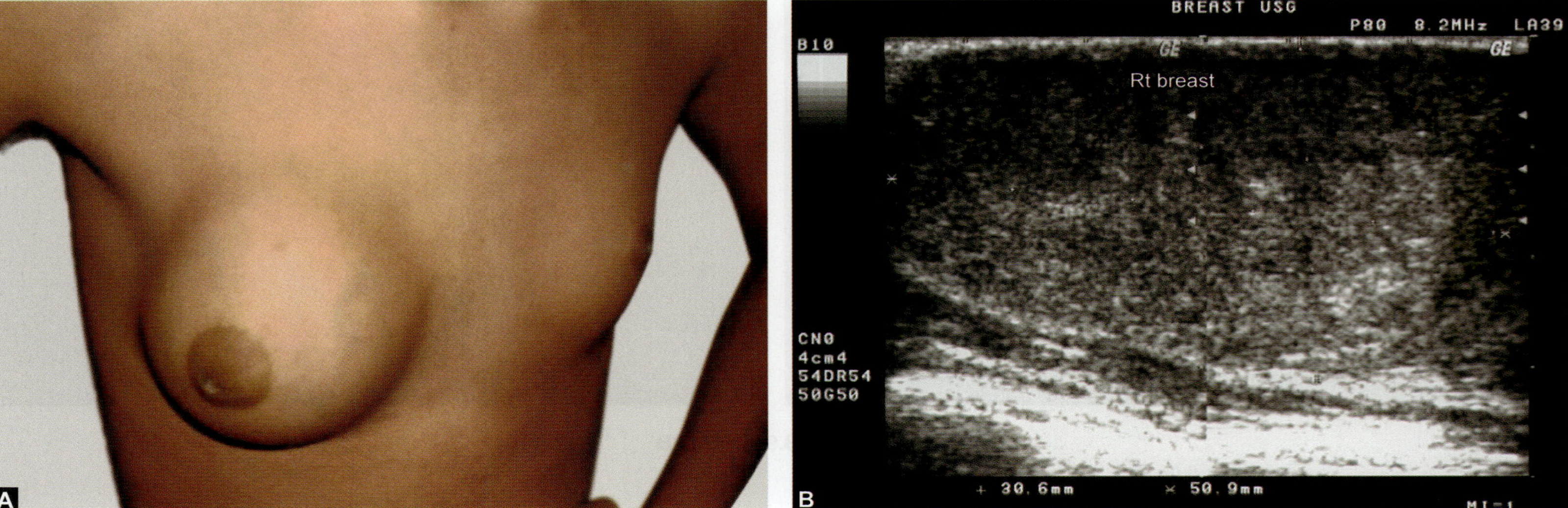

FIGURES 8.95A and B

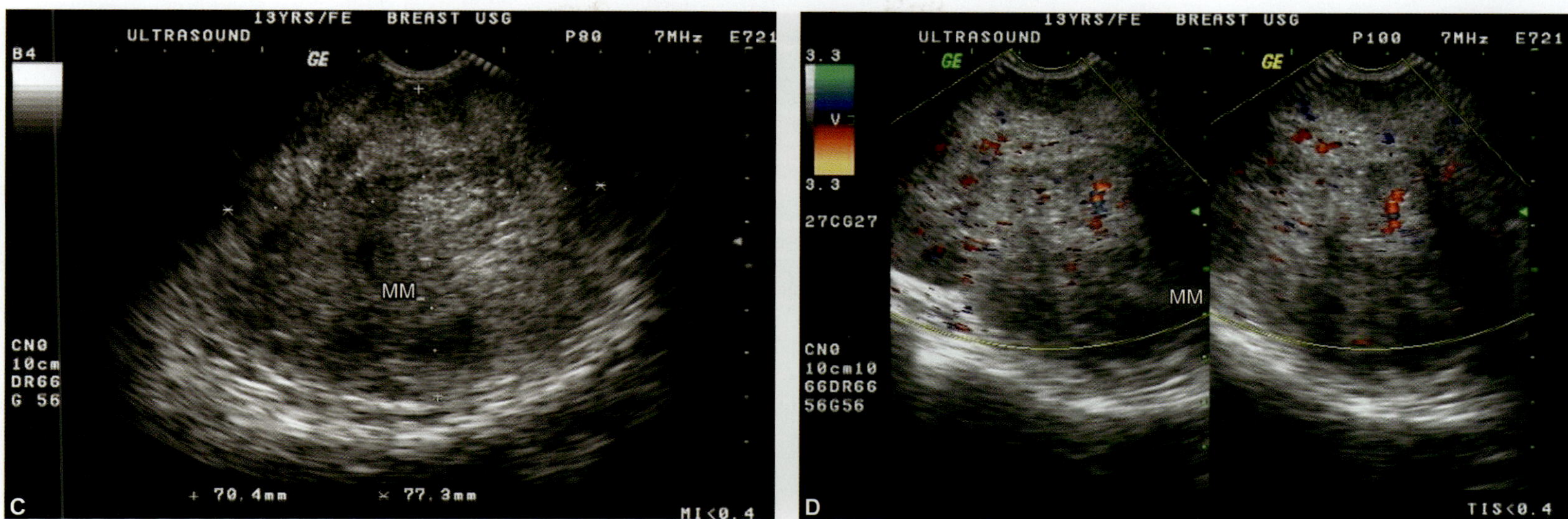

FIGURES 8.95C and D

FIGURES 8.95A to D: Breast sarcoma. A 13-year-old young girl presented with soft tissue mass in the right breast. The mass was slowly growing and it was not painful. HRSG shows a big soft tissue mass in the breast. Normal texture of the breast is lost. However, it is homogeneous in texture. No calcification is seen in it. No cystic degeneration is seen. Biopsy of the mass confirmed breast sarcoma.: On color flow imaging, low flow was seen in the mass.

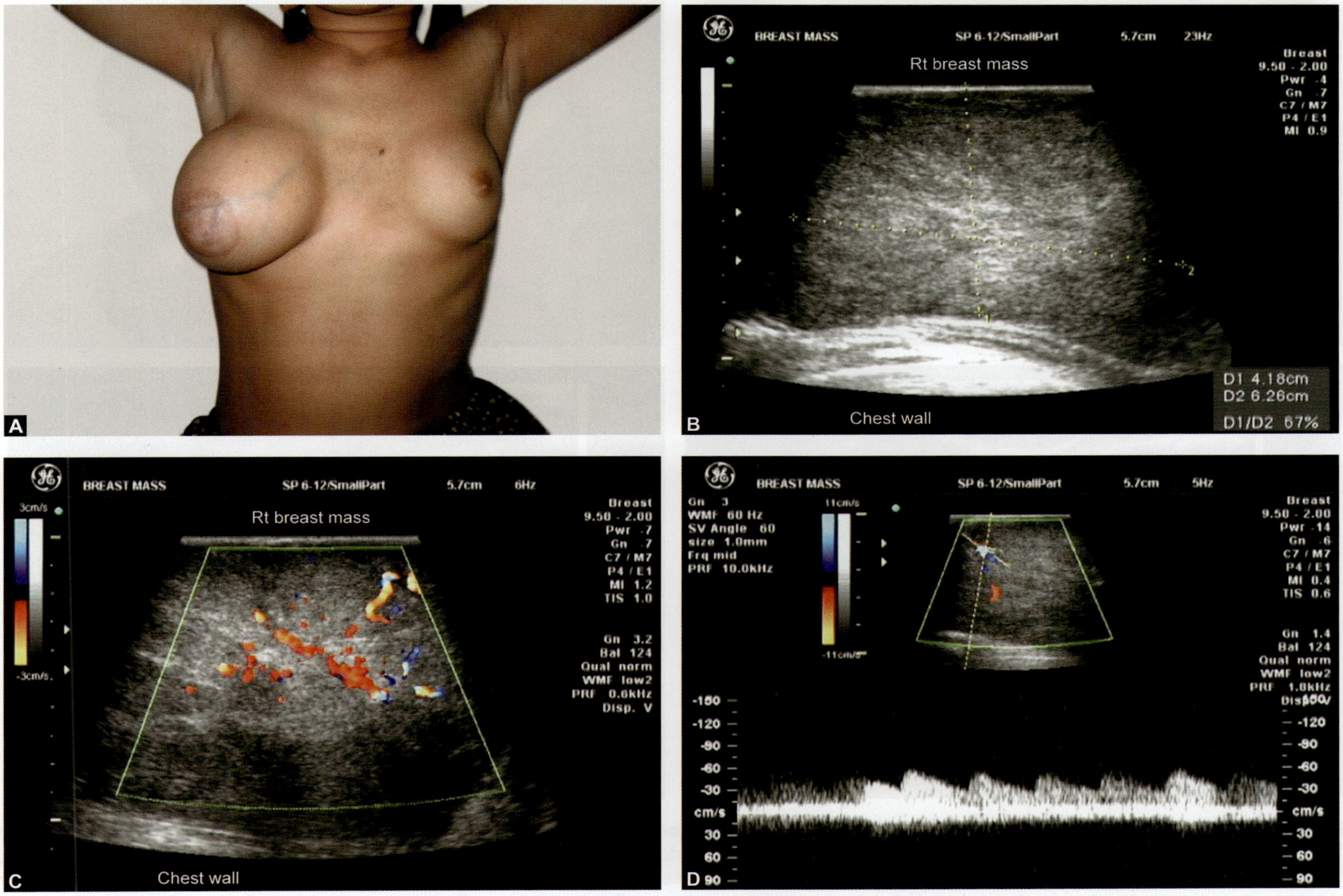

FIGURES 8.96A to D

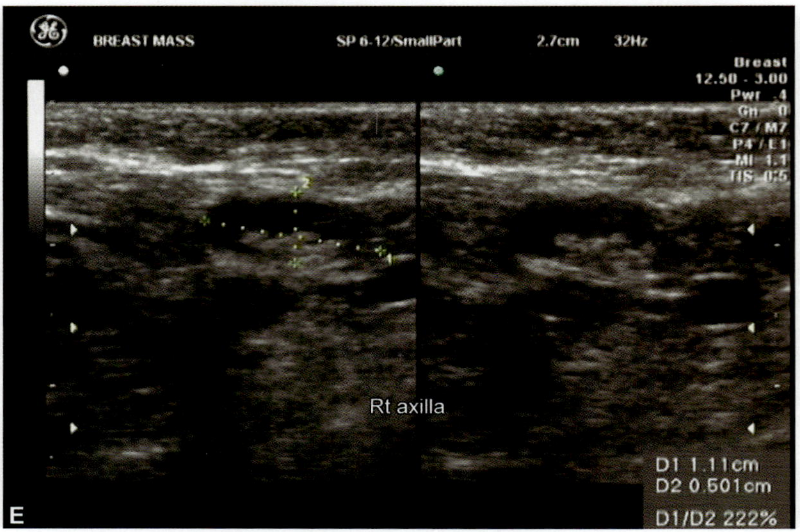

FIGURE 8.96E

FIGURES 8.96A to E: Sarcoma breast. A 12-year-old girl presented big mass in the right breast. The mass was rapidly growing. Venous congestion is also seen on the surface of the breast. HRSG shows big mass in the breast. Normal breast texture is lost. The mass is seen fixed with the chest wall. However, it is homogeneous in texture. **On color flow imaging,** multiple vessels are seen feeding the mass. **On spectral Doppler tracing** moderate flow seen in the mass. The right axilla also shows enlarged nodes with malignant changes in the nodes.

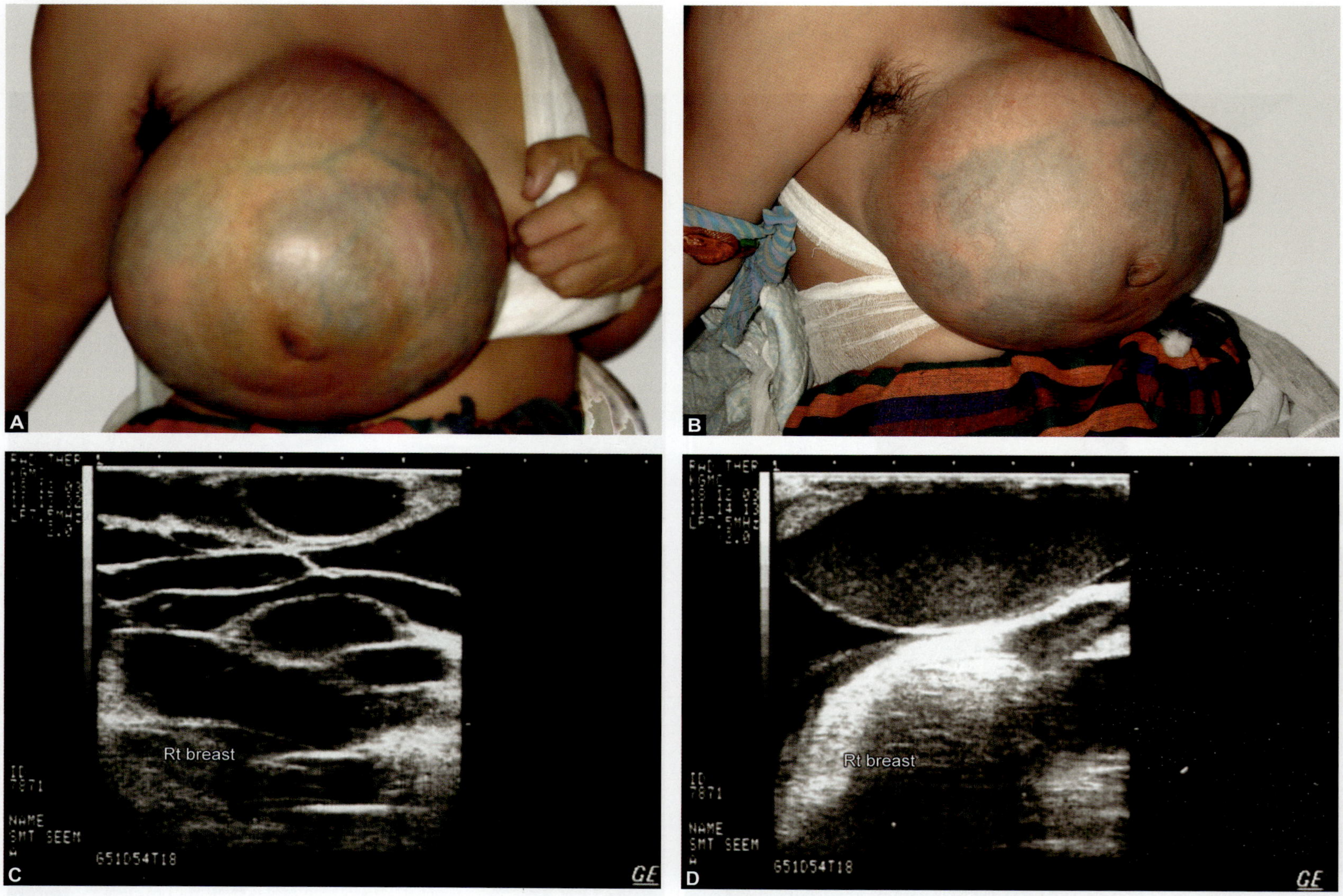

FIGURES 8.97A to D: Huge sarcoma breast. A 22-year-old girl presented with rapidly increasing mass in the breast. The mass is seen whole of the anterior chest wall. It is seen grossly enlarged and hanging. The surface of the mass shows multiple dilated veins. HRSG shows a big mass in the breast with predominantly solid texture. Few cystic areas are also seen in the mass with echogenic septa due to big size of the mass, lower frequency transducer was used for evaluation of tumor mass. High-resolution ultrasound shows the cystic areas in much clear detail. Multiple cysts are seen in the solid tumor with fine echogenic septa. Thick collection was seen in the cysts. Biopsy of the tumor confirmed malignant sarcoma.

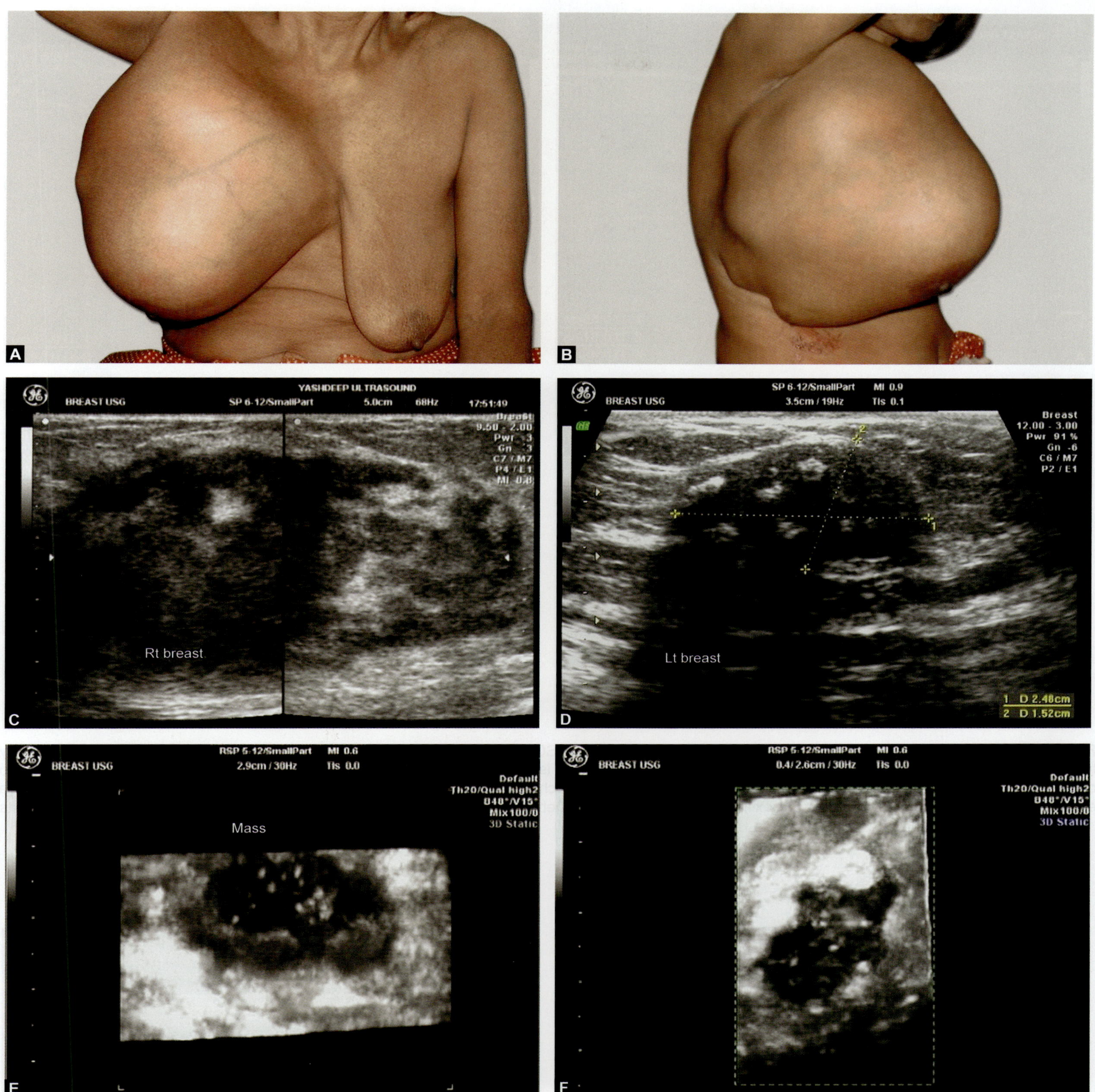

FIGURES 8.98A to F: Phyllodes tumor. A lady presented with huge mass coming out from the right breast. The mass shows lobulated surface. It is seen extending anteroposteriorly and also going on the backside. HRSG shows big mass in the breast. The mass could not be wholly asseed on ultrasound, as it was not properly covered even on 3 MHz transducer. The details of the mass were well appreciated on HRSG. It was predominantly solid with variegated texture. Few areas show degeneration. Biopsy of the mass confirmed malignant phyllodes tumor. HRSG shows a big heterogeneous mass in the breast. It shows lobulations. Echogenic calcified shadows are also seen in the mass. They are accompanied with acoustic shadowing. **3D imaging** of the same mass shows details of the mass with multiple calcified shadows embedded in the mass. The mass shows crenated margins and it is confined to the mammary zone.

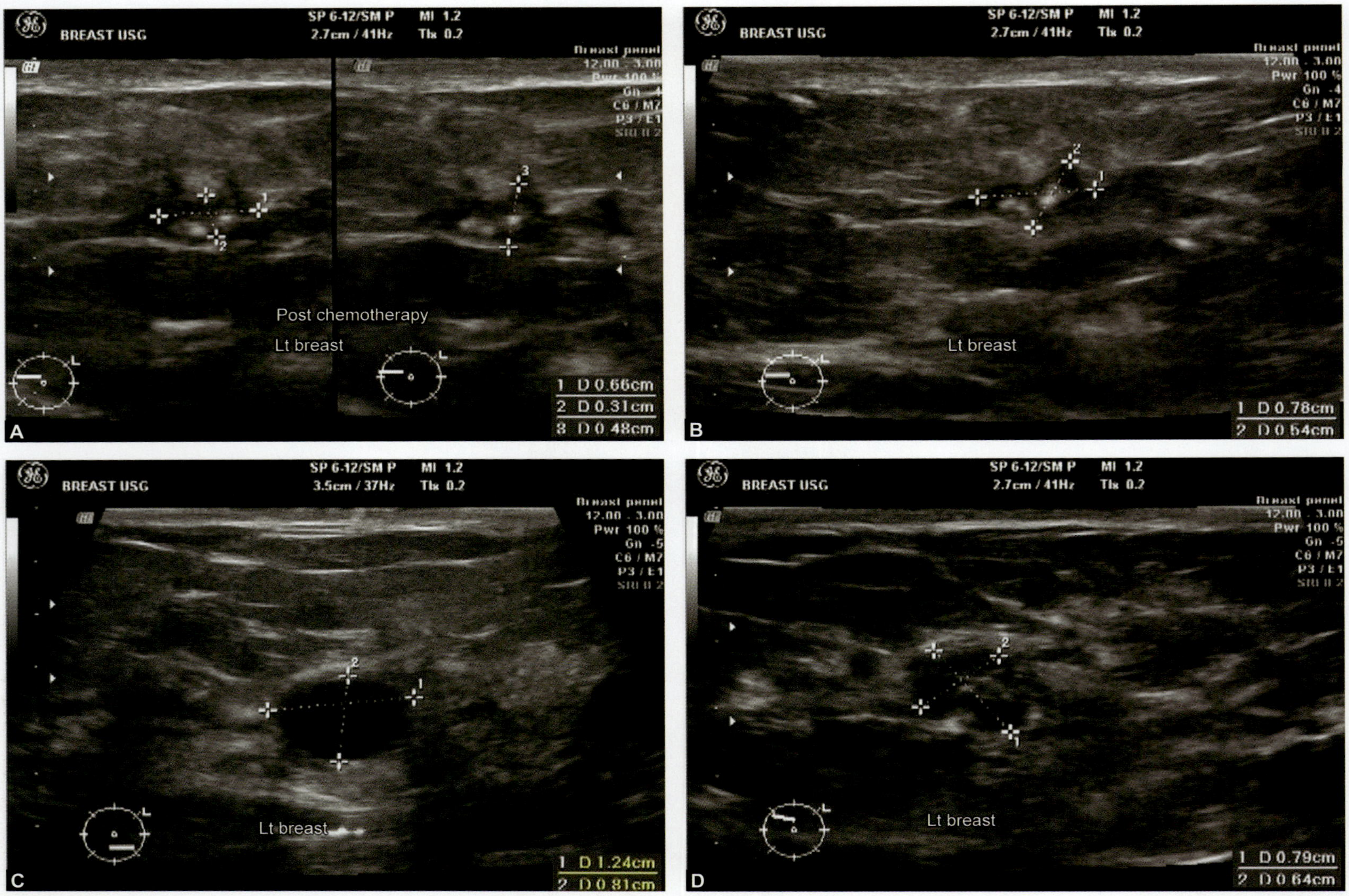

FIGURES 8.99A to D: Chemo reduction of the carcinoma breast. HRSG is very good modality for evaluation of mass after giving chemotherapy. It can give proper assessment of the mass after chemoreduction. There is evidence of an irregular ill-defined soft tissue mass seen in a patient of carcinoma breast after chemotherapy. The mass has reduced in size. Echogenic shadows are seen in the mass. But no evidence of any perifocal edema is present. The lymph nodes in the axilla also reduced in size. Debulking and chemo reduction of the mass helps into good surgical results.

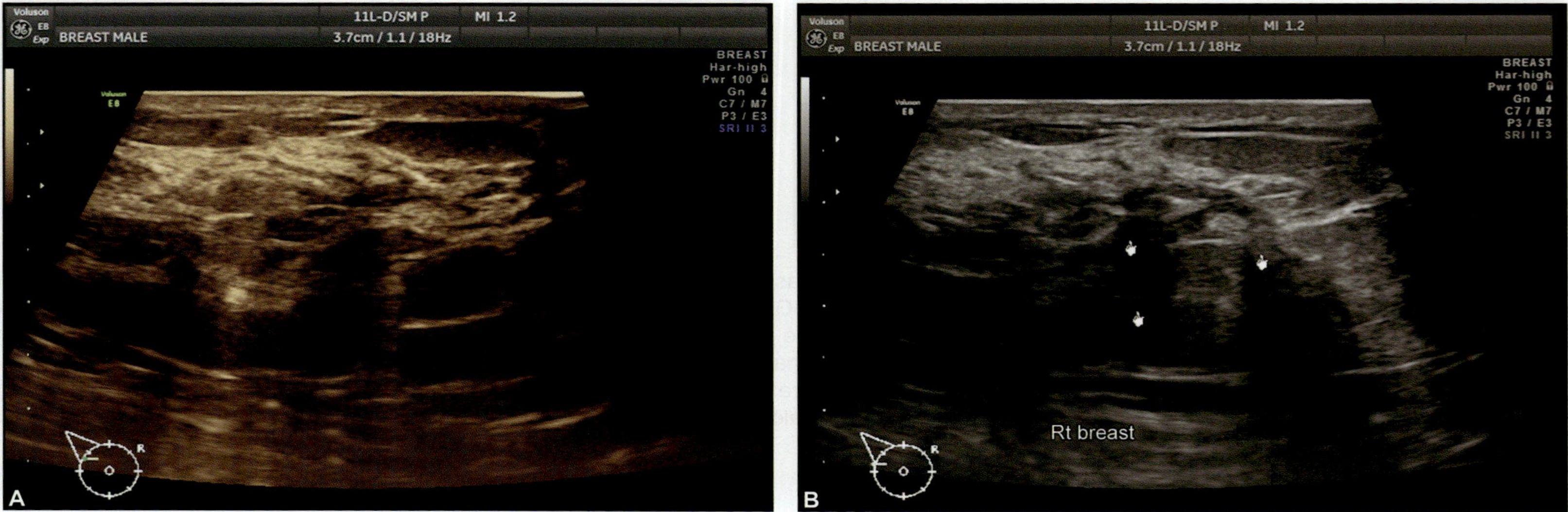

FIGURES 8.100A and B

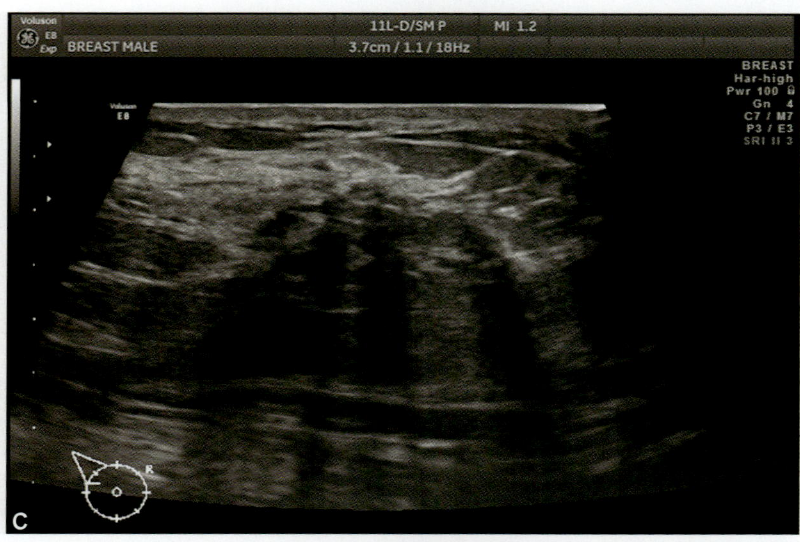

FIGURE 8.100C

FIGURES 8.100A to C: Male breast CA. A male patient presented with soft tissue mass in the right breast. HRSG shows irregular ill-defined echogenic foci seen in right breast. They are seen at 9 and 11 o'clock position in the right breast. The echogenic foci appear to be macrocalcification. They are accompanied with acoustic shadowing. Biopsy of the mass confirms carcinoma breast.

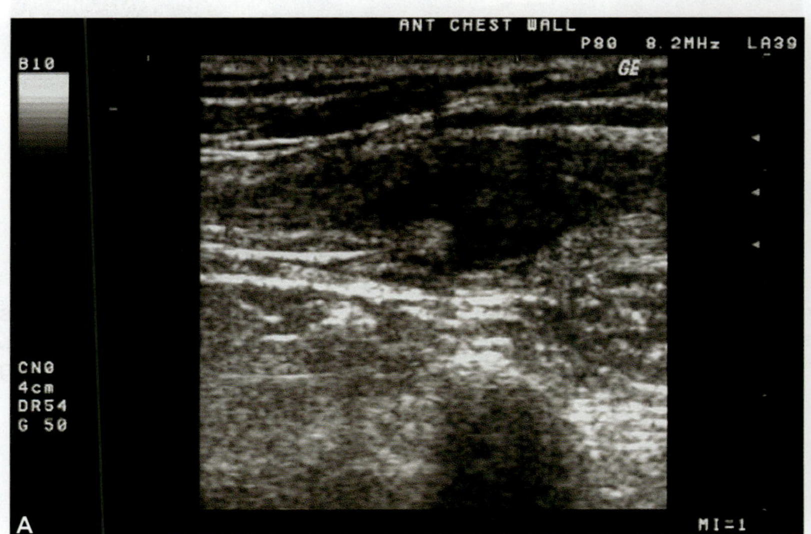

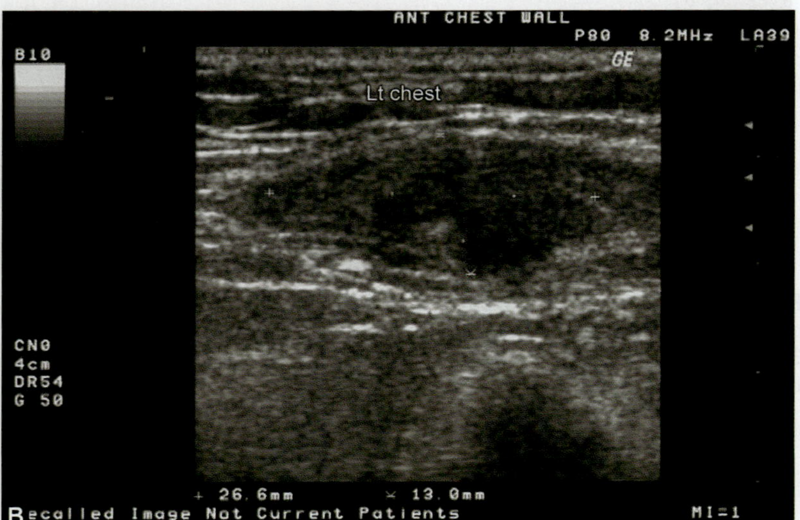

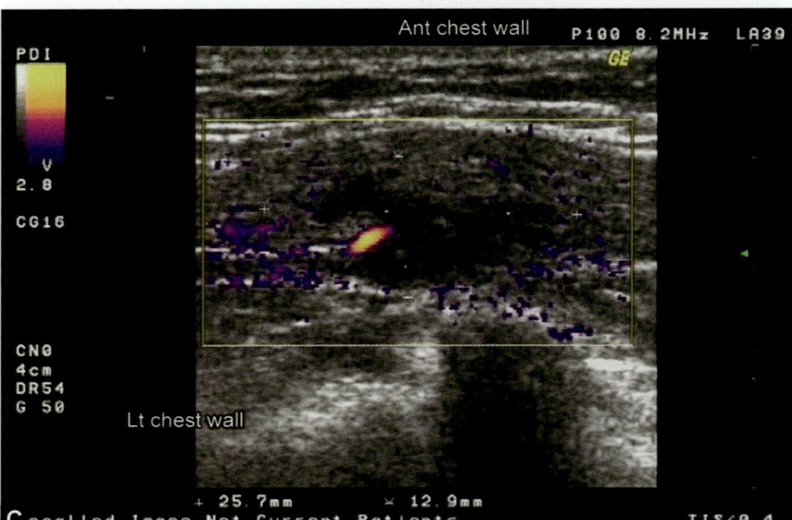

FIGURES 8.101A to C: Male breast carcinoma. A patient presented with irregular lump in the periareolar area. HRSG shows heterogeneous irregular mass in the periareolar area. **On color flow imaging**, vessel is seen feeding the mass. Biopsy of the mass confirmed carcinoma breast.

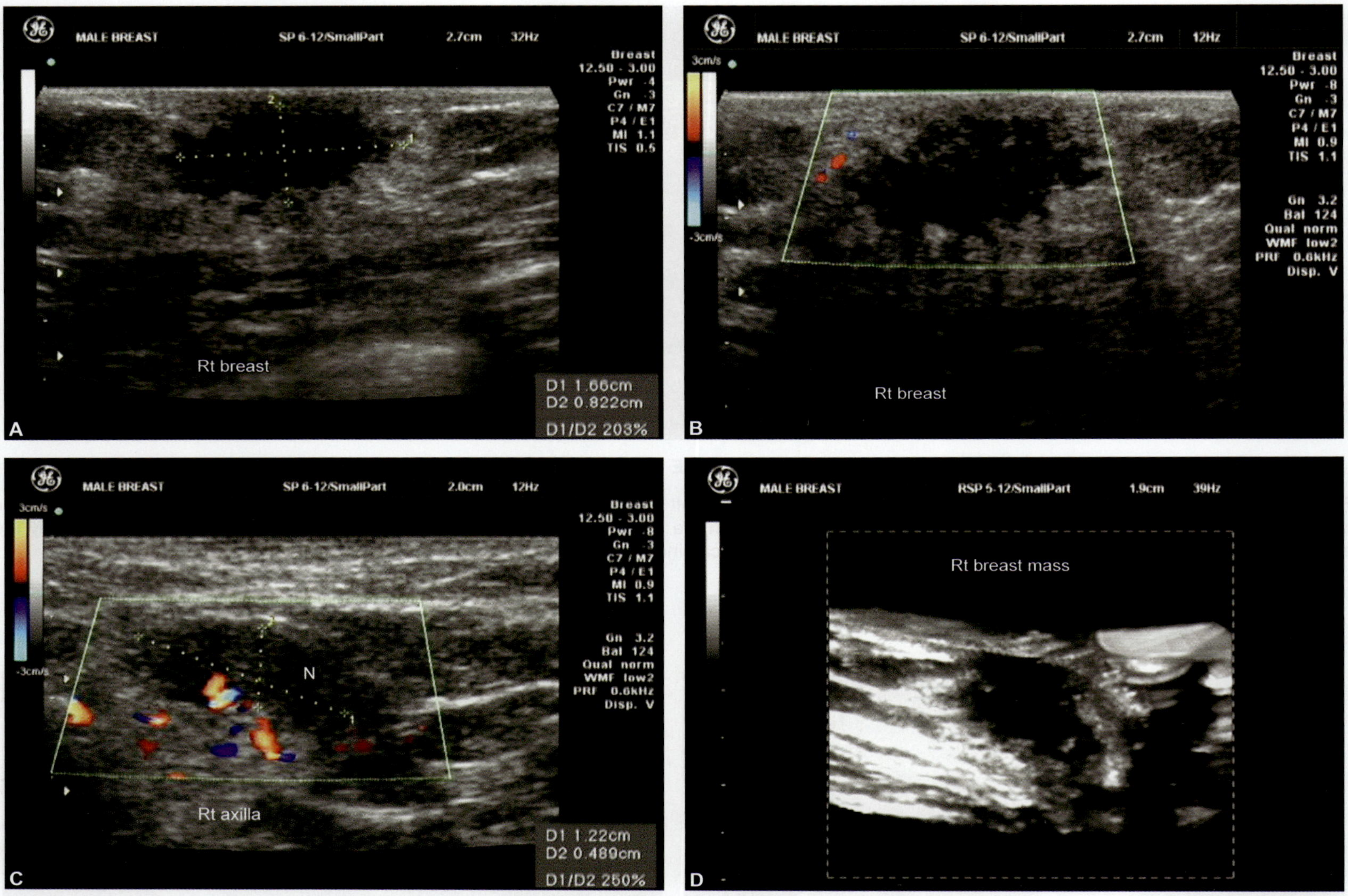

FIGURES 8.102A to D: Carcinoma male breast. An old man presented with heterogeneous mass in the right breast periareolar area. HRSG shows irregular heterogeneous mass in the subareolar region. The mass shows branching pattern running in all the directions. Biopsy confirmed carcinoma. **3D imaging** of the mass shows details of the invasion of the mass in the chest muscle. **On color flow imaging**, multiple vessels are seen feeding the mass.

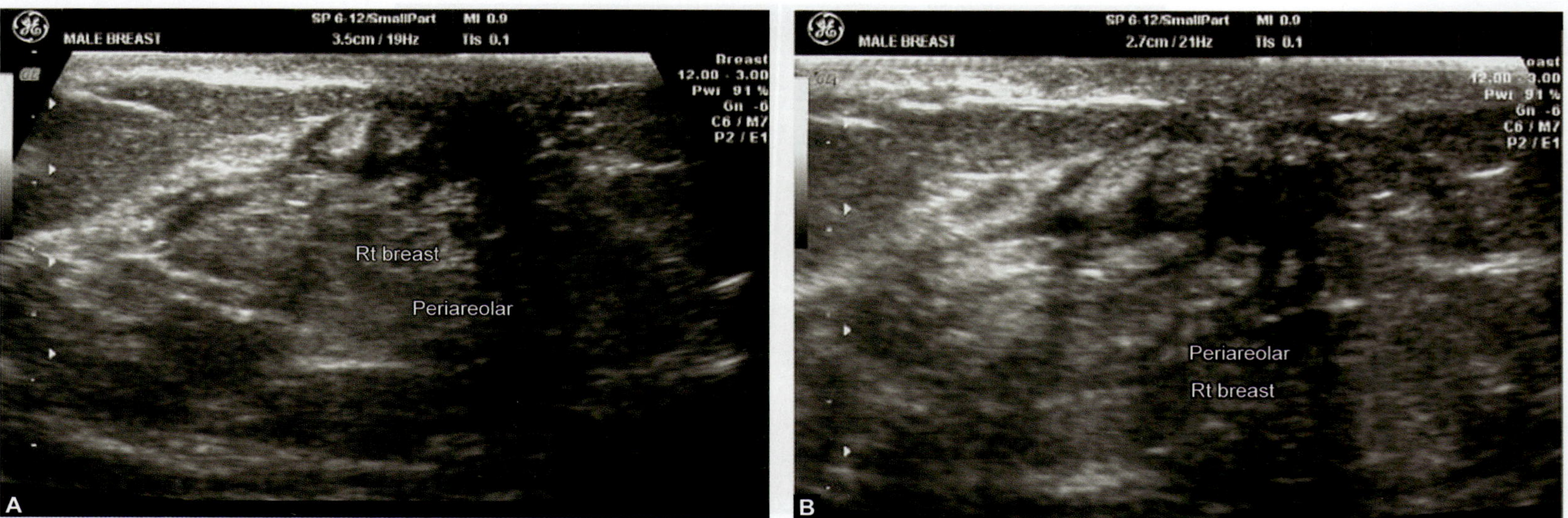

FIGURES 8.103A and B

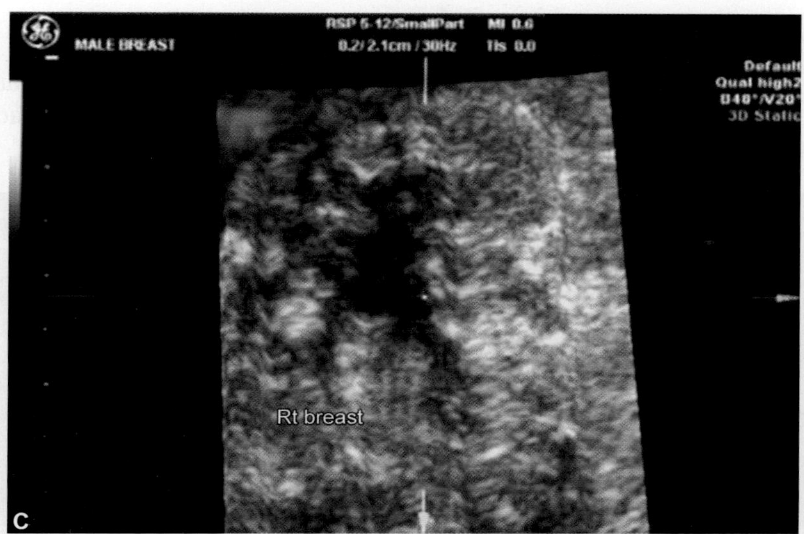

FIGURE 8.103C

FIGURES 8.103A to C: Carcinoma male breast. An old patient presented with irregular heterogeneous mass in the right breast in periareolar area. HRSG shows irregular heterogeneous mass in the periareolar area. Multiple branches are seen coming out from the mass. The mass is seen areolar tissue and invading the chest wall muscle. **3D imaging** of the mass shows typical branching pattern of malignant mass.

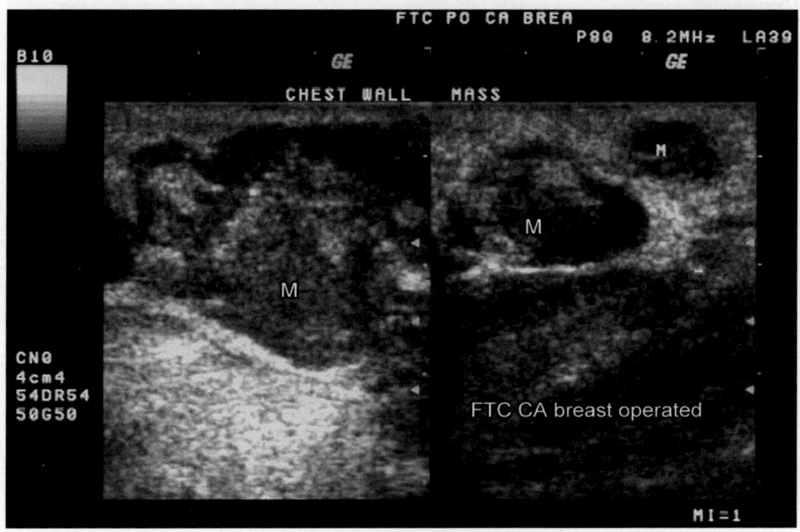

FIGURE 8.104: Recurrence of operated carcinoma breast. HRSG shows multiple irregular heterogeneous mass over the right chest wall in an operated case of carcinoma breast. Chest wall muscle invasion is also seen.

BREAST IMPLANT

High-resolution sonography (HRSG) is very good for evaluation of breast implant, which are used for augmentation of breast for cosmetic value and also after breast surgery. HRSG can show implant in position as anechoic fluid containing sac. The 3D imaging shows the global view of implant. HRSG is also very good for evaluation of rupture of implant.

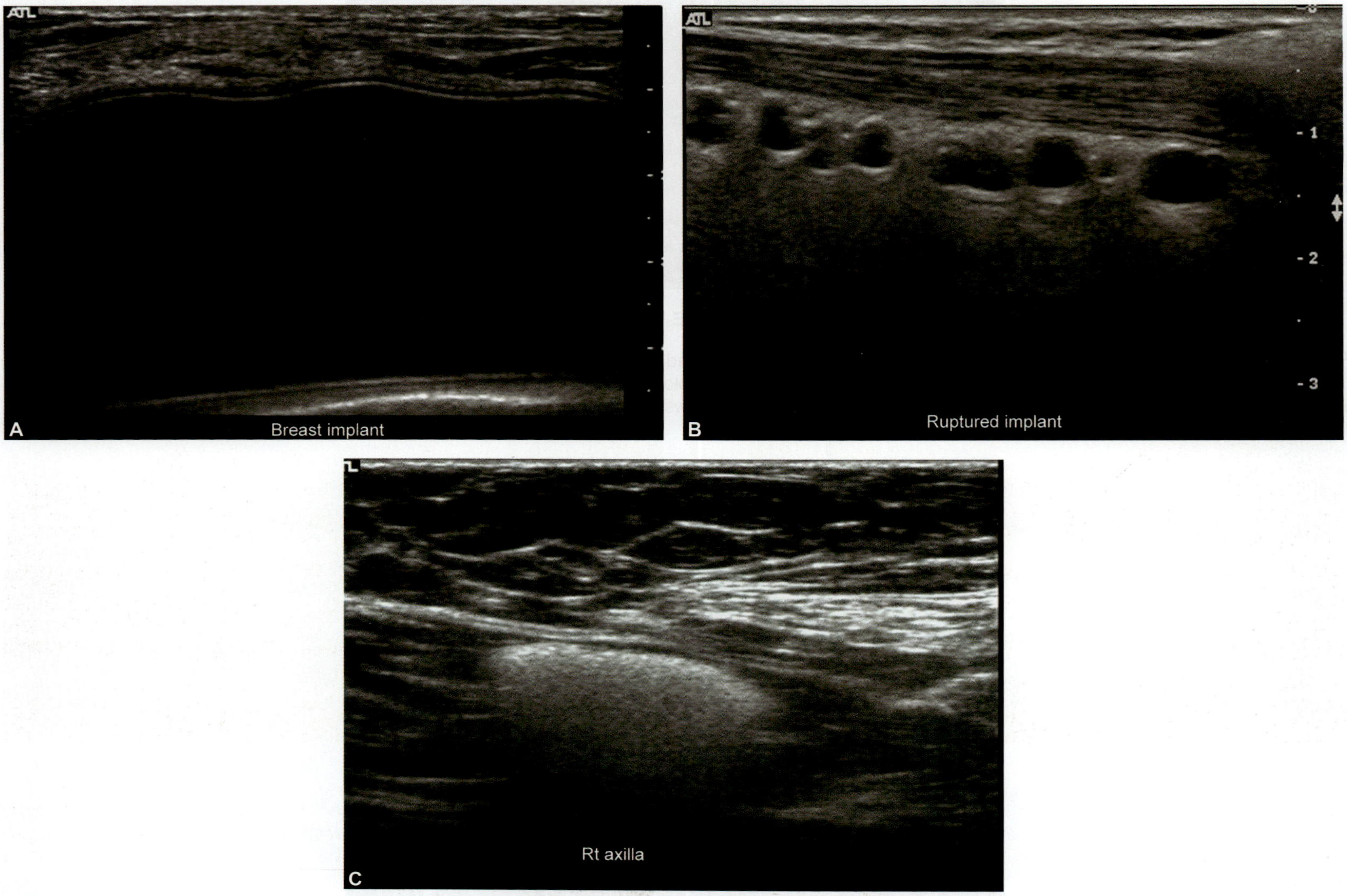

FIGURES 8.105A to C: HRSG shows breast implant in position in Figure A. Echogenic capsule of the implant is seen at the periphery. Internal texture of implant is anechoic. Figure B and C shows rupture of implant. The smooth margins of the implant shows irregular outline with interrupted pockets of collection. Echogenic fluid collection is also seen seeping in right axilla.

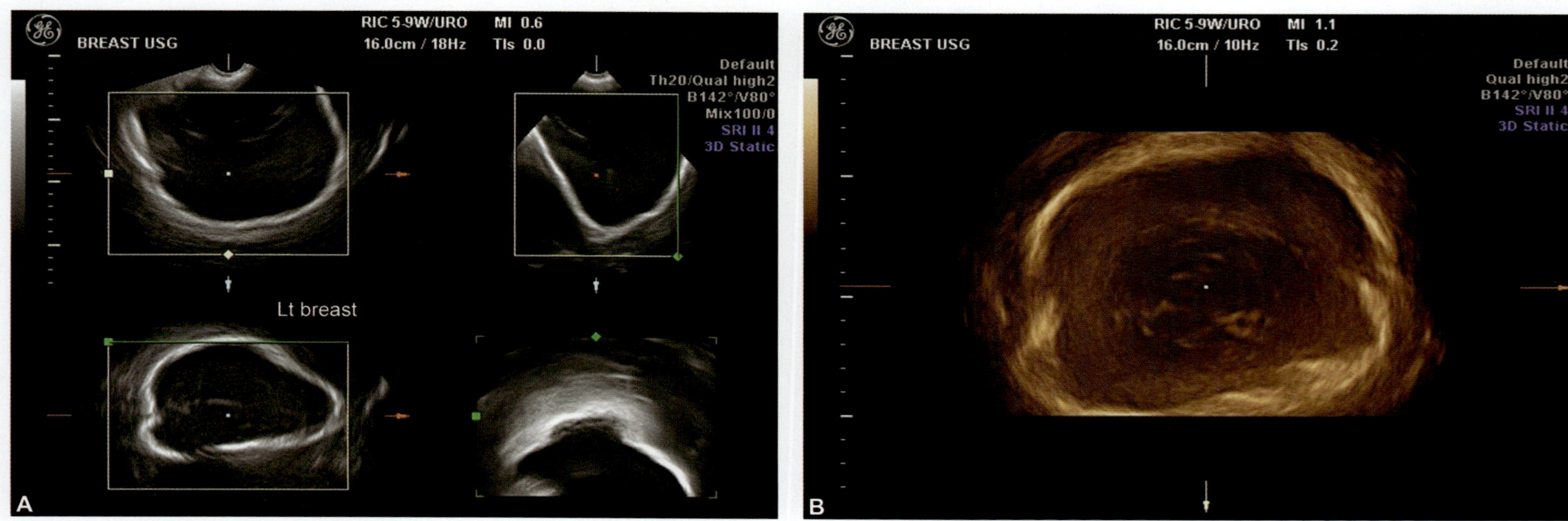

FIGURES 8.106A and B

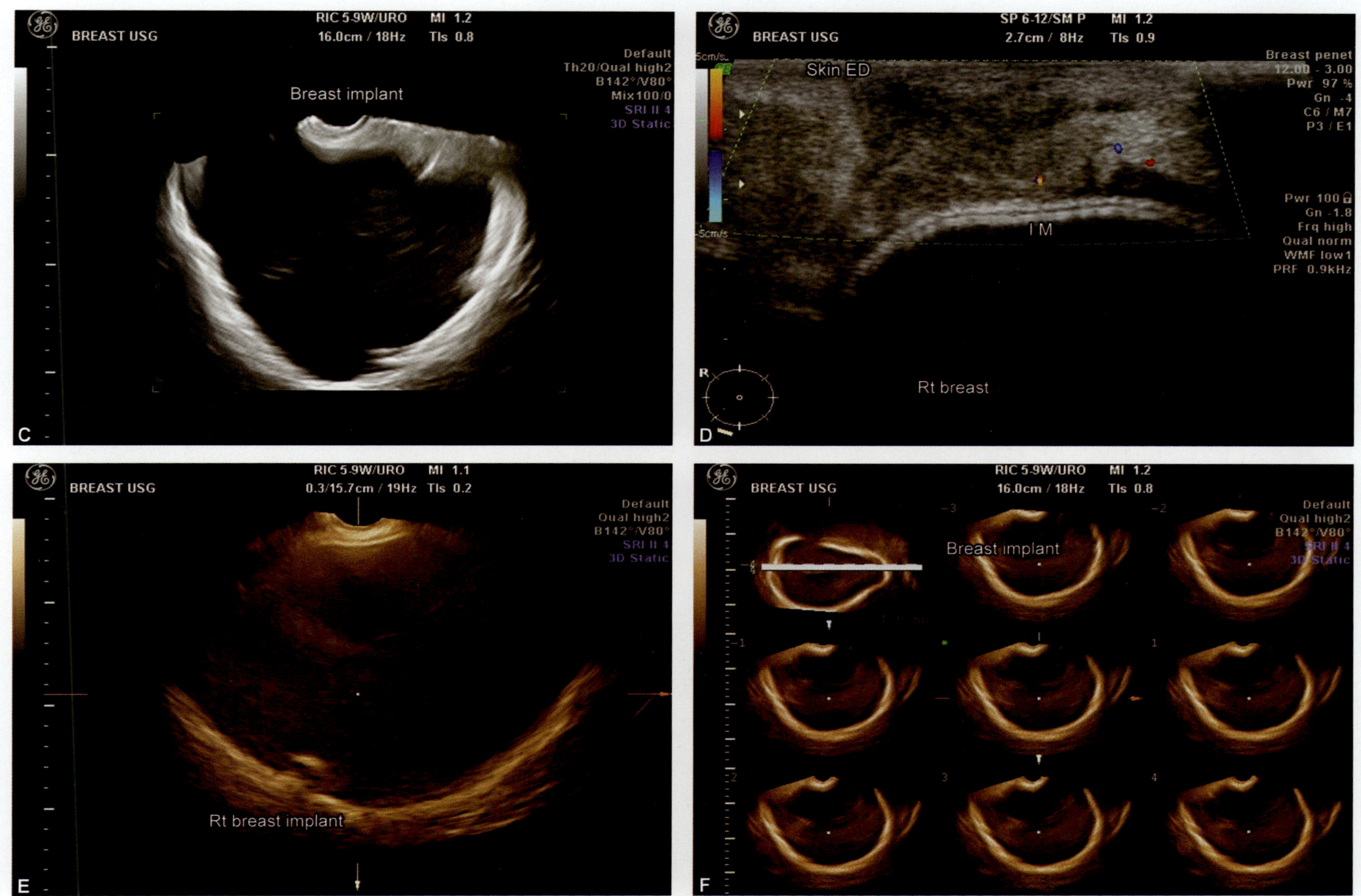

FIGURES 8.106C to F

FIGURES 8.106A to F: A patient underwent augmentation breast surgery with placement of implant in both the breasts. She presented with asymmetrical lump in the left breast. HRSG with 3D imaging shows rupture of the implant at 3 and 9 o' clock position, which is seen clearly on TUI imaging. However, the right breast shows implant is intact and seen in position with smooth capsule. The entire implant with intact capsule is seen on 3D ultrasound with TUI imaging.

SUMMARY

High resolution ultrasound in an excellent modality for evaluation of breast masses. It is cost effective. Multiplaner imaging modality in comparison to CT MR. The 3D imaging enhances the diagnostic accuracy. The best result can be achieved when it is used in conjunction with the X-ray and the combined sensitivity of sono and X-ray mammography can go up to 97% in detection of the breast cancer in preoperative patients.

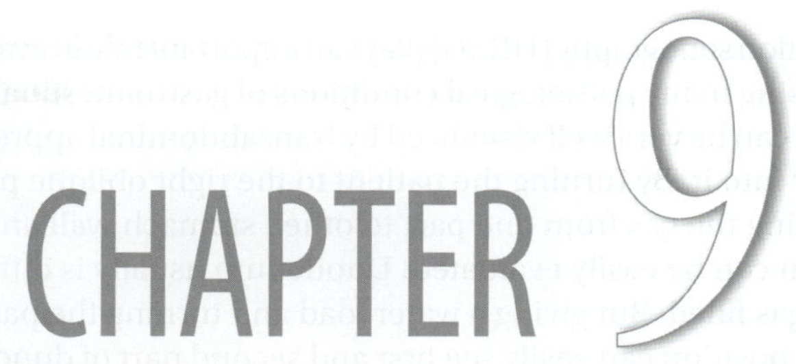

CHAPTER 9

Gastrointestinal Tract

PK Srivastava

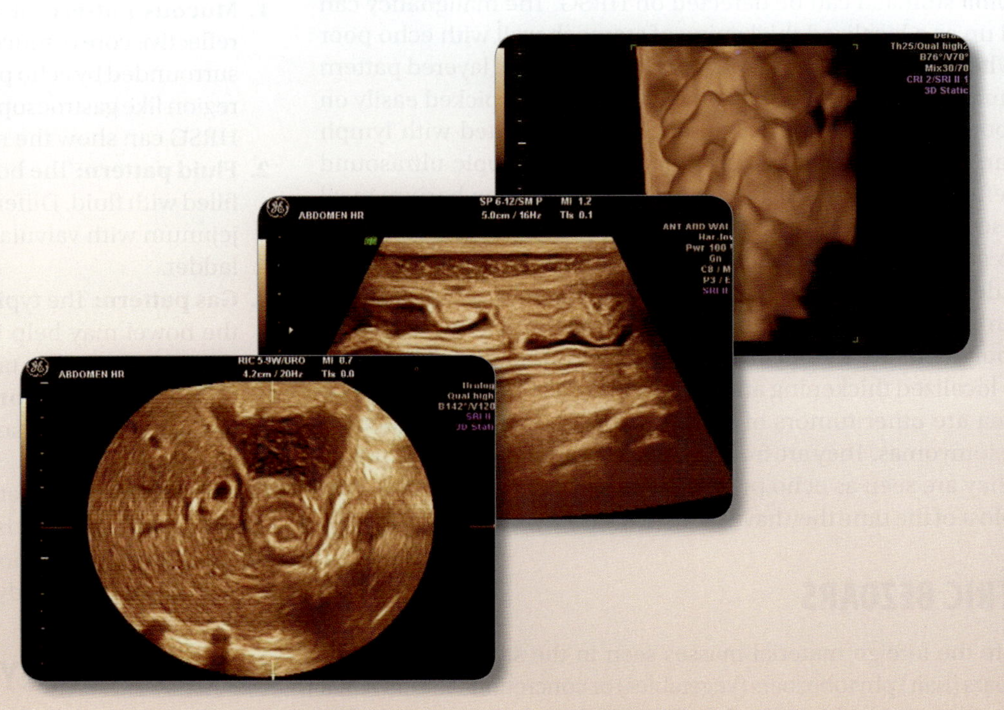

INTRODUCTION

High-resolution sonography (HR SG) plays an important role in evaluating and diagnosing many pathological conditions of gastrointestinal tract.

Stomach can be very well visualized by transabdominal approach by filling water into it. By turning the patient to the right oblique position and displacing the gas from one part to other, stomach wall and mass adhered to it can be easily evaluated. Duodenum usually is difficult to see, as it is gas filled. But giving a water load and turning the patient to right lateral position can easily see first and second part of duodenum. Duodenal cap is seen lying posterior to gall bladder when scanning done through liver and seen contracting and relaxing.

SONOGRAPHIC FEATURES OF GUT WALL

The gut wall is a multi-layered structure. It is seen as many layers of echogenic and hypoechoic layers parallel to mucosal and serosal surfaces. The five-layer structure is seen in good scanning technique. However, most of the time only three-layered gut wall structure is seen: (i) mucosal surface, (ii) middle echo poor muscularis mucosa, (iii) outer echogenic serosal surface.

PATHOLOGICAL CONDITIONS

Stomach

Normal stomach wall is 3–5 mm in thickness when distended. If it is more than 10 mm in thickness, malignancy should be suspected. However, inflammatory pathology can also lead to thickening. Majority of carcinoma stomach can be detected on HRSG. The malignancy can be picked up as a localized thickening of stomach wall with echo poor texture. When the tumor spreads there is loss of normal layered pattern of the stomach wall. Lymph node enlargement can be picked easily on HRSG. About 80% of carcinoma stomachs are presented with lymph node enlargement, when clinically detected. Endoscopic ultrasound is very useful in picking up early gastric lymphoma when barium meal and endoscopic findings are in conclusive.

Benign gastric tumors are much less common than the malignant tumors. Adenomatous polyp is thought to be a premalignant condition. It arises from mucosal or submucosal layer. Hyperplastic polyps are not true polyp but are more common than adenomatous polyp. They appear as localized thickening and usually multiple. Carcinoid tumors, hamartoma are other tumors of stomach. The most common benign tumor is leiomyomas. They are from muscle layer and seen as polypoidal growth. They are seen as echo poor mass coming out from muscularis propria. Most of the time they have ulcerated surface and seen on HRSG.

GASTRIC BEZOARS

Bezoars are the foreign material masses seen in the stomach. They are trichobezoars (hair) phytobezoars (vegetables) or concretions like cow milk in infants and antacid tablets in adult. On HRSG they are seen as highly reflective masses in stomach. The trichobezoar is seen as solid echogenic mass with total acoustic shadowing suggestive of calcified surface.

HYPERTROPHIC PYLORIC STENOSIS

Hypertrophic pyloric stenosis is usually seen in male infants at birth or up to 6 month of age. HRSG is choice of investigation for diagnosing it. It shows the pyloric muscle thickening. If it is more than 4mm in thickness, it is abnormal. The total thickness of pyloric muscle from one surface to other surface should be more than 15 mm and length of pyloric canal is less than 17 mm in pyloric stenosis.

GASTRIC DIAPHRAGM

The gastric diaphragm is the congenital membrane. It is also known as web. It is seen extending into the gastric antrum and partially obstructing it. Most of the time it is 2 cm before the pylorus. When it is complete it is thought to be one of the types of gastric atresia. However, most of the diaphragm are incomplete and results into various form of obstruction.

DUODENAL ATRESIA

Typical double bubble sign is seen in duodenal atresia on HRSG. The common causes of duodenal obstruction are bands, atresia and stenosis. The other less common causes are annular pancreas, preduodenal and portal vein. The distal small bowel obstruction or volvulus can also result in duodenal obstruction.

The duodenal hematoma can occur due to blunt trauma to abdomen. It is seen a hypoechoic or echo free mass indenting the wall of duodenum. It is to be differentiated from pseudo pancreatic cyst.

BOWEL

Normal bowel shows may patterns on HRSG. It depends upon the part of bowel seen on HRSG, amount of fluid in bowel, gas in the bowel, and peristalsis present in bowel. The different bowel patterns are as follows:

1. **Mucous pattern:** It is having the classical target pattern. Highly reflective core of mucous with entrapped gas is seen in the center. It is surrounded by echo poor halo of bowel wall. It is typical of a sphincter region like gastroesophageal region, pyloric antrum or in duodenum. HRSG can show the multi-layered structure of bowel wall.
2. **Fluid pattern:** The bowel is seen as tubular organ on long axis when filled with fluid. Different portion of bowel can be seen on HRSG. The jejunum with valvulae conniventes usually give an appearance of a ladder.
3. **Gas pattern:** The typical gas pattern of bowel and its distribution in the bowel may help in tracking down the disease. The typical ring down artifact often tapers and described as "**comet tail pattern**".
4. **Colon pseudotumor pattern:** At time colonic contents trapped in gas can give rise Pseudo tumor pattern. It may be caused due to faecolith.

Bowel pathology: Variation for normal bowel pattern is known as bowel pathology. Therefore, it is mandatory to assess the normal bowel pattern, distribution of gas, amount of fluid in bowel and evaluation of bowel wall thickness and study of peristalsis and man movement.

PSEUDOKIDNEY SIGN

Normal bowel wall thickness is around 5 mm in nondistended state and 3 mm in distended state. If it is greater than the normal limits it should be treated as abnormal. When bowel wall is thickened the mucous pattern changes to thickened irregular halo of bowel wall, central echogenic complex thinned and compressed and become irregular, pathological changes should be suspected and known as **pseudokidney sign. The various conditions which may show pseudo kidney signs are as listed below:**

Inflammatory Disease

1. Tuberculosis of bowel.
2. Ruptured appendix with appendiceal mass.
3. Chronic granulomatous disease.
4. Crohn's disease.
5. Antibioma.
6. Diverticulosis.

Tumors

1. Adenocarcinoma.
2. Lymphoma.
3. Leiomyosarcoma.
4. Carcinoid tumor.
5. Metastatic deposits.

INTUSSUSCEPTION

HRSG shows typical crescentric triple layer appearance of intussusceptum in transverse axis. The longitudinal scan shows trident sign representing intussusceptum and intussuscipiens.

MUCOVISCIDOSIS

Mucoviscidosis or cystic fibrosis is uncommon condition involving small bowel loops, pancreas, kidney and the lungs. The bowel loops are seen dilated. Thick low-level collection is seen filling the bowel loop. It is thick jelly-like. In consistency the thick echogenic bands are seen crisscrossing the bowel loops and cause the intestinal obstruction. Specks of calcification are also seen in kidneys.

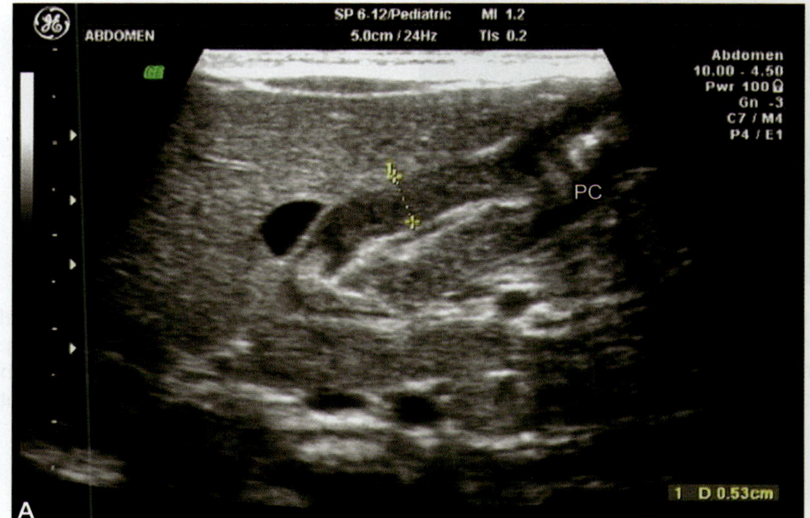

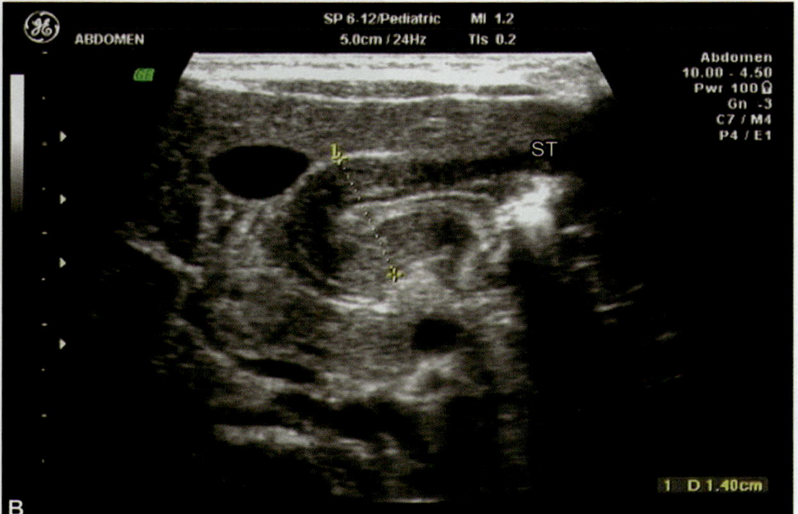

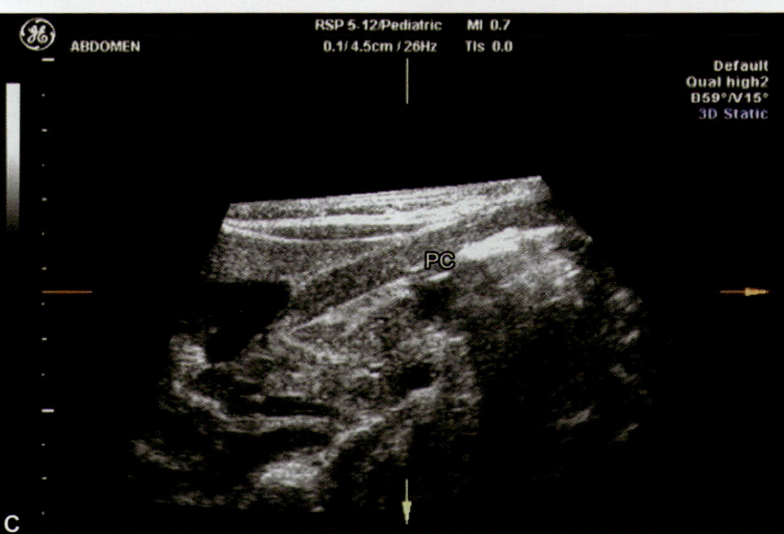

FIGURES 9.1A to C: Hypertrophic pyloric stenosis. High-resolution sonography (HRSG) shows markedly thickened pyloric muscle in a 1-month-old infant. The pyloric muscle is 6 mm in thickness. Pyloric canal is collapsed and a thick mucus line is seen in the pyloric canal. In the transverse axis, typical target sign is seen on HRSG.

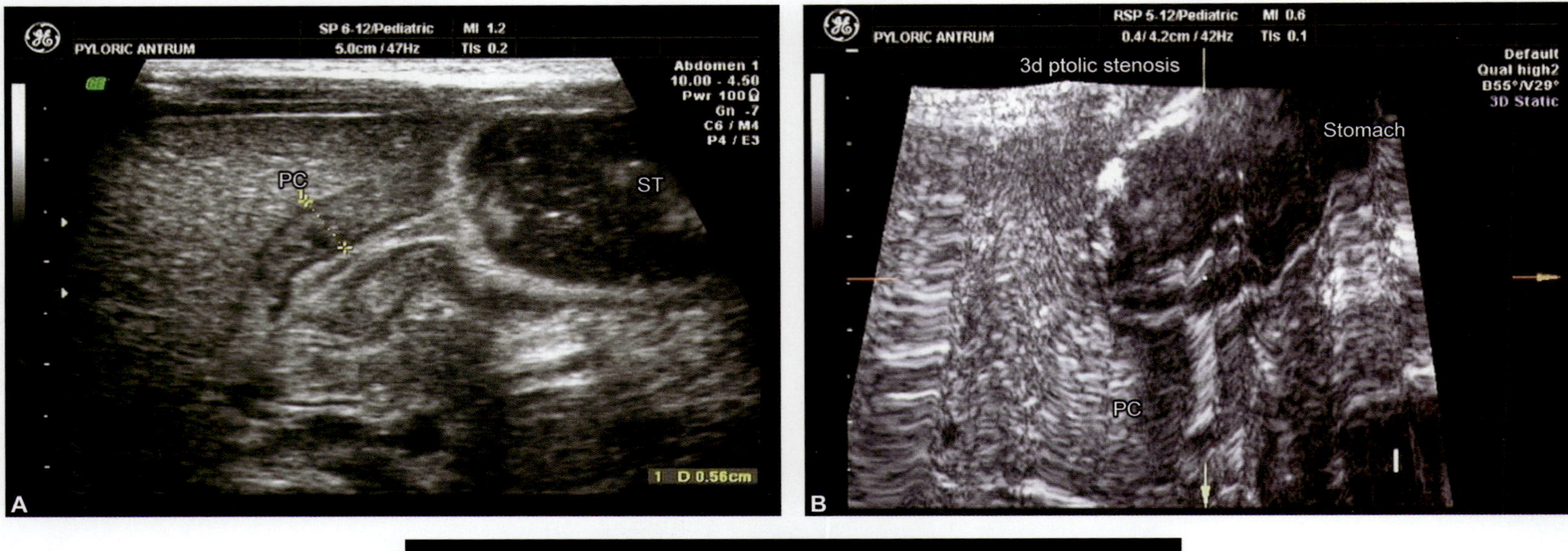

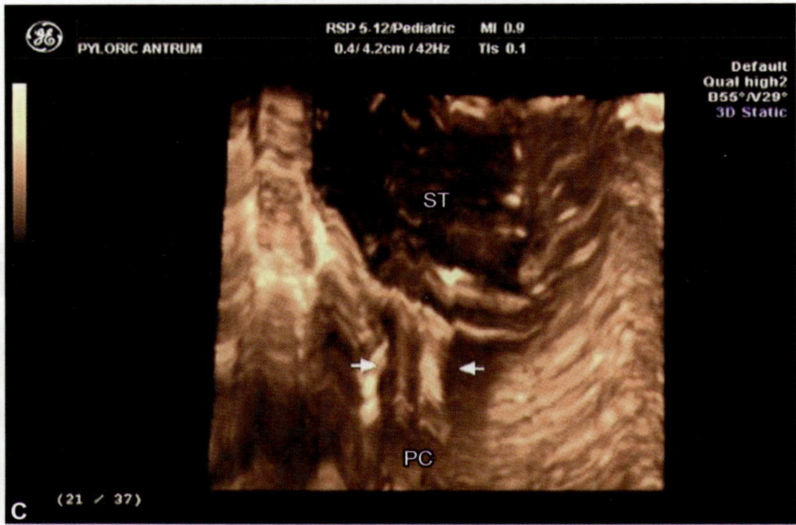

FIGURES 9.2A to C: Gross pyloric muscle hypertrophy. High-resolution sonography shows gross hypertrophy of the muscle. The pyloric canal seen obliterated in its proximal part. The stomach is seen distended with sudden obliteration of the proximal part of pyloric canal with marked beaking. 3D imaging through the pyloric canal and stomach shows the details of the hypertrophy of the pyloric muscle and stomach. The distended stomach show thickened mucosal folds. The pyloric muscle hypertrophy is well appreciated on 3D. The obliterated canal is also seen beautifully in the cut section on 3D imaging.

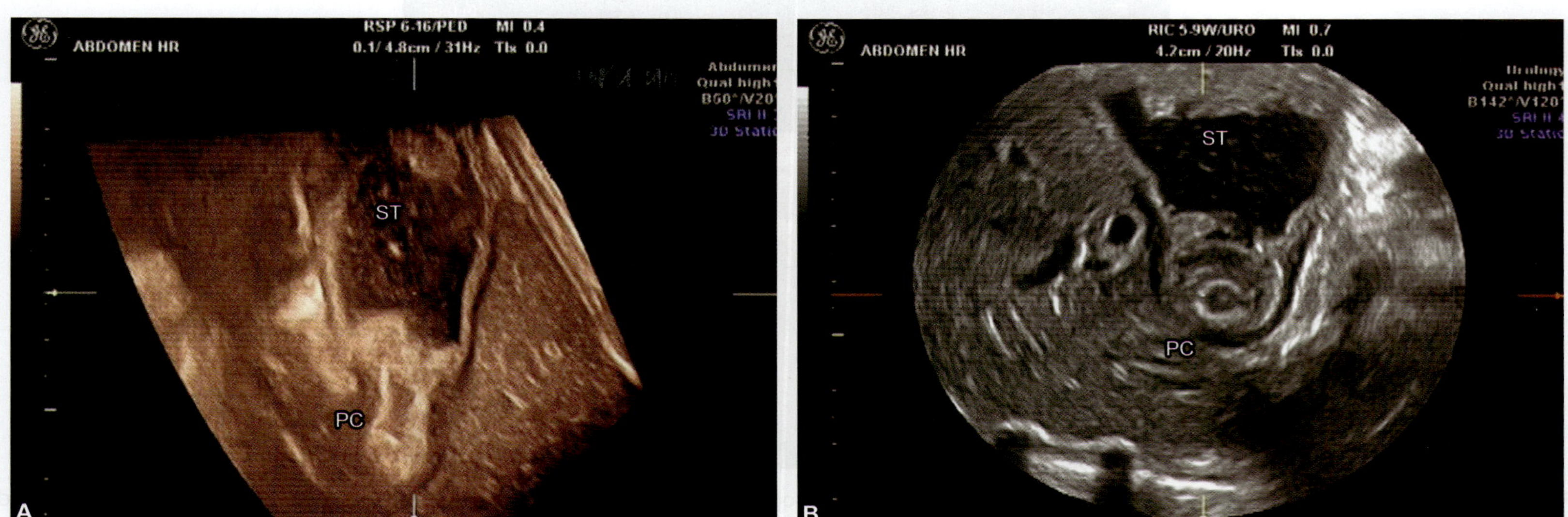

FIGURES 9.3A and B

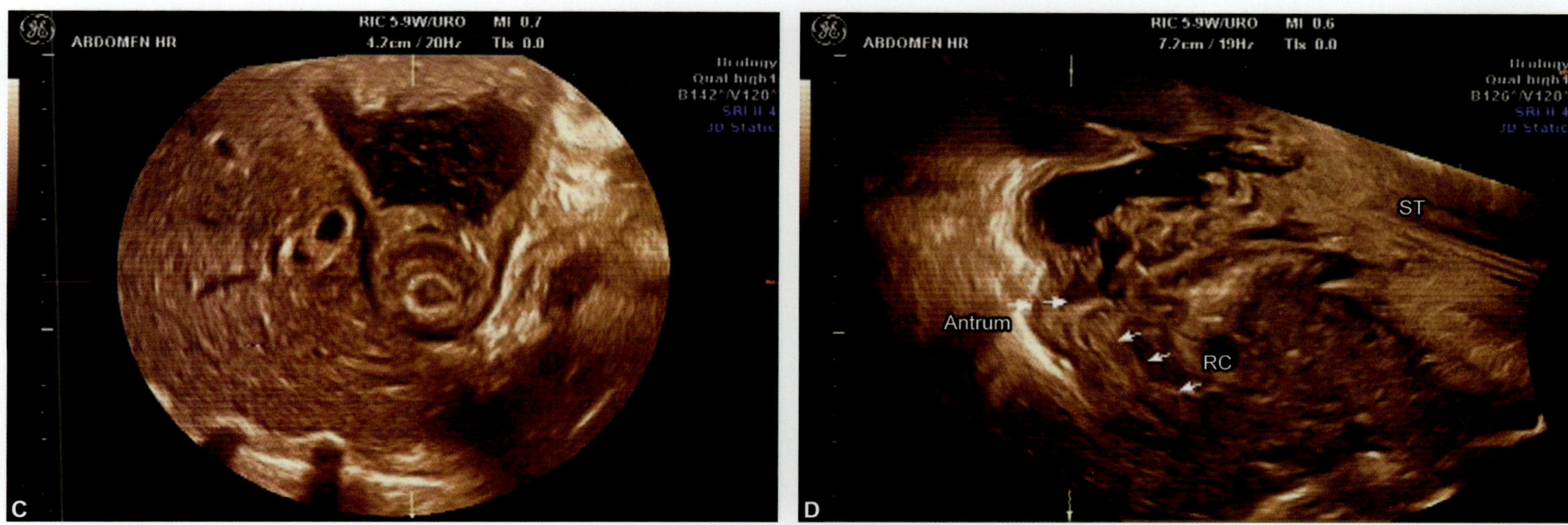

FIGURES 9.3C and D

FIGURES 9.3A to D: Pyloric stenosis with 3D imaging (Sonoendoscopy). A newborn baby presented with persistent vomiting. HRSG shows diffuse thickening of pyloric muscle. The pyloric canal is seen obliterated. On 3D sonoendoscopic imaging, concentric rings of thickened pyloric muscle are seen obliterating the pylori canal. 3D imaging shows cut pictures of pyloric antrum known as sonoendoscopy.

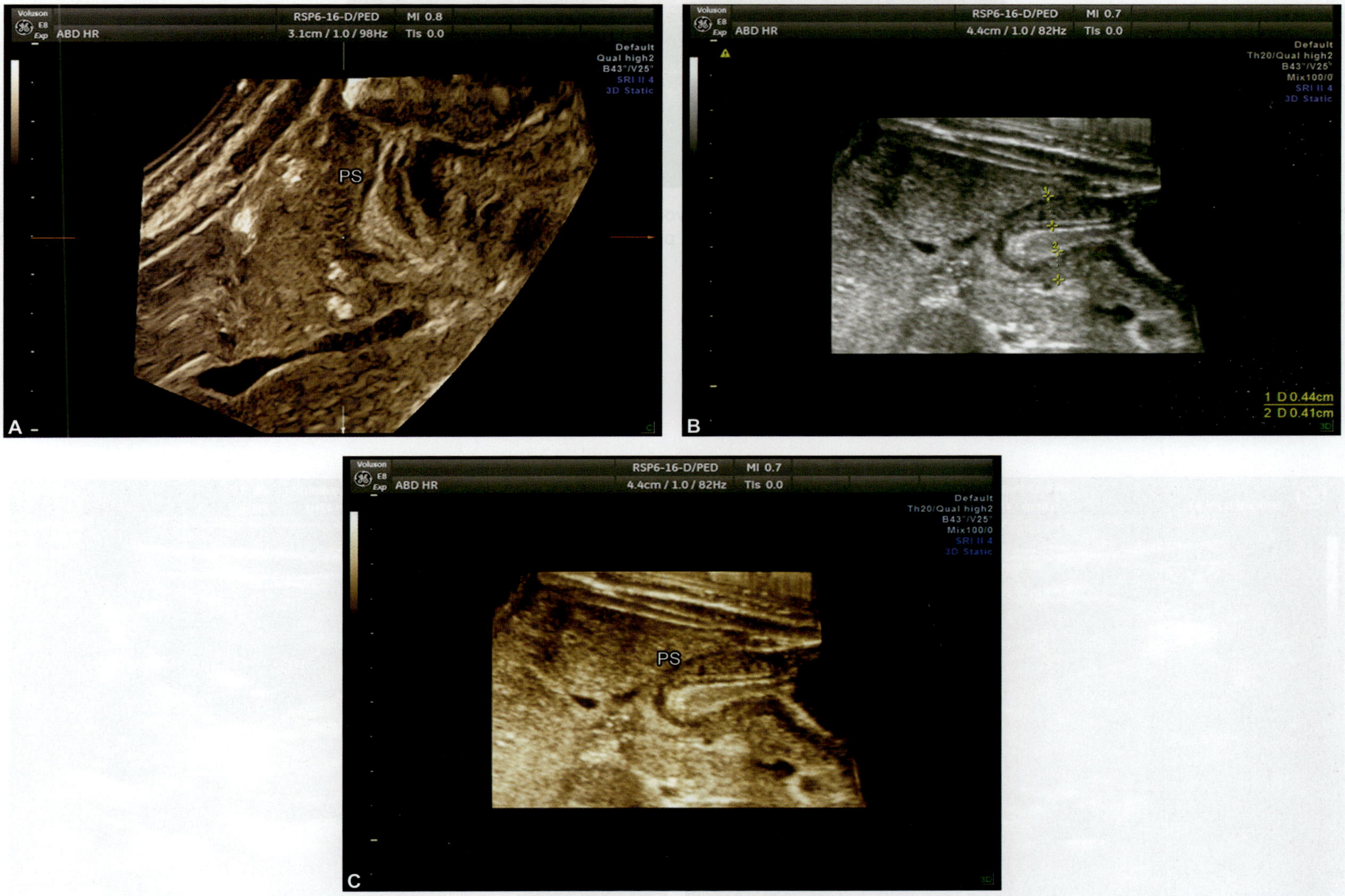

FIGURES 9.4A to C: Pyloric stenosis. A 23-day-old baby presented with persistent vomiting. HRSG shows markedly thickened pyloric muscle. The pyloric canal is obliterated. The pyloric muscle is 4.4 mm in thickness on one side (normal <1.2 mm).

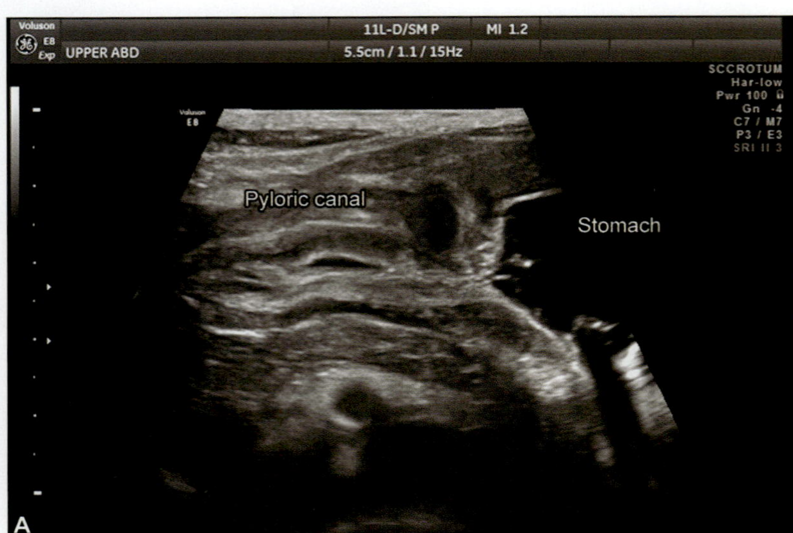

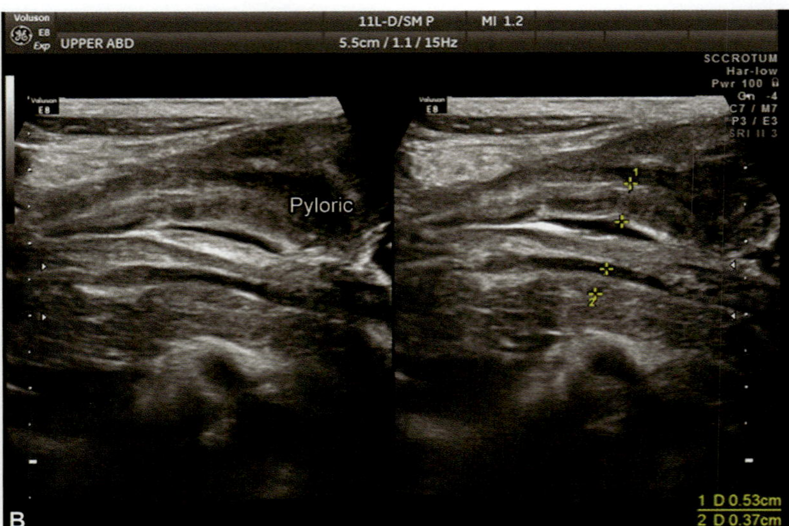

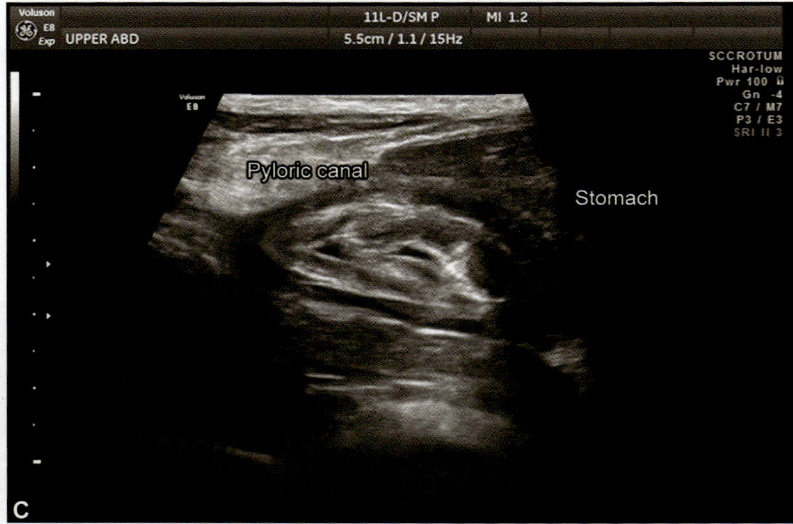

FIGURES 9.5A to C: Pyloric spasm. A baby presented with intermittent vomiting. HRSG shows sluggish opening of the pyloric canal. Small amount of fluid is also seen going through the pyloric canal. On contraction, the pyloric muscle is seen thickened. However, the contraction gets released after sometime suggestive of pyloric spasm.

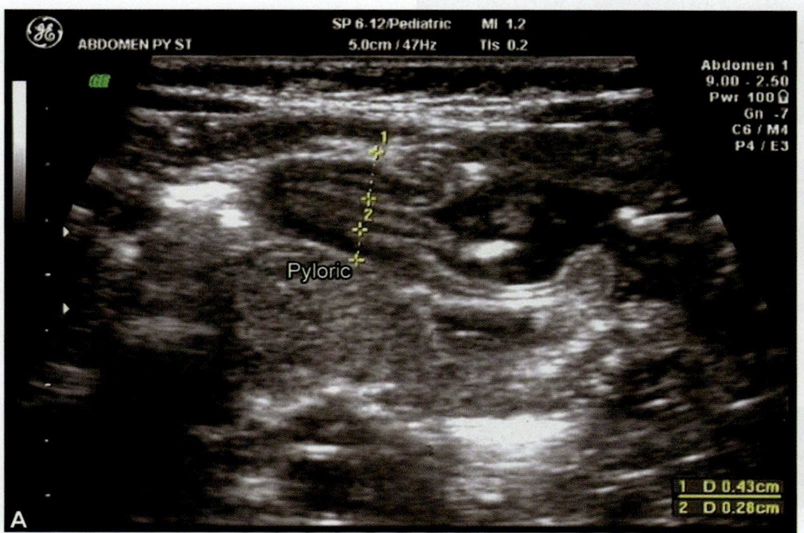

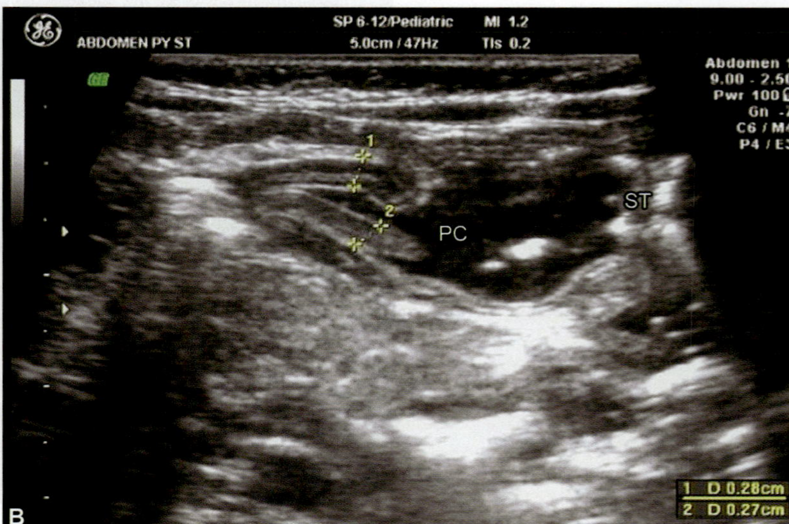

FIGURES 9.6A and B

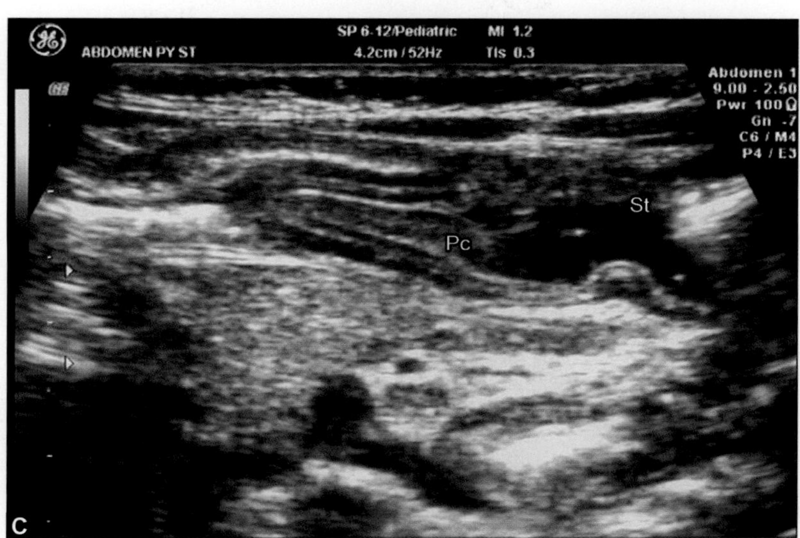

FIGURE 9.6C

FIGURES 9.6A to C: Moderate muscular hypertrophy with pylorospasm. HRSG shows moderate pyloric muscle hypertrophy with persistent pyloric spasm partial opening of the pyloric canal seen. Small fluid is seen in the canal.

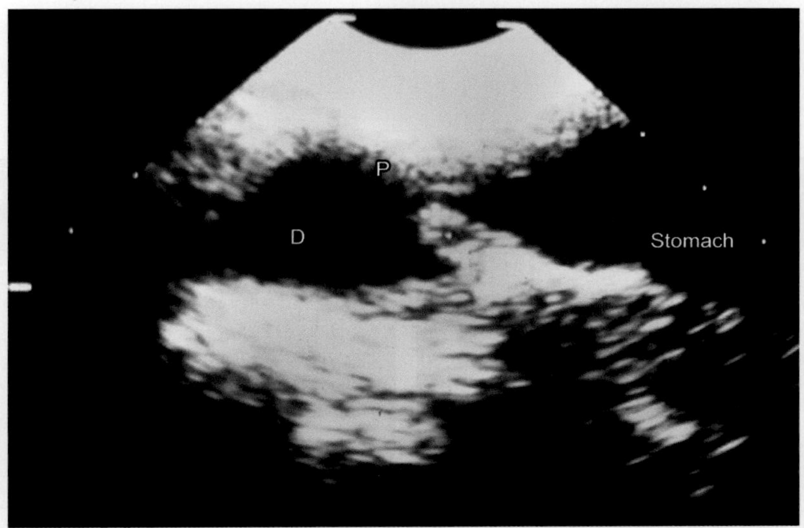

FIGURE 9.7: Gastric diaphragm. Echogenic bulging membrane is seen in the antrum before the pylorus suggestive of a gastric diaphragm. The fold is seen partially obliterating the pyloric canal. First part of duodenum is seen distended.

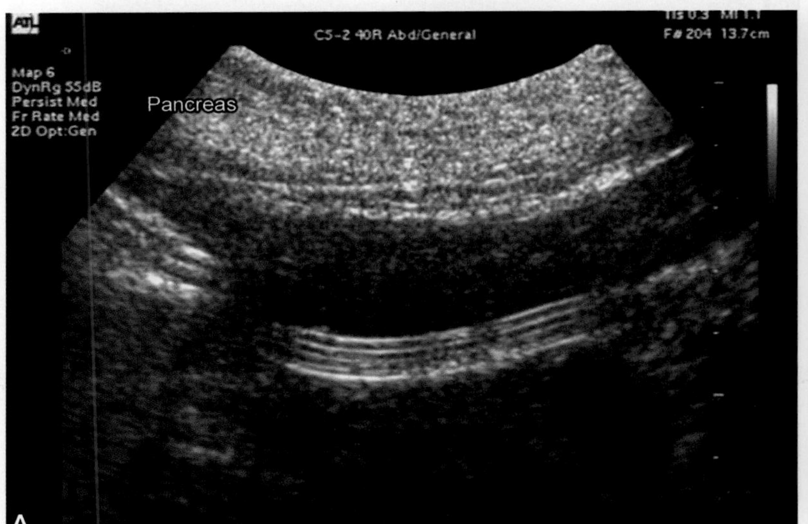

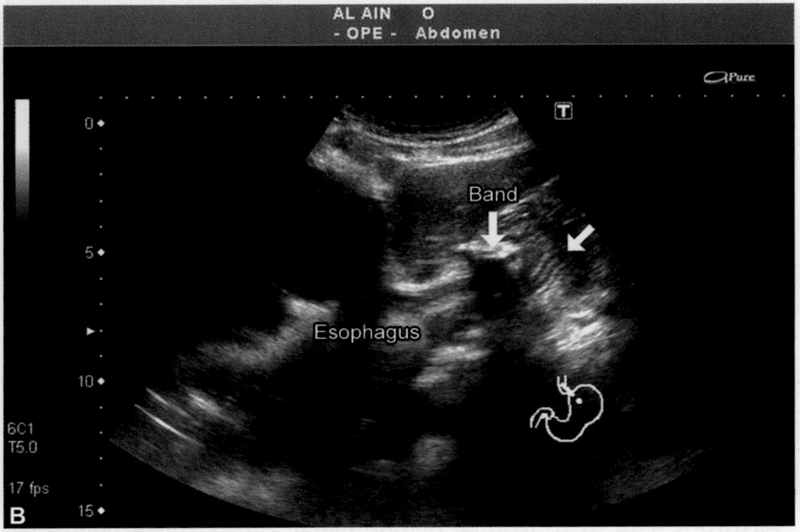

FIGURES 9.8A and B

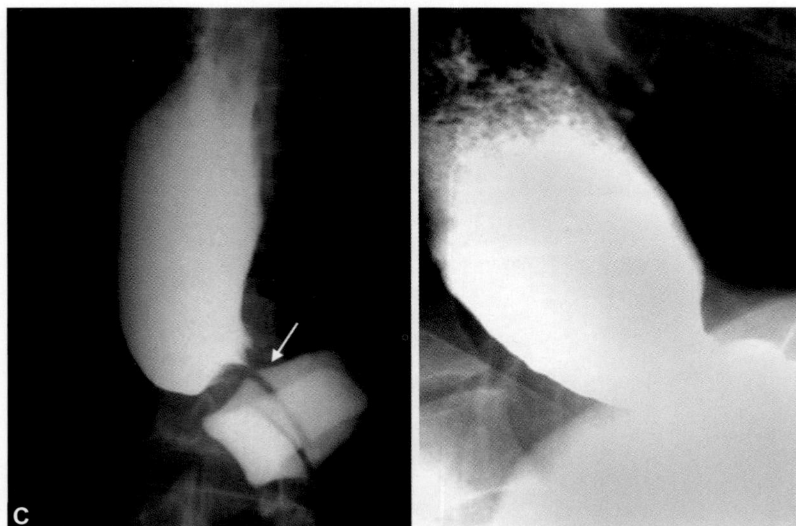

FIGURE 9.8C

FIGURES 9.8A to C: Gastric band. A patient underwent bariatric surgery with gastric band application to reduce stomach size. HRSG shows echogenic linear shadows seen in the upper part of stomach suggestive of gastric band in position. Barium meal of the same patient shows constriction at the site of gastric band application (*Courtsey:* Dr Shlomo Gobi, Tel Aviv, Isreal).

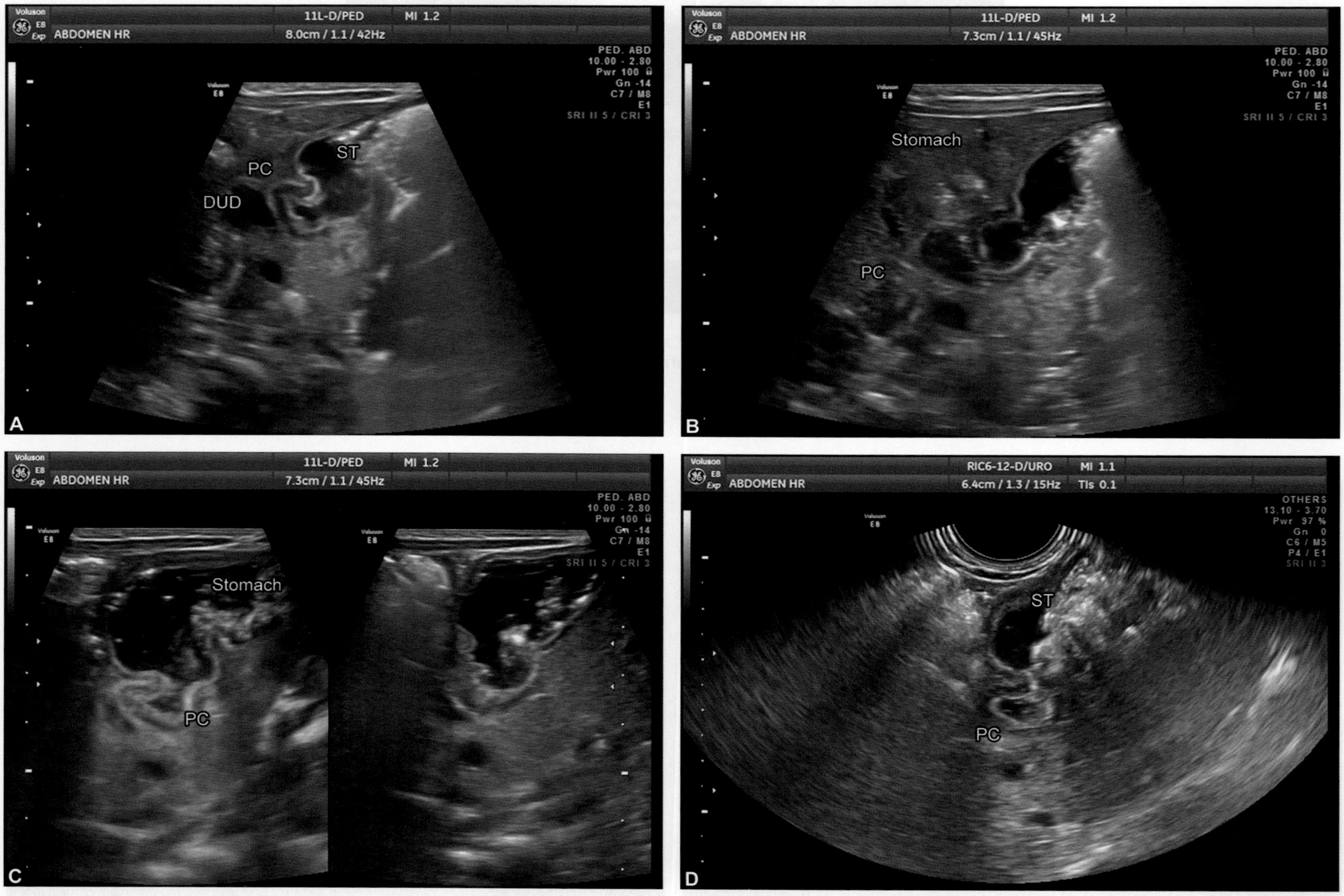

FIGURES 9.9A to D: Normal pyloric canal. HRSG shows normal pyloric canal and its opening. Opening of pyloric canal and fluid movement through it is seen on dynamic scanning.

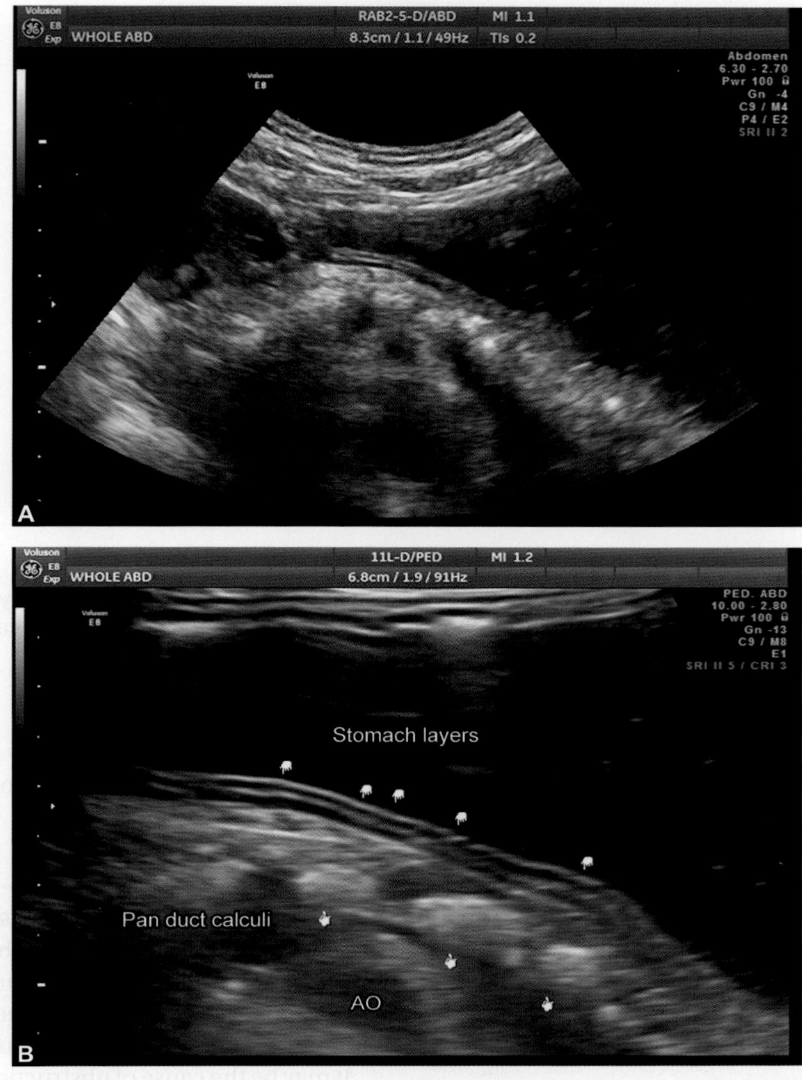

FIGURES 9.10A and B: Normal stomach layer. High-resolution sonography shows beautifully the mucosal layer of stomach, which are seen as hypoechoic and echogenic bands. Posterior to the stomach wall multiple echogenic calculi are seen in the pancreatic duct in the same patient, a known case of chronic calcific pancreatitis.

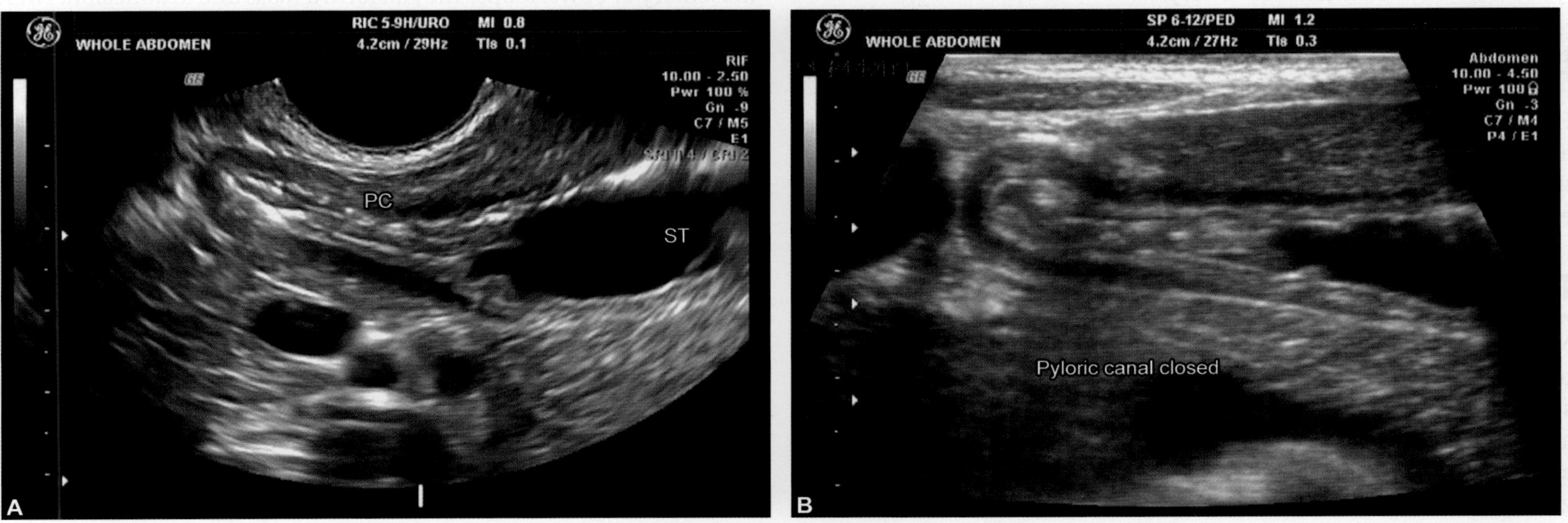

FIGURES 9.11A and B

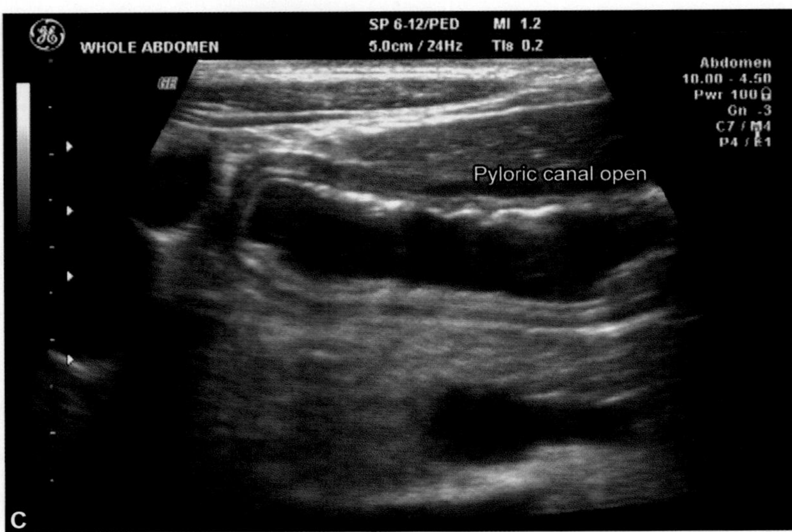

FIGURE 9.11C

FIGURES 9.11A to C: Normal opening of pyloric antrum and pyloric canal. High-resolution sonography shows normal opening of pyloric antrum and fluid movement is seen going through it, and normal opening of pyloric canal is seen.

APPENDIX

Acute appendicitis is one of the most common causes of acute abdomen. Although the clinical diagnosis of classical acute appendicitis can be made easily, however, most of the time the patient presents with vague symptoms and a typical presentation. In such settings, HRSG is a good tool to study appendicular pathology. The hallmark of the modality is to visualize inflamed appendix directly and also to detect any other pathology, which mimics appendicitis clinically. Appendix can be visualized in almost every position except when it is present retrocaecal, it cannot be seen on HRSG.

Normal Anatomy

Appendix is seen as a blind ended aperistaltic tube with typical "gut signature" in appendicular fossa. The normal appendix is usually not visualized. However, in few patients, it can be seen as a thin compressible blind-ended tubular structure. Its wall obliterate with graded compression, as it is easily compressible, mobile tube. It is seen lying anterior to common iliac artery.

Equipment

High-resolution transducers of 5 and 7.5 MHz are required to see the appendix. At times 10 MHz transducer is also required to see it in very thin patients and in children. Appendix can be seen in every position except in retrocaecal or aberrant position of appendix.

Technique and Preparation

No specific preparation is required to see the appendix. A special technique of "graded compression" with transducer head is applied to see the appendix with slowly increasing pressure applied on anterior abdominal wall in appendicular or right iliac fossa. The fat and bowel are displaced and compressed. This reduces the artifacts from bowel gas and its contents. It also brings transducer near to the appendix. Full urinary bladder displaces bowel loops in appendicular fossa; therefore, urinary bladder should be empty prior to examination. Gentle graded compression should be applied to avoid pain.

Acute Appendicitis

The biggest advantage of HRSG is the direct visualization of inflamed appendix, which appears to be a thick-walled incompressible, sausage-like tube with concentric layers on HRSG. It is an elongated tube with one end blind. When wall thickness exceeds 6 mm, it is suggestive of inflammation. Many a times, faecolith is seen in the lumen of appendix.

It may be the cause of obstruction. A small amount of fluid collection may be seen in appendicular fossa due to inflammation. The adjacent bowel loop may show dilatation due to local inflammation and irritation. Local adynamic ileus may result due to inflammation.

Appendiceal Mass

Perforation of appendix leads to peritoneal spill. It leads to peritonitis. The spill of pus may be limited due to sealing of perforation by omentum, mesentery or bowel loops. They all form a mass due to adhesion. HRSG shows a non-compressible mass. It is predominantly echo poor with heterogeneous texture. However, secondary infection may lead to an abscess formation with fluid collection and debris. When appendiceal mass is formed, immediate surgery is not required and these patients are treated conservatively. Cecum and ileum also show muscle thickening and they can be easily identified in thin patients. An abscess can develop in appendiceal mass following secondary infection. HRSG can very well identify the abscess. Most of the abscess resolves on conservative treatment, or they may drain in adjacent bowel loops.

Differential Diagnosis

Many clinical conditions may present as acute appendicitis. They may include right ureteric colic, perforated peptic ulcer, right-sided twisted ovarian cyst, right-sided ectopic tubal pregnancy, acute cholecystitis or right iliac fossa abscess. Therefore, in 50% cases presented as acute appendicitis, the reason is found to be something else rather than acute appendicitis. Therefore, HRSG is also helpful in diagnosing the above conditions by excluding acute appendicitis.

Limitations

Failure to visualize inflamed appendix may lead to erroneous diagnosis in inexperienced hands. An inflamed appendix can be seen in 90% of the cases in nonperforated cases, 80–85% in appendiceal mass and 50–55% in free perforation of appendix. However, in over 80% of the cases, a positive diagnosis of appendicitis can be made on HRSG. But non-visualization of appendix does not rule out appendicitis particularly when it is aberrantly placed or retrocecal in position. It these situations, indirect signs of local ileus, small fluid in appendicular fossa or an abscess formation may lead to diagnosis.

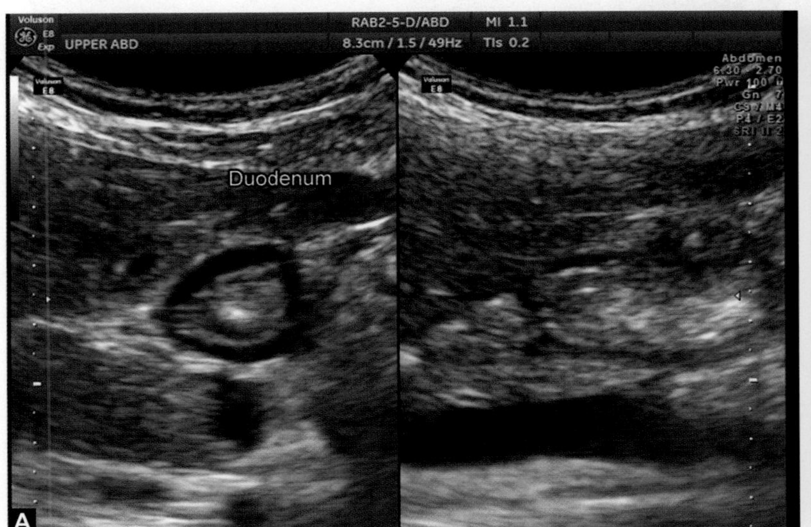

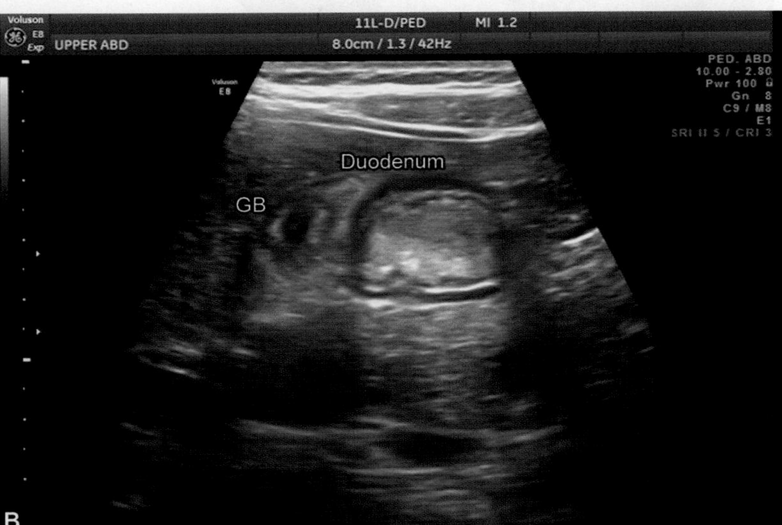

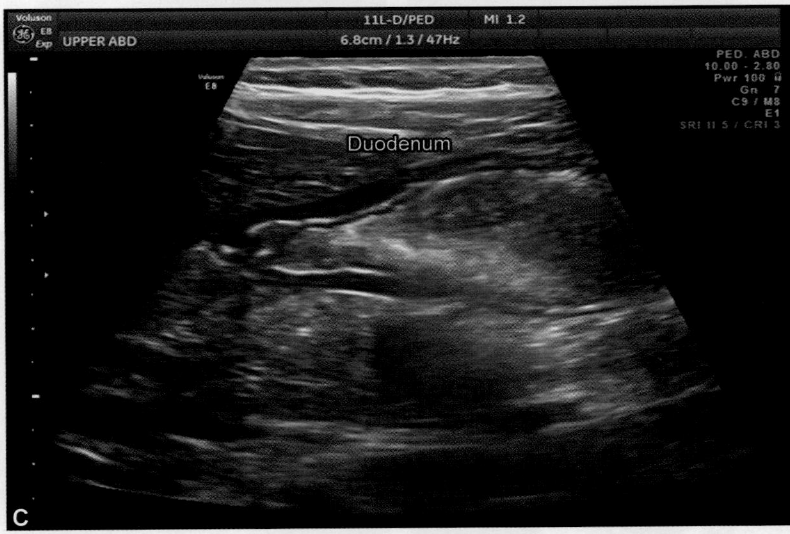

FIGURES 9.12A to C: Inflammatory duodenum. A patient presented with pain in abdomen and vomiting. HRSG shows distended duodenum. The duodenal wall is edematous. Perifocal edema is also present. The fluid content is seen stagnated in the duodenum. The duodenal walls show mucosal edema suggestive of duodenitis.

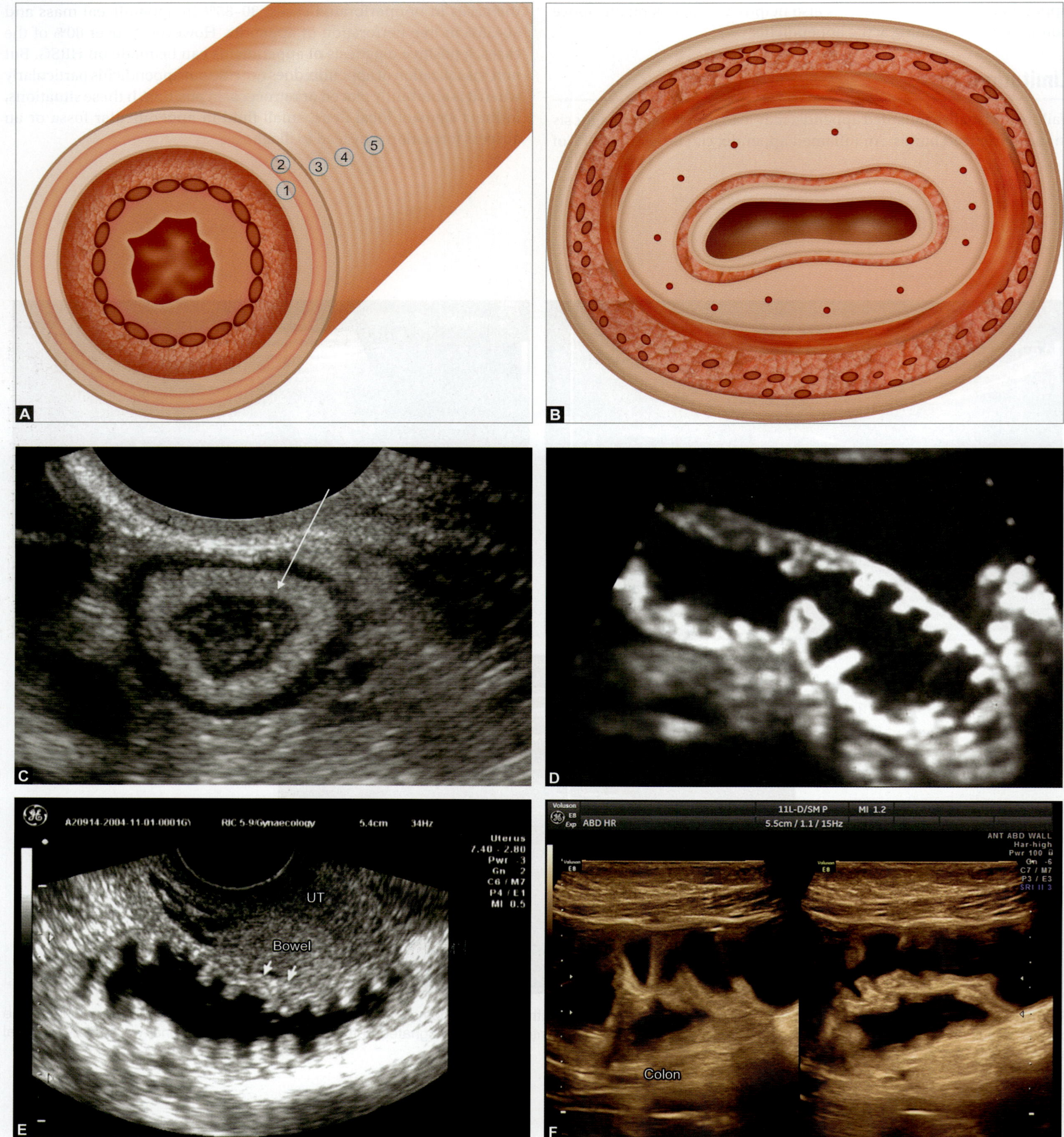

FIGURES 9.13A to F

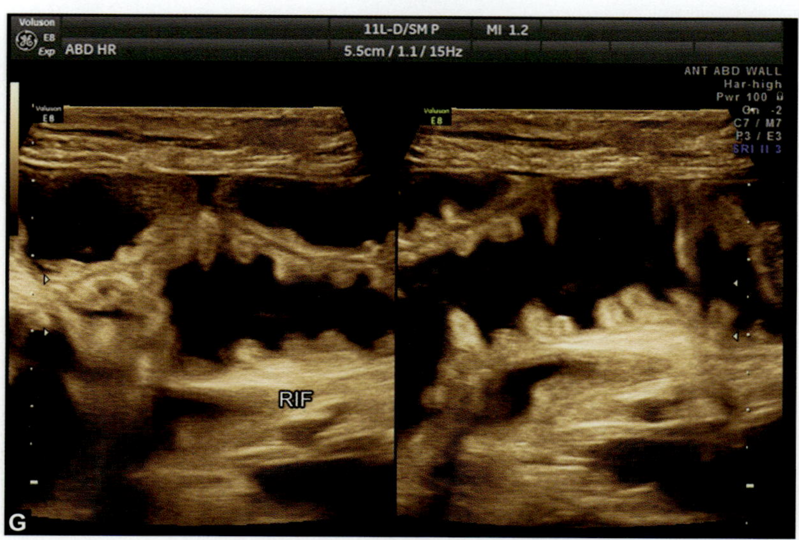

FIGURE 9.13G

FIGURES 9.13A to G: Normal sonographic bowel anatomy and mucosal folds. Figures A and B show diagrammatic representation of bowel muscle layers. Figure C shows different layers in cross section on High-resolution sonography. Figures D to G shows the mucosal fold in small bowel and in the large bowel. HRSG is an excellent modality to show the mucosal folds in gastrointestinal tract.

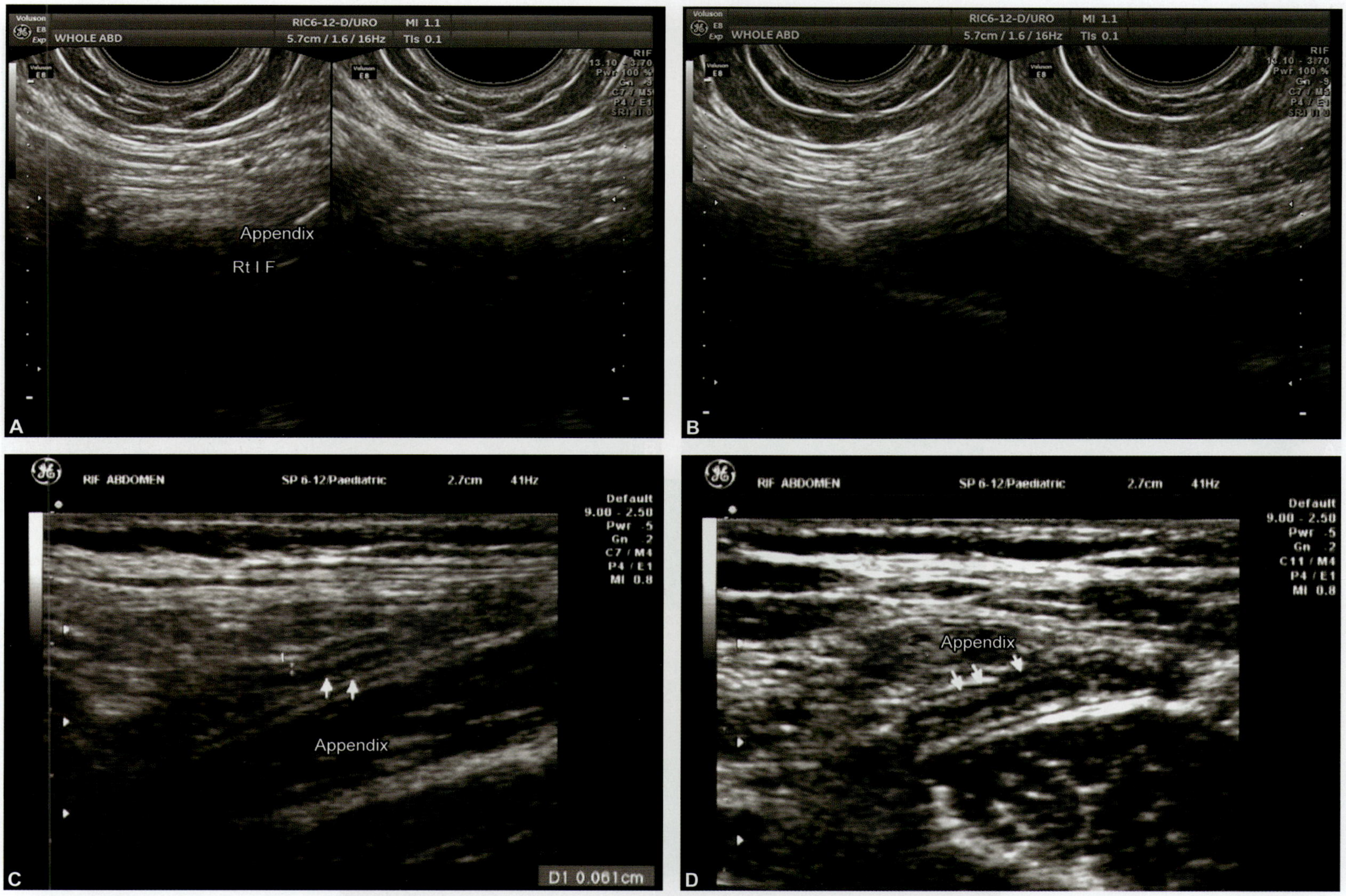

FIGURES 9.14A to D: Normal appendix. High resolution ultrasound is an excellent modality for visualization of normal appendix. High-resolution sonography (HRSG) shows a normal appendix in appendicular fossa. Appendix is seen as an echogenic tubular shadow having blind one end. The lumen is anechoic. Normal wall thickness is 3 mm. Normal appendix—High-resolution sonography shows normal appendix in the right iliac fossa. It is seen anterior to the iliac vessels. Walls are normal. Lumen is free. No internal echo is seen in the lumen

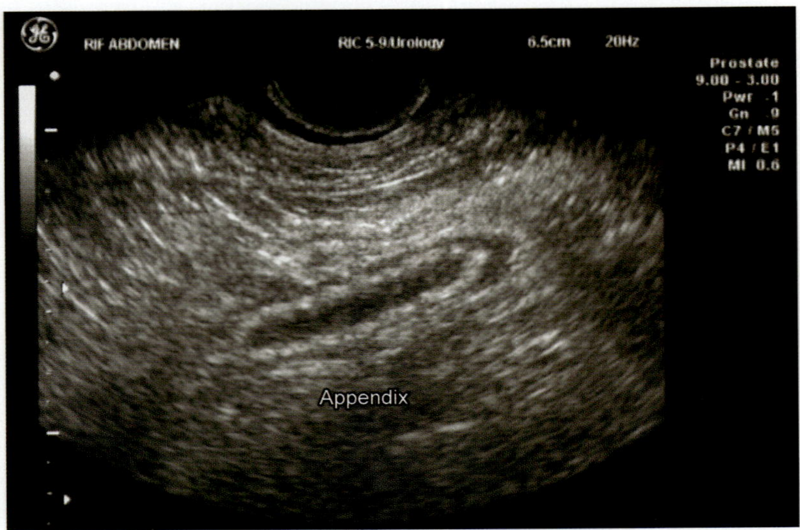

FIGURE 9.15: Acute appendicitis. High-resolution sonography (HRSG) shows inflamed thickened edematous appendix anterior to the iliac vessels. The appendix is seen as thickened echogenic tubular shadow. Small amount of fluid is also seen in appendicular fossa suggestive of reactionary fluid collection

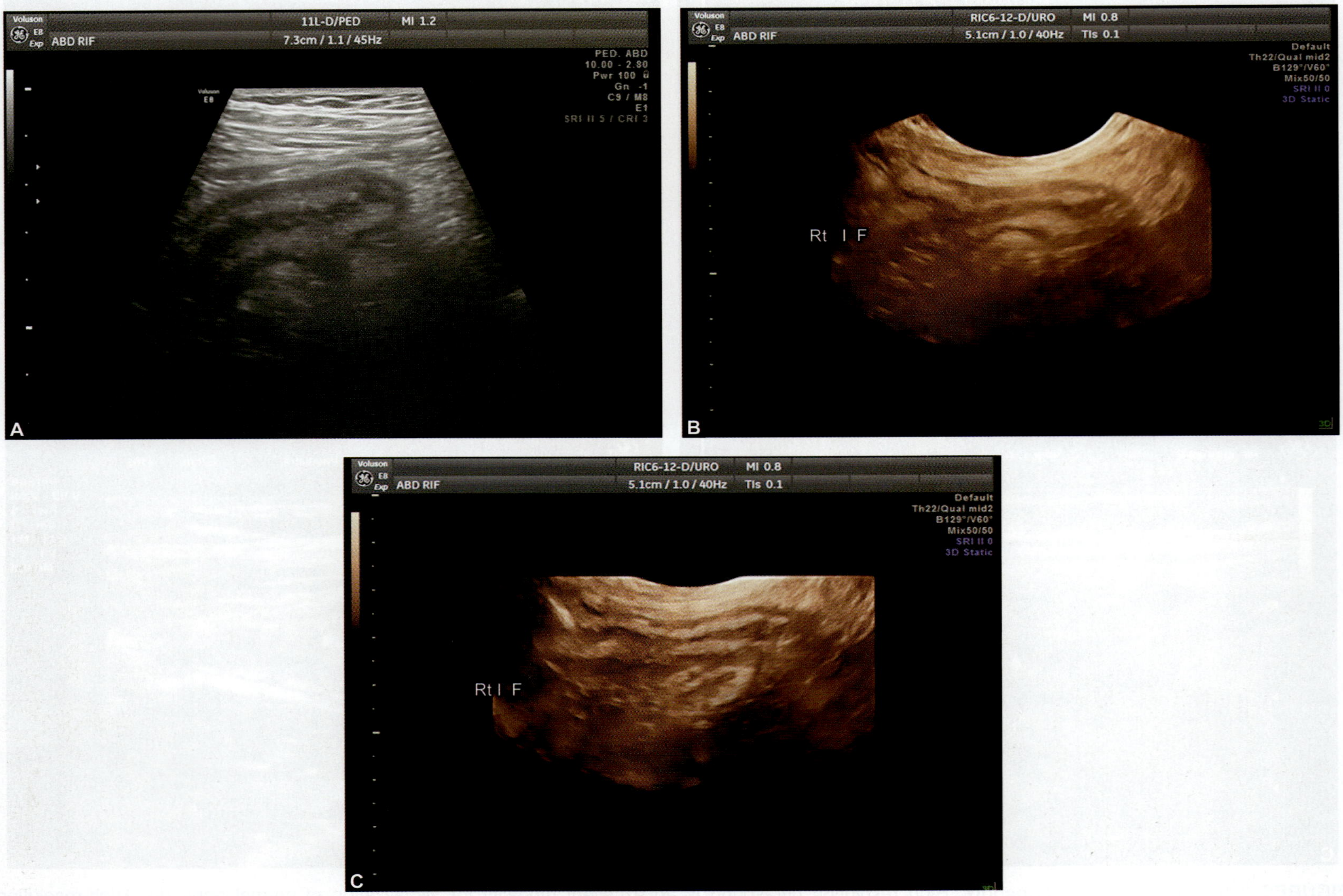

FIGURES 9.16A to C: Acute appendicitis. High-resolution sonography (HRSG) shows thickened edematous appendix in the right iliac fossa. It is seen anterior to the iliac vessels. Walls are thickened and edematous. Periappendicular fat is also inflamed. However, no fluid is seen in appendicular fossa. Findings are suggestive of acute appendicitis.

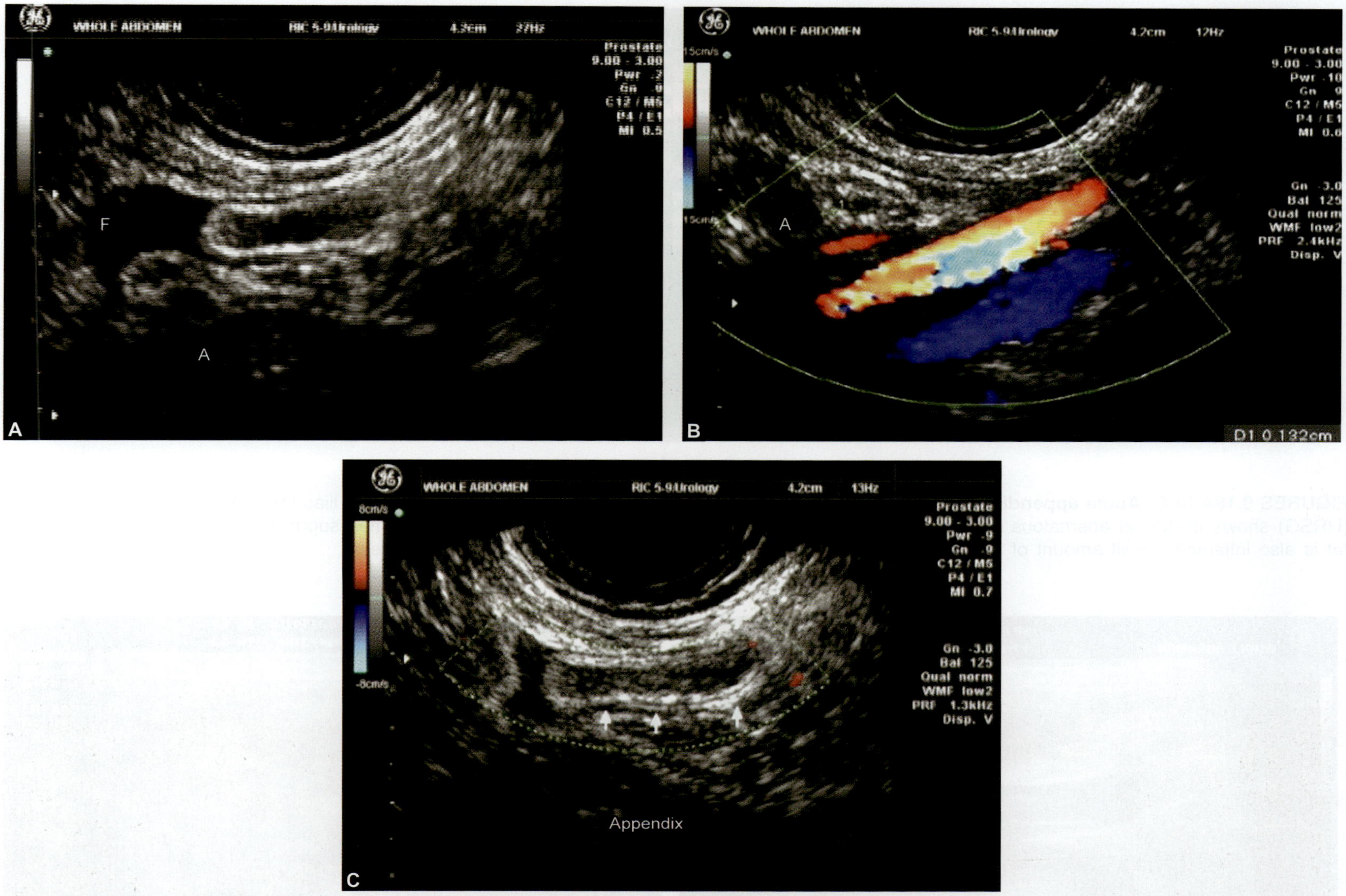

FIGURES 9.17A to C: Acute Appendicitis. The appendix is seen as an inflamed edematous tubular shadow in appendicular fossa in a young girl. Wall edema is also present. Perifocal edema is present. Low-level echo collection is seen in the lumen of the appendix. Small amount of fluid collection is seen in the appendicular fossa. Appendix is seen to the iliac vessels. High-resolution sonography (HRSG) also shows subserosal edema in the wall of appendix.

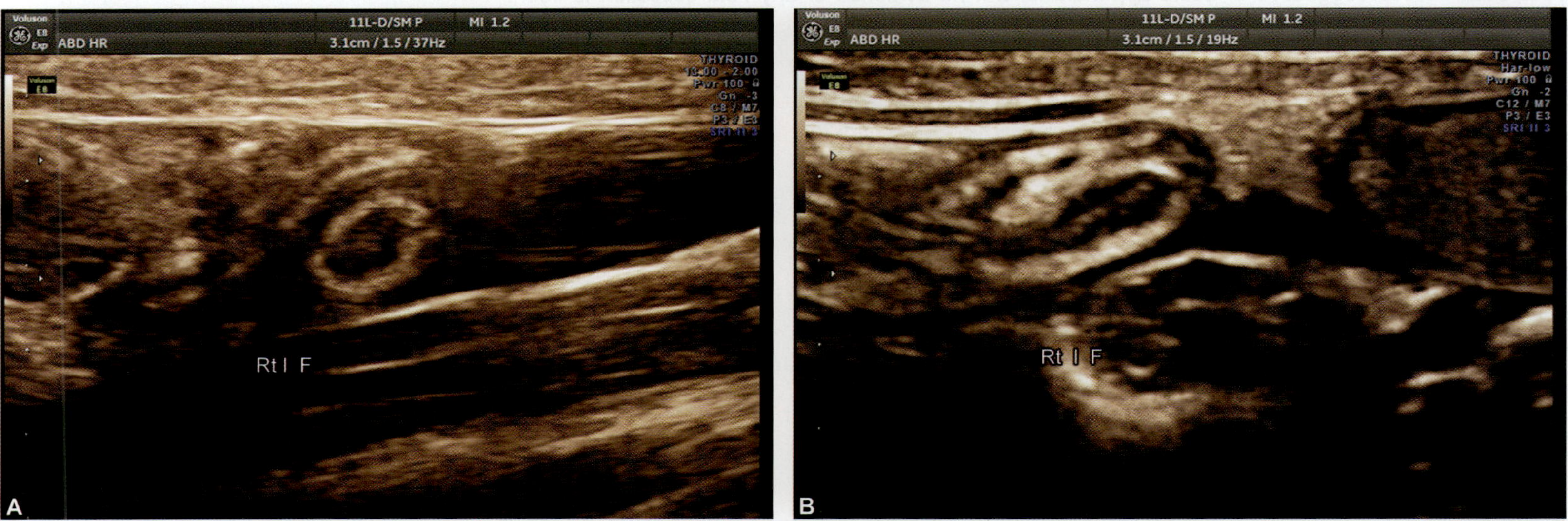

FIGURES 9.18A and B

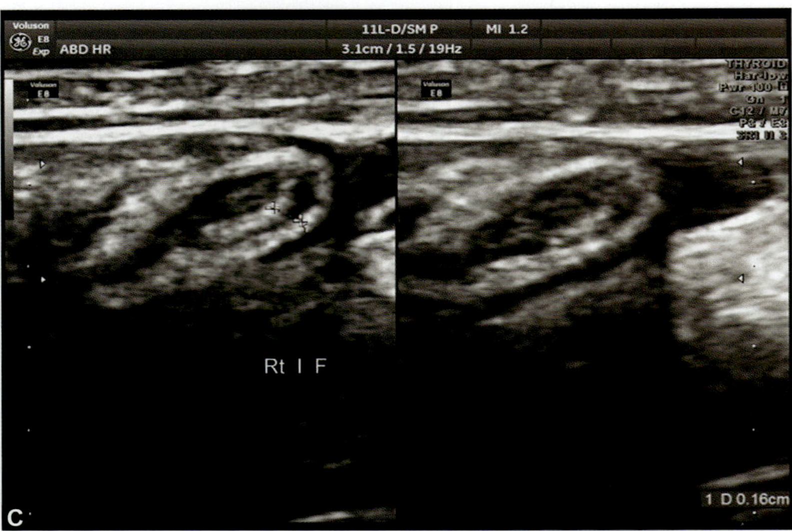

FIGURE 9.18C

FIGURES 9.18A to C: Acute appendicitis with appendicular leak. A patient presented with acute pain in right iliac fossa. High-resolution sonography (HRSG) shows thickened edematous appendix in right iliac fossa. Low-level echo collection is seen in lumen suggestive of debris. Periappendicular fat is also inflamed. Small amount of fluid is also seen in appendicular fossa suggestive of appendicular leak.

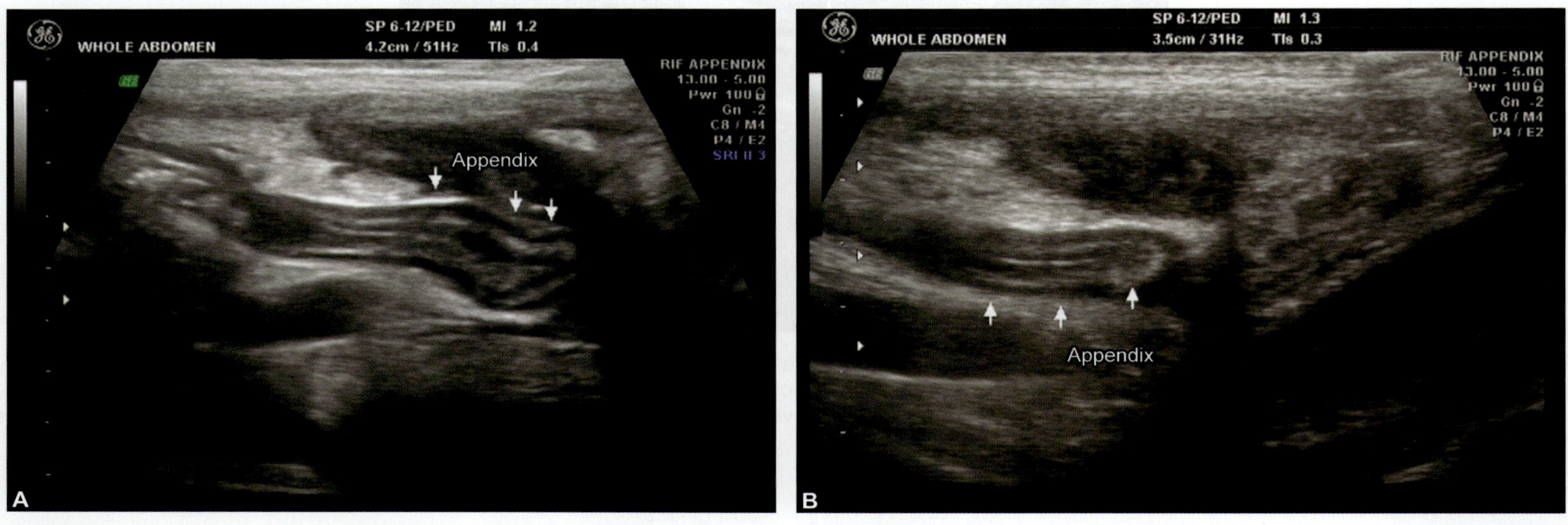

FIGURES 9.19A and B: Acute appendicitis with long appendix. A patient presented with acute pain in right iliac fossa with vomiting. High-resolution sonography (HRSG) shows elongated edematous appendix in right iliac fossa. Marked perifocal edema is present. Echogenic fat is seen in the appendicular fossa suggestive of acute appendicitis. But no evidence of any fluid collection is seen.

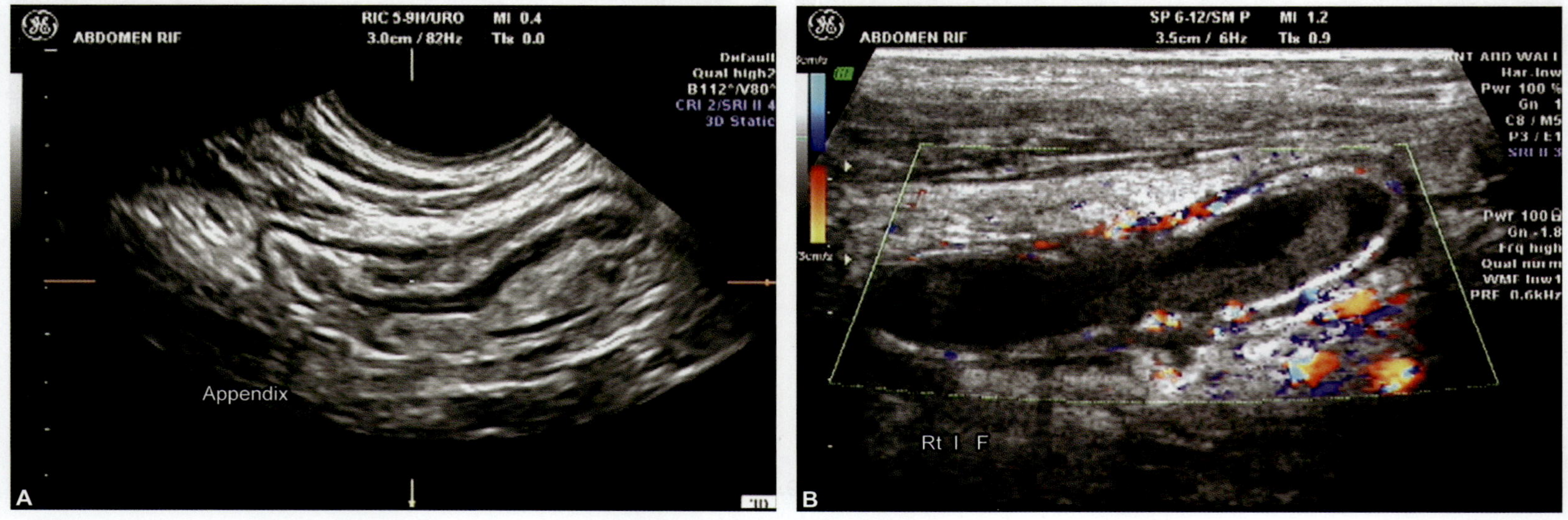

FIGURES 9.20A and B

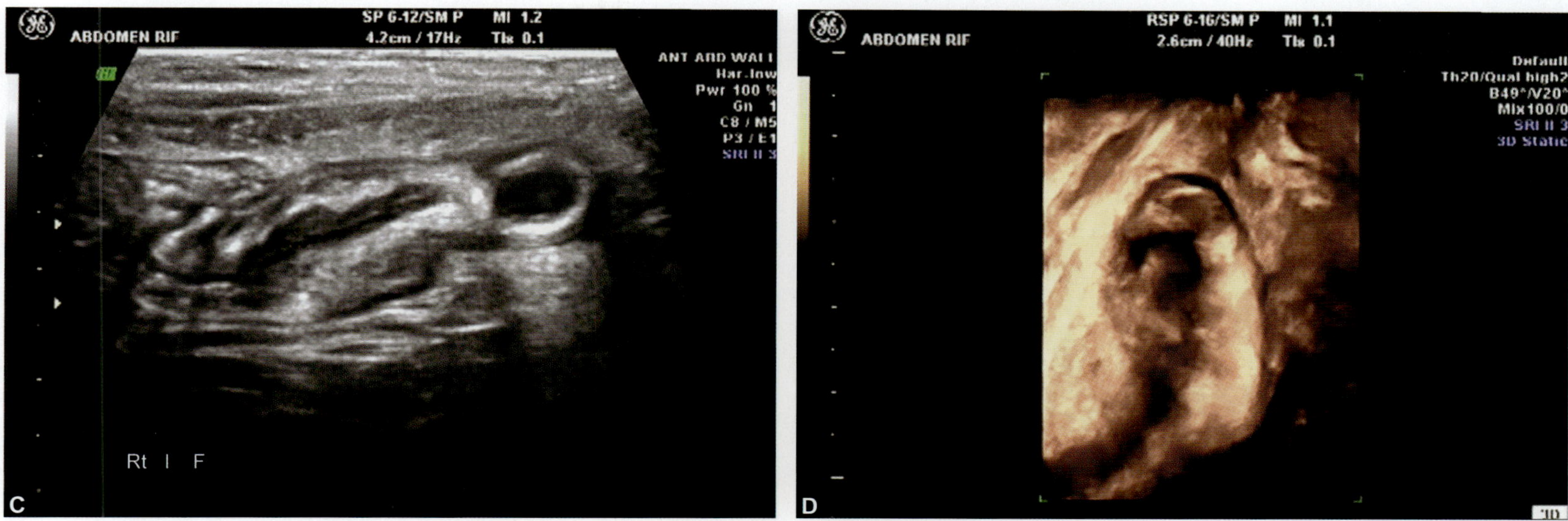

FIGURES 9.20C and D

FIGURES 9.20A to D: Acute appendicitis with pus collection. A patient presented with high fever and acute pain in right iliac fossa. High-resolution sonography (HRSG) shows markedly thickened appendix. Low-level echoes are seen in the appendix lumen suggestive of pyogenic collection. Marked perifocal edema is present. On 3D imaging, the inflamed appendix is clearly seen with distended lumen suggestive of pyogenic appendix. On color flow imaging, increased flow is seen in appendicular wall.

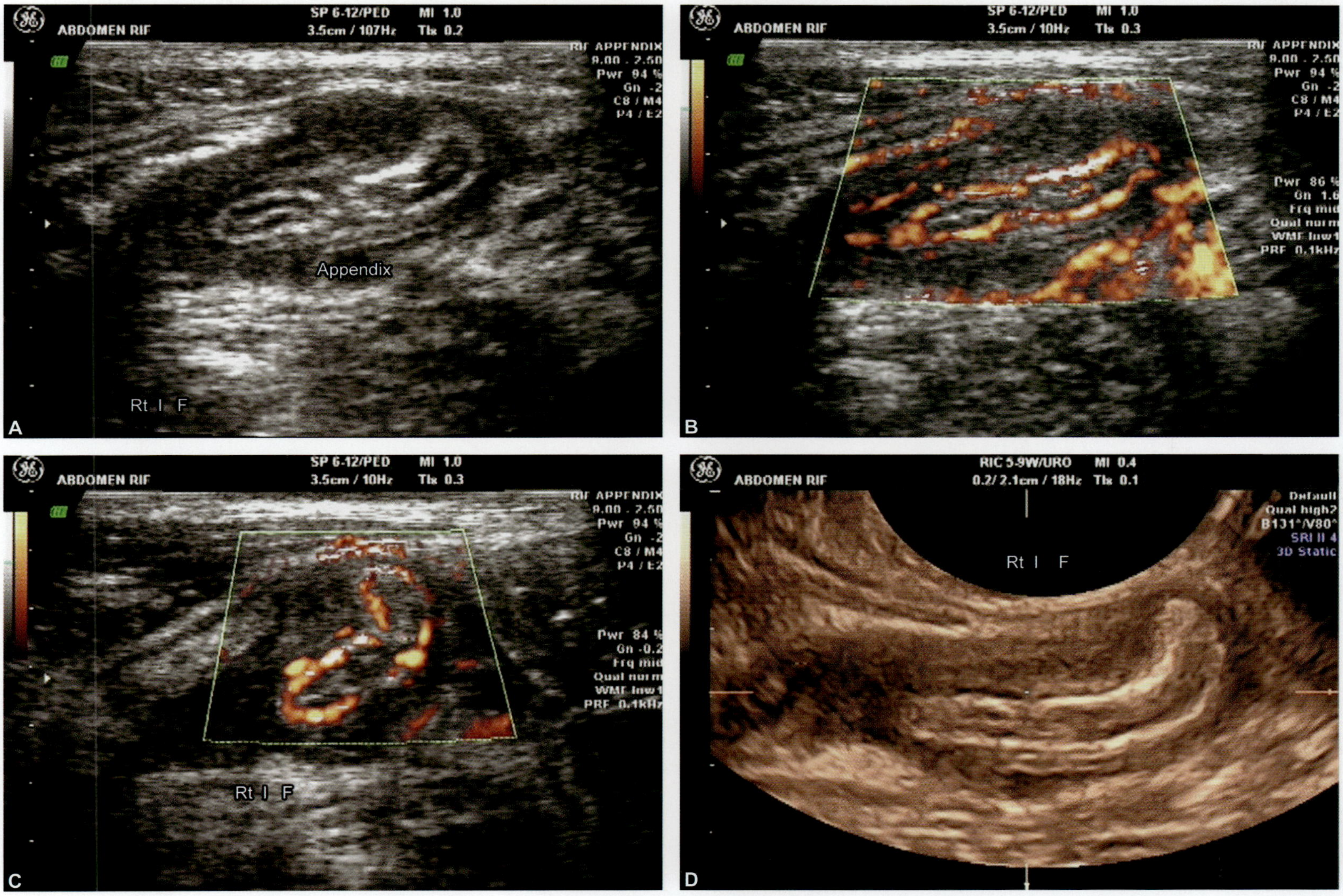

FIGURES 9.21A to D

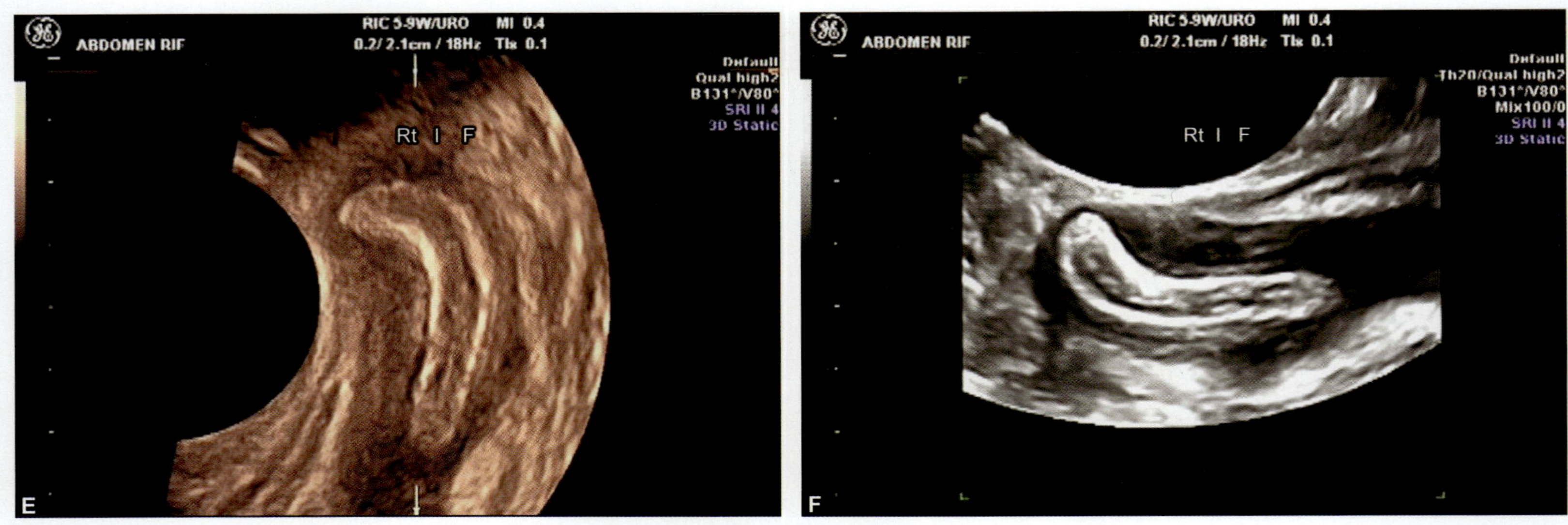

FIGURES 9.21E and F

FIGURES 9.21A to F: Inflamed appendix with pyocele. A patient presented with acute pain with vomiting. HRSG shows markedly thickened edematous appendix in right iliac fossa. Lumen is edematous. Low-level echo collection is seen in the lumen. Marked perifocal edema is present with inflamed periappendicular fat. On color flow imaging, marked increased flow is seen in the appendicular wall. On 3D and volume contrast imaging, the edematous appendix is clearly seen with multiple internal echoes suggestive of pyocele.

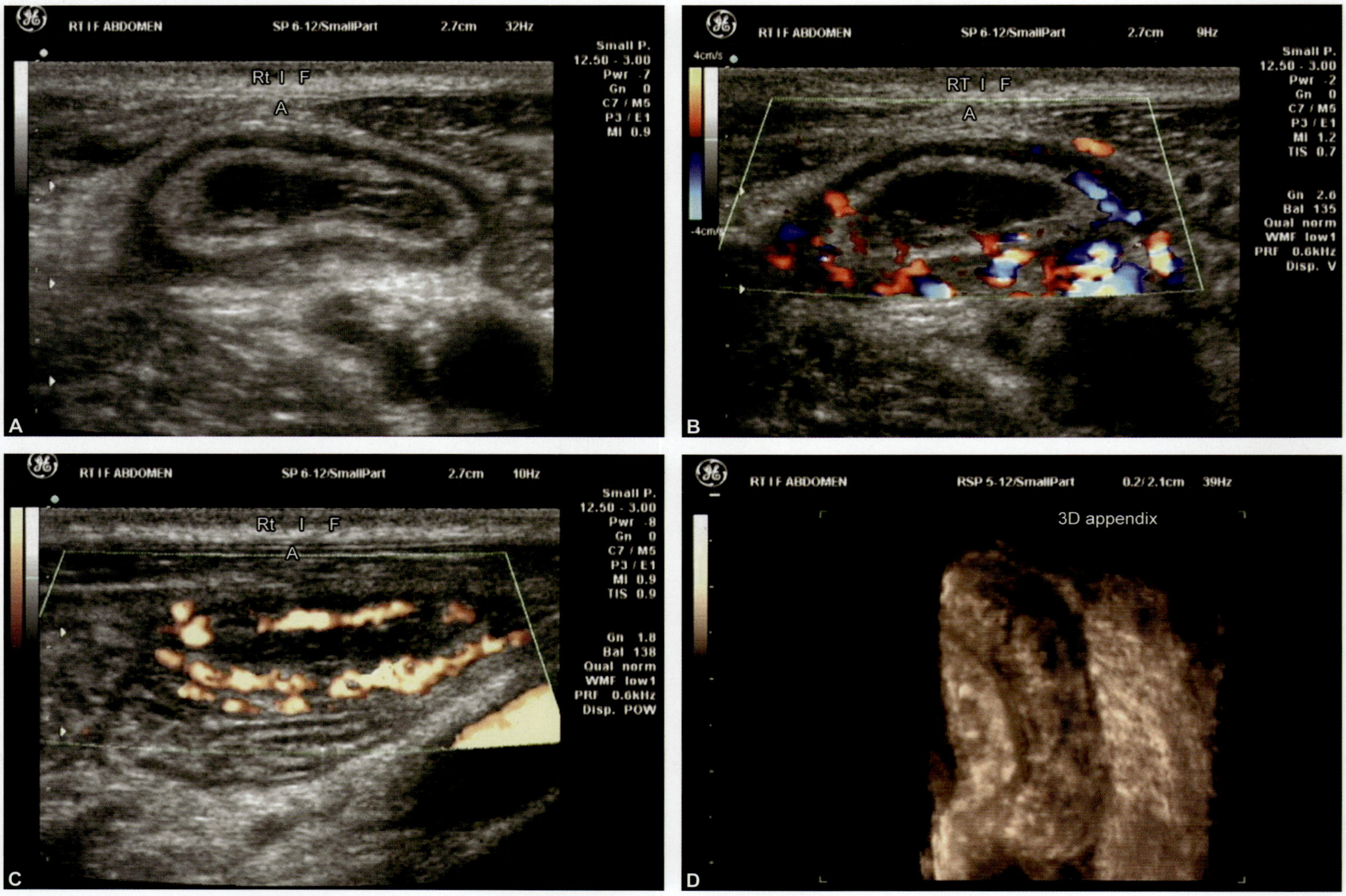

FIGURES 9.22A to D

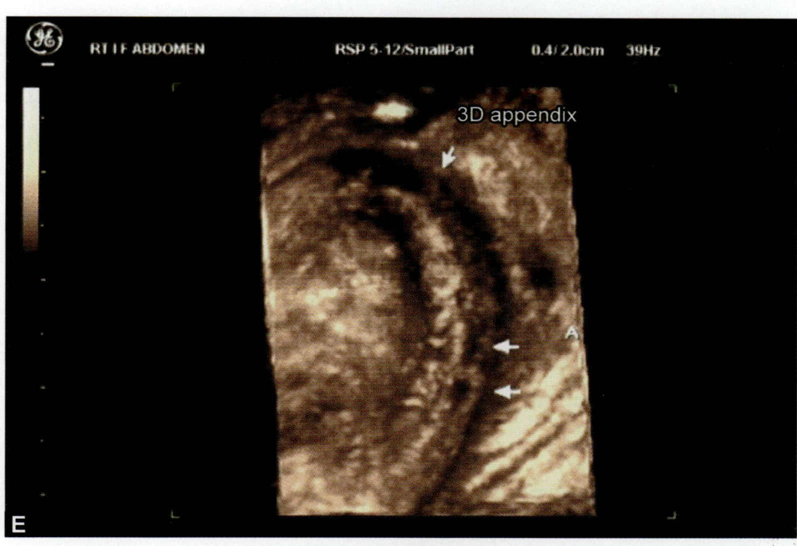

FIGURE 9.22E

FIGURES 9.22A to E: Necrotising appendicitis. HRSG shows acutely inflamed appendix. Appendicular walls are edematous. Small amount of collection is seen in appendicular fossa. On color flow imaging increased flow is seen in appendicular wall suggestive of hyperemia. Power Doppler imaging shows appendicular wall flow. It is seen as ring of fire suggestive of acute inflammation. 3D surface rendering imaging of the appendix shows grossly edematous appendicular walls. Multiple hypoechoic areas are seen on the surface of the appendix suggestive of micro abscesses.

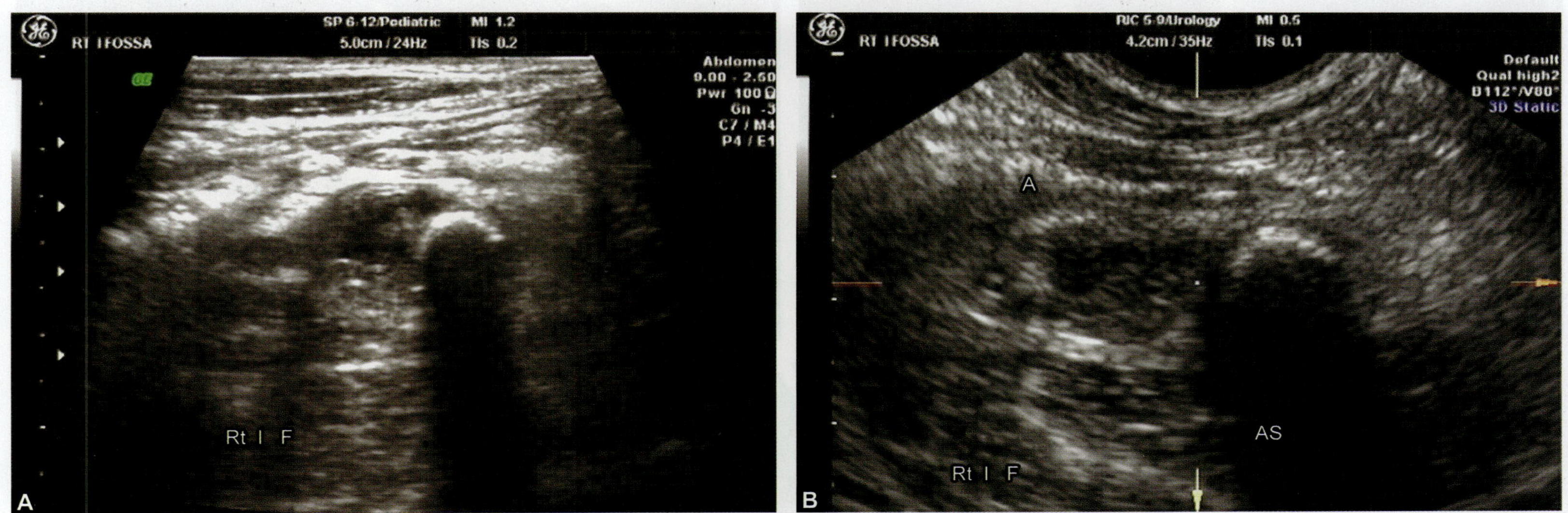

FIGURES 9.23A and B: Obstructed appendix with appendicolith. High-resolution sonography (HRSG) shows edematous thickened appendix. The lumen is distended. Low-level echoes are seen in the lumen of appendix. Big echogenic shadow is seen blocking of the mouth of the appendix. It is accompanied with acoustic shadowing suggestive of appendicolith. Perifocal edema is also seen. Walls of appendix also show edema.

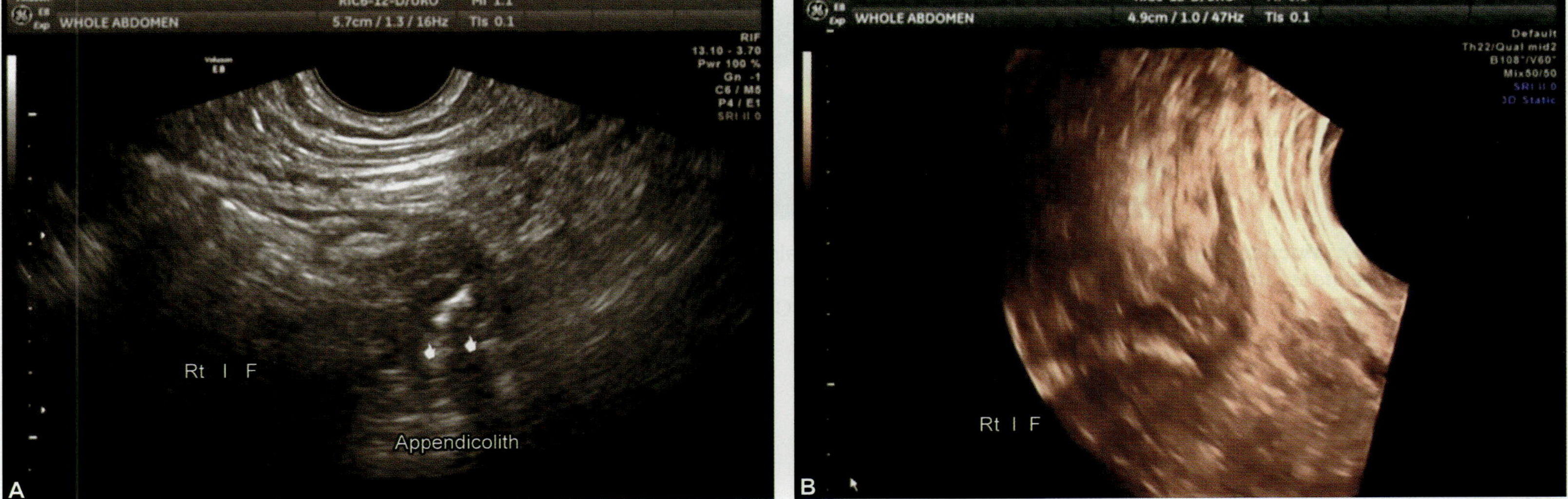

FIGURES 9.24A and B: Obstructed appendix with appendicolith. A patient presented with acute pain with vomiting. HRSG shows inflamed edematous appendix in right iliac fossa. An echogenic shadow is seen impacted in the mouth of appendix, which is accompanied with acoustic shadowing suggestive of appendicolith. On 3D imaging, the inflamed obstructed appendix with appendicolith is clearly seen.

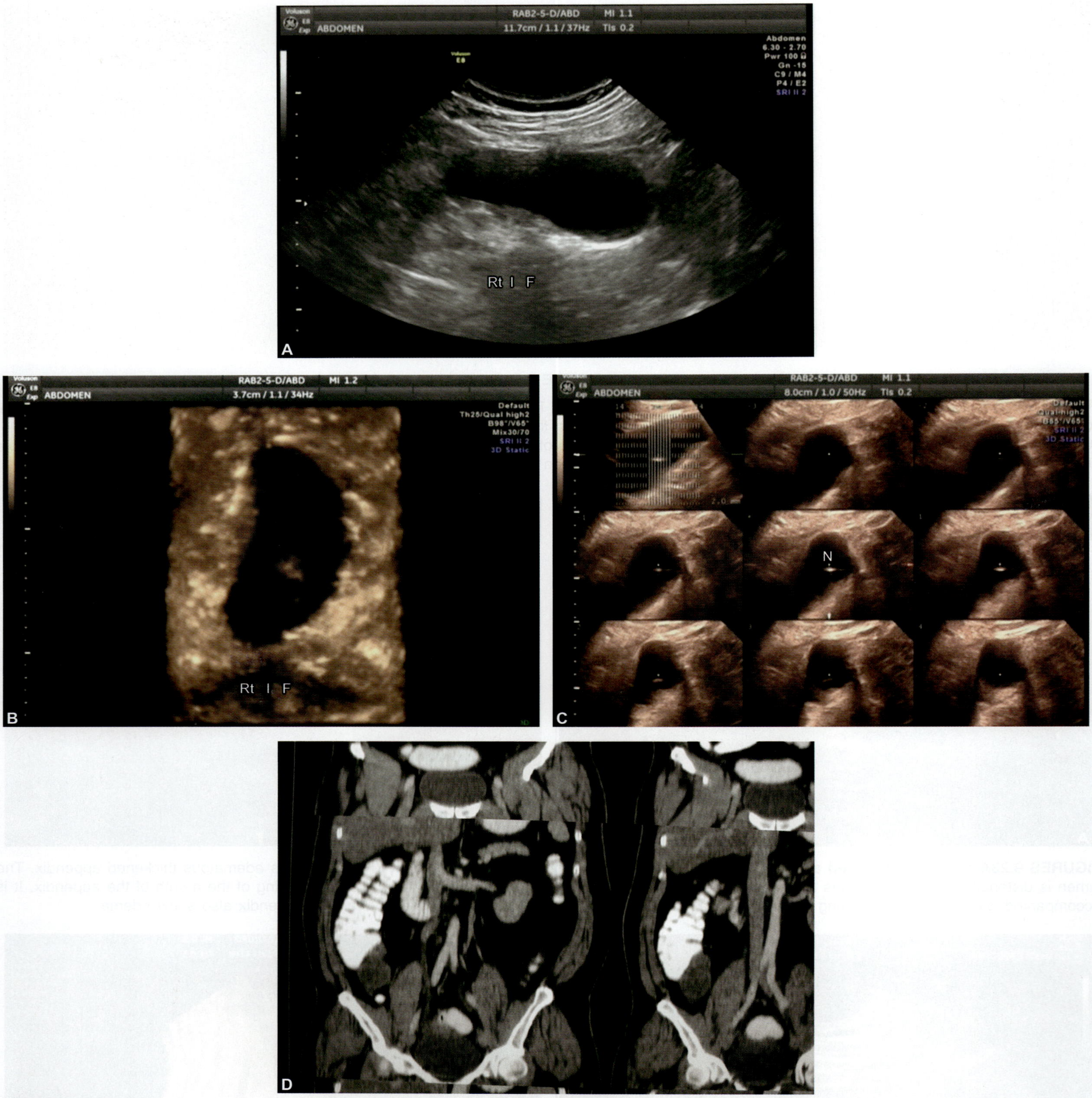

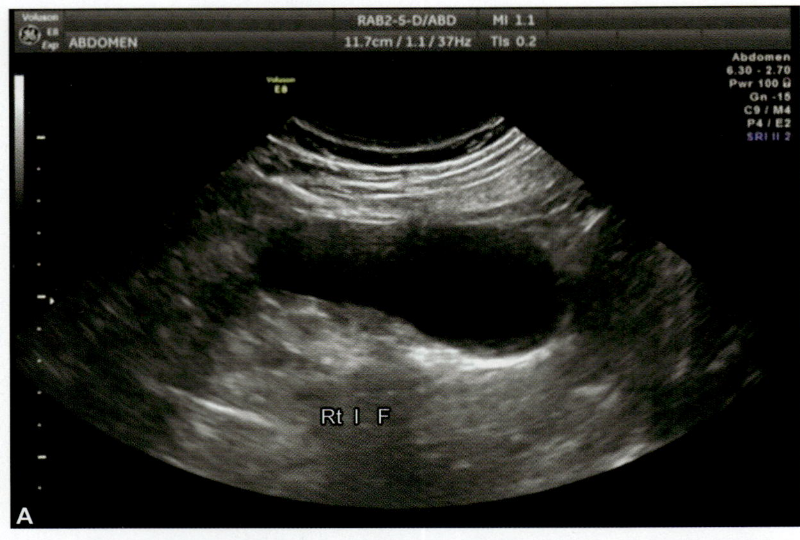

FIGURES 9.25A to D: Mucocele appendix. A patient presented with pain in right iliac fossa with a soft lump. HRSG shows markedly distended appendix. Low-level echoes are seen in it. But no septation or calcification is seen. Associated perifocal edema is present. But no free fluid is seen in appendicular fossa. Findings are consistent with mucocele of appendix. CT scan of the same patient shows distended appendix with homogeneous collection. Findings are suggestive of mucocele appendix.

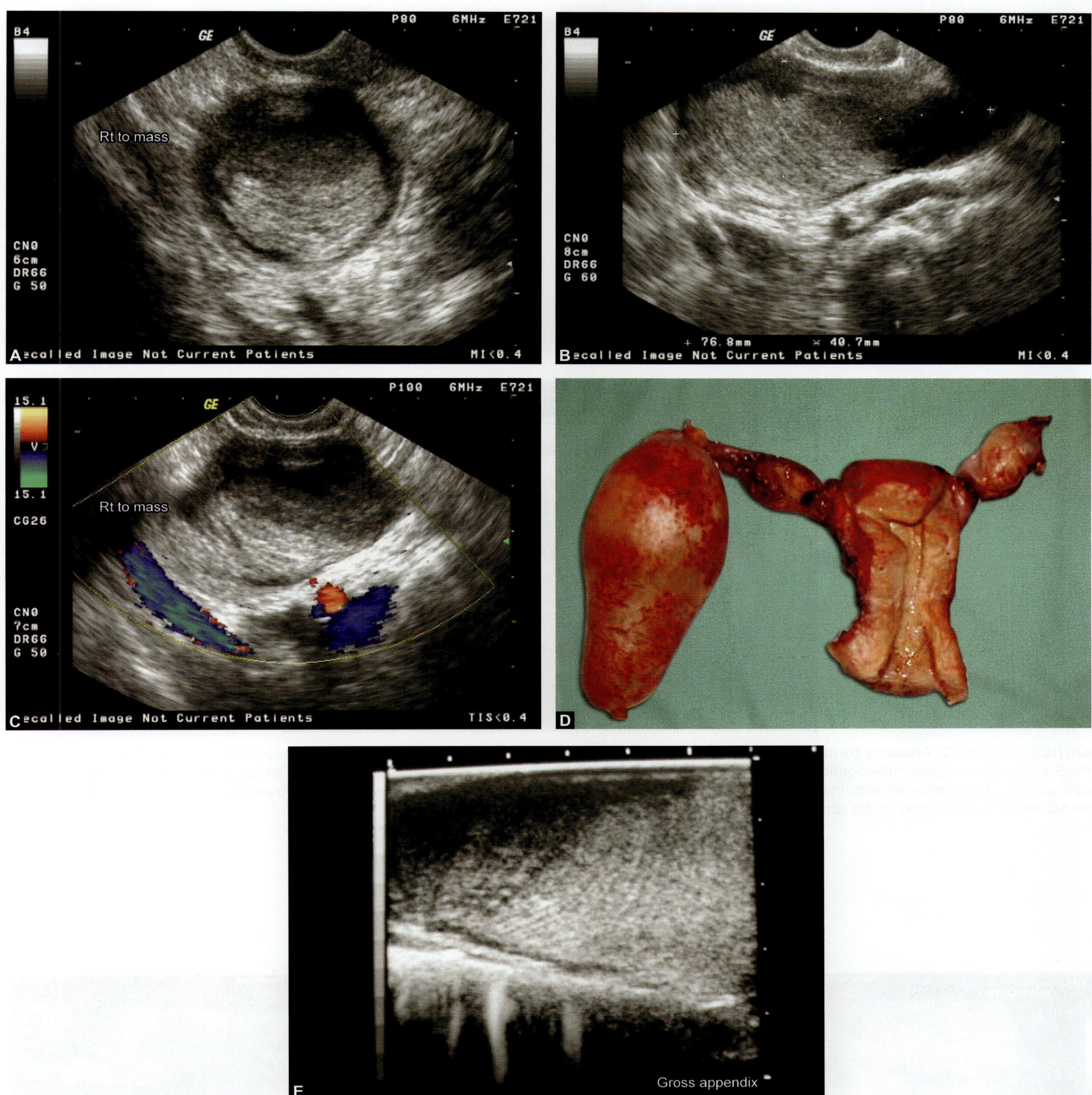

FIGURES 9.26A to E: Mucocele of appendix. A patient presented with palpable lump in the right iliac fossa. It was mistaken as ovarian cyst. High-resolution sonography (HRSG) shows a thick walled cystic mass in cross section. Multiple internal echoes are seen in it with positive layering sign. The longitudinal imaging shows a tubular fusiform shadow in the right iliac fossa. Thick debris is seen filling the lumen of it suggestive of mucocele of appendix. On color flow imaging poor flow is seen in the wall of appendix. "The gross specimen" after surgery shows the mucocele appendix. The right ovary is seen normal. Uterus and left ovary are also seen with the specimen. HRSG of the "gross specimen" of mucocele shows thick collection with positive layering sign confirming the findings of HRSG of the patient.

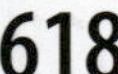

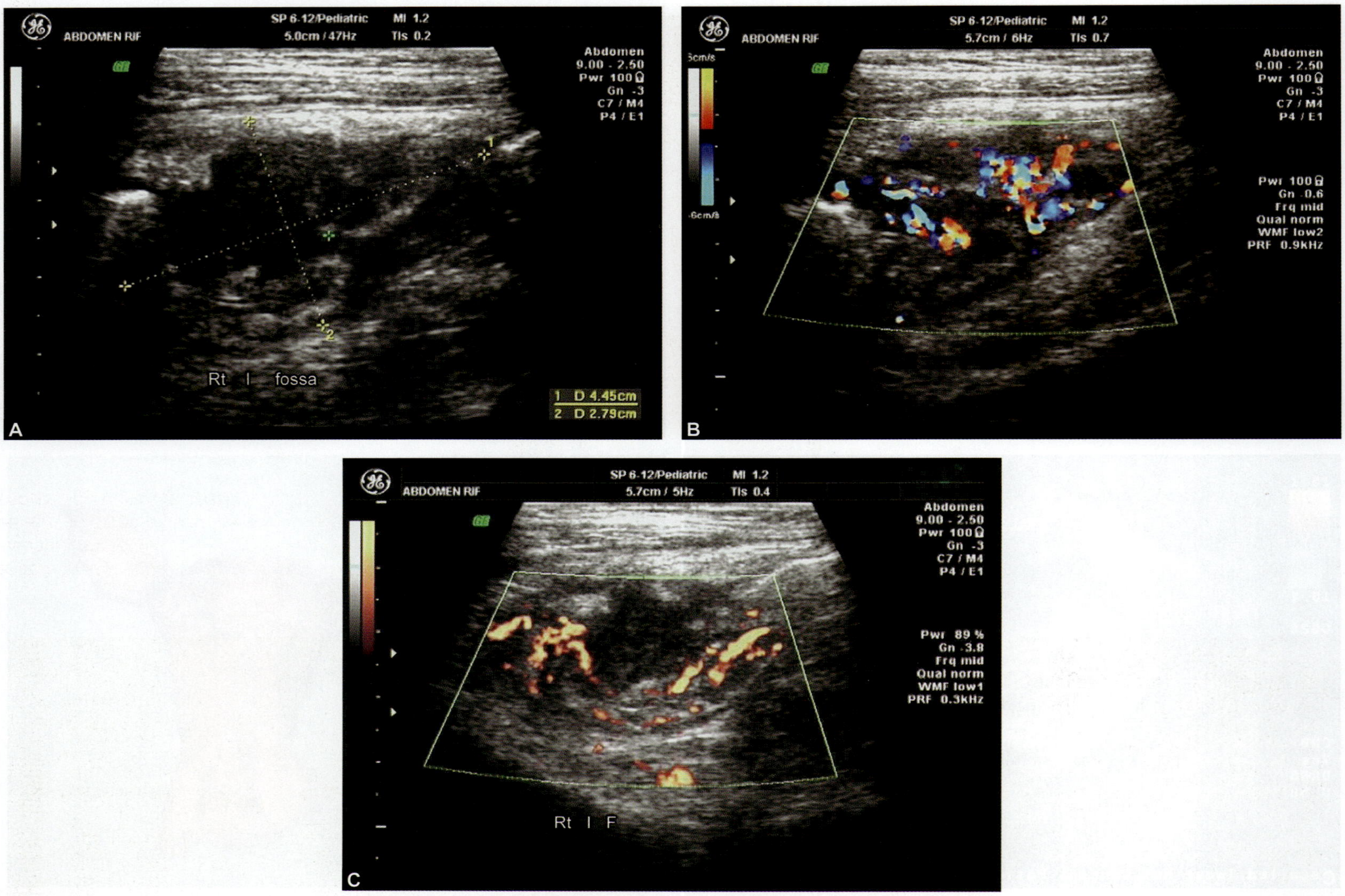

FIGURES 9.27A to C: Abscess formation in appendicular fossa. A patient operated for acute appendicitis presented with a lump in right iliac fossa. HRSG shows an irregular heterogeneous low-level echo complex mass in the right iliac fossa suggestive of an abscess formation. Adjacent bowel loops are also seen adherent with the mass. On color flow imaging, the abscess wall shows increased flow around it suggestive of acute hyperemia. Internal debris is also seen in the abscess.

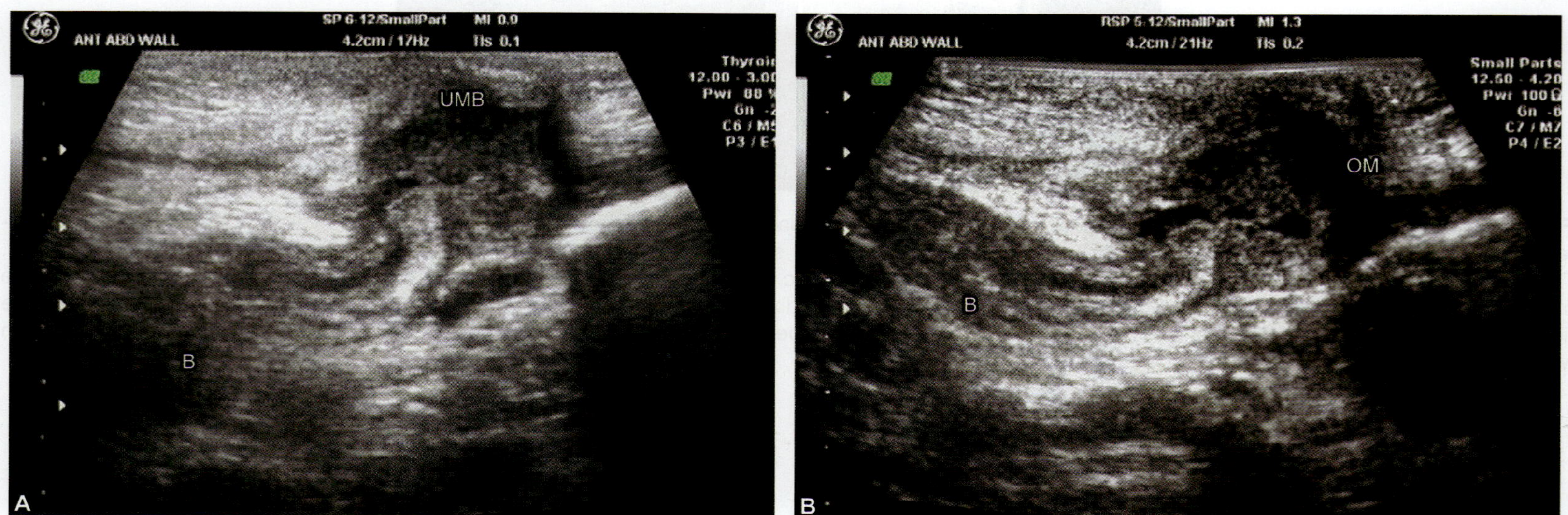

FIGURES 9.28A and B

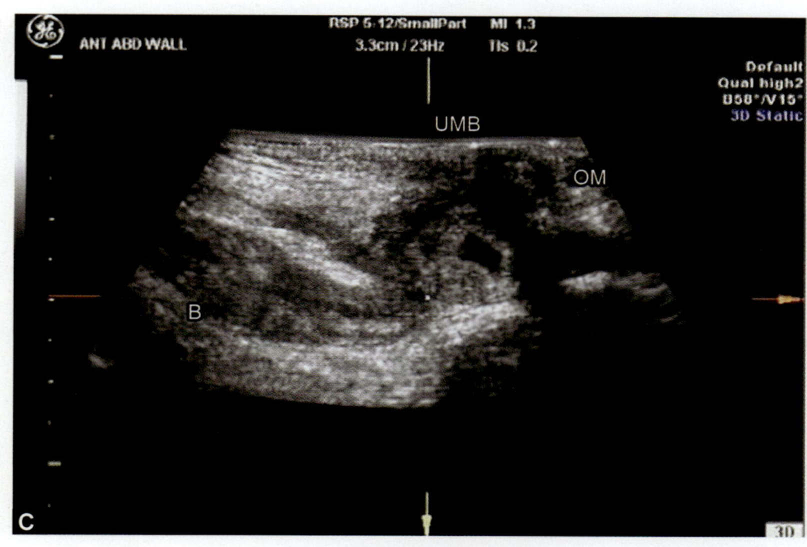

FIGURE 9.28C

FIGURES 9.28A to C: Obstructed Meckel's diverticulum. A young child presented with pain in the abdomen. HRSG shows an elongated edematous tubular shadow running in the paraumblical area and going towards the umbilicus. The neck of the diverticulum is seen torsed. Marked perifocal edema is present. Fluid is also seen in the peridiverticulum area suggestive of obstruction of the diverticulum. HRSG shows clearly the edematous mucosal folds of the diverticulum. Small abscess is also seen in the floor of the diverticulum. Partial herniation is seen in the umblical region. Postoperative findings confirmed obstructed torsed Meckel's diverticulum.

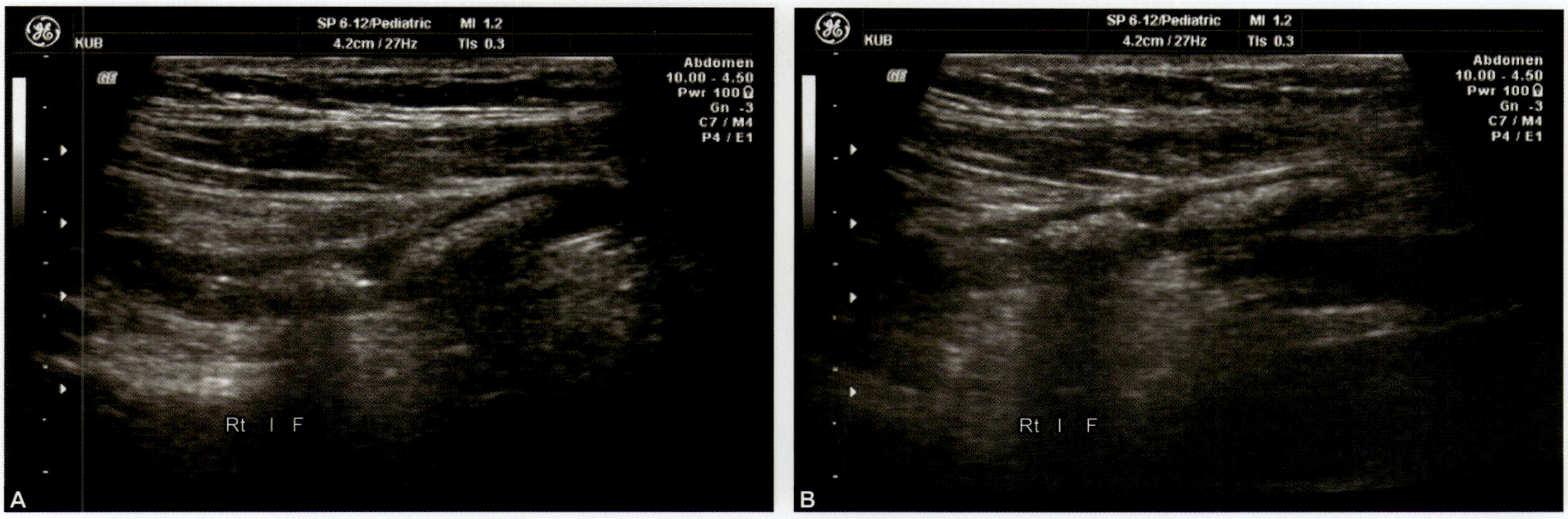

FIGURES 9.29A and B: Inflamed Meckel's diverticulum. A young patient presented with pain in the right iliac fossa. HRSG shows thickened edematous tube. It was rigid and noncompressible on transducer pressure. Echogenic shadows are seen filling the lumen with gas entrapment. It was mistaken as inflamed appendix. However, postoperative findings confirmed inflamed Meckel's diverticulum.

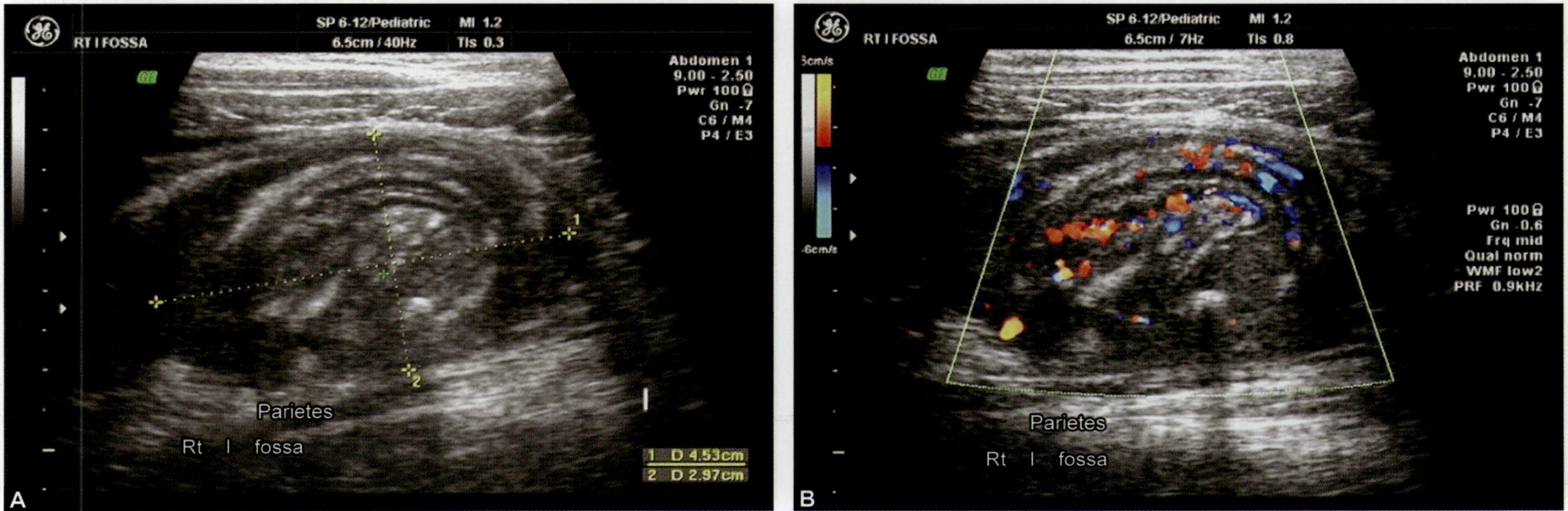

FIGURES 9.30A and B

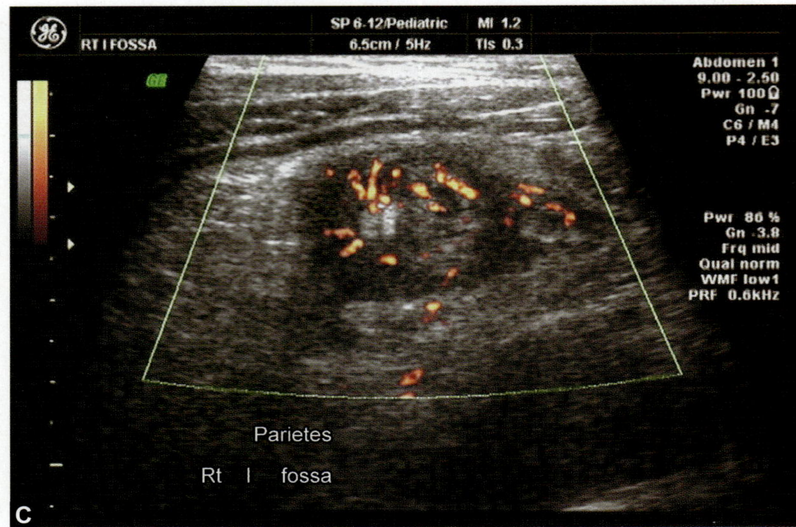

FIGURE 9.30C

FIGURES 9.30A to C: Parietal abscess in right iliac fossa. HRSG shows well-defined parietal abscess in the right iliac fossa. The abscess is seen confined to the parietes. Layering sign is positive. Perifocal edema is present. It was mistaken as appendicitis on clinical examination. On color flow imaging, wall hyperemia is seen in the abscess. Multiple vessels are seen feeding the abscess.

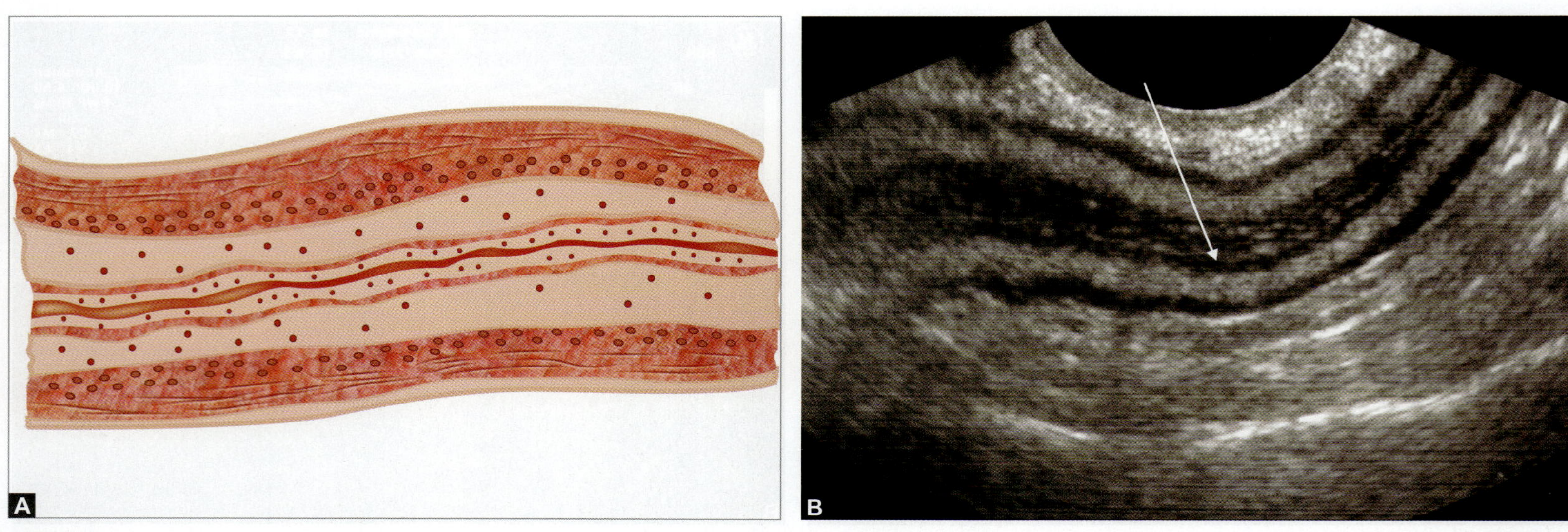

FIGURES 9.31A and B: Normal ultrasound appearance of colon of large bowel. Figure A shows diagrammatic representation of normal large bowel layers and the lumen. Figure B shows normal sonographic appearance of large bowel, which matches with the normal muscle layers

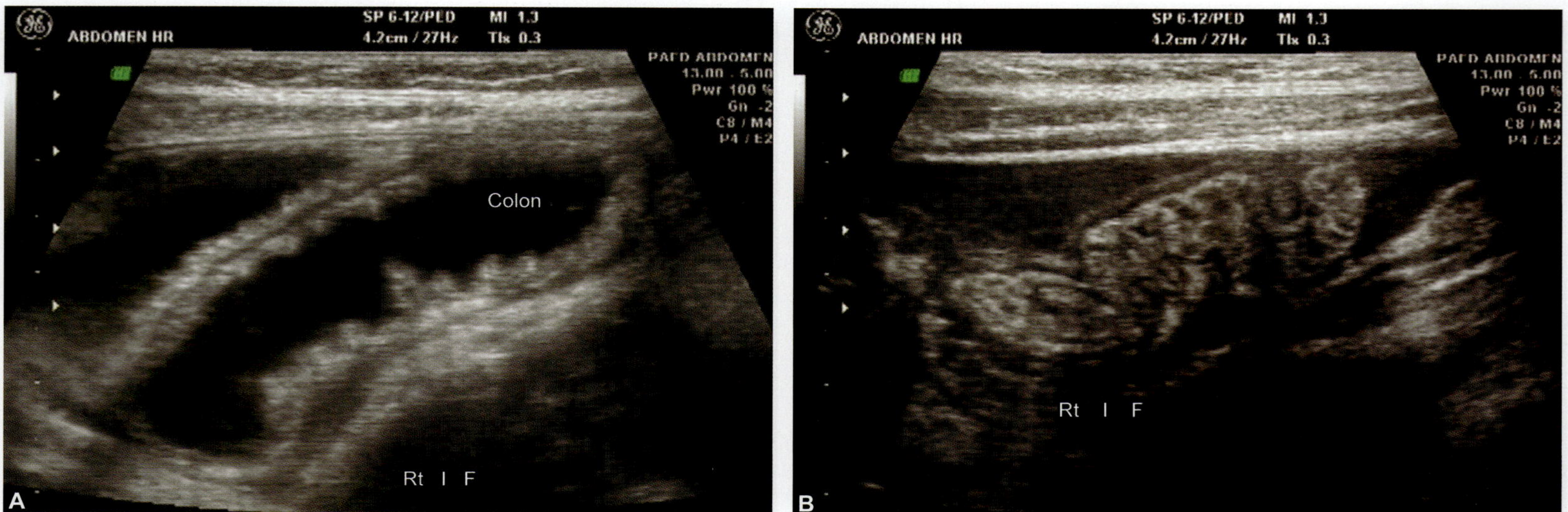

FIGURES 9.32A and B

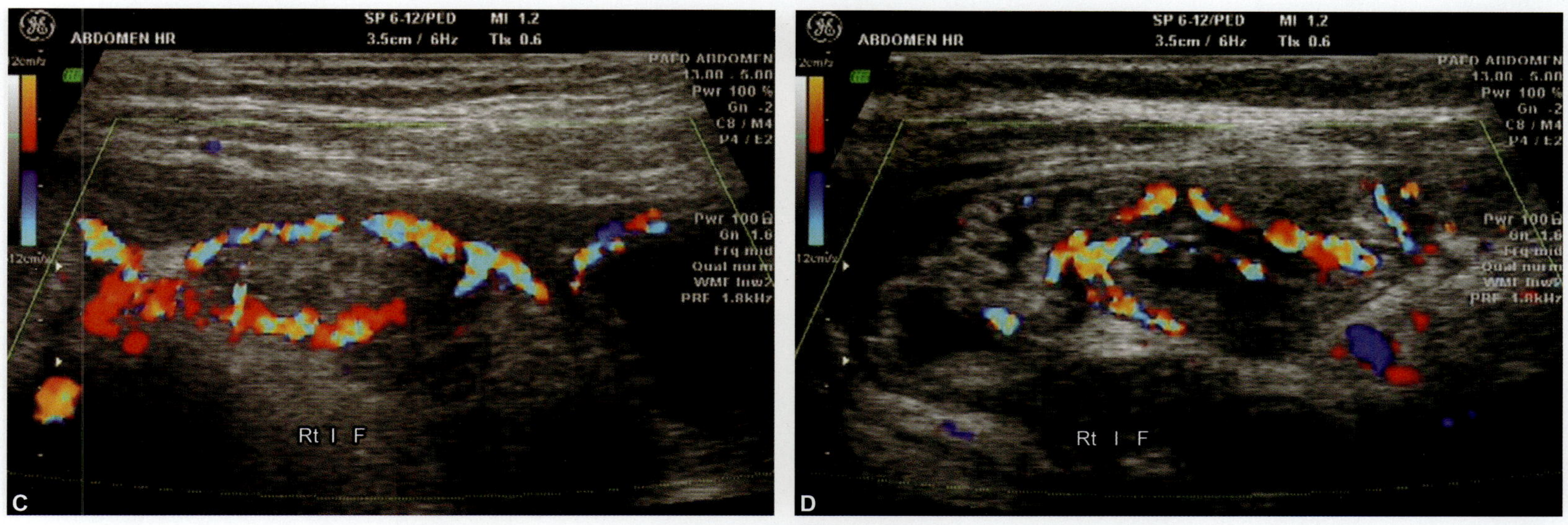

FIGURES 9.32C and D

FIGURES 9.32A to D: Acute inflammation of the colon. A patient presented with pain in the abdomen. HRSG shows dilated colon. The colonic wall is edematous. Low-level echo collection is seen in the colon. Fluid movement is sluggish suggestive of acute colitis. On color flow imaging, marked increased flow is seen in the colonic wall due to secondary infection.

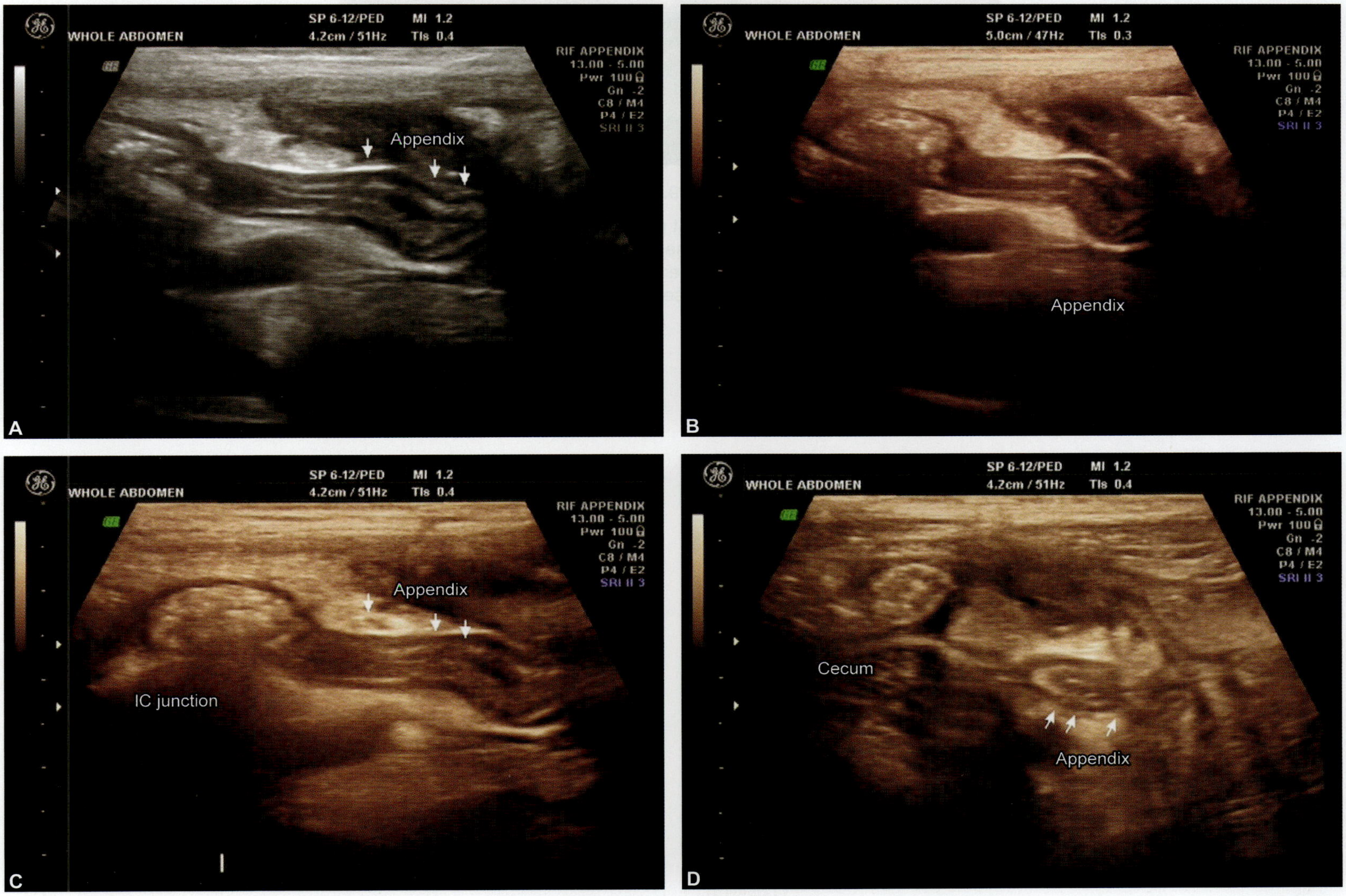

FIGURES 9.33A to D

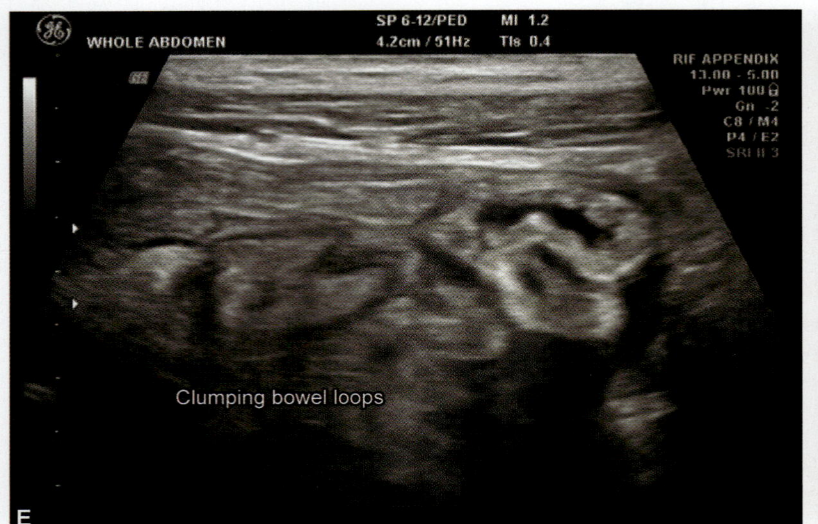

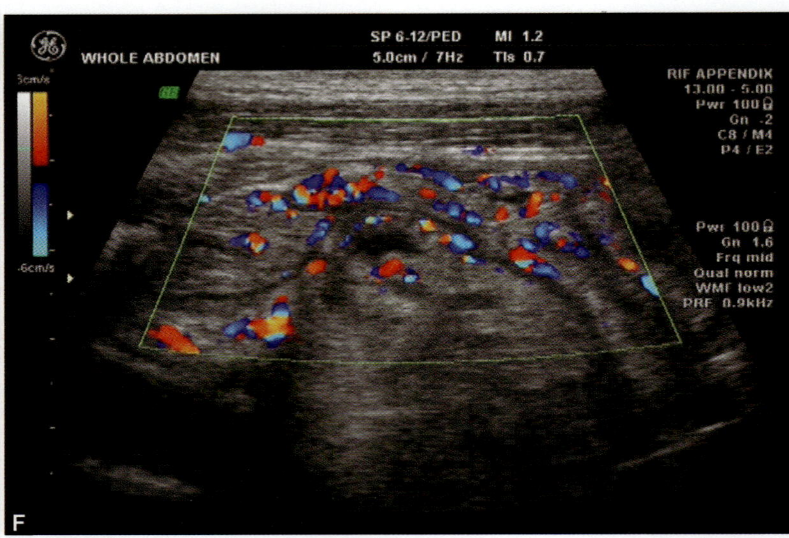

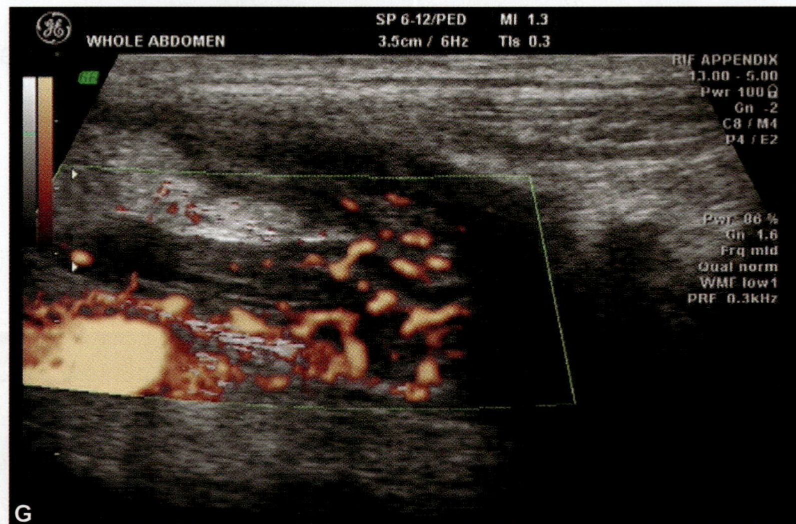

FIGURE 9.33E to G

FIGURES 9.33A to G: Inflamed cecum with acute appendicitis. A patient presented with pain in right iliac fossa with vomiting. HRSG shows markedly edematous appendix suggestive of acute appendicitis. The cecum is also seen edematous. Perifocal edema is present in cecum. The ileocecal junction shows dilated bowel loops with clumping. Bowel loop edema is also presented suggestive of acute inflammatory disease involving ileocecal junction, bowel loops and the appendix. On color flow imaging, increased flow is seen in the walls of inflamed bowel loops.

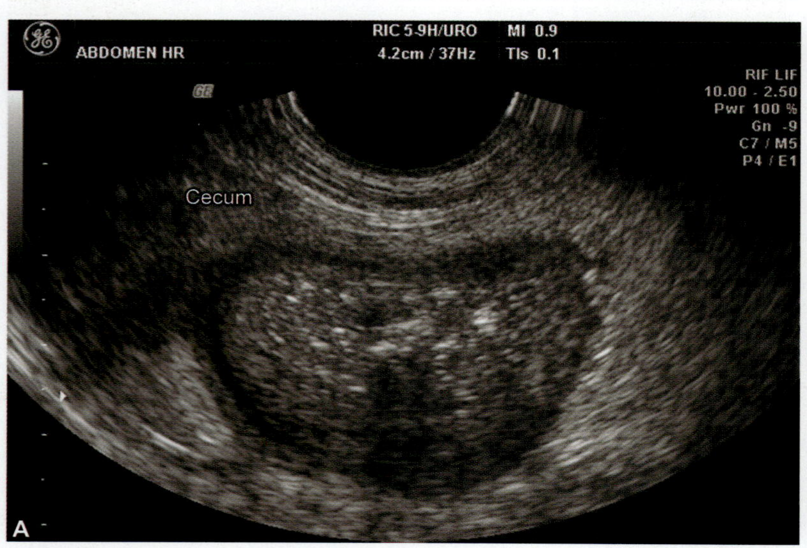

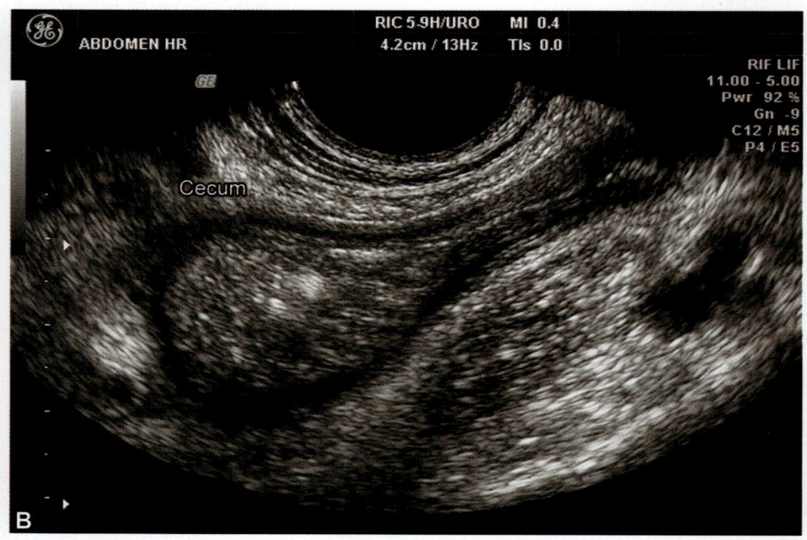

FIGURES 9.34A and B

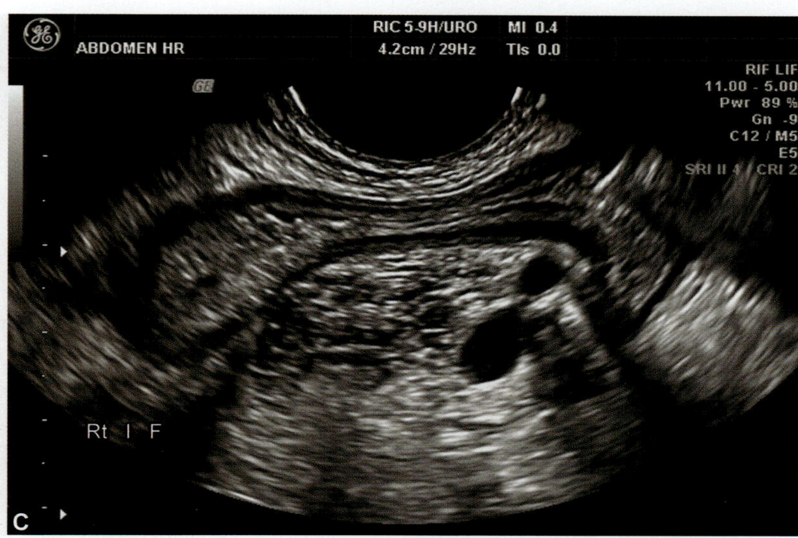

FIGURE 9.34C

FIGURES 9.34A to C: A patient presented with recurrent pain in abdomen. High-resolution sonography (HRSG) shows thickened edematous cecum. Thick collection is seen in cecum with slow fluid movement. The proximal bowel loops are dilated. There is also evidence of multiple multiple enlarged nodes seen in right iliac fossa suggestive of chronic ileocecal disease

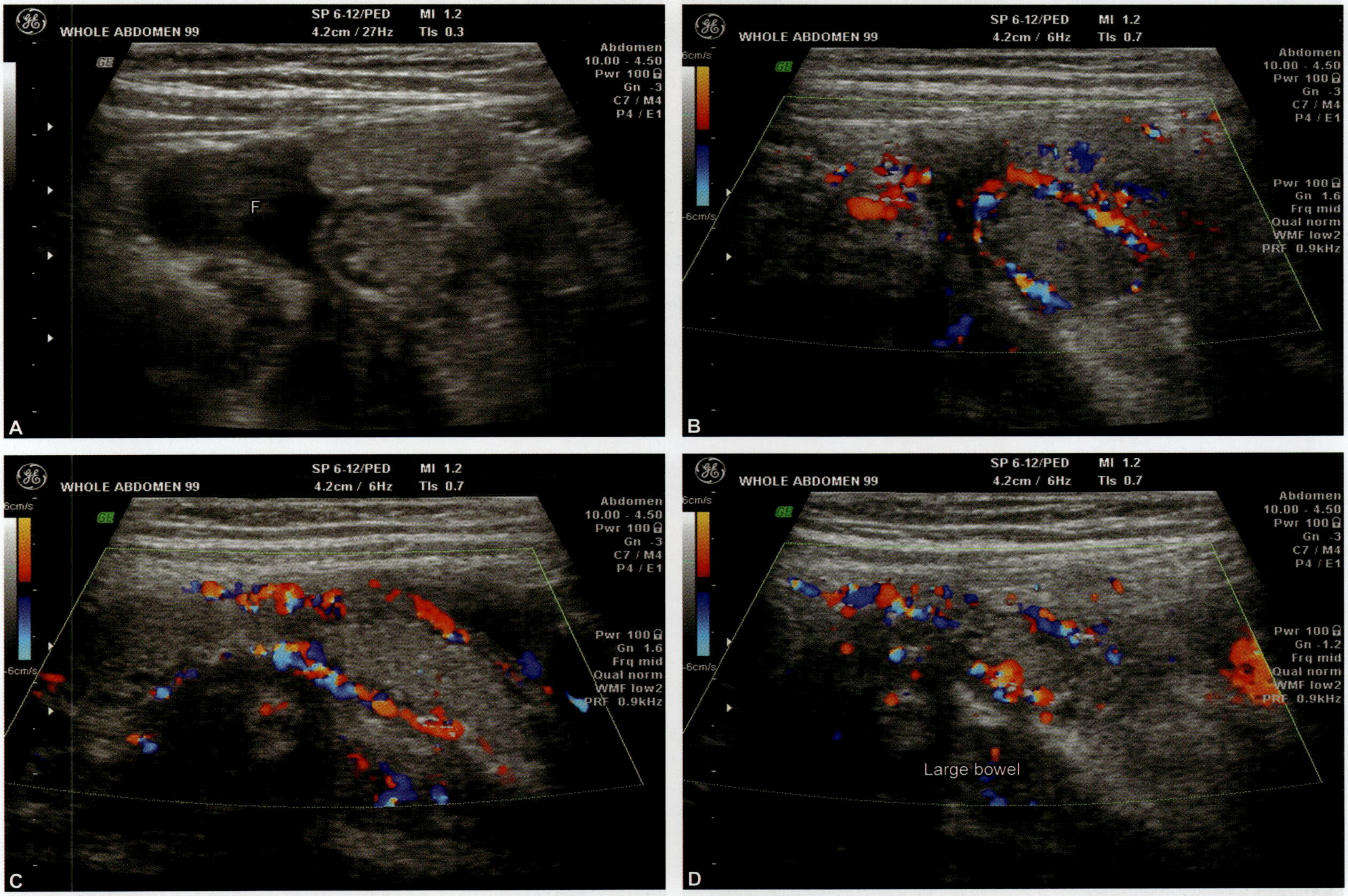

FIGURES 9.35A to D: Acute necrotizing colitis. A young girl presented with high fever and vomiting. High-resolution sonography (HRSG) shows distended bowel loops. Low- level echo collection is seen in the bowel loops. Air is also seen in the wall. On color flow imaging, marked increased flow is seen in the wall of the loops. Small amount of fluid collection is also seen in the peritoneal cavity. Findings are suggestive of acute necrotizing enterocolitis. Air in the muscle of bowel is the cardinal sign of necrotizing enterocolitis.

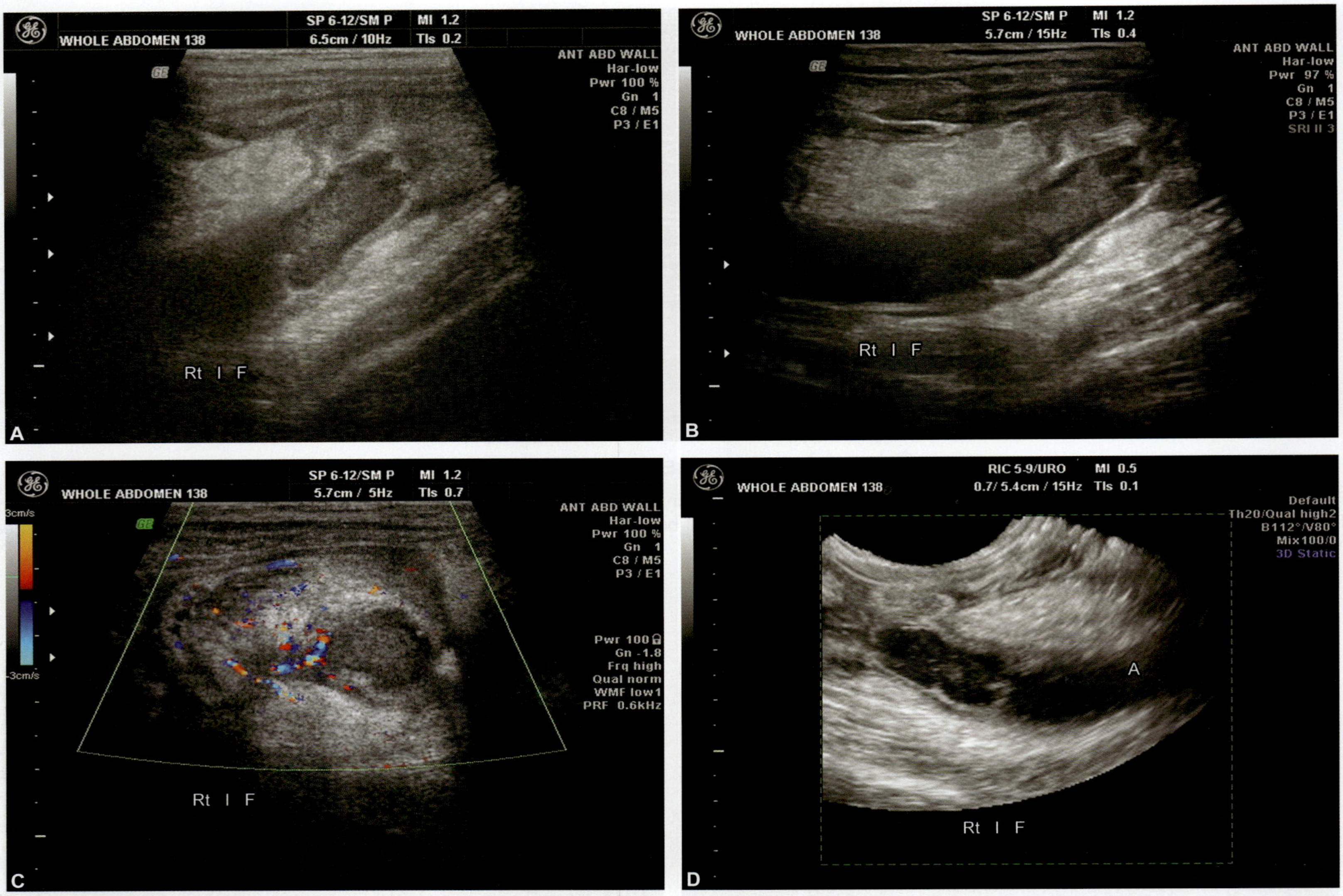

FIGURES 9.36A to D: Empyema appendix. A patient presented with high fever and vomiting. High-resolution sonography (HRSG) shows a thickened tubular shadow in the right iliac fossa. It shows low-level echo collection. Perifocal edema is also present. Multiple enlarged lymph nodes are also seen in the iliac fossa. On 3D imaging, the pyogenic collection is seen clearly in the appendix. Findings are suggestive of empyema appendix.

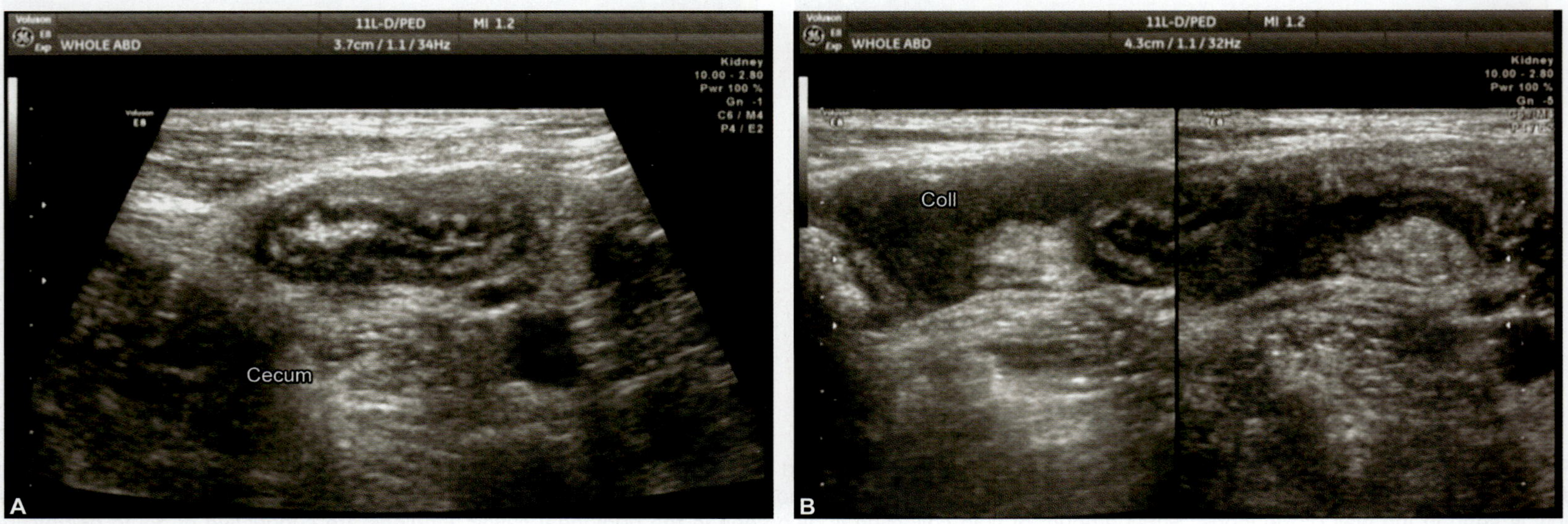

FIGURES 9.37A and B

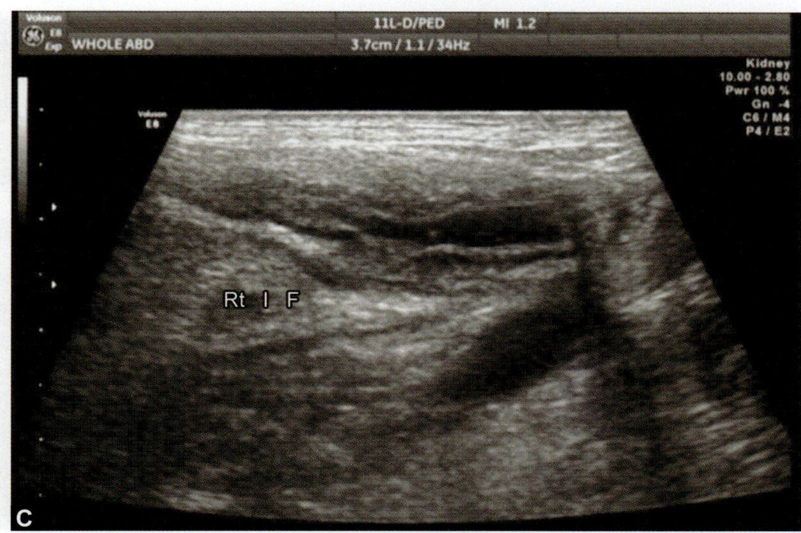

FIGURE 9.37C

FIGURES 9.37A to C: Thickened cecum. A patient presented with recurrent pain in abdomen in right iliac fossa. High-resolution sonography (HRSG) shows markedly thickened cecum. Low-level echo collection is seen in the lumen of caecum. Small collection is also seen around the cecum suggestive of chronic inflammation of cecum

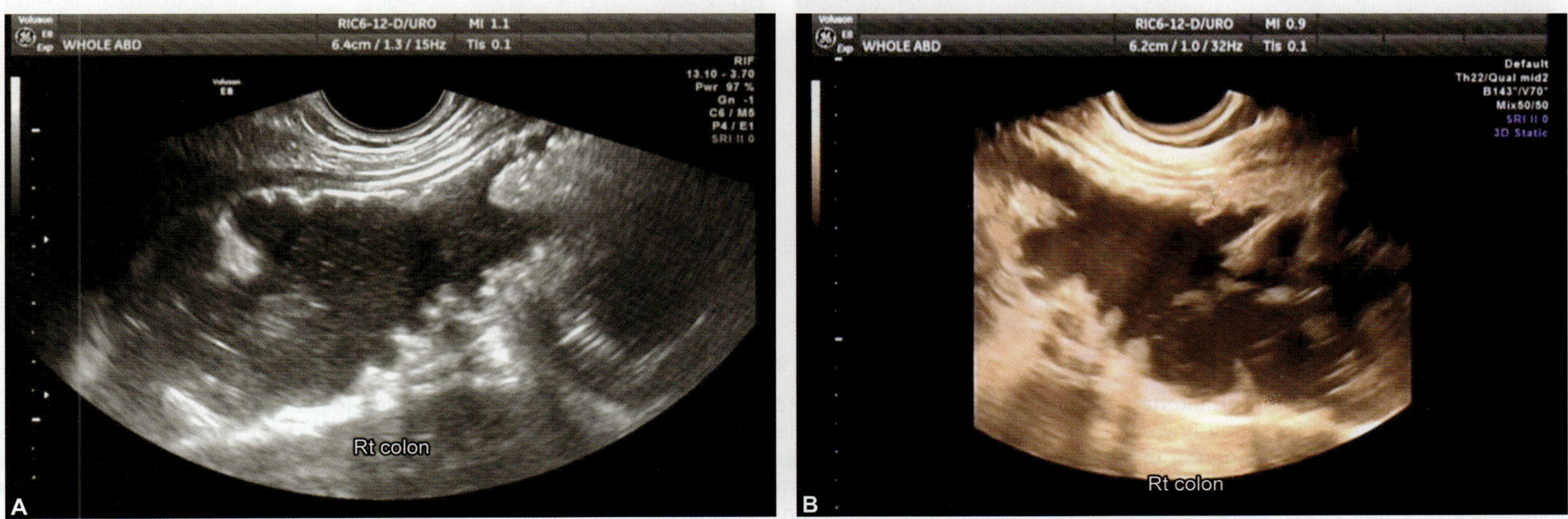

FIGURES 9.38A and B: Toxic dilatation of the colon. A young girl presented with acute pain in abdomen with vomiting. HRSG shows markedly dilated colon. Low-level echo collection is seen in colon. Fluid movement is sluggish and almost absent. Colonic mucosal fold is also edematous. Findings are suggestive of toxic dilatation of colon.

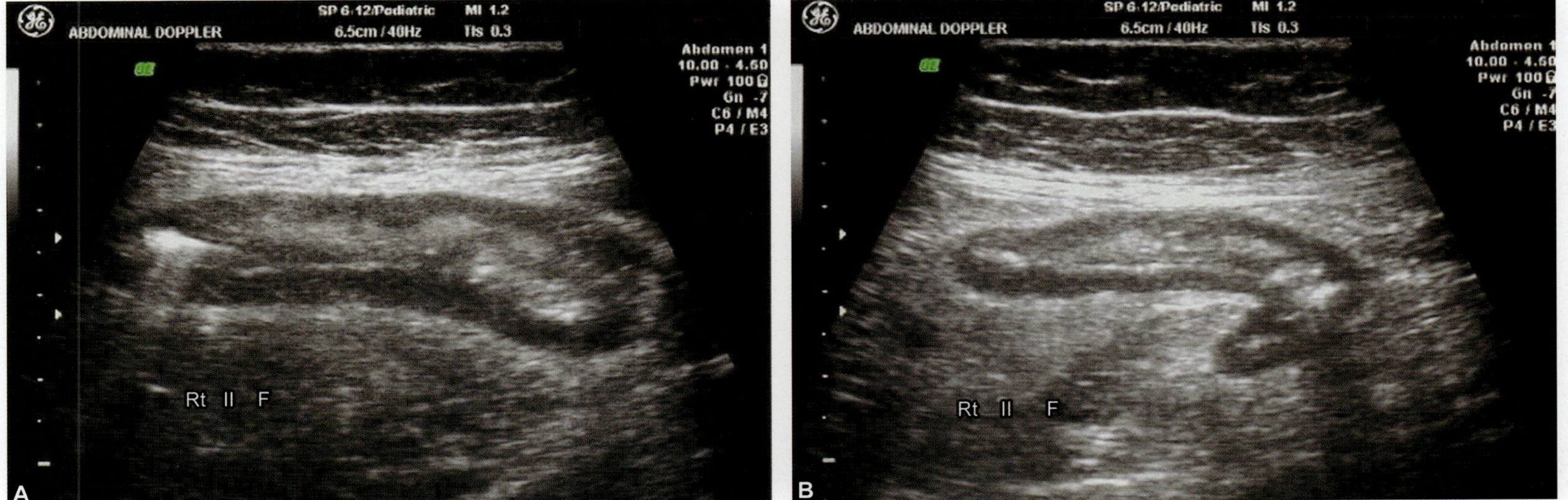

FIGURES 9.39A and B

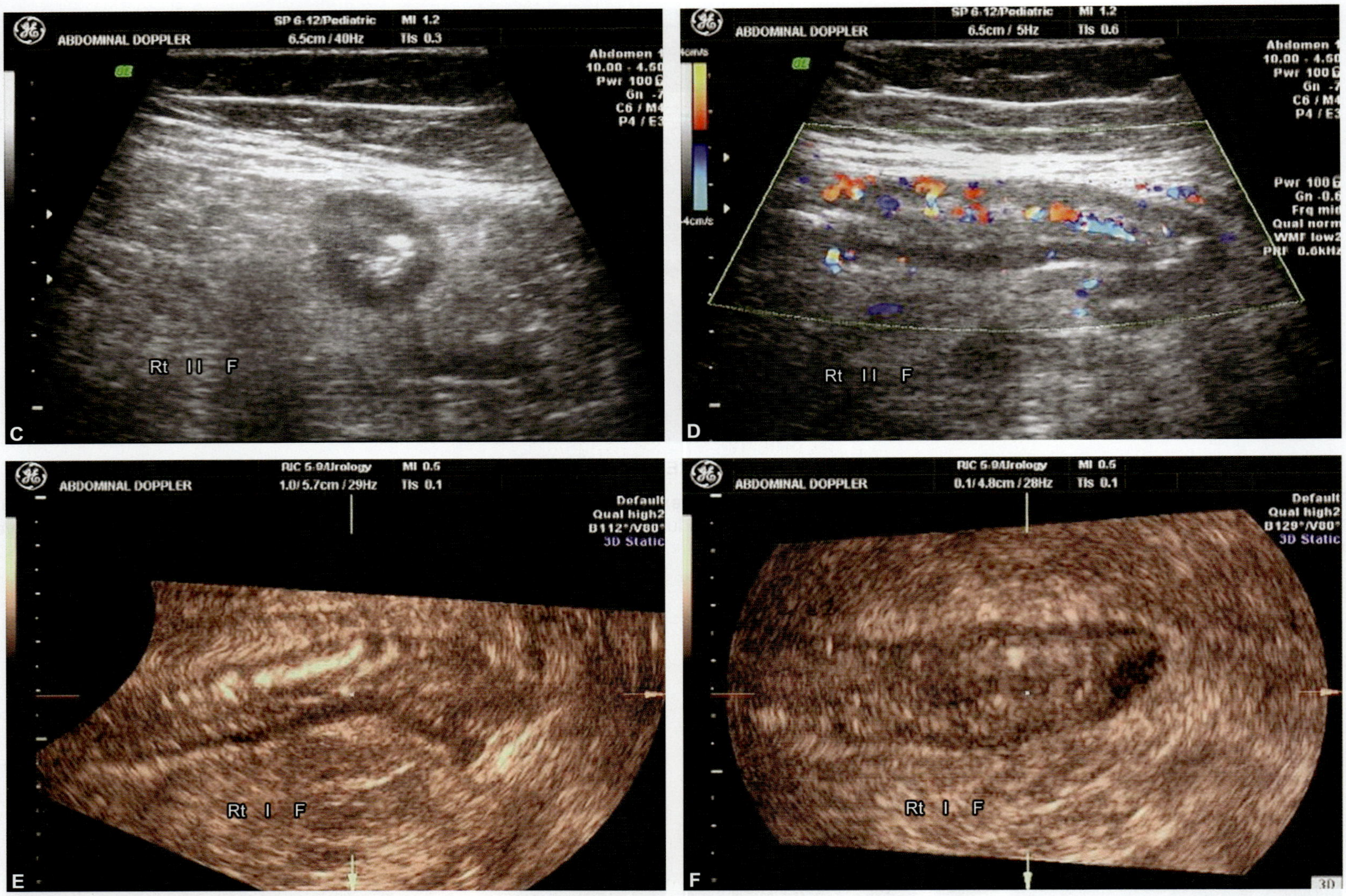

FIGURES 9.39C to F

FIGURES 9.39A to F: Grossly thickened ascending colon. A patient presented with recurrent pain in right iliac fossa. High-resolution sonography (HRSG) shows markedly thickened bowel loop in the right iliac fossa. Walls are edematous. Lumen is obliterated. Gas entrapment is seen. On color flow imaging, moderate flow is seen in the wall of the thickened bowel loop. Power Doppler imaging shows blood flow in much better way suggestive of chronic inflammation. No evidence of any fluid collection seen in the lumen of the loop. 3D surface rendering imaging of the bowel shows marked thickening of the wall of the bowel. Postoperative findings confirmed chronic inflammatory disease.

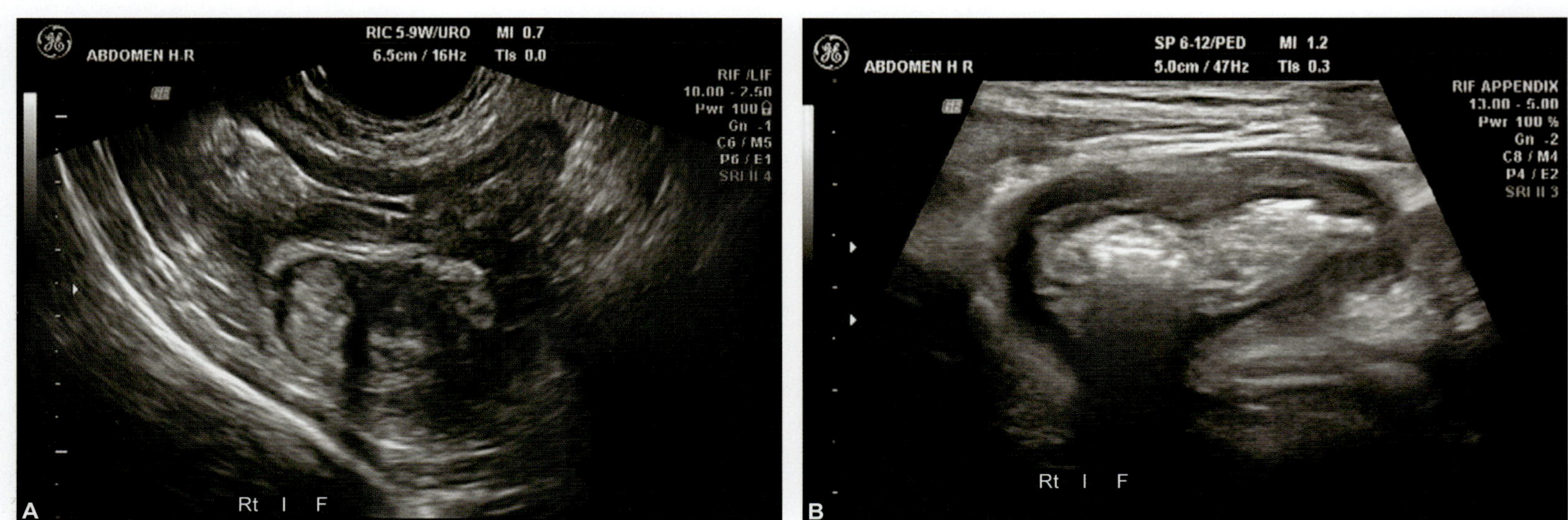

FIGURES 9.40A and B

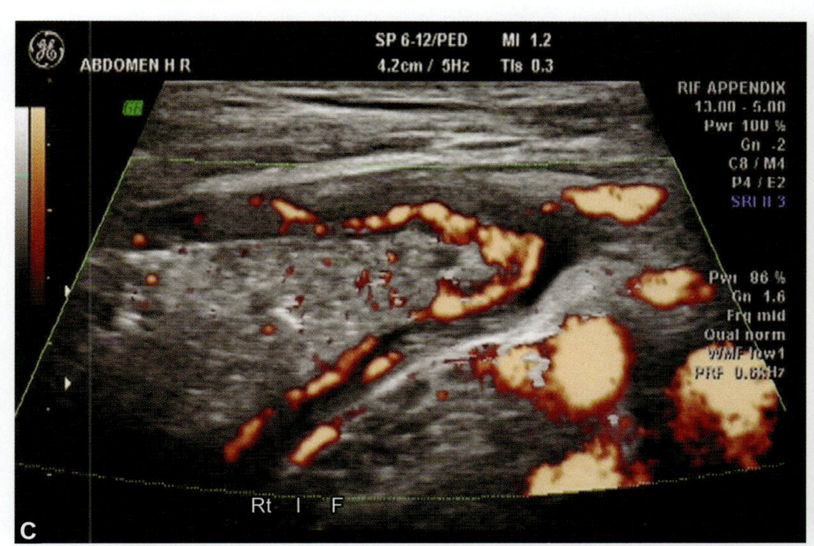

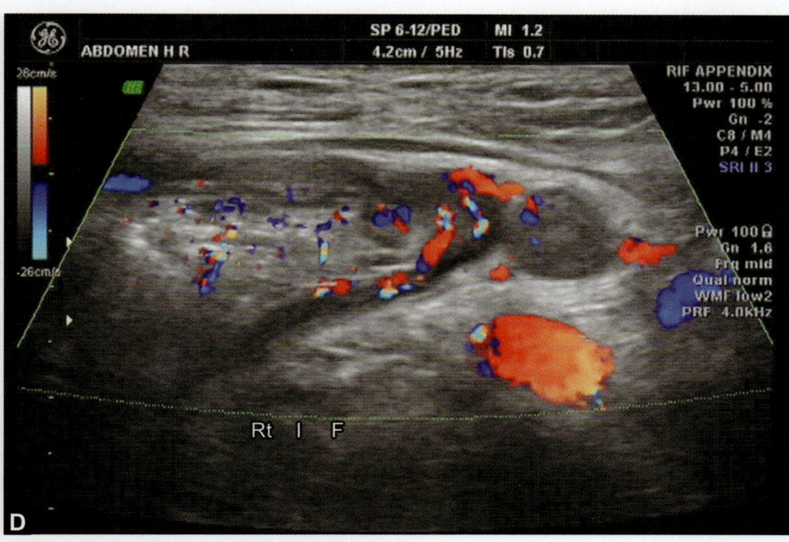

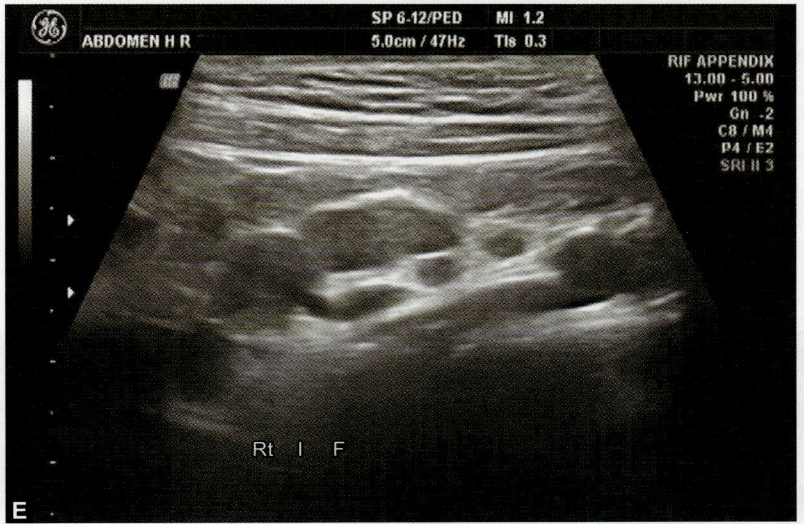

FIGURES 9.40C to E

FIGURES 9.40A to E: Ileocecal tuberculosis. A young boy presented with recurrent pain in abdomen. High-resolution sonography (HRSG) shows clumping of bowel loops. They are thickened. The cecum is markedly thickened. Gas entrapment is seen in the cecum. Pseudokidney sign is positive. Fluid movement is sluggish. Multiple enlarged nodes are also seen in right iliac fossa. On color flow imaging, increased flow is seen in cecal wall. Findings are suggestive of chronic inflammatory disease of tubercular bowel.

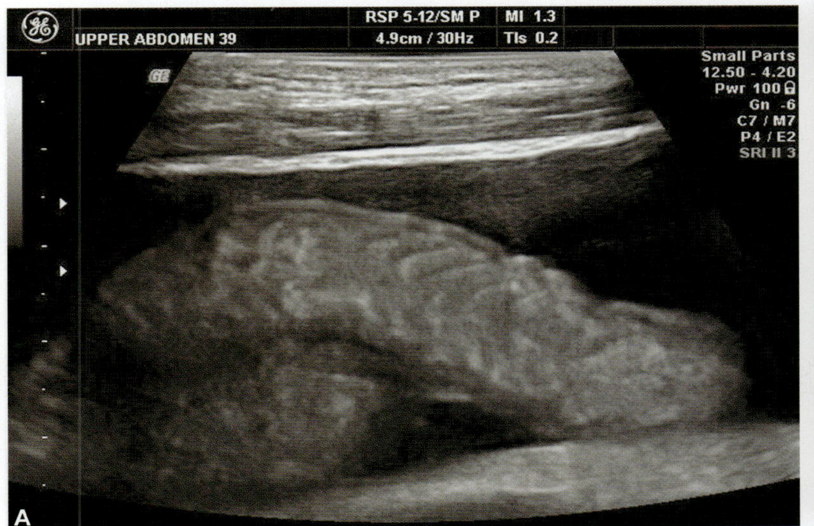

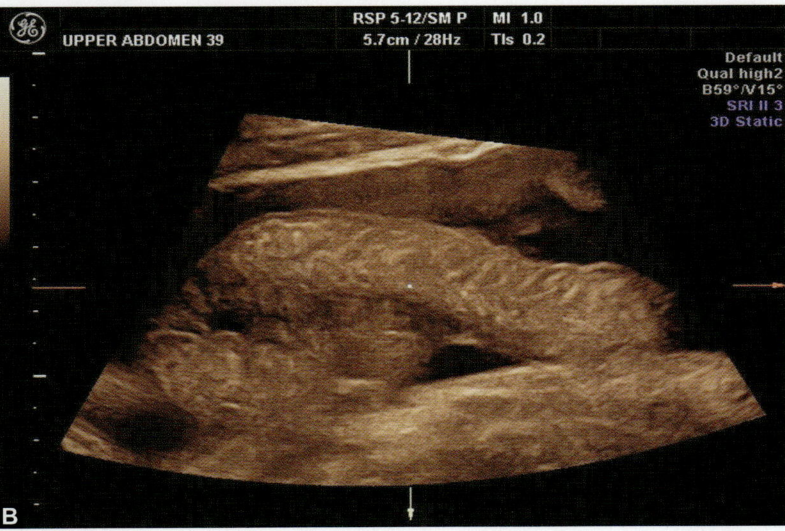

FIGURES 9.41A and B

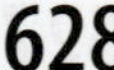

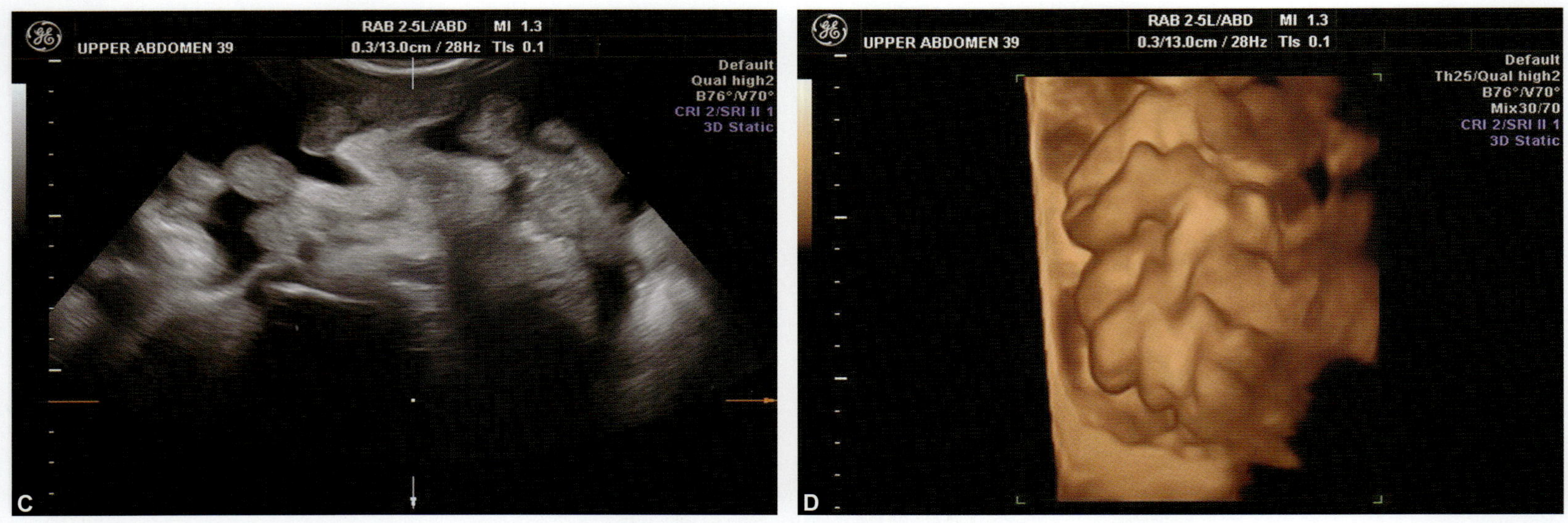

FIGURES 9.41C and D

FIGURES 9.41A to D: Bowel tuberculosis with cocoon formation. A patient presented with ascites with loss of weight. HRSG shows edematous bowel loops with clumping of bowel loops. On 3D imaging, clumped bowel loops are clearly seen. They are jumbled together and forming a cocoon suggestive of chronic bowel disease due to tuberculosis.

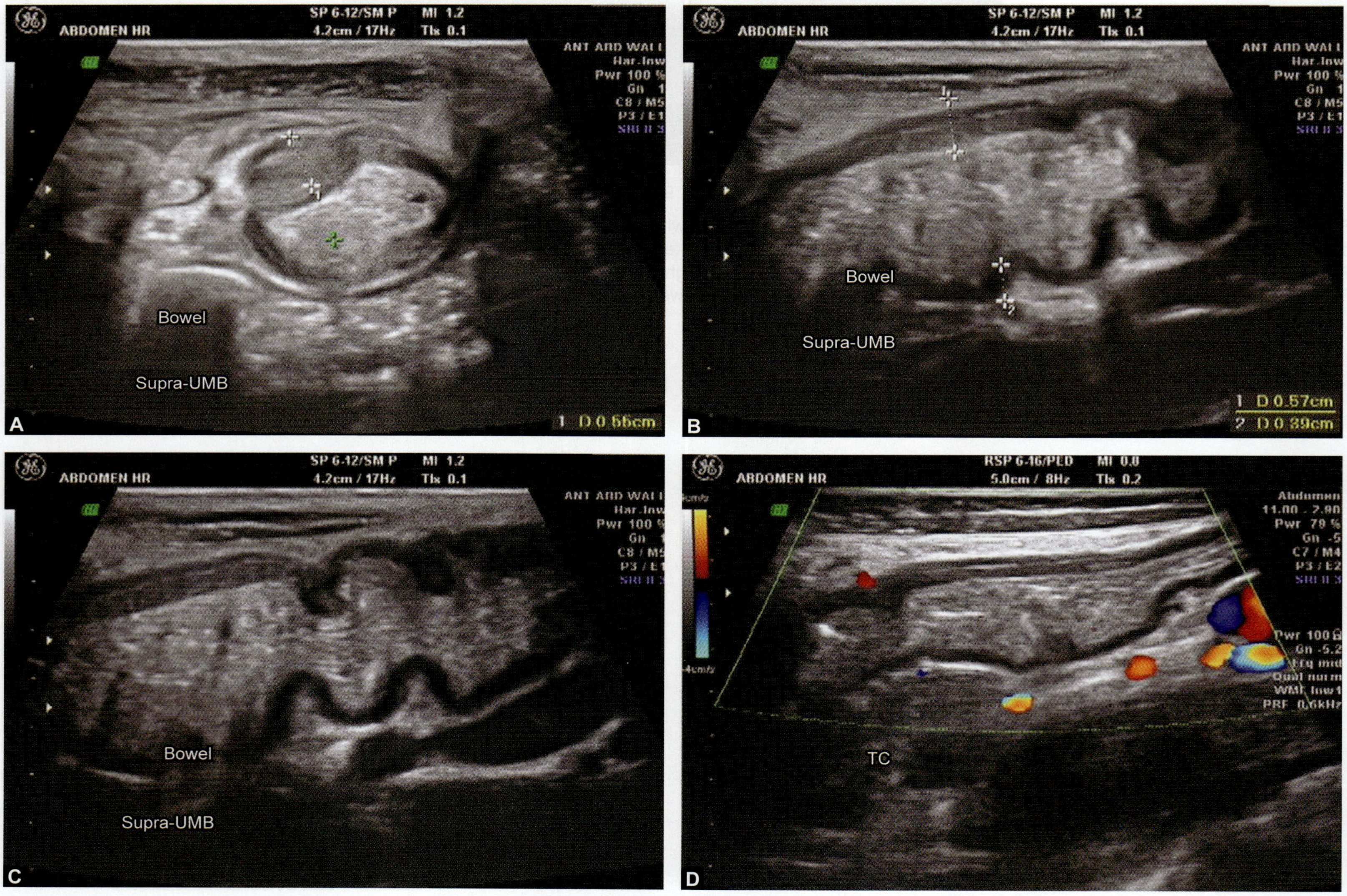

FIGURES 9.42A to D

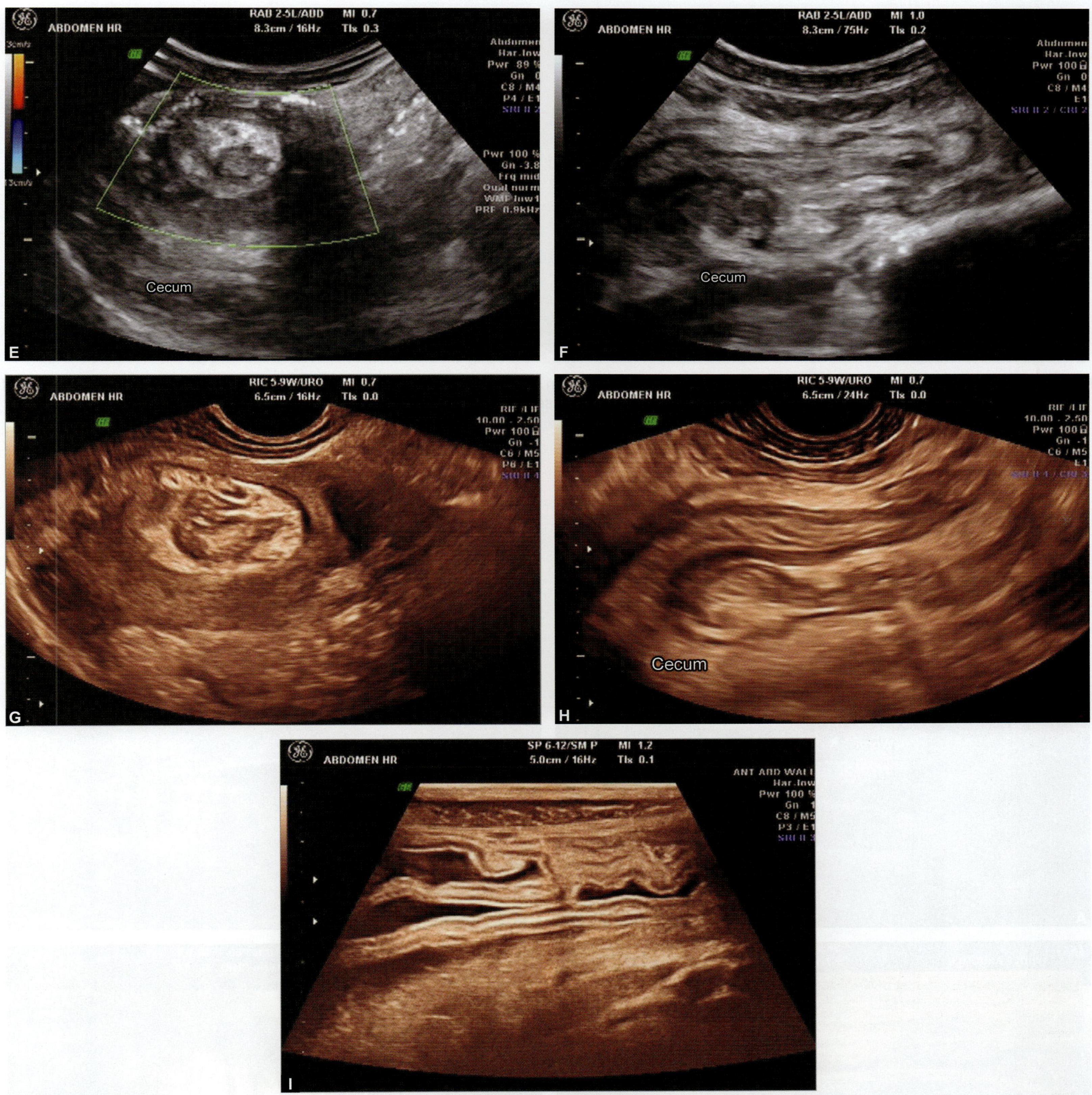

FIGURES 9.42E to I

FIGURES 9.42A to I: Bowel tuberculosis. High-resolution sonography (HRSG) shows bowel loops in supraumbilical region. The proximal small bowel loops and jejunum are dilated. Rapid fluid movement is seen in them. But no focal mass is seen in the bowel loops. However, the transverse colon shows diffused wall thickening. It is more than 5.5 mm in thickness. Slow fluid movement is seen through the bowel loops. The ileocecal junction is also thickened. Diffuse thickening of the cecum wall is seen. Lumen is obliterated. Slow fluid movement is seen in cecum. Bowel loop formation is seen in the cecal region. **On color flow imaging**, increased flow is seen along the bowel wall. Findings are suggestive of bowel tuberculosis.

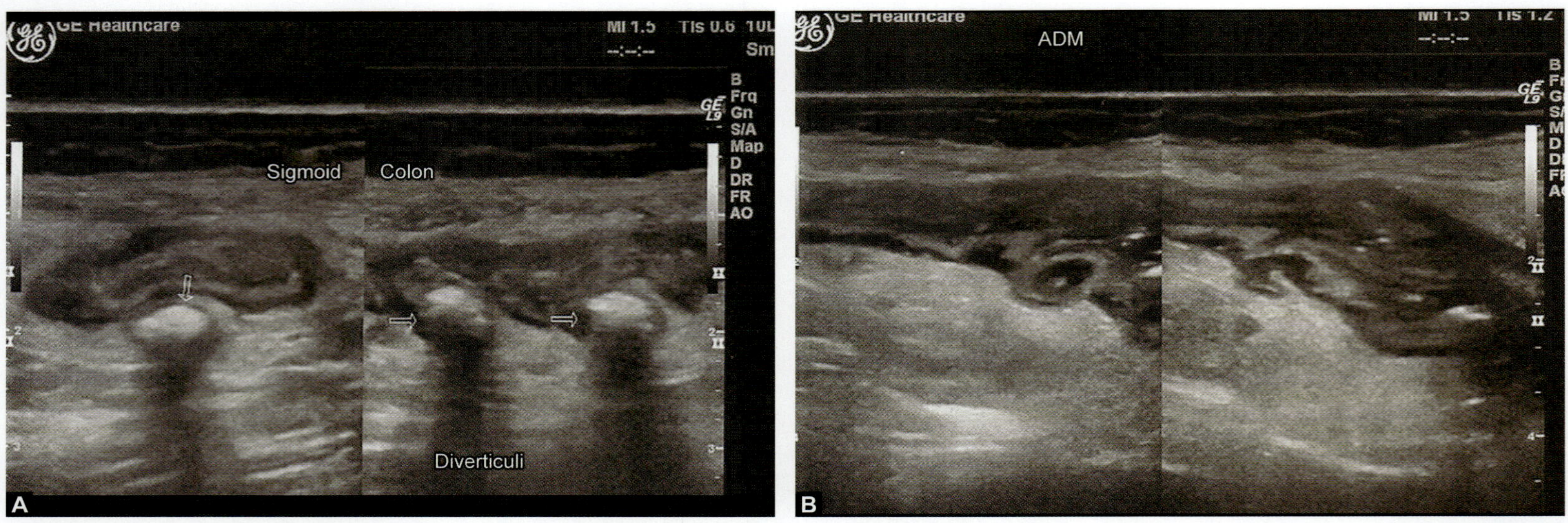

FIGURES 9.43A and B: Bowel diverticuli. A patient presented with pain in abdomen. High-resolution sonography (HRSG) shows out pouching of posterior wall of sigmoid colon. Air entrapment is seen in the pouch suggestive of multiple diverticuli.

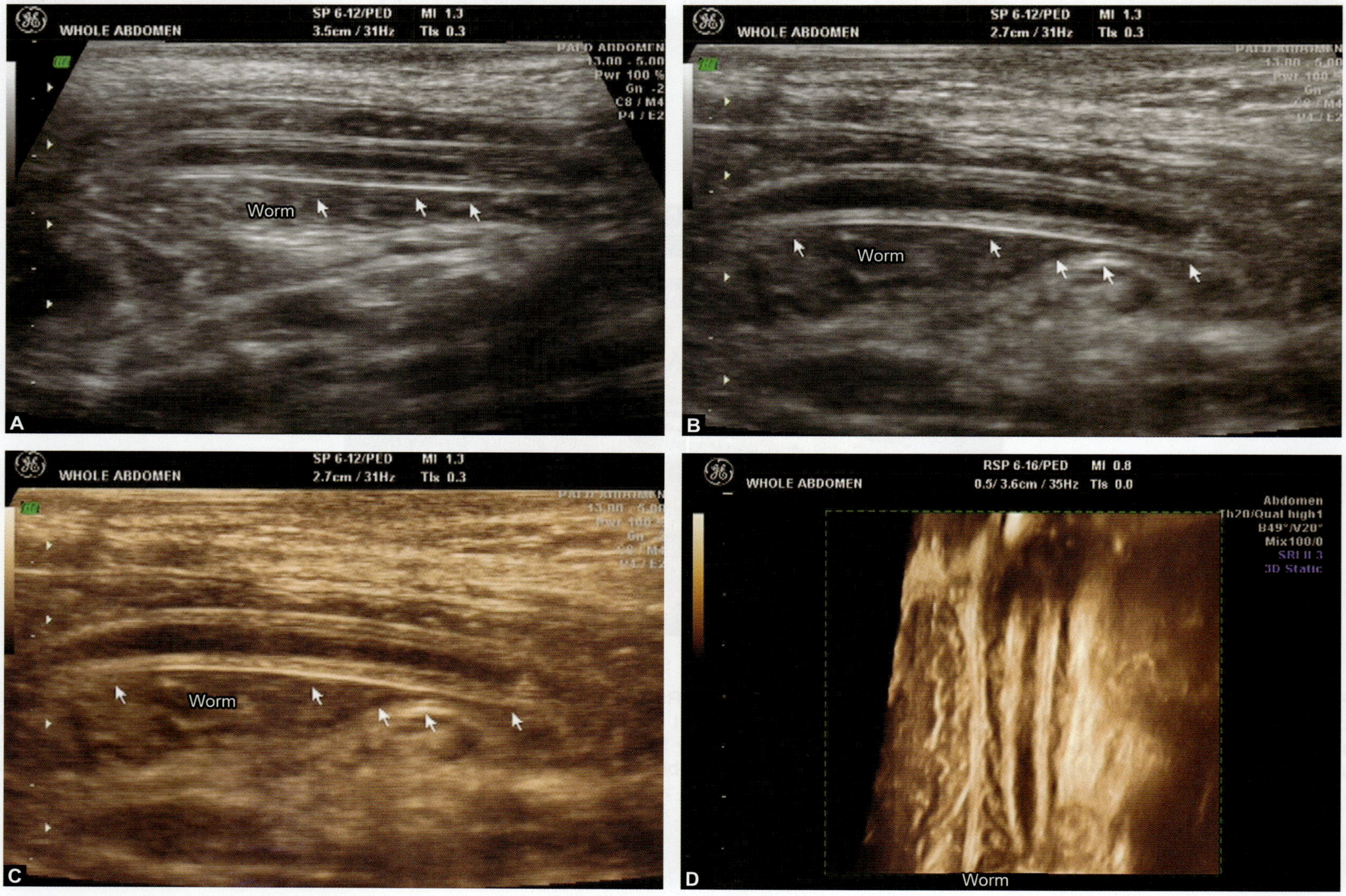

FIGURES 9.44A to D: Roundworm (Ascaris) in gastrointestinal tract (GIT). High-resolution sonography (HRSG) shows moving roundworm in the colon. The intestine of the worm is beautifully seen on 3D imaging; entire length of the worm is seen.

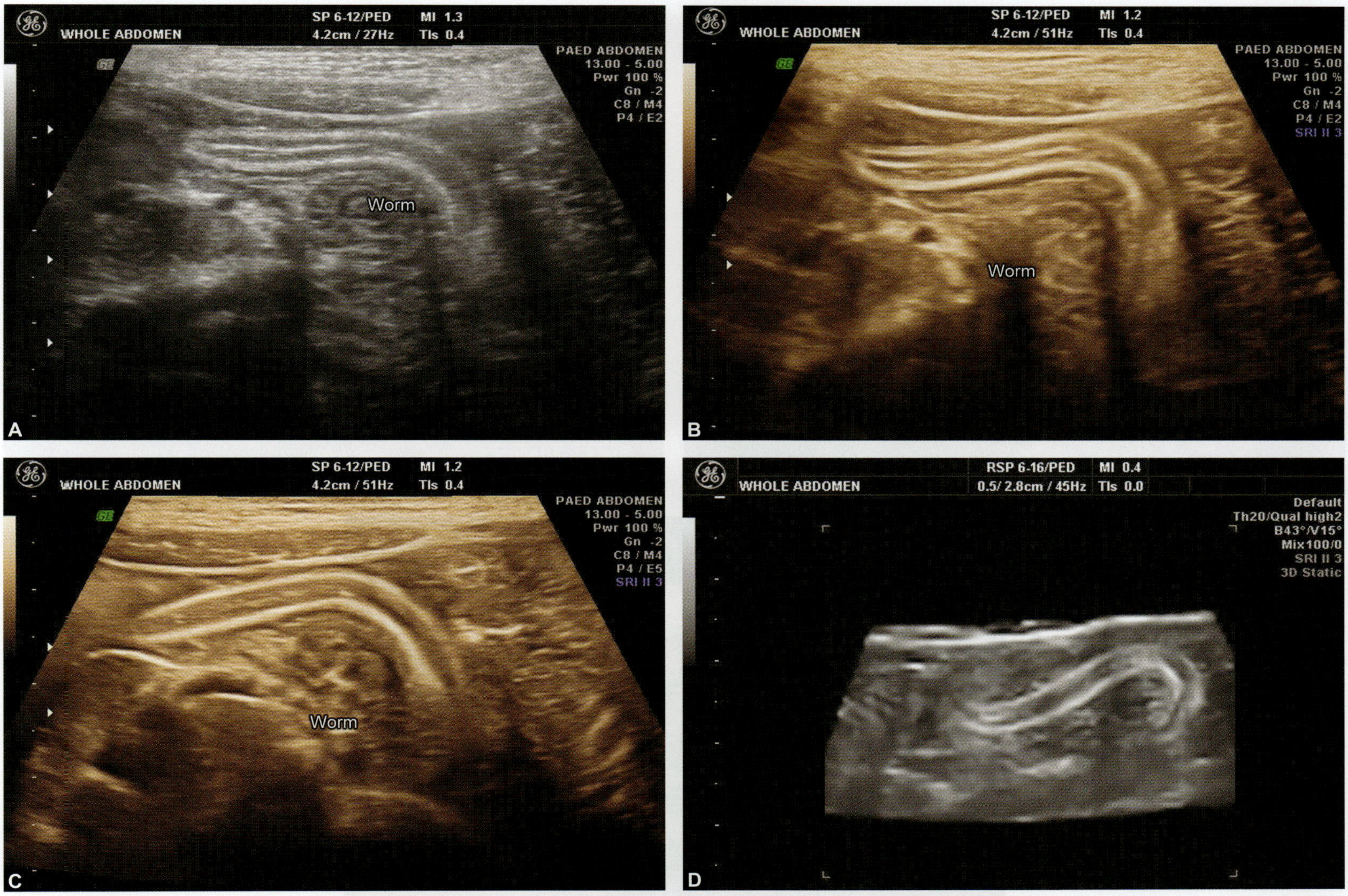

WHOLE ABDOMEN SP 6-12/PED 4.2cm / 27Hz MI 1.3 TIs 0.4
PAED ABDOMEN 13.00 - 5.00 Pwr 100 % Gn -2 C8 / M4 P4 / E2
Worm
A

WHOLE ABDOMEN SP 6-12/PED 4.2cm / 51Hz MI 1.2 TIs 0.4
PAED ABDOMEN 13.00 - 5.00 Pwr 100 % Gn -2 C8 / M4 P4 / E2 SRI II 3
Worm
B

WHOLE ABDOMEN SP 6-12/PED 4.2cm / 51Hz MI 1.2 TIs 0.4
PAED ABDOMEN 13.00 - 5.00 Pwr 100 % Gn -2 C8 / M4 P4 / E5 SRI II 3
Worm
C

WHOLE ABDOMEN RSP 6-16/PED 0.5/ 2.8cm / 45Hz MI 0.4 TIs 0.0
Default Th20/Qual high2 B43°/V15° Mix100/0 SRI II 3 3D Static
D

FIGURES 9.45A to D: Moving roundworm in gastrointestinal tract (GIT). High-resolution sonography (HRSG) shows moving roundworm in GIT. On dynamic scanning, movement of the roundworm and coiling of the worm is seen. On 3D volume contrast imaging, the worm is clearly seen

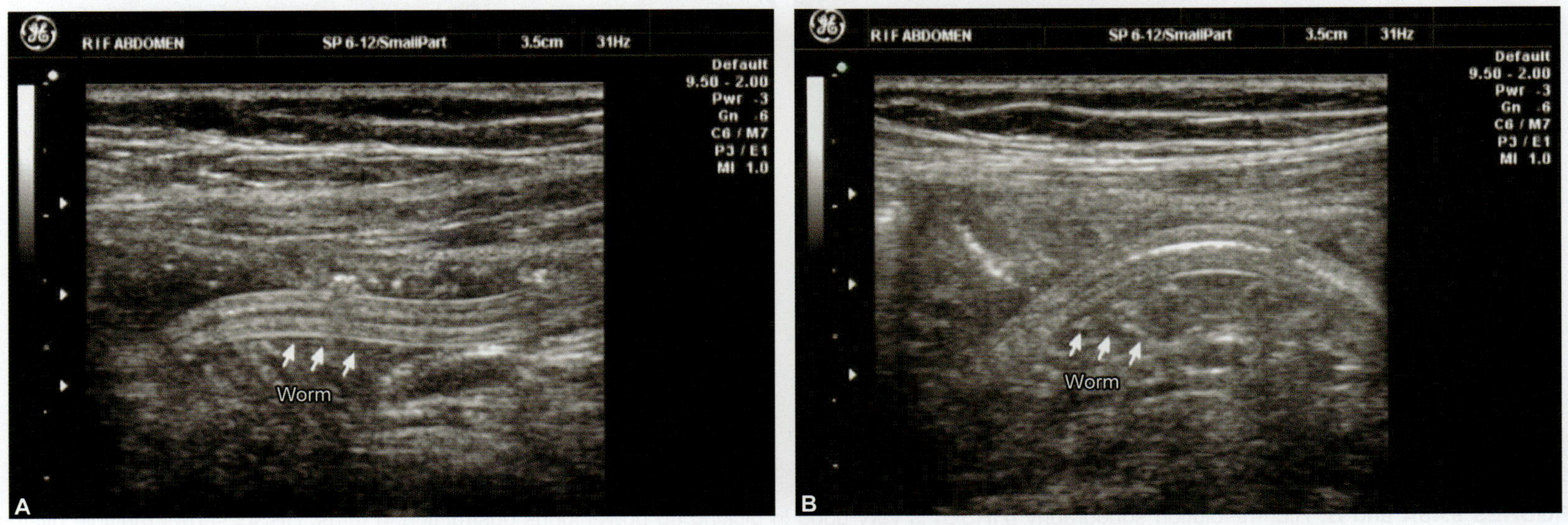

FIGURES 9.46A and B: Ascaris in the bowel loops. A young child presented with recurrent pain in the abdomen. High-resolution sonography (HRSG) show moving tapeworm (*Ascaris*). The details of the worm are beautifully resolved on HRSG.

GASTROINTESTINAL TRACT OBSTRUCTION

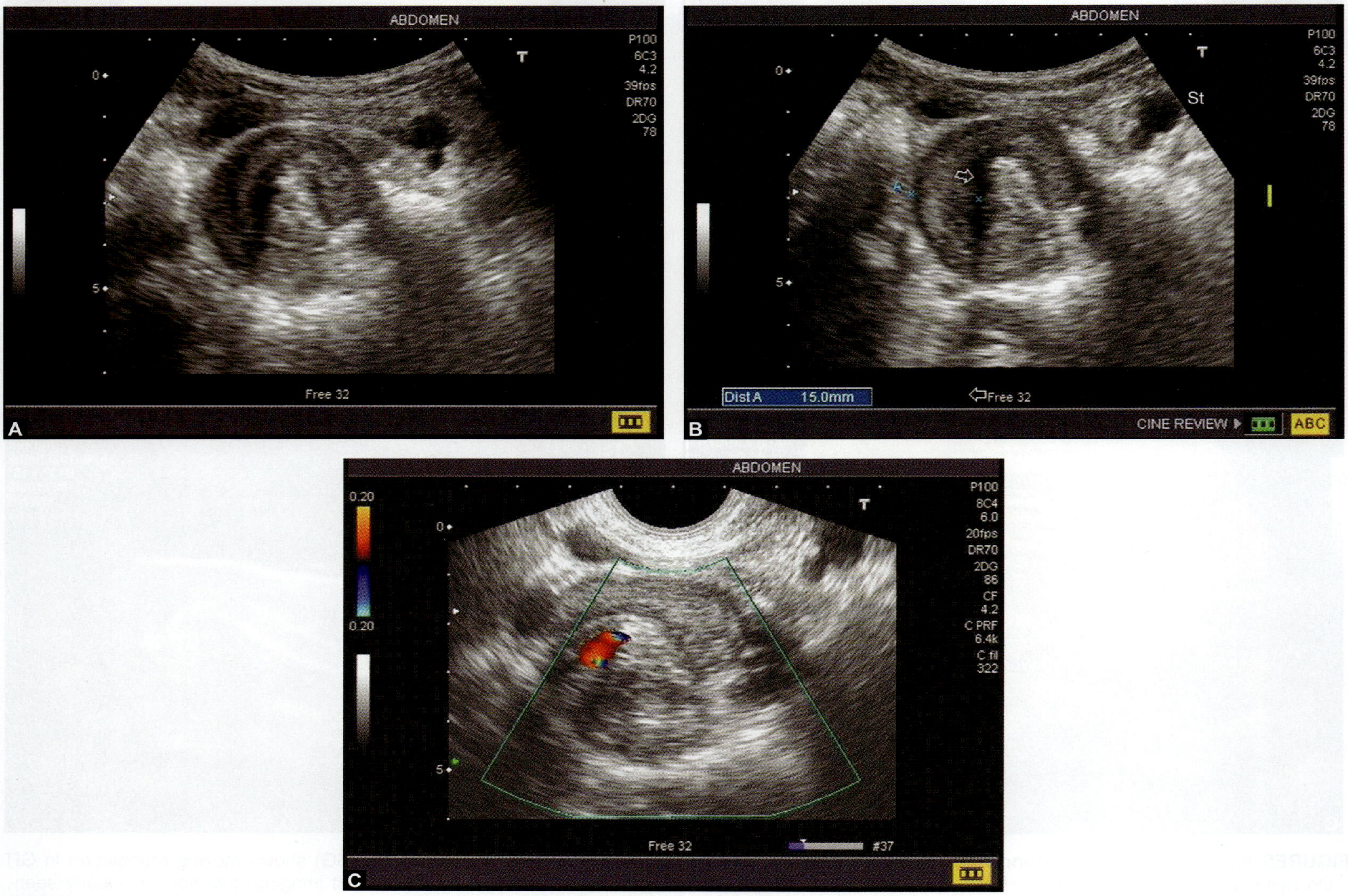

FIGURES 9.47A to C: Pyloric spasm. A 13-year-old boy presented with recurrent vomiting. HRSG shows thickened edematous pylorus. The pyloric muscle is inflamed and edematous. Gas entrapment is seen in the lumen. Target sign is positive. However, small amount of fluid is seen passing through the lumen, which is picked up on color flow imaging. Findings are suggestive of acute pyloric spasm.

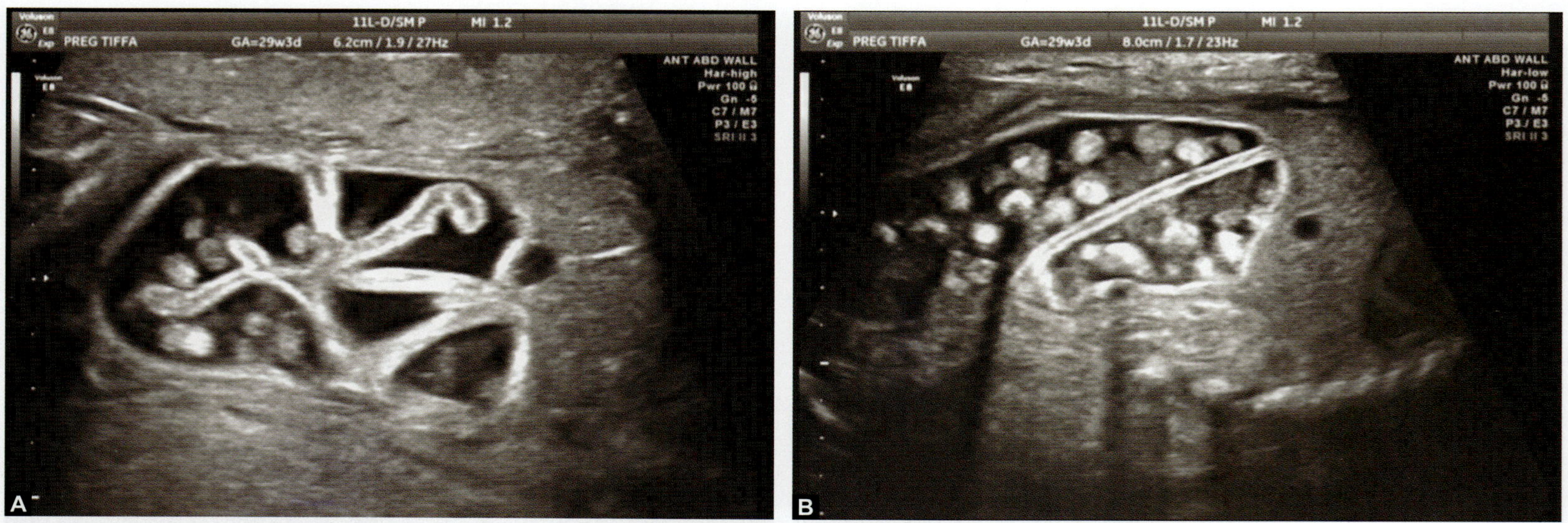

FIGURES 9.48A and B: High-resolution sonography (HRSG) is very good in picking up bowel loops obstruction in fetus. HRSG shows multiple dilated bowel loops in the fetus. The echogenic shadows are seen in the lumen of the fetus suggestive of meconium beads. Thick echogenic meconium is also seen in the bowel loops.

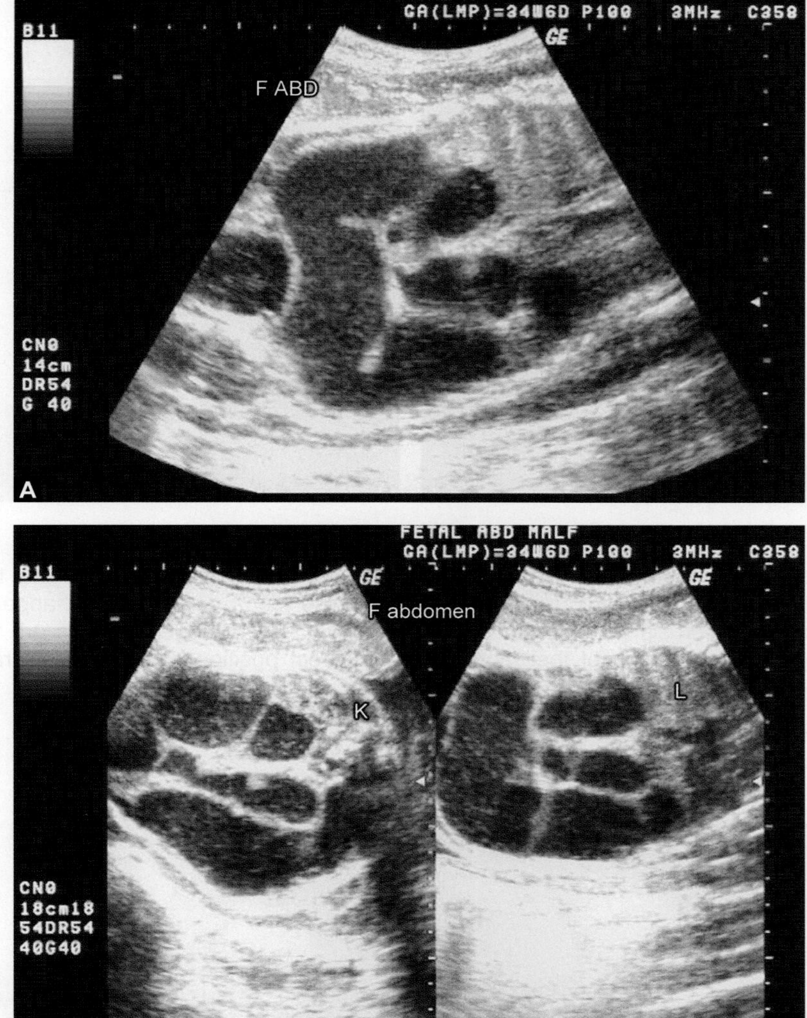

FIGURES 9.49A and B: Large bowel loop obstruction in fetus. High-resolution sonography (HRSG) shows dilated large bowel loops in the fetus. The colonic bands are seen clearly in the dilated bowel loops.

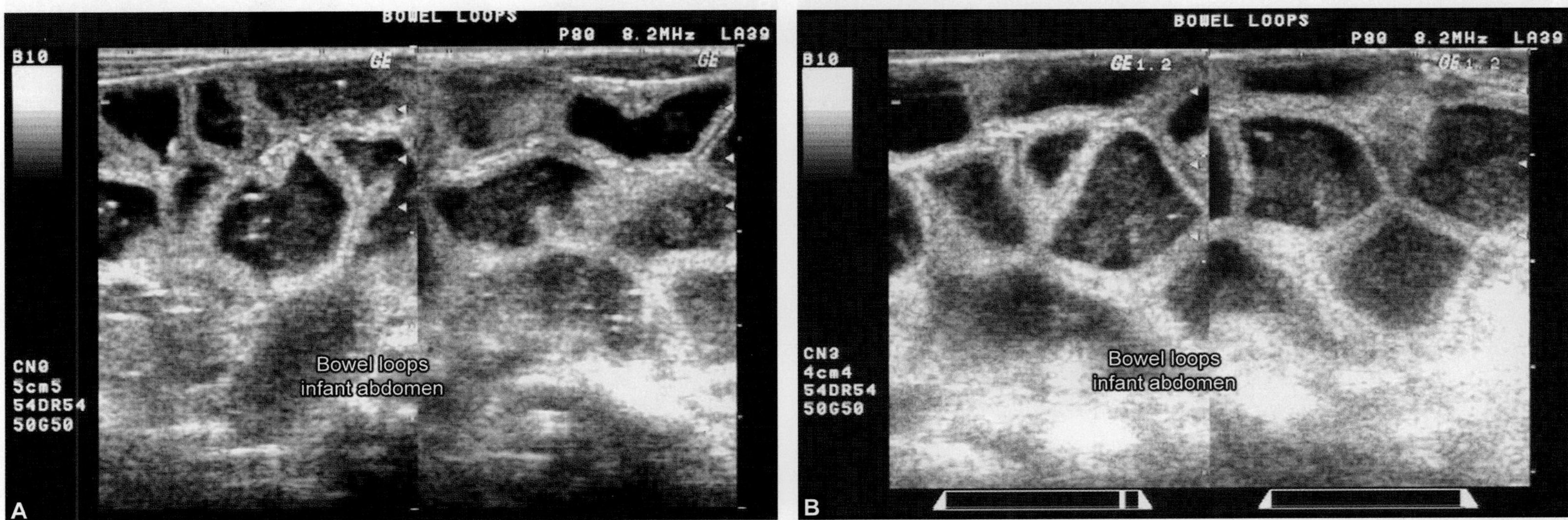

FIGURES 9.50A and B

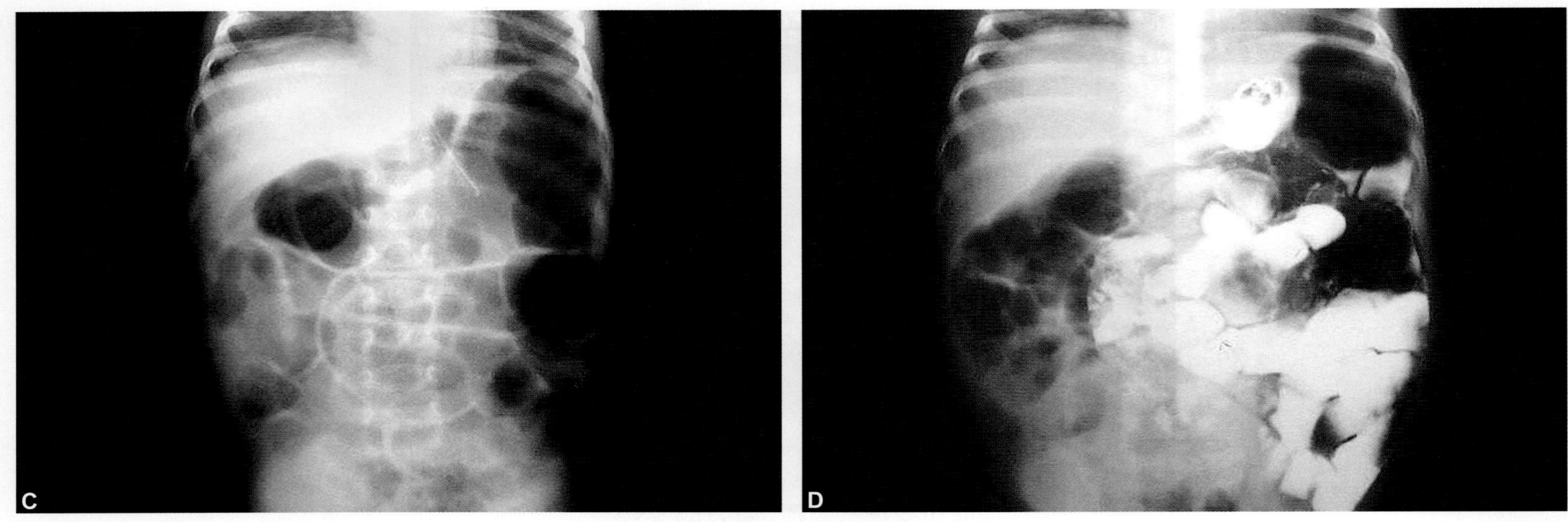

FIGURES 9.50C and D

FIGURES 9.50A to D: Mucoviscidosis. A 3-month-old child presented with persistent vomiting and failure to thrive. High-resolution sonography (HRSG) shows dilated bowel loops with multiple echogenic bands crisscrossing the loops giving fish net appearance. Thick echogenic collection is also seen in bowel loops suggestive of cystic fibrosis (Mucoviscidosis) of the bowel. The echogenic bands are fibrosed septa. The sweat test of the same patient was positive. Plain X-ray of the abdomen of the same patient in erect position shows multiple radio opaque bands in the abdominal cavity. No fluid level is seen in the bowel loops.

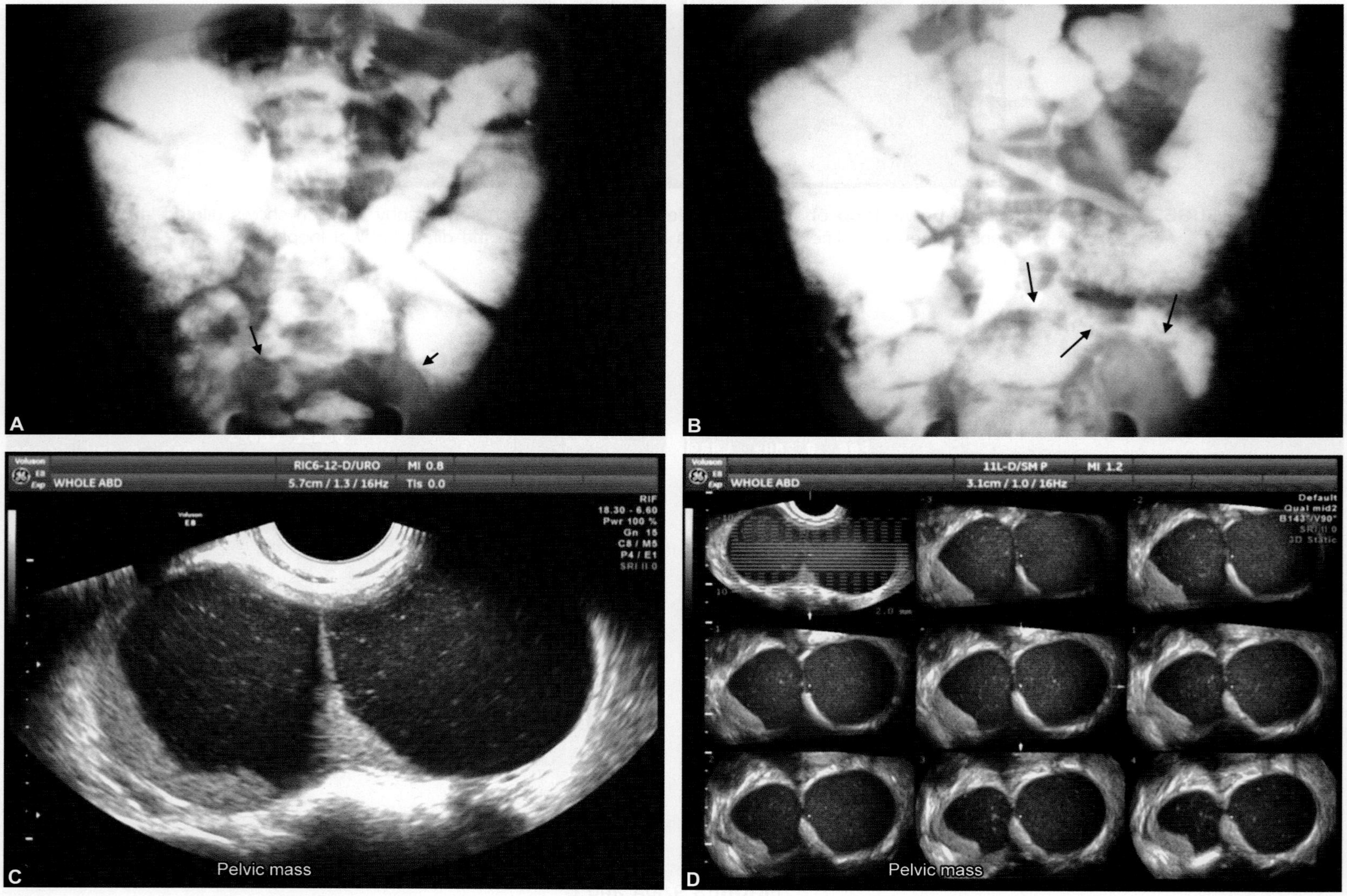

Pelvic mass

Pelvic mass

FIGURES 9.51A to D

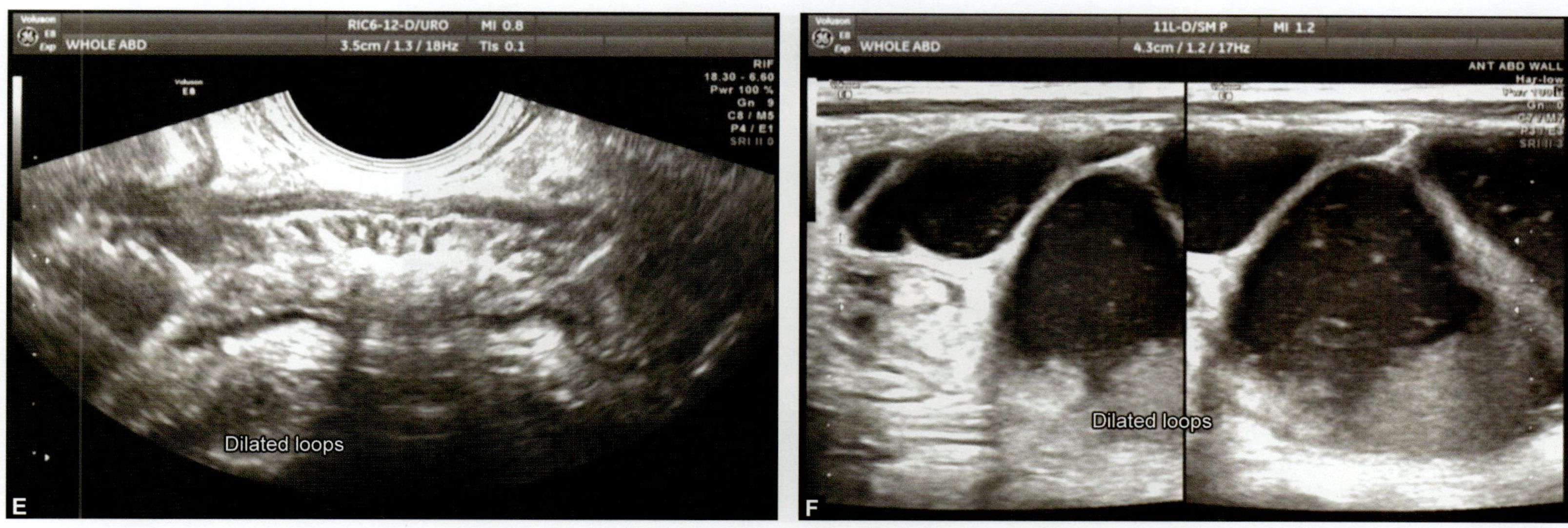

FIGURES 9.51E and F

FIGURES 9.51A to F: Enteric duplication cyst. A 5-year-old girl presented with pain in abdomen with vomiting. The barium meal shows soft indentation over the bowel loops in the pelvis. High-resolution sonography (HRSG) shows well defined loculated cystic mass in the pelvis. It is seen pressing over the bowel loops. A thin septum is seen in the cyst suggestive of duplication cyst. The proximal bowel loops are also dilated.

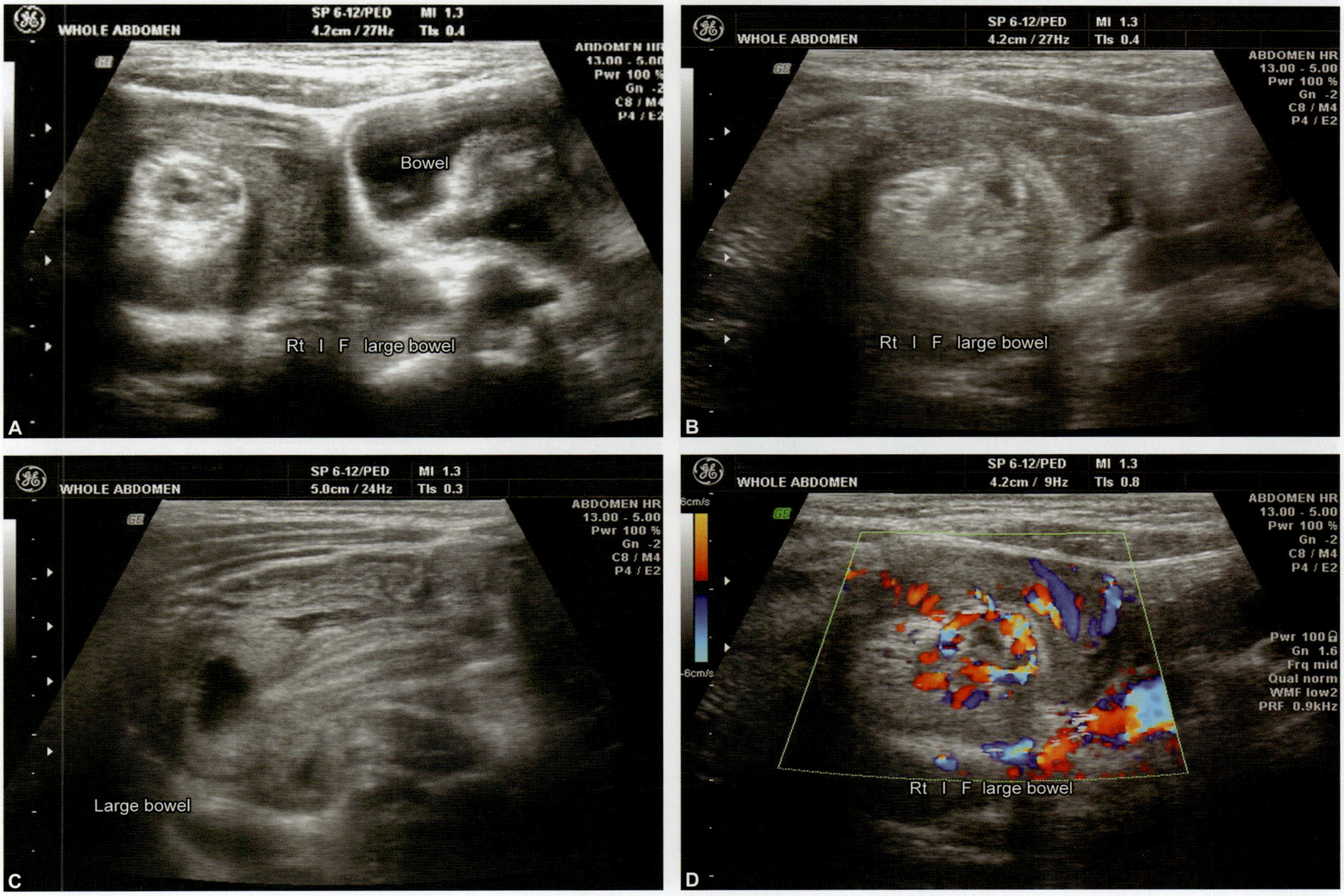

FIGURES 9.52A to D

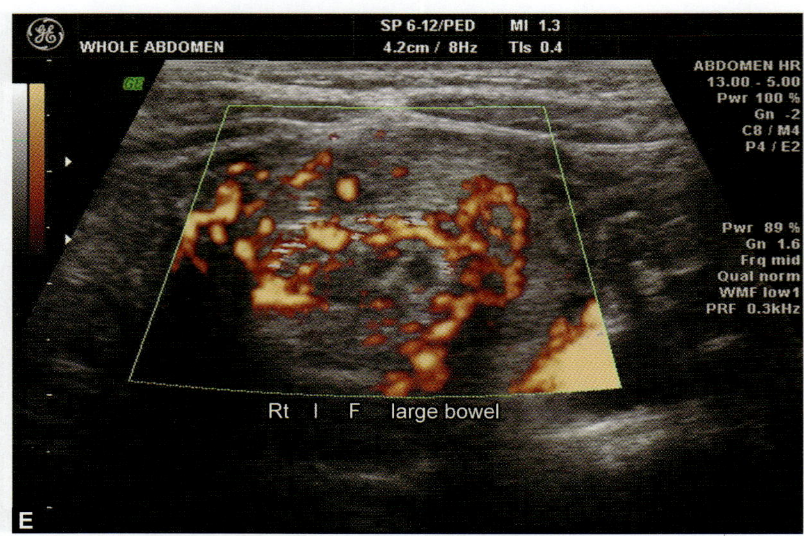

FIGURE 9.52E

FIGURES 9.52A to E: A young boy presented with pain with abdomen with vomiting. High-resolution sonography (HRSG) shows multiple dilated bowel loops in right iliac fossa and right paraumbilical region suggestive of dilated small bowel loops. One bowel loop is seen going into another bowel loop. Multiple layers are seen in the outer bowel ring. The outer bowel is edematous. Crescentic rings are seen into it. The inner bowel loop shows echogenic central portion suggestive of intussusception. The proximal bowel loops are dilated. On color flow imaging, marked flow is seen in the inner bowel ring due to the edema. Fluid is seen trapped in the bowel loops.

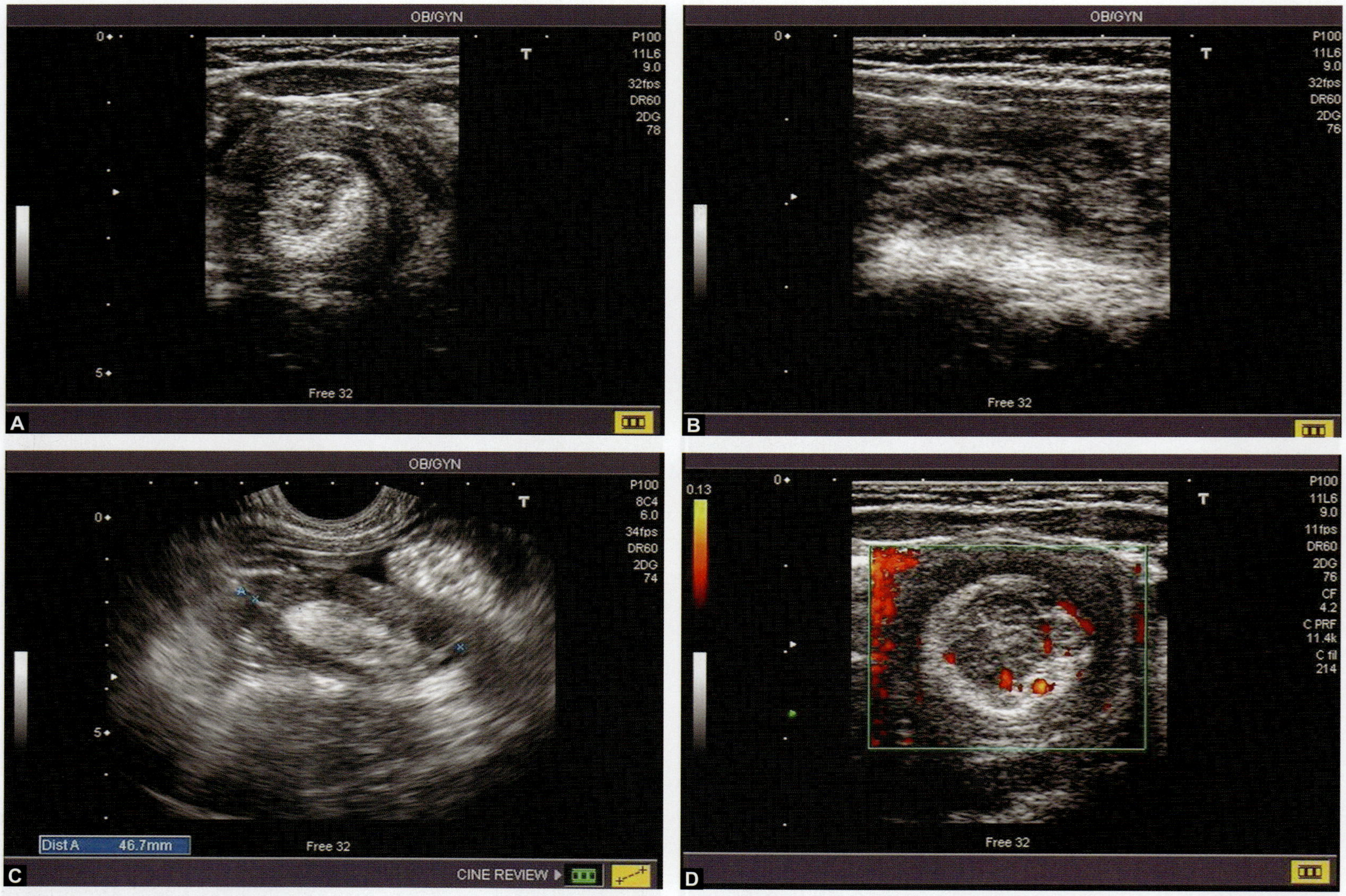

FIGURES 9.53A to D: Intussusception. A 4-month-old baby presented with vomiting. High-resolution sonography (HRSG) shows dilated proximal bowel loops. A bowel loop is seen going in another bowel loop. Doughnut sign is positive suggestive of intussusception. On color flow imaging, increased flow is seen around the bowel loops.

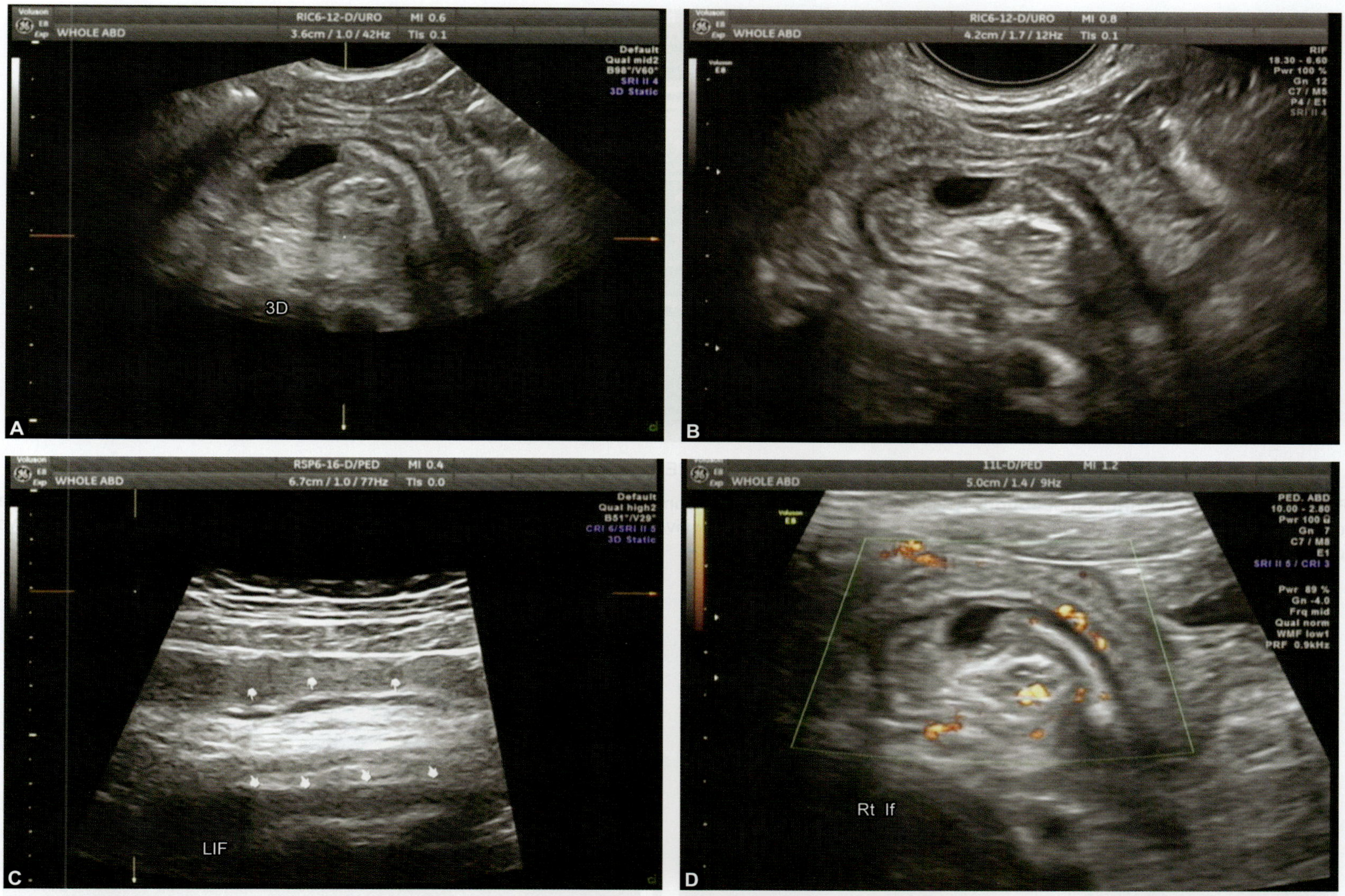

FIGURES 9.54A to D: An 8-year-old boy presented with vomiting. High-resolution sonography (HRSG) shows a bowel loop seen going in another bowel loop suggestive of intussusception. However, it is seen reduced on ultrasound pressure suggestive of transient intussusception. On color flow imaging, increased flow is seen around the outer wall.

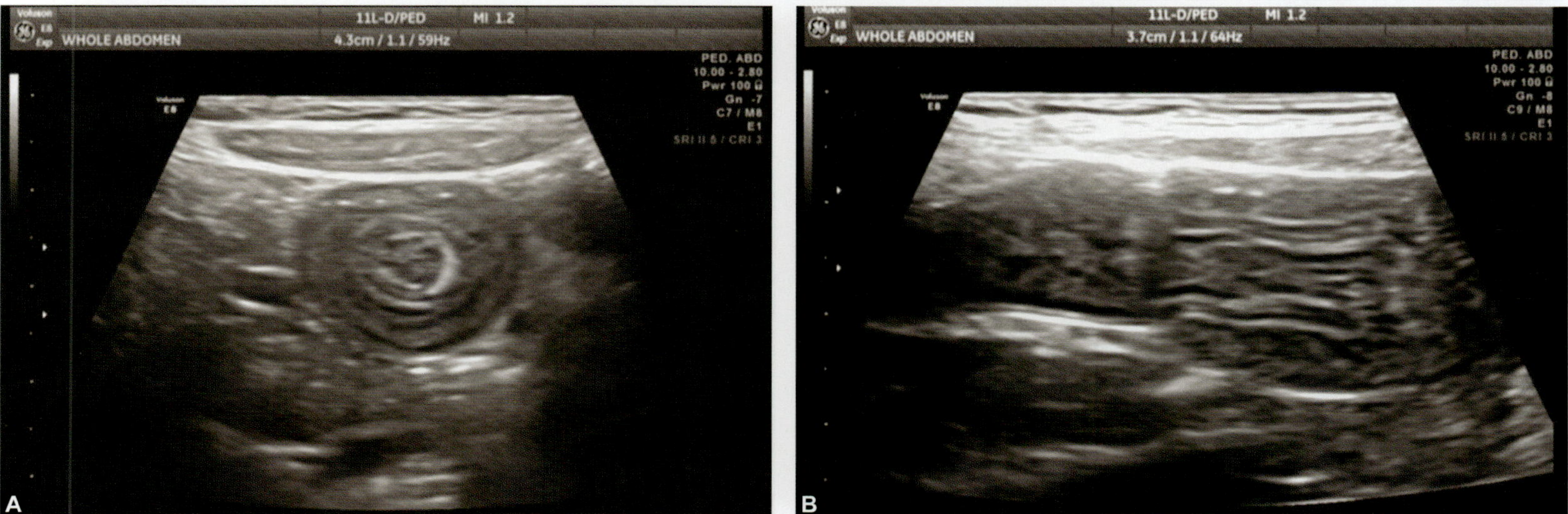

FIGURES 9.55A and B

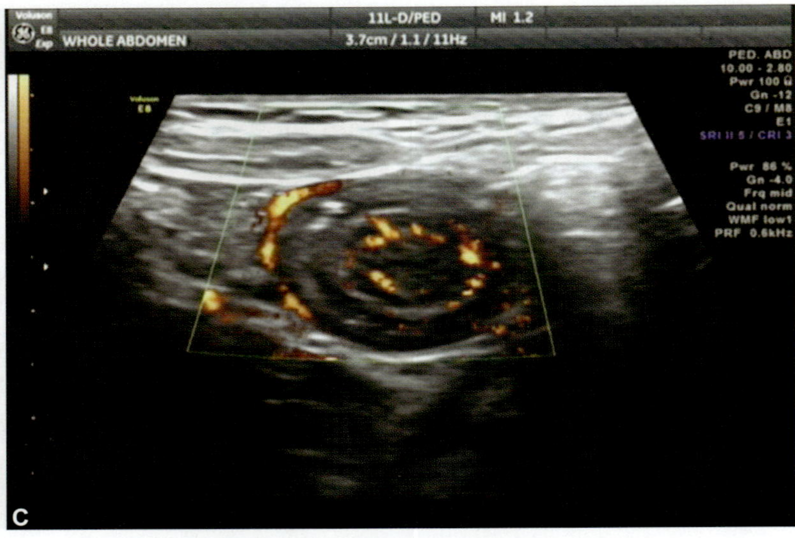

FIGURE 9.55C

FIGURES 9.55A to C: Intussusception. A young child presented with vomiting and acute pain. High-resolution sonography (HRSG) shows a bowel loop seen invaginating in another bowel loop. The doughnut sign is positive. On color flow imaging, increased flow is seen in the edematous bowel loop suggestive of intussusception

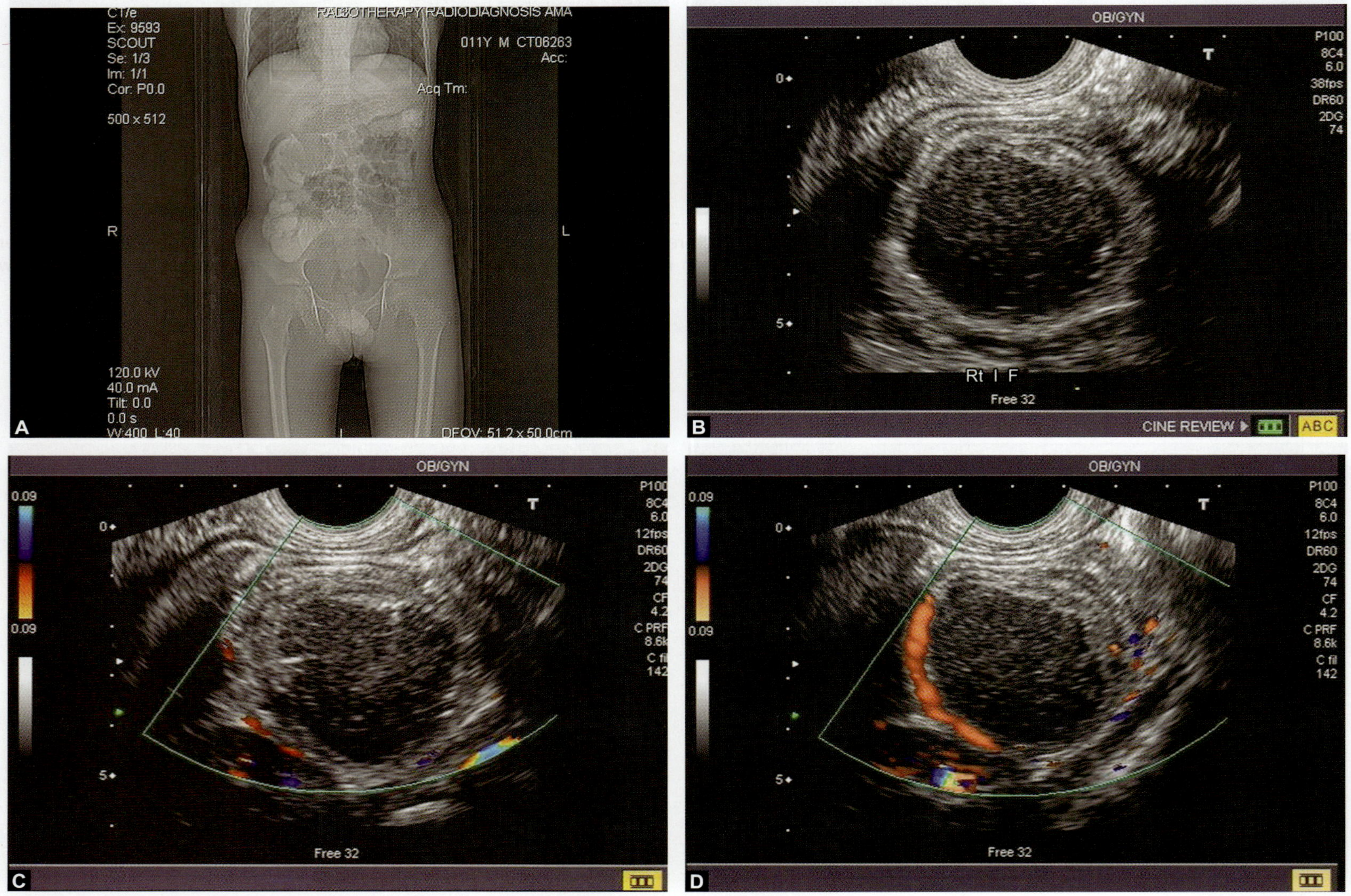

FIGURES 9.56A to D

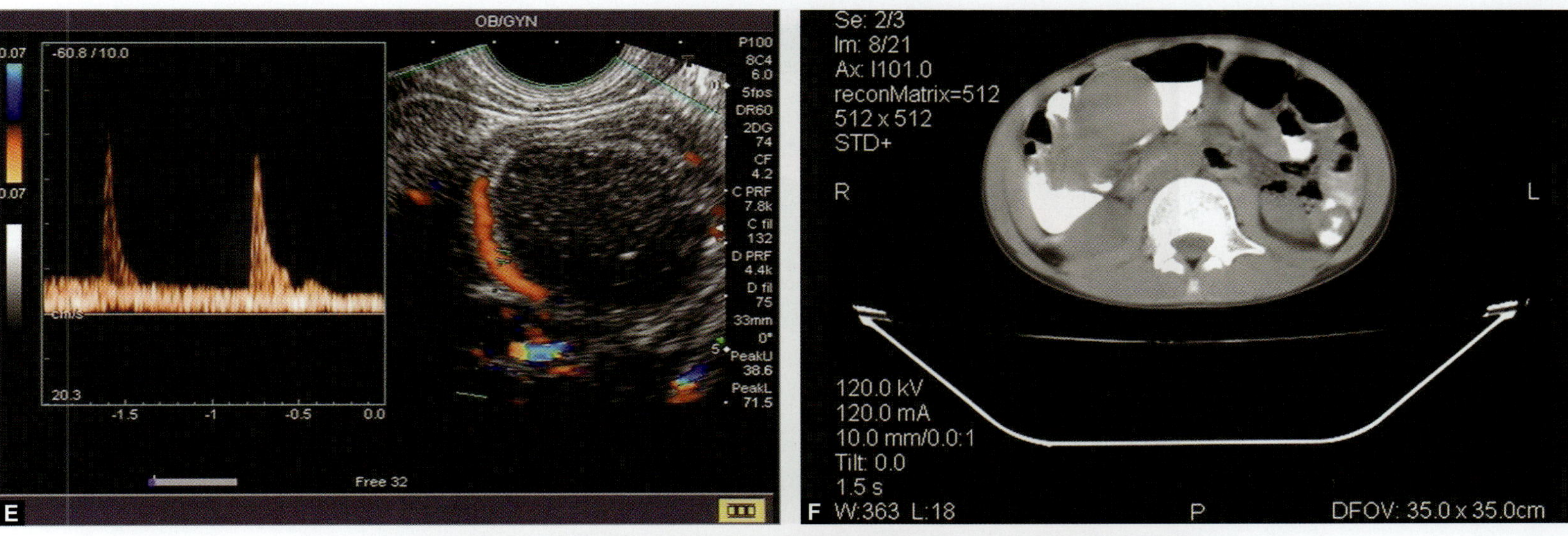

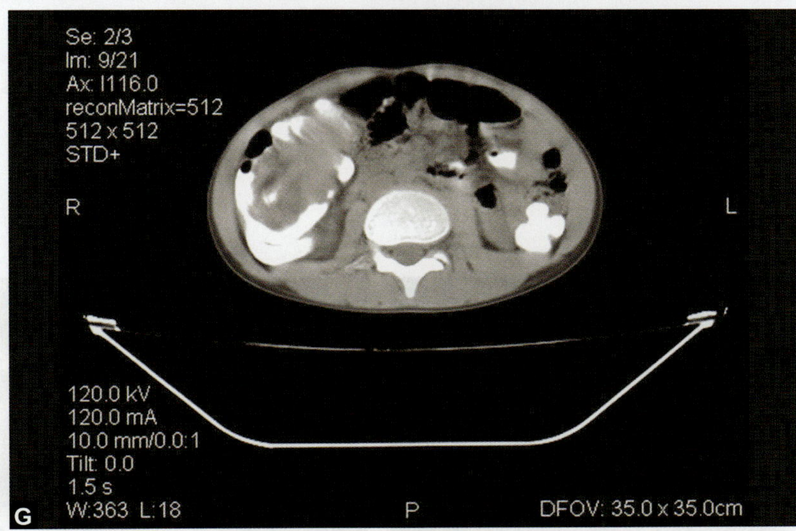

FIGURES 9.56E to G

FIGURES 9.56A to G: Volvulus. A patient presented with acute pain with vomiting. Plain X-ray abdomen does not show any remarkable finding. However, high-resolution sonography (HRSG) shows a twisted bowel loop in the right iliac fossa. Low-level echo collection is seen in the distended bowel loops. On color flow imaging, an artery is seen in the twisted bowel loop. On spectral Doppler tracing, high resistance flow is seen in the artery suggestive of volvulus. CT scan of the same patient confirms the ultrasound findings.

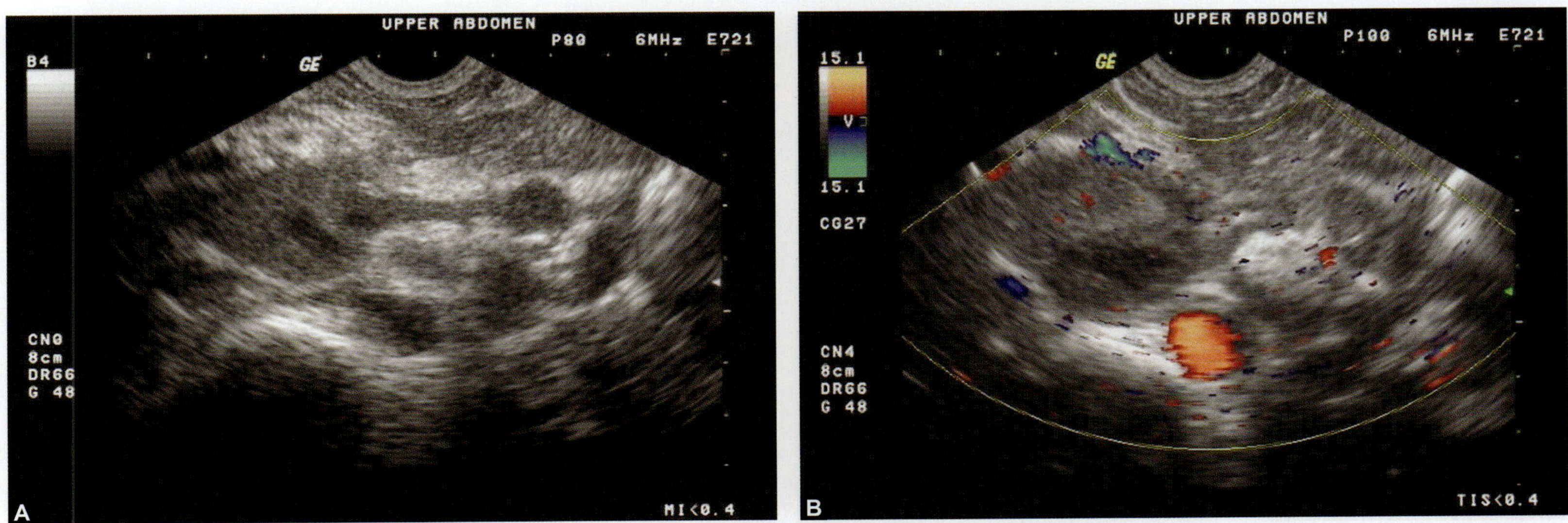

FIGURES 9.57A and B

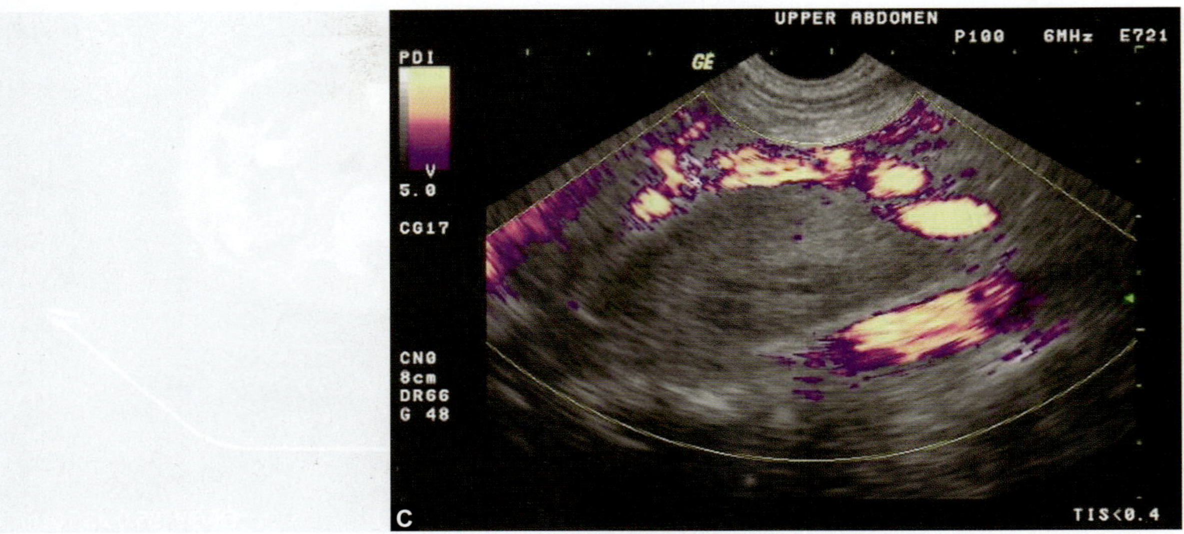

FIGURE 9.57C

FIGURES 9.57A to C: Small intestine volvulus. HRSG shows volvulus of small intestine. The bowel loop is edematous and hypoechoic. Perifocal edema is present. On color flow imaging peripheral flow is seen around the bowel loop. A vascular band is running around the volvulus. It is seen as a ring around the constricting bowel loop. Power Doppler imaging shows the vascular band beautifully.

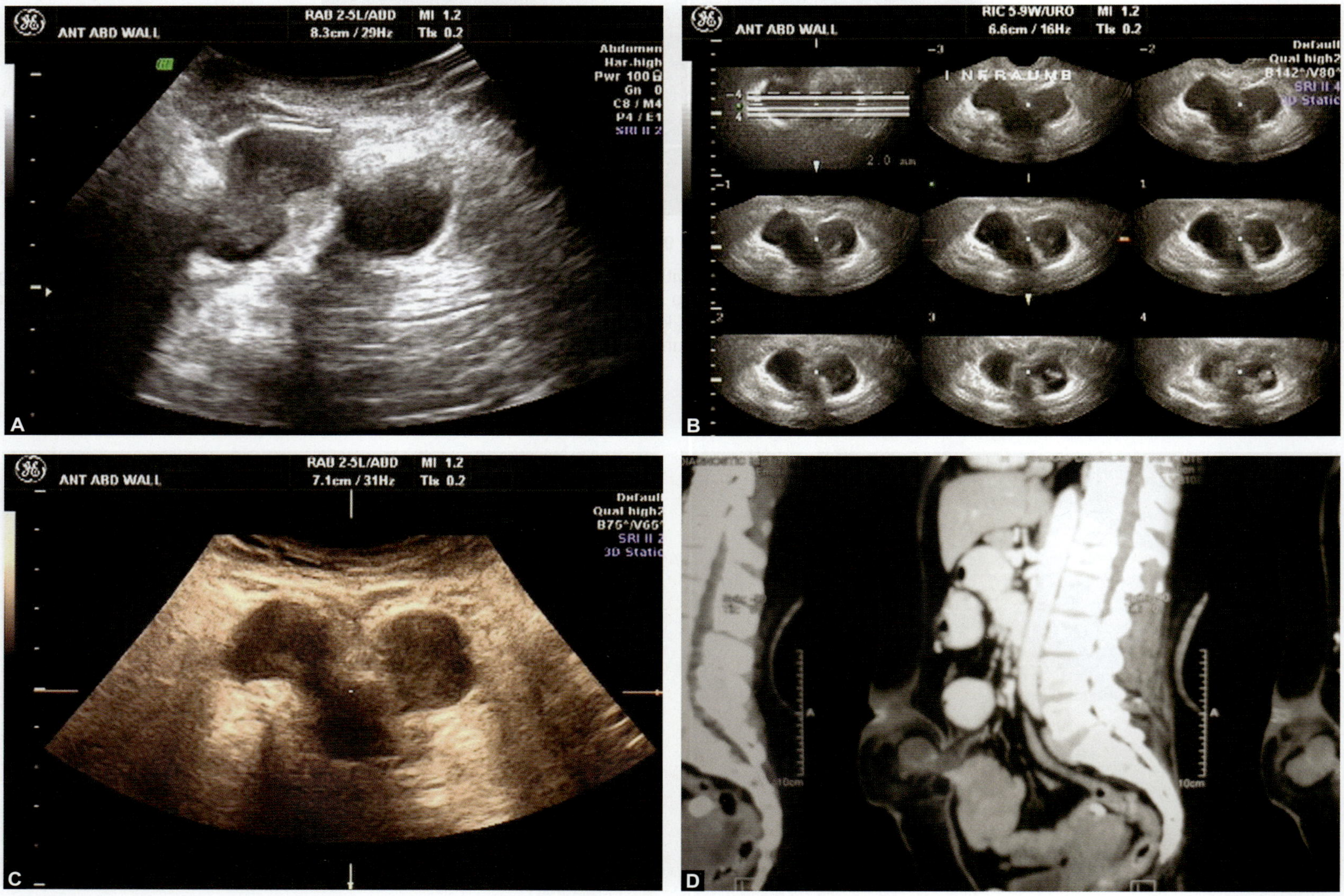

FIGURES 9.58A to D

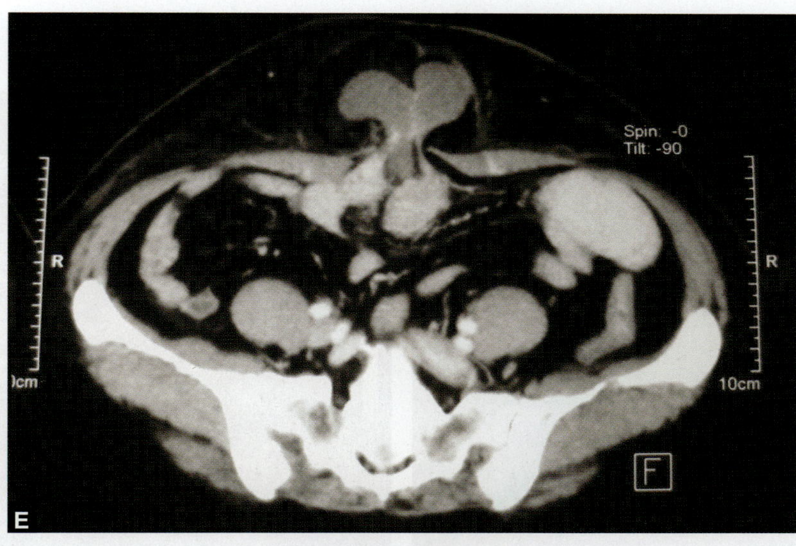

FIGURE 9.58E

FIGURES 9.58A to E: Obstructed infraumbilical hernia. A patient presented with acute pain with vomiting. High-resolution sonography (HRSG) shows a defect in the anterior abdominal wall in infraumbilical region. A bowel loop is seen coming out from the defect. An echogenic band is seen in the bowel loop, which is not allowing loop to be reduced suggestive of obstructed hernia. CT scan of the same patient also shows infraumbilical hernia with obstructed bowel loops

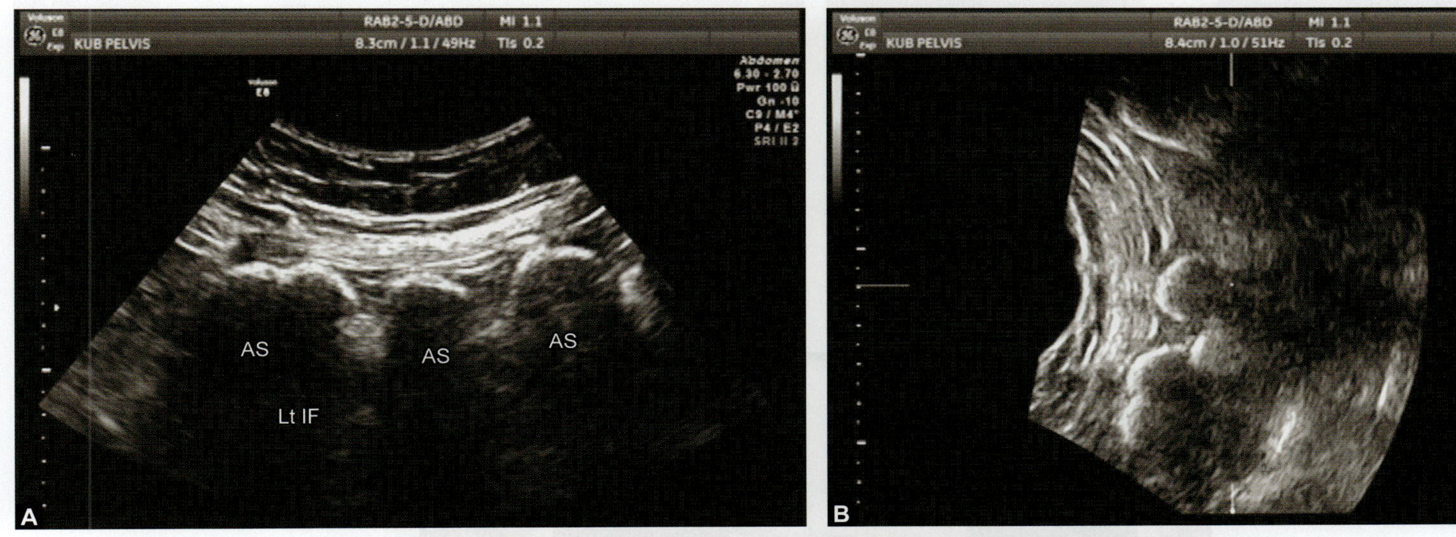

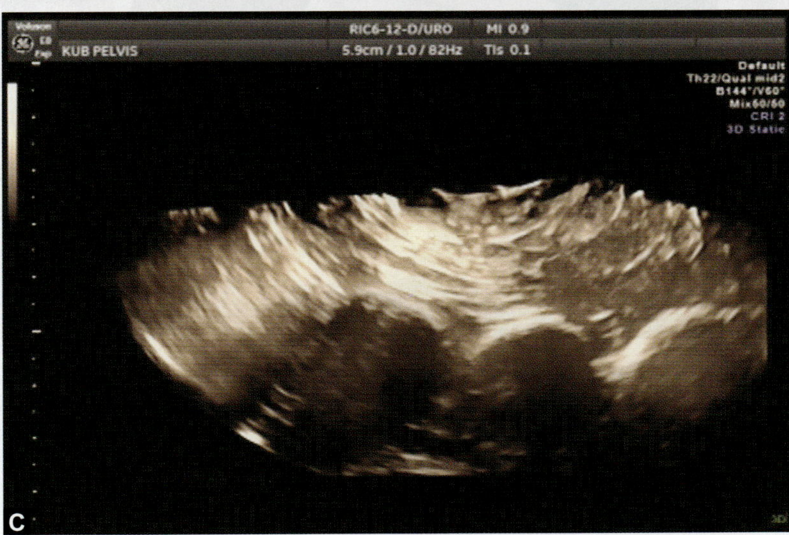

FIGURES 9.59A to C: Fecaliths in the large bowel. A patient presented with pain in the abdomen. HRSG shows multiple nodular masses in the descending colon and part of sigmoid colon. They show rim calcification and accompanied with acoustic shadowing. 3D imaging clearly shows the masses suggestive of fecaliths.

MALIGNANT GASTROINTESTINAL MASSES

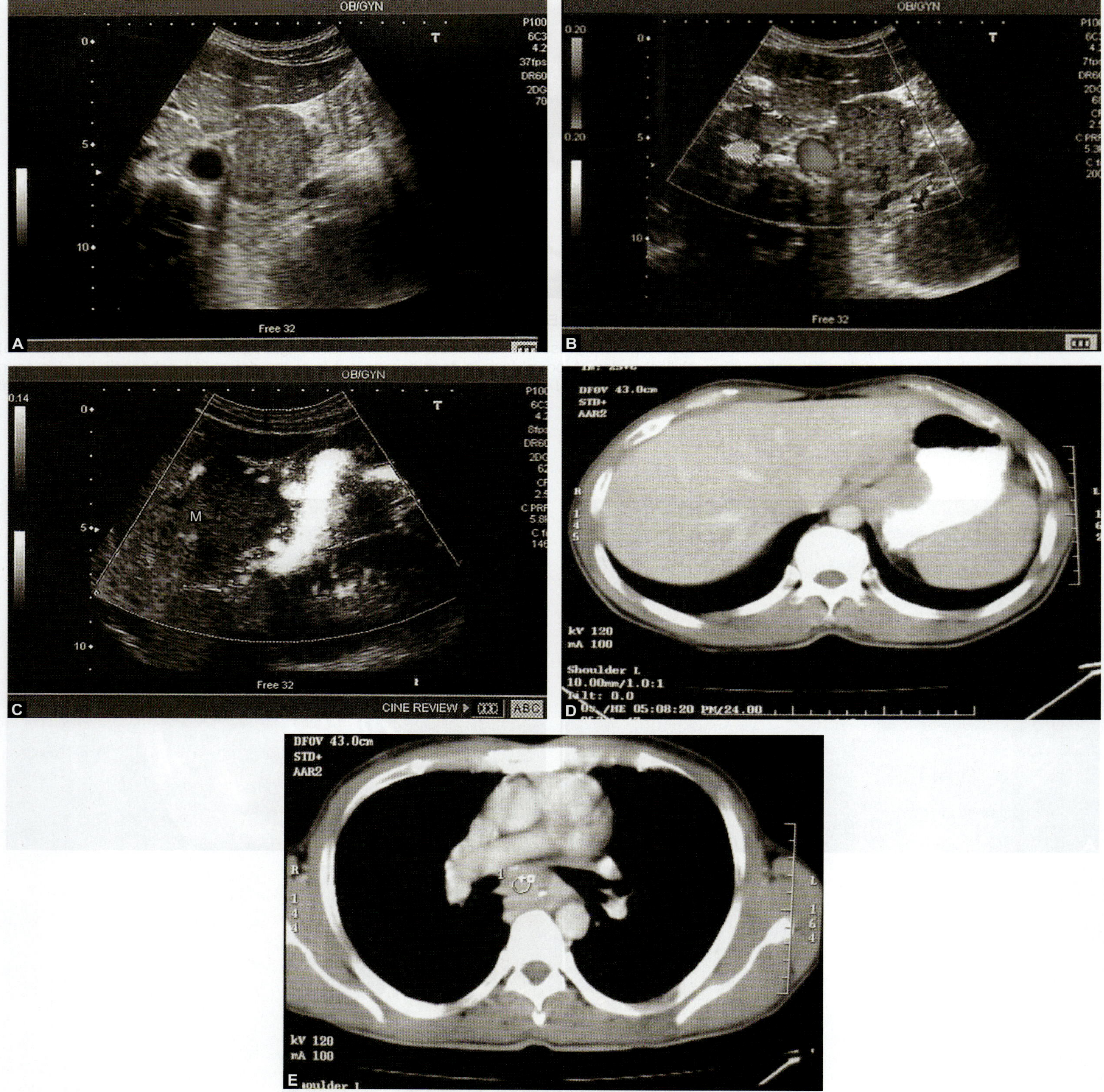

FIGURES 9.60A to E: CA esophagus. A patient presented with dysphagia. High-resolution sonography (HRSG) shows a hypoechoic mass in the region of lesser sac and anterior to aorta. The mass is seen extending to the lower end of esophagus and also seen involving the gastroesophageal junction. On color flow imaging, poor flow is seen in the mass. CT scan of the same patient confirms the ultrasound findings. Biopsy of the mass confirms CA lower end of esophagus invading the gastroesophagus junction.

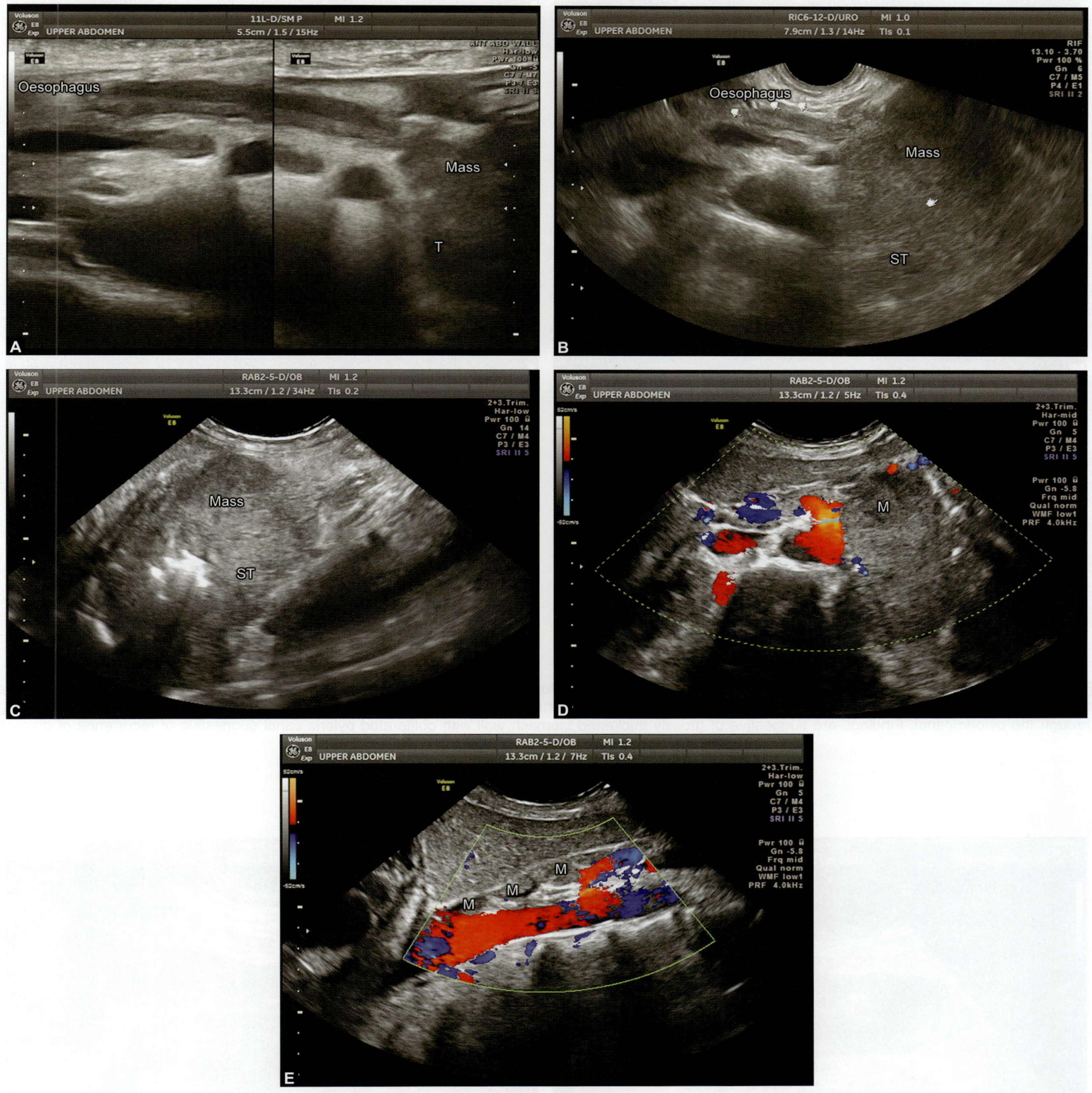

FIGURES 9.61A to E: CA lower end of esophagus invading gastroesophageal junction and stomach. A patient presented with dysphagia. High-resolution sonography (HRSG) shows a soft tissue mass in the lower end of esophagus. The entire lumen is seen invaded by the mass. The mass is also seen invading the gastroesophageal junction and lower part of stomach. The stomach wall is markedly thickened and lumen is seen invaded by the mass. On color flow imaging, poor flow is seen in the mass. Multiple enlarged nodes are also seen in the retroperitoneum suggestive of highly malignant mass.

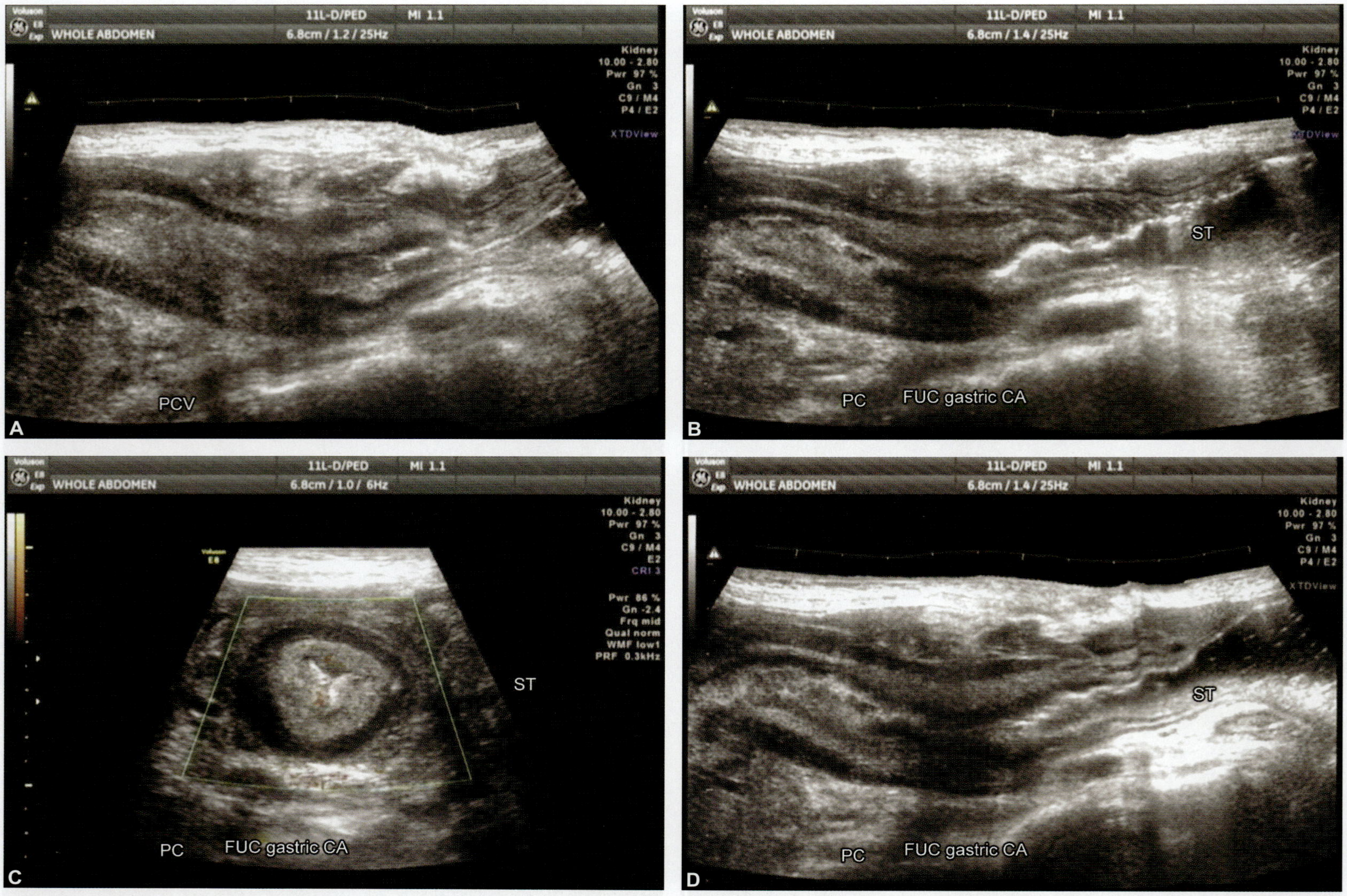

FIGURES 9.62A to D: FUC gastric CA. A patient known case of CA stomach presented with vomiting and loss of appetite. HRSG shows diffuse thickening of stomach wall. The lumen is seen obliterated. The pyloric antrum is grossly thickened. Target sign is positive. The fluid is not seen going through the pyloric canal. Findings are suggestive of grossly thickened stomach wall with obliterated pyloric canal suggestive of recurrence of disease

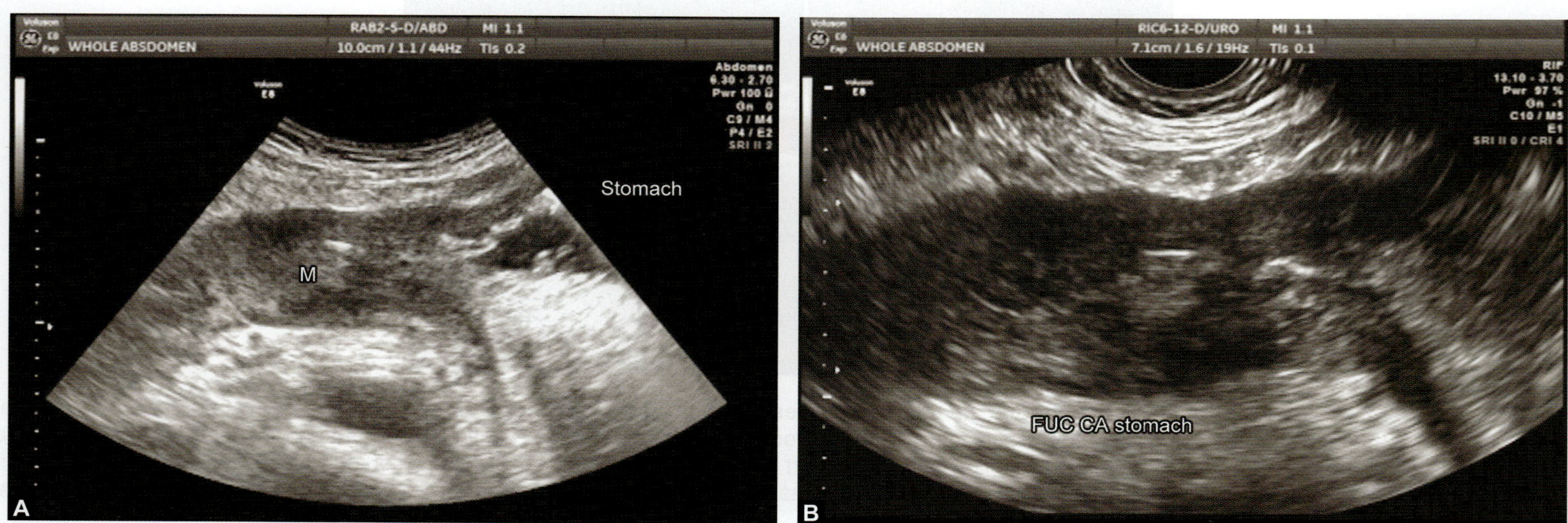

FIGURES 9.63A and B

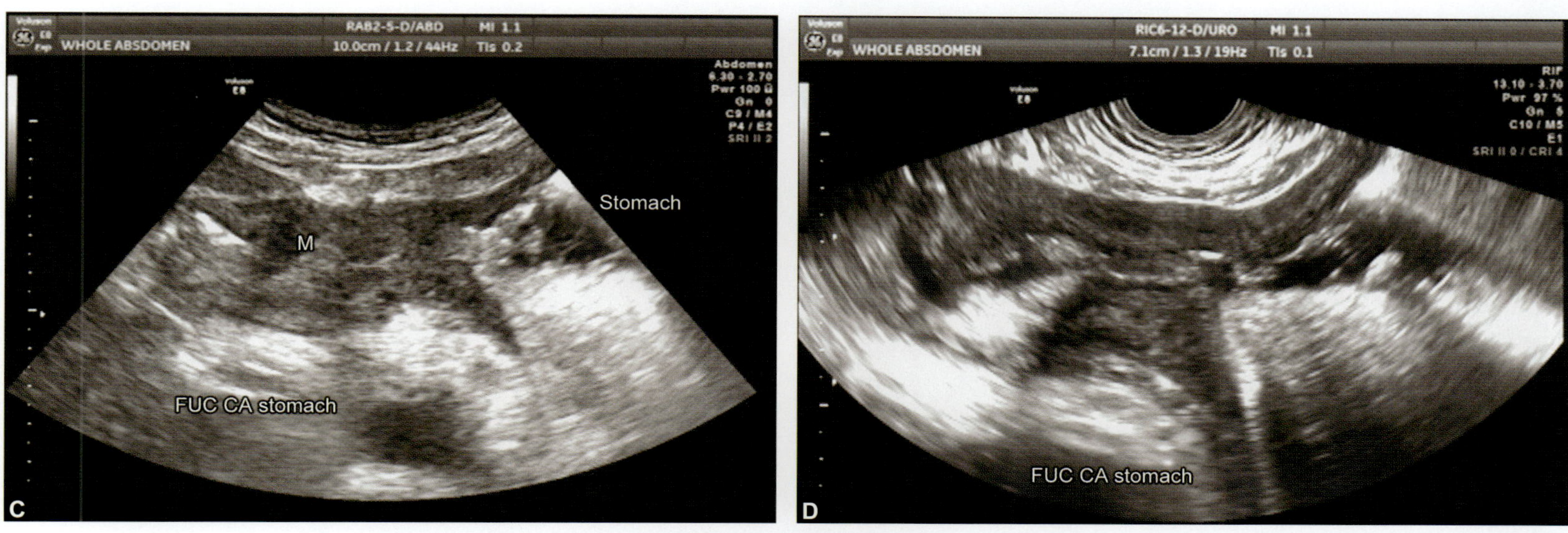

FIGURES 9.63C and D

FIGURES 9.63A to D: CA stomach presented with loss of appetite. High-resolution sonography (HRSG) shows stomach walls are grossly thickened. Lumen is obliterated in its lower part. Gas entrapment is seen. Findings are suggestive of grossly thickened stomach wall with obliterated lumen as described above suggestive of malignancy

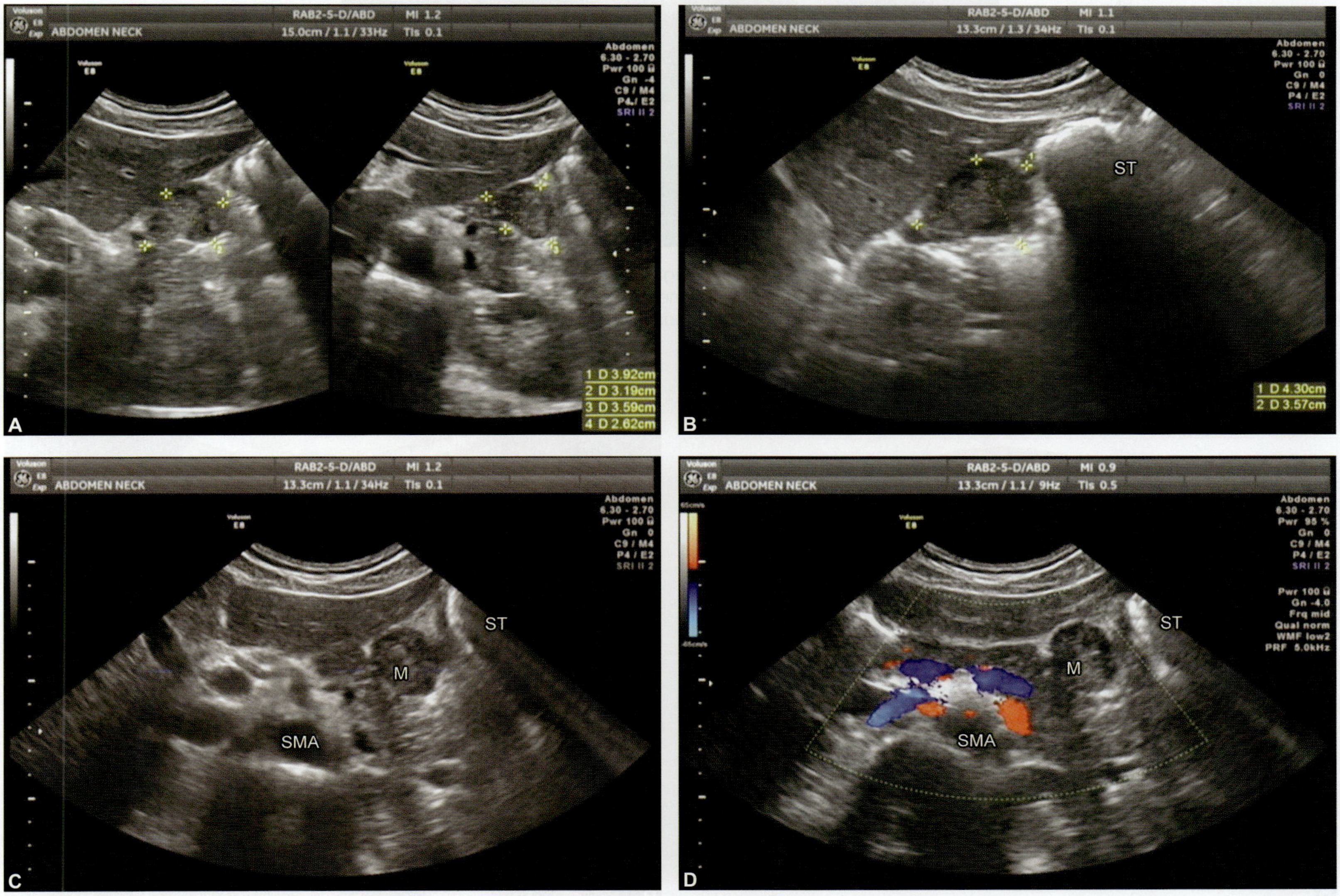

FIGURES 9.64A to D: High-resolution sonography (HRSG) shows a well defined homogeneous hypoechoic mass anterior to the laser curvature of stomach. The mass shows sharp margins. It is well encapsulated. It measures 45 x 35 mm in size. No evidence of any cystic degeneration is seen in the mass. No calcification is seen. It is separate from the pancreas. On color flow imaging, poor flow is seen in the mass. Biopsy of the mass confirms CA stomach.

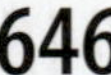

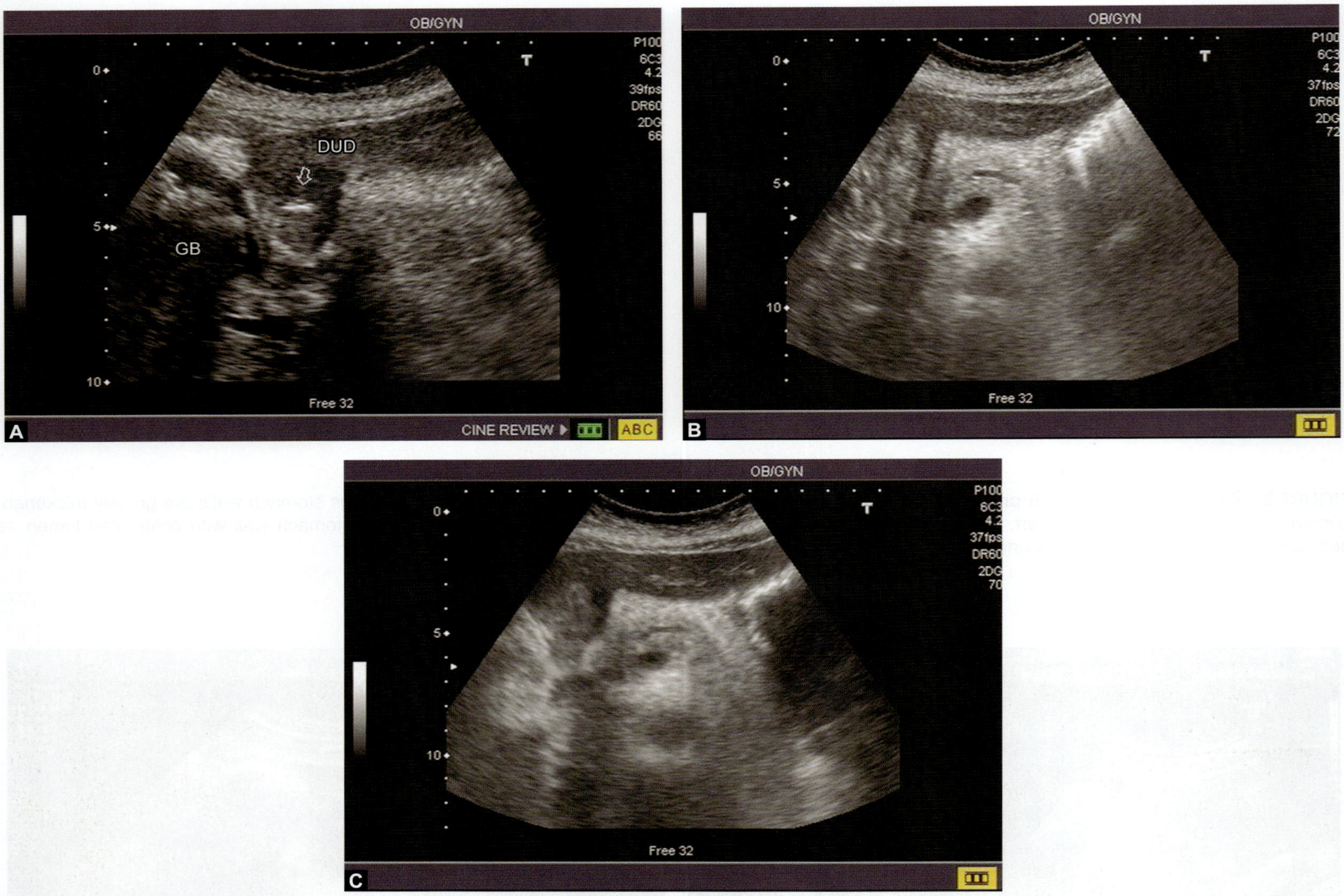

FIGURES 9.65A to C: Duodenal mass. A patient presented with vomiting. HRSG shows obliterated lumen of the duodenum. A soft tissue mass is seen filling the duodenum. The air is seen entrapped in the obliterated lumen. No fluid movement is seen going through the duodenum. The stomach is seen dilated. Findings are suggestive of malignant mass in the duodenum. Biopsy of the mass confirms ultrasound findings.

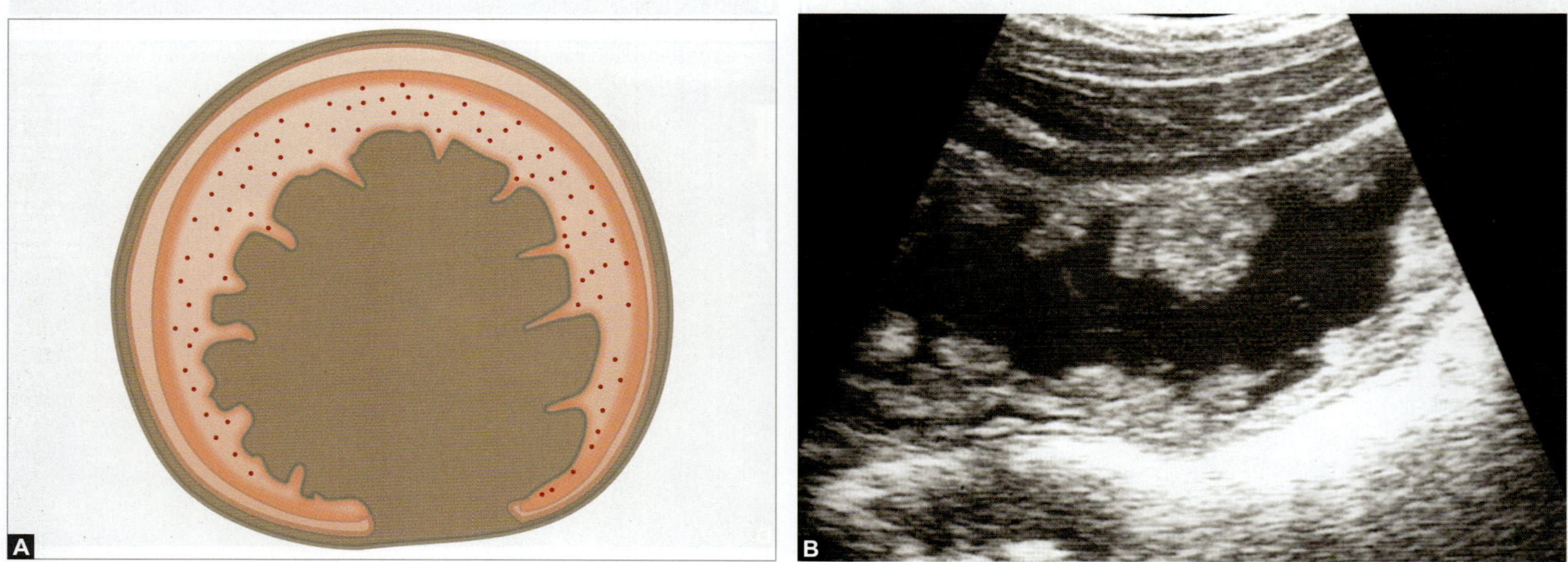

FIGURES 9.66A and B: High-resolution sonography (HRSG) is very good in evaluating bowel masses and they stand out clearly if the bowel loops are distended. Figure A shows diagrammatic representation of the bowel mass in the lumen of gallbladder. It is endophytic in nature. Figure B shows a endophytic soft tissue mass shows a large bowel loop.

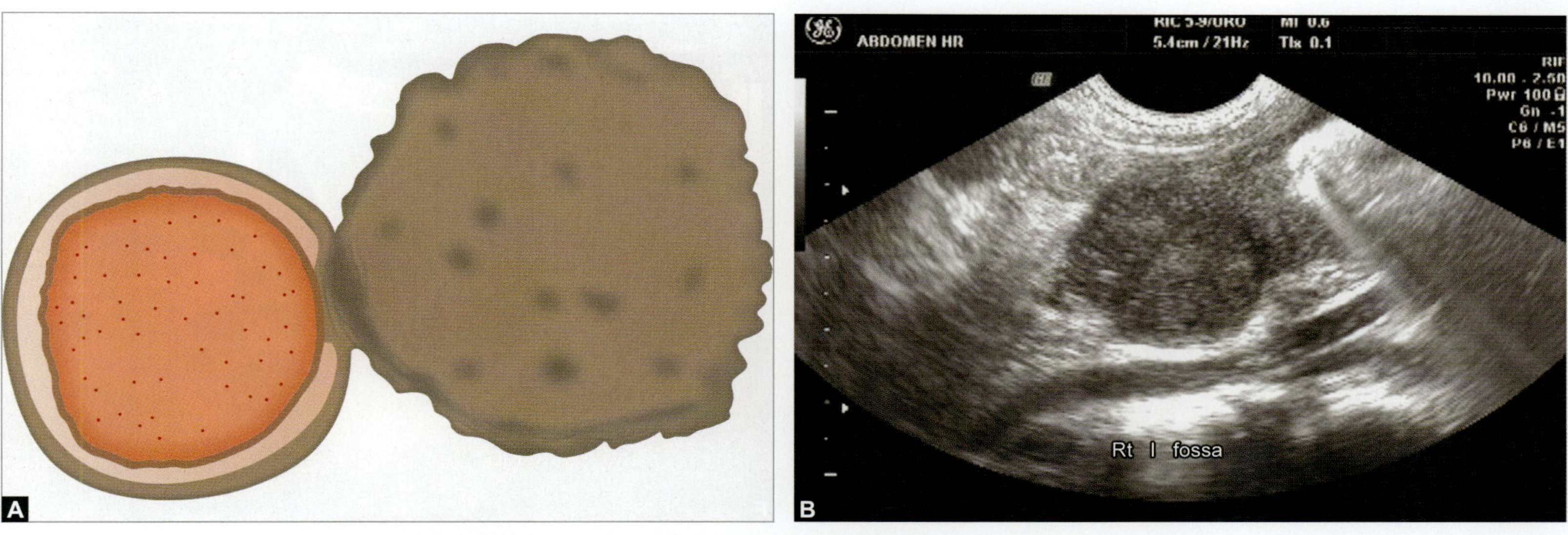

FIGURES 9.67A and B: Exophytic bowel mass. High-resolution sonography (HRSG) shows exophytic mass coming out from the bowel. It is hypoechoic in texture. Biopsy of the mass confirms malignant mass.

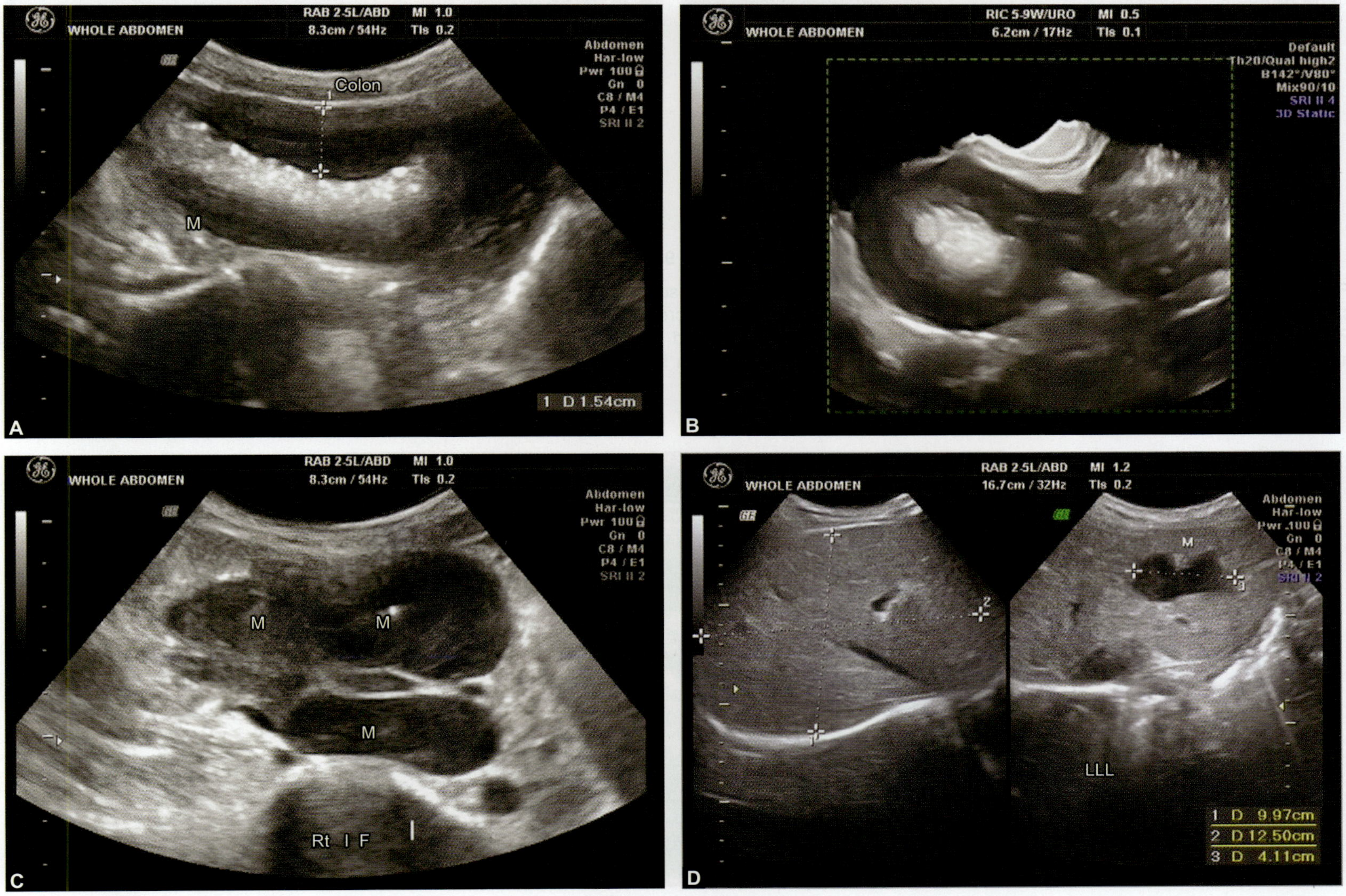

FIGURES 9.68A to D

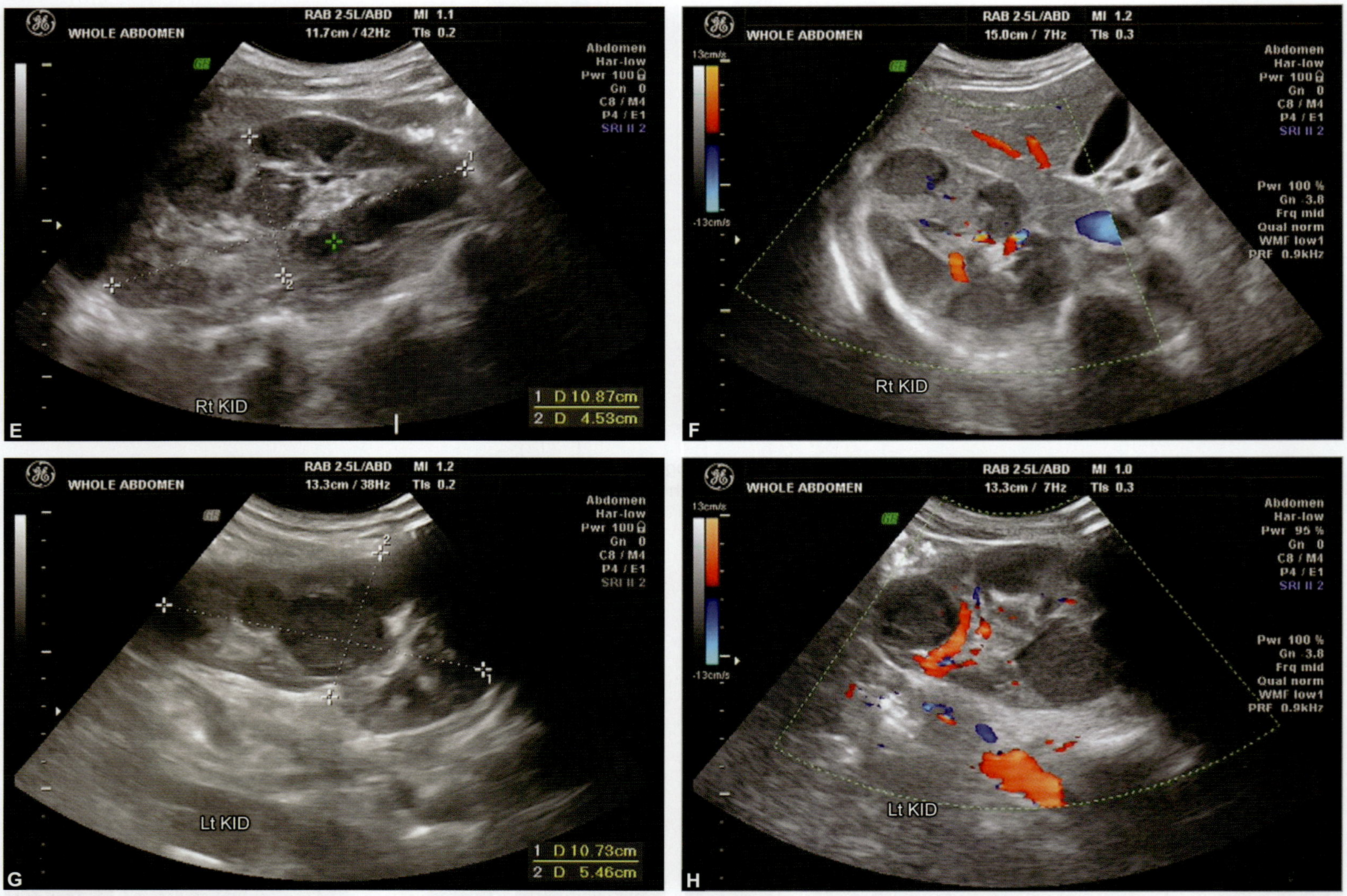

FIGURES 9.68E to H

FIGURES 9.68A to H: Bowel lymphoma with metastasis. A patient presented with obstructive bowel disease. High-resolution sonography (HRSG) shows diffuse thickening of bowel involving the large bowel. Marked increased thickening is seen. Lumen is obliterated. Gas is seen entrapped. Pseudo-kidney sign is positive suggestive of lymphoma. Multiple enlarged nodes are also seen in the iliac fossa. The liver and both kidneys show metastatic deposits of lymphoma. On color flow imaging, low flow is seen in it

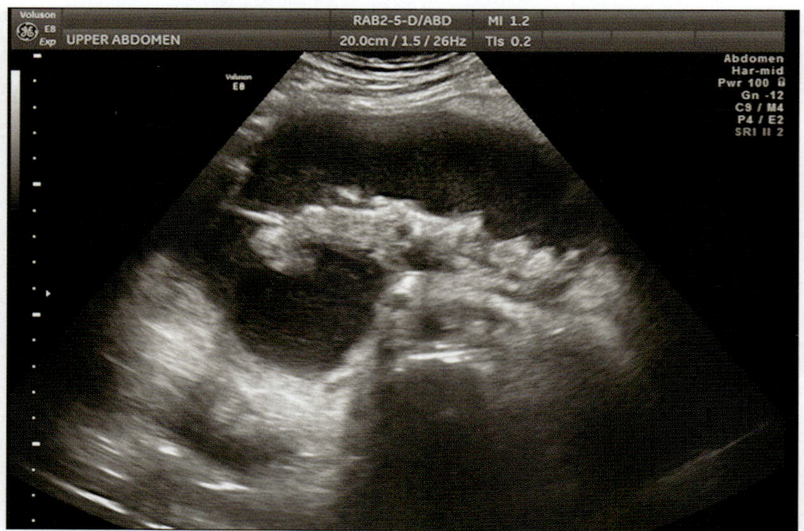

FIGURE 9.69: A patient presented with **obstructive bowel features.** HRSG shows irregular mass involving the large bowel. Diffuse thickening of the bowel loops is seen. Pseudokidney sign is positive suggestive of lymphoma.

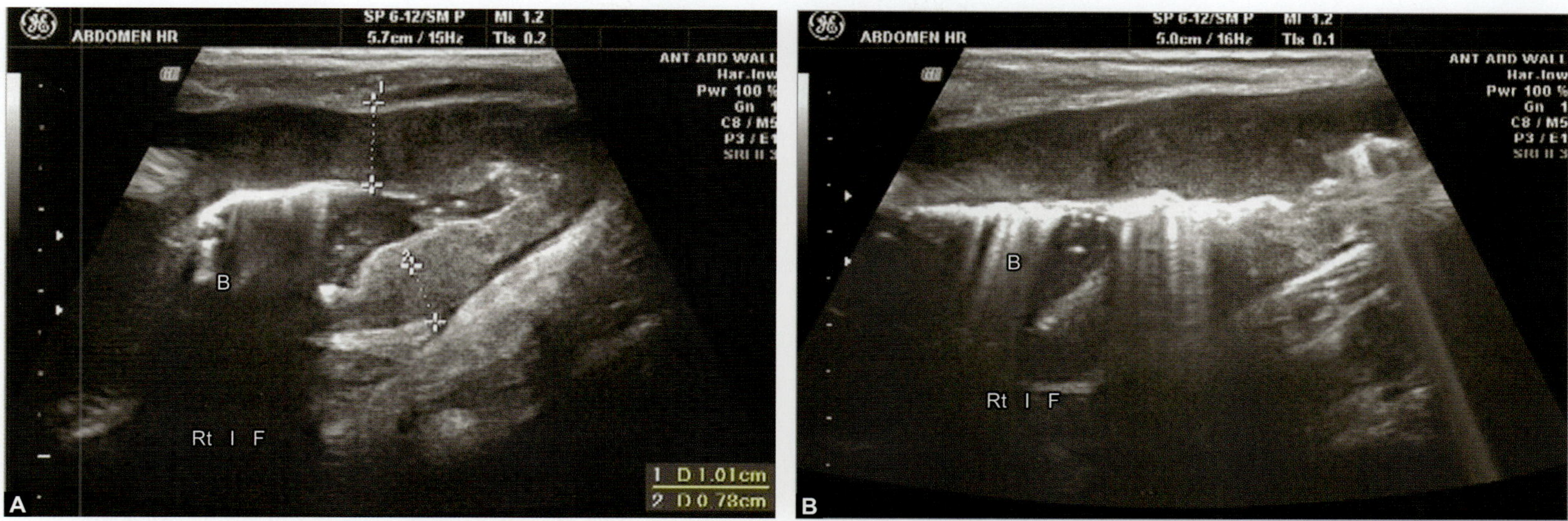

FIGURES 9.70A and B: A young boy presented with **fever and lump in abdomen.** High-resolution sonography (HRSG) shows a soft tissue mass seen in the abdomen. The mass is seen in relation to the large bowel. It is seen engulfing the bowel loop. Air entrapment is seen into it. Pseudo kidney sign is positive. Multiple enlarged nodes are also seen in both iliac fossae. They are hypoechoic in texture but homogeneous in echo pattern. Biopsy of the nodes confirms lymphoma.

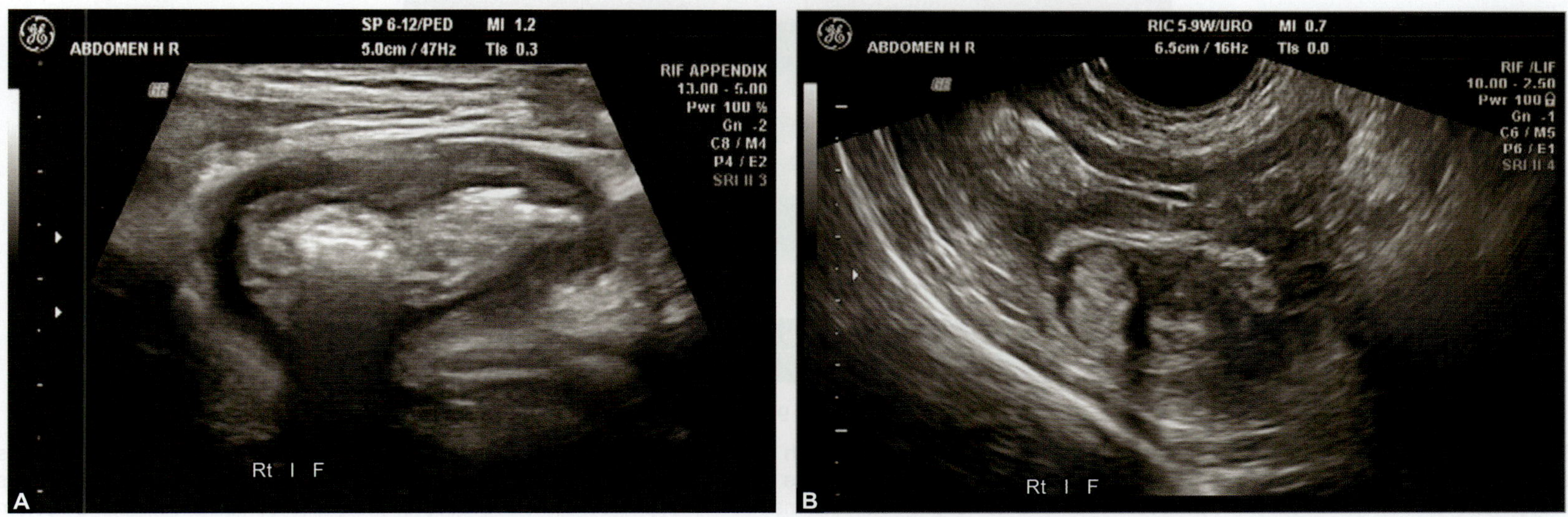

FIGURES 9.71A and B: A 14-year-old boy presented with **lump in abdomen in right iliac fossa**. High-resolution sonography (HRSG) shows diffuse thickening of the bowel loop. Gas entrapment is seen. Pseudokidney sign is positive. Proximal bowel loops are dilated. Multiple enlarged nodes are also seen in the iliac fossa suggestive of lymphoma.

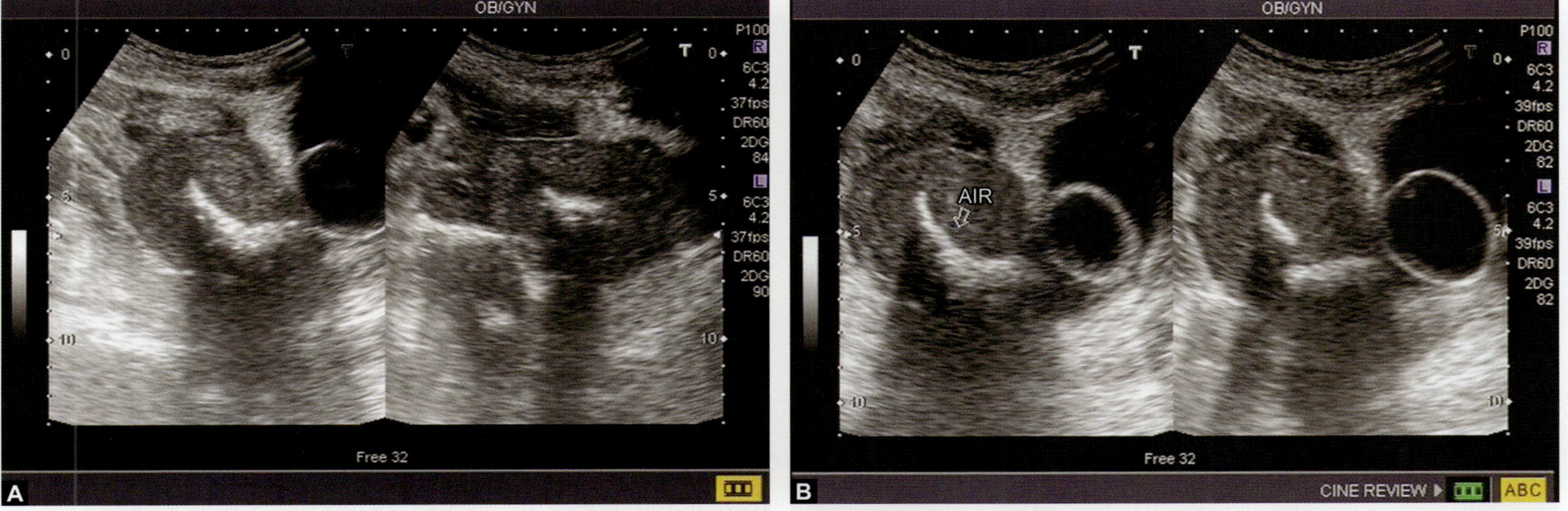

FIGURES 9.72A and B

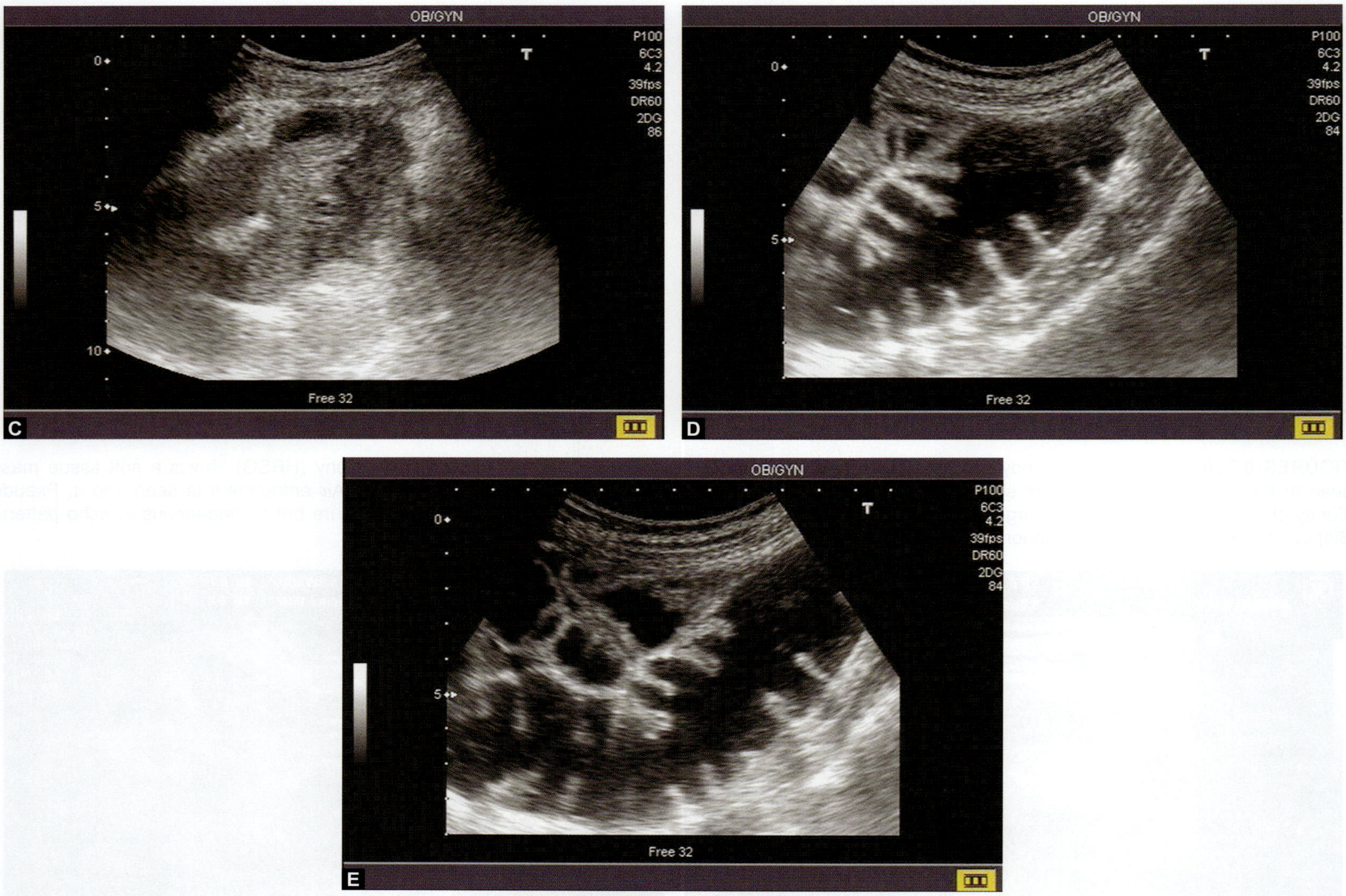

FIGURES 9.72C to E

FIGURES 9.72A to E: A patient presented with **bleeding per rectum with gastrointestinal obstruction**. High-resolution sonography (HRSG) shows a big heterogeneous mass involving the rectum and anal canal. The mass is involving the rectal wall from all sides. Lumen is seen obliterated. Gas entrapment is seen in it. Muscle layer rectal wall are not seen. The proximal bowel loops are dilated. Biopsy of the mass confirms carcinoma rectum

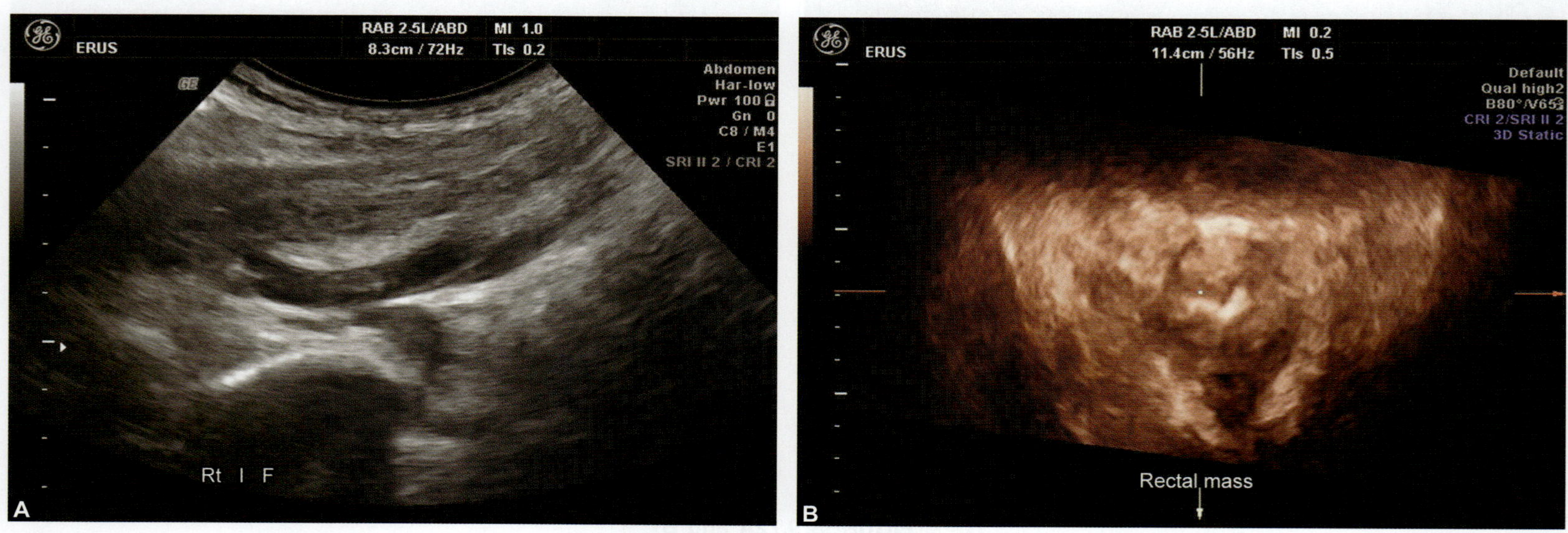

FIGURES 9.73A and B

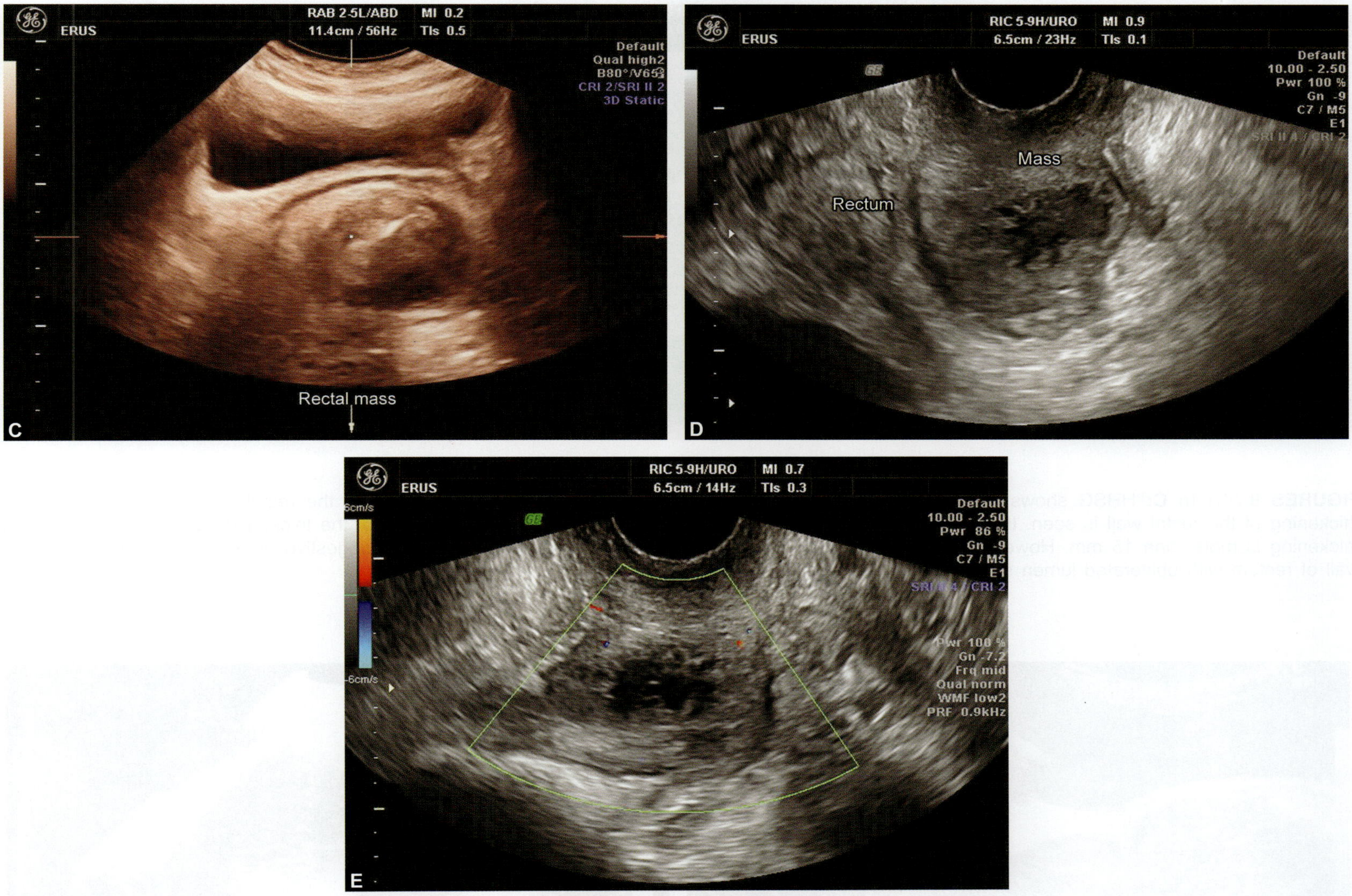

FIGURES 9.73C to E

FIGURES 9.73A to E: A patient presented with **bleeding per rectum with bowel obstruction**. High-resolution sonography (HRSG) shows an irregular heterogeneous mass seen in the rectum. The mass is seen extending into the anal canal. It is seen obliterating the lumen of the rectum and it is also seen invading the mucosa and the muscle layer of the rectum. However, the no extraluminal spread is seen. The recto vesicle space is maintained. No free fluid is seen in the peritoneal cavity or in the pelvis. The mass is separate from the prostate. The facial plane is maintained. Biopsy of the mass confirms carcinoma rectum and anal canal.

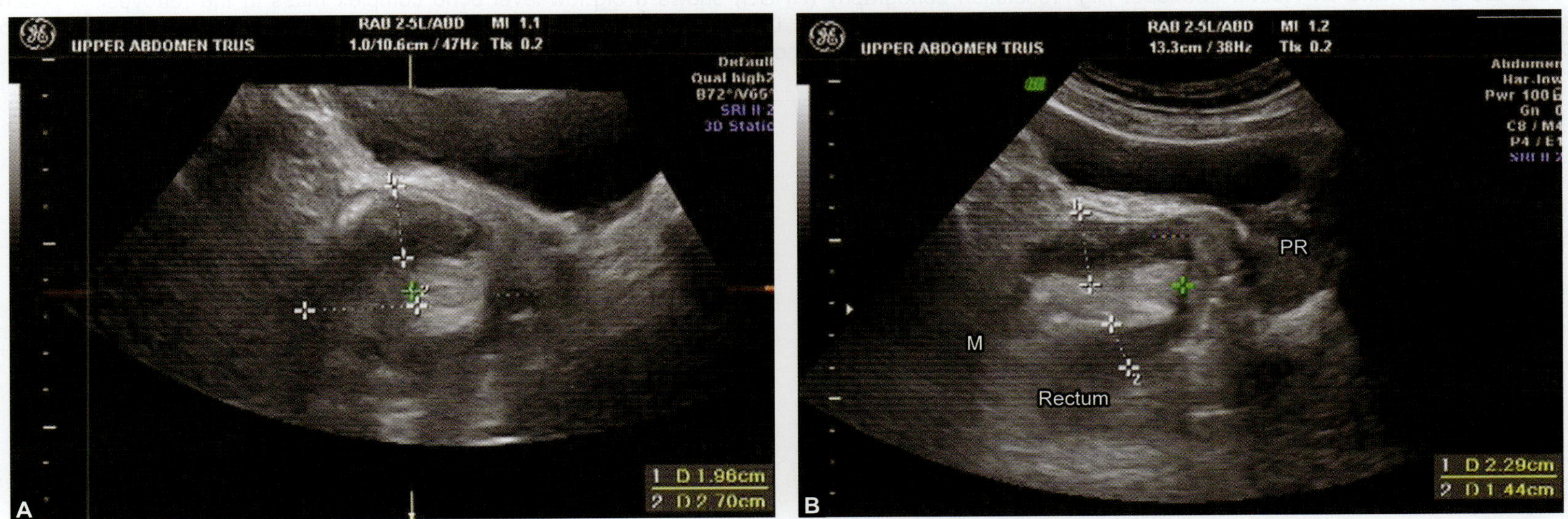

FIGURES 9.74A and B

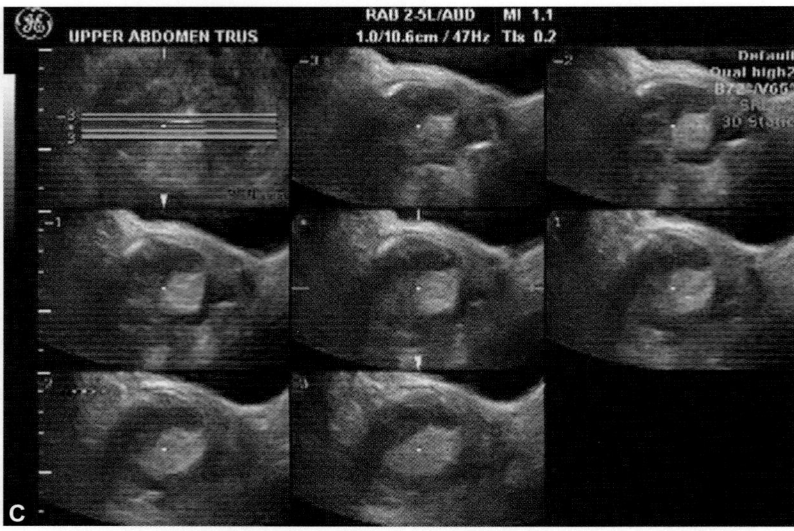

FIGURE 9.74C

FIGURES 9.74A to C: HRSG shows a **soft tissue mass in the rectal canal**. The mass is seen invading the rectal wall from all sides. Gross thickening of the rectal wall is seen. It is circumferential in nature. The rectal lumen is obliterated. Length of the thickened wall is 25 mm. The wall thickening is more than 15 mm. However, no evidence of any extraluminal growth is seen. Findings are suggestive of circumferential thickening of wall of rectum with obliterated lumen suggestive of carcinoma rectum.

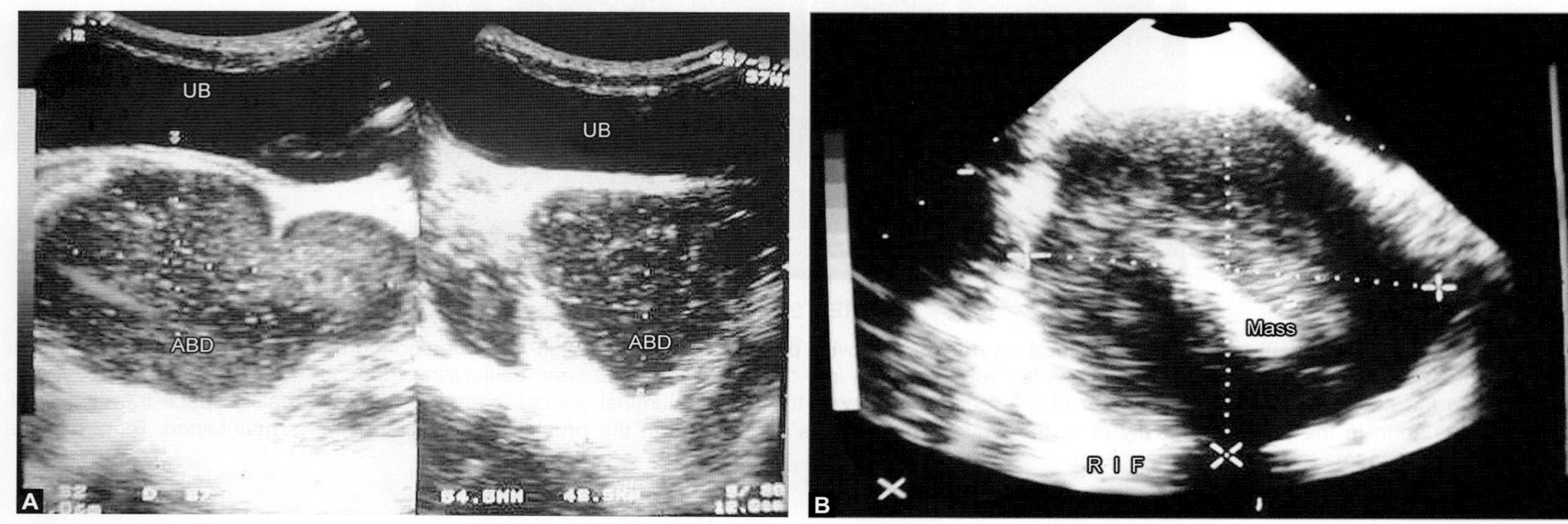

FIGURES 9.75A and B: Rectal abscess. High-resolution sonography (HRSG) shows a big low-level echo complex mass in the retrovesicle pouch suggestive of an abscess. Homogeneous low-level echoes are seen in it. Layering is also seen, typical feature of an abscess. A big low-level echo complex mass is seen in the rectum. The mass shows homogeneous echoes. The gas entrapment is seen in it in the collapsed rectal lumen.

CHAPTER 10

Prostate

Mukund Joshi, PK Srivastava

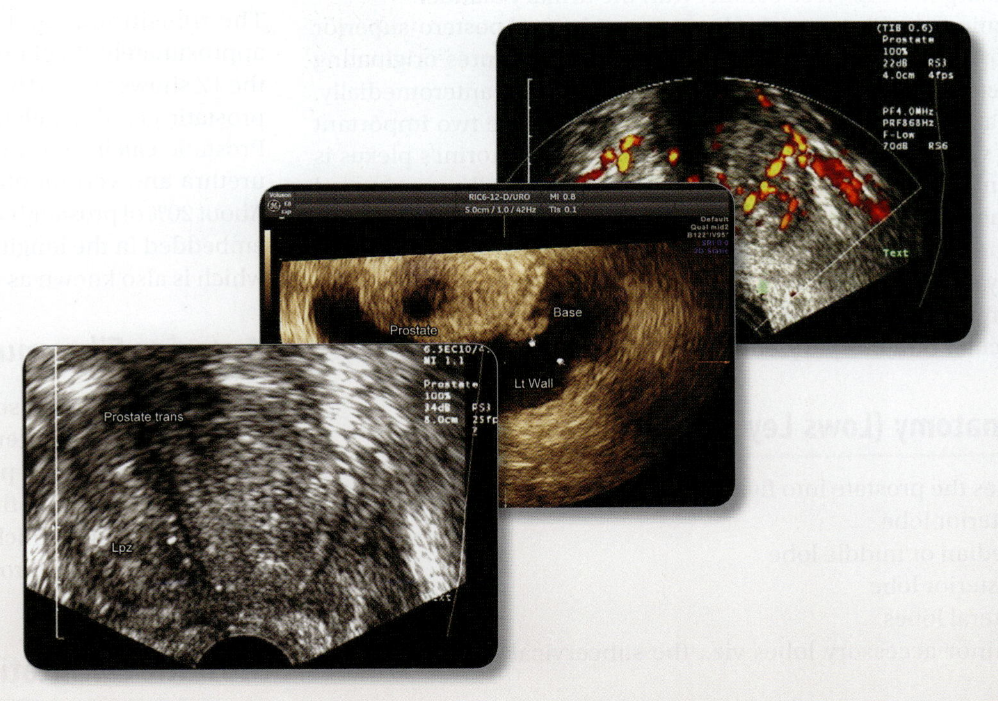

PROSTATE

The approach to the diagnosis of prostatic disease has changed over the last two decades. Apart from digital rectal examination (DRE), Transabdominal ultrasound and the development of serum assays, the availability of transrectal ultrasound with biopsy has revolutionized the thought process in prostatic pathology. Transrectal ultrasonography (TRUS) of the prostate is a dynamic study and needs to be carried out systematically. In order to understand the pathologies, it is quite essential to know the internal US anatomy of the prostate in great details. The availability of excellent quality color Doppler facilities has added a new dimension to the diagnosis of prostatic cancer.

Gross Anatomy

The normal prostate in a young adult has a triangular or conical shape and a weight of about 12–20 g. The gland progressively enlarges with age. The average measurements of a normal prostate are 4.0–4.5 cm (transverse) × 2.5–3.0 cm (AP) × 3.0–4.0 (cephalo caudad). The prostate is surrounded by a thin "pseudo-capsule" which consists of dense fibrous tissue and smooth muscle, which is connected with the muscular layers of the prostatic urethra. This pseudocapsule has a few areas of weakness.

- At the insertion of the neurovascular bundle
- At the insertion of the ejaculatory duct
- At the insertion of the internal sphincter
- At the apex and external sphincter

The prostate is situated immediately superior to the urogenital diaphragm. Its anterior relation is the symphysis pubis and the pubis bone. Laterally, the obturator internus and levator ani border the gland. Posteriorly, the 'Denonvilliers' fascia separates the prostate and its superior margin are in close contact with the urinary bladder.

The seminal vesicles are paired structures situated postero-superior to the prostate. The vas deferens is also paired structures originating from the epididymis and joining the seminal vesicles anteromedially. The prostatic urethra traverses the prostate. There are two important groups of vessels that surround the prostate. The Santorini's plexus is situated anterior to the prostate. The neurovascular bundles are situated postero-laterally in the prostate and course from the apex of the gland towards the seminal vesicles. The importance of neurovascular bundles is that they can be involved by tumor extension. They are also important during surgical interference for prostatic cancer. The branches from the neurovascular bundles perforate the capsule and enter the prostate.

Lobar Anatomy (Lows Ley's Classification)

This divides the prostate into five major and two minor lobes:

- The anterior lobe
- The median or middle lobe
- The posterior lobe
- Two lateral lobes
- Two minor accessory lobes viz., the subcervical and subtrigonal lobes.

However, the newer classification depending upon the histopathology of various prostatic disorders is now the accepted standard and not lobar anatomy.

Zonal Anatomy of Prostate

McNeal in 1968, first introduced the concept of zonal prostatic anatomy. He defined three glandular zones, which are covered anteriorly by a fibromuscular stroma. The urethra and the ejaculatory ducts form the network for these glandular zones. The three zones described are:

- The central zone
- The transition zone
- The peripheral zone

Each zone has significant implications related to the origin of the various disease processes.

Central Zone

The central zone (CZ) is pyramidal in shape and contains approximately 25% of glandular tissue at the base of the prostate. Its apex is at the verumontanum. Ducts from the CZ radiate form the base of the gland and terminate into the proximal urethra. The ejaculatory ducts pass through the CZ and terminate into the urethra at the verumontanum. The CZ is resistant to disease process. It is the site of origin of 10% of all prostatic cancers.

Peripheral Zone

The peripheral zone (PZ) is the largest of the glandular zones and contains 70% of prostatic glandular tissue and surrounds the distal urethra. It occupies the posterolateral and apical regions of the prostate and extends anteriorly. The ducts of the PZ enter the distal urethra, distal of the verumontanum. The PZ is homogeneous in echotexture. About 70% of prostatic cancers originate in the PZ. The majority of these are located in close proximity of the prostatic capsule. They are separated from the central and transition zones by the surgical capsule.

Transition Zone

The transition zone (TZ) in the earlier years of the life contains approximately 5% of prostatic glandular tissue. In the ageing prostate, the TZ shows marked hyperplasia and constitutes the majority of overall prostatic glandular elements. It is located on both sides of the urethra. Prostatic calcification within the periurethral glands in the proximal urethra and verumontanum produce of typical "Eiffel tower" effect. About 20% of prostatic cancers arise within the transition zone. These are embedded in the longitudinal smooth muscle of the proximal urethra, which is also known as the internal prostatic sphincter.

Anterior Fibromuscular Stroma

The anterior fibromuscular stroma (AFMS) is non-glandular tissue, which forms the anterior surface of the prostate. It is situated in anterior surface of the prostate. It is situated anterior to the urethra and is composed of smooth muscle that is continuous with the detrusor muscle fibers. It is thickest just distal to the verumontanum where it mainly consists of fibrous tissue. It becomes thinner as it reaches the apex of the prostate.

Prostatic Calcifications

Calcifications within the gland may form denovo or represent sequelae secondary to inflammatory conditions. Pathologically, they usually represent calcifications of the corpora amylacea, a proteinaceous material present within the gland. Dahnert et al. showed in a sonographic-xeroradiographic-histopathologic correlation study that calcifications within the gland and especially within the corpora amylacea cause bright reflections with or without acoustic shadowing. Calcification in this study was not associated with cancer of the prostate. The distribution of calcifications was either in the central portion of the gland immediately adjacent to the urethra or at the margins of the internal and external gland in an arc/wing-shaped configuration.

A more recent study, however, reported that occasionally tumors may contain echogenic foci, which at a pathological level correspond either to high-grade tumors with extensive central comedonecrosis and calcifications, or unusual deposits of small intraluminal crystalloid within tumor glands. These however, were never as bright or large as calcified corpora amylacea and usually were central in location within the tumor.

Clinical Indications for Transrectal Ultrasound Plug (TRUS)

The following are the indications for the use of transrectal ultra sonography:

1. *Patients with abnormal digital rectal examination (DRE):* Sonography should be performed when the DRE is abnormal. Sonography can differentiate a benign process (e.g. a cyst or calculus) from a neoplastic process. A neoplastic lesion would require further evaluation by biopsy. However, no every palpable lesion (seen on DRE) can be identified using sonography.
2. *Biopsy guidance:* TRUS is an accurate, safe approach for obtaining tissue from a focal abnormality in the gland especially from non-palpable lesions.
3. *Abnormal laboratory studies:* Men who have normal DRE may still harbor unsuspected prostatic cancer. Abnormally elevated levels of the prostate specific antigen (PSA) and value, the more likely it is that malignancy exists. TRUS can evaluate such occult neoplasms and a transrectal biopsy can be easily performed.
4. *Prostatic inflammation:* Ultrasonography of the prostate is generally not required in acute prostatitis. However, in patients who do not respond to antibiotics, US may delineate a fluid collection/abscess.
5. *Infertility:* Occasionally, male infertility may be due to agenesis and atresia of the seminal vesicles or ejaculatory duct obstruction. TRUS can be used to identify these anatomic abnormalities.
6. *Staging of prostate cancer:* TRUS can only detect local extension of the disease. Once cancer is diagnosed, magnetic resonance imaging (MRI) performs staging.
7. *Deflation of a Foley's catheter.*
8. *Evaluation of carcinoma of cervix.*
9. *Brachytherapy.*
10. *Screening.*

Cancer of prostate is one of the most prevalent malignancies in the world and is the second most common cause of related morbidity in the United States. Should screening be used to detect prostate cancer, earlier than is now possible by DRE, and if so, should sonography be the technique used? The statistics of prostatic cancer suggest that early diagnosis is beneficial. It has been shown that the cancer becomes more aggressive with associated increased metastatic potential when the tumor screening tests with TRUS have shown a small but significant yield of carcinoma in patients without clinical suspicion. US is complementary to DRE, but cannot stand alone as a screening tool. When combined with DRE, and routing PSA/PAP, TRUS helps in detecting more cancers at an earlier stage in high-risk age groups.

Procedure (Technique of TRUS)

When Watanabe and coworkers first introduced TRUS in Japan in 1967, the patients were examined in the lithotomy position following a routine urologic examination. In the early 1970s however, a sitting position with a chair mounted 3.5 transrectal probe was used for more efficient examination. Most investigators today prefer equipment using hand-held transducers with frequencies ranging from 4.5 -7.5 MHz. The patient is usually examined in a left side down decubitus position. In this fashion, the operator has more control over the endorectal probe position. An enema prior to the examination ensures adequate evacuation of the rectum. A rectal examination done just before the study gives the sonologist a "feel" of the prostatic nodularity, its firmness and the size of the prostate.

With the advancement of technology multiplanar imaging is now possible with accurate localization of abnormalities and extent of the disease. Three major planes are imaged-axial (transverse), sagittal and oblique coronal. The transaxial plane encompasses views made transversely across the gland. Moving the probe cephalocaudally and angling the transducer posteriorly allows all of the prostate and seminal vesicles to be visualized in multiple obtained by moving the probe from side to side within the rectum. Transverse images yield more information concerning the lateral margins and symmetry of the prostate, while longitudinal images show the base and apex of the gland more clearly. The transverse images are easier to understand than the longitudinal images. The sonographer must adopts a standardized examination technique in order to evaluate the prostate and the periprostatic issue completely. By moving the transrectal probe in a cephalocaudally direction, the entire prostate can be visualized. The apex, the base and the intervening can be well-delineated, but the bladder is not well-evaluated in this plane. The seminal vesicles appear as symmetrically paired structures (bow-tie appearance) at the base of the prostate. On the longitudinal section, the bladder neck and the urethra are well-identified. The ejaculatory duct is then seen to traverse through the prostate to the verumontanum.

SONOGRAPHIC APPEARANCES OF NORMAL AND ABNORMAL PROSTATE

Normal Prostate

On transrectal sonography, the normal prostate appears as a symmetrical, triangular, ellipsoid structure that is covered by a continuous prostatic capsule. The internal texture of the prostate is composed of multiple, fine, diffuse, homogeneous echoes. The true capsule of the prostate is not identified on US. However, the demarcations between the edge of the prostate and the surrounding periprostatic tissue are usually well-visualized on TRUS. The surgical capsule of the prostate is comprised of the peripheral and central zones, which becomes compressed into a thin layer by benign hyperplasia of the transition zones. The surgical capsule represents the demarcation between the transition zone and the two outer zones viz. the central and peripheral zones.

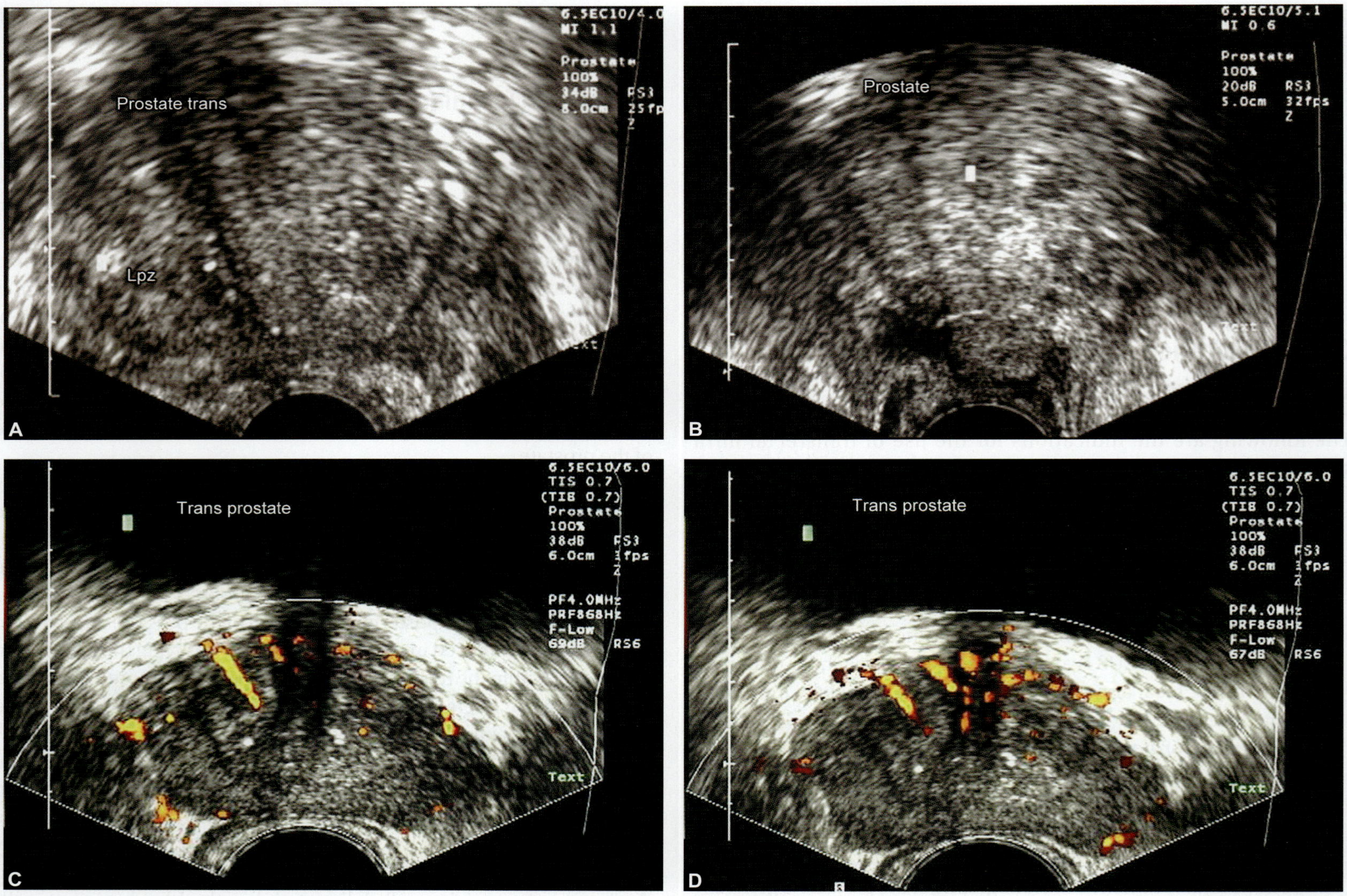

FIGURES 10.1A to D: Normal prostate. TRUS shows normal prostate gland. The lateral lobes are seen as a medium level echoes. The left and right peripheral zones are seen. Transrectal ultrasound (TRUS) shows normal prostate gland. The central zone and peripheral zones are seen very clearly on high-resolution sonography (HRSG). HRSG shows normal flow of the prostate gland. The vessels show low flow.

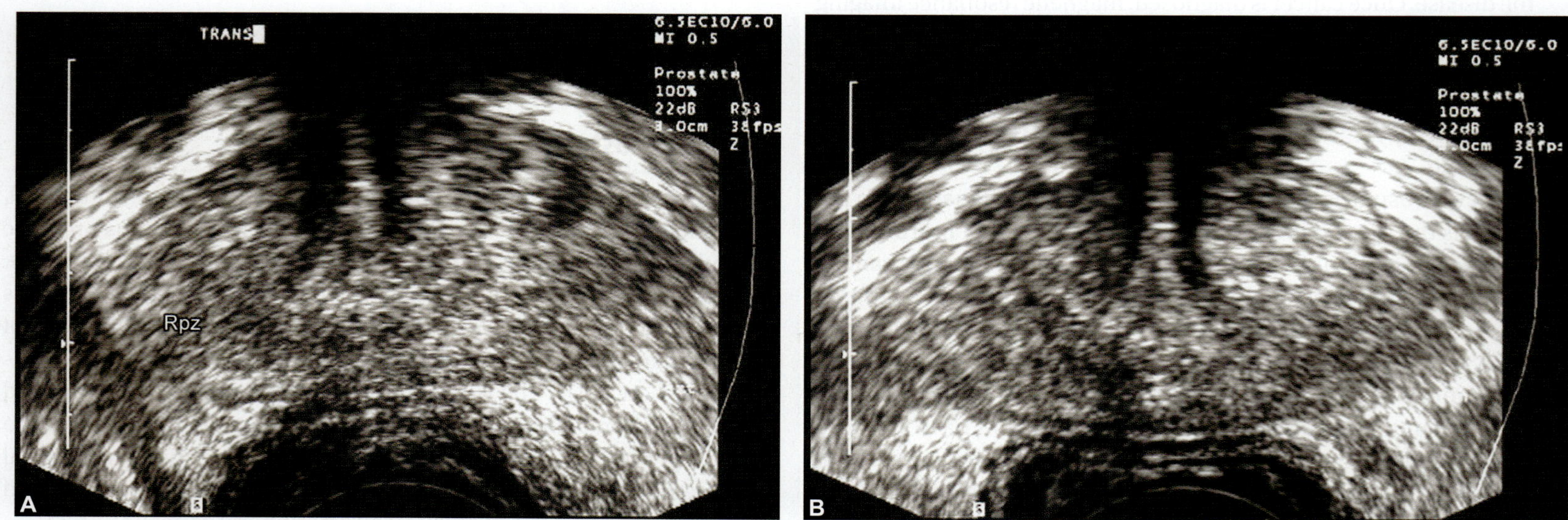

FIGURES 10.2A and B: Normal Eiffel tower. High-resolution sonography (HRSG) shows transition zone in the gland. Typical Eiffel tower appearance of gland is seen in transition zone due to urethra and periurethral glands.

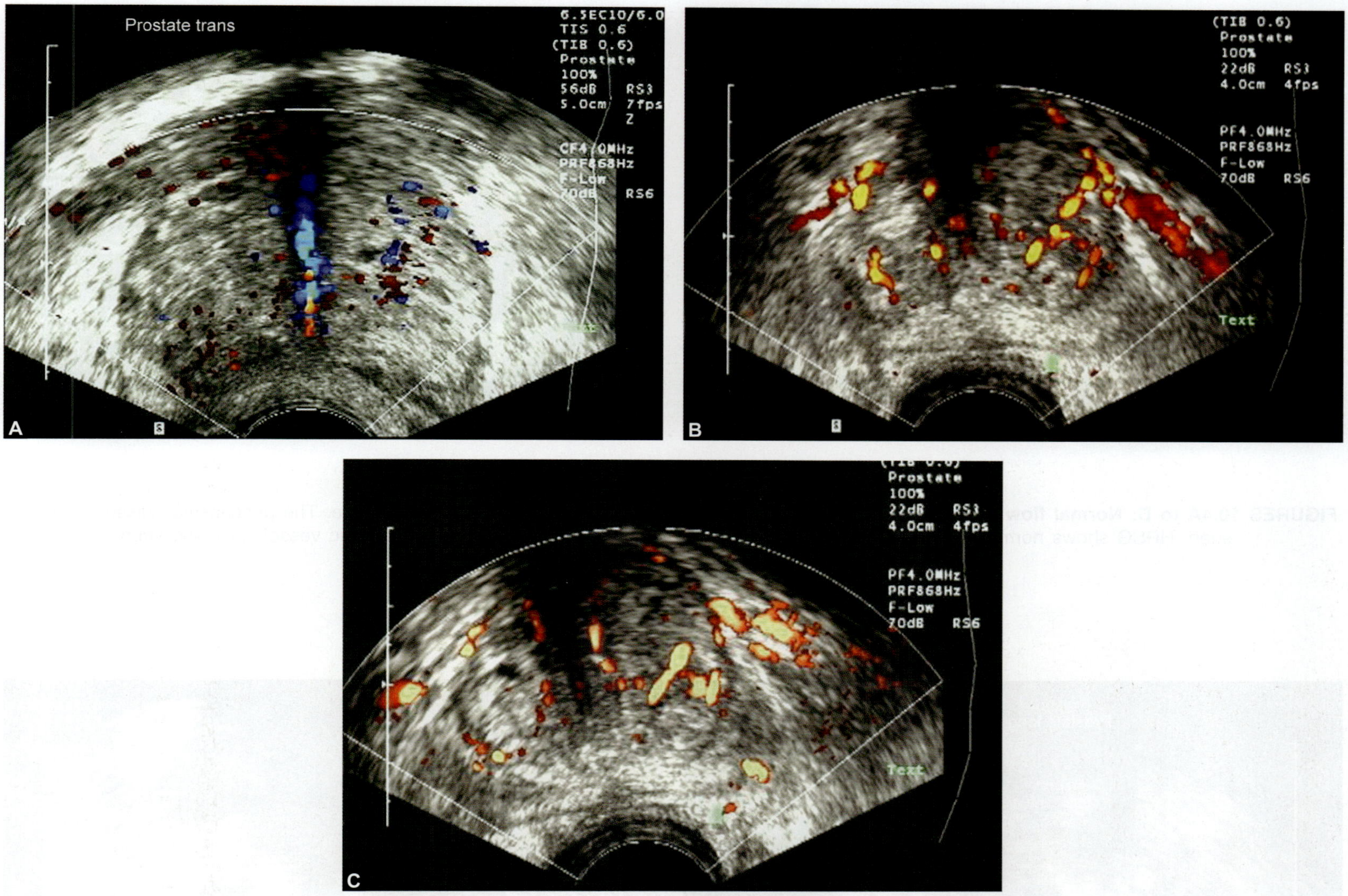

FIGURES 10.3A to C: High-resolution sonography (HRSG) and color flow imaging show normal flow in the peripheral zone on both sides. Low flow is also seen in the central zone.

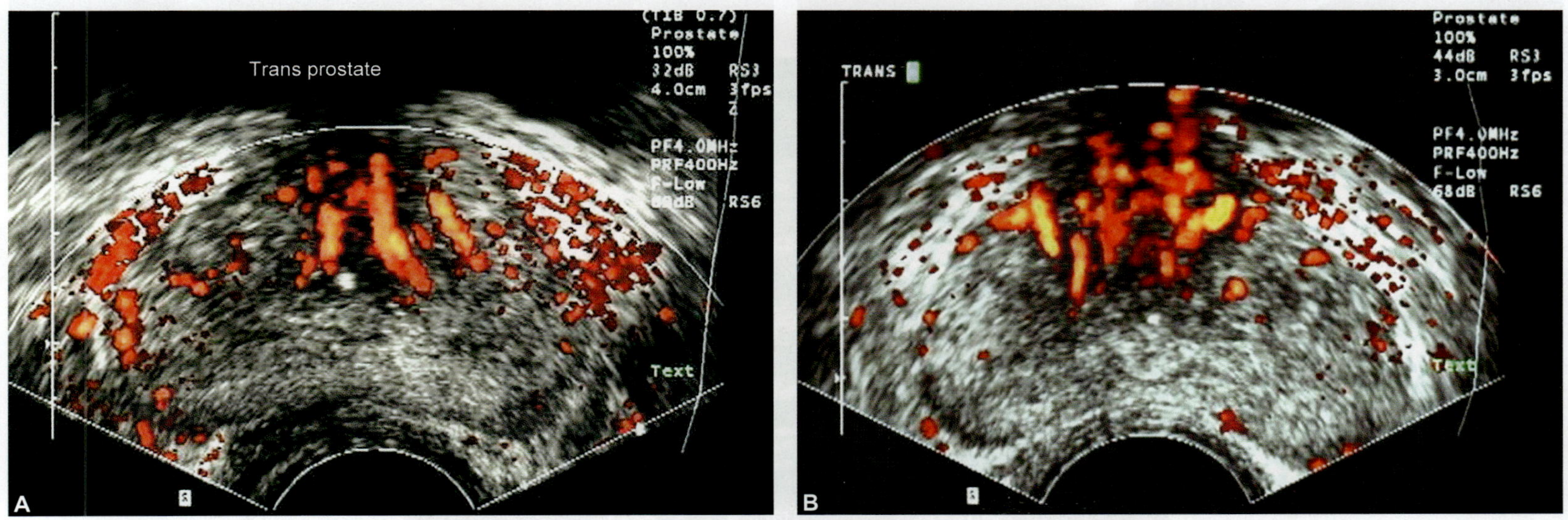

FIGURES 10.4A and B

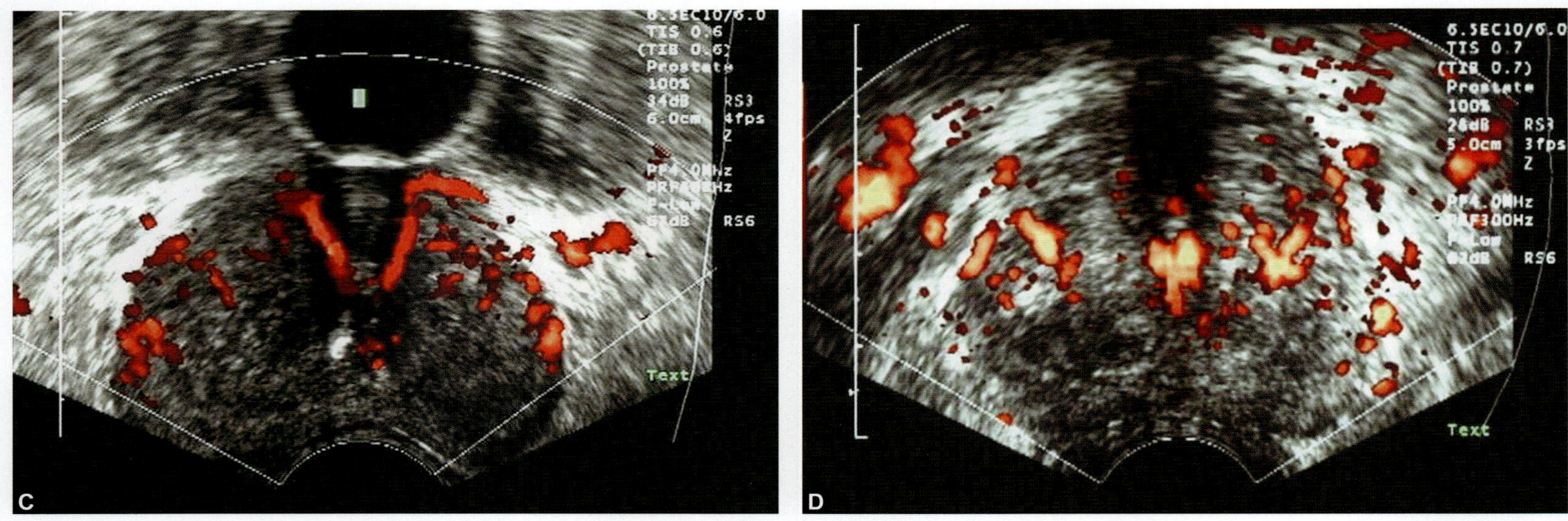

FIGURES 10.4C and D

FIGURES 10.4A to D: Normal flow. Power Doppler imaging shows multiple vessels feeding the central zone. The pericapsular vessels are also seen. HRSG shows normal flow in the gland in central and peripheral zones. Multiple periprostatic vessels are also seen.

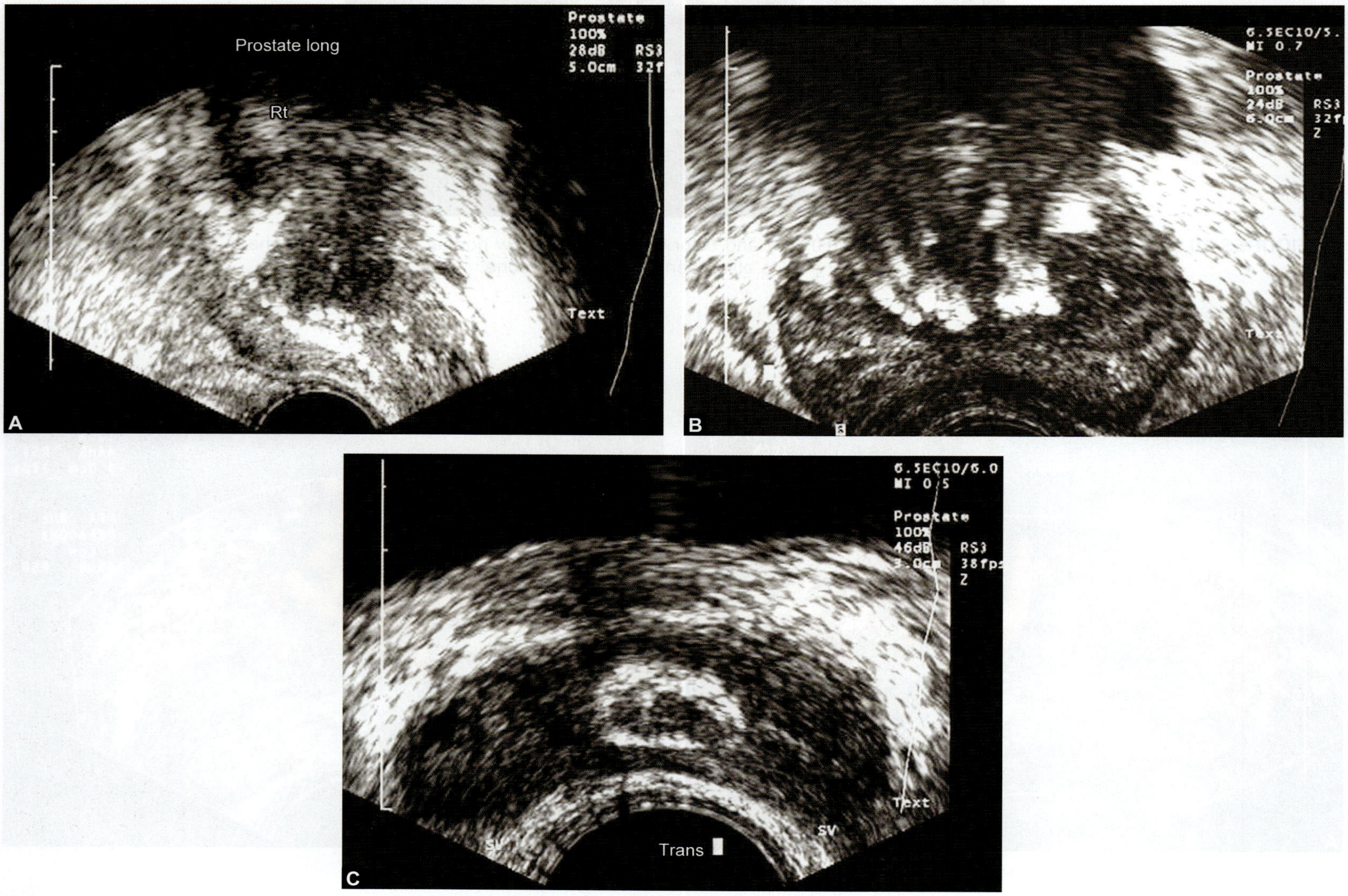

FIGURES 10.5A to C: Corpora amylacea. High-resolution sonography (HRSG) shows echogenic-calcified specks between the peripheral and central zones of the gland. It is curvilinear calcification between peripheral and central zone and presents corpora amylacea calcification. HRSG shows corpora amylacea calcification. Specks of calcification with calcified rim are seen. Color flow imaging shows normal flow.

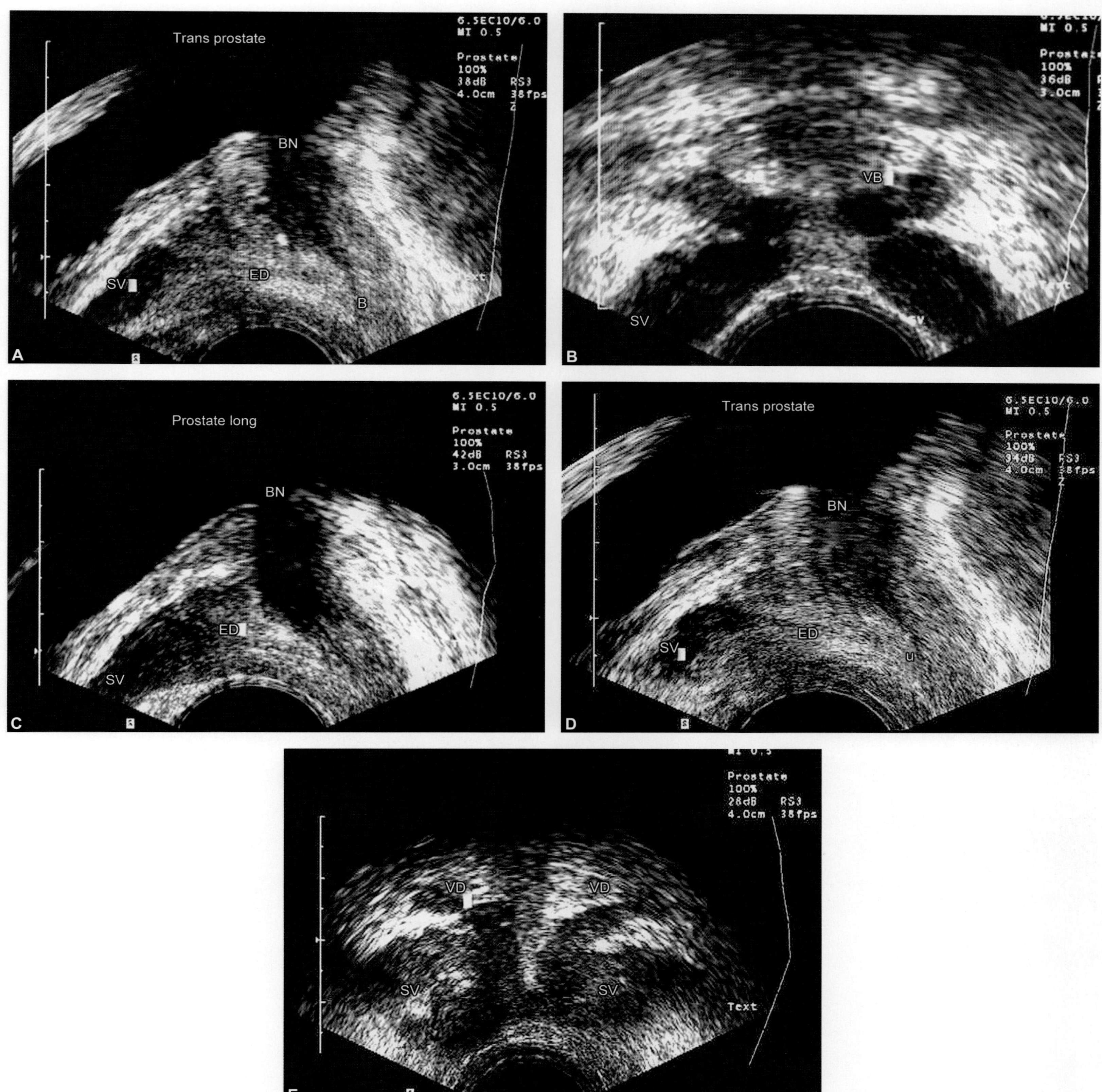

FIGURES 10.6A to E: HRSG shows normal gland. The seminal vesicles (SV) are seen partially on the left side. The ejaculatory duct (ED) and urethra are also seen. HRSG shows normal seminal vesicle. The vas deferens (VD) is seen anterior to the seminal vesicle on either side. They have similar appearance of seminal vesicle. The ejaculatory duct is also seen running in central zone and opening the verumontanum.

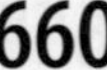

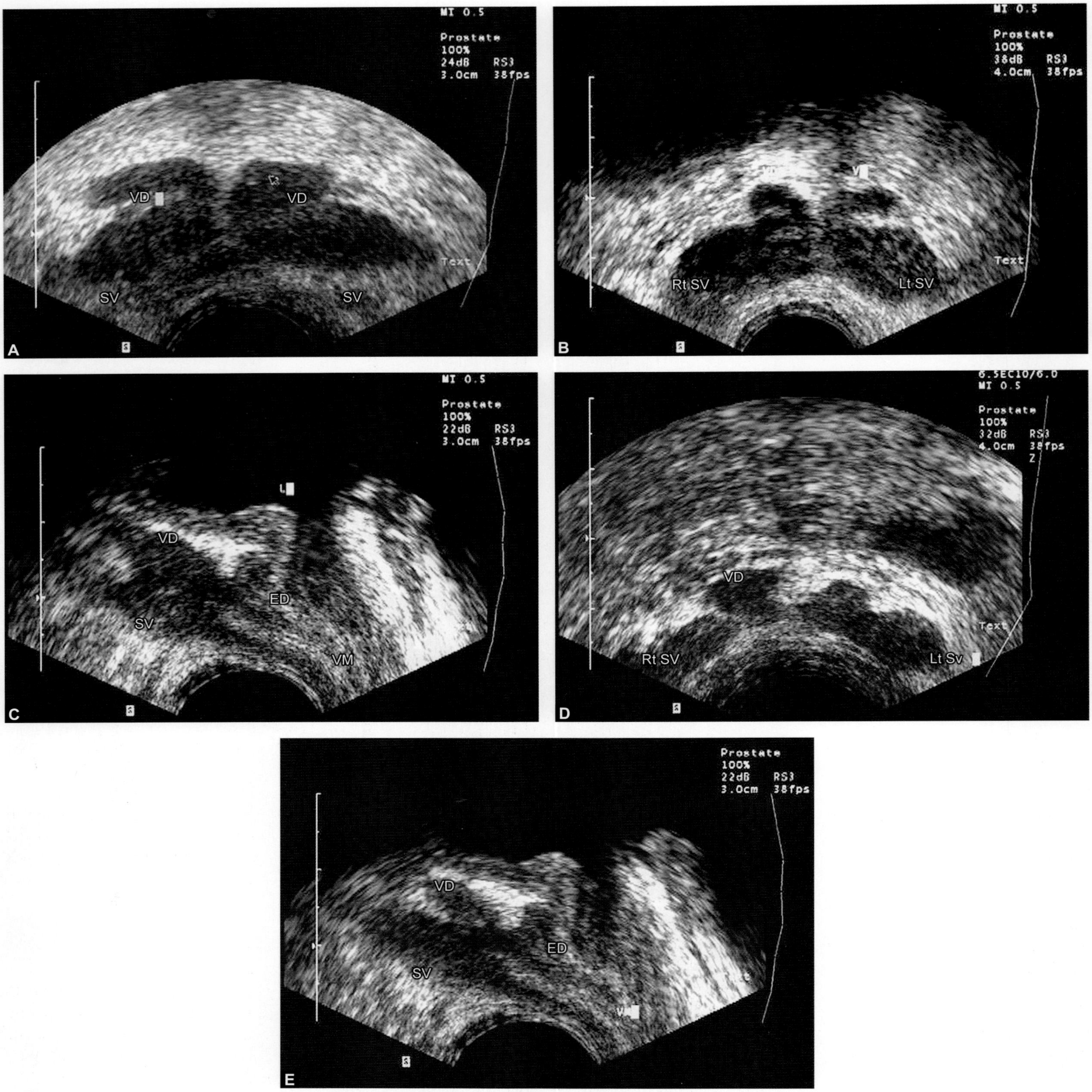

FIGURES 10.7A to E: Normal seminal vesicle and vas deferens in transverse plane. HRSG shows normal vas deferens (VD) and seminal vesicle (SV) in transverse plane. Ejaculatory duct is also seen. HRSG shows normal seminal vesicles on either side. The vas deferens are seen anterior to the seminal vesicles. Ejaculatory duct is also seen in the central zone and terminating at verumontanum (VM). HRSG shows normal seminal vesicle, vas deferens and ejaculatory duct.

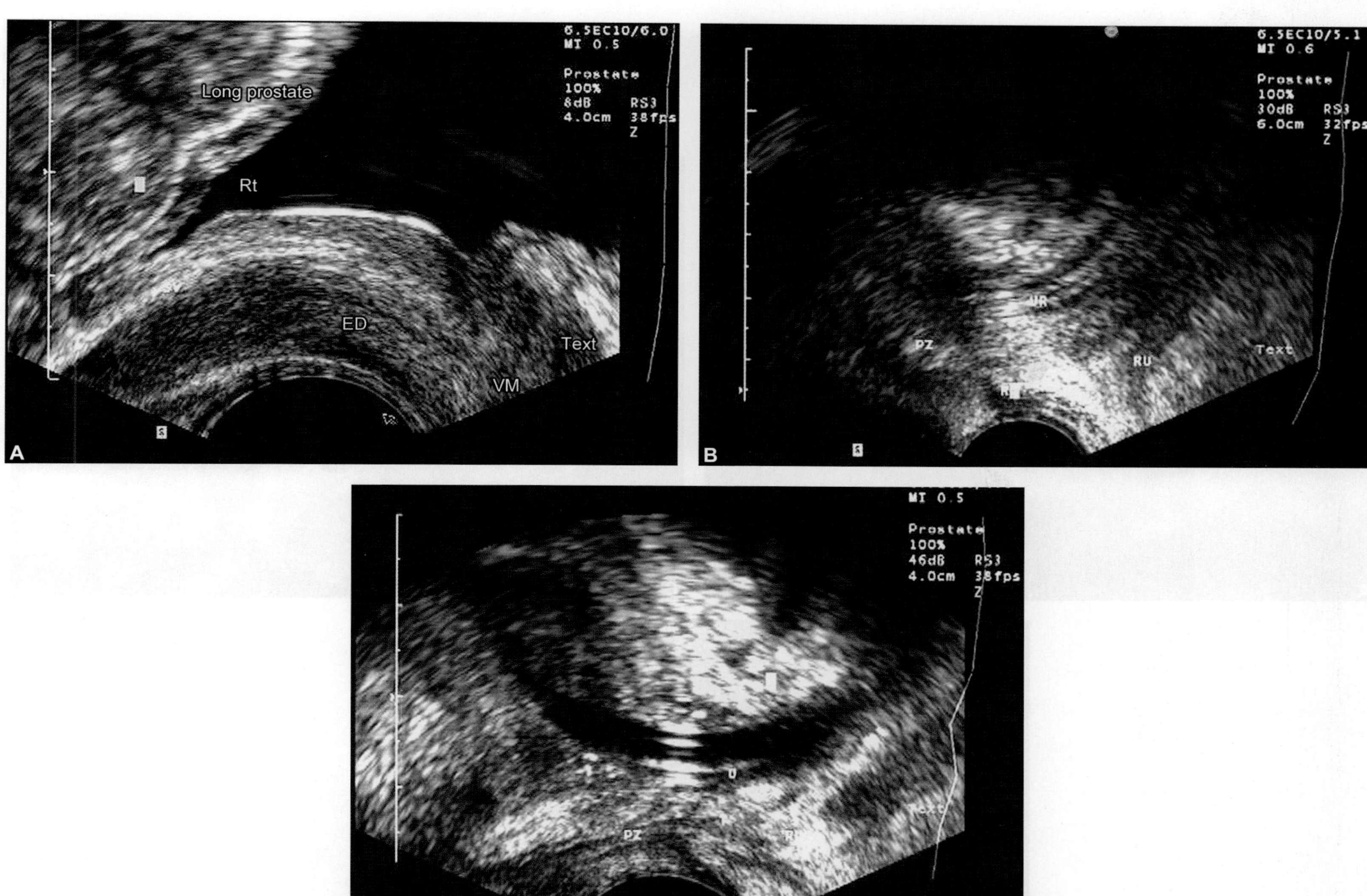

FIGURES 10.8A to C: HRSG shows normal ejaculatory duct running in central zone and opening in the urethra at verumontanum. Normal upper limit of ejaculatory duct is 2 mm. HRSG shows normal trapezoid area. The catheters tube is seen in position passing through prostate.

Benign Prostatic Hypertrophy

Most men with benign prostatic hypertrophy (BPH) see an urologist because of obstructive and irritative symptoms. These manifestations have been grouped together as 'prostatism'. DRE demonstrates a smooth firm and soft enlargement of the prostate. However, depending upon the anatomical site of the adenoma, the gland may feel normal. Abnormal uroflowmetry suggests decrease in stream and force of the urine stream.

Transrectal ultrasound (TRUS) is used very commonly for the evaluation of the prostate. Periurethral enlargement is noticed as intravesical extension of the gland. The AP and the lateral dimensions of the gland appear normal, but there is cephalad extension of the prostate. Approximately, 95% of cases of BPH arise from the transition zone and 5% from periurethral glandular tissue. Distinct nodules or diffuse enlargement can be present. The US appearance of BPH varies depending upon histopathologic changes. Typically, the central gland enlarges of BPH. Often with BPH the inner gland remains hypoechoic. On TRUS, it is frequently seen as a hypoechoic or heterogeneous, well-delineated mass involving the periurethral regions. Occasionally, BPH may compress the central zone as well as the peripheral zone to only a few millimeters in thickness. The surgical capsule is the line of demarcation between the central BPH changes and the peripheral zone. Often, a halo and/or calcifications may be seen. In normal young men, there is usually no clear differentiation between the central and peripheral glands. However, when BPH develops, those two areas can usually be identified separately. Focal BPH nodules can bulge the capsule of the gland or compress the lateral margins, but they should not disrupt the capsule or periprostatic fat. If diffuse involvement with BPH is present, the zonal anatomy of the gland can no longer be discerned.

Prostatitis—Prostatic Abscess

Prostatitis is an acute inflammatory condition that can involve either the peripheral zones or the central, periurethral areas. It can be seen in men of all ages. Prostatitis, when not due to surgical manipulation, develops nearly exclusively in the acinar prostate. Therefore, the distribution of hematogeneous spread of infection is predominantly in the peripheral zone resembling prostate cancer. When prostatitis is secondary to post-surgical instrumentation or manipulation, the central gland can be infected. Unless abscess formation occurs, the US features of prostatitis are rather nonspecific. Focal or diffuse hypo-or hyperechoic areas may be seen, often mimicking cancers of the gland. In chronic prostatitis, the TRUS findings are variable, usually showing a heterogeneous echotexture with an irregular appearance resulting in difficulties with the diagnosis. Dystrophic calcifications can develop in the peripheral gland due to chronic inflammation (chronic prostatitis). Additional US features than can be seen in chronic prostatitis include focal masses of different echogenicities that, if hypoechoic can mimic cancer, ejaculatory duct calcifications, capsular thickening or periurethral glandular irregularities. Occasionally, enlarged blood vessels creating a translucent zone around the prostate have been described in patients with chronic prostatitis. Color Doppler US may help in the detection of increased vascularity in the inflammatory phase of prostatitis. Complications of prostatitis, i.e. abscess formation may be seen as hypoechoic or fluid filled areas within the central or peripheral gland. US guided aspiration and instillation of antibiotic into the abscess can be performed via a transperineal or transrectal route.

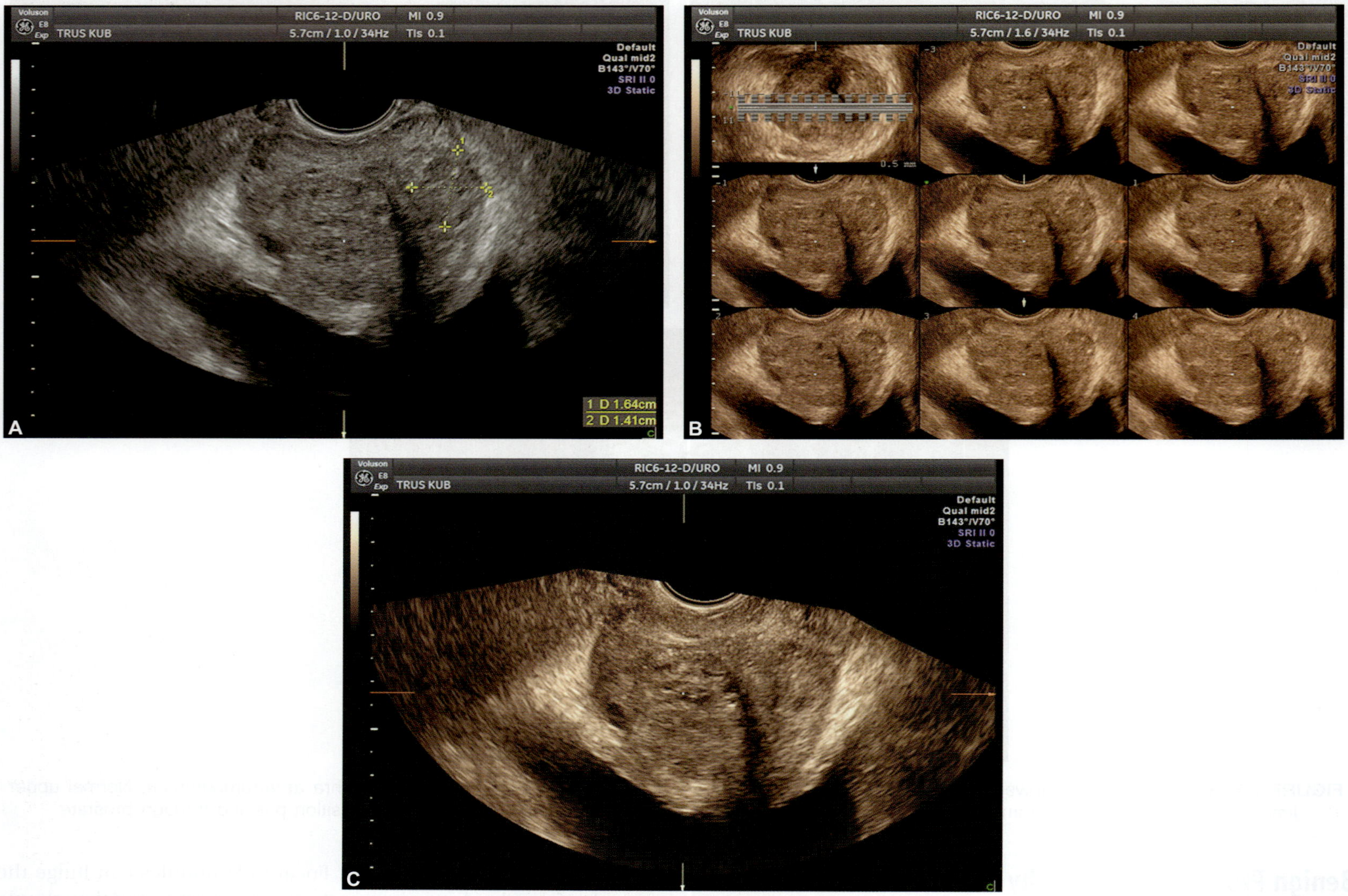

FIGURES 10.9A to C: HRSG shows diffuse hypertrophy of all the three lobes of prostate. A small hypoechoic nodule is seen in the left transitional zone. But it is smooth in outline. No suggestion of any calcification is seen in it. The capsule of the gland is seen intact. Tomographic ultrasound (TUI) imaging shows details of the nodule.

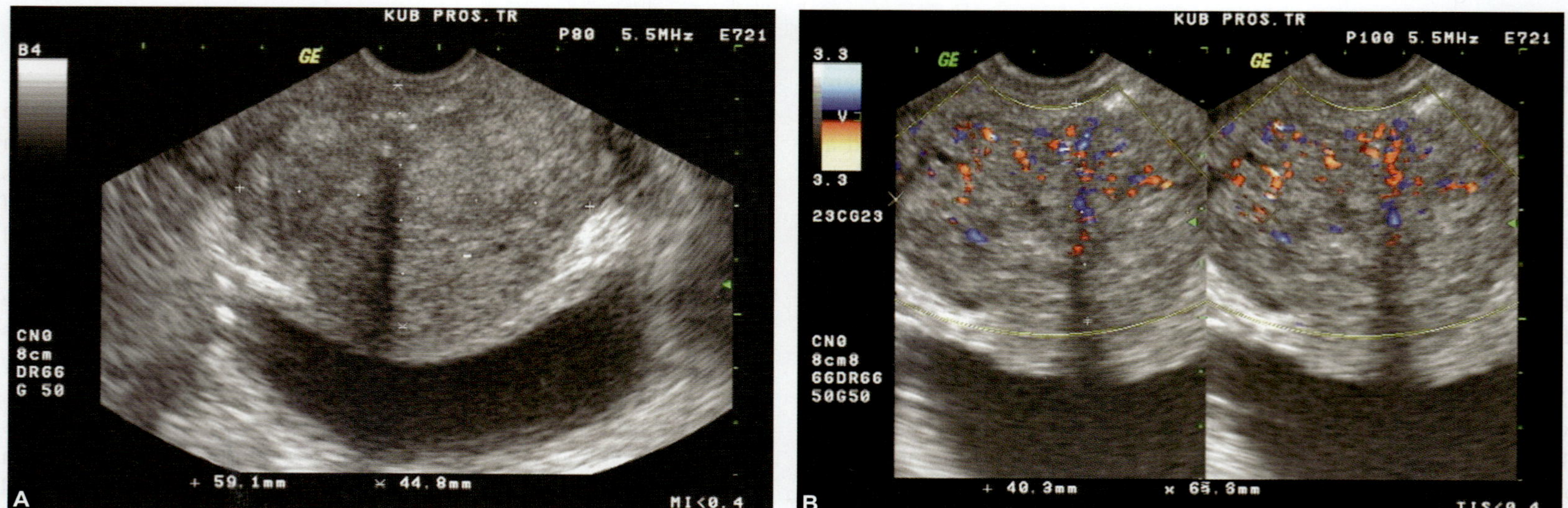

FIGURES 10.10A and B: Diffuse enlargement of prostate. HRSG shows diffuse prostatic enlargement involving all the lobes. However, the right lateral lobe more enlarged than the left lateral lobe. No evidence of any calcification or necrosis is seen in it. On color flow imaging, normal flow is seen in the gland.

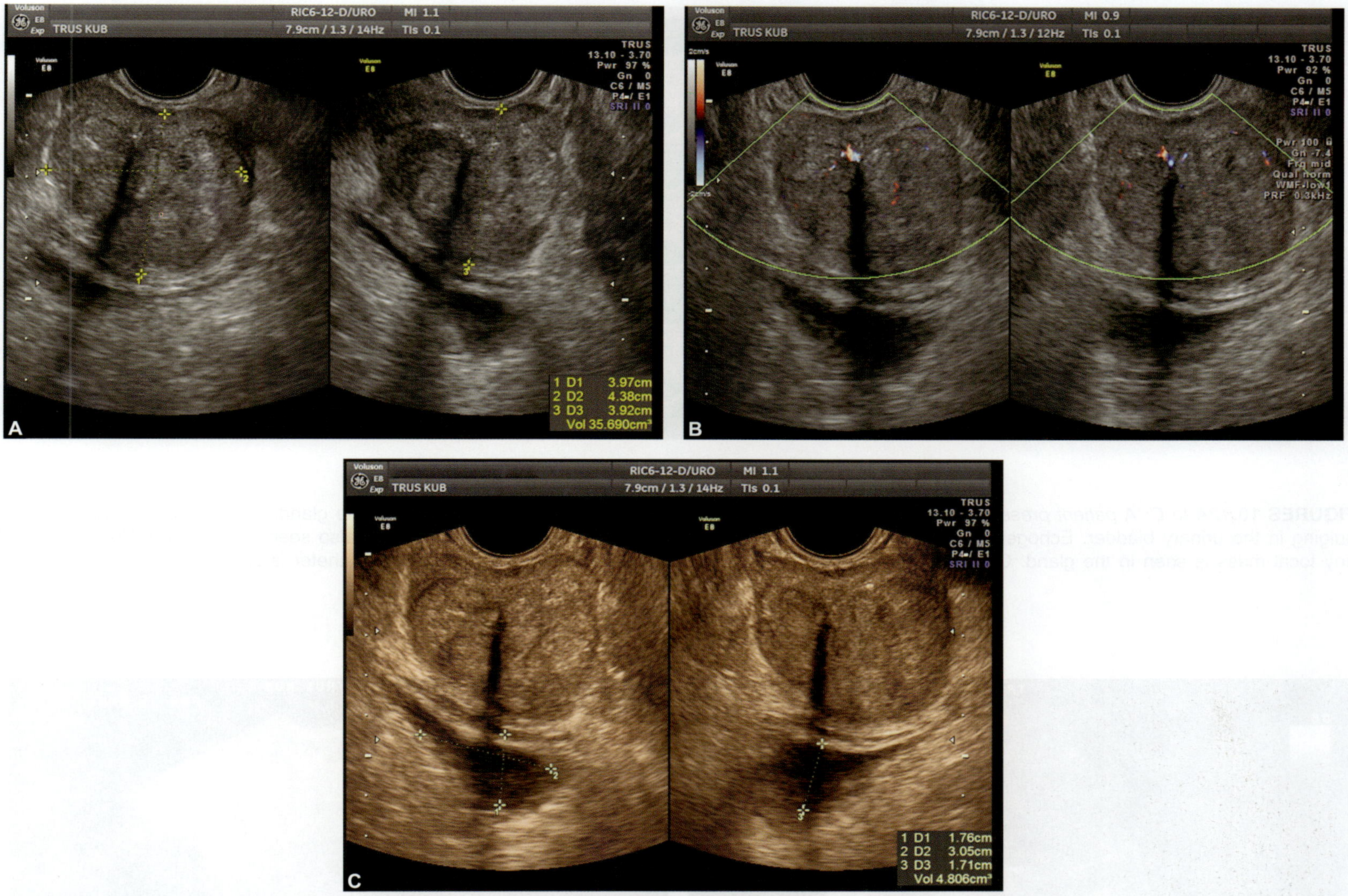

FIGURES 10.11A to C: Benign prostatic hypertrophy. A patient presented with retention of urine. HRSG shows diffuse hypertrophy of both lateral lobes of the prostate. The gland texture is homogeneous. Capsule of the gland is intact. Small punctate calcification is seen in the gland. But no focal mass is seen in the gland.

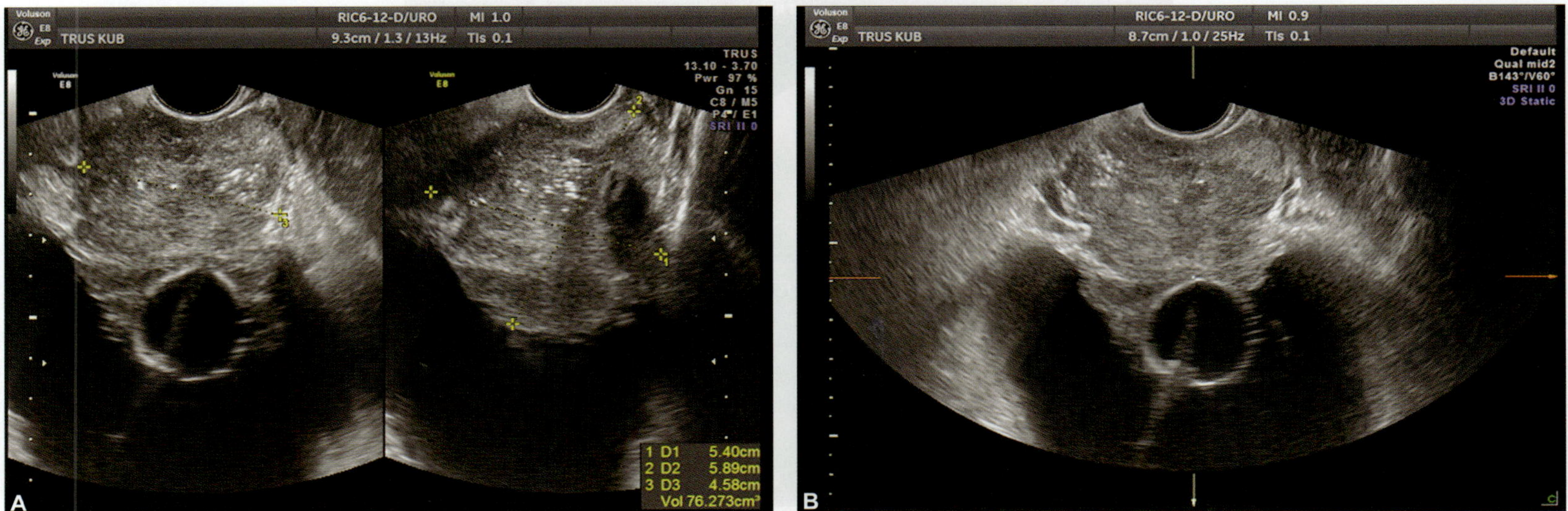

FIGURES 10.12A and B

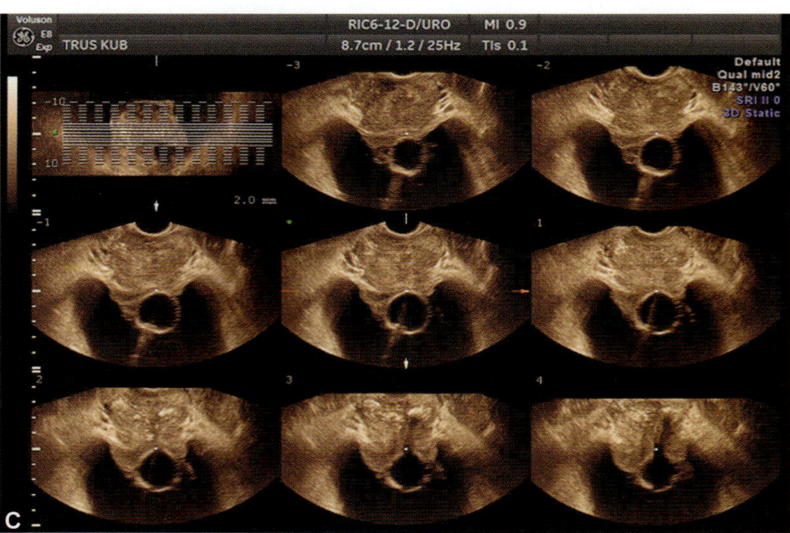

FIGURE 10.12C

FIGURES 10.*12A to C: A patient presented with retention of urine.* HRSG shows diffuse enlargement of prostate gland. Median lobe is prominent and bulging in the urinary bladder. Echogenic calcified specks are also seen in the gland. Hypoechoic areas are also seen in the gland. No evidence of any focal mass is seen in the gland. On color flow imaging, low flow is seen in the prostate gland. Foley's catheter is seen in position.

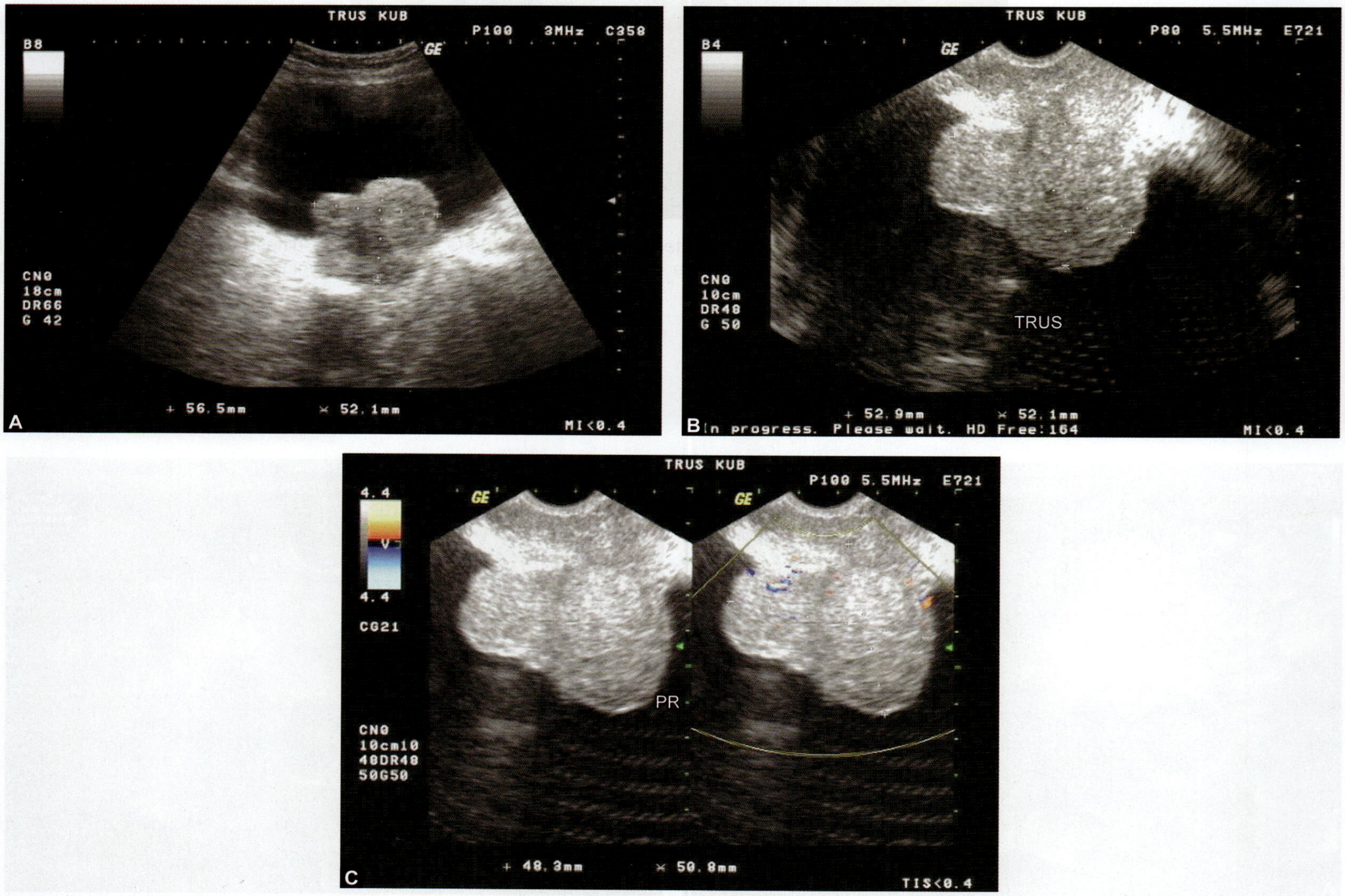

FIGURES 10.13A to C: Marked median lobe enlargement. HRSG shows marked enlargement of the median lobe of the gland. It is seen bulging in the posterior wall of urinary bladder. However, the lobe shows smooth bulging. Transrectal ultrasonography (TRUS) shows well-defined lobulated structure of the enlarge lobe with smooth outline. The lateral lobes are not significantly enlarged.

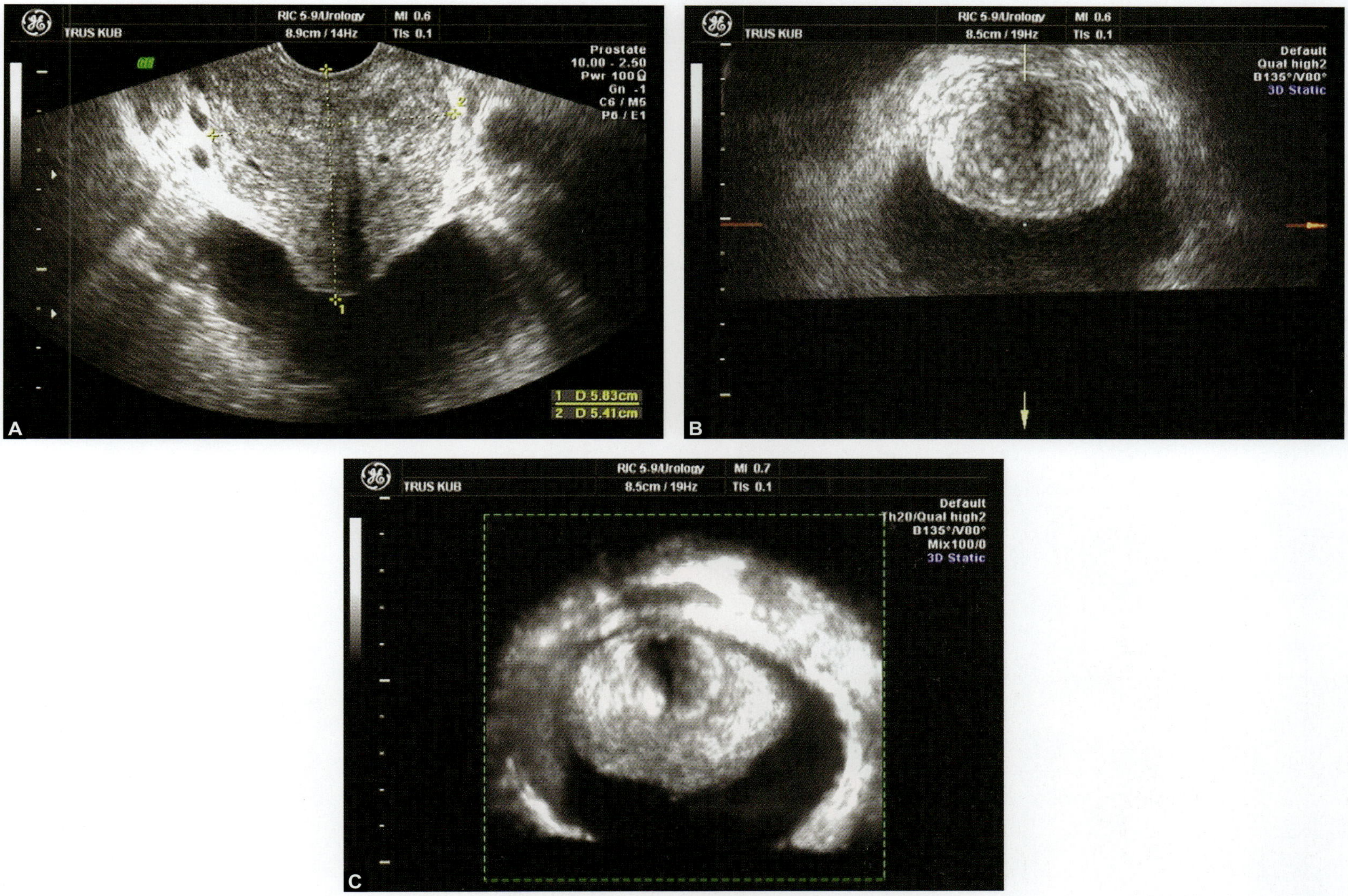

FIGURES 10.14A to C: Diffuse enlargement of prostate with prominent median lobe. HRSG shows diffuse enlargement of the prostate gland involving all the lobes. However, the median lobe is more marked than the lateral lobes. 3D imaging of the enlarged median lobe shows better anatomic details of the median lobe. No evidence of any mass lesion is seen in the lobe. It is seen projecting in the posterior wall of urinary bladder.

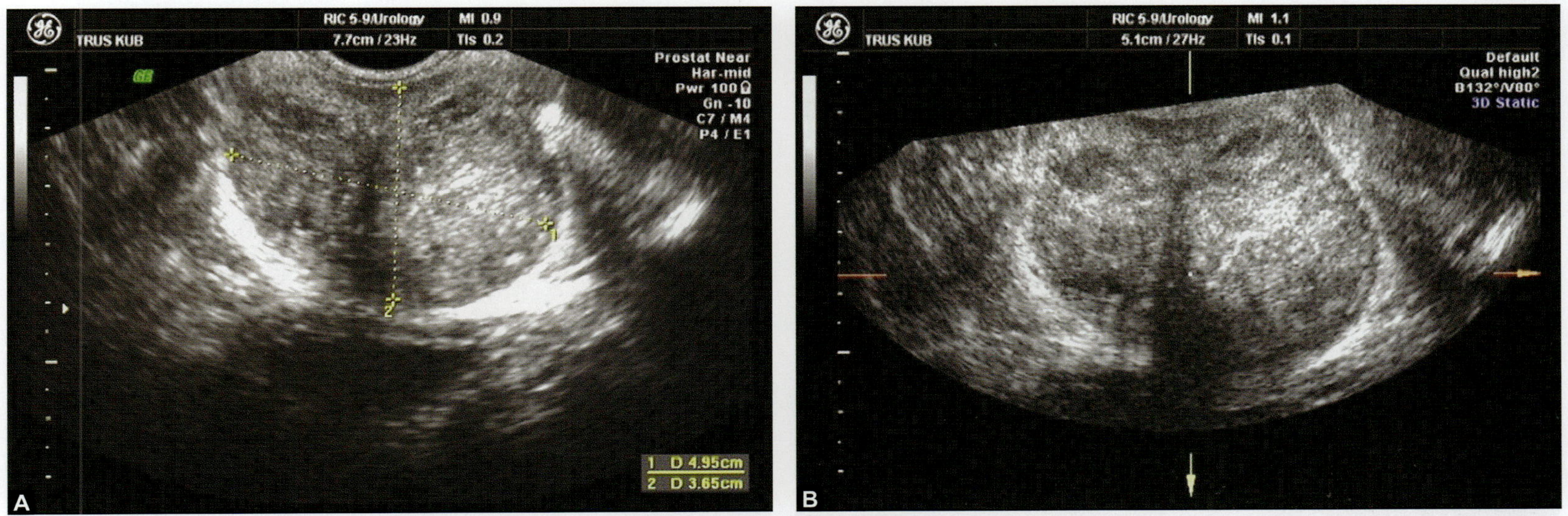

FIGURES 10.15A and B

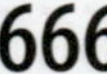

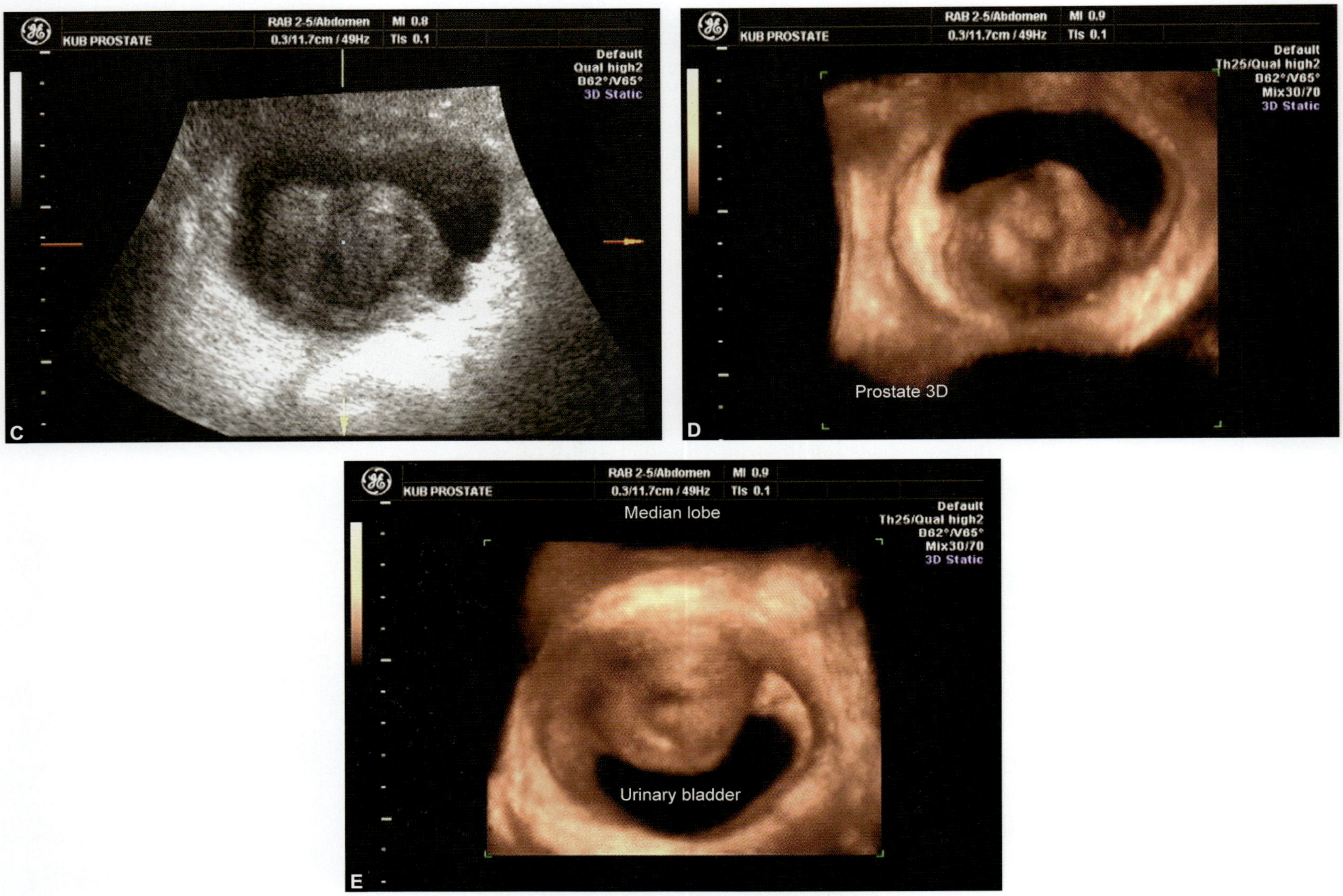

FIGURES 10.15C to E

FIGURES 10.15A to E: Diffuse enlargement of the lateral lobes. HRSG shows homogeneous smooth enlargement of both lateral lobes of the gland. The median lobe is not enlarged. No evidence of any necrosis is seen in the lobes. 3D imaging of the gland shows better anatomic details of the enlarged lobes the left lobe is more enlarged than the right lobe. 3D imaging of the prostate shows diffuse lobulated enlargement of the gland with homogeneous in texture. 3D surface rendering of the gland shows well-defined lobulated appearance of the gland. No evidence of any mass lesion is seen in the gland.

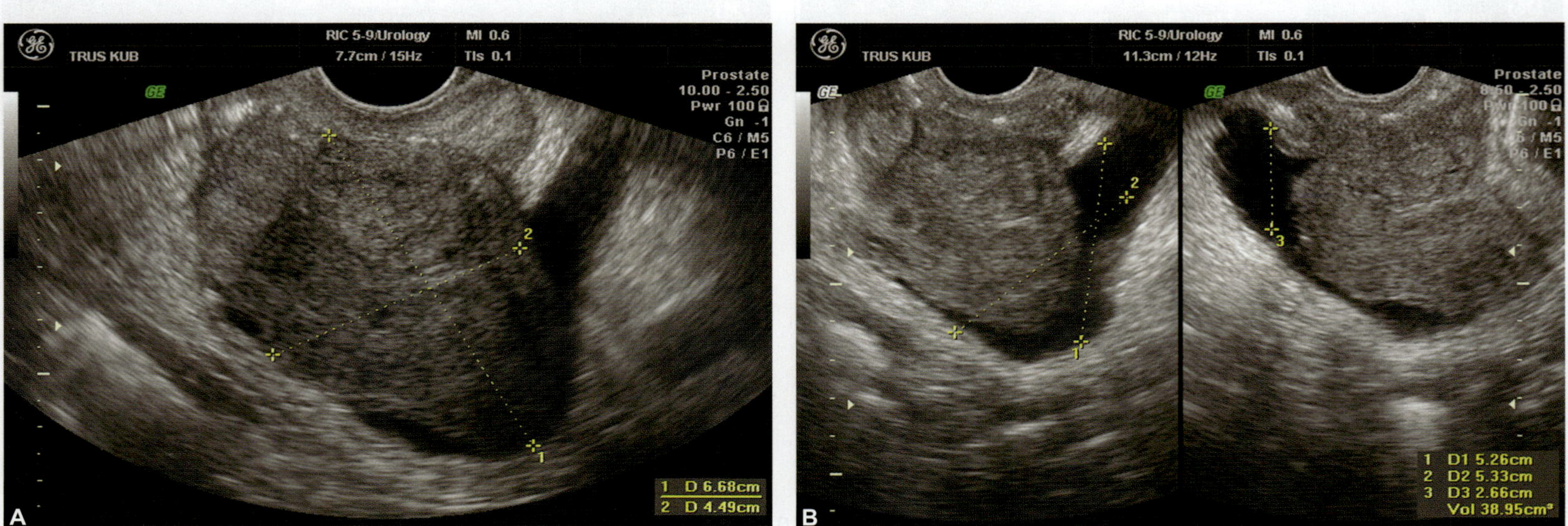

FIGURES 10.16A and B

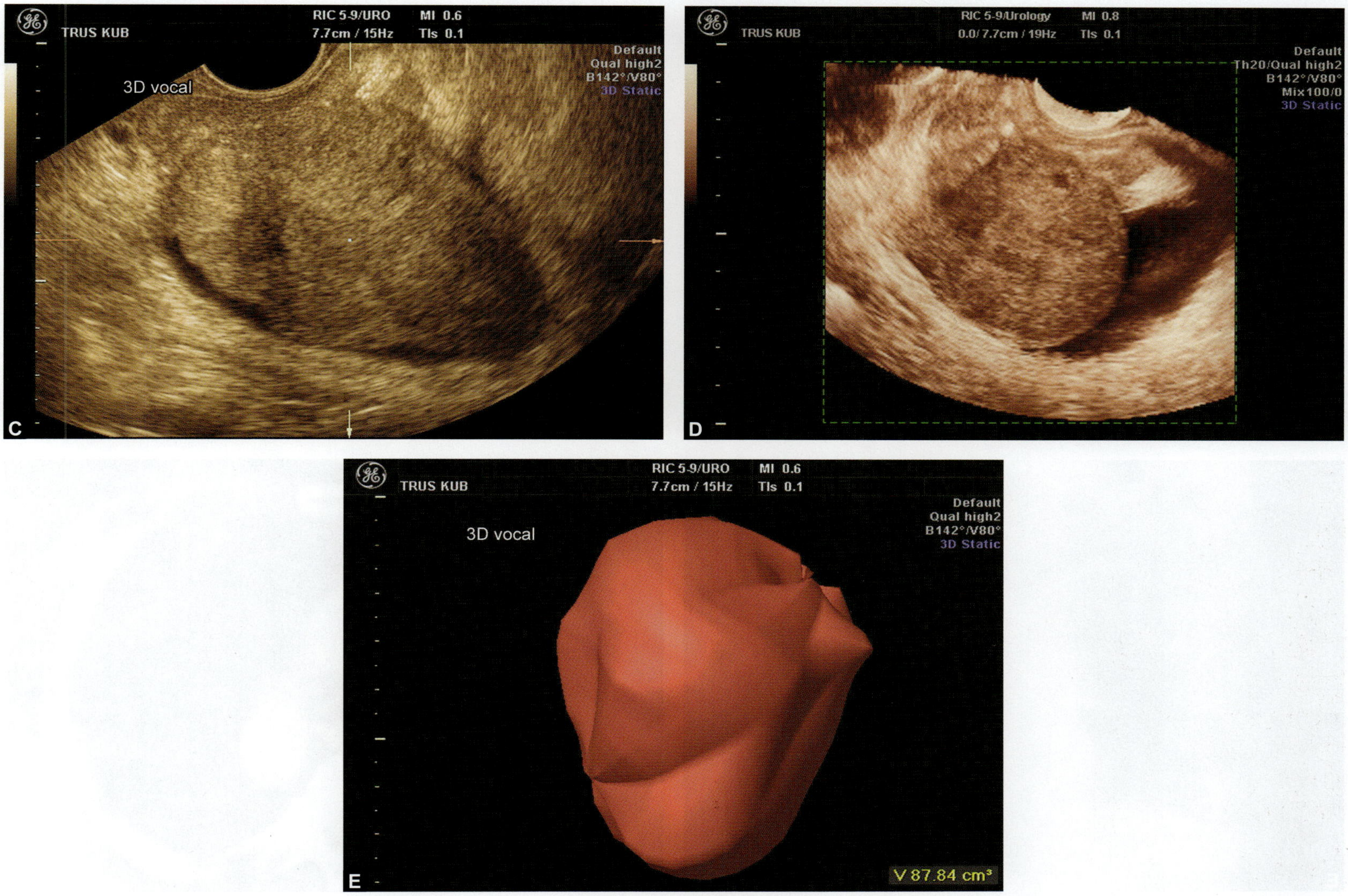

FIGURES 10.16C to E

FIGURES 10.16A to E: Marked enlargement of median lobe. HRSG shows marked conical enlargement of median lobe of the gland. The median lobe is seen coming out from the gland displacing the lateral lobe. However, the facial planes are seen intact. It is seen projecting in the urinary bladder wall. The lobe shows homogeneous texture. However, few small cysts are seen in the lobe. 3D surface rendering of the lobes show better clinical details of the lobe. The margins are well-defined with smooth outline. However, macrolobulation are seen at the margins suggestive of macronodular texture of the lobe. 3D volume imaging shows the whole gland taken out and shows marked enlargement of the median lobe.

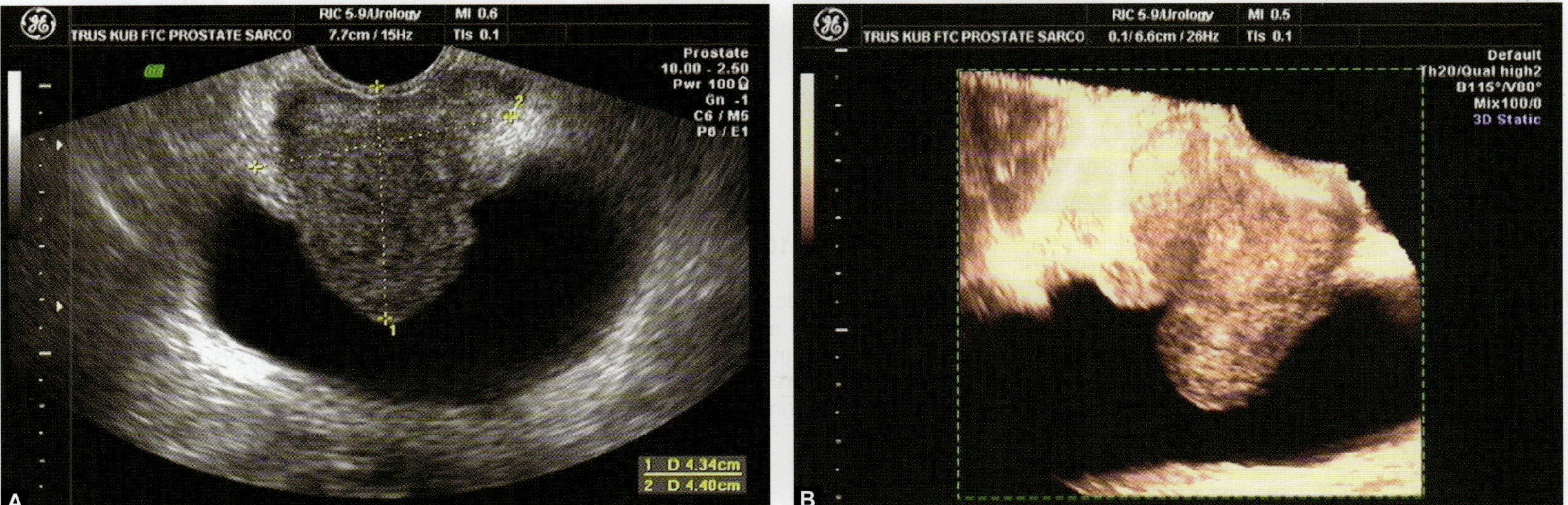

FIGURES 10.17A and B

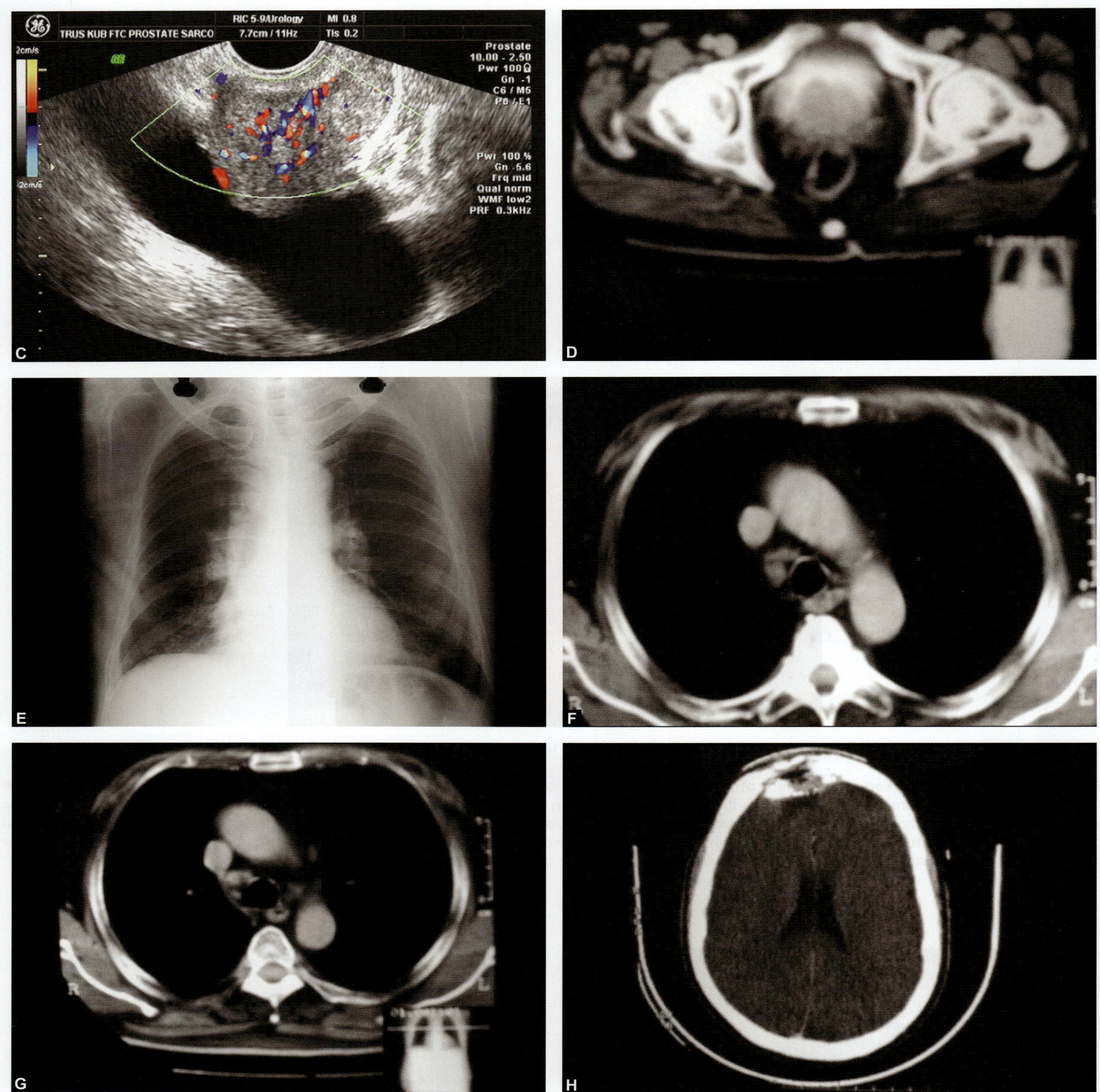

FIGURES 10.17C to H

FIGURES 10.17A to H: Prostate sarcoidosis. A known patient of sarcoidosis presented with obstructed uropathy. HRSG shows marked enlargement of the gland. The lobe is hypoechoic in texture with smooth outline. The median lobe is seen as cone. No necrosis is seen in it. The lateral lobes are also enlarged. On color flow imaging increased flow is seen in the gland. 3D surface rendering of the enlarged lobes shows better clinical details of the gland. The cone shape enlarged median lobe is well-appreciated on 3D imaging. Biopsy of the enlarged lobe confirmed sarcoidosis. CT of the pelvis of the same patient shows enlarged median lobe indenting over urinary bladder wall. X-ray and CT of the same patient shows enlarged hilar shadows suggestive of hilar lymphadenopathy.

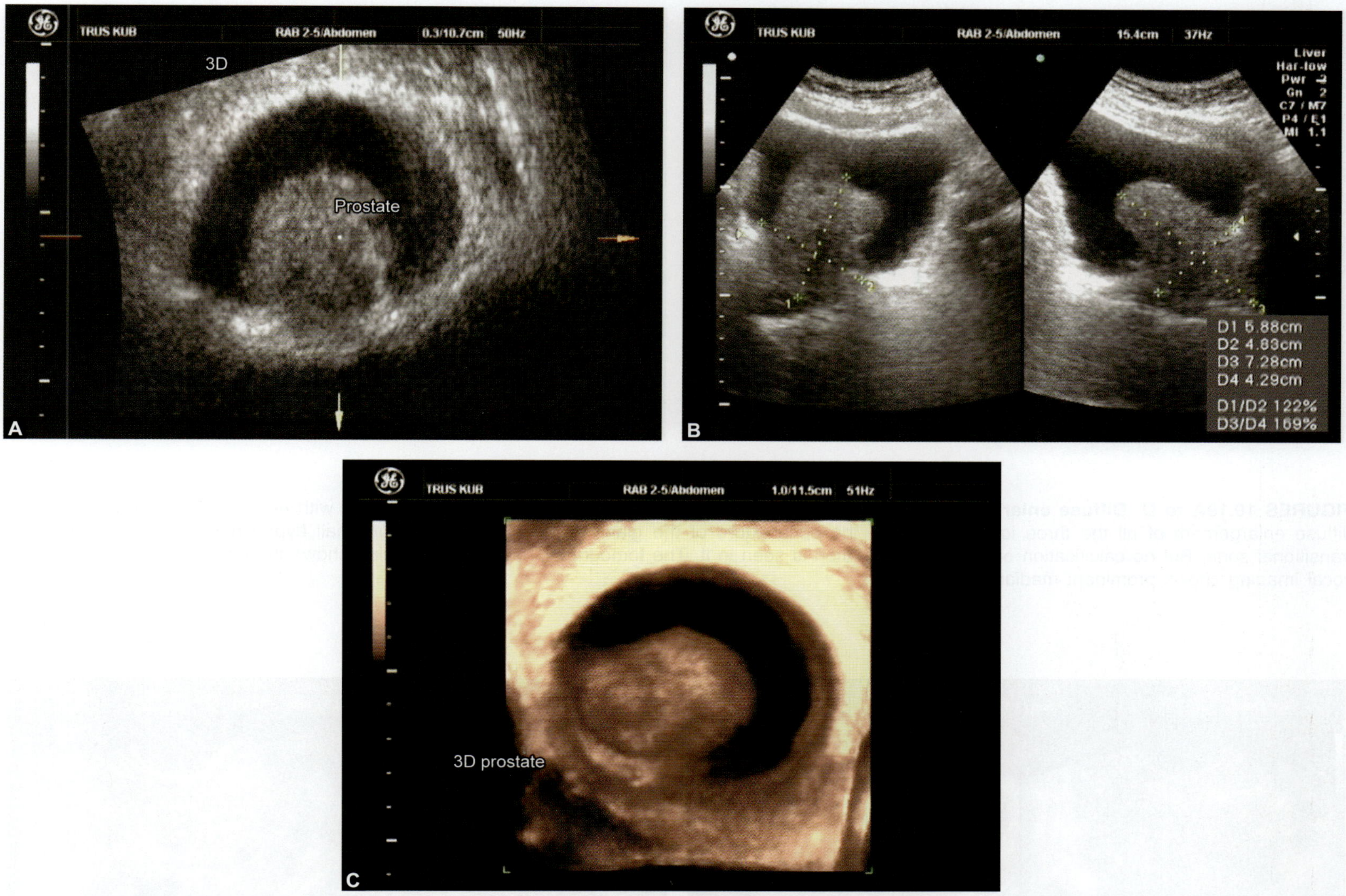

FIGURES 10.18A to C: A patient presented with retention of urine. HRSG shows markedly enlarged median lobe. It is seen projecting in the posterior wall of urinary bladder (UB). However, echotexture is homogeneous. No mass lesion is seen in the median lobe. The 3D imaging clearly shows enlarged median lobe bulging in posterior wall of UB.

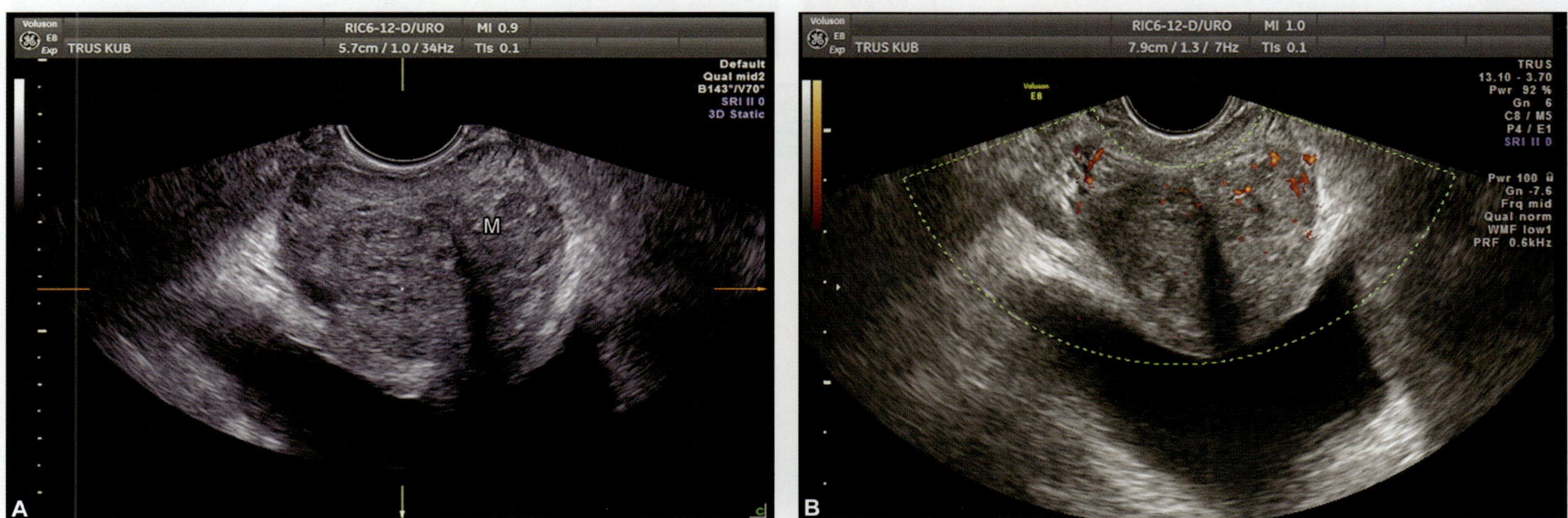

FIGURES 10.19A and B

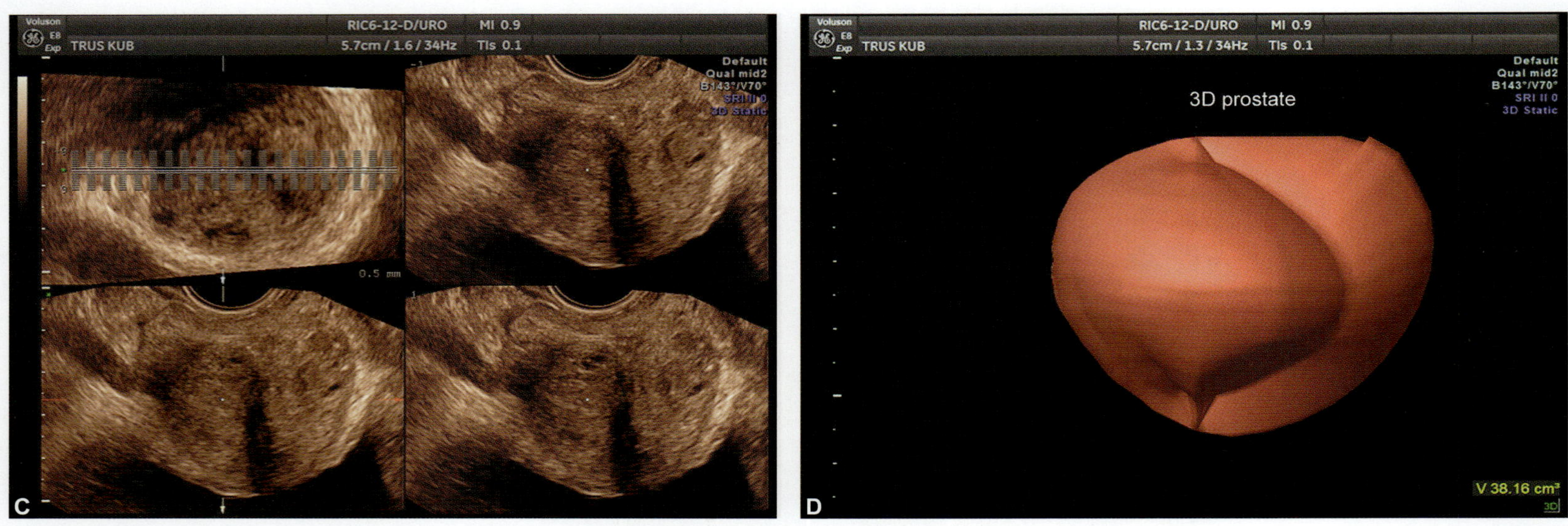

FIGURES 10.19C and D

FIGURES 10.19A to D: Diffuse enlargement of prostate with prominent median lobe. A patient presented with retention of urine. HRSG shows diffuse enlargement of all the three lobes. However, the echotexture of the gland is inhomogeneous. But small hypoechoic nodule is seen in left transitional zone. But no calcification or cystic degeneration is seen in it. The tomographic ultrasound imaging shows the nodule very clearly. The 3D vocal imaging shows prominent median lobe.

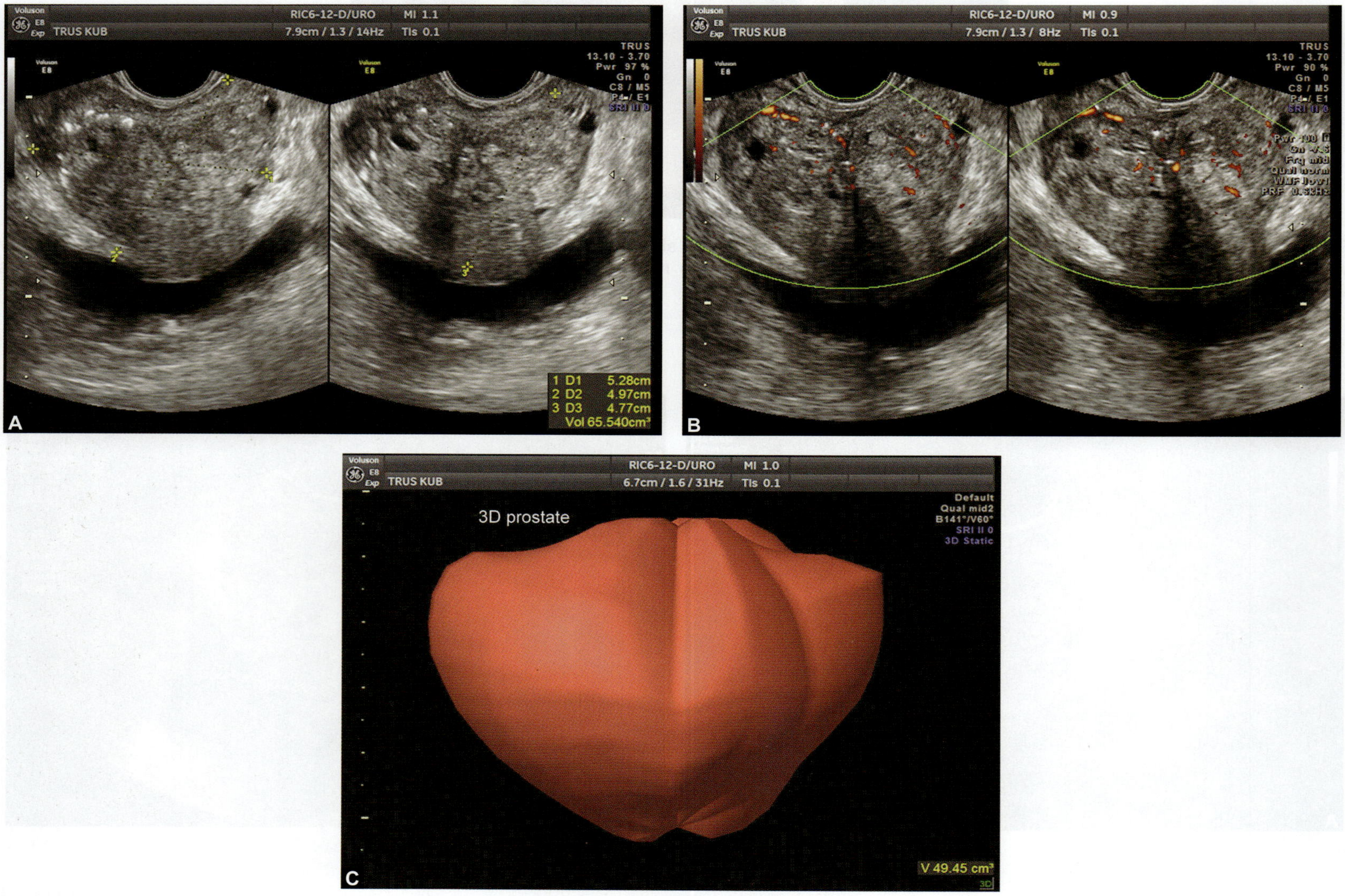

FIGURES 10.20A to C: HRSG shows diffuse enlargement of prostate gland. Median lobe is prominent and bulging in posterior wall of urinary bladder. Small cysts are seen in the transitional zone of the gland on both sides. Peripheral calcification is seen in the gland. On 3D volume imaging, the whole gland shows enlargement of three lobes.

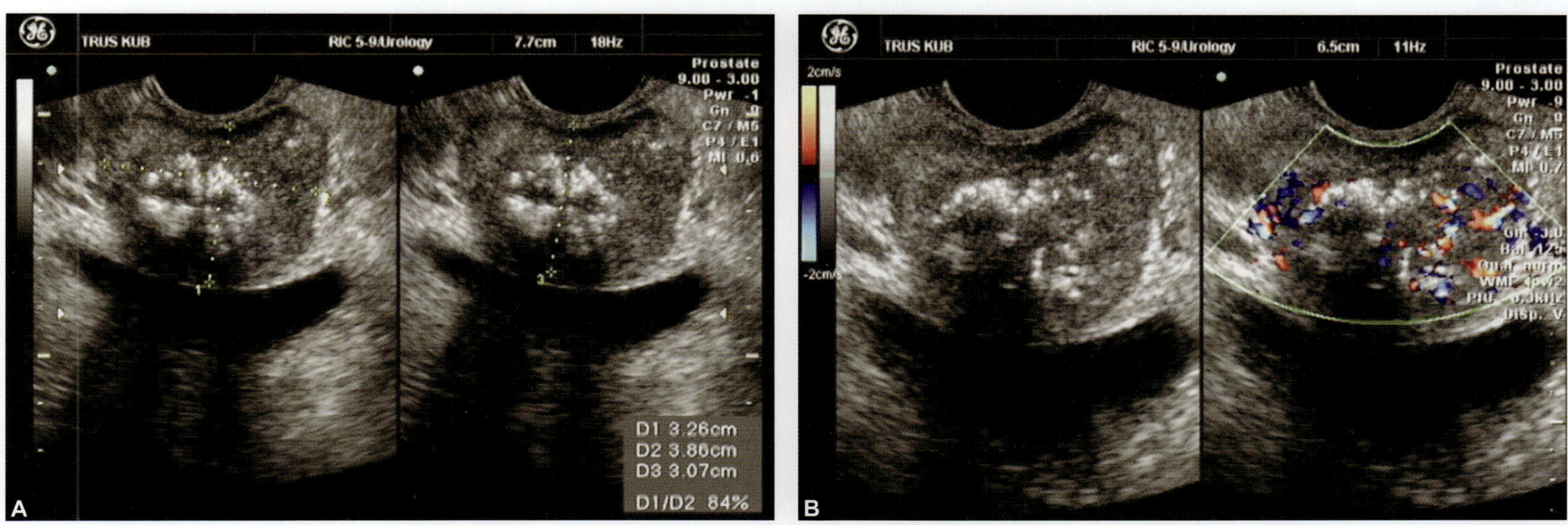

FIGURES 10.21A and B: Corpus amylacea. HRSG shows dense calcification in the inner gland, which is accompanied with acoustic shadowing. But no evidence of any focal mass is seen in the gland. On color flow imaging, low flow is seen in the gland.

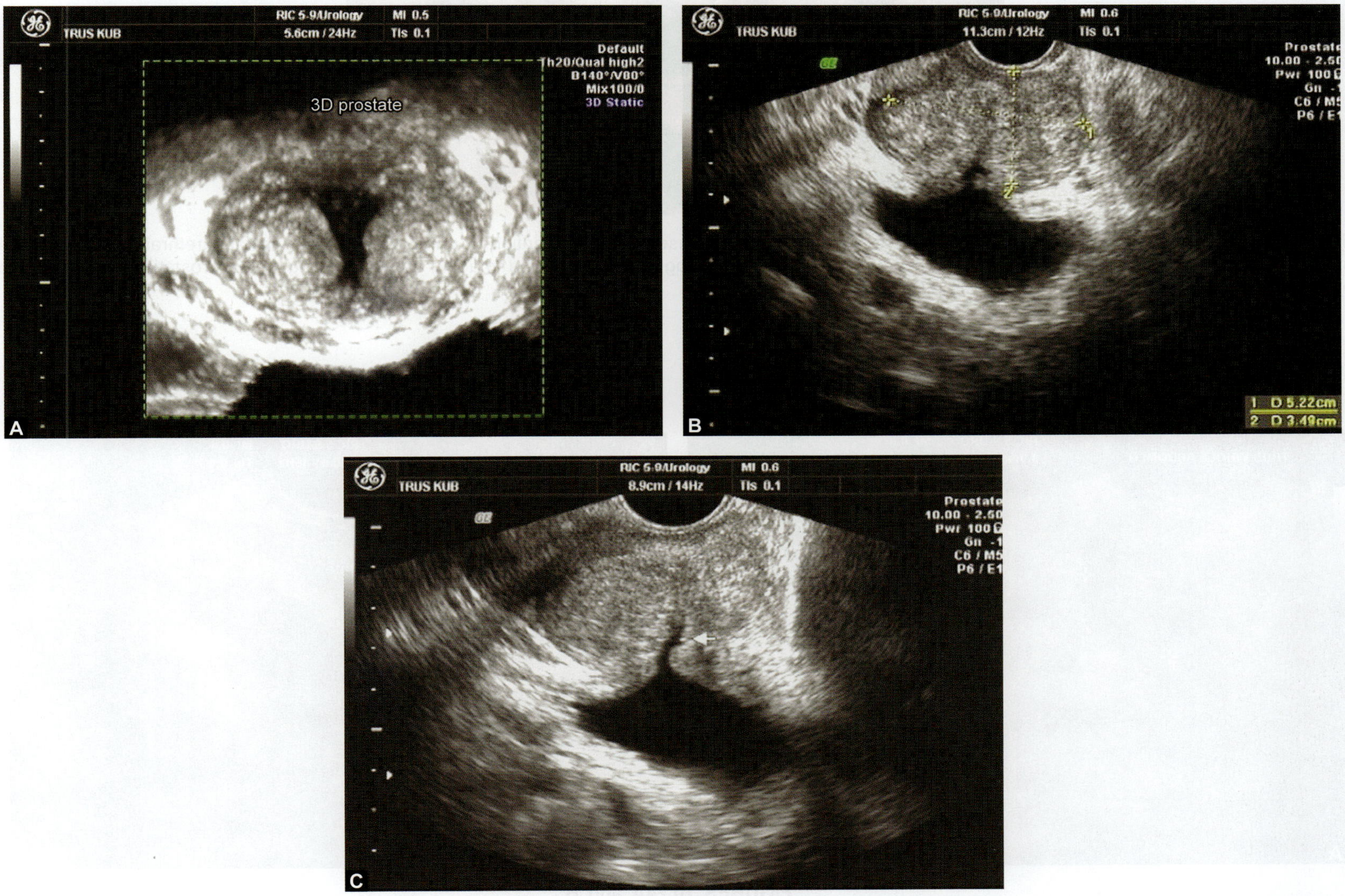

FIGURES 10.22A to C: Patent prostatic tunnel after TURP. Transrectal ultrasonography (TRUS) is very good modality for evaluating patency of the prostatic tunnel. HRSG shows patent prostatic tunnel in a patent underwent TURP.

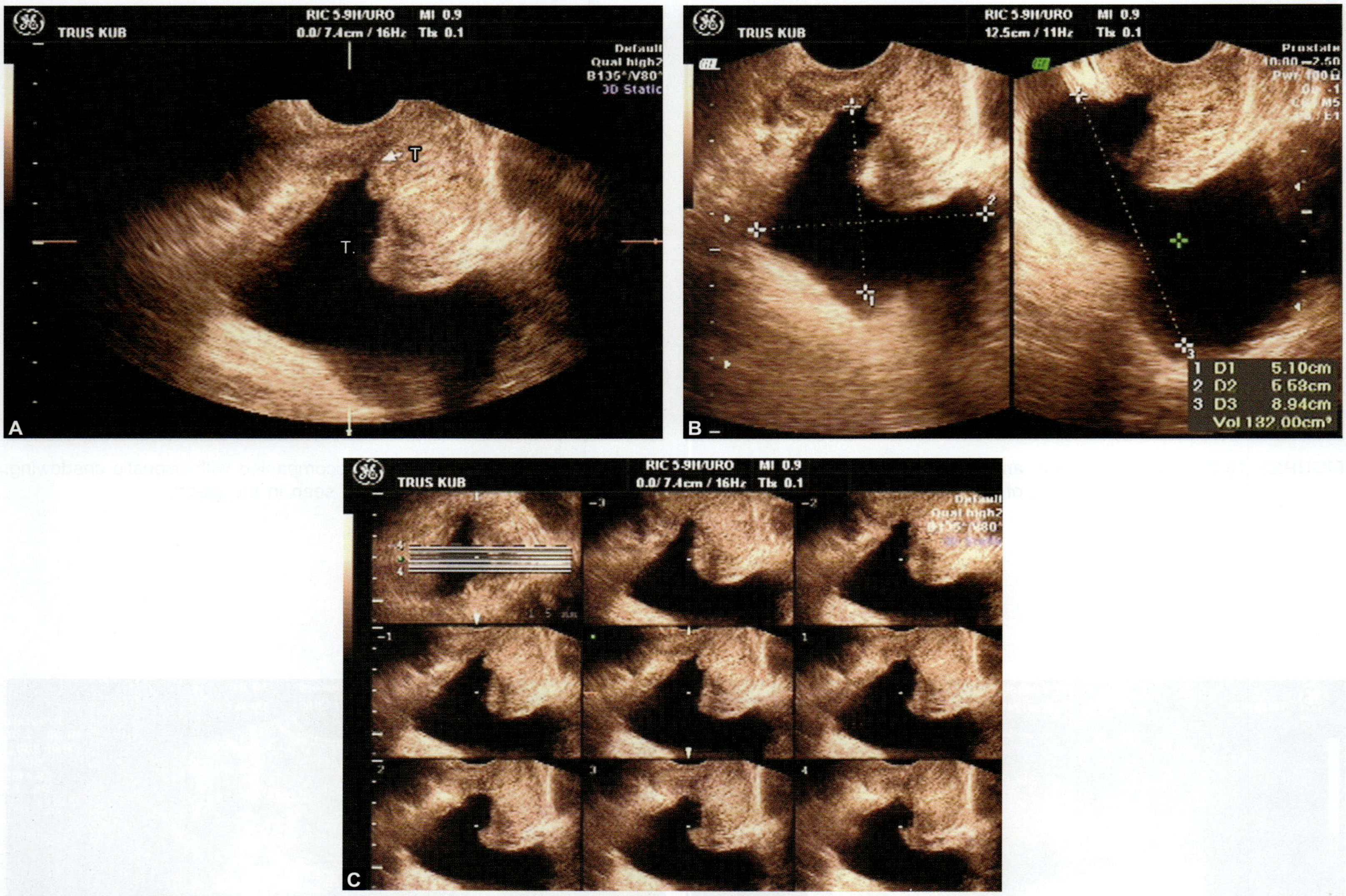

FIGURES 10.23A to C: Narrowing of the prostatic tunnel. A patient presented with retention of urine after underwent transurethral resection of the prostate (TURP). HRSG shows narrowing of the prostatic tunnel. 3D tomographic ultrasound imaging shows beaking of the prostatic tunnel because of fibrosis. Ballooning of the bladder neck is also seen.

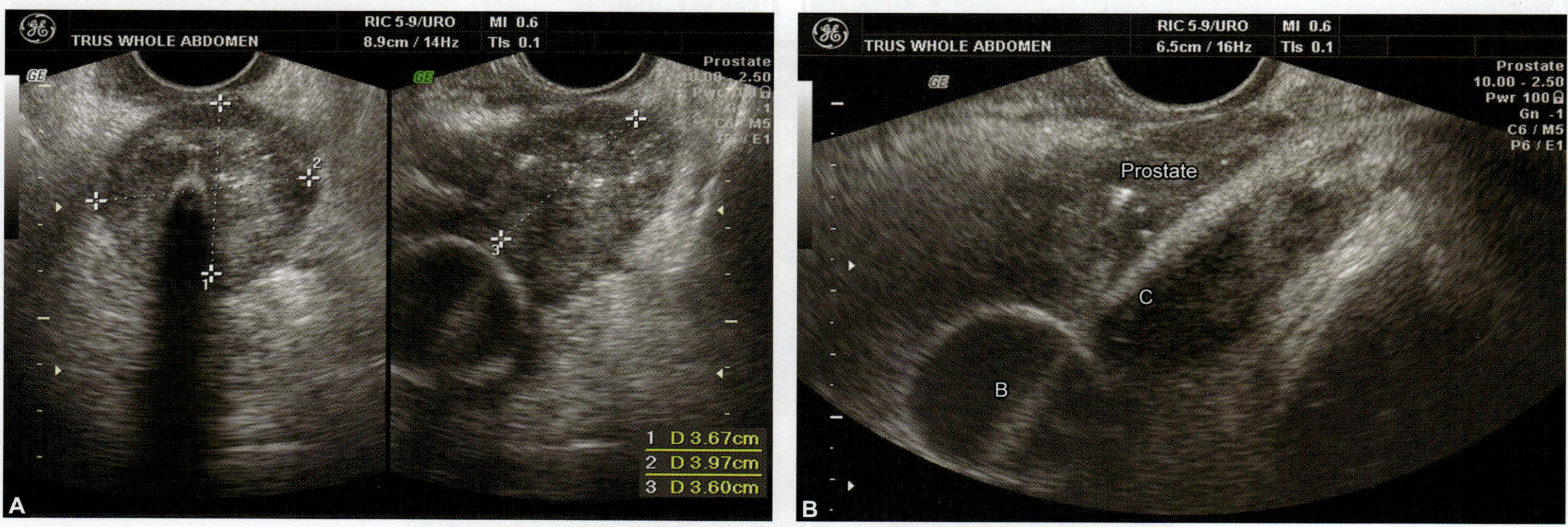

FIGURES 10.24A and B

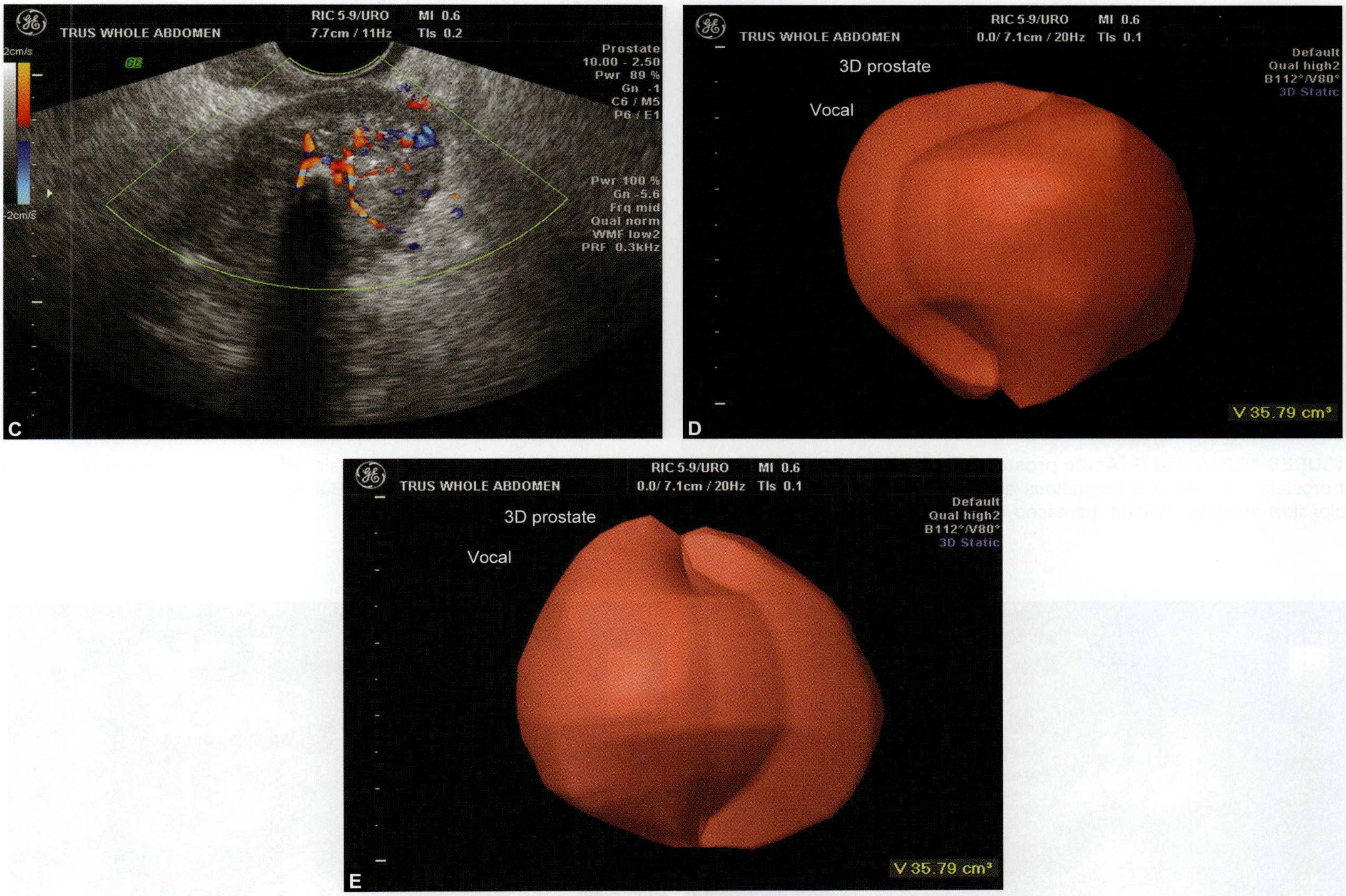

FIGURES 10.24C to E

FIGURES 10.24A to E: BPH with Foleys' catheter in position. A patient presented with retention of urine. HRSG show diffuse enlargement of prostate gland. The Foleys' catheter is seen in urinary bladder (UB). The bulb is seen in UB and the catheter tube is seen passing through prostatic urethra and clearly seen in long axis of the gland. 3D vocal imaging shows all the three lobes enlarged.

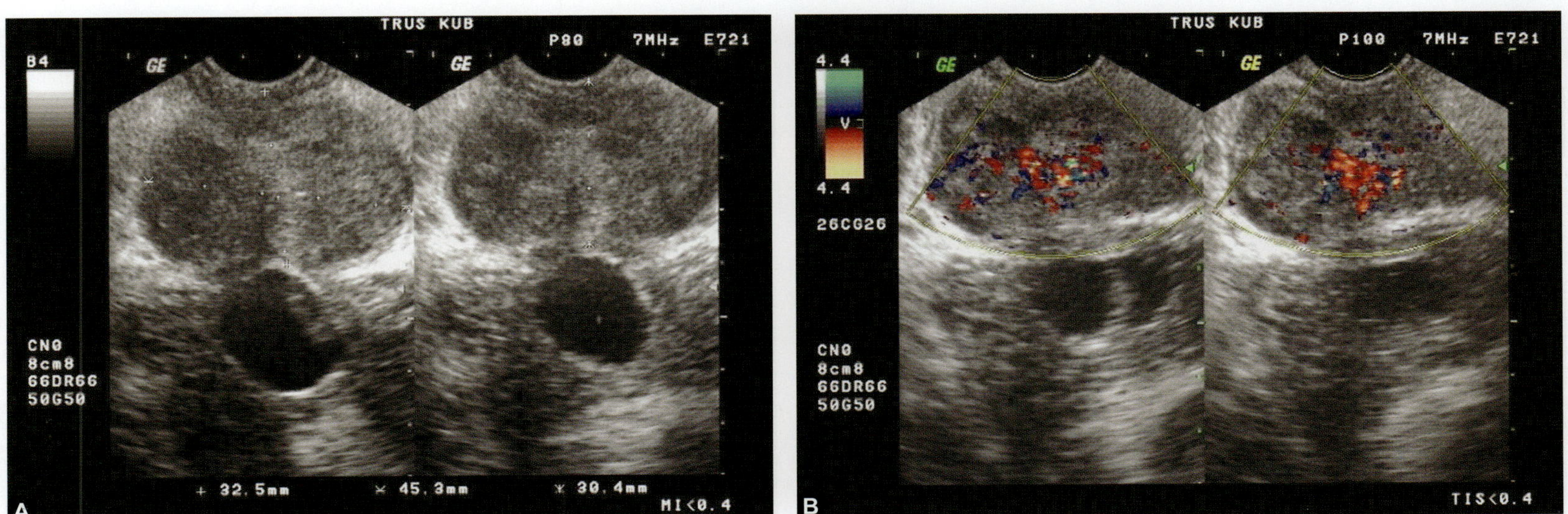

FIGURES 10.25A and B: BPH with prostatitis. HRSG shows benign prostatic enlargement. However, multiple hypoechoic areas are seen in the gland. Small abscess is also seen on right side. On color flow imaging increased flow is seen in the gland suggestive of hyperemia indicating prostatitis. On power Doppler imaging marked increased flow is seen in the inflamed prostate.

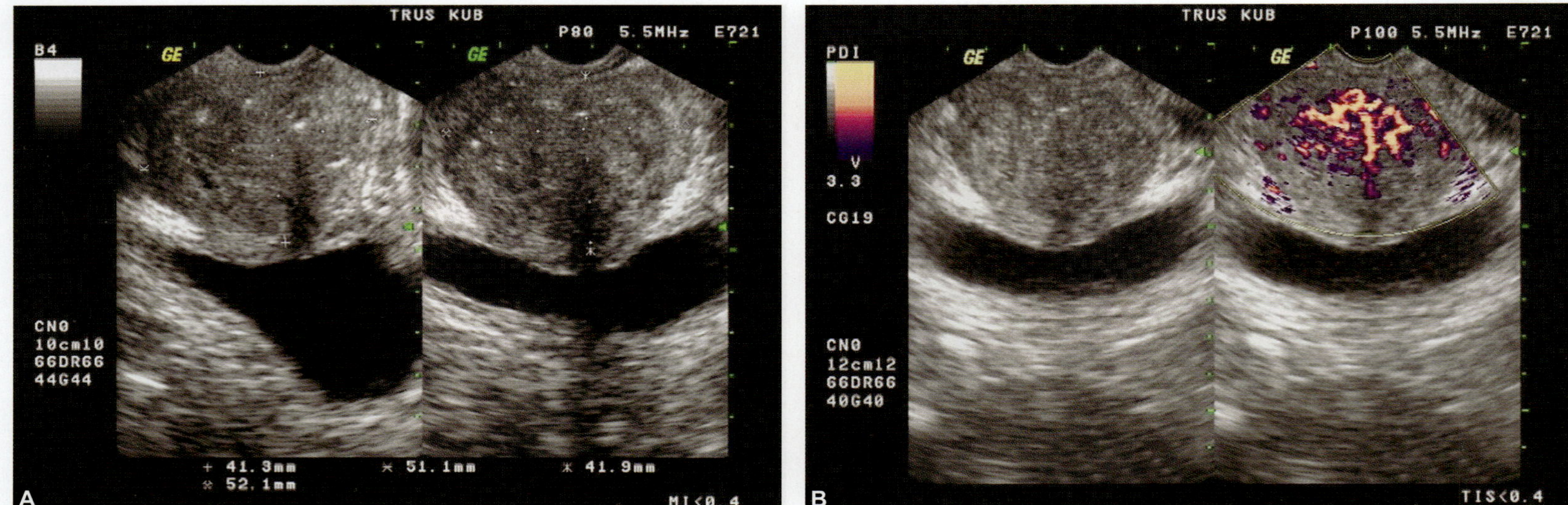

FIGURES 10.26A and B: Acute prostatitis with BPH. A patient presented with retention of urine with perineal pain. HRSG shows diffuse enlargement of prostate. The gland is edematous and inhomogeneous in texture. Hypoechoic areas are seen in the gland. But no abscess formation is seen. On color flow imaging, marked increased flow is seen in the gland suggestive of acute prostatitis with BPH.

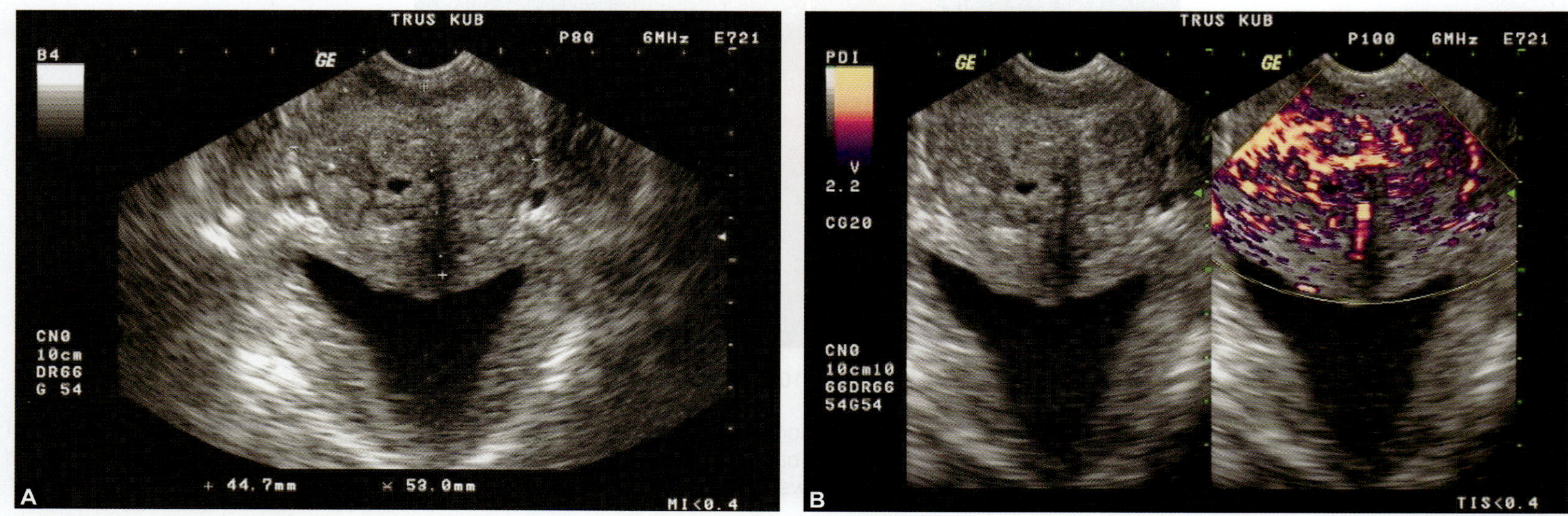

FIGURES 10.27A and B: Acute prostatitis with BPH. A patient presented with retention of urine with BPH with fever. HRSG shows prostatic gland enlargement. The gland is edematous. Hypoechoic areas are seen in the gland. On color flow imaging, increased flow is seen in the gland.

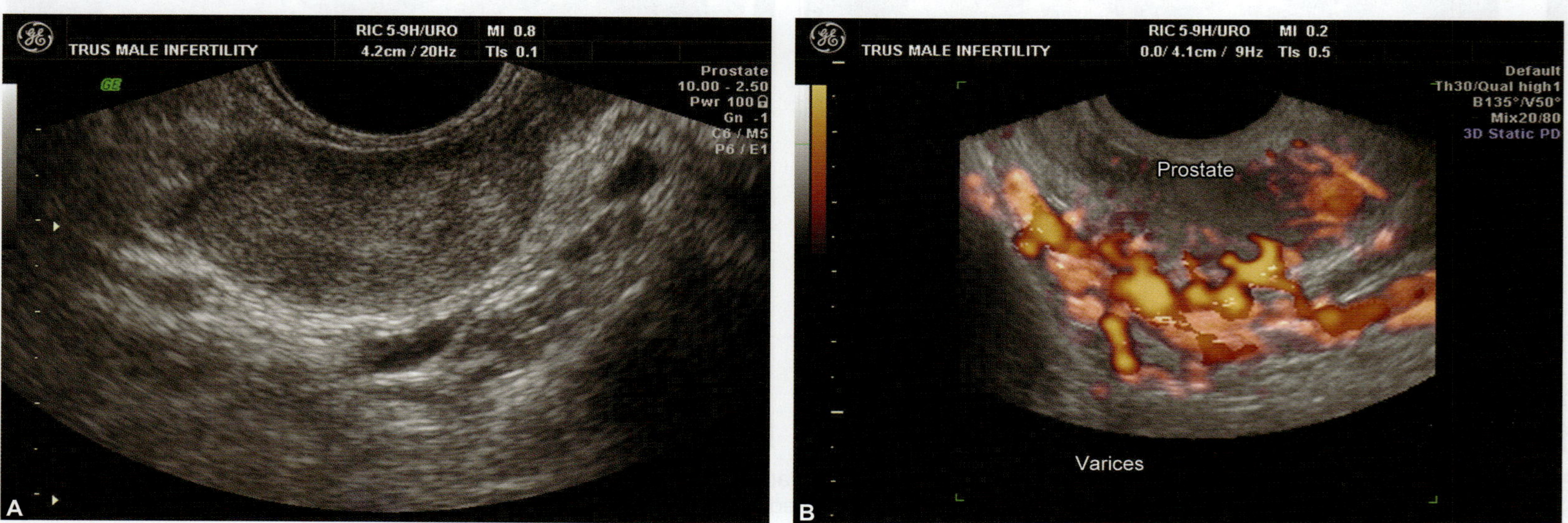

FIGURES 10.28A and B

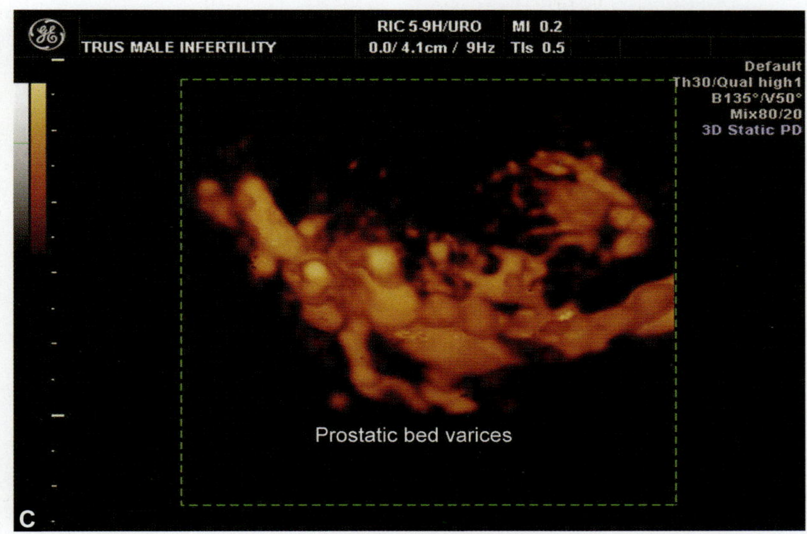

FIGURE 10.28C

FIGURES 10.28A to C: Acute prostatitis with very prostatic varices. A patient presented with persistent perineal pain with dysuria. Transrectal ultrasound (TRUS) shows edematous hypoechoic prostate gland. The margins are shaggy. Ill defined areas are seen in the gland. On color flow imaging, multiple vessels are seen feeding the gland. Multiple dilated vessels are seen in the periprostatic area suggestive of periprostatic varices. On 3D power angio, the varices are seen prominently.

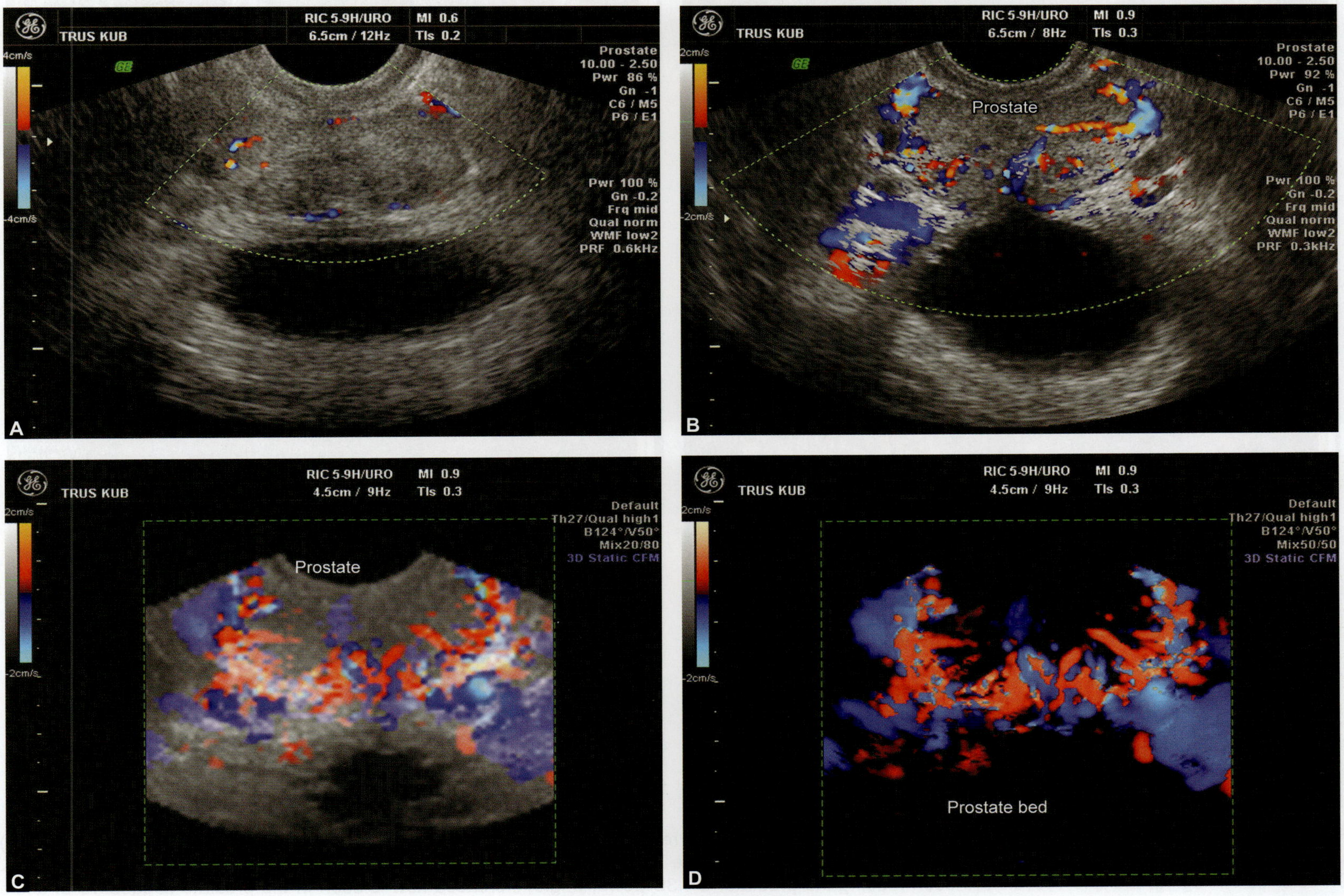

FIGURES 10.29A to D

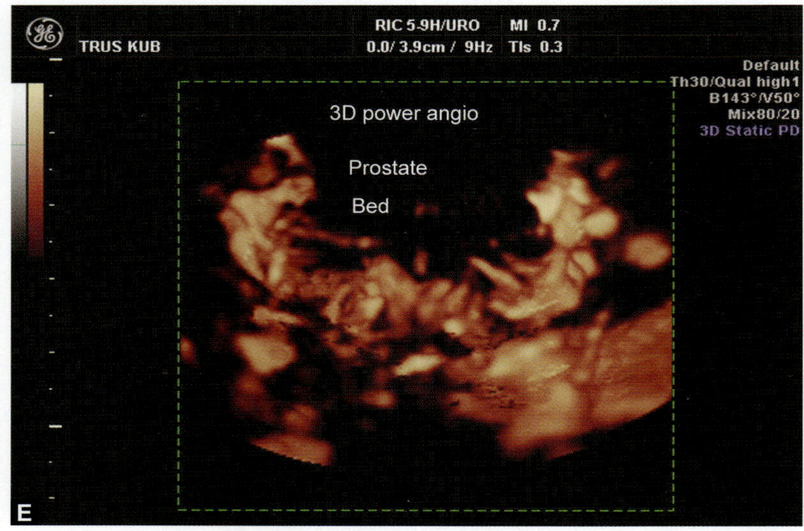

FIGURE 10.29E

FIGURES 10.29A to E: Acute prostatitis. A patient presented with fever and retention of urine. Transrectal ultrasound (TRUS) shows edematous hypoechoic prostate gland. On color flow imaging, multiple dilated vessels are seen in the prostate. On 3D power angio, the vessels are seen feeding the peripheral and the inner gland. Multiple dilated periprostatic varices are also seen.

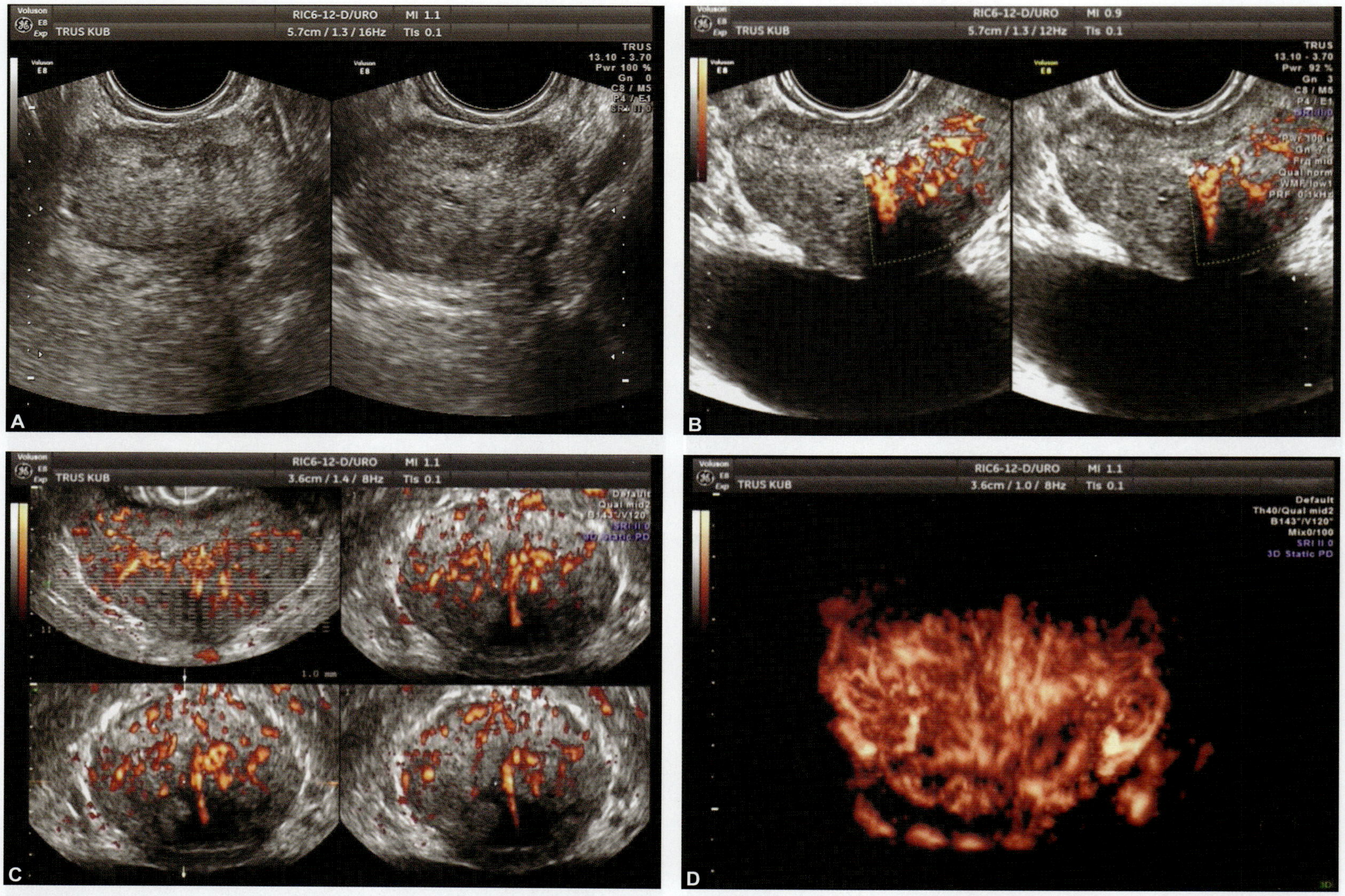

FIGURES 10.30A to D: Acute prostatitis. A patient presented with acute retention of urine with lower abdominal pain. Transrectal ultrasound (TRUS) shows markedly edematous enlarged prostate gland. Hypoechoic areas are also seen in the gland. A small abscess formation is seen in the prostate. On color flow imaging, multiple vessels are seen feeding the prostate. On 3D power angio, increased flow is seen in the prostate suggestive of acute prostatitis.

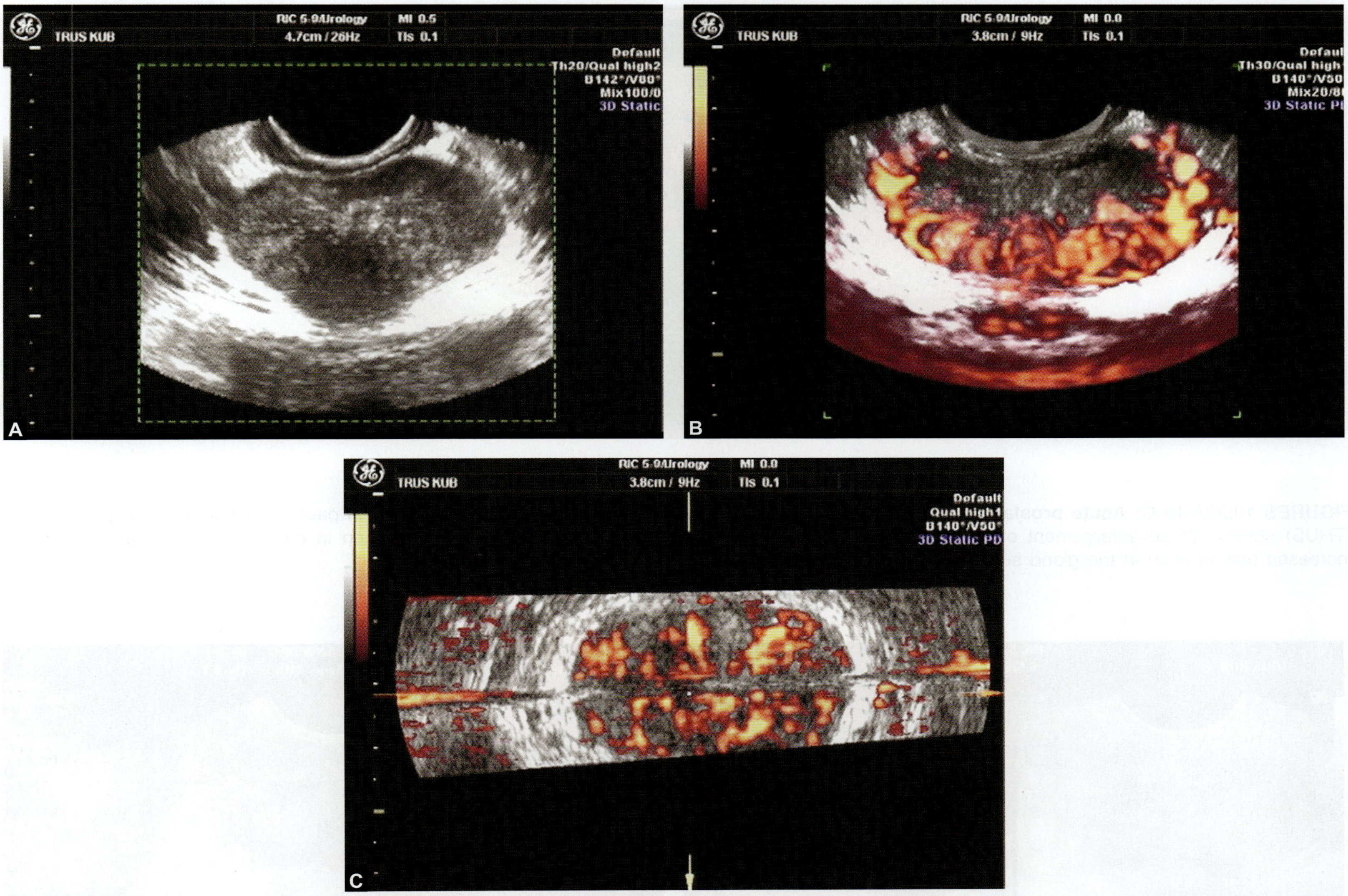

FIGURES 10.31A to C: Acute prostatitis. A patient presented with acute pain with dysuria. Transrectal ultrasound (TRUS) shows diffuse enlargement of prostate. An irregular ill defined area is seen in the prostate suggestive of abscess formation. On power Doppler imaging, marked increased flow is seen in the gland suggestive of acute prostatitis.

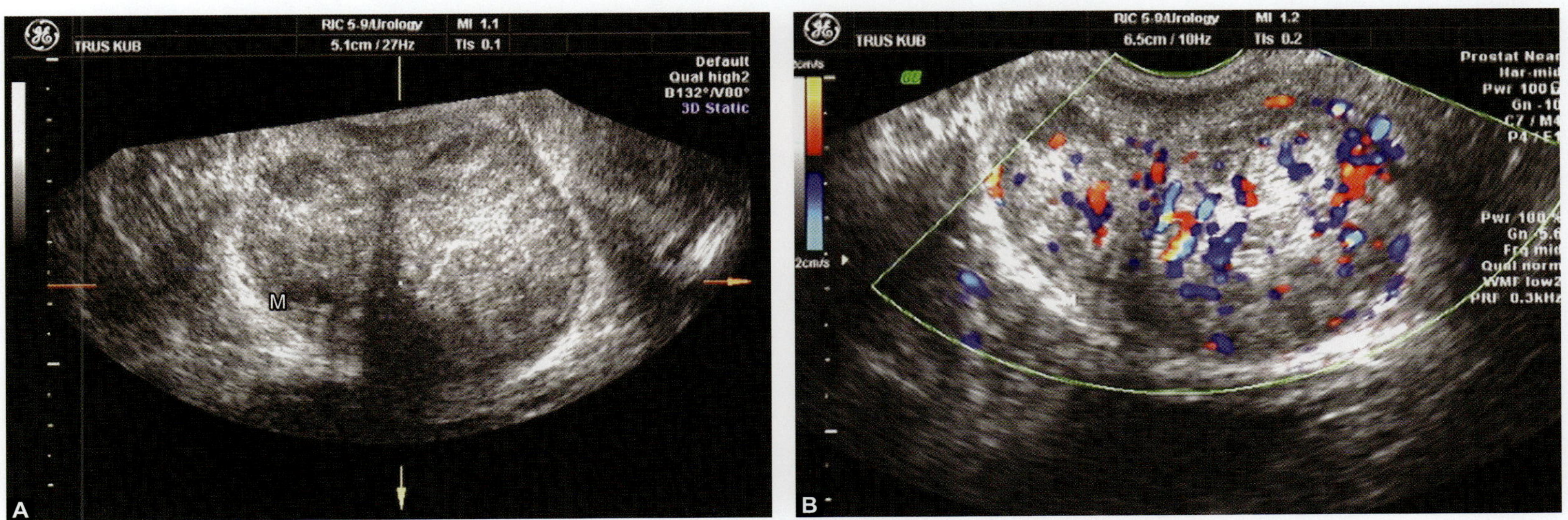

FIGURES 10.32A and B

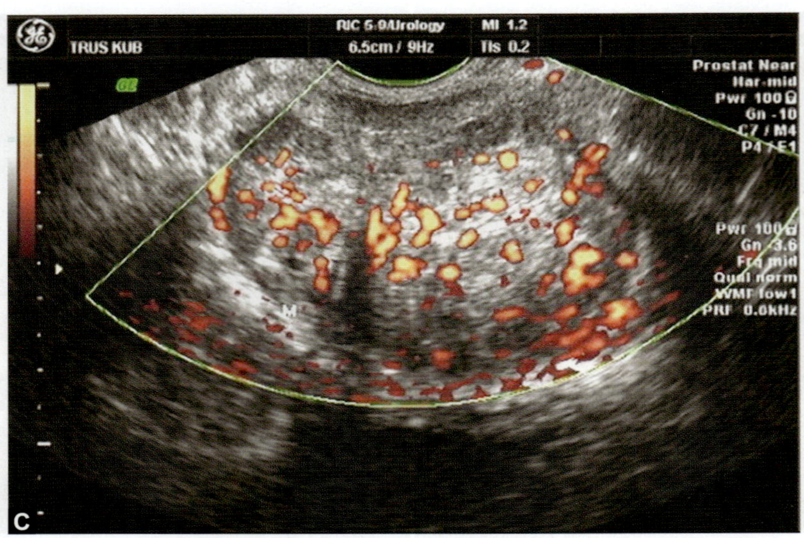

FIGURE 10.32C

FIGURES 10.32A to C: Acute prostatitis with BPH. A patient presented with retention of urine with perineal pain and fever. Transrectal ultrasound (TRUS) shows diffuse enlargement of the prostate. The margins are ill-defined. Hypoechoic areas are seen in the gland. On color flow imaging, increased flow is seen in the gland suggestive of acute prostatitis with prostatomegaly.

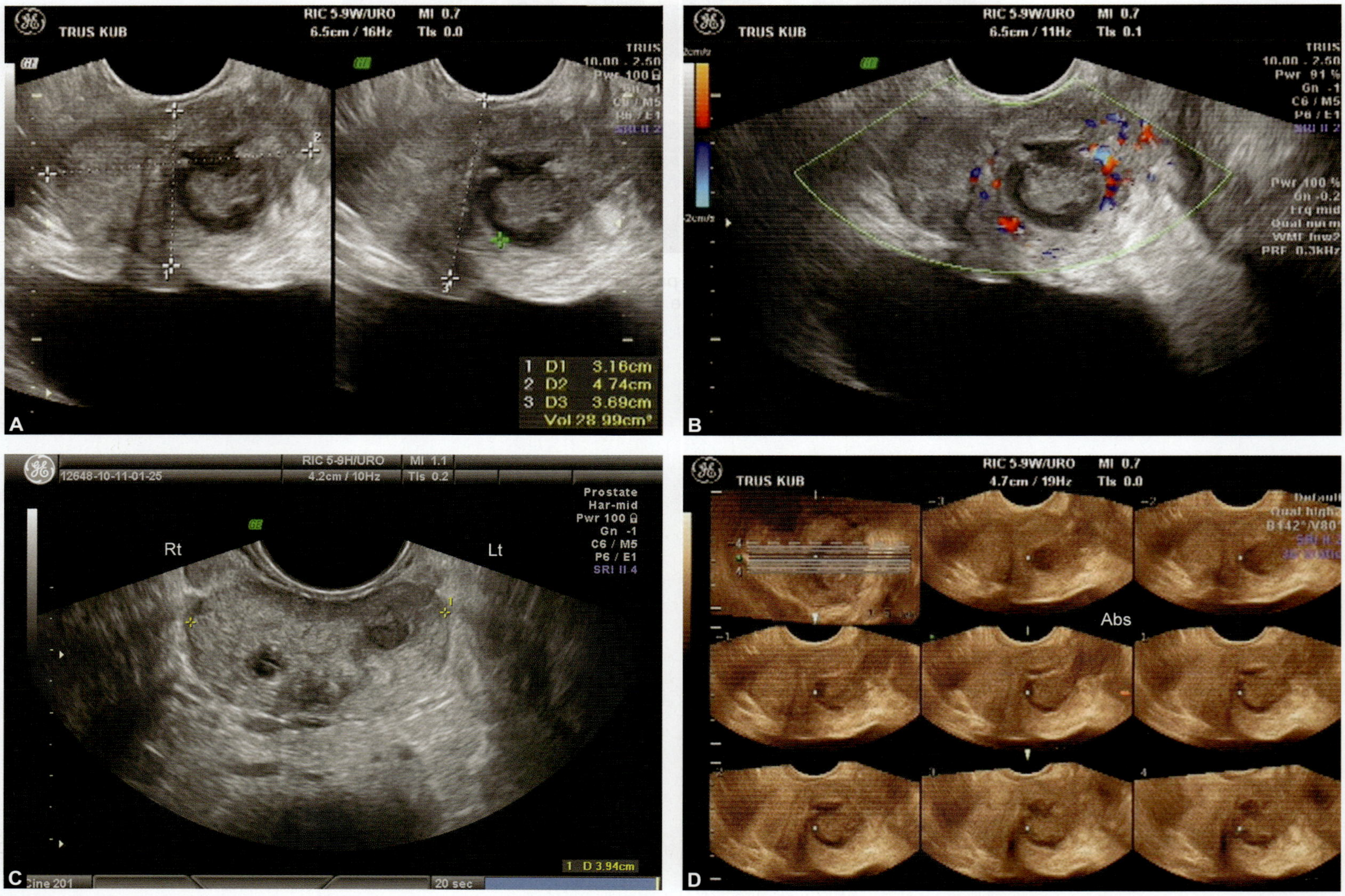

FIGURES 10.33A to D: Prostatic abscess. A patient presented with acute perineal pain with marked dysuria. TRUS shows a thick walled hypoechoic pocket in the left lobe of the gland. Central area of necrosis is seen in it with internal debris. On color flow imaging, increased flow is seen around it. The tomographic ultarsound (TUI) imaging shows the abscess cavity. Findings are suggestive of acute abscess formation in the prostate.

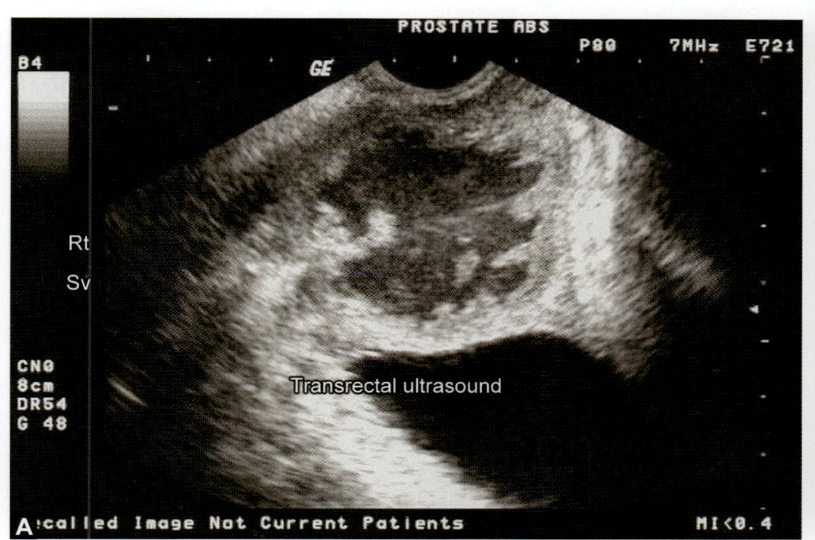

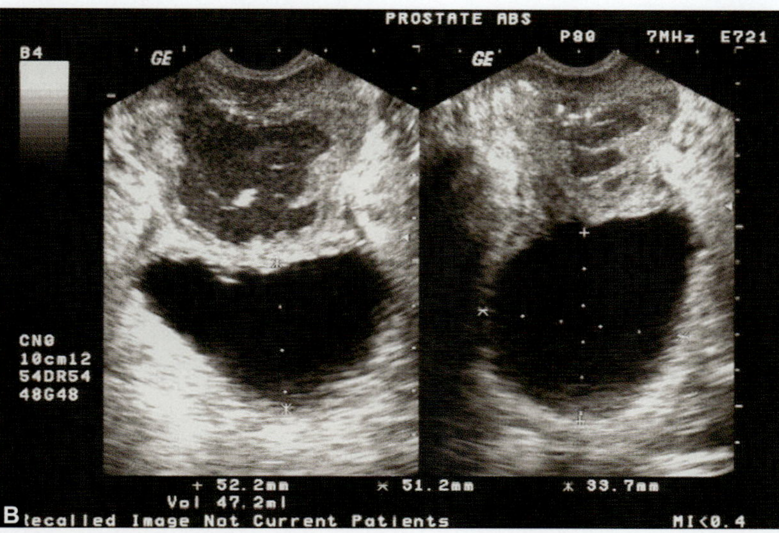

FIGURES 10.34A and B: Pyogenic abscess in the prostate. HRSG shows an irregular heterogeneous low-level echo complex mass in the substance of gland. Central area of necrosis is also seen. Normal prostatic gland texture is lost suggestive of abscess. Patient was having severe pyuria.

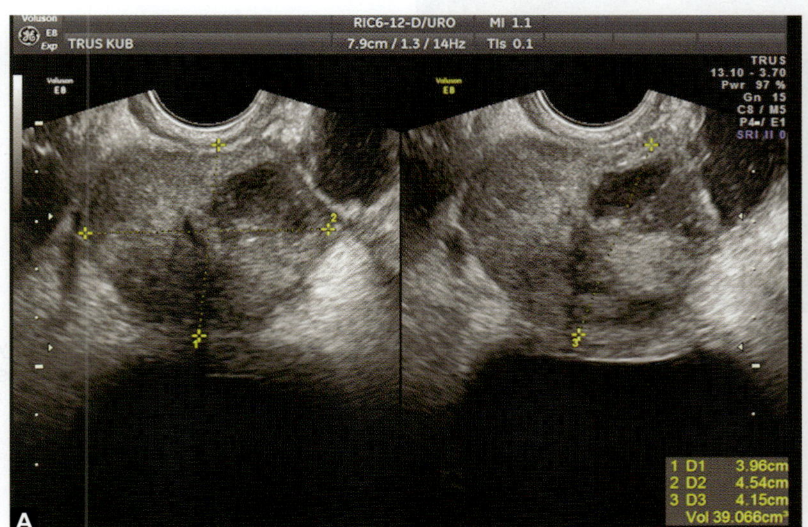

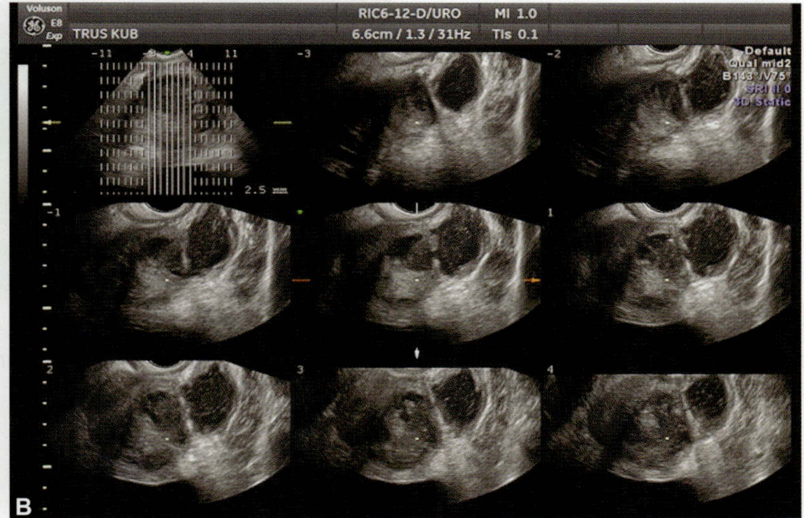

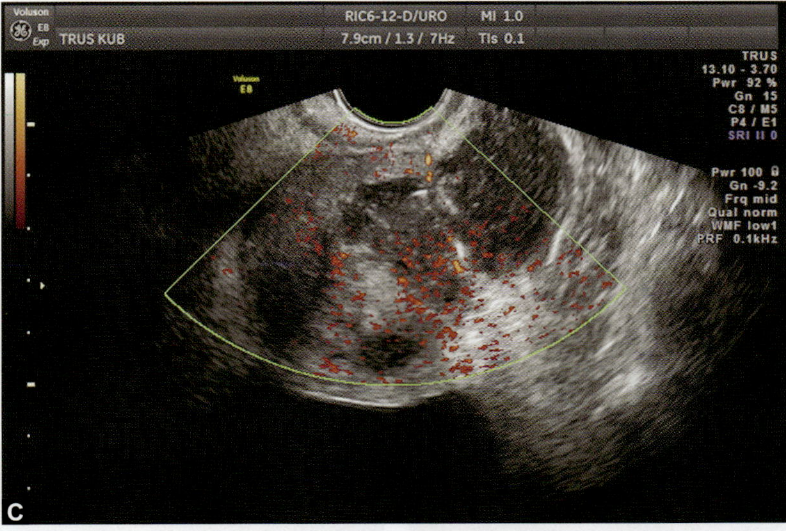

FIGURES 10.35A to C: Big abscess in the left lobe of prostate. A patient presented with acute pain in perineum with high fever with dysuria. TRUS shows enlarged prostate gland. A thick walled low level echo complex mass seen involving the left lateral lobe. It is also seen extending in the adjacent tissue. Thick echoes are seen in it with internal debris. Perifocal edema is seen. On color flow imaging, no flow is seen in it. Findings are suggestive of a big prostatic abscess extending into surrounding tissue.

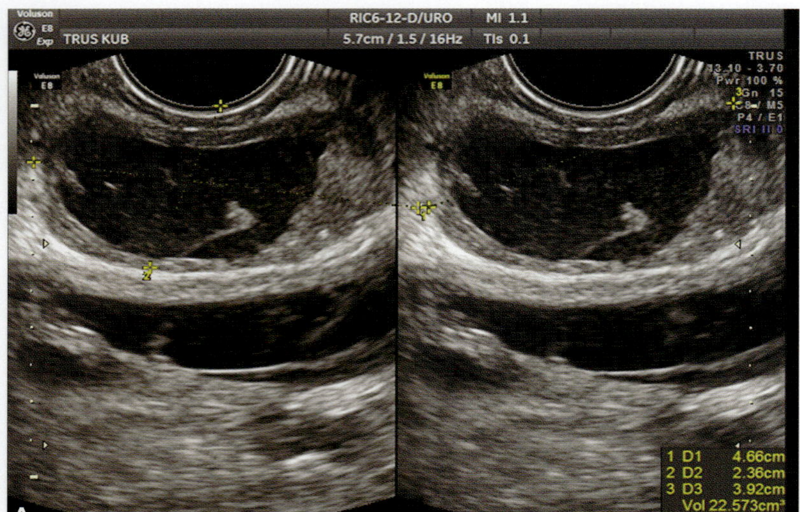

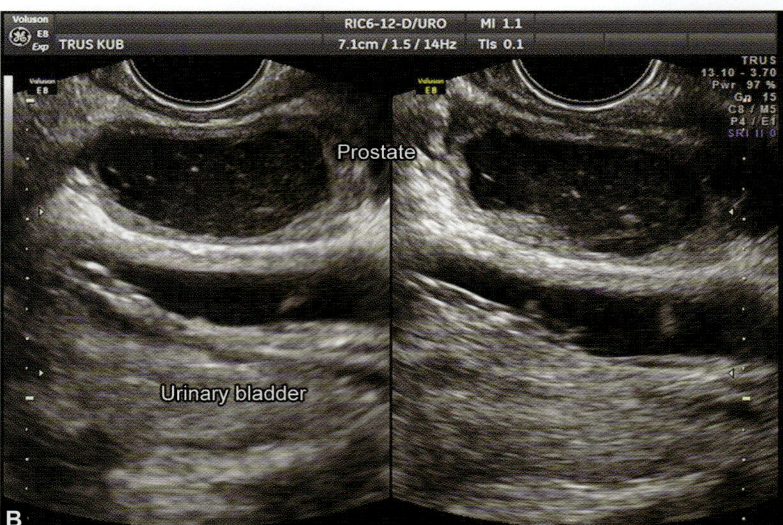

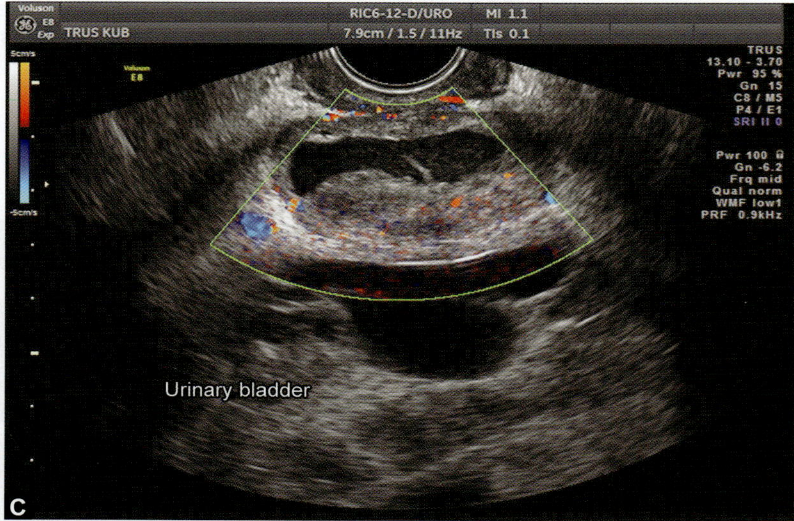

FIGURES 10.36A to C: Big prostatic abscess. A patient presented with retention of urine and dysuria. Transrectal ultrasound (TRUS) shows markedly enlarged prostate. A big pocket of thick collection is seen in the substance of prostate. Thick echoes are seen in it with central area of necrosis suggestive of a big prostatic abscess.

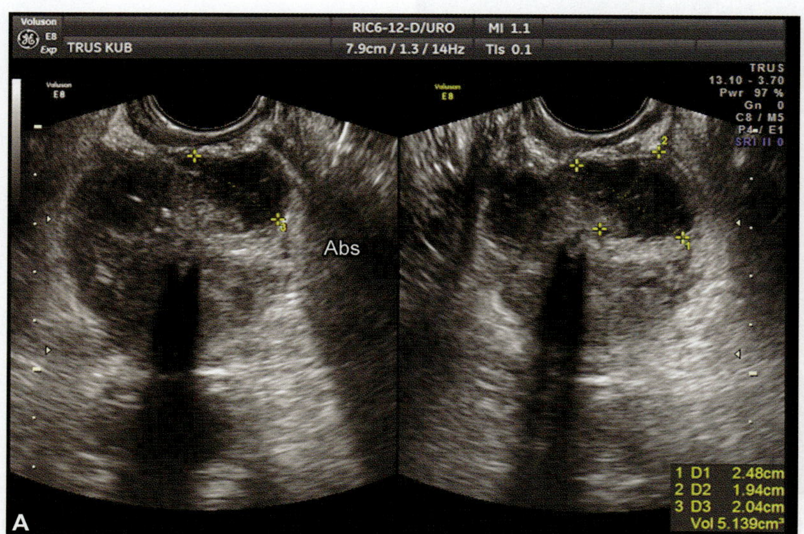

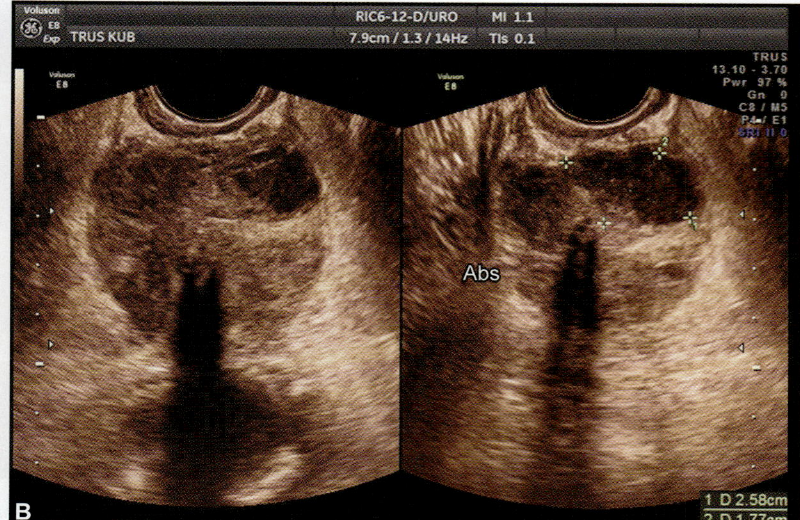

FIGURES 10.37A and B

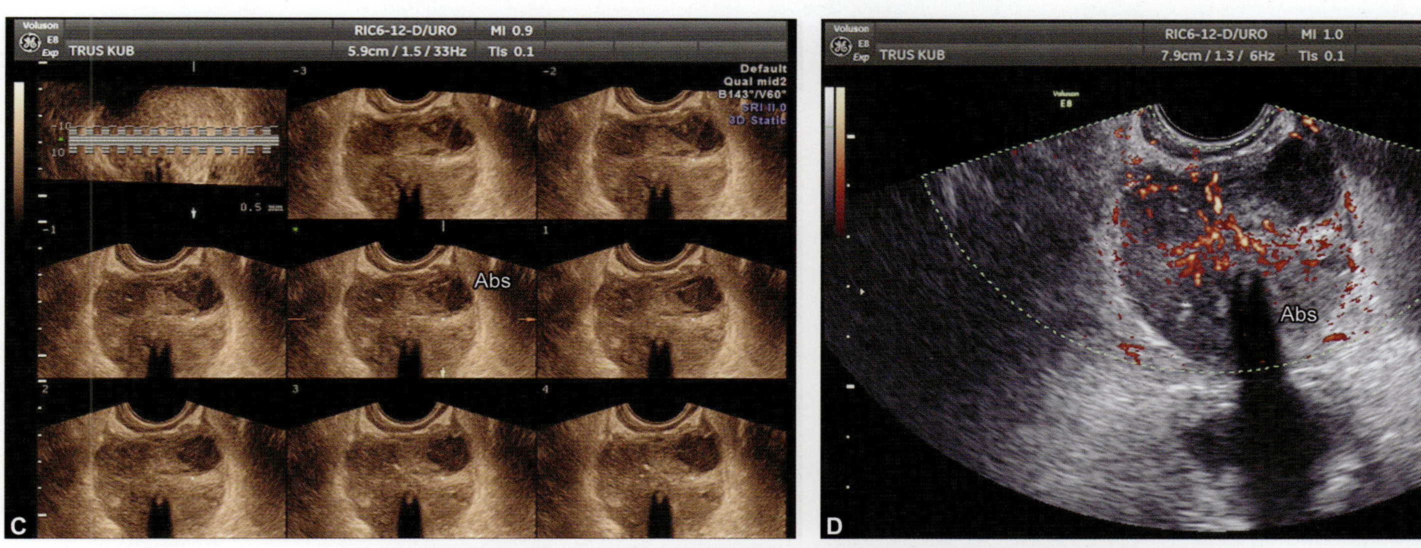

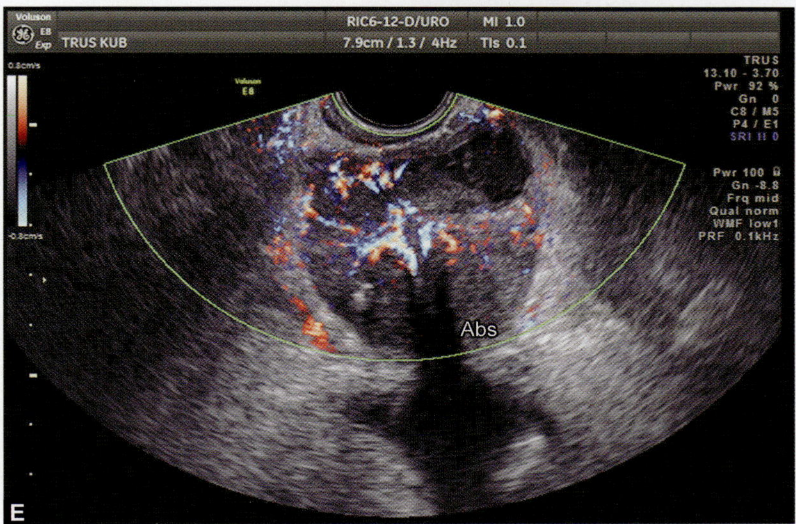

FIGURES 10.37C to E

FIGURES 10.37A to E: Multiple prostatic abscesses. TRUS shows enlarged prostate gland. Pockets of loculated collection seen in both peripheral zones. The thick capsule is seen around them. Associated edema is also present in the gland suggestive of multiloculated prostatic abscesses (Abs). The tomographic ultrasound imaging shows the abscesses cavity clearly. On color flow imaging, increased flow is seen in the inflamed prostate. But no flow is seen in the abscess cavity.

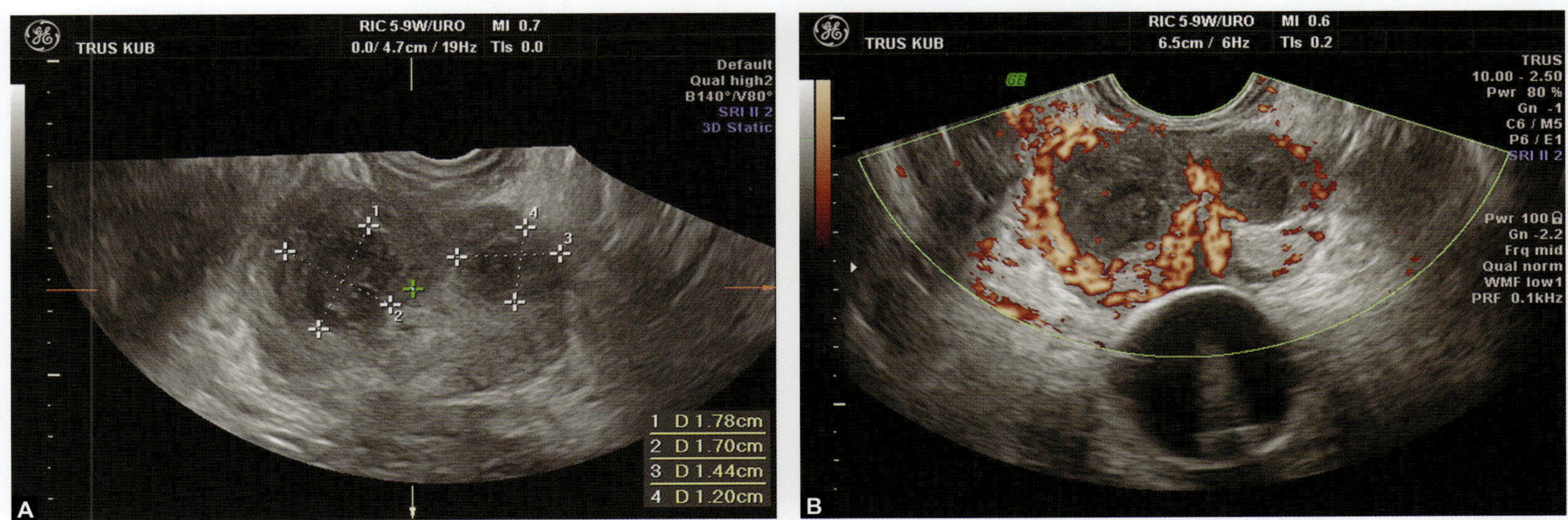

FIGURES 10.38A and B

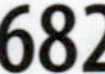

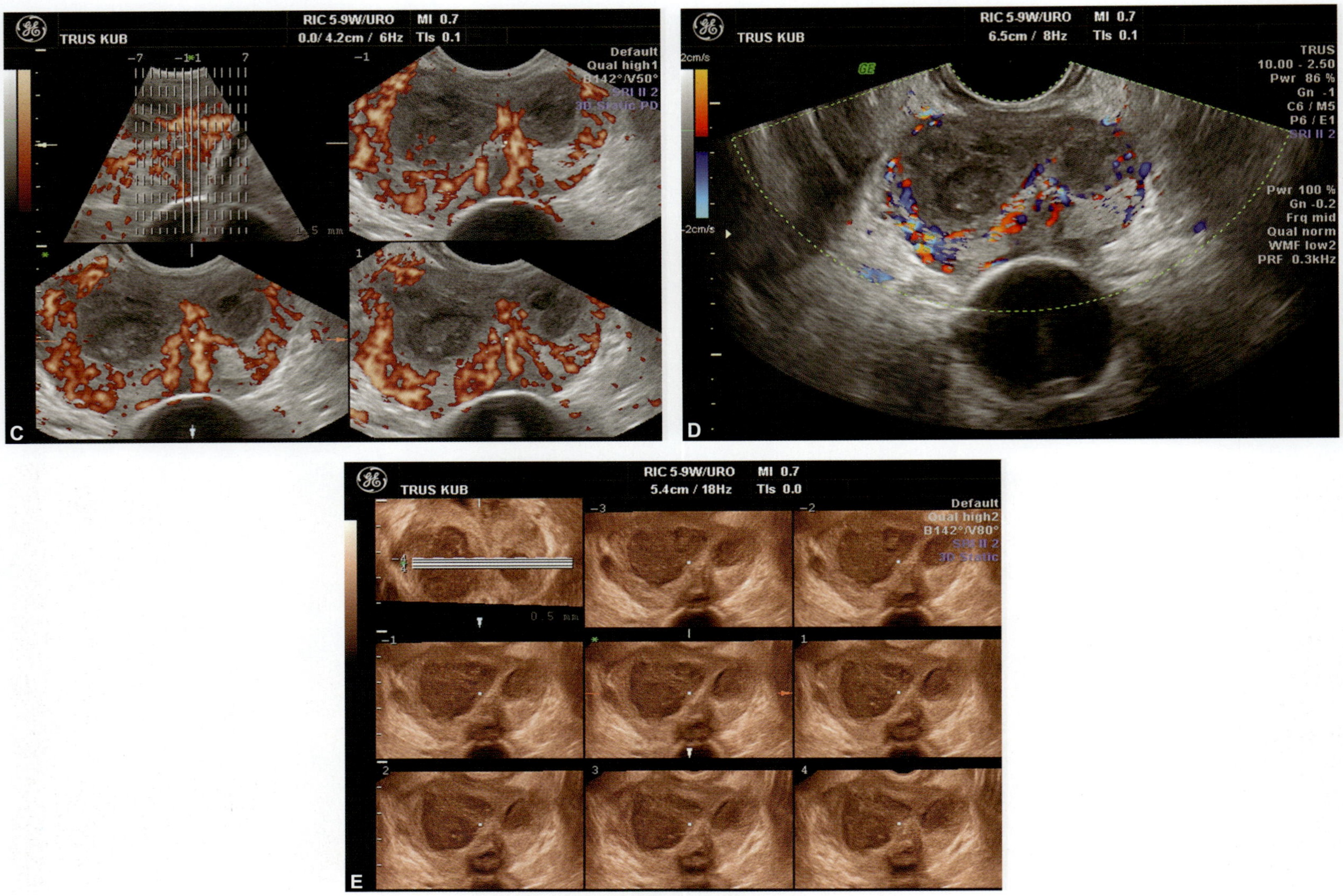

FIGURES 10.38C to E

FIGURES 10.38A to E: Multiple prostatic abscesses. A 41-year-old male presented with high fever and retention of urine with pain in the lower abdomen. TRUS shows diffuse enlargement of the prostate. Thick pocket of collection is seen in both the lobes. Increased flow is seen in around them. But no flow is seen in the cavity. Findings are suggestive of multiple prostatic abscesses. 3D tomographic ultrasound imaging clearly shows the prostatic abscesses.

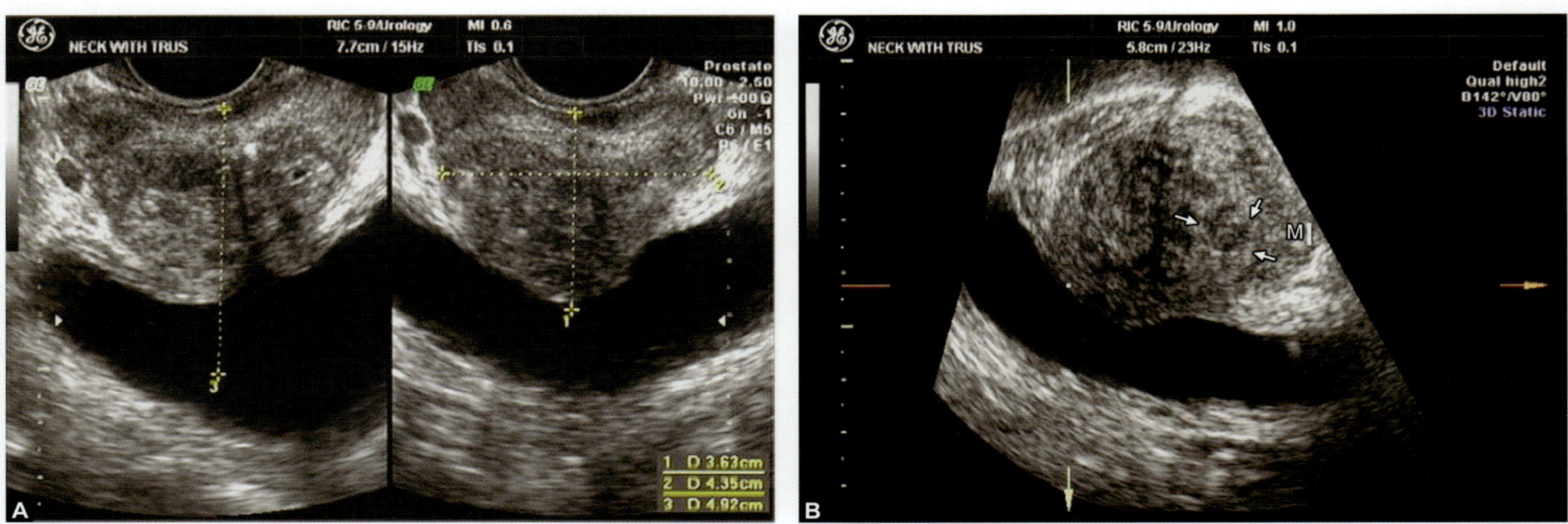

FIGURES 10.39A and B

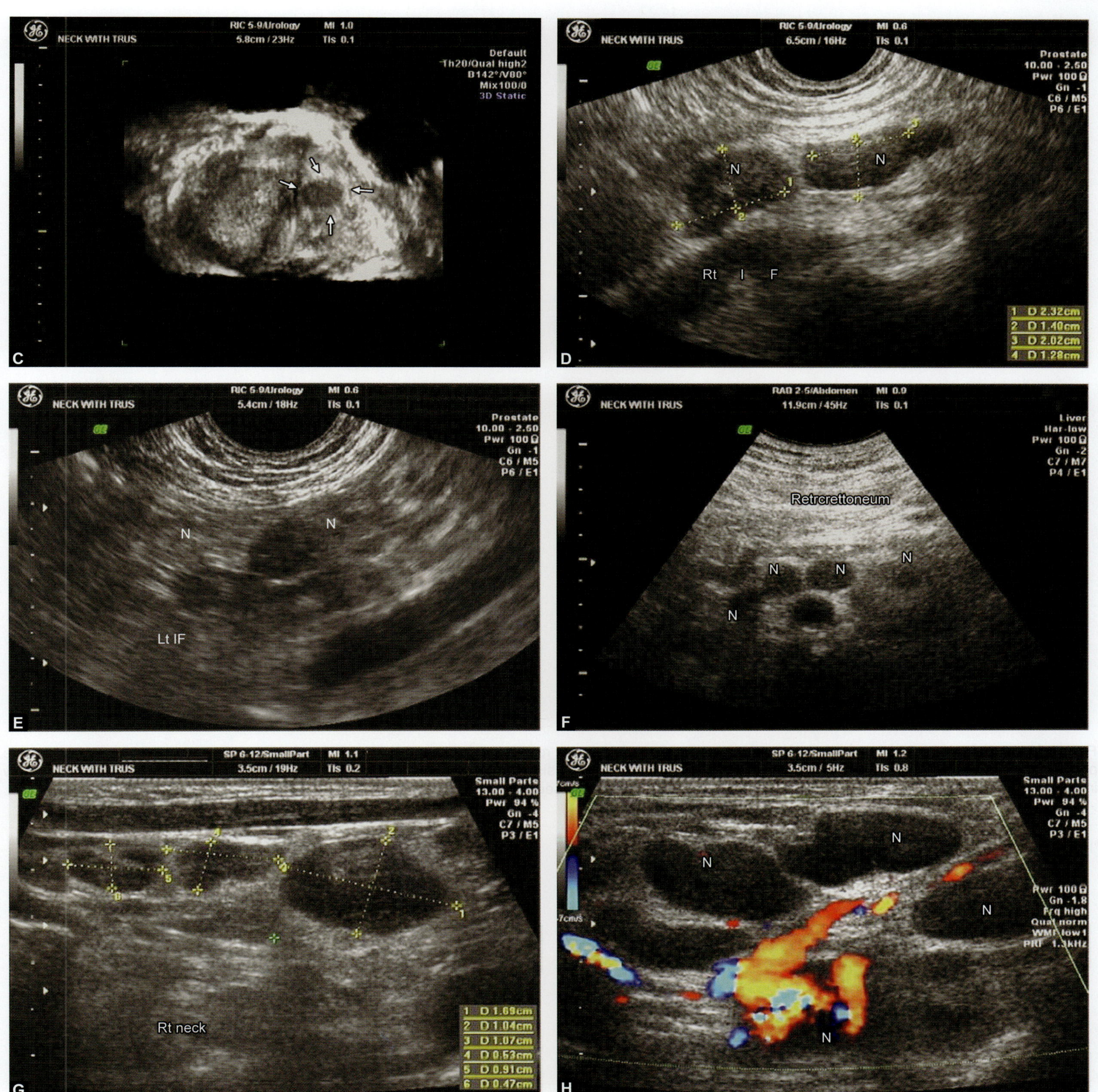

FIGURES 10.39C to H

FIGURES 10.39A to H: Tubercular prostatitis. An old man presented with gradual loss of weight and signs of prostatism. HRSG shows enlarged inhomogeneous gland. The glandular texture is hypoechoic small nodules are seen in the gland. They are discrete in position. 3D imaging of the gland shows the nodules in the central zone of the gland. Biopsy of the nodules confirmed tuberculosis. Abdominal imaging shows multiple enlarged nodes in both iliac fossa. Enlarged nodes are also seen in the retroperitoneum of the same patient. HRSG of the neck of the same patient shows multiple enlarged nodes in the supraclavicular regions. Biopsy of the nodes confirmed tuberculosis.

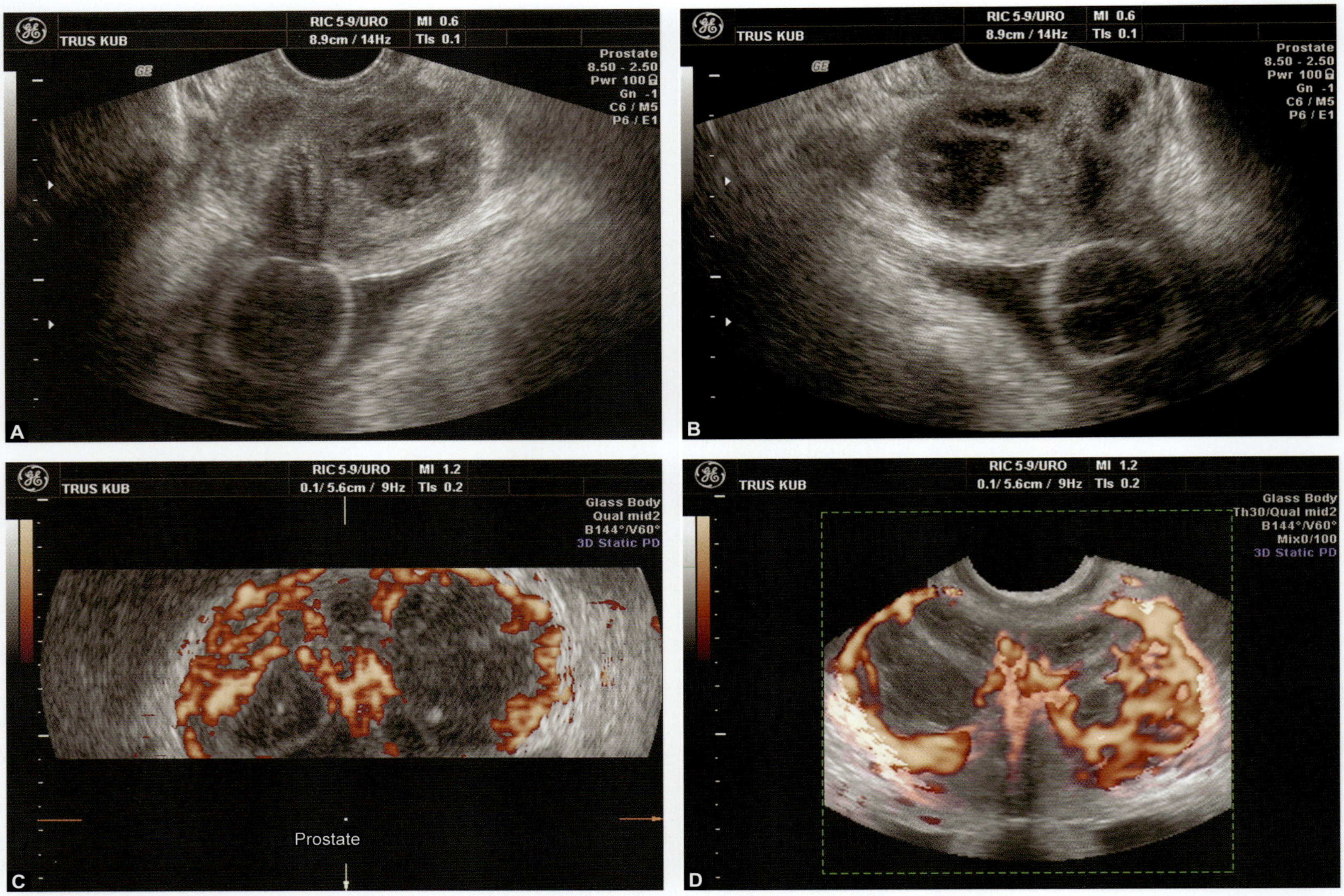

FIGURES 10.40A to D: Big prostatic abscess. A patient presented with retention of urine with acute pain. TRUS shows enlarged prostate. Multiple pockets of thick collection is seen in the prostate. Central area of necrosis is also seen suggestive of multiple prostatic abscesses. On color flow imaging, marked peripheral increased flow is seen. However, no flow is seen in abscess cavity.

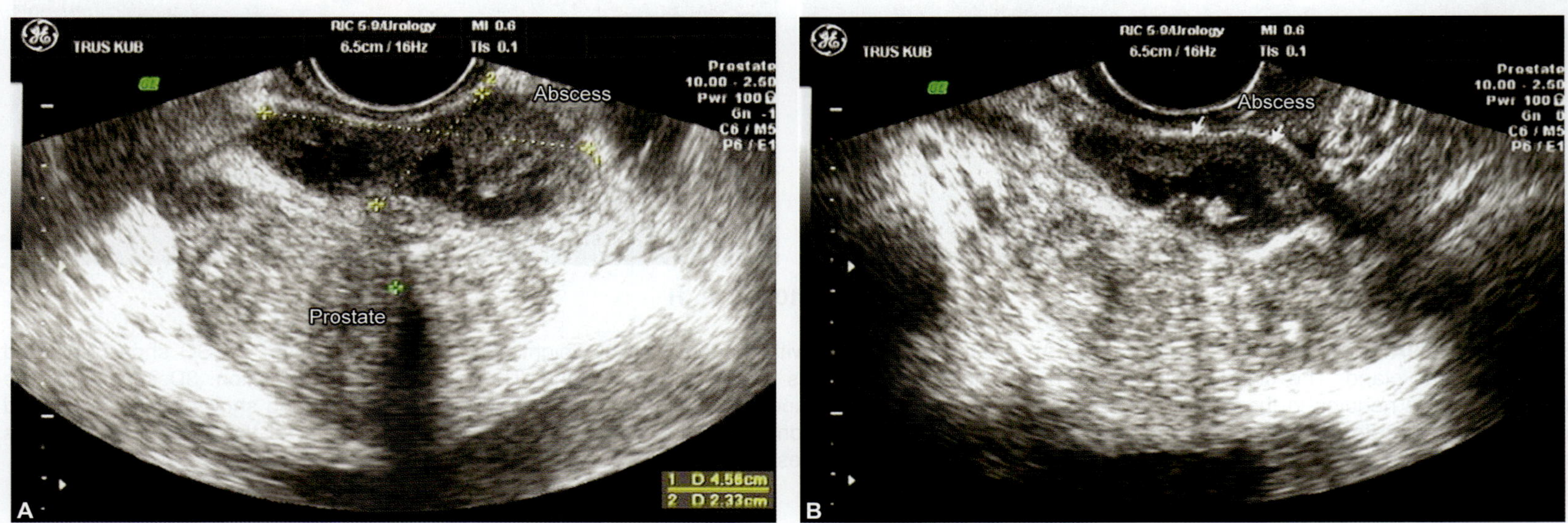

FIGURES 10.41A and B

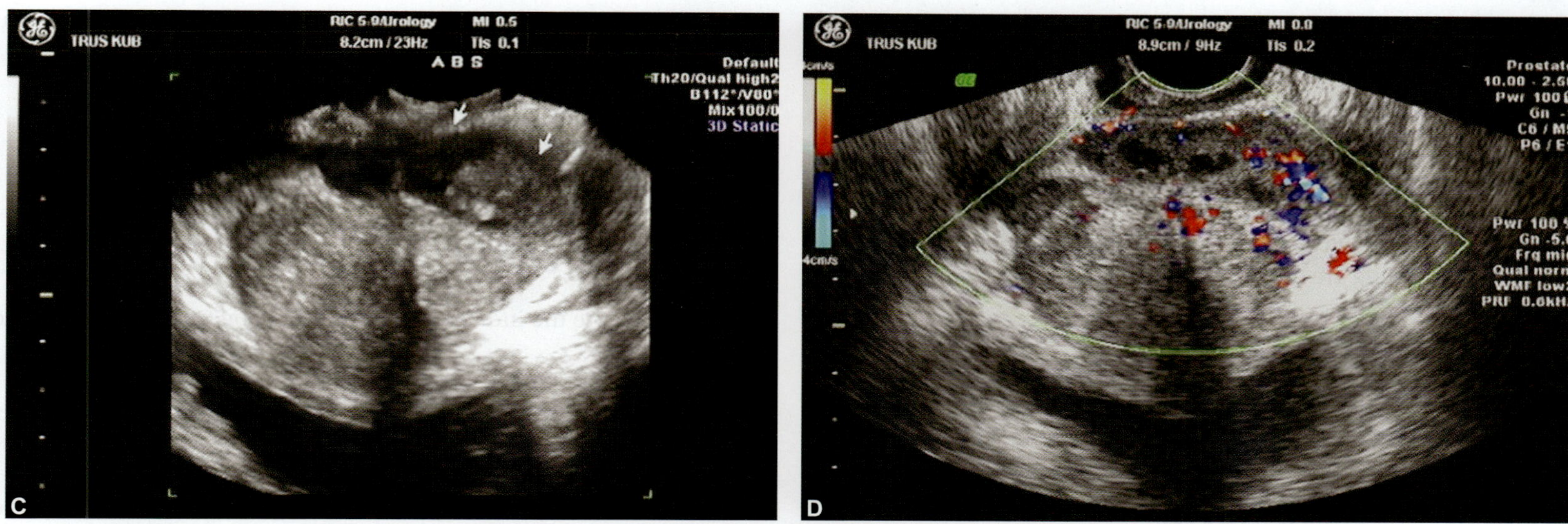

FIGURES 10.41C and D

FIGURES 10.41A to D: Abscess in the prostatic bed. Patient presented with high fever with chills and riggers and tender perineum. HRSG shows low-level echo complex mass in the prostatic bed. Thick echoes are seen in it. The abscess is seen pressing over the prostate. However, the prostatic capsule is intact. No evidence of any breaking down of the capsule is seen. On color flow imaging, multiple vessels are seen around the capsule of the abscess. 3D imaging of the abscess clearly demarcated the abscess separate from the prostate. Echogenic debris is also seen.

Carcinoma of the Prostate

Localized prostatic cancer classically presents as a hypoechoic lesion with ill-defined or well-defined borders in the peripheral zone of the prostate. Contrast between the echotexture of the tumor and that of the normal, evenly echogenic surrounding peripheral zone allows easy detectability. Sonographic-pathologic correlation studies of radical prostatectomy specimens have shown that approximately 70–75% of tumors have this classical US appearance, while; about 30% of cancers are isoechoic and flush with the surrounding tissue. These cannot be identified by TRUS unless secondary sonographic signs of cancer, such as a bulge of the capsule or distortion of the periprostatic fat are present. A smaller number of cancers have a heterogeneous echotexture with subtle areas of hyperechogenicity or stippled small echogenic foci scattered within the hypoechoic lesion.

The reasons for the variable sonographic appearance of prostate carcinoma are incompletely understood. Well-differentiated tumors tend to be hypoechoic. Higher-grade lesions are more heterogeneous perhaps due to a higher degree of stromal fibrosis and desmoplastic reaction or invasion of areas of prostate hyperplasia by larger cancers. Hyperechogenic foci within the tumor correspond pathologically to comedo calcification within highly undifferentiated anaplastic tumors. Echogenic areas located in the periphery of the tumor are usually calcified corpora amylacea is adjacent benign prostatic tissue.

Factors which Affect the Detectability

Two factors affect the detectability of a tumor on TRUS.

Tumor echogenicity: Hypoechoic tumors are readily visible, whereas isoechoic lesions blend with the surrounding tissues.

Tumor size: Small cancers (less than 5 mm) are often undetected. Very extensive cancers involving the entire peripheral zone are difficult to identify because comparison with normal tissue is impossible. Almost 50% of cancers are found in the anterior half of the prostate, and either arises from the central or transition zone, or from the anterolateral portion of the peripheral zone. These tumors are often located beyond the focal zone of the transducers, or blend in with areas of prostatic hyperplasia. Stage A cancers (cancers not palpable clinically), are specifically difficult to detect, even in retrospect unless they extend into the posterior portion of the peripheral zone, or appear as irregular hypoechoic extend into the posterior portion of the peripheral zone, or appear as irregular hypoechoic mass adjacent to the TURP defect.

Accuracy of Diagnosis

Estimation of tumor volume by TRUS: *It is often inaccurate for two reasons:* Tumor size is usually underestimated particularly in large cancers, which tend to infiltrate into and spread through the gland to invade areas of benign prostate hyperplasia. Prostatic cancer is often multifocal. Only approximately half of contralateral tumor foci were prospectively identified by TRUS in one study comparing preoperative TRUS and sections of radical prostatectomy specimens.

Accuracy of TRUS in the diagnosis of prostatic cancer: The US appearance of early prostate cancer is not specific. The positive predictive value (PPV) for a hypoechoic lesion to be cancer increases with the size of the lesion, presence of a palpable nodule, and elevated PSA. Overall, the use of TRUS can also determine glandular volume accurately. The most commonly used method to measure prostatic or tumor volume is the formula for a prostatic ellipse (length × width × height x 0.523). Volumes can then be easily converted to weight because of 1 mass lesion of prostatic tissue is equivalent to 1 g.

PROSTATE SPECIFIC ANTIGEN

Prostate specific antigen (PSA) is a low-molecular weight glycoprotein, which is produced exclusively by the prostate and to a smaller extent by the seminal vesicular tissue. It is normally present in small amounts in all postpubertal males and is absent in women. The two techniques for measuring PSA are:

- Polyclonal assay (Yang method)
- Monoclonal assay (Hybritech method)

The monoclonal assay is the most commonly used method the world over.

PSA levels have been evaluated as normal borderline and abnormal values. The following are the accepted levels.

- <4 ng/cc—normal
- 4.0–10.0 ng/cc—borderline
- >10 ng/cc—abnormal

However, the diagnosis of prostatic malignancy is not specific or absolute with PSA studies. A normal PSA does not necessarily mean that the patient has no cancer. Similarly, abnormal values are not definitive for the presence of prostatic malignancy. There are several entities, which can increase the PSA values. These are:

- Prostate cancer
- Benign prostatic hypertrophy
- Prostatic inflammation
- Prostatic infarct
- Post digital rectal examination.

In view of the limitations of the role of PSA in detecting prostatic cancer, newer parameters are being evolved. Some of these are as follows:

Free Prostate Specific Antigen

This is one of the parameters, which is now being advocated since the absolute PSA is not definitive of prostatic cancer. Evaluation of free versus bound PSA may provide additional information for the evaluation of prostatic cancer. However, further work is needed to confirm the role of free PSA in prostatic pathology.

Prostate Specific Antigen Density

It has been suggested that a measure of the volume of the prostate may correlate with PSA level to a specific disease. It has now been shown that men who have PSA levels >4 ng/cc with no palpable lesion on digital rectal examination, but have a PSAD>0.10 and .12/.15 have cancer.

Prostate Specific Antigen Velocity

It had been suggested that the changing levels of PSA especially increasing values, even if within the normal range may be significant and require further evaluation. A PSA level that doubles or triples in the course of a single year should raise suspicion that the patient may be harboring prostatic cancer.

Age-related Prostate Specific Antigen

As men age, their prostate also enlarge due to BPH. It has been suggested that the normal PSA values may relate to the age of the individual and the range may vary with the age. The following parameters may be useful for "normal age-related PSA".

40–50 years	0.0–2.5 ng/cc
50–60 years	0.0–3.5 ng/cc
60–70 years	0.0–4.5 ng/cc
>70 years	0.0–6.5 ng/cc

PROSTATIC BIOPSY

The following are the indications for undertaking transrectal prostatic biopsies.

- A suspicious lesion, i.e. a peripheral, ill-defined lesion in the PZ
- Focal bulge in the prostate
- Capsular or pericapsular irregularity
- Rising PSA levels.

Biopsies of the prostate gland can be performed either by the transperineal route or the transrectal approach. The transrectal biopsy is a relatively simple procedure carried out under antibiotic cover. A true-cut 18-gauge spring-loaded needle is used. The position of the transducer is adjusted until the puncture guideline, superimposed on the image, transects the area of biopsy. The tip of the needle is visualized as it penetrates the rectal wall and enters the prostate. Transrectal biopsies are performed without anesthesia and are well-tolerated in most patients.

Hypoechoic lesions that are larger and exist with significantly elevated PSA levels have a higher risk of malignancy. Lesions that are smaller and are in patients with lower or normal PSA levels have a lower risk of being malignant. Lesions in the TZ and the CZ or other gland have much lower rates of malignancy than those with similar lesions in the PZ.

COLOR DOPPLER OF THE PROSTATE

In general, cancer anywhere in the body has the following characteristics on color Doppler:

- An increased number of visualized vessels
- An increase in the size of the vessels
- Increase in the irregularity and contours of the vessels
- Increased diastolic flow indicating a low resistance system.

The normal prostate has abundant surrounding vasculature. The two largest collections of vessels are the Santorini's plexus and the neurovascular bundles.

In BPH, there is increased vascularity within the inner gland and the surgical capsule. However, the flow may vary from patient to patient. In prostatitis, there is increased high velocity and low resistance flow. In diffuse prostatitis, there is diffuse increase in prostatic vascularity throughout the gland. Early studies in prostatic cancer have suggested increased blood flow in cancers greater than 5 mm in size. However, recent studies have demonstrated that only 50% of patients with cancer have increased flow. Three different patterns have been identified. All have low resistance patterns; diffuse flow, focal flow or surrounding flow. The most frequently encountered pattern is diffuse flow within the lesion. When there is focal flow it is not pathognomonic of cancer. In general, color Doppler has not been of great help in distinguishing between benign and malignant lesions.

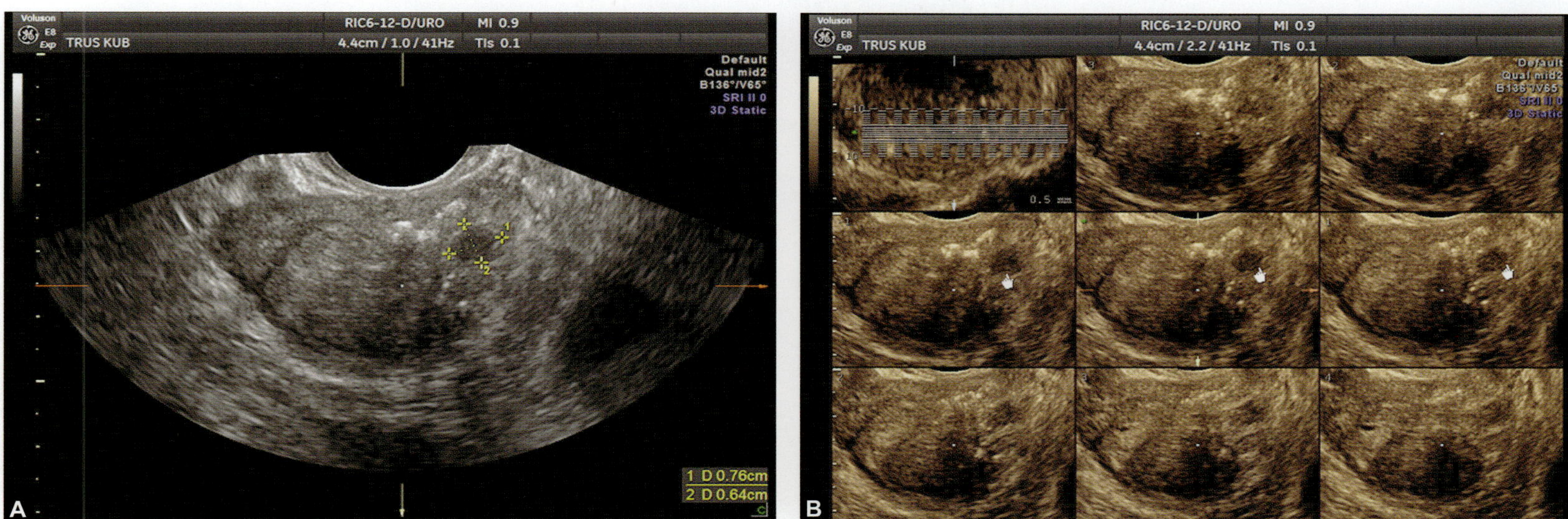

FIGURES 10.42A and B: Hypoechoic nodule in left transitional zone. A patient presented with increased prostate specific antigen (PSA) above the normal limits. TRUS shows a small irregular hypoechoic nodule in the left transitional zone. Margins are irregular and ill-defined. But no necrosis is seen in it. TUI imaging shows the details of the nodule.

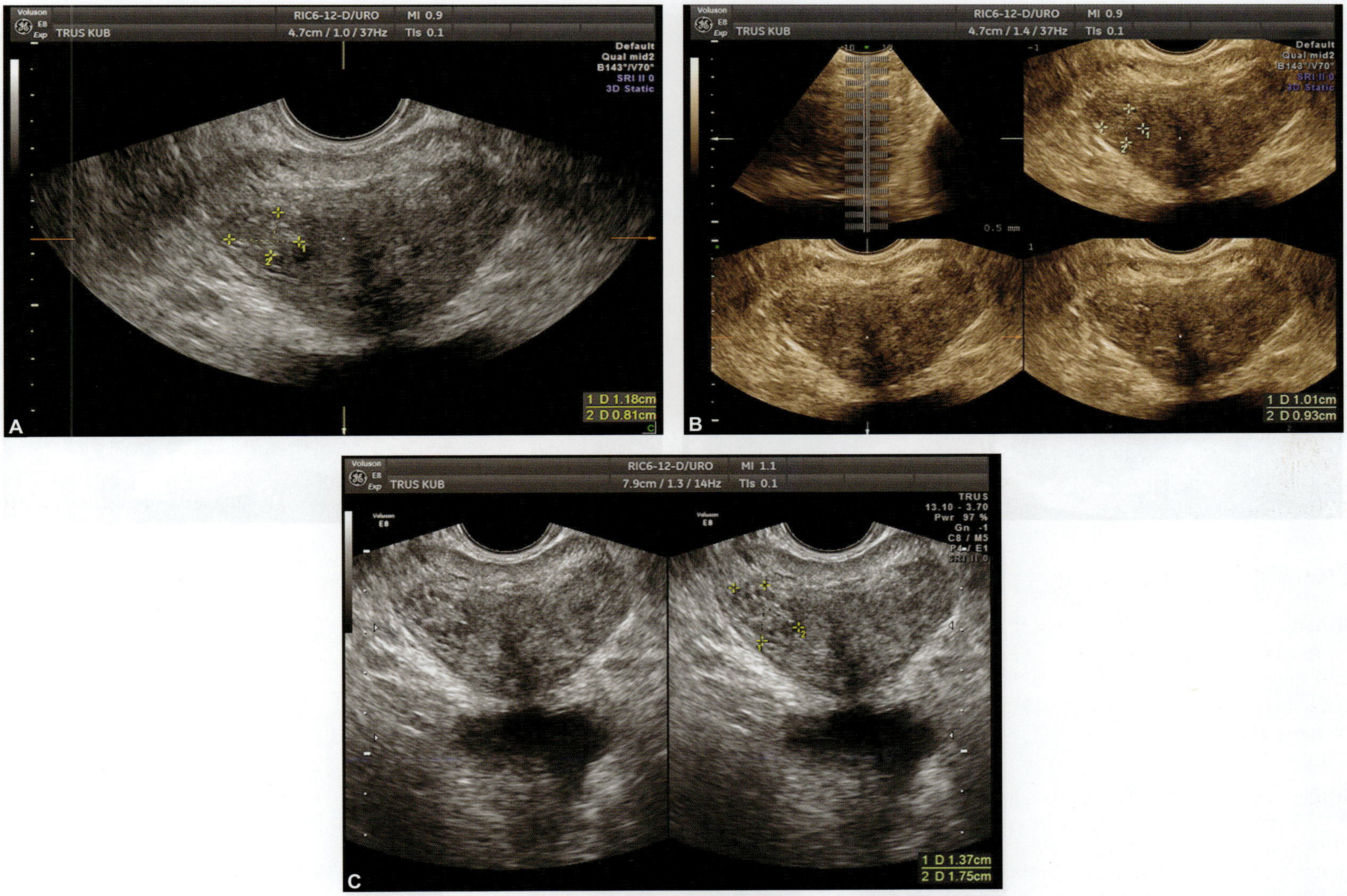

FIGURES 10.43A to C: Isoechogenic nodule in the right transitional zone. A patient presented with PSA at the borderline at the upper limit. Transrectal ultrasound (TRUS) shows an isoechogenic nodule in the right transitional zone. A hypoechoic halo is seen around the nodule. These type of the nodule should be kept under observation and to be followed periodically with PSA estimation.

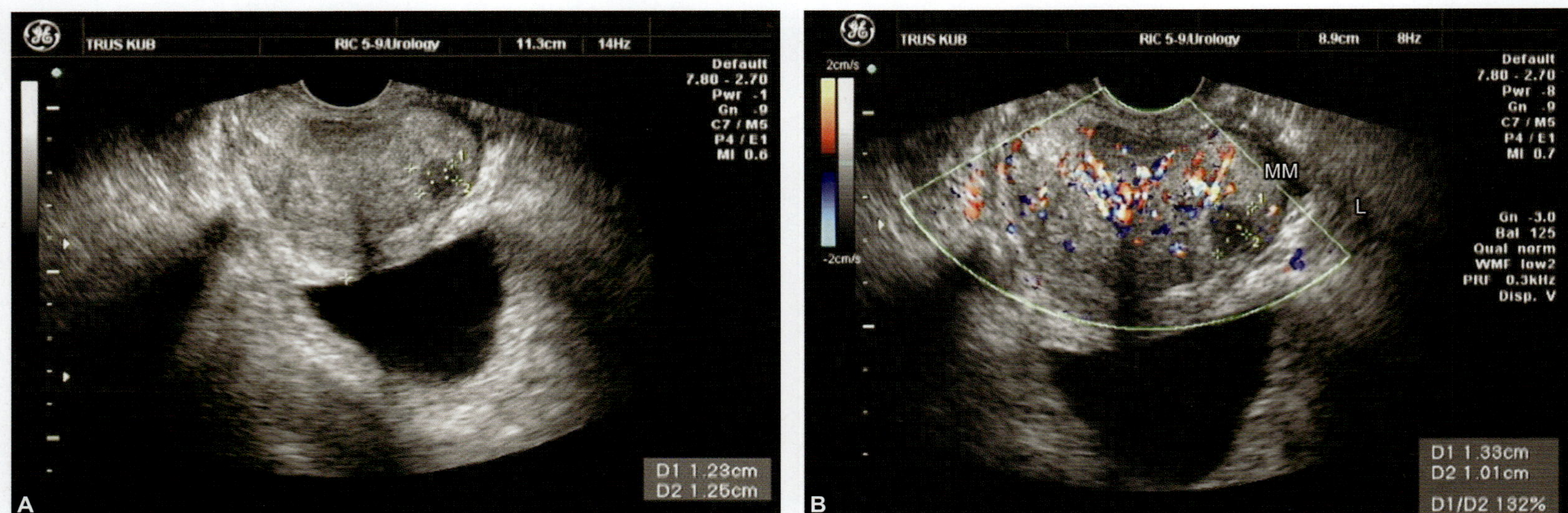

FIGURES 10.44A and B: Mass in the left peripheral zone. HRSG shows an irregular hypoechoic mass in the left peripheral zone. The margins are irregular in outline. No necrosis is seen in the mass. Biopsy of the mass confirms adenocarcinoma. On color flow imaging, there is evidence of increased flow which is seen around the nodule.

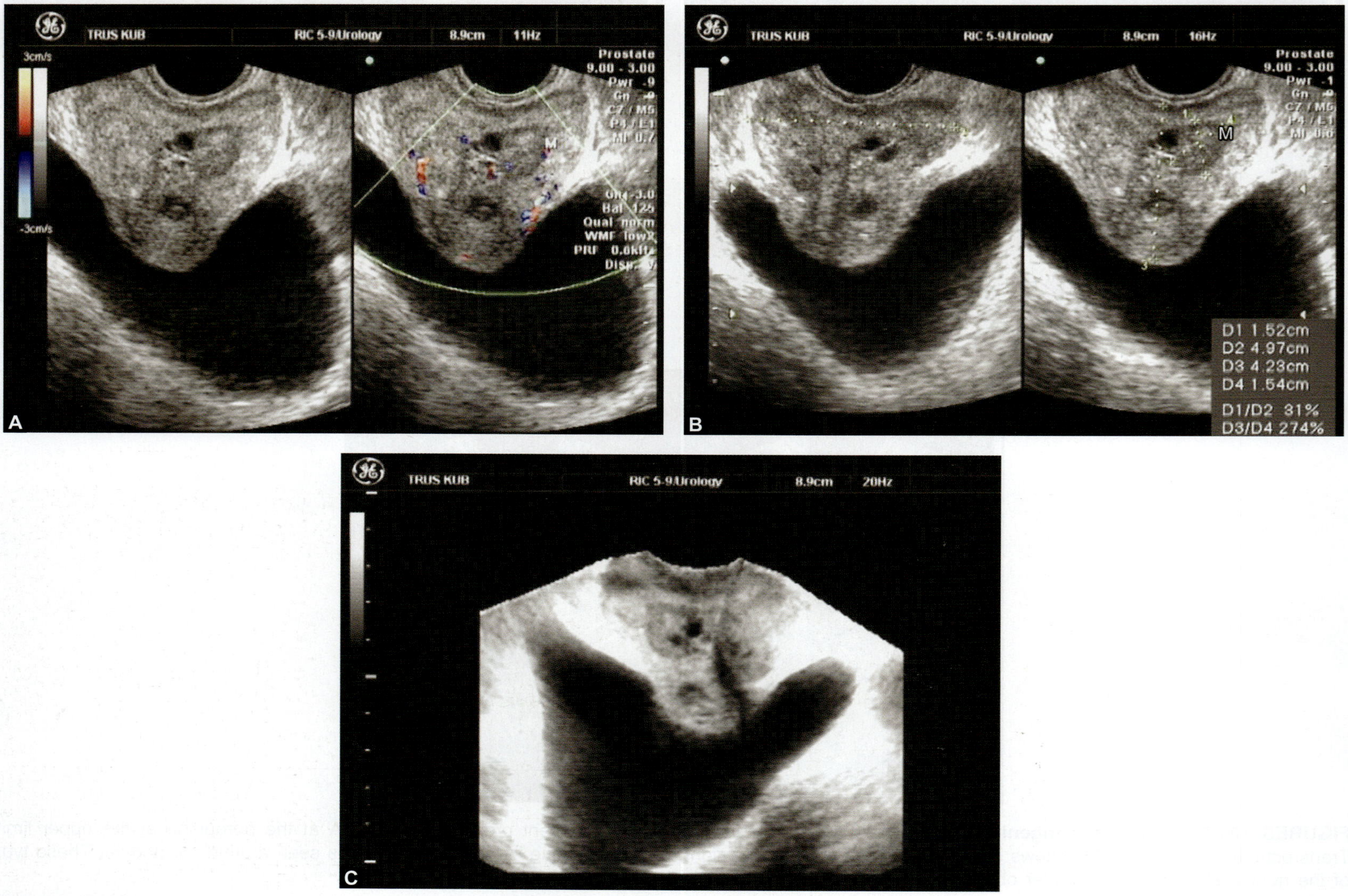

FIGURES 10.45A to C: Irregular hypoechoic mass in the left peripheral zone. HRSG shows irregular hypoechoic nodular mass in the left peripheral zone. The mass is seen encroaching the central zone. Few cystic areas are seen in the mass. But no calcification is seen. Bulging of the lateral margins of the lobe is also seen. On 3D Imaging multiple nodules are seen in the gland. Another hypoechoic nodule is also seen in the median lobe. 3D imaging is good technique to look for hidden nodules in the prostate gland.

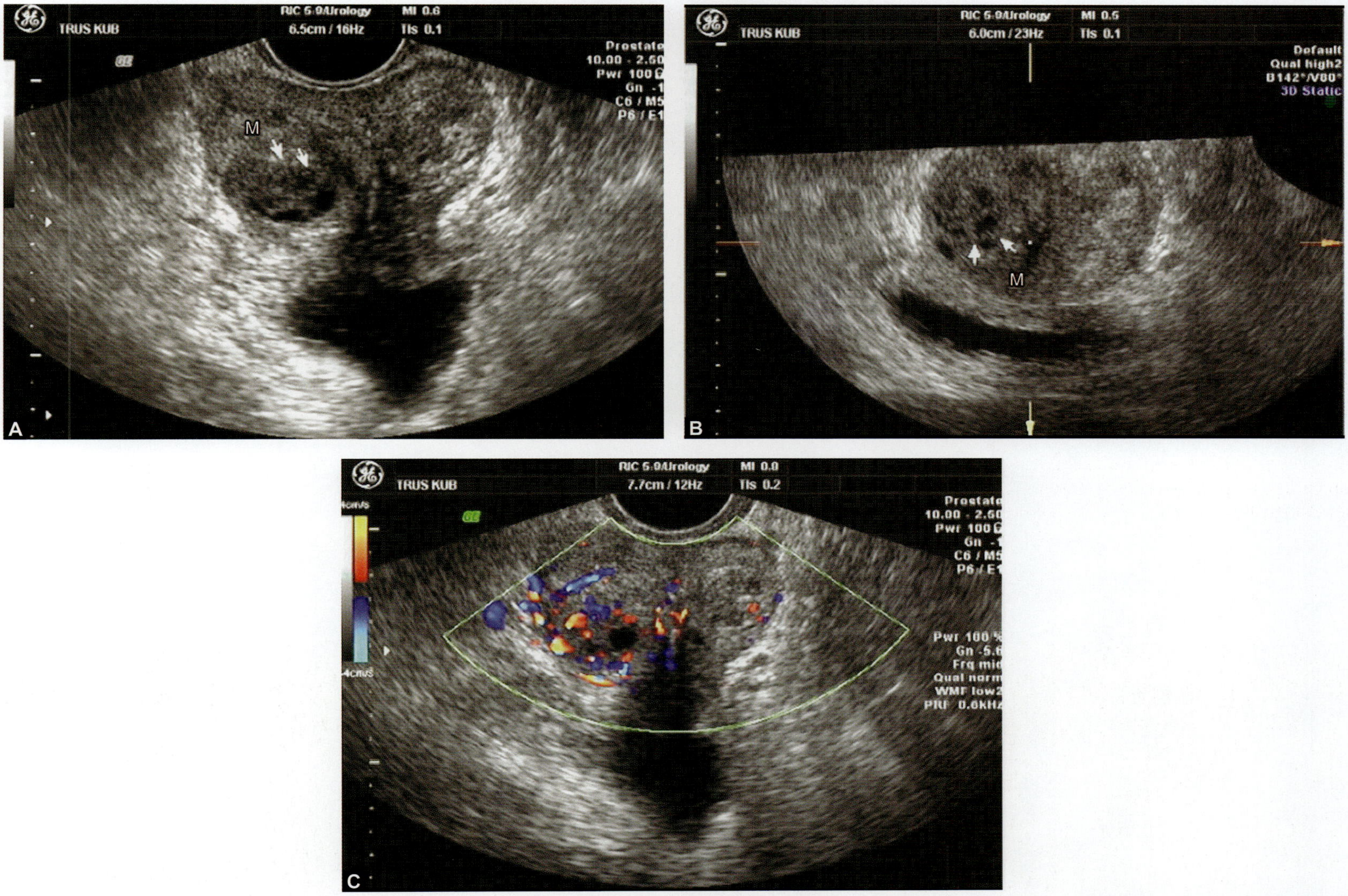

FIGURES 10.46A to C: Hypoechoic nodular mass in the right peripheral zone. HRSG shows well-defined hypoechoic mass in the right peripheral zone. The mass shows variegated texture. No calcification is seen in it. No cystic necrosis is seen in it. 3D imaging of the prostate shows irregular heterogeneous texture of the mass in much better view. Multiple hypoechoic areas are seen in the mass. The margins are ill-defined. Biopsy of the mass confirms adenocarcinoma. On color flow imaging, the mass shows increased flow around the nodule.

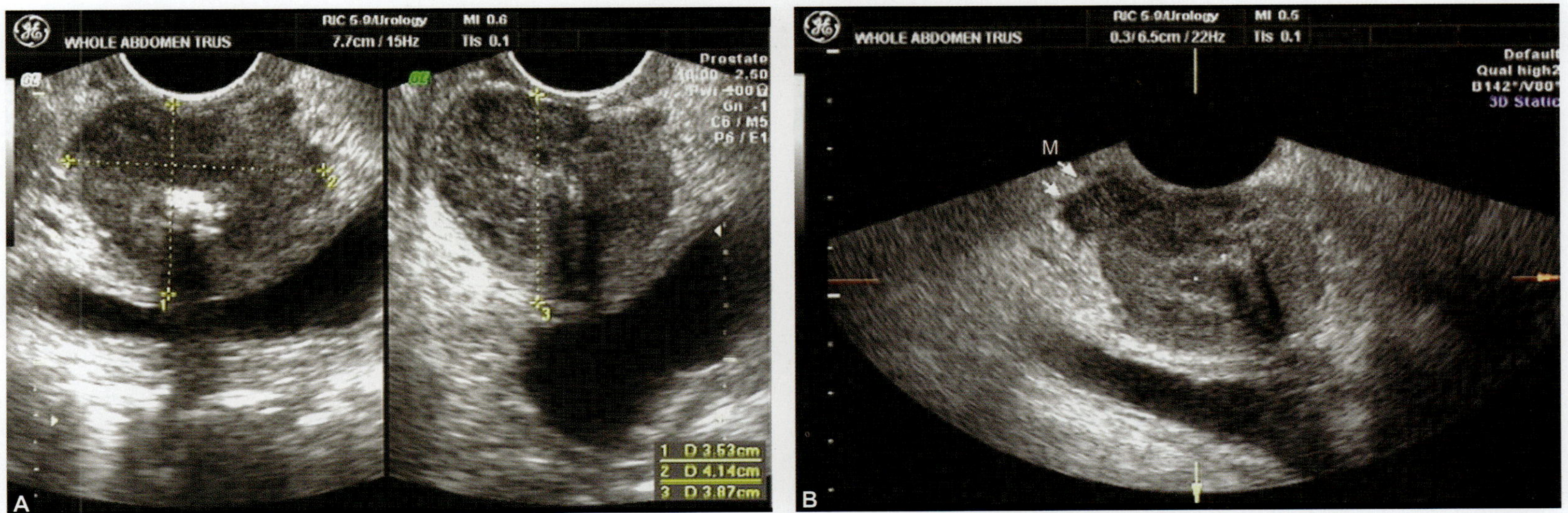

FIGURES 10.47A and B

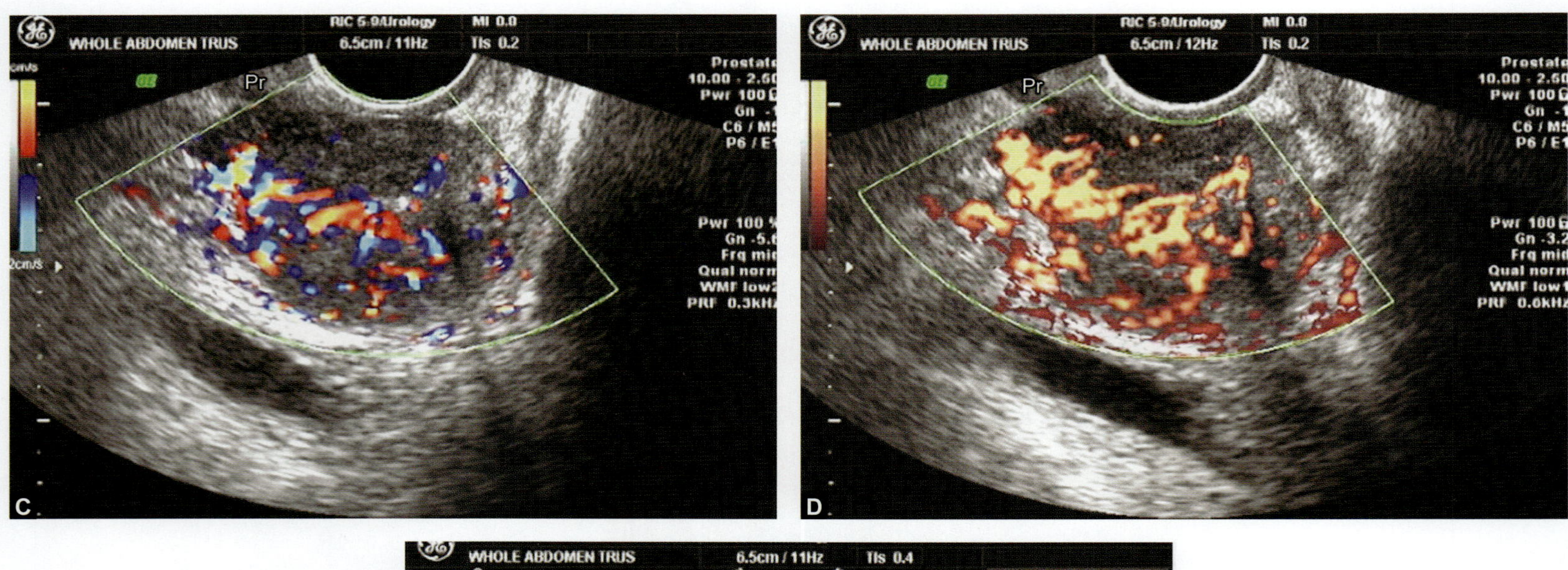

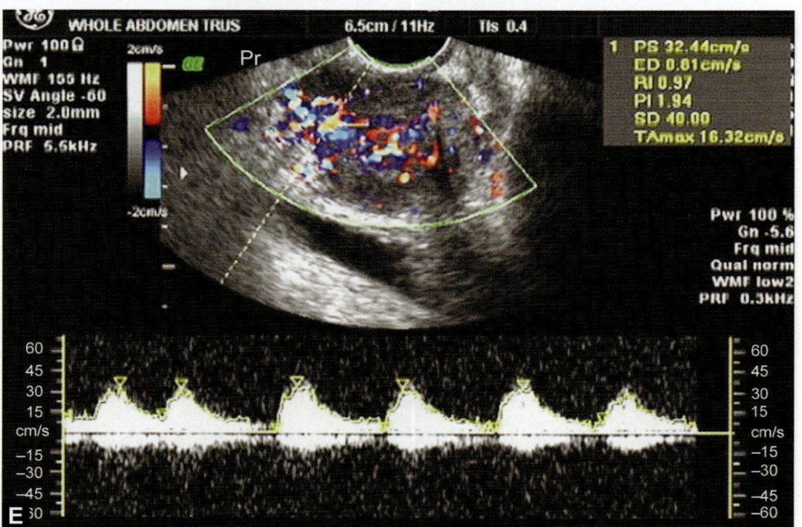

FIGURES 10.47C to E

FIGURES 10.47A to E: An old man presented with markedly increased PSA with nodular prostate on clinical examination. HRSG shows an irregular hypoechoic mass in the transition zone. The mass is seen bulging toward the right lateral lobe. 3D imaging of the mass shows broken capsule of the gland in the right lateral lobe. The mass is seen growing beyond the capsule and invading the periphrastic area. On color flow imaging, high flow is seen in the gland. Marked increased flow seen in the left peripheral zone on power Doppler imaging. On spectral Doppler tracing, high flow is seen in the mass.

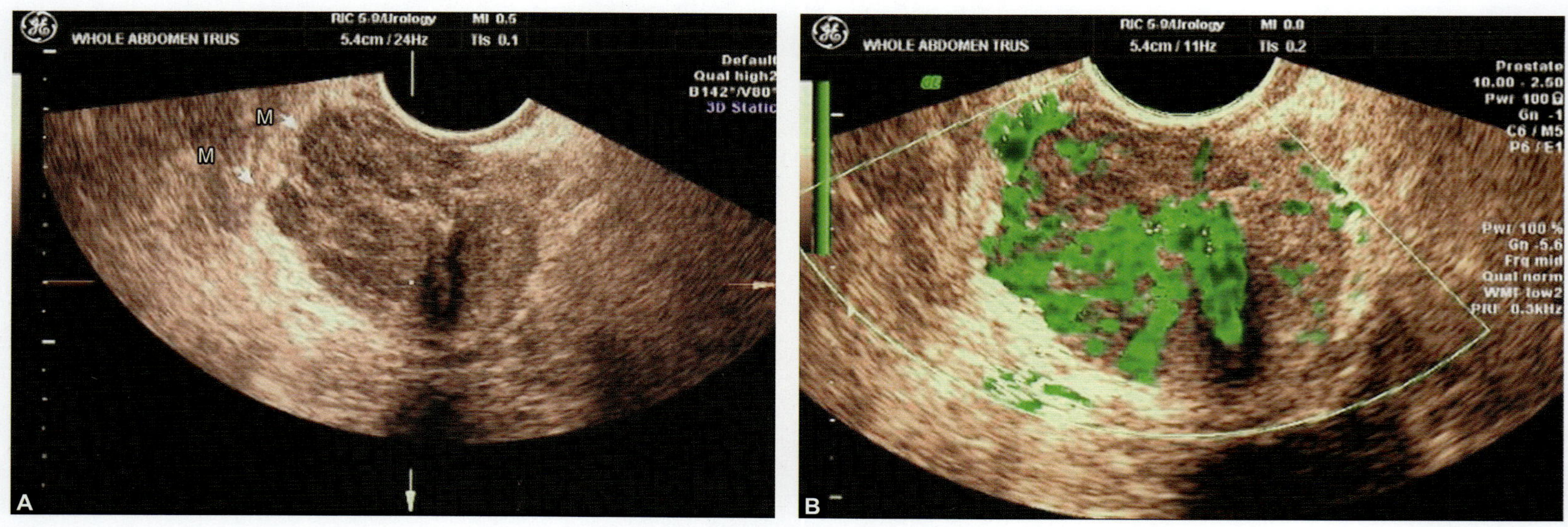

FIGURES 10.48A and B

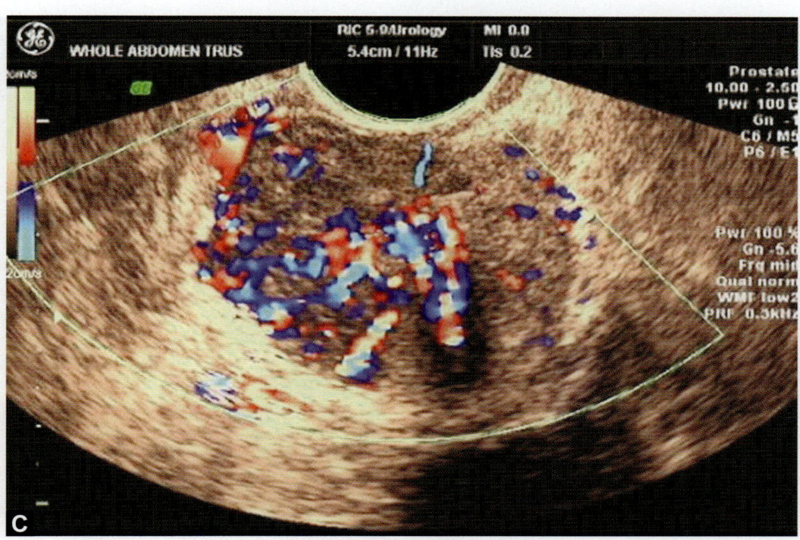

FIGURE 10.48C

FIGURES 10.48A to C: 3D imaging of the prostate shows multiple heterogeneous nodules in the right peripheral zone. They are seen bulging out. On directional power Doppler imaging, high flow is seen around the mass. Biopsy of the mass confirms adenocarcinoma prostate.

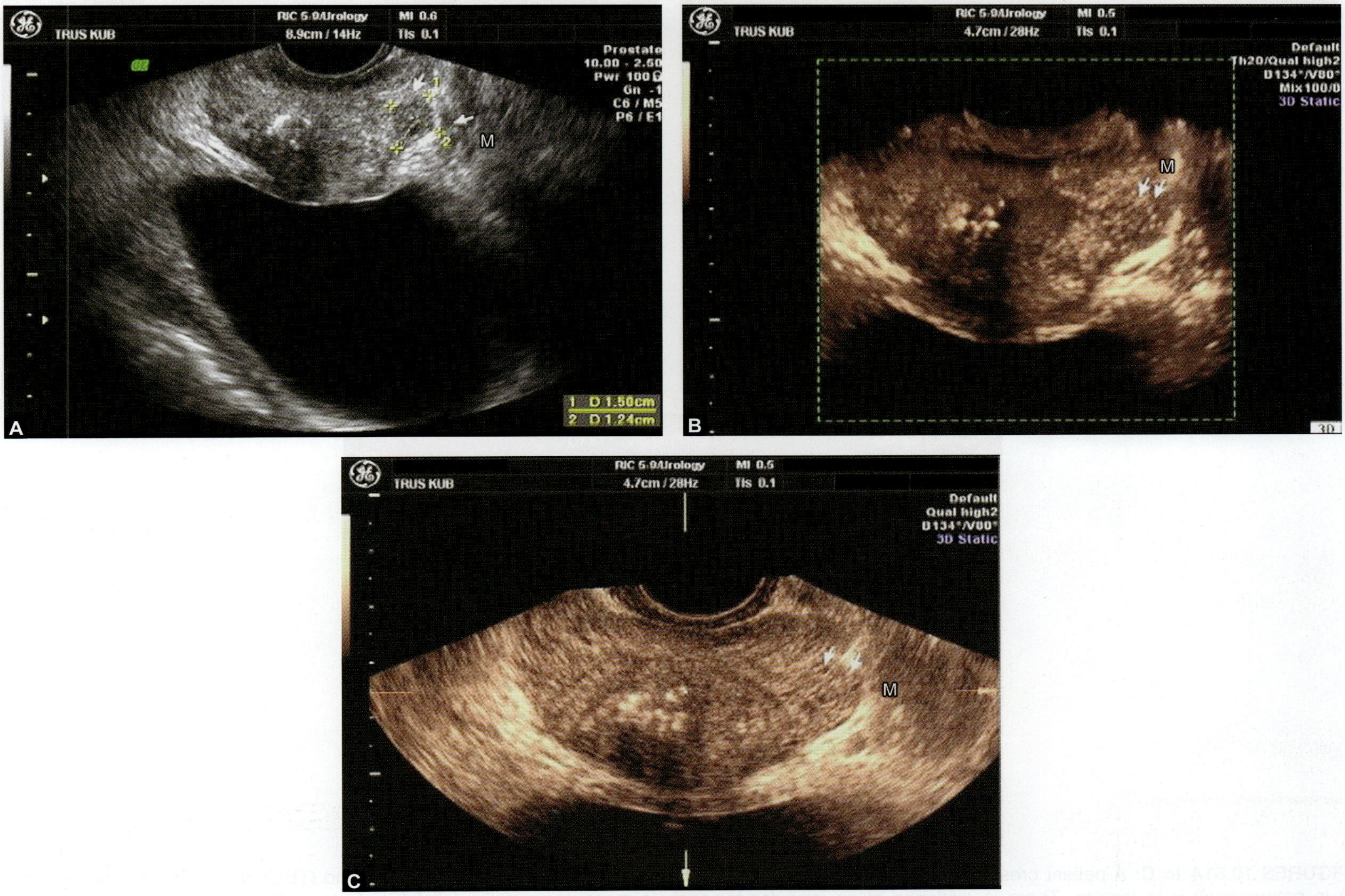

FIGURES 10.49A to C: Nodular mass in the left peripheral zone. HRSG shows irregular hypoechoic mass in the left peripheral zone. The mass is seen pressing over the capsule. Capsular bulge is seen. But no evidence of any breaking of the capsule is seen. 3D surface rendering of the prostate shows the mass in much clear details with capsule bulge.

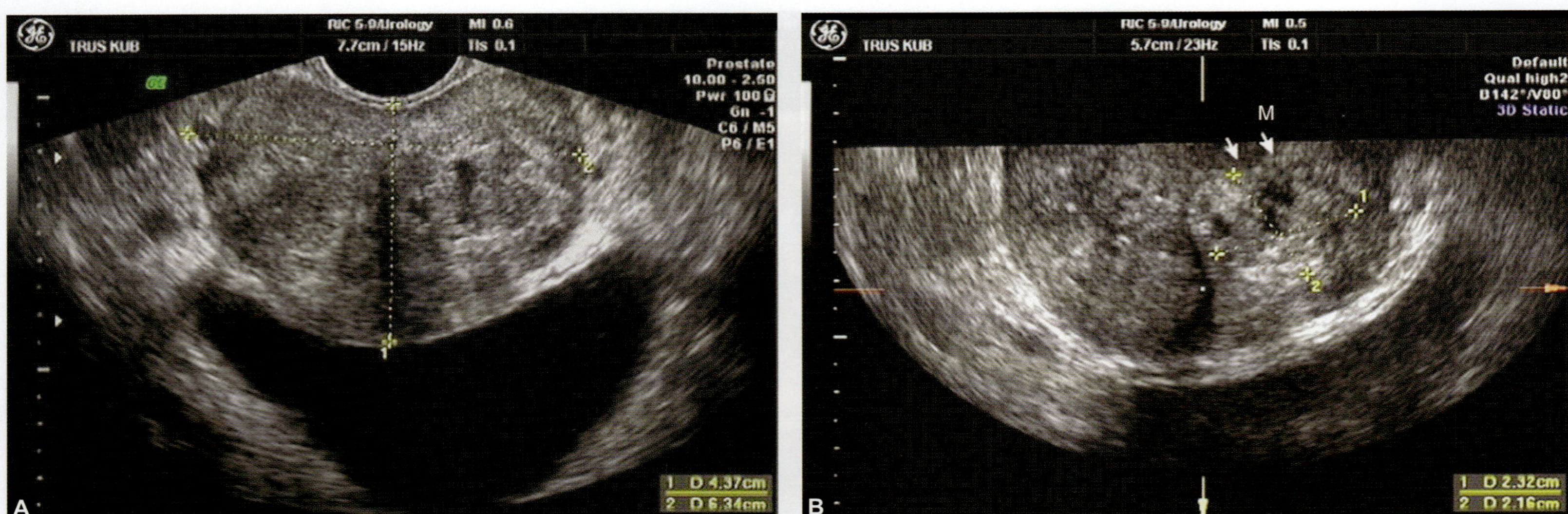

FIGURES 10.50A and B: Heterogeneous mass in the left peripheral zone. Irregular heterogeneous mass is seen in the left peripheral zone. The mass is confined to the zone. No pressure is seen on capsule. 3D imaging of the prostate shows the mass in much better clearity.

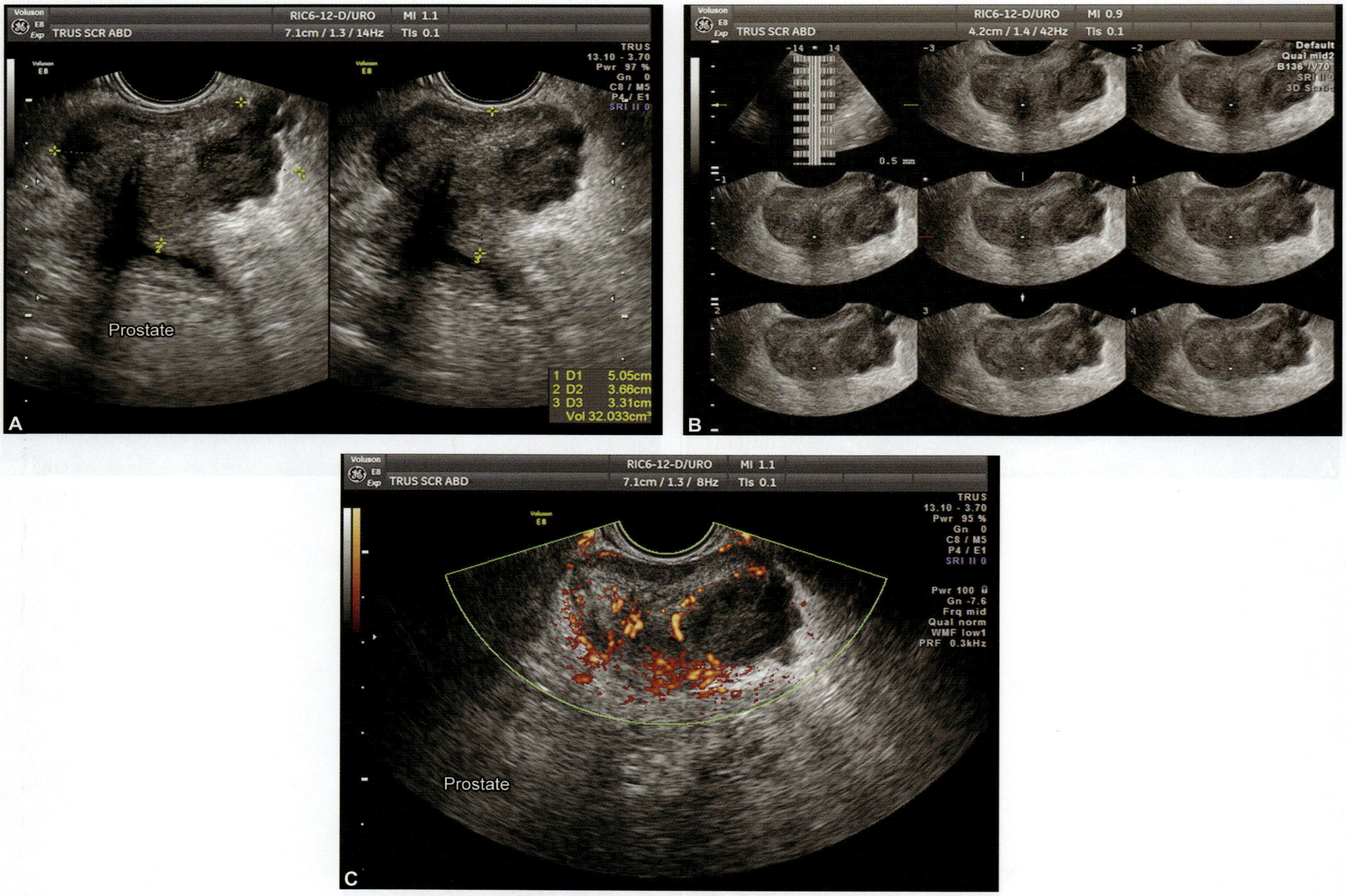

FIGURES 10.51A to C: A patient presented with difficulty in urination and increased PSA. Transrectal ultrasound (TRU) shows the enlarged prostate. It is heterogeneous in texture. There is evidence of an irregular hypoechoic mass seen in the left lobe of gland. The mass is seen invading the left peripheral zone and the transitional zone. It is also seen invading the left capsule of the gland and seen invading the surrounding tissue. The tomographic ultrasound imaging (TUI) shows markedly heterogeneous mass invading the prostatic capsule and adjacent tissue. On color flow imaging, poor flow is seen in the mass. However, moderate flow is seen in the peripheral gland. Biopsy of the mass confirms invasive carinoma prostate.

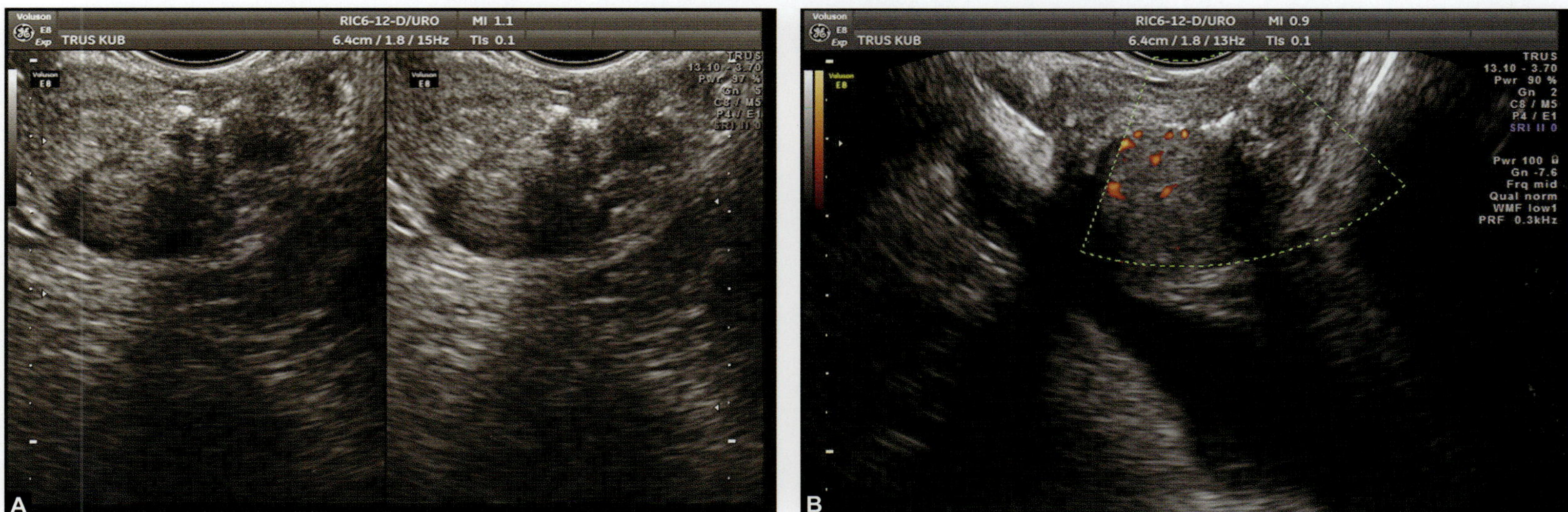

FIGURES 10.52A and B: Transrectal ultrasound (TRUS) shows an irregular ill-defined hypoechoic mass in the left peripheral zone. It is also seen invading the transitional zone. Peripheral calcification is seen in it. On color flow imaging, poor flow is seen in the mass. Transrectal ultrasound (TRUS) guided biopsy confirms malignancy.

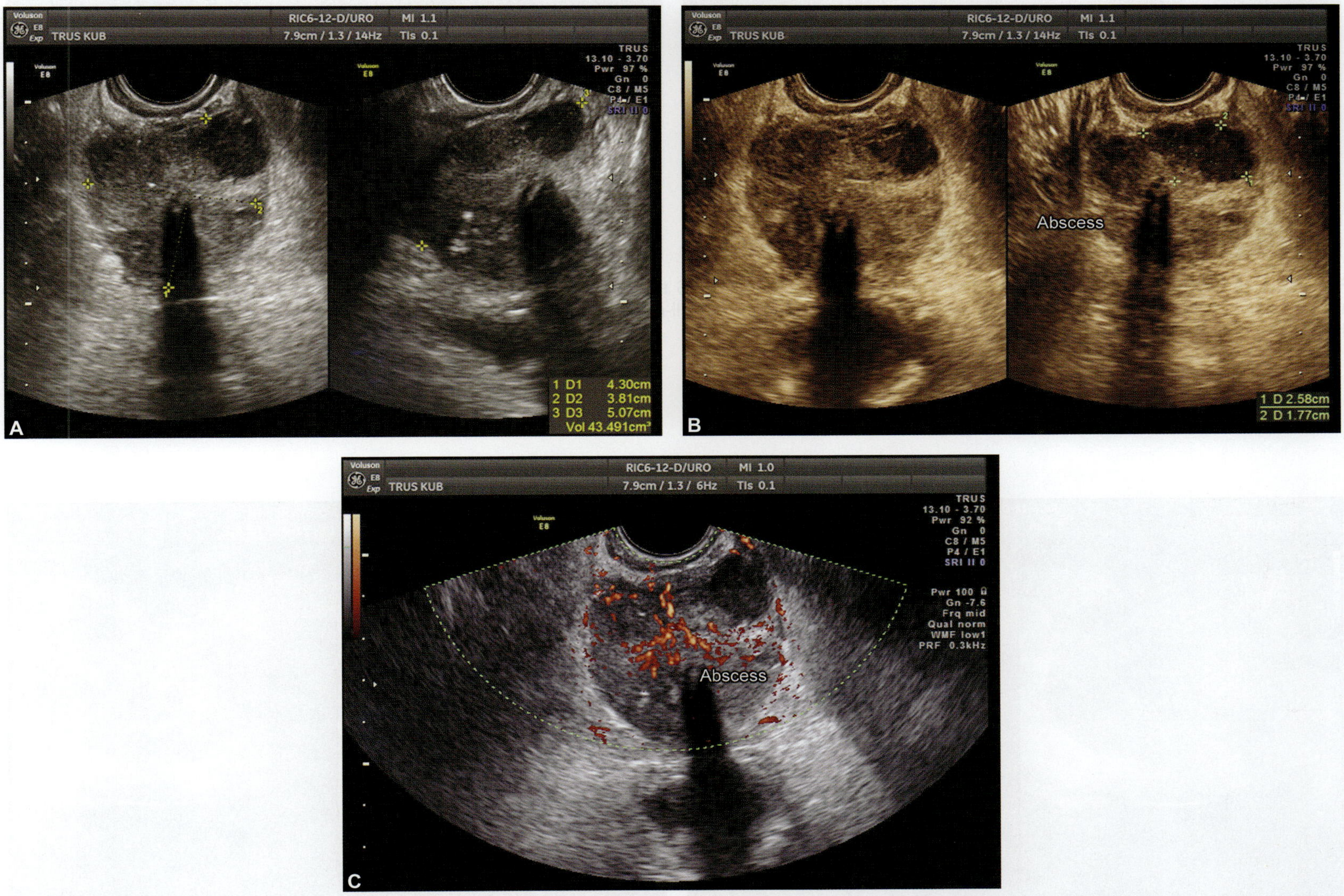

FIGURES 10.53A to C: Tubercular abscess. A patient presented with retention of urine. Transrectal ultrasound (TRUS) shows enlarged prostate. There is also evidence of a hypoechoic nodular shadow seen in the left peripheral zone. Margins are irregular and ill-defined. Biopsy of the mass confirms chronic tubercular abscess.

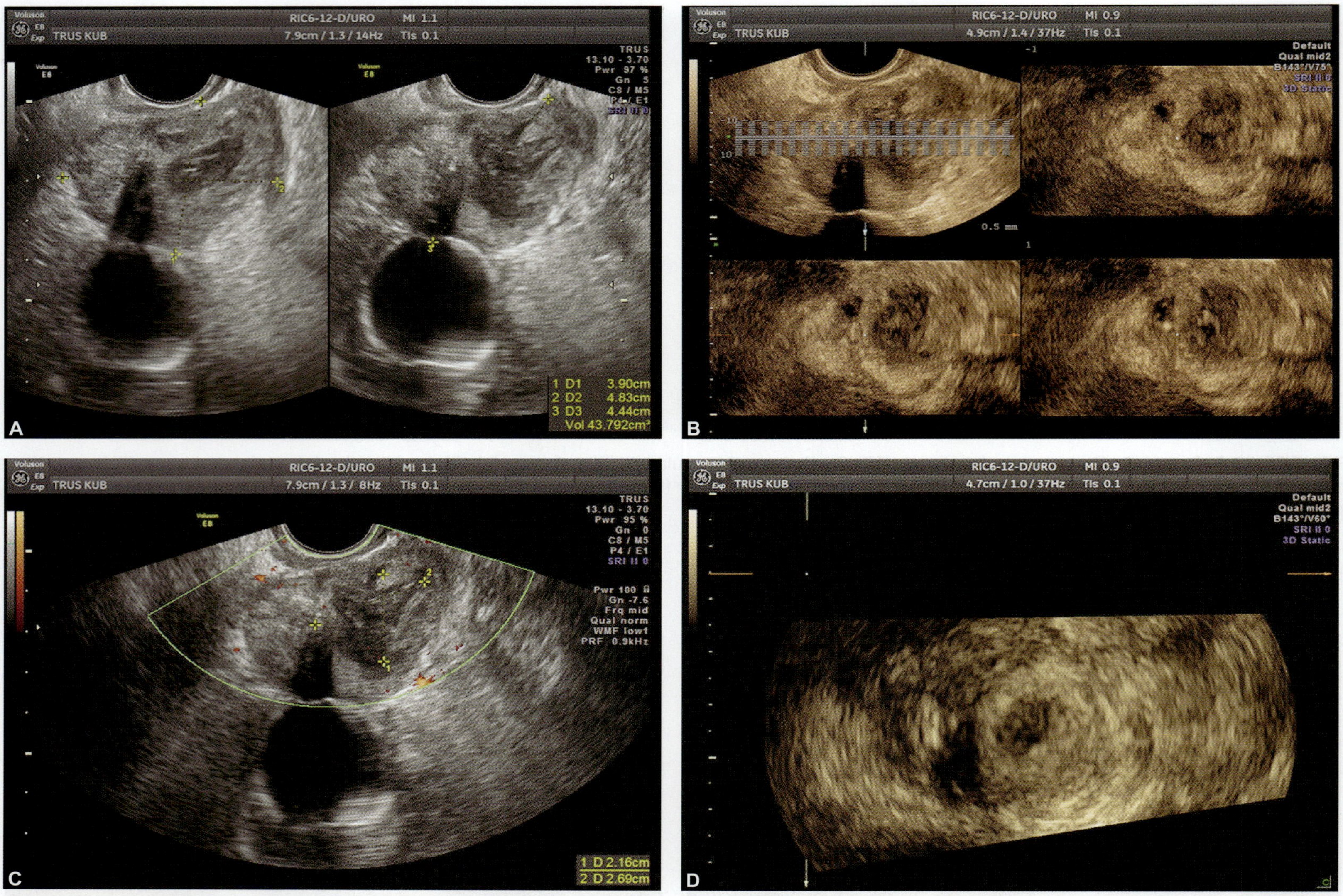

FIGURES 10.54A to D: A patient presented with retention of urine. TRUS shows heterogeneous texture and enlarged prostate. There is evidence of an irregular soft tissue mass seen in the left lobe of gland. Margins are ill-defined and inhomogeneous. No necrosis is seen in the mass. Biopsy of the mass confirms carcinoma prostate.

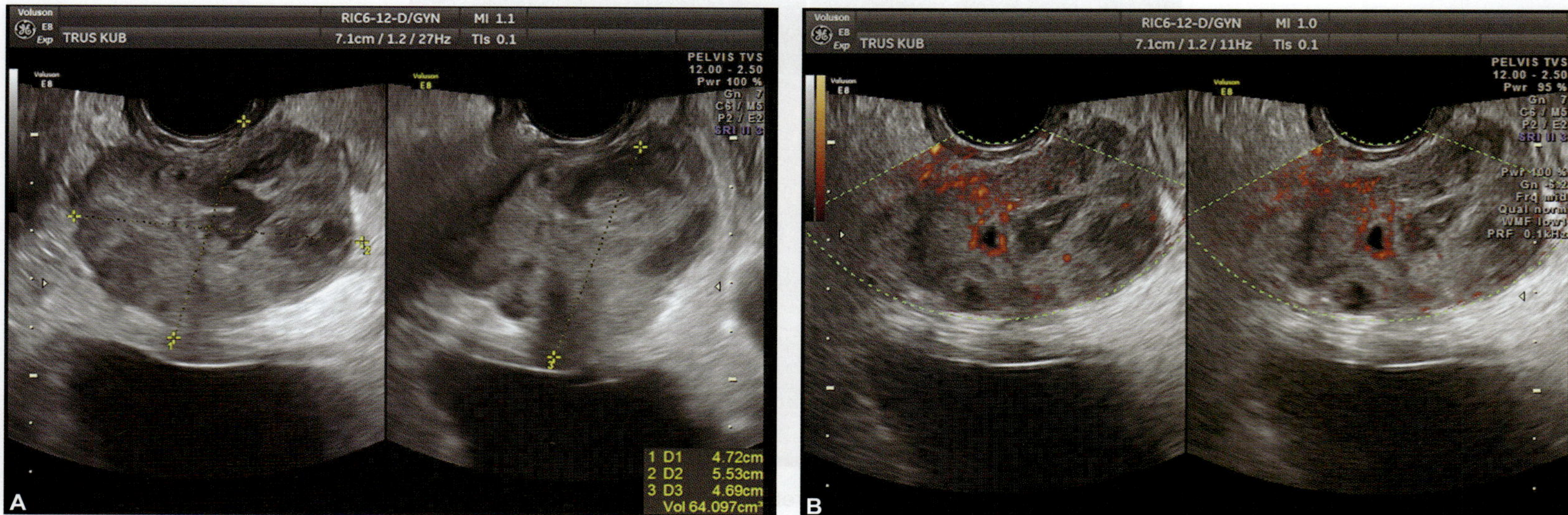

FIGURES 10.55A and B

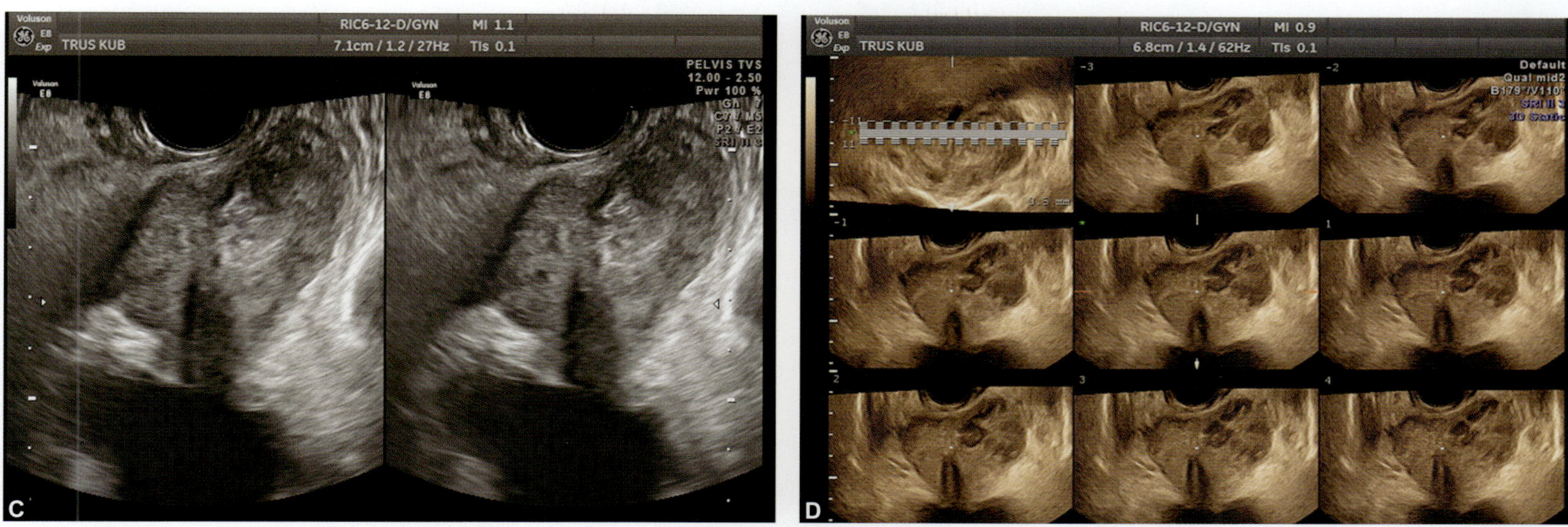

FIGURES 10.55C and D

FIGURES 10.55A to D: A patient presented with high PSA. Transrectal ultrasound (TRUS) shows heterogeneous enlarged prostate. There is also evidence of a big irregular heterogeneous mass seen in the left lobe of the gland. It is seen invading the transition zone and the peripheral zone. No necrosis is seen in the mass. The capsule of the gland is also seen invaded by the mass. TRUS guided biopsy confirms malignant mass. 3D tomographic ultrasound imaging (TUI) shows invasion of the capsule by the mass.

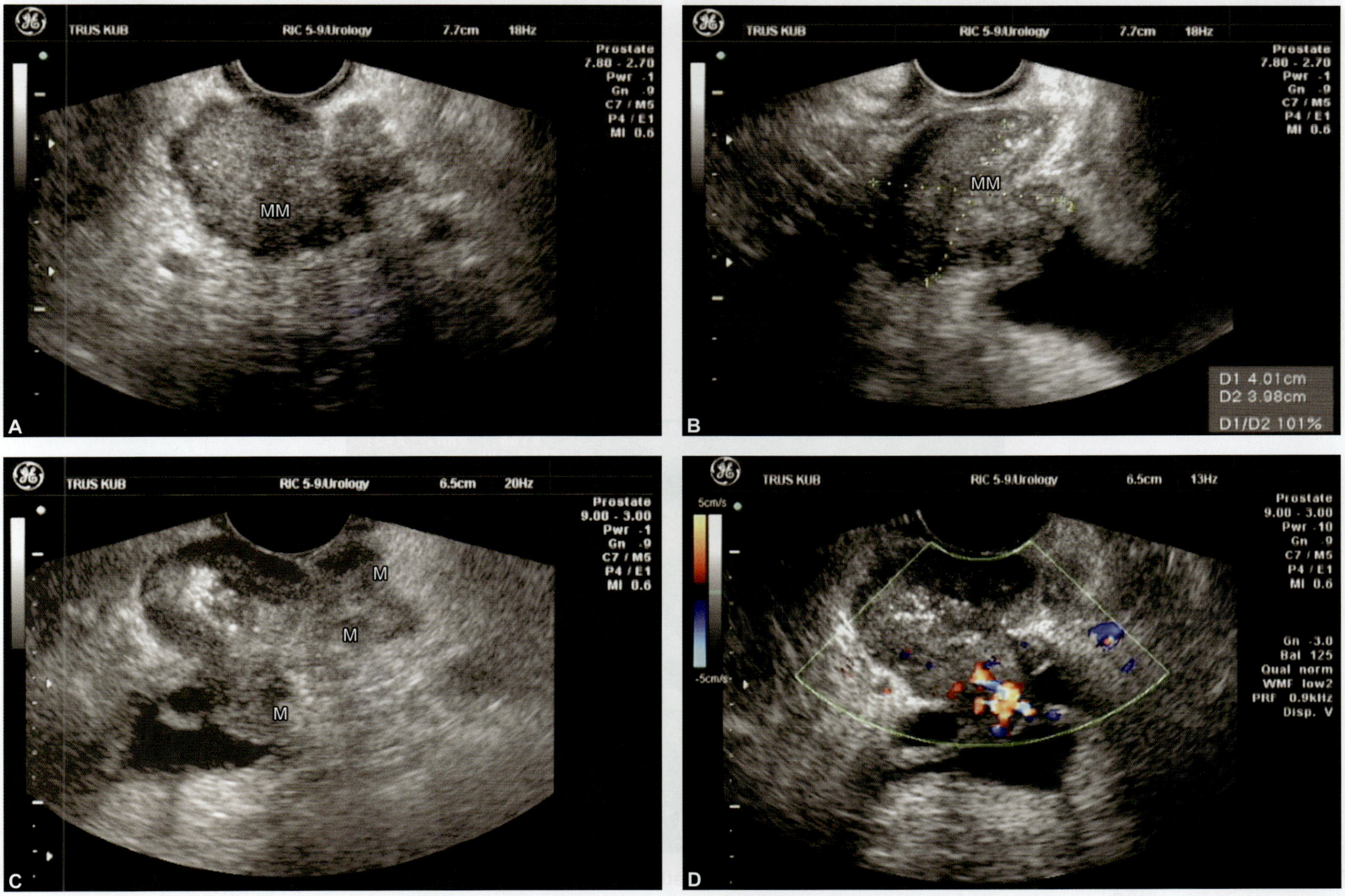

FIGURES 10.56A to D: Heterogeneous mass in the prostate with broken capsule and local invasion. HRSG shows big heterogeneous mass in the gland involving the left peripheral zone. The mass is seen breaking the capsule of the gland and invading the surrounding tissue. The inner mass of the gland is also seen invaded by the mass. On color flow imaging, increased flow is seen in the mass.

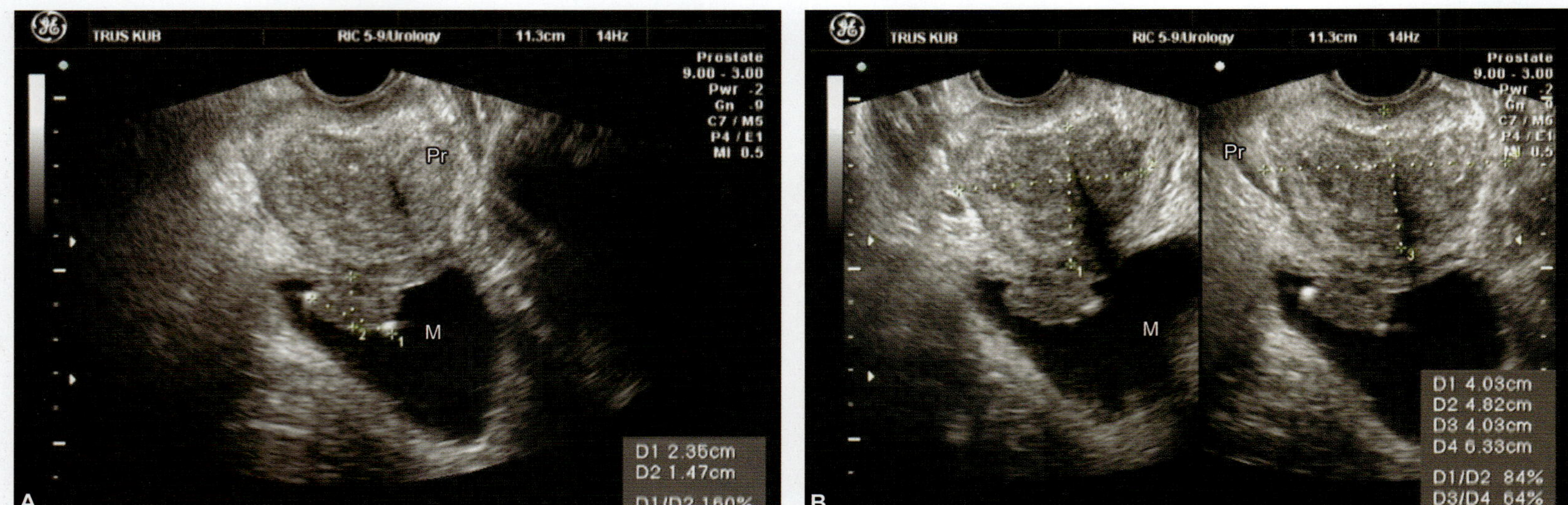

FIGURES 10.57A and B: Malignant mass of the median lobe. HRSG shows irregular hypoechoic mass coming out from the median lobe of the gland. The mass shows heterogeneous texture. No calcification is seen in the mass. Another mass is also seen in the inner mass of the gland and more confined to the right side. Biopsy of the mass confirms malignancy.

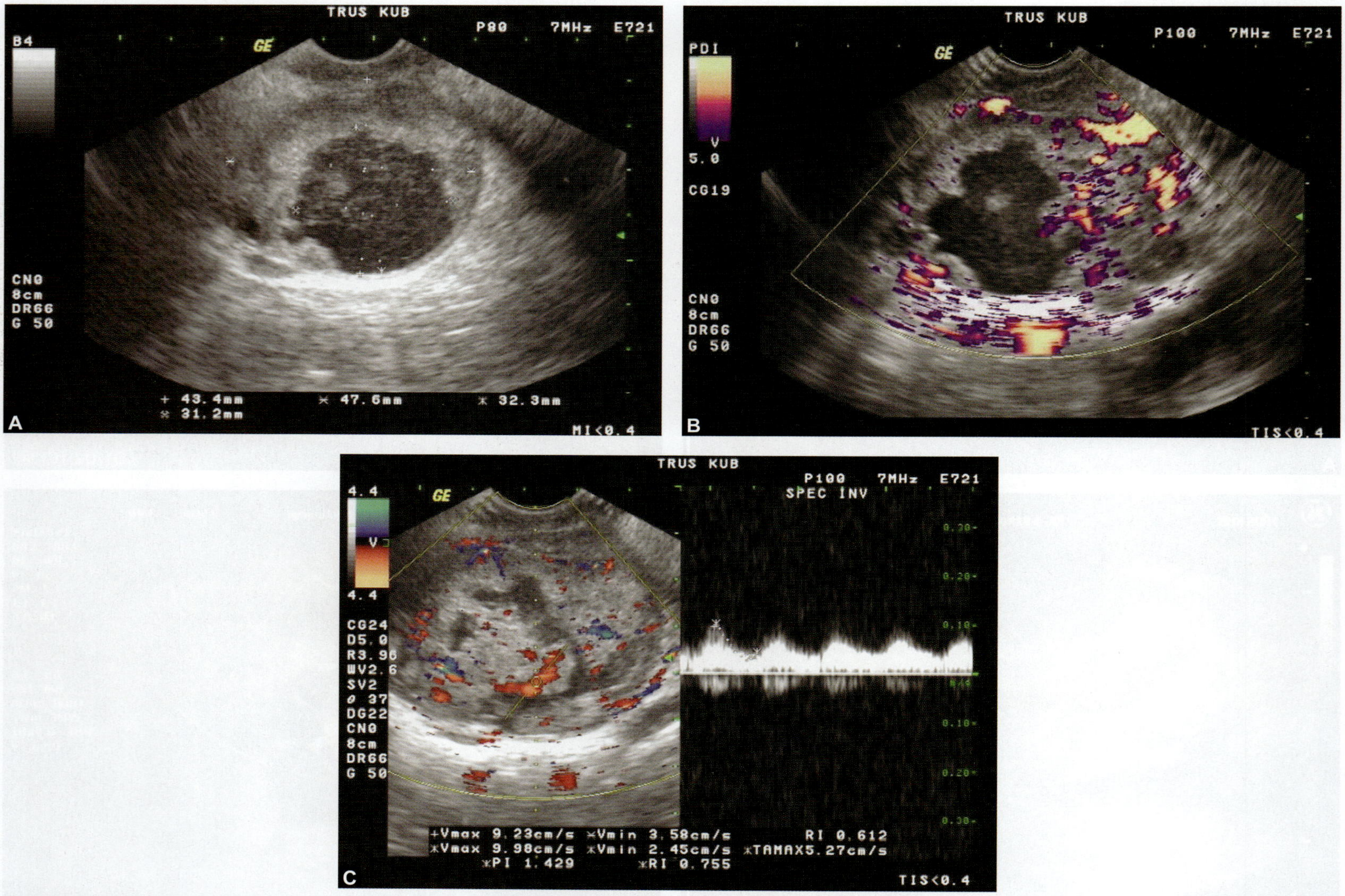

FIGURES 10.58A to C: Adenocarcinoma prostate with cystic degeneration. An old patient presented with heterogeneous prostomegaly. The PSA titer was very high. HRSG shows grossly heterogeneous prostate gland. Irregular cystic degeneration was also seen in the gland. The big mass is seen in the inner gland. Central area of necrosis is seen in it. On color flow imaging, high flow is seen in the gland. On spectral Doppler tracing, increased arterial flow is seen in the gland. Biopsy of the mass confirms adenocarcinoma.

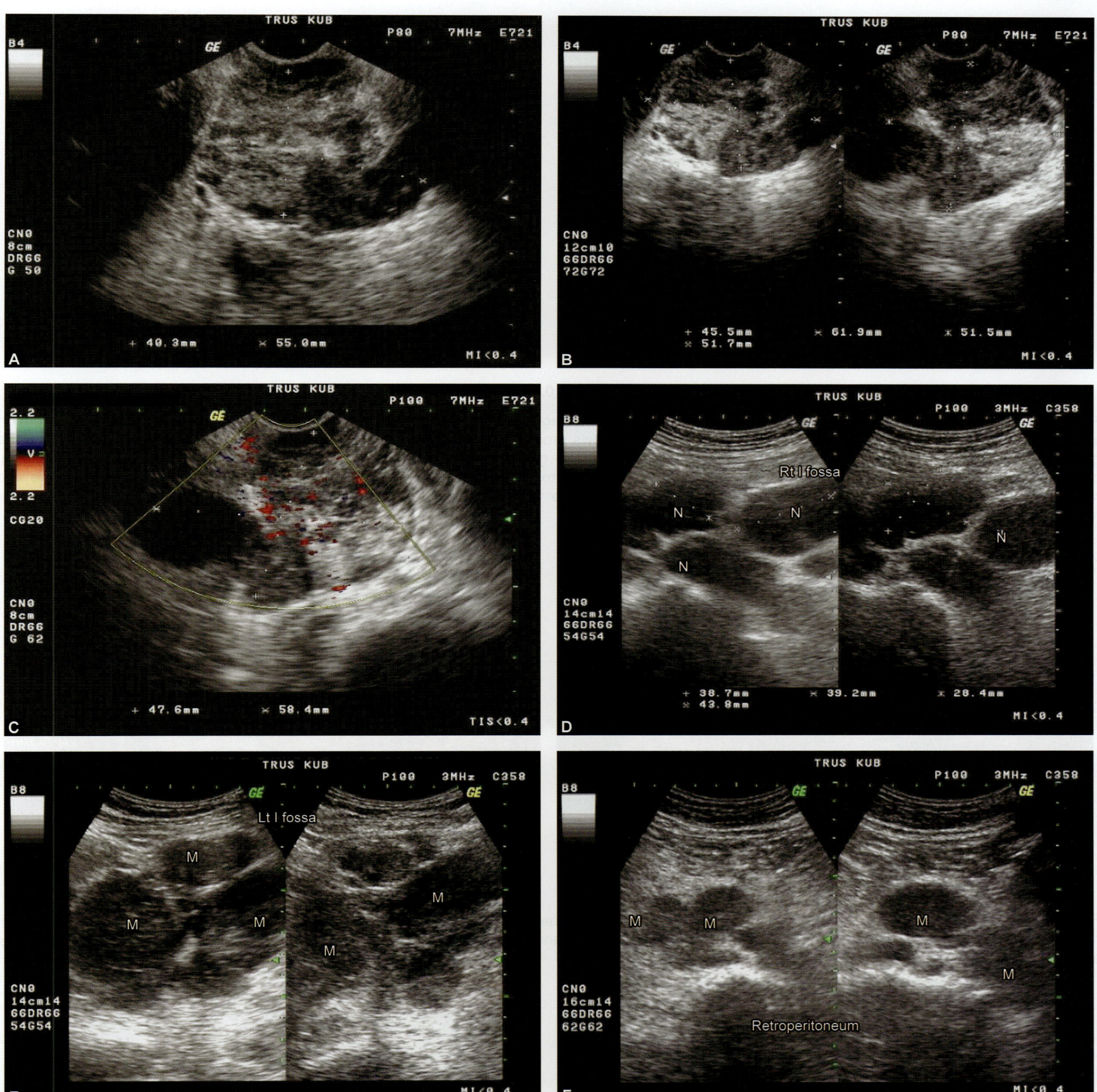

FIGURES 10.59A to F

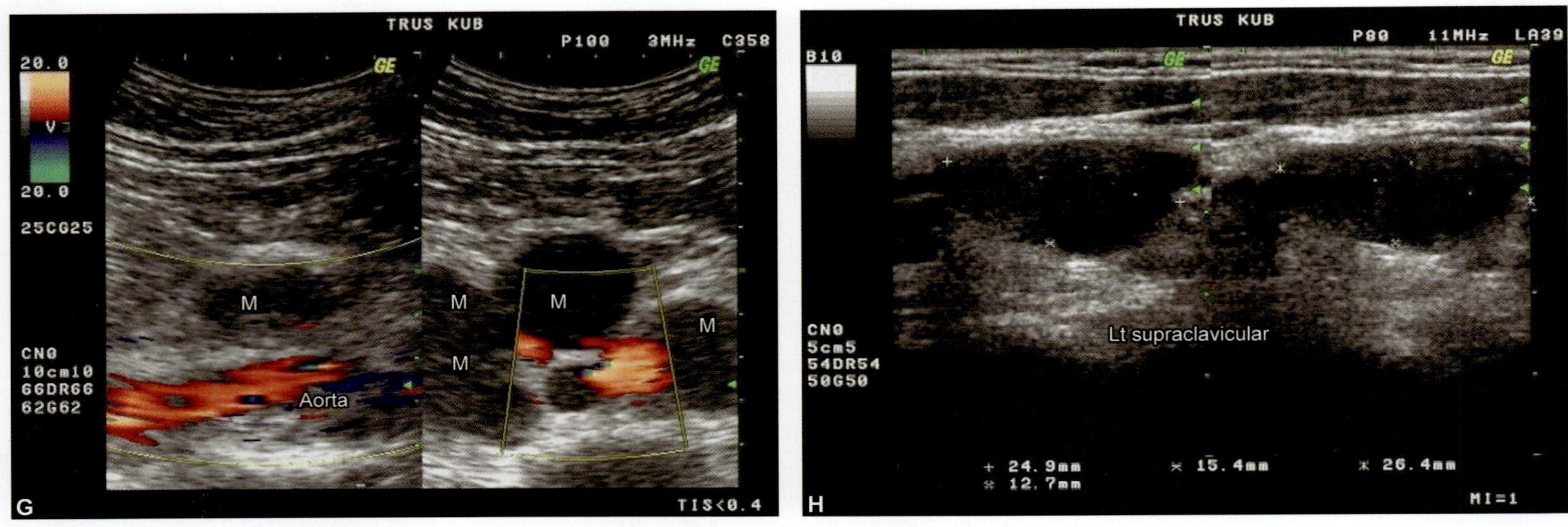

FIGURES 10.59G and H

FIGURES 10.59A to H: Invasive adenocarcinoma of prostate. A middle aged patient presented with markedly enlarged PCA with fever and discomfort in urination. HRSG shows enlarged prostate whole of the gland shows grossly distorted texture. Multiple irregular hypoechoic areas are seen in the gland. Cystic degeneration is seen in it. Capsule was seen broken. The gland was seen invading the surrounding tissues. On color flow imaging, poor flow was seen in the gland. Abdominal and neck imaging of the same patient showed multiple enlarged lymph nodes in both iliac fossae and retroperitoneum. Lymph node hilum was seen destroyed. Normal texture was lost. Multiple enlarged nodes were also seen in the supraclavicular region. Biopsy of the nodes confirms invasive adenocarcinoma.

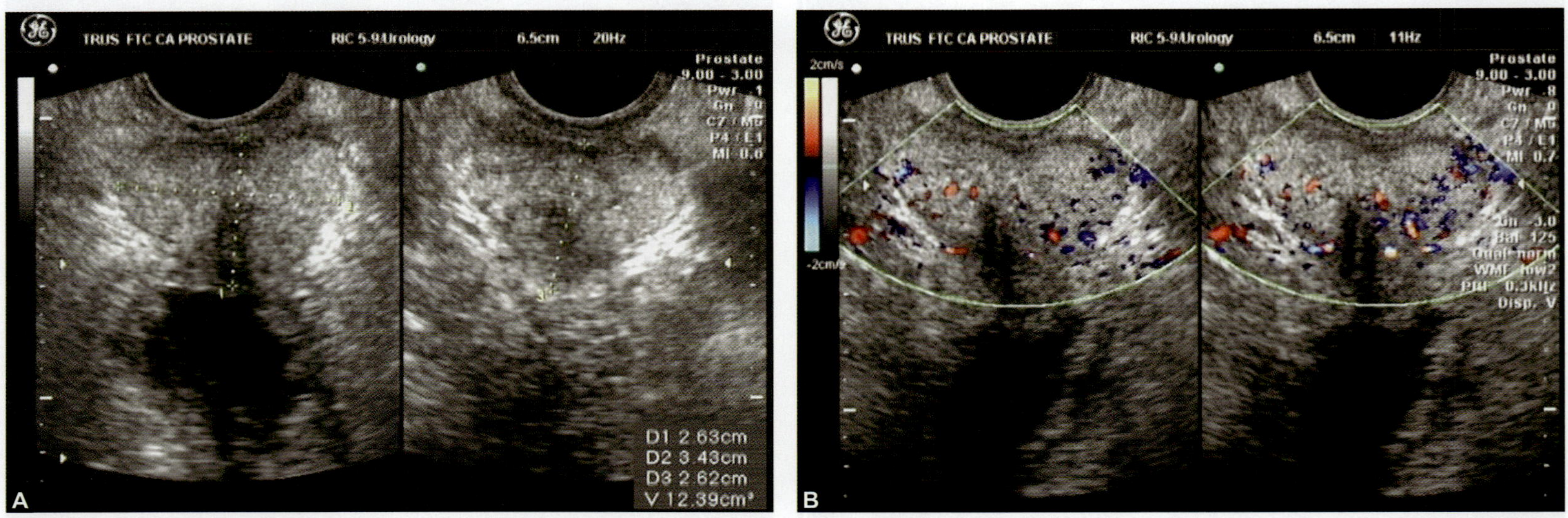

FIGURES 10.60A and B: The same patient after 6 months of hormone therapy for carcinoma prostate was examined. The prostate gland was seen reduced in size. Echotexture has become almost homogeneous. The gland got shrunk in size. The iliac, retroperitoneal and supraclavicular nodes also regressed in size. Patient responded well to the treatment.

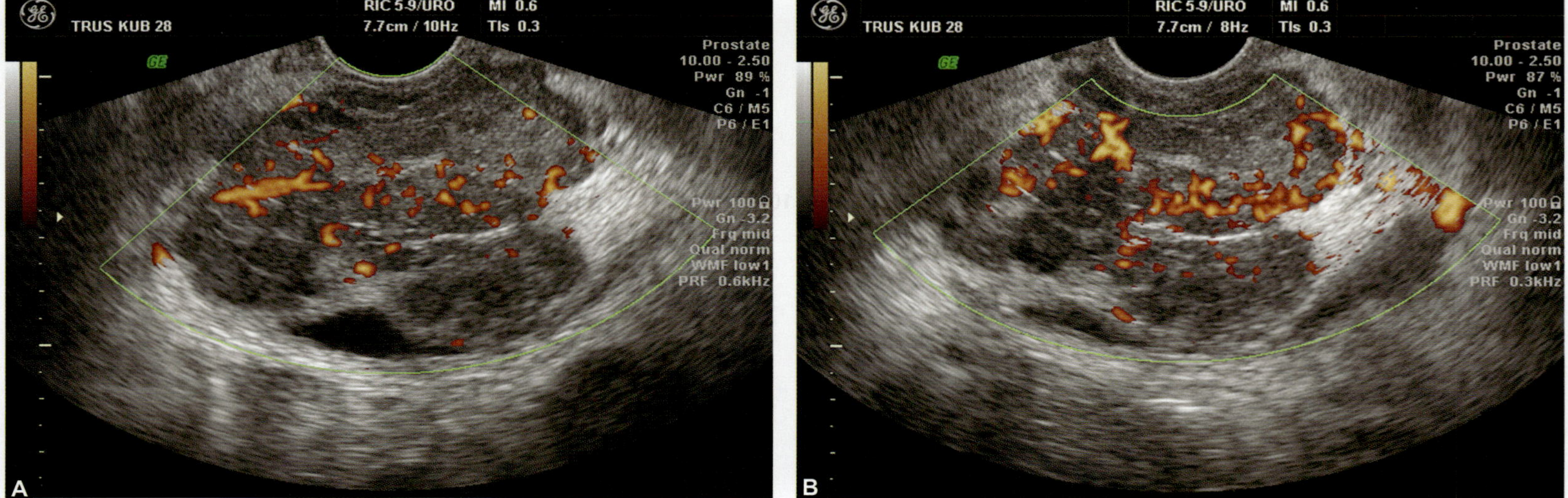

FIGURES 10.61A and B

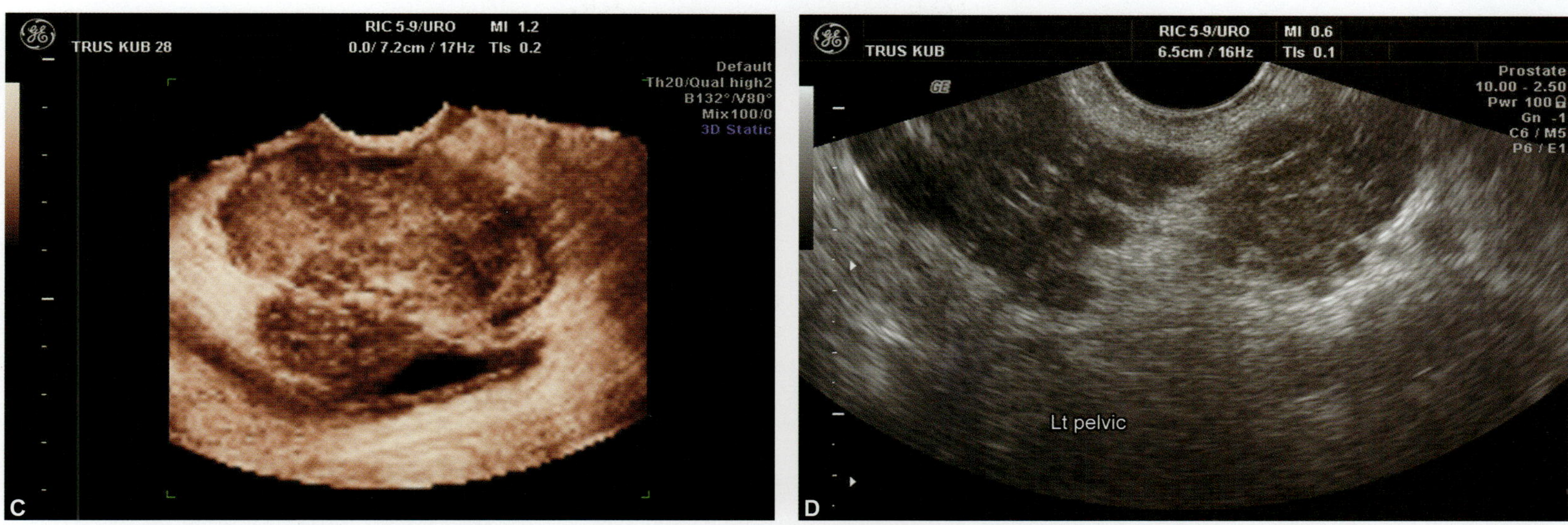

FIGURES 10.61C and D

FIGURES 10.61A to D: Invasive adenocarcinoma prostate with local spread. TRUS shows a grossly heterogeneous prostate gland which is enlarged in size. Margins are irregular in outline. Heterogeneous masses are seen in the gland. The capsule is seen broken. A big heterogeneous mass is seen in the median lobe. There is also evidence of nodal enlargement seen in the pelvis mainly on the left side. On color flow imaging, increased flow is seen in the gland. 3D imaging shows the details of the mass with capsular invasion. On color flow imaging, moderate flow is seen in the mass. Biopsy of the mass confirms invasive adenocarcinoma with local spread.

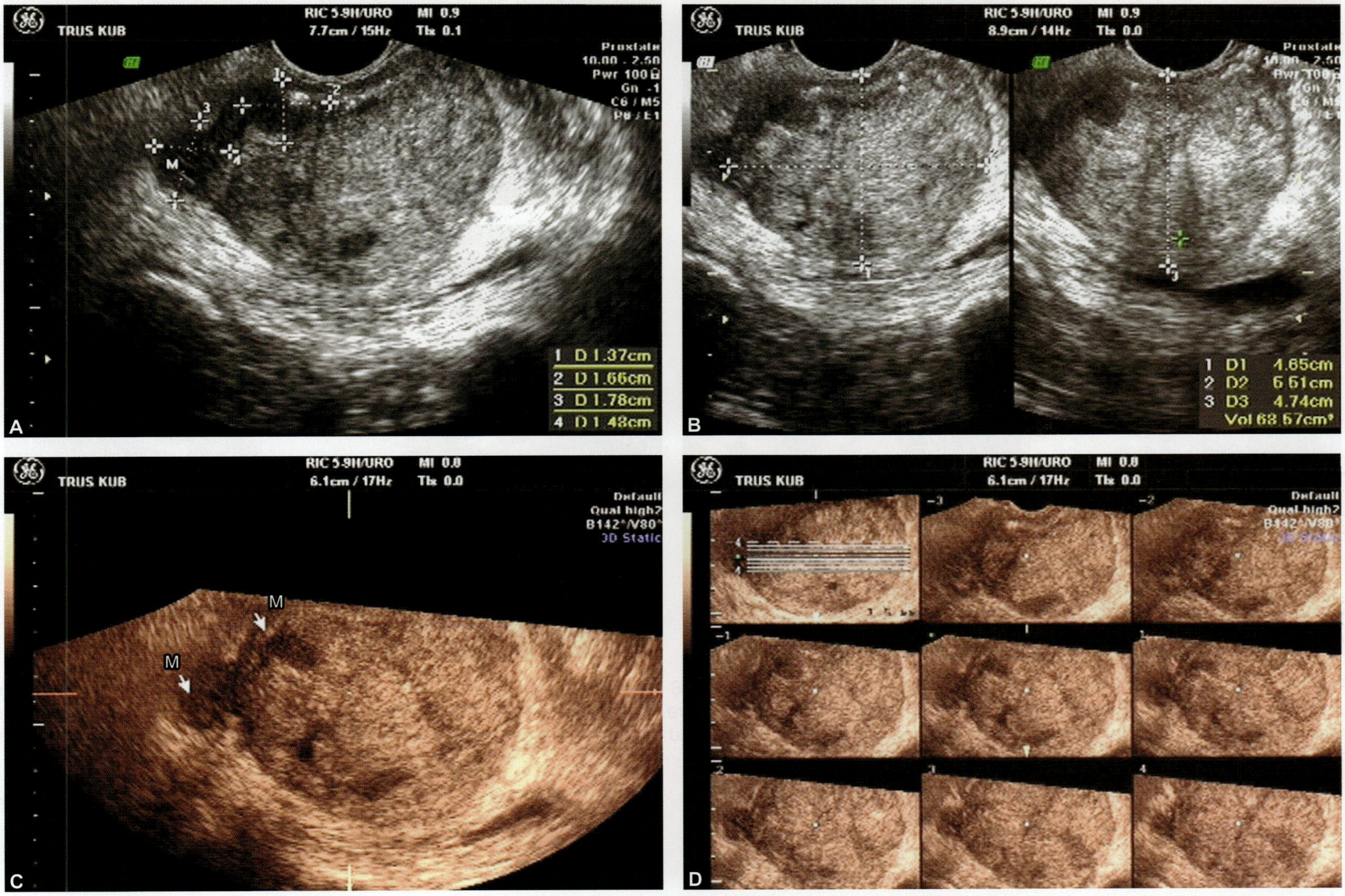

FIGURES 10.62A to D: Heterogeneous nodular mass with broken capsule. Transrectal ultrasound (TRUS) shows enlarged prostate with heterogeneous texture. Hypoechoic nodules are seen in the right transitional zone. The nodules are seen invading the capsule of the gland and extracapsular spread is seen. The 3D ultrasound with tomographic ultrasound imaging (TUI) clearly shows broken capsule and surrounding tissue invasion.

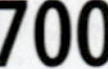

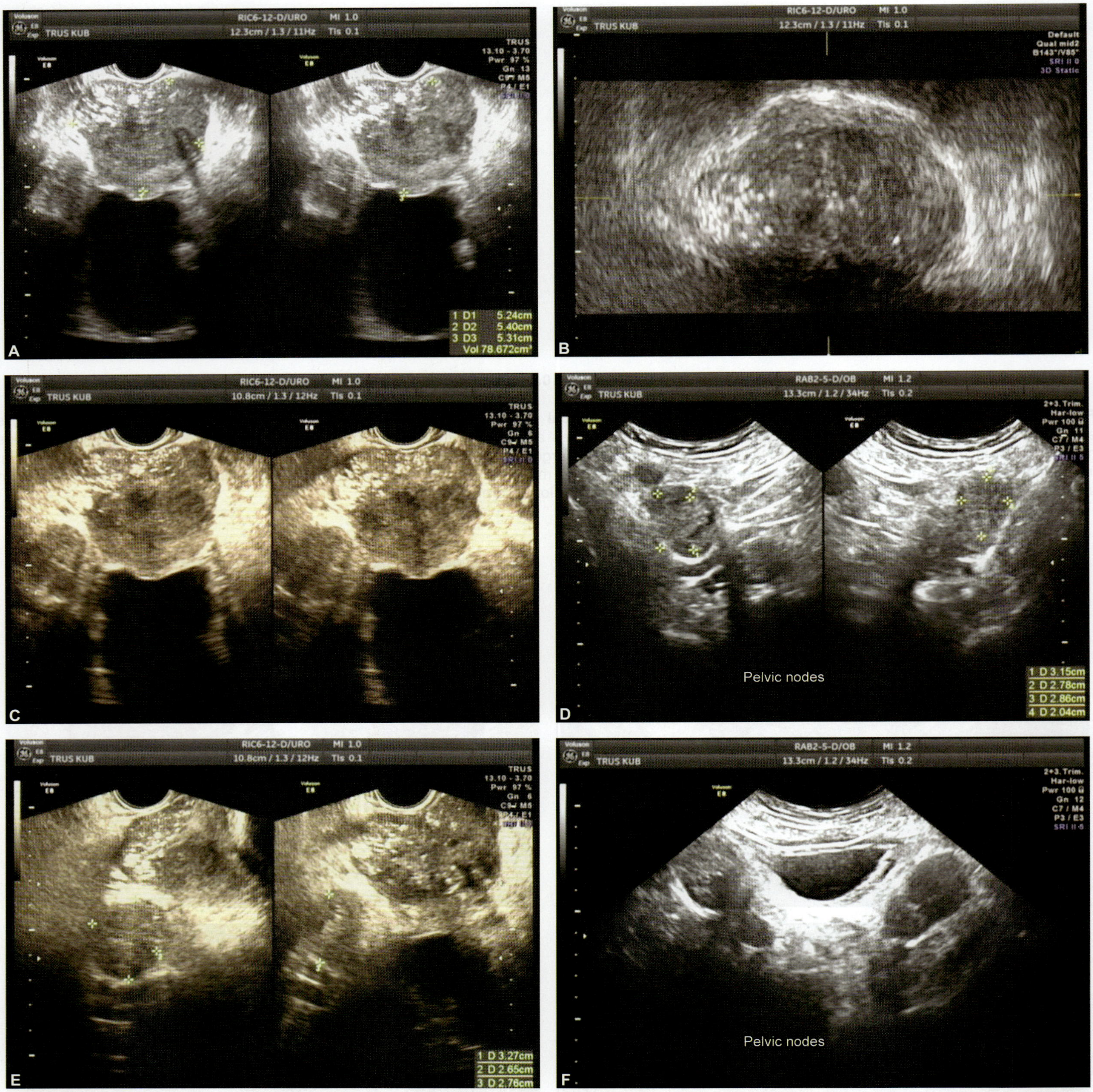

FIGURES 10.63A to F: A patient presented with enlarged prostate. TRUS shows heterogeneous enlargement of the gland. Multiple nodular masses are seen in the gland, which are ill-defined and inhomogeneous in texture. An echogenic nodular shadow is seen in the right peripheral zone. It is seen invading the capsule. Another nodal mass is seen in the inner gland. Multiple enlarged nodes are also seen in the pelvis. Biopsy of the mass confirms invasive adenocarcinoma with local spread.

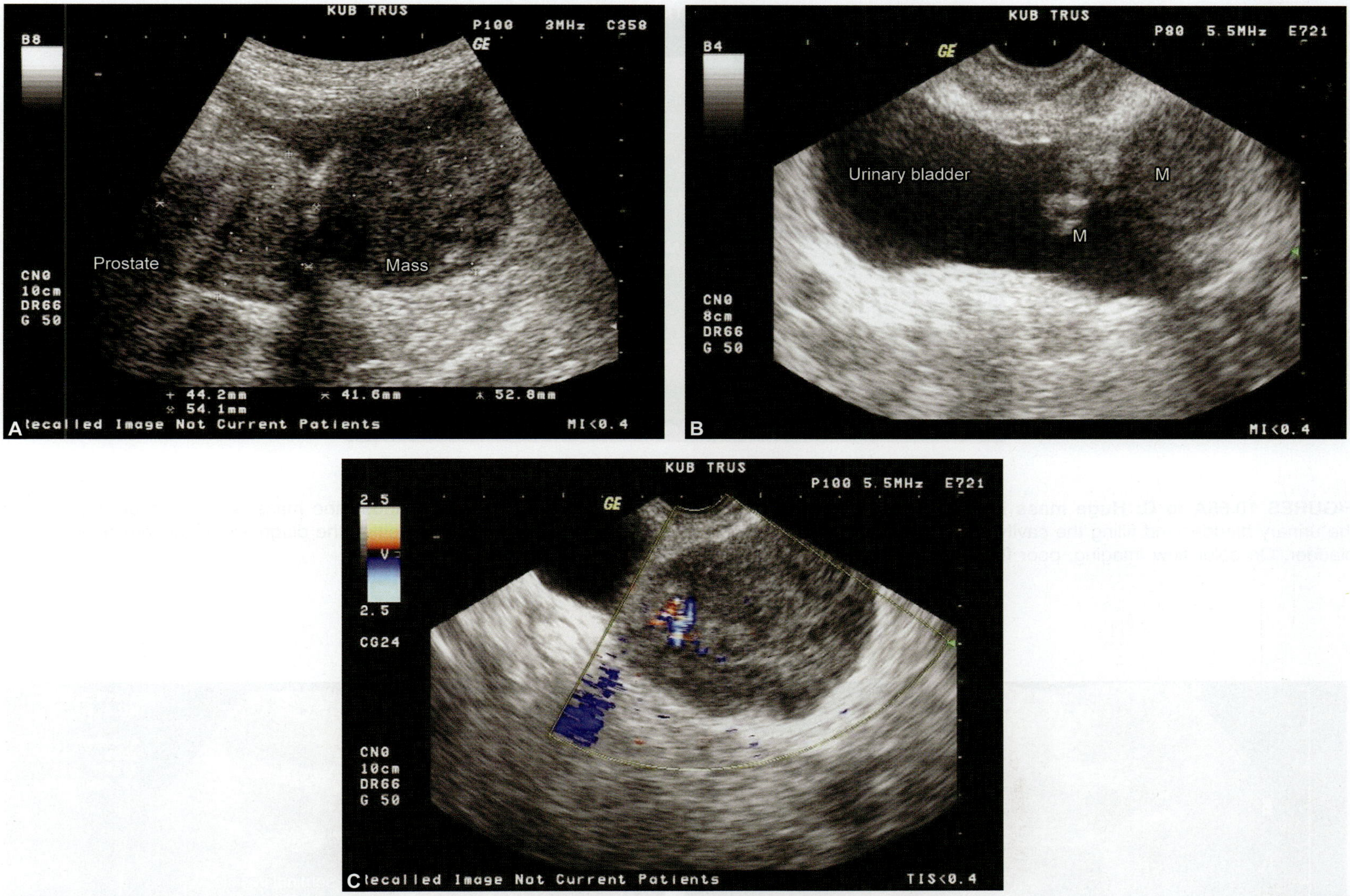

FIGURES 10.64A to C: Carcinoma urinary bladder presented with retention of urine. A patient presented with retention of urine. HRSG shows enlarged prostate gland. However, the gland was homogeneous in texture. No evidence of any focal mass was seen in the gland. But there was a growth seen hanging from the apex of the urinary bladder. It was irregular in outline. The growth is seen invading the urinary bladder wall. A big hypoechoic mass was also seen in the extra vasicle space. It was irregular in outline. However, it was separate from prostate gland. The biopsy of the mass confirms carcinoma urinary bladder with enlarged nodal spread to the pelvis.

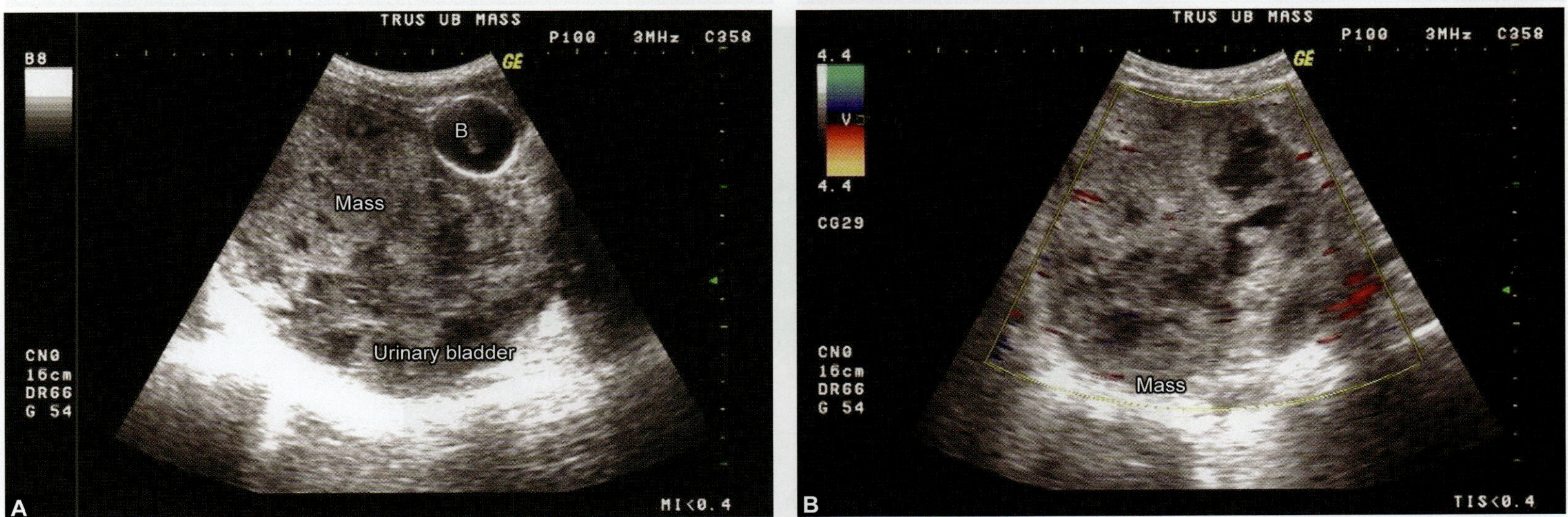

FIGURES 10.65A and B

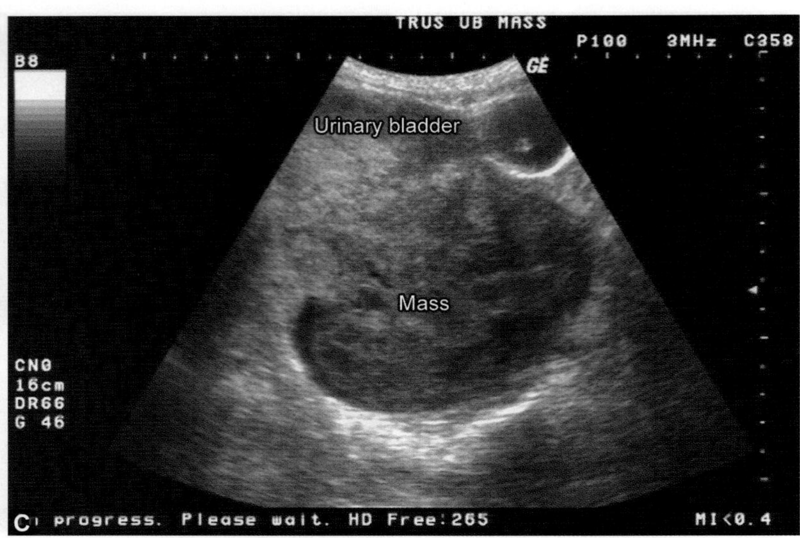

FIGURE 10.65C

FIGURES 10.65A to C: Huge mass in urinary bladder. HRSG shows a huge mass in the urinary bladder, the mass is seen occupying whole of the urinary bladder and filling the cavity. Clinically it was thought to be prostate mass. However, HRSG settled the diagnosis to be carcinoma urinary bladder. On color flow imaging, poor flow was seen in the mass.

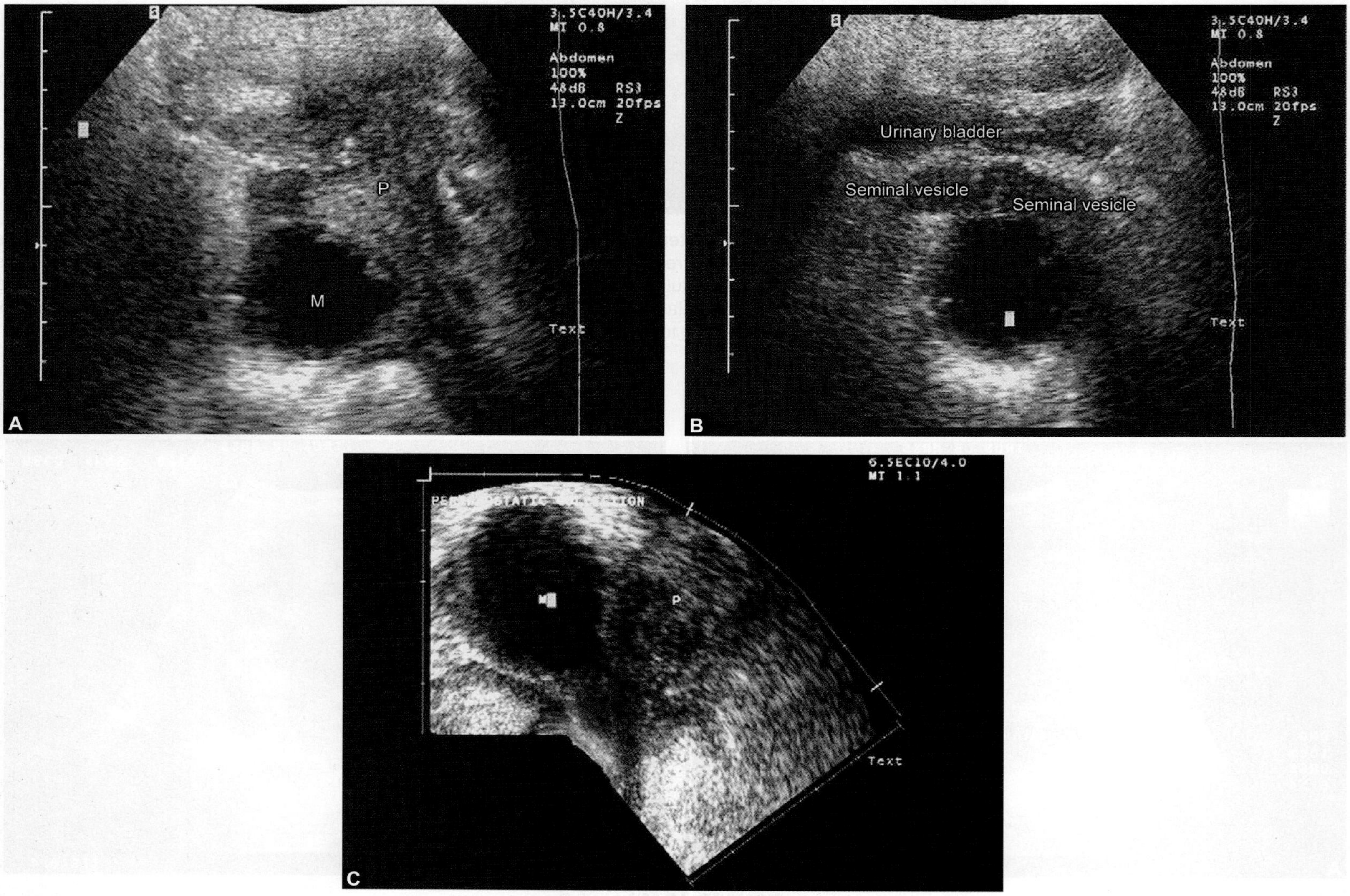

FIGURES 10.66A to C: Periprostatic fluid collection. HRSG shows low-level echo collection in periprostatic area. No septation or loculation is seen in collection. It is seen pressing over the prostate. The prostate gland is well-visualized. The fluid collection is seen separate from the prostate. Prostate seems to be normal in texture.

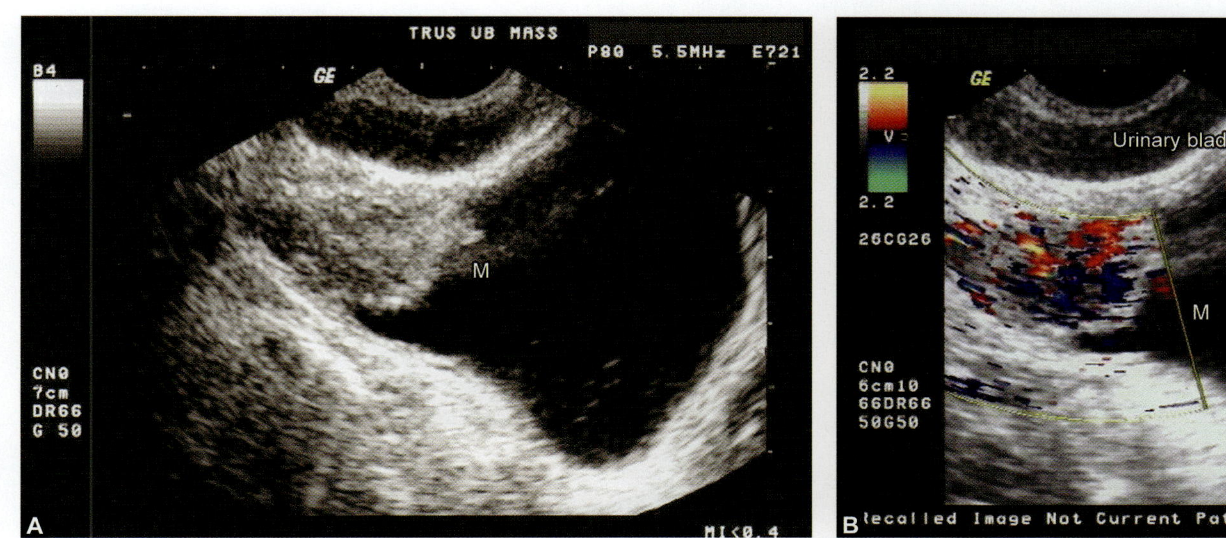

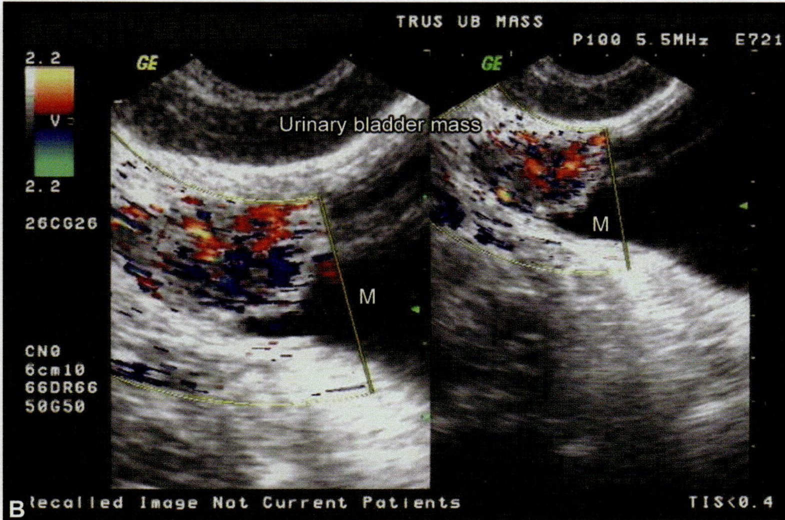

FIGURES 10.67A and B: Urinary bladder mass. High resolution TRUS shows mass hanging from the superior wall of urinary bladder. It is homogeneous in texture and well-defined in shape. No extra vesicle spread is seen. On color flow imaging, moderate flow is seen in the mass. Biopsy of the mass shows carcinoma urinary bladder.

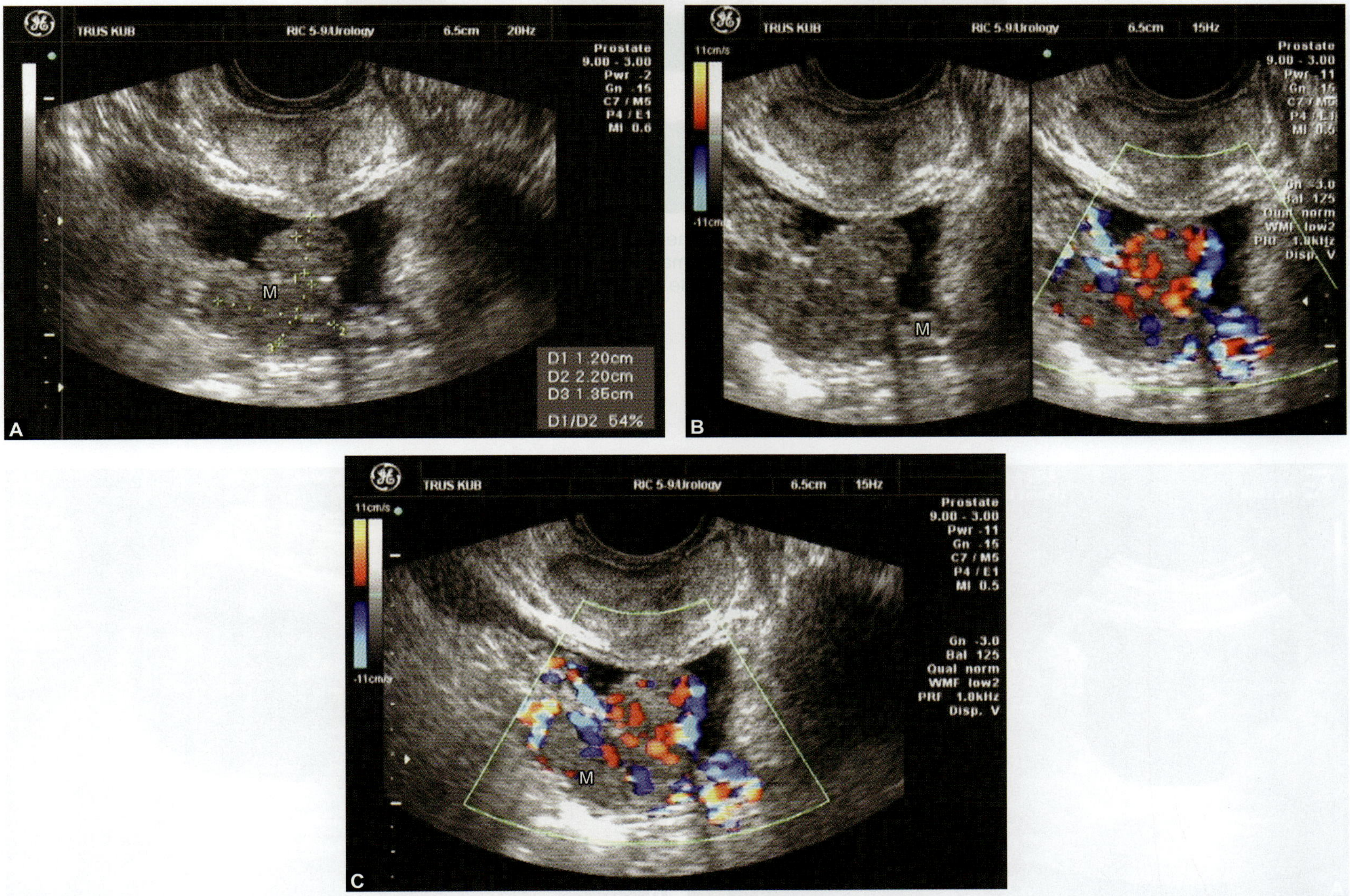

FIGURES 10.68A to C: Urinary bladder mass with bladder wall invasion. HRSG shows a polypoidal growth hanging in the UB. The mass is seen invading the UB wall and shows extra vesicle spread. No calcification or necrosis is seen in the mass. On color flow imaging, high flow is seen in the mass.

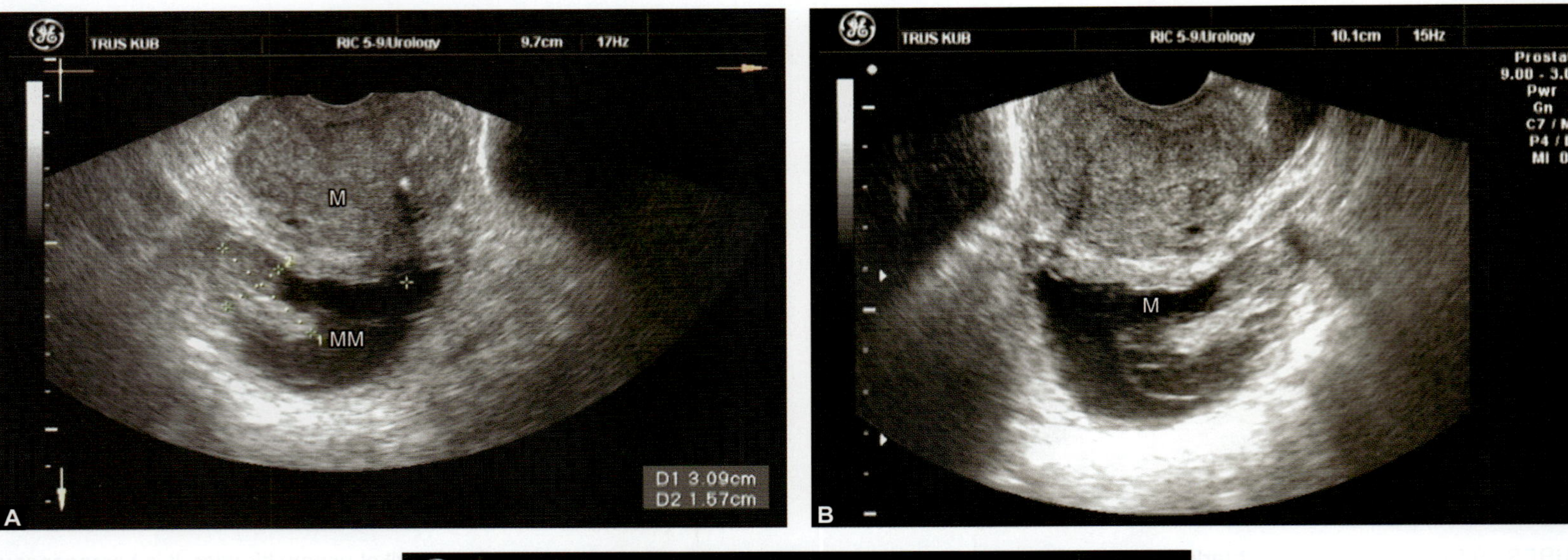

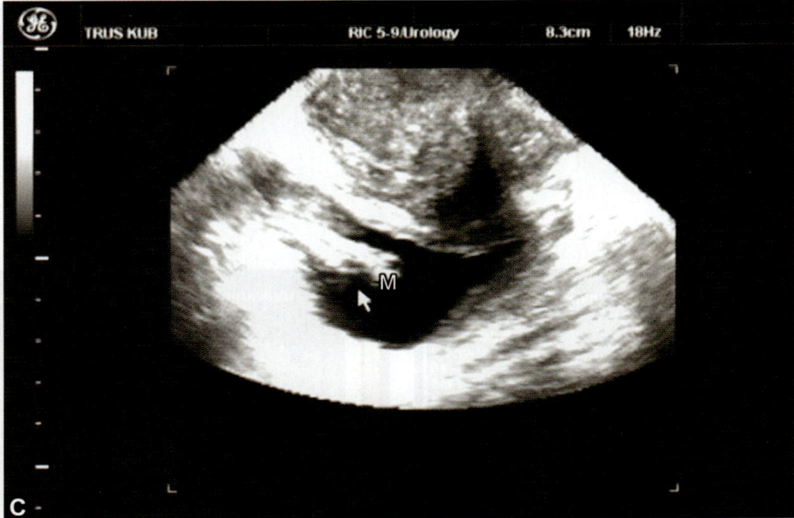

FIGURES 10.69A to C: Urinary bladder mass. A patient presented with hematuria and prostomegaly. HRSG shows an irregular heterogeneous mass fixed with the urinary bladder mass. Finger-like projection is seen in the mass. The mass is seen fixed with the urinary bladder wall. No calcification necrosis is seen in the mass. 3D imaging of the mass shows it separate from the prostate. Prostate shows homogeneous enlargement. No focal mass is seen in the prostate.

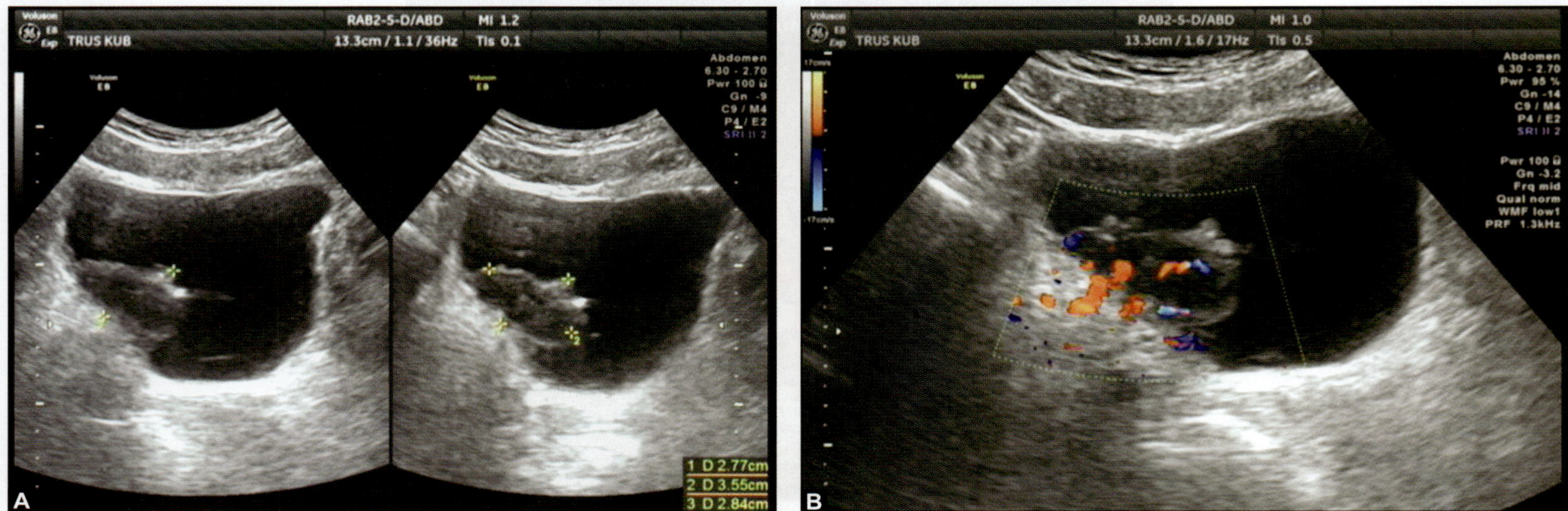

FIGURES 10.70A and B

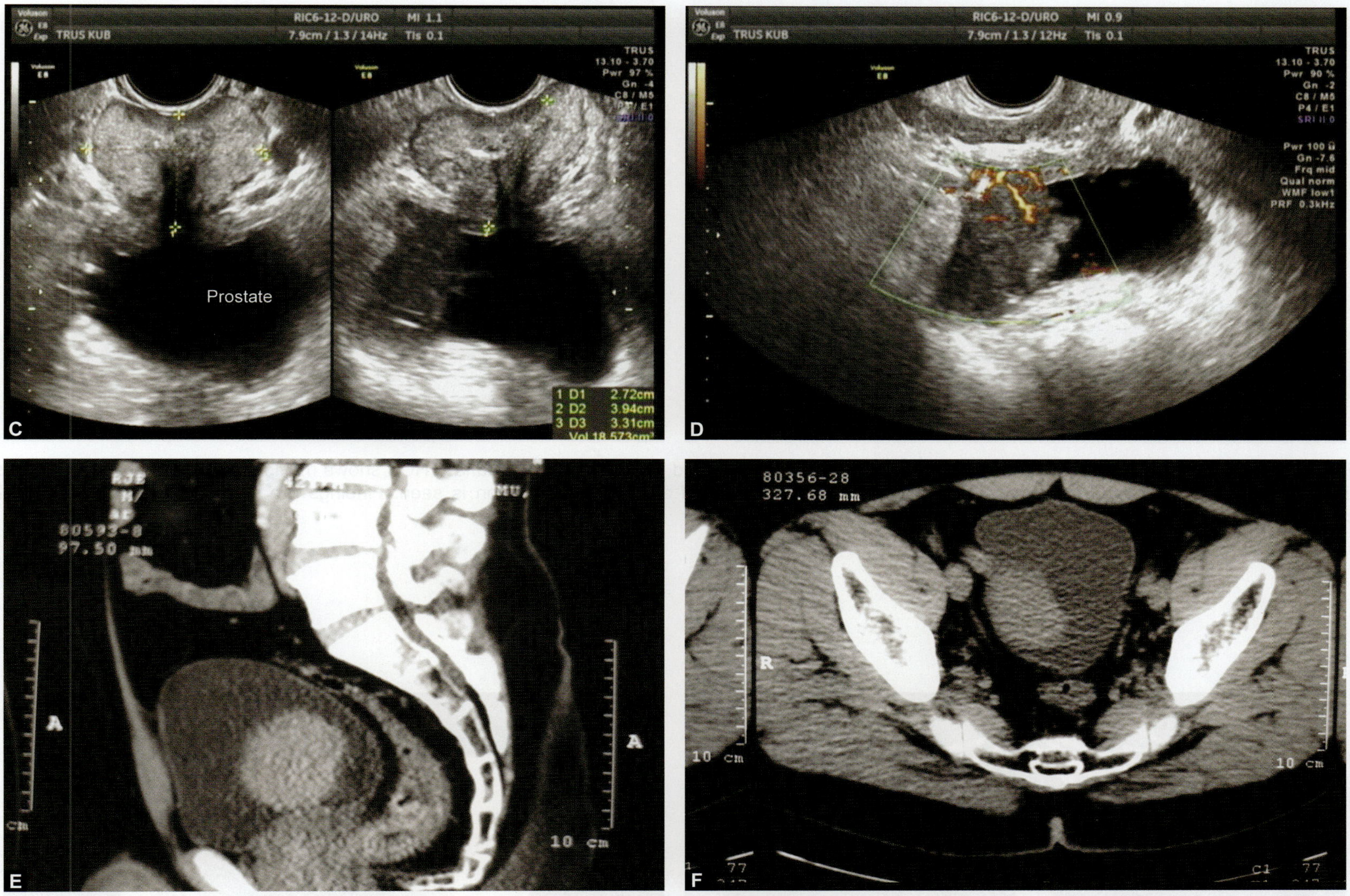

FIGURES 10.70C to F

FIGURES 10.70A to F: Urinary bladder mass with urinary bladder wall invasion. A patient presented with irregular hematuria. HRSG shows a big heterogeneous polypoidal mass fixed with the right lateral wall of urinary bladder. Transrectal ultrasound (TRUS) shows the mass invading the UB wall. On color flow imaging, multiple vessels are seen feeding the mass and also invading the UB wall. CT scan of the same patient also shows a soft tissue fixed with the right UB wall and also invading the UB muscle.

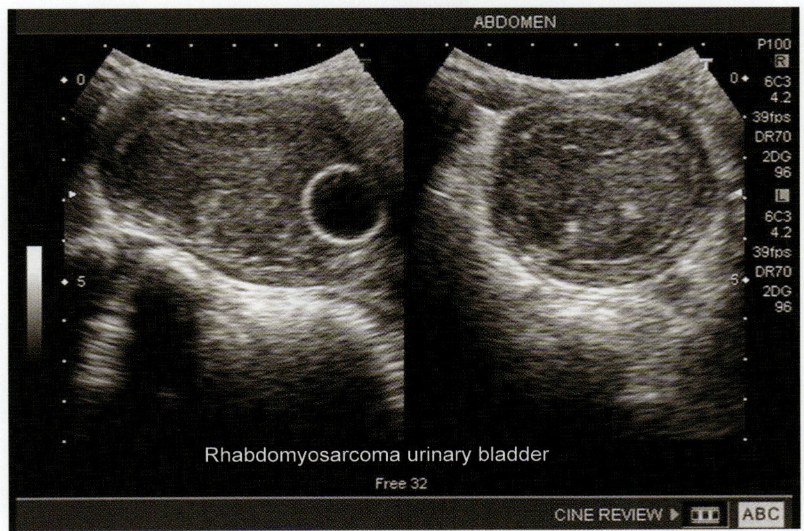

FIGURE 10.71: Rhabdomyosarcoma of urinary bladder. A 6-year-old boy presented with hematuria. HRSG shows a big heterogeneous mass in urinary bladder. It is seen invading the urinary bladder wall and also obliterating the lumen. Biopsy of the mass confirms rhabdomyosarcoma urinary bladder.

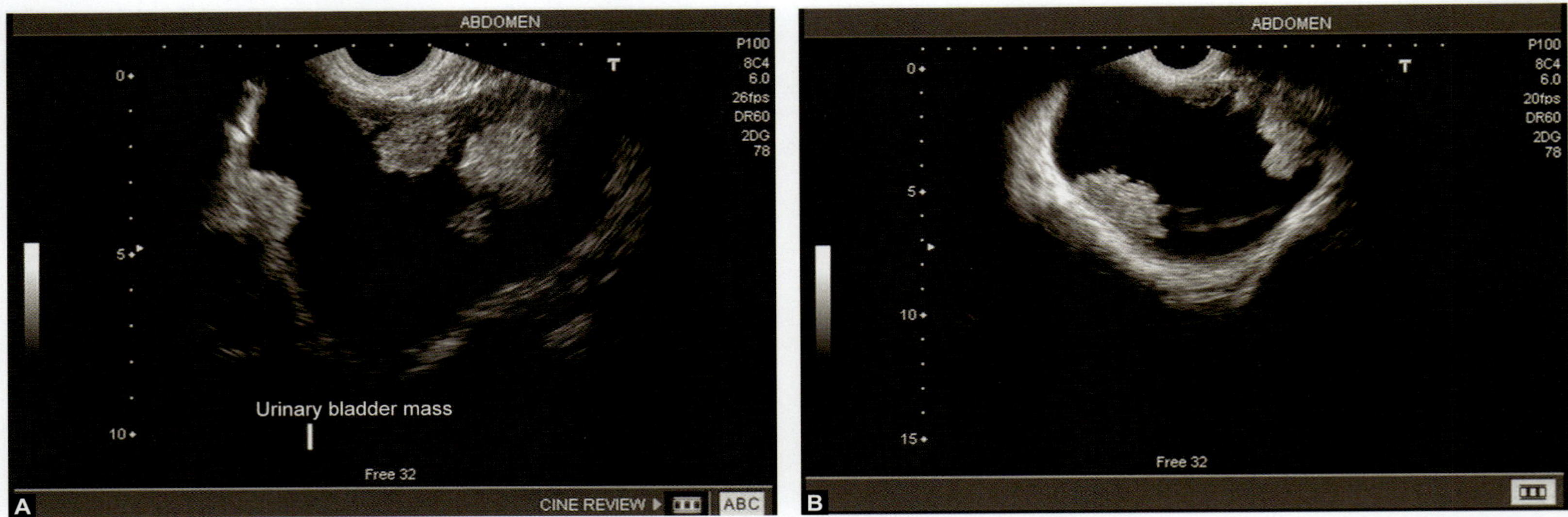

FIGURES 10.72A and B: Carcinoma urinary bladder. A patient presented with painless hematuria. TRUS shows multiple irregular soft tissue masses fixed with the UB wall. They show small projections. But no evidence of any UB wall invasion is seen. Findings are suggestive of transitional cell carcinoma urinary bladder.

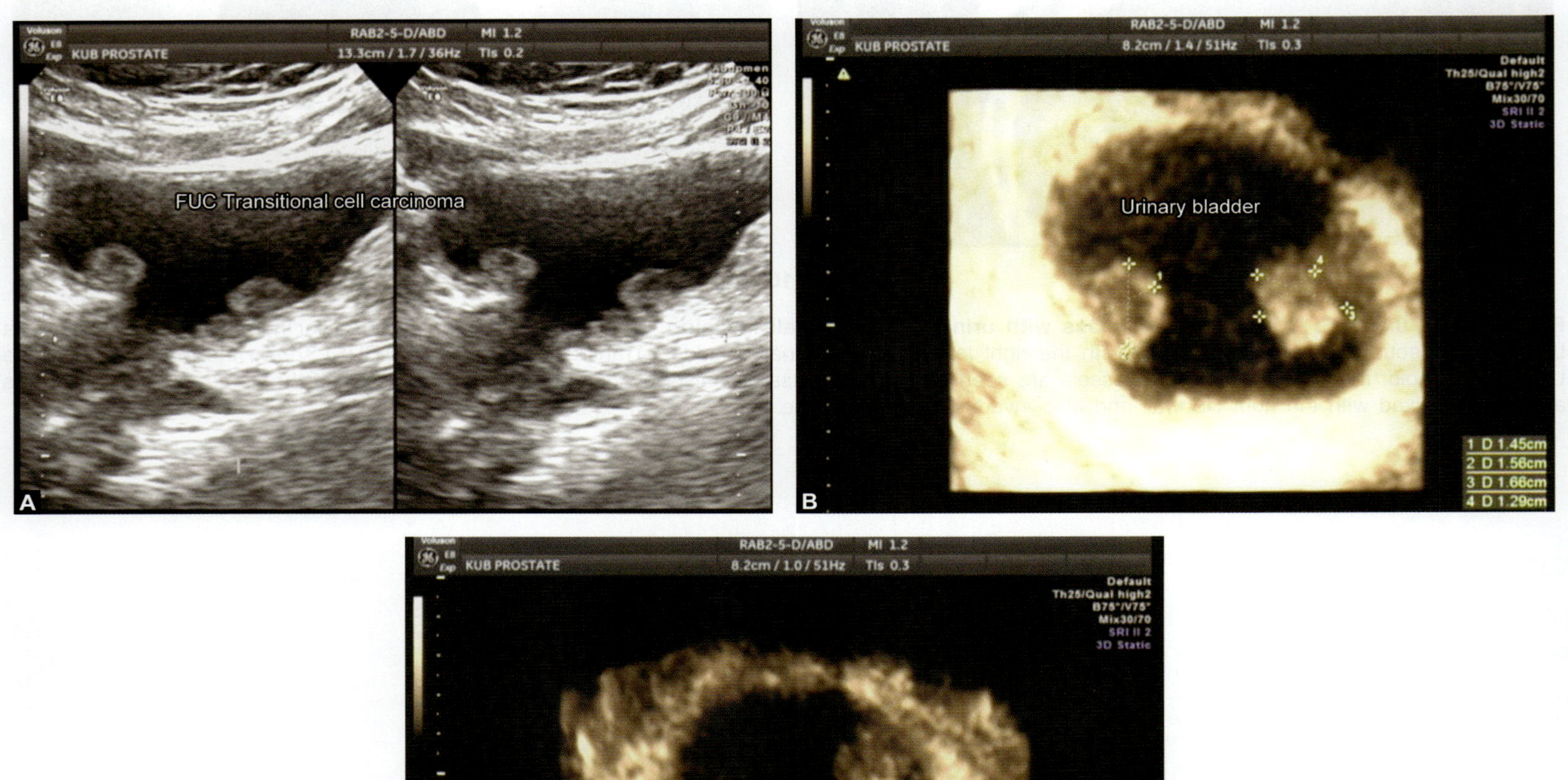

FIGURES 10.73A to C: FUC of transitional cell carcinoma. A known case of transitional cell carcinoma urinary bladder presented with hematuria. Transrectal ultrasound (TRUS) shows multiple cauliflowers growth fixed with the UB wall suggestive of recurrence of disease.

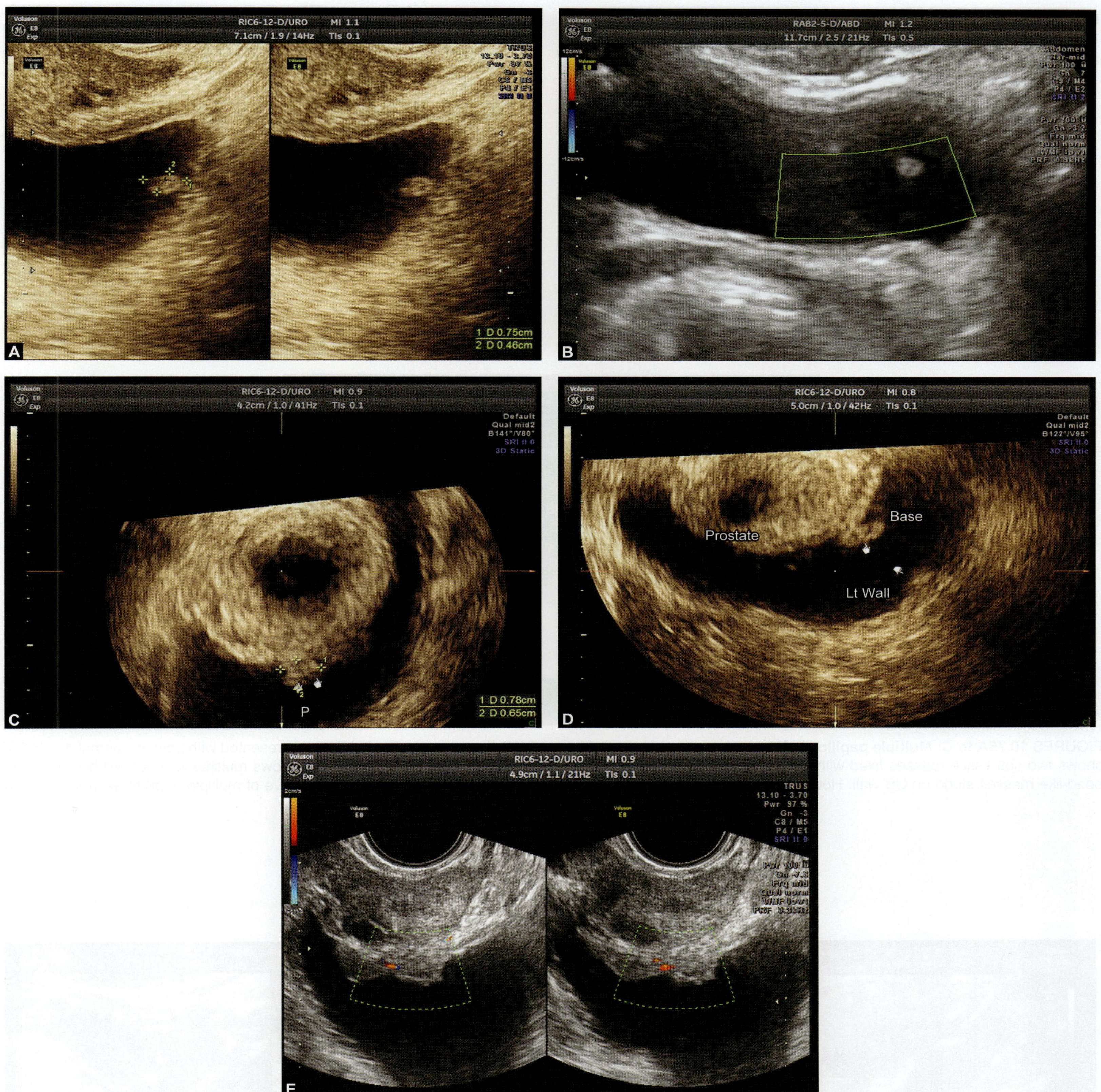

FIGURES 10.74A to E: UB wall papilloma (3D sonocystoscopy). A patient presented with painless hematuria. TRUS with 3D imaging shows three well-defined soft tissue masses. They are small in size and smooth in outline. They are seen fixed with the urinary bladder wall at the base and on left lateral wall and right lateral wall of carcinoma urinary bladder (UB). 3D imaging shows the masses very clearly. On color flow imaging, low flow is seen in them. The masses are confined to the mucosal wall. But no UB wall invasion is seen. Findings are suggestive of multiple small papilomas in UB.

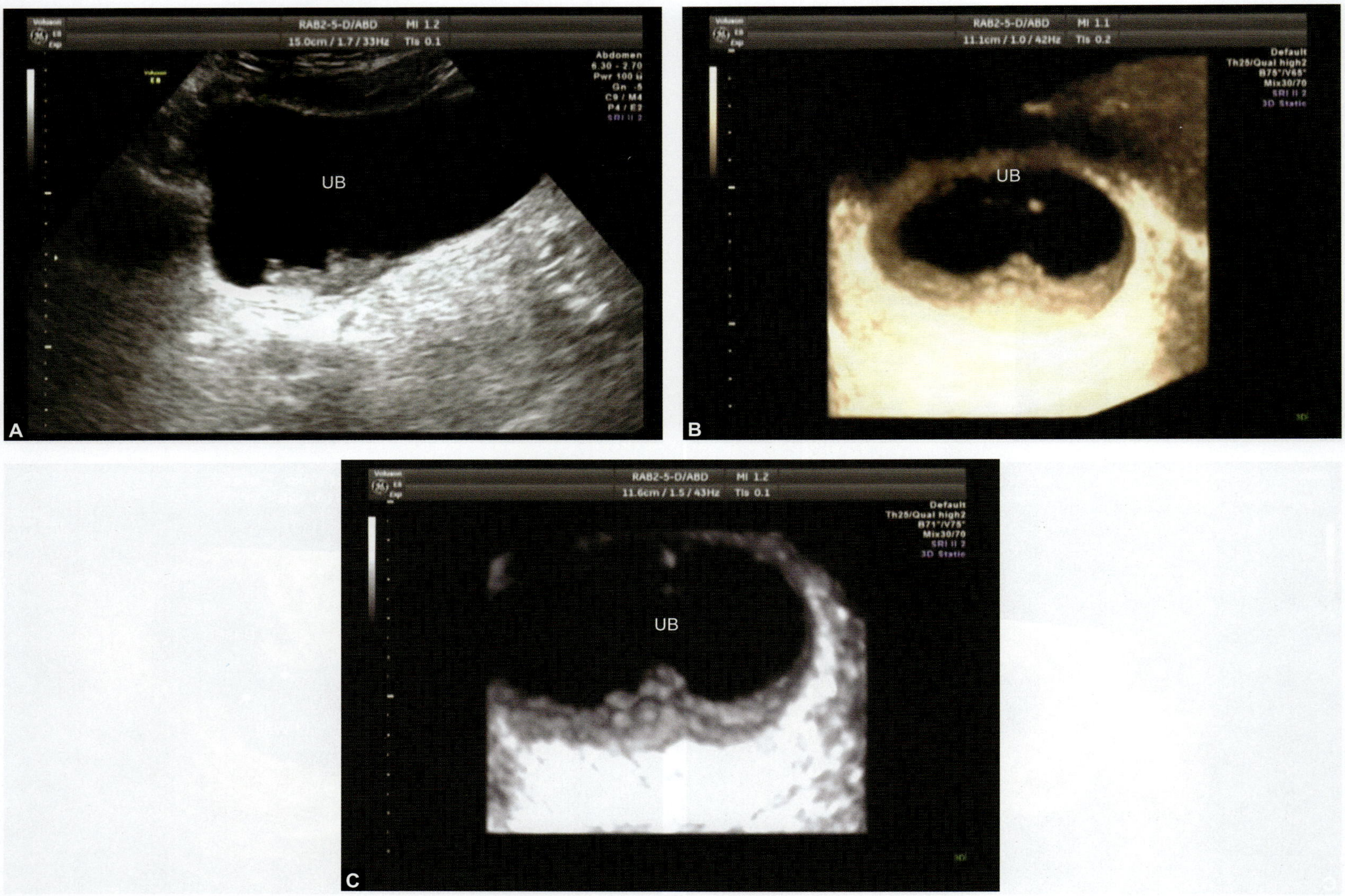

FIGURES 10.75A to C: Multiple papillomas in carcinoma urinary bladder wall (3D sonocystoscopy). A patient presented with painless hematuria. HRSG shows two soft tissue masses fixed with carcinoma urinary bladder wall. Transrectal ultrasound with 3D imaging shows multiple well-defined homogeneous bead-like masses studd on UB wall. However, no suggestion of any UB wall invasion is seen. Findings are suggestive of multiple papillomas in the UB wall.

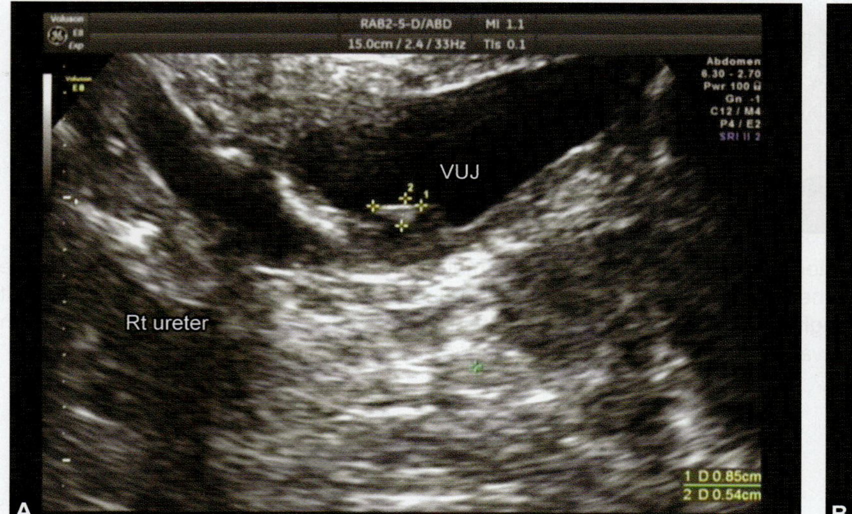

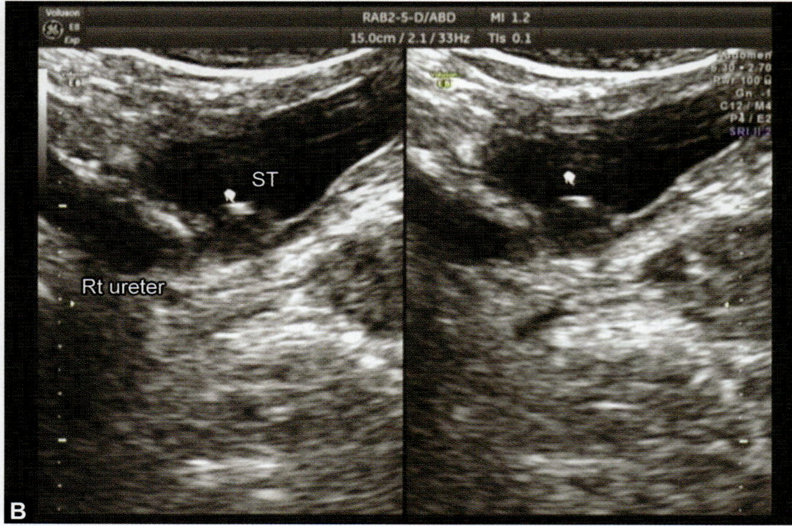

FIGURES 10.76A and B

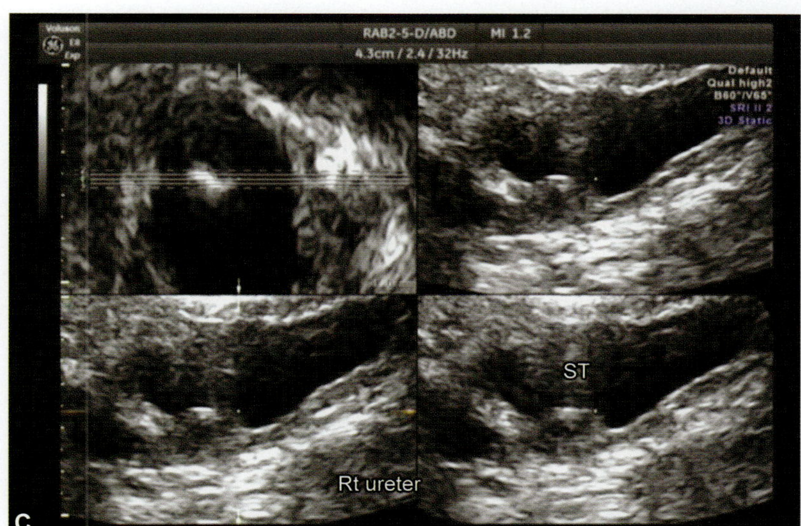

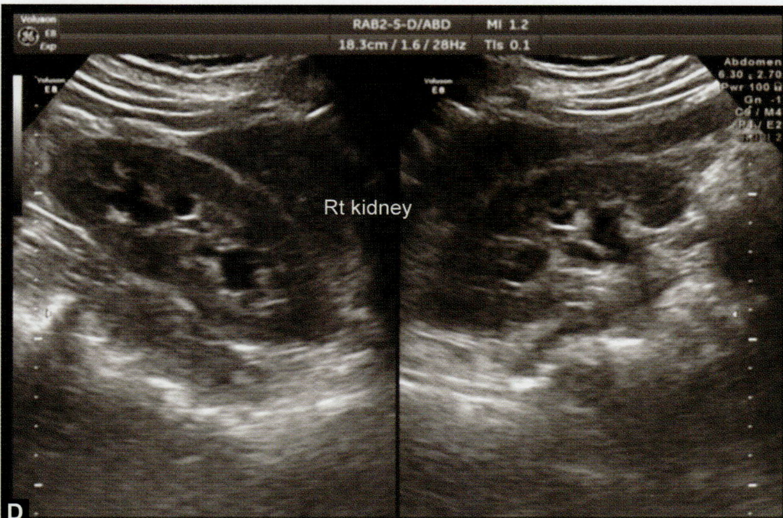

FIGURES 10.76C and D

FIGURES 10.76A to D: A patient presented with painless hematuria. Transrectal ultrasound with 3D imaging shows irregular of right vesicoureteric junction (VUJ). An echogenic shadow suggestive of a calculus seen impacted in it. A soft tissue shadow is seen invading the UB wall and right VUJ. It is seen extending in the distal part of the right ureter resulting into right side hydroureter. Mild fullness of right renal collecting system is also seen. The biopsy of the mass confirms transitional cell CA invading the UB wall, right VUJ and extending in the distal part of right ureter. HRSG with TRUS is a very good modality in picking up the early masses in UB.

SUMMARY

Transrectal ultrasound of prostate is now a well-established procedure in the diagnosis of prostatic pathologies, especially for prostatic cancer. Transrectal biopsies under ultrasound guidance have been of great value in establishing diagnosis.

Evaluation of the seminal vesicles by transrectal sonography has enabled to evaluate patients with infertility. However, it is vital to understand the limitations of this procedure especially for diagnosing prostatic lesions.

CHAPTER 11

Sperm Transport System

PK Srivastava

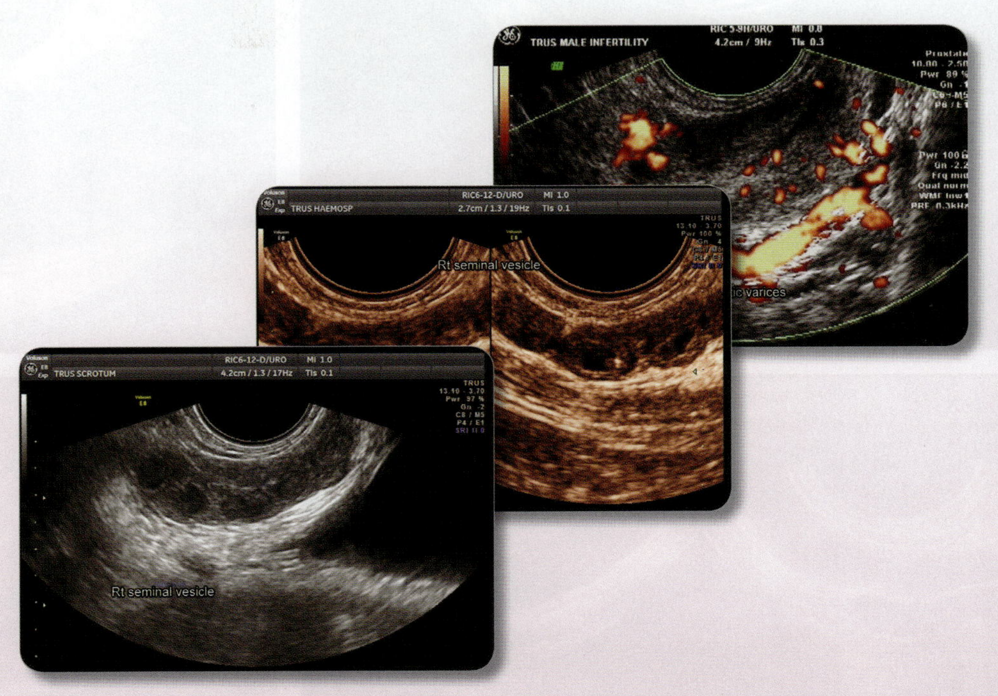

Sperm transport system in the males consists of seminal vesicle, VAS deference, ejaculatory duct, prostatic urethra and penis and penile urethra. HRSG is very good noninvasive imaging modality for evaluation of sperm transport system. High resolution transrectal ultrasound is the choice of investigation for evaluation of sperm transport system.

SEMINAL VESICLES

The normal seminal vesicles are paired, well defined, saccular and elongated structures situated cephalad to the prostate and posterior to the urinary bladder. They present a classical "bow-tie" appearance in transverse imaging. The seminal vesicles (SV) have internal septations giving rise to the saccular convoluted structure. There are marked variations in the size, shape and degree of distension of the seminal vesicles. They are usually symmetric and measure 3.0–1.5 cm in size. When the seminal vesicles are not identified on more than one occasion with abstinence, the diagnosis of absent seminal vesicles is made. If the seminal vesicles are smaller than 30 percent of normal volume (13–17 ccs), the diagnosis of hypoplastic seminal vesicles is made.

The vas differentia including their Ampula is normally well visualized on a transrectal study, cephalad to the seminal vesicles. They have appearances similar to those of the seminal vesicles and are usually bilaterally symmetrical. The confluence of the seminal vesicles and the ampullary portion of the vas deferens join together to form the ejaculatory duct, which crosses the prostate through the central zone and terminates at the level of the verumontanum. On an average the normal ejaculatory ducts have a lumen of about 2 mm. With good technique and meticulous examination, the ejaculatory ducts can be visualized in most of the patients.

US have become a major aid in the evaluation of male infertility. Seminal vesicles abnormalities are reported to occur in 90 percent of patients with agenesis of the vas deferens. Congenital unilateral absence of the vas deferens occurs in 1–7 men per thousand individuals. Congenital bilateral absence of the vas deferens occurs in approximately 1 percent of patients. A good few of these patients also have associated renal anomalies such as renal agenesis and crossed renal ectopic pelvic kidney commonly seen on the left side.

Seminal vesicle cysts may be either congenital or acquired in association with obstructive lesions. The congenital variety is rare in midline cysts or Mullerian duct cysts or urogenital sinus cysts. The orifices of the ejaculatory ducts enter into the cysts. These cysts contain sperms. On US, they are easy to identify and have the characteristics of other benign cyst in the body. Stone formation is seen in the ejaculatory duct as a sequelae to inflammation and are well visualized on the trans rectal study.

In all congenital anomalies of the seminal vesicles, the vas deferens or the ejaculatory ducts it is mandatory to evaluate the rest of the urinary tract to rule out other congenital anomalies.

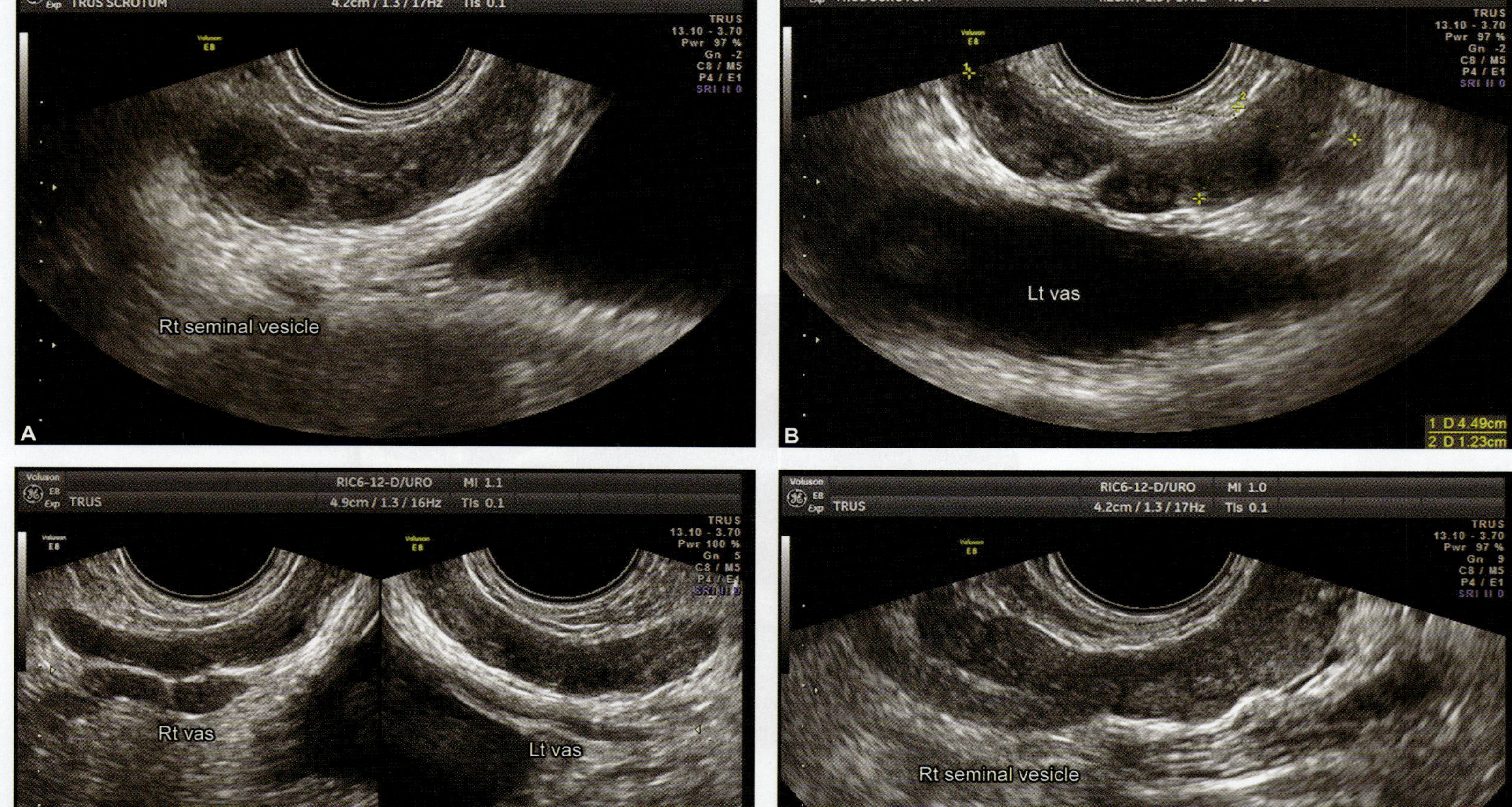

FIGURES 11.1A to D: Normal SV and vas deferens. HRSG shows normal seminal vesicles on both sides. They are seen as hypoechoic convoluted saccular tubal shadows. They give typical "Bow Tie" appearance. On color flow imaging, low or no flow is seen in them. Normal vas deferens are seen as hypoechoic tubular shadows running posterior to the seminal vesicle in parallel fashion.

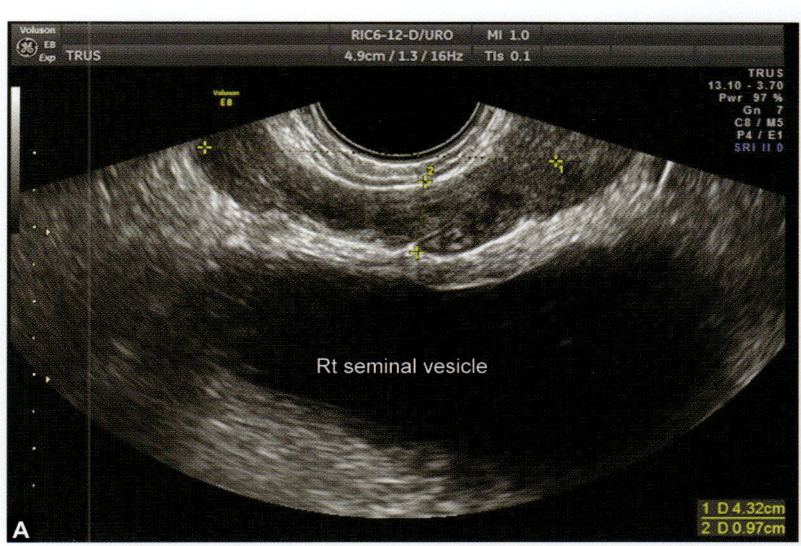

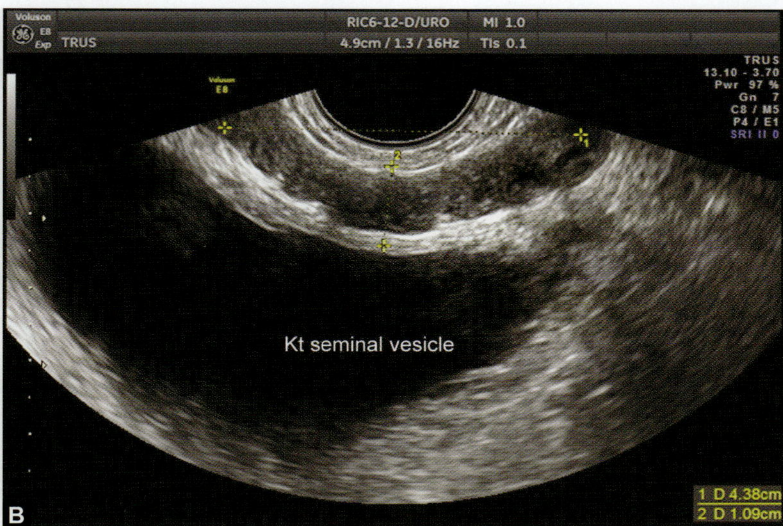

FIGURES 11.2A and B: Normal seminal vesicle. HRSG shows normal right and left seminal vesicle with typical "Bow Tie" appearance. Low level echoes are seen in the seminal vesicle.

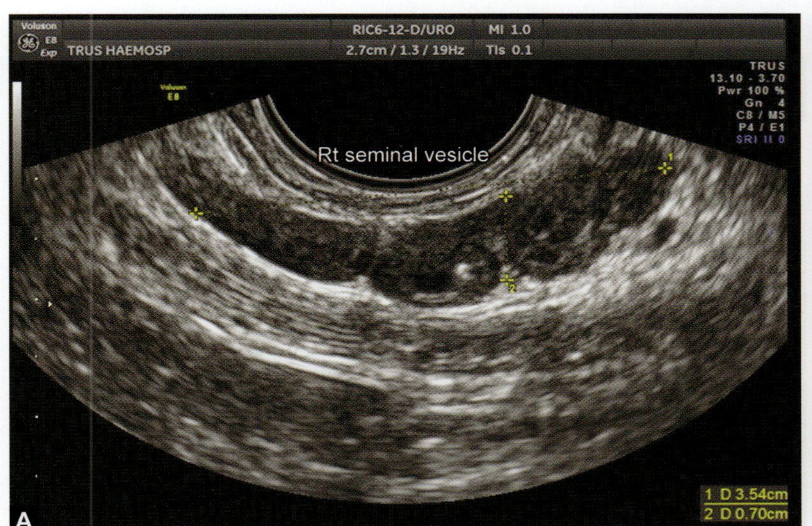

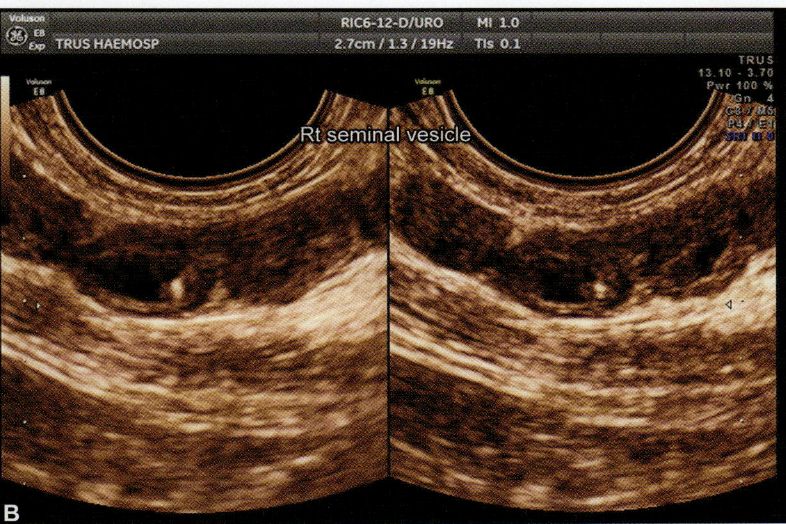

FIGURES 11.3A and B: Engorged seminal vesicle. Normal engorged seminal vesicles is seen as distended tubular shadows. Multiple internal echoes are seen in them because of the seminal vesicle fluid. Distended seculae are seen in them.

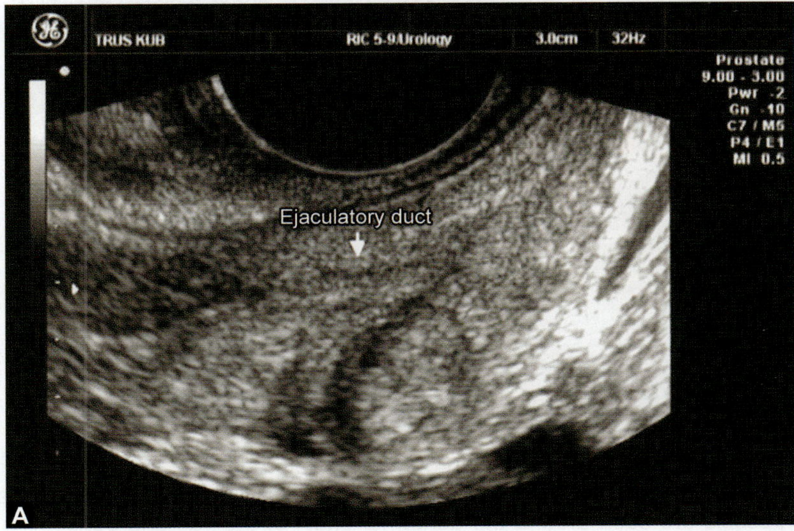

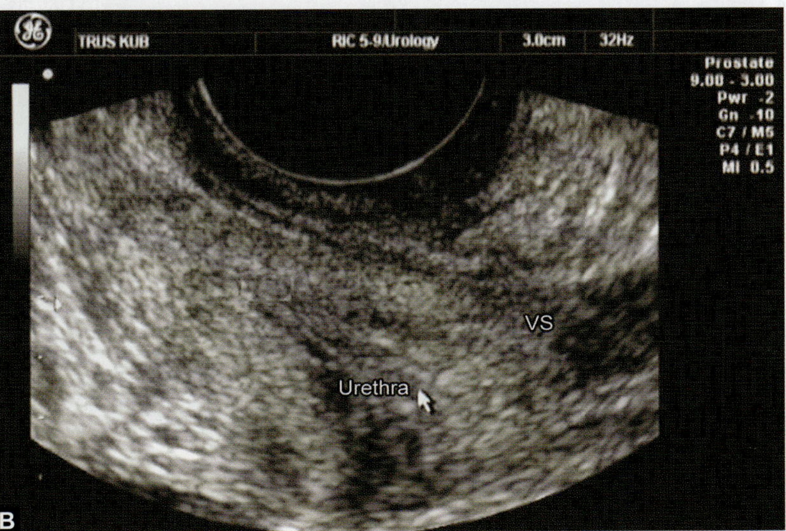

FIGURES 11.4A and B: Normal ejaculatory ducts. HRSG shows normal ejaculatory ducts in longitudinal section of the prostate. It is seen as thin hypoechoic line in the running obliquely and opening in the prostatic part of urethra.

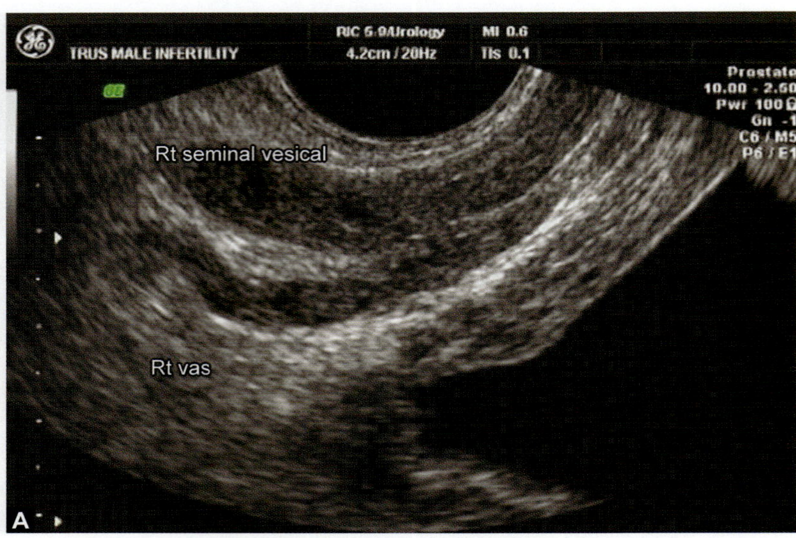

FIGURE 11.5A: Normal ampulla of seminal vesicle. The ampulla of seminal vesicles are seen as at distal of the seminal vesicle. They are seen as flared reservoirs. Thick echo low-level collection is seen in them suggestive of seminal vesicle fluid.

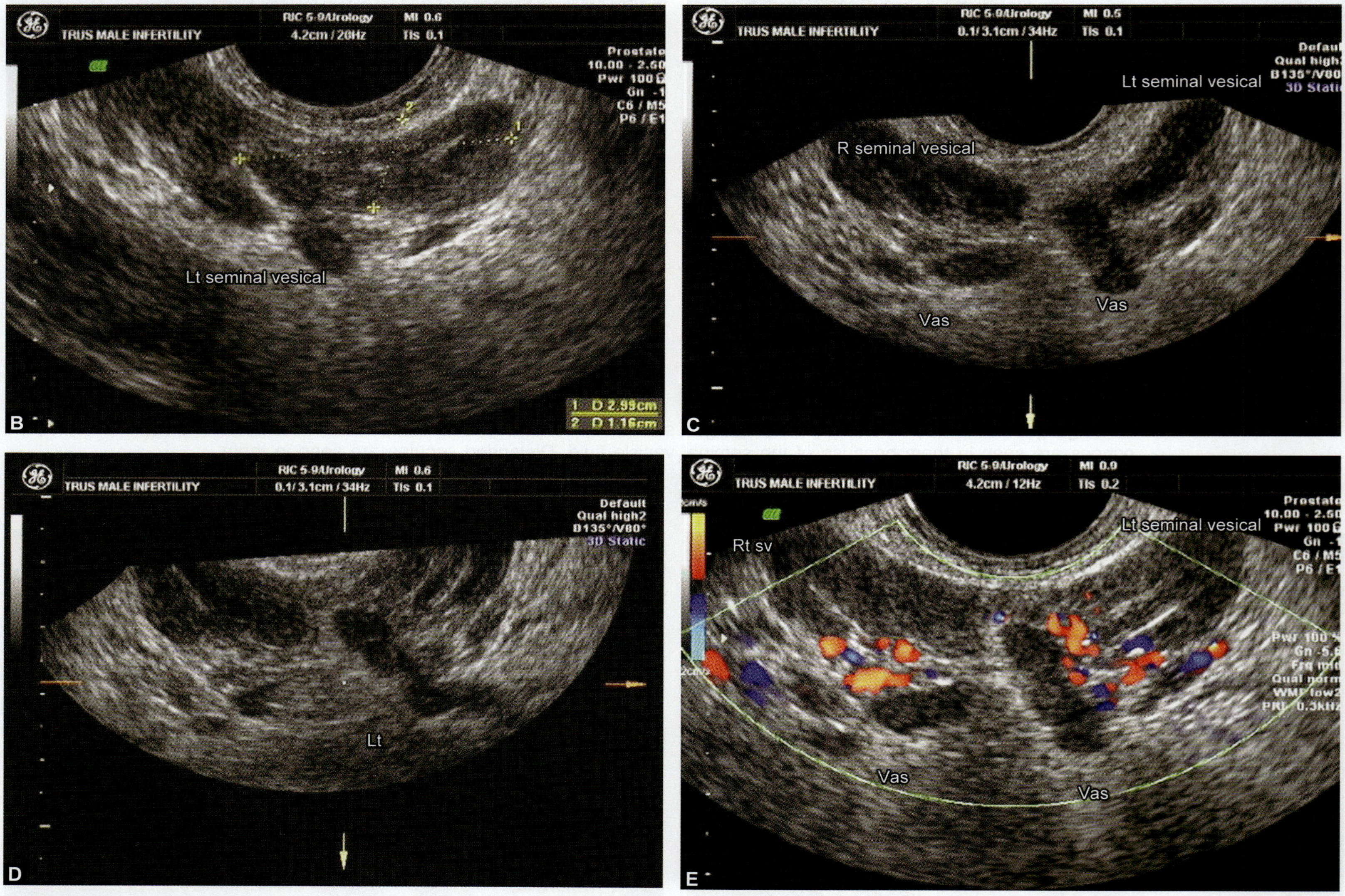

FIGURES 11.5B to E: A patient of male infertility presented with oligospermia. HRSG shows aberrant origin of left vas deferens. The left vas is seen coming out vertically from the left SV and runs down in an abnormal fashion. The right Vas is seen normal in position. **3D imaging** of vas shows abnormal origin of left vas in better details. **On color flow imaging,** multiple vessels are seen around the abnormal origin of the vas and periseminal vesicle area.

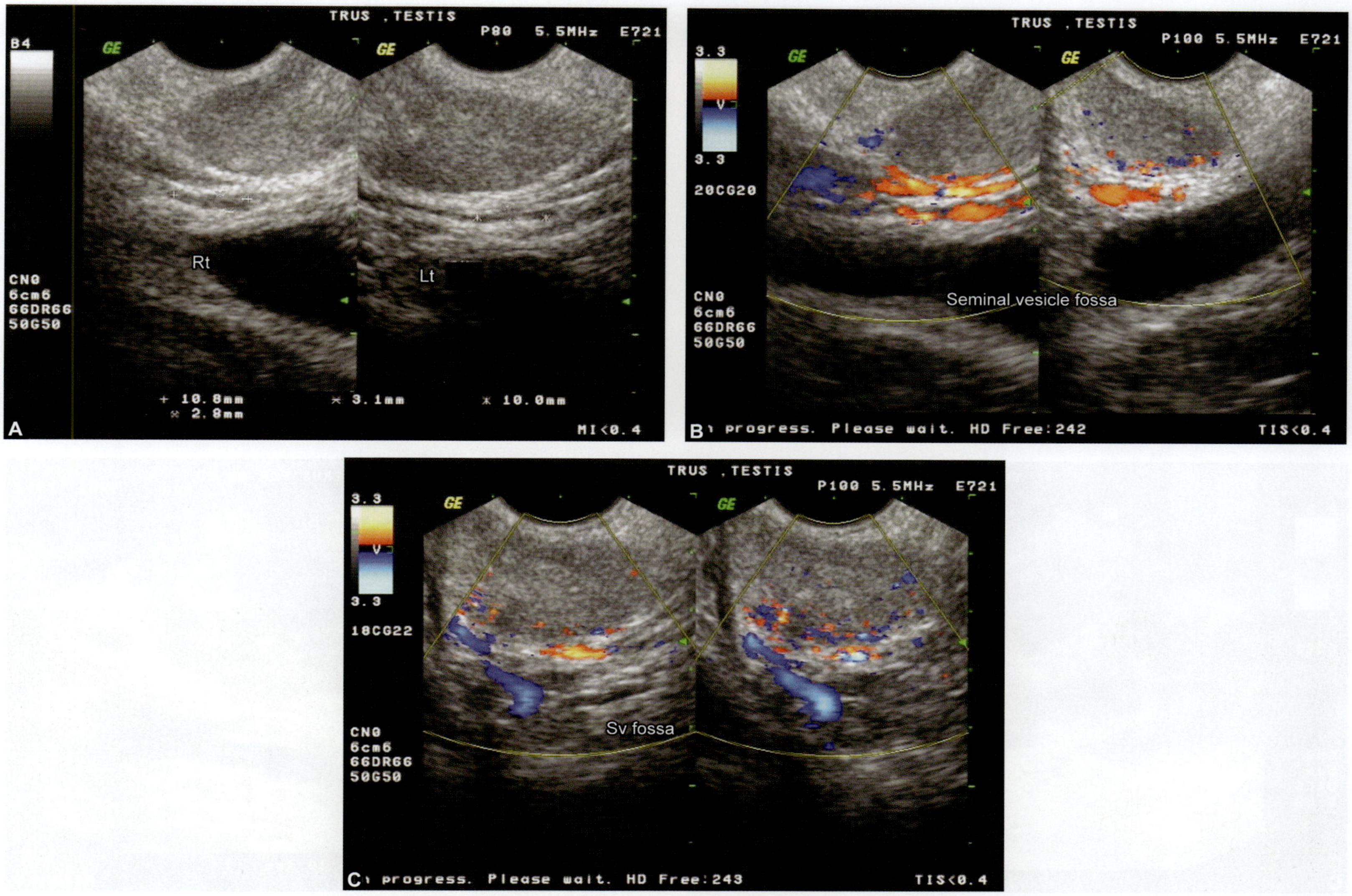

FIGURES 11.6A to C: Absent seminal vesicles. A patient presented with azoospermia. HRSG shows absent seminal vesicles on either side. On color flow imaging, dilated vessels are seen filling the seminal vesicle fossa. They are confirmed on color Doppler imaging.

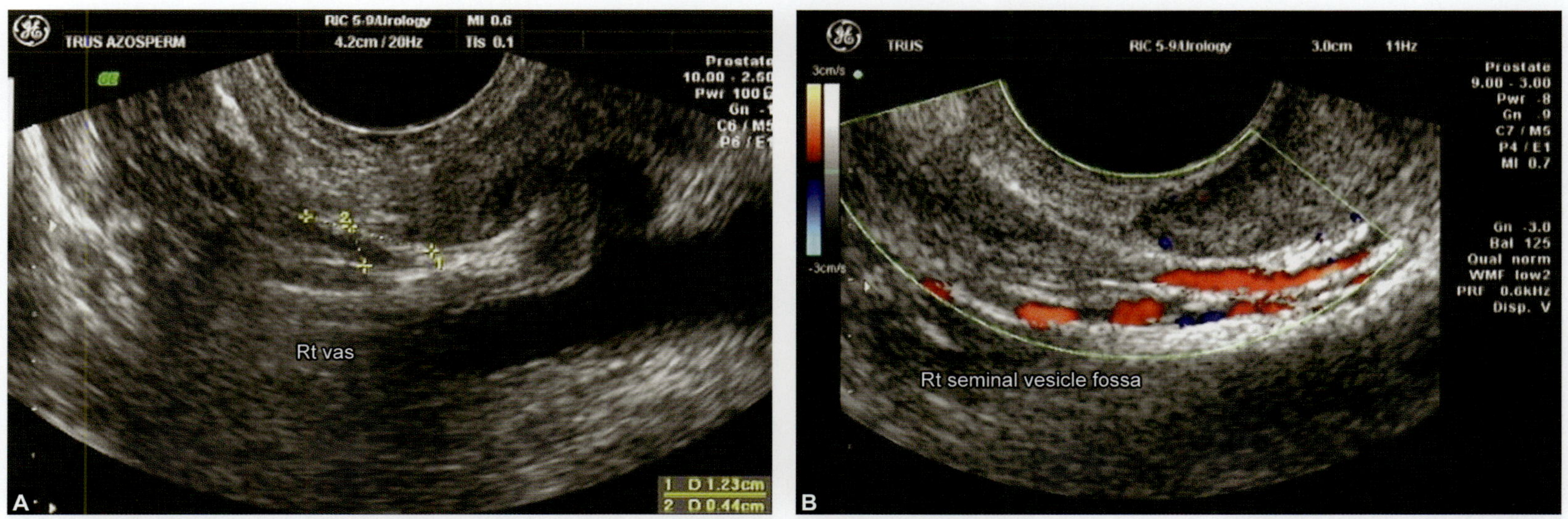

FIGURES 11.7A and B: Absent right seminal vesicle and small left seminal vesicle. HRSG shows absent right seminal vesicle. However, left seminal vesicle is small in size. On color Doppler imaging, vessels are seen in the right seminal vesicle fossa. The patient presented as azoospermia. left seminal vesicle was normal.

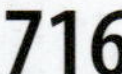

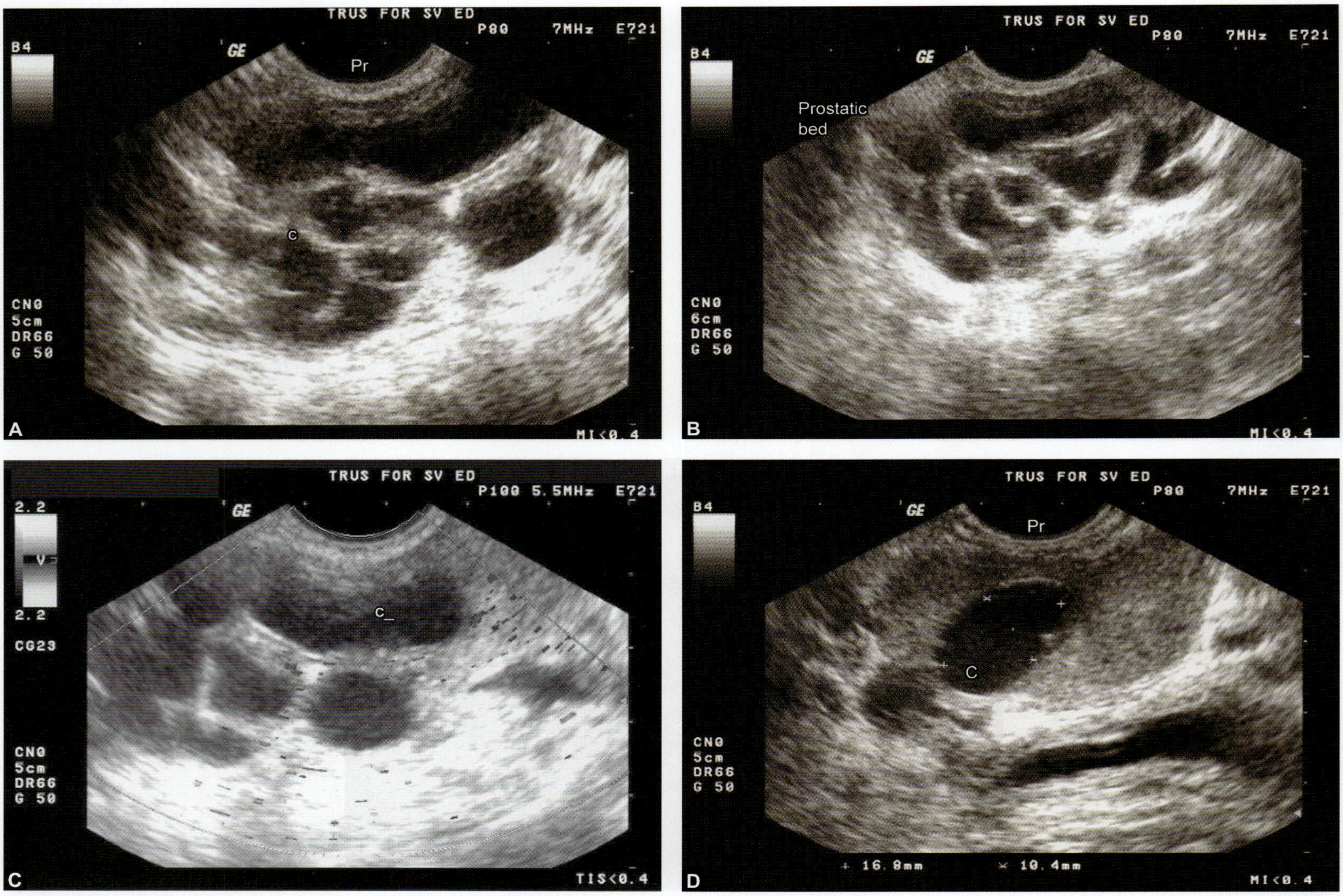

FIGURES 11.8A to D: Abnormal seminal vesicle cysts. A patient of male infertility presented with azoospermia. TRUS shows abnormal multiple cysts in both seminal vesicle fossae. The cysts are noncommunicating. Thick echogenic septa are seen in the cysts. Multiple cysts are seen in the prostatic bed in the same patient. A big cyst is seen in the substance of prostate suggestive of a big utricular cyst. Biopsy confirmed congenital cyst.

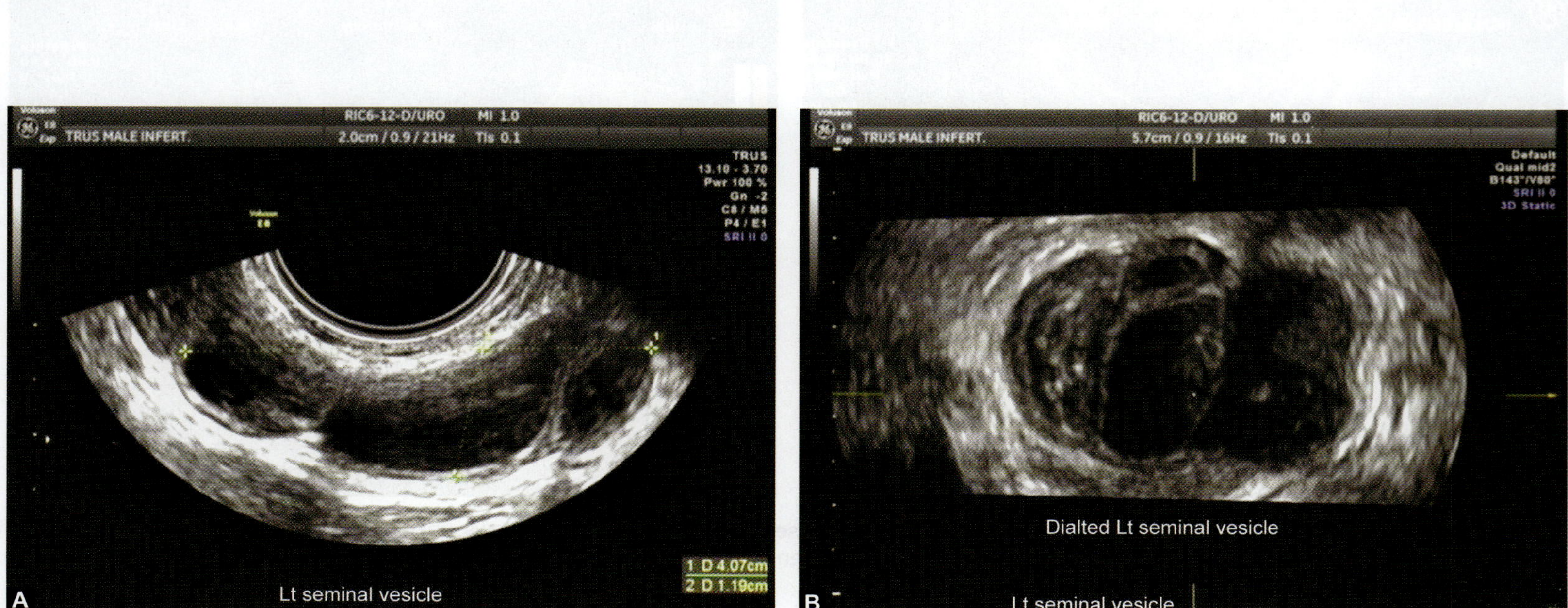

FIGURES 11.9A and B

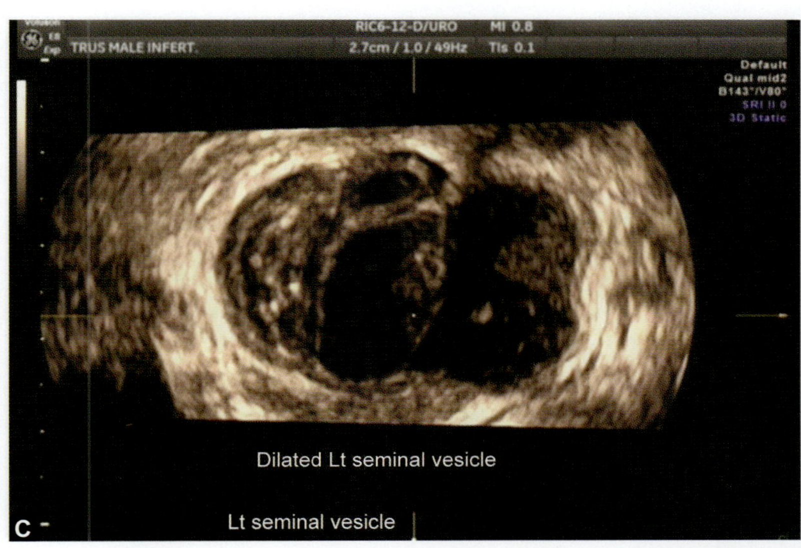

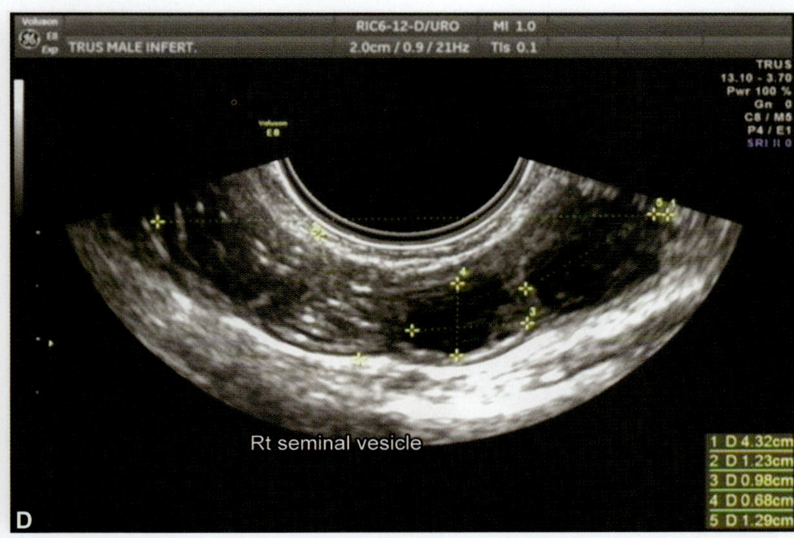

FIGURES 11.9C and D

FIGURES 11.9A to D: Seminal vesicle cyst. A patient presented with oligospermia with male infertility. Both seminal vesicle show multiple cysts. The cysts are non-communicating. Internal echoes are seen in the cyst. On 3D ultrasound the cyst are seen in coronal plane with multiple internal echocardiogram.

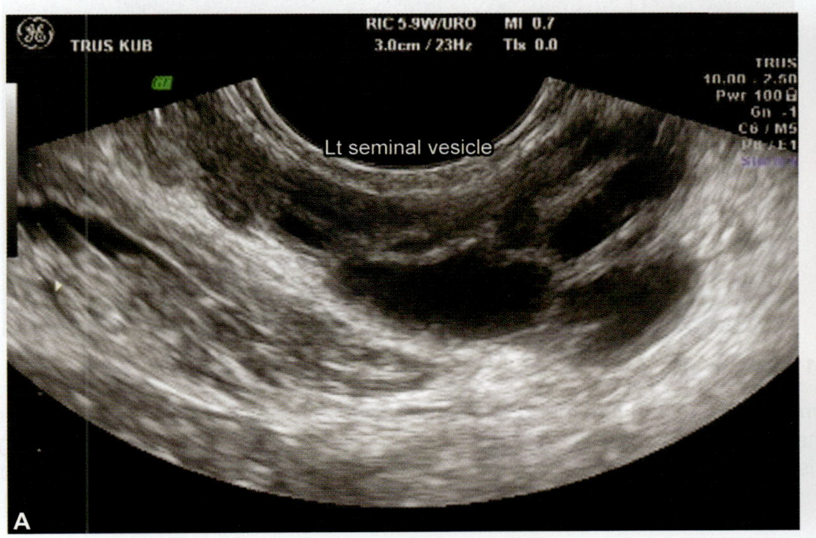

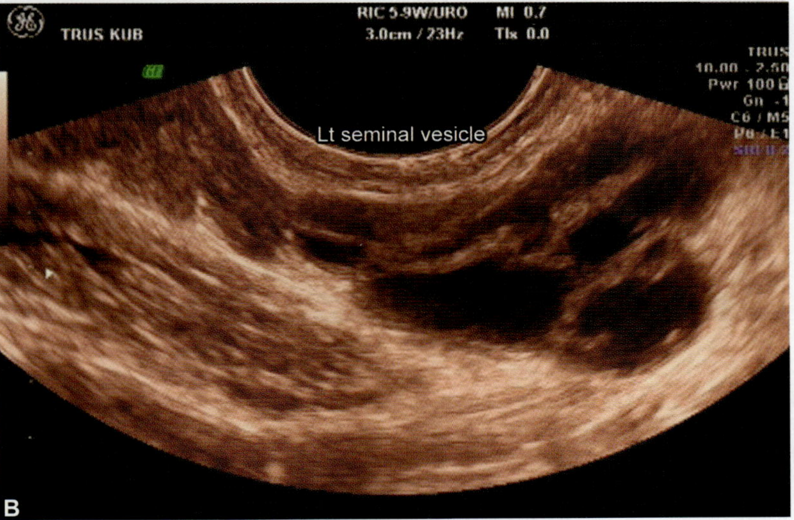

FIGURES 11.10A and B: Dilated engorged seminal vesicle. HRSG shows distended seminal vesicle. The seminal vesicle seculae are distended. Distended seminal vesicle are seen in the people, who abstain from sex from 3 to 4 days resulting into distended seminal vesicle.

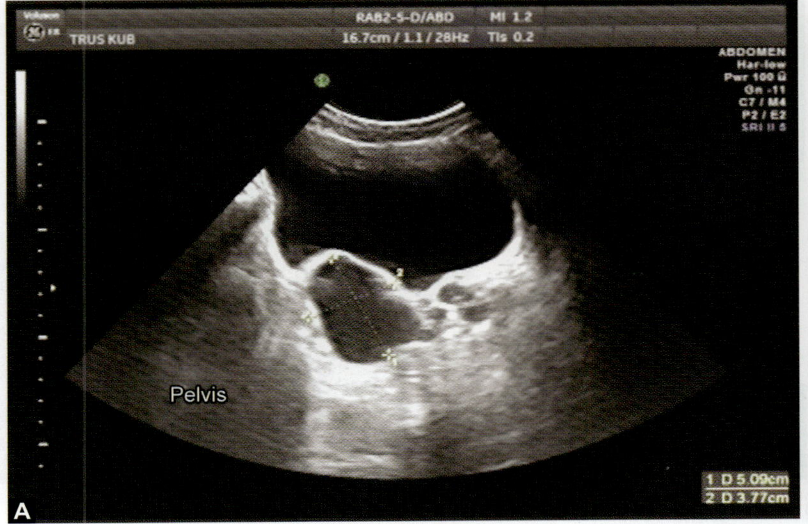

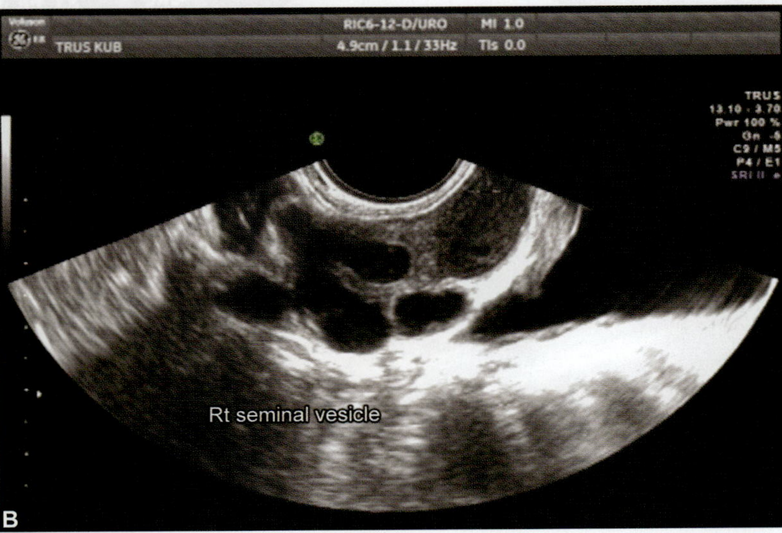

FIGURES 11.11A and B

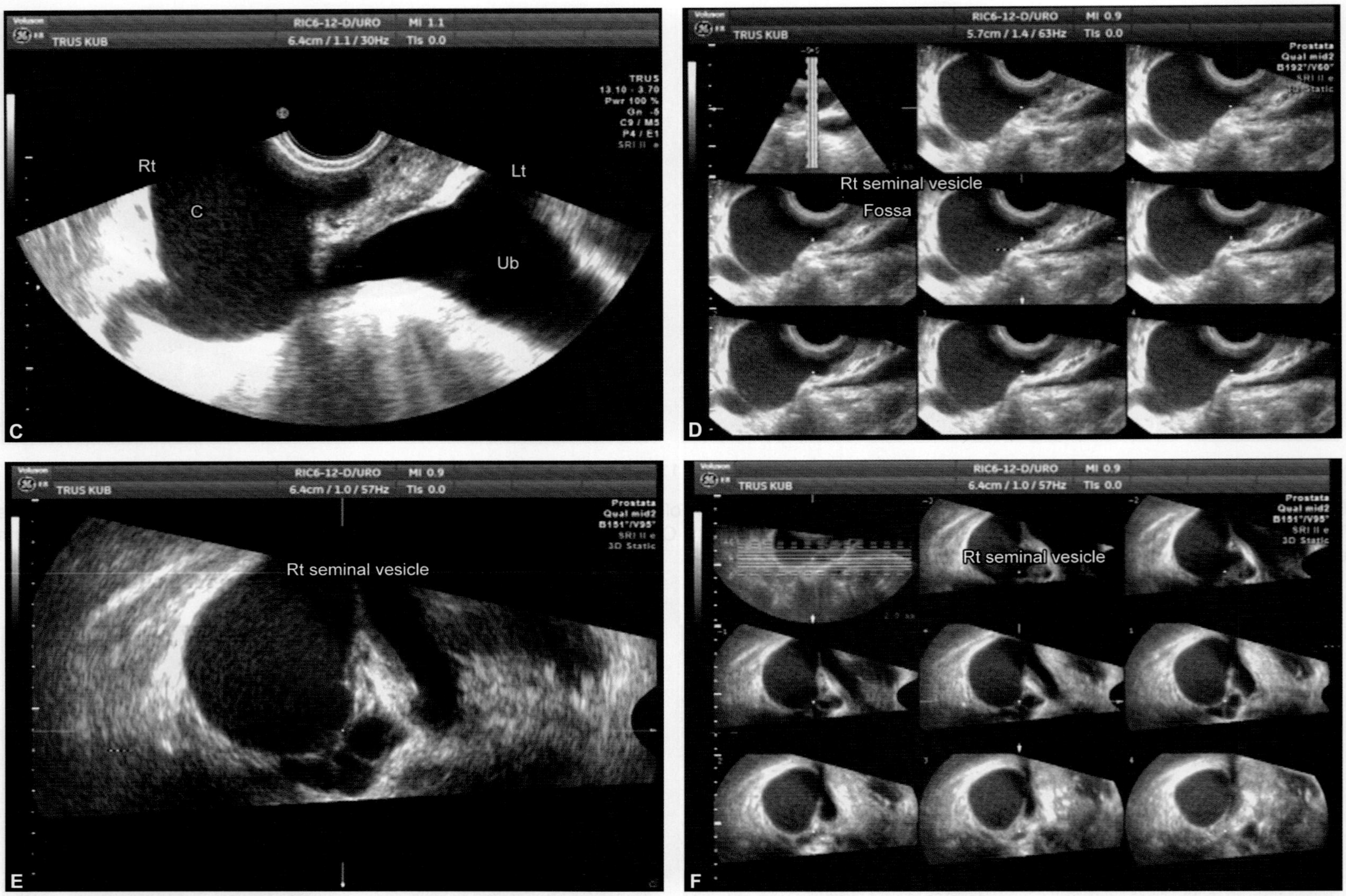

FIGURES 11.11C to F

FIGURES 11.11A to F: A patient of male infertility presented with azoospermia. Transrectal ultrasound shows big cystic masses in both seminal vesicle fossae. Normal seminal vesicle are not seen on either side. Big cystic shadows are seen. Thick echoes are seen in the cyst. On 3D TUI imaging, the cyst shows communication with ejaculatory duct. Left seminal vesicle is seen posterior to the cystic mass. It also shows noncommunicating cyst.

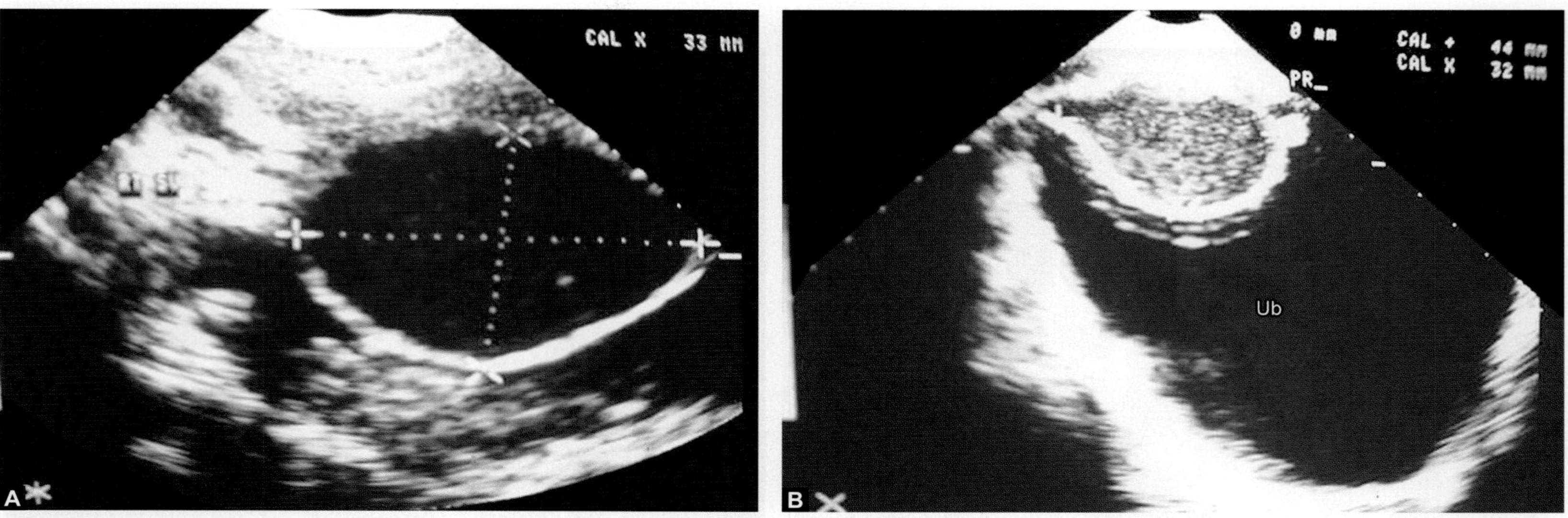

FIGURES 11.12A and B

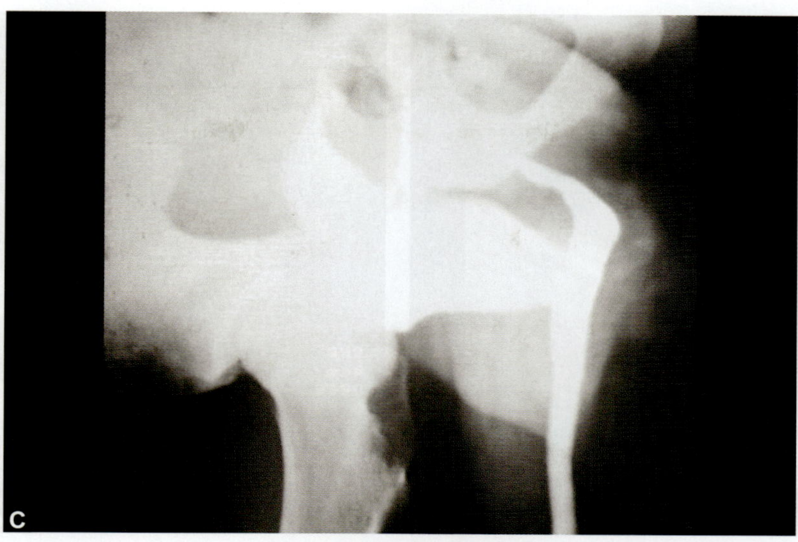

FIGURE 11.12C

FIGURES 11.12A to C: Seminal vesicle cyst. A patient presented with pyo-oligospermia. Retrograde urethrogram shows pressure over the prostatic part of the urethra with indentation. Transabdominal ultrasound shows a cyst bulging in the urinary bladder. TRUS shows a well-defined cyst in relation to the right seminal vesicle. Multiple internal echocardiograms are seen in it. USG-guided aspiration showed an infected seminal vesicle cyst.

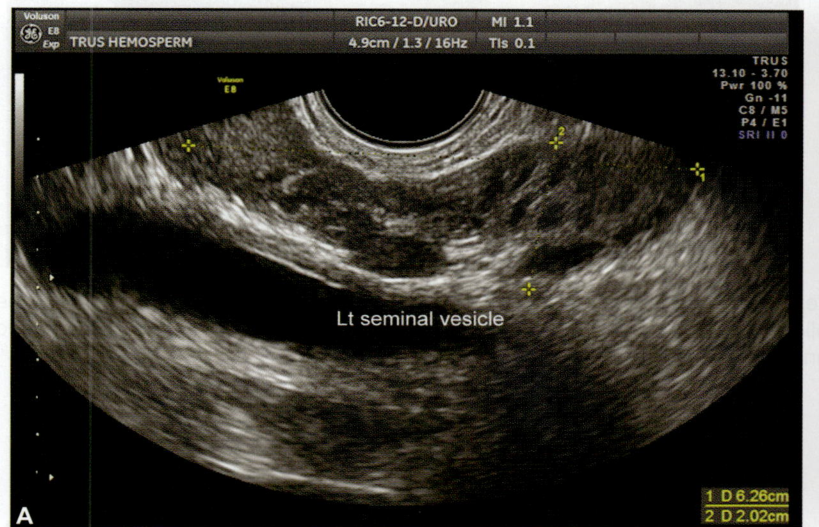

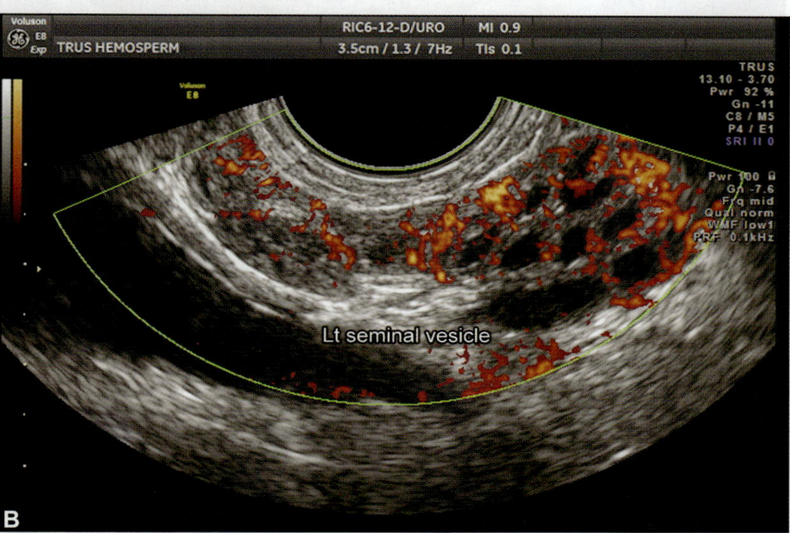

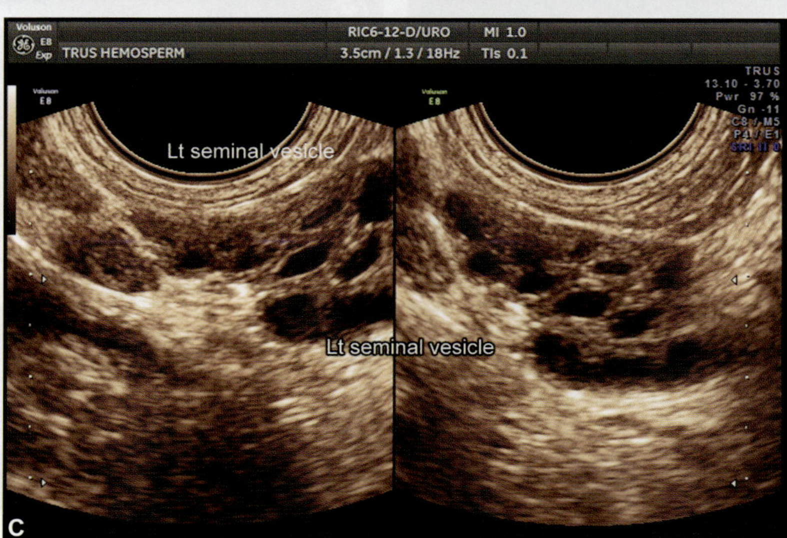

FIGURES 11.13A to C: Hemospermia. A patient presented with hemospermia. TRUS shows thick echo collection in both seminal vesicle. The seculae are thickened and edematous. On color flow imaging, increased flow is seen in them suggestive of infection.

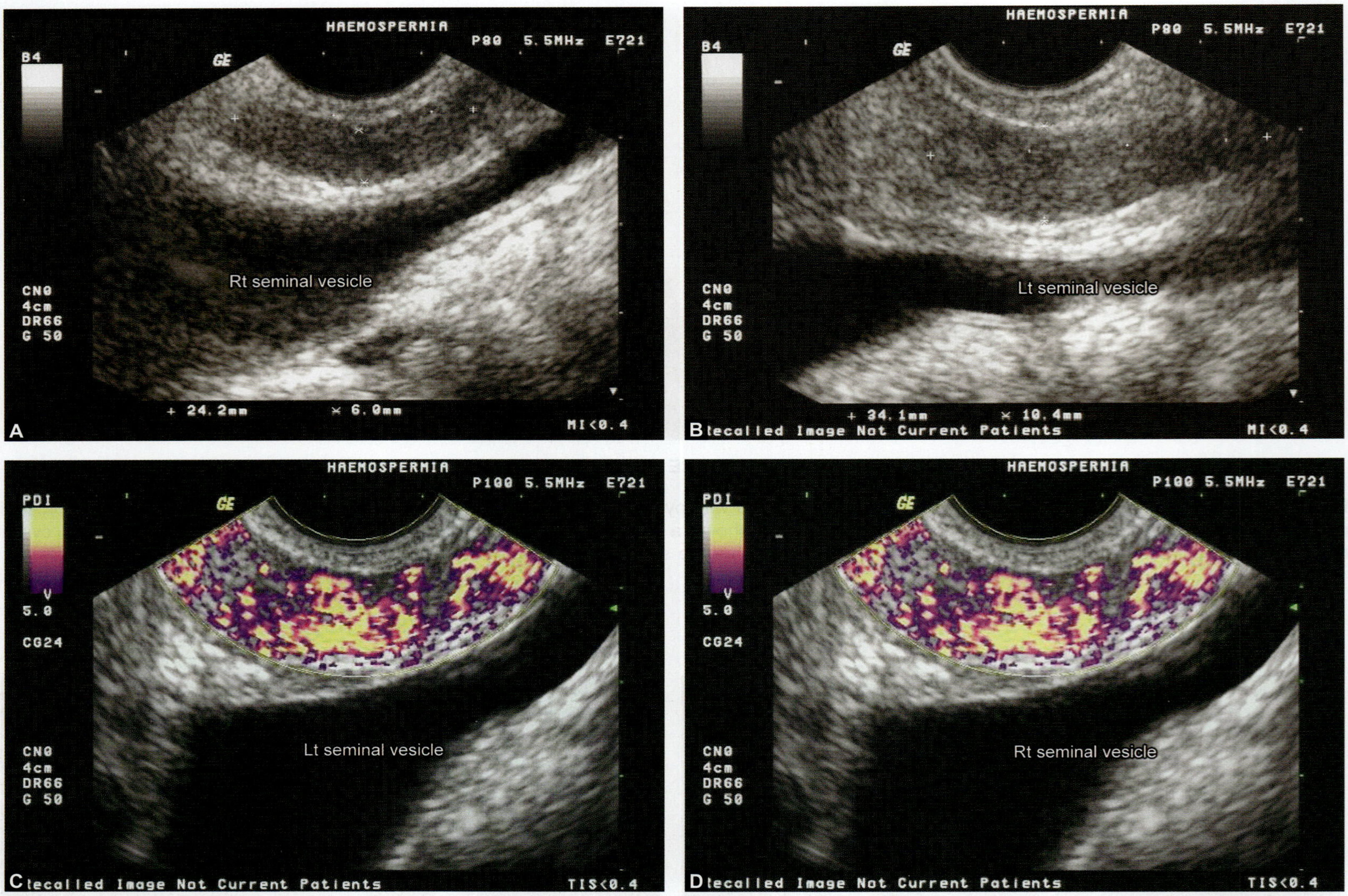

FIGURES 11.14A to D: Bilateral seminal vesiculitis. HRSG shows low-level echocardiogram collection in a patient presented with pyospermia. The collection shows multiple homogeneous echoes suggestive of pyogenic collection. Perifocal edema is also seen. On color Doppler imaging, increased flow is seen in seminal vesicle suggestive of hyperemia indicating acute inflammation of the seminal vesicles.

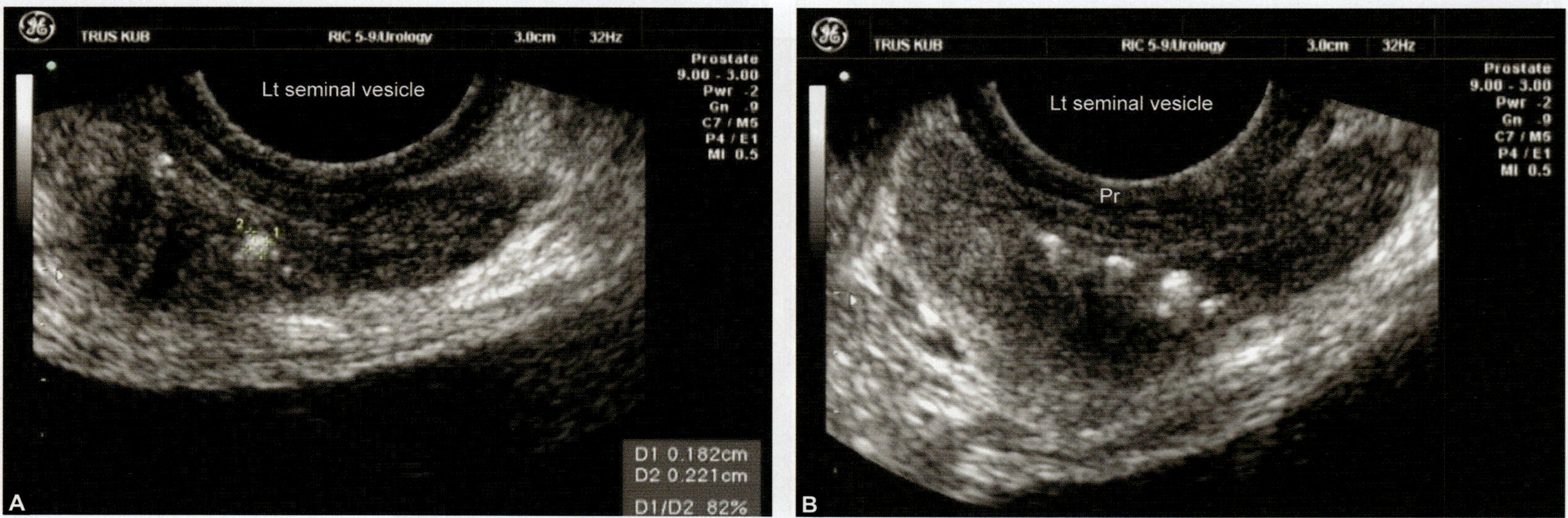

FIGURES 11.15A and B

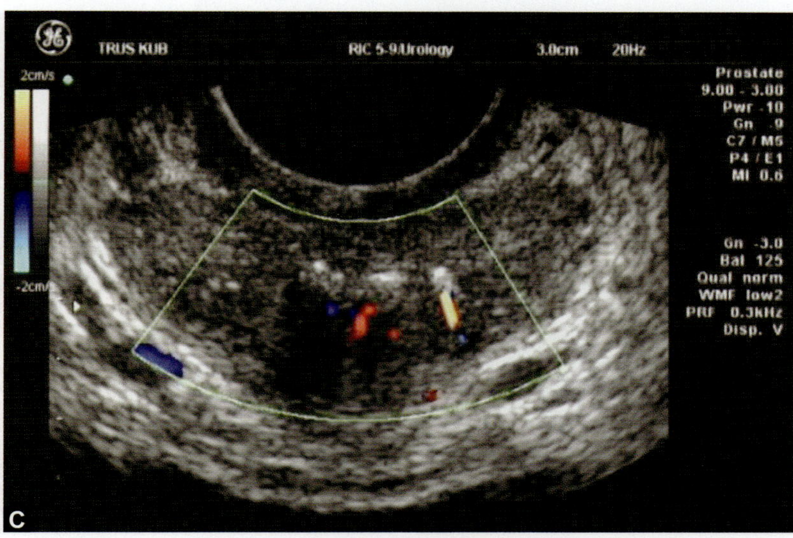

FIGURE 11.15C

FIGURES 11.15A to C: Chronic seminal vesiculitis. A patient presented with pyospermia. HRSG shows hypoechoic distended seminal vesicle. Thick collection is seen in the seminal vesicle. Echogenic calcified specks are also seen in the wall of the seminal vesicle. Echogenic calcified shadows are also seen in the prostate.

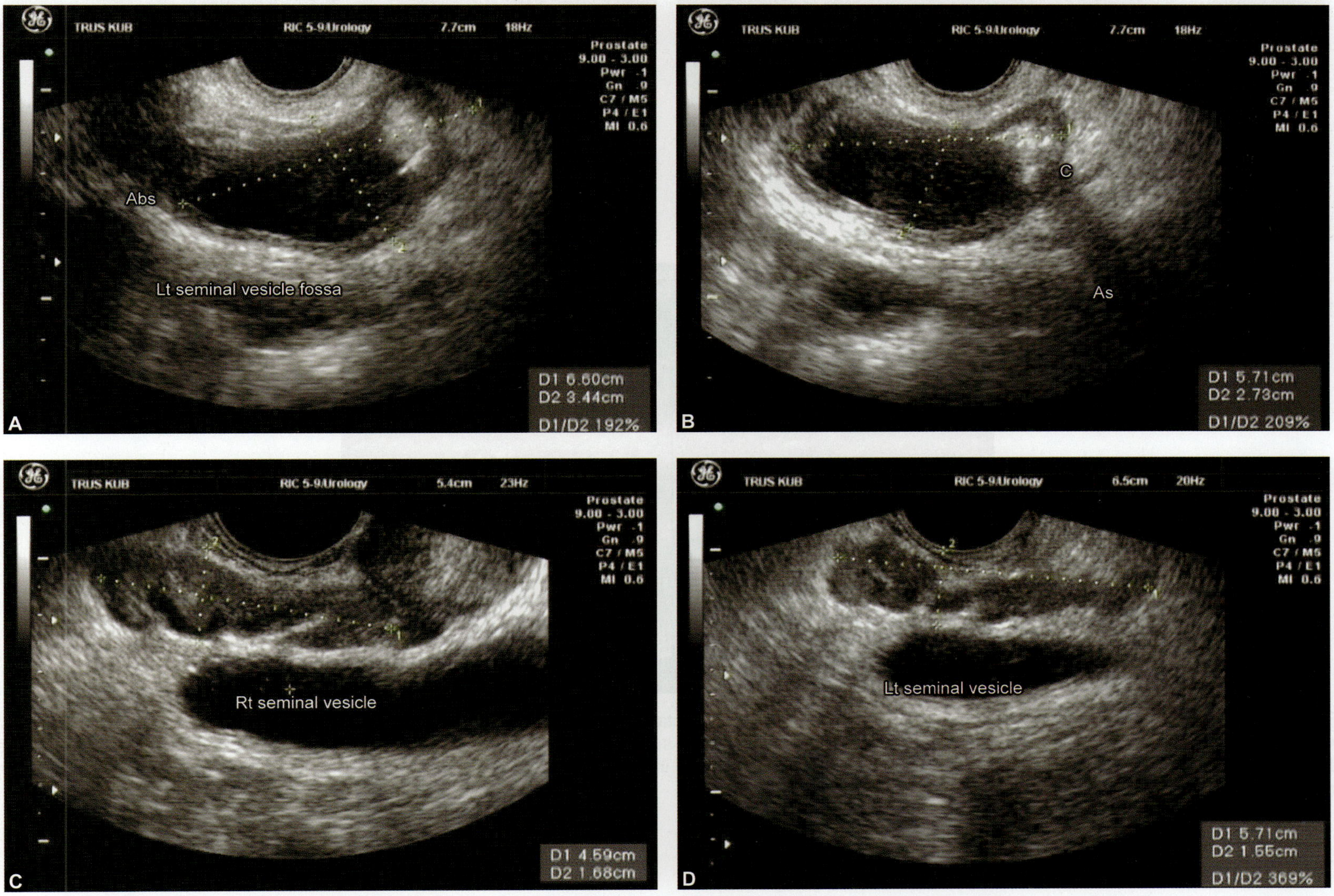

FIGURES 11.16A to D: Seminal vesicles abscess. A patient presented with pyospermia with fever. HRSG shows thick low-level echocardiogram collection in the right seminal vesicle. Echogenic floating shadows are seen in it suggestive of abscess. Echogenic debris is also seen in the seminal vesicle. Calcification is seen in it suggestive of chronic abscess. Right seminal vesicle also shows echogenic collection. The seminal vesicle walls are irregular in outline.

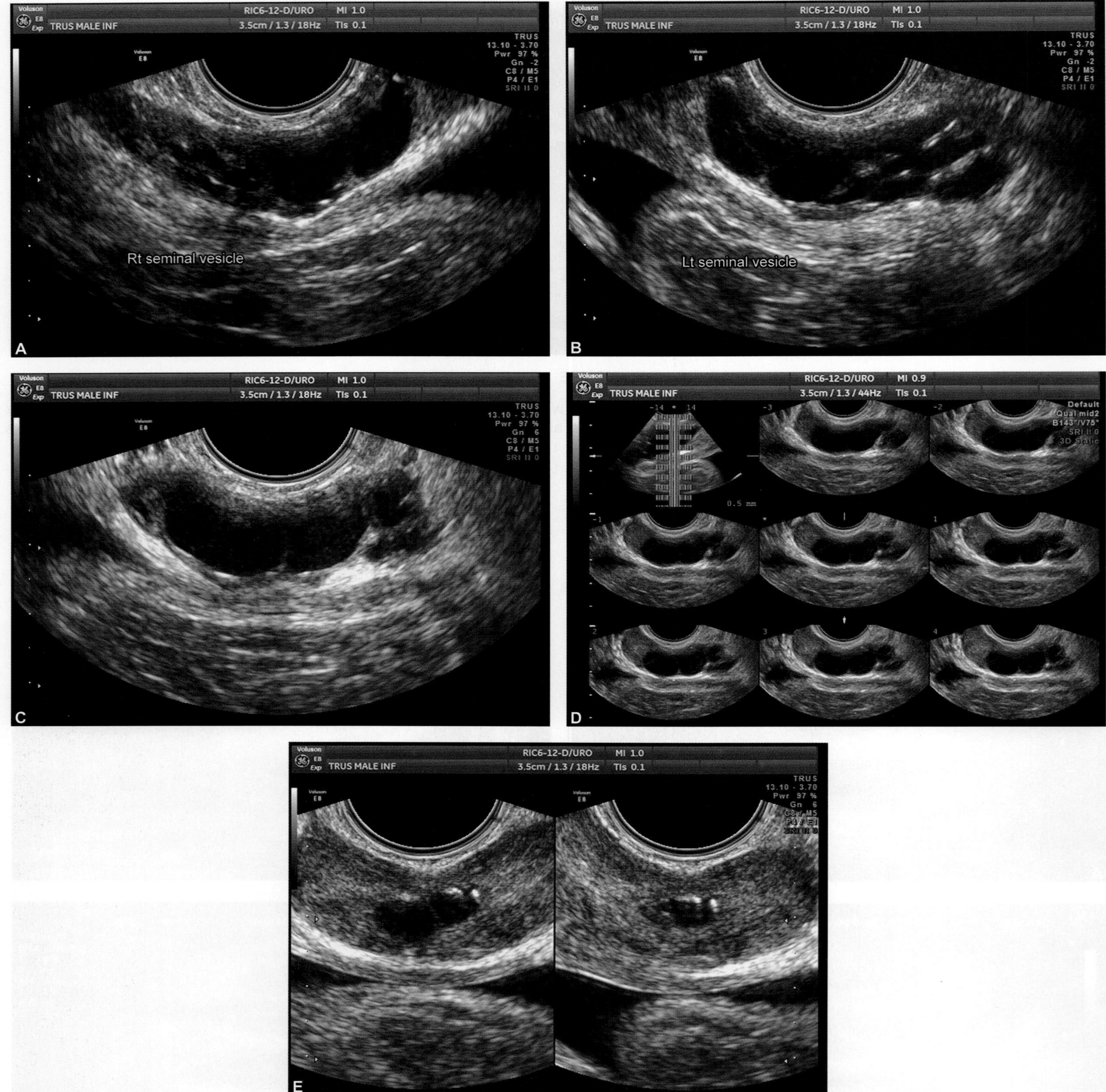

FIGURES 11.17A to E: A patient presented with oligospermia. Transrectal ultrasound shows a well-defined cystic mass in the prostate. The cyst wall shows echogenic calcification. Internal echoes are seen in the cyst suggestive of utricle cyst with chronic infection. Both seminal vesicles are distended and they are engorged. Multiple echogenic shadows are seen in the seminal vesicle. TUI imaging shows distended seminal vesicle with internal echoes and thin septa suggestive of chronic infection.

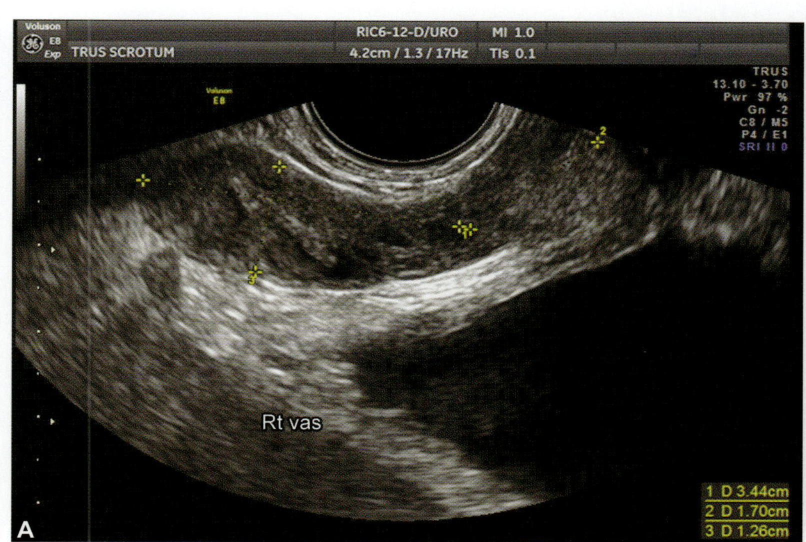

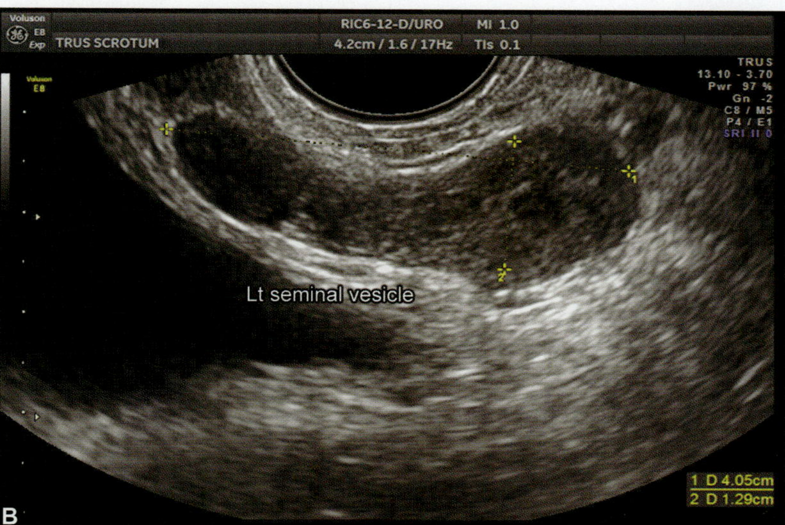

FIGURES 11.18A and B: Pyospermia. The TRUS shows distended seminal vesicle on both sides. Multiple internal echoes are seen in the seminal vesicle with thick collection suggestive of exudative collection resulting into pyospermia.

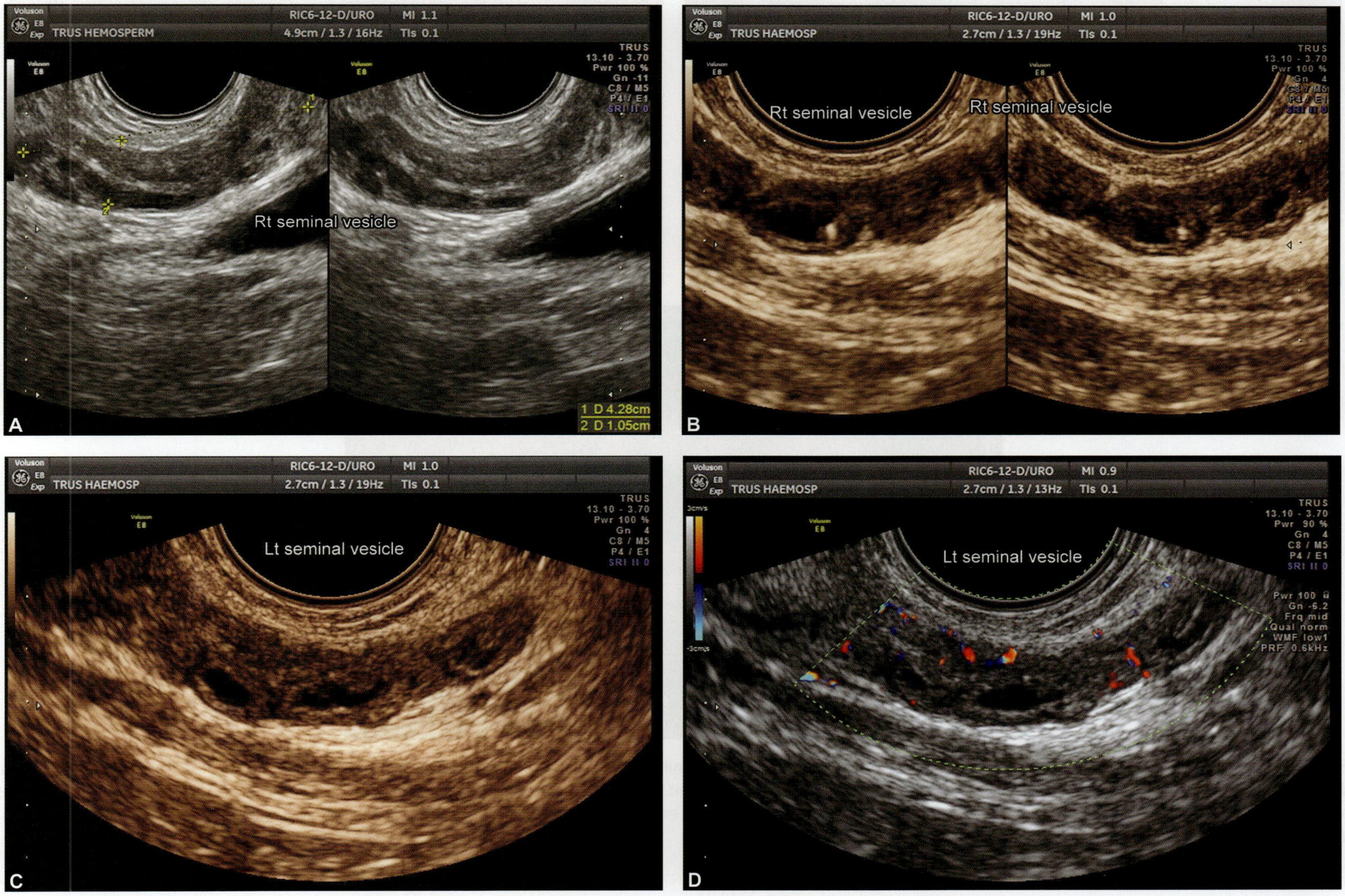

FIGURES 11.19A to D: Pyospermia. A patient presented with pyospermia. HRSG shows bilateral distended seminal vesicle. Echogenic foci are seen in the collection. On color flow imaging, few vessels are seen in the seminal vesicle wall suggestive of inflammation.

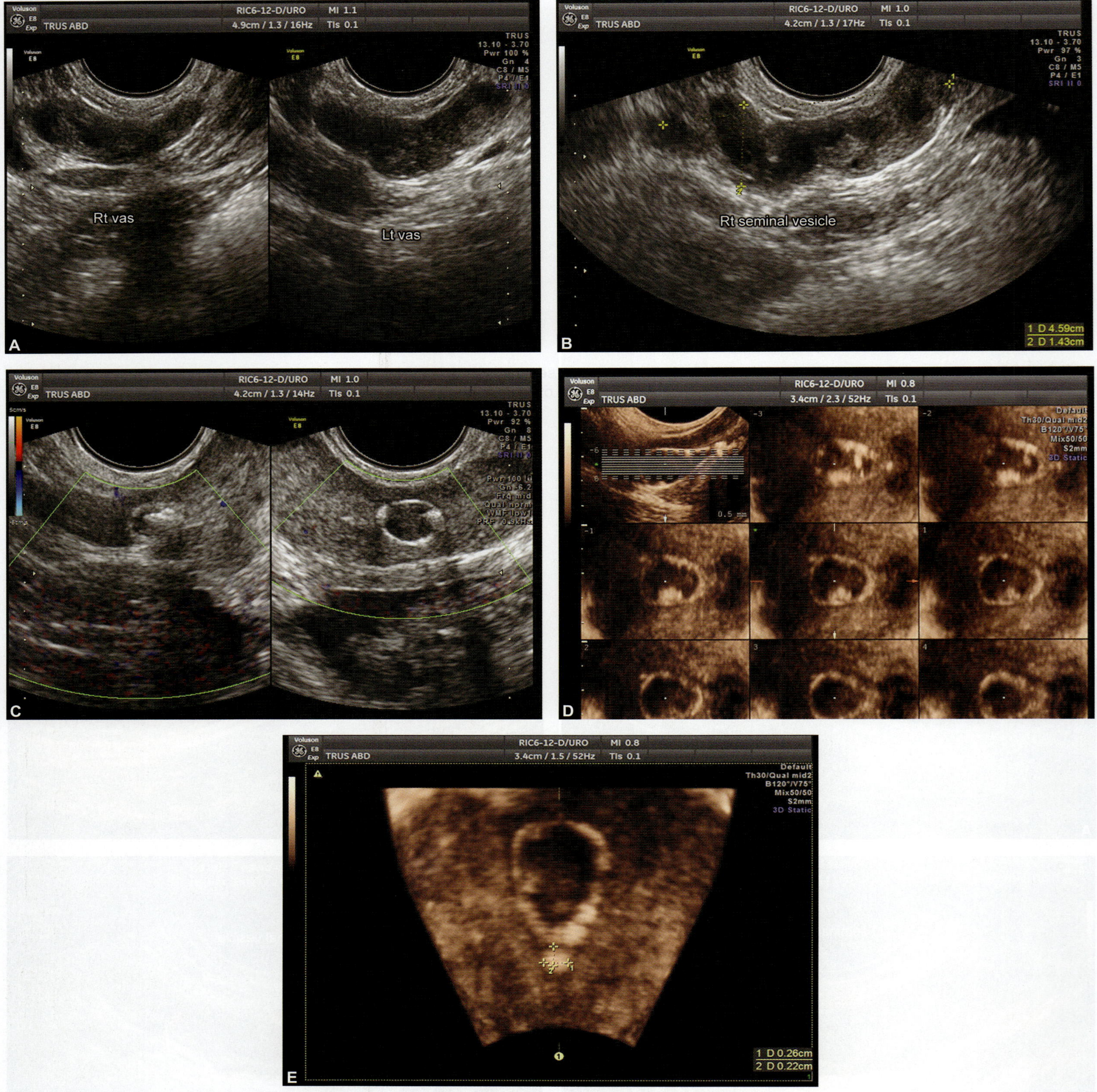

FIGURES 11.20A to E: Pyospermia. TRUS shows bilateral distended seminal vesicle. Thick echocardiogram collection is seen in the SV with internal debris suggestive of pyogenic collection. There is also evidence of a cystic shadow seen in the prostate. The cyst wall is echogenic. Multiple specks are seen in the cyst wall. 3D ultrasound with TUI imaging shows a small echogenic shadow at the mouth of the cyst suggestive of a small calculus. Internal echoes are also seen in it suggestive of infective collection.

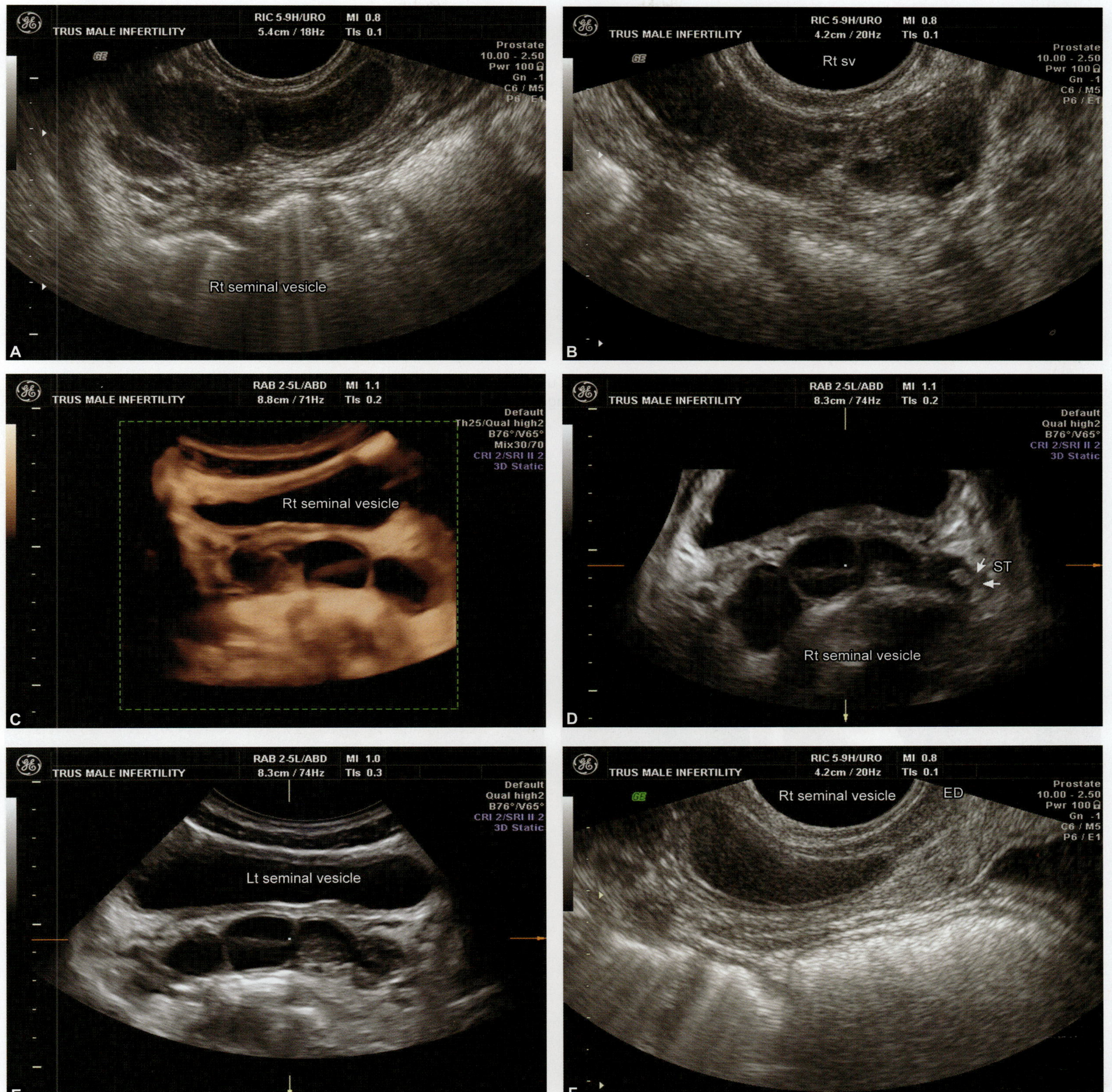

FIGURES 11.21A to F: Pyospermia. A patient of male infertility presented with pyospermia. Transrectal ultrasound shows bilateral distended seminal vesicle. Thick echocardiogram collection is seen in the seminal vesicle. Thin echogenic septa are also seen in the collection. On 3D ultrasound imaging, both seminal vesicle shows internal echocardiogram with thin septa. Right seminal vesicle shows small echogenic shadow at it ampulla suggestive of small calculus. Findings are consistent with chronic infection with small stone.

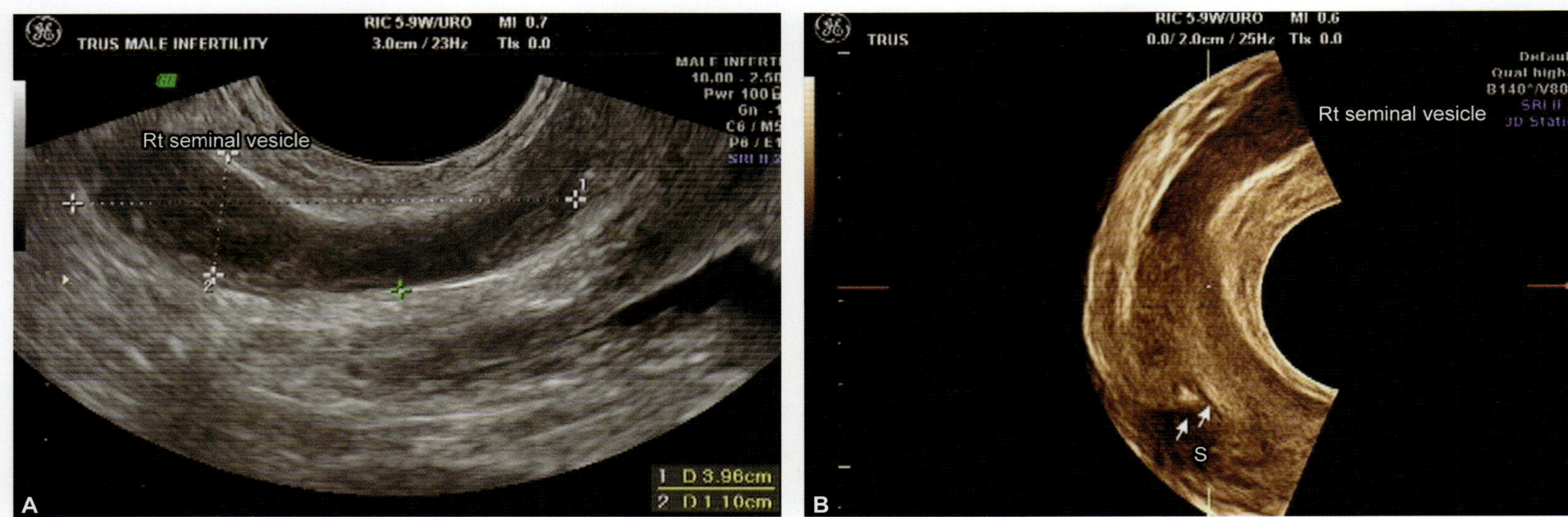

FIGURES 11.22A and B: Right seminal vesicle calculus. Transrectal ultrasound with 3D imaging shows an echogenic shadow at the mouth of right seminal vesicle, which is accompanied with acoustic shadowing. The 3D volume contrast imaging, shows the calculus very clearly.

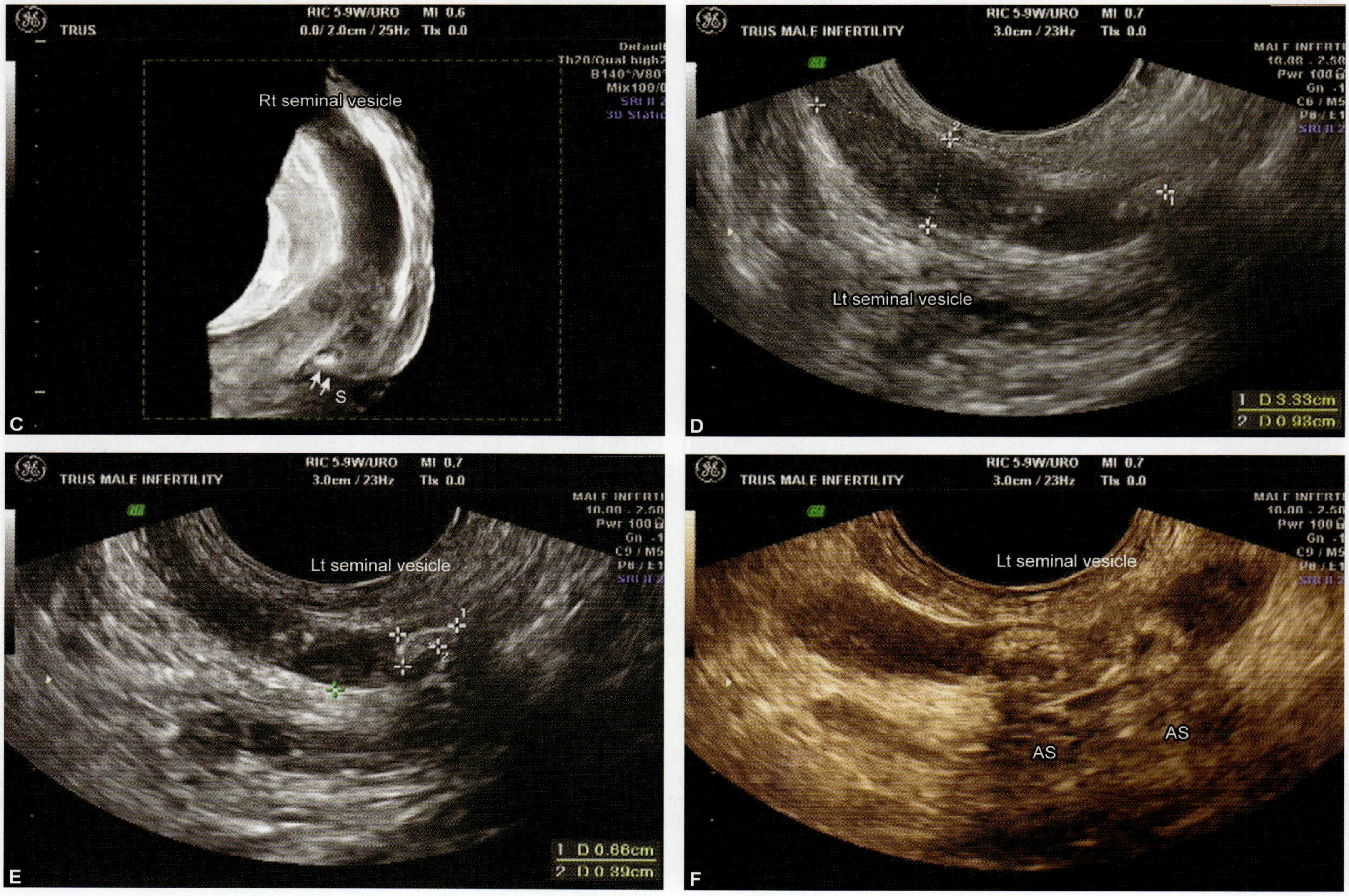

FIGURES 11.22C to F

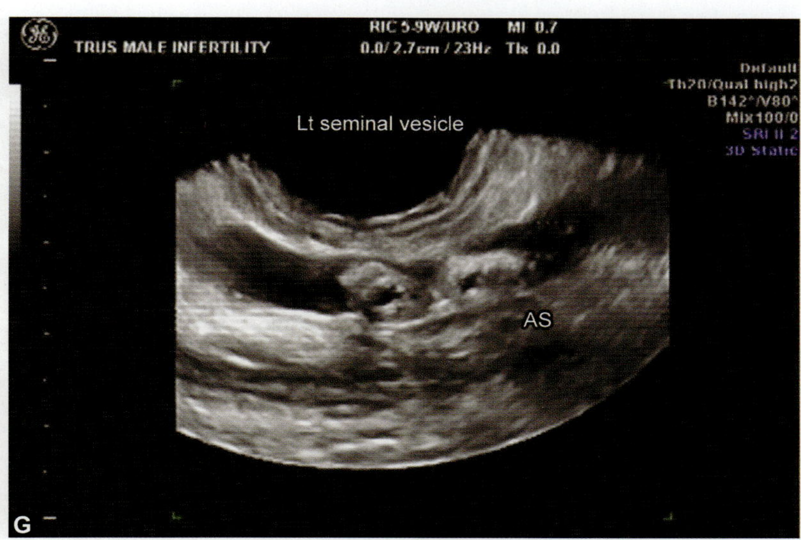

FIGURE 11.22G

FIGURES 11.22C to G: Multiple seminal vesicle calculi. A patient presented with oligospermia. HRSG shows distended seminal vesicle. Internal echoes are seen in them. There is evidence of echogenic shadows seen in both seminal vesicle. On 3D volume contrast imaging, the stones are seen beautifully. On further investigation the patient was having tubercular infection.

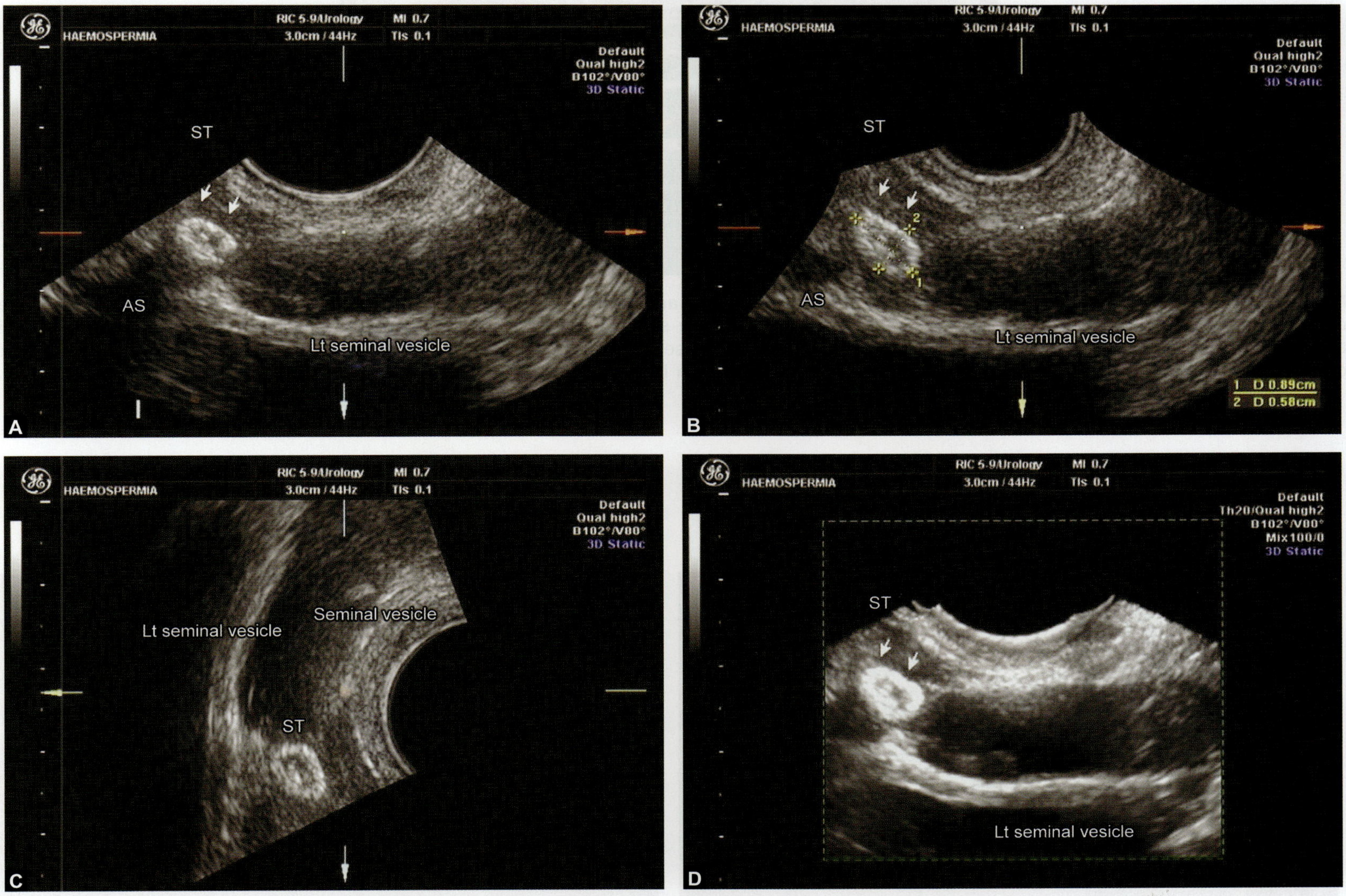

FIGURES 11.23A to D: Left seminal vesicle calculus. A patient presented with oligospermia. HRSG shows dilated left seminal vesicle. A big echogenic calculus shadow is seen impacted at the mouth of seminal vesicle. It is well defined and accompanied with acoustic shadowing. **3D surface rendering imaging**, shows the calculus in much better view. Echogenic floating collection is also seen in the seminal vesicle.

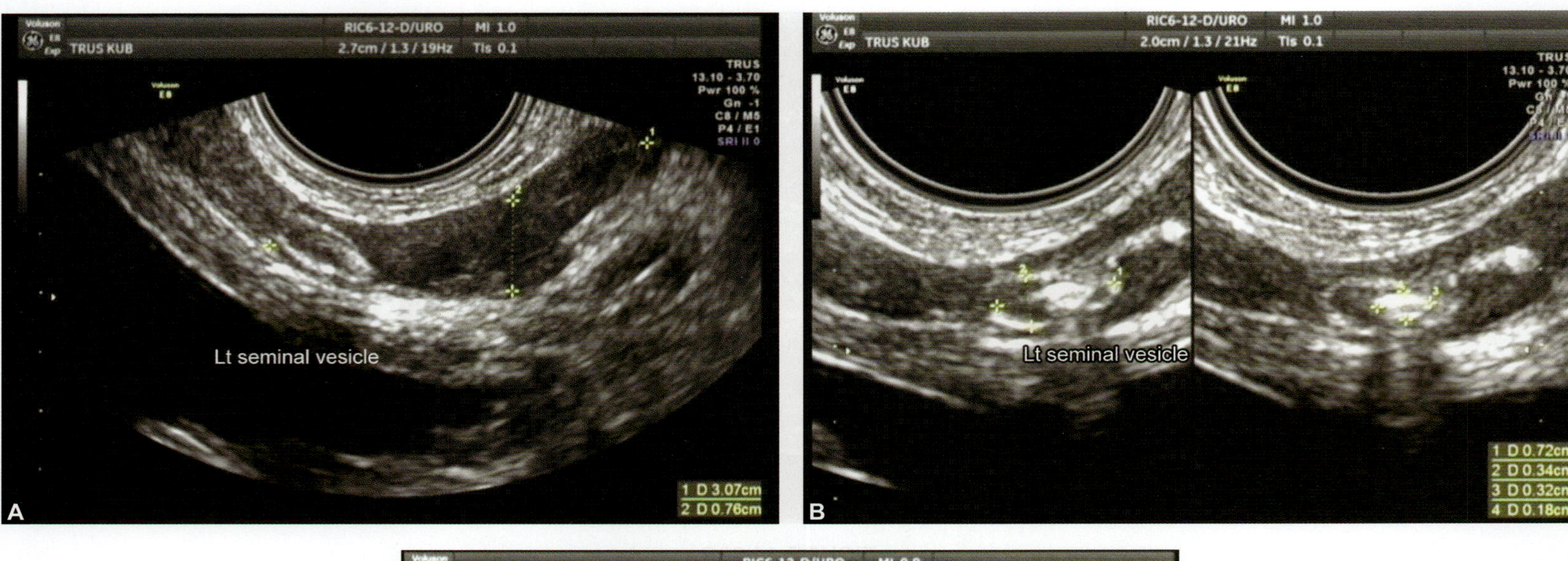

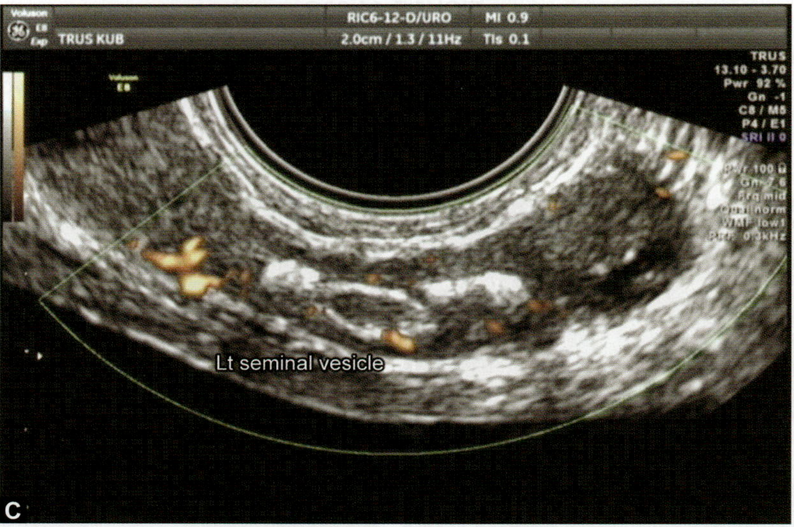

FIGURES 11.24A to C: Tubercular seminal vesiculitis with granulomas formation. TRUS shows distended left seminal vesicle. Internal echoes are seen in the seminal vesicle. Multiple echogenic foci are seen in the seminal vesicles. The big echogenic shadow shows calcification, which is accompanied with acoustic shadowing. On color flow imaging, few vessels are seen in inflamed seminal vesicle wall. Findings are suggestive of chronic granulomatous infection. The patient also had tubercular infection in the chest.

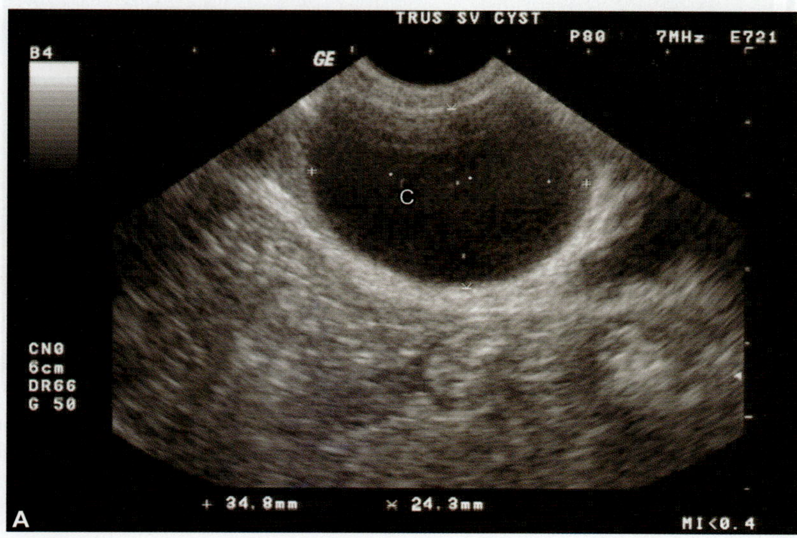

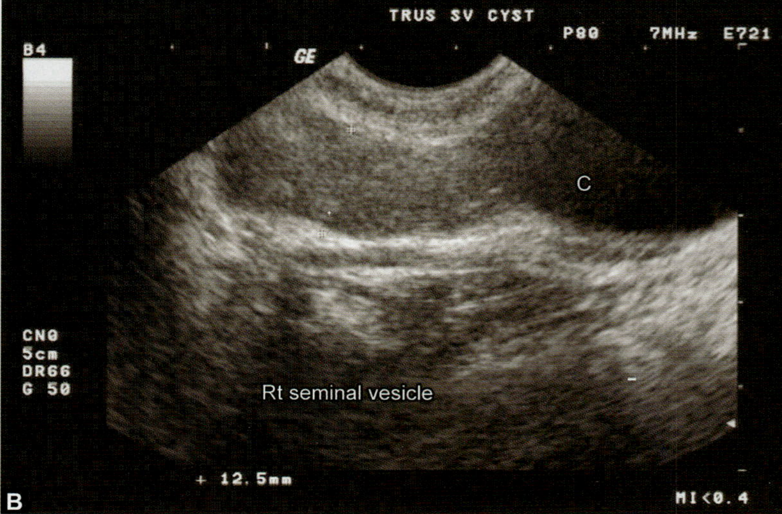

FIGURES 11.25A and B

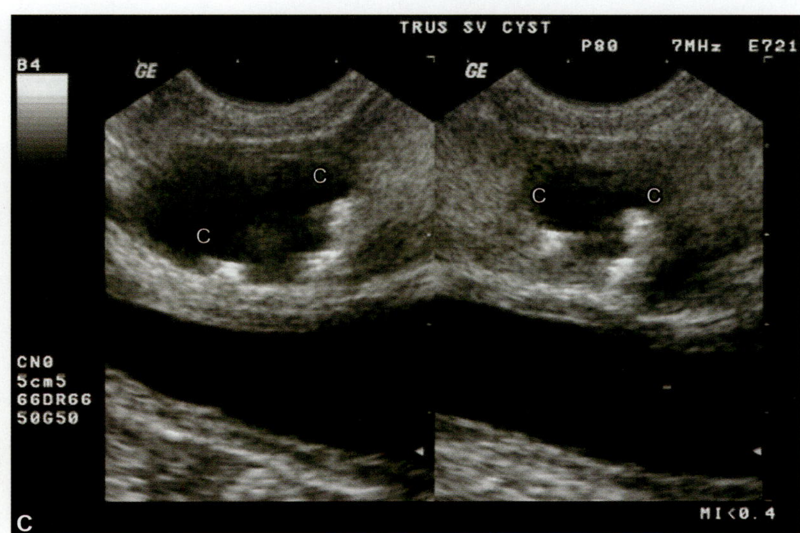

FIGURE 11.25C

FIGURES 11.25A to C: Right seminal vesicle cyst. HRSG shows a big cystic mass in relation to the right seminal vesicles in a patient of oligospermia. The cyst is seen blocking the mouth of the seminal vesicle. Echogenic calcified specks are also seen fixed with the cyst wall suggestive of chronicity.

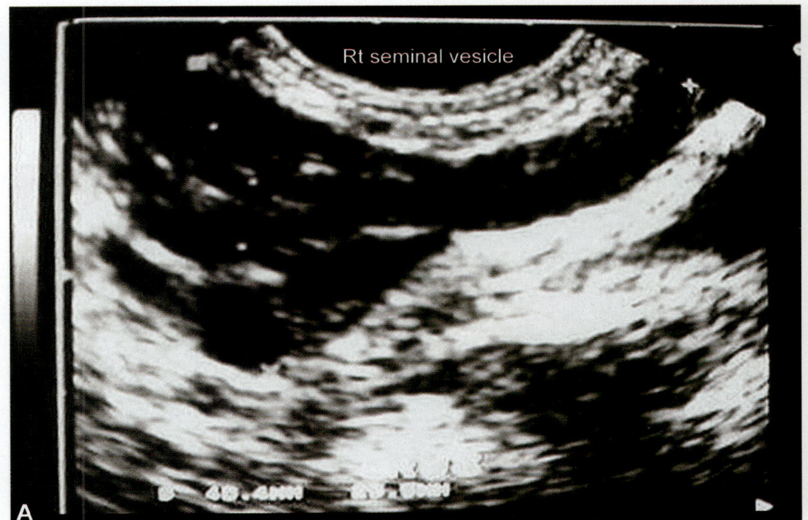

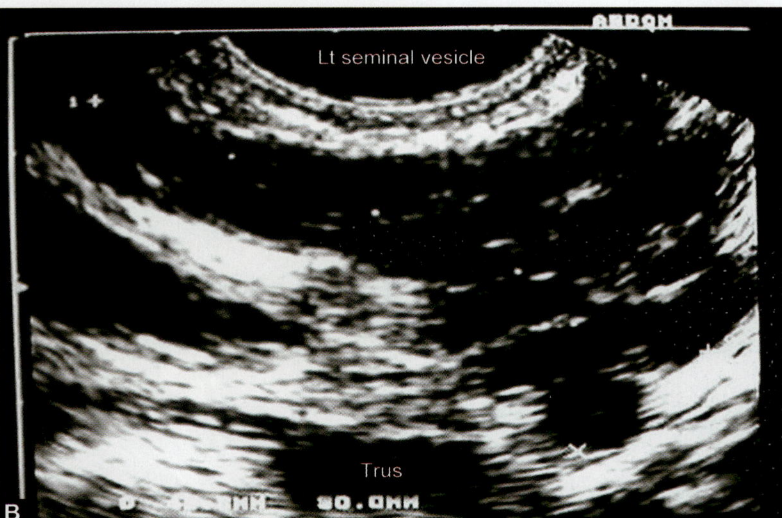

FIGURES 11.26A and B: Tubercular seminal vesiculitis. HRSG shows bilateral dilated seminal vesicles. Multiple echogenic septa are seen in the seminal vesicles. Septation and honeycombing is seen on both sides. Low-level echocardiogram collection is seen in them. The patient presented with oligospermia. On fine needle aspiration cytology (FNAC) chronic granulomatous infection is seen in both the seminal vesicle suggestive of tubercular infection.

EJACULATORY DUCT PATHOLOGIES

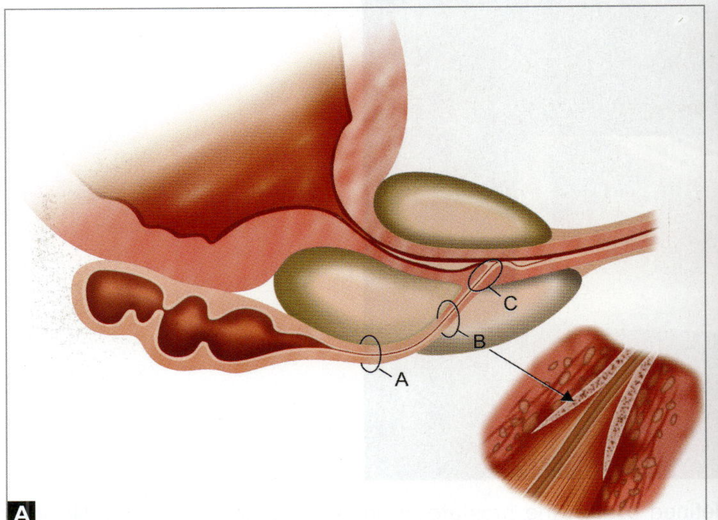

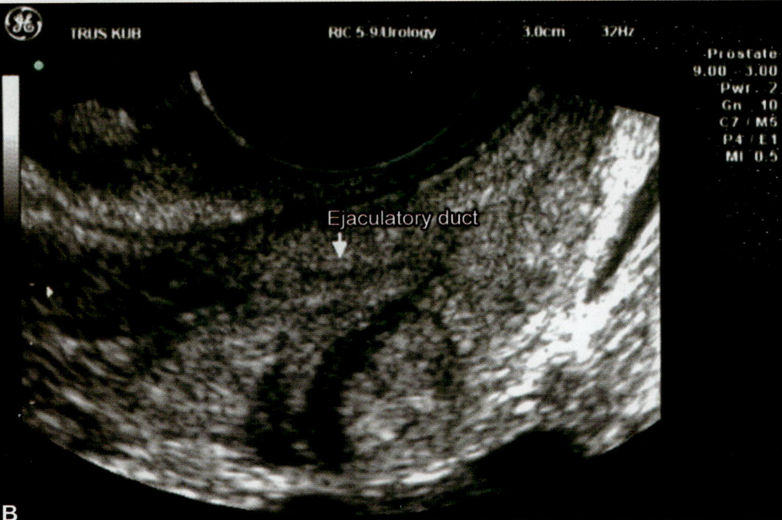

FIGURES 11.27A and B

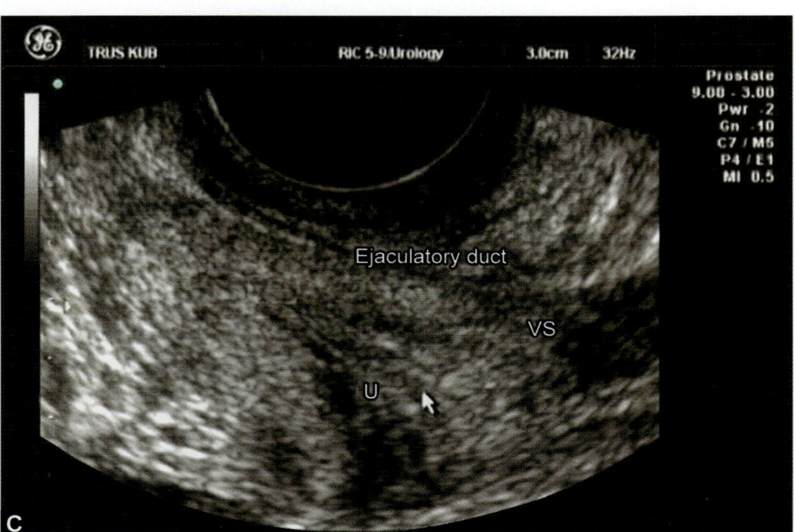

FIGURE 11.27C

FIGURES 11.27A to C: Diagrammatic representation shows normal relationship of seminal vesicle, VAS deferens and ejaculatory duct. Oblique view of the prostate in TRUS shows relationship of the seminal vesicle and ejaculatory duct.

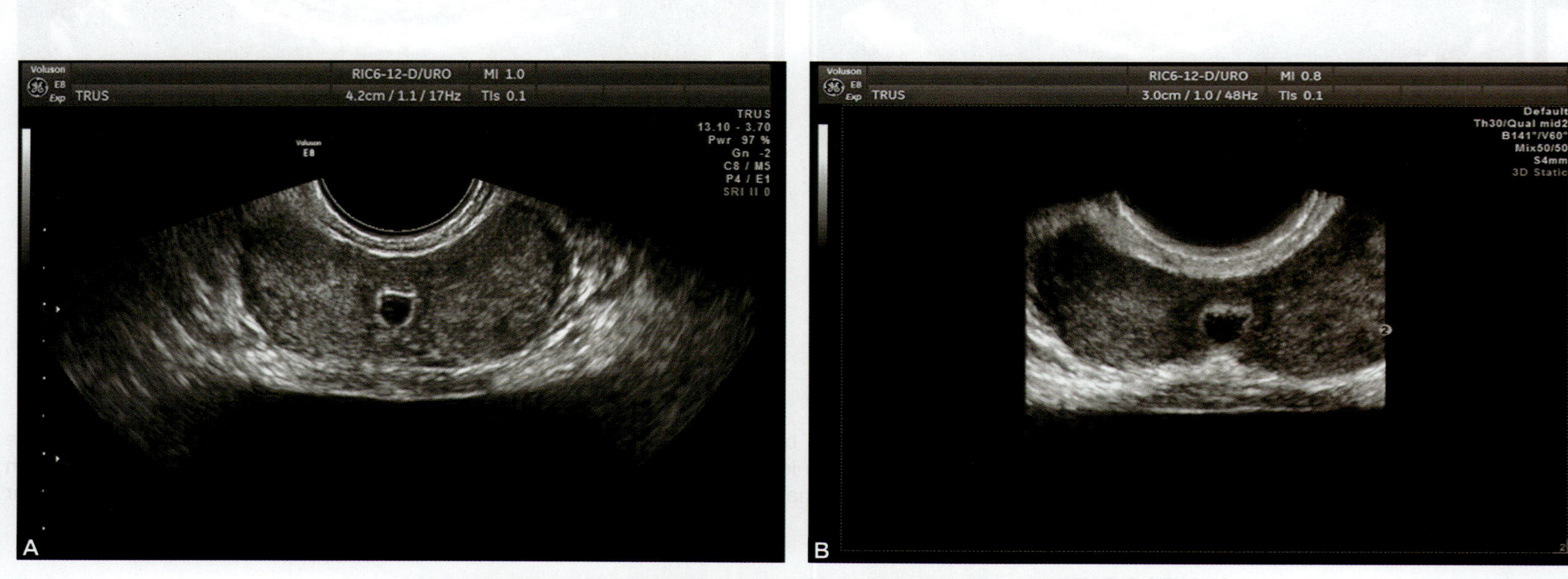

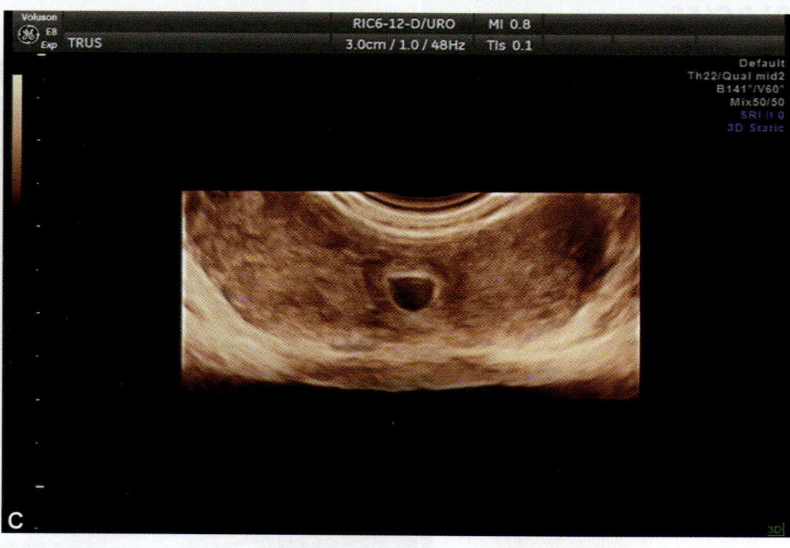

FIGURES 11.28A to C: Utricle cyst. Transrectal ultrasound shows a well-defined cyst in the prostate. It shows echogenic margins. No internal echocardiograph is seen in it suggestive of utricle cyst. 3D imaging shows the utricle cyst.

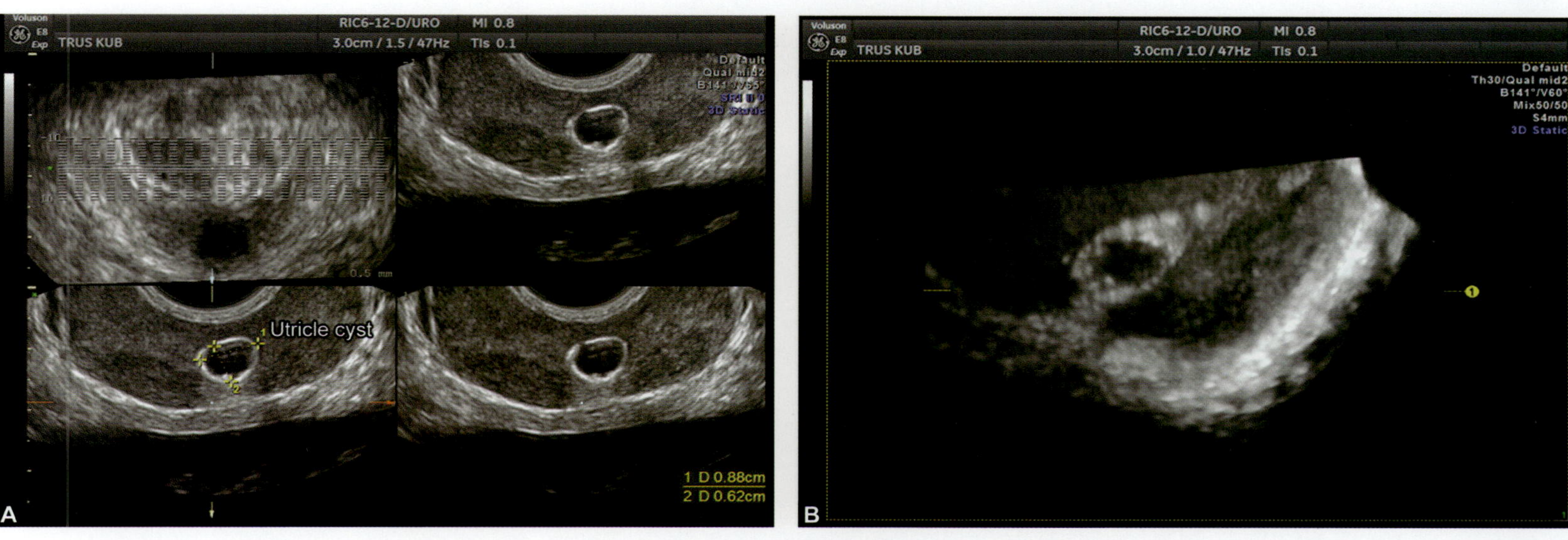

FIGURES 11.29A and B: Utricle cyst in the prostate. Transrectal ultrasound with TUI imaging shows well-defined cyst in the prostate with echogenic margins suggestive of utricle cyst.

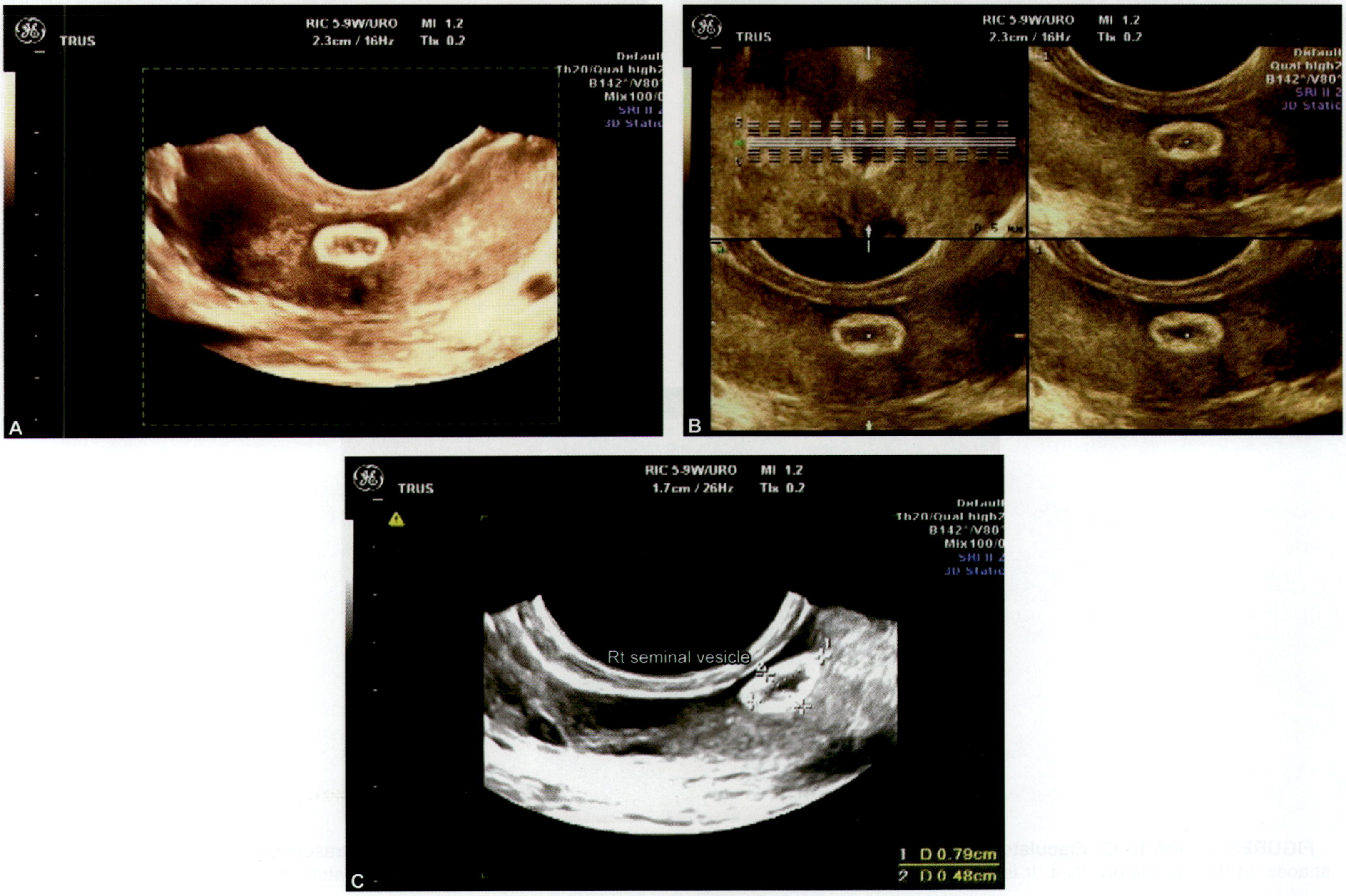

FIGURES 11.30A to C: Transrectal ultrasound shows a calcified utricle cyst in the prostate. TUI with 3D volume contrast imaging shows the cyst very clearly. It is seen blocking the mouth of right seminal vesicle.

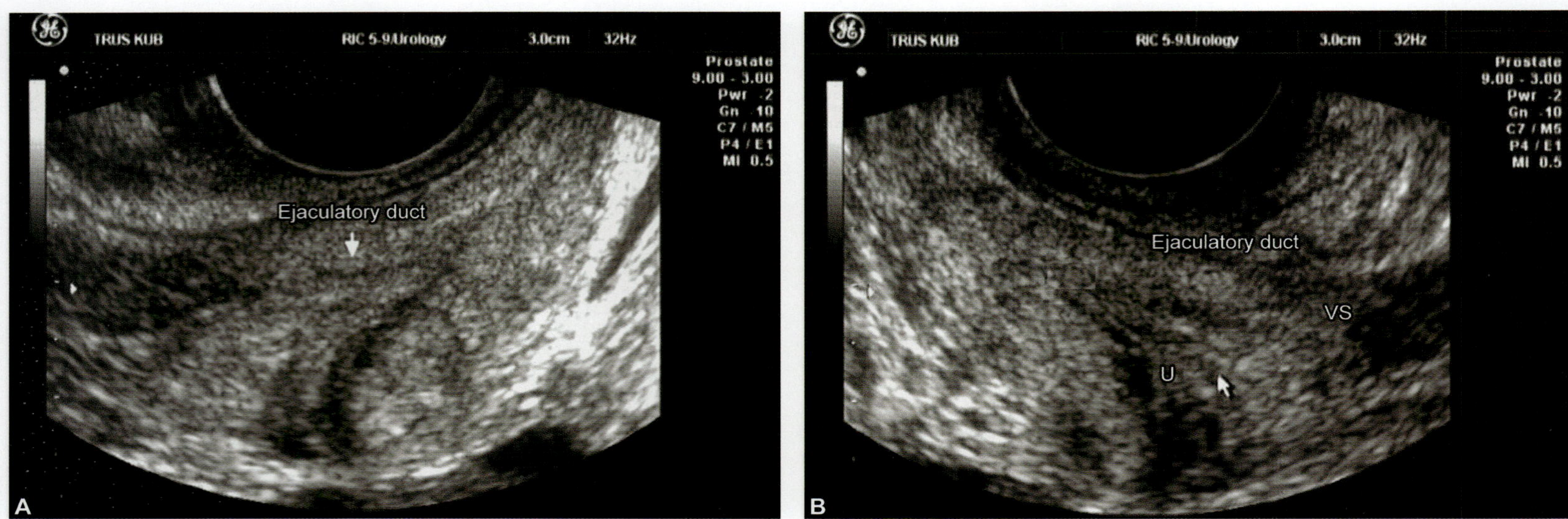

FIGURES 11.31A and B: Normal ejaculatory duct. Transrectal ultrasound shows normal ejaculatory duct as a hypoechoic tubular shadow. It is seen clearly in the oblique plane of the prostate.

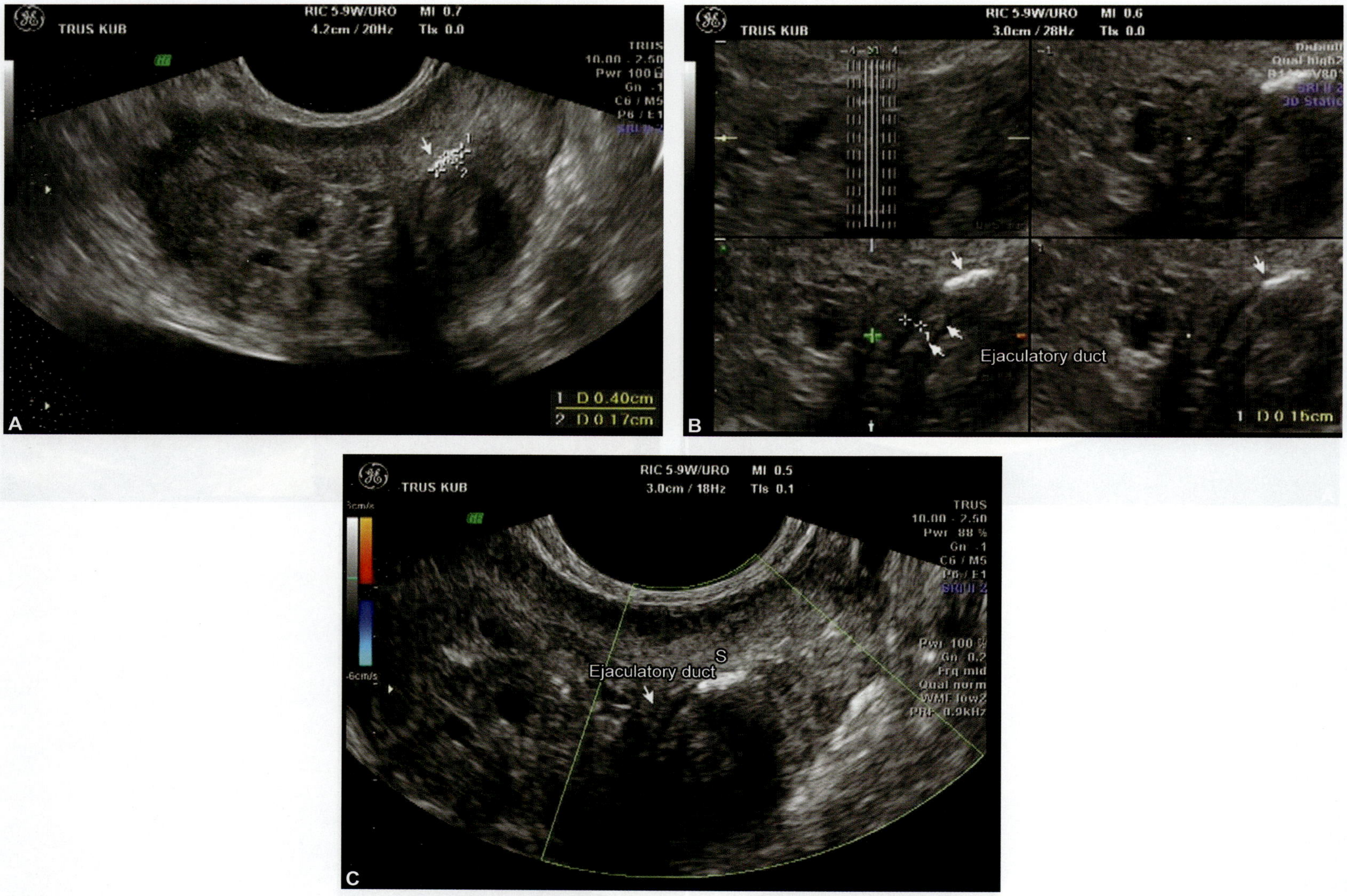

FIGURES 11.32A to C: Ejaculatory duct calculus. A patient presented with oligospermia. Transrectal ultrasound shows a linear echogenic shadow in the ejaculatory duct. It is accompanied with acoustic shadowing. It is seen obstructing the ejaculatory duct. The duct is seen dilated.

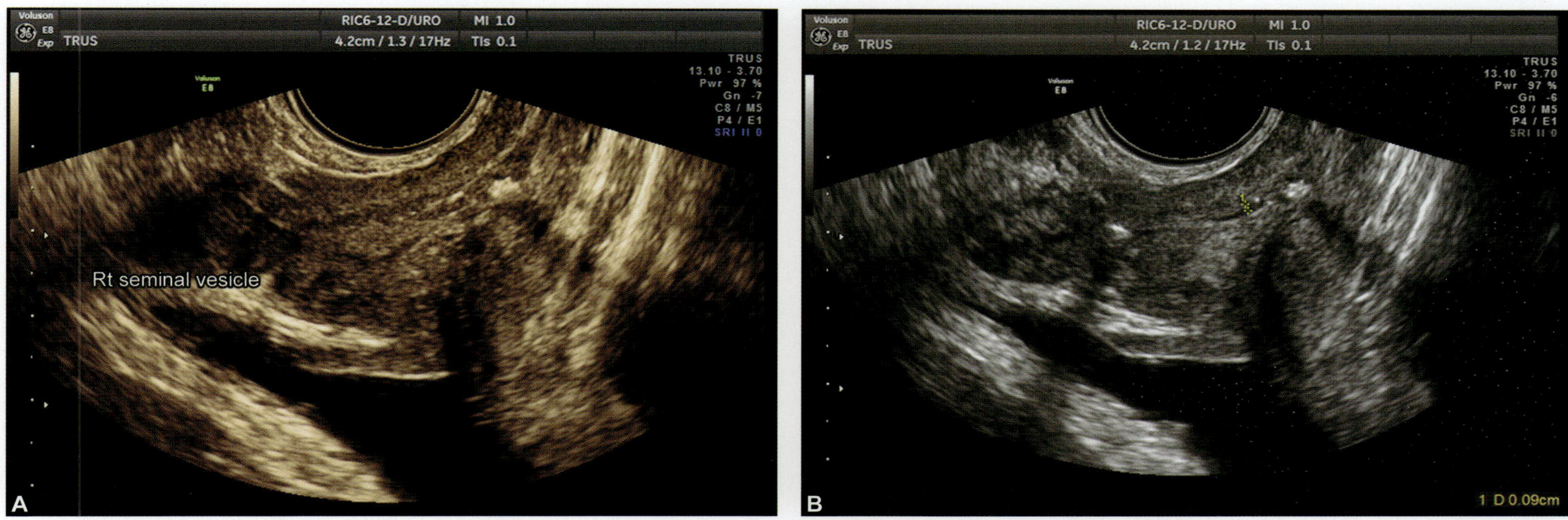

FIGURES 11.33A and B: Ejaculatory duct calculus. A patient presented with decreased amount of ejaculate. TRUS shows two echogenic shadows in the ejaculatory duct. One in the proximal part and another in the distal part suggestive of ejaculatory duct calculi. They are accompanied with acoustic shadowing.

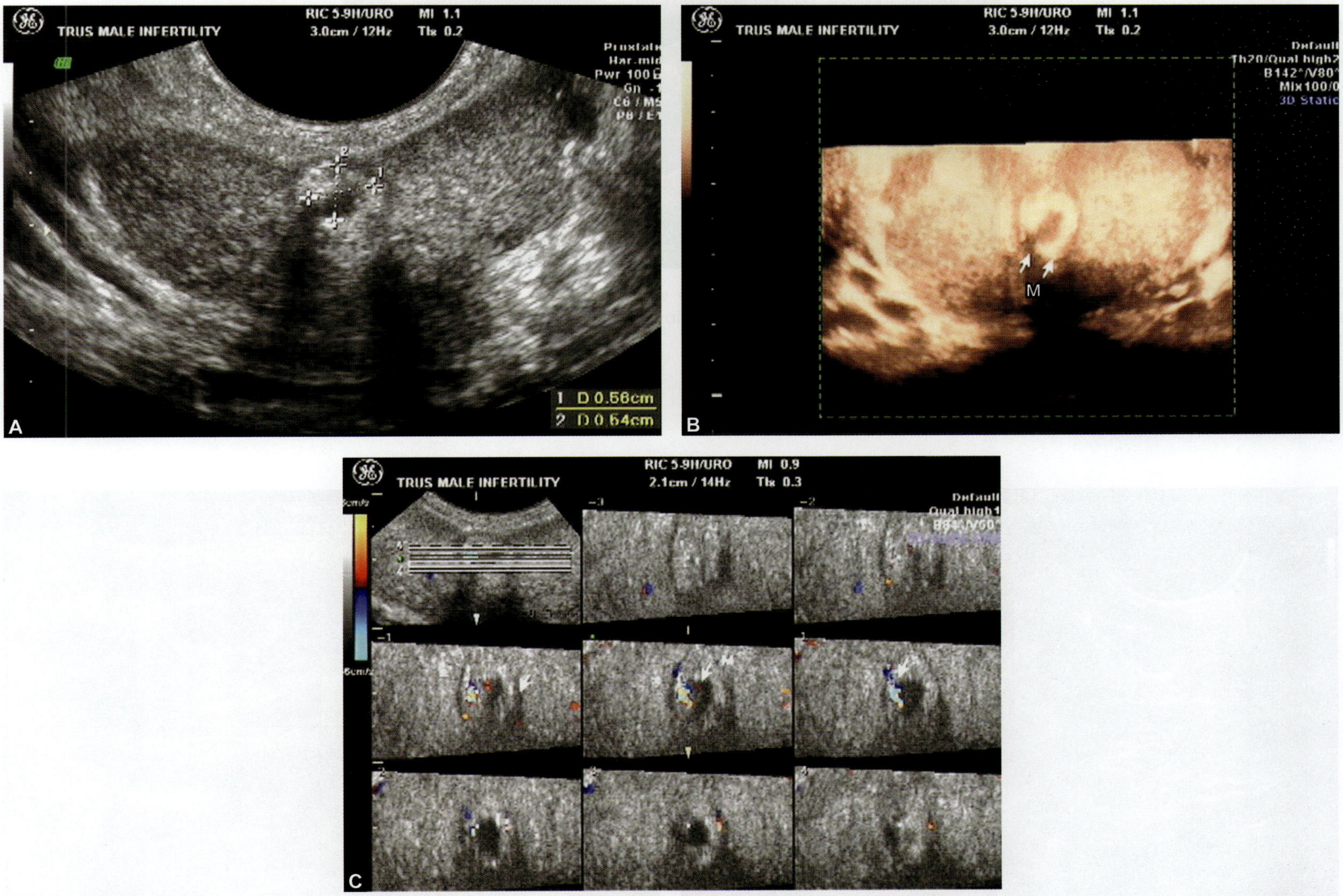

FIGURES 11.34A to C: Calcified utricle cyst. Transrectal ultrasound with 3D imaging shows calcified utricle cyst. On 3D ultrasound in coronal plane, the cyst is seen clearly. The dense calcification is seen in the cyst wall.

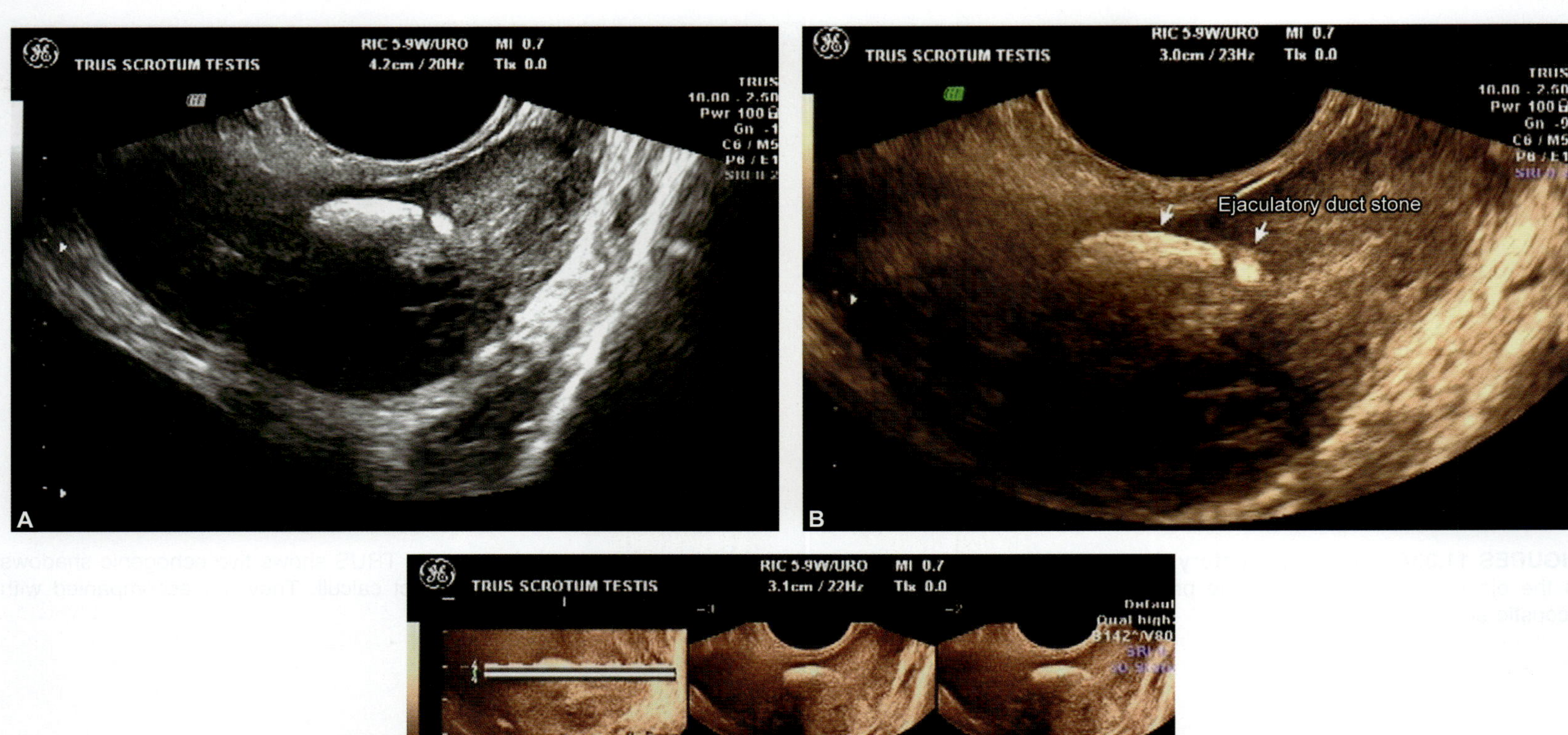

FIGURES 11.35A to C: Big ejaculatory duct calculus. A patient came with the history of scanty ejaculate with oligospermia. TRUS shows a big echogenic shadow in the ejaculatory duct. It is accompanied with acoustic shadowing. On 3D TUI imaging, another small calculus is seen near the big calculus.

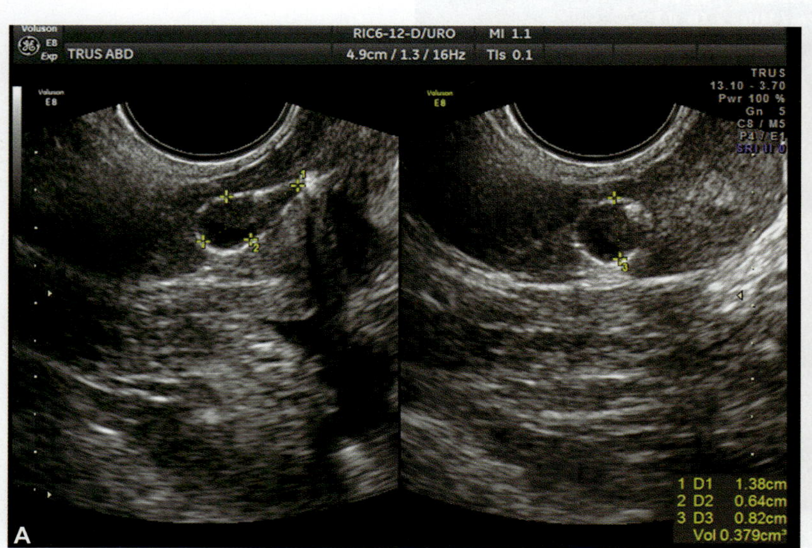

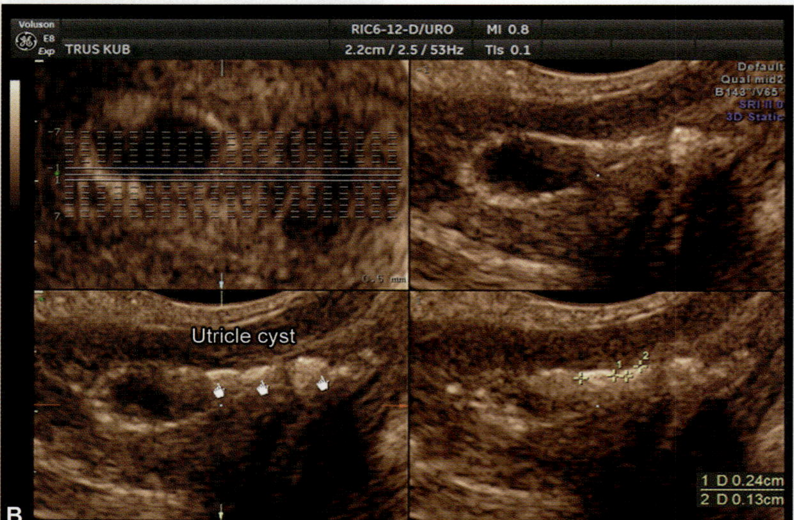

FIGURES 11.36A and B

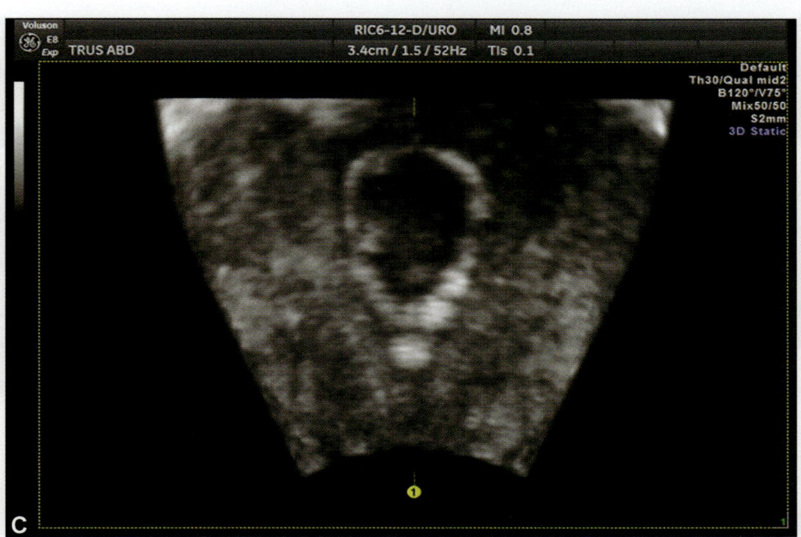

FIGURE 11.36C

FIGURES 11.36A to C: Utricle cyst with small calculi in ejaculatory duct. TRUS shows a well-defined cyst in the prostate. It shows echogenic calcification in its wall. Small echogenic shadows are also seen in the proximal part of ejaculatory duct suggestive of ejaculatory duct calculi. On 3D ultrasound in coronal plane shows the calculi very clearly.

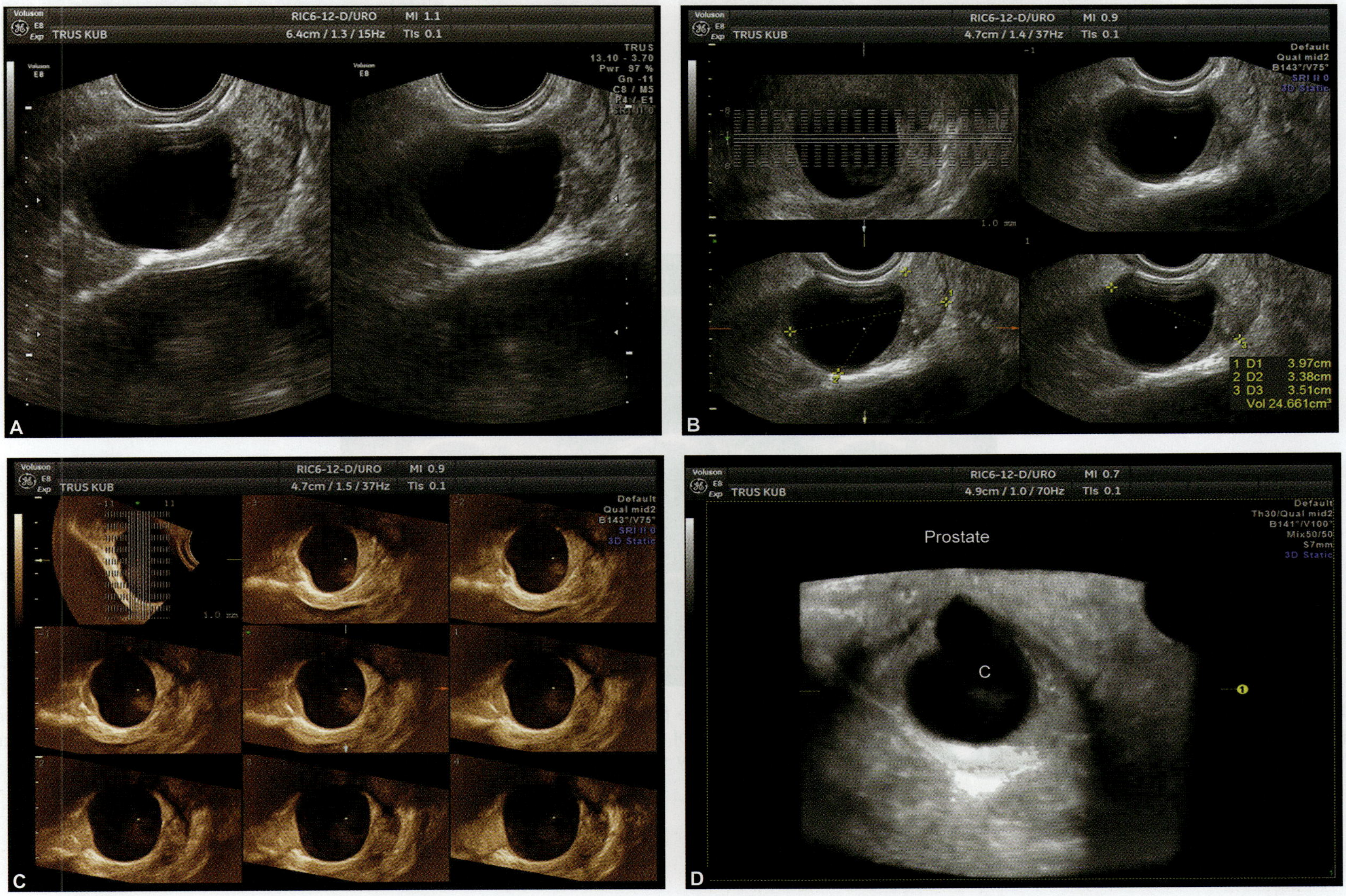

FIGURES 11.37A to D: A patient presented with scanty ejaculate. HRSG shows a big cyst in the prostate suggestive of big utricle cyst. 3D ultrasound with volume contrast imaging, clearly shows the cyst.

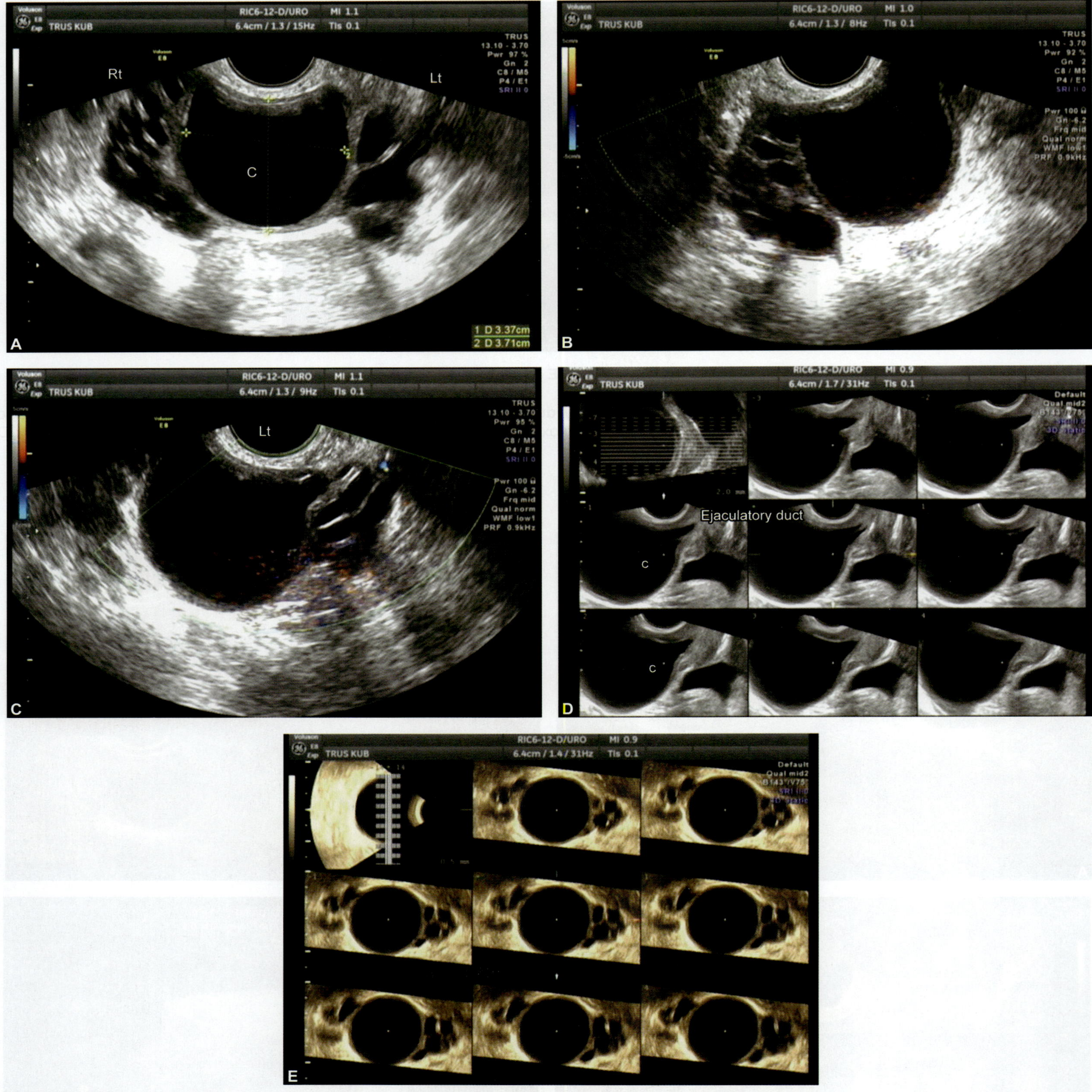

FIGURES 11.38A to E: A patient presented with big cystic shadow in the prostate. It is seen in relation to the ejaculatory duct on transverse oblique plane. Sharp beaking of the cyst is seen suggestive of acute obstruction of the cyst. There is also evidence of backpressure seen on both the seminal vesicle resulting into engorgement of the seminal vesicle, which is clearly seen on 3D ultrasound with TUI imaging.

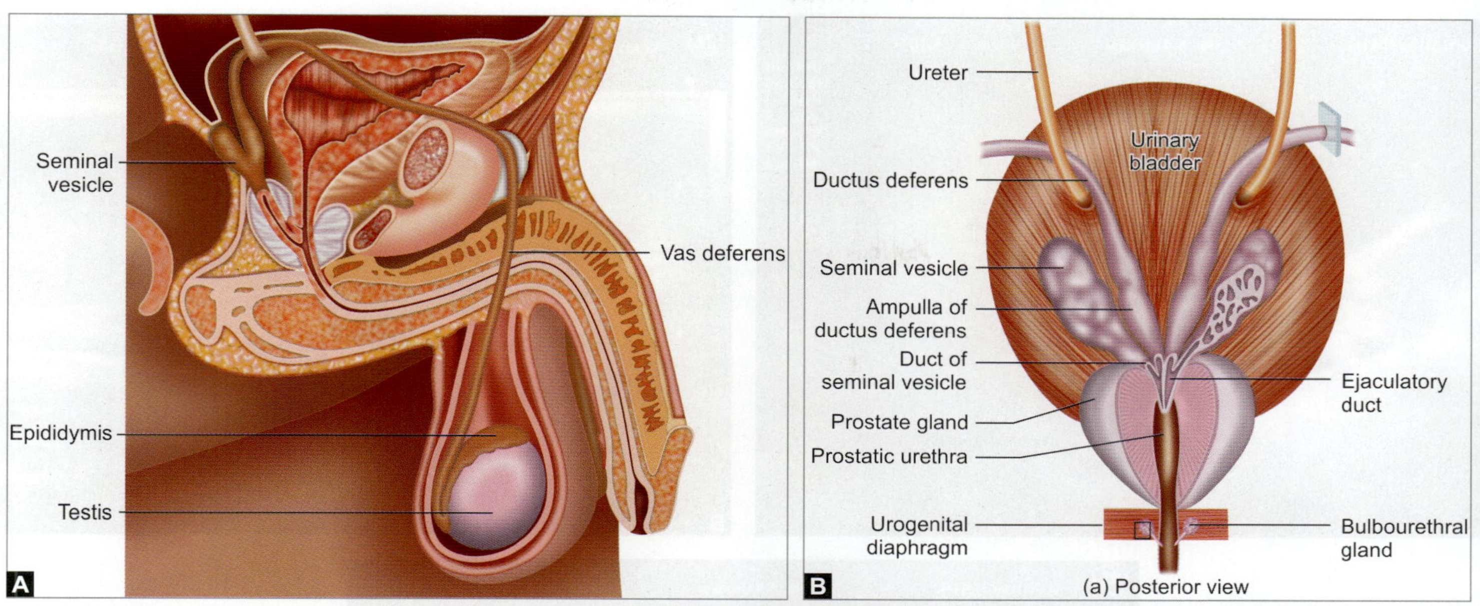

FIGURES 11.39A and B: The figure shows normal relations of seminal vesicle, vas deferens and ejaculatory duct in longitudinal and coronal plane with diagrammatic representation of the ejaculatory duct opening into prostatic urethra.

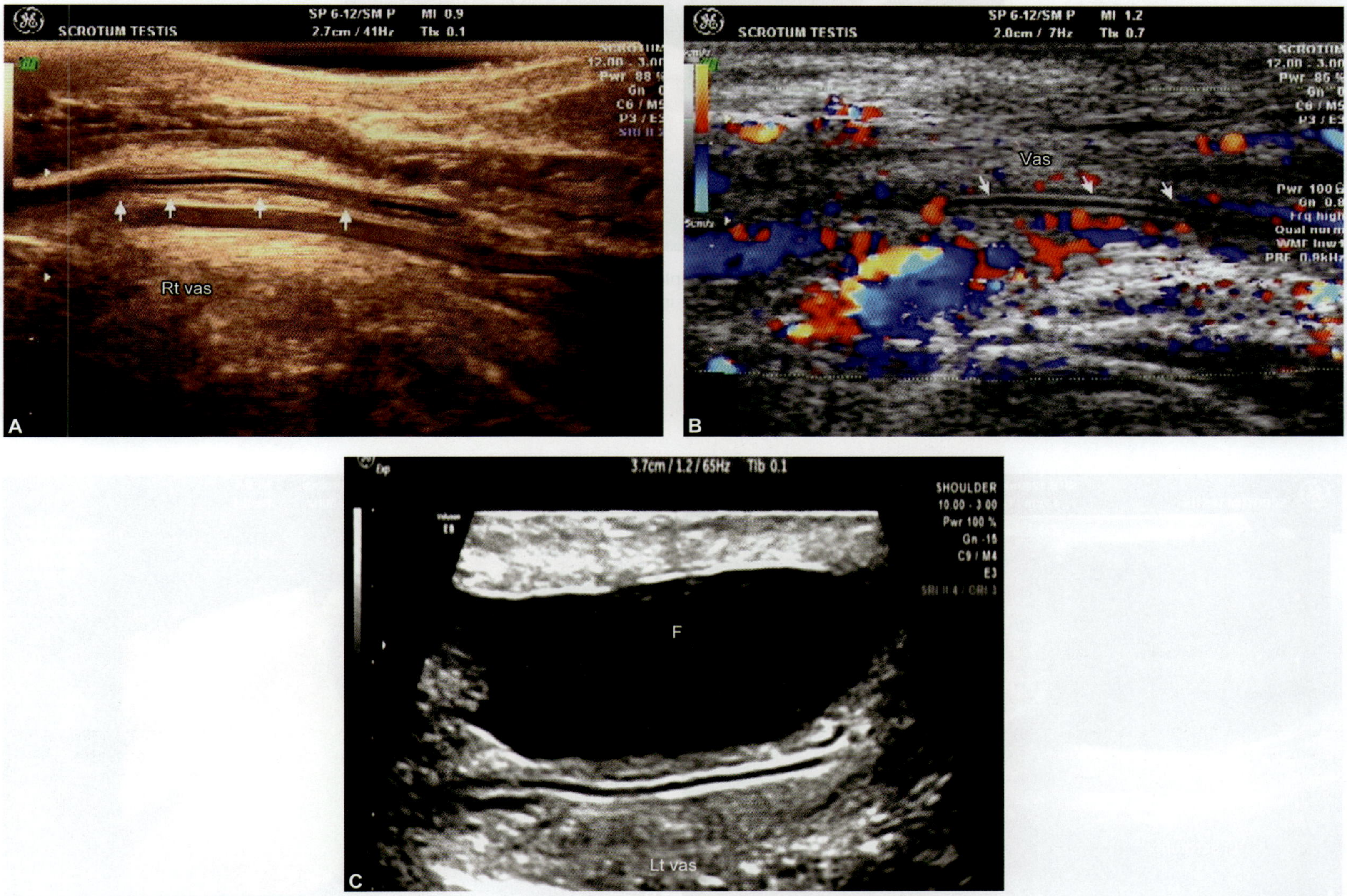

FIGURES 11.40A to C: Normal vas deferens. HRSG shows normal vas deferens in the inguinal canal. It is seen as thin echogenic tubular shadow, which may be mistaken as vessel. However, color flow imaging, does not show any flow in it. Figure 11.40B shows intrascrotal part of vas deferens.

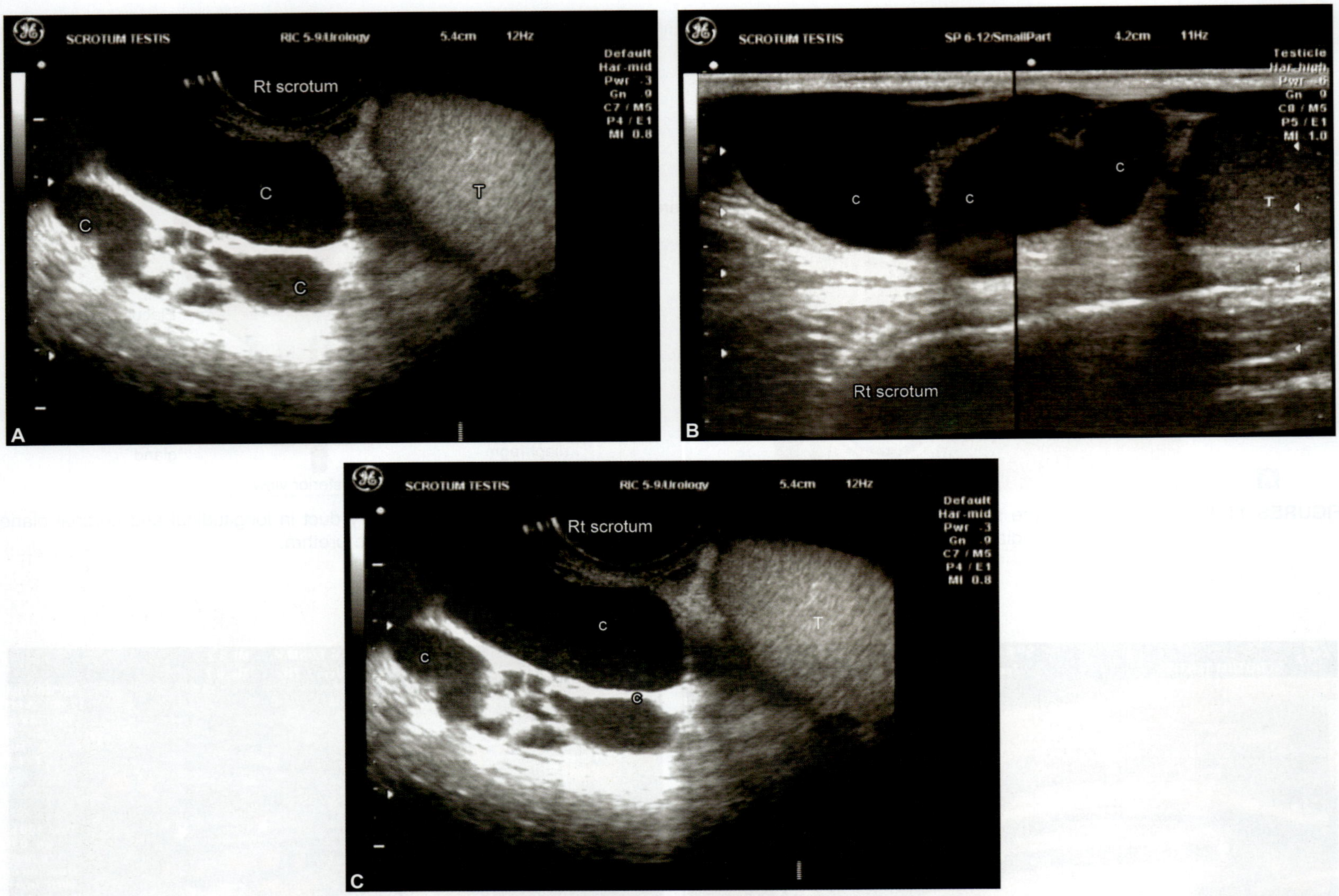

FIGURES 11.41A to C: Epididymis and cord cyst. HRSG shows multiple cysts along the cord. Normal cord tissue replaced by the cysts. These cord cysts are known as spermatocele. The arrest of the sperm is seen in the cord resulting into oligo or azoospermia. Small cyst is also seen in the epididymal head.

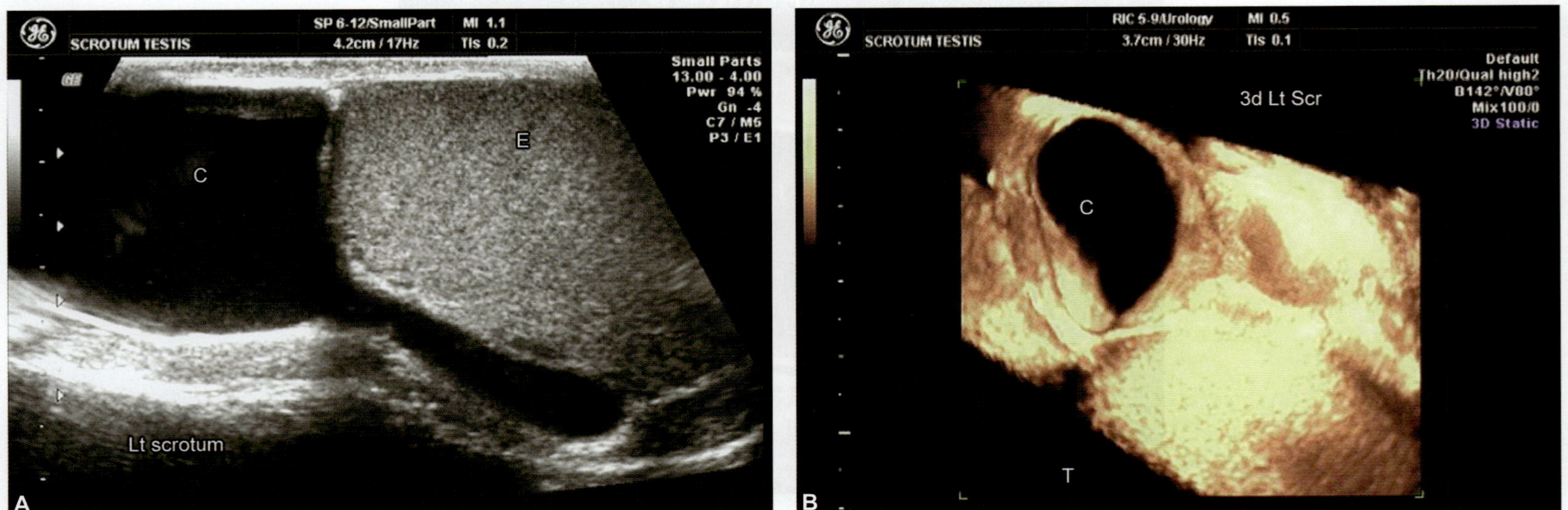

FIGURES 11.42A and B: Big epididymal cyst extending in the body and the tail. HRSG shows a big cystic mass in the head of the epididymis. The cyst is seen extending in the body in the tail of epididymis. It is seen replacing the normal structure. 3D surface rendering imaging of the scrotum shows the cyst in much clear detail.

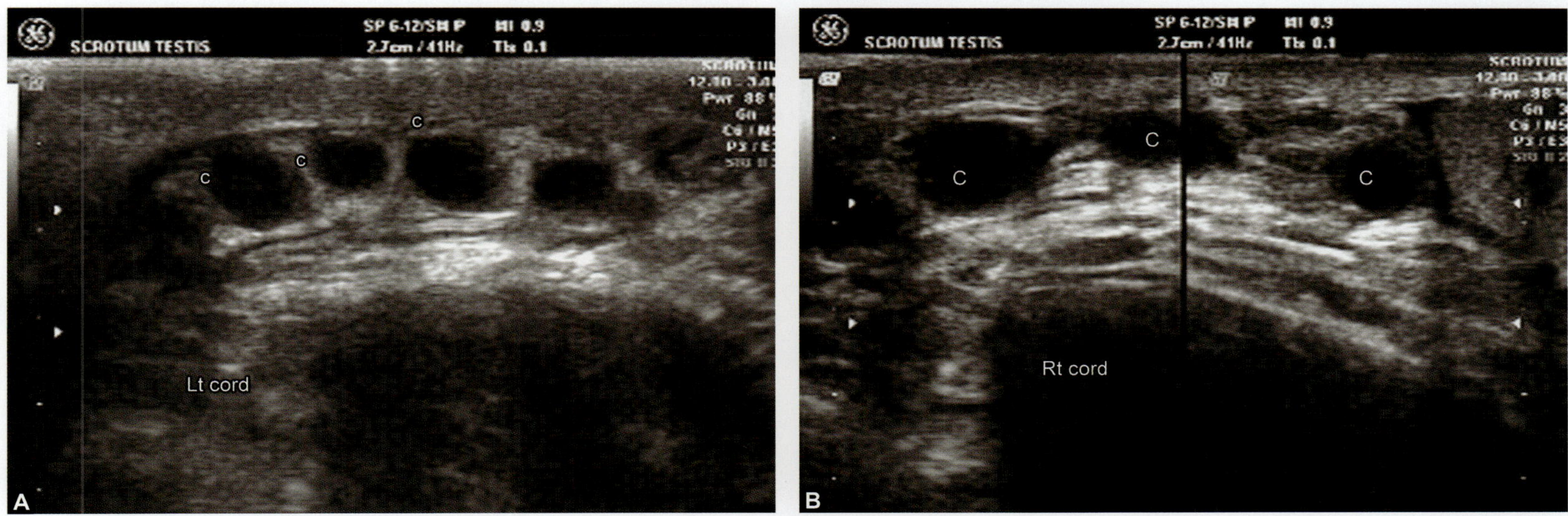

FIGURES 11.43A and B: Multiple cord cysts. HRSG shows multiple cyst in the left spermatic cord. The cysts are noncommunicating.

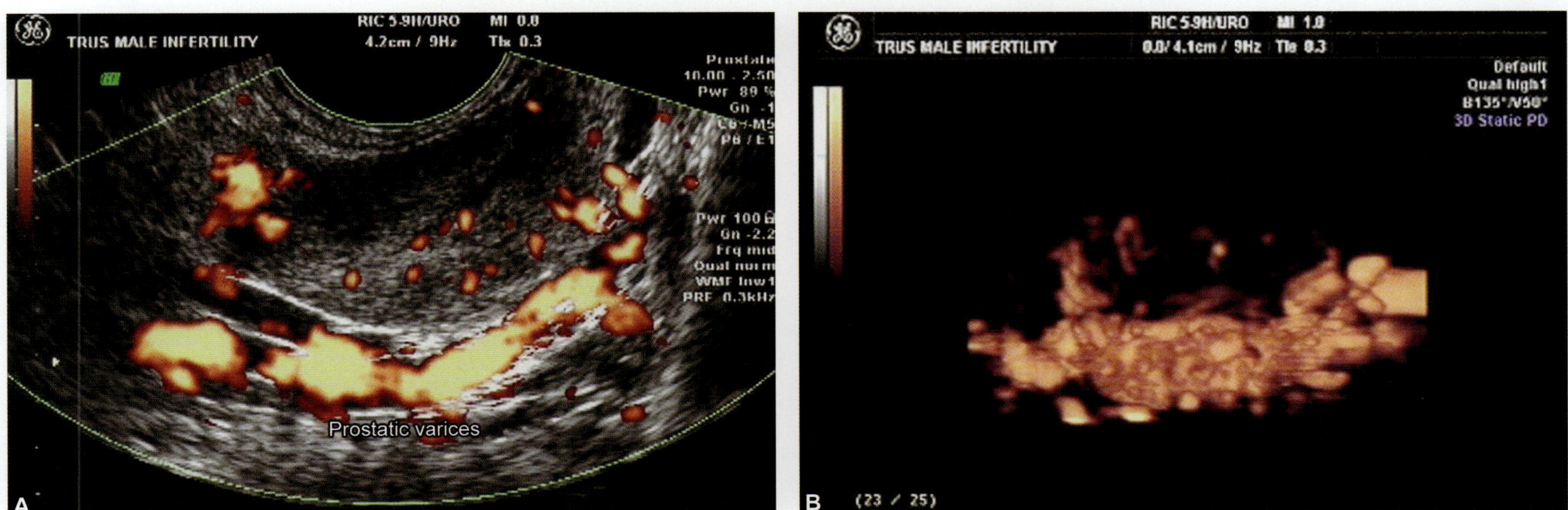

FIGURES 11.44A and B: Prostatic varices. A patient presented with oligospermia with perineal pain. TRUS shows multiple dilated vessels in the prostatic bed suggestive of prostatic varices. 3D power angio shows bunch of varices in the prostatic bed. The prostatic varices increased the temperature of the prostatic bed, which results into oligospermia and also affects motility of the sperm.

CONCLUSION

High resolution transrectal ultrasound is an excellent modality for evaluation of sperm transport system. It has high accuracy, rapid to perform. The 3D ultrasound with color flow imaging increases the diagnostic accuracy of investigation. It is 1st line of investigation to evaluate sperm transport system in cases of male infertility.

CHAPTER 12

Testes

PK Srivastava

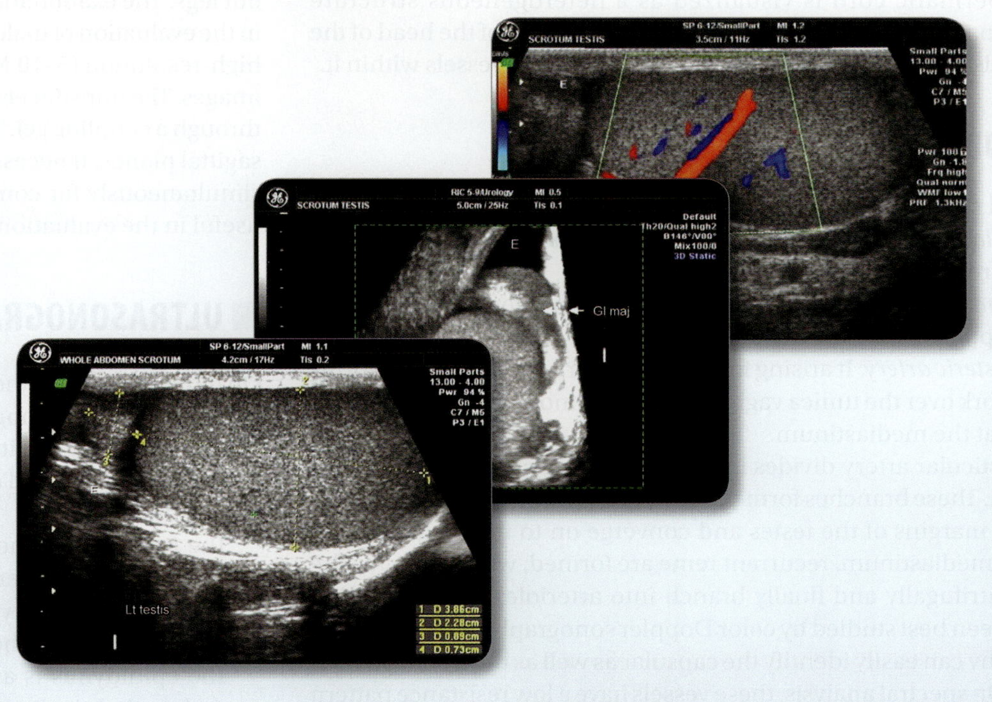

INTRODUCTION

At one time, diagnosis of scrotal pathologies was dependent not only on clinical manifestation but to a large extent on the palpatory examination of the scrotum. Today the advent of newer high-resolution ultrasonographic machines has revolutionized imaging of the scrotum. Further addition of color Doppler imaging has increased the efficiency of diagnosis of scrotal pathologies especially in acute scrotum. In fact probably the single most important advantage of ultrasonography is its ability of distinguish between intra- and extratesticular mass lesions.

In general, the initial confusion of overlapping signs and symptoms in many conditions is now significantly made easy due to the availability of sonography. Ultrasonography allows the clinician to treat a patient early with no delays and confirms the clinical diagnosis with relative ease, and yields adequate information in most cases.

NORMAL ANATOMY

The testes is symmetrical, ovoid structures measuring about 2 to 3 cm in diameter and 3 to 5 cm in length. Each testes is encased in a dense white membrane called tunica albuginea. The epididymis is a tortuous tubular structure located superolaterally over the posterior aspect of the testes. It is round or triangular in shape with two expansions, the head (globus major) at the lower pole. The testes, epididymis and proximal segment of spermatic cord are invested in the visceral layer of tunica vaginalis, which covers the entire testes except for a small area posteriorly where it folds on itself. This bare area, the mediastinum testes, is where the spermatic cord and its contents, i.e. the blood and lymphatic vessels, the nerves and epididymal ducts join the testicle. The parietal layer of tunica vaginalis lines the inner wall of the scrotum.

The spermatic cord is visualized as a heterogeneous structure (predominantly echogenic) arising in close proximity of the head of the Epididymis. Color Doppler studies show presence of vessels within it.

BLOOD SUPPLY

The blood supply to the scrotum and its contents is as follows:

1. *Testicular artery:* It supplies mainly the testes and epididymis and arises from the abdominal aorta.
2. *Differential artery:* It arises from the superior or inferior vesicle artery and supplies to the vas deferens.
3. *Cremasteric artery:* It arising from the inferior epigastric artery forms a network over the tunica vaginalis to anastomose with the testicular artery at the mediastinum.

The testicular artery divides into branches, which pierce the tunica albuginea. These branches form the centripetal branches, which course along the margins of the testes and converge on to the mediastinum. From the mediastinum, recurrent reme are formed, which traverse the testes centrifugally and finally branch into arterioles and capillaries. This has been best studied by color Doppler sonography. Color Doppler sonography can easily identify the capsular as well as the intratesticular arteries. On spectral analysis, these vessels have a low resistance pattern with high diastolic flow.

VENOUS DRAINAGE

The pampiniform plexus exits from the mediastinum and converges into the testicular vein, which drains into the renal vein on the left side and inferior vena cava on the right. The deferential vein drains into the pelvic veins, and cremasteric vein drains into tributaries of the inferior epigastric and deep pudendal veins.

Indications for Scrotal Sonography

1. Evaluation of acute scrotal disorders
   - Torsion
   - Inflammation
   - Trauma
2. Evaluation of scrotal fluid collections
   - Hydrocele
   - Pyocele/hematocele
3. Evaluation of a scrotal mass
   - Extratesticular
   - Intratesticular
4. Evaluation of metastatic disease
   - Retroperitoneal lymphadenopathy
   - Testicular involvement—lymphoma, leukemia
5. Unexplained abdominal mass
   - Malignant change in an undescended testis
6. Evaluation of undescended testes
7. Exclusion of occult testicular neoplasm
   - Leydig cell tumor
8. Evaluation of infertility
   - Varicocele.

TECHNIQUE

The examination of the scrotum is normally done in supine position with the patient's scrotum supported by towels or other means with spread-out legs. The examination may also be done in erect position especially in the evaluation of male infertility for visualizing varicoceles. A real-time high-resolution (5–10 MHz) linear array transducer provides excellent images. The transducer is normally applied directly to the scrotal surface through a coupling gel. The testes is scanned in both transverse as well as sagittal planes. If necessary a transverse section to visualize both testes simultaneously for comparison is undertaken. Valsalva's maneuver is useful in the evaluation of varicocele.

ULTRASONOGRAPHIC APPEARANCES

On ultrasonography, the normal testes is an ovoid structure with smooth contours and a homogeneous echo texture—medium level echoes. In fact the echogenicity of the testes simulates that of the thyroid. A bright echogenic band extending craniocaudally in the testes indicates mediastinum testes.

The tunica albuginea is not well identified normally while linear hypoechoic areas traversing through the testes indicate testicular septa. The rete testes, not very commonly seen, presents as a hypoechoic area in close proximity of the epididymal head.

The epididymis is an elongated structure measuring about 6 to 7 cm in length. It is situated posterolateral to the testes. The head of the epididymis is the largest portion of the epididymis and is situated in close proximity of the upper pole of the testes. The body of the Epididymis is thinner and lies along the lateral surface of the testes. The tail is situated in the region of the lower pole of the testes but is not usually visualized. The appendicular testis is a remnant of the mullerian duct and is best visualized in the presence of hydrocele. On an average, the epididymis is relatively hypoechoic compared to the testes.

With the use of color Doppler sonography, arterial flow is normally demonstrated in the testes and in the spermatic cord. However, the arterial flow in the epididymis is seldom or never seen because of the small size of the vessels and very slow flow (any detectable flow in the epididymis is usually considered abnormal) within the testes the capsular, centripetal and centrifugal arteries are well identified.

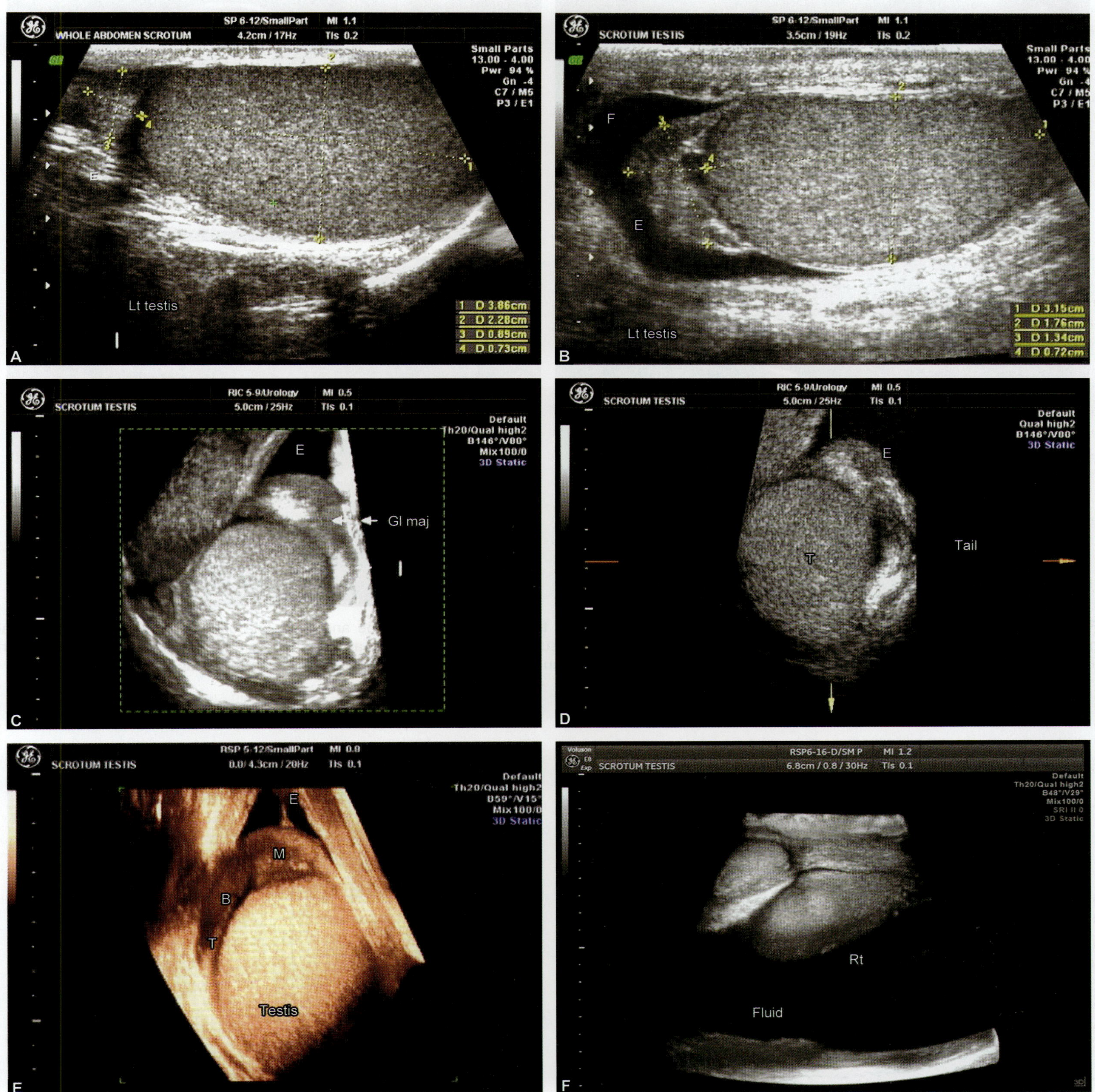

FIGURES 12.1A to F: HRSG shows normal testis. The testes is ovoid in shape with fine granular echoes and homogeneous texture. Head of the epididymis is seen in proximity to the upper pole of the testes. It is less echogenic than the testes. HRSG shows a small well-defined Iso echogenic nodular shadow fixed with upper pole of the testes is appendix testes. Small amount of fluid is seen in the scrotal sac and the appendix is seen clearly in fluid background. 3D surface rendering of the testes clearly shows the testes. Head of epididymis body and tail of the epididymis are well appreciated on 3D imaging. 3D view of the scrotum shows both testes the raphe is seen dividing the scrotal cavity into two. Each testes is well visualized in each scrotal sac.

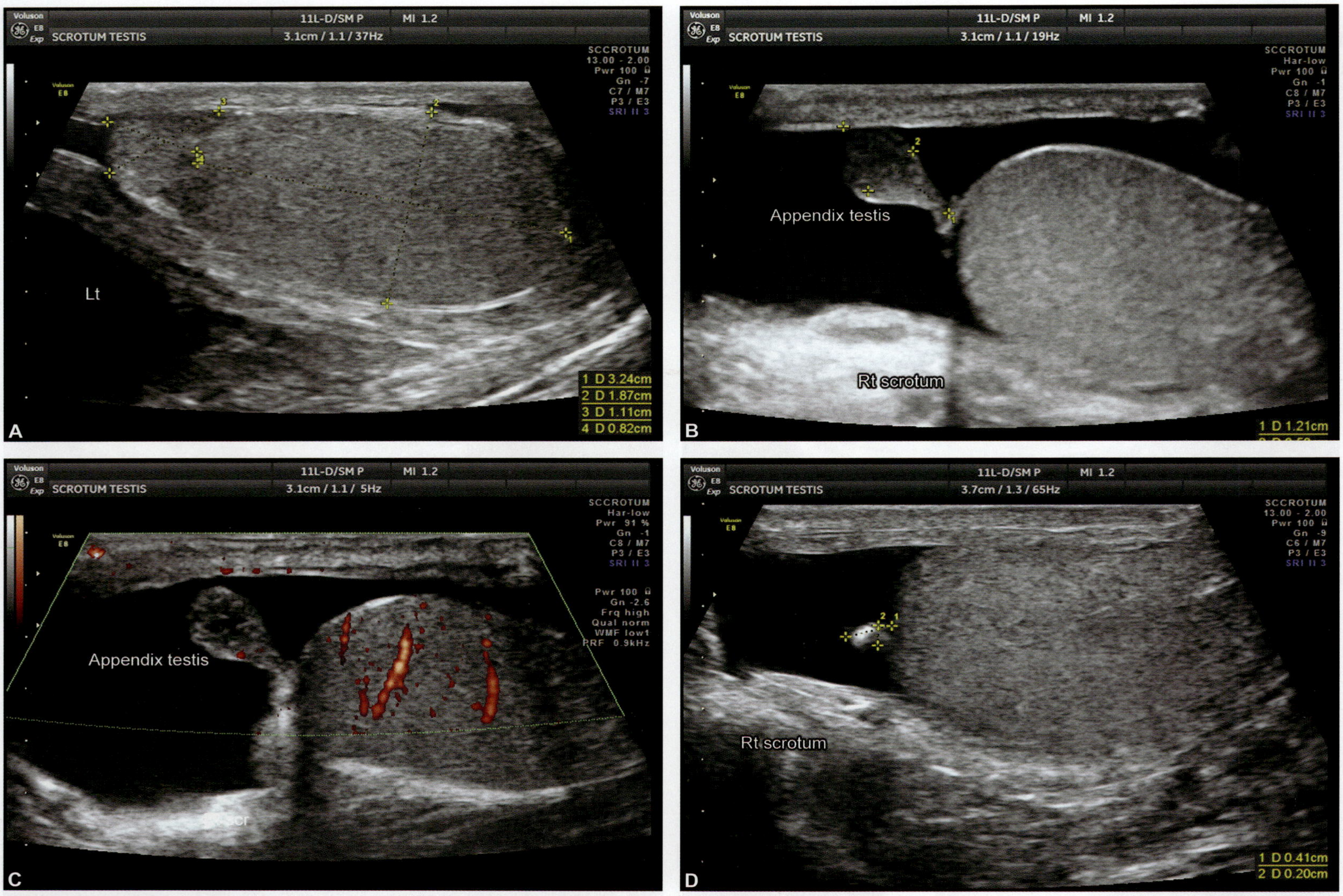

FIGURES 12.2A to D: Normal testes. HRSG shows normal testes. The testes are ovoid in shape and show fine granular texture. The epididymal head is seen sitting at the upper pole of right epididymis. A small soft tissue shadow is seen fixed at the upper pole of right testes, which is smooth in outline and homogeneous in texture suggestive of appendix testes. Figure C also shows echogenic calcification in the appendix testes.

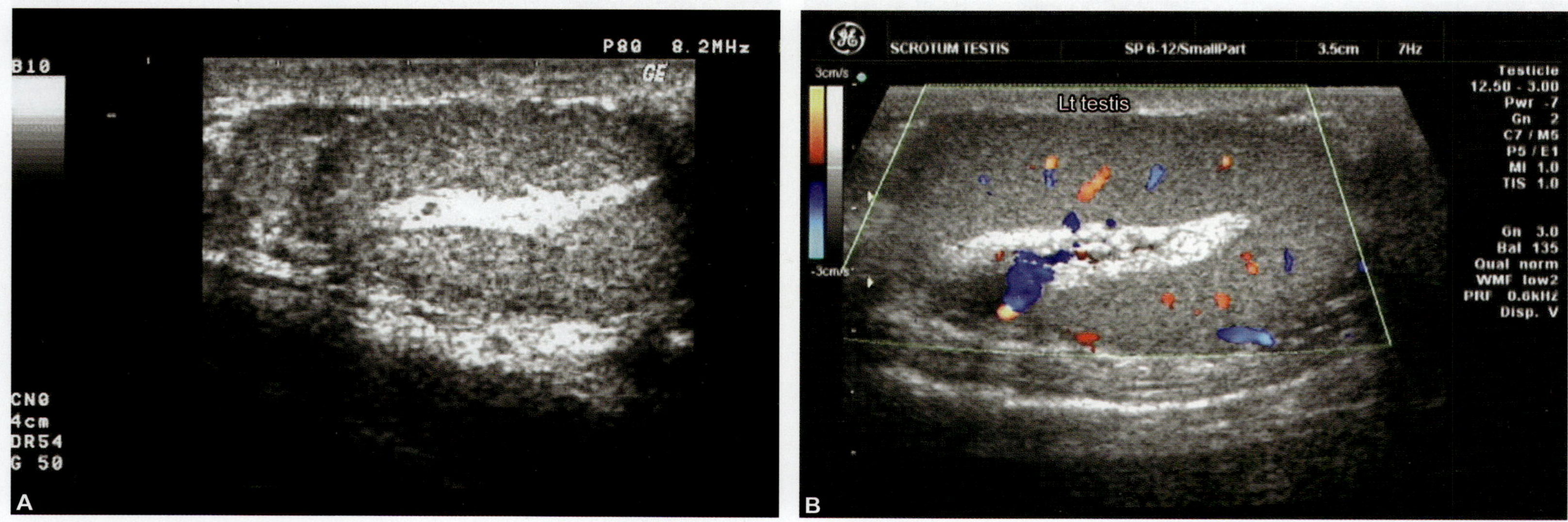

FIGURES 12.3A and B: Normal mediastinum testes. Longitudinal image shows an echogenic band running in the substance of the testes is mediastinum testes. On color flow imaging, few vessels are seen feeding the testes.

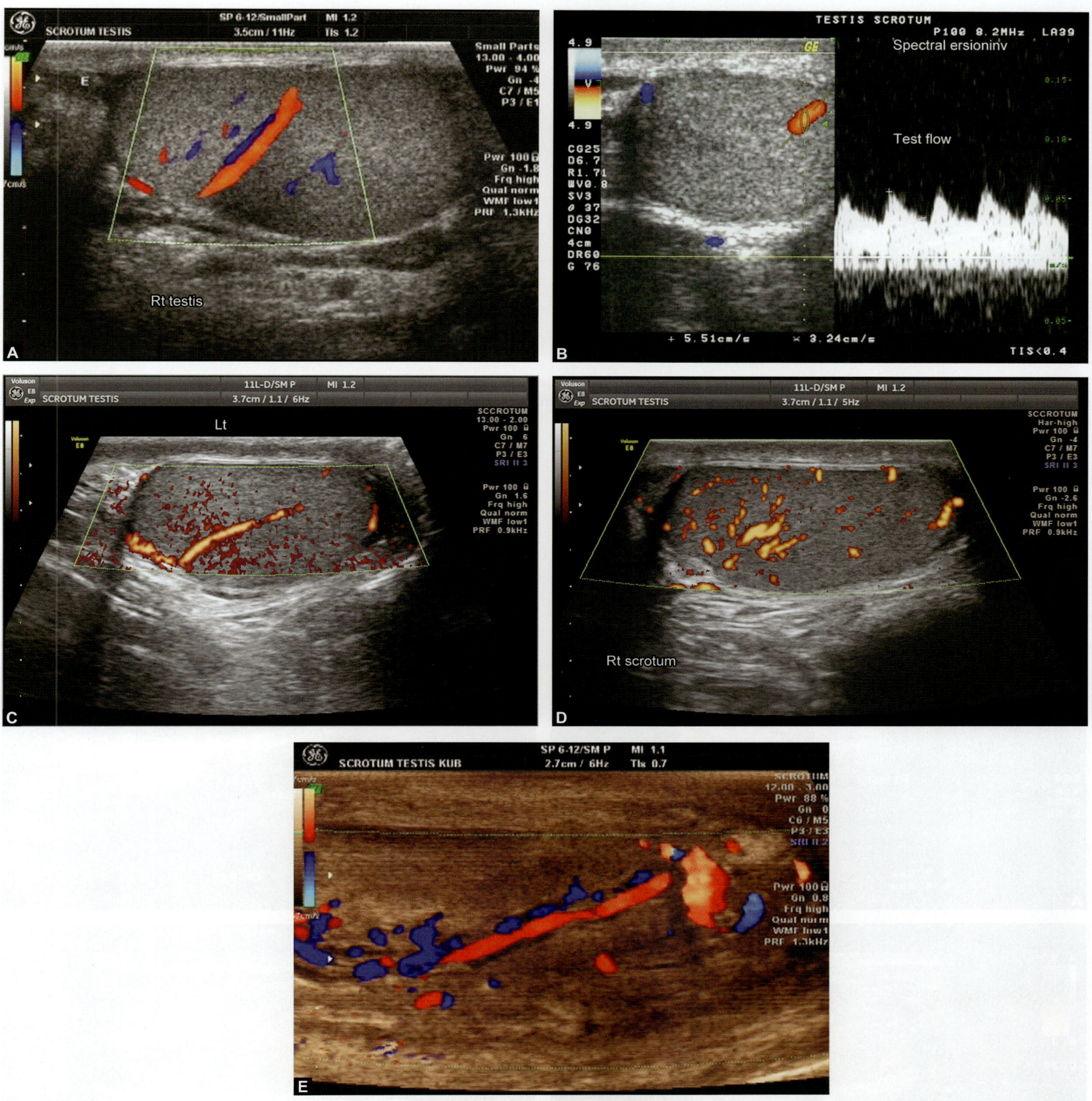

FIGURES 12.4A to E: Normal testicular flow. The testes is supplied by testicular artery. Color Doppler shows the artery supplying the testes. On spectral Doppler tracing, low systolic and prolonged diastolic flow is seen in inter testicular artery. Typical of low arterial flow pattern.

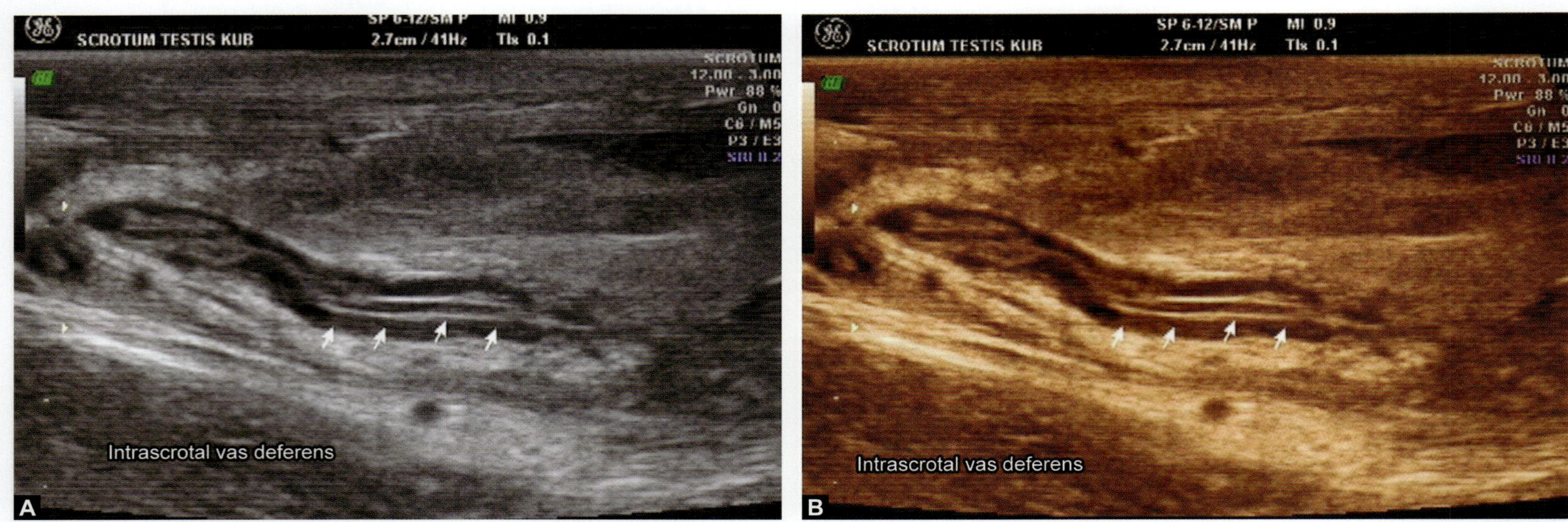

FIGURES 12.5A and B: Normal intrascrotal VAS deferens. HRSG shows the intra scrotal part of VAS deferens. A thin echogenic tubular shadow is seen running posterior to the testes. It shows bright echogenic wall. It may be confused with the vessel. Therefore, color flow imaging is important to differentiate it from the vessel.

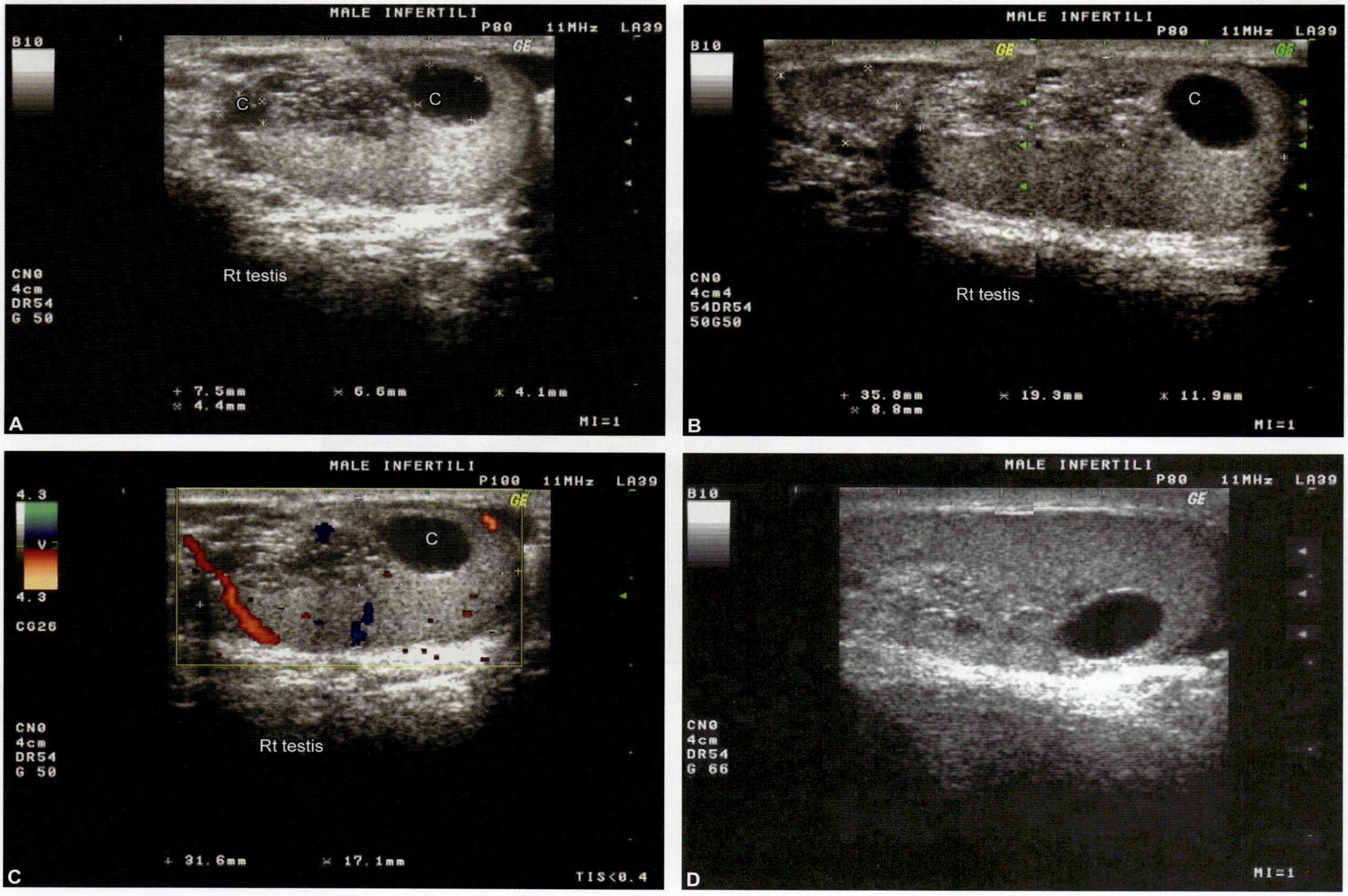

FIGURES 12.6A to D: Cysts of rete testes. A patient presented with male infertility azoospermia. HRSG of testes show multiple cysts running through the mediastinum testes in the substance of the testes. Few medium size cysts are also seen in the testes. They are dispersed in the testicular substance suggestive of cysts of rete testes. On color flow imaging, no flow is seen in the cysts.

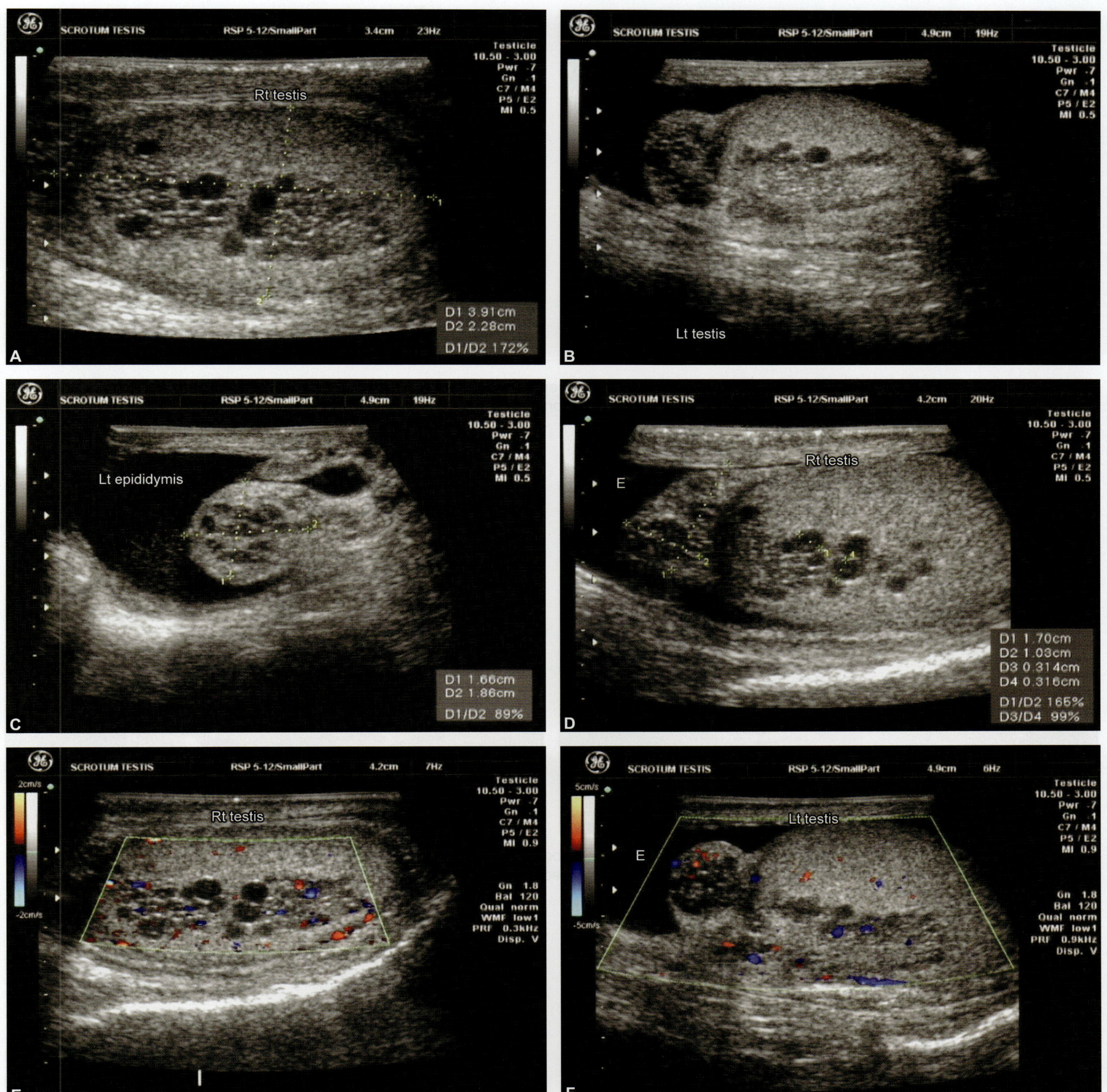

FIGURES 12.7A to F: Bilateral rete testes cysts. A patient of male infertility shows bilateral cysts in the testes. The cysts are diffuse in distribution suggestive of rete testes cysts. The cysts are also seen in the epididymis of both testes. On color flow imaging, no flow is seen in the cyst.

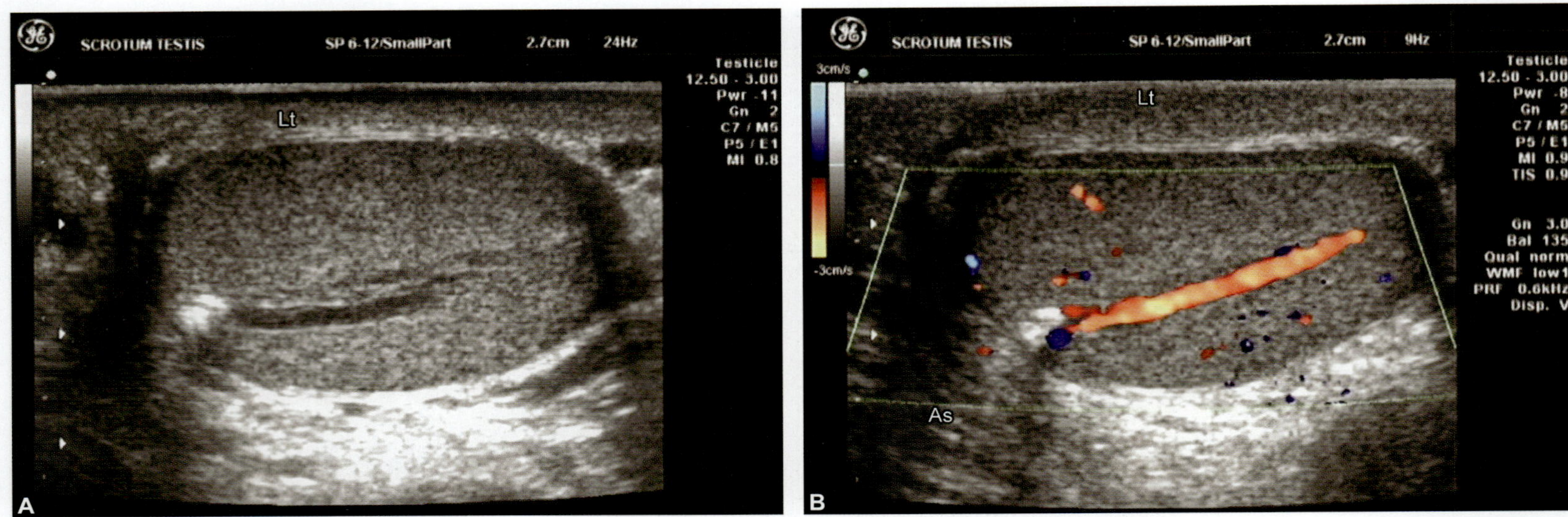

FIGURES 12.8A and B: Scrotal calcification. HRSG shows well defined calcified shadow in the testes. It is seen along the vascular band. On color flow imaging, vessel is confirmed. Scrotal calcifications are not very uncommon and they are benign in nature.

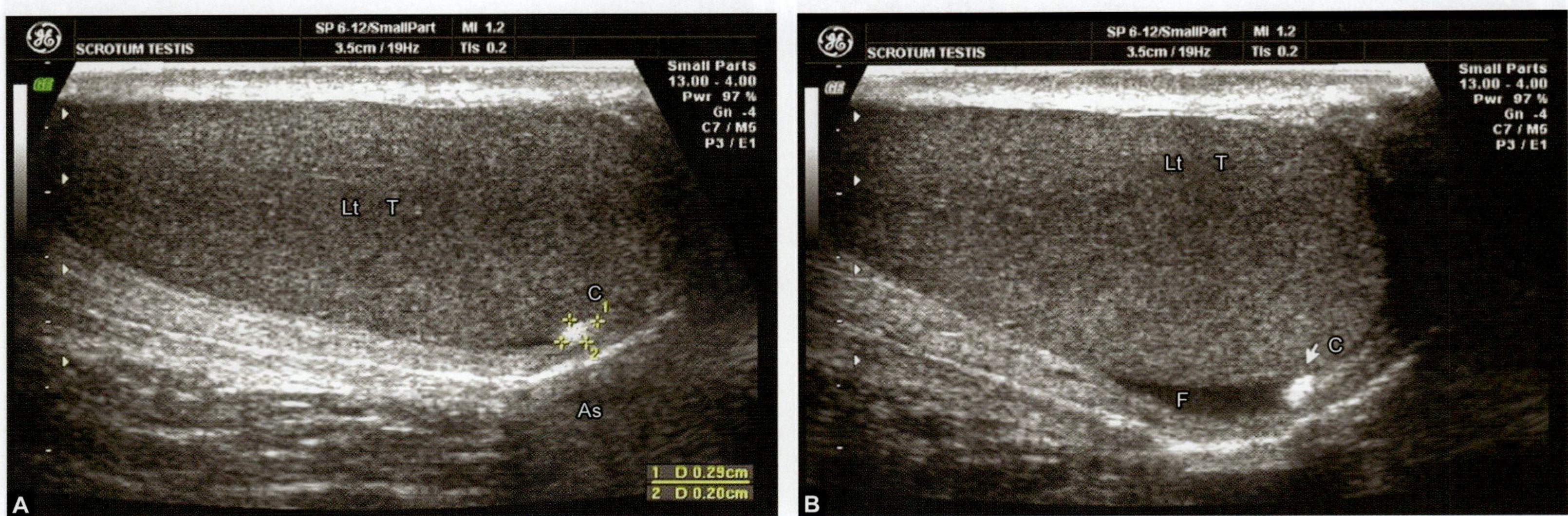

FIGURES 12.9A and B: Scrotal mouse. Scrotal mouse are calcified nodules, which is seen in tunica albuginea. They move on palpation that is why known as scrotal mouse. On HRSG they are seen echogenic calcified shadow between tunica and the testes.

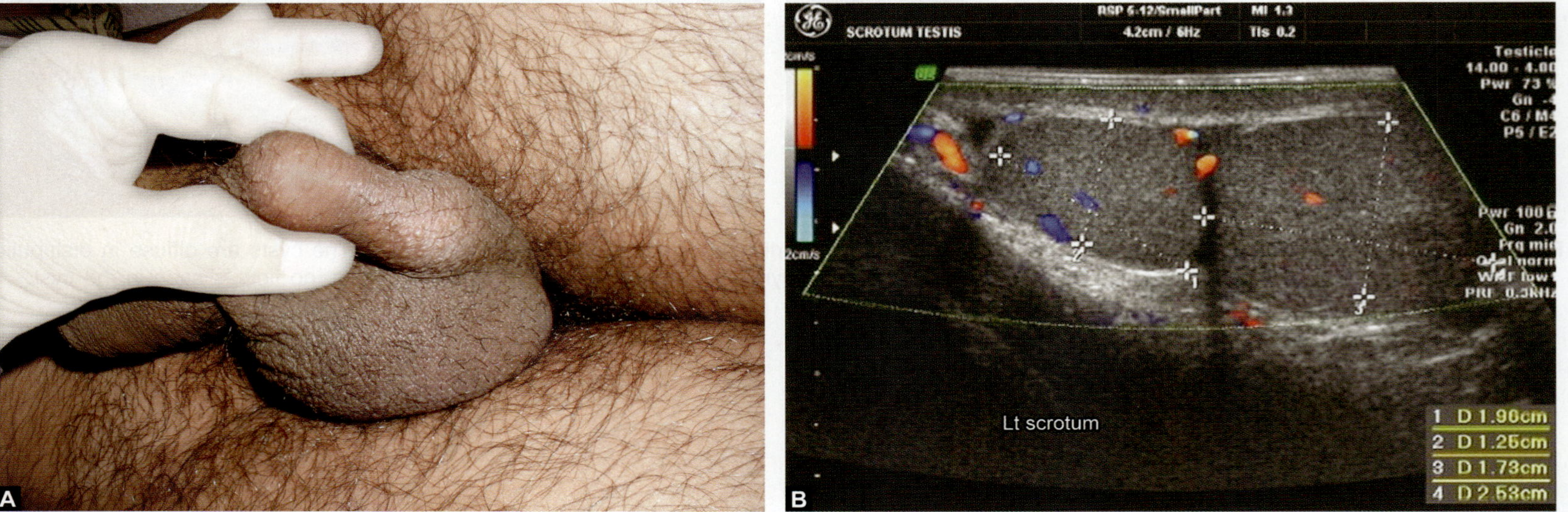

FIGURES 12.10A and B

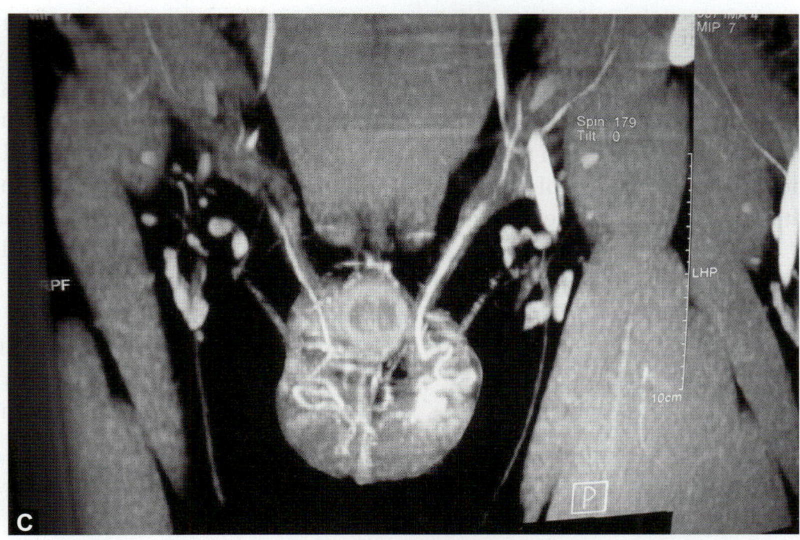

FIGURE 12.10C

FIGURES 12.10A to C: Triorchidism (supernumerary testis). A young patient presented with palpable lump in the left scrotum. Clinical examination shows lobulated mass at the upper pole of the left testes. HRSG shows well-defined homogeneous lobulated mass similar to testicular texture in relation to the left testes. It appears to be another testes in the left scrotum suggestive of supernumerary testes. Surfaces rendering imaging shows the supernumerary testes and the normal testes with better sonographic details. The testes shows the same texture. A single epididymis is seen in the left scrotum. On color Doppler imaging, normal flow is seen in the normal testes and supernumerary testes. Normal intratesticular flow is seen. CT angio and MRI of the same case shows single testicular artery supplying the both testes. MRI image shows normal signals in both the testes confirming the sonographic findings. Triorchidism is a rare phenomenon and only hundred cases are reported in world literature. Modern imaging techniques confirmed the triorchidism without any interventional procedures.

ACUTE SCROTAL PATHOLOGIES

Acute scrotum is a general term used to indicate various pathologies which present with a triad of symptoms and signs, viz. (i) acute pain, (ii) swelling and (iii) redness. Ultrasonographic studies help significantly in aiding the clinician's decision of "surgery or no surgery". Some of the major causes of acute scrotum are as follows:

1. Testicular torsion
2. Testicular inflammation (epididymitis, orchitis)
3. Testicular trauma
4. Torsion of the appendix, epididymis and testes
5. Strangulated hernia
6. Testicular vasculitis and infarction

Testicular (Spermatic Cord) Torsion

Testicular torsion is defined as "rotation of the testes" on the longitudinal axis of the spermatic cord. The events that take place when the spermatic cord is twisted are as follows:

1. Blocked venous drain (edema and hemorrhage)
2. Impaired arterial flow (hemorrhage necrosis of testes).

Depending upon the site of twisting, torsion has been classified as extravaginal, intravaginal and mesorchial.

Intravaginal torsion is more common and occurs at 12 to 18 years of age. It occurs in patients with absent or short mesenteric attachment of the testes to the scrotal sac, allowing excess mobility of the testes and cord. This in turn results in twisting of the vascular pedicle, which results in complete, incomplete or recurrent obstruction to venous flow and eventually the arterial flow. Initially thin walled drainage veins are compressed by the twisted cord leading to congestion and edema, thereby, elevating pressure in the cord. Subsequently, it causes occlusion of the arteries leading to ischemia and infarction of the testes. In the early phase (with 4 hours), there is ischemia of the testes, a little reactive hydrocele and hyperemia of the scrotum. Sonography may be normal at this stage. However, color Doppler studies will show no detectable flow in the affected testis.

In the mid phase (5 to 24 hours), there is increasing congestion, edema and hemorrhage in the testes. Ultrasonography in this phase shows an abnormal testes that is enlarged and hypoechoic. As congestion, hemorrhage and ischemia progress, the testicle becomes heterogeneous with areas of decreased echogenicity. Color Doppler shows no flow in the affected testes, but flow is seen in the peritesticular area and in the scrotal wall due to reactive hyperemia.

In the late phase (more than 24 hours), infarction sets in. The testes is enlarged and shows heterogeneous texture. The epididymis is thickened, there is reactive hydrocele and thickened scrotal walls. If an abscess develops it is seen as a focal, complex, fluid-filled collection.

Color Doppler sonography has been of immense value in distinguishing between testicular torsion and inflammation. While there is no testicular flow in torsion with associated peritesticular flow, marked hyperemia is noticed in testicular inflammation. However, it is often difficult to differentiate between a spontaneously detorsed testes and testicular inflammation, when both pathologies show evidence of increased intratesticular vascularity.

Detorsion of the cord must be achieved as early as possible. If surgery is performed within six hours, the testicular viability is significantly high. If performed within 24 hours, the salvage rate is 60 to 70%. It fails to be less than 20% when surgery is undertaken after 24 hours. Scintigraphy is very useful in patients with torsion when reduced or absent perfusion is demonstrated (94 to 90%).

It may also be remembered that the sensitivity of the machine for detecting low flows is vital in visualizing intratesticular flows. With a situation like a detorsed testes or a poor sensitivity machine, the surgeon cannot depend only on color flow imaging to decide the line of therapy.

Testicular Inflammation

Epididymitis and orchitis are the most common infections involving the scrotum. The presenting symptom is acute scrotal pain.

There is considerable overlap of clinical findings between testicular torsion and acute inflammatory disorders. Color Doppler is of immense value in distinguishing one from the other especially since the treatment is completely different.

Scrotal infections are usually secondary to prostatitis or bladder infections. Orchitis can also be the result of viral infection sonographic features.

1. Enlargement of the testes.
2. Hypoechoic testes with involvement being diffuse or focal.
3. Abscess formation may show a totally heterogeneous epididymis.
4. Color Doppler studies reveal hypervascular pattern.

These vessels have a low vascular resistance and more venous flow indicating hyperemia. Normally the epididymis is avascular, but increased flow pattern in the epididymis is diagnostic of inflammatory changes. The common pitfalls in the diagnosis of acute epididymo-orchitis are as follows:

1. Diffuse increase in vascularity is often seen in infiltrative lesions like leukemia or lymphoma.
2. A distorted testes may also have increased vascular pattern. Commonly a hydrocele and thickening of the scrotal wall are noted in inflammations rather than a neoplasm.
3. Focal orchitis may be mistaken for an occult neoplasm.

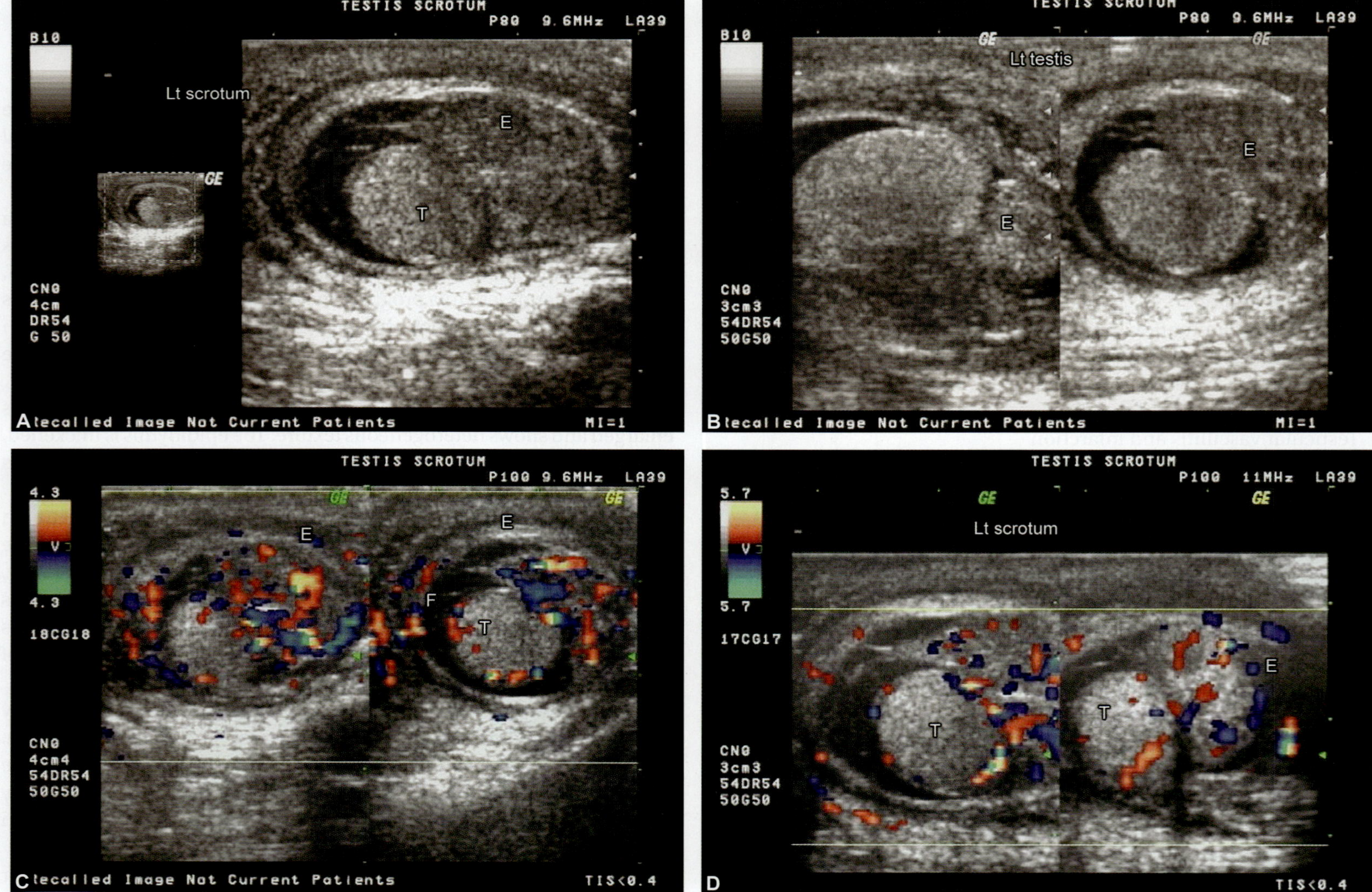

FIGURES 12.11A to D: Acute epididymitis. HRSG shows irregular hypoechoic enlarged epididymis suggestive of acute epididymitis. However, the testis is seen normally. Reactionary collection is seen in the scrotal sac. Color flow imaging of the same patient shows increased flow in the epididymis. The flow is seen in bizarre fashion. Normal flow is seen in the testes.

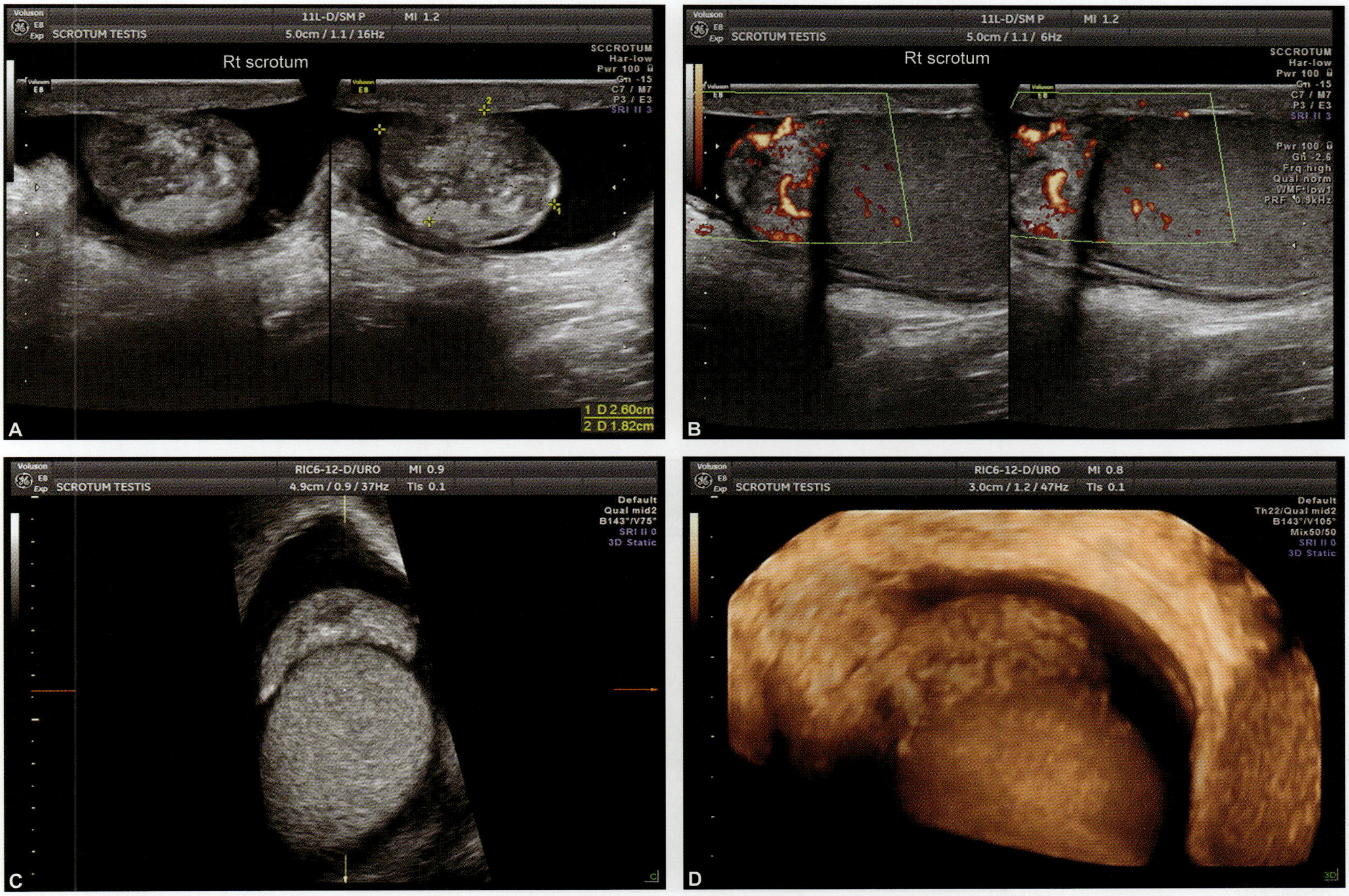

FIGURES 12.12A to D: Acute epididymitis. A patient presented with acute pain in right scrotum. HRSG shows enlarged edematous inhomogeneous right epididymis. Hypoechoic areas are seen in the epididymis. But no cystic degeneration is seen. On color flow imaging, increased flow is seen in the epididymis. The 3D ultrasound shows the inflamed epididymis clearly and surface rendering shows multiple hypoechoic areas in the epididymis.

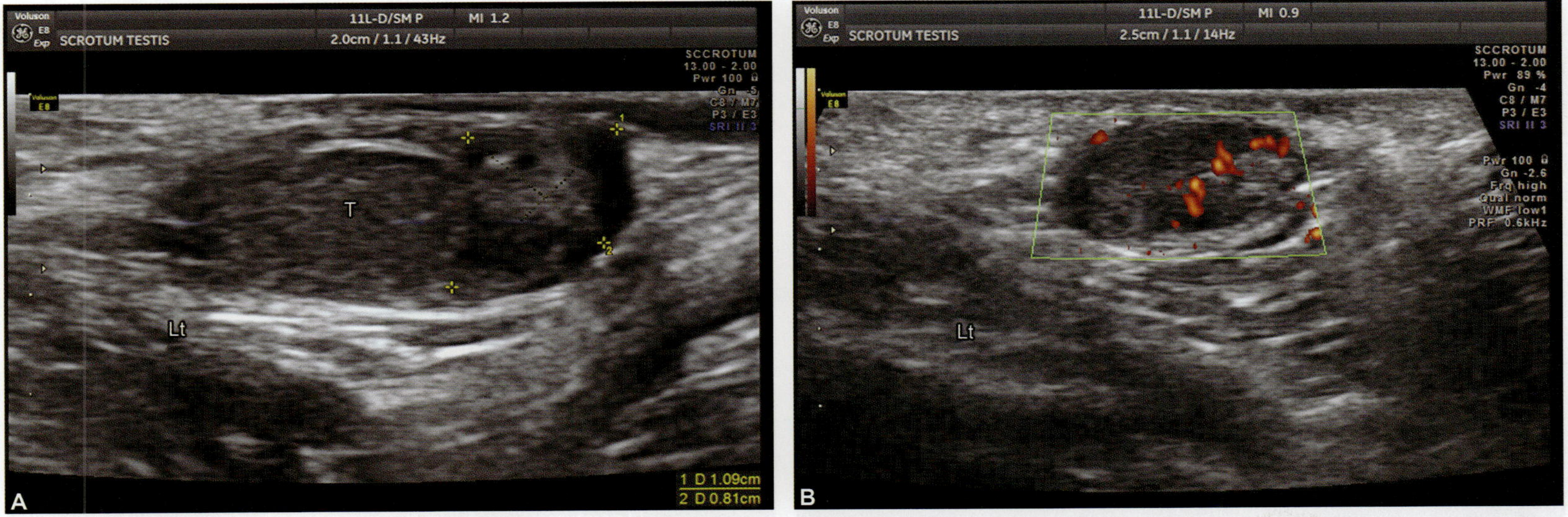

FIGURES 12.13A and B: Acute epididymitis. A 1-year-old baby presented with pain and swelling in left scrotum. HRSG shows inflamed edematous hypoechoic left epididymis. It shows hypoechoic texture. On color flow imaging, increased flow is seen in it. But testes is normal.

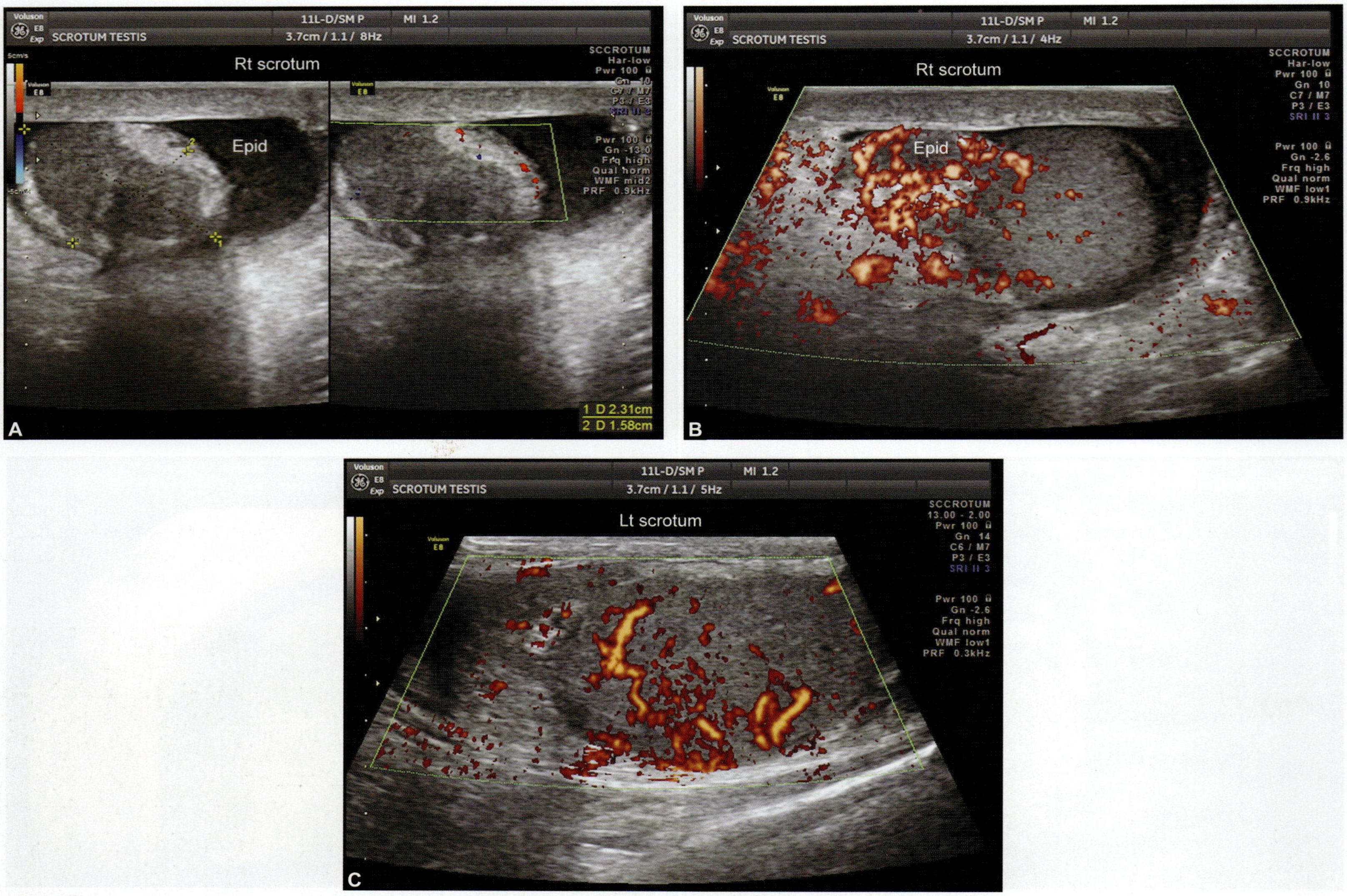

FIGURES 12.14A to C: Acute epididymitis. A patient presented with painful swelling in right scrotum. HRSG shows enlarged edematous right epididymis. It is hypoechoic in texture. Small amount of fluid is also seen in the right scrotal sac. On color flow imaging, increased flow is seen in the epididymis. However, the testes does not show any sign of inflammation and it is normal in texture.

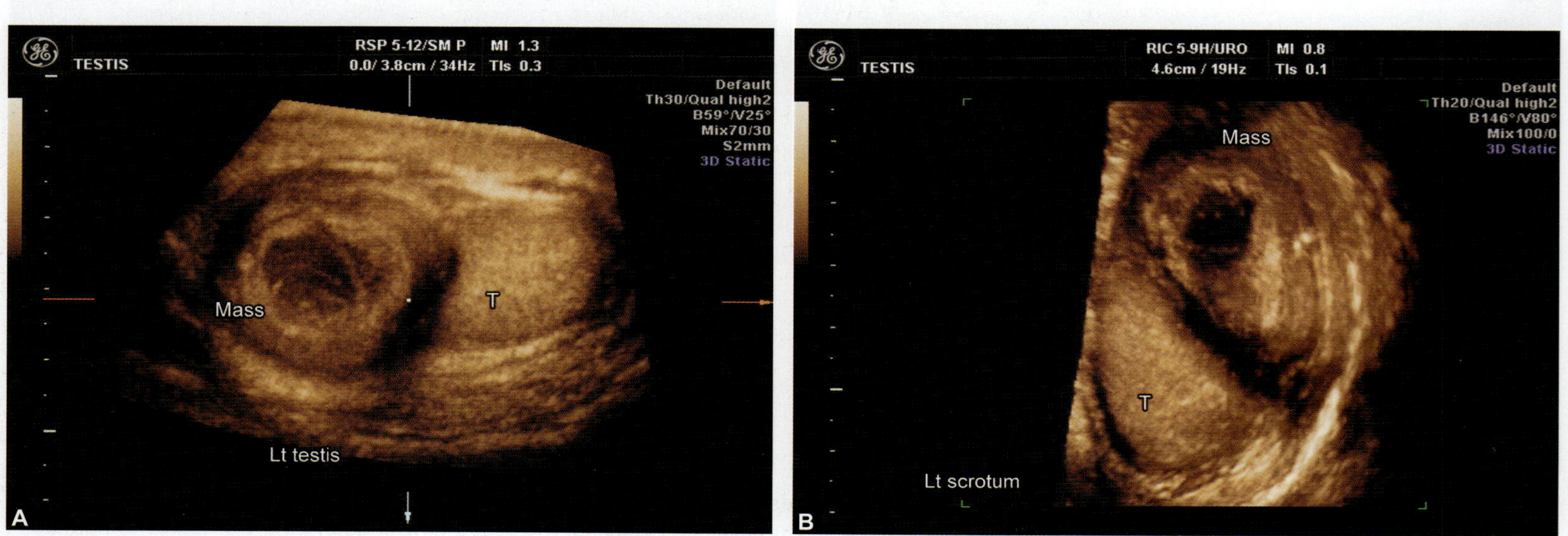

FIGURES 12.15A and B

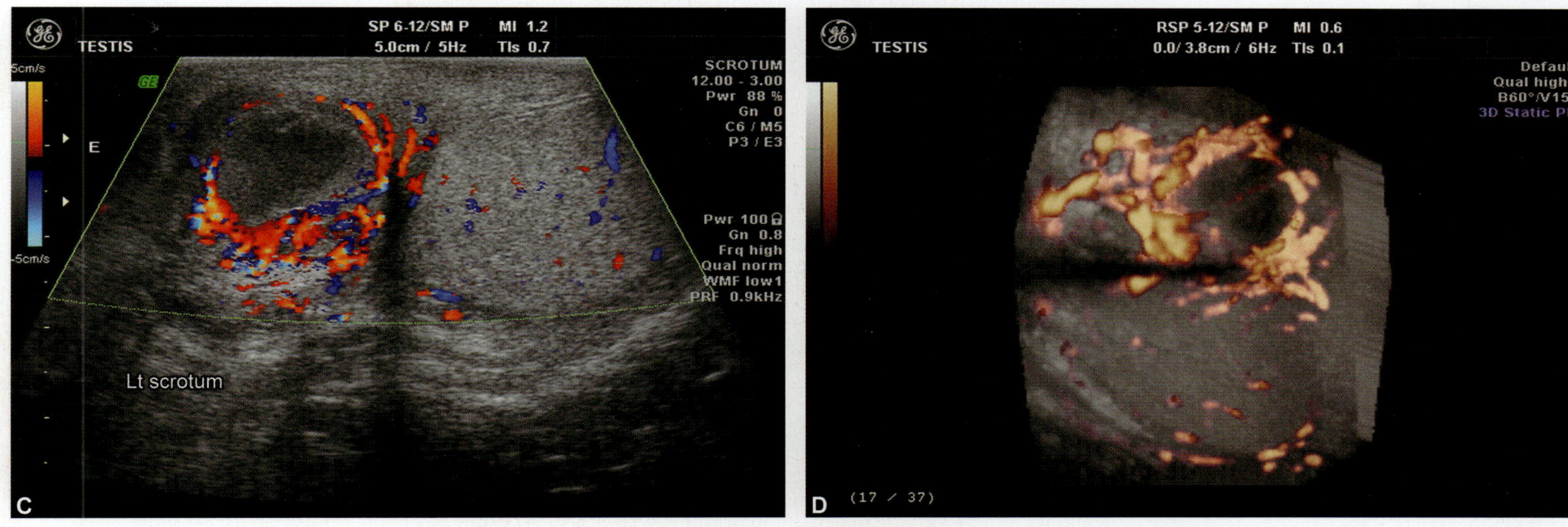

FIGURES 12.15C and D

FIGURES 12.15A to D: Epididymis abscess. A patient presented with acute pain in the left scrotum with a nodular mass. HRSG shows enlarged edematous left epididymis. A hypoechoic pocket is seen in the left epididymis. Central area of necrosis is seen in it. Perifocal edema is also presented suggestive of an abscess. 3D imaging clearly shows the abscess. On color flow imaging, increased flow is seen around the epididymis. But no flow is seen in abscess. The testes is normal in appearance.

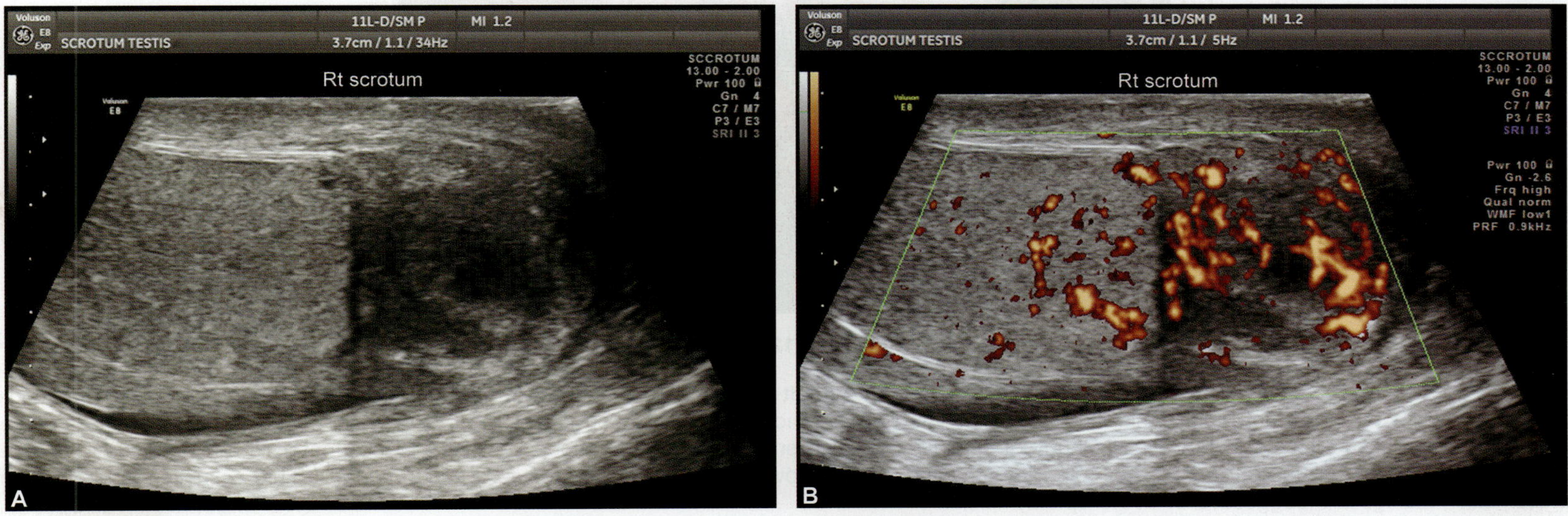

FIGURES 12.16A and B: Abscess in the tail of epididymis. A patient presented with nodular mass in the right scrotum. HRSG shows a hypoechoic nodular mass at the tail of epididymis. Margins are shaggy. Perifocal edema is present. But no cystic degeneration is seen. On color flow imaging, increased flow is seen in it. It is separate from the left testes. Findings are suggestive of chronic abscess

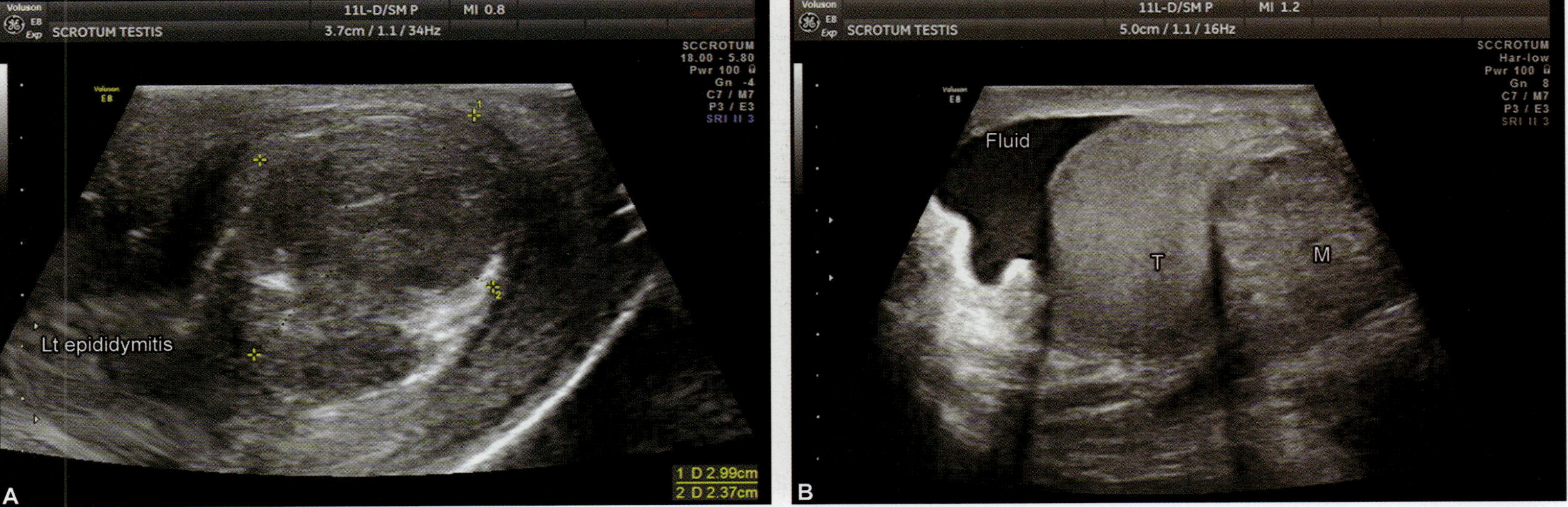

FIGURES 12.17A and B

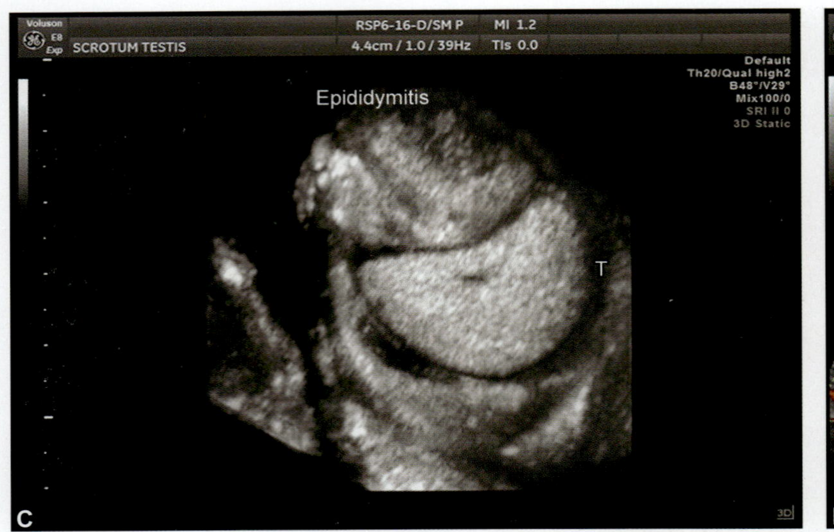

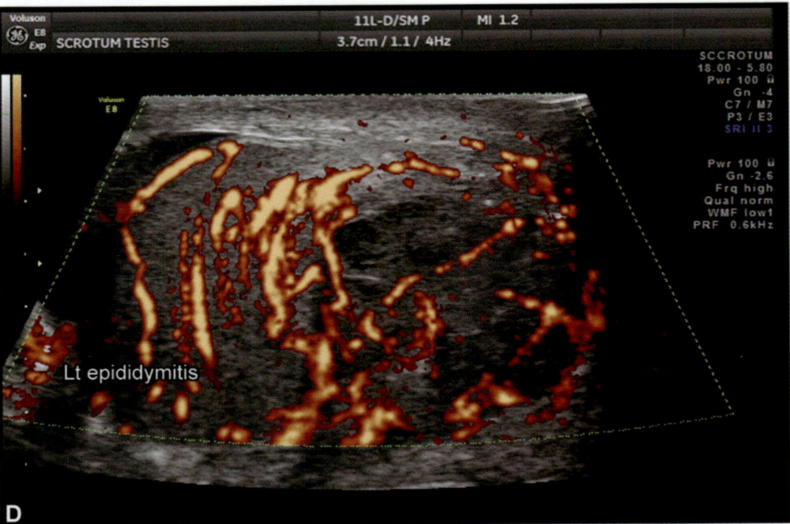

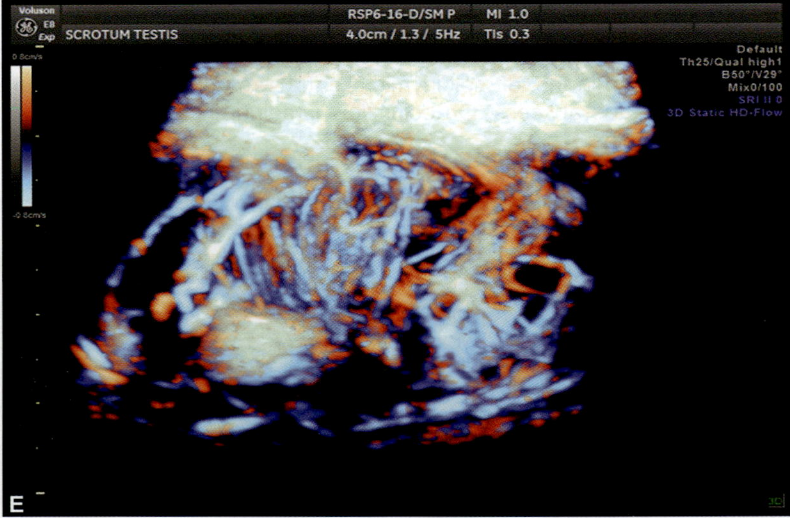

FIGURES 12.17C to E

FIGURES 12.17A to E: A patient presented with painful swelling in the left scrotum. HRSG shows an irregular ill-defined inhomogeneous hypoechoic mass seen at the tail of the left epididymis. It shows variegated appearance. No calcification is seen in it. No cystic degeneration is seen. On color flow imaging, increased flow is seen in it. The body of epididymis is also enlarged and edematous. Left testes is normal. It is homogenous in texture. No focal mass is seen in the left testes. On color flow imaging, normal flow is seen in the left testes. Small amount of fluid collection is seen in left scrotal sac. Findings are suggestive of acute epididymitis.

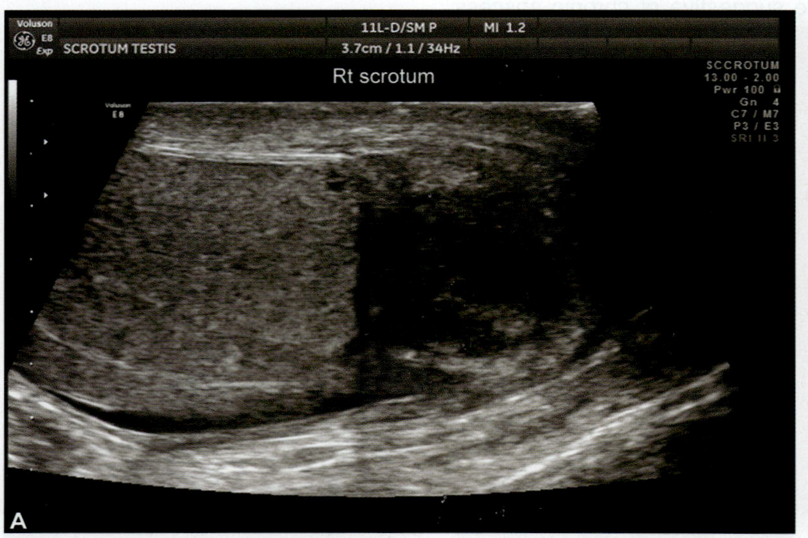

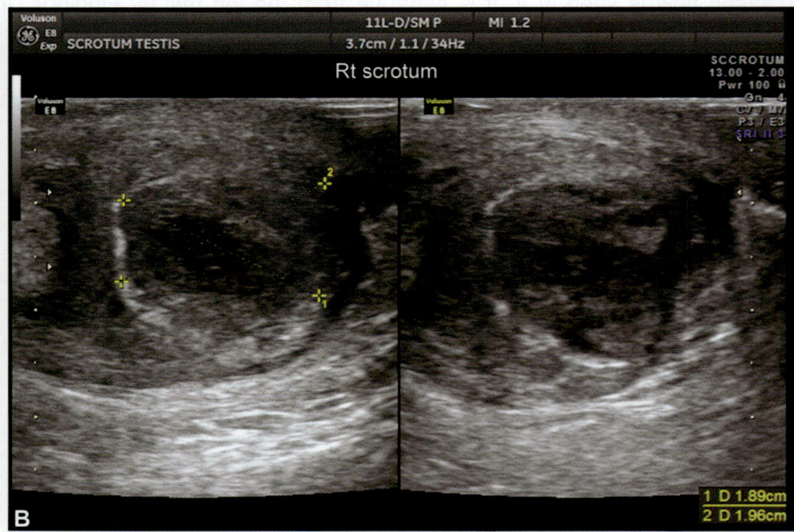

FIGURES 12.18A and B

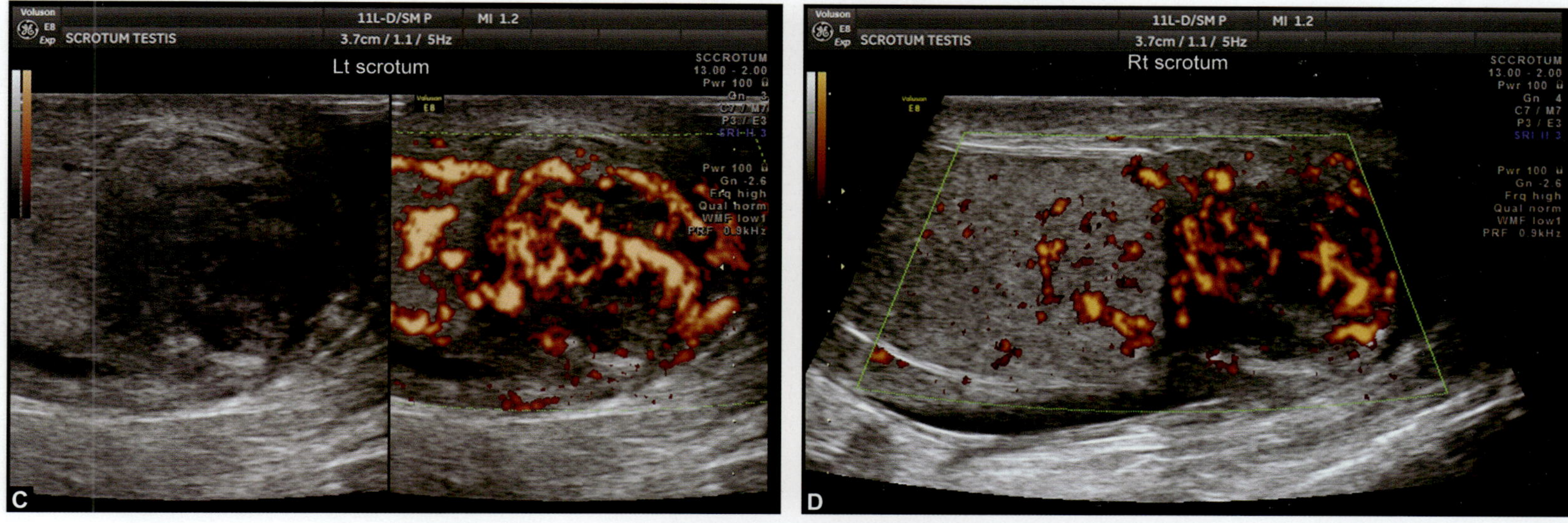

FIGURES 12.18C and D

FIGURES 12.18A to D: Acute epididymo-orchitis. A patient presented with pain in right scrotum. HRSG shows enlarged right testes. Epididymis is also enlarged and inhomogeneous. Body and tail of the epididymis is also inhomogeneous. On color flow imaging, increased flow is seen in testes and epididymis. But tail of the epididymis shows inhomogeneous hypoechoic mass. It is irregular in outline suggestive of inflammatory mass. On color flow imaging, marked increased flow is seen in it. Scrotal wall edema is also present. Small amount of fluid is also seen in right scrotal sac. Findings are suggestive of acute epididymo-orchitis.

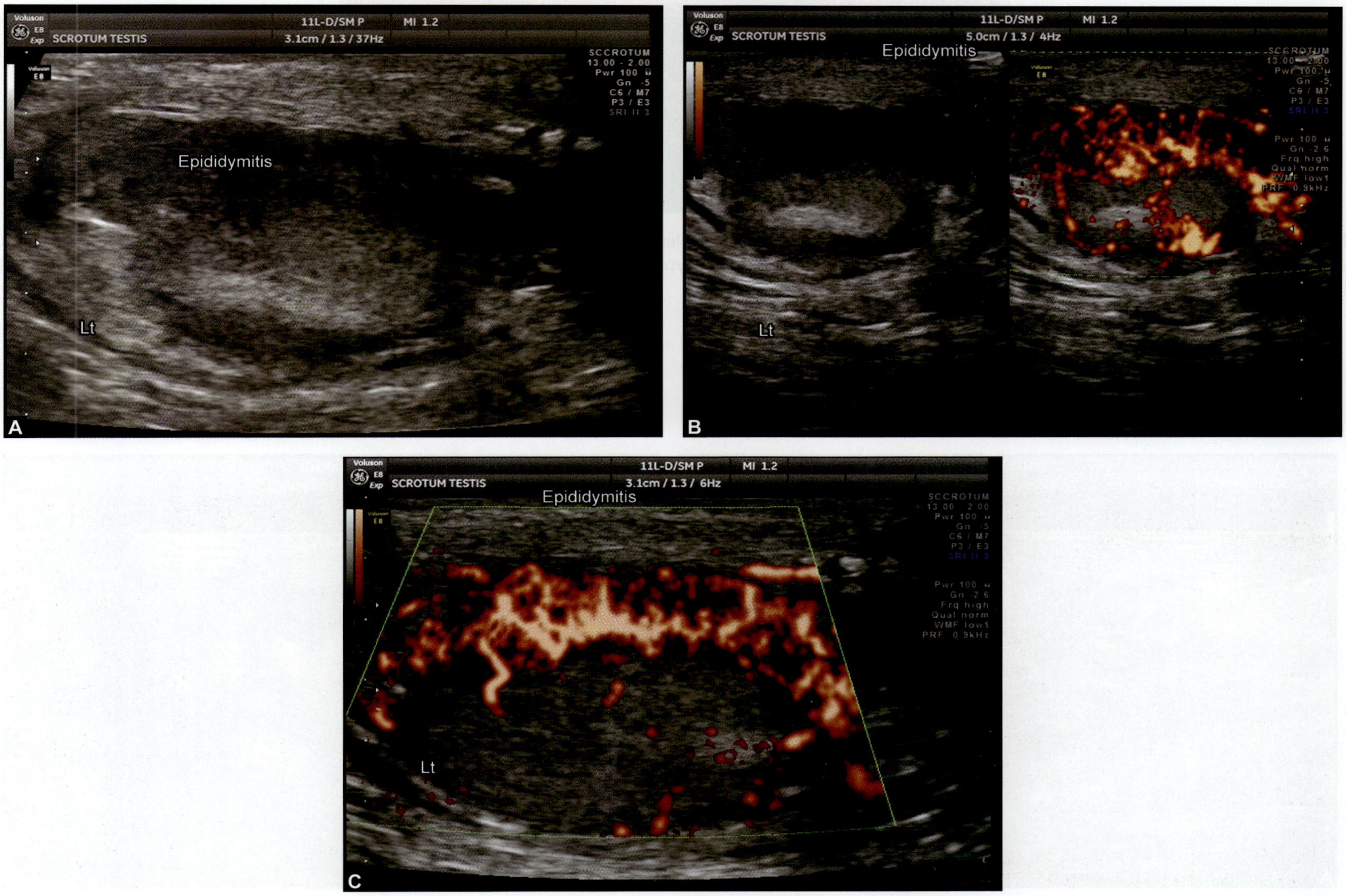

FIGURES 12.19A to C: Acute epididymitis. HRSG shows enlarged edematous inhomogeneous left epididymis. The body and tail of the epididymis are thickened. A hypoechoic irregular ill-defined shadow is seen in the tail of the epididymis. No calcification is seen into it. No cystic degeneration is seen. On color flow imaging, increased flow is seen in the left epididymis suggestive of left epididymitis.

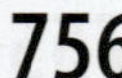

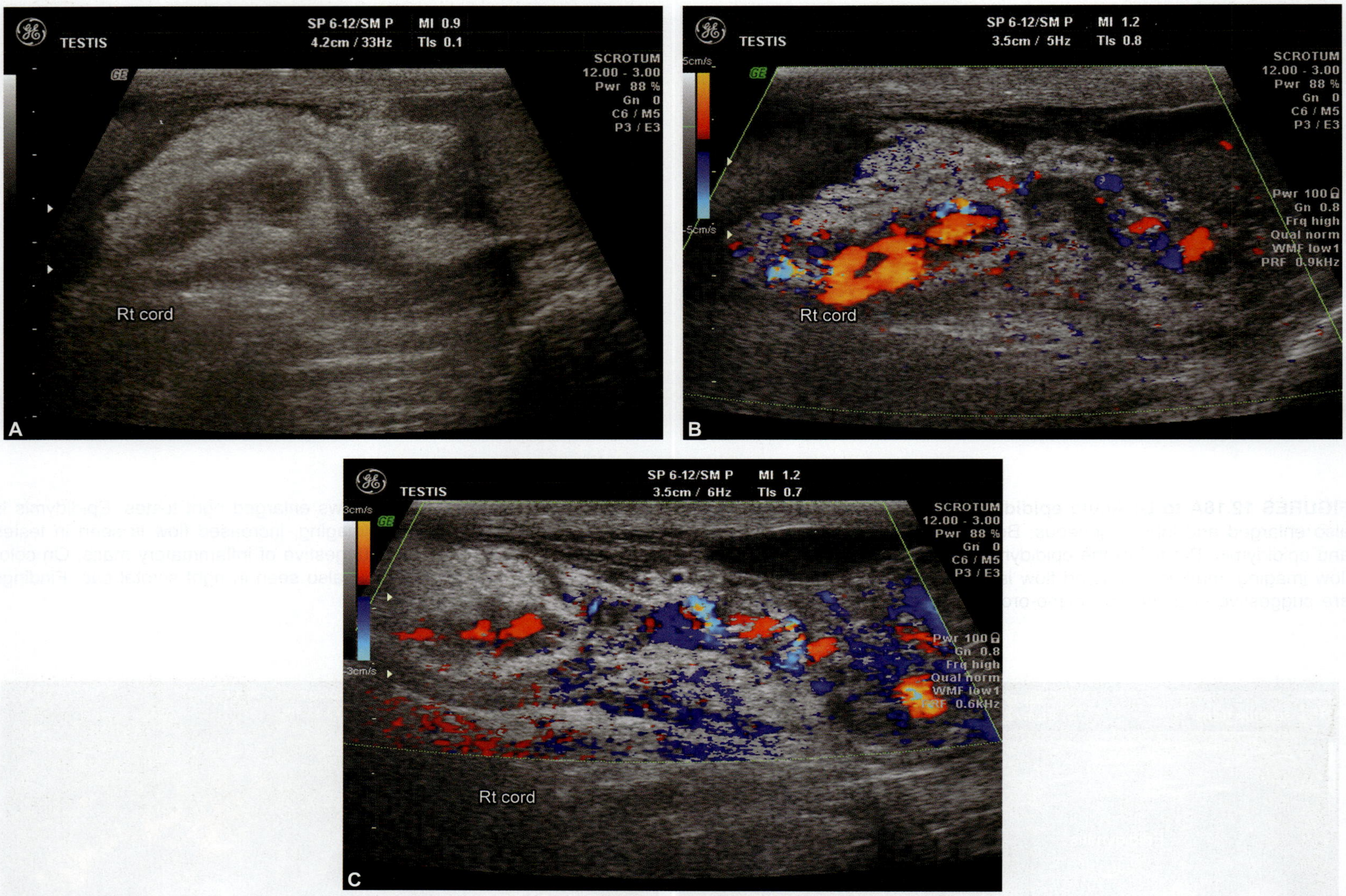

FIGURES 12.20A to C: Funiculitis. A patient presented with painful swelling in the right cord and right scrotum. HRSG shows thickened edematous cord. Cord edema is present. The fat is also inflamed and edematous. Hypoechoic areas are seen in the cord. On color flow imaging, increased flow is seen in cord suggestive of funiculitis.

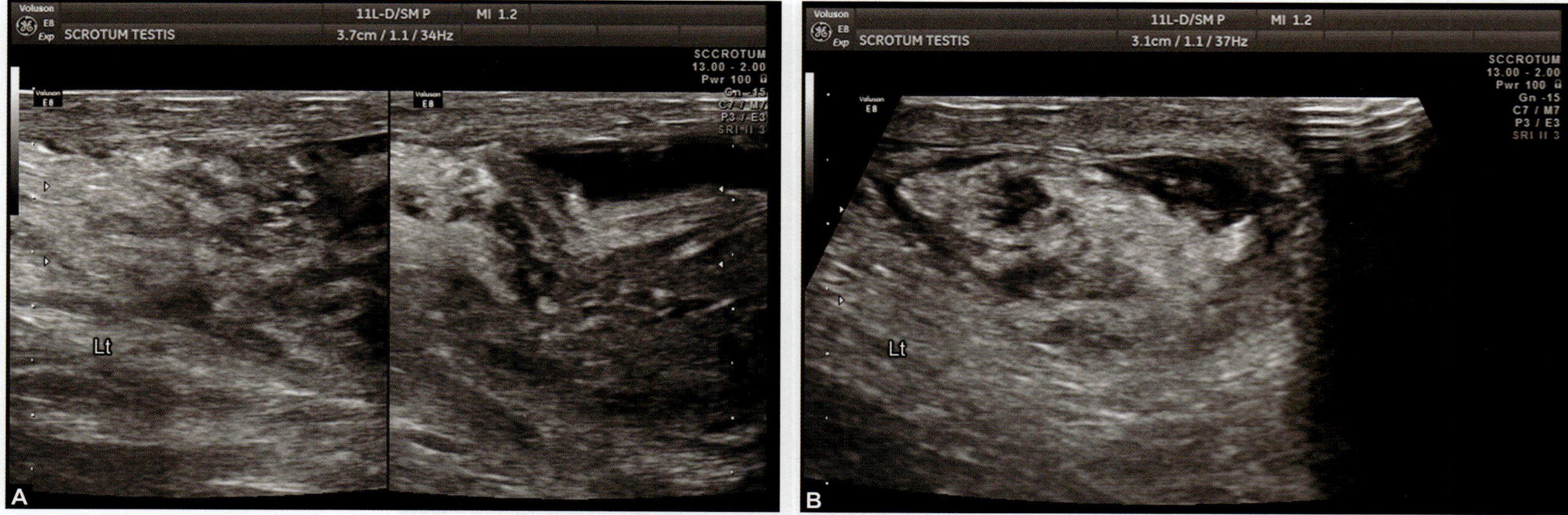

FIGURES 12.21A and B

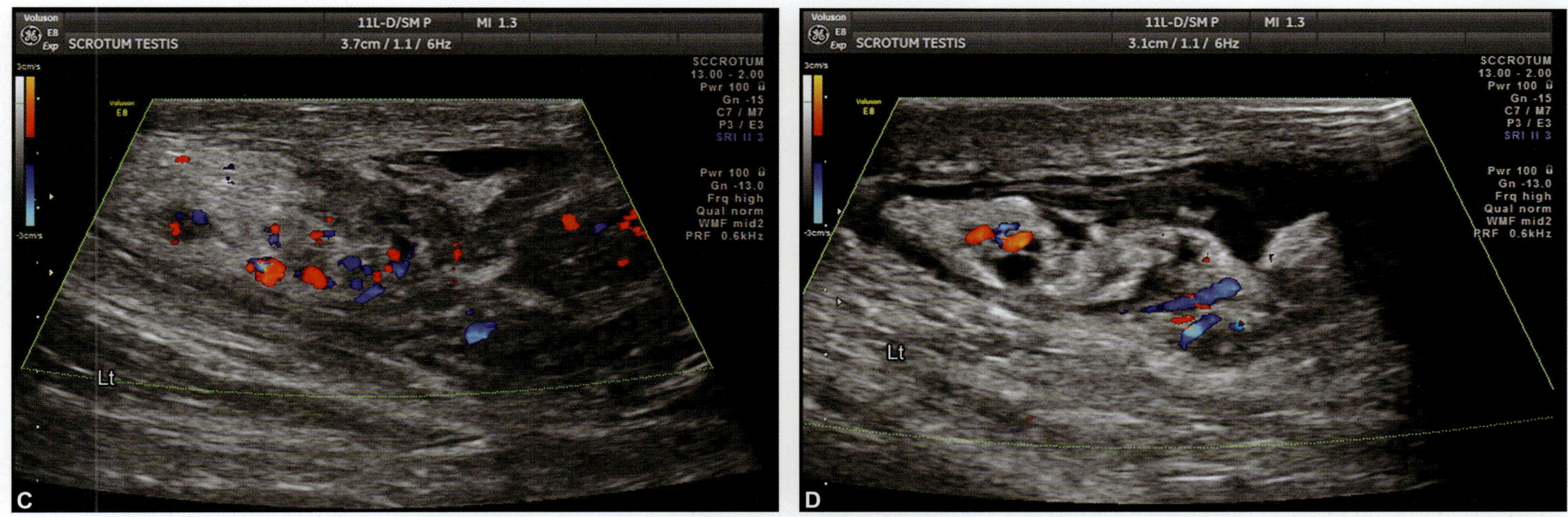

FIGURES 12.21C and D

FIGURES 12.21A to D: Funiculitis with small hydrocele. A patient presented with painful swelling in the right cord. HRSG shows thickened edematous left cord. Fat inflammation is also seen. Hypoechoic areas are also seen in the cord. On color flow imaging, few vessels are seen in the cord. Findings are suggestive of acute funiculitis. Small amount of fluid is also seen in cord suggestive of reactionary fluid.

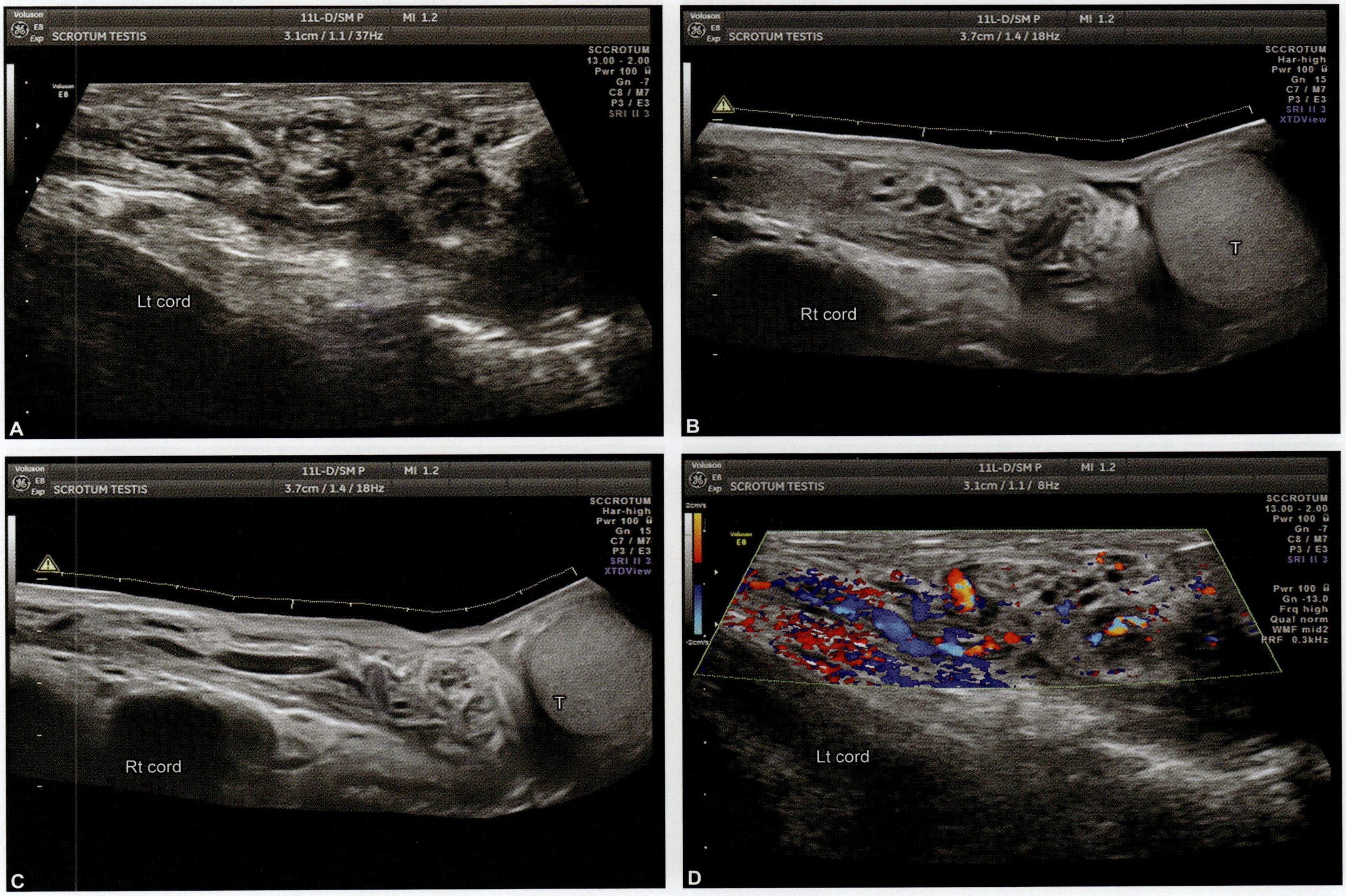

FIGURES 12.22A to D: Funiculitis—Extended field of view. HRSG shows thickened edematous cord in the left scrotum. Multiple hypoechoic areas are seen in the cord. The cord fat is also seen inflamed. Extended field of view shows entire length of edematous cord. On color flow imaging, multiple vessels are seen feeding the cord.

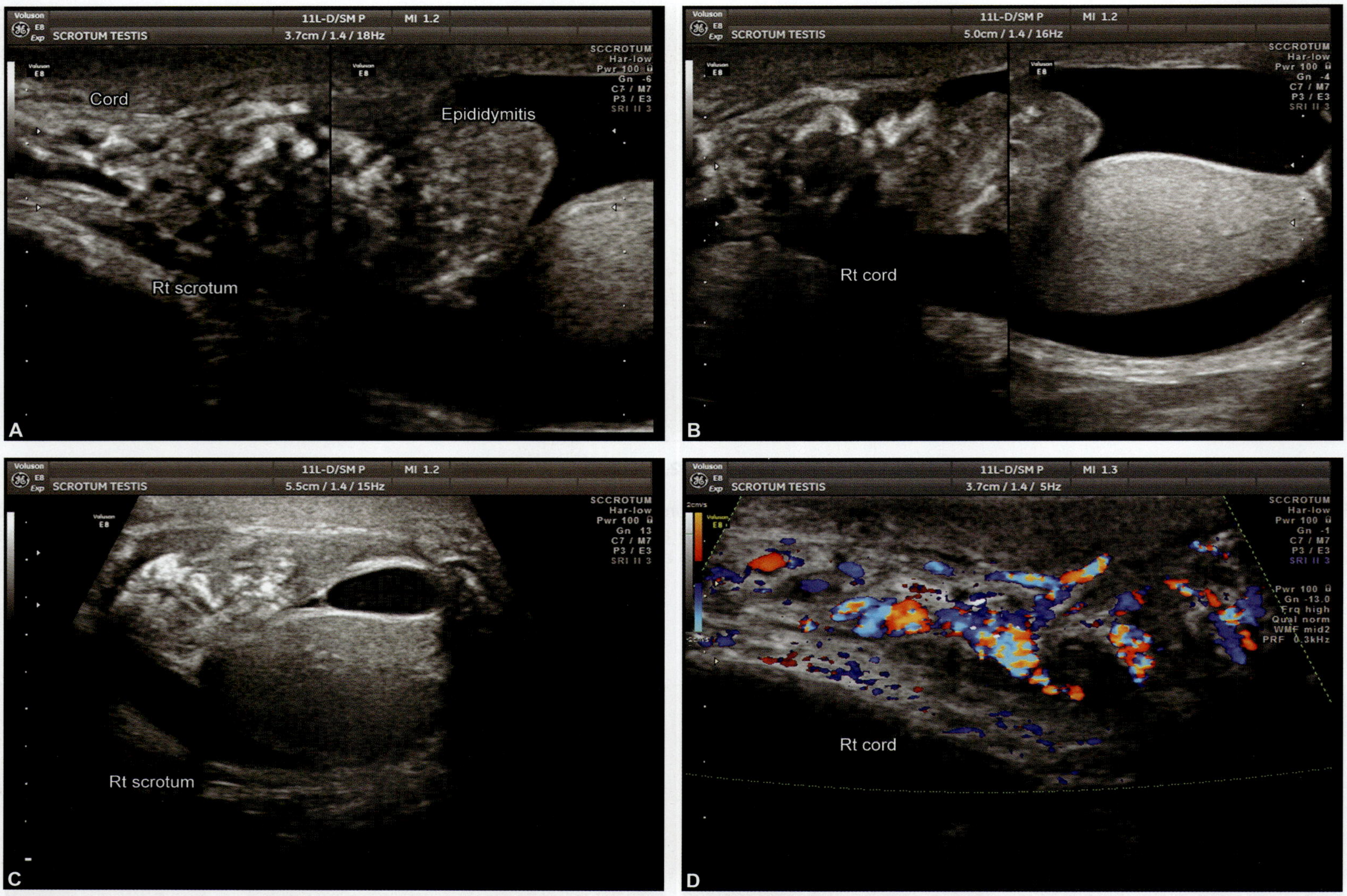

FIGURES 12.23A to D: Chronic epididymitis with funiculitis. HRSG shows thickened head, body and tail of the epididymis. Echogenic foci are seen in head and body. But no necrosis is seen. Moderate amount of collection is seen in right scrotal sac. Right cord is thickened. It is inhomogeneous in texture. Multiple dilated vessels are also seen along the right cord suggestive of right cord varices. No other focal mass seen. On color flow imaging, increased flow is seen in it.

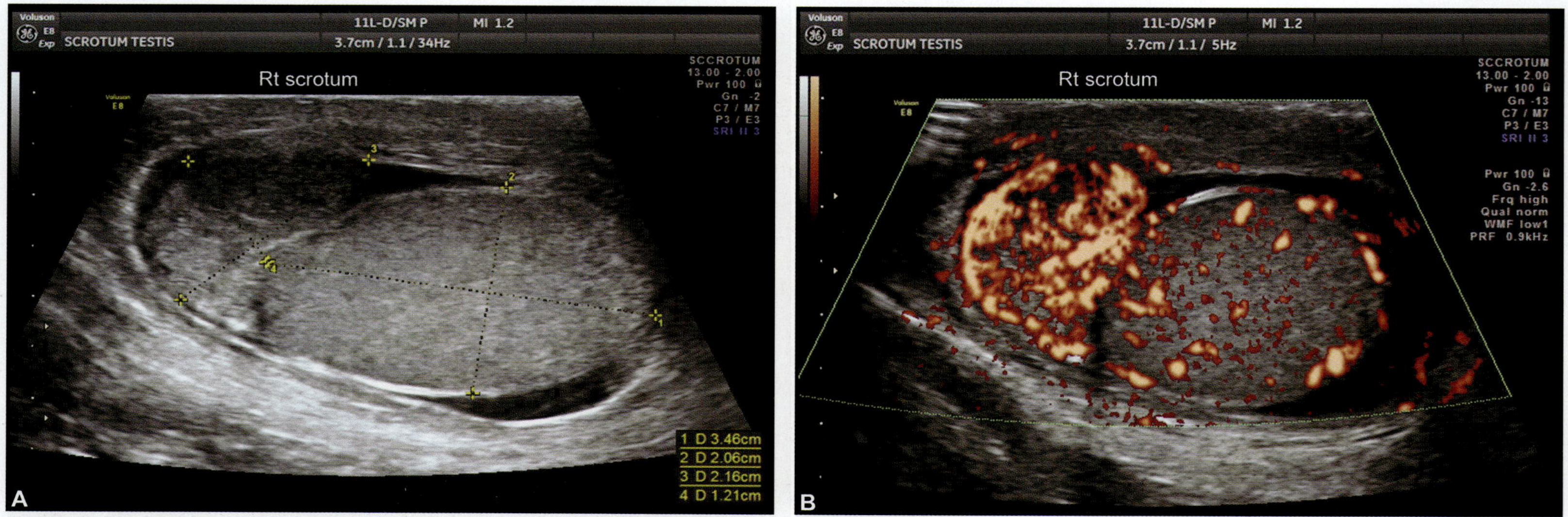

FIGURES 12.24A and B

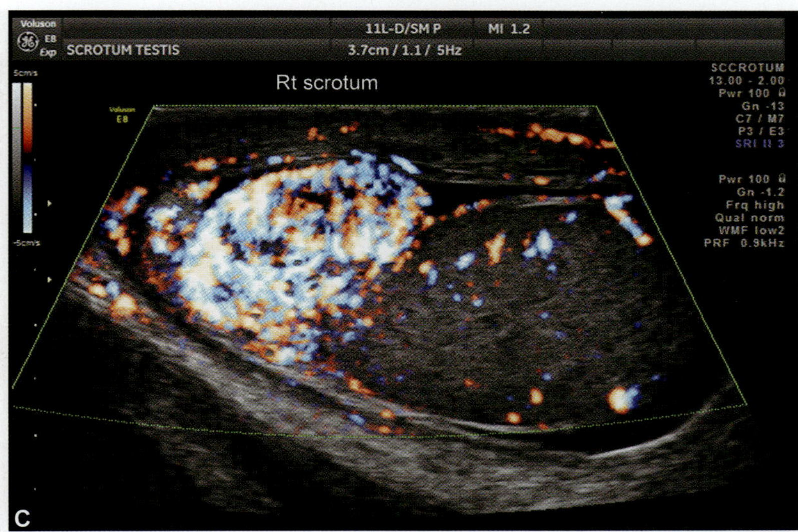

FIGURE 12.24C

FIGURES 12.24A to C: Acute epididymitis. HRSG shows enlarged and swollen epididymis. Hypoechoic areas are seen in the epididymis. No calcification is seen. No abscess formation is seen. On color flow imaging, marked increased flow is seen in the epididymis. Small amount of collection is also seen in the right scrotal sac. Findings are suggestive of acute epididymitis

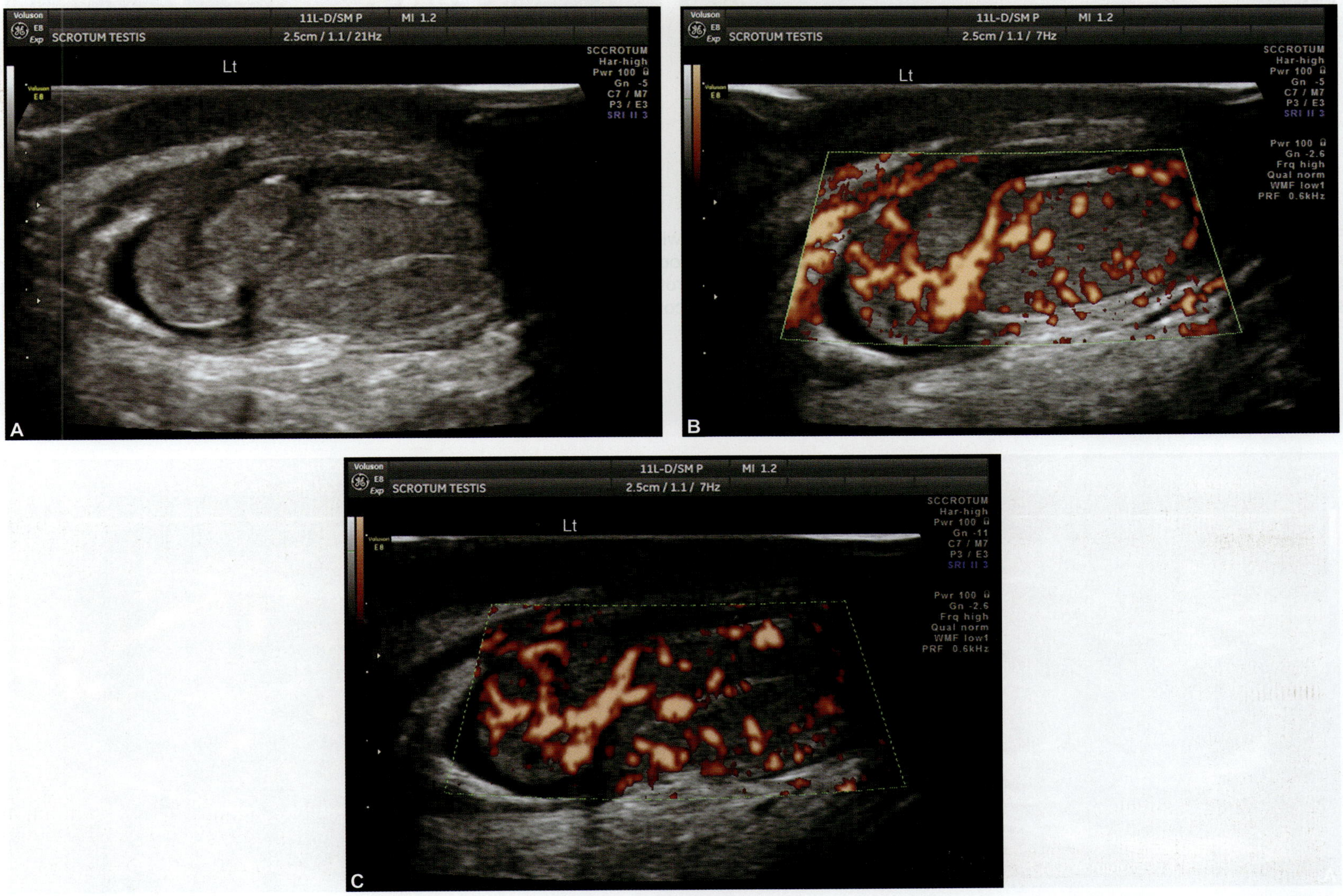

FIGURES 12.25A to C: Acute epididymo-orchitis. A 5-year-old boy presented with acute pain in left scrotum. HRSG shows enlarged edematous left epididymis. The testes is also edematous and hypoechoic in texture. But no focal mass is seen in them. On color flow imaging, high flow is seen in the left testes and the epididymis suggestive of acute epididymo-orchitis.

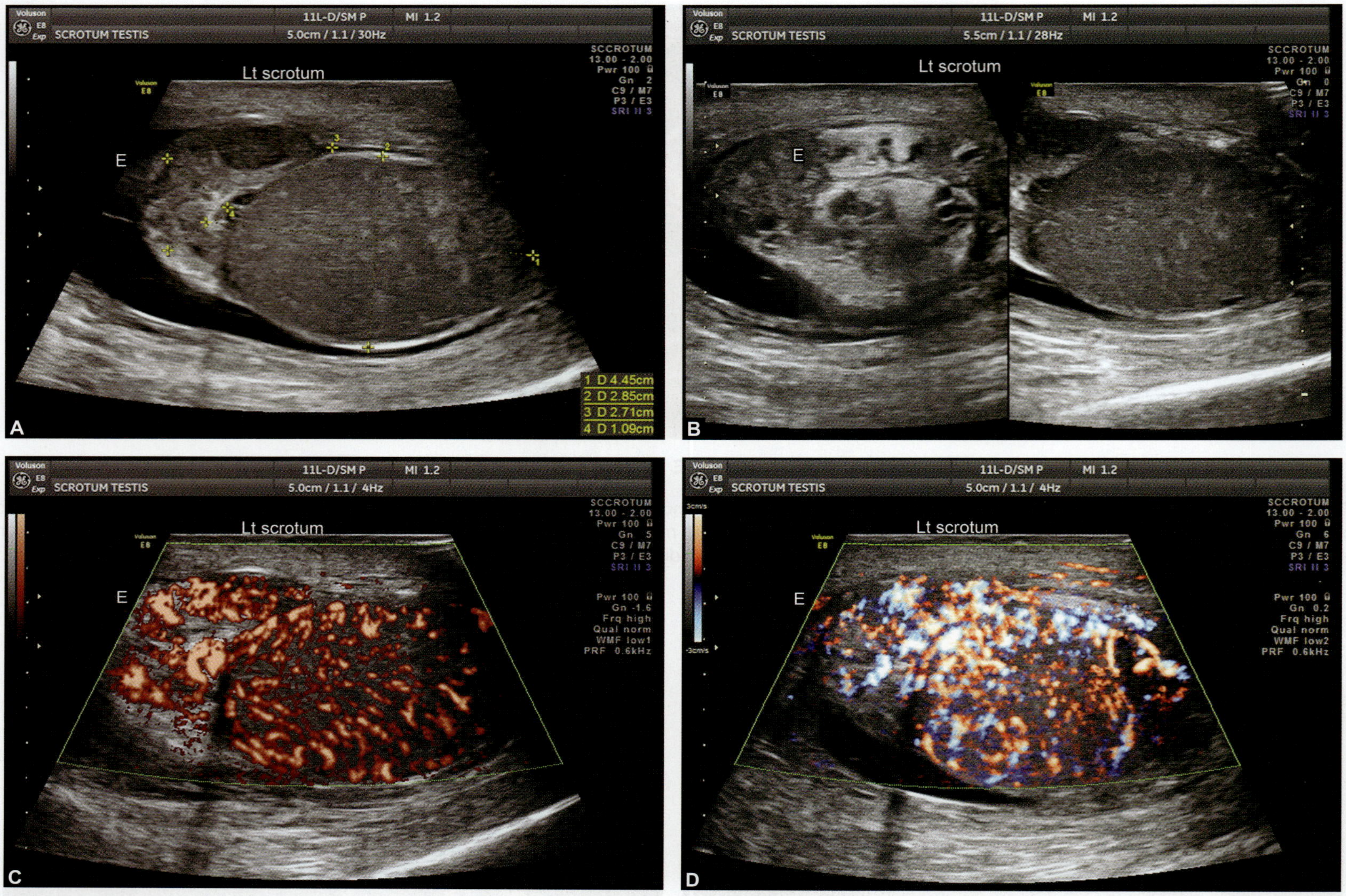

FIGURES 12.26A to D: Acute epididymo-orchitis. A patient presented with swollen, edematous and hypoechoic left testes. Left epididymis is also swollen, edematous and hypoechoic. It shows echogenic foci. The head, body and tail of the epididymis are also swelled up. But no abscess formation is seen. On color flow imaging, high flow is seen in the left testes and scrotum. There is evidence of low level echo collection seen in the left scrotal sac. Echogenic foci are seen in the collection suggestive of exudative collection. Left scrotal wall is also edematous suggestive of inflamed wall. Findings are suggestive of acute epididymo-orchitis.

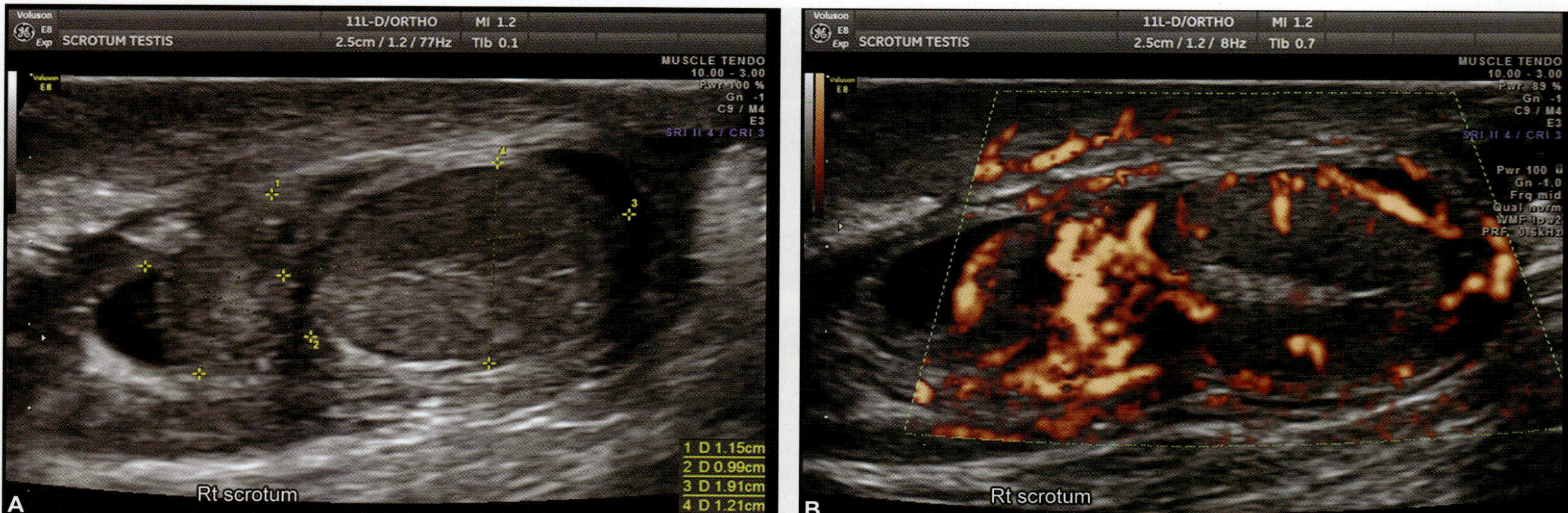

FIGURES 12.27A and B

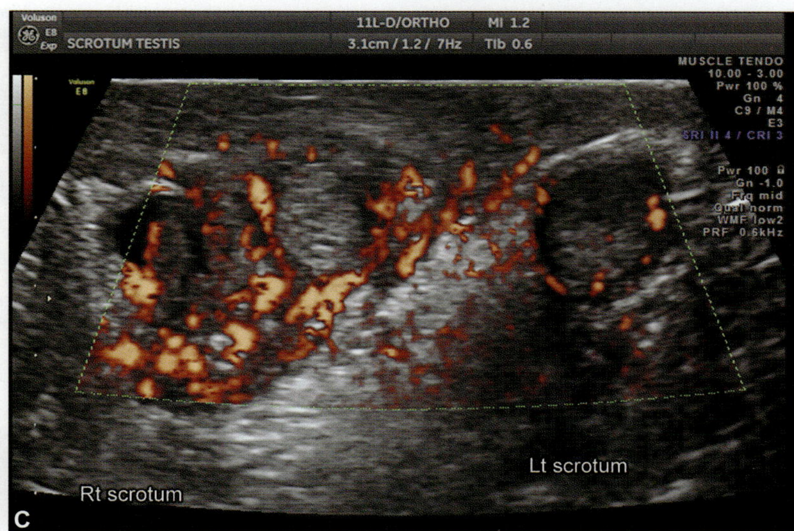

FIGURE 12.27C

FIGURES 12.27A to C: Acute epididymo-orchitis. An 8-year-old boy presented with painful swelling in the right scrotum. HRSG shows diffuse scrotal wall edema. The right epididymis and the testes are hypoechoic and edematous. But no focal mass is seen in them. On color flow imaging, marked increased flow is seen in the epididymis and scrotum suggestive of right epididymo-orchitis.

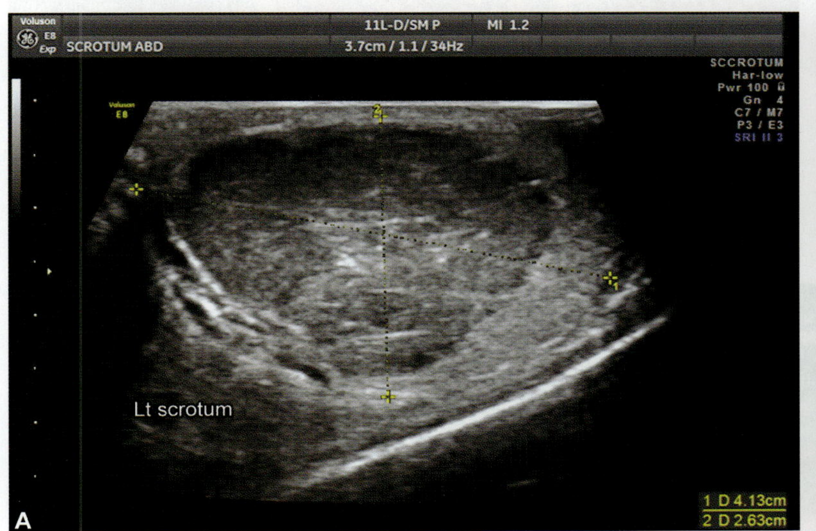

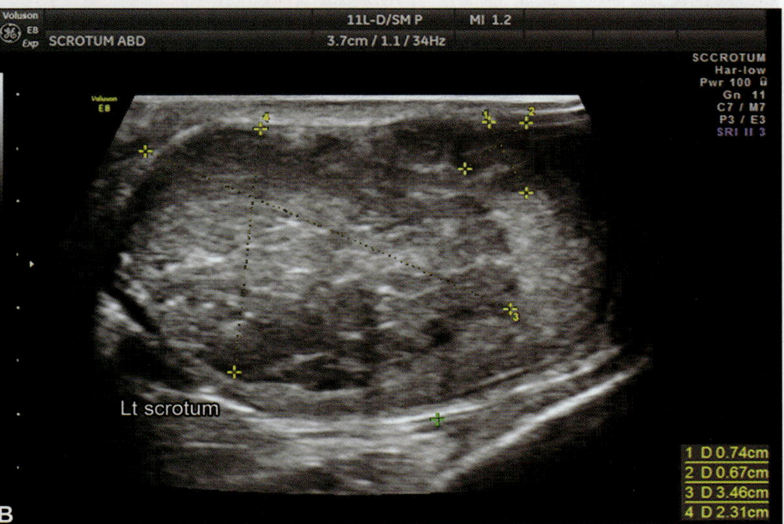

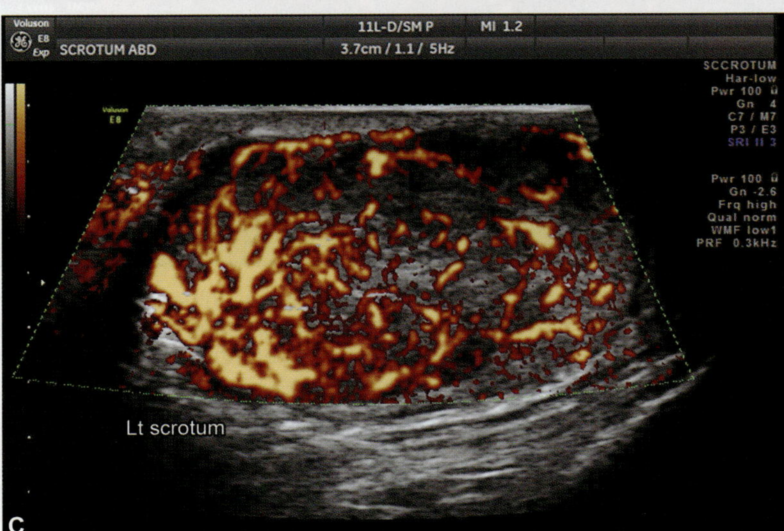

FIGURES 12.28A to C: Acute epididymo-orchitis. A patient presented with painful swelling in the left scrotum. HRSG shows enlarged edematous hypoechoic left testes. Irregular ill-defined hypoechoic area is seen in the left testes. But no focal mass is seen. On color flow imaging, marked increased flow is seen in the left testes suggestive of left epididymo orchitis.

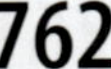

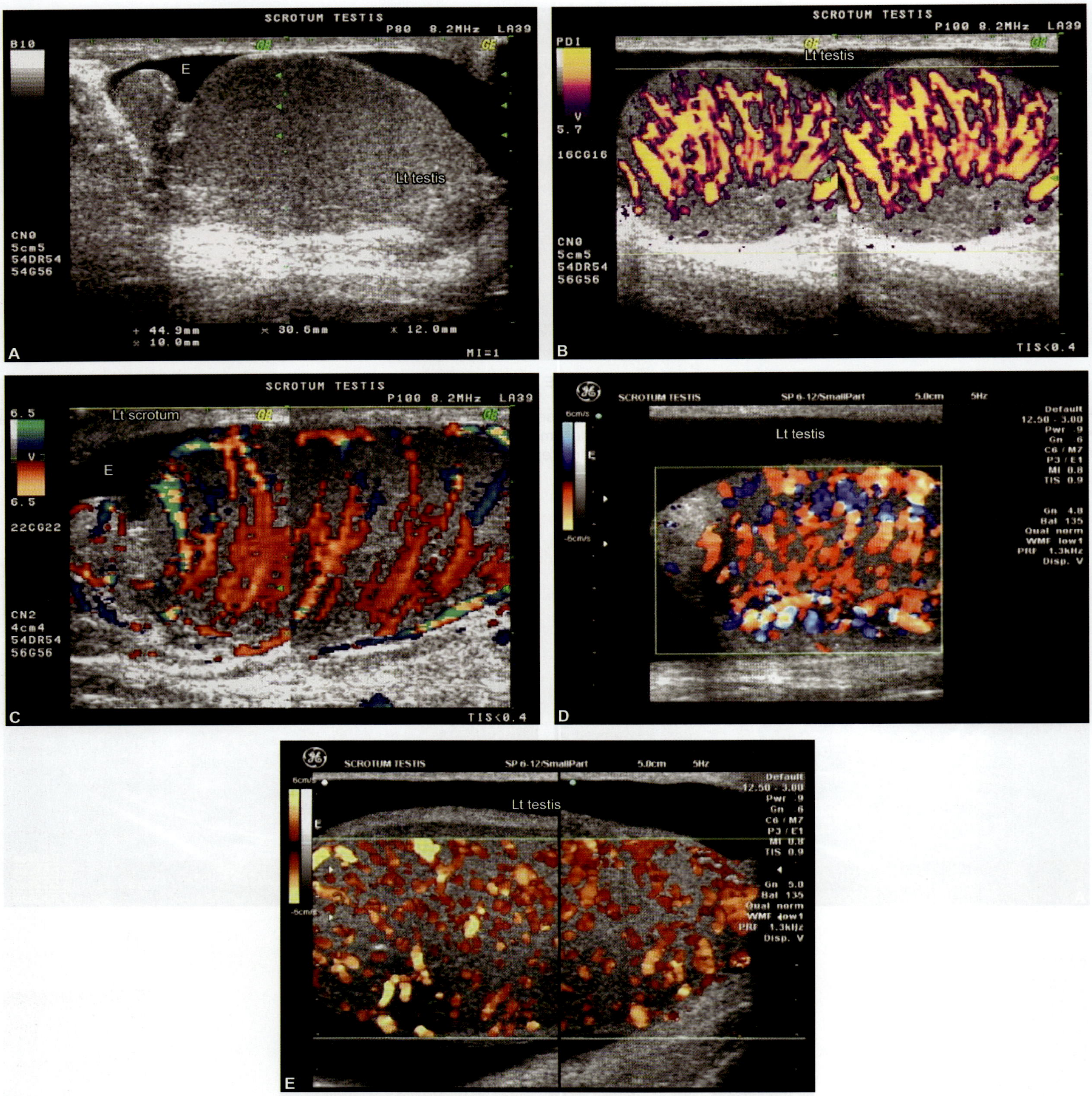

FIGURES 12.29A to E: Acute epididymo-orchitis. A patient presented with acutely painful left scrotal swelling. HRSG shows diffusely hypoechoic-enlarged testes. Echo texture is homogeneous. However, the testes is swollen. On color flow imaging, the testes shows marked increased flow. On power Doppler imaging, it looks like “testes on fire”. The epididymis is also enlarged and hypoechoic. It also shows increased flow. The sonographic signs are suggestive of acute epididymo-orchitis.

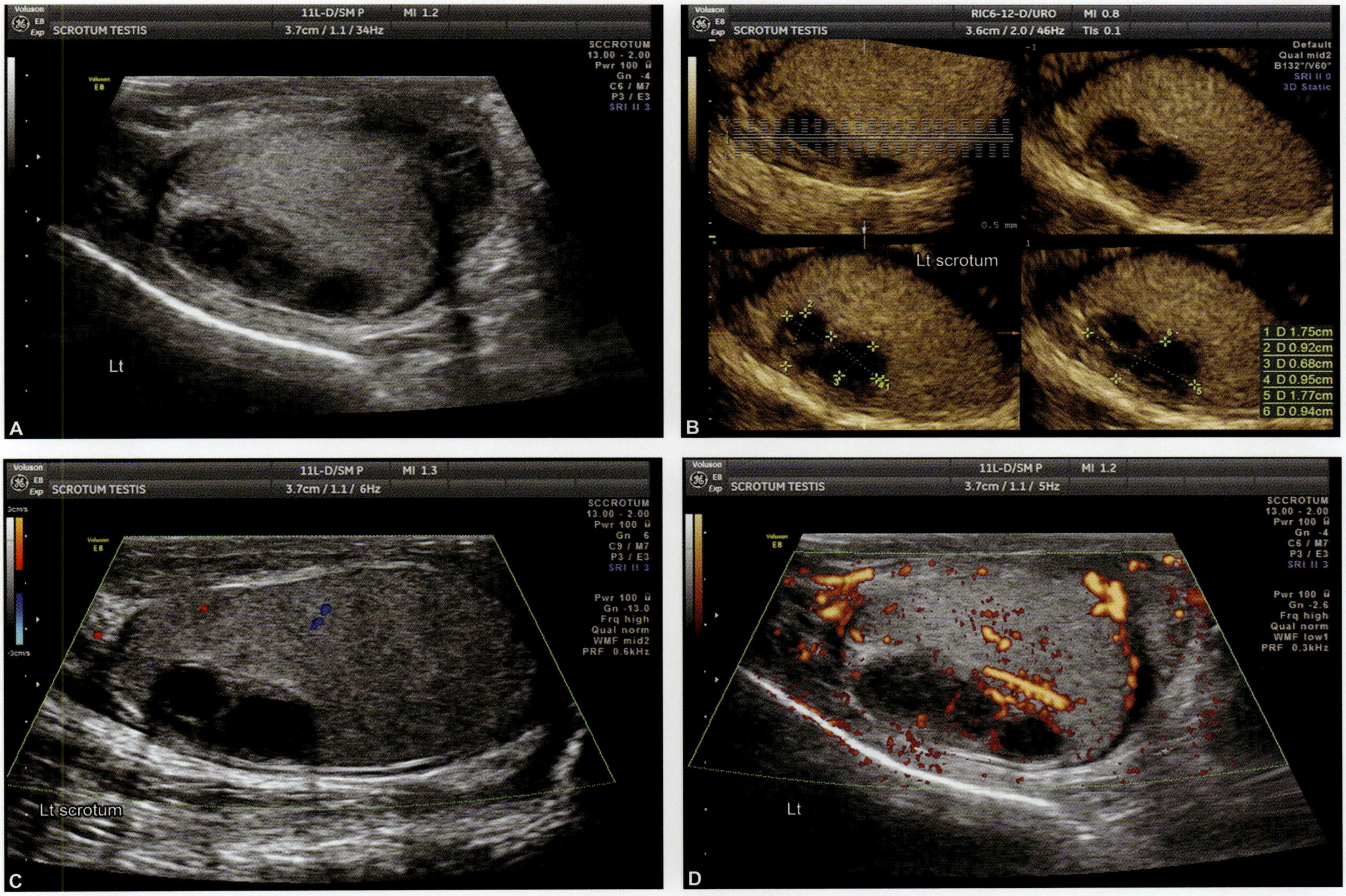

FIGURES 12.30A to D: Testicular infarcts. HRSG is very good in picking up the testicular infarcts. A patient presented with pain in the left scrotum. HRSG shows edematous left testis. Irregular hypoechoic foci are seen in the left testis at the periphery. No evidence of any necrosis is seen in them. No cystic degeneration is seen. On color flow imaging, no flow is seen in the hypoechoic areas. However, normal flow is seen in rest of testicular parenchyma. Findings are suggestive of testicular infarcts.

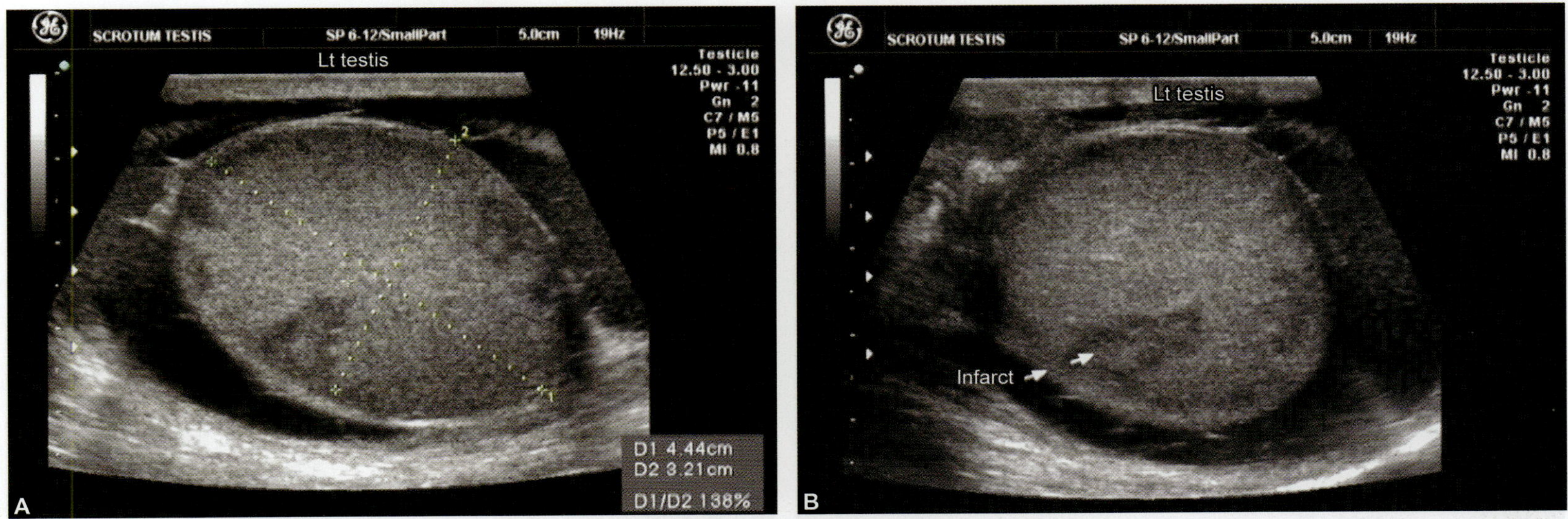

FIGURES 12.31A and B

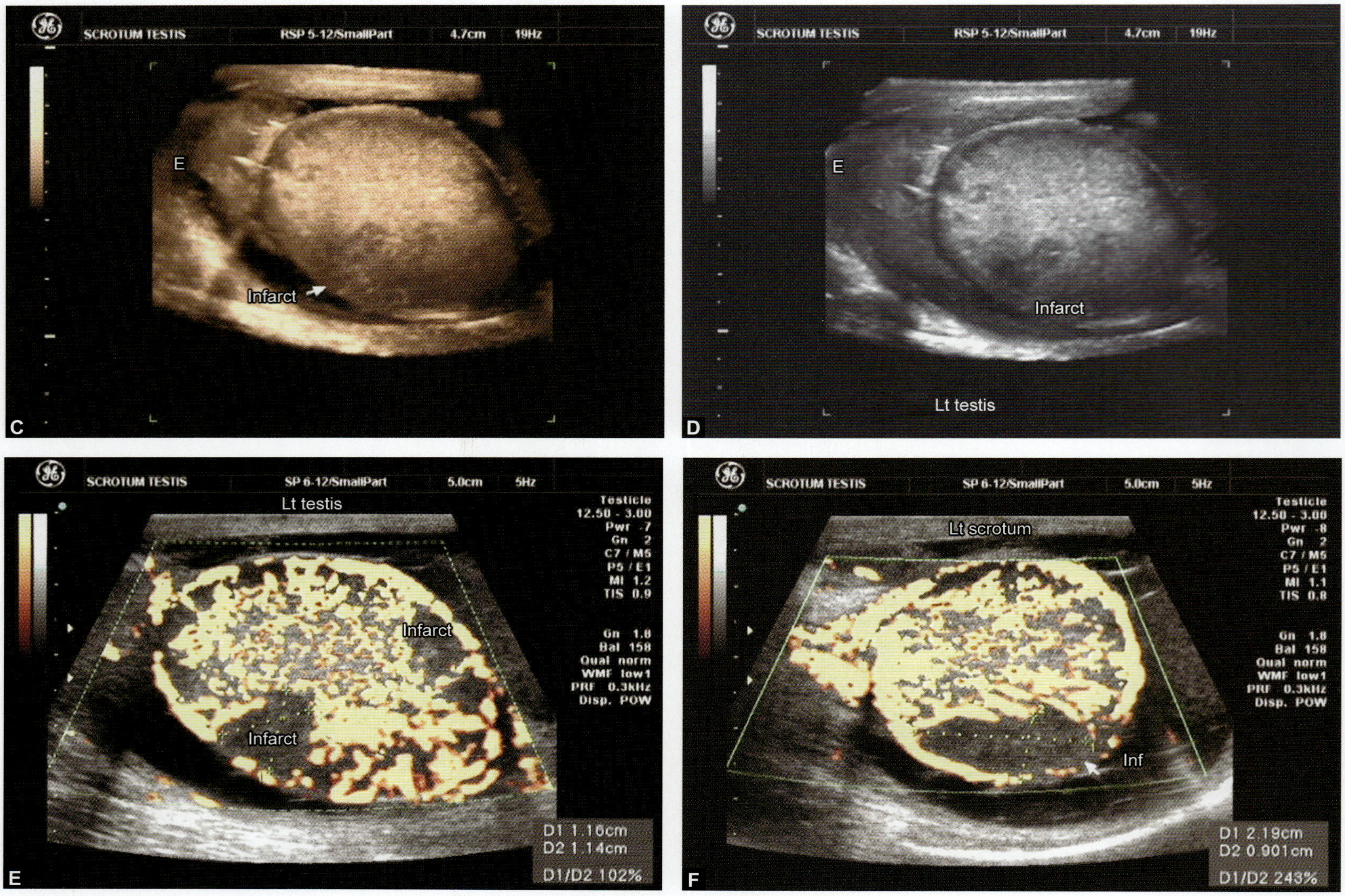

FIGURES 12.31C to F

FIGURES 12.31A to F: Testicular infarcts. A patient presented with painful swelling in the left scrotum. HRSG shows enlarged swollen left testis. Multiple wedge shaped areas are seen in the testes. They are coming from the periphery suggestive of infarctions. 3D surface rendering of the testes shows infarcts in much better view. They are seen as hypoechoic triangular areas. On power Doppler imaging, the infarcted areas are seen devoid of blood supply. The normal testicular parenchyma shows high flow.

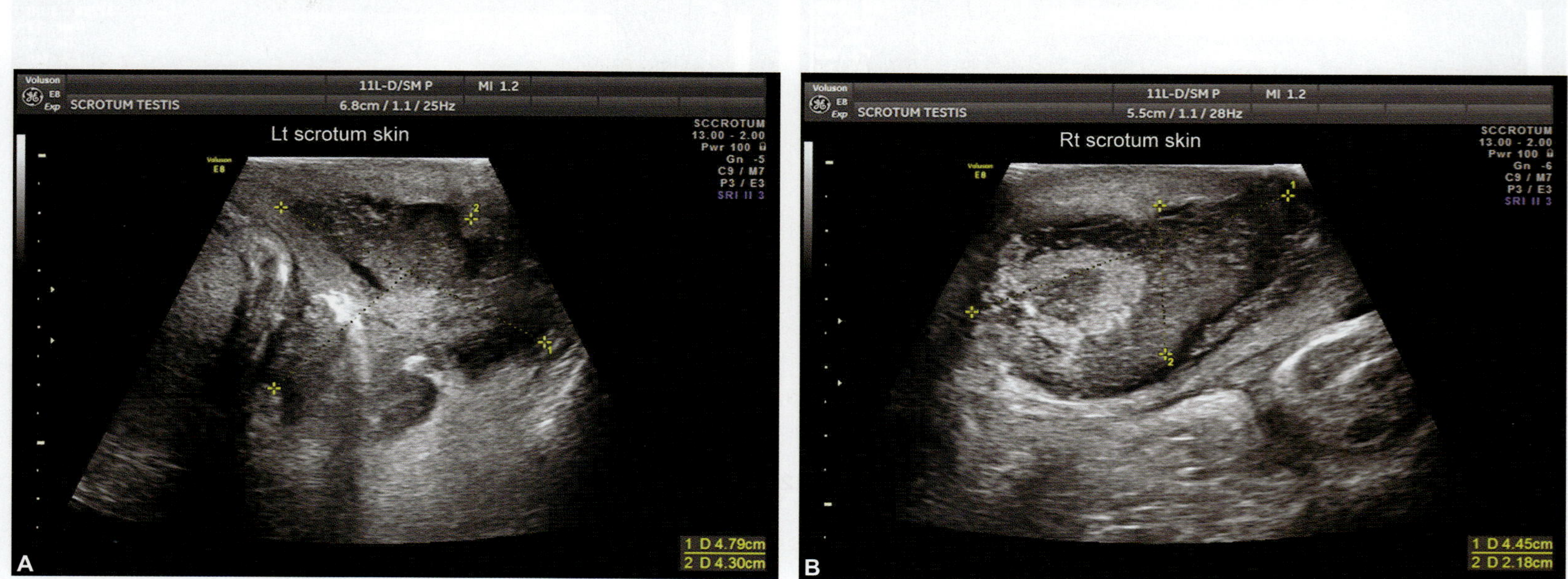

FIGURES 12.32A and B

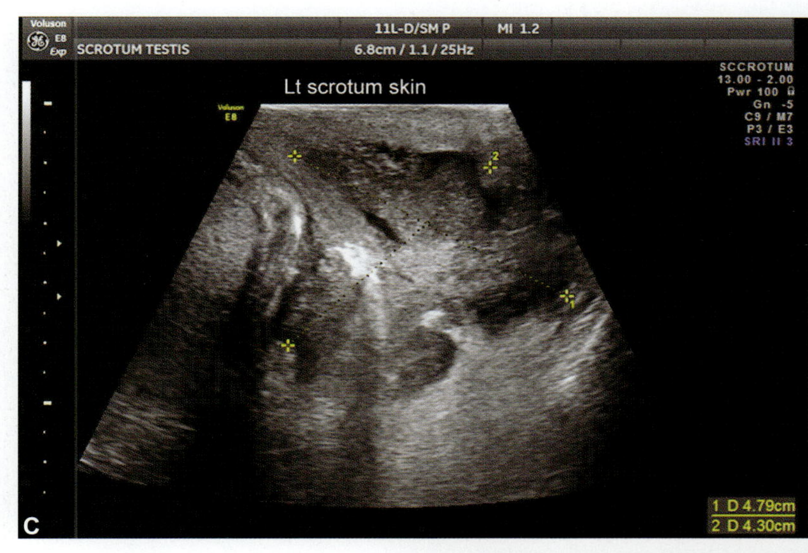

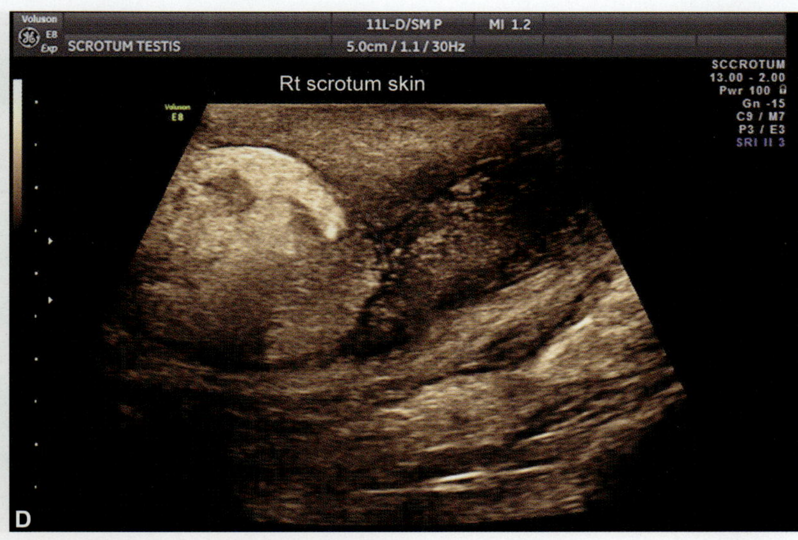

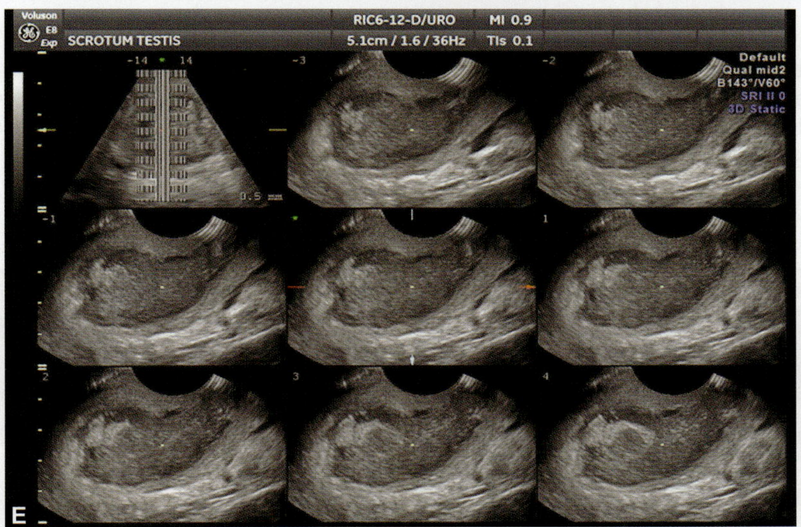

FIGURES 12.32C to E

FIGURES 12.32A to E: A patient presented with diffuse painful swelling of left scrotum. HRSG shows a thick pocket of collection in right scrotal skin. It is seen extending to the lower pole. Area of necrosis is also seen. But no cystic degeneration is also seen. Marked soft tissue edema is also seen suggestive of associated cellulitis. TUI imaging shows the normal testes.

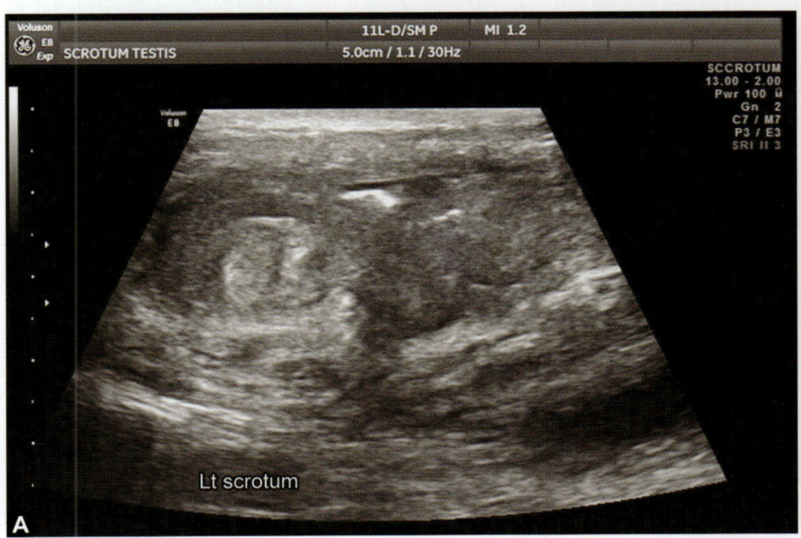

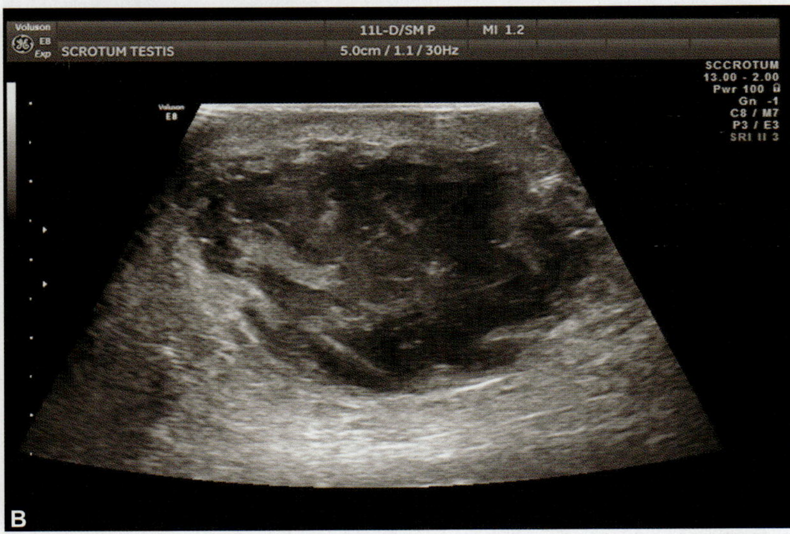

FIGURES 12.33A and B

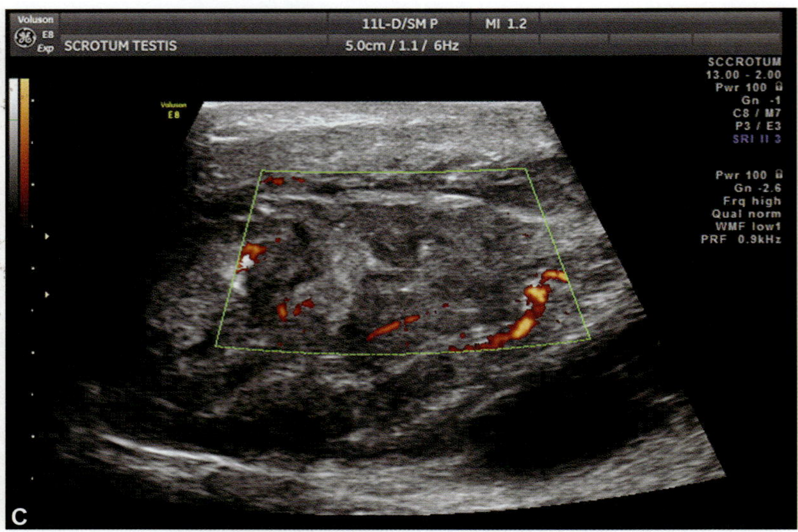

FIGURE 12.33C

FIGURES 12.33A to C: Left scrotal abscess. HRSG shows markedly edematous left scrotal wall. Soft tissue scrotal edema is present. The pocket of thick collection is also seen in the left scrotum. Thick echoes are seen in it. Left testis is hypoechoic in texture. Echogenicity has reduced. On color flow imaging, low flow is seen in the testes. Thick echogenic shadows are also seen filling the scrotum suggestive of exudative collection. Pressure is seen on testes. Findings are suggestive of left scrotal abscess with left epididymo-orchitis.

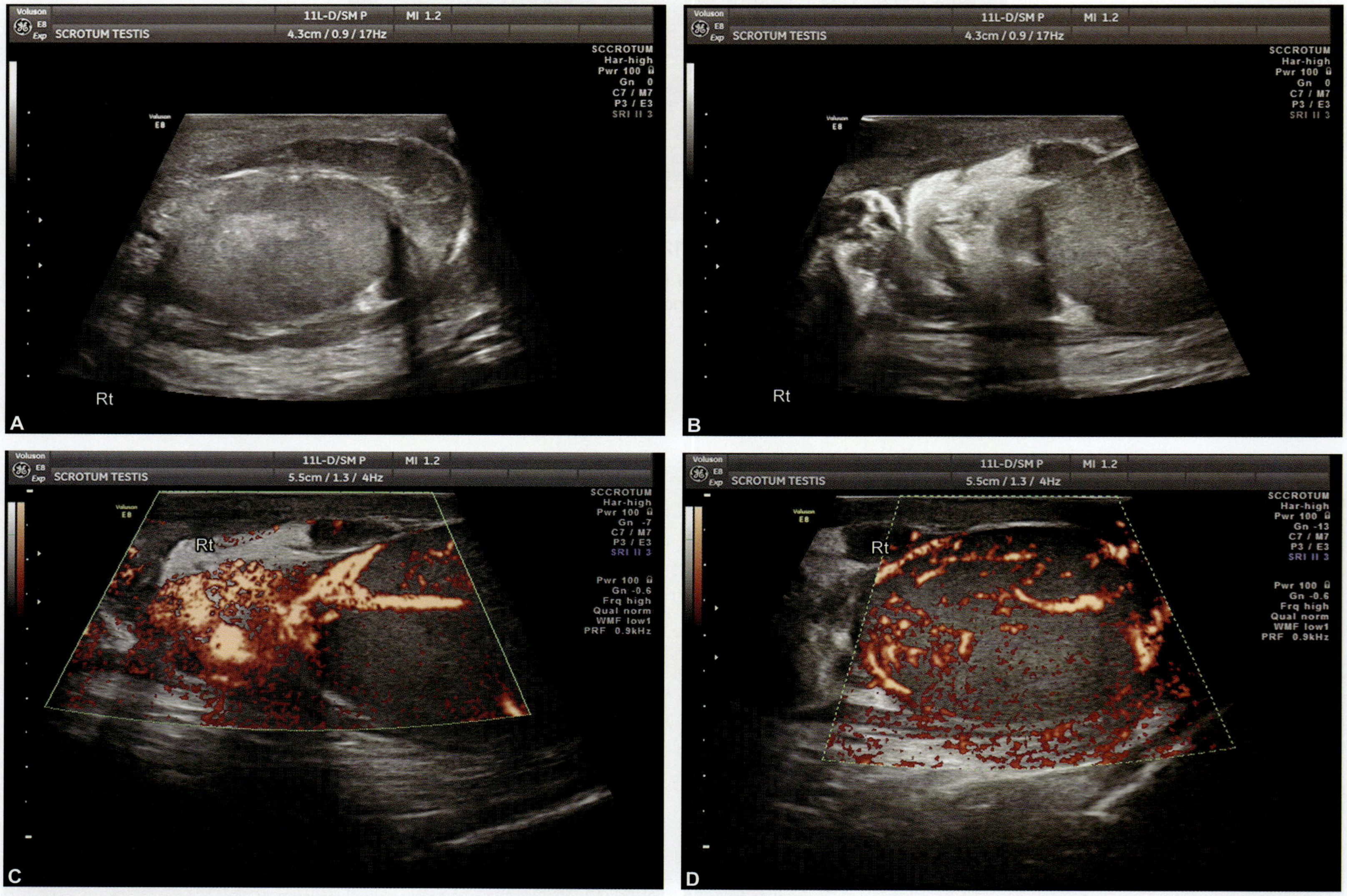

FIGURES 12.34A to D: Acute epididymo-orchitis. HRSG shows enlarged and edematous right testes. Echo texture is hypoechoic and inhomogeneous. No focal mass is seen in the testes. Right epididymis is also enlarged. Echogenic shadows are also seen in the epididymis. On color flow imaging, increased flow is seen in the epididymis. Right cord is also edematous. Cord edema is present. Fat inflammation is also seen. On color flow imaging, multiple vessels are seen feeding the cord. Right scrotal wall is also edematous

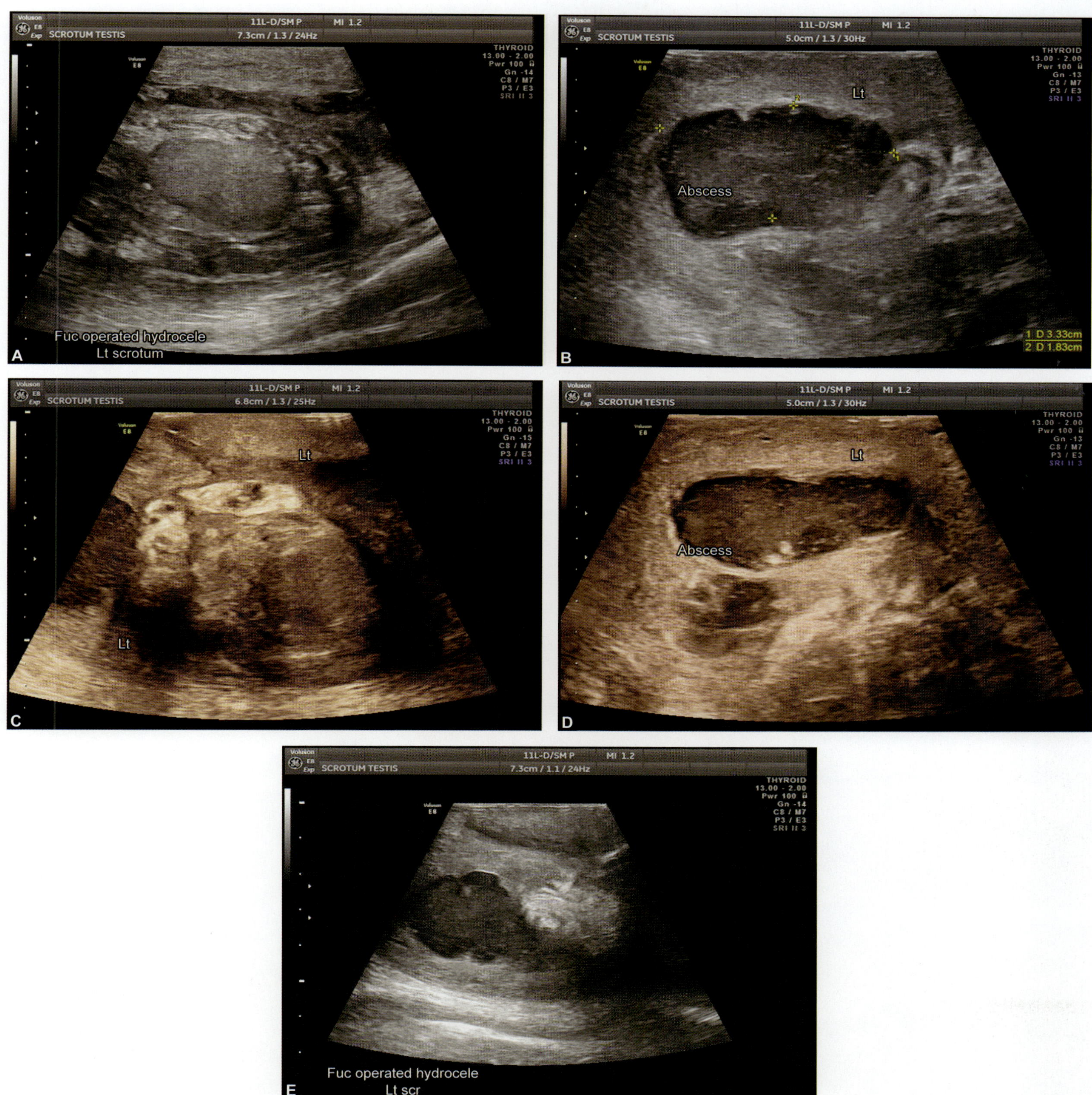

FIGURES 12.35A to E: Post-surgery scrotal abscess. A patient operated for left side hydrocele. HRSG shows hypoechoic but homogeneous testes. Epididymis is hypoechoic and inhomogeneous in texture. It is edematous. Echogenic foci are seen in the epididymis. On color flow imaging, increased flow is seen in left epididymis and testes. There is evidence of a pocket of thick collection seen in the left scrotal wall lateral to the median raphe. Thick echo collection is seen suggestive of an abscess. Marked scrotal wall edema is also presented suggestive of cellulitis.

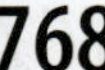

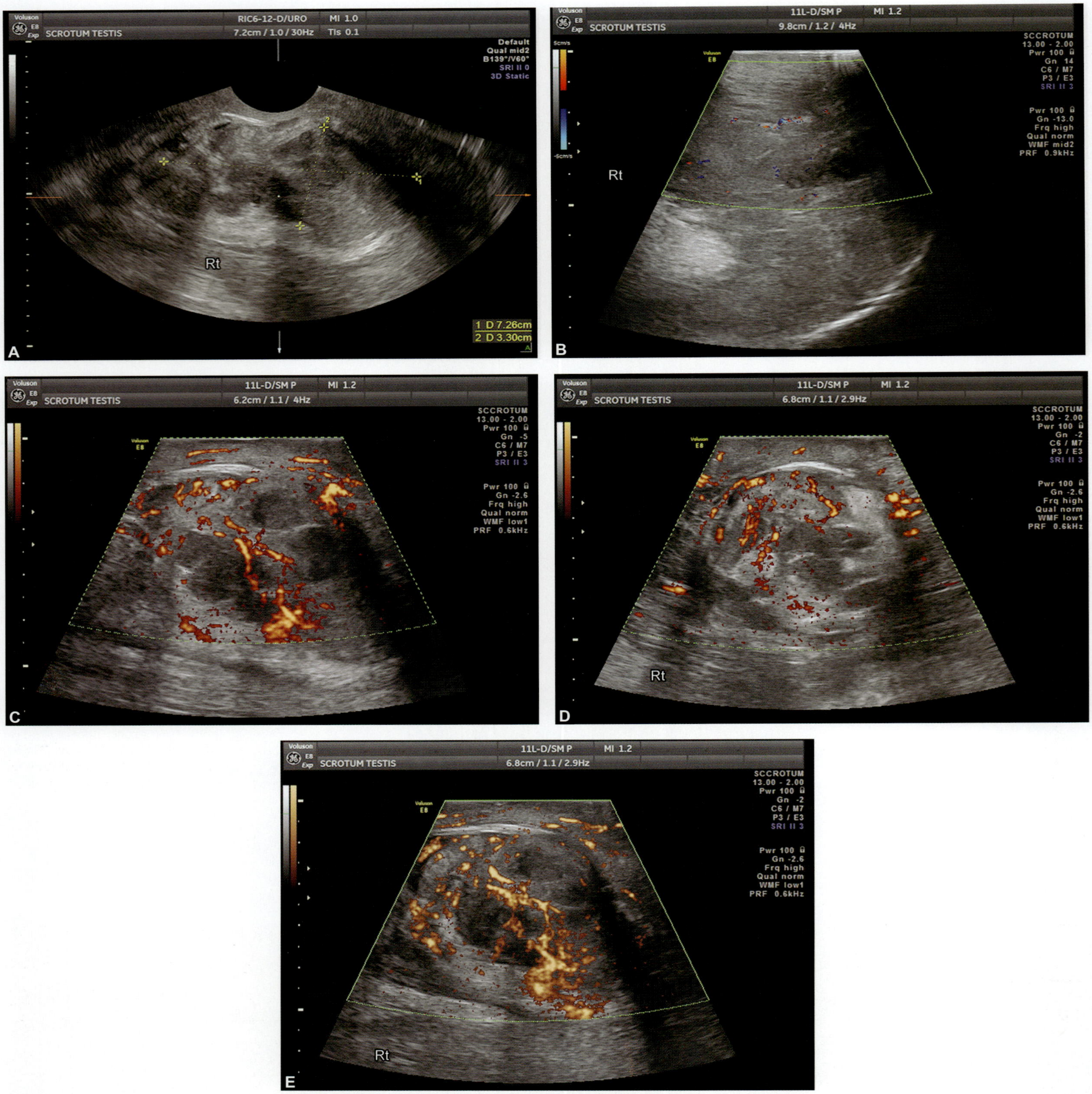

FIGURES 12.36A to E: Intratesticular abscess with acute epididymo-orchitis. HRSG shows marked scrotal wall edema involving both the scrotum. The testes are grossly inhomogeneous and edematous. It is hypoechoic in texture. Irregular ill-defined hypoechoic pockets are seen in the substance of testes suggestive of small abscess. On color flow imaging, increased flow is seen in the testes. However, the necrotic part of the testes does not show any flow. Increased flow is seen in the epididymis. Findings are suggestive of acute epididymo-orchitis with intratesticular abscess.

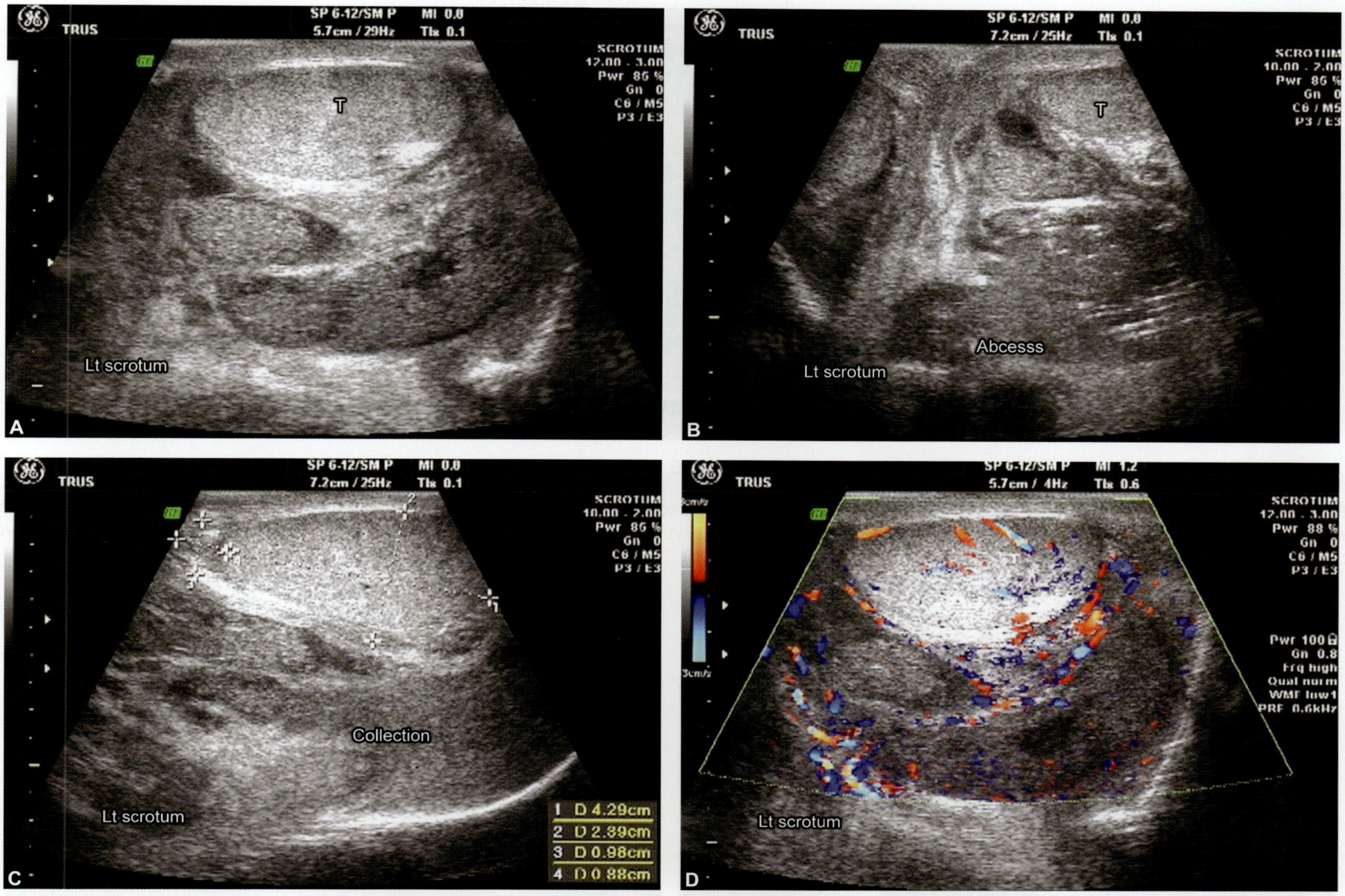

FIGURES 12.37A to D: Anaerobic scrotal abscess. A patient presented with acute swelling in left scrotum. HRSG shows marked scrotal wall edema involving left scrotal sac. Thick echo collection is also seen suggestive of abscess formation. Floating air bubbles is also seen suggestive of anaerobic abscess. But no cystic degeneration is seen. There is also evidence of soft tissue edema seen over the perineum. Subcutaneous edema is present.

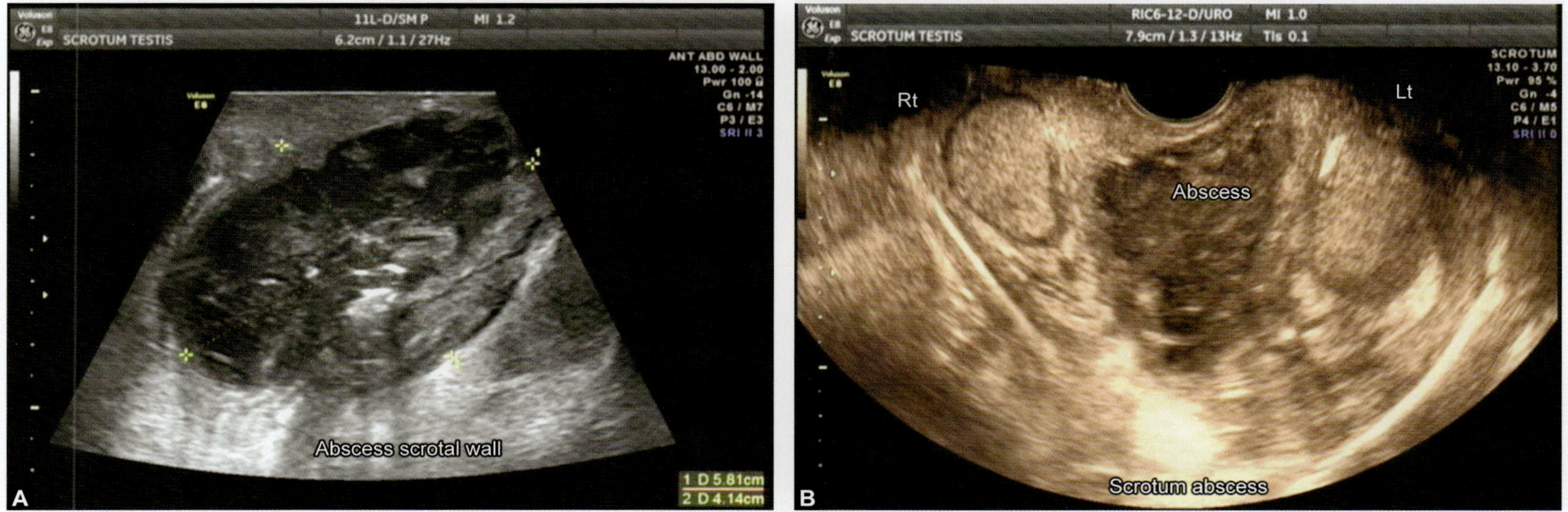

FIGURES 12.38A and B

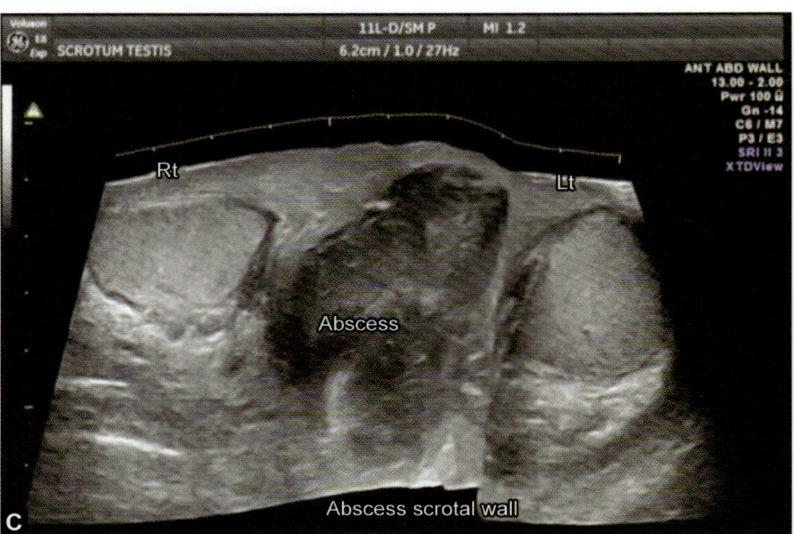

FIGURE 12.38C

FIGURES 12.38A to C: Anaerobic scrotal abscess. HRSG shows marked scrotal. A thick pocket of collection is seen in the mid line of the scrotal wall. It is extratesticular in nature. Thick echoes are seen into it suggestive of an abscess. Air is also seen floating in the abscess cavity suggestive of anaerobic abscess.

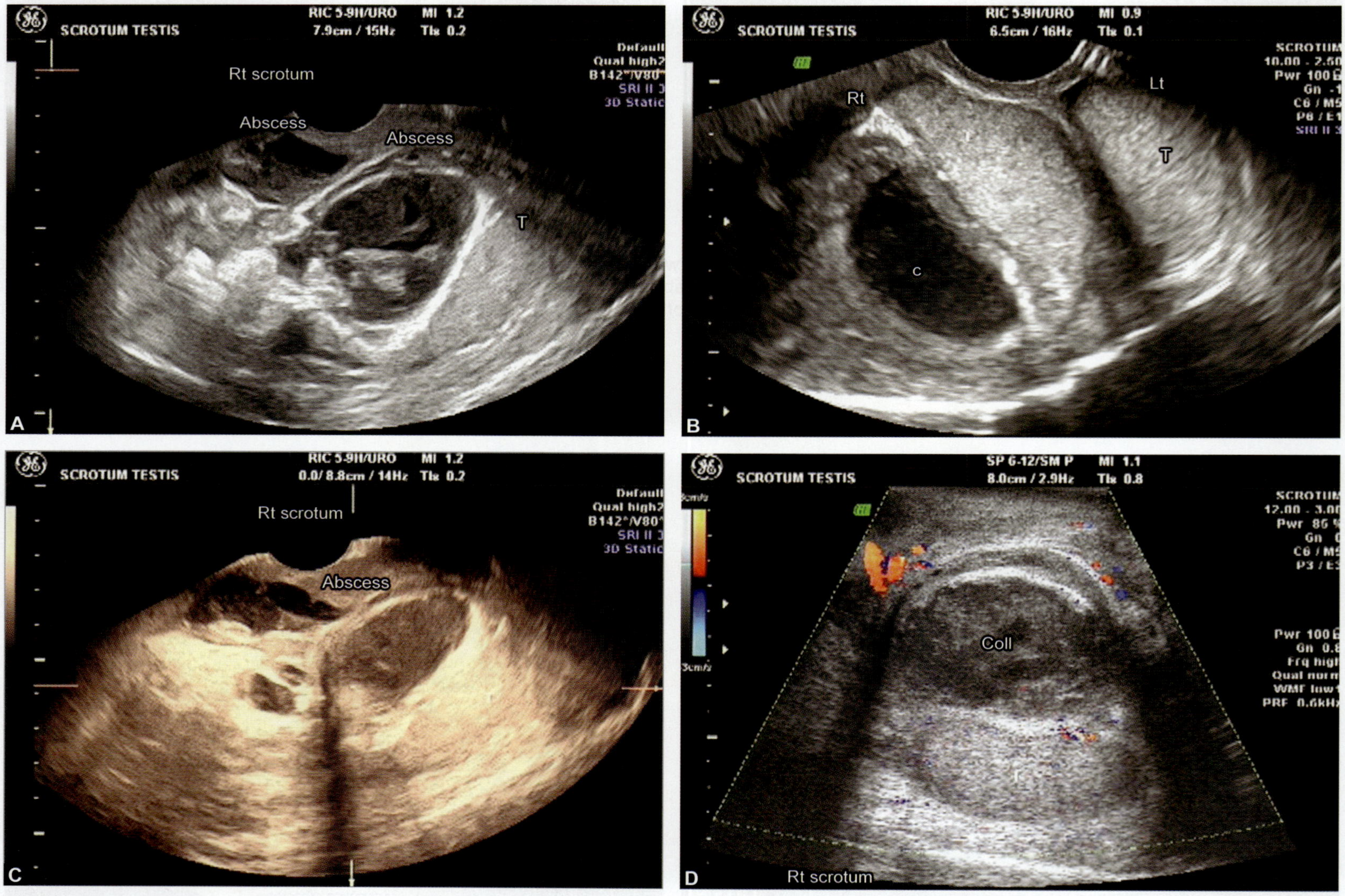

FIGURES 12.39A to D: Scrotal abscess. HRSG shows enlarged and edematous right scrotum. Scrotal wall edema is present. There is evidence of a thick loculated collection seen in the scrotum. Internal echoes are also seen into it suggestive of scrotal abscess. Echogenic septum is seen into it. It is seen pushing the right testes down and compressed it. However, the testes is normal in appearance. Echo texture is homogeneous. On color flow imaging low flow is seen in the testes. Echogenic floating shadows are seen in the collection. Findings are suggestive of scrotal abscess.

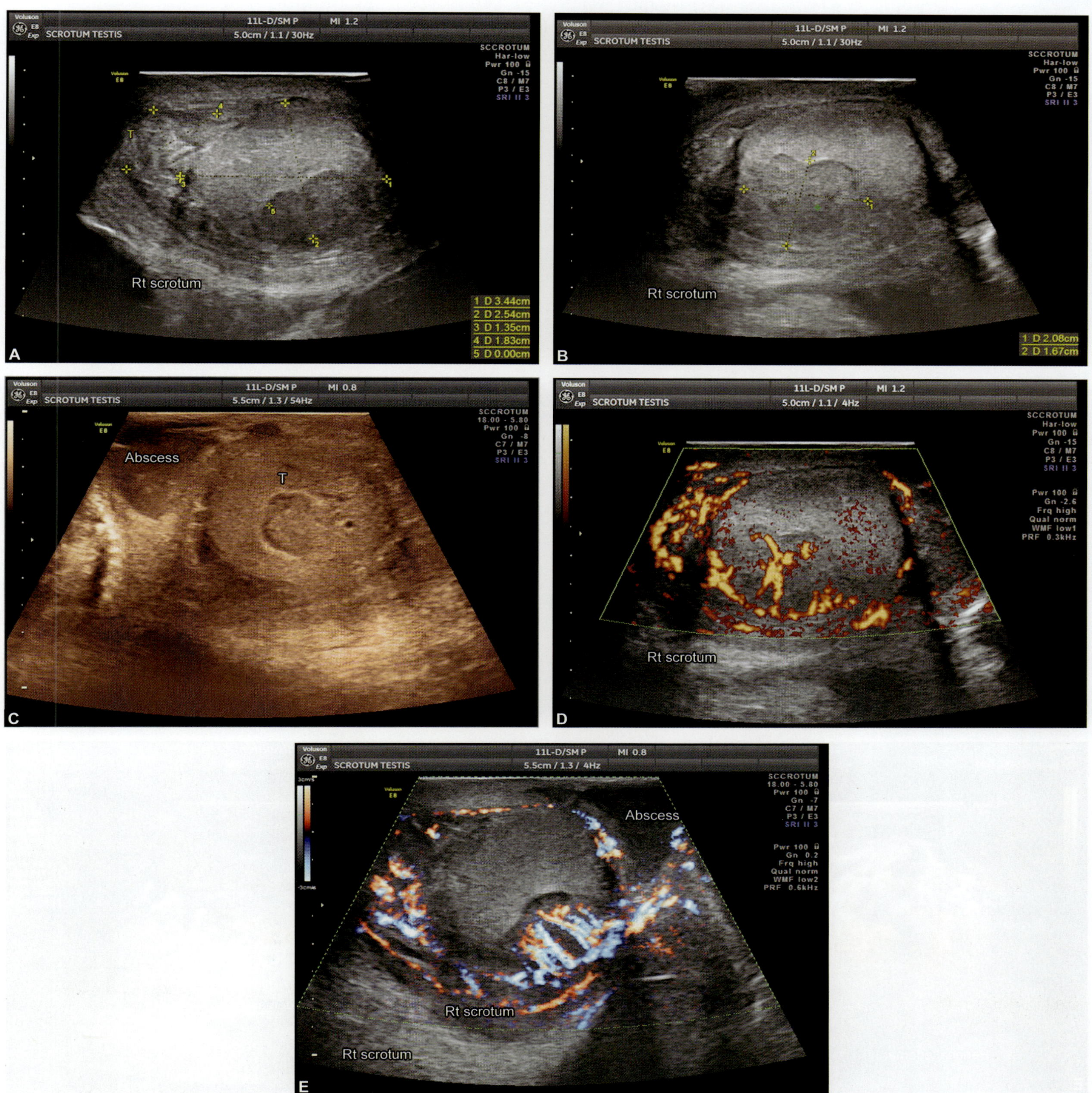

FIGURES 12.40A to E: Acute epididymo-orchitis with testicular abscess. HRSG shows enlarged, hypoechoic and edematous right testes. Epididymis is also enlarged and hypoechoic. There is evidence of hypoechoic irregular shadow is seen in the right testes. On color flow imaging, marked increased flow is seen in the epididymis and testes. Right cord is also thickened. Cord edema is present. Scrotal wall edema is also present. There is evidence of low level echo collection is also seen in right scrotal wall suggestive of abscess formation.

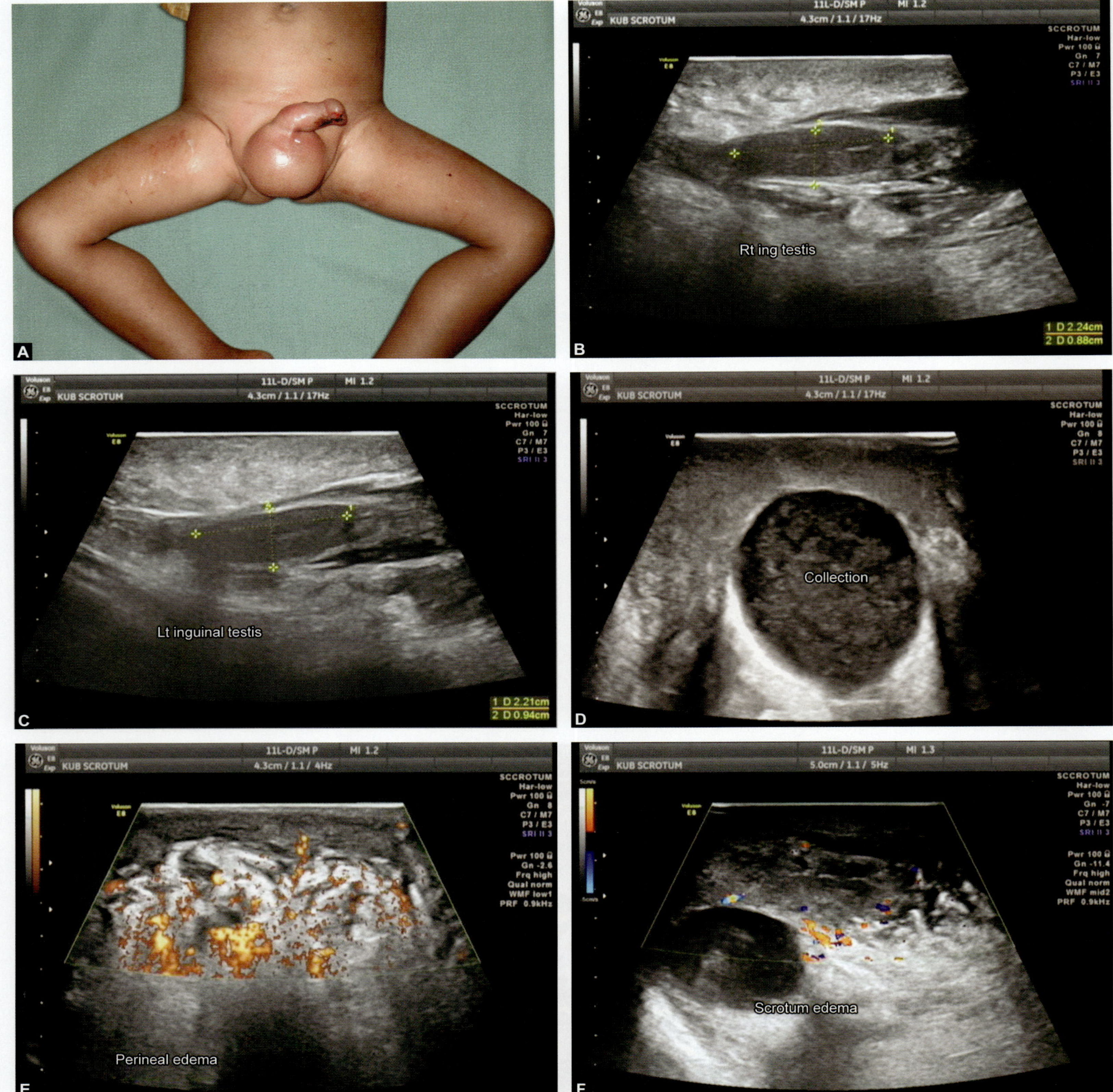

FIGURES 12.41A to F: Diffuse cellulitis of scrotum with penile edema. A 3-year-old boy presented with retention of urine and acute painful scrotal swelling. HRSG shows gross soft tissue edema over the both scrotal wall inguinal region, perineum and over the penile shaft. Dermis and hypodermis edema is present with breaking down of the fat lobules suggestive of diffuse cellulitis. There is also evidence of thick low level echo collection seen in the right scrotum. Collection shows multiple internal echoes. No septation is seen into it. On color flow imaging, no flow is seen. However, multiple vessels are seen feeding the skin and perineal region.

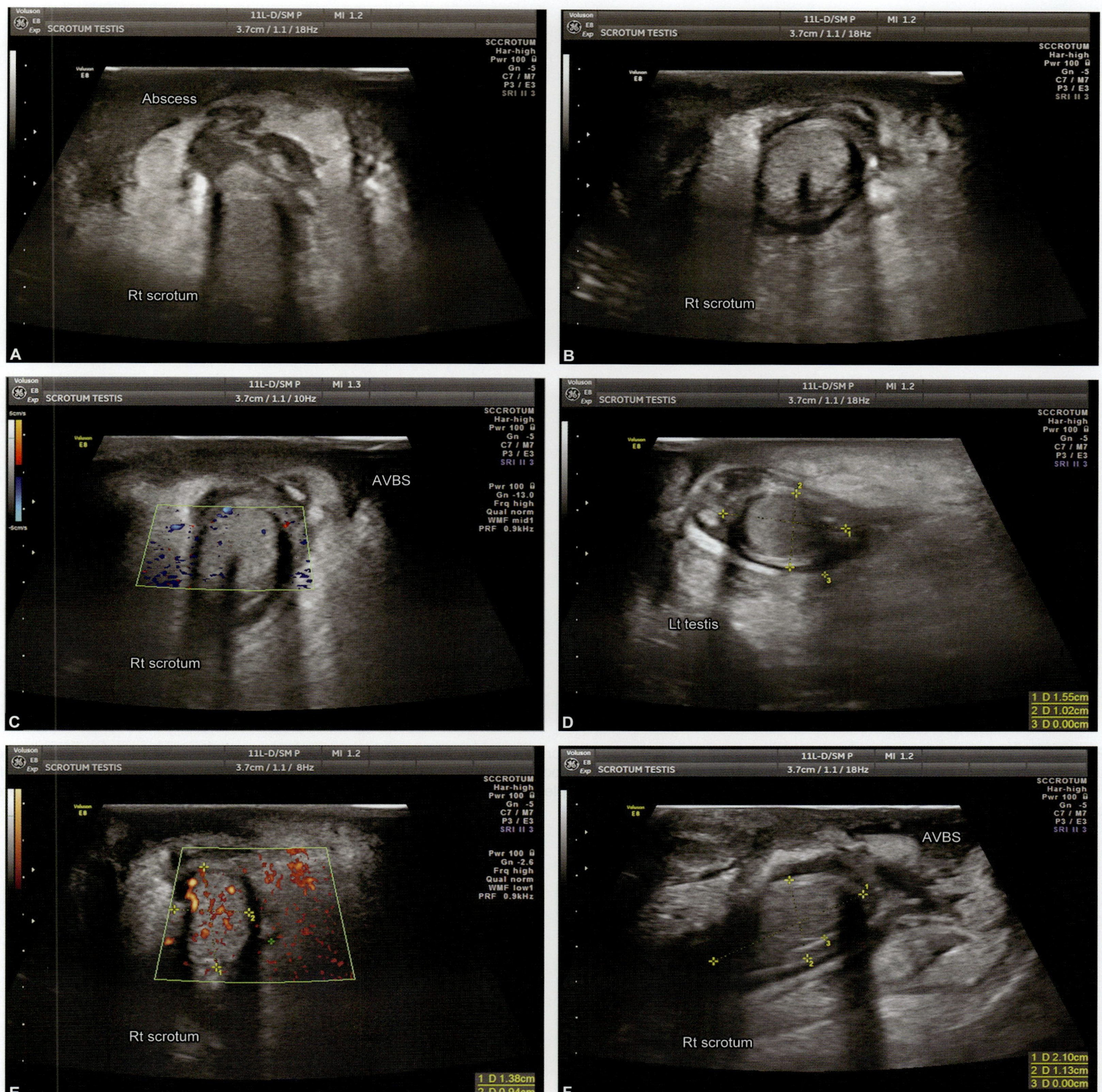

FIGURES 12.42A to F: A 10-month-old baby presented with both scrotal swelling more on the right side. HRSG shows marked scrotal wall edema. Abscess formation seen in the right scrotal wall. Breaking down of the tissue is seen. But no cystic degeneration is seen. However, both testes are normal in size and shape. On color flow imaging, normal flow is seen in the testes. No necrosis is seen. Findings are suggestive of acute scrotal wall abscess with cellulitis.

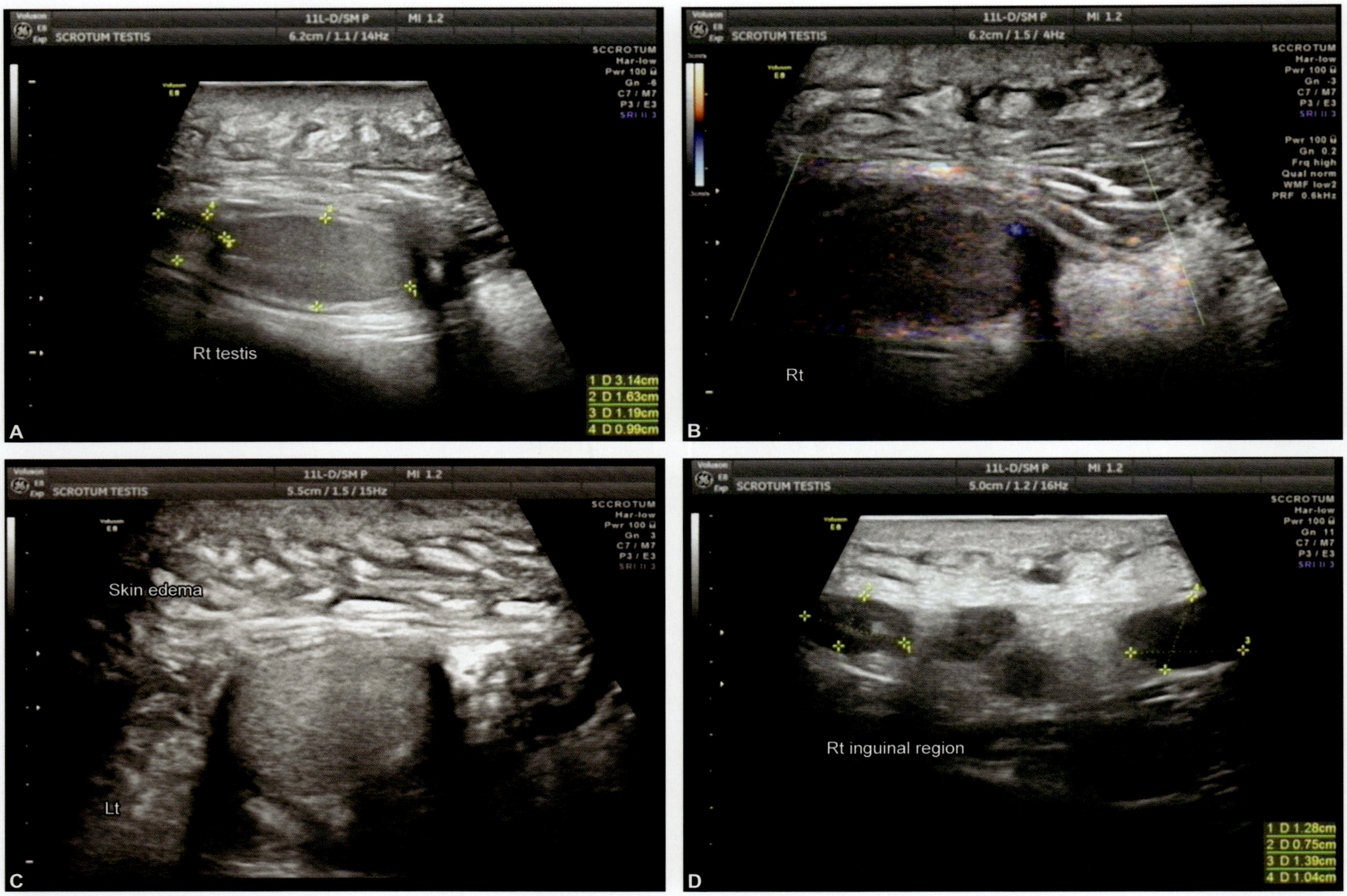

FIGURES 12.43A to D: Scrotal wall cellulitis. HRSG shows marked scrotal wall thickening on both sides. It is 25 mm in thickness on right side and 30 mm on the left side. Soft tissue edema is seen. Dermis and hypodermis edema is present. No evidence of any mass lesion is seen. Soft tissue edema is also seen over the inguinal region on both sides. Multiple enlarged nodal shadows are seen in both inguinal regions. Findings are suggestive of scrotal wall cellulitis.

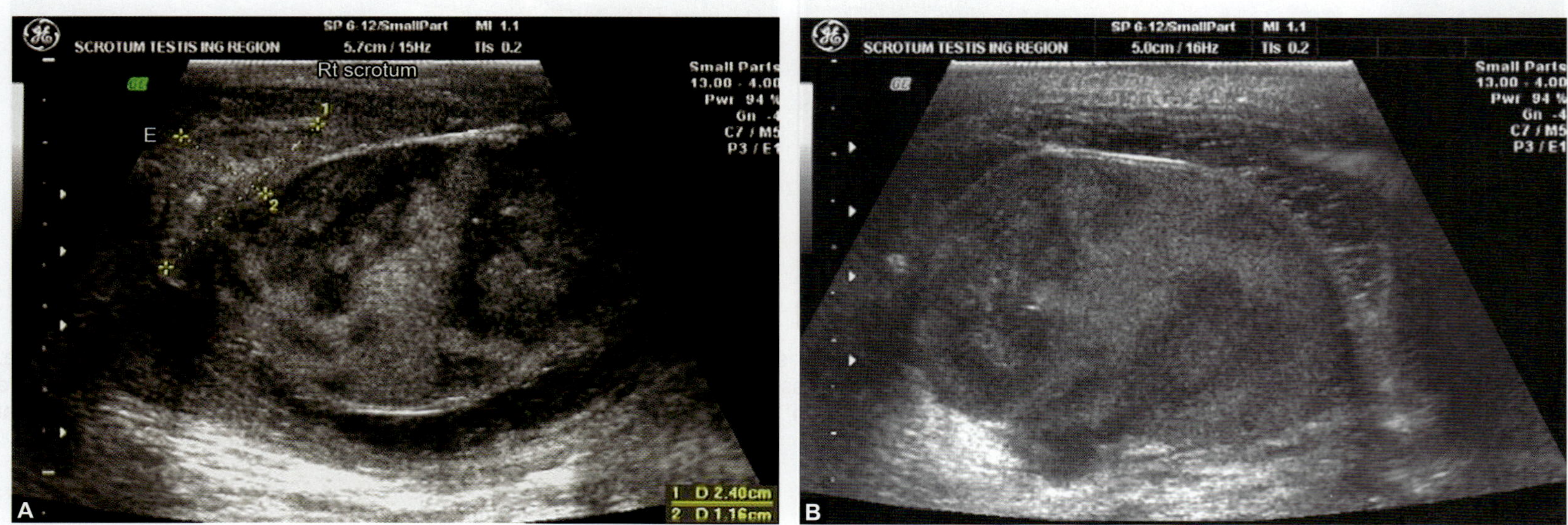

FIGURES 12.44A and B

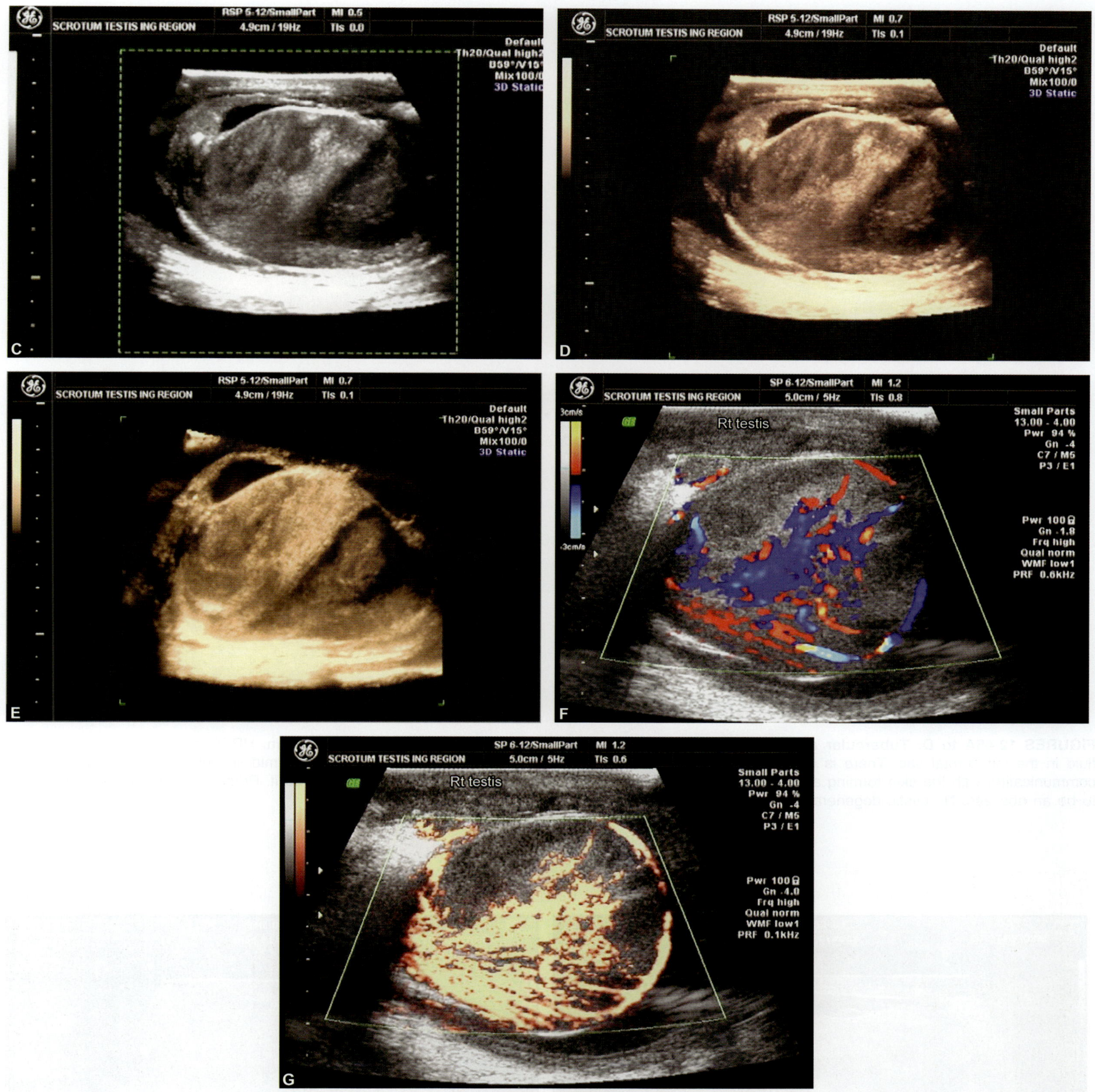

FIGURES 12.44C to G

FIGURES 12.44A to G: Epididymo-orchitis with infected tubercular abscess. A patient presented with Red Hot right scrotal swelling with acute pain with high fever. Marked scrotal skin edema was present. HRSG shows diffusely enlarged testes. Multiple irregular hypoechoic areas are seen in the testes suggestive of abscess formation. Low-level echoes are seen in them. 3D surface rendering of the image shows the testes in much better view. The abscess cavity is well marked on 3D imaging. On color flow and power Doppler imaging marked increased flow seen in the testes. On surgical exploration it came out to be infected tubercular abscess.

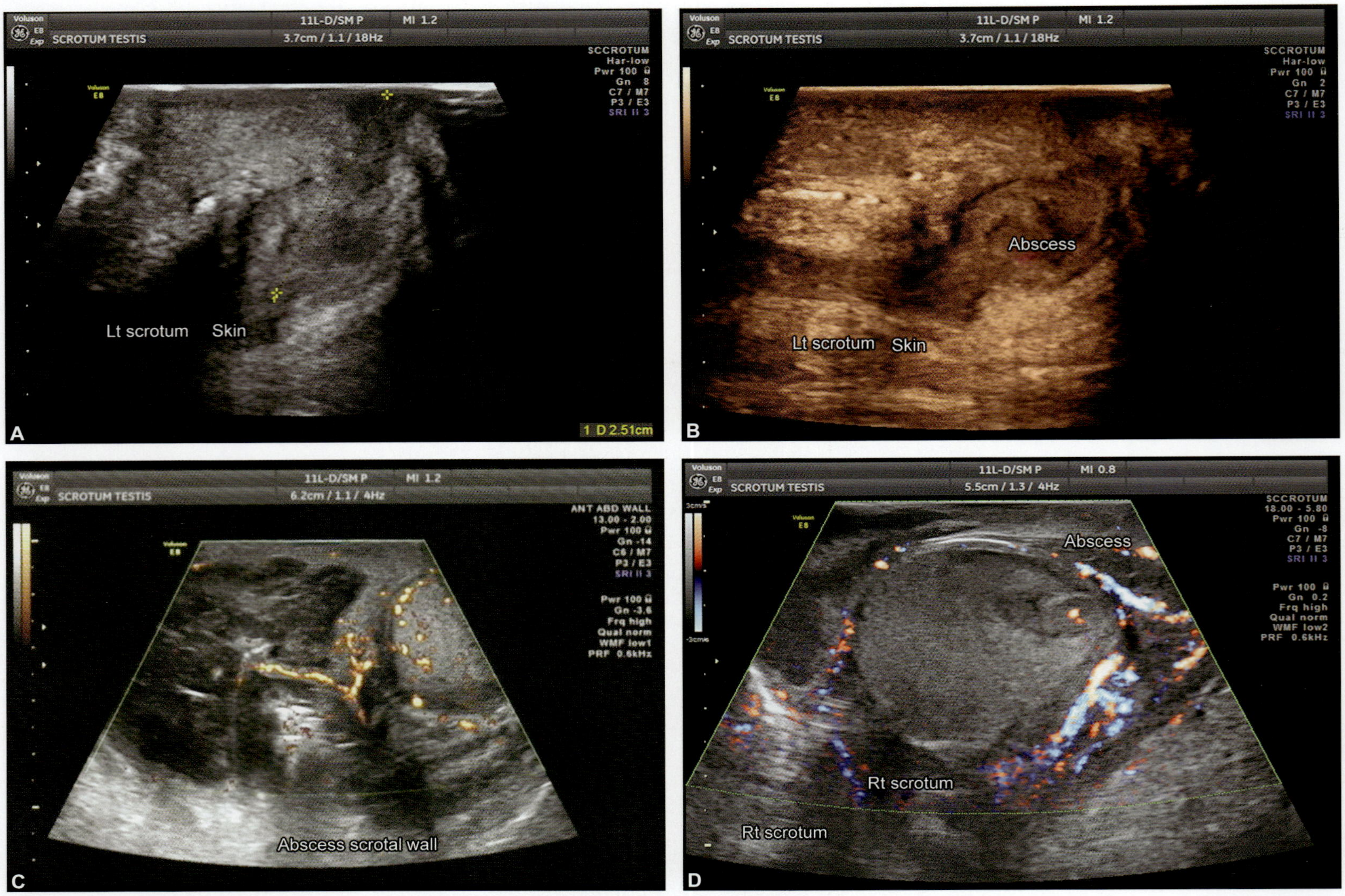

FIGURES 12.45A to D: Tubercular abscess with sinus formation. A patient presented with painful scrotum. HRSG shows moderate amount of fluid in the left scrotal sac. There is evidence of a low level echo complex shadow seen at the skin of the mid line of the scrotal sac. It is seen communicating with the skin forming a sinus. It is 2.5 cm deep from the skin. Low level echoes are seen into it. Perifocal edema is seen. It appears to be an abscess. No cystic degeneration seen.

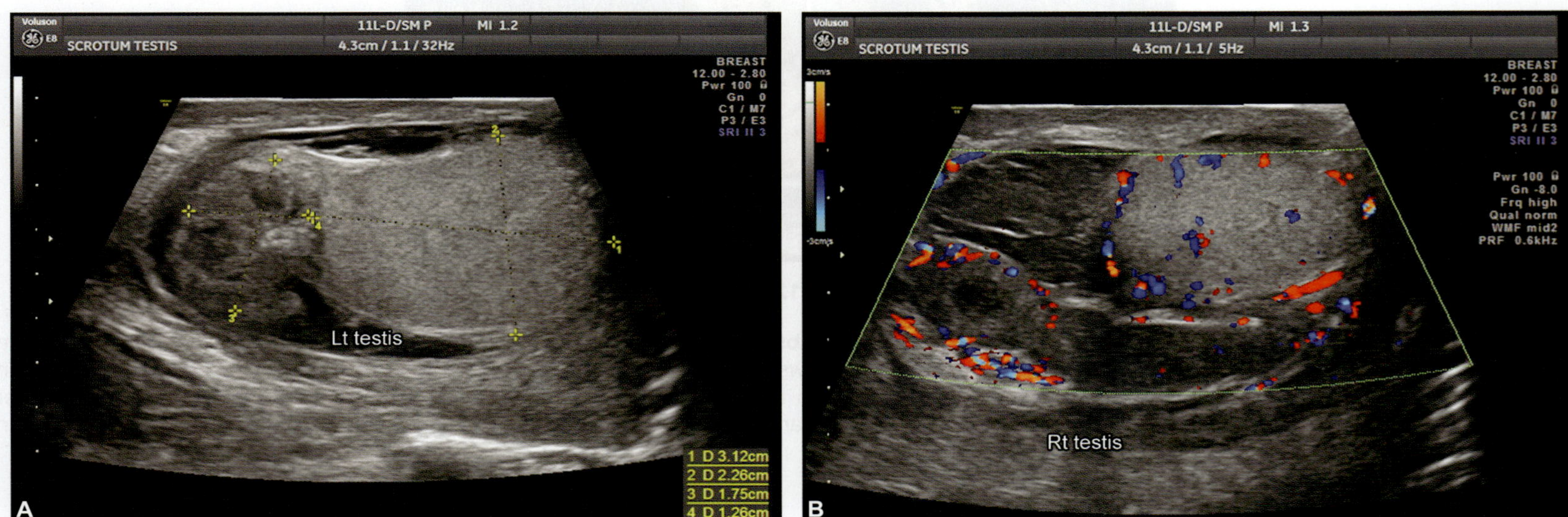

FIGURES 12.46A and B

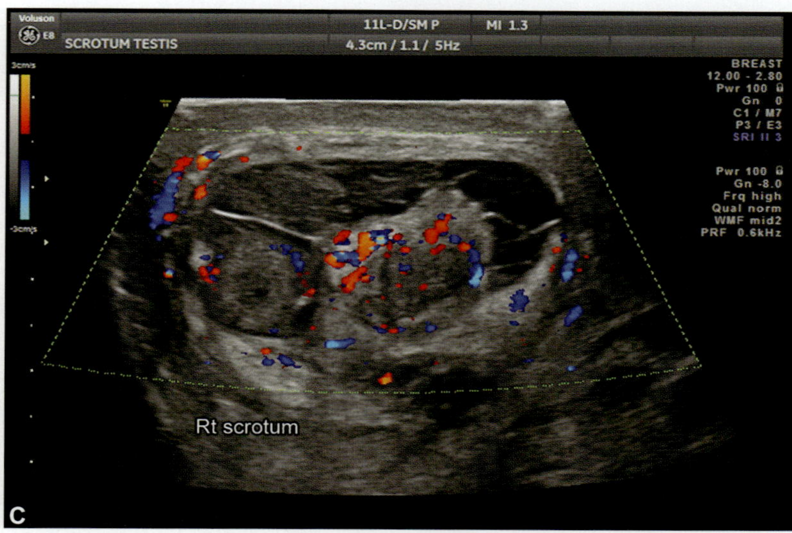

FIGURE 12.46C

FIGURES 12.46A to C: Bilateral epididymo-orchitis. HRSG shows enlarged and inhomogeneous both epididymis. Thick collection is seen in both scrotal sac more on the right side. Echogenic bands are also seen in the collection. On color flow imaging high flow is seen in the testes and epididymis on both sides. Findings are suggestive of bilateral epididymo-orchitis.

Testicular Trauma

The common causes of testicular trauma are sport injuries and vehicular accidents.

Sonographic Features

Several sonographic features are seen. There is thickening of the scrotal skin as a result of edema. The thickness can also be due to hemorrhage and extravasations. It there is associated bladder rupture; a multilayered pattern of the scrotal wall is seen. Hemorrhage is generally echo poor, and low-level mobile echoes are seen within the fluid.

Hematocele may have a complex or echogenic pattern. In the presence of hematoceles, the testes must be thoroughly scanned for an intratesticular hematoma or a fracture.

Acute hematomas in any location are heterogeneous masses often with increased echogenicity. As hematoma resolves in 1 to 2 weeks, it becomes smaller and anechoic cystic mass with septations replacing the heterogeneous lesion.

Intratesticular hematomas have an appearance similar to extra-testicular ones, but because of their position they may mimic a tumor. These cases require close observation as hematomas will become cystic and change their appearance rapidly over the course of several days, whereas a tumor will remain unchanged for a long-time.

Testicular rupture leads to loss of normal smooth contours of testes with interruption of bright capsule of the tunica albuginea and protrusion of parenchyma. Echo poor and heterogeneous areas will be seen in the testicle as a result of hemorrhage and parenchymal disruption.

Testicular contusion or fracture without tunical rupture will have a smooth and remain surrounded by bright tunica albuginea. The fracture will be seen as a linear hypoechoic area within the testes. There are associated changes in the epididymis in the form of enlargement, reduced echogenicity or abnormal position in relation to the testes.

Fluid Collections

Hydrocele is the most common cause of an enlarged scrotum for a patient presenting to the surgeon. It is an abnormal fluid collection between the two layers of the tunic vaginalis.

Most commonly hydrocele are idiopathic. In the neonates, this can be the result of the processes vaginalis being open. It invariably closes by about 2 years. In the adults, the other causes of hydrocele are inflammation, torsion and trauma. Hydroceles are not commonly encountered with testicular tumors.

Sonographic Features

Hydroceles are present as hypoechoic/anechoic fluid collections surrounding the testes. The testes as often displaced posteriorly and medially.

Septations may be present and indicate old hemorrhage or infections. Thick septations are often seen in tuberculosis. Diagnosis of hydrocele is usually straightforward. There may be fine debris within the fluid in long-standing hydroceles; these indicate cholesterol crystals, some of these patients where the hydroceles are tense may even suggest solid lesion clinically. This may be associated with thickening of the scrotal wall in longstanding hydroceles. Parietal calcifications are also noted.

Other Fluids

Hematoceles and pyoceles are usually secondary to trauma and inflammation. They present as scrotal swelling. Sonography reveals fluid surrounding the testes. The fluid contains low level echoes, debris and internal septations. There may be associated air.

Scrotal lymphoceles are secondary to renal transplantation. They are the result of lymphatic dissection with perirenal lymphocele tracking down to the scrotum. It presents as any other fluid with low-level echoes and septations.

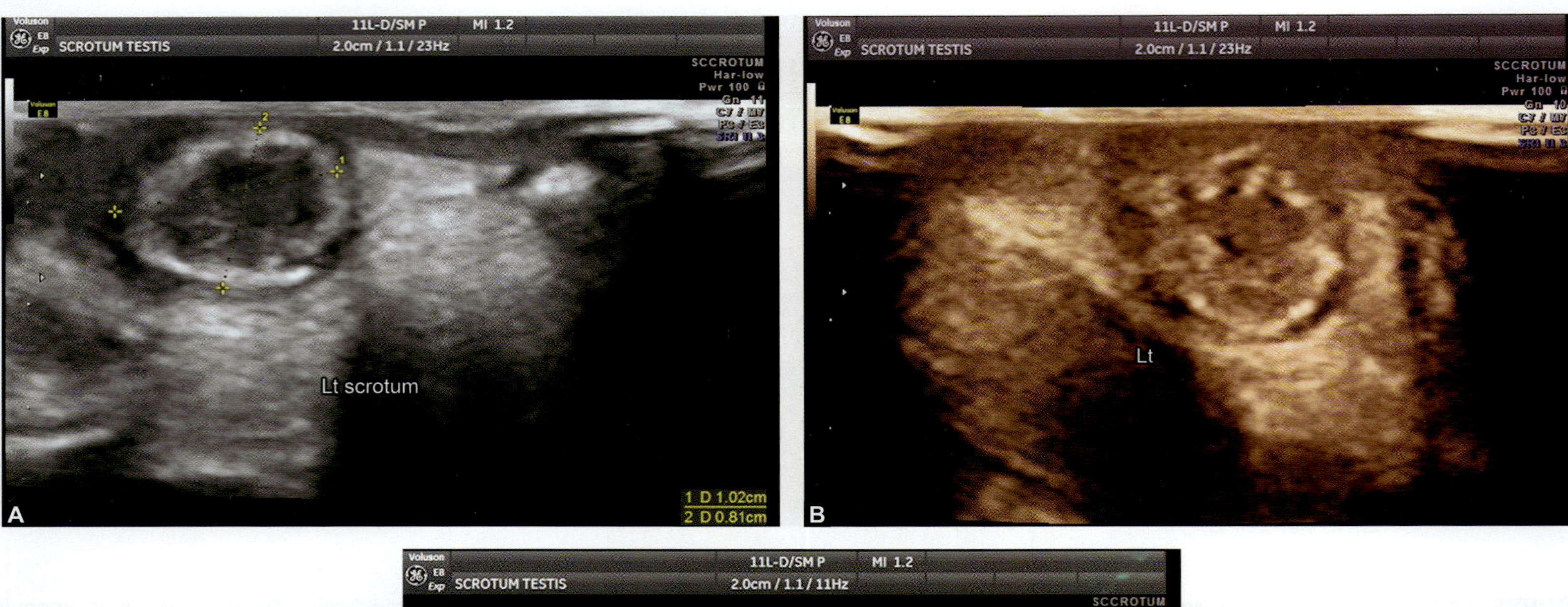

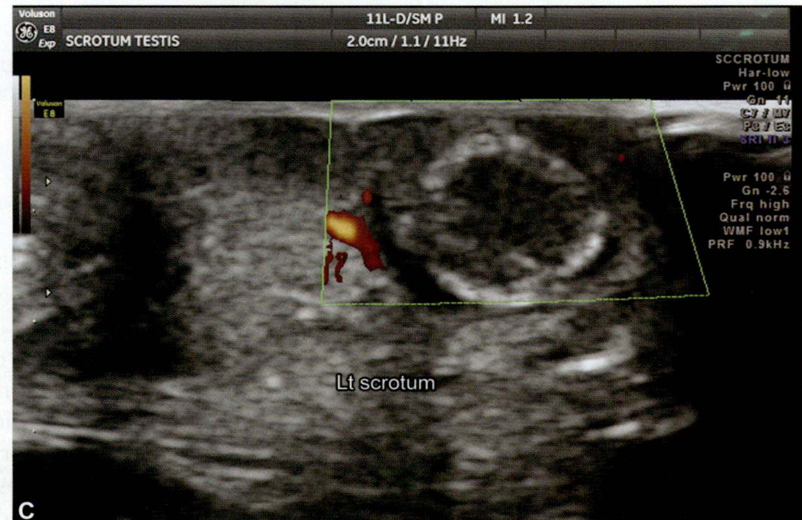

FIGURES 12.47A to C: Neonatal testicular torsions. A 17-day-old baby presented with acute painful swelling of left scrotum. HRSG shows enlarged edematous left testes. It is hypoechoic in texture. The margins are echogenic. On color flow imaging, no flow is seen in the testes. Findings are suggestive of acute torsion of the testes.

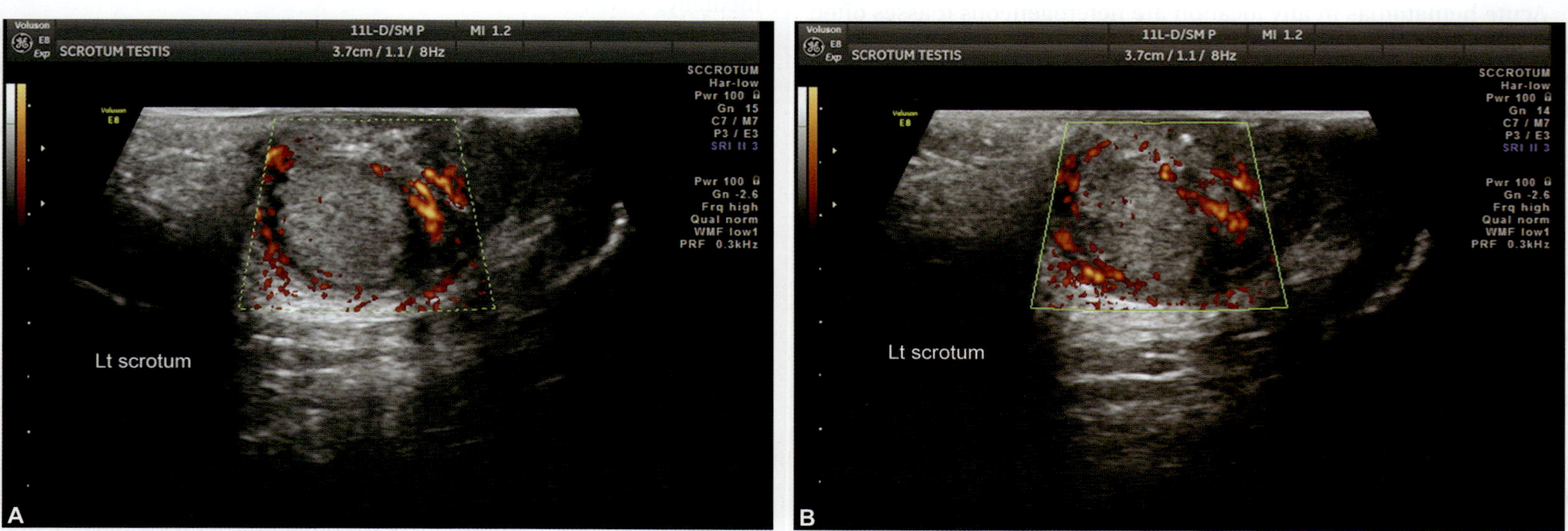

FIGURES 12.48A and B

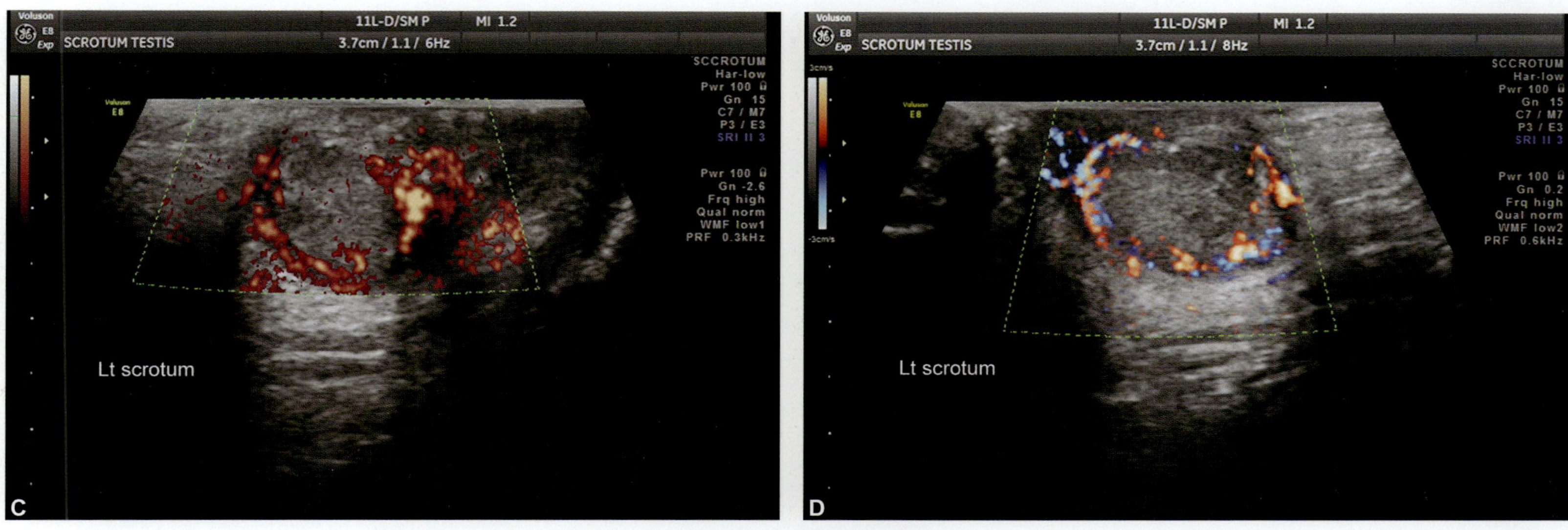

FIGURES 12.48C and D

FIGURES 12.48A to D: Partial torsion of the testes. A 1-year-old baby presented with painful swelling of left scrotum. HRSG shows enlarged edematous left testes. However, the testes is hypoechoic but homogeneous. On color flow imaging, increased peripheral flow is seen in the testes. But no intra testicular flow is seen. On peroperative findings partial torsion of the testes is seen and testes was salvage.

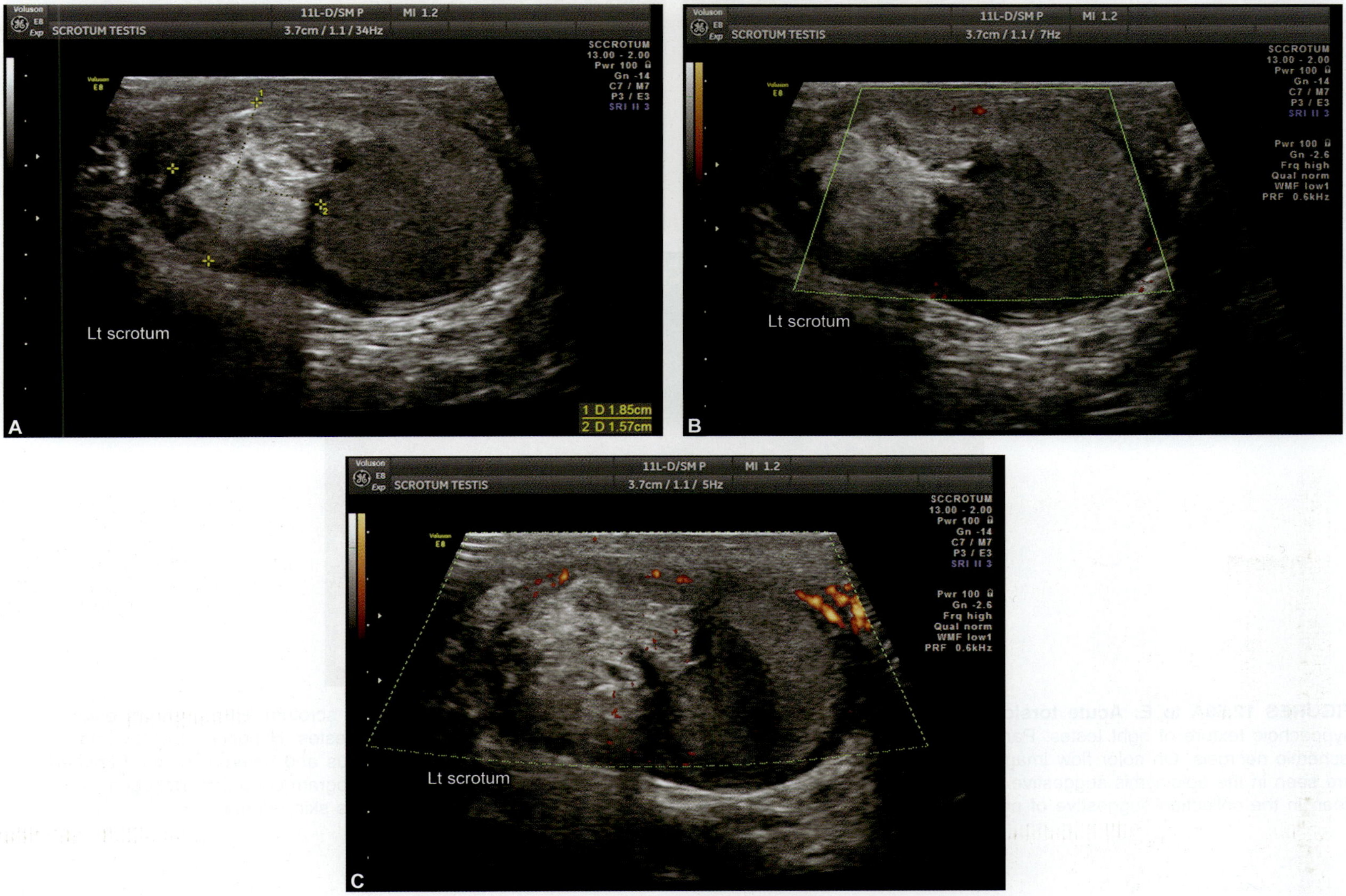

FIGURES 12.49A to C: Acute torsion of left testes. A patient presented with hard swelling in the left scrotum, which was associated with acute pain. HRSG shows enlarged edematous left testes. The echo texture is inhomogeneous and hypoechoic. On color flow imaging, no flow is seen in the testes. The left epididymis is also enlarged. It is irregular in outline and echogenic in texture. Echogenic areas are seen in the left epididymis suggestive of hemorrhagic epididymitis.

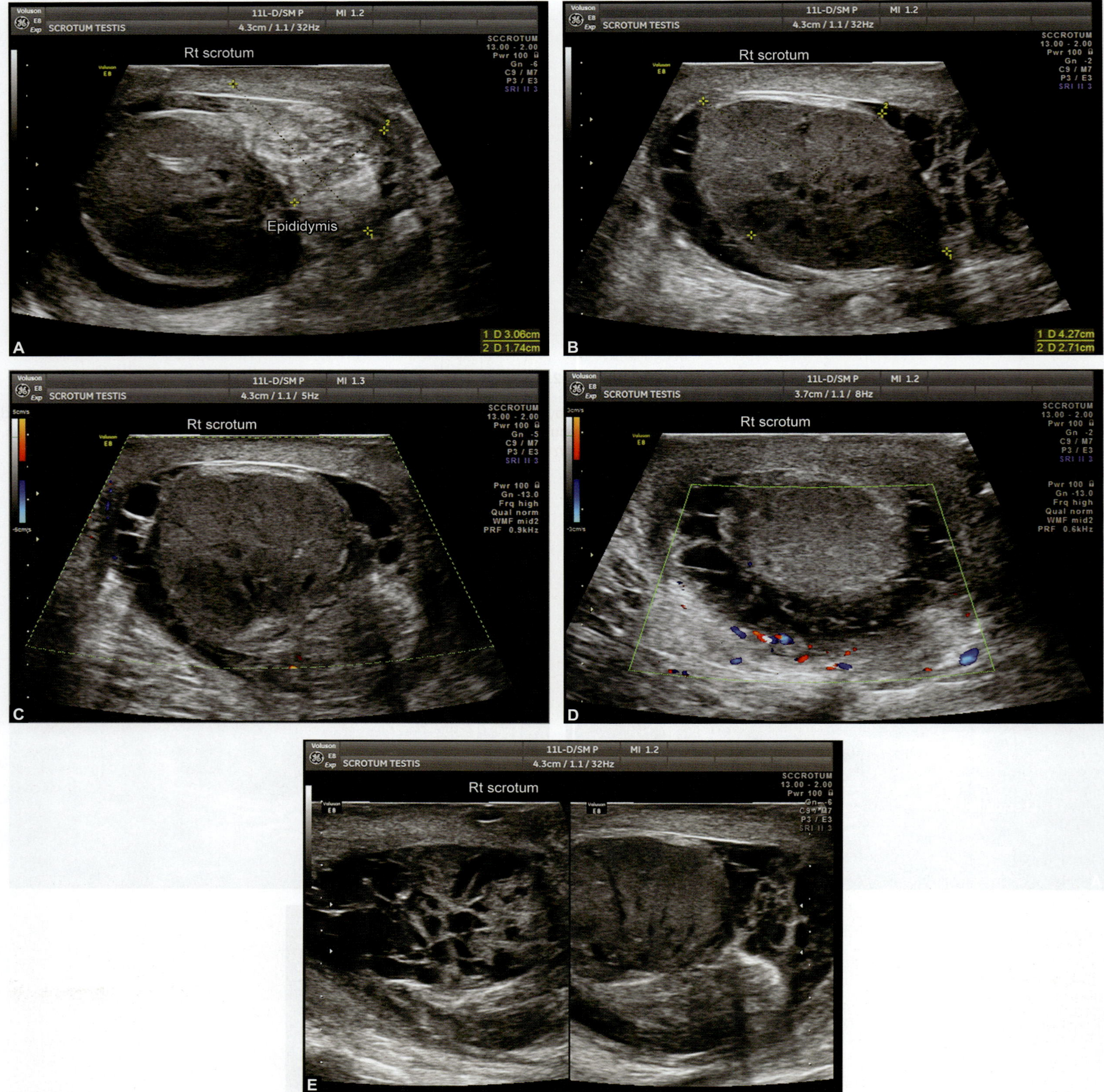

FIGURES 12.50A to E: Acute torsion with hematocele formation. A patient presented with acute pain in scrotum. HRSG shows enlarged and hypoechoic texture of right testes. Parenchyma is heterogeneous. Multiple hypoechoic areas are seen in the testes. Hypoechoic areas appear to be ischemic necrosis. On color flow imaging, no flow is seen in the testes. The epididymis is enlarged, edematous and heterogeneous. Echogenic foci are seen in the epididymis suggestive of hemorrhagic epididymitis. Right scrotal sac shows low level echocardiogram collection. Echogenic bands are seen in the collection suggestive of protein bands because of chronic hematocele. The scrotal wall also shows skin edema.

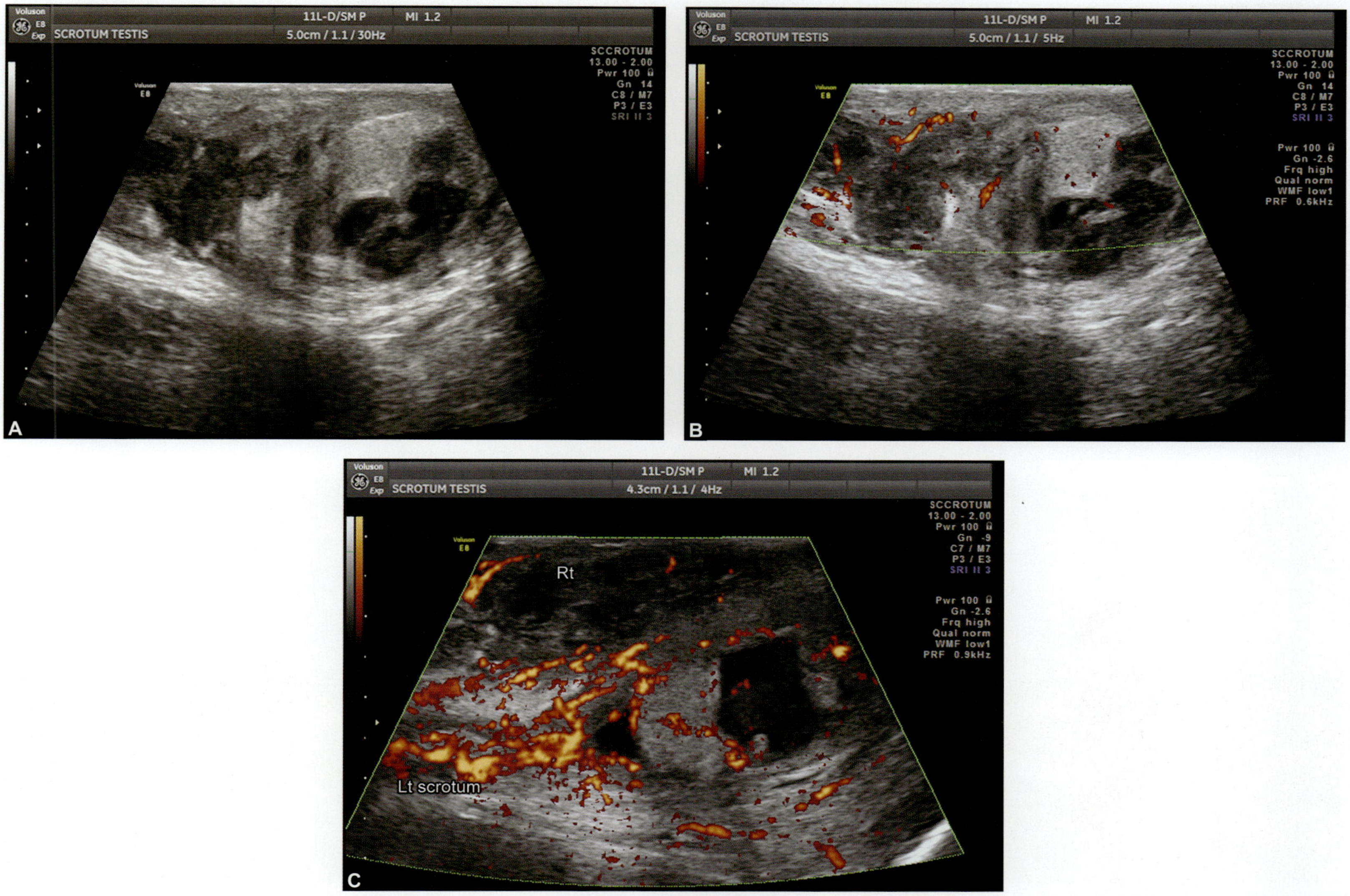

FIGURES 12.51A to C: Chronic torsion with necrosis. A patient presented with hard mass in right scrotum. HRSG shows heterogeneous testes. Normal texture is lost. On color flow imaging no flow is seen in the testes. Area of necrosis is seen in the testes because of chronic torsion and ischemia. The epididymis is enlarged and edematous. Scrotal wall edema is also present. On color flow imaging, increased flow is seen in edematous scrotal wall and epididymis.

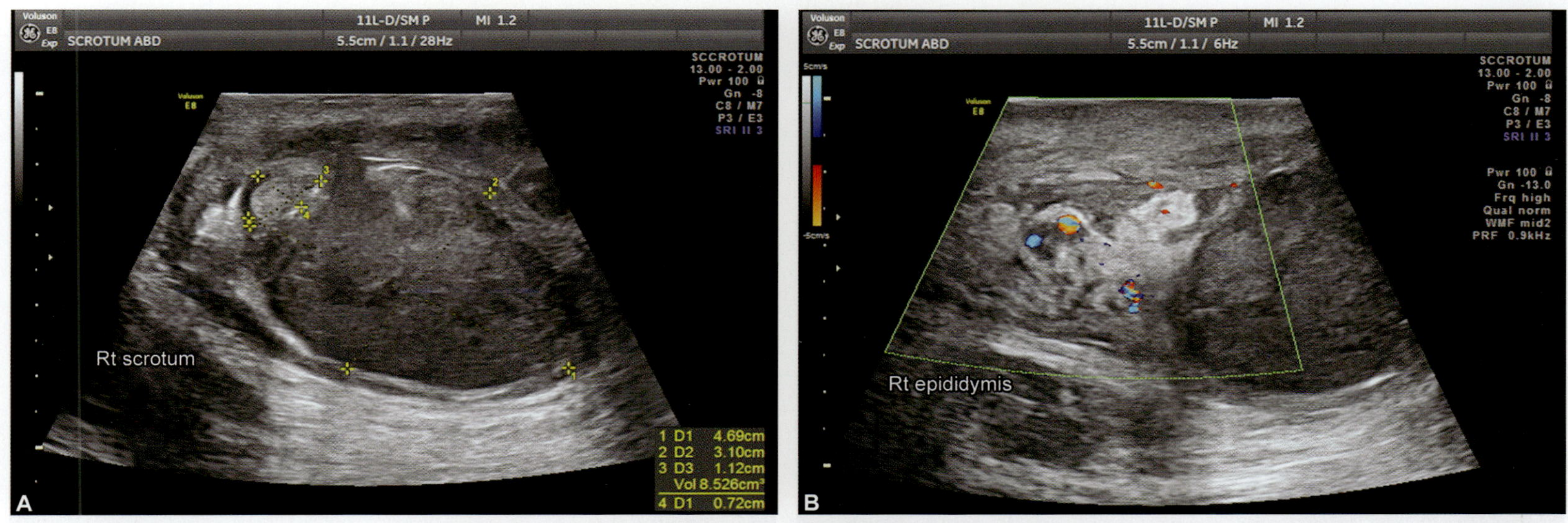

FIGURES 12.52A and B

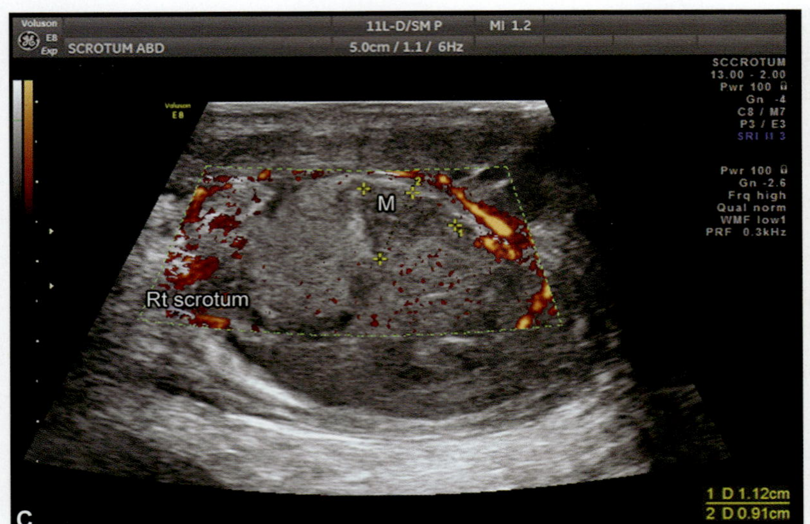

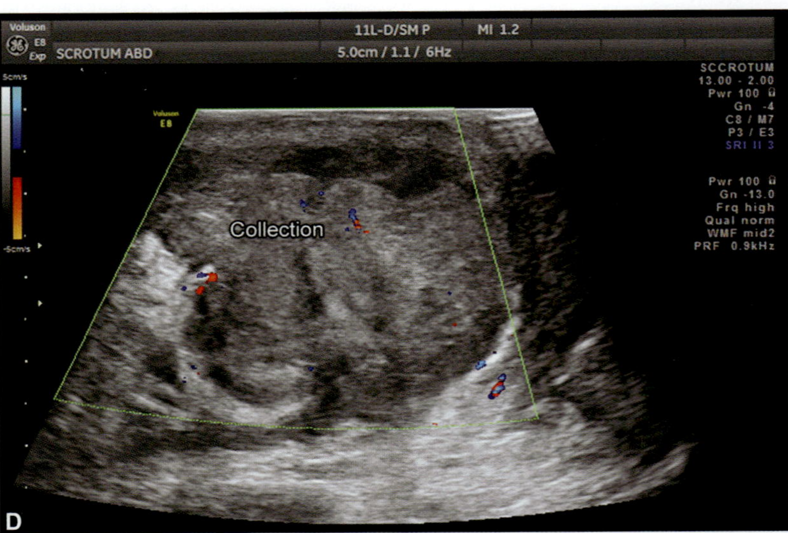

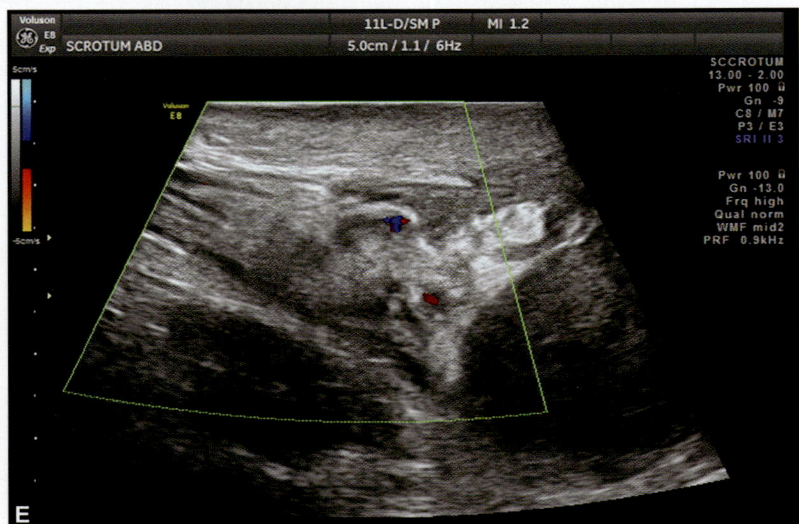

FIGURES 12.52C to E

FIGURES 12.52A to E: Partial torsion of the testes. A 22-year-old man presented with acute painful swelling in the right scrotum. HRSG shows enlarged edematous right testes. It shows inhomogeneous texture. Hypoechoic areas are seen in it. On color flow imaging, increased peripheral flow is seen in the testes. Few vessels are also seen feeding the testicular parenchyma. The epididymis is also edematous and inhomogeneous in texture. Findings are suggestive of partial torsion of testes. Patient underwent emergency surgery and testes was detorsed and salvaged.

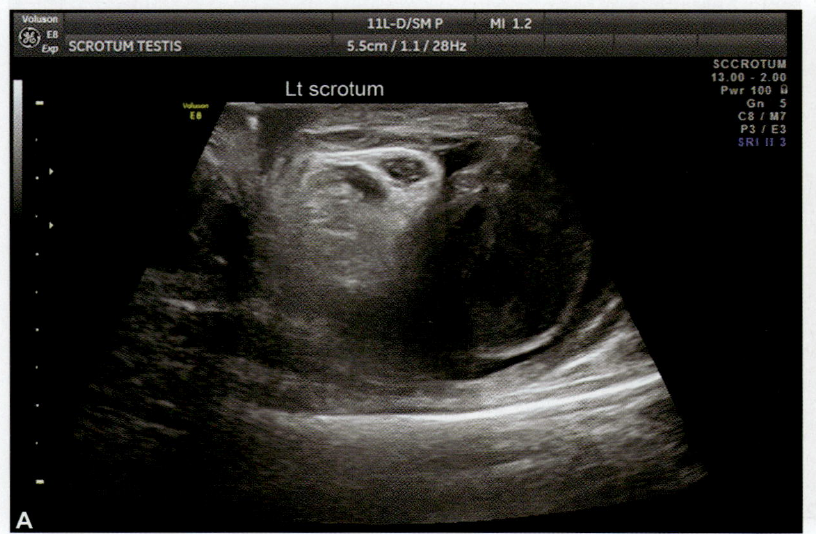

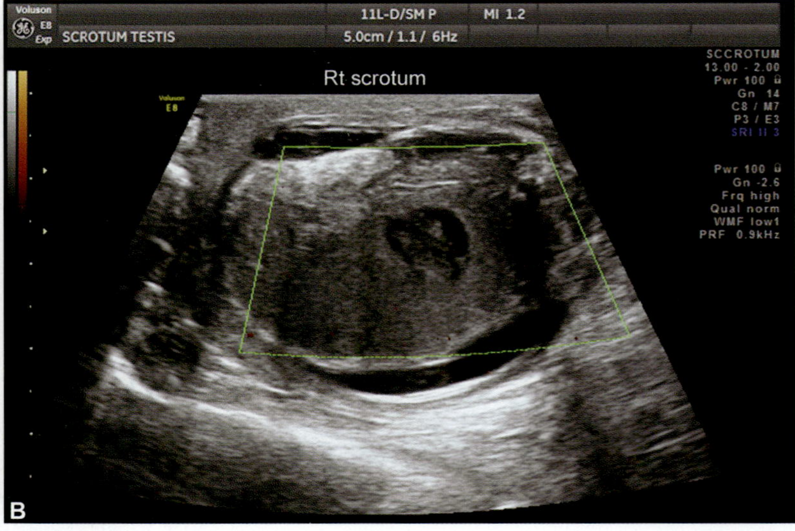

FIGURES 12.53A and B

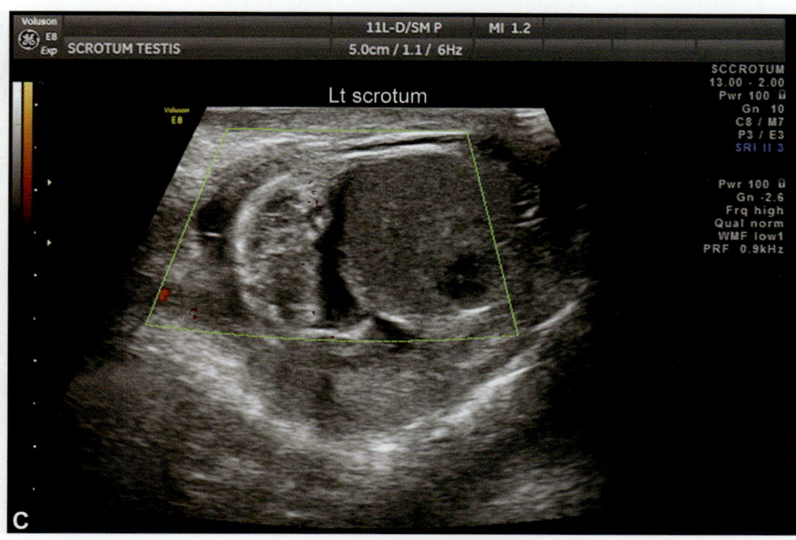

FIGURE 12.53C

FIGURES 12.53A to C: Testicular torsion with necrosis. A patient presented with hard swelling in the left scrotum. HRSG shows enlarged edematous hypoechoic left testes. Echo texture is heterogeneous. On color flow power Doppler imaging, no flow is seen in the testes suggestive of torsion of the testes. Central area of necrosis is also seen in the testes. The epididymis is also enlarged and echogenic. Multiple calcified specks are seen in the epididymis.

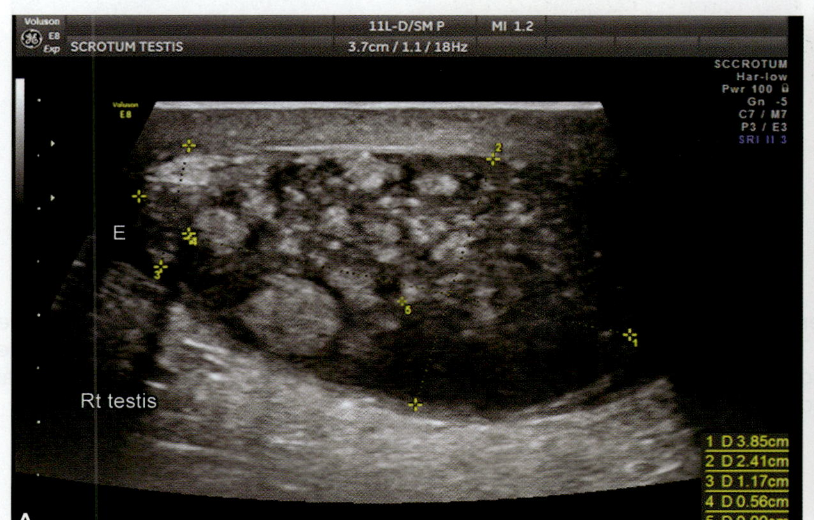

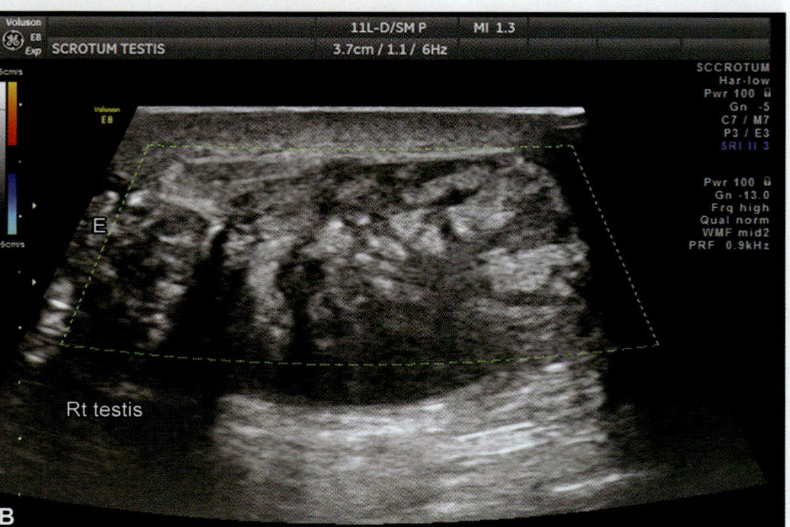

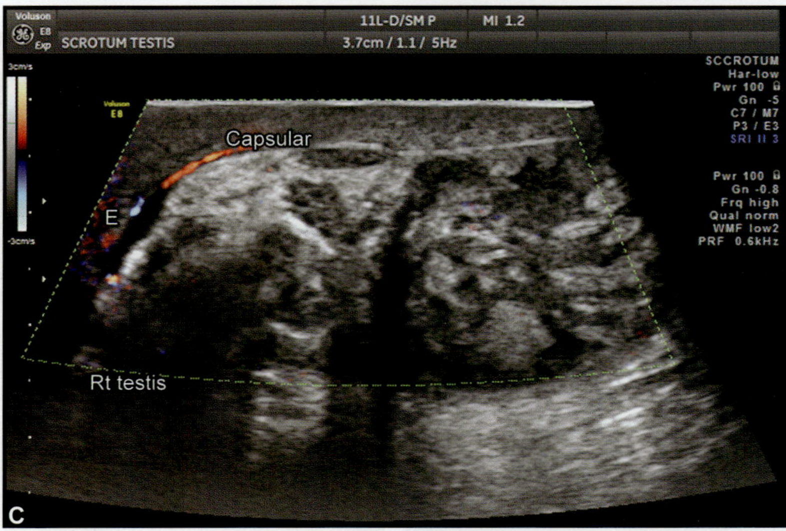

FIGURES 12.54A to C: Chronic torsion of the testes. HRSG shows enlarged and edematous right testes. Echo texture is inhomogeneous. Irregular hypoechoic echogenic foci are seen in the testes. They are discrete in distribution. Normal texture is lost. Epididymis is also enlarged and swollen. It is heterogeneous in texture. Echogenic foci are seen in the epididymis. On color flow imaging no flow is seen in the testes. Findings are suggestive of chronic testicular torsion.

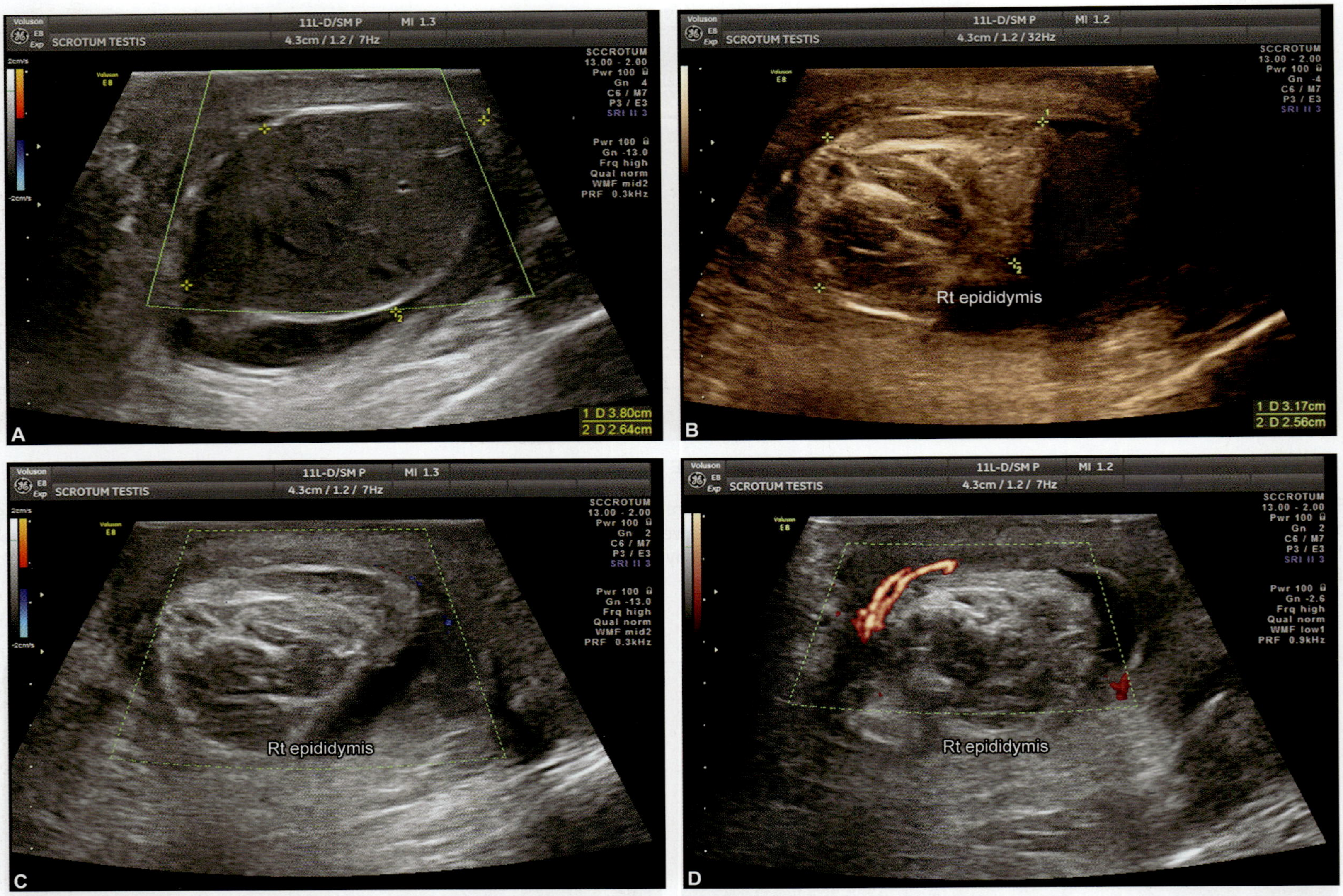

FIGURES 12.55A to D: Chronic torsion. HRSG shows enlarged and edematous right testes. It is inhomogeneous in texture. Hypoechoic areas are seen in the testes. On color flow imaging, no flow is seen in the testes. The right epididymis is also enlarged and edematous. Echogenic foci are seen in the epididymis. On color flow imaging, no flow is seen in the epididymis. The scrotal wall is also edematous. Poor flow is seen in the scrotal wall. A small vessel is seen in the scrotal wall with low flow. Echogenic collection is also seen in right scrotal sac.

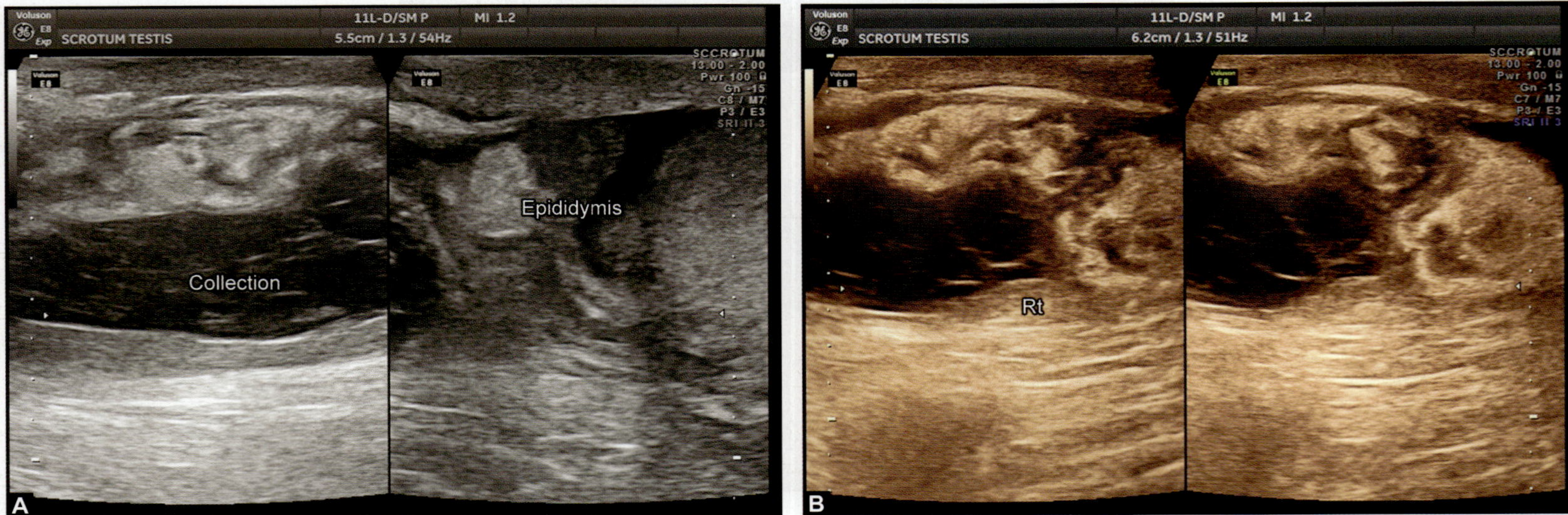

FIGURES 12.56A and B

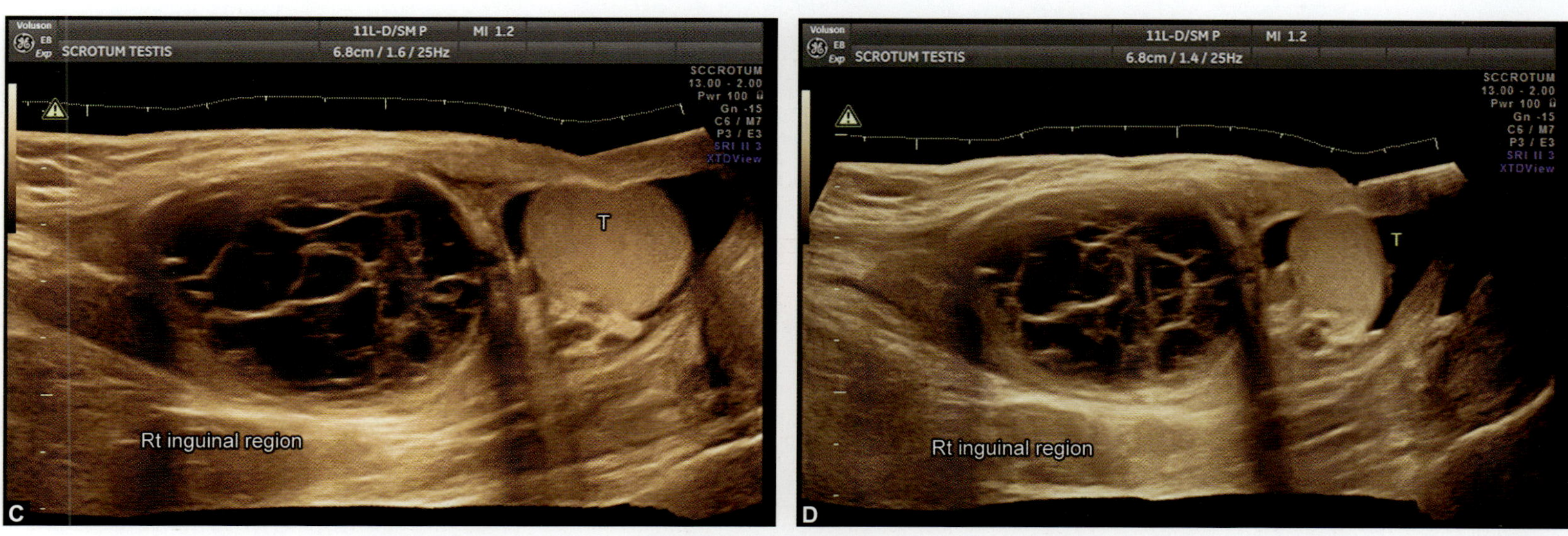

FIGURES 12.56C and D

FIGURES 12.56A to D: Inguinal hematoma. A patient presented with soft tissue swelling in the inguinal region after sustaining trauma. HRSG shows markedly edematous right cord. Hypoechoic areas are seen in the cord. Thick echogenic collection is seen in the cord with multiple echogenic bands suggestive of cord hematoma. However, the epididymis and the testes are normal.

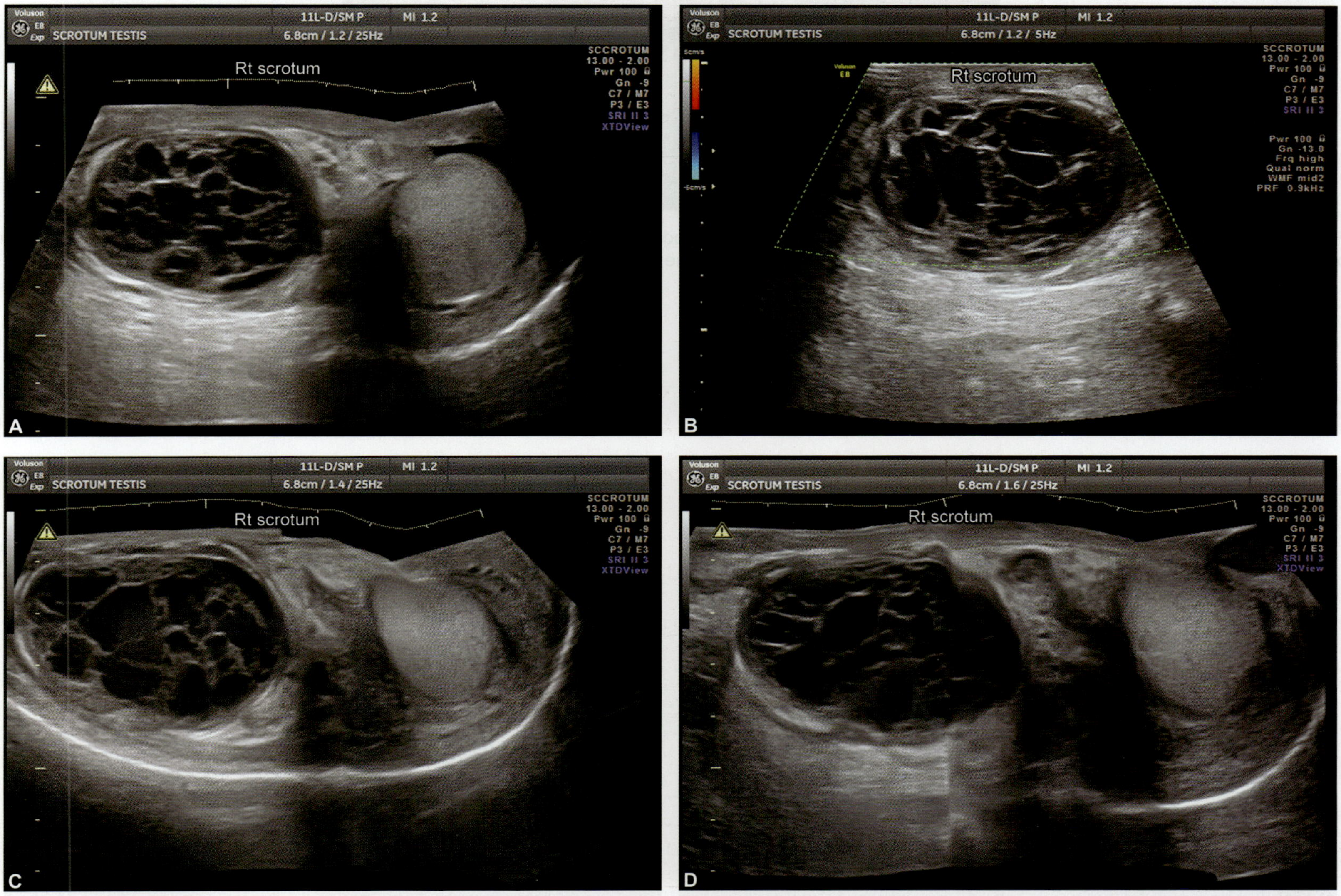

FIGURES 12.57A to D: Cord hematocele formation. A patient presented with painful swelling in right inguinal region. HRSG shows edematous right cord. A loculated pocket of collection is seen in it. Echogenic bands are also seen in the pocket. On color flow imaging, no flow is seen in it. However, the testes and epididymis are normal. Findings are suggestive of posttraumatic cord hematoma with hematocele formation.

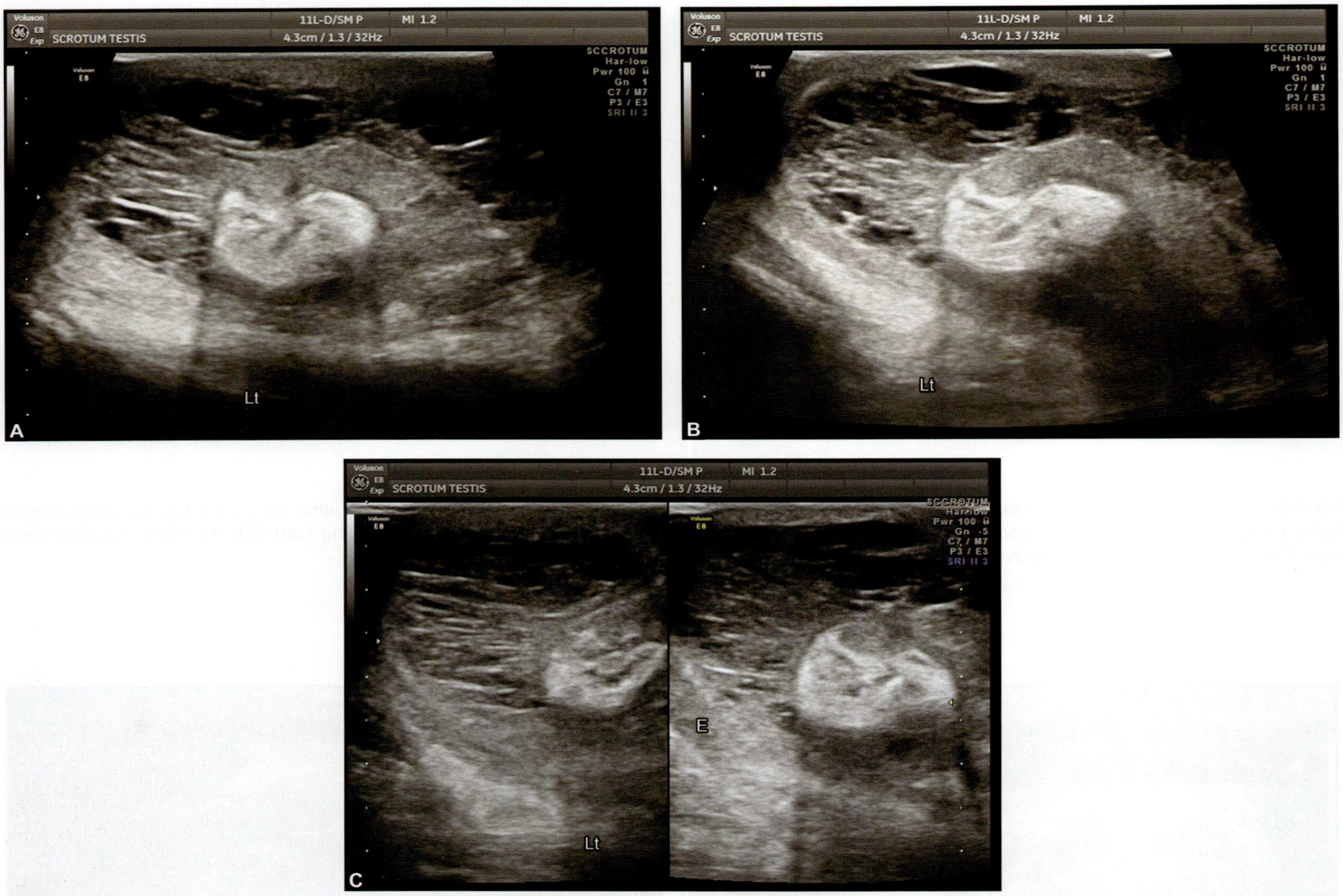

FIGURES 12.58A to C: Fresh cord hematoma. HRSG shows markedly edematous left cord. Echogenic foci are seen in the cord suggestive of fresh blood. There is also evidence of low level echo collection seen around the cord with echogenic bands suggestive of hematocele formation.

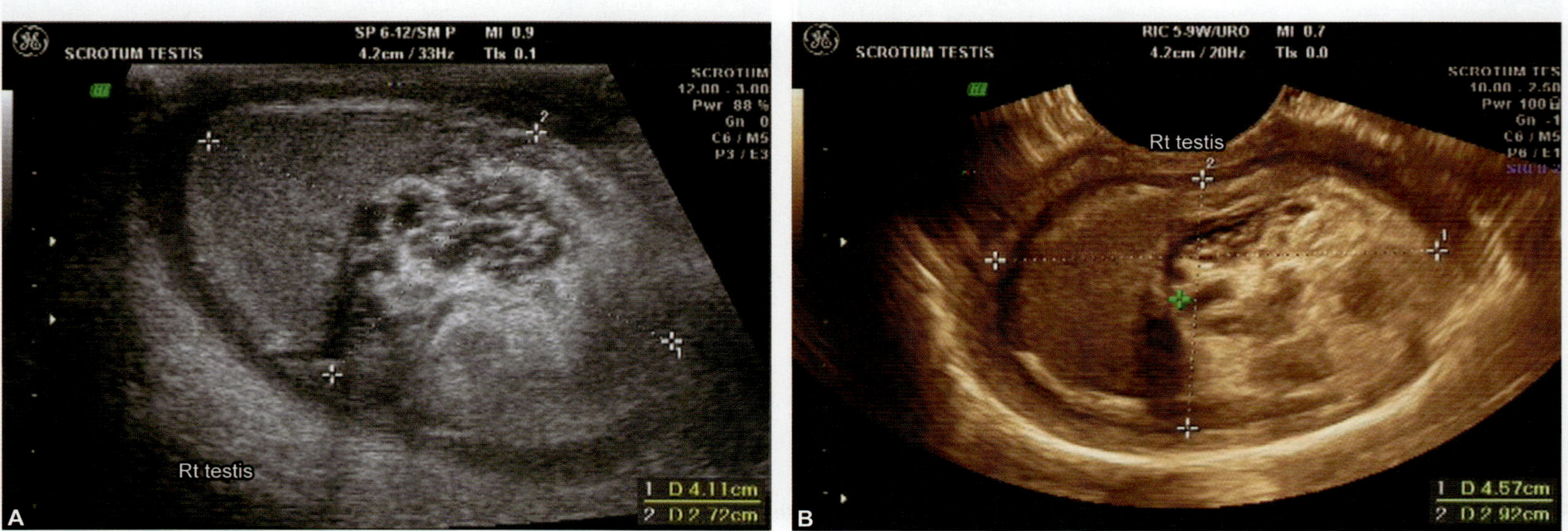

FIGURES 12.59A and B

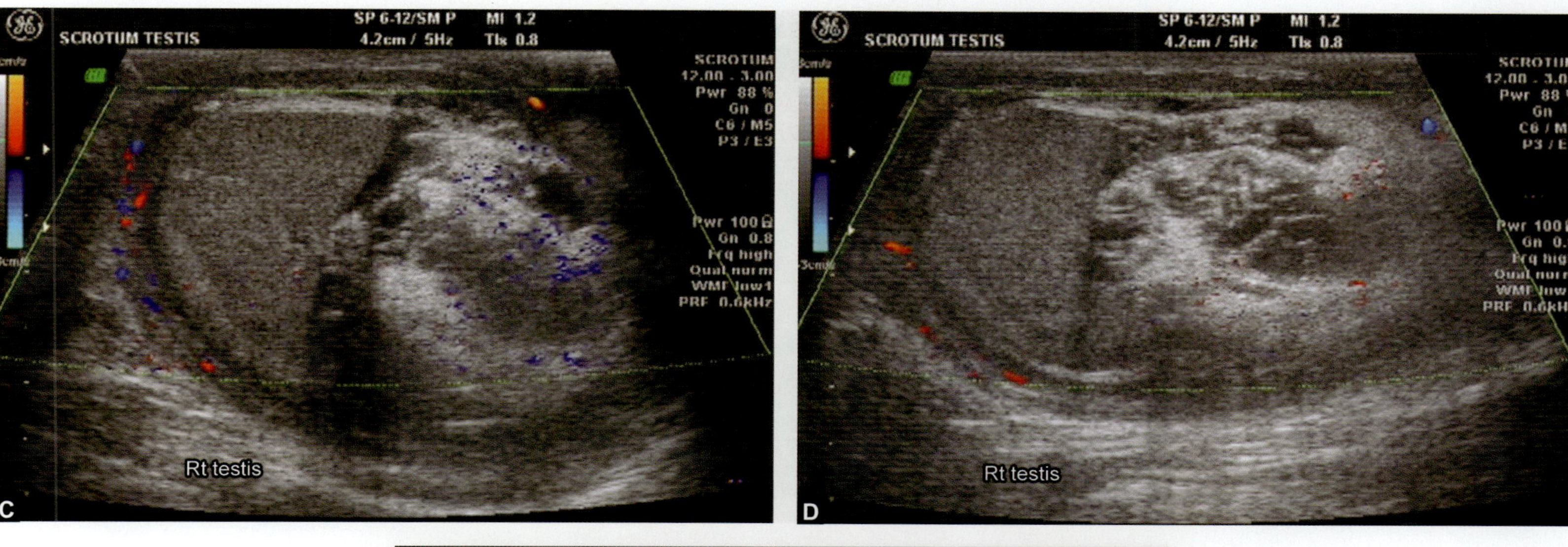

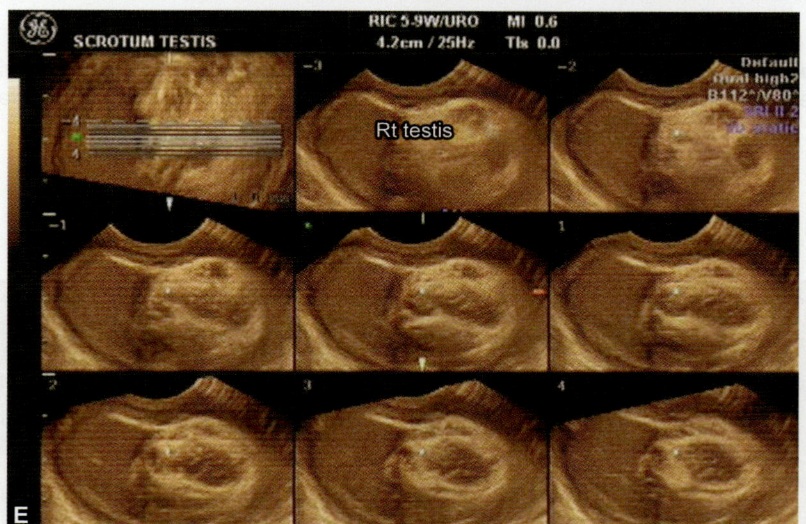

FIGURES 12.59C to E

FIGURES 12.59A to E: Fracture of testes. A patient presented with acute pain in right scrotum after sustaining trauma. HRSG shows markedly edematous right testes. It is inhomogeneous in texture. A hypoechoic vertical cleft is seen in the testes, which is running in its entire length. Half of the testes shows normal granular echoes. But other half of testes shows heterogeneous texture with echogenic foci suggestive of fractured testes with haematoma formation. 3D ultrasound and TUI imaging clearly shows the fracture line. On color flow imaging, no flow is seen in the testes.

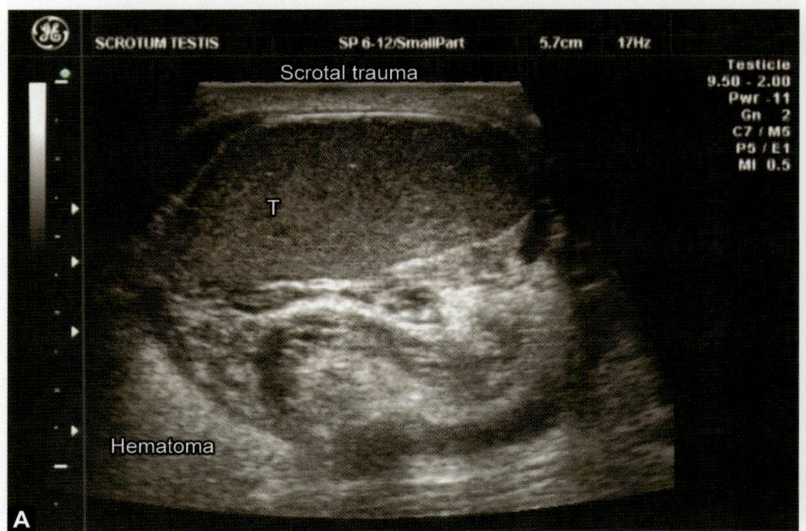

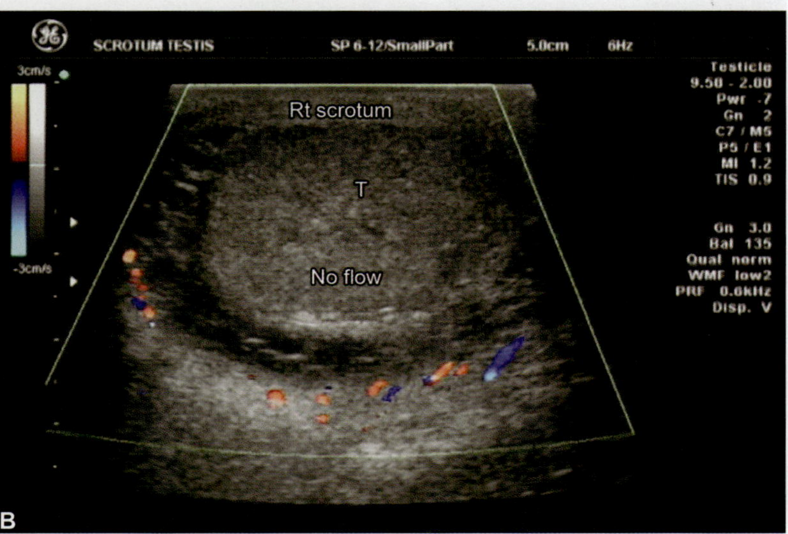

FIGURES 12.60A and B

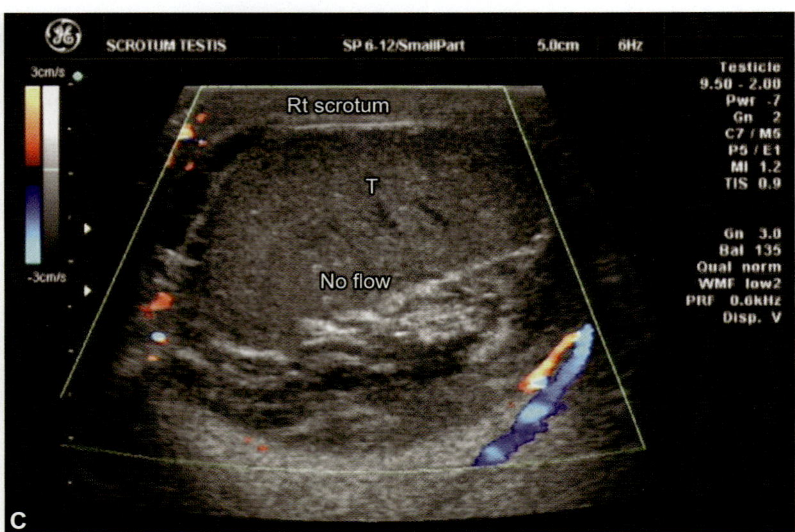

FIGURE 12.60C

FIGURES 12.60A to C: Testicular trauma with hematoma formation. A patient presented with trauma to the right scrotum. HRSG shows edematous hypoechoic right testes. A big echogenic pocket of collection is seen in the scrotum suggestive of hematocele formation. On color flow imaging, no flow is seen in the testes.

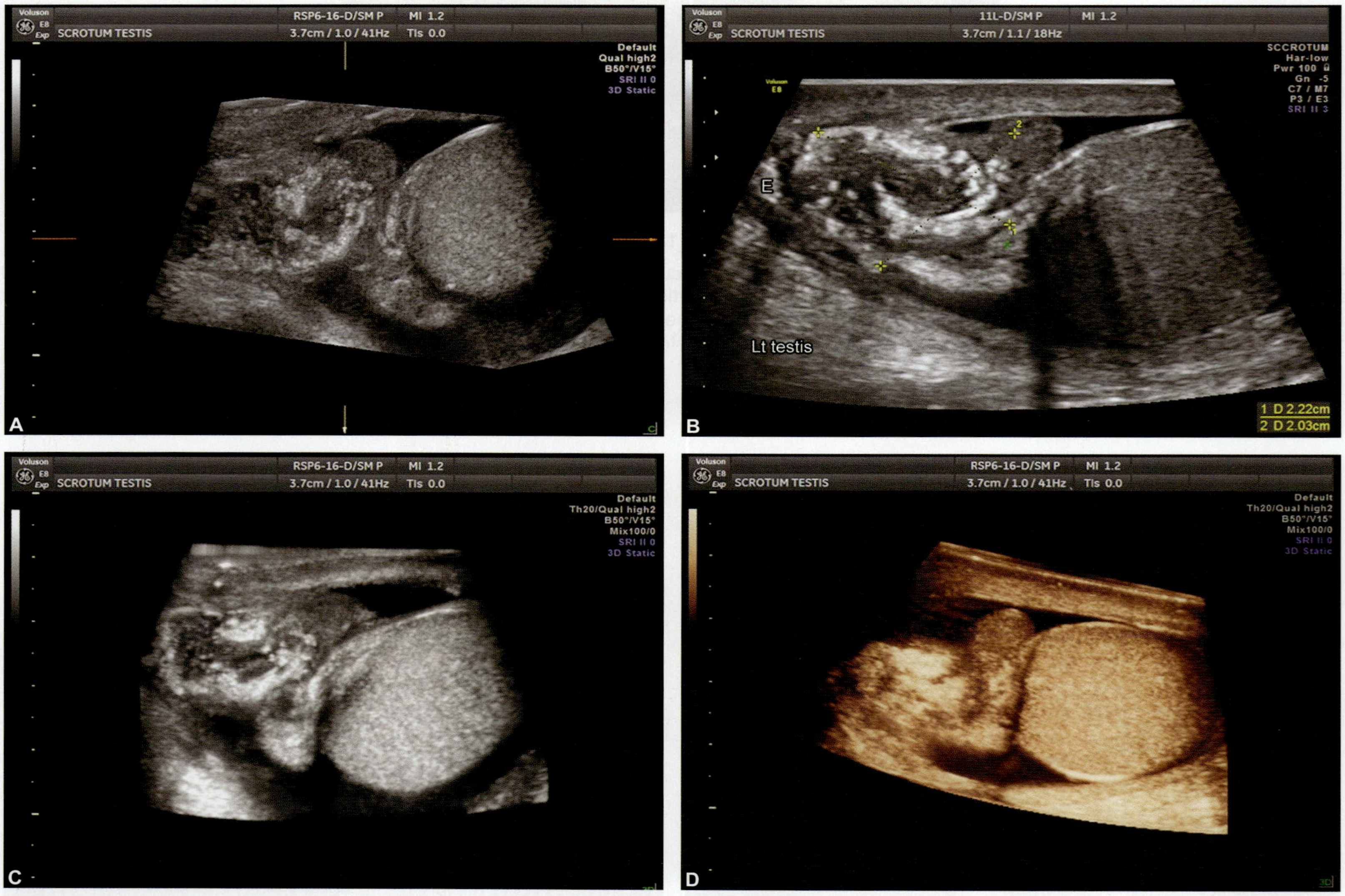

FIGURES 12.61A to D: Traumatic hemorrhagic epididymitis. A patient sustained trauma to the scrotum and perineum. HRSG shows markedly edematous and heterogeneous left epididymis. Multiple echogenic foci are seen in the epididymis suggestive of hemorrhagic epididymitis. On 3D imaging, it is seen clearly. However, the testes is normal.

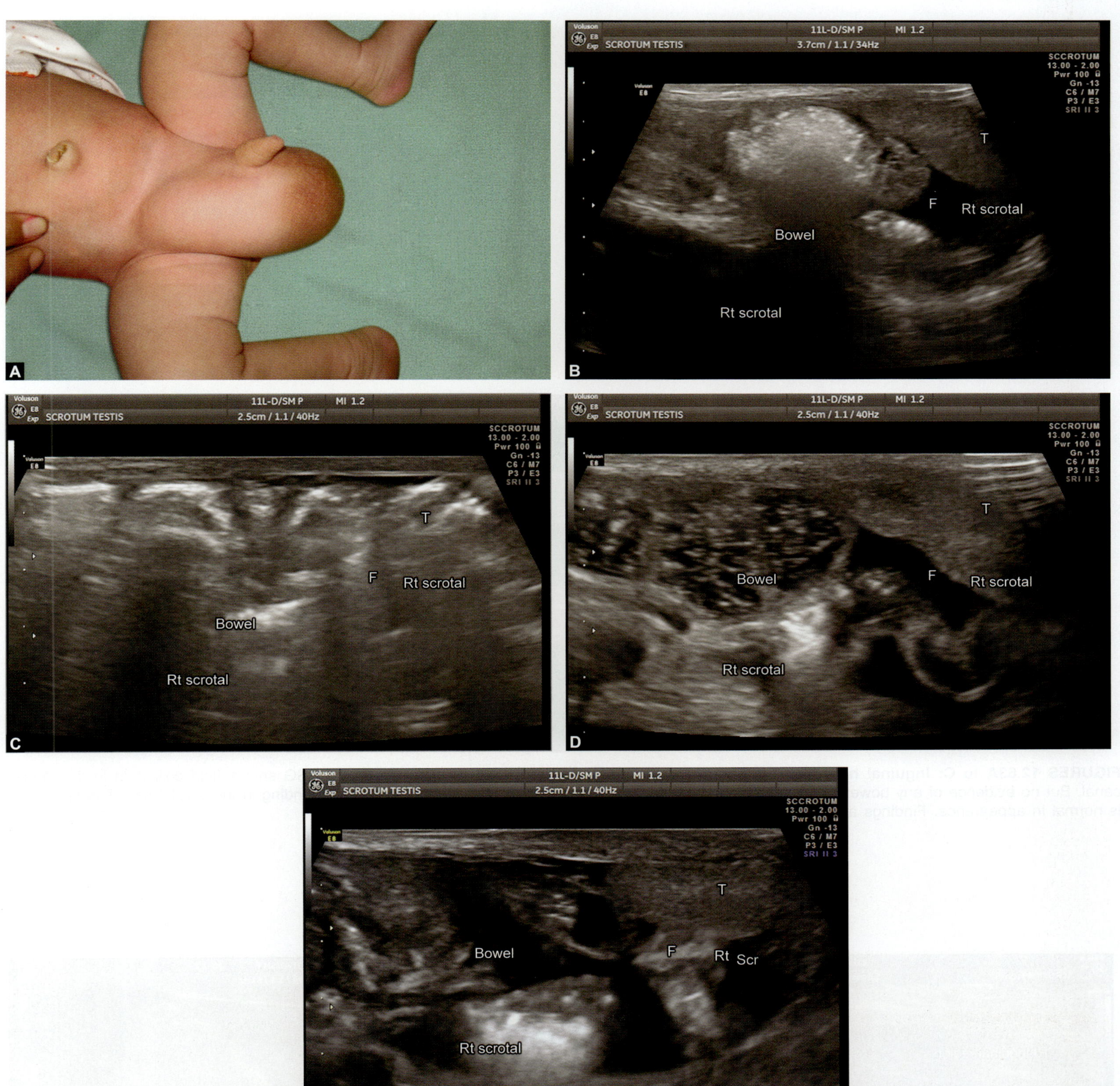

FIGURES 12.62A to E: Inguinoscrotal hernia. A newborn baby presented with big welling in the right inguinoscrotal region. HRSG shows right sided inguinoscrotal hernia. A bowel loop is seen herniating in the inguinal canal. It is also seen going in the right scrotal sac. Fluid movement is seen in the bowel loops. Small amount of fluid is also seen in the right scrotum suggestive of inguinoscrotal hernia.

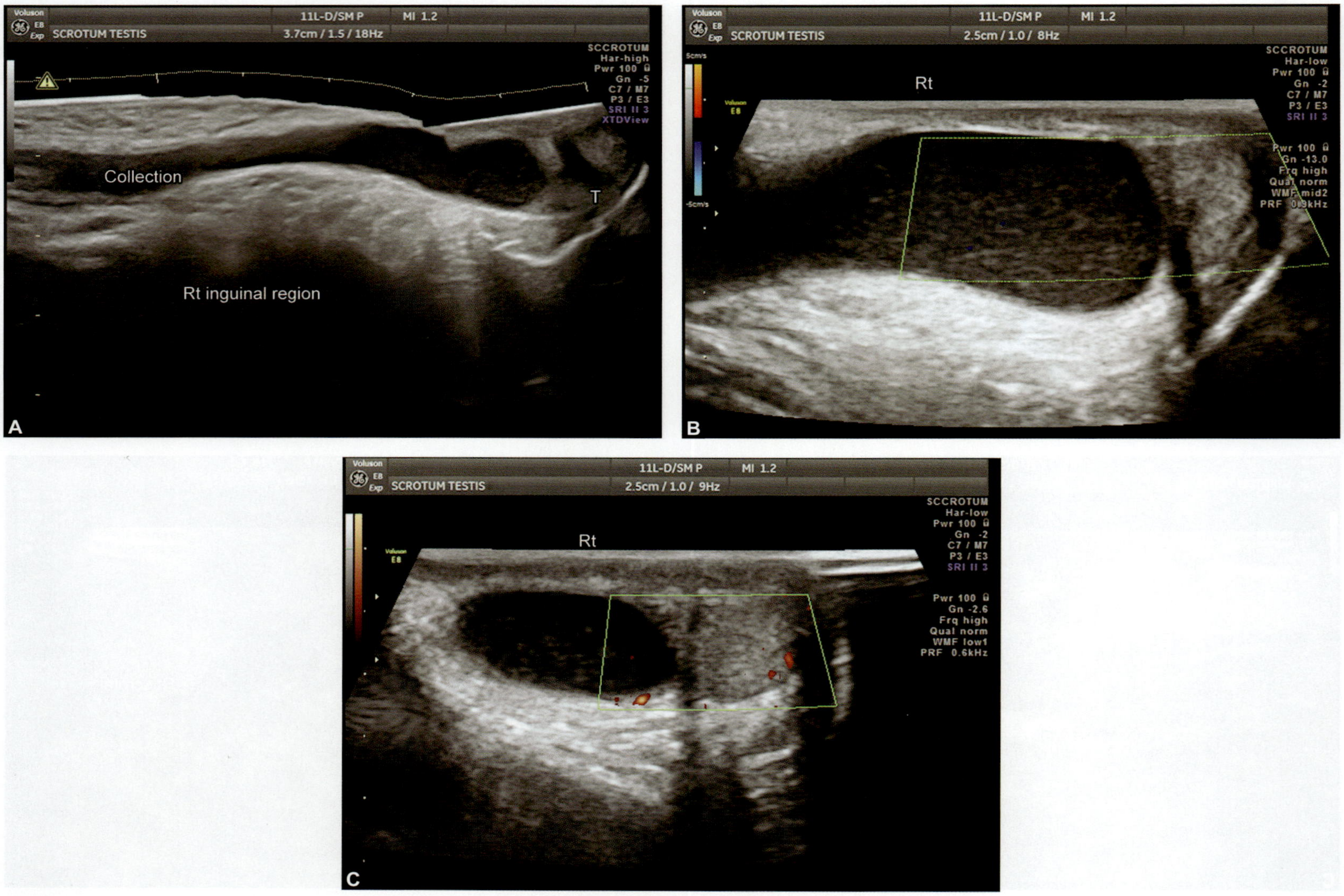

FIGURES 12.63A to C: Inguinal hydrocele. A 2-year-old child presented with right inguinal swelling. HRSG shows fluid collection in the inguinal canal. But no evidence of any bowel loop herniation is seen in the inguinal region. The fluid is not seen extending in the scrotal sac. The right testes is normal in appearance. Findings are suggestive of inguinal hydrocele.

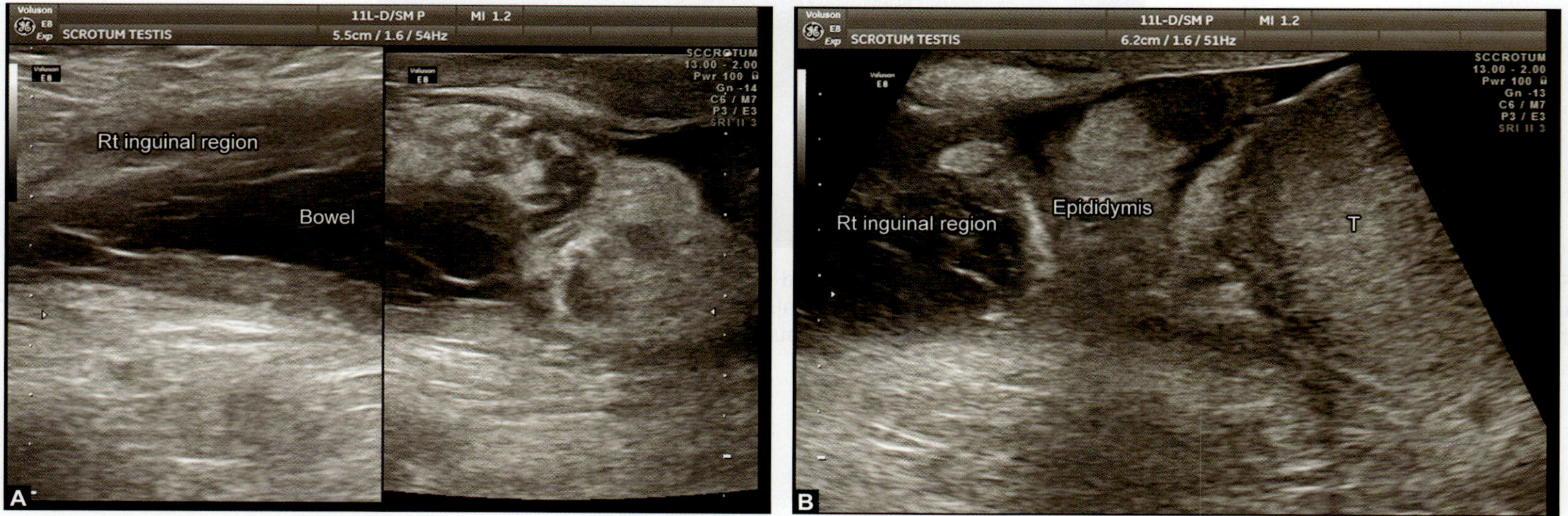

FIGURES 12.64A and B

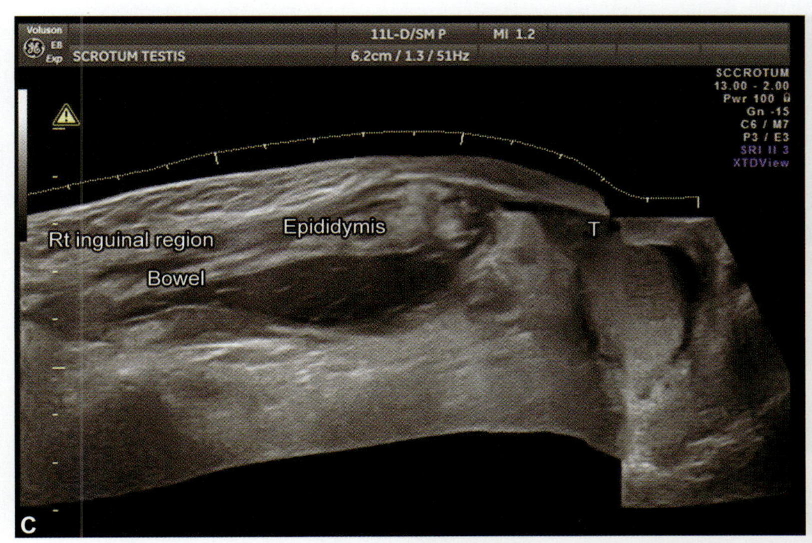

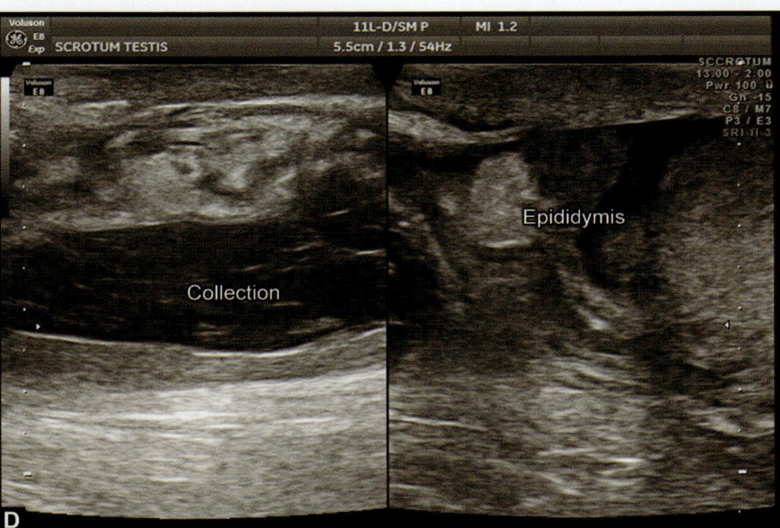

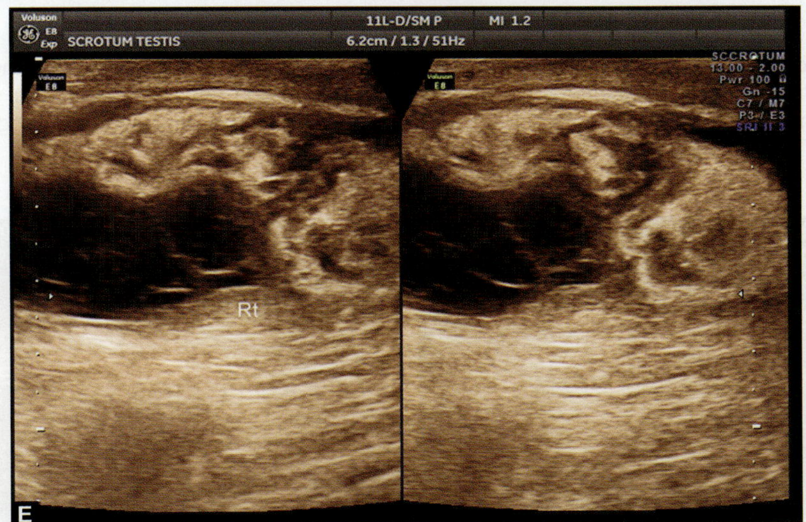

FIGURES 12.64C to E

FIGURES 12.64A to E: Inguinal hernia. A patient presented with soft tissue swelling in the right inguinal region. HRSG shows fluid collection in the right inguinal canal. A bowel loop is seen herniating into it. However, it is not seen going into the scrotal sac suggestive of inguinal hernia. The right testes and epididymis are normal. The extended field of view shows the entire length of hernia.

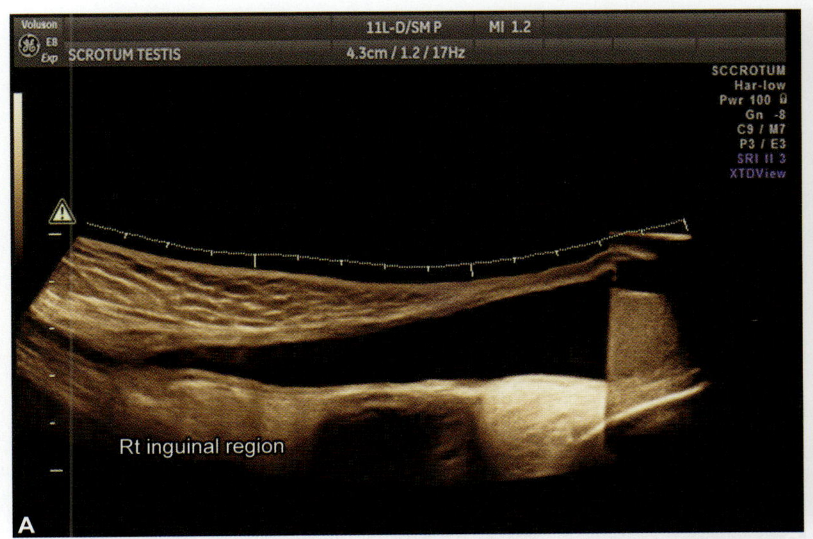

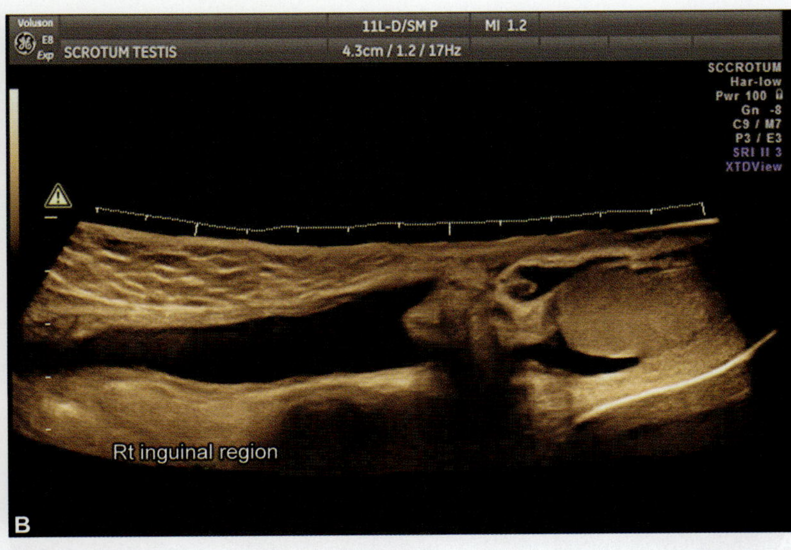

FIGURES 12.65A and B

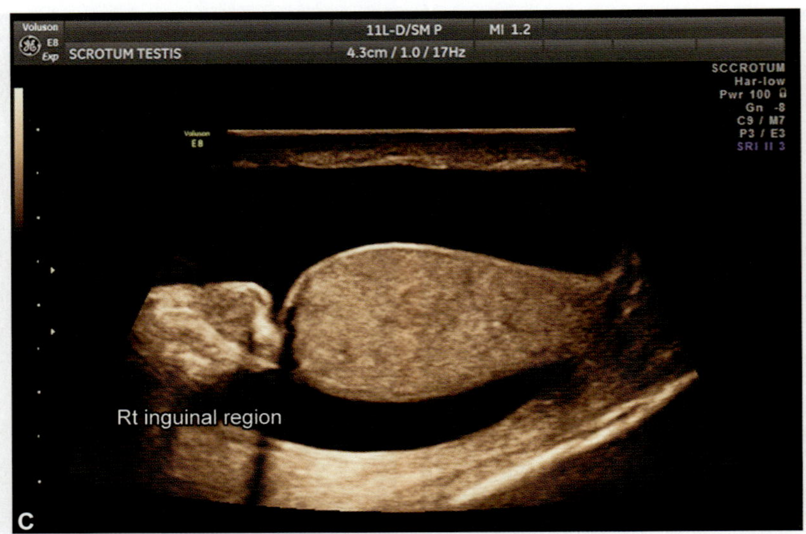

FIGURE 12.65C

FIGURES 12.65A to C: Right inguinoscrotal hernia. A patient presented with right side inguinoscrotal swelling. HRSG shows fluid collection in the inguinal canal. A bowel loop is seen herniating in the inguinal canal. It is also seen going into the scrotal sac. Fluid movement is seen in the bowel loop. However, the right testes is normal. Moderate amount of fluid collection is seen in the right scrotum suggestive of inguinoscrotal hernia.

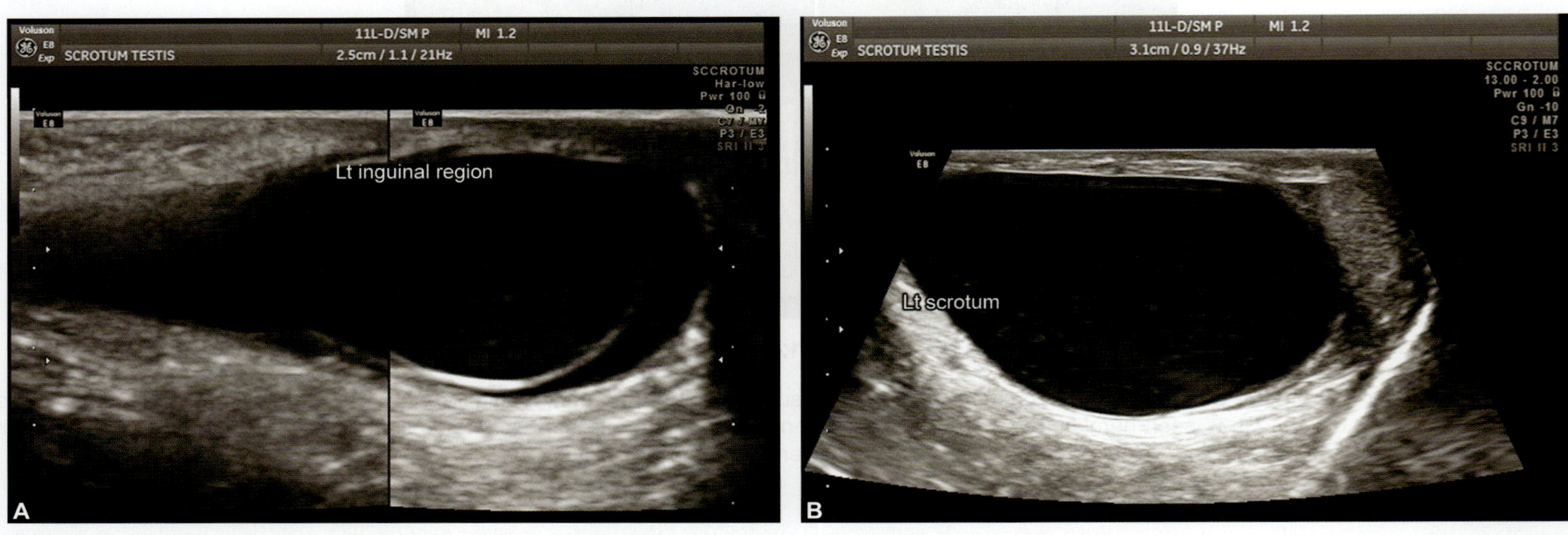

FIGURES 12.66A and B: Inguinal hydrocele. A 4-year-child presented with left inguinal swelling. HRSG shows a pocket of collection in the left inguinal canal. However, no bowel loop herniation is seen in it. No septation is seen.

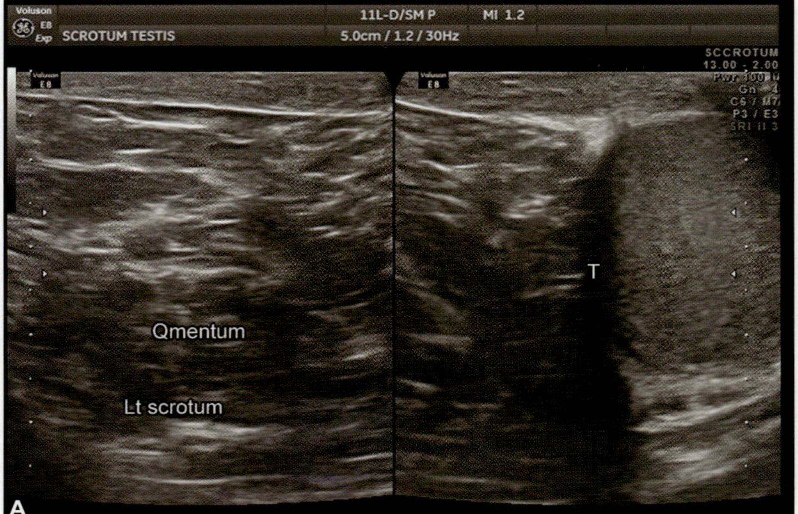

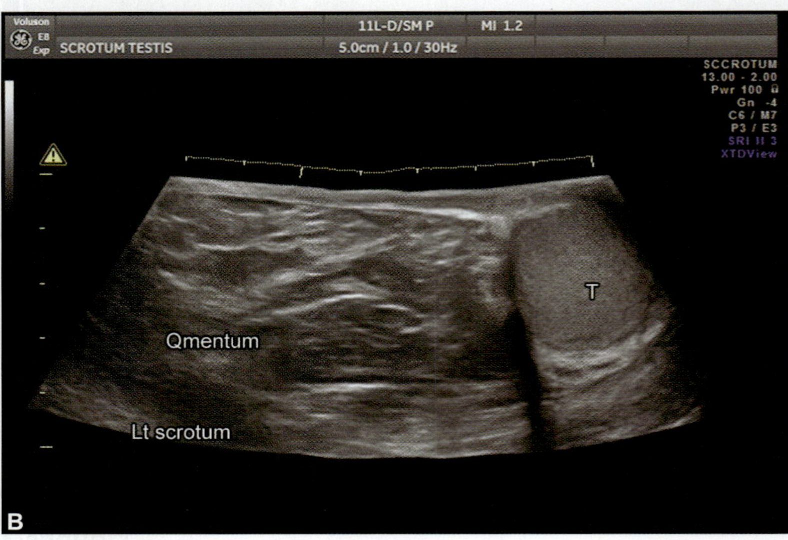

FIGURES 12.67A and B

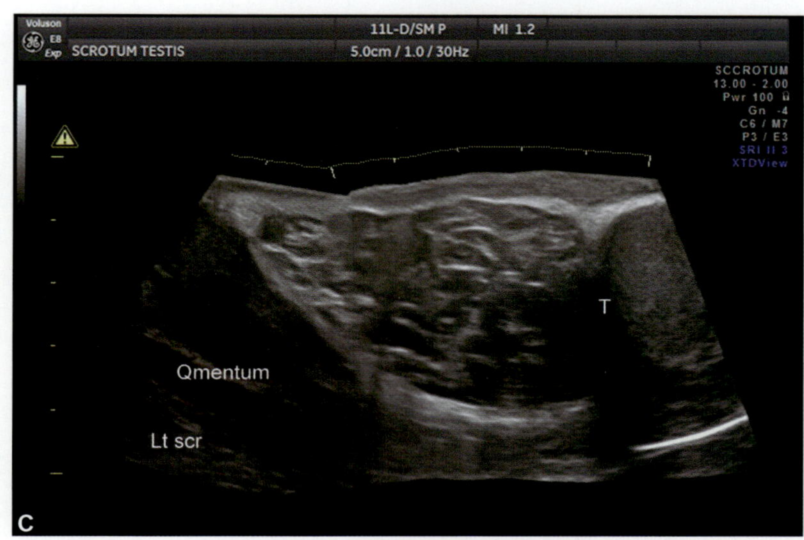

FIGURE 12.67C

FIGURES 12.67A to C: Omental hernia. A patient presented with soft tissue swelling in the left inguinoscrotal region. HRSG shows a membranous shadow seen herniating in the left inguinal region suggestive of omentum. No bowel loop is seen herniating with omentum. No evidence of omental hernia seen in the right scrotal sac. 3D imaging clearly shows huge omental hernia.

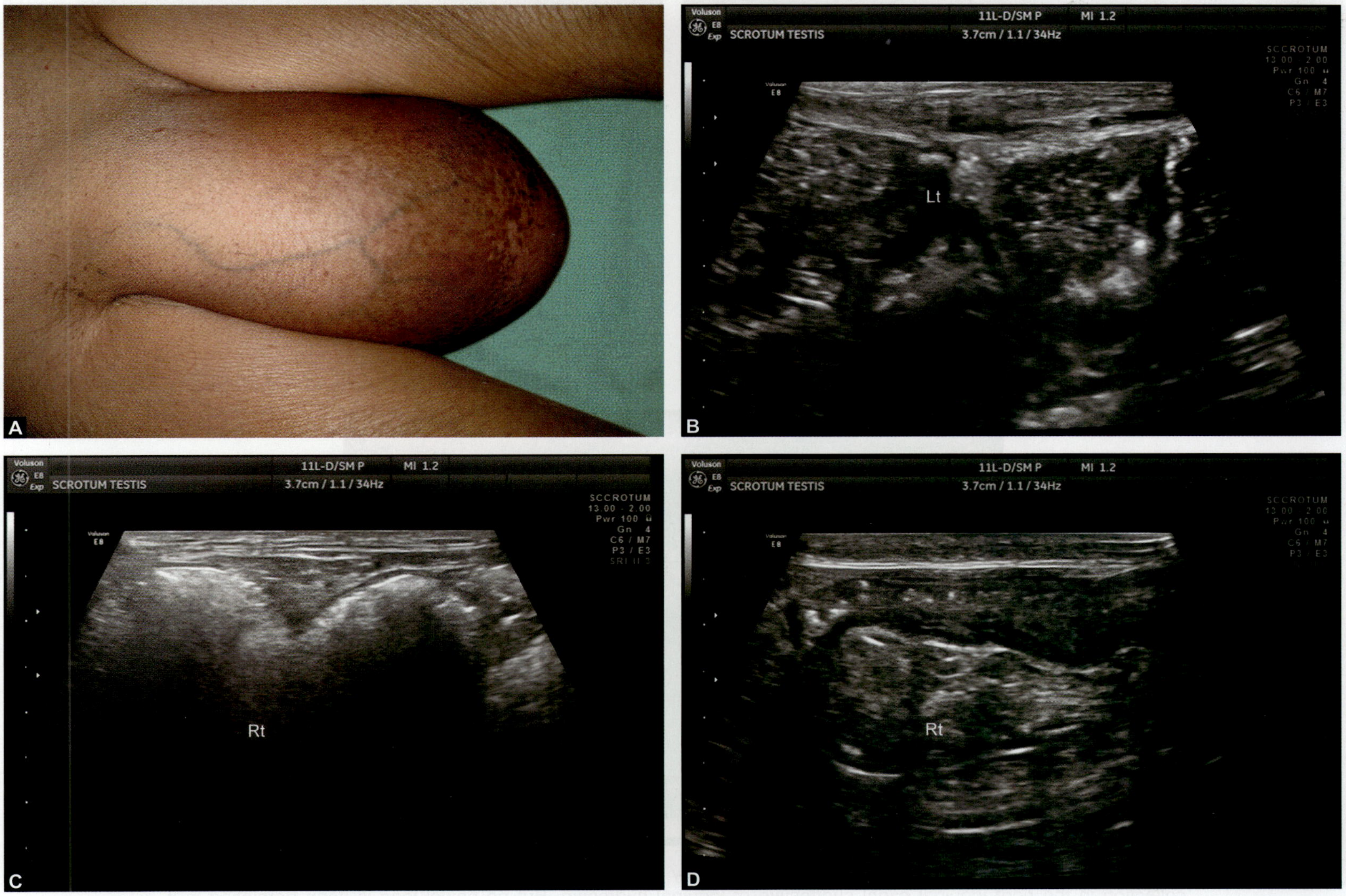

FIGURES 12.68A to D

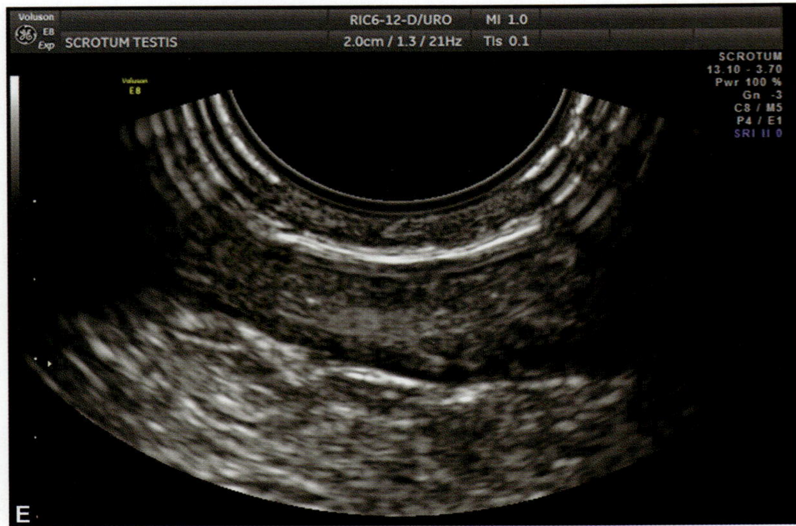

FIGURE 12.68E

FIGURES 12.68A to E: Huge right side inguinal hernia. A patient presented with huge inguinoscrotal swelling. The penis is seen buried in the swelling. HRSG shows bowel loop herniating in the inguinoscrotal region, which is seen herniating in the scrotal sac. Omentum is also seen herniating with the bowel loop. However, the both testes appear to be normal. No focal mass is seen in the testes.

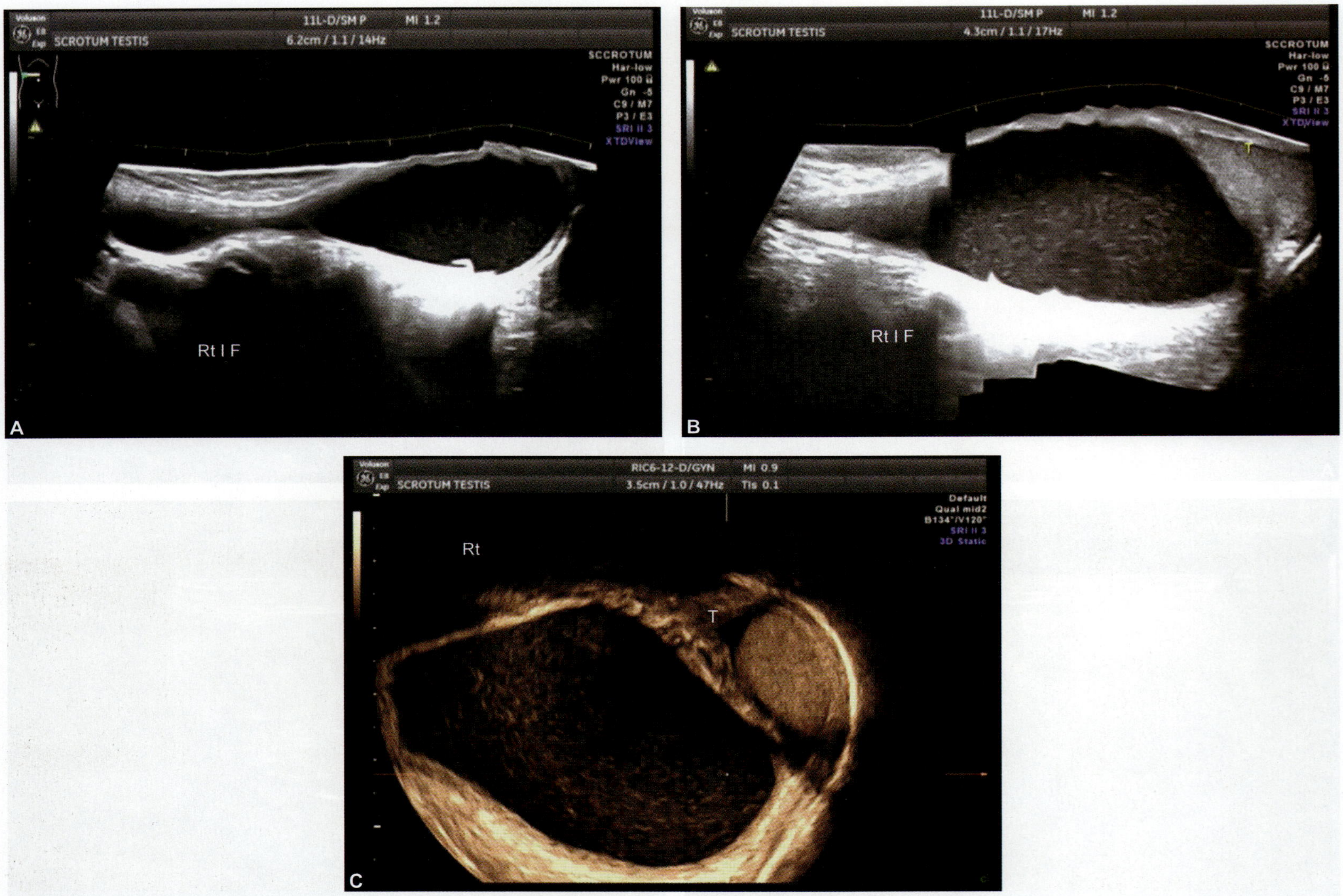

FIGURES 12.69A to C: Big right inguinal collection. A nine years boy presented with big right inguinal swelling. HRSG shows a big pocket of collection in the right inguinal canal suggestive of inguinal hydrocele. But no bowel loop is seen herniating in it.

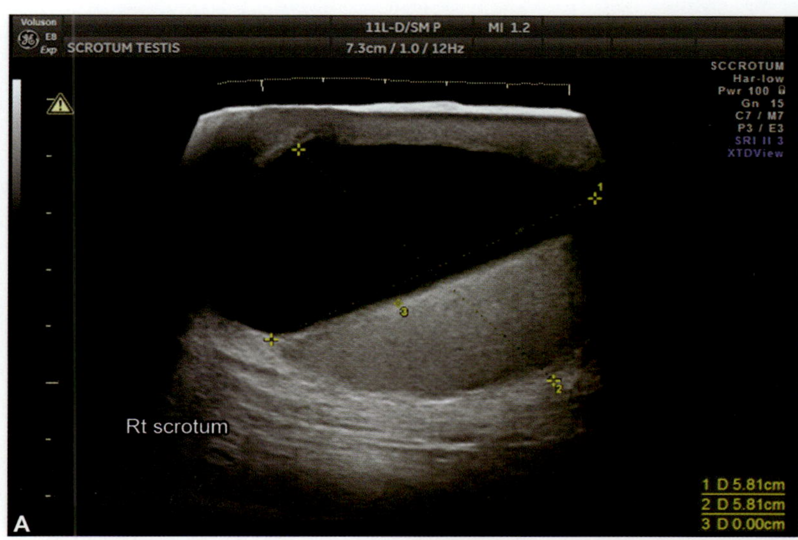

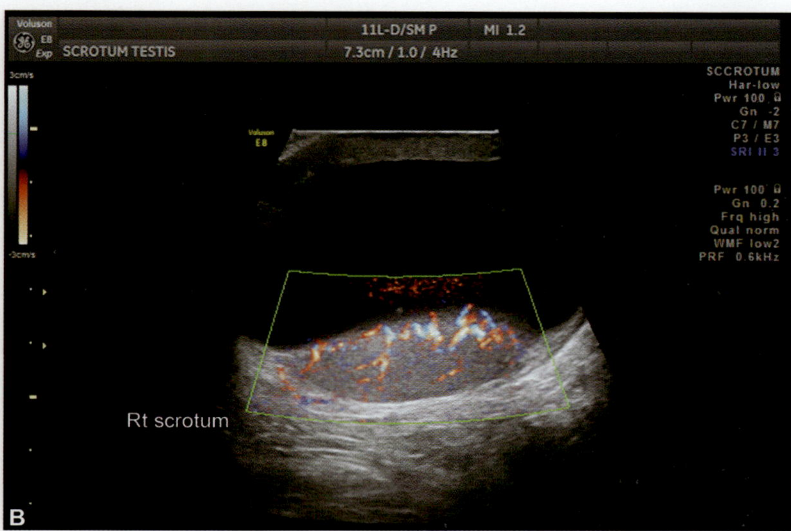

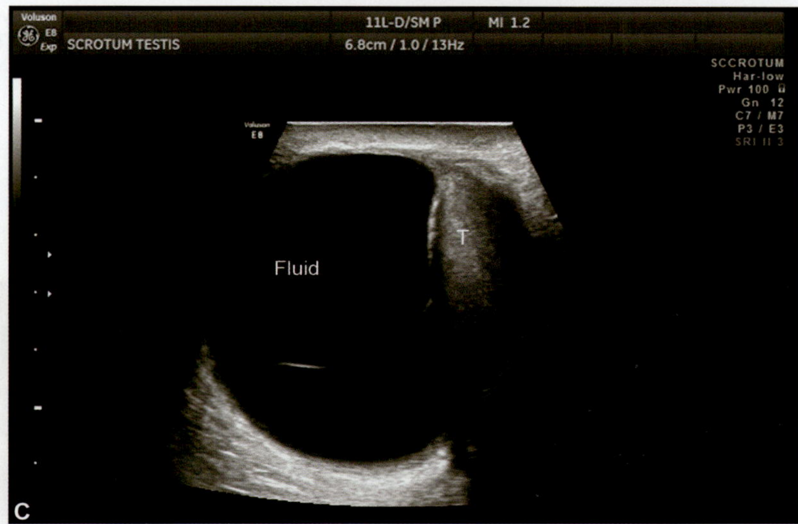

FIGURES 12.70A to C: Right extratesticular fluid collection. A patient presented with big right scrotal swelling. HRSG shows a big pocket of fluid collection in the extratesticular space. The fluid is seen compressing the testes. However, the testes appears to be normal. No evidence of any focal mass is seen in the testes.

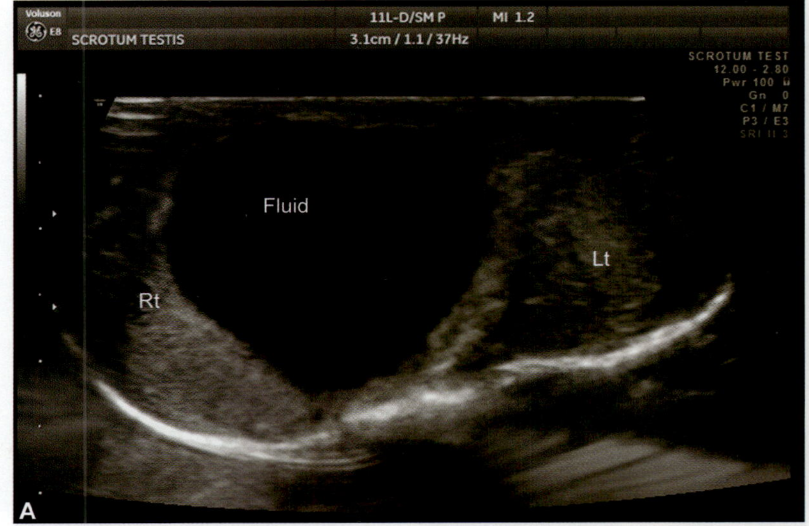

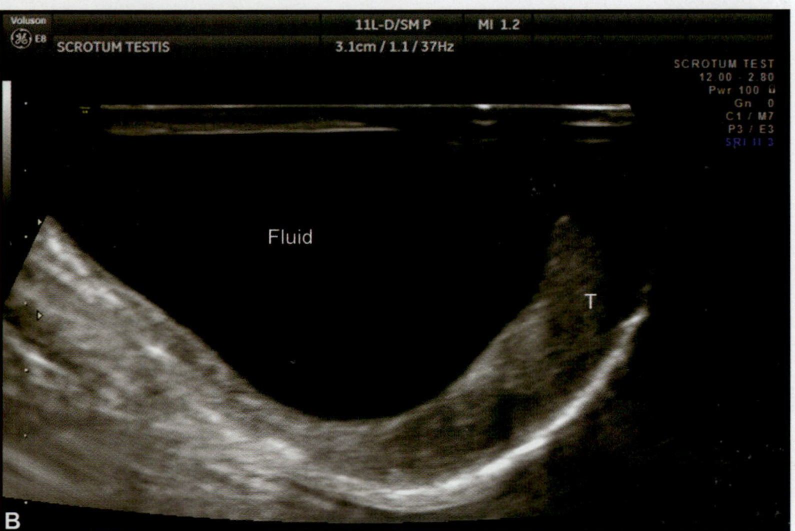

FIGURES 12.71A and B: Huge hydrocele. A patient presented with big swelling in the right scrotum. HRS shows a big pocket of extra testicular collection in the right scrotal sac. It is seen displacing and pressing the testes.

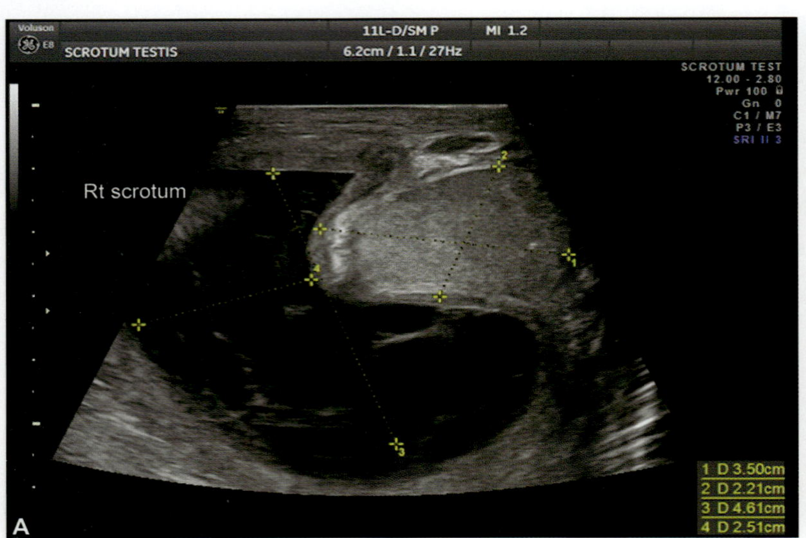

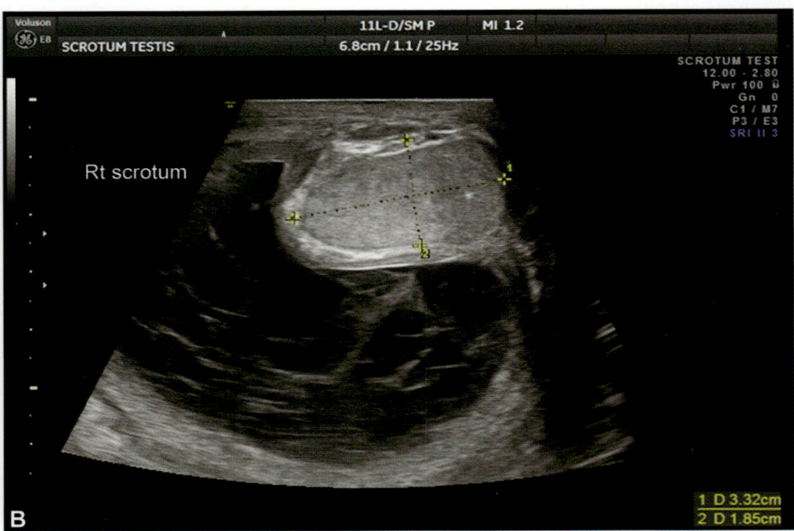

FIGURES 12.72A and B: Chronic extratesticular collection. A patient presented with large right scrotal swelling. HRSG shows a big pocket of collection in the right scrotal sac. Multiple thin echogenic bands are seen in the collection forming loculations. The testes is seen displaced. However, it is normal in appearance suggestive of chronic collection.

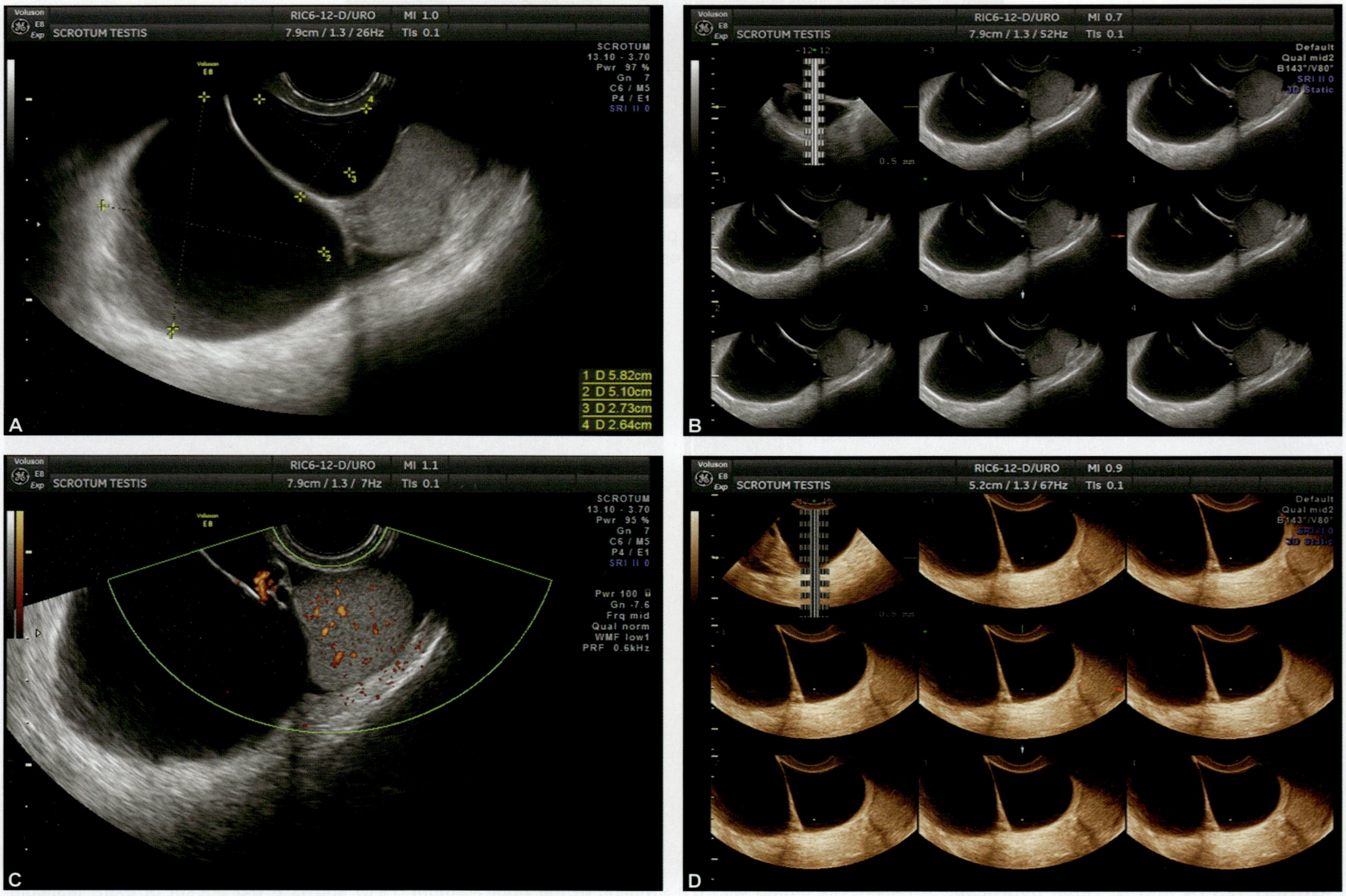

FIGURES 12.73A to D: Loculated testicular collection. HRSG shows a big loculated testicular collection in the right testes. A thick band is seen in the collection. The testes is seen displaced and compressed. Echotexture is normal. On color flow imaging, normal flow is seen in the testes.

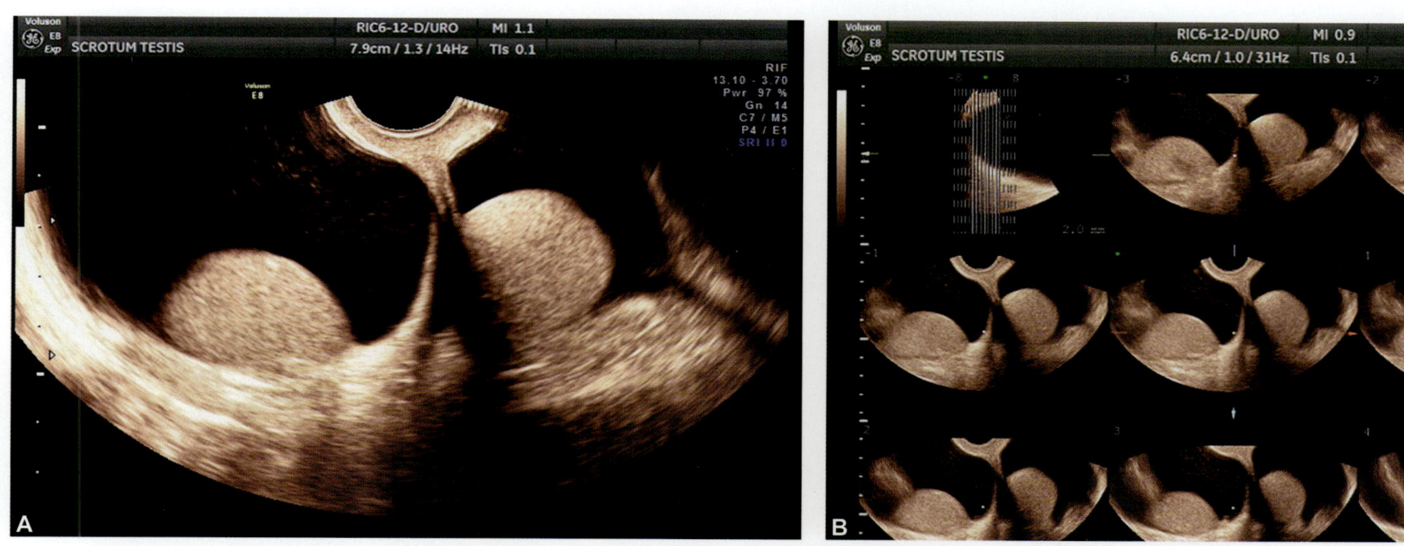

FIGURES 12.74A and B: Bilateral hydrocele. HRSG shows fluid collection in both scrotal sac. Both testes appear to be normal.

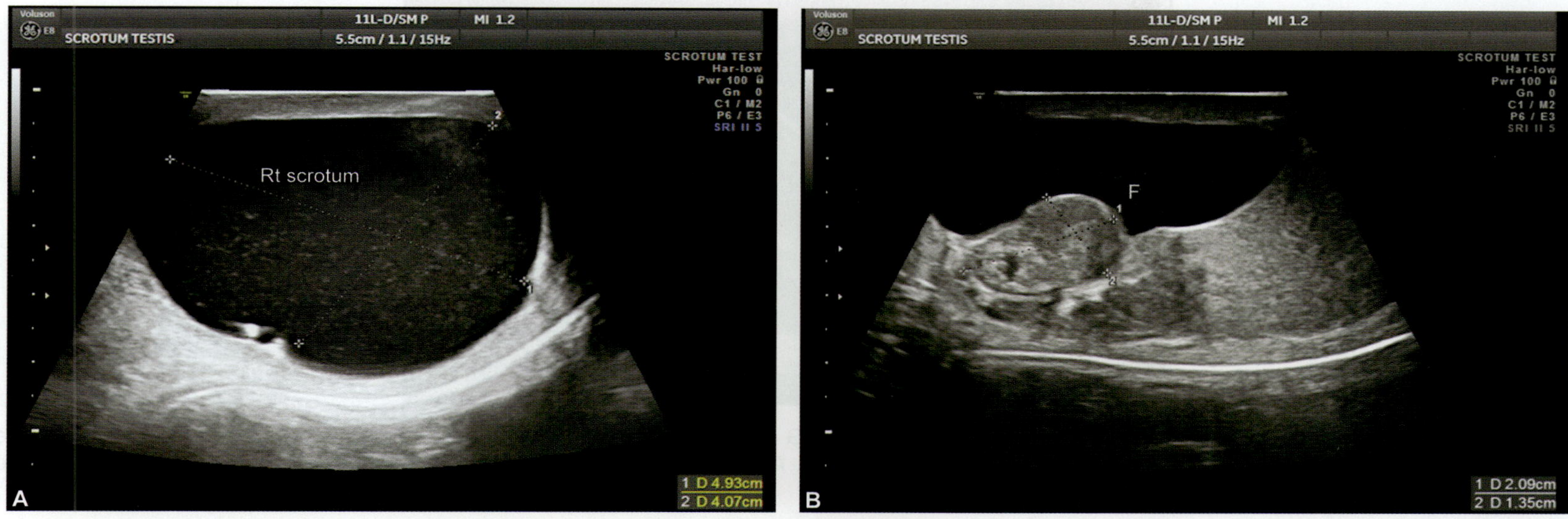

FIGURES 12.75A and B: Big tunica albuginea cyst. A patient presented with soft tissue swelling in the right scrotum. HRSG shows a big cystic mass seen coming out from the superior part of tunica albuginea. Well defined cystic wall is seen in it. But no septation or loculation is seen. The cyst is seen pressing over the right testes. Findings are suggestive of tunica albuginea cyst.

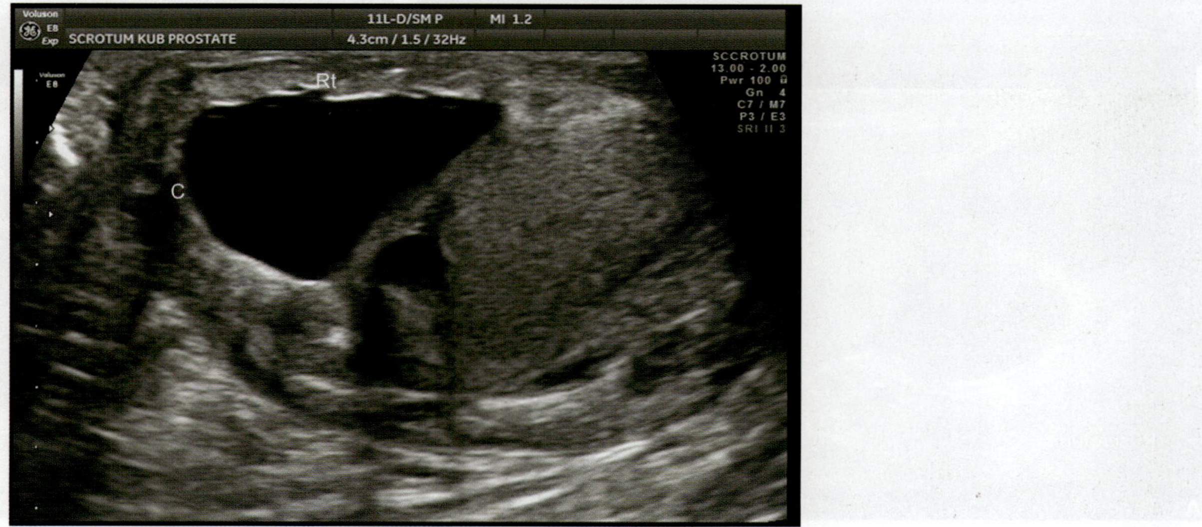

FIGURE 12.76: Tunica albuginea cyst. HRSG shows a big cystic mass coming out from upper part of tunica albuginea. Walls are echogenic and thickened. But no evidence of any septation is seen. The testes appears to be normal in size.

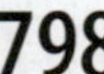

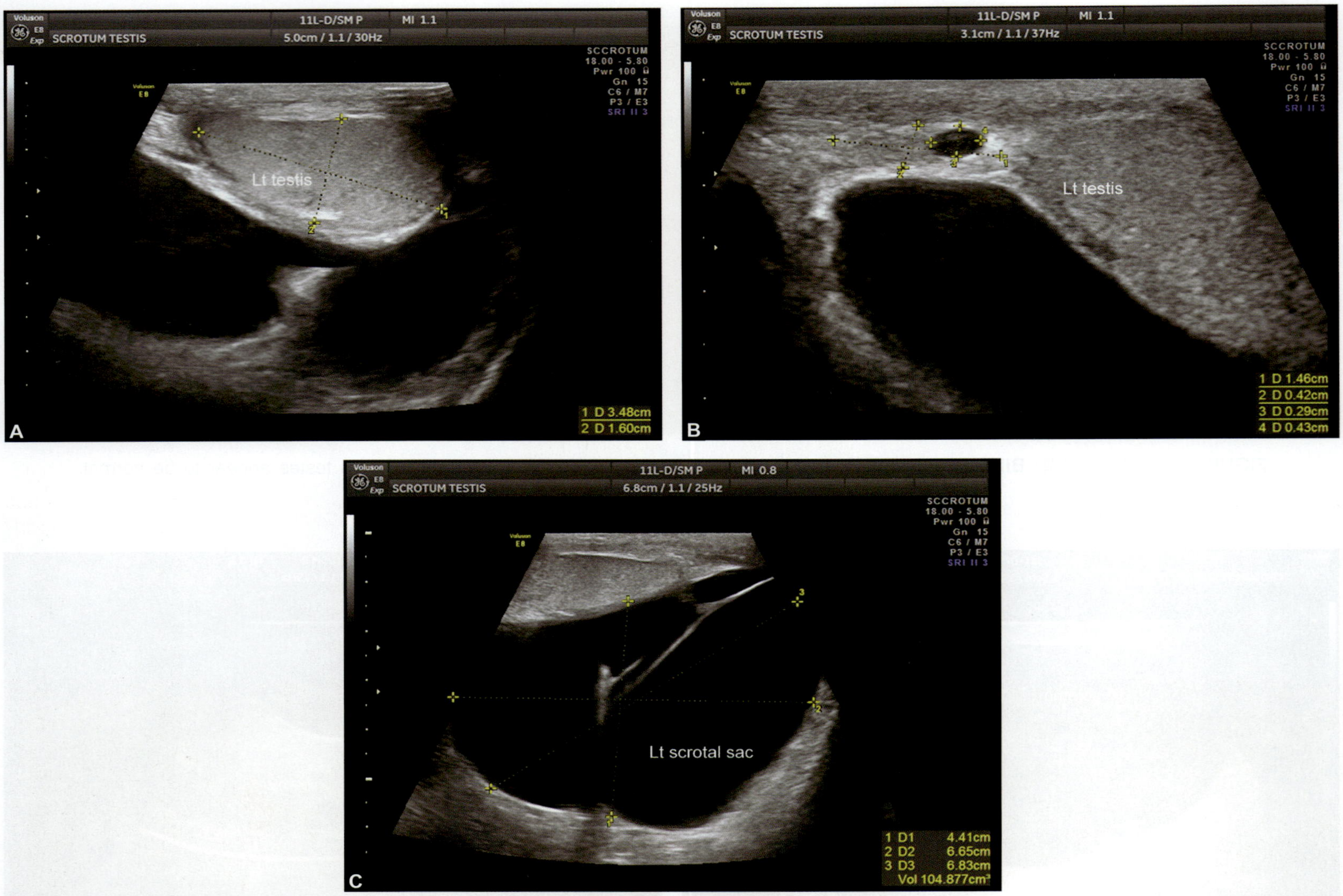

FIGURES 12.77A to C: A patient presented with left side swelling. HRSG shows moderate amount of fluid collection in the left scrotal sac. Multiple small strands are also seen in the collection suggestive of protein bands. A small cyst is seen at the superior border of tunica albuginea suggestive of small tunica albuginea cyst.

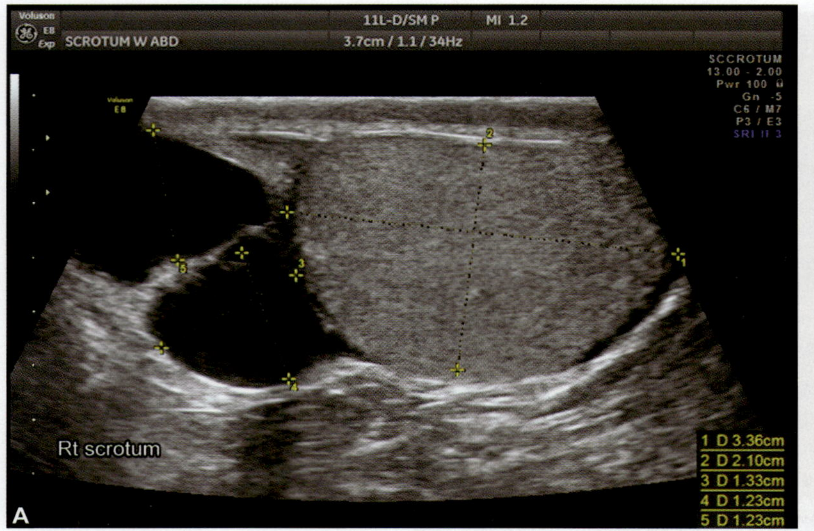

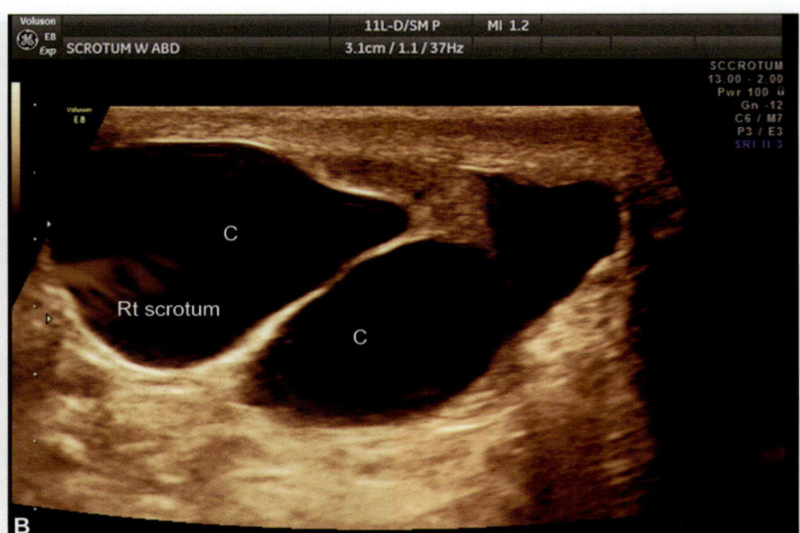

FIGURES 12.78A and B

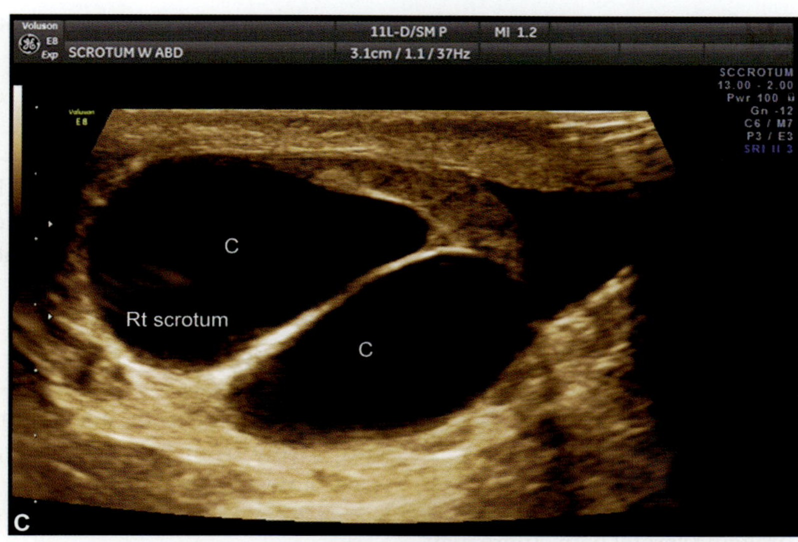

FIGURE 12.78C

FIGURES 12.78A to C: Multiple tunic albuginea cysts. HRSG shows multiple cystic shadows in the right scrotum. They are seen coming out from the superior surface of tunica albuginea. Echogenic bands are seen in them. However, the testes are normal. Findings are suggestive of multiple tunica albuginea cysts.

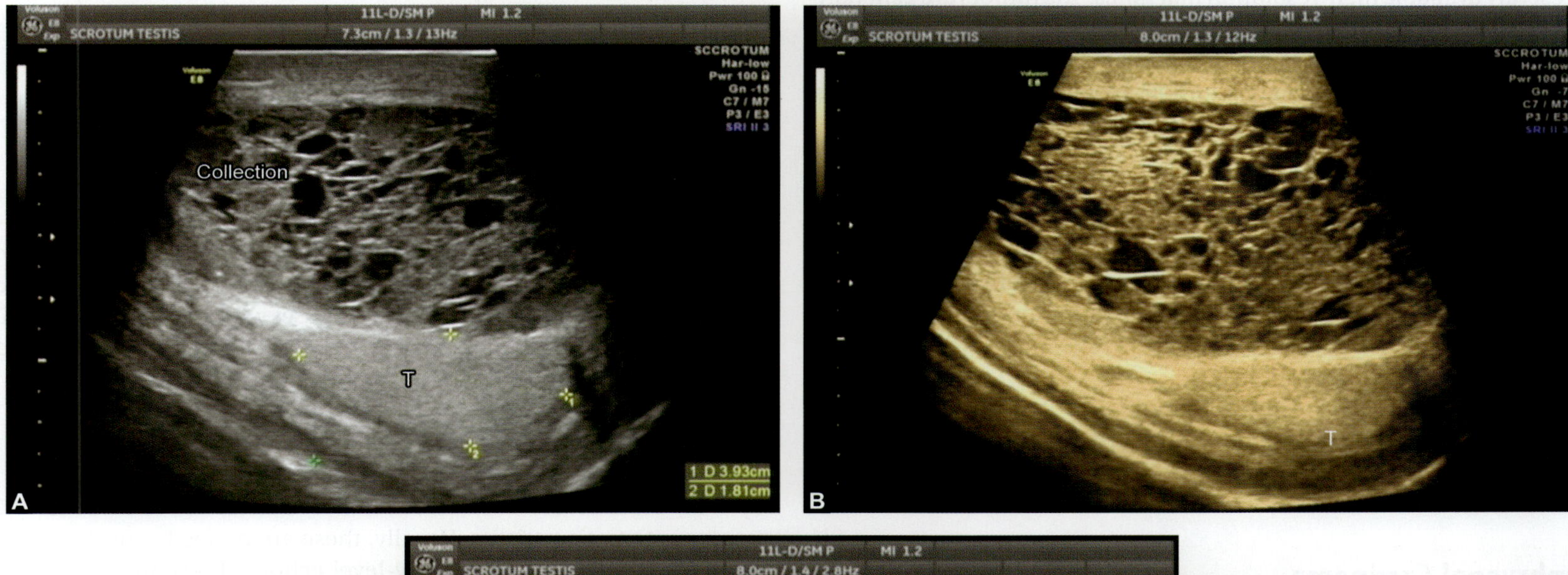

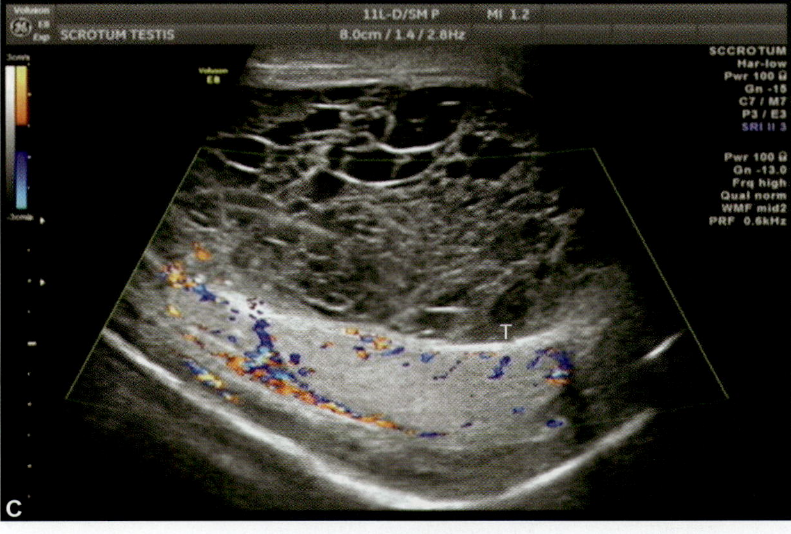

FIGURES 12.79A to C: Chronic hematocele. A patient presented with hard swelling in the left scrotal sac. HRSG shows thick collection in the scrotal sac. Multiple echogenic strands are seen in it. Typical honey comb appearance is seen. The collection is seen pressing and compressing the testes. However, the testes appears to be normal suggestive of chronic hematocele.

Scrotal Masses

Unless proved otherwise an intratesticular mass must be considered to be malignant. The small number (5% benign tumors include epidermoid cyst, leiomyomas, gonadostromal tumors, lipoma, fibroma, hamartoma and neurofibroma).

The following are the commonly encountered neoplasms of the testes.

1. Seminomatous germ cell tumors
   - Seminoma—40 to 50%
2. Nonseminomatous germ cell tumors
   - Embryonal cell carcinoma—15 to 20%
   - Teratocarcinoma
   - Choriocarcinoma
3. Metastatic tumors—0.6 to 3.6%.

   Most tumors are of germ cell origin.

   Most patients of testicular tumors present as painless testicular masses. Some of them complain of dragging scrotal pain. There may be associated symptoms of metastatic disease.

   The commonly encountered sonographic appearances are as follows:

Focal Alteration in Testicular Echo Texture (100% Sensitivity)

Nodules as small as 5.0 mm can be resolved with great accuracy due to presently available high-resolution machines. The tumors are generally hypoechoic when under 8 to 10 mm in size. The margins are usually regular, and the tumors are well defined in comparison to the rest of the testicular echo texture. Larger tumors are invariably heterogeneous showing areas of calcifications, necrosis (cystic areas) and dysembryogenetic components.

Seminoma

Seminoma in 40 to 50% are the most common testicular tumor in the adult age group of 40–50 years. It is more common in undescended testes. Sonography findings include:

i. Hypoechoic solid mass
ii. Homogeneous echo texture of tumor,
iii. Round or oval shape of tumor with sharp delineation from normal testicular parenchyma, and
iv. Multifocal involvement.

Embryonal Carcinoma

Embryonal cell carcinoma is more aggressive than a typical seminoma. Pure embryonal cell carcinoma is rare. Commonly it is a component of mixed tumors mainly in association with teratoma or teratocarcinoma. Sonographically, it demonstrates heterogeneous echo texture secondary to necrosis or hemorrhage, but often-cystic components and possibly calcification may occur.

Choriocarcinoma

Choriocarcinoma is a highly malignant tumor prone to hematogeneous metastasis.

Teratoma

Teratoma occurs commonly in infants and children. Sonographically, these lesions are markedly heterogeneous with multiple cystic areas and echogenic foci with or without acoustic shadowing, secondary to bone, fibrosis or hair.

Non-germ Cell Tumor

Non-germ cell tumors are usually benign, but may secrete steroids such as estrogen leading to endocrinological syndromes. These tumors may be malignant in 10% of the cases, and include those of Sertoli cell, Leydig cell or mesenchymal origin.

Metastasis

Metastasis to the testes may occur from renal and prostatic carcinoma, and rarely from bronchogenic, urinary bladder, melanoma and gastrointestinal neoplasms.

Adrenal Rest Tumors

Adrenal rest tumors of the testes may occur in cases of congenital adrenal hyperplasia or Cushing's syndrome leading to increased circulating adrenocorticotrophic hormone (ACTH).

Color Doppler studies show increased vascularity. However, differentiation between benign tumors and neoplasms cannot be distinguished with certainty of color flow studies. However, the final answer is obtained either by an orchidectomy or a fine-needle aspiration cytology study.

Lesions of the Epididymis

Tumors

Tumors are very rare and are almost benign. They appear as well-outlined and demarcated solid mass usually of increased echogenicity. Adenomatoid tumors are most common epididymal tumors. These are rounded, homogeneous and isoechoic masses with adjacent epididymal tissue. Adenomatoid tumors may arise from the tunica albuginea and may be hyper or hypoechoic.

Cysts

Cysts are the most common scrotal masses and are seen with 20 to 40% are asymptomatic patients. Usually, these are perfectly anechoic, but some contain homogeneous low-level echoes. These may represent spermatocele and are usually seen in patients with previous history of vasectomy and contain spermatozoa.

Calcifications

Calcifications may be seen in the tunica of the testes near the epididymis or free floating within the scrotal sac. These are also called as "scrotal calculi" or scrotal pears and are always benign.

Scrotal Lymph Edema

In scrotal lymph edema, there is marked thickening of the scrotal skin and median raphe. The skin can by up to 4 cm in thickness and shows evidence of tubular channels of varying dimensions. There should be no confusion with varicoceles lymphatics are within the scrotal wall. Whereas, varicoceles are inside the scrotal sac. Filariasis is one of the common causes of lymph edema in India. Some workers have been successful in isolating live filarial worm from lesion recently.

Tuberculosis

The common ultrasonographic features noted in chronic inflammatory disease as in tuberculosis of the scrotum are as follows:

1. An enlarged deformed epididymis especially in the tail.
2. Heterogeneous echo texture with associated calcification.
3. Extra testicular nodules.
4. Associated hydrocele, which is invariably septate.

Epididymis is the main site of tubercular involvement in the scrotum. There is enlargement of the epididymis followed by abscess formation. Adjacent scrotal wall is thickened with sinus formation and coarse thickening of tunica vaginalis. Involvement of contra lateral epididymis (Probably by lymphatic route) is involvement of testes. Resolution of tubercular epididymitis may leave residual extra testicular masses with large area of calcification.

Though tuberculosis primarily involves the epididymis, there is a definite entity where there is primary involvement of the testes. The testes is then enlarged, hypoechoic and the epididymis is completely normal. An FNAC (fine-needle aspiration cytology) is of great help. Primary testicular tuberculosis is commonly found in patients who are on immunochemotherapy for generalized diseases like leukemia or lymphoma. The color flow study does not show any significant increase in vascularity.

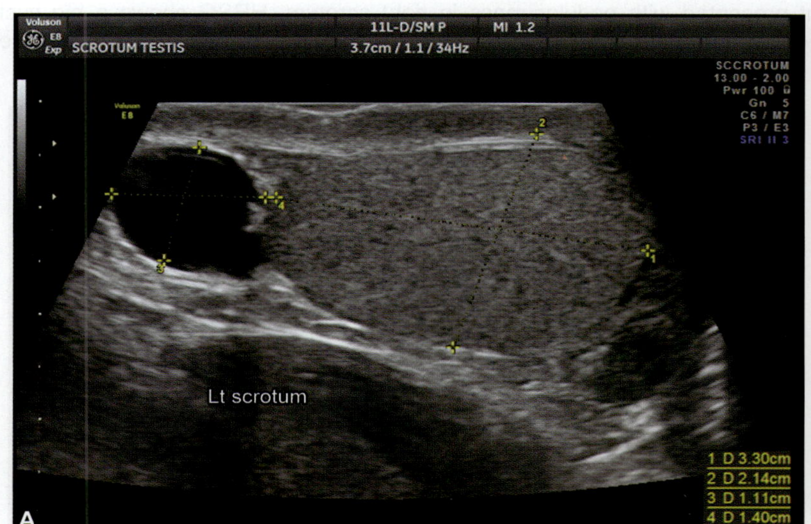

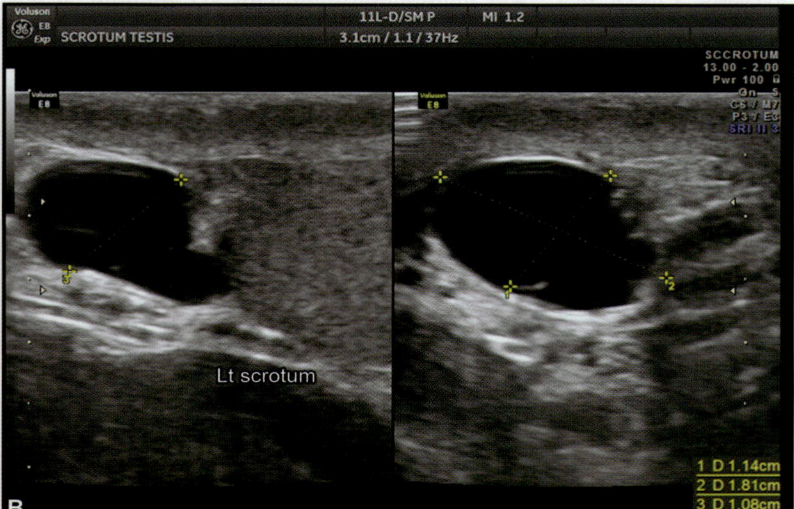

FIGURES 12.80A and B: Epididymal cyst. HRSG shows a well defined cyst in left epididymis. No internal echo is seen in the cyst. No septation is seen in the cyst.

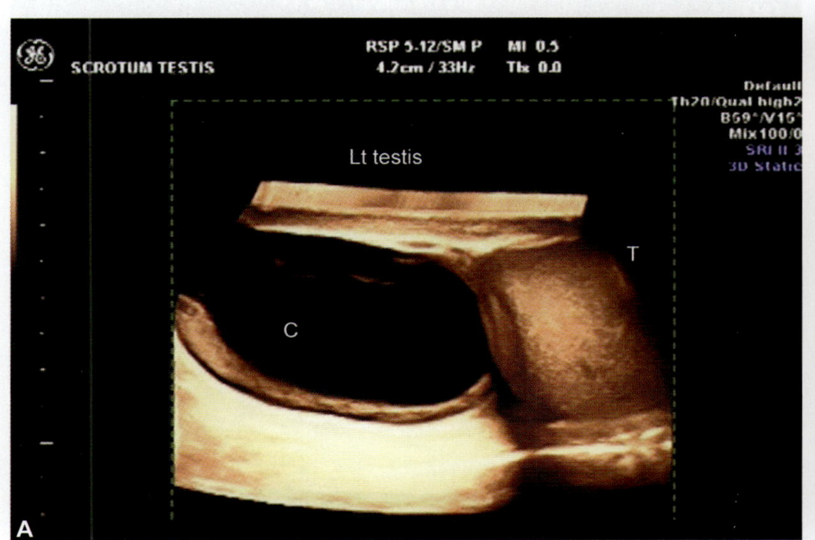

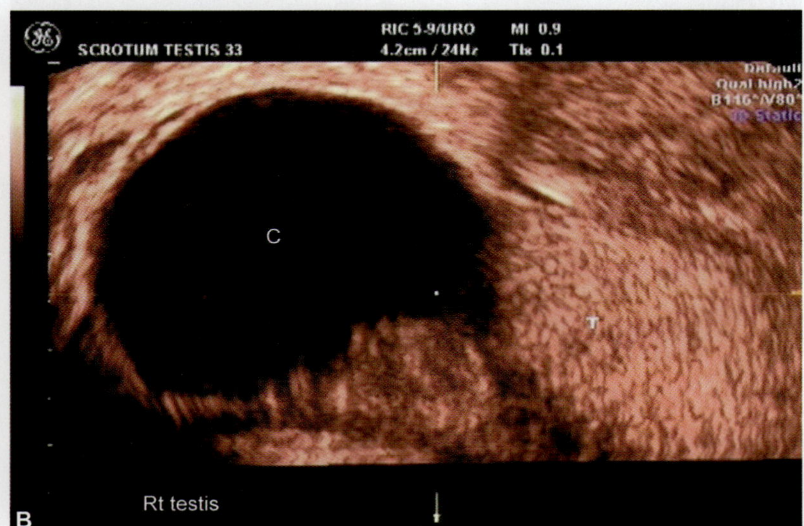

FIGURES 12.81A and B

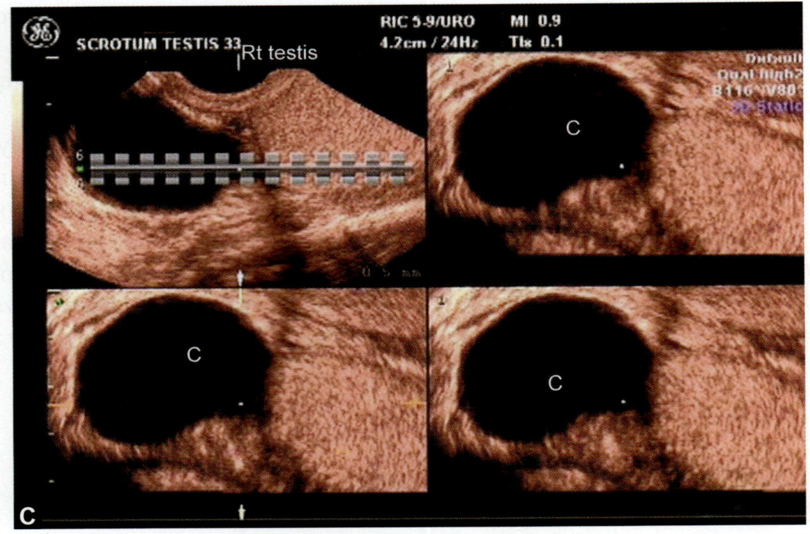

FIGURE 12.81C

FIGURES 12.81A to C: Big epididymal cyst with 3D imaging. A patient presented with nodular mass in right scrotum. HRSG shows a big cyst in right epididymis. The cyst is seen separate from the testes. No internal echocardiogram is seen in the cyst. No septation is seen in the cyst. The testes is normal.

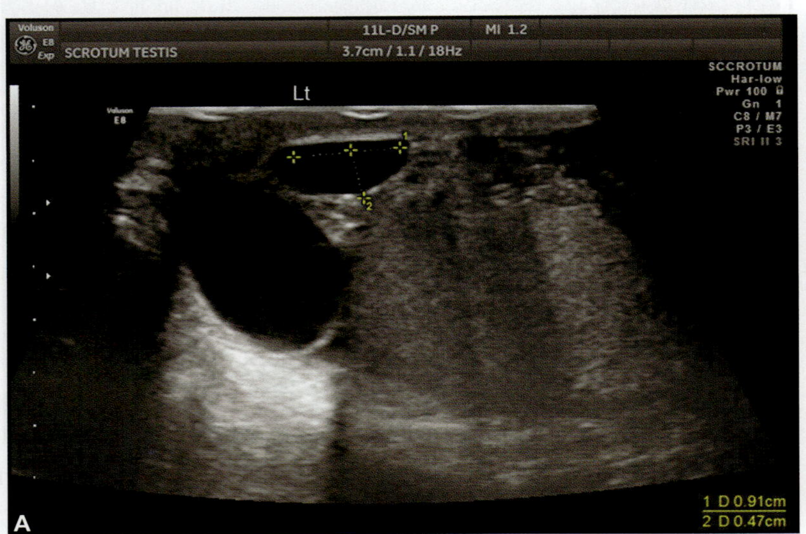

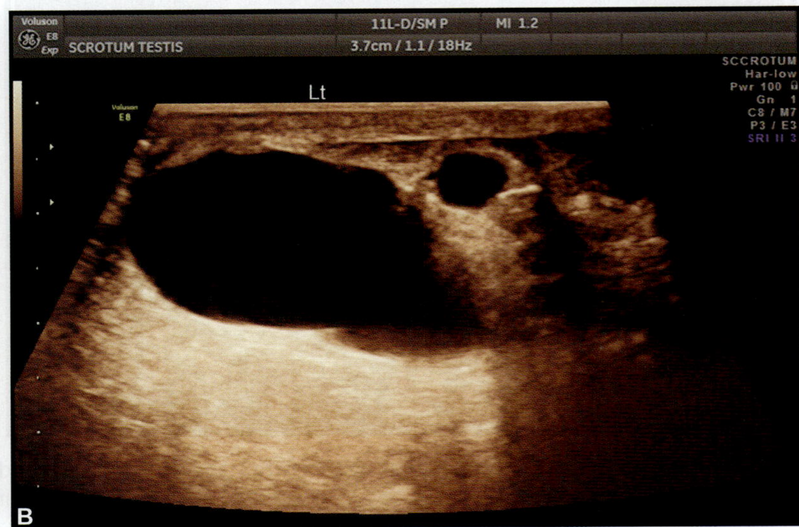

FIGURES 12.82A and B: Big epididymal cyst with a small cyst. HRSG shows a well defined cyst in the epididymis. It is smooth in outline. No septation or loculation is seen in the cyst. Another small cyst is seen near the big cyst.

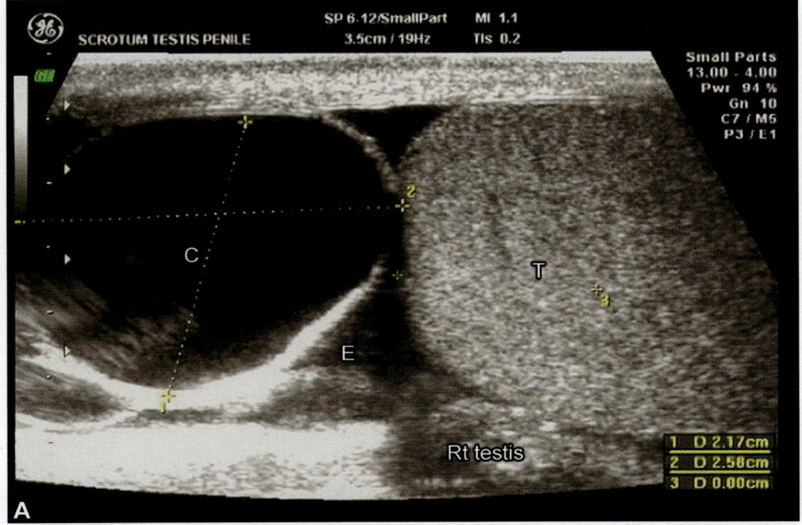

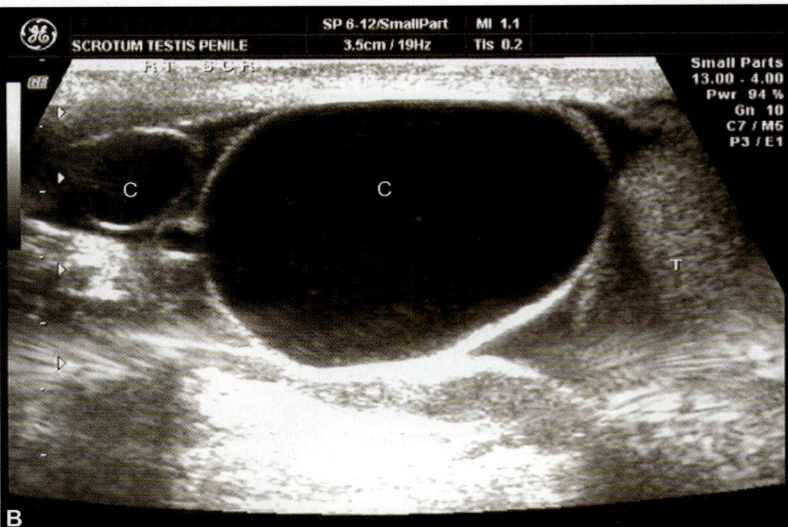

FIGURES 12.83A and B: Big epididymal cyst. A patient presented with palpable mass in the right scrotum. HRSG shows big cyst in the epididymis. No internal echo seen in the cyst. The cyst is seen replacing whole of the epididymis. Small proximal cord cyst is also seen with the big cyst. Global view of the scrotum shows the cyst and the testes. The cyst is seen separate from the testes.

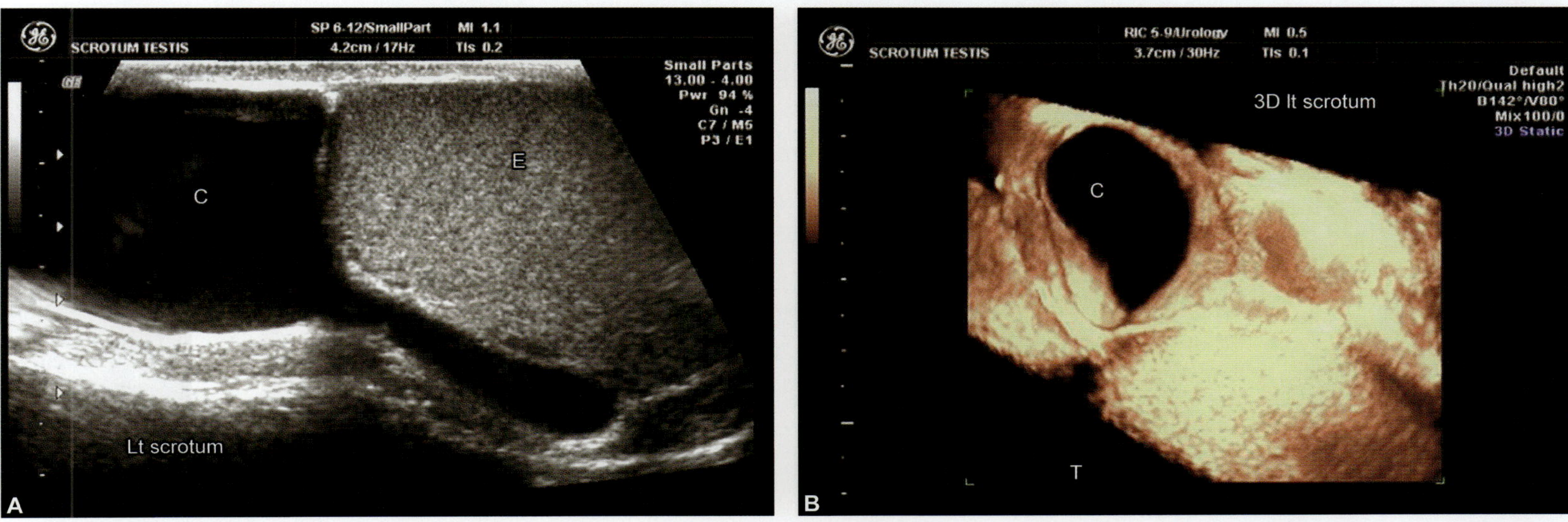

FIGURES 12.84A and B: Big epididymal cyst extending in the body and the tail. HRSG shows a big cystic mass in the head of the epididymis. The cyst is seen extending in the body in the tail of epididymis. It is seen replacing the normal structure. 3D Surface rendering imaging of the scrotum shows the cyst in much clinical detail.

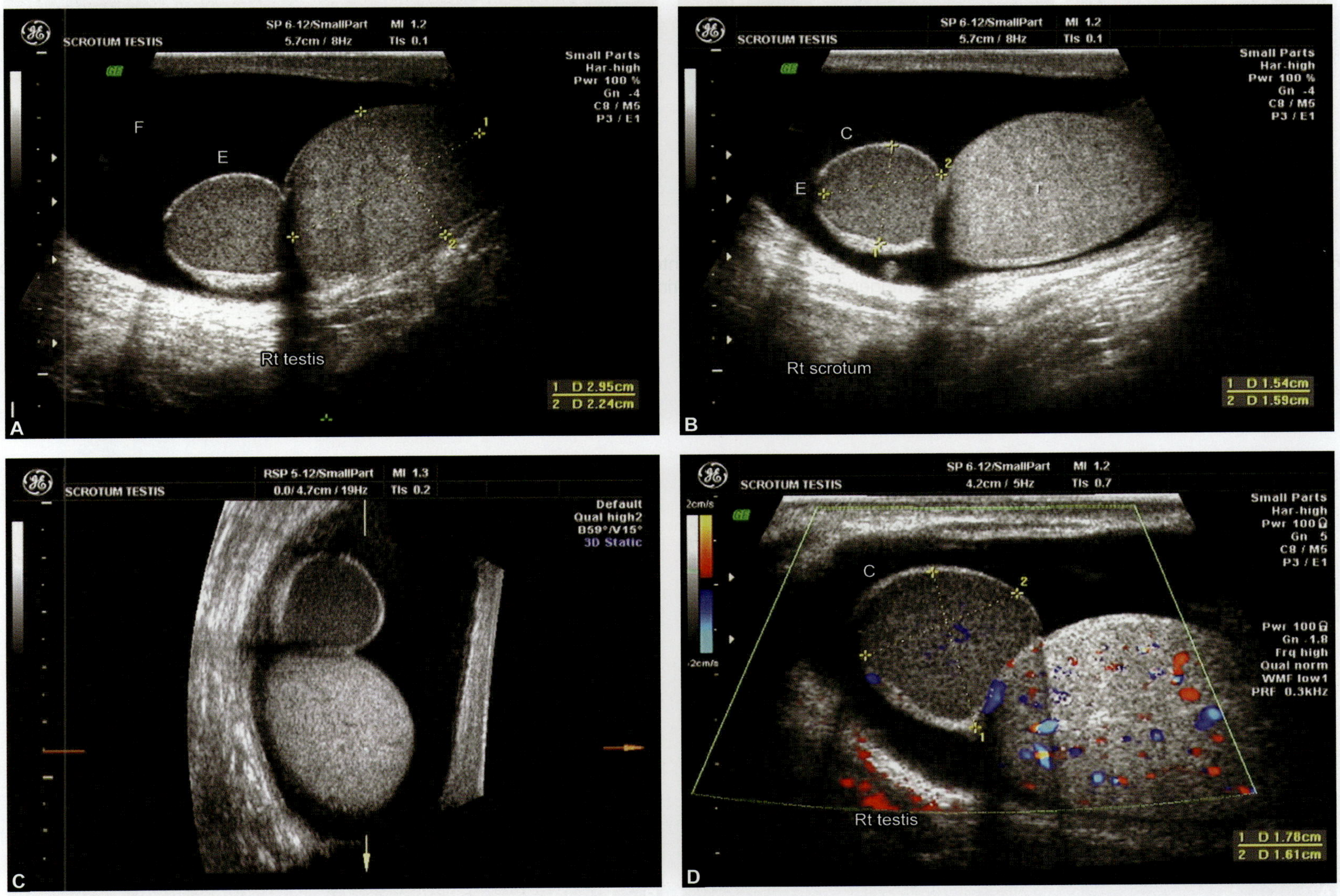

FIGURES 12.85A to D: Epididymal spermatocele. HRSG shows a thick walled cyst in the right scrotum. The cyst shows homogeneous echoes with "ground glass appearance". No septation is seen in the cyst suggestive of spermatocele. 3D surface-rendering image shows the cyst in much better view. On color flow imaging, no flow is seen in the cyst.

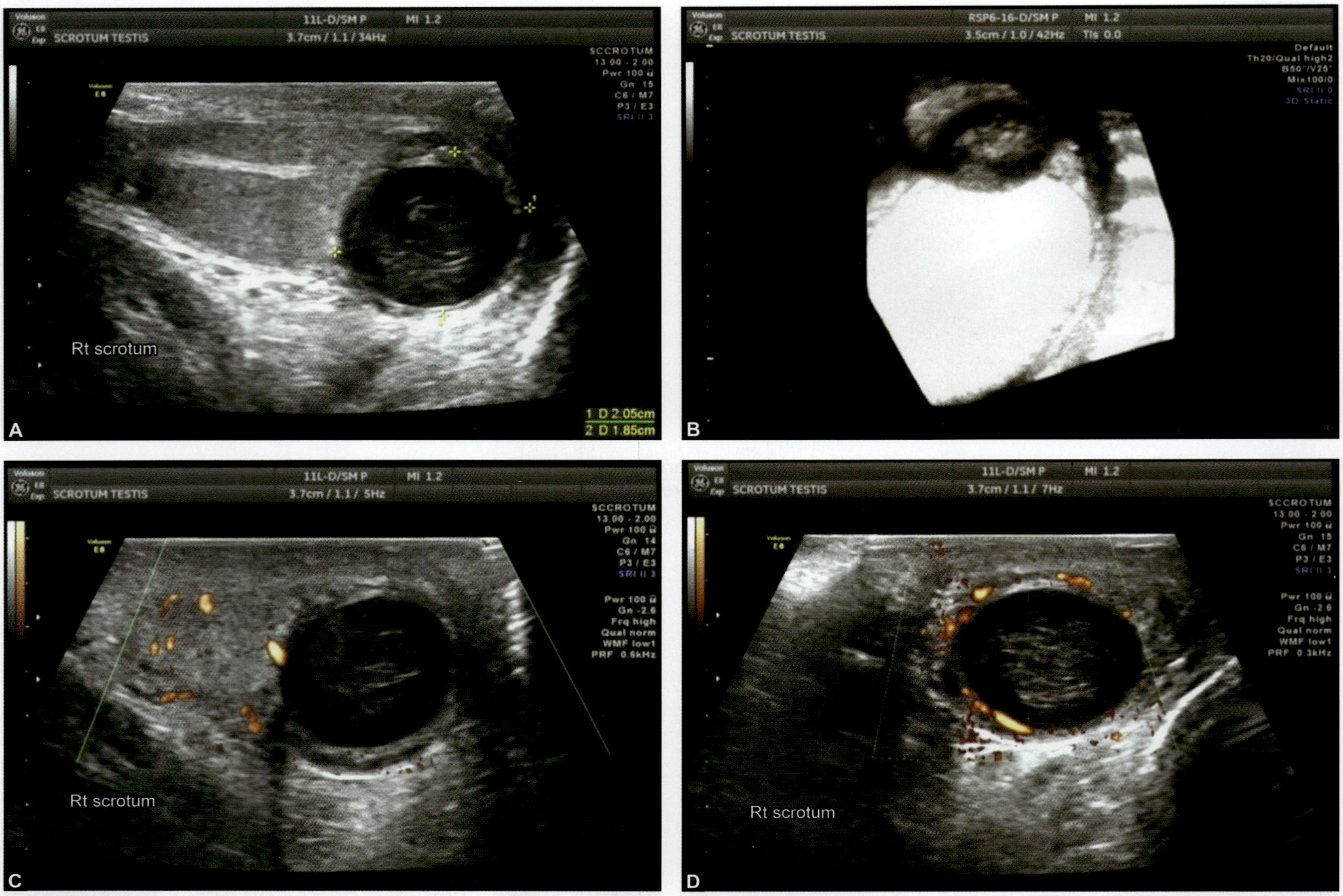

FIGURES 12.86A to D: Epidermoid cyst in epididymis. A patient presented with soft nodular shadow in the right scrotum. HRSG shows a complex cyst at the lower pole of epididymis. It shows homogeneous echoes. Layering sign is positive. On color flow imaging, no flow is seen in it. 3D imaging shows the cyst clearly. Findings are suggestive of epidermoid cyst.

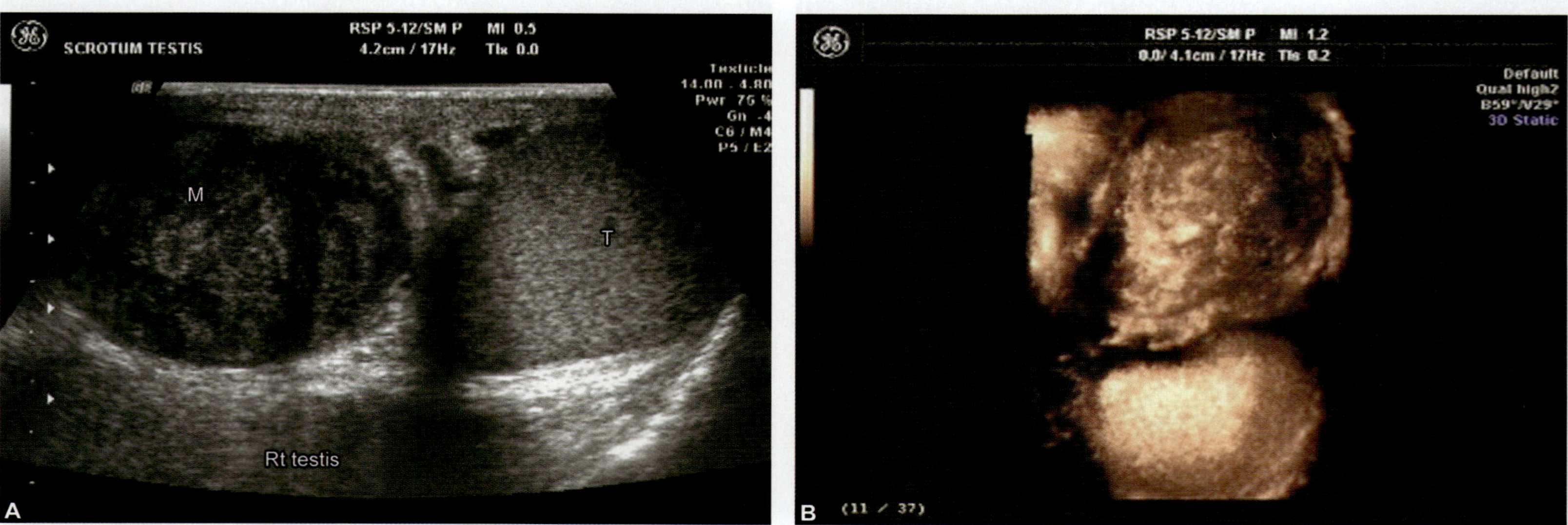

FIGURES 12.87A and B

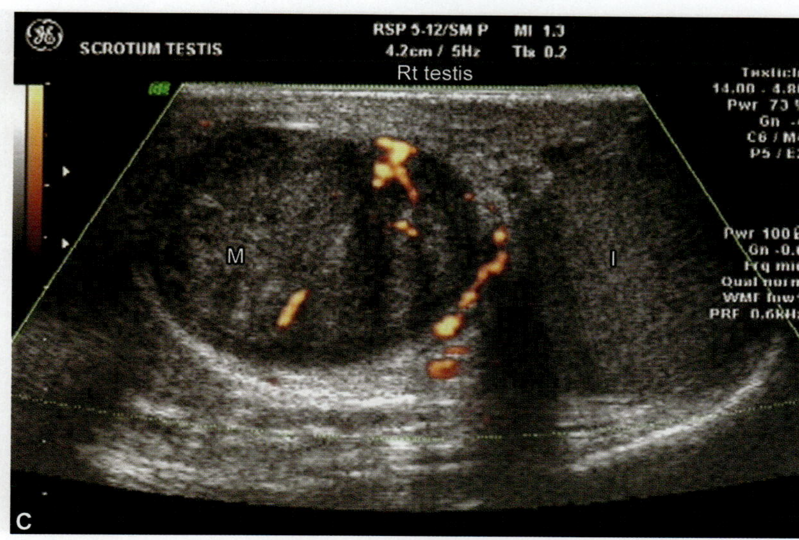

FIGURE 12.87C

FIGURES 12.87A to C: Adenomatoid tumor of epididymis. A patient presented with hard swelling in the right scrotum. HRSG shows a complex echo mass. It is well defined and well encapsulated. No calcification is seen in it. On color flow imaging, few vessels are seen feeding the mass. It is separate from testes. Per-operative finding confirms adenomatoid epididymis.

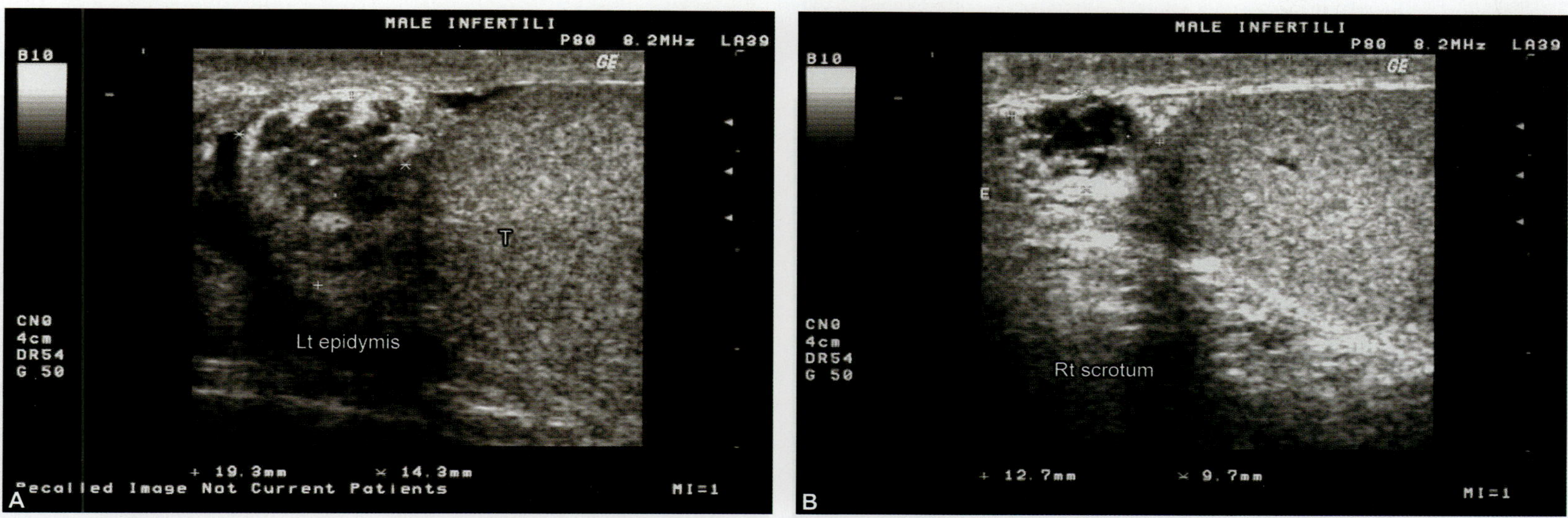

FIGURES 12.88A and B: Tubercular epididymitis. Irregular hypoechoic areas are seen in the right and left epididymis. Multiple calcified specks are also seen in it. Biopsy of the mass shows tubercular infiltration.

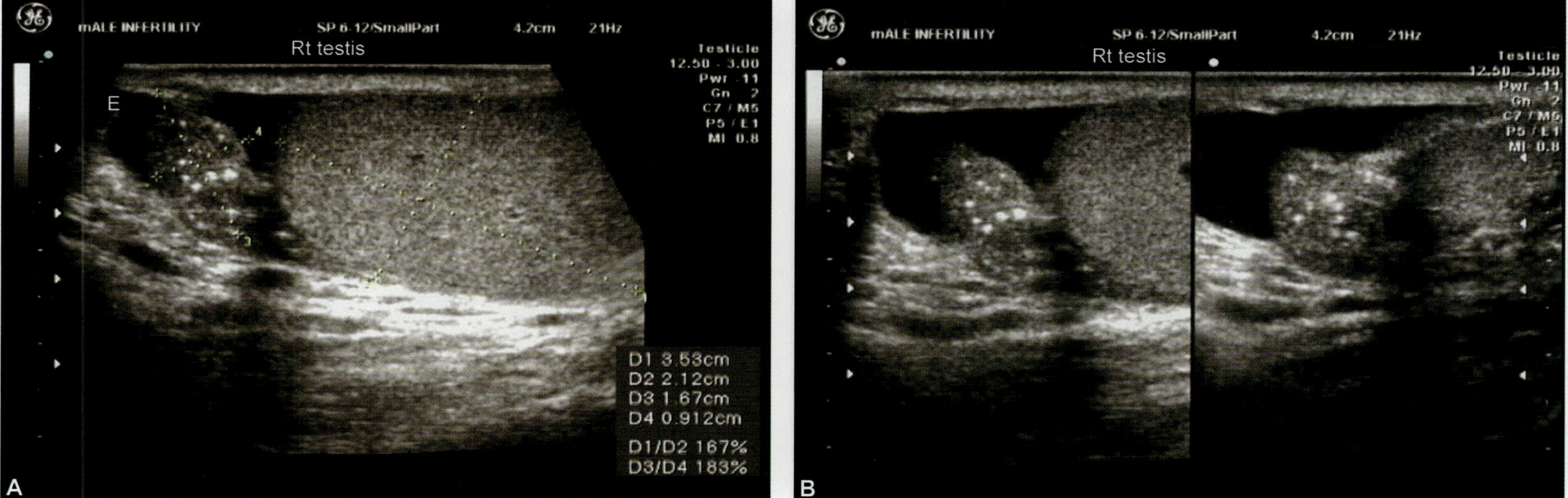

FIGURES 12.89A and B

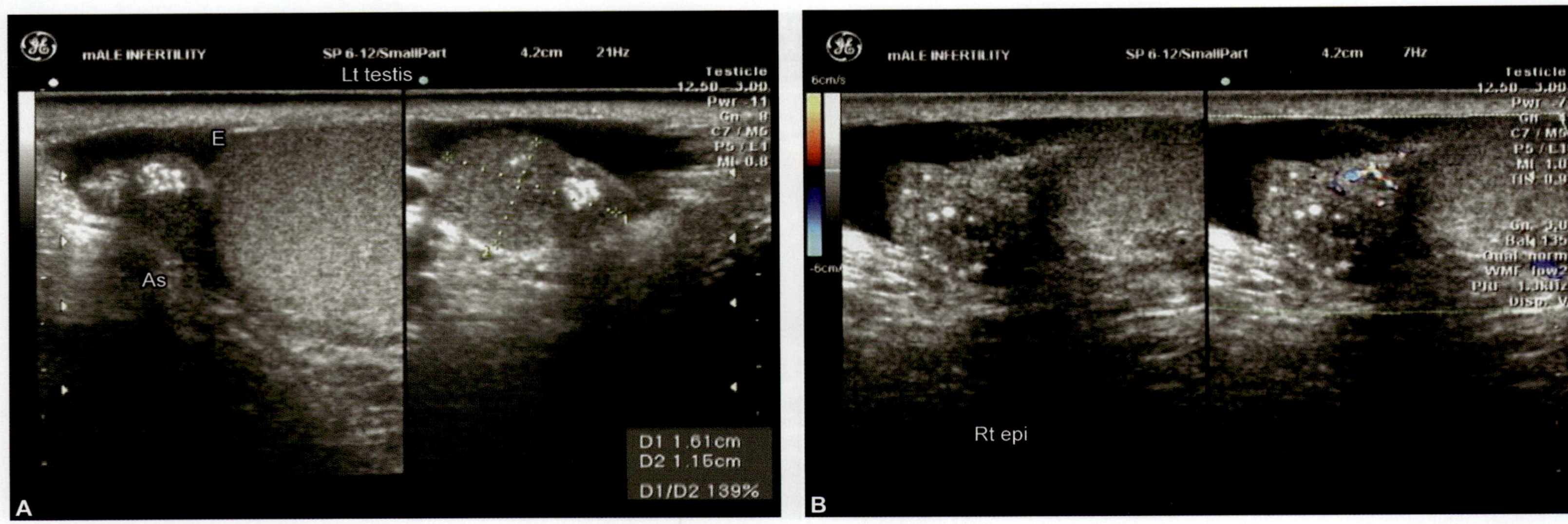

FIGURES 12.90A and B

FIGURES 12.89 and 12.90: Tubercular epididymitis. A patient presented of male infertility presented with oligoasthenospermia. HRSG shows irregular heterogeneous epididymis in both scrotal sac. Multiple calcified specks are seen in the epididymis. Epididymis is irregular in outline. On color flow imaging, no flow is seen in them. Biopsy of the epididymis confirms tubercular epididymitis.

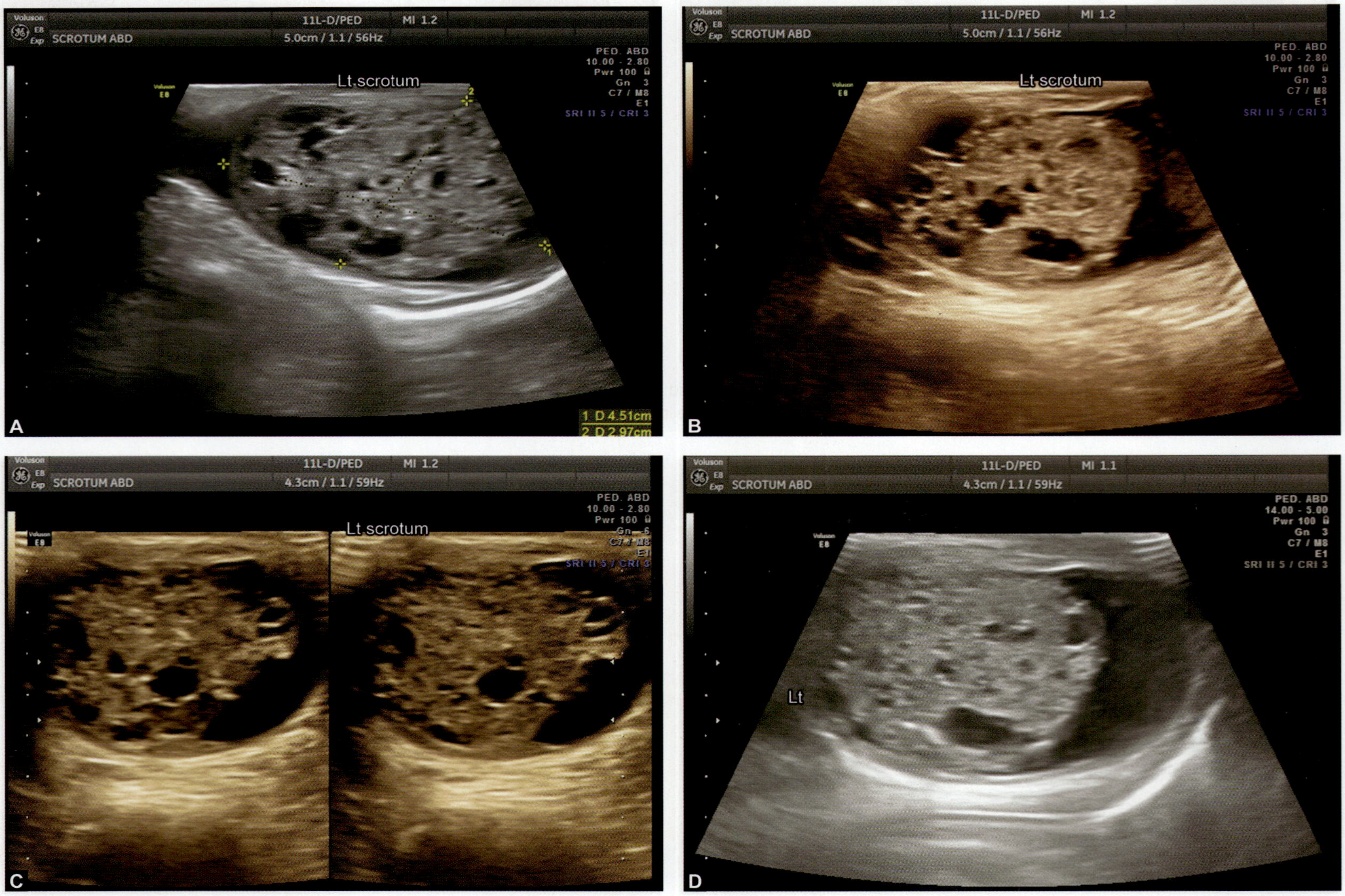

FIGURES 12.91A to D: Germ cell tumor. A small baby presented with left testicular mass. HRSG shows enlarged heterogeneous left testes. Normal texture is lost. Multiple hypoechoic areas are seen in the testes with area of necrosis. Small amount of fluid is also seen in left scrotal sac. Peroperative findings confirms germ cell tumor.

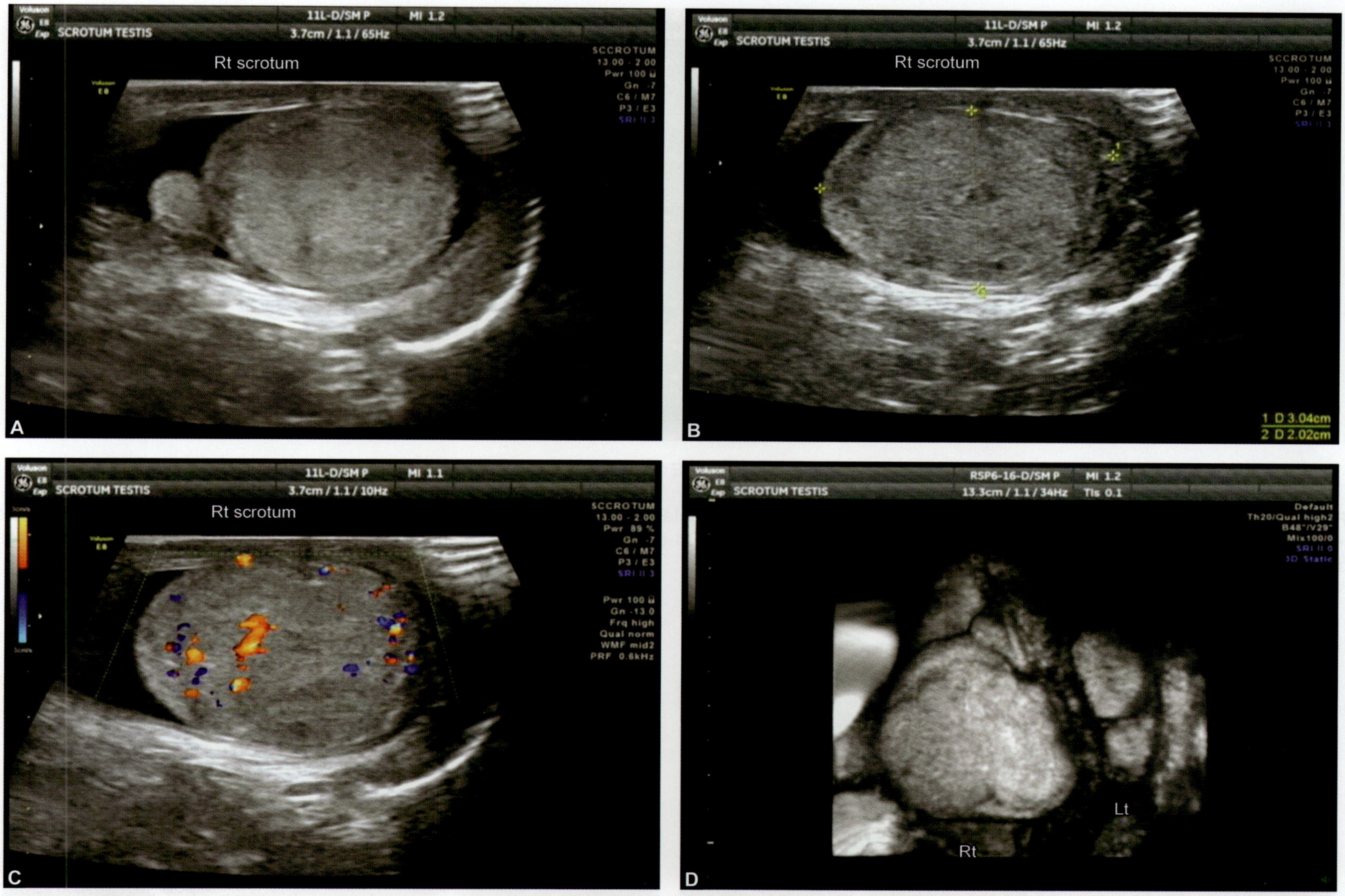

FIGURES 12.92A to D: Germ cell tumor. A 4-month-old baby presented with hard right scrotal mass. HRSG shows enlarged heterogeneous right testes. Normal texture is lost. hypoechoic areas are seen in it. On color flow imaging, few vessels are seen feeding it. The 3D ultrasound shows heterogeneous texture of the mass. Findings are suggestive of germ cell tumor.

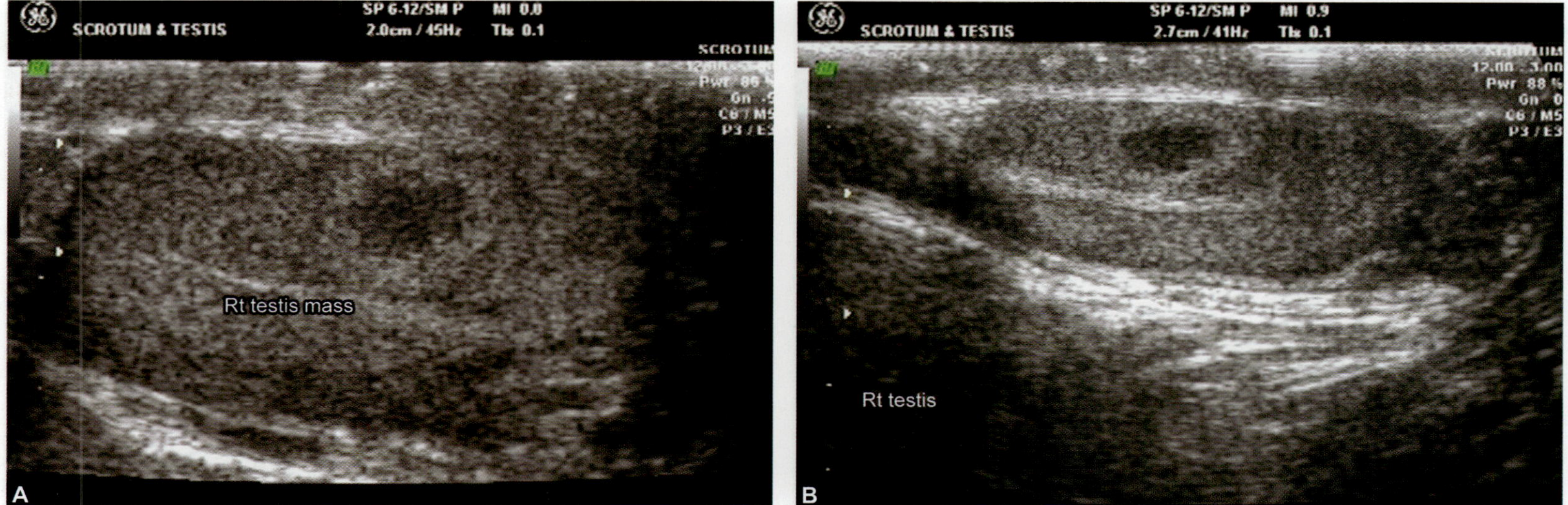

FIGURES 12.93A and B

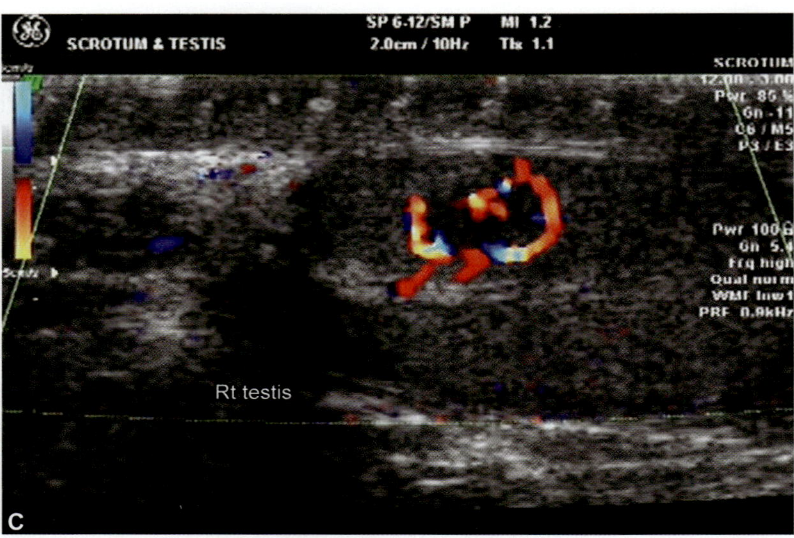

FIGURE 12.93C

FIGURES 12.93A to C: Small germ cell tumor. HRSG shows small irregular ill defined mass in the right testes. It is irregular in outline and hypoechoic in texture. No calcification is seen in it. No cystic degeneration is seen. On color flow imaging, peripheral flow is seen around it. Per-operative findings confirms germ cell tumor.

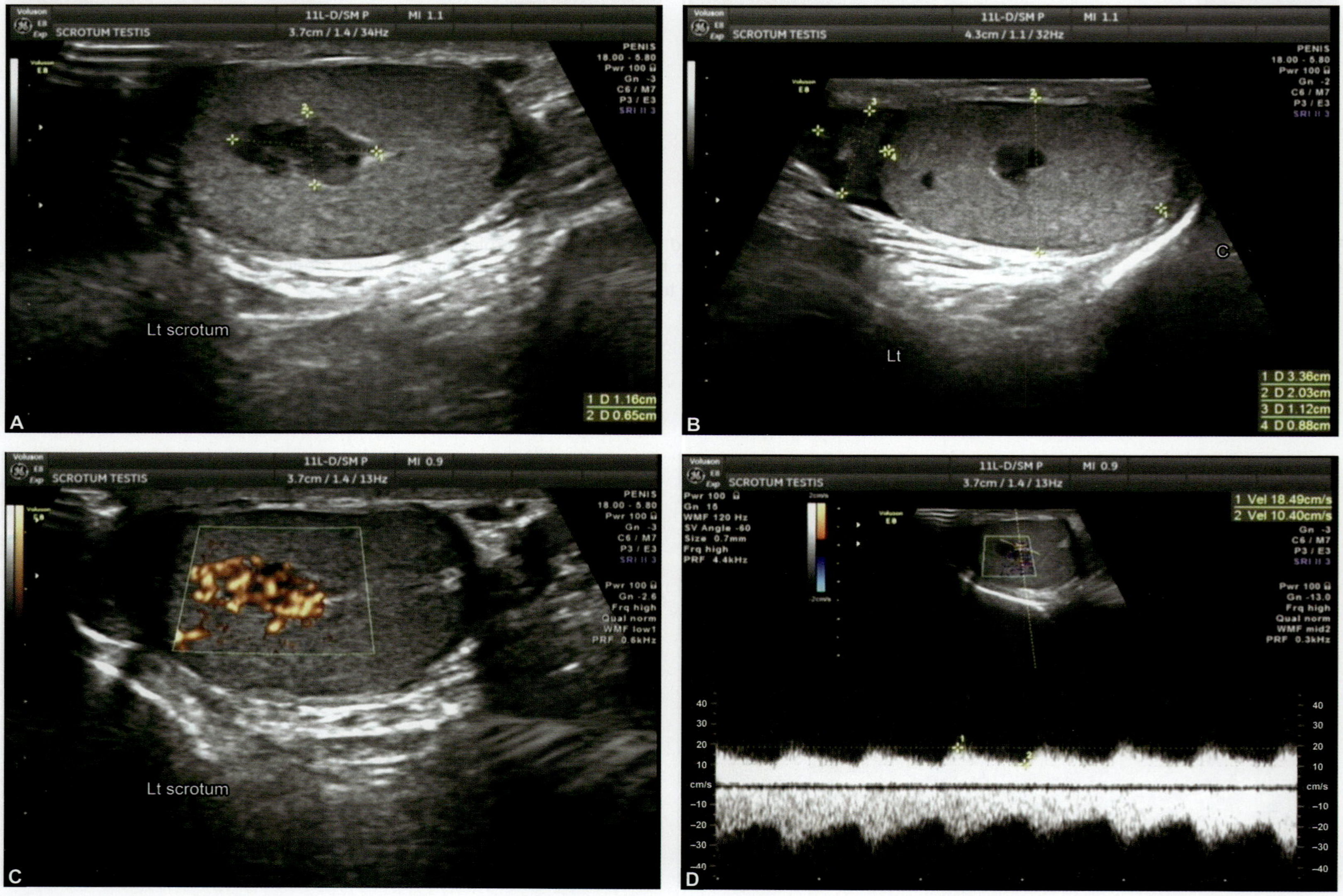

FIGURES 12.94A to D: Small seminoma testes. A patient presented with enlarged left testes. HRSG shows diffuse enlargement of testes. An irregular hypoechoic mass is seen in left testes. It shows heterogeneous texture. On color flow imaging increased flow is seen in the mass. Multiple vessels are seen feeding the mass. On spectral Doppler tracing, moderate flow is seen in the mass. Findings are suggestive of seminoma testes.

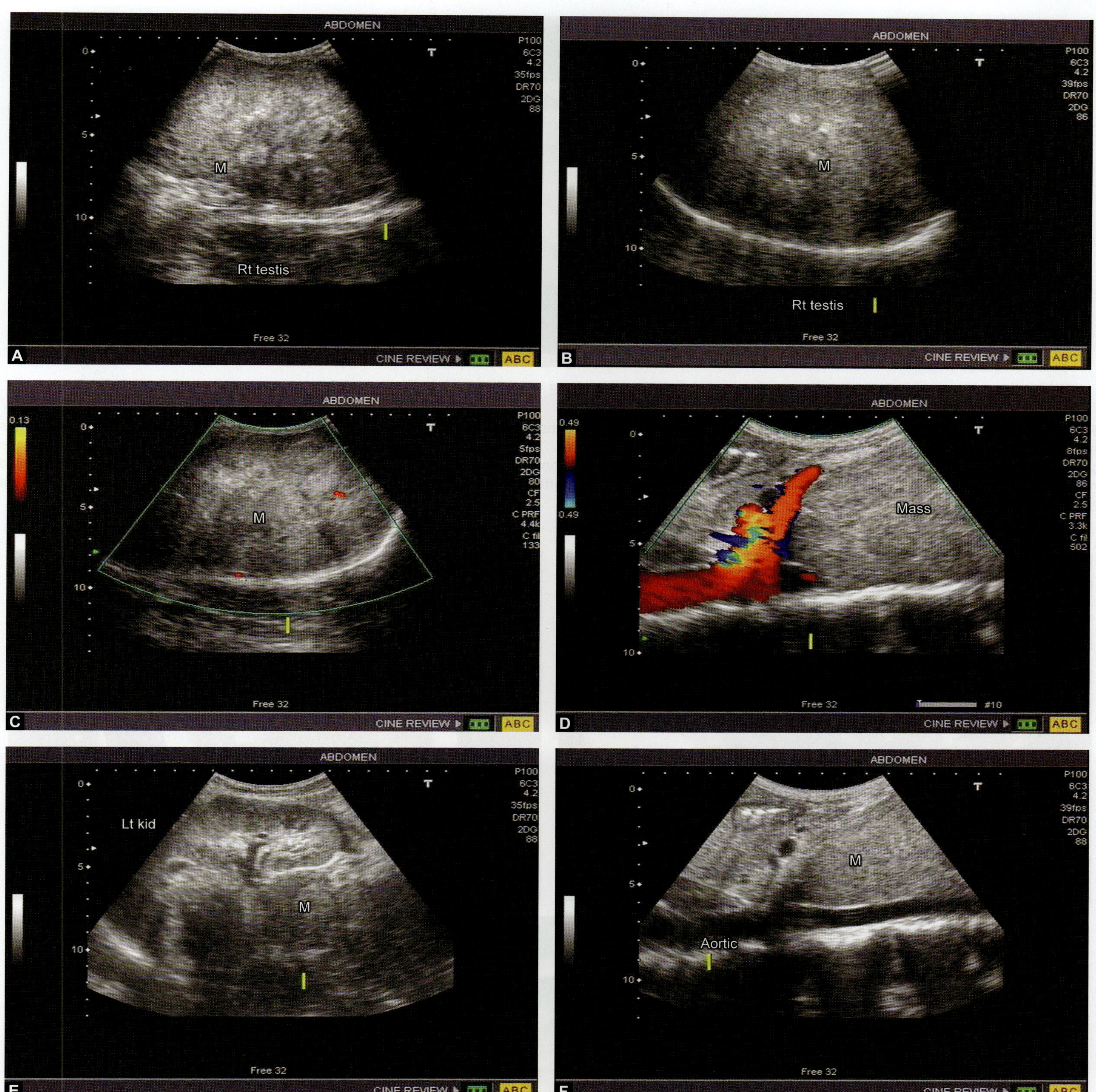

FIGURES 12.95A to F

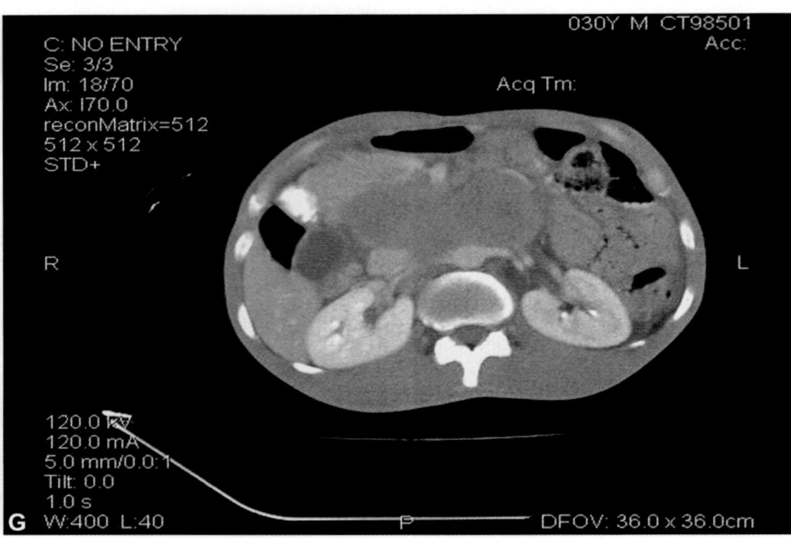

FIGURE 12.95G

FIGURES 12.95A to G: Seminoma testes with metastasis. A patient presented with huge right scrotal swelling. HRSG shows a big heterogeneous mass in the right testes. The mass is seen involving the whole of testes. Area of necrosis is also seen in the mass. But no cystic degeneration is seen in the mass. Normal anatomy is distorted. On color flow imaging, poor flow is seen in the mass. There is also evidence of multiple enlarged nodal shadows seen in the retroperitoneum. They are seen in the para aortic region. Splaying of the artery is also seen. CT scan of the same patient shows retroperitoneal lymph node mass.

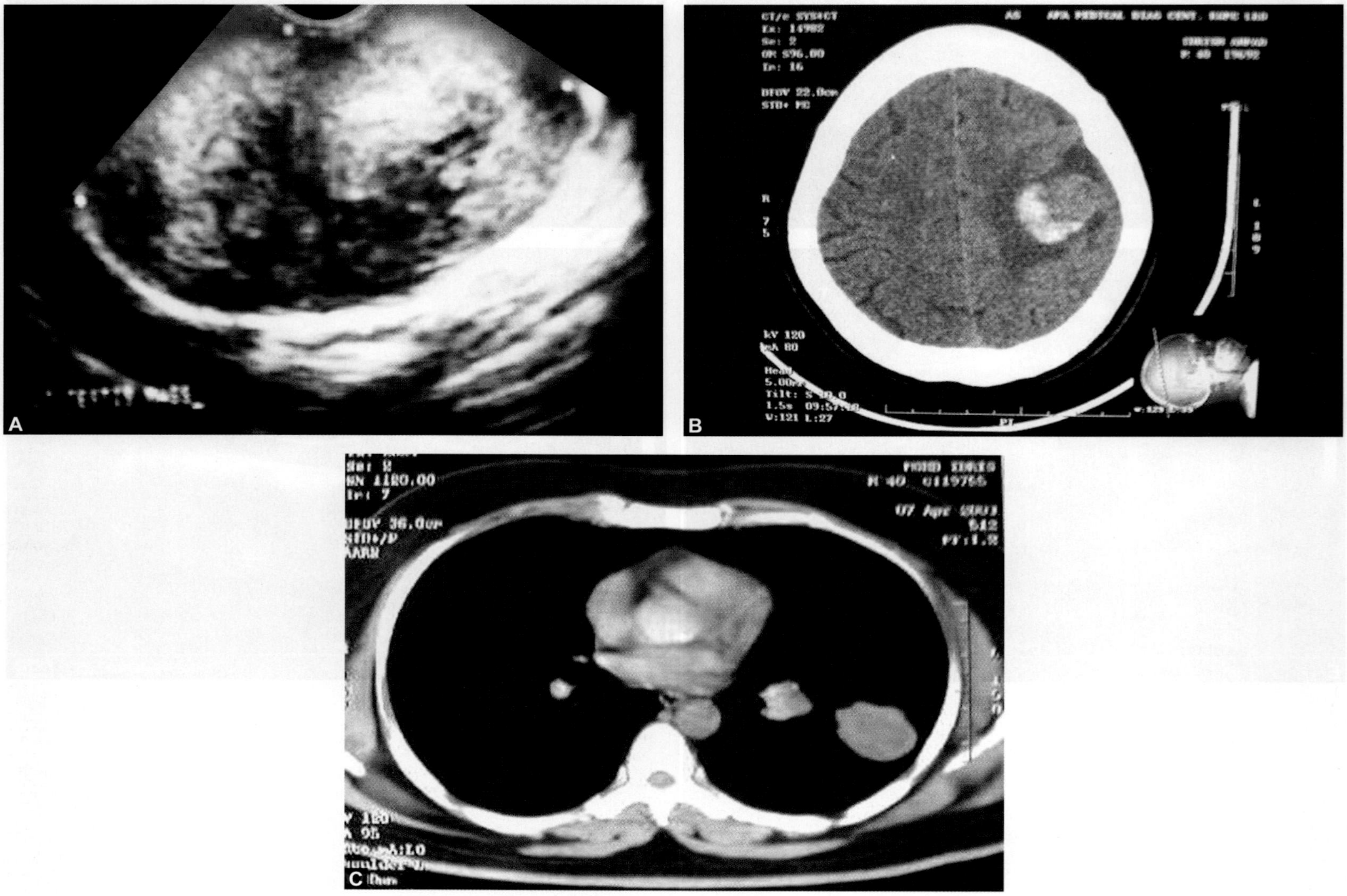

FIGURES 12.96A to C: Seminoma testes with distant metastasis. A patient presented with soft tissue mass in the right scrotal sac. HRSG shows a big heterogeneous mass invading the testes. The capsule of the testes is also seen broken. The same patient presented with seizure disorder. CT scan of the head shows a big metastatic deposit in the left parietal lobe with internal hemorrhage. CT thorax also shows big nodular masses in the left lung suggestive of secondaries.

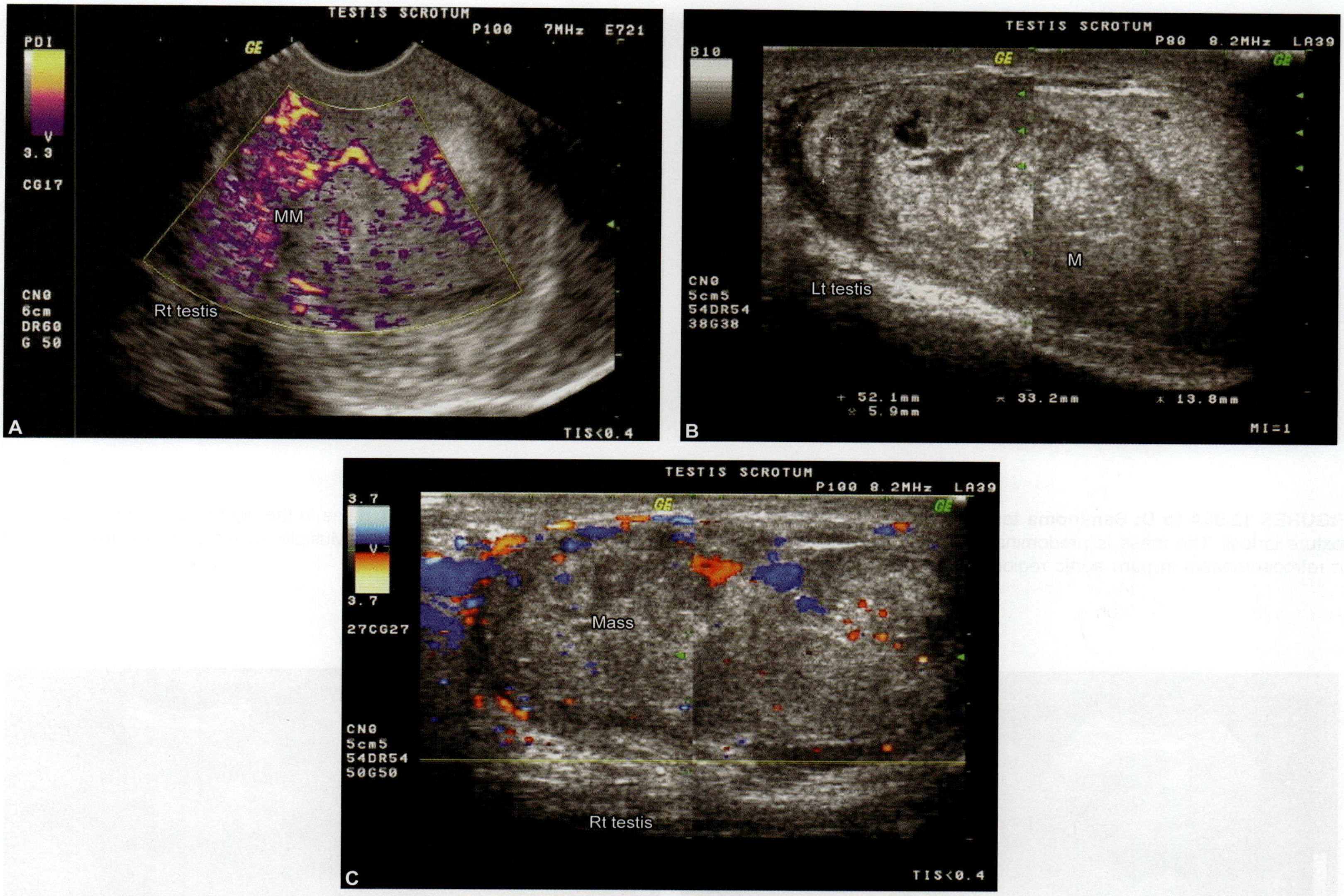

FIGURES 12.97A to C: Seminoma testes. Right scrotum shows a big heterogeneous mass in the testes. The mass has destroyed normal testicular texture. Multiple hypoechoic areas are seen in the mass. But no cystic degeneration is seen. The mass is seen confined to the tunica albuginea. Color flow-imaging shows increased flow in the mass. Biopsy of the mass shows seminoma.

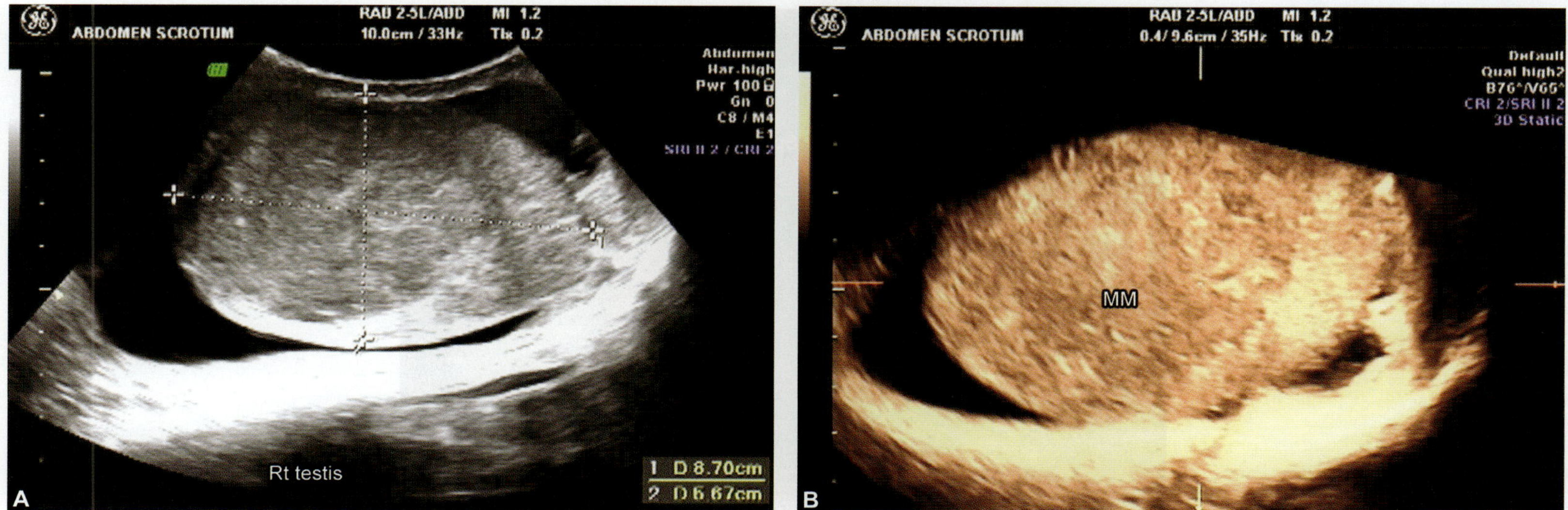

FIGURES 12.98A and B

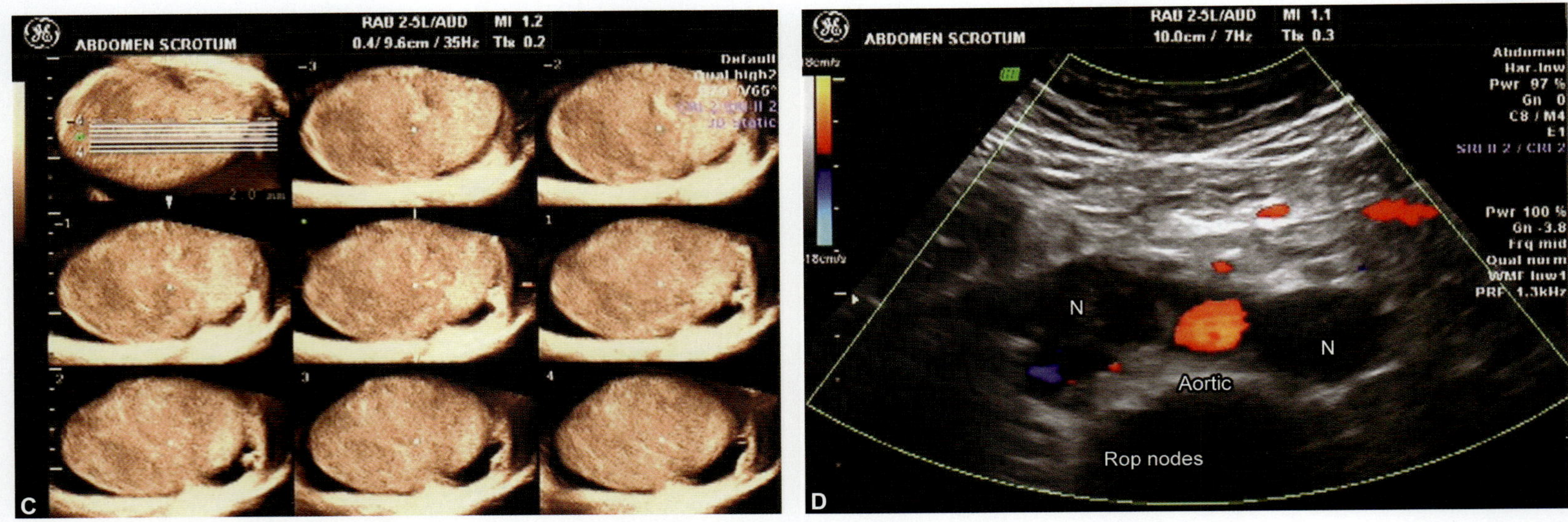

FIGURES 12.98C and D

FIGURES 12.98A to D: Seminoma testes with retroperitoneal nodes. HRSG shows a big heterogeneous mass in the right testes. Normal testicular texture is lost. The mass is predominately solid. No calcification or cystic degeneration is seen in the mass. Multiple enlarged nodes are also seen in retroperitoneum in para aortic region. They are hypoechoic in texture.

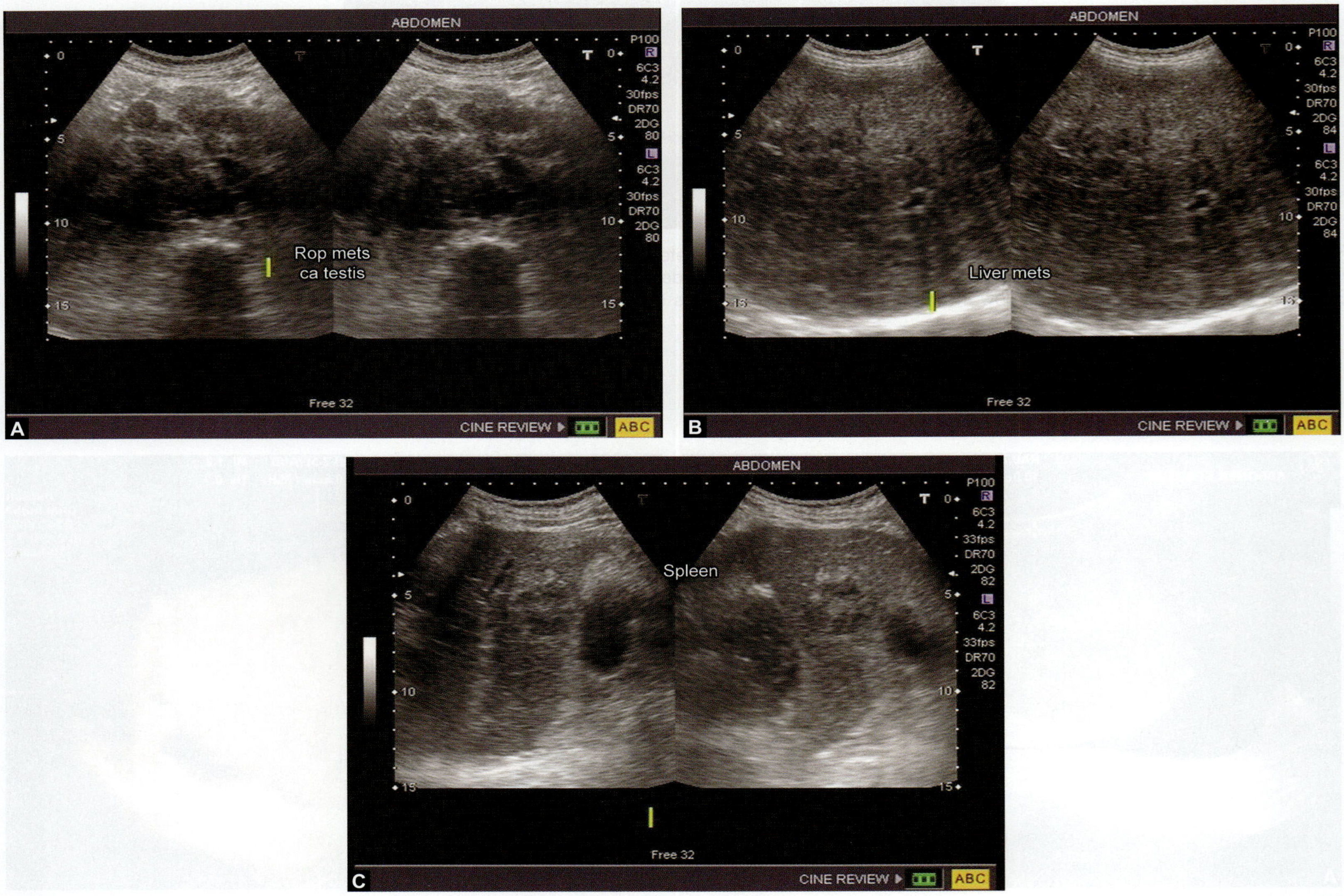

FIGURES 12.99A to C: Seminoma testes with metastasis. An operated case of seminoma testes presented with multiple mets. HRSG shows multiple retroperitoneal nodes. The liver also shows multiple heterogeneous mass suggestive of metastatic deposits. Spleen also shows metastatic deposits suggestive of disseminated metastasis disease.

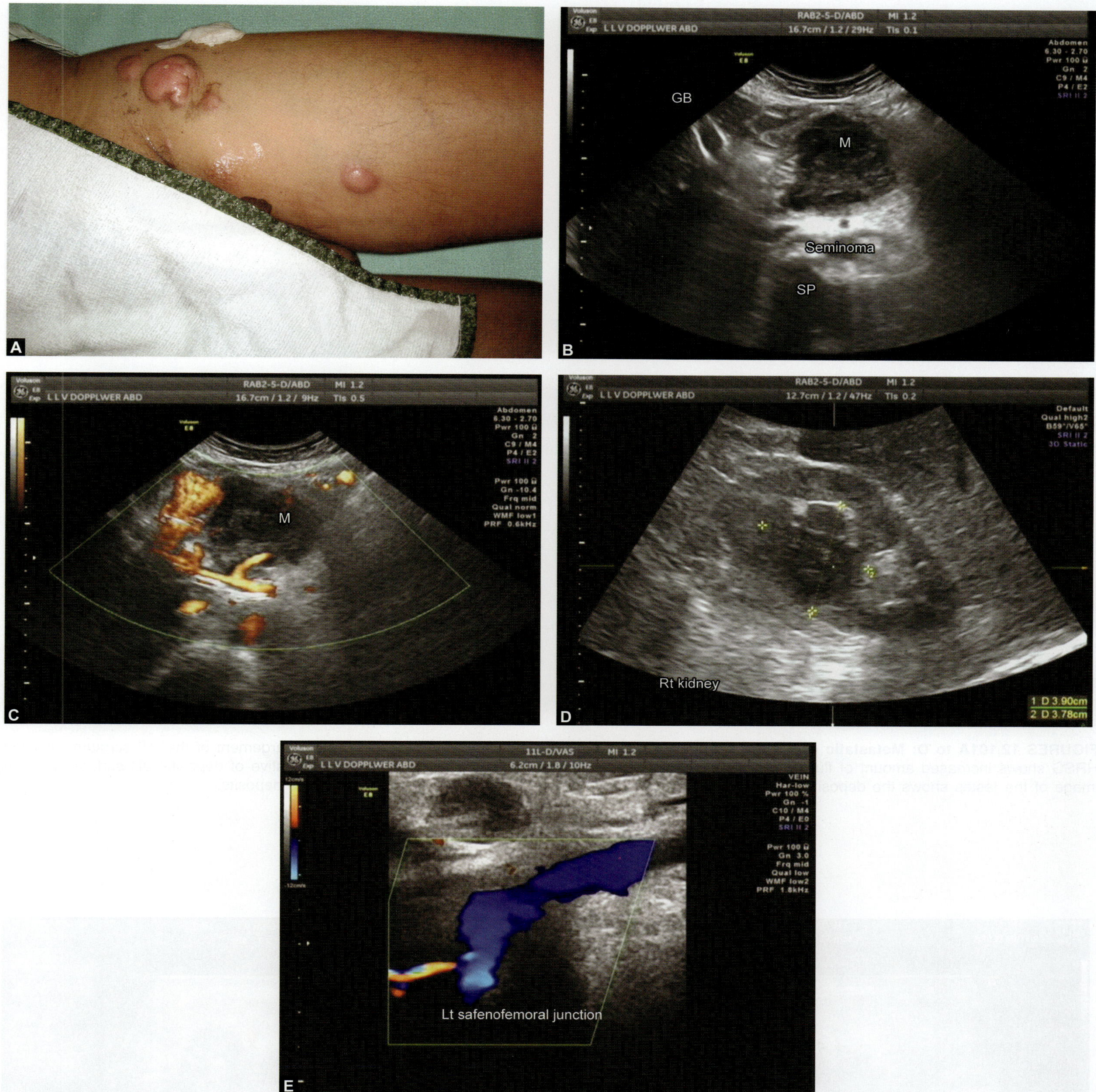

FIGURES 12.100A to E: Seminoma testes with multiple metastasis. An operated case of seminoma testes presented with disseminated metastasis. The clinical image shows multiple cutaneous metastatic deposits. Multiple nodes are also seen in retroperitoneum splaying the vessels. Right kidney also shows metastatic deposits. There is also evidence of enlarged nodal shadows seen in the left inguinal region.

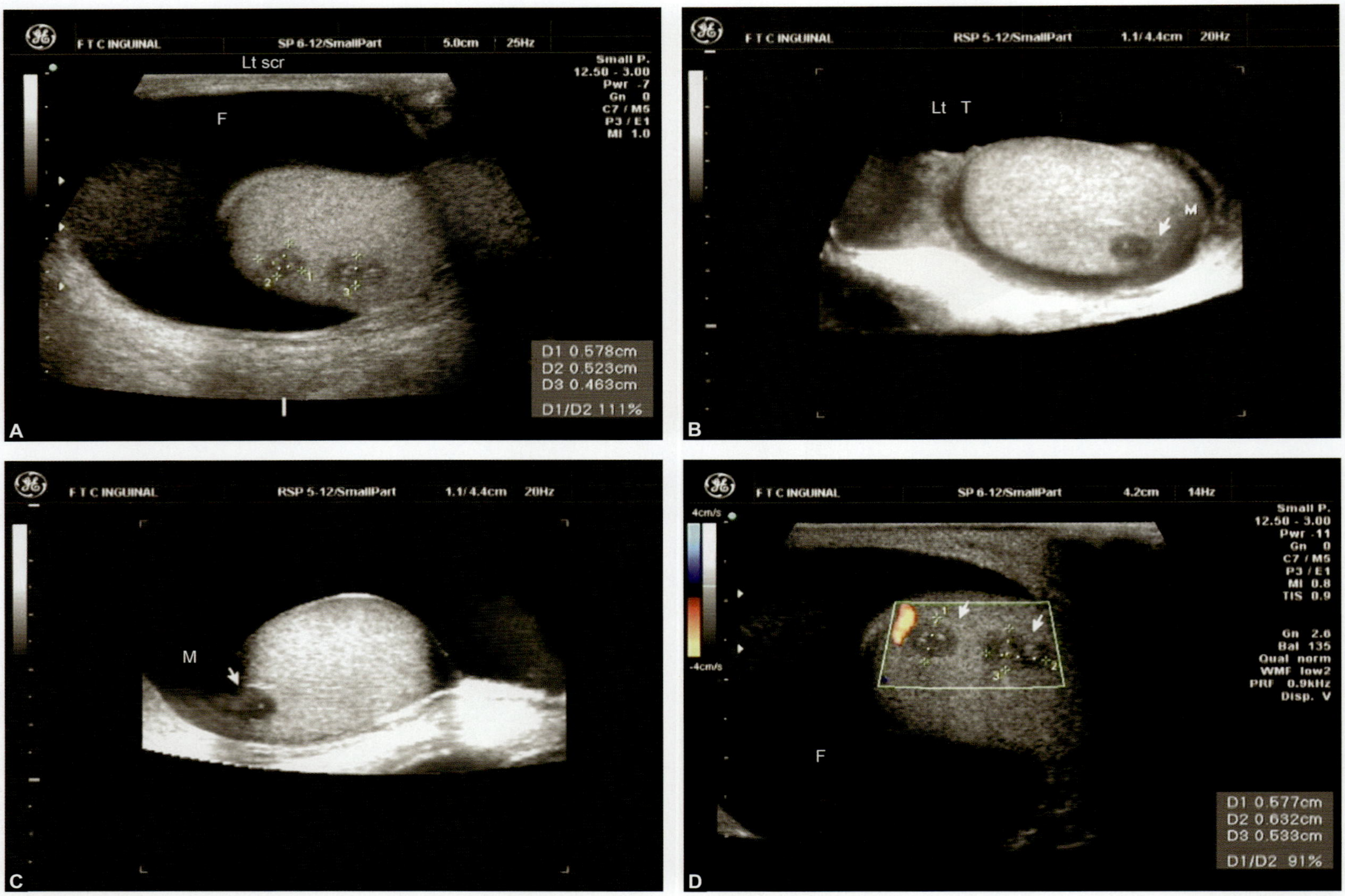

FIGURES 12.101A to D: Metastatic deposits of leukemia. A known patient of leukemia presented with enlargement of the left scrotum with pain. HRSG shows increased amount of fluid in the scrotal sac. The testes shows irregular hypoechoic foci suggestive of deposits. 3D surface rendering image of the testes shows the deposits clearly. On color Doppler imaging shows poor flow in the metastasis deposits.

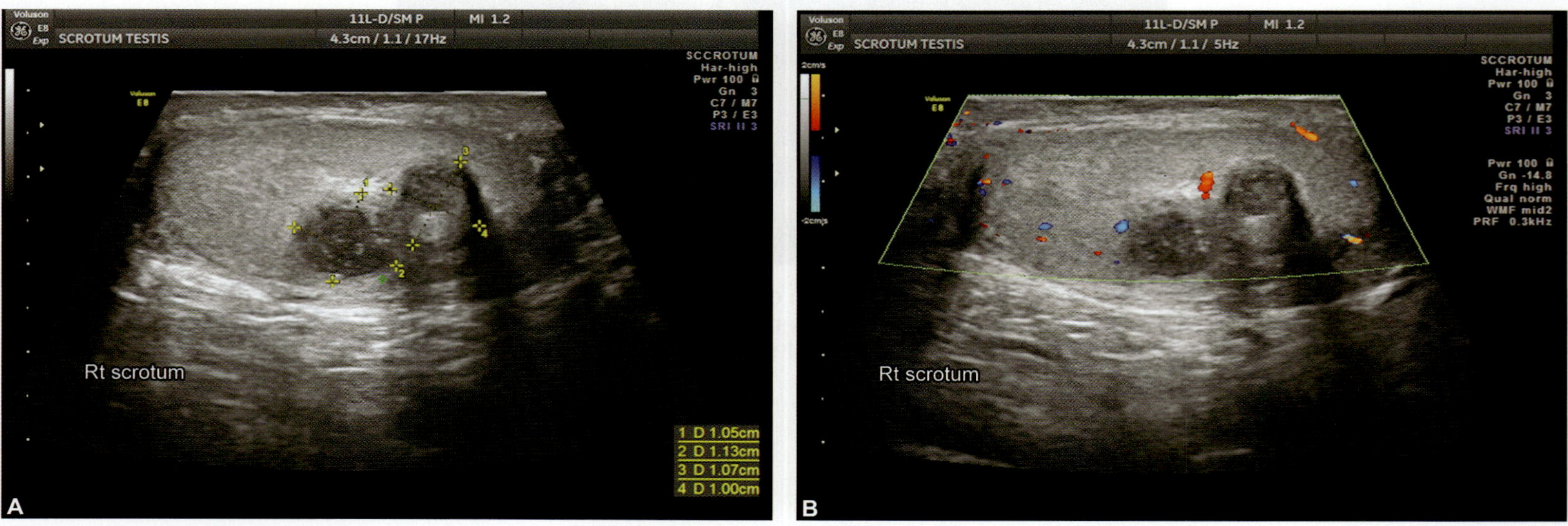

FIGURES 12.102A and B

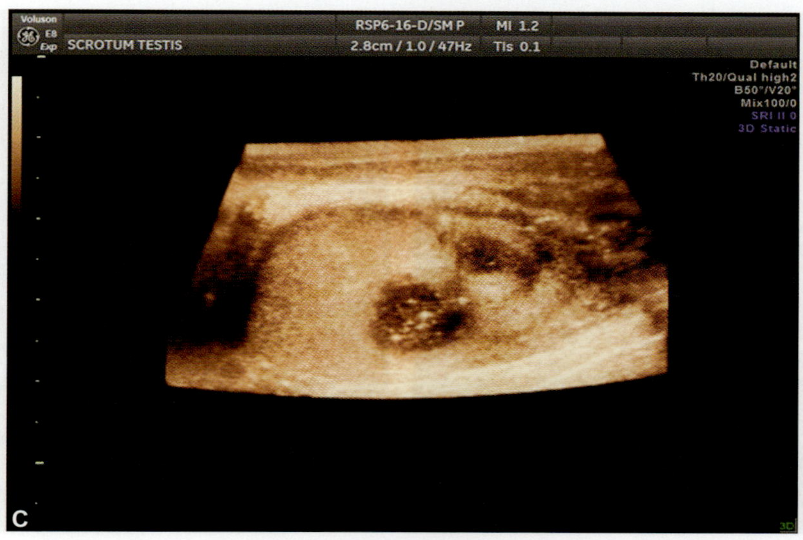

FIGURE 12.102C

FIGURES 12.102A to C: Metastatic deposits in the testes. HRSG shows hypoechoic nodular masses in the right testes in a patient of malignant melanoma. Hypoechoic ill defined masses are seen in the testes. But no necrosis is seen in them. 3D imaging shows metastatic deposits.

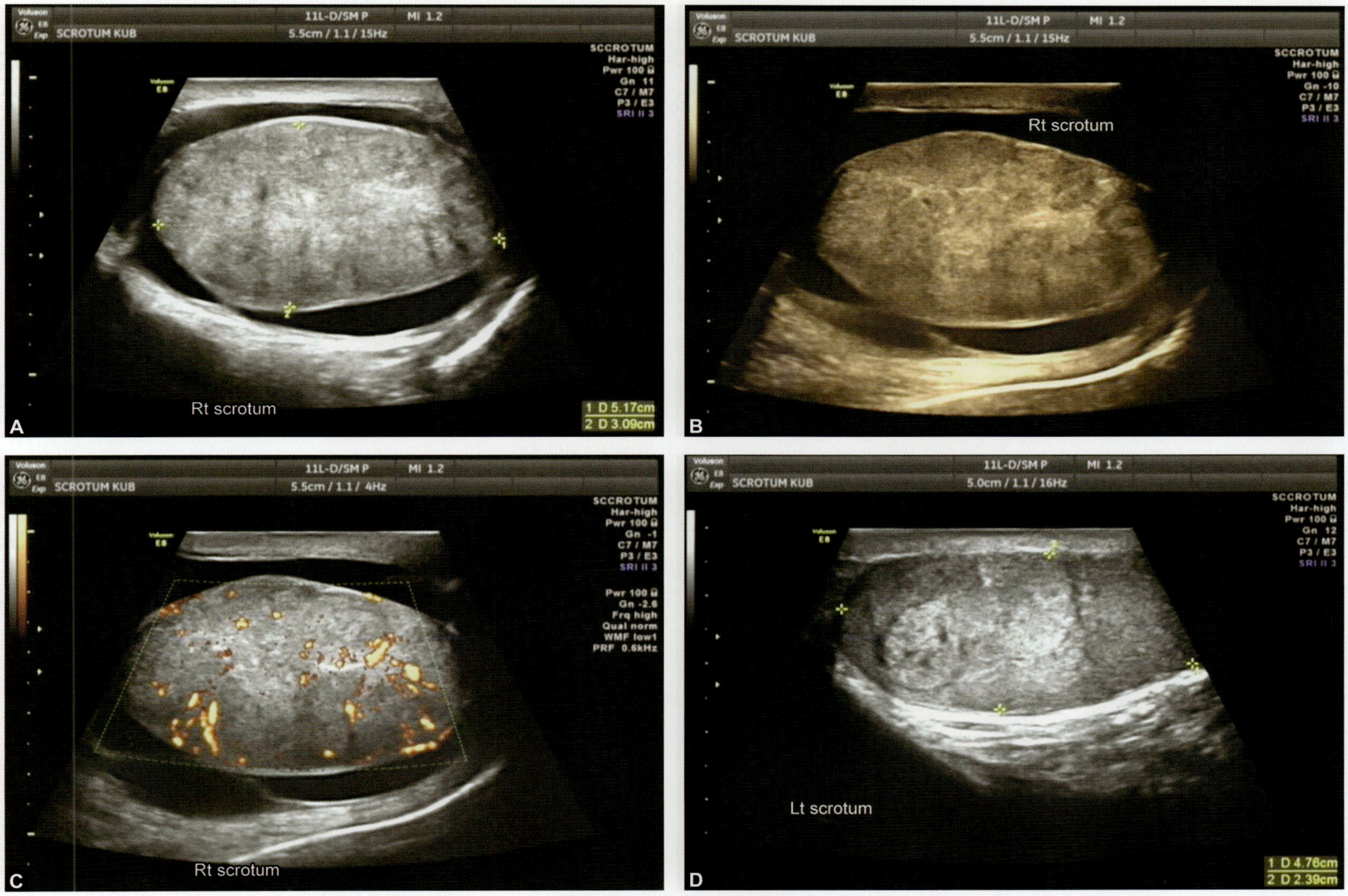

FIGURES 12.103A to D

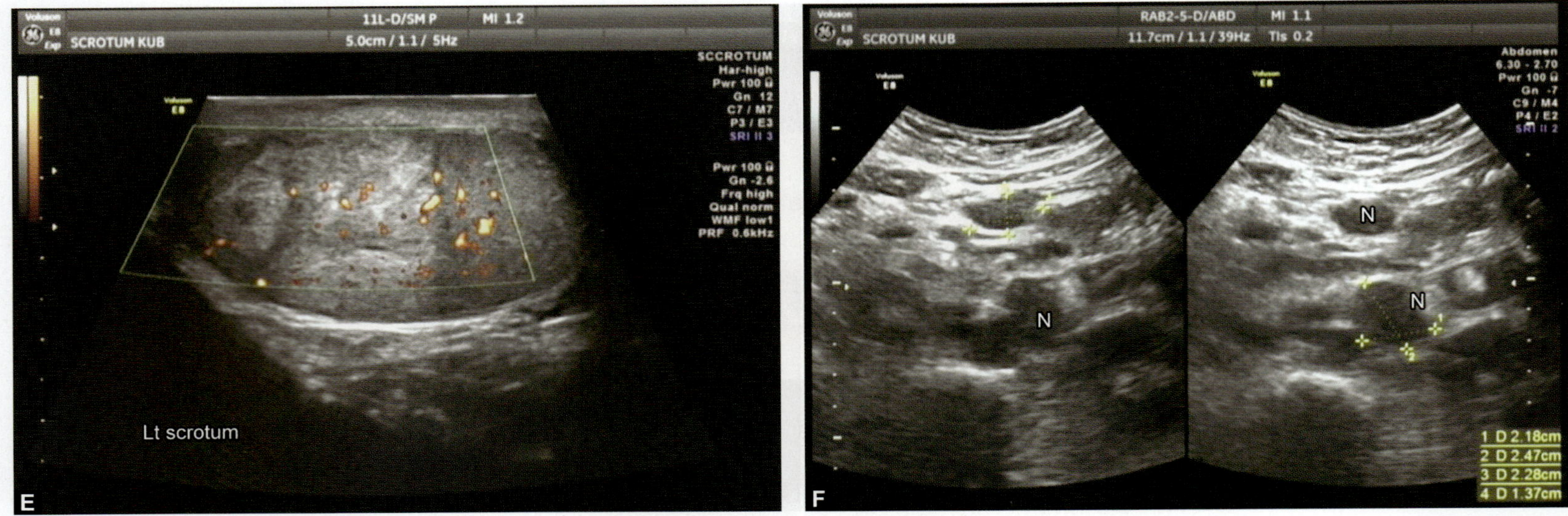

FIGURES 12.103E and F

FIGURES 12.103A to F: Lymphoma testes. A patient presented with disuse enlargement of both testes. HRSG shows heterogeneous enlargement of both testes. Normal granular texture is lost on both sides. Irregular ill defined areas are seen in the testes. But no necrosis is seen in them. On color flow imaging, poor flow is seen in both the testes. On abdominal ultrasound, multiple enlarged lymph nodes seen in retroperitoneum. Biopsy of node confirms lymphoma. Lymphoma is one of the main causes of bilateral testicular enlargement.

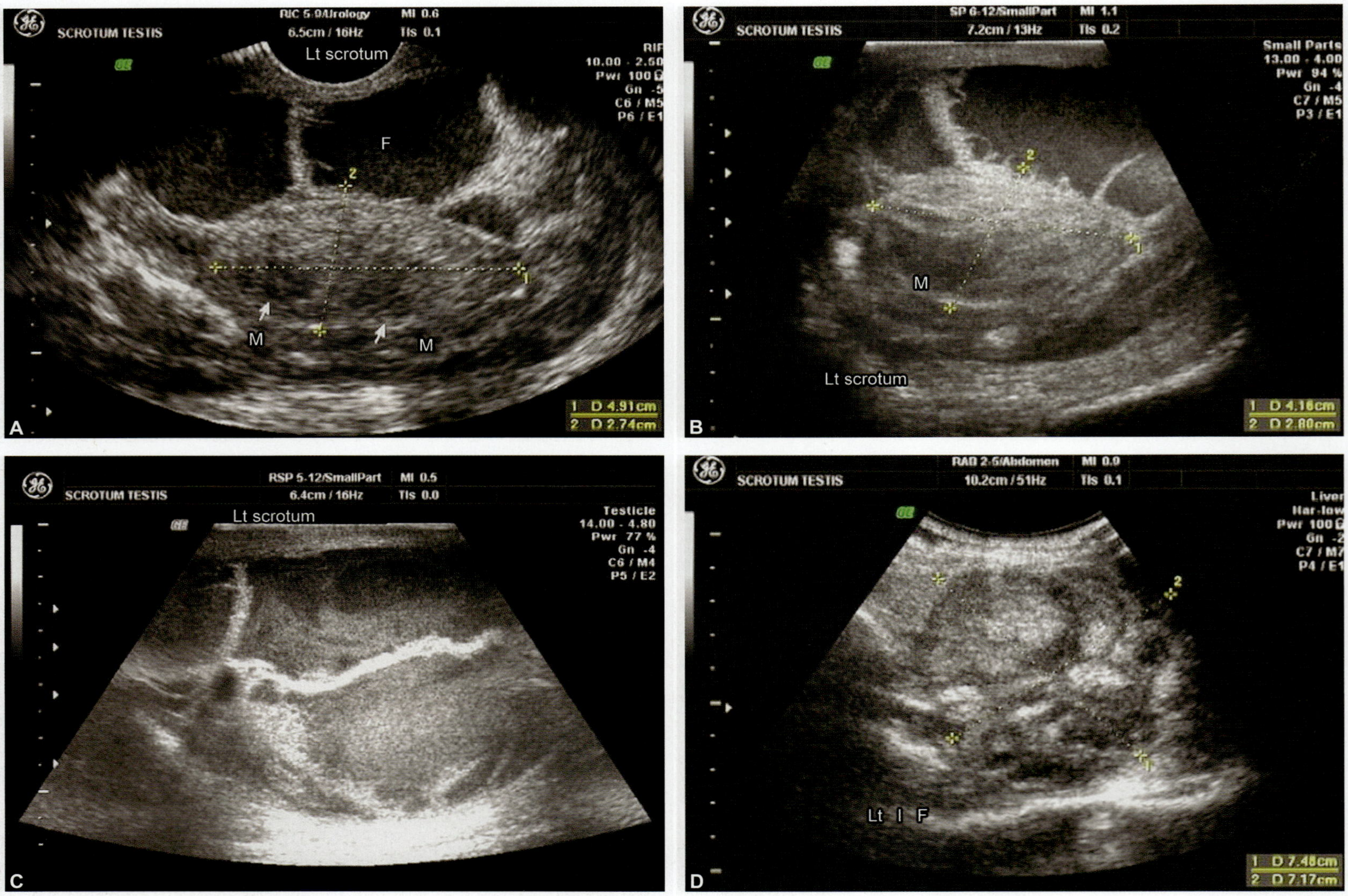

FIGURES 12.104A to D

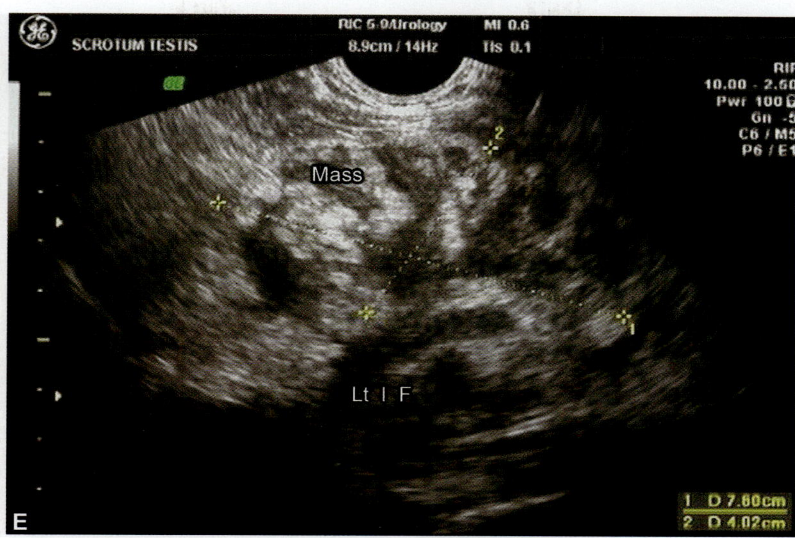

FIGURE 12.104E

FIGURES 12.104A to E: Lymphoma testes. A known patient of lymphoma presented with left scrotal swelling. HRSG shows low-level echo collection in the left scrotum. Echogenic bands are also seen in the scrotal sac. The left testes shows irregular hypoechoic foci, which are seen in the testes suggestive of deposit. Thick collection is also seen in the testes. Heterogeneous masses are also seen in the left iliac fossa. They are seen invading the bowel loops. Nodal masses are also seen in the left inguinal region. Biopsy of the mass confirms lymphoma.

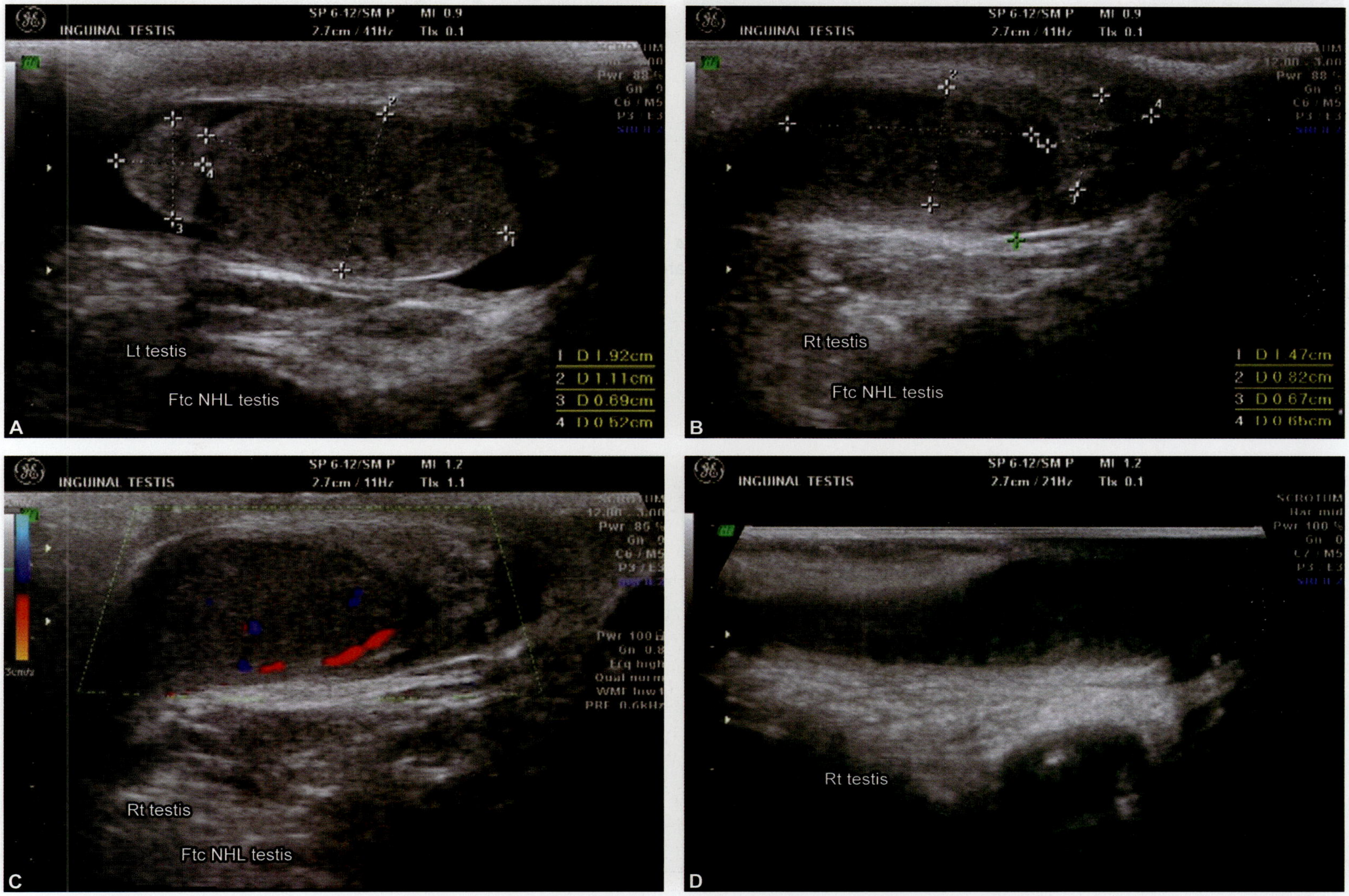

FIGURES 12.105A to D: FUC of NHL. A known case of NHL presented with left testicular swelling. HRSG shows diffuse enlargement of left testes. The testes shows inhomogeneous texture and coarse parenchyma. Hypoechoic areas are seen in the testes. But no evidence of any focal mass is seen in the testes. On color flow imaging, low flow is seen in the testes. The right testes is normal in appearance. No focal mass is seen in the testes.

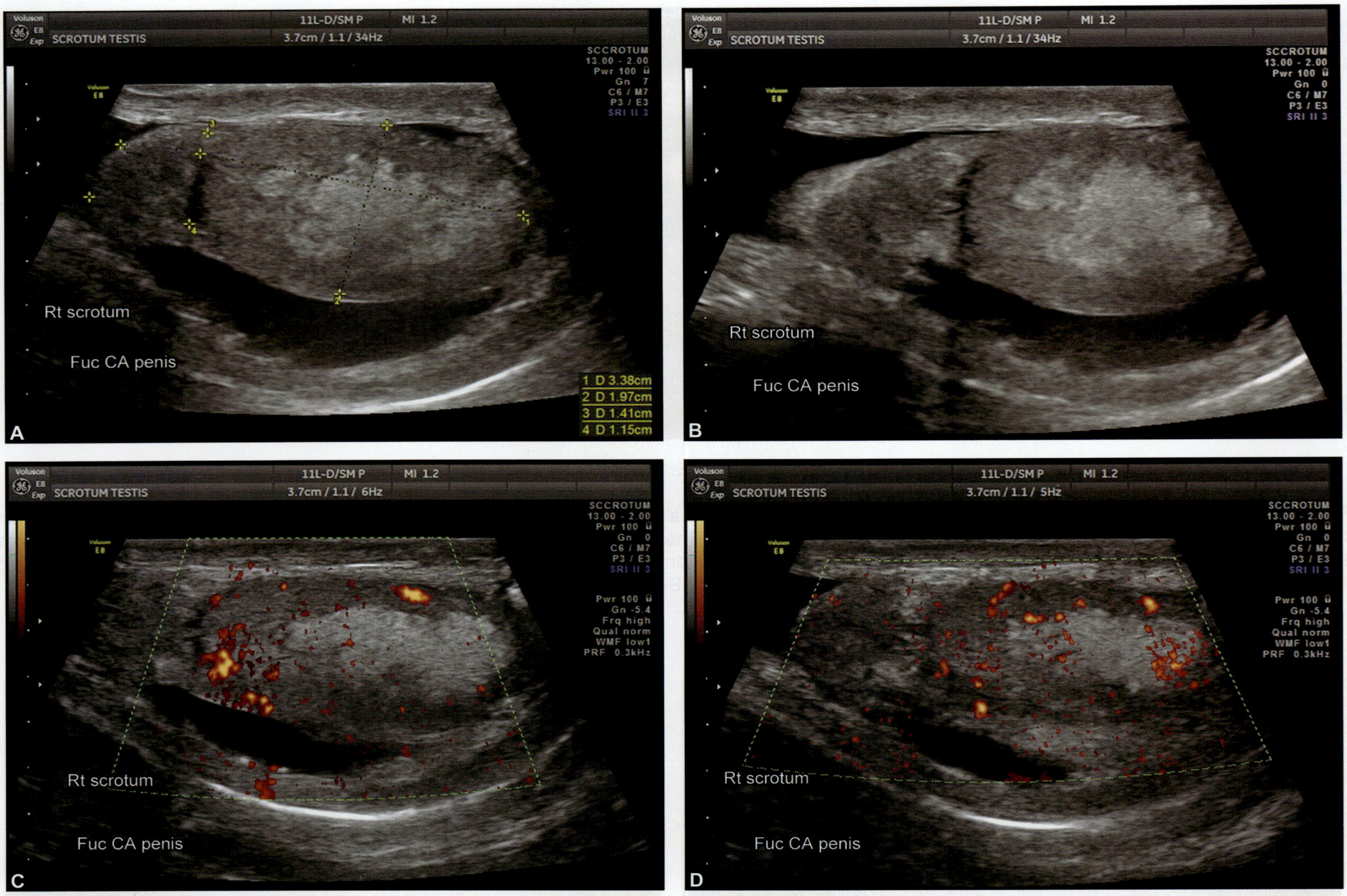

FIGURES 12.106A to D: Testicular mets CA penis. A known case of CA penis presented with testicular swelling. HRSG shows diffuse enlargement of the testes. The testicular texture is heterogeneous. Hypoechoic areas are seen in the testes. The epididymis is also edematous and enlarged. On color flow imaging, moderate flow is seen in the testes.

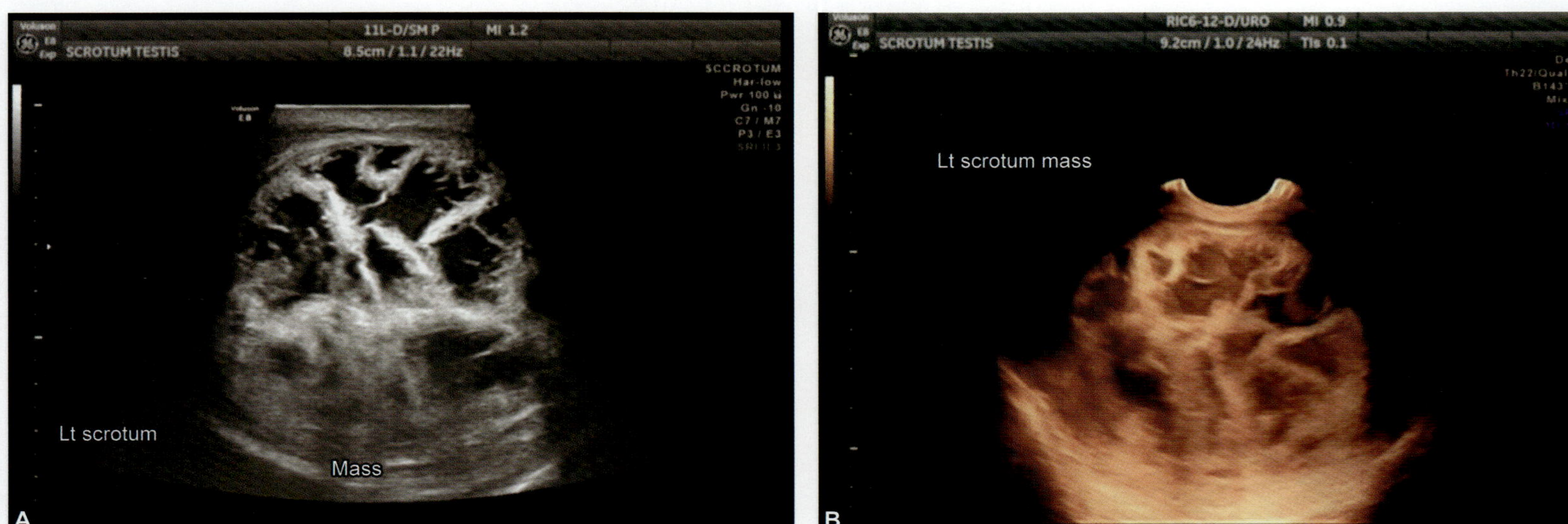

FIGURES 12.107A and B

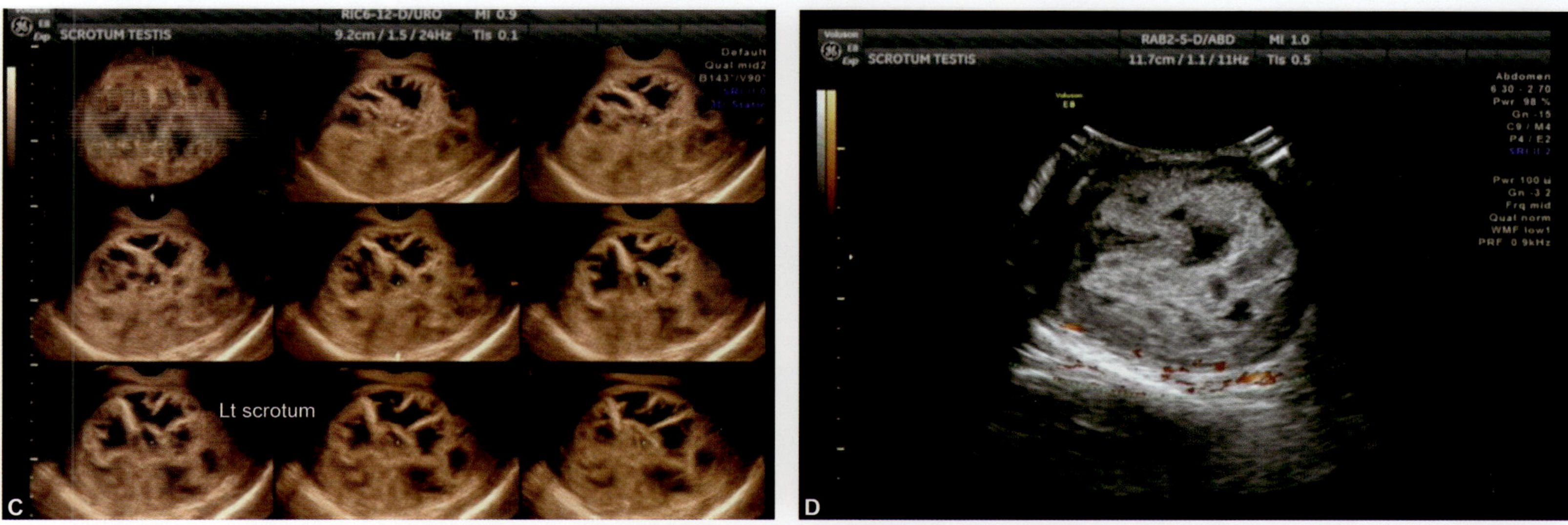

FIGURES 12.107C and D

FIGURES 12.107A to D: Teratoma testes. A patient presented with hard swelling in the left scrotum. HRSG shows a big heterogeneous mass in the left scrotum. It shows multiple cystic areas. Thick septa are seen in the mass. Normal testicular texture is lost. The TUI imaging shows heterogeneous texture of the mass. Biopsy of the mass confirms teratoma testis.

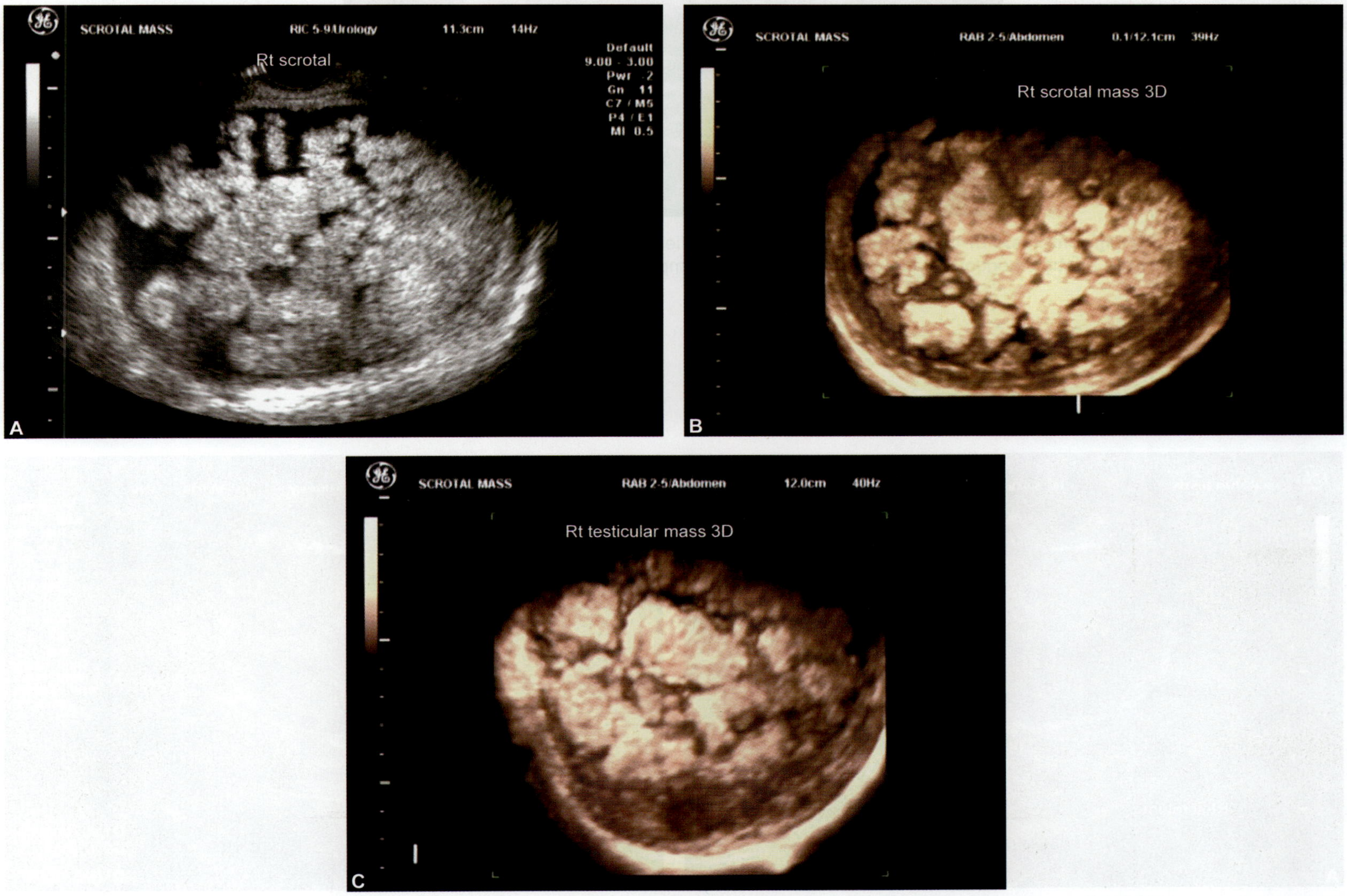

FIGURES 12.108A to C: Huge testicular hematoma presented as mass. A patient with huge right scrotal mass. HRSG of the scrotal shows big heterogeneous disorganized mass-filling whole of the scrotal sac. No evidence of any calcification or cystic degeneration is seen in it. Initially the mass was mistaken as testicular tumor. However, the testes was seen lying at the root of the scrotum. It was displaced and small in size. 3D surface-rendering image of the mass shows lobulated structure of the mass. The biopsy of the mass confirmed disorganized chronic hematoma.

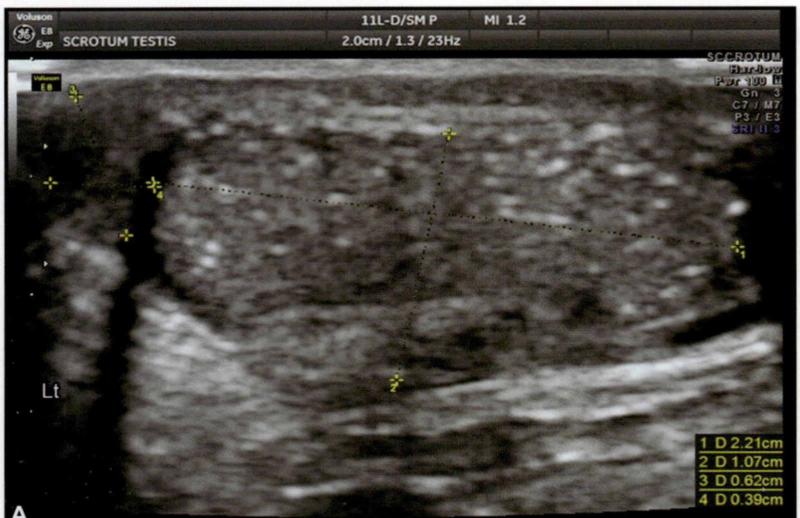

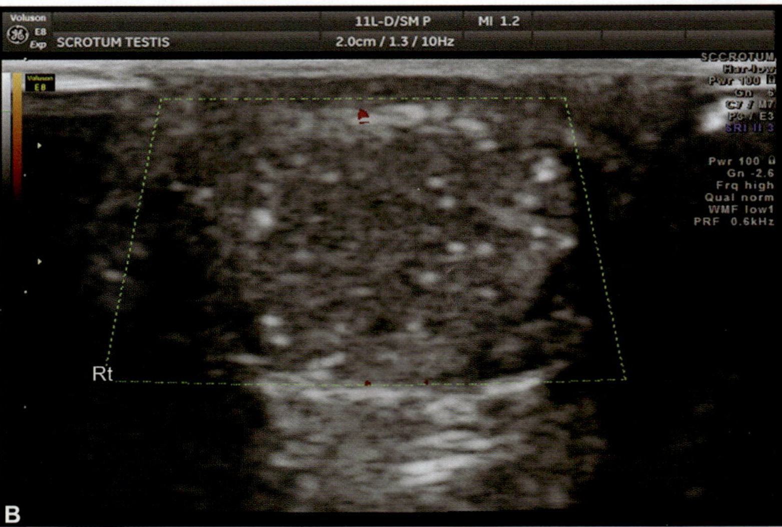

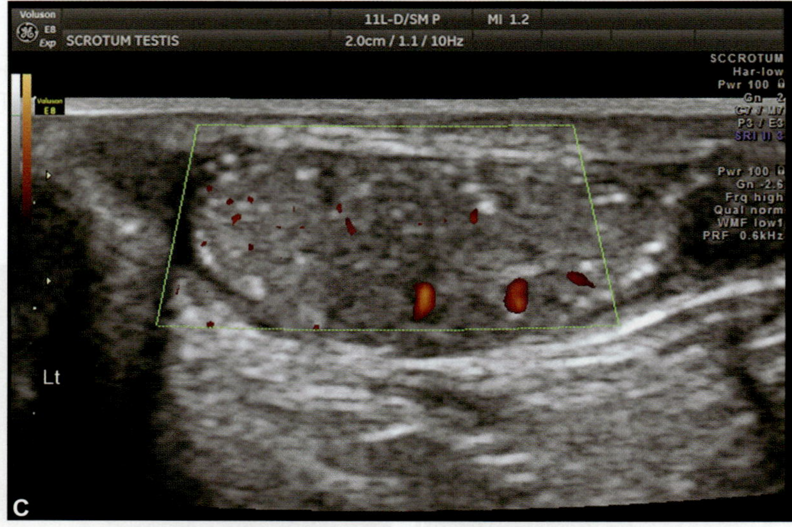

FIGURES 12.109A to C: Microlithiasis of the testes. Multiple small-calcified specks are seen distributed in both the testes parenchyma suggestive of micro-calcification. They are bright echogenic shadows, which are not accompanied acoustic shadowing. Micro-calcification is known to be precancerous condition of the testes.

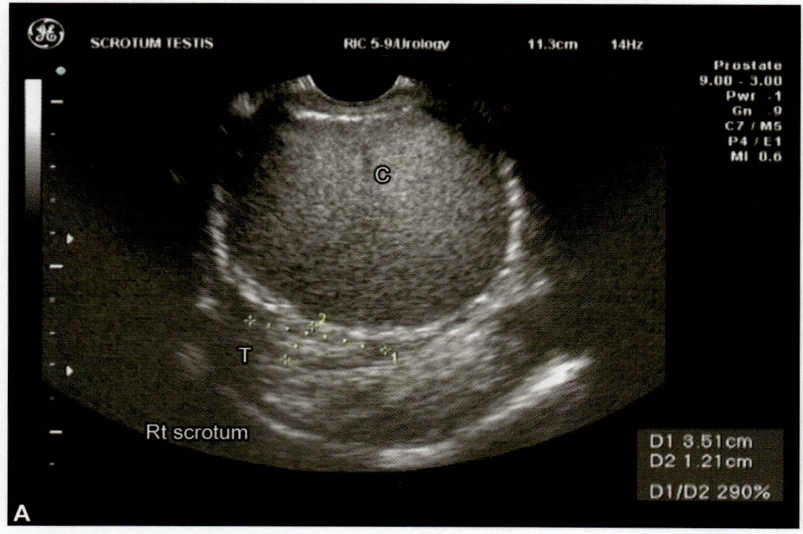

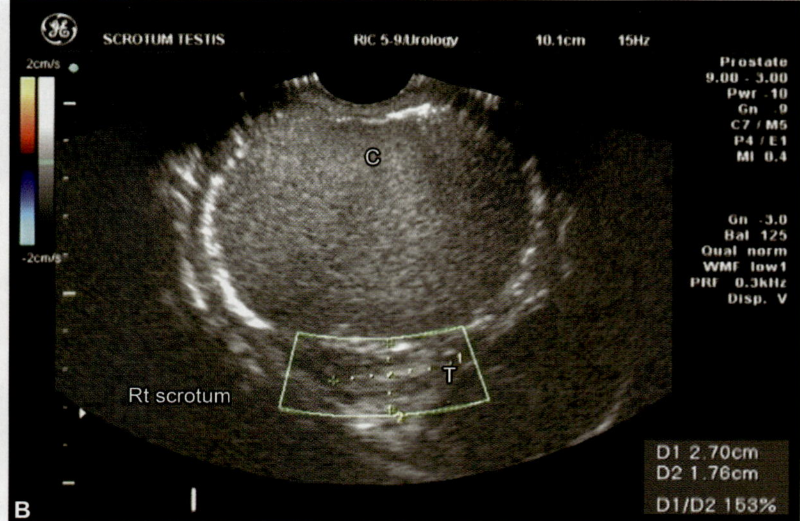

FIGURES 12.110A and B

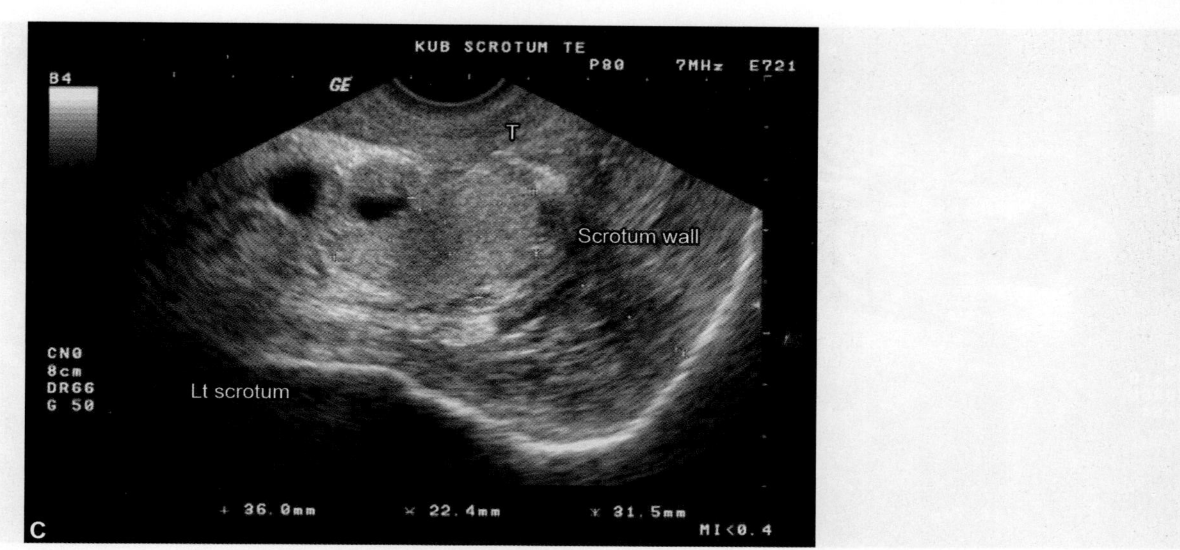

FIGURE 12.110C

FIGURES 12.110A to C: Chronic scrotal collection. HRSG shows large amount of fluid collection in the scrotal sac. It is seen in the extra testicular space. The periphery of the collection shows echogenic calcified specks fixed with the peripheral wall. The testes is seen displaced down and compressed by the fluid.

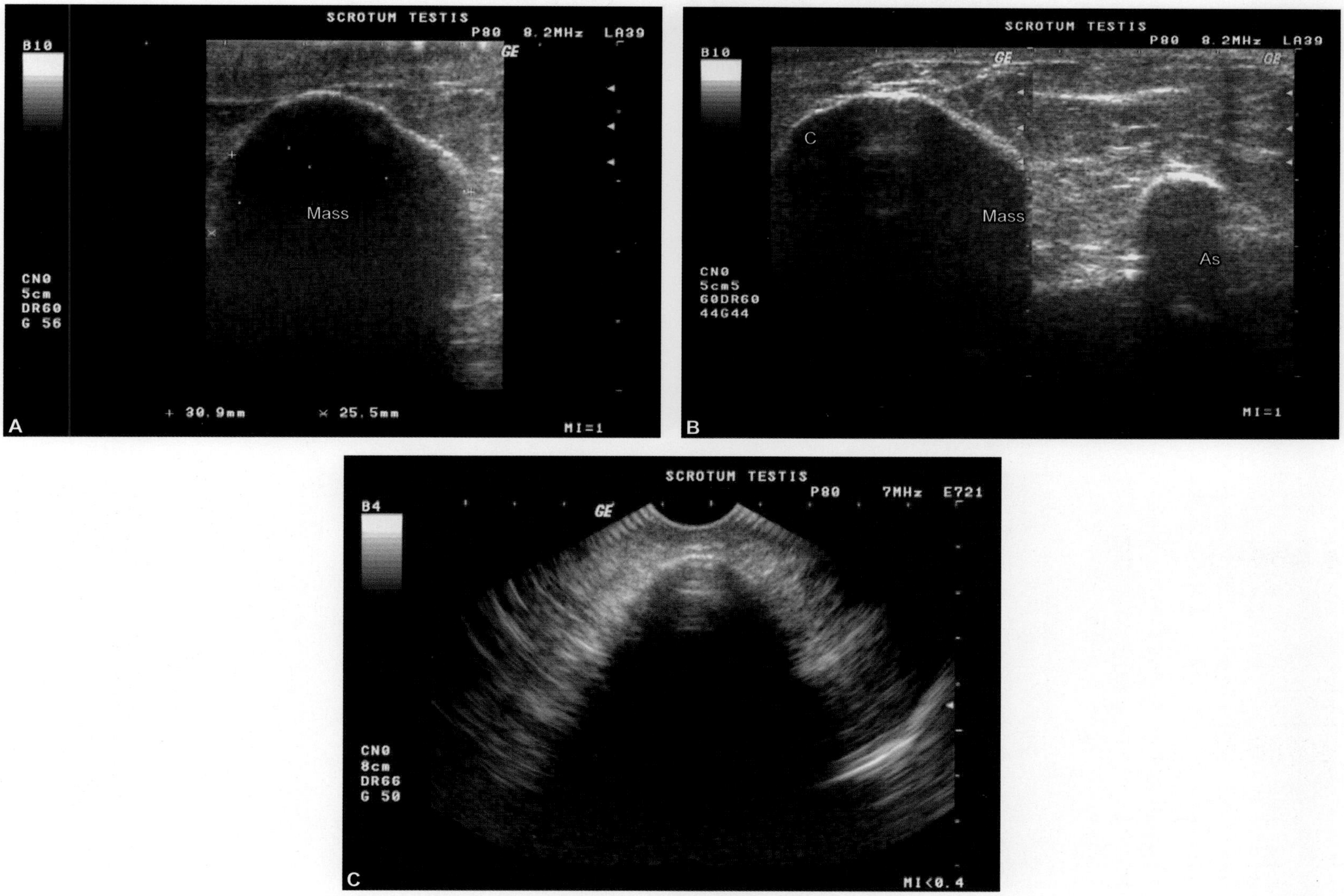

FIGURES 12.111A to C: Calcified hematoma in the scrotal wall. A patient presented with mass in the left scrotal wall. HRSG shows densely calcified mass. The mass shows dense calcification. The calcification makes strong acoustic shadowing, masking the mass. Peripheral ring calcification is seen in the mass. Postoperative findings confirmed calcified hematoma.

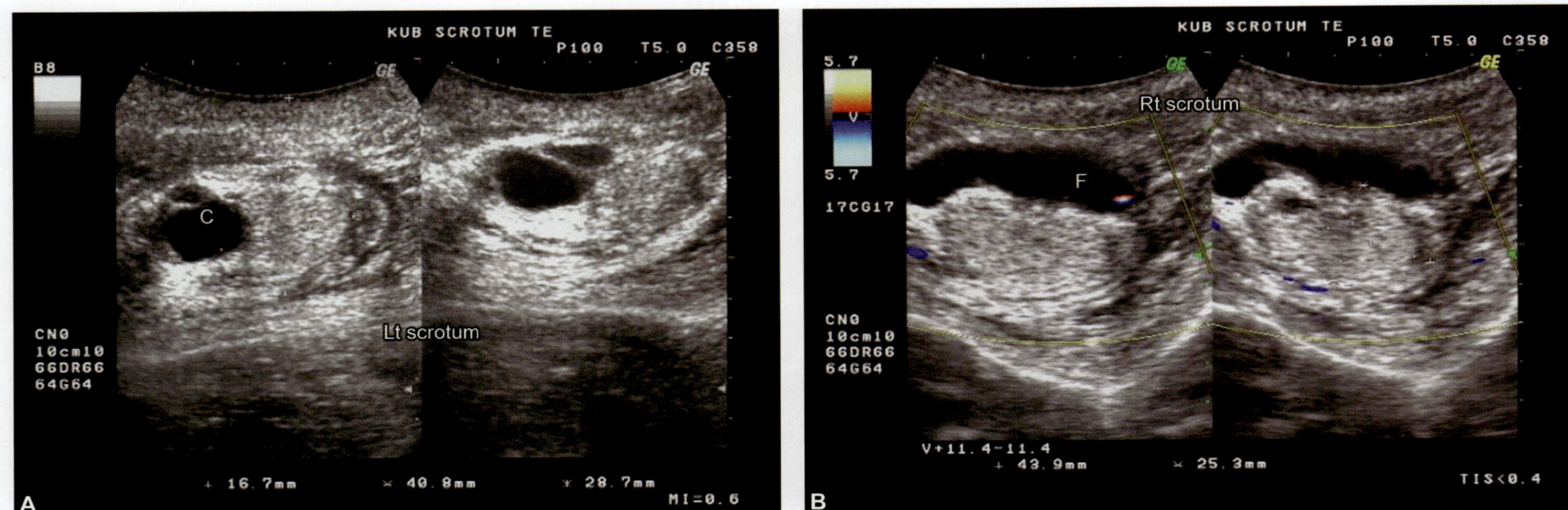

FIGURES 12.112A and B: Bilateral atrophic testes. HRSG shows bilateral small testes. They are irregular in outline. Cystic necrosis is also seen in them. The scrotal wall shows marked thickening. Therefore the testes was not clinically palpable. There is also evidence of cystic degeneration seen in the left testes. On color flow imaging poor flow seen in the testes. Small amount of fluid collection is also seen.

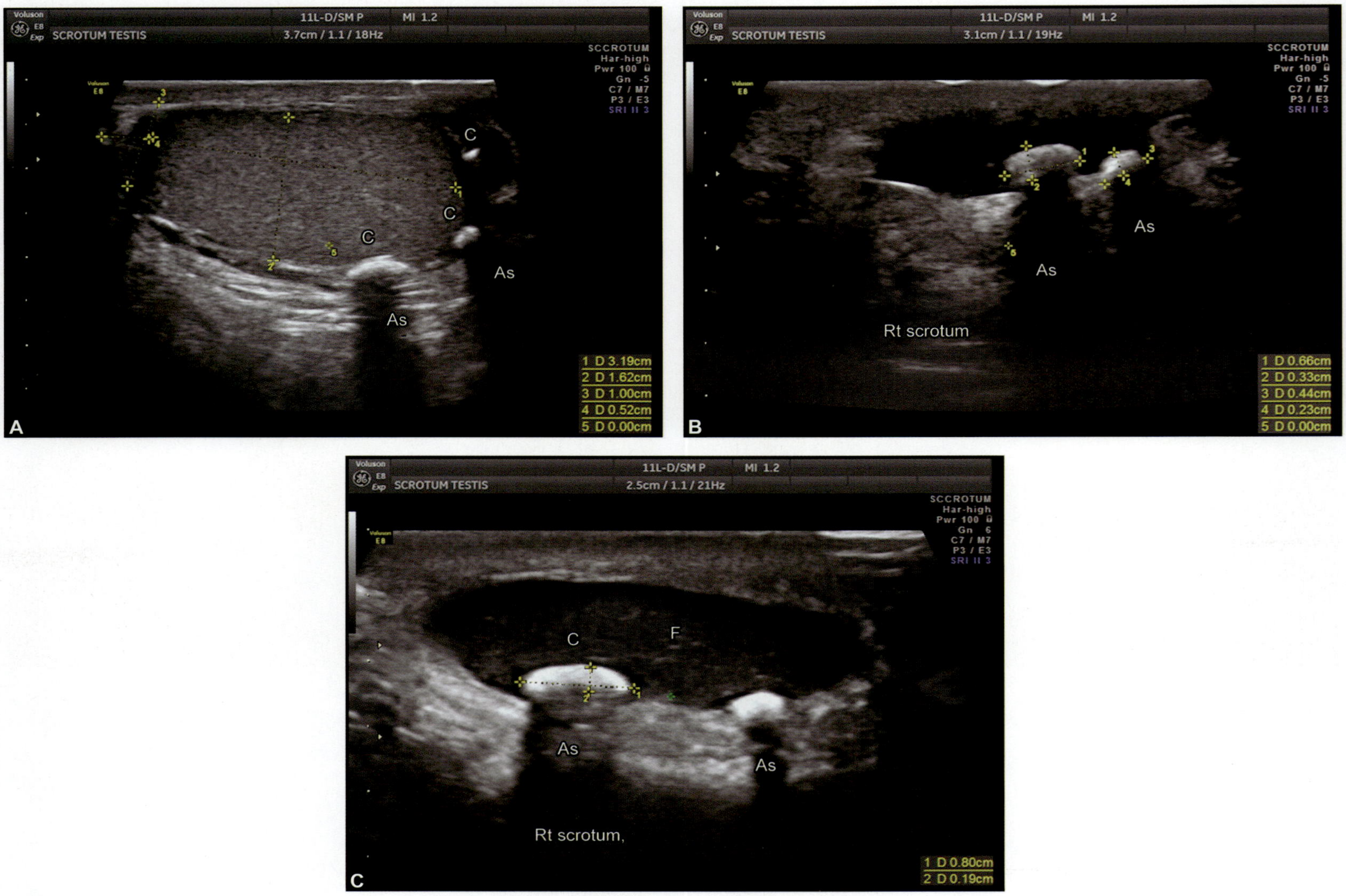

FIGURES 12.113A to C: Scrotal pearls. HRSG shows multiple echogenic calcified shadows in tunica vaginalis. They are accompanied with acoustic shadowing suggestive of scrotal pearls.

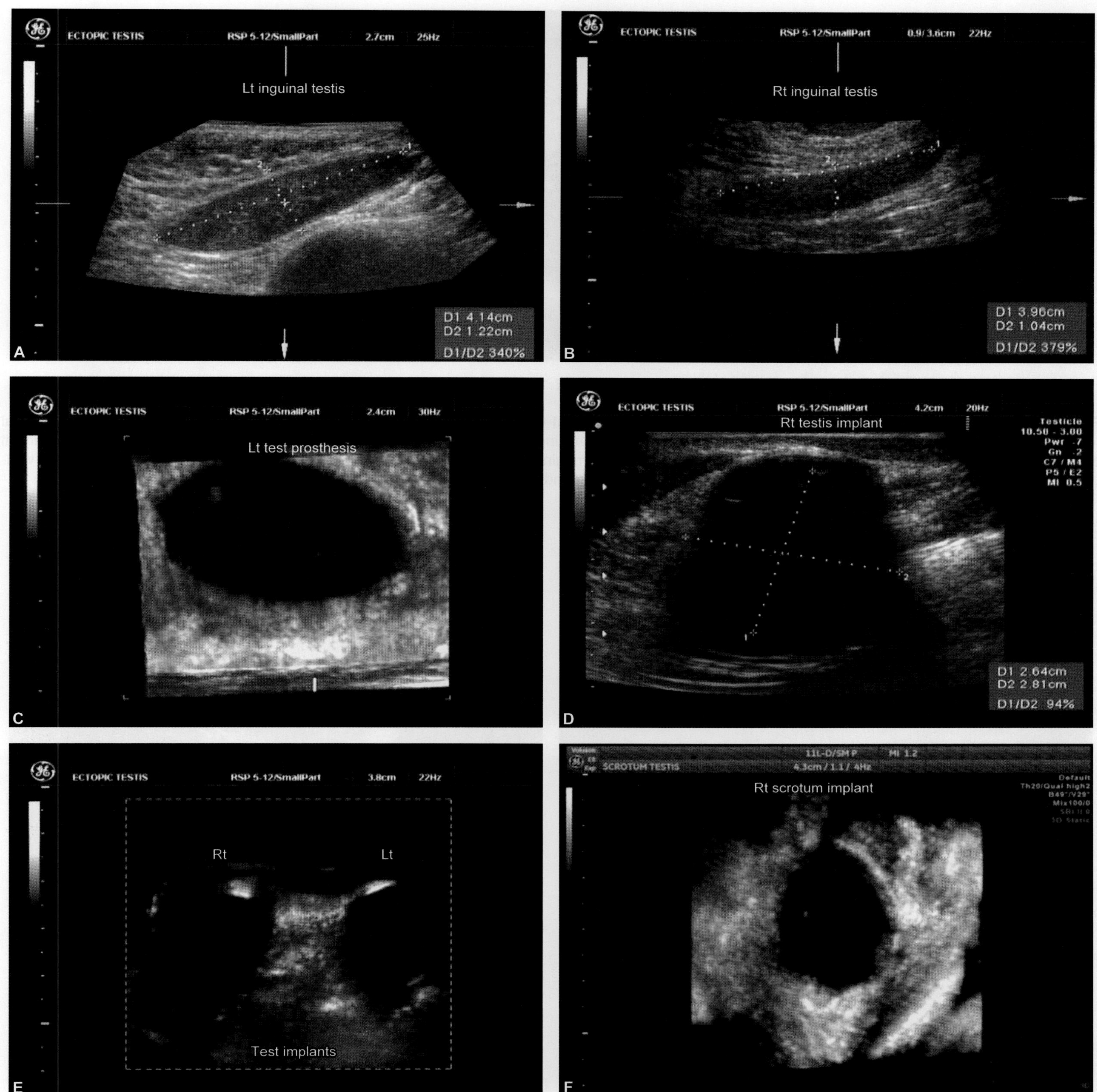

FIGURES 12.114A to F

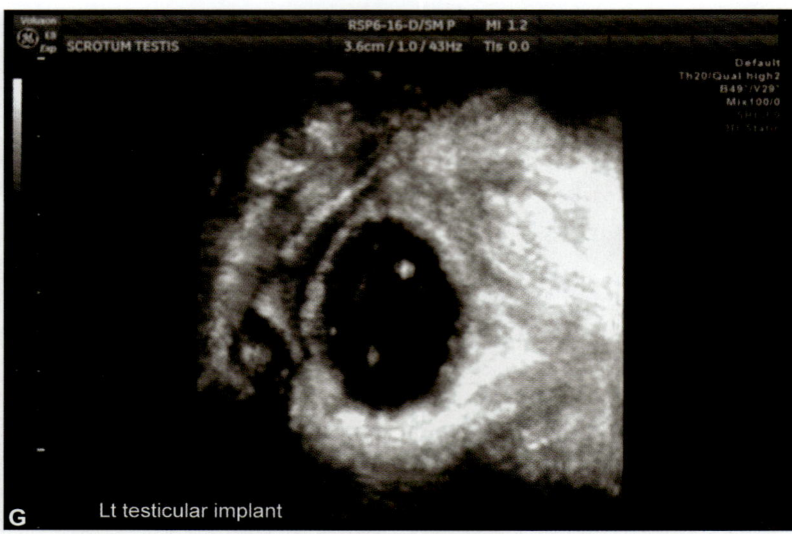

FIGURE 12.114G

FIGURES 12.114A to G: Atrophic inguinal testes with bilateral scrotal testes implants. A patient presented with bilateral small atrophic inguinal testes. The testes is seen as hypoechoic flat band like shadows in the inguinal canal. 3D imaging of the testes shows the testes in much clinical details. On color Doppler imaging, low flow is seen in the testes. 3D imaging of the both scrotum show the testicular implant. They are seen as well-defined homogeneous anechoic masses. The implants attenuate the sound beam making them anechoic on HRSG.

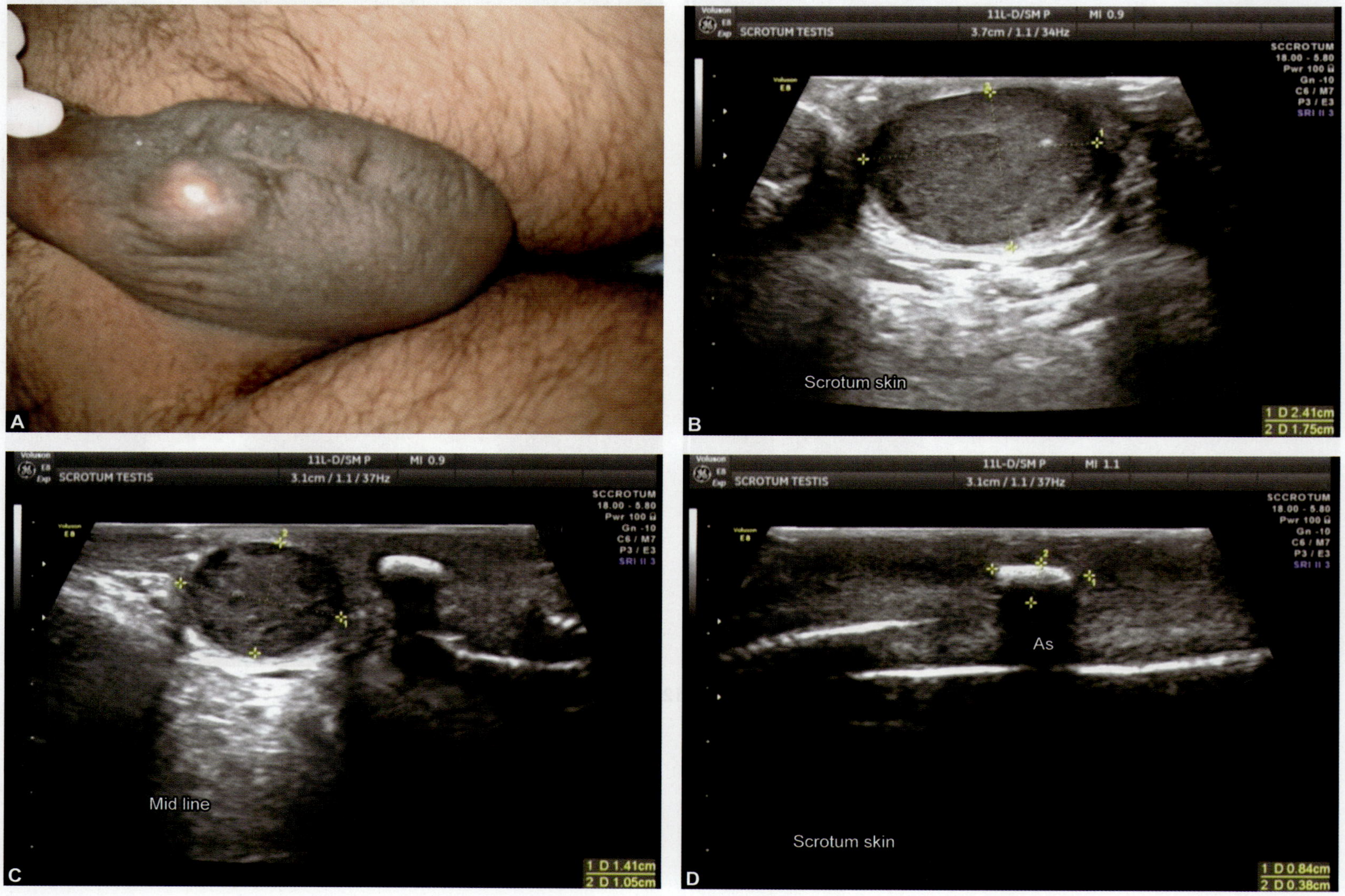

FIGURES 12.115A to D

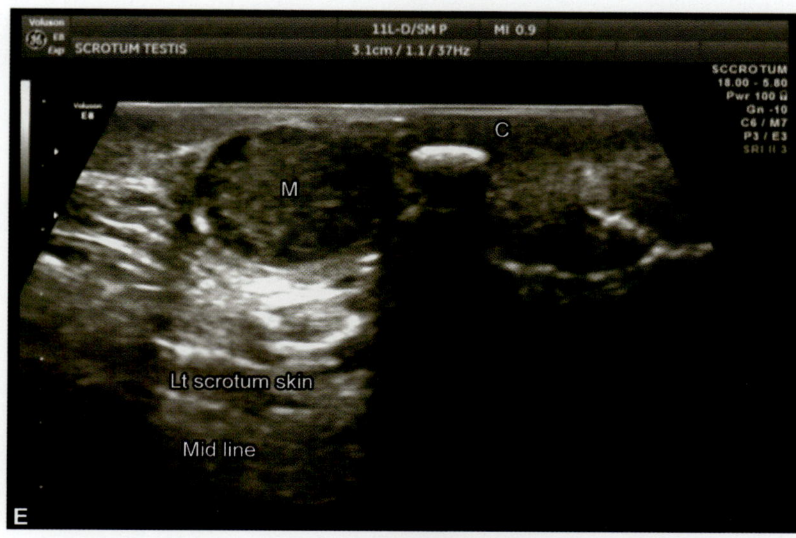

FIGURE 12.115E

FIGURES 12.115A to E: Sebaceous cyst. HRSG shows well defined low level echo complex masses in the mid line along the raphe. Homogeneous echoes are seen in them. On color flow imaging, no flow is seen in them. No septation is seen. There is also evidence of echogenic calcified nodular shadow seen in the subcutaneous tissue plane in left scrotal skin. It is accompanied with dense acoustic shadowing. They are separate from the testes. No other focal mass seen. Both testes are normal in size. A thin walled cyst is seen in the left scrotum coming out form the tunica albuginea. On color flow imaging normal flow is seen in testes.

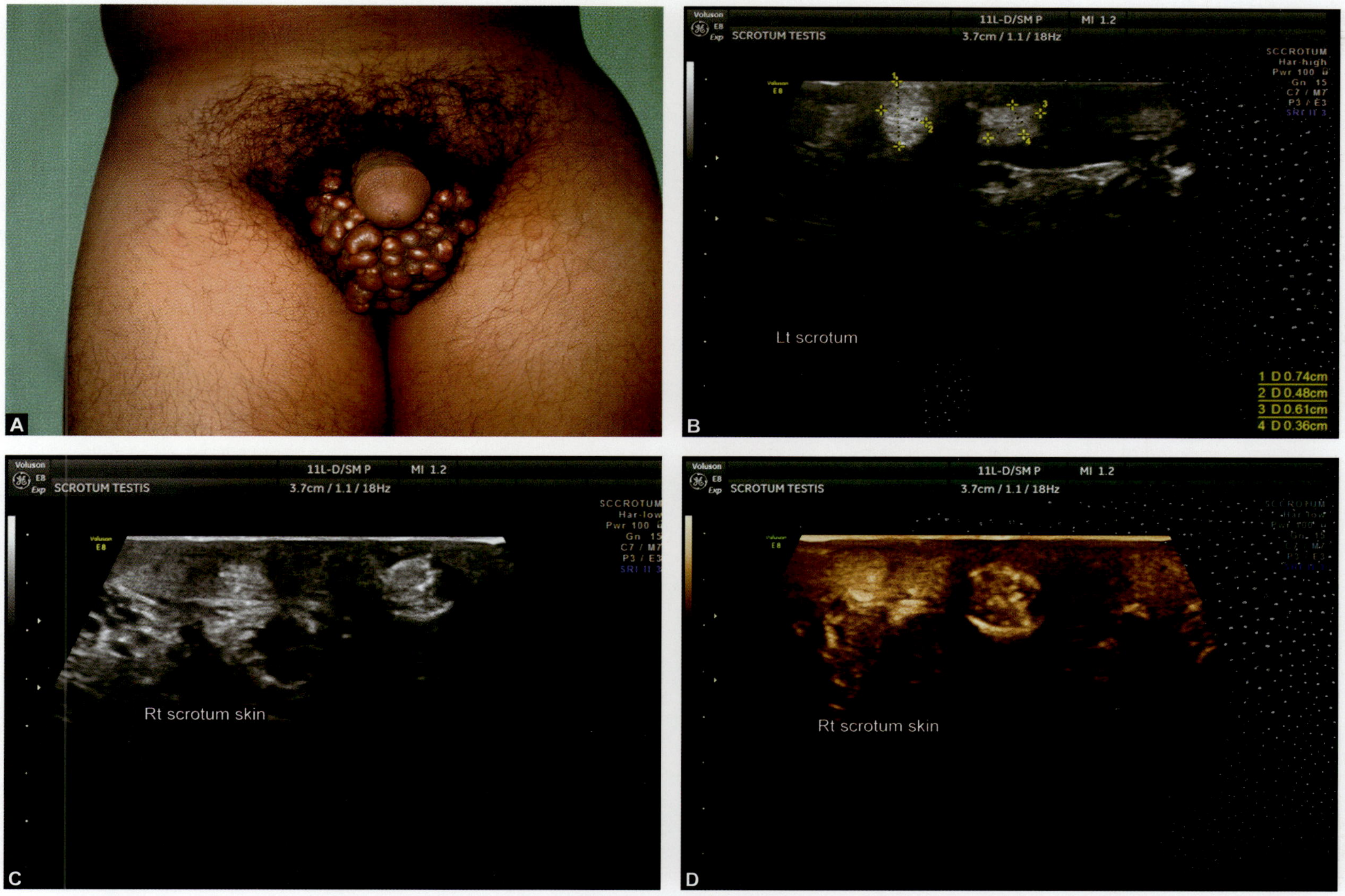

FIGURES 12.116A to D

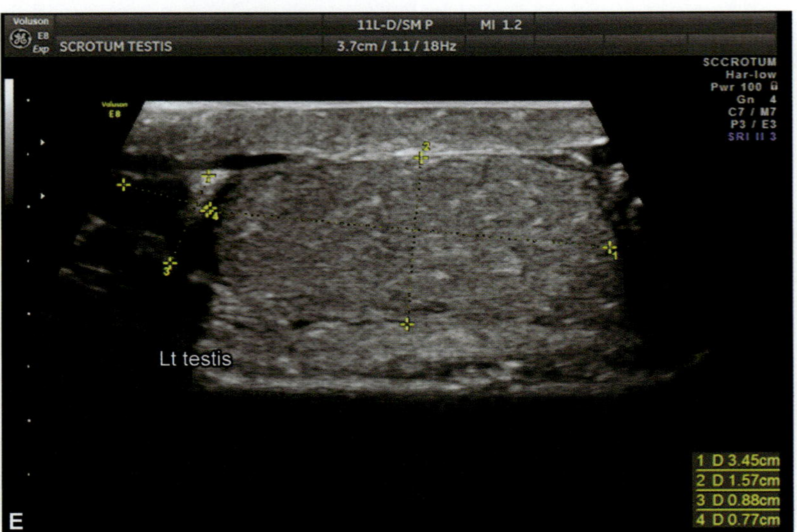

FIGURE 12.116E

FIGURES 12.116A to E: Chronic granulomatous wart. HRSG shows multiple echogenic foci on the scrotal skin on both sides. Echogenic punctate calcification is seen in them. No necrosis is seen. No cystic degeneration is seen. However, both testes are normal.

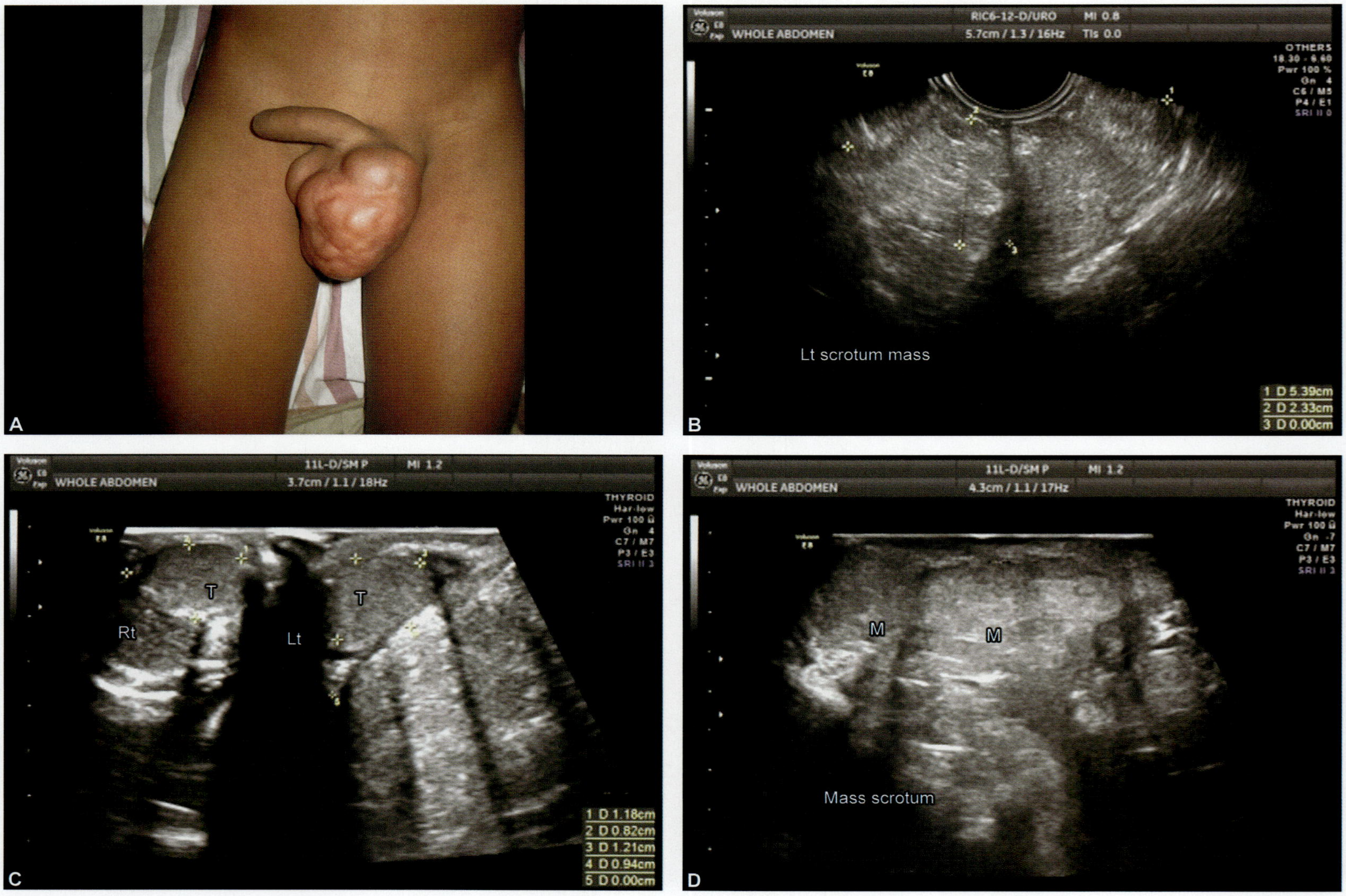

FIGURES 12.117A to D: Lipoma scrotum. A 7-years-old boy presented with multiple soft tissue masses over the scrotum. HRSG shows well defined echogenic masses in the scrotal wall. The echo texture is similar to the fat. No suggestion of any calcification is seen in them. They are confined to the skin. However, both testes are normal in appearance. Findings are suggestive of multiple lipomas.

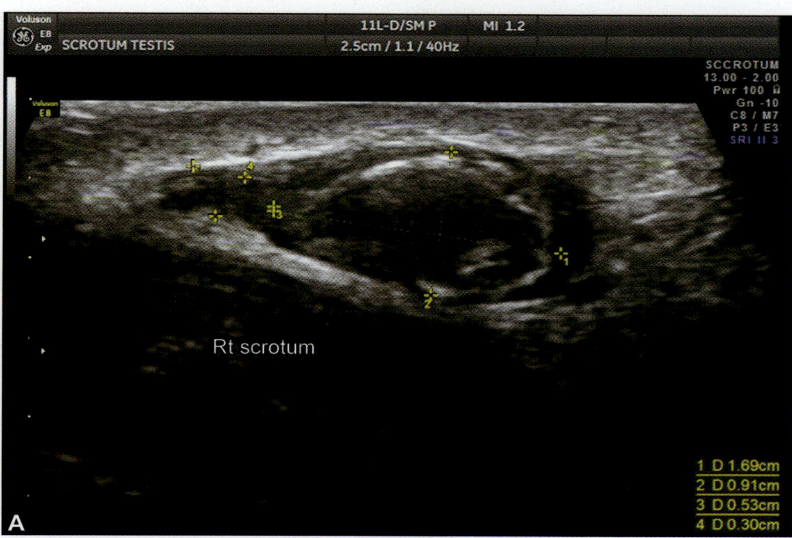

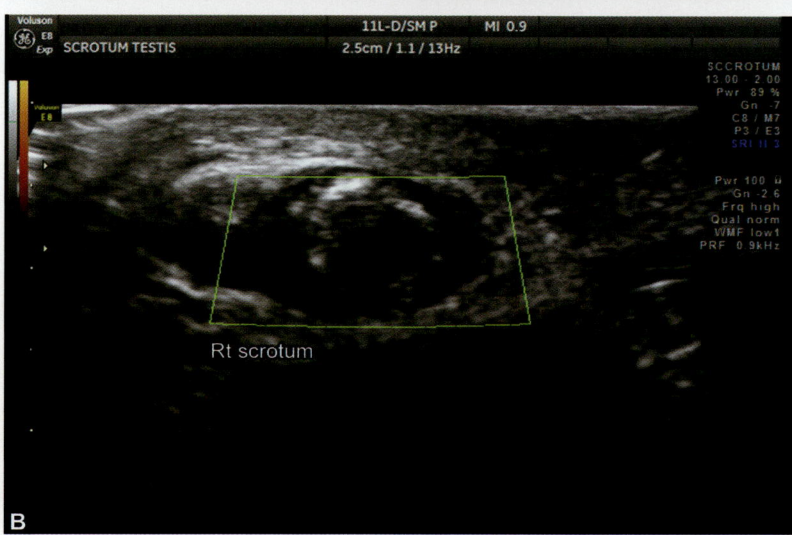

FIGURES 12.118A and B: Atrophic testes. A patient presented with non palpable testes in the Rt scrotum. HRSG shows an irregular ill defined hypoechoic nodular shadow in the Rt scrotum. It shows dense echogenic calcification. Hypoechoic areas are seen in it. On color flow imaging, no flow is seen in it. Findings are suggestive of atrophic testes because of chronic ischemia.

Cord Pathology

Varicoceles occur in 2 to 20% of the normal adult population. Varicocele is a potential cause of male infertility due to increased scrotal temperature as a result of venous stasis. Varicocele is more common on the left side due to its direct drainage in the left renal vein. It is bilateral in 10–15% of the cases. However, this incidence will surely increase with the advent of color Doppler sonography. The causes of varicoceles are the incompetence of the spermatic vein valves, left renal vein thrombosis or tumoral compression and neoplastic involvement of the retroperitoneum and pelvis.

Ultrasonographic Features

Ultrasonographic diagnosis is usually easy. The spermatic cord is normally examined in supine and erect positions at rest and with Valsalva's maneuver.

Dilated spermatic vessels giving rise to a "bag of worms" appearance is the most common feature. With color Doppler, a varicocele is diagnosed when the vessel has diameter of more than 3 mm. With Valsalva maneuver, the diameter increases significantly, and greater number of dilated vessels are identified. Presence of reflux is seen in varicoceles. Color Doppler studies have been used to grade the venous reflux.

- Grade I — Venous stasis
- Grade II — Intermittent stasis
- Grade III — Continuous stasis
- Ligation of the varicosed vessels often improves the sperm quality, and increased conception rates are reported.

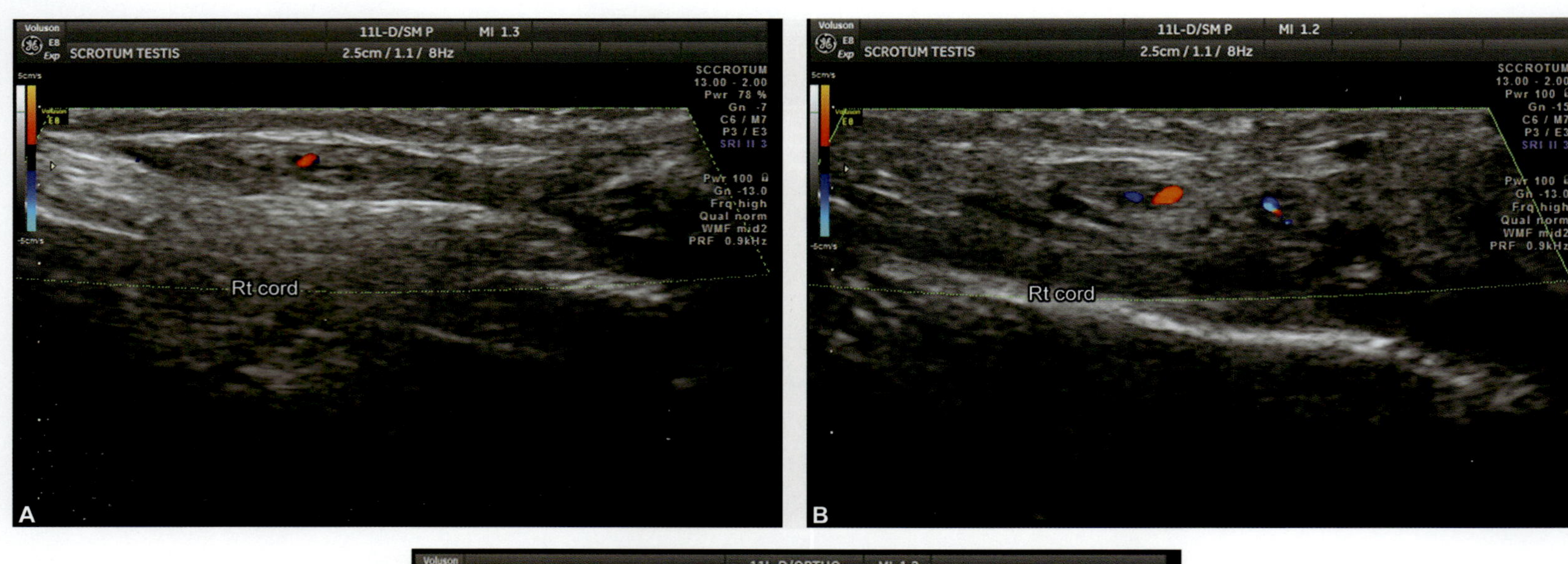

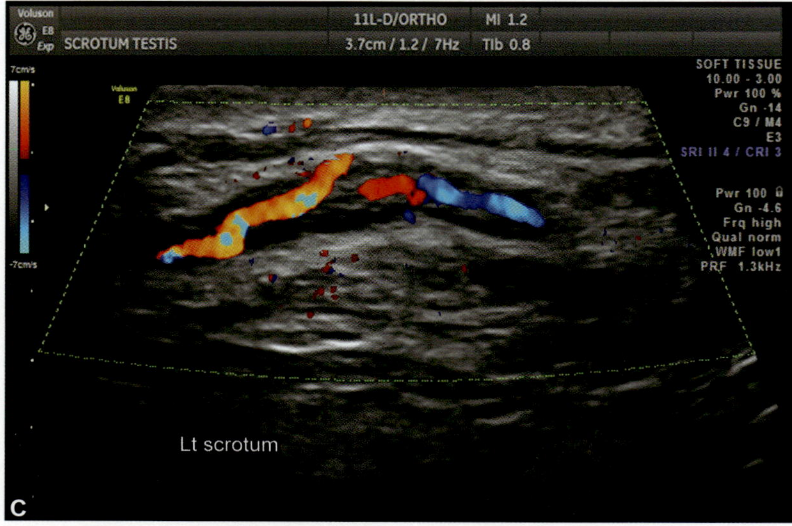

FIGURES 12.119A to C: Normal cord. HRSG shows normal cord. Fat and the vessels are predominant part of cord. The Vas deferens is seen as a tubular shadow.

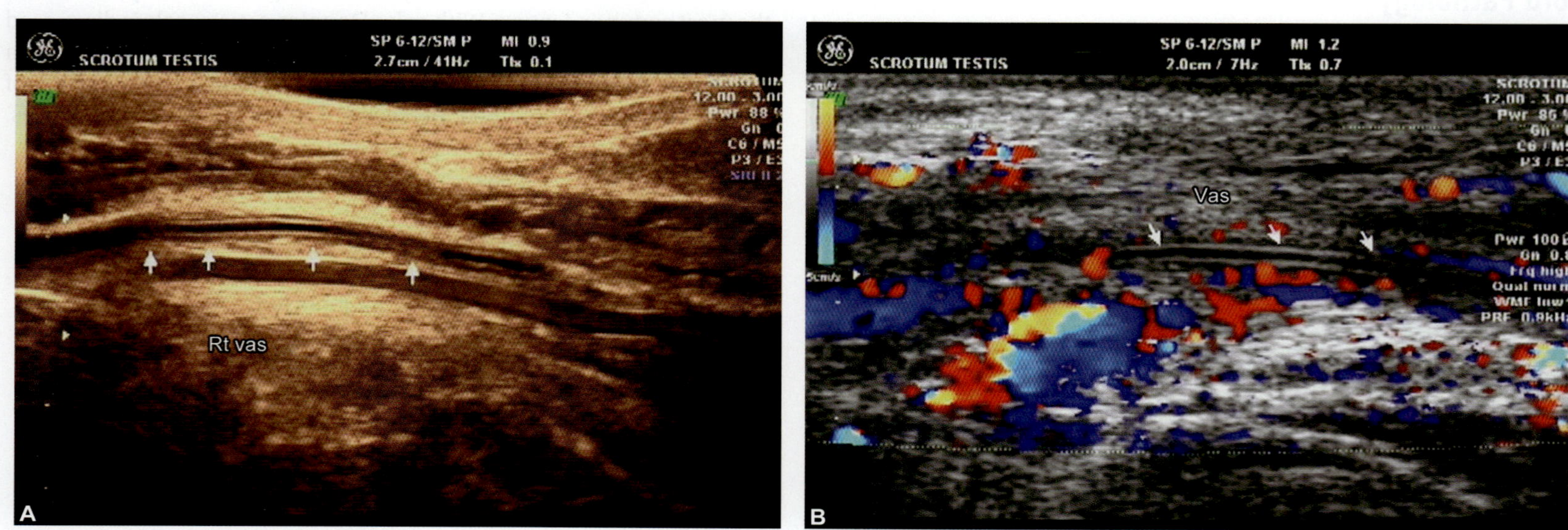

FIGURES 12.120A and B

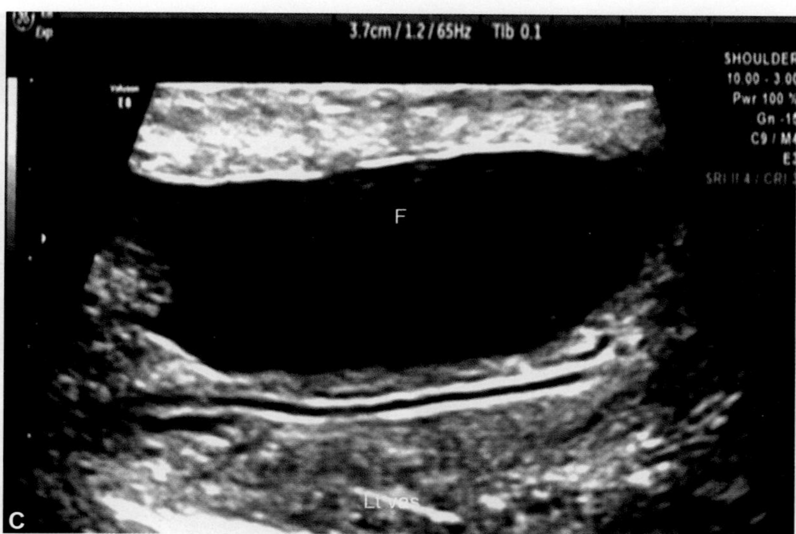

FIGURE 12.120C

FIGURES 12.120A to C: Normal vas deferens. HRSG shows normal vas deferens in the inguinal canal. It is seen as thin echogenic tubular shadow, which may be mistaken as vessel. However, color flow imaging, does not show any flow in it. Figure B shows intrascrotal part of vas deferens.

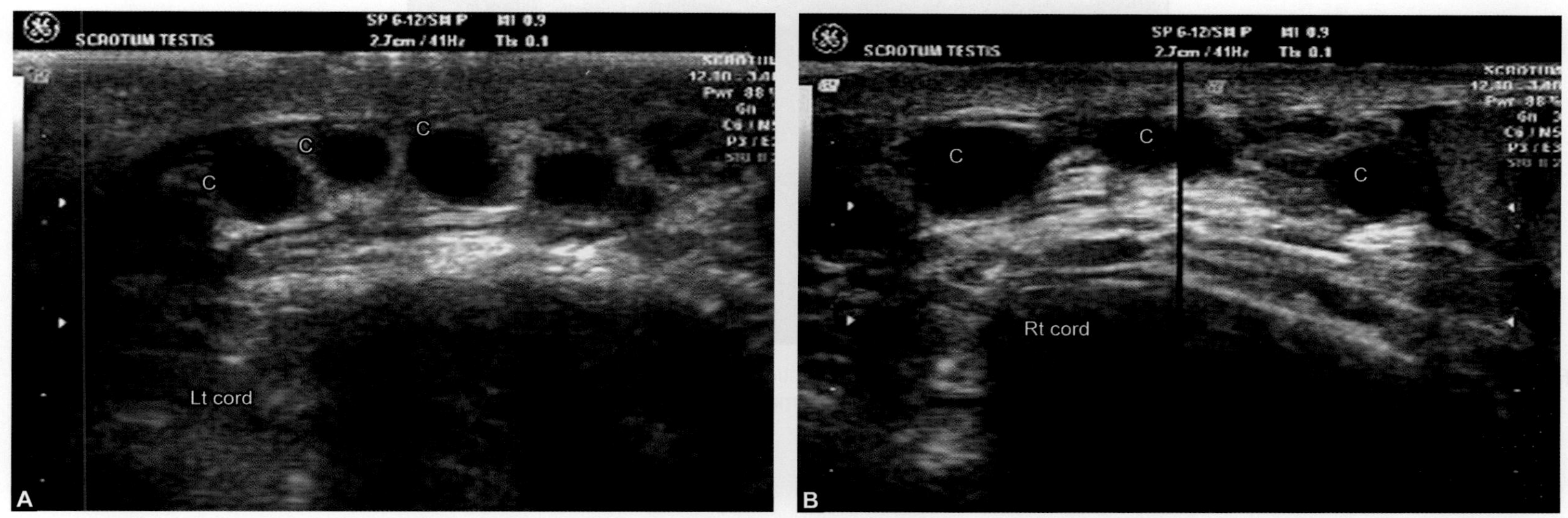

FIGURES 12.121A and B: Multiple cord cysts. HRSG shows multiple cyst in the left spermatic cord. The cysts are non communicating.

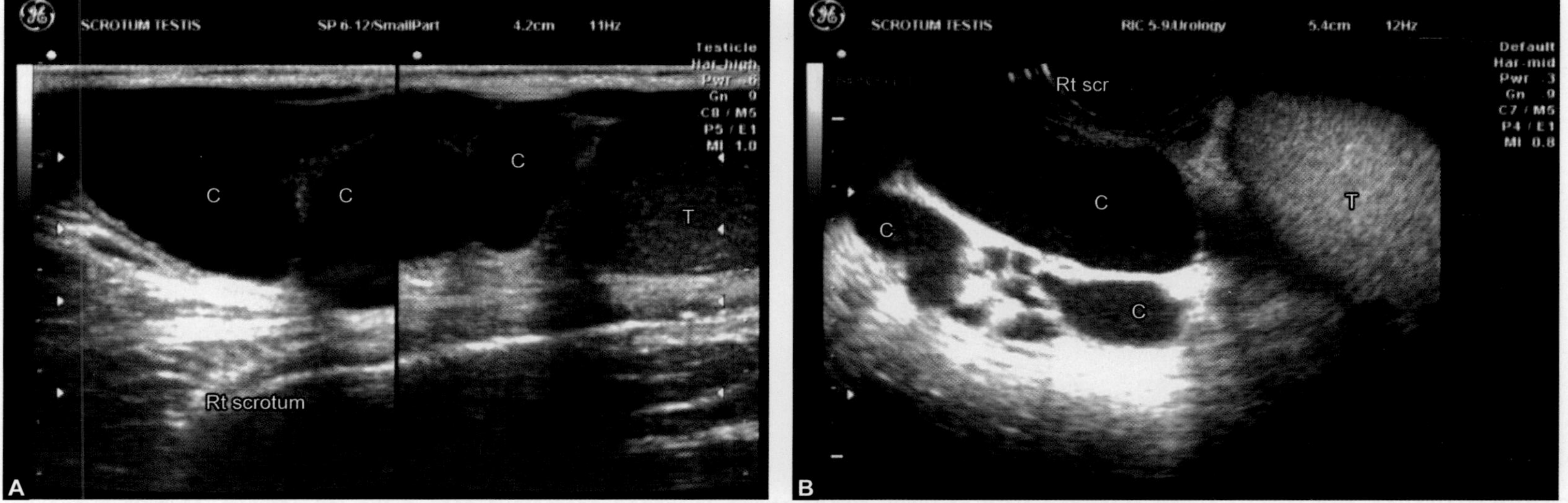

FIGURES 12.122A and B: Epididymis and cord cyst. HRSG shows multiple cysts along the cord. Normal cord tissue replaced by the cysts. These cord cysts are known as spermatocele. The arrest of the sperm is seen in the cord resulting into oligo or azoospermia. Small cyst is also seen in the epididymal head.

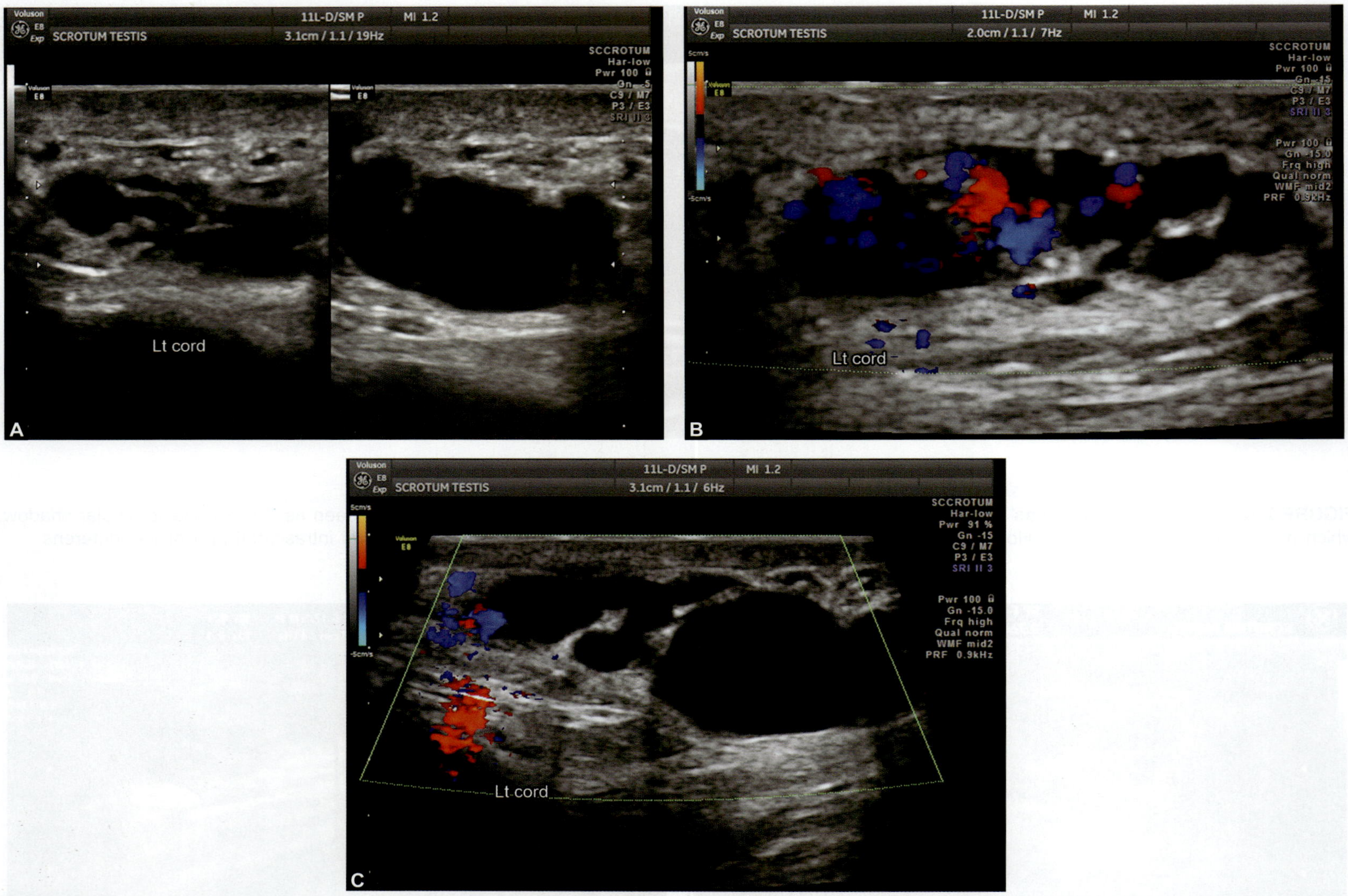

FIGURES 12.123A to C: **Multiple cord cysts.** HRSG shows multiple cystic shadows in the left cord. They are seen in the inguinal canal and non-communicating. On color flow imaging, no flow is seen in them.

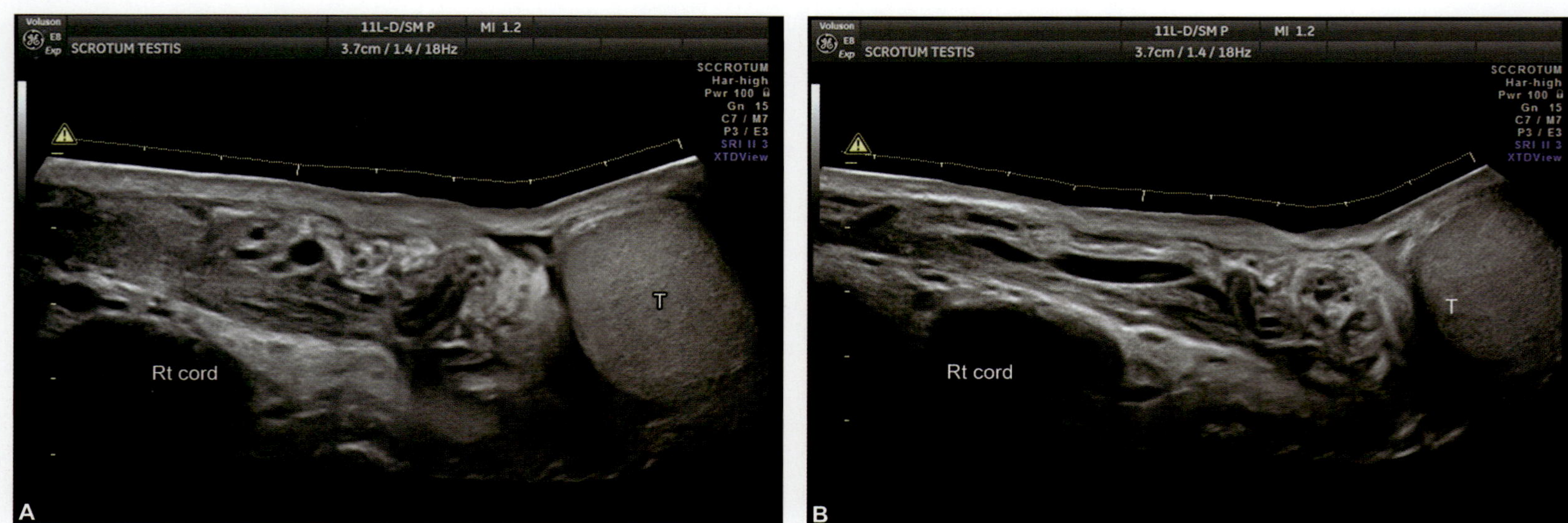

FIGURES 12.124A and B: Funiculitis-extended field of view. HRSG shows thickened edematous cord in the left scrotum. Multiple hypoechoic areas are seen in the cord. The cord fat is also seen inflamed. Extended field of view shows entire length of edematous cord. On color flow imaging, multiple vessels are seen feeding the cord.

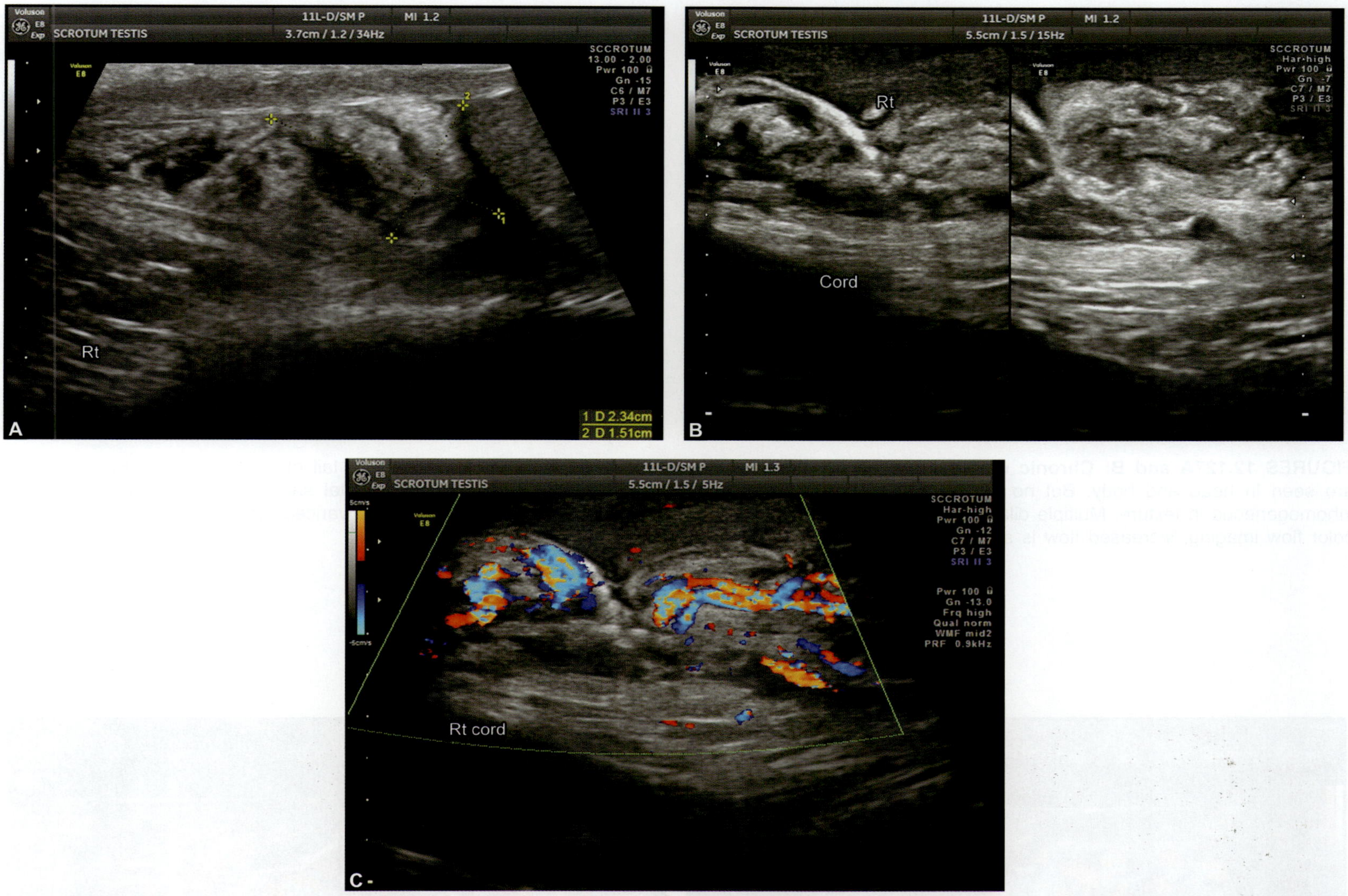

FIGURES 12.125A to C: Funiculitis with small hydrocele. A patient presented with painful swelling in the right cord. HRSG shows thickened edematous Lt cord. Fat inflammation is also seen. Hypoechoic areas are also seen in the cord. On color flow imaging, few vessels are seen in the cord. Findings are suggestive of acute funiculitis. Small amount of fluid is also seen in cord suggestive of reactionary fluid.

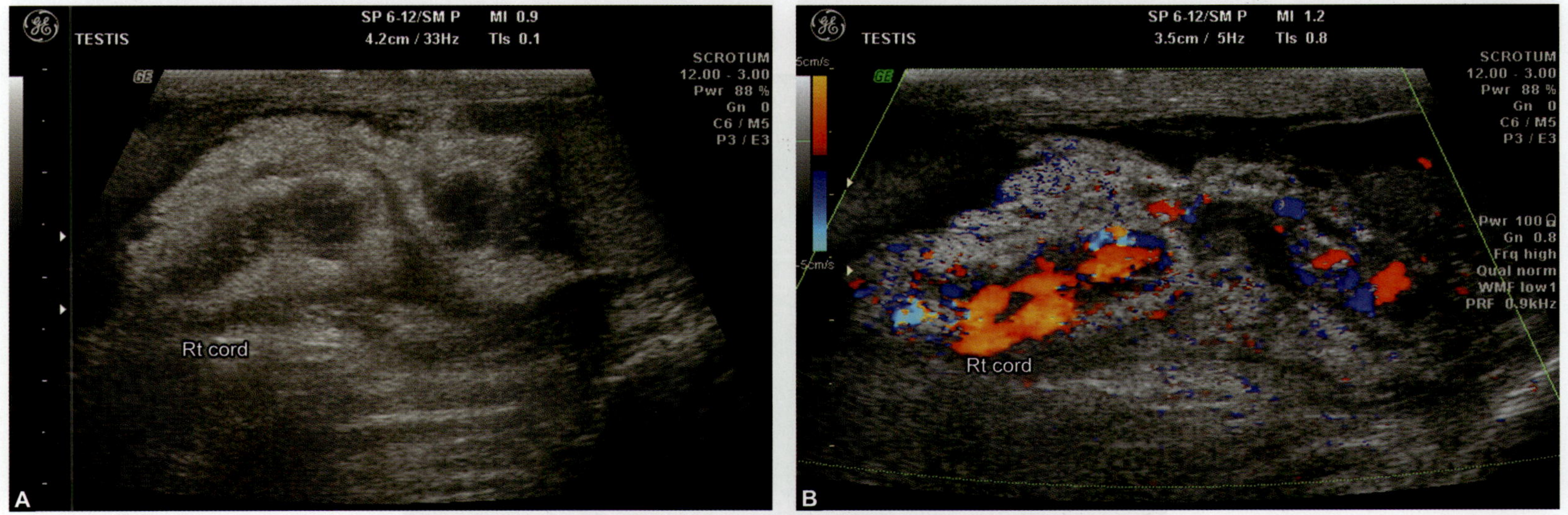

FIGURES 12.126A and B: Funiculitis. A patient presented with painful swelling in the right cord and right scrotum. HRSG shows thickened edematous cord. Cord edema is present. The fat is also inflamed and edematous. Hypoechoic areas are seen in the cord. On color flow imaging, increased flow is seen in cord suggestive of funiculitis.

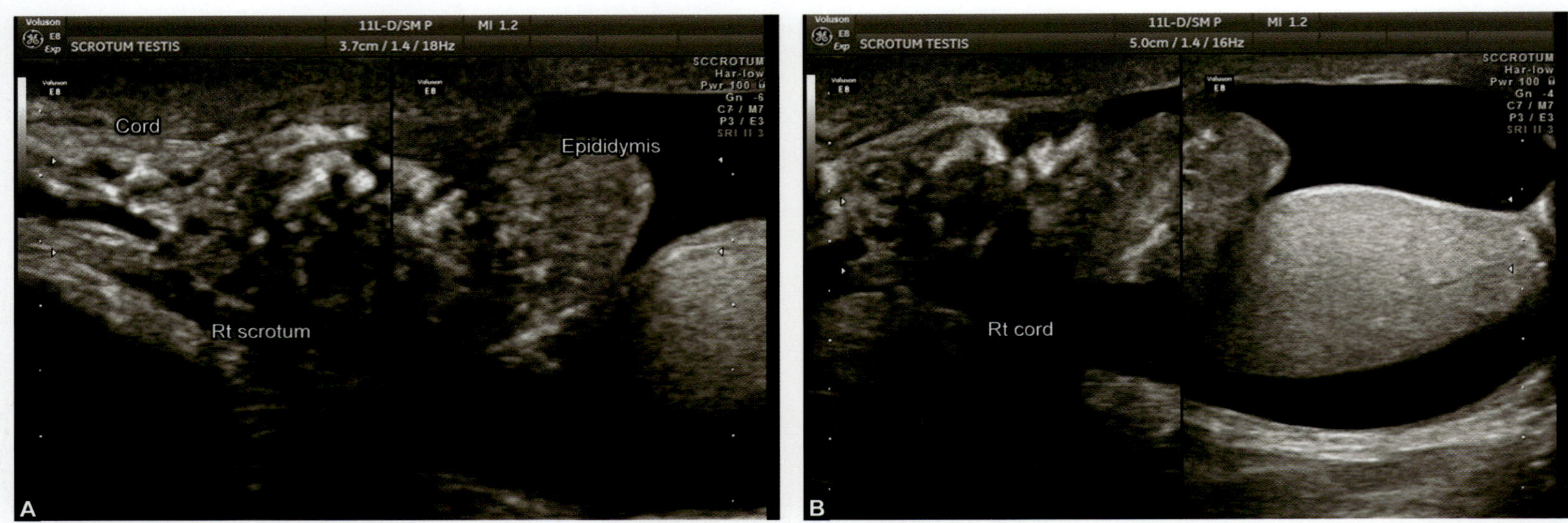

FIGURES 12.127A and B: Chronic epididymitis with funiculitis. HRSG shows thickened head, body and tail of the epididymis. Echogenic foci are seen in head and body. But no necrosis is seen. Moderate amount of collection is seen in right scrotal sac. Right cord is thickened. It is inhomogeneous in texture. Multiple dilated vessels are also seen along the right cord suggestive of right cord varices. No other focal mass seen. On color flow imaging, increased flow is seen in it.

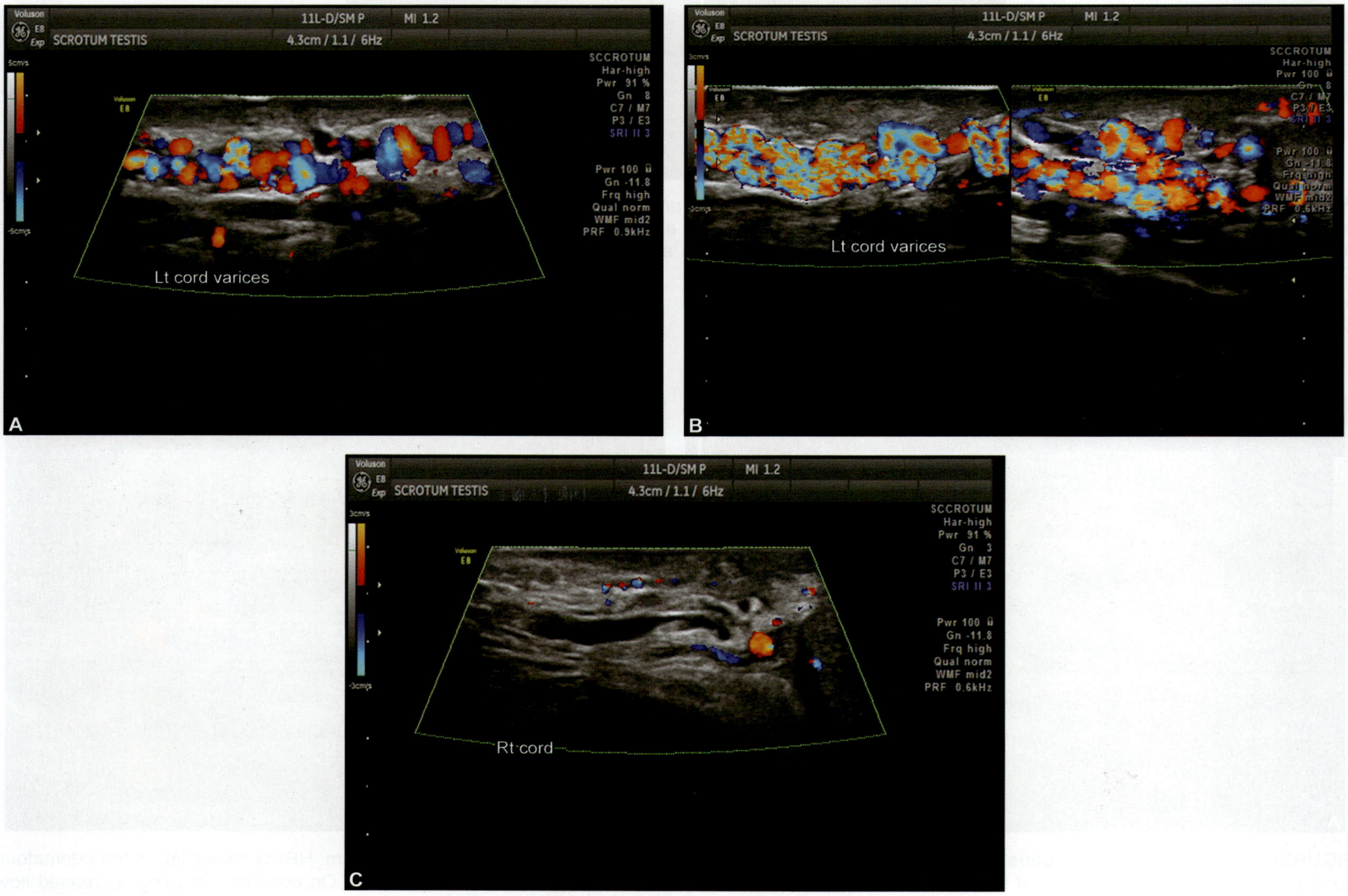

FIGURES 12.128A to C: Grade I cord varices. HRSG shows multiple dilated vessels along the left cord suggestive of cord varices. They get distended on valsalva maneuver suggestive of varicocele. Right cord is normal. No cord varices is seen on right side.

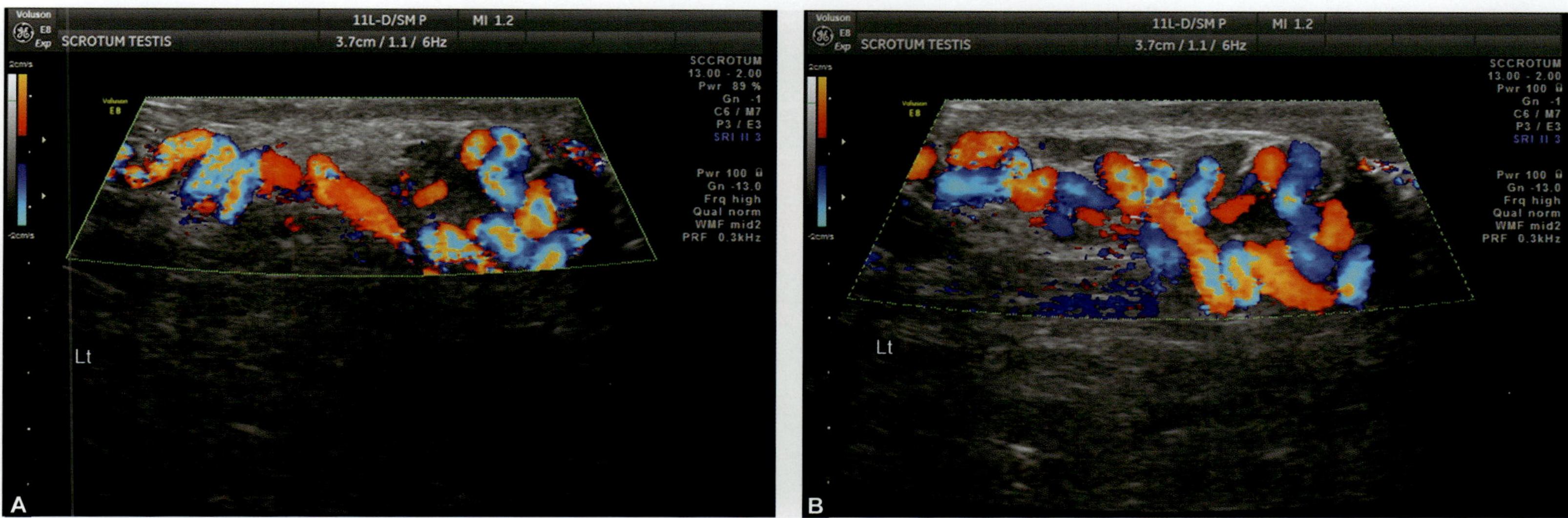

FIGURES 12.129A and B: Grade II cord varices. HRSG shows multiple dilated vessels along the left cord. They get distended on valsalva maneuver. The champagne effect is seen on valsalva maneuver.

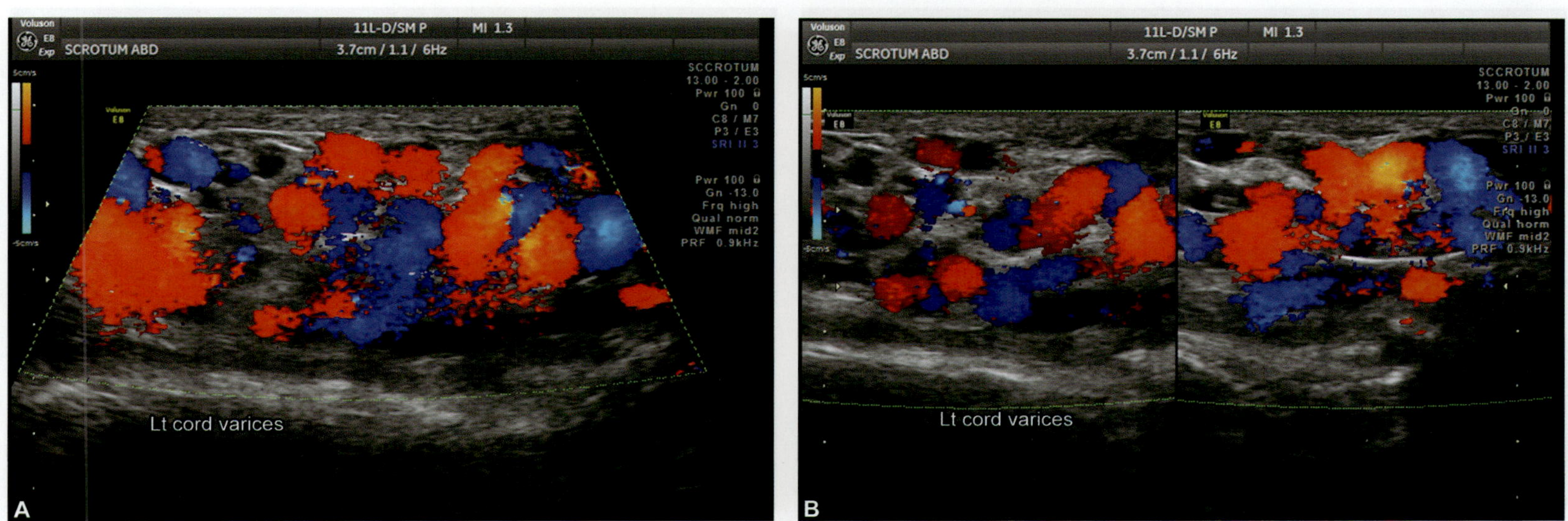

FIGURES 12.130A and B: Grade III cord varices. HRSG shows multiple dilated vessels in neutral position in the left cord. Marked reversal of flow is seen in them on valsalva maneuver suggestive of grade III cord varices.

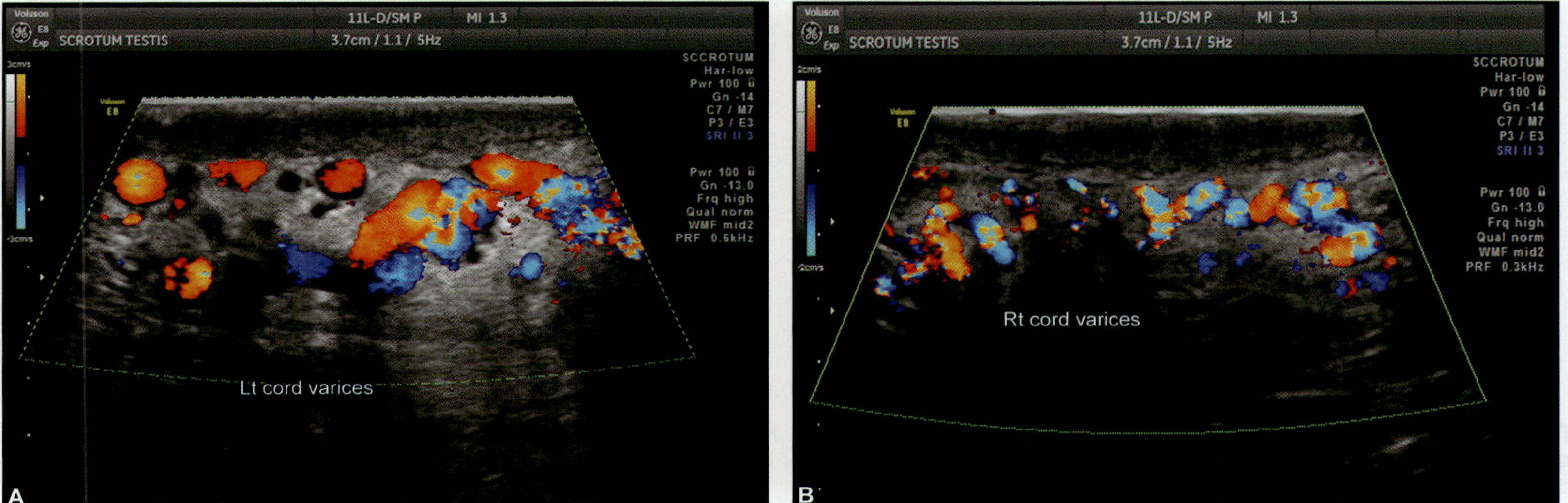

FIGURES 12.131A and B

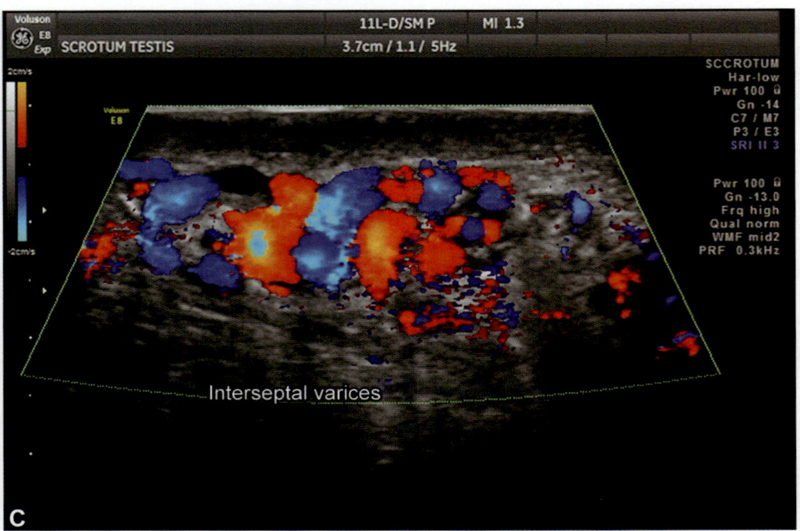

FIGURE 12.131C

FIGURES 12.131A to C: Bilateral cord varices. HRSG shows multiple dilated vessels along both the cords. However, they are more prominent on the left side. Reflux is seen in them on valsalva maneuver.

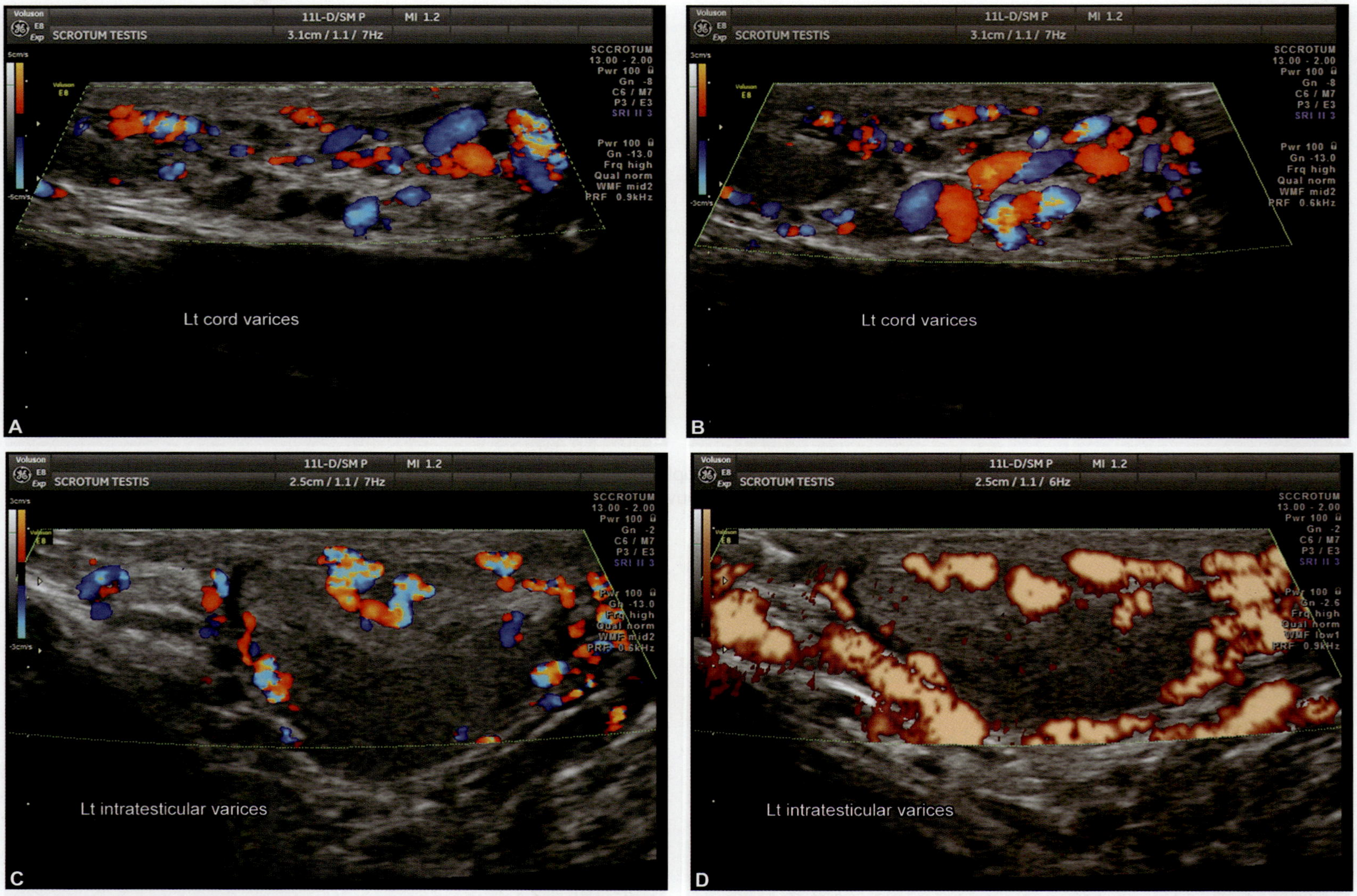

FIGURES 12.132A to D: Left cord varices with intratesticular varices. HRSG shows multiple dilated vessels along the left cord suggestive of left cord varices. Dilated vessels are also seen along the septum suggestive of interseptal varices. There is also evidence of multiple vessels seen feeding the testes. Reflux is seen in them suggestive of intratesticular varices.

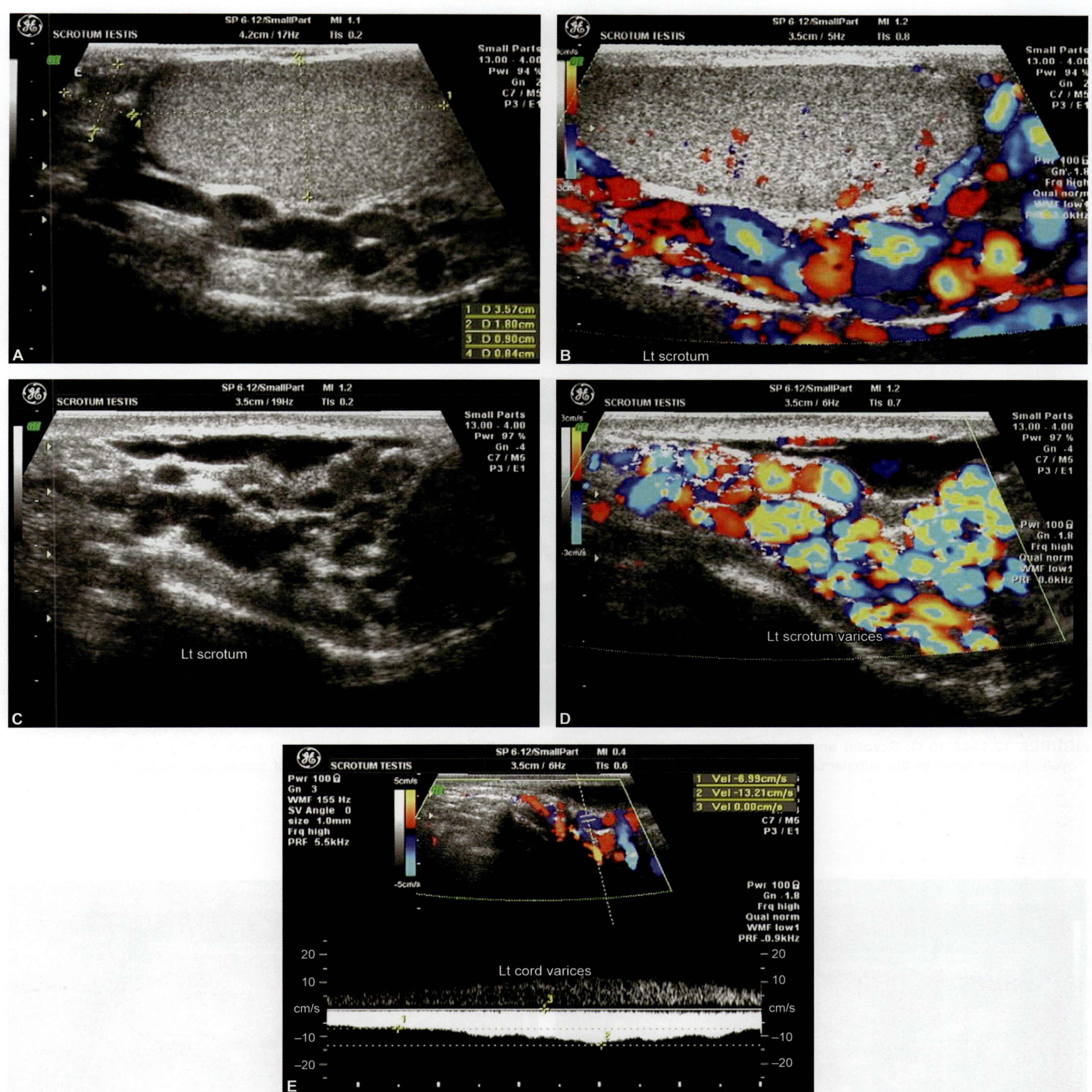

FIGURES 12.133A to E: Left scrotal varices. HRSG shows multiple dilated veins in the left scrotum posterior to the testes. They are seen as a bag of worm. Color Doppler imaging shows low flow in the varices. Reflux is also seen in them. Marked reflux is seen on valsalva maneuver. Dilated vessels are also seen along the cord in the same patient suggestive of cord and scrotal varices. Cord and scrotal varices. HRSG shows multiple dilated vessels along the left cord. The dilated vessels look like fine net on gray scale imaging. On color Doppler imaging the vessels are seen having low venous flow, which is confirmed on spectral Doppler tracing on valsalva maneuver. High reflux is seen in them.

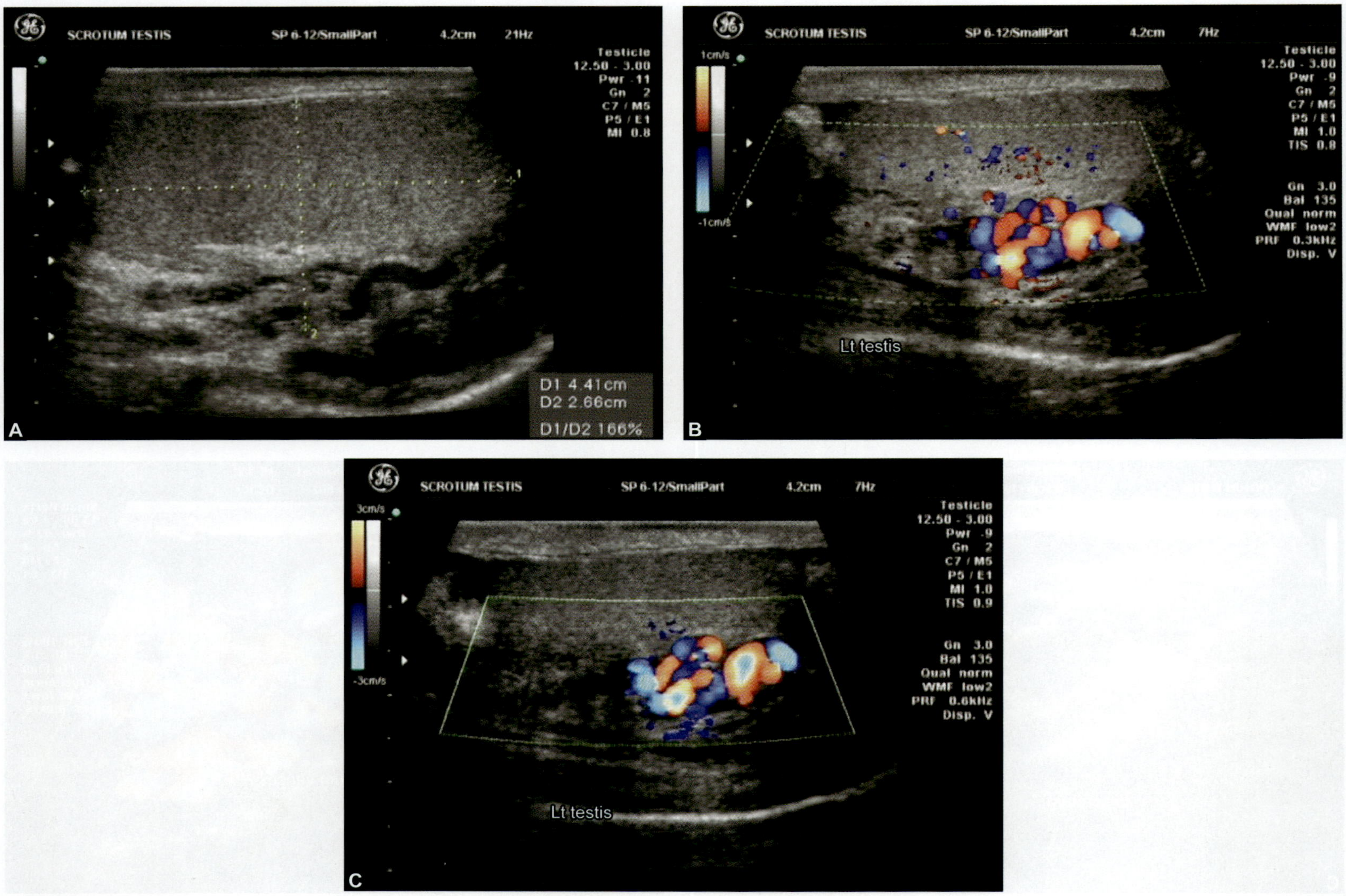

FIGURES 12.134A to C: Scrotal and intratesticular varices. HRSG shows multiple dilated vessels in the left scrotum. There is also evidence of cystic spaces seen in the substance of testes. On color flow imaging they are filled with blood suggestive of scrotal and intratesticular varices.

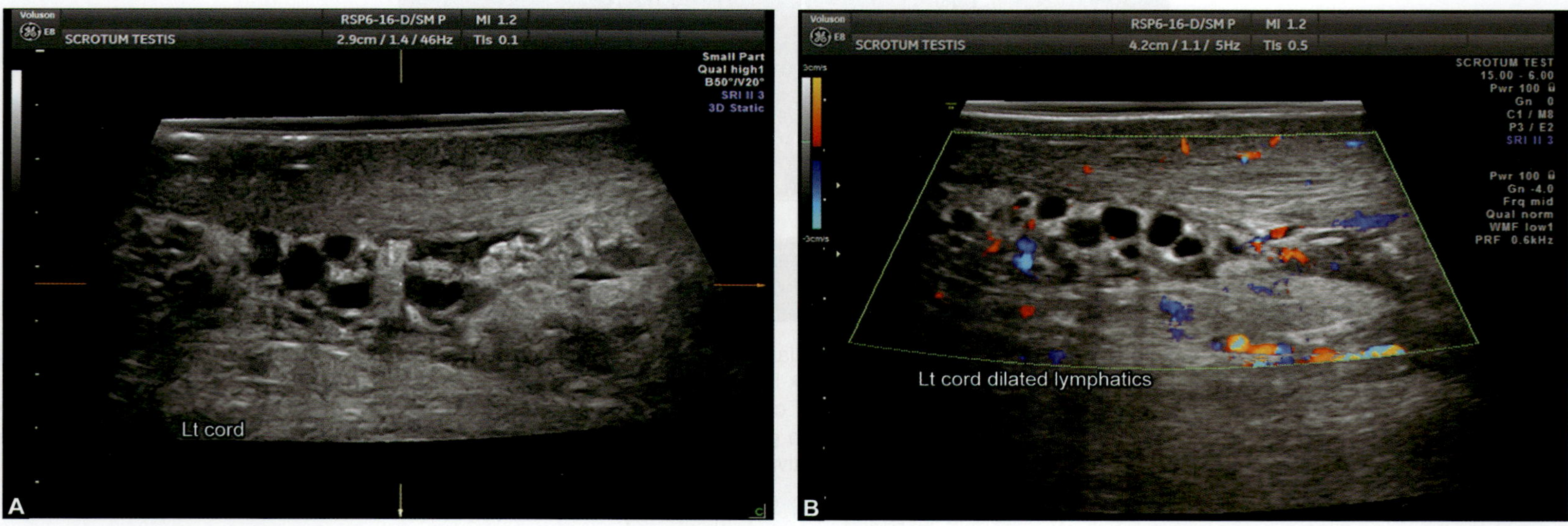

FIGURES 12.135A and B

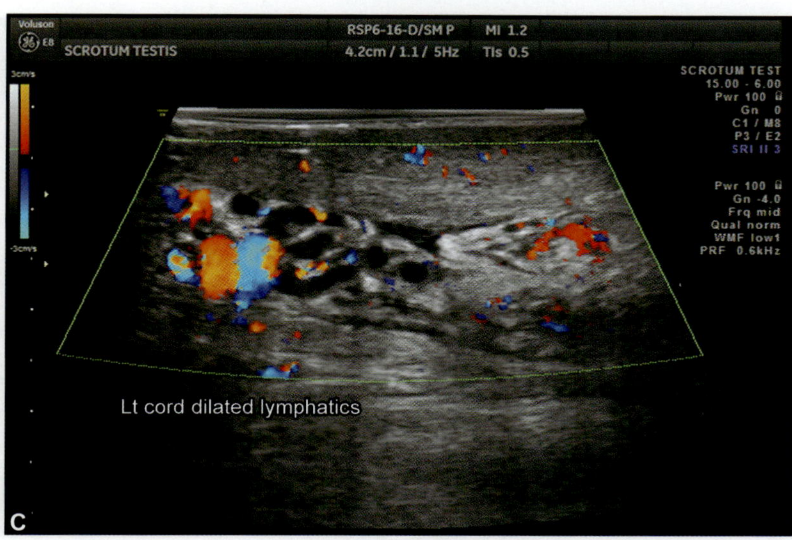

FIGURE 12.135C

FIGURES 12.135A to C: Dilated lymphatics. HRSG shows multiple dilated vessels under the scrotal skin. On color flow imaging, no blood flow is seen in them suggestive of dilated lymphatics.

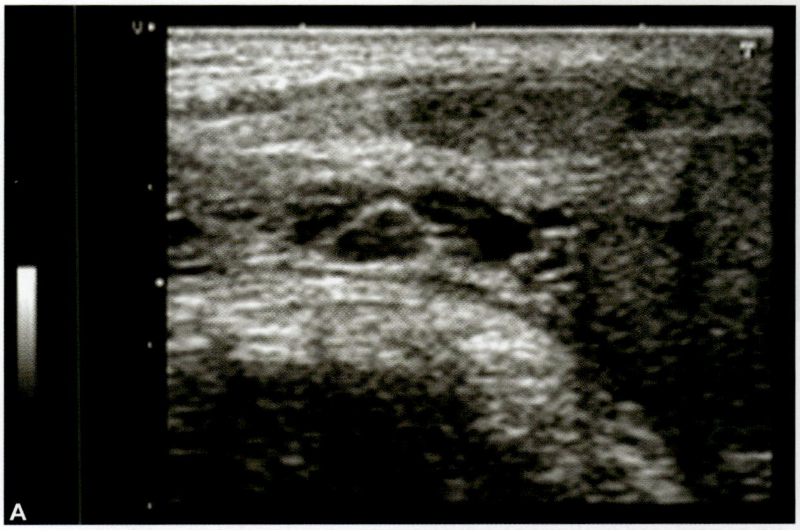

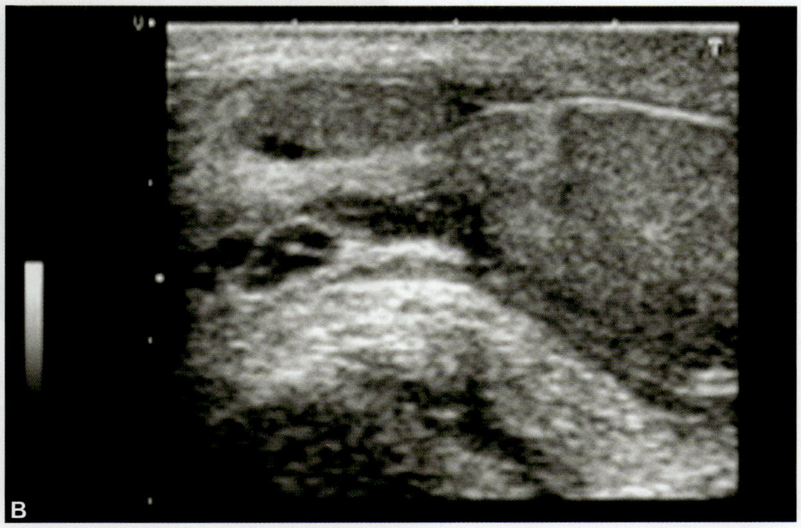

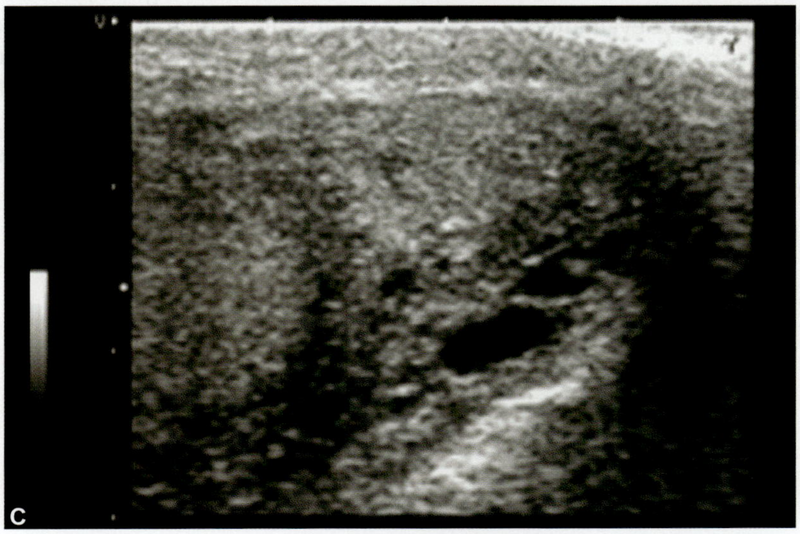

FIGURES 12.136A to C: Dilated lymphatics with filarial dance. HRSG shows multiple dilated lymphatics. On real time imaging, multiple tiny echogenic shadows seen moving in it suggestive of microfilaria moving in the lymphatics also known as filarial dance.

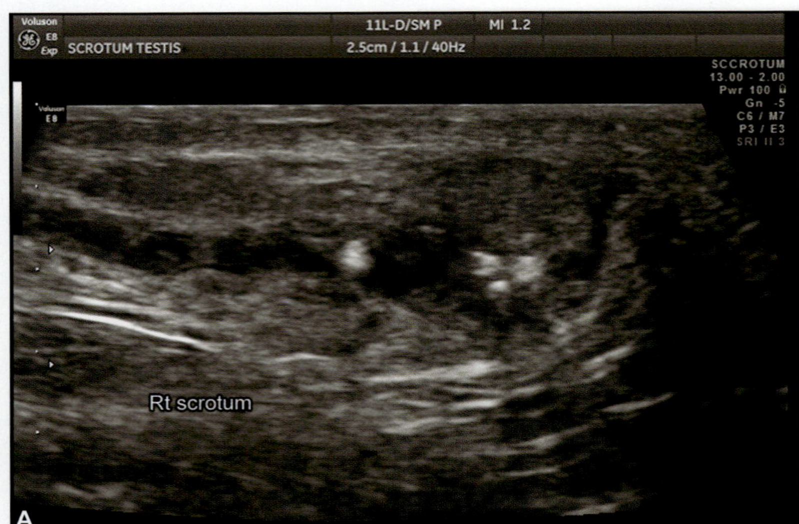

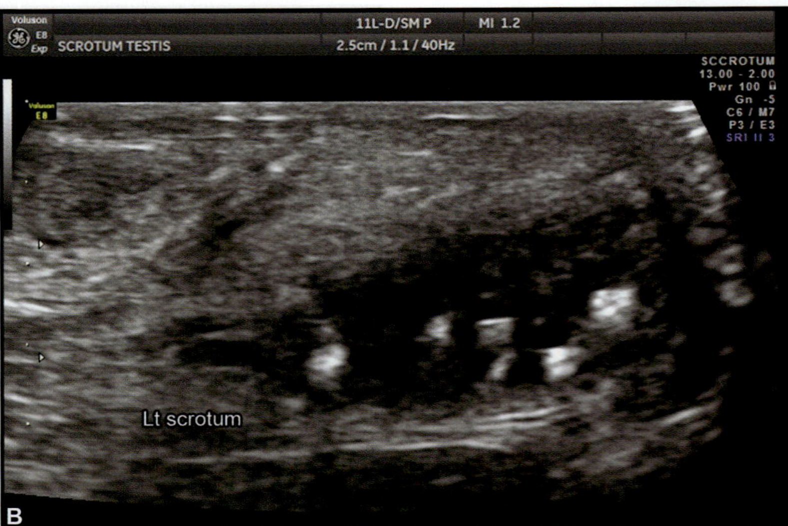

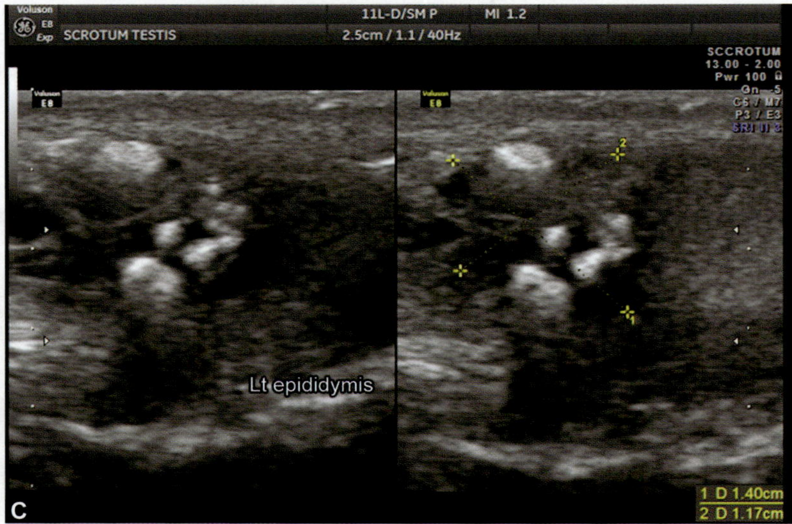

FIGURES 12.137A to C: HRSG shows thickened cord. The epididymis is also inhomogeneous in texture. Multiple echogenic foci are seen in the epididymis. They are also seen in the proximal spermatic cord. Perifocal edema is present suggestive of chronic epididymitis with cord infection.

CONCLUSION

High-resolution sonography has been a boon in the evaluation of scrotal pathologies especially after the advent of color Doppler imaging. It might be in order to say that visualizing the intra scrotal structures and deciphering pathologies of the scrotal contents have greatly facilitated the clinical approach to acute scrotal disorders. As mentioned earlier, the greatest advantage of ultrasonography is to distinguish between intra and extratesticular abnormalities, since most intrascrotal masses should be considered malignant, while extratesticular abnormalities are more commonly benign. An abdominal sonography helps in the evaluation of metastatic disease in the abdomen and also helps in following up of patients after surgery. Though MRI has been of help in assessing the scrotum, ultrasonography will not only remain the primary screening modality but adds good information in making a specific diagnosis in majority of cases.

CHAPTER 13

Ambiguous Genitalia and Intersex

PK Srivastava

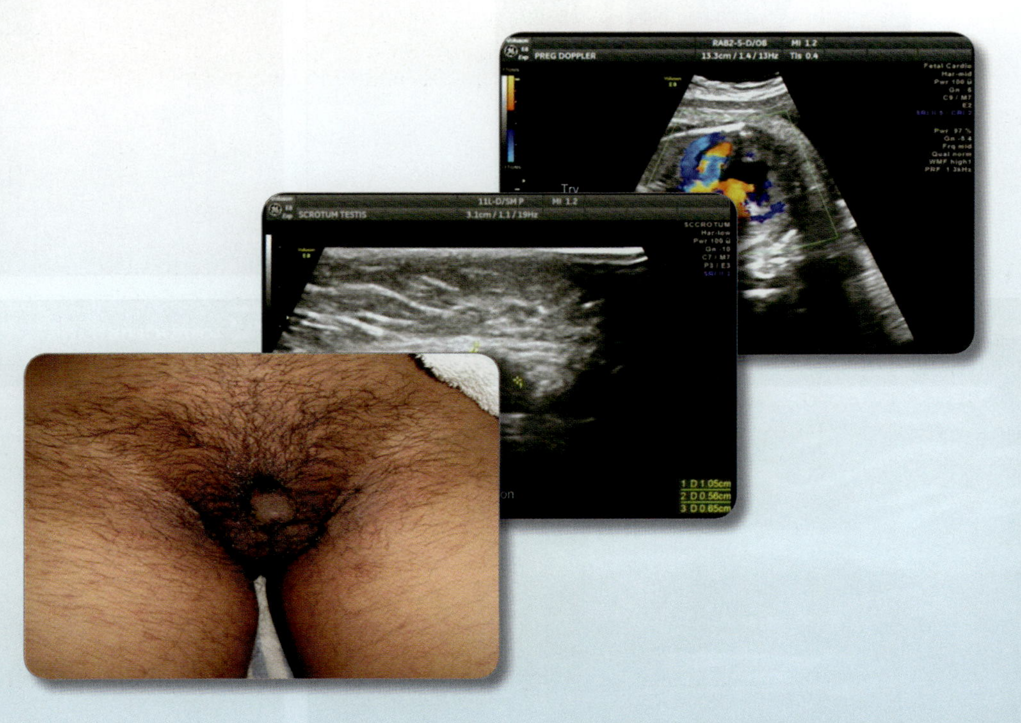

INTRODUCTION

High-resolution ultrasound is an important modality for evaluation of ambiguous genitalia and intersex. The disorder of sex development is known as DSD. The main causes are development of abnormal chromosome results into gonadal and anatomical sex abnormalities. Four types of disorders of sex development is found on gonadal histology.

- Male pseudohermaphroditism—46, XY with two testes.
- Female pseudohermaphroditism—46XX with to ovaries.
- True hermaphroditism DSD—both ovarian and testis tissue
- Gonadal dysgenesis—either mixed a testes and one streak

Imaging is important for evaluation of disorders of the sex development. Ultrasound is the primary imaging modality. The disorder of sex development has got physiological and psychological impact on the child affected by it. The evaluation of ambiguous genitalia requires:

1. Presence or absence of palpable testes, its position and position of the urethral meatus and phallus.
2. Presence of Müllerian structure seen on ultrasound.
3. Estimation of serum 17 OH progesterone and progesterone
4. Karyotyping of the child.

On clinical examination, ambiguous genitalia is suspected in the absence of palpable testis or the presence of one testis with hypospadias is suspected case of intersex disorder until proven otherwise.

Unilateral palpable undescended testis is seen 15% intersex. Unilateral impalpable undescended testis is seen in 50% intersex. Bilateral undescended testis and hypospadias is seen 32% intersex patients. Therefore, role of imaging is very important. The diagnosis is made by ultrasound and magnetic resonance imaging (MRI), Laproscopy and gonadal biopsy, culture of the genital skin and fibroblast and contrast study of urogenital sinus. The ultrasound protocol is to look for pelvis, inguinal canal, perineal region, renal and adrenal regions and to size of adrenals.

Intersex is a general term and used for variety of conditions in which a person is born with a reproductive or sexual anatomy that does not seem to fit the typical definitions of female or male. The intersex conditions are also known as disorders of sex development or DSD.

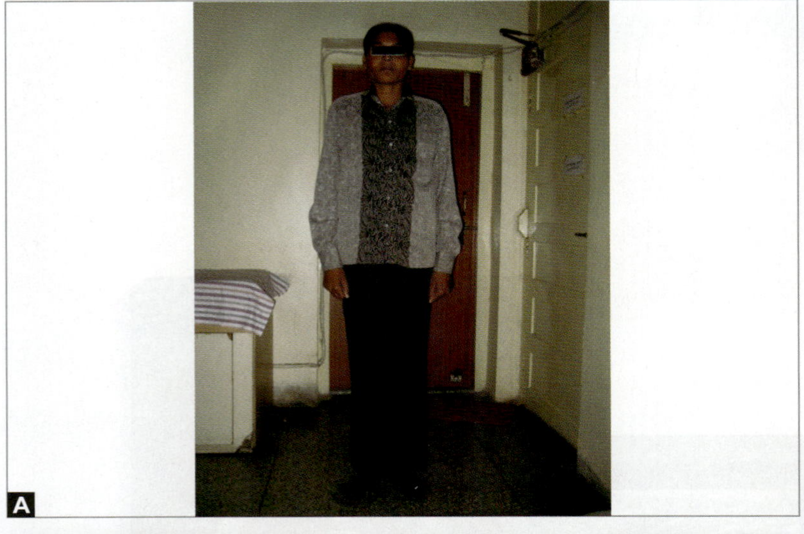

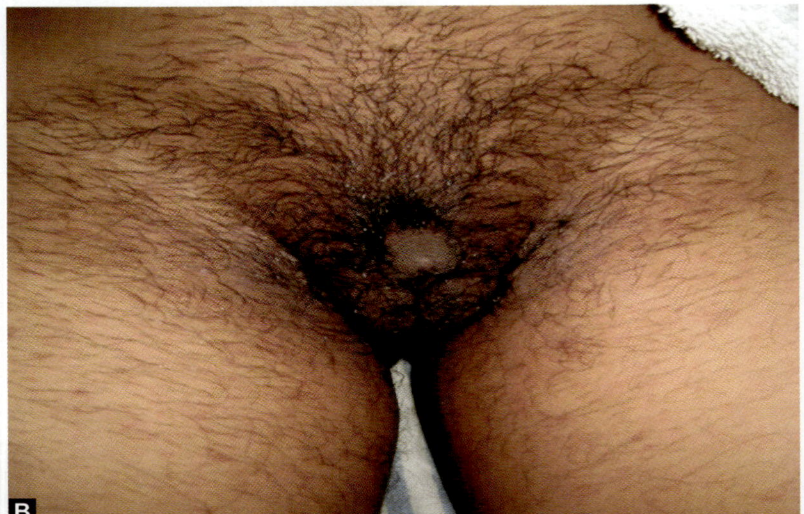

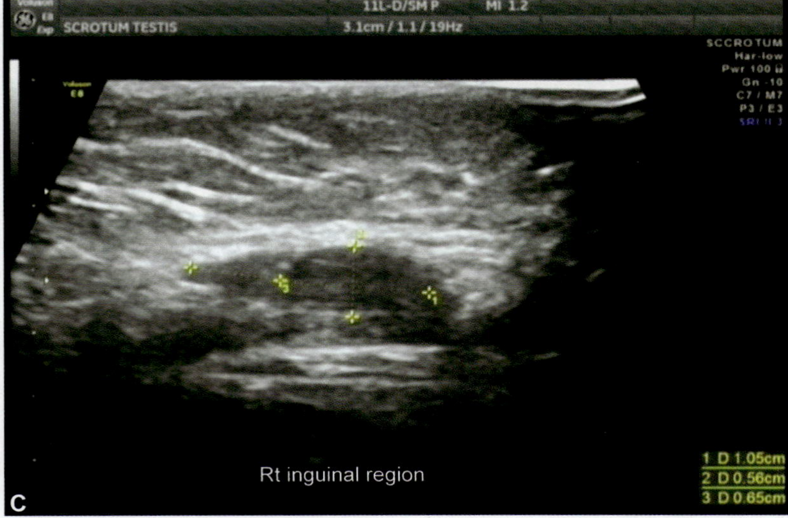

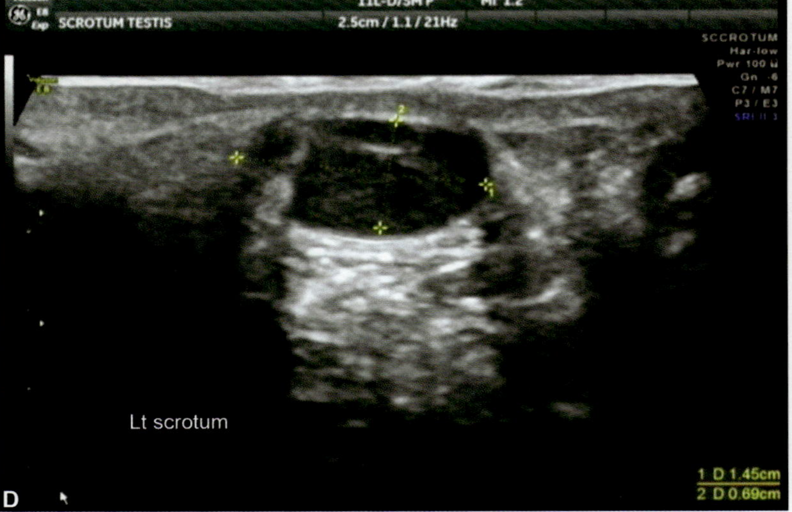

FIGURES 13.1A to D: Klinefelter syndrome. A patient presented with increase height and high-resolution sonography (HRSG) shows small phallus. The scrotums are also small in size. Both testis are small and hypoechoic in texture. The chromosome analysis shows 47XXY.

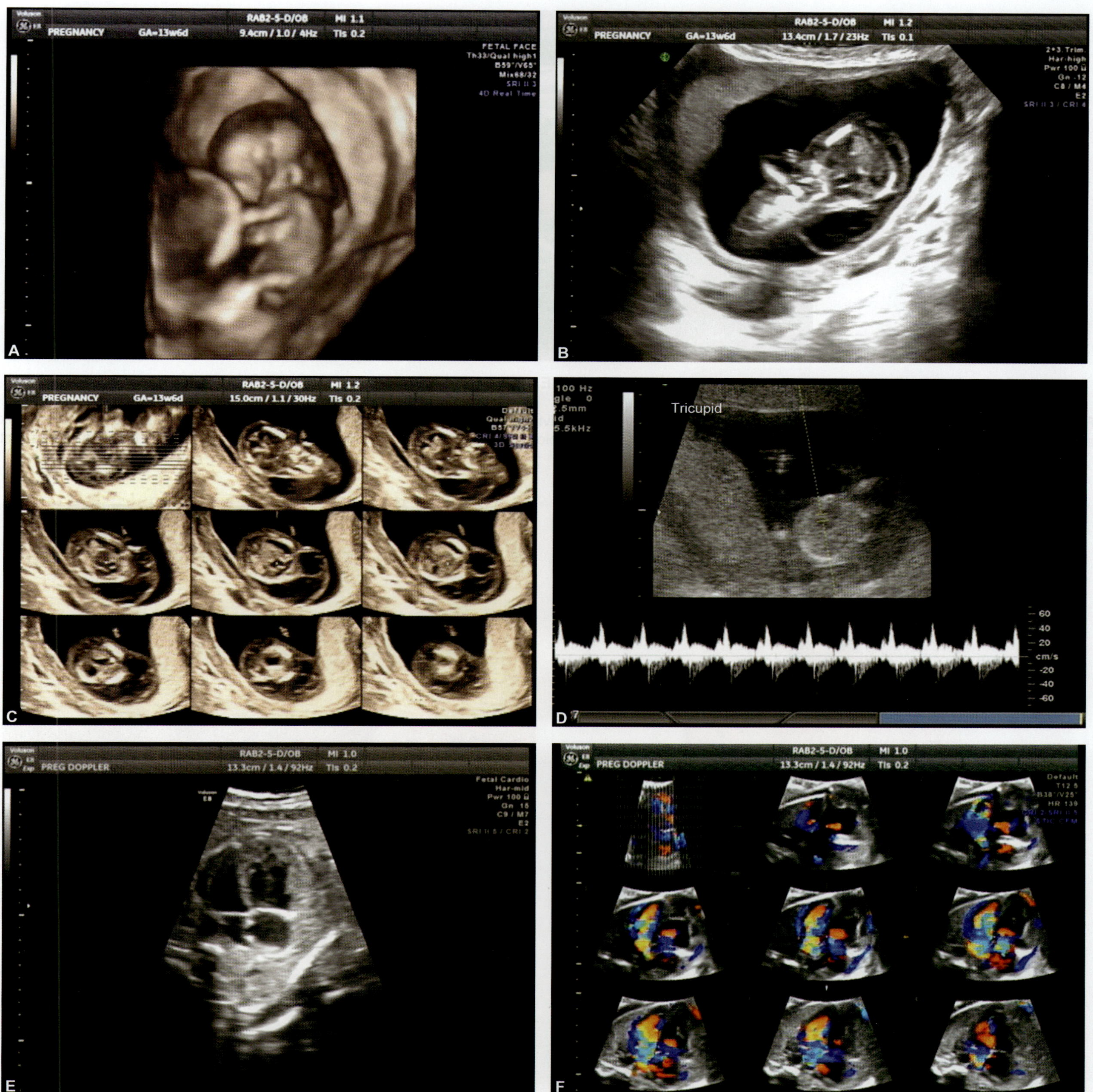

FIGURES 13.2A to F

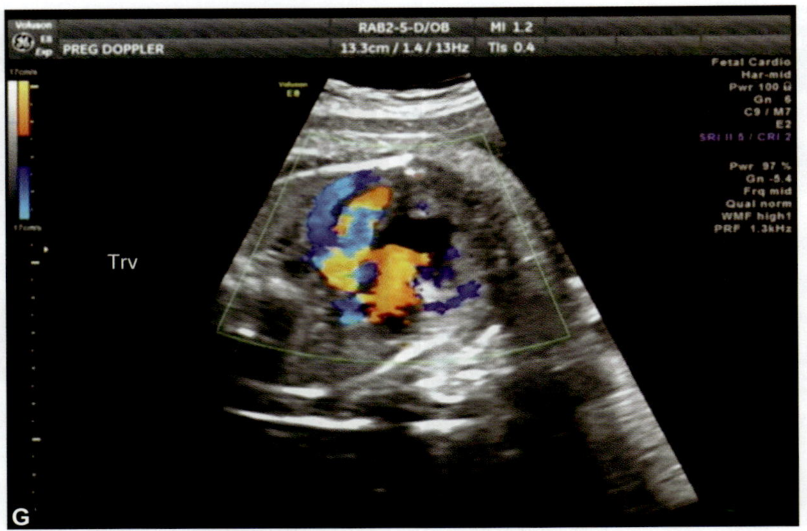

FIGURE 13.2G

FIGURES 13.2A to G: Turner's syndrome. The Turner's syndrome is having classic 45X0. A patient presented with Turner's syndrome has multiple anomalies. HRSG shows cystic hygroma. There is also evidence of tricuspid renegotiation, which is seen on color Doppler of fetal heart to the patient.

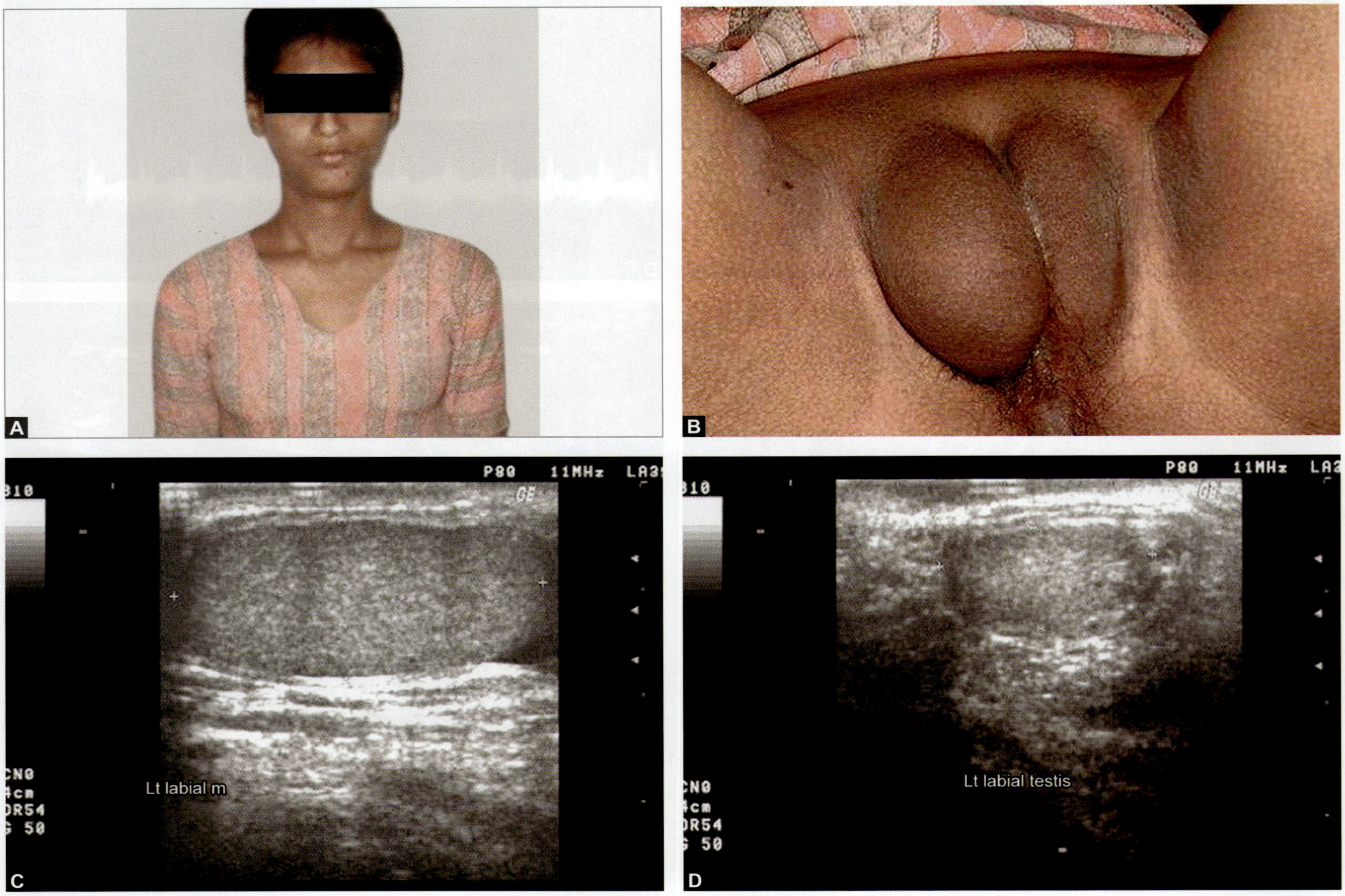

FIGURES 13.3A to D

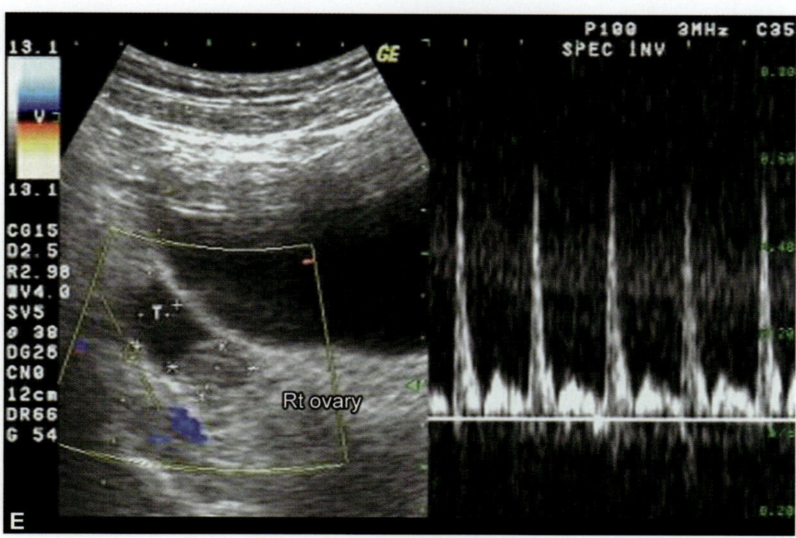

FIGURE 13.3E

FIGURES 13.3A to E: True hermaphrodite. A young girl presented with bilateral labial masses. The serum testosterone was very high. Then girl was having well-developed breasts. HRSG shows well-defined homogeneous ovoid masses in both labia. They show fine granular texture similar to the testis. Biopsy of the mass confirmed labial testis. After surgery of the testis the serum testosterone came to normal range. The patient was also having well-developed ovaries. Therefore, it was true hermaphrodite.

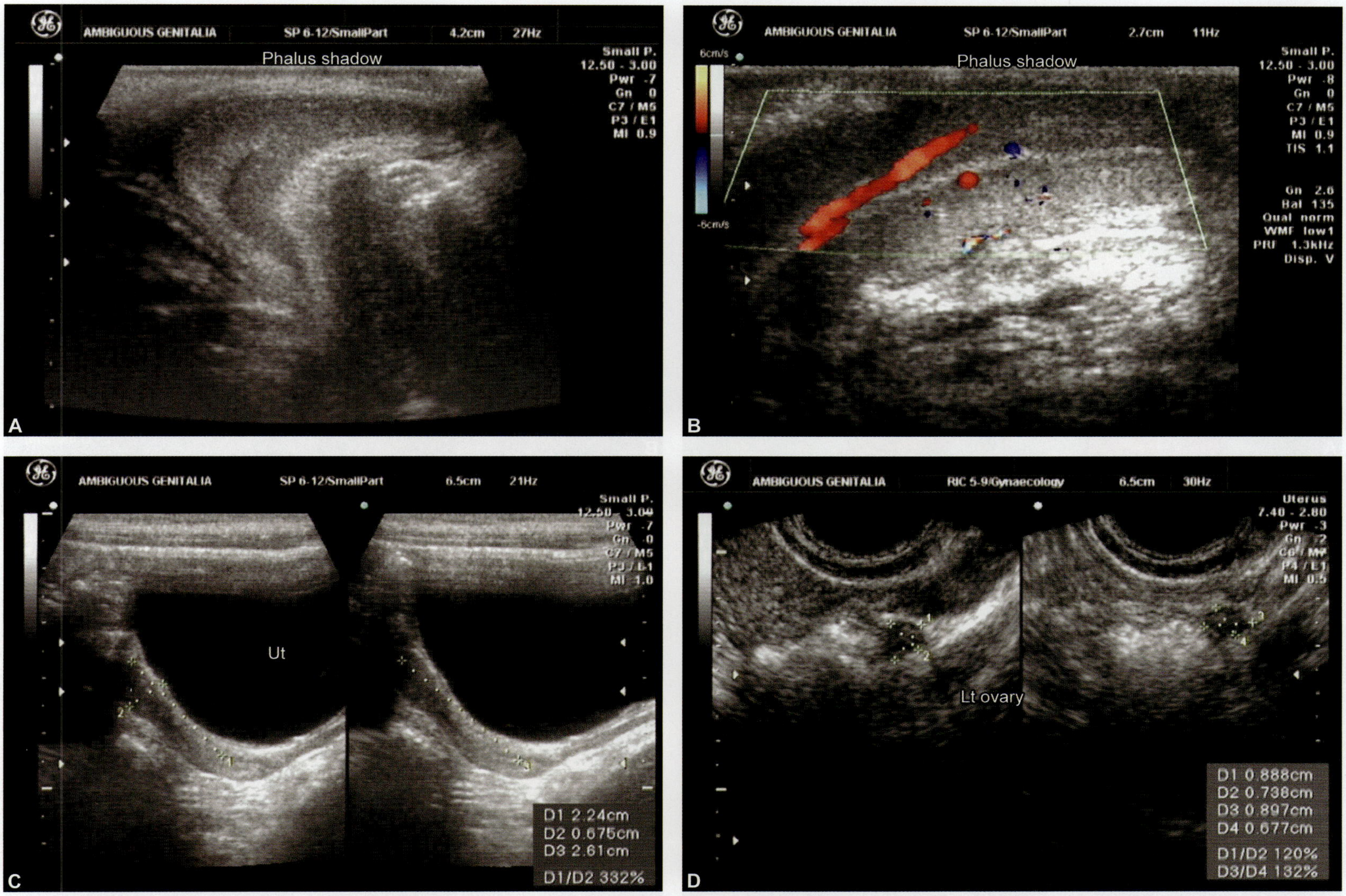

FIGURES 13.4A to D

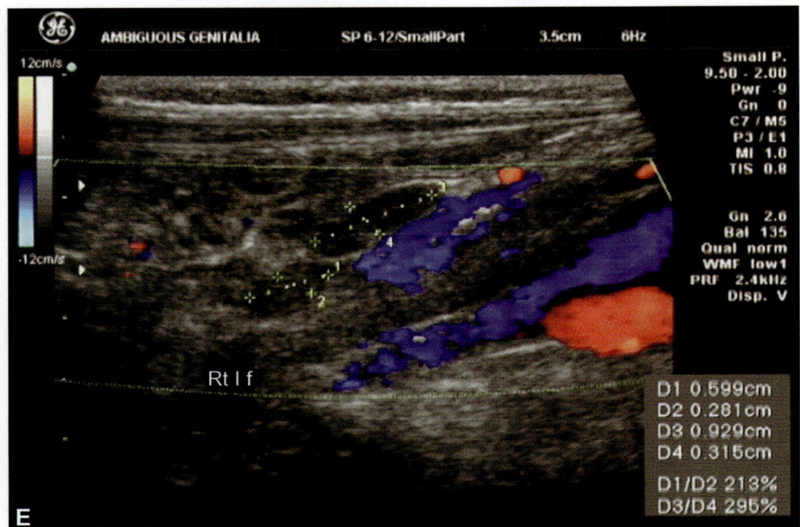

FIGURE 13.4E

FIGURES 13.4A to E: True hermaphrodite. A patient presented with disorder of sex. HRSG shows phallus shadow seen buried in the skin. Uterus is also seen in the pelvis. The left ovary is seen in the left ovarian fossa and the left ectopic testis is seen in the left iliac fossa anterior to the iliac vessels suggestive of true hermaphrodite.

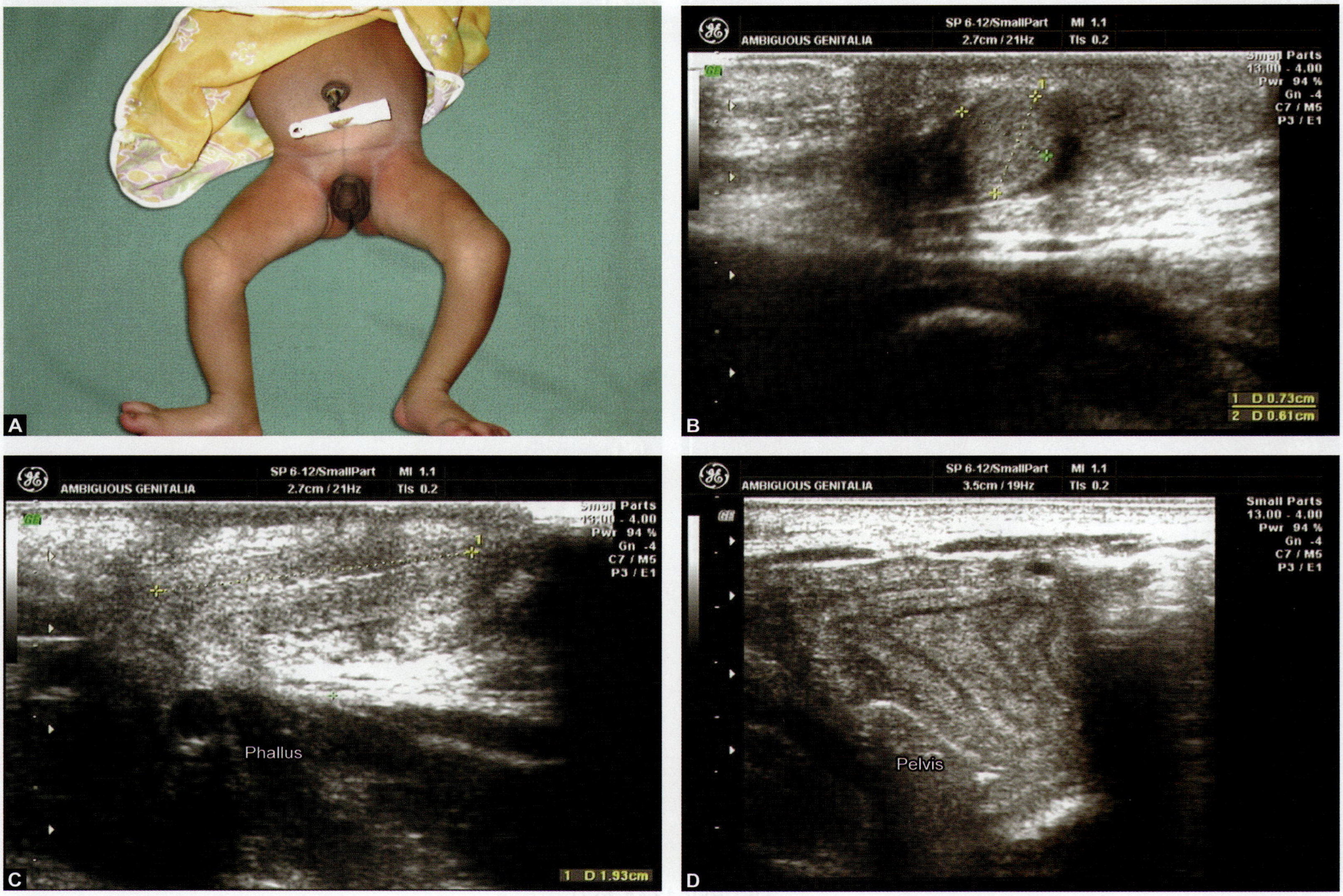

FIGURES 13.5A to D

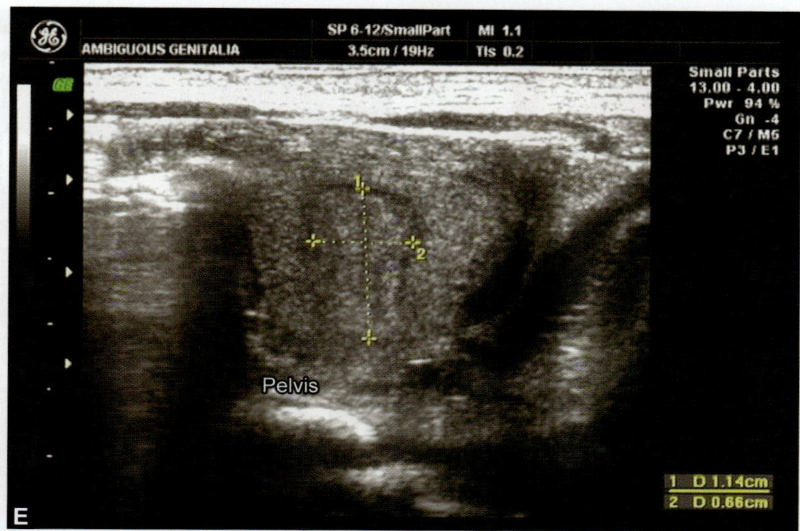

FIGURE 13.5E

FIGURES 13.5A to E: True hermaphrodite. A young baby presented with disorder of sex. HRSG shows phallus shadow. The right testis is seen in the right iliac fossa. But left testis is not seen. The infantile uterus is well-visualized in the pelvis suggestive of true hermaphrodite.

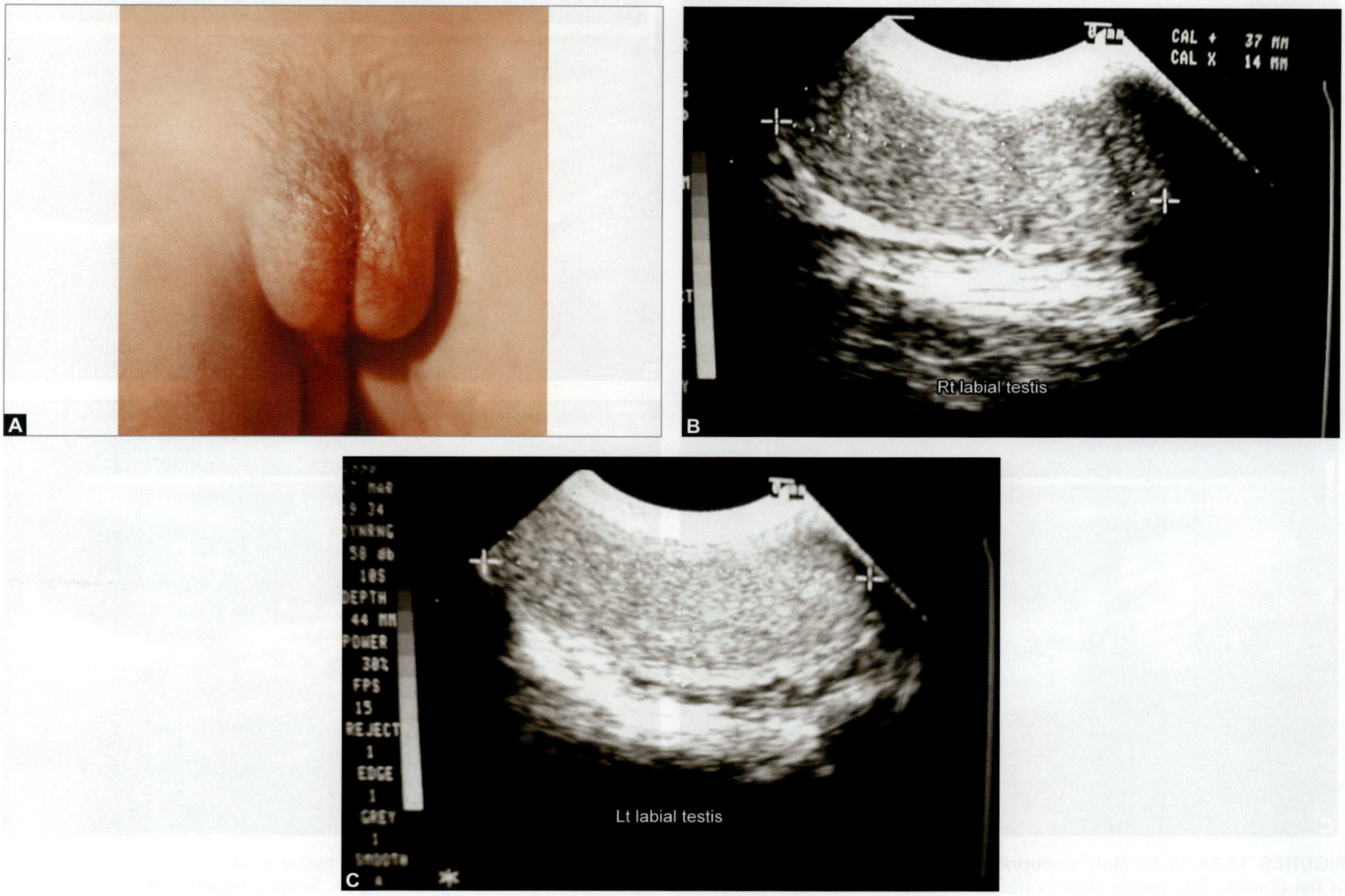

FIGURES 13.6A to C: Male pseudohermaphroditism. A newborn baby presented with disorder of sex. The clinical examination does not show the phallus shadow. HRSG shows well-defined ovoid shadows in both labia. They show granular texture similar to the testis suggestive of male pseudohermaphroditism.

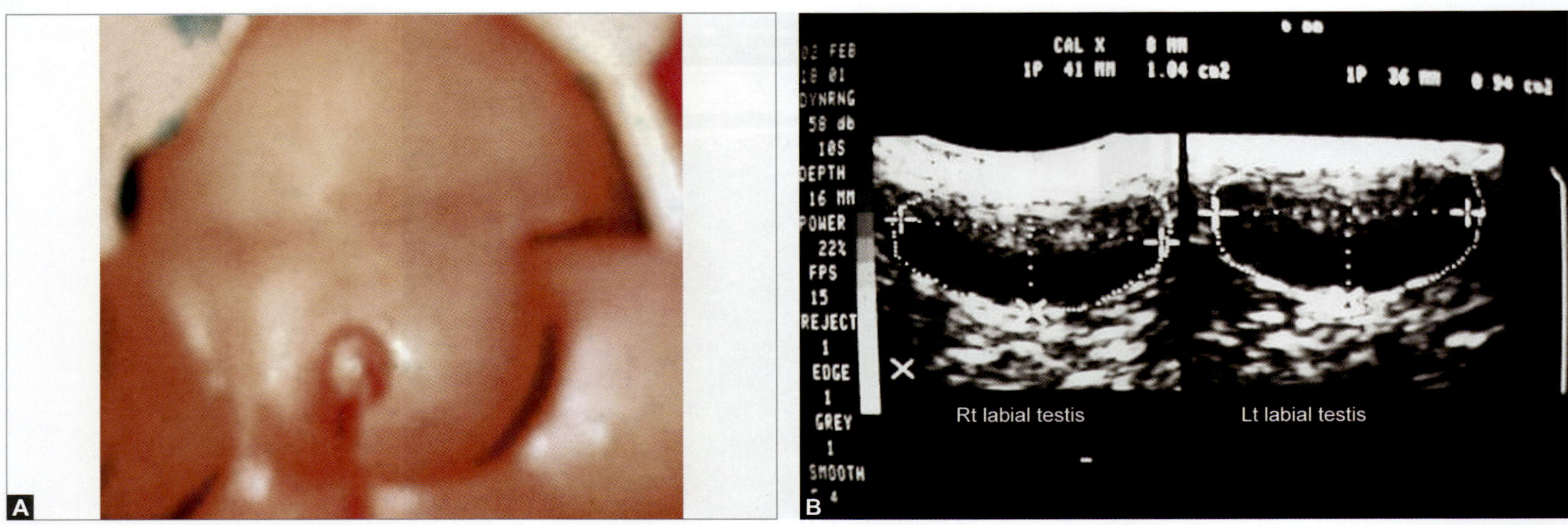

FIGURES 13.7A and B: Disorder of the sex. A newborn baby presented with disorder of sex. Small phallus shadow is seen in the baby. Scrotal shadows are not seen. However, well-defined ovoid shadows are seen in both labia, which show granular texture similar to the testis suggestive of disorder of sex.

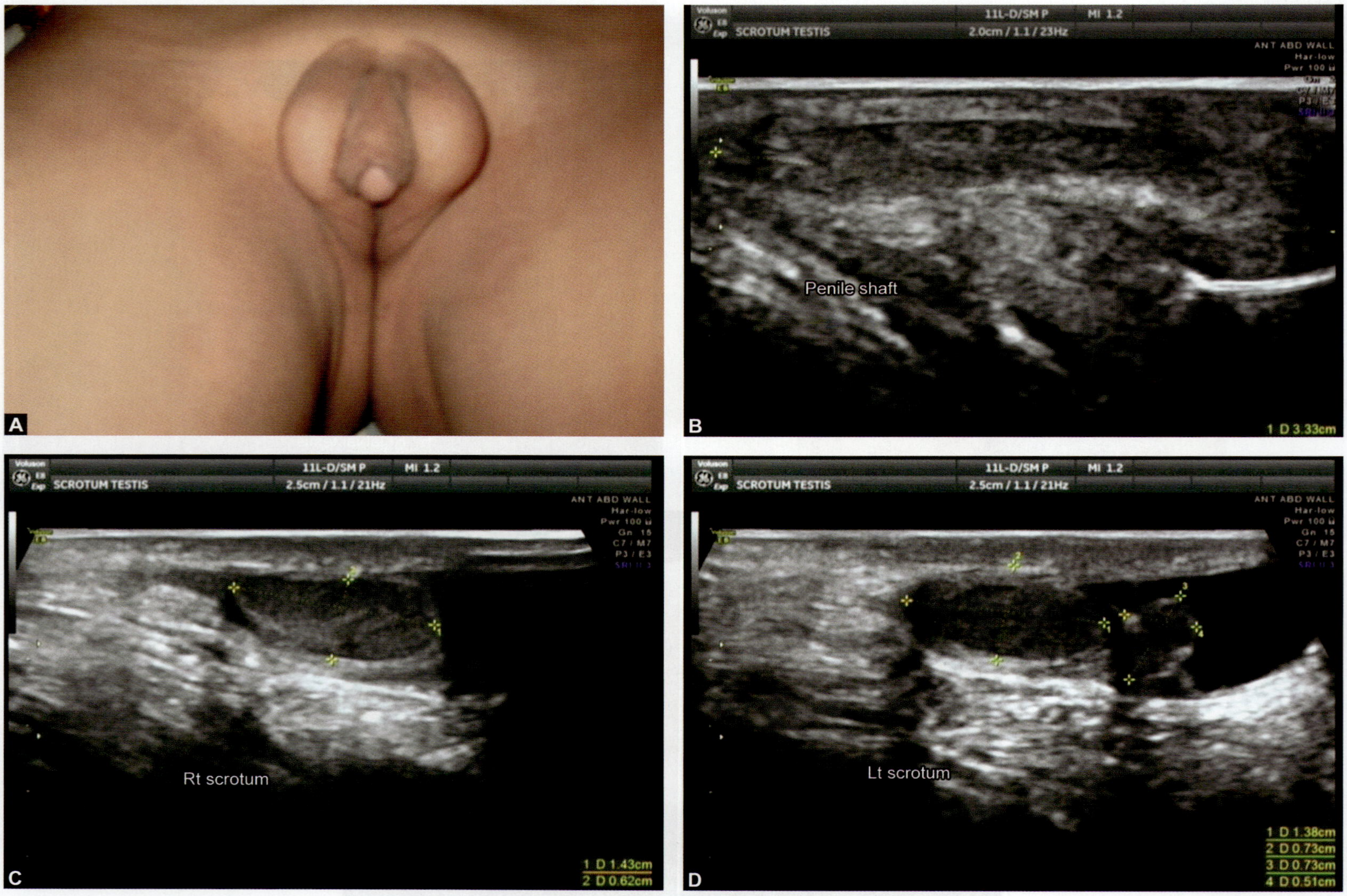

FIGURES 13.8A to D: Male pseudohermaphroditism. A patient presented with small scrotal shadows. Soft tissue swelling is seen on either side of the phallus. The penile shaft is normal in size and appearance. Both testis are seen in both inguinal region. Small amount of fluid is seen in the left scrotal sac. The echotexture is normal suggestive of male pseudohermaphroditism.

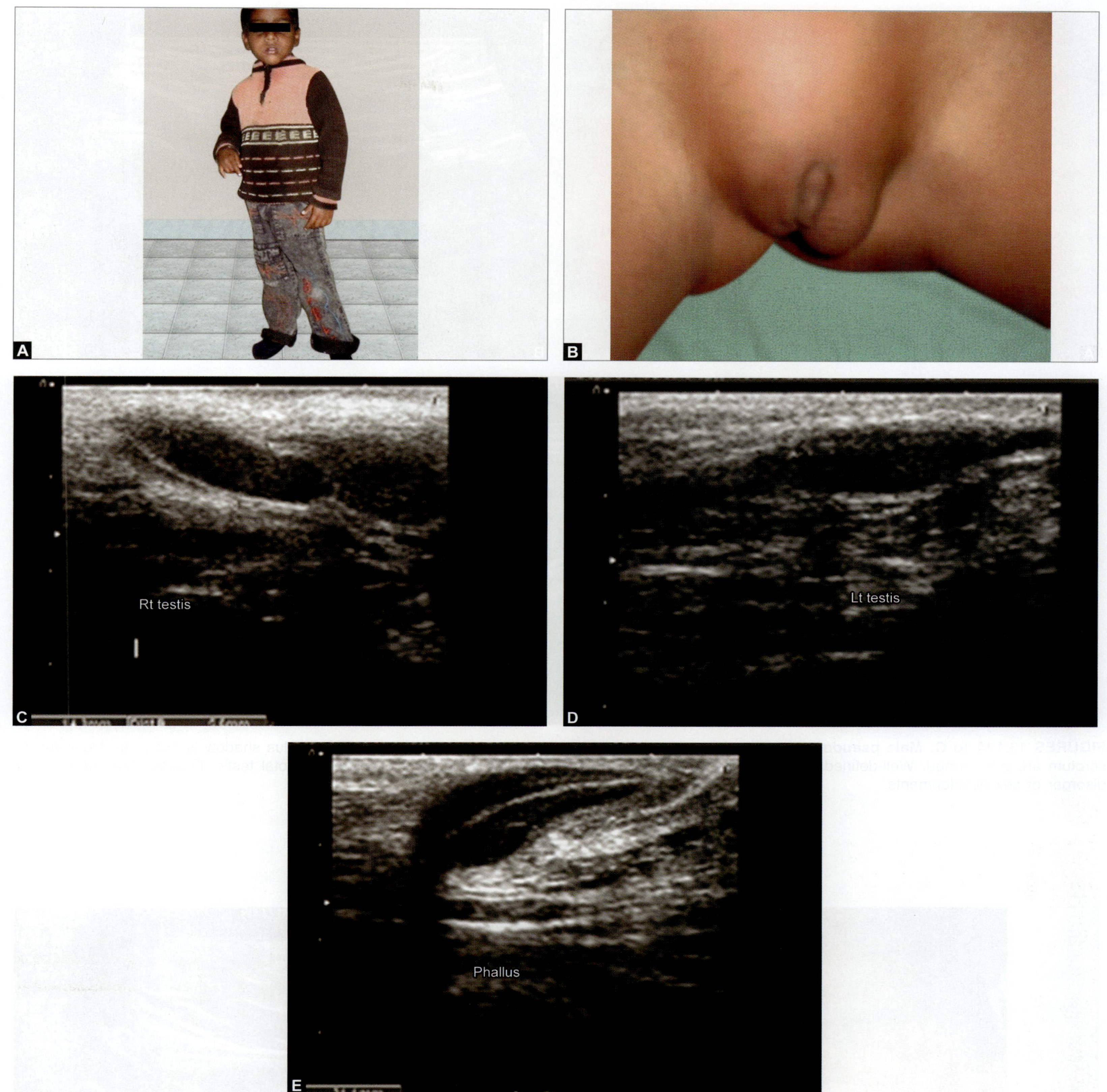

FIGURES 13.9A to E: A young boy present with small phallus shadow. HRSG shows small phallus. There is evidence of small hypoechoic shadow seen in both inguinal region. Normal scrotal shadow is not seen. The testis are hypoechoic but homogeneous in texture. On color flow imaging, low flow is seen in the testis suggestive of bilateral inguinal testis with small phallus.

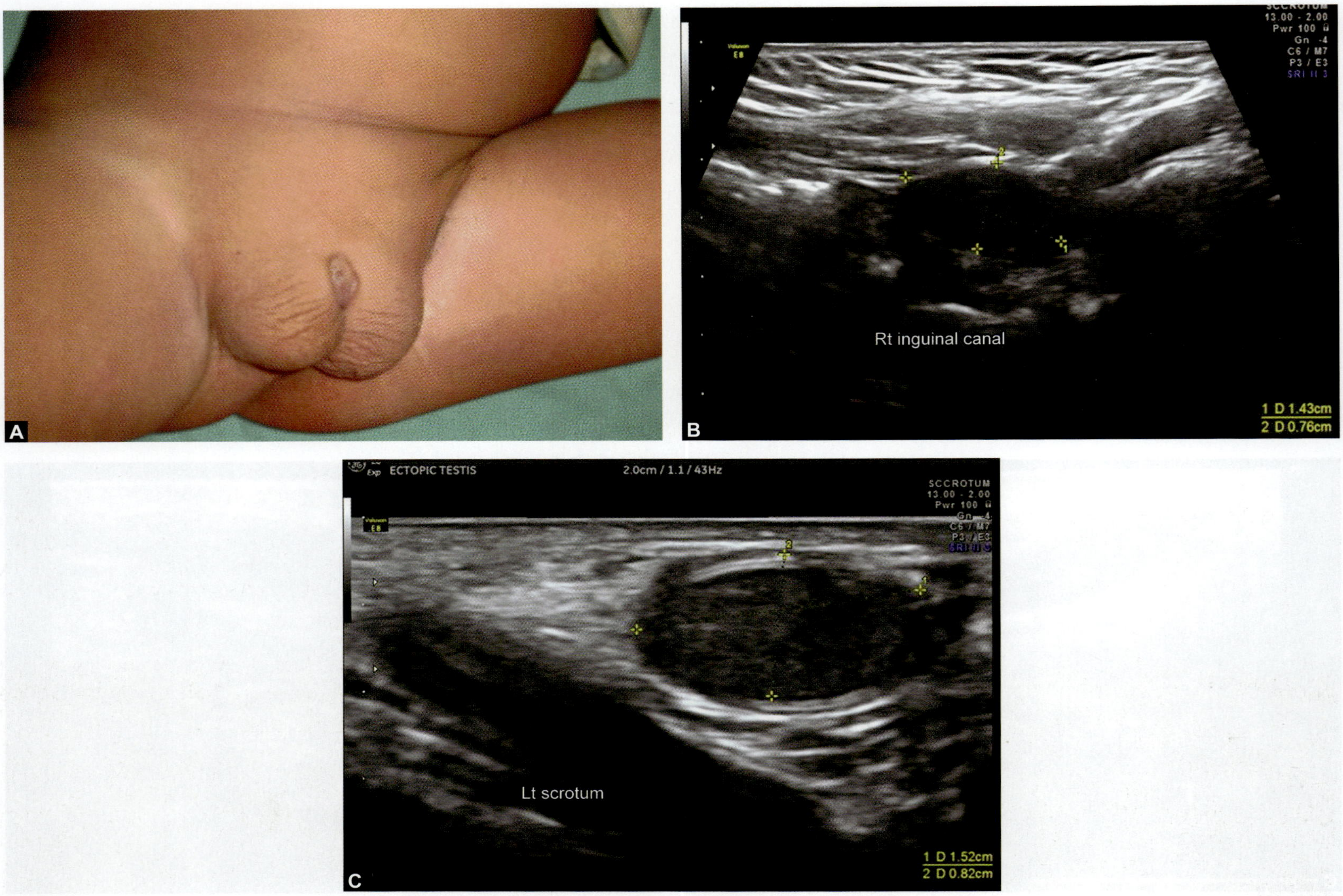

FIGURES 13.10A to C: Male pseudohermaphroditism. A baby was born with genitals abnormality. The phallus shadow is not seen. However, the scrotum are well-formed. Well-defined ovoid shadows are seen in both scrotal sac suggestive of bilateral scrotal testis. Findings are suggestive of disorder of sex developments.

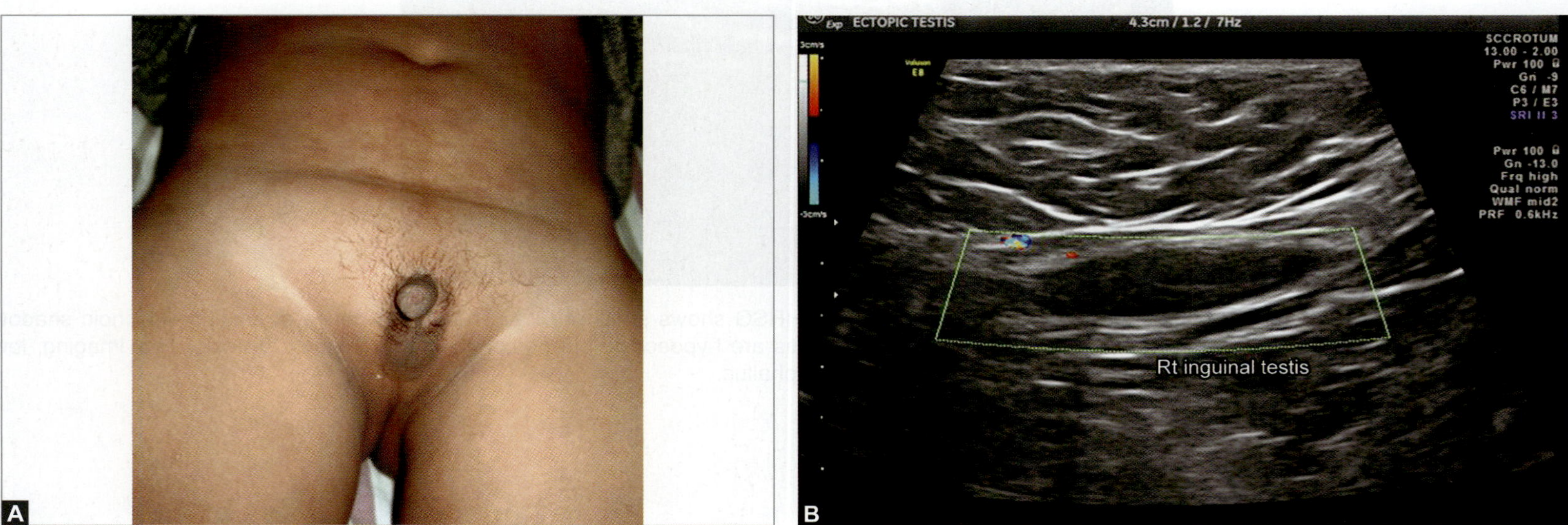

FIGURES 13.11A and B

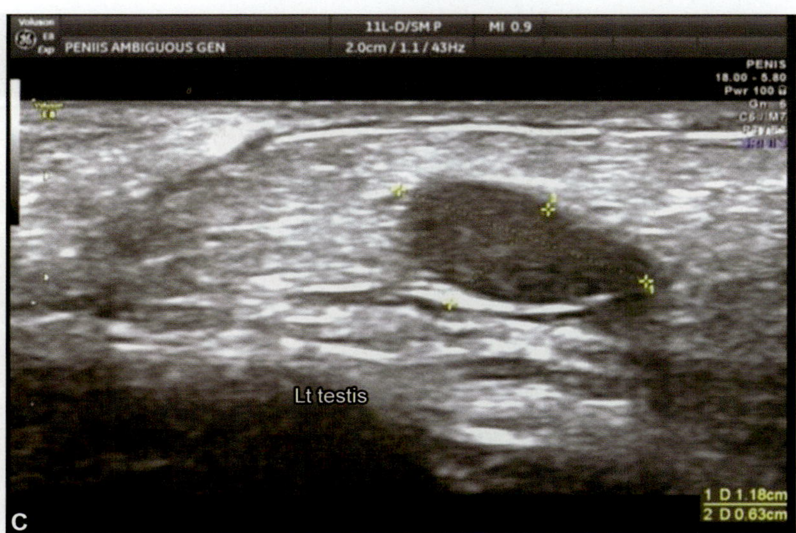

FIGURE 13.11C

FIGURES 13.11A to C: Male pseudohermaphroditism. A baby was born with ambiguous genitalia. The phallus is small. The scrotum are not formed. HRSG shows hyperechoic nodular shadows in both inguinal region suggestive of bilateral ectopic testis. They are small in size but show normal granular pattern of testis.

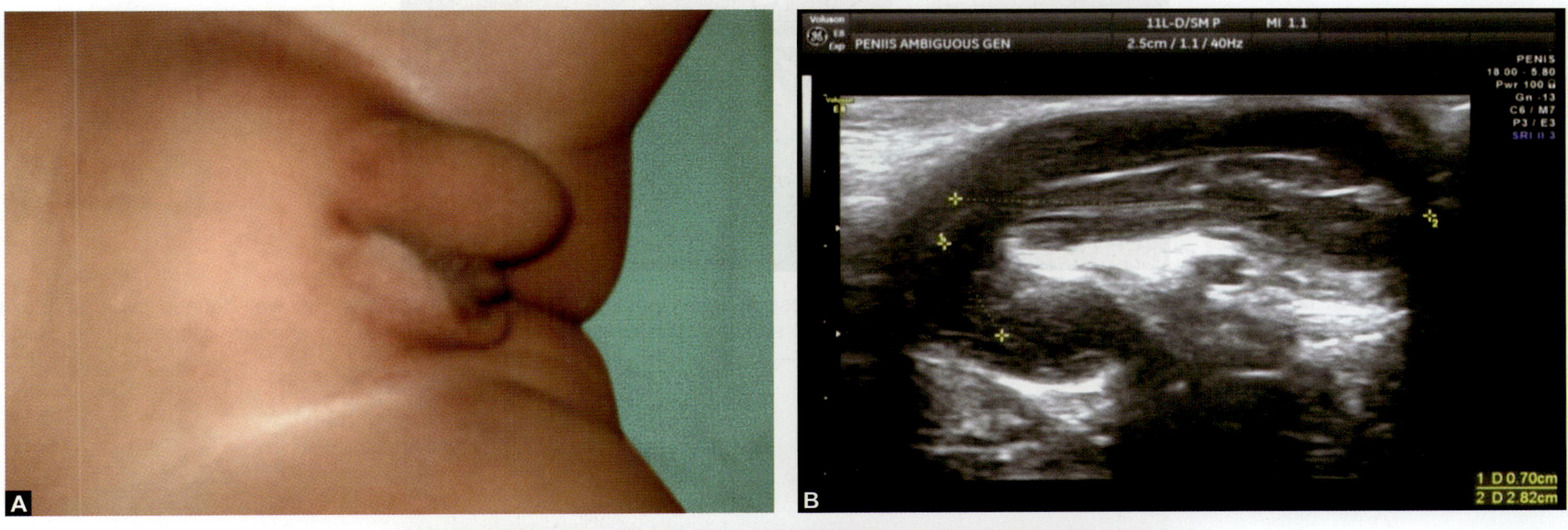

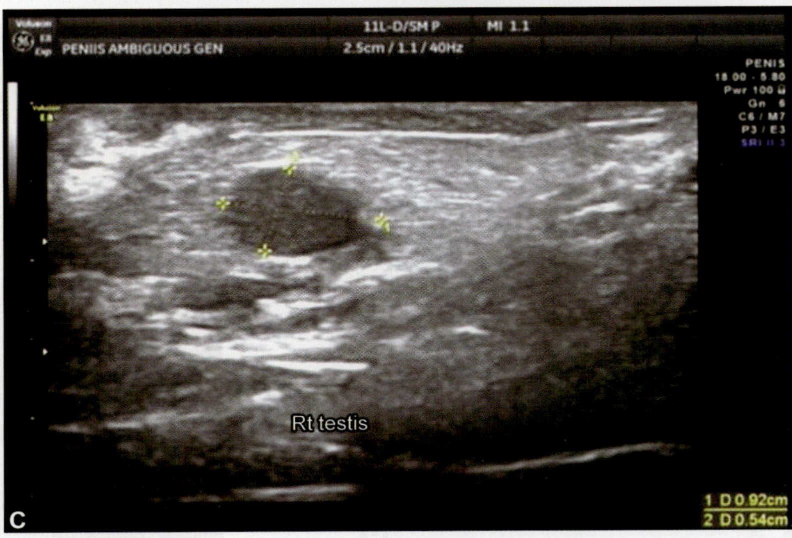

FIGURES 13.12A to C: Male pseudohermaphroditism. A 2-year-baby presented with bilateral small scrotal sac. The phallus is well-formed and appears to be normal. HRSG shows normal size phallus. However, both testis are not seen in both scrotal sacs. Well-defined ovoid shadow is seen in both inguinal regions. Right testis is seen in right inguinal region but left testis is not visualized.

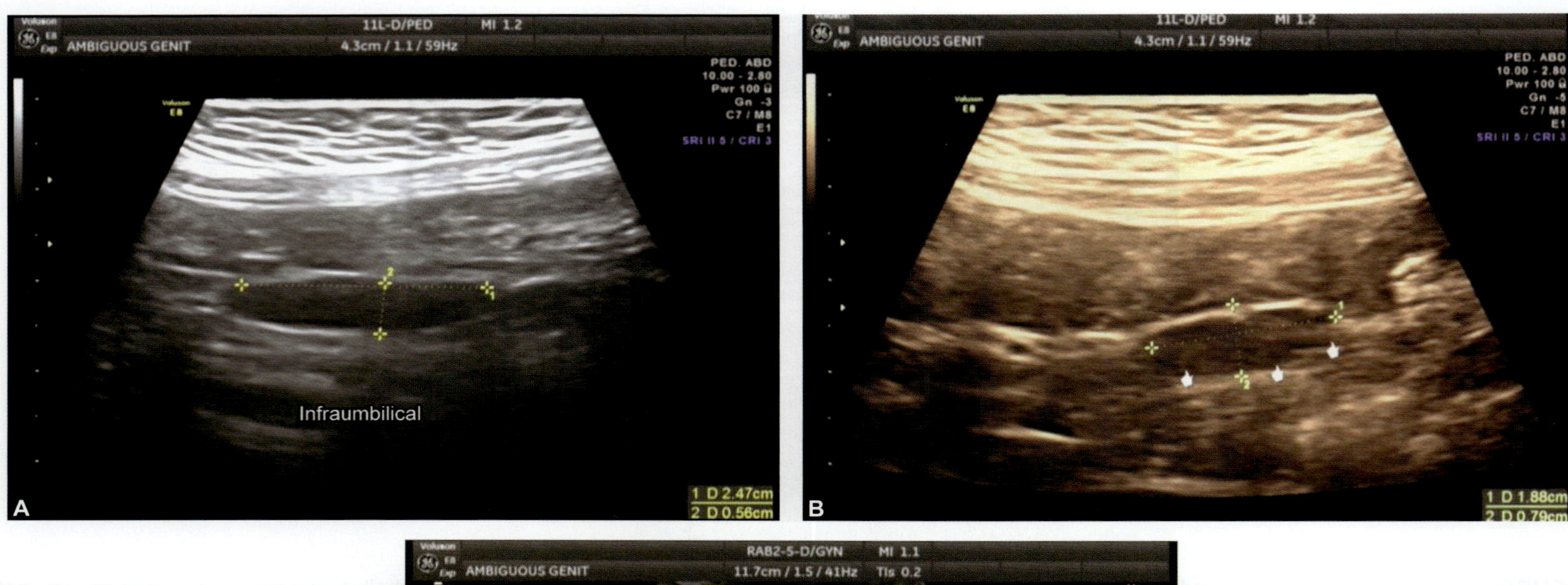

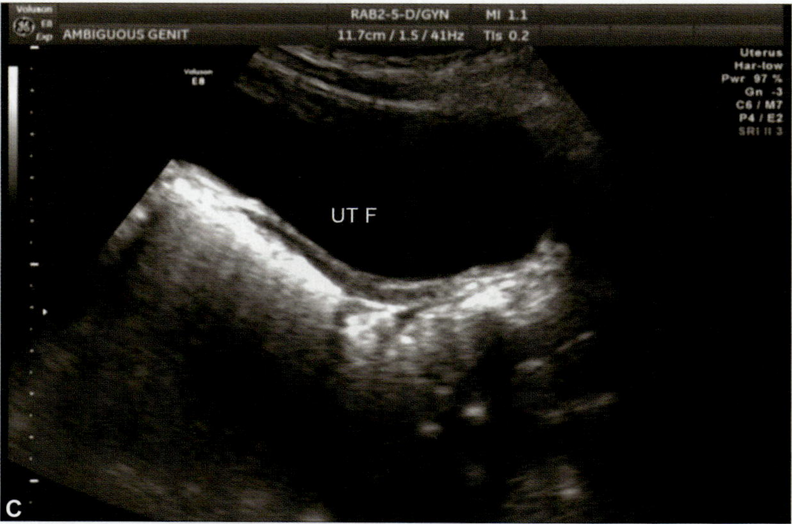

FIGURES 13.13A to C: Male pseudohermaphroditism. A male child presented with ambiguous genitalia. HRSG shows well-defined ovoid shadows in infraumbilical region suggestive of ectopic testis. The pelvic ultrasound shows a streak-like shadow. But no uterine shadow is seen in the pelvis. No ovarian shadow is seen.

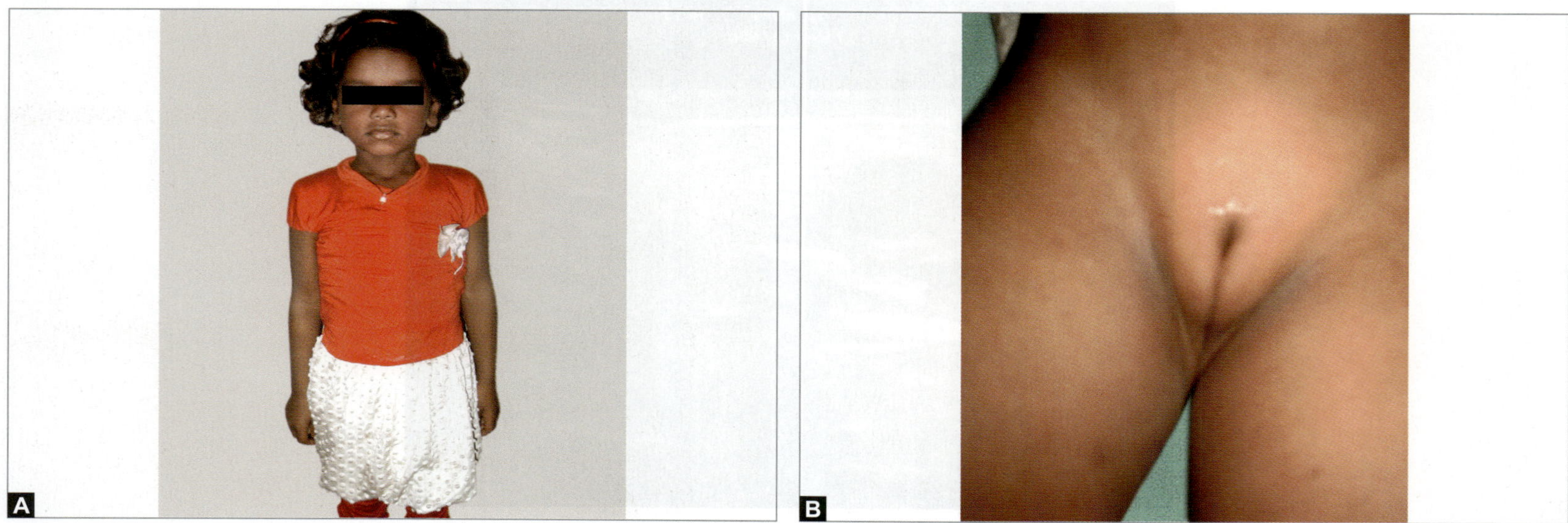

FIGURES 13.14A and B

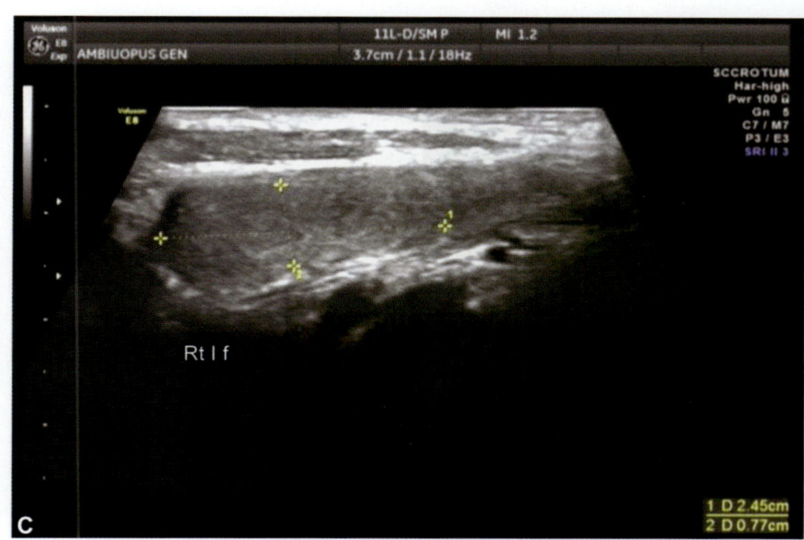

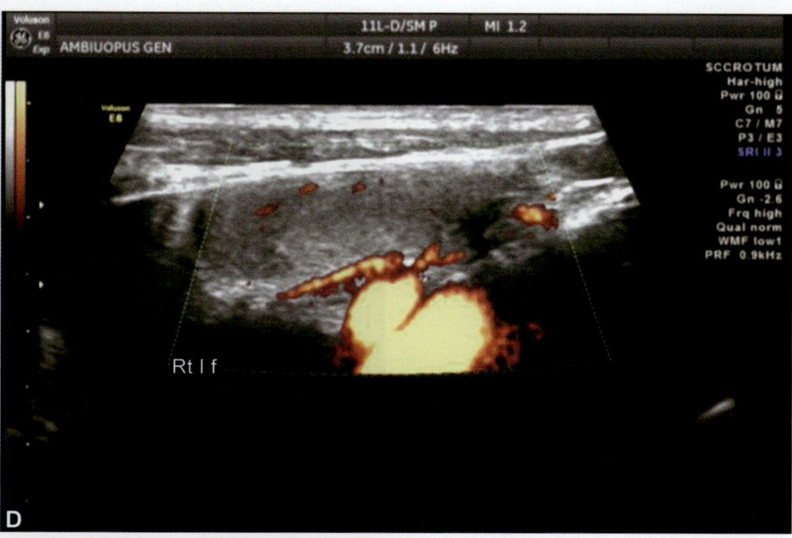

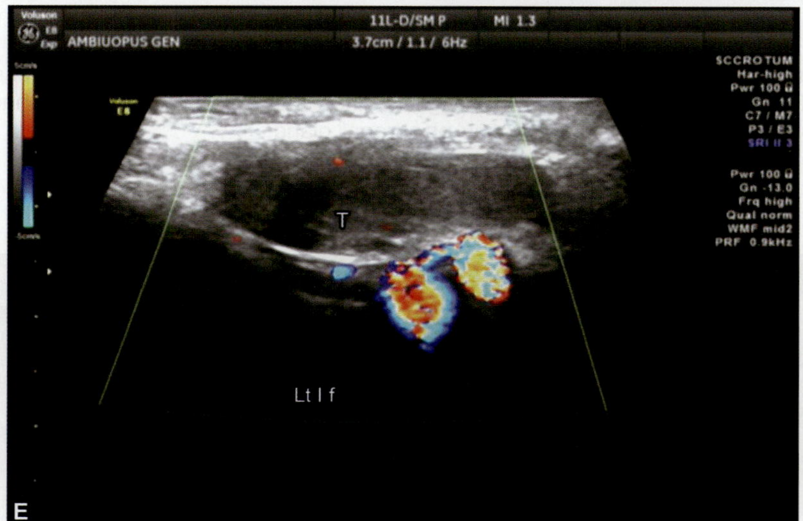

FIGURES 13.14C to E

FIGURES 13.14A to E: Male pseudohermaphroditism. A 6-year-old girl presented with ambiguous genitalia. The clinical image shows labial folds. No phallus shadow is seen. HRSG shows well-defined ovoid shadows in right and left iliac fossae. They are hypoechoic in texture with granular echo pattern suggestive of arrest of the testis. No suggestion of uterine or ovarian shadow is seen in the pelvis.

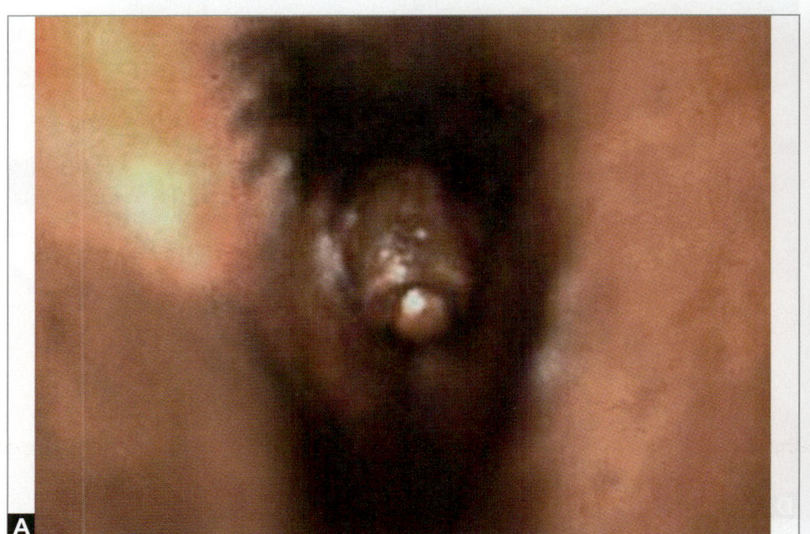

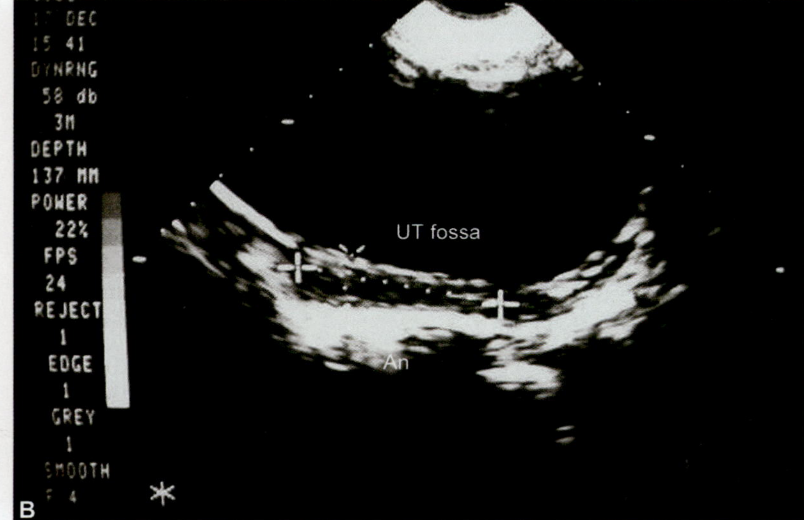

FIGURES 13.15A and B

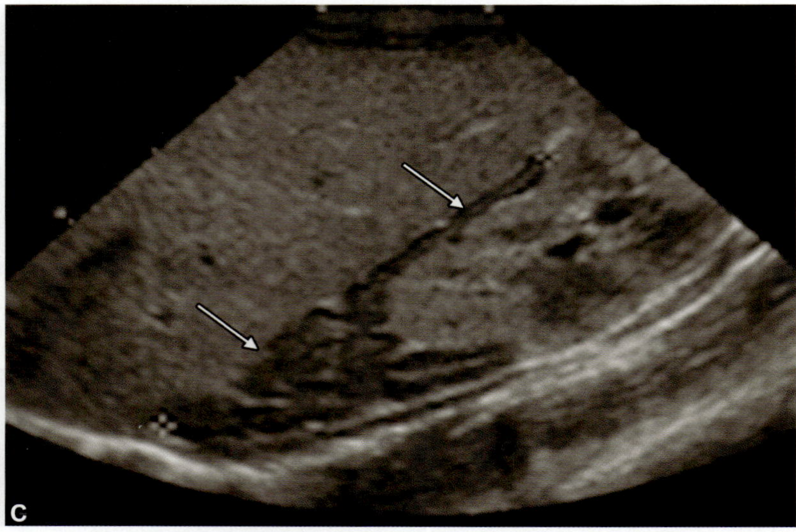

FIGURE 13.15C

FIGURES 13.15A to C: Female pseudohermaphroditism (Congenital adrenal hypertrophy). A patient presented with hypertrophy clitoris. HRSG shows uterine shadow in the pelvis. The right ovary is also seen in right ovarian fossa. But no testicular shadow is seen suggestive of congenital adrenal hypertrophy. The abdominal ultrasound shadows hypertrophy of adrenal gland.

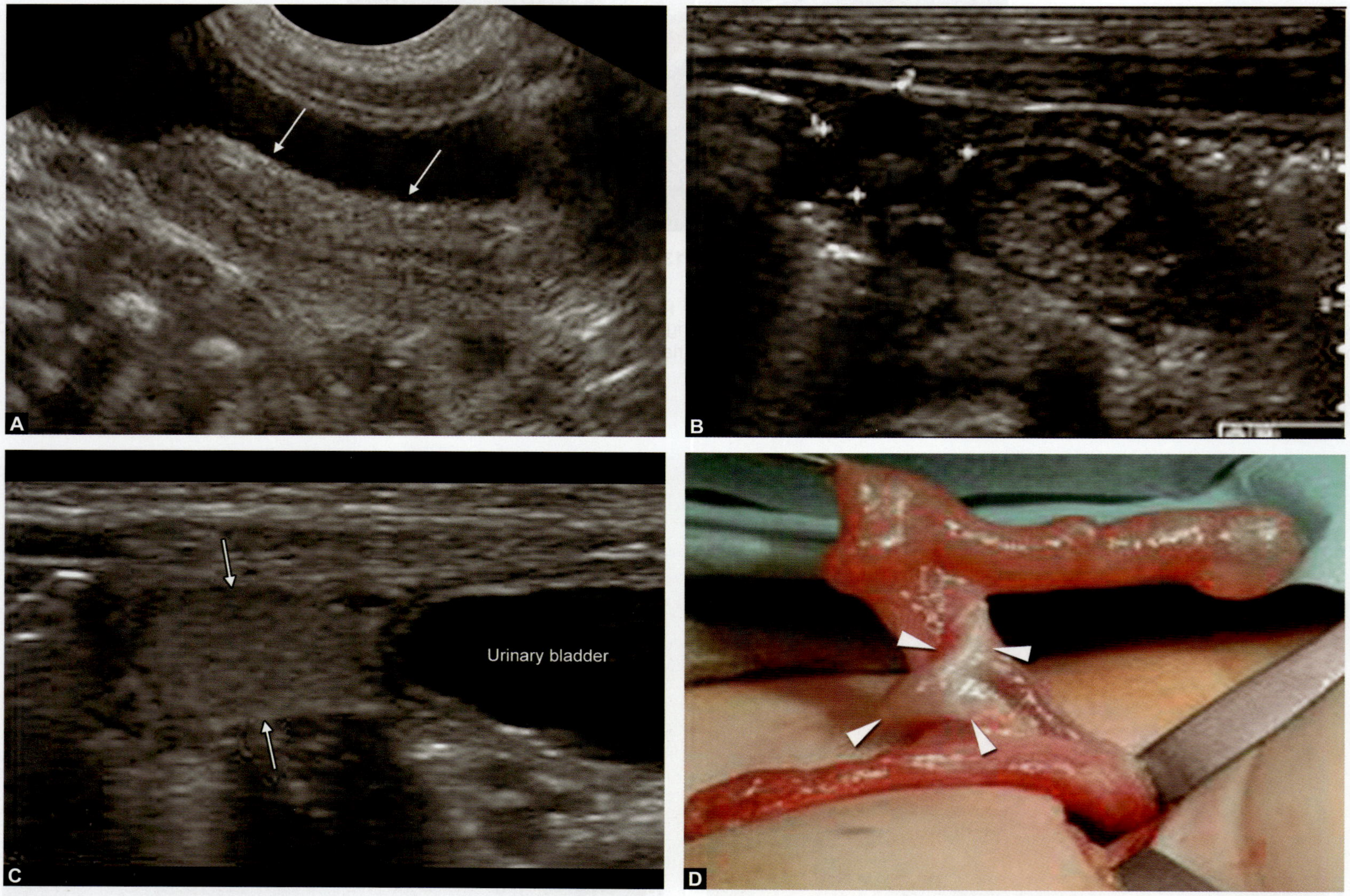

FIGURES 13.16A to D: Mixed gonadal dysgenesis. A baby presented with ambiguous genitalia. HRSG shows well-defined uterus in the pelvis. Right ovary is also seen in the right ovarian fossa. There is also evidence of a ovoid shadow seen on the anterosuperior aspect of UB suggestive of testis. Perioperative findings show streak gonad on one side and one testis is seen on other side. The phallus was buried in the skin.

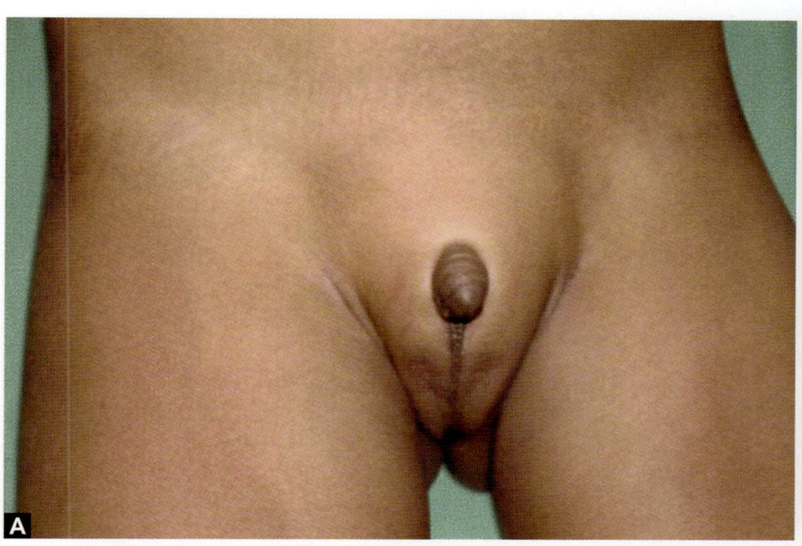

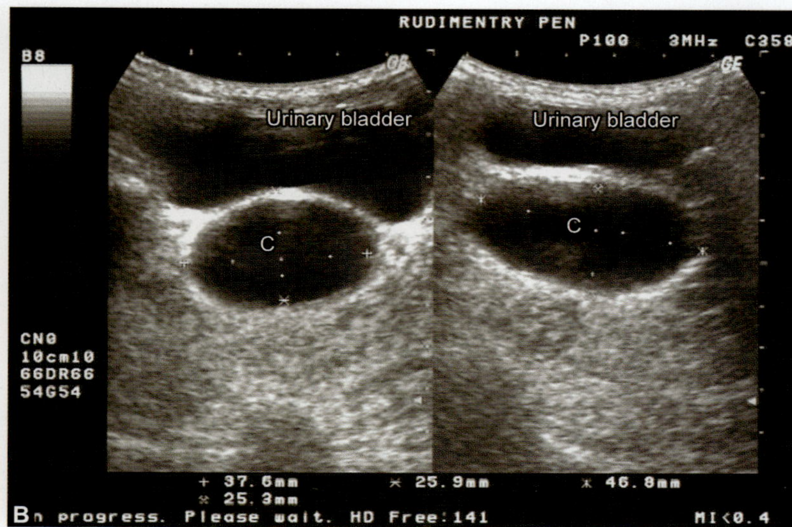

FIGURES 13.17A and B: Pure gonadal agenesis. A 4-year-old baby presented with ambiguous genitalia. The clinical image shows hypertrophy of clitoris. But no scrotal shadow is seen. On ultrasound, no evidence of uterus and ovaries is seen in the pelvis. The testes are also not seen in inguinal canal or in abdomen. However, a well-defined cystic shadow is seen in the pelvis suggestive of pure gonadal agenesis.

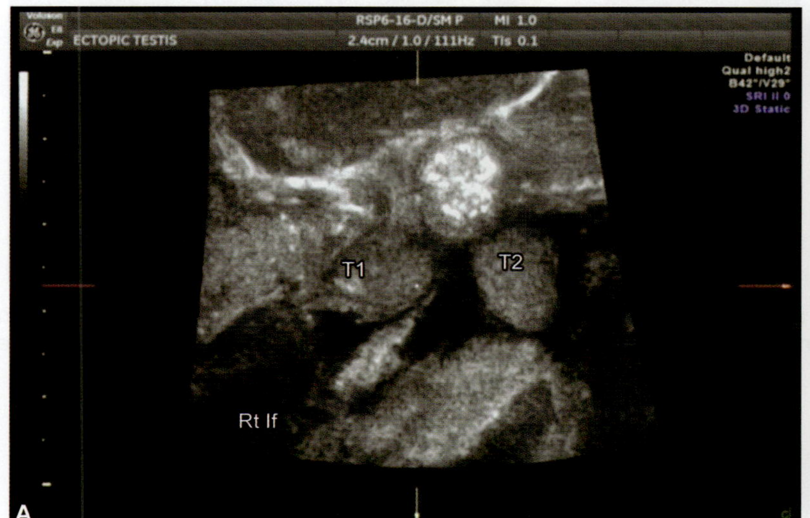

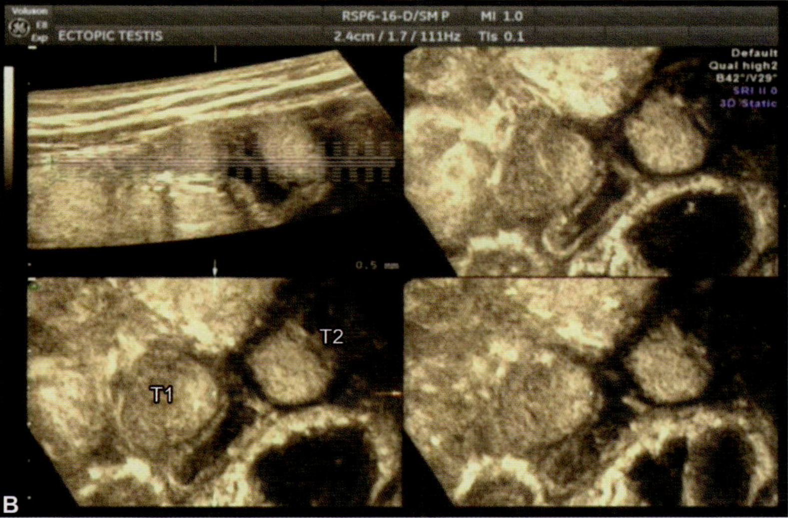

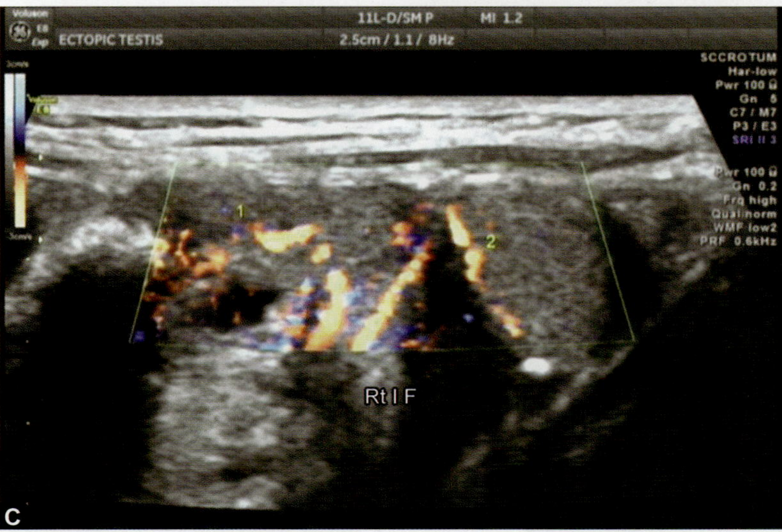

FIGURES 13.18A to C: Ambiguous genitalia with crossed testis. A baby was born with ambiguous genitalia. The clinical image shows small phallus. The scrotal shadows are not seen. HRSG shows small phallus. There is also evidence of well-defined ovoid shadows seen in right iliac fossa anterior to iliac vessels. They show granular texture similar to testes. On color flow imaging, low flow is seen in them suggestive of bilateral crossed ectopic testis.

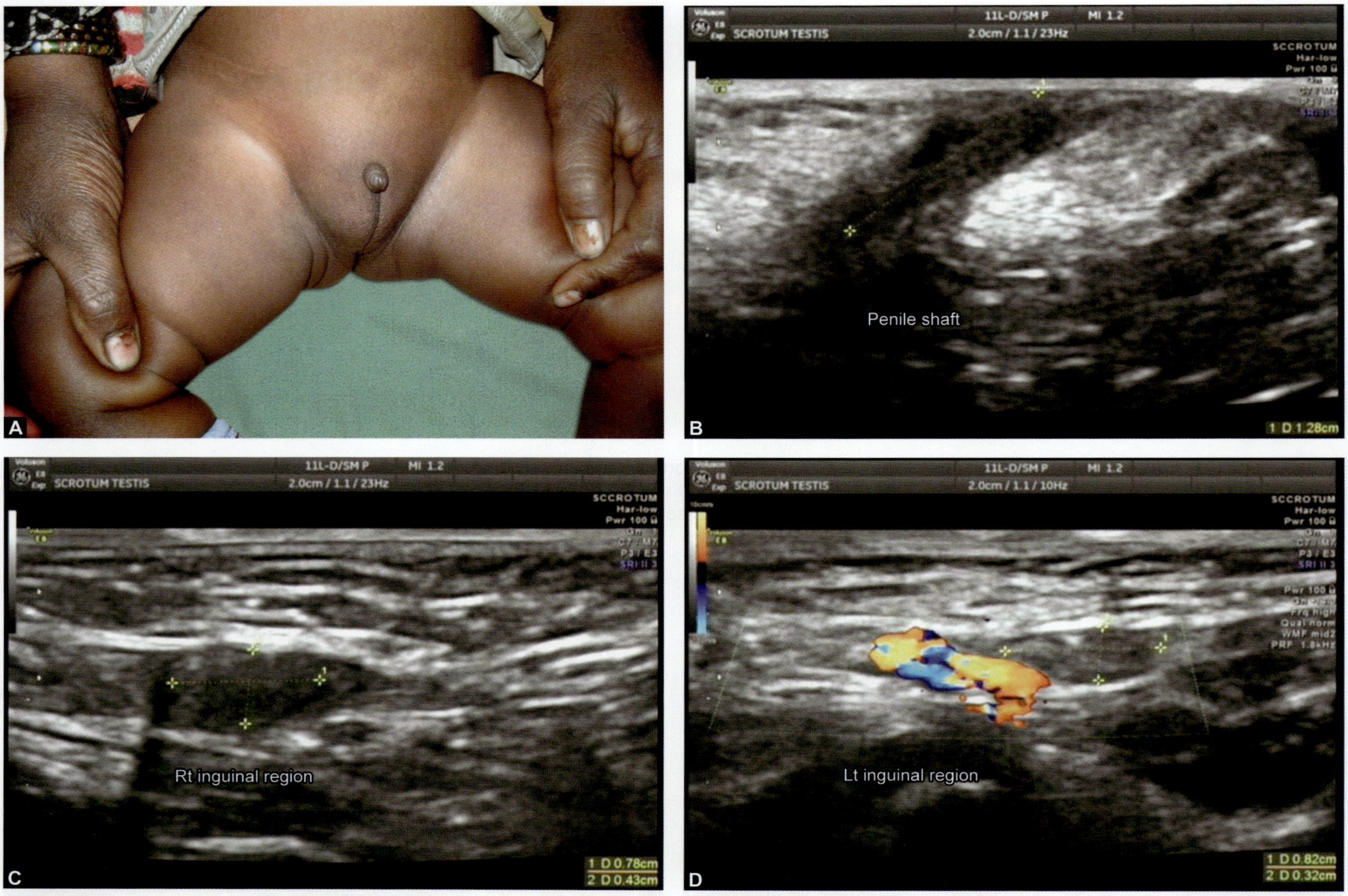

FIGURES 13.19A to D: Small rudimentary penis. A baby presented with ambiguous genitalia. HRSG shows small rudimentary penis, which is seen buried in the skin. Both testes are seen in both inguinal canal. They are small in size. But they show granular texture similar to the testes suggestive of bilateral ectopic testes.

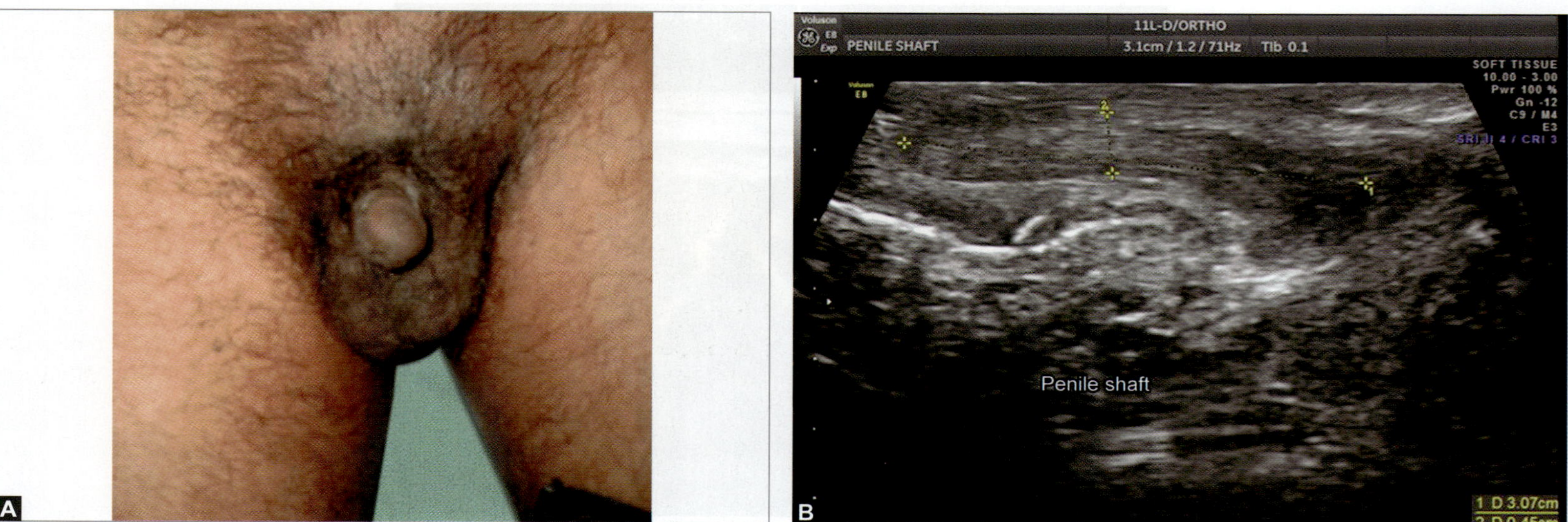

FIGURES 13.20A and B

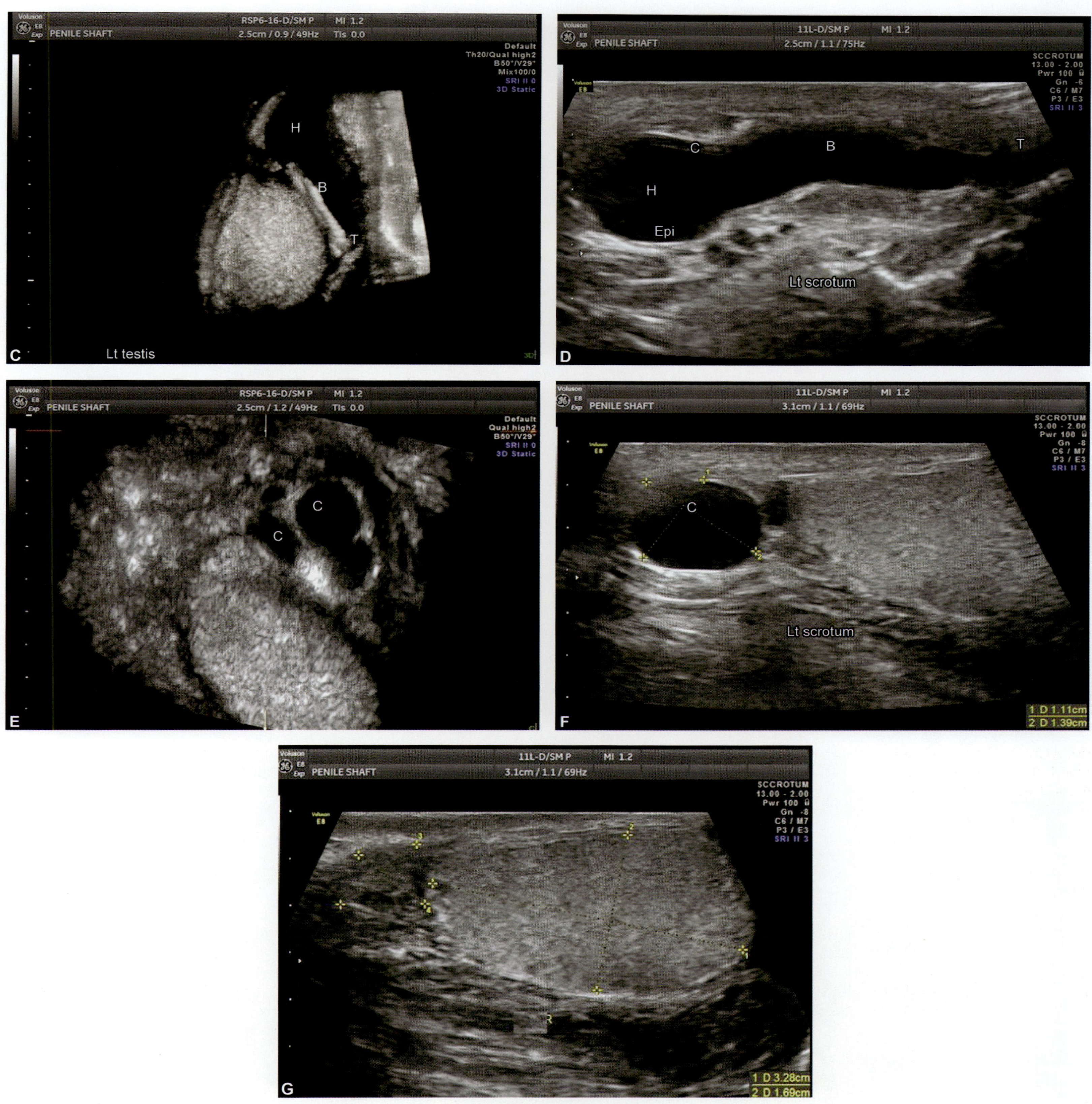

FIGURES 13.20C to G

FIGURES 13.20A to G: A patient presented with small penis. HRSG shows small penile shaft. However, echotexture of penile shaft is normal. Both testes are normal. Big cyst is seen in left epididymis. It is seen extending to the body and tail of epididymis. Right testis is normal. No cyst is seen in body and tail of right epididymis.

CONCLUSION

High-resolution ultrasound is the first line investigation of disorders of sex development (DSD). It can detect all the four categories of DSD with other associated anomalies. It is noninvasive, cost effective and multiplanar modality. It does not require sedation or medication. Color Doppler ultrasound with 3D imaging enhances the diagnostic accuracy.

CHAPTER 14

Penis

PK Srivastava

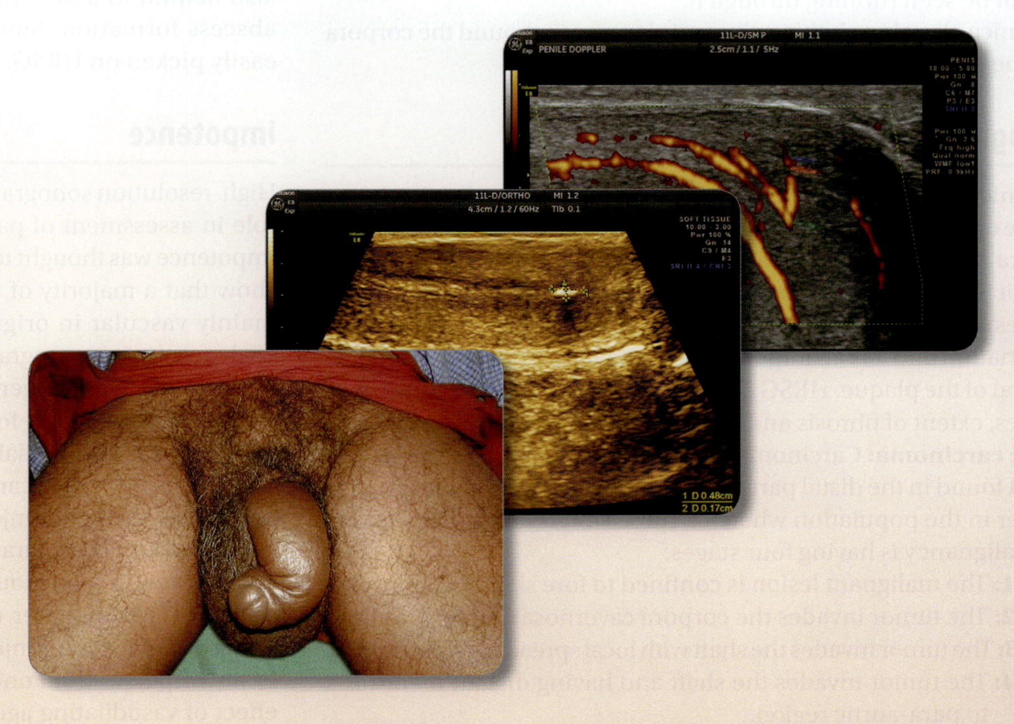

PENIS

Penis, the male genital organ is an important part of the body to do dual role of providing excretion of urine and also semen, vital for natural human reproduction. In the past, investigation of penis was limited to plain X-ray films, micturating or retrograde urethrography and cavernography. Recently, high-resolution sonography (HRSG) of penis and Doppler flow imaging of penile vasculature and blood vessels have made study of penile anatomy, physiological, pathological erectile functional study a practical proposition. Sono urethrography with the saline solution or water as contrast agents, has made HRSG an exciting modality for assessment of penile urethra. Assessment of penile erectile dysfunction with color Doppler study is the most exciting development in field of impotence.

Anatomy

Penis has three major components. They are two paired dorsal columns of corpora cavernosa and one ventral column of corpus spongiosum. They are highly vascular structures and having paired dorsal arteries lying superficially and two deep arteries each running through corpora cavernosa known as cavernosal arteries. These corpora are covered with a much dense connective tissue known as tunica albuginea. The penile urethra runs through the penile shaft through the corpora spongiosa. The venous drainage takes place through the corpora and dorsal vein of penis. It is situated between the two dorsal arteries. HRSG shows normal corpora cavernosa as medium level echo complex bodies running longitudinally. They are best assessed in cross section. In normal situation low blood flow is seen in the cavernosal arteries. The corpora spongiousm is less echogenic than corpora cavernosa. The urethral lumen can be seen running through it.

The tunica albuginea is thin echogenic layer seen around the corpora and can be easily resolved on HRSG.

Pathological Conditions

1. **Peyronie's disease:** This is an idiopathic condition usually seen in 4th decade onward. There is deposition of fibrous and calcified plaques in corpora cavernosa and tunica albuginea. HRSG shows these plaques. When it is calcified it is accompanied with acoustic shadowing. These plaques can be better assessed and resolved on HRSG than clinical examination and it is an important investigation prior to the surgical removal of the plaque. HRSG can specially tells about the number of plaques, extent of fibrosis and tunica involvement by the disease.
2. **Penile carcinoma:** Carcinoma of penis is epithelial carcinoma. It is almost found in the distal part of penis. The incidence of malignancy is lower in the population where circumcision is common practice. The malignancy is having four stages:
   Stage 1: The malignant lesion is confined to fore skin or glans only.
   Stage 2: The tumor invades the corpora cavernosa and penile shaft.
   Stage 3: The tumor invades the shaft with local spread to lymph nodes.
   Stage 4: The tumor invades the shaft and having distant metastasis to para-aortic region.

Almost 50% patients report when tumor spreads to regional inguinal lymph nodes HRSG can very well tell the extent of the primary tumor and its invasion to corporal tissue. Distant metastasis to para-aortic region or to other distant location can be easily assessed on HRSG.

URETHRA

The male urethra is having three parts.
1. Prostatic
2. Membranous
3. Penile or spongy urethra.

Posterior urethra is about 3 cm long and seen passing through prostate gland. It is also known as prostatic part of urethra. The membranous urethra is about 1.5 cm in length and narrowest part of urethra. It lies at the level of external urethral sphincter. The penile urethra is the longest part of urethra and measures 15–20 cm in length. It is about 6 mm in diameter. The proximal bulbar and intrabulbar part and the distal part of urethra near the meatus show slight dilatation. HRSG shows all the three part of urethra. Prostatic part of urethra is seen through trans abdominal, transperineal approach. However, it is best seen with trans rectal approach.

The penile urethra is seen with high frequency transducers having frequency from 7–10 MHz. It is seen with direct contact scanning technique. Urethrography is done to evaluate rupture of urethra, urethral fistula and urethral structures. It is done with 8 no. Foley's catheter with balloon inflated in the navicular fossa. The antegrade urethrography is done by asking the patient to void the urine against distally blocked urethral meatus. The retrograde urethrography is done by sterile saline solution through the Foley's catheter. The urethral pathology can very well be evaluated on HRSG. The urethral structure can be identified. Extent of the fibrosis in the surrounding corpus spongiousm can be easily evaluated on HRSG than by conventional X-ray urethrography. HRSG shows narrowing of the lumen with structure of urethra. The fibrosis is seen as an irregular echogenic shadow extending or involving in the spongiosum. It is also helpful in assessing the urethral diverticulam and periurethral abscess formation. Small urethral calculi in the diverticula can be easily picked on HRSG.

Impotence

High-resolution sonography and color flow imaging plays an important role in assessment of pathological causes of impotence. Till recently impotence was thought to be a psychological problem. However, studies show that a majority of the cases were having pathological problems mainly vascular in origin-like arterial insufficiency or venous leak. High-resolution sonography plays an important role in assessment in both types of vasculogenic impotence. The duplex color flow imaging is an accurate method for the assessment of arterial flow in the dorsal penile artery, cavernosal artery and venous flow in dorsal penile vein. The arterial flow study can be done before and after injecting vasodilating agents like papaverine injection. The longitudinal examination of corpora cavernosa is done in parasagittal axis. In a flaccid stage, cavernosal artery can be seen in a tortuous course. However, in erect stage it becomes straight. The diameter of cavernosal arteries can also be assessed. 60 mg of papaverine is injected in either of corpora cavernosum. The drug easily disperses from one corpus cavernosum to other. The maximum effect of vasodilating agent is achieved between 5 to 20 minutes after the injection. However, in standard protocol, the study is carried out up to 45 minutes after the injection depending upon the patient response. The velocity measurements are taken at 5 minutes interval for at least 30 minutes after the injection. The normal peak systolic and diastolic measurements should be recorded in both cavernosal arteries at 5 minutes interval.

There are five phases of spectral waveform in the cavernosal arteries after the injecting. These 5 phases are seen within 5–20 minutes after the injection. However, in a patient having vasculogenic impotence, all the normal five phases cannot be achieved due to arterial insufficiency or venous leak.

Arteriogenic Impotence

The normal peak systolic velocity which is achieved after intracavernosal injection of vasodilating agent is >30 cm/sec. Most of the patients are having moderate to good response on injection have peak systolic velocity >25 cm/sec. However, those patient who are having arterial insufficiency, the peak systolic velocity is <25 cm/sec. This indicates an arterial disease. The peak systolic value between 25 and 30 cm per second should be considered as borderline response. However, value more than 30 cm/sec should be taken as normal. If there is difference of 10 cm/sec between the values of both cavernosal arteries, unilateral arterial disease should be suspected. The diastolic flow in the cavernosal artery may be reversed and should be taken as normal phenomena in latter stages of erection. Collateral vessels to the cavernosal artery may present as a normal variant.

Vengeance Impotence

The vasculogenic impotence may be due to excessive venous leak from the corpora cavernosa. Although, the exact cause of this excessive venous leak is not known however, it is assumed that tunica albuginea stretches beyond the normal limit thus cannot obliterate the emissary veins draining the sinusoids during the erection. Due to the inadequate compression of emissary veins the venous outflow continuous and erection is never fully obtained. A venous leak is suspected when persistent high diastolic flow is seen in the cavernosal arteries and the diastolic flow is >3 cm/sec.

CONCLUSION

High-resolution sonography and color flow imaging are an excellent modality for evaluation of penis and its pathological conditions. The biggest advantage of modality is the study of physiological and pathological erectile function of penis in impotence. It is reliable, cost effective and noninvasive in technique for assessment of vasculogenic impotence.

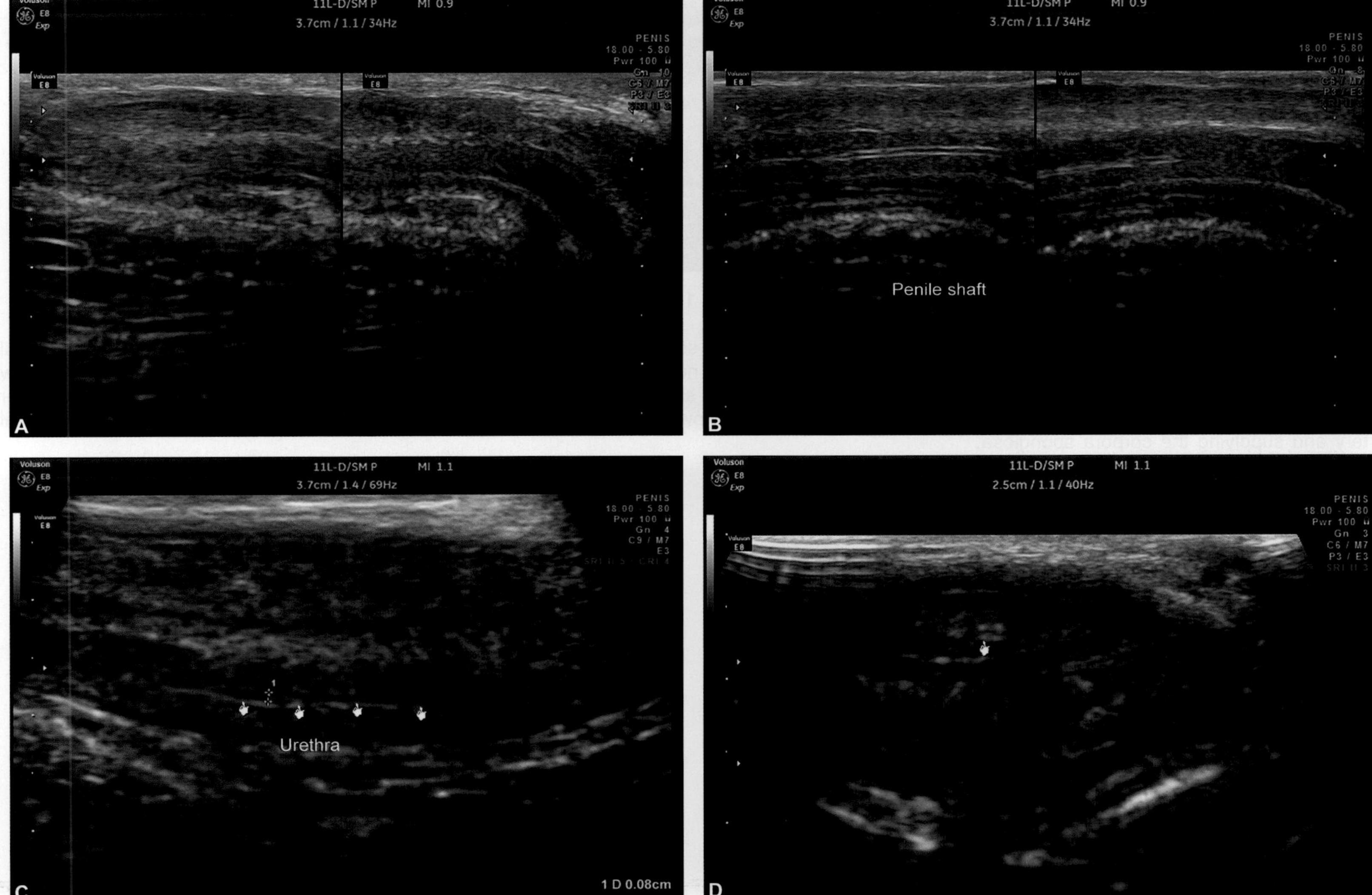

FIGURES 14.1A to D

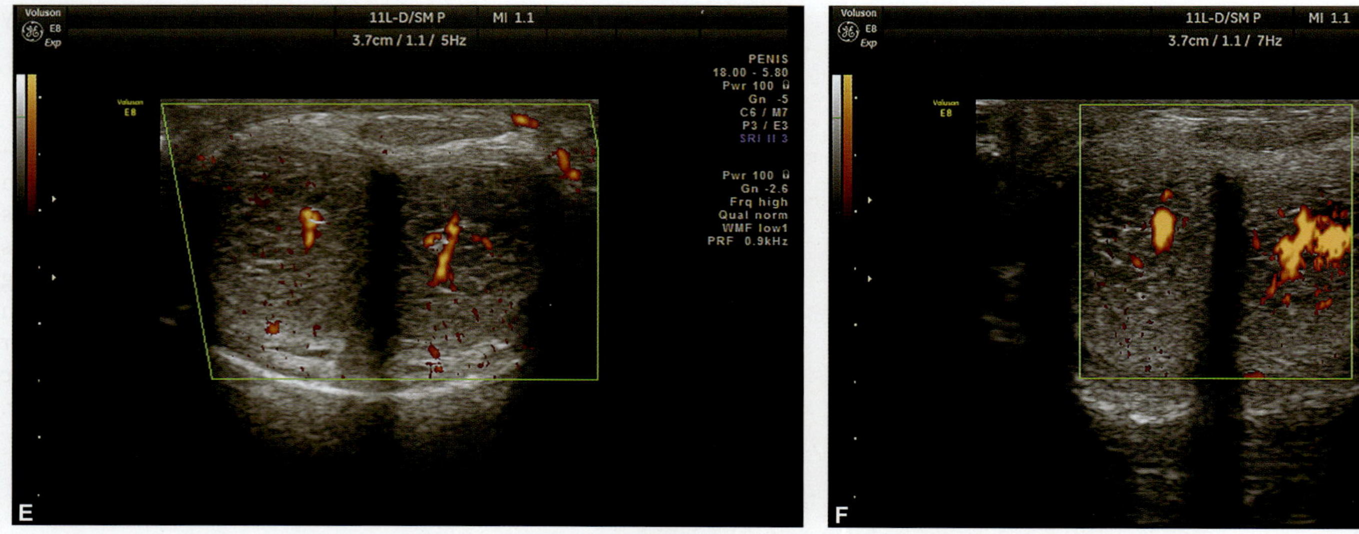

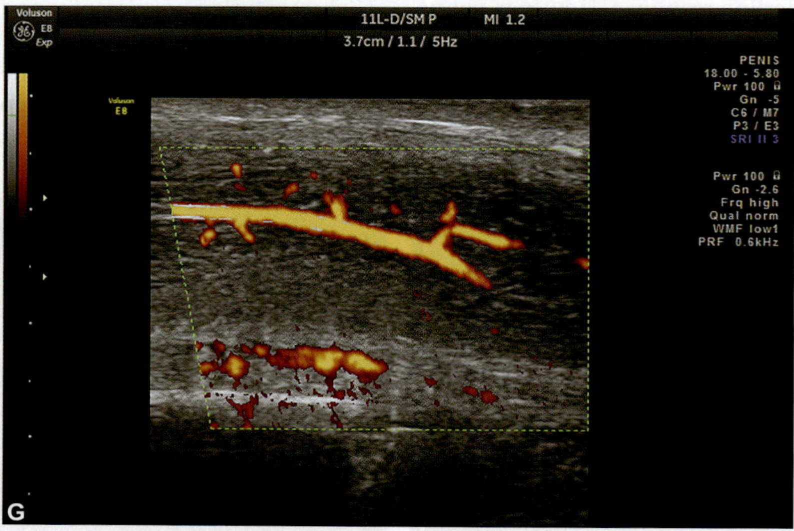

FIGURES 14.1E to G

FIGURES 14.1A to G: Normal anatomy (Penile shaft). High-resolution sonography (HRSG) shows the normal penile shaft. Homogeneous medial level echoes are seen in the corpora. On color flow imaging very low or no flow is appreciated in penile vessel. Color flow imaging shows low flow in the dorsalis penile artery and cavernosal arteries. Color flow imaging shows low flow in cavernosal artery in longitudinal axis. Spectral Doppler tracing of cavernosal arteries shows the low arterial flow pattern. Color flow imaging shows multiple small branches coming out from the cavernosal artery and supplying the corpora spongiosa.

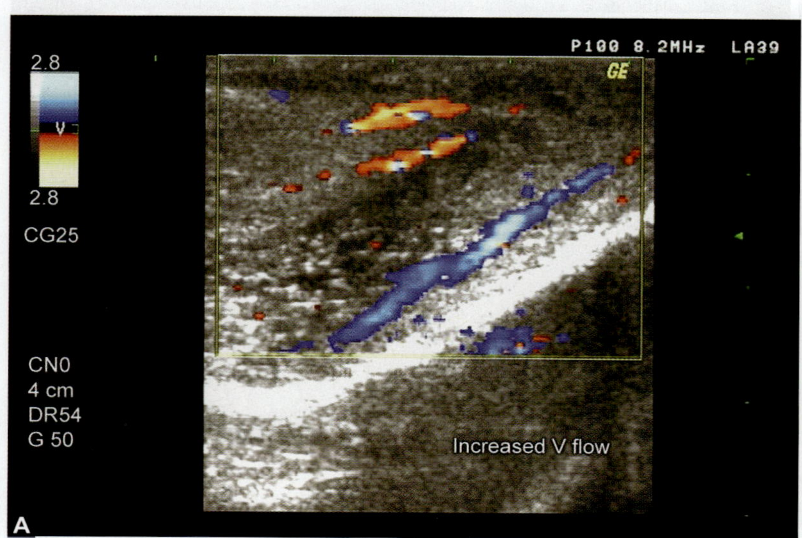

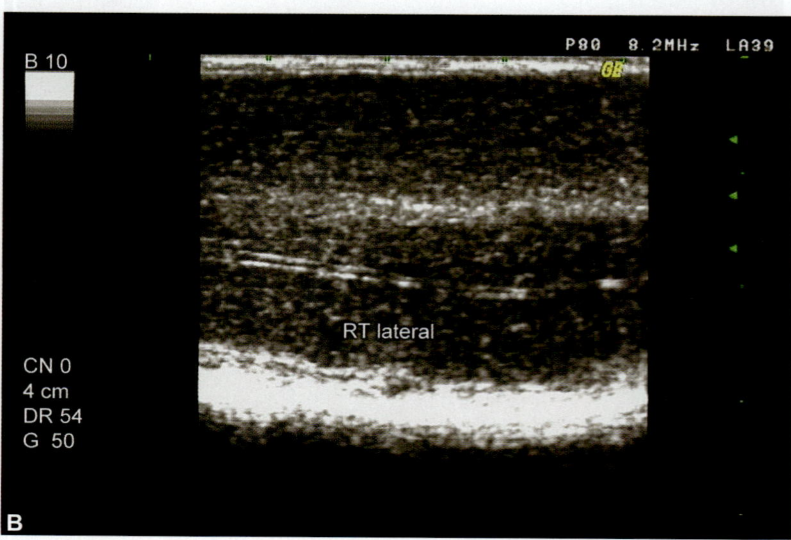

FIGURES 14.2A and B

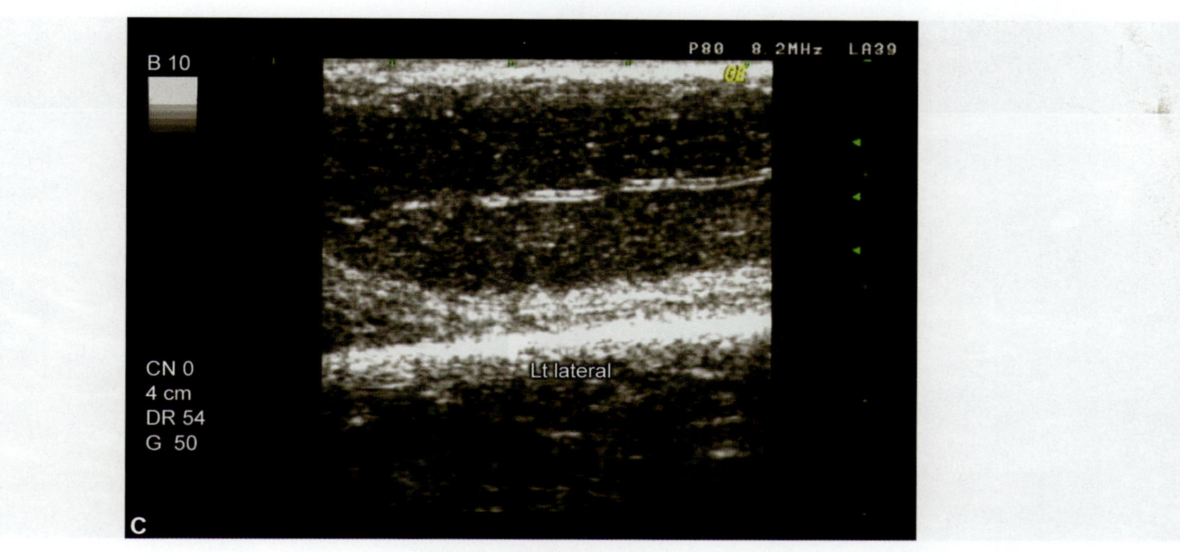

FIGURE 14.2C

FIGURES 14.2A to C: The dorsal vein of penis. HRSG shows dorsal vein of penis running in the substance of penile shaft. Urethra is seen as well-defined echogenic tubular shadow running on the ventral side of penis on HRSG.

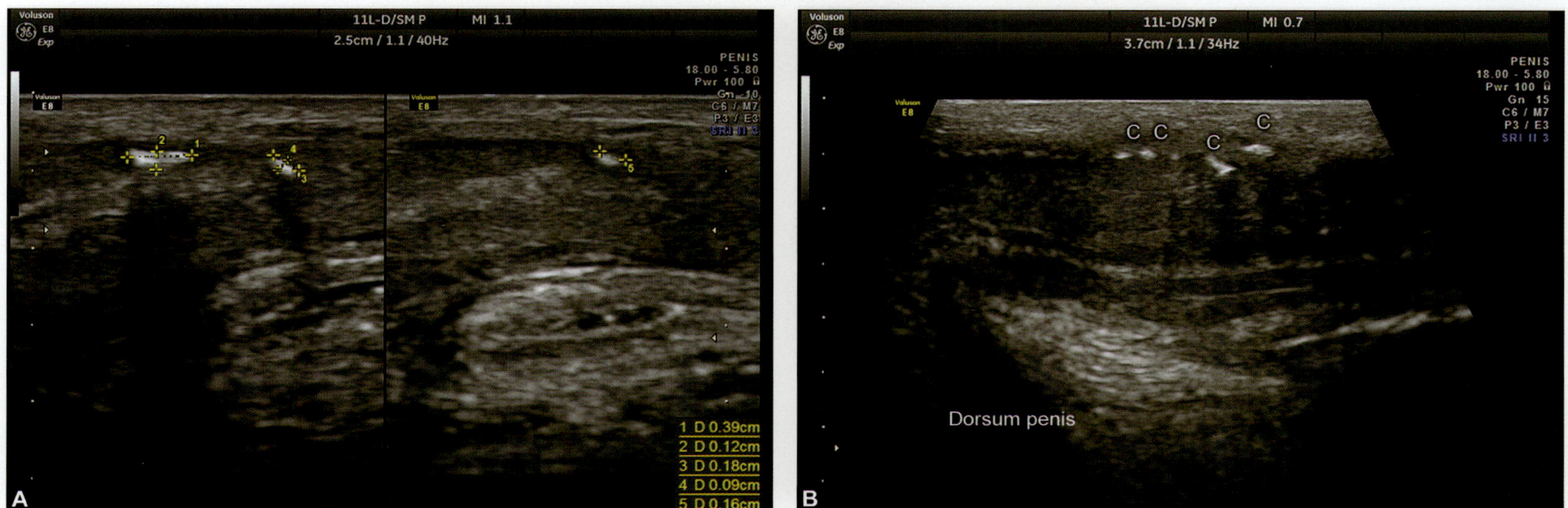

FIGURES 14.3A and B: Tunica albuginea calcification. HRSG shows fine echogenic calcified plaque seen on the anterior aspect of tunica albuginea in a patient of peyronie's disease.

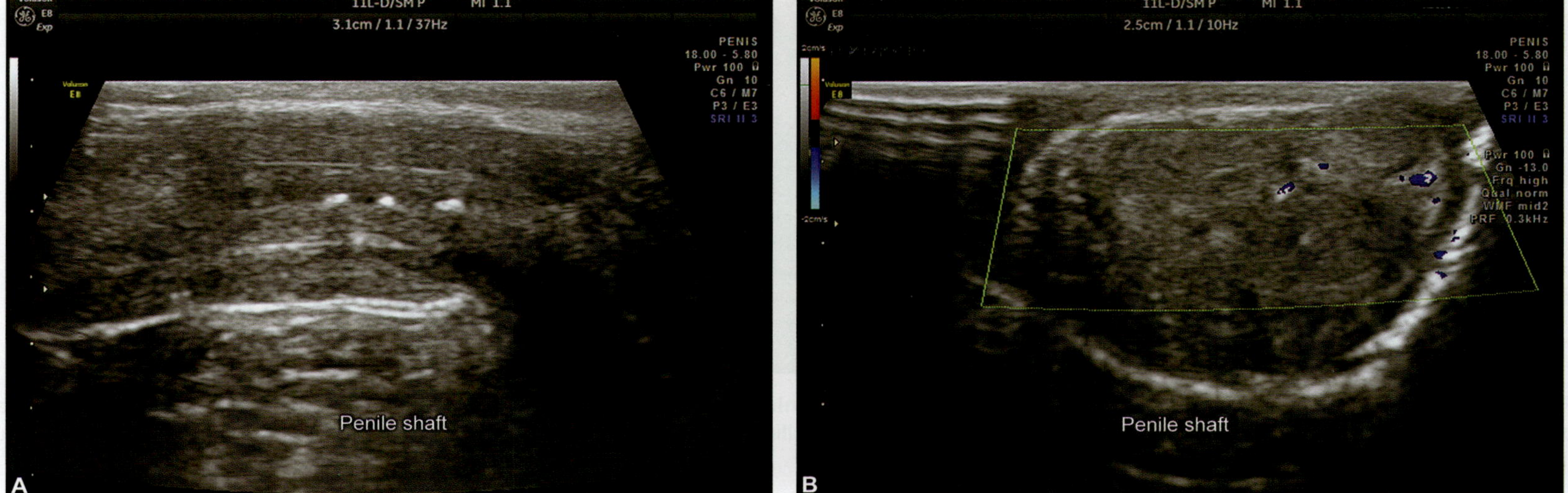

FIGURES 14.4A and B: Rim calcification in tunica albuginea and calcified plaques in corpora cavernosa. HRSG shows dense calcified rim in tunica albuginea. Echogenic calcified plaques are also seen in corpora cavernosa.

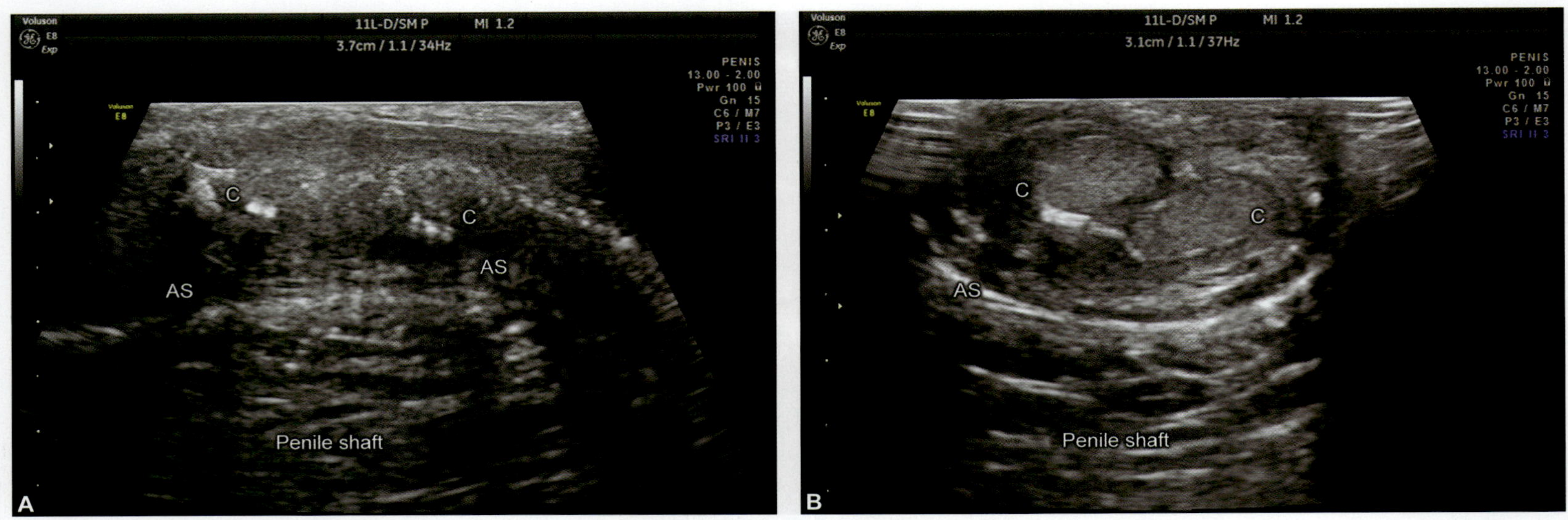

FIGURES 14.5A and B: Discrete calcified plaque in corpora cavernosa with fibrosis. HRSG shows multiple echogenic calcified plaques in corpora cavernosa, which are accompanied with acoustic shadowing. Irregular hypoechoic areas are seen around the plaque suggestive of fibrosis.

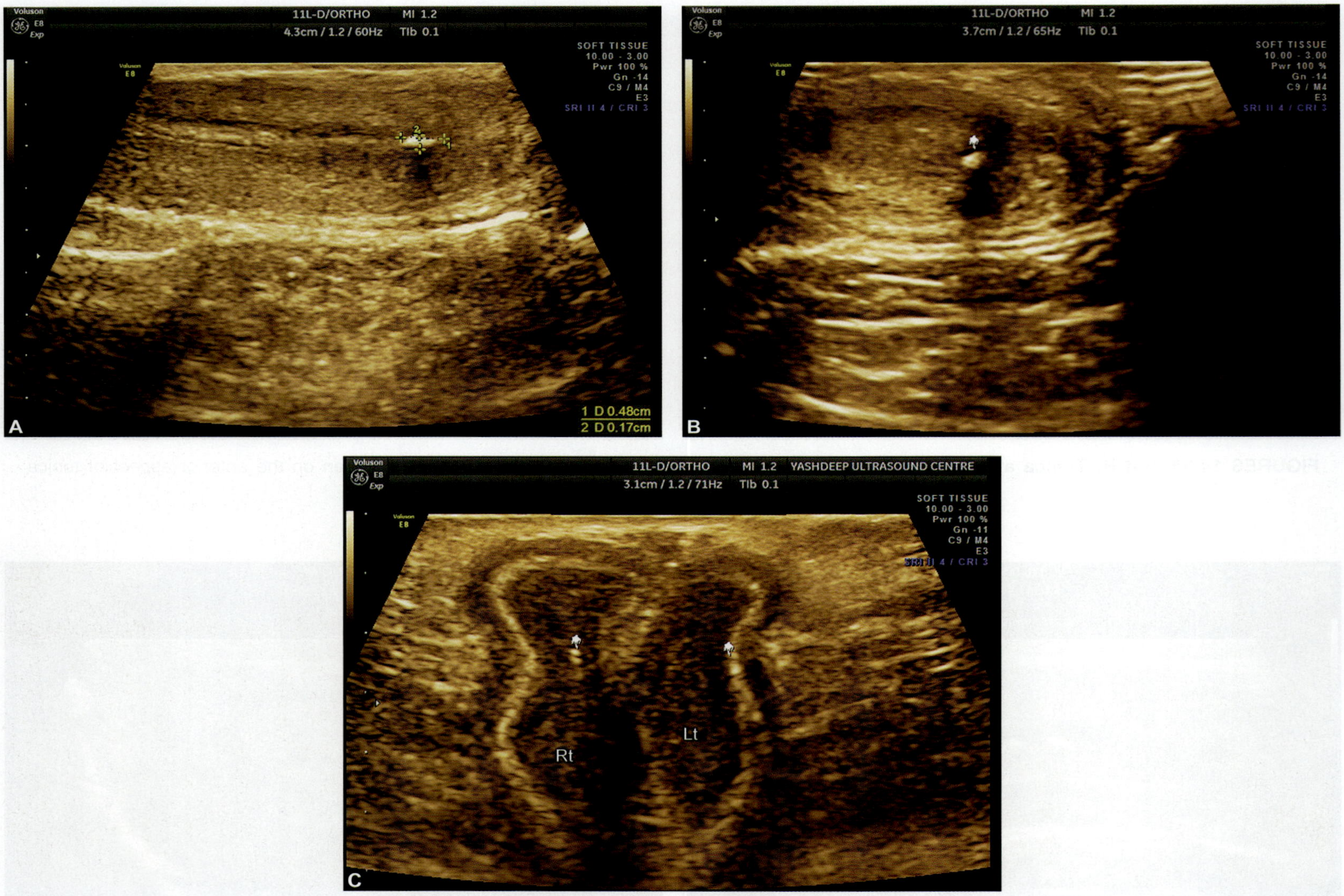

FIGURES 14.6A to C: Calcified plaque in corpora cavernosa and tunica albuginea calcification. A patient presented with echogenic calcified plaque in corpora cavernosa. There is also evidence of echogenic calcification seen in tunica albuginea on dorsal and ventral side. 3D coronal ultrasound shows the calcified tunica albuginea clearly.

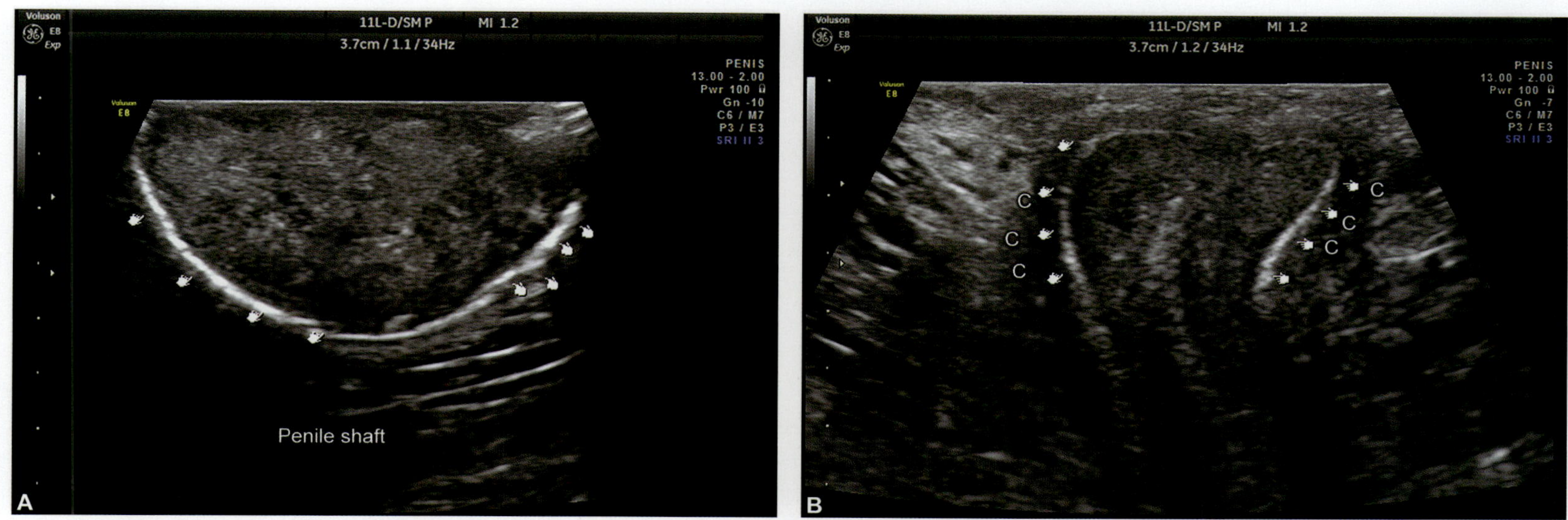

FIGURES 14.7A and B: Rim calcification in tunica albuginea. HRSG with 3D imaging shows dense rim calcification in tunica albuginea. 3D coronal imaging shows the rim very clearly.

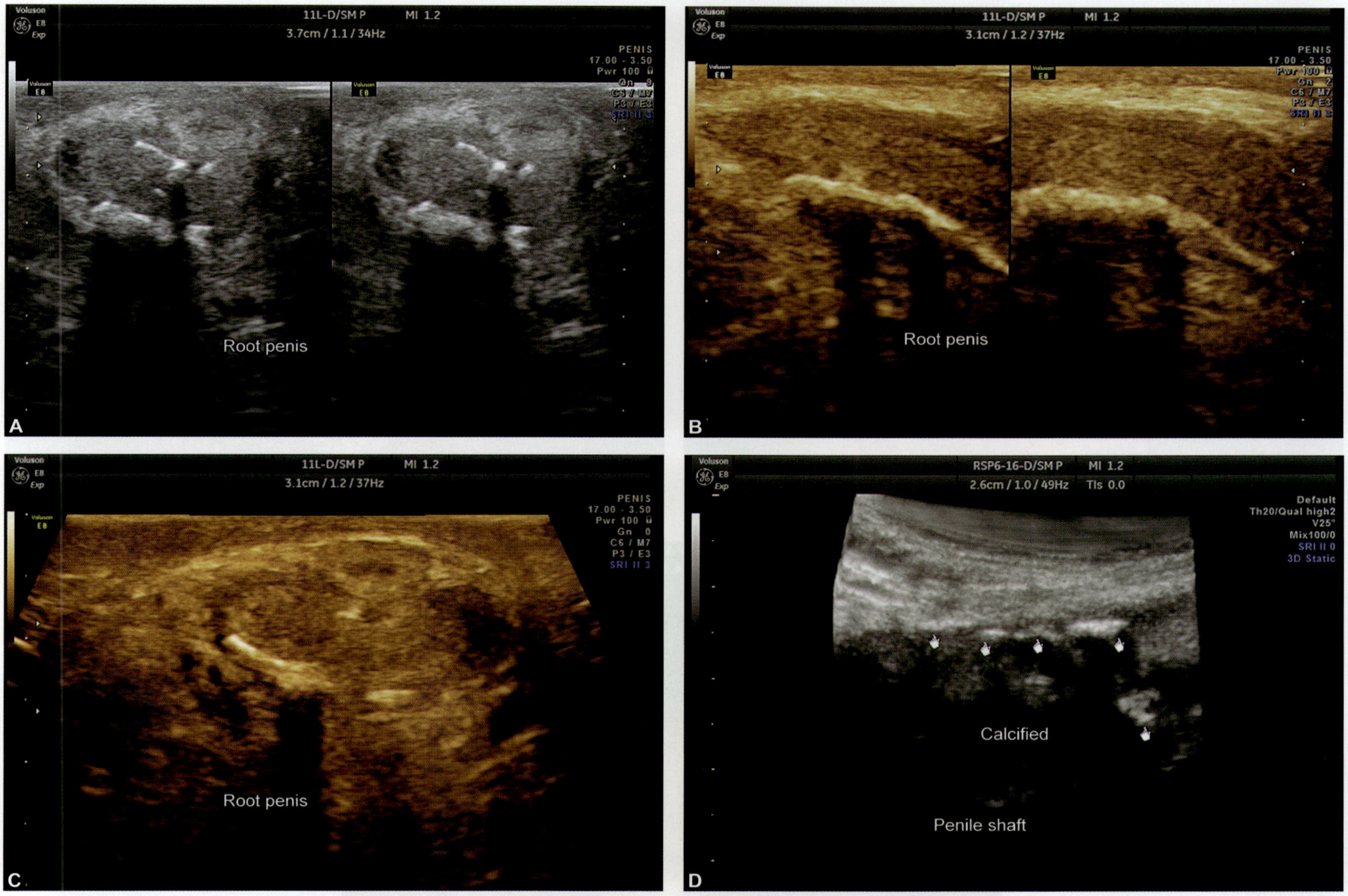

FIGURES 14.8A to D

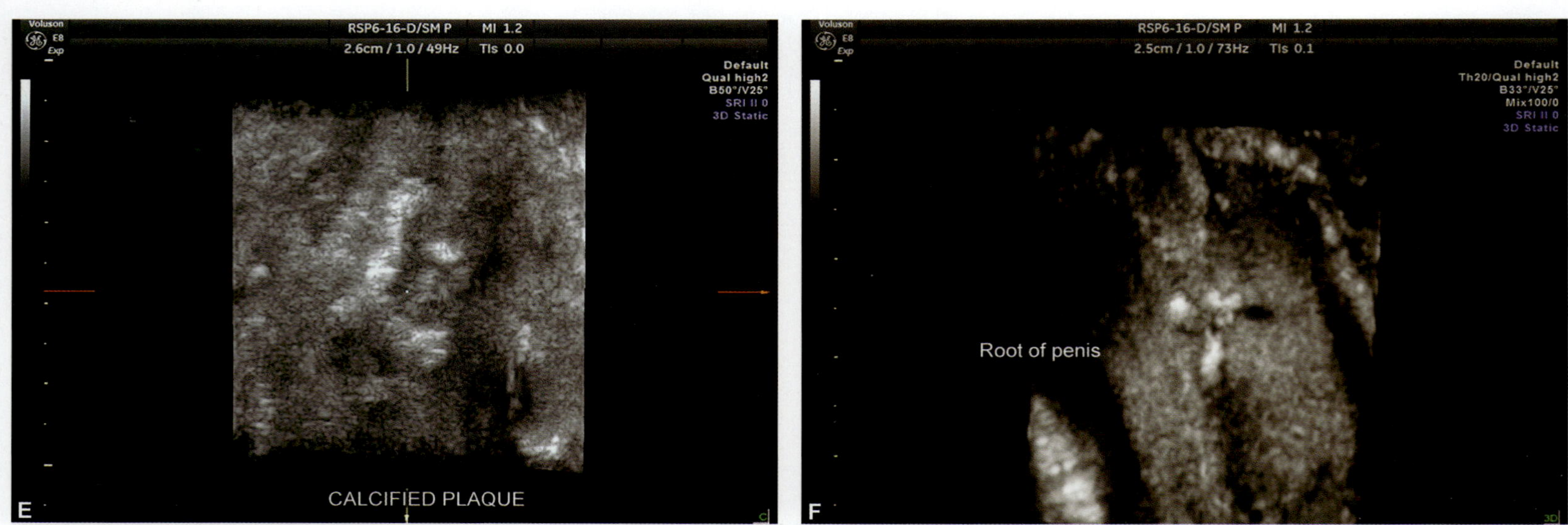

FIGURES 14.8E and F

FIGURES 14.8A to F: Dense calcification in corpora cavernosa and tunica albuginea calcification. A patient presented with hard nodule at the root of penis. HRSG shows a dense calcified plaque at the root of penis. It is accompanied with acoustic shadowing. In long axis, the plaque is seen extending to the proximal part of the penile shaft. On 3D ultrasound, the calcified plaque is seen clearly involving both corpora cavernosa and mid part of the shaft in a case of peyronie's disease.

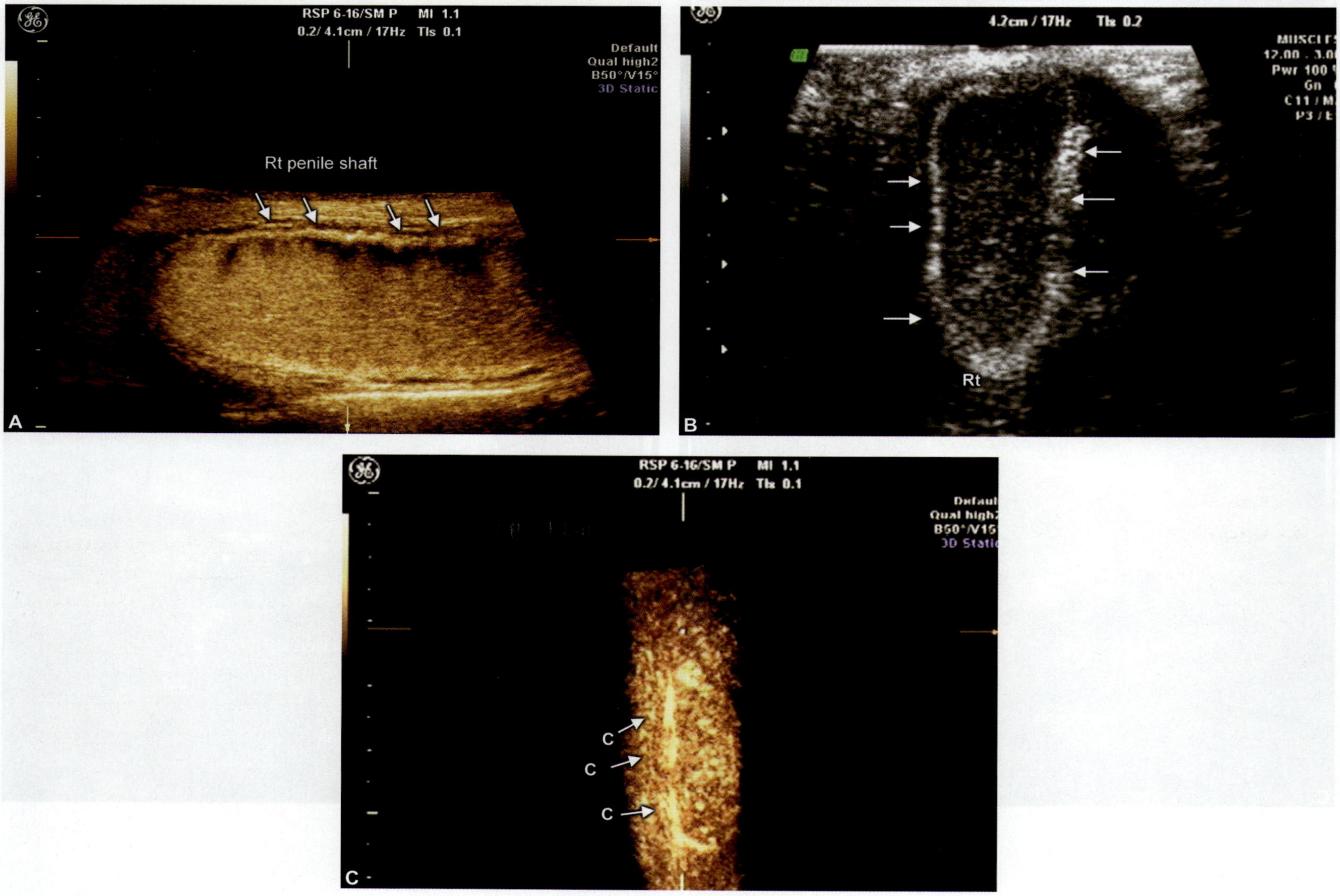

FIGURES 14.9A to C: HRSG shows dense calcification in tunica albuginea from all sides. On 3D ultrasound, the entire tunica albuginea is calcified. On surface rendering image, calcified tunica albuginea is seen cord-like calcification.

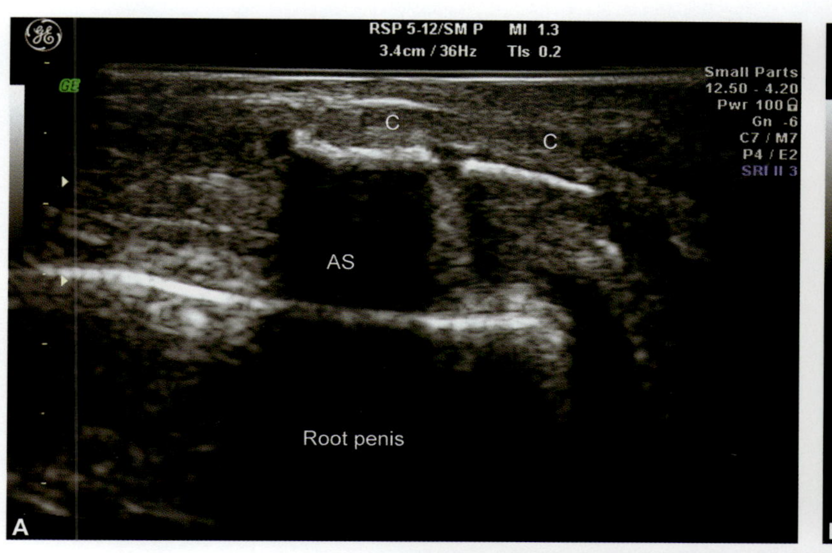

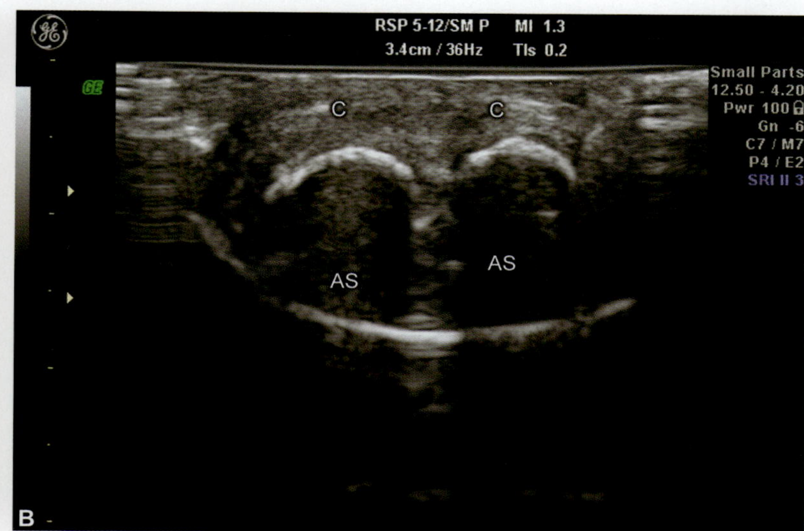

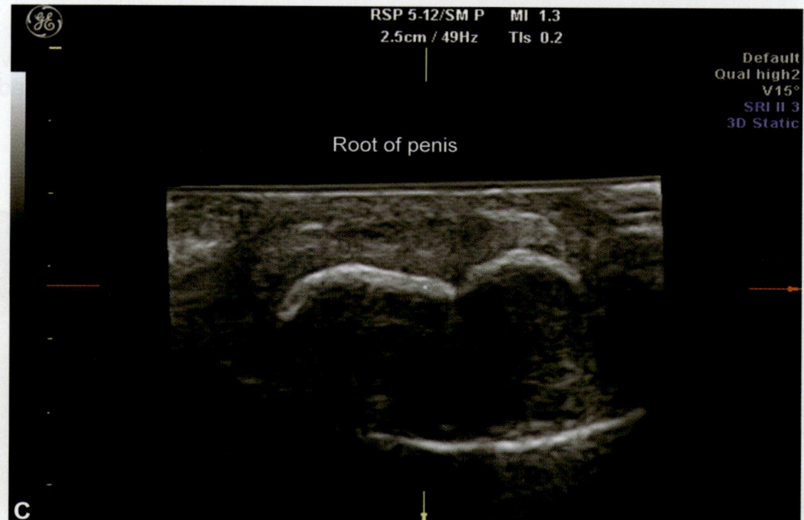

FIGURES 14.10A to C: Dense calcified plaques at root of penis. HRSG shows dense echogenic calcified plaques in both corpora cavernosa. They are accompanied with acoustic shadowing in a case of peyronie's disease.

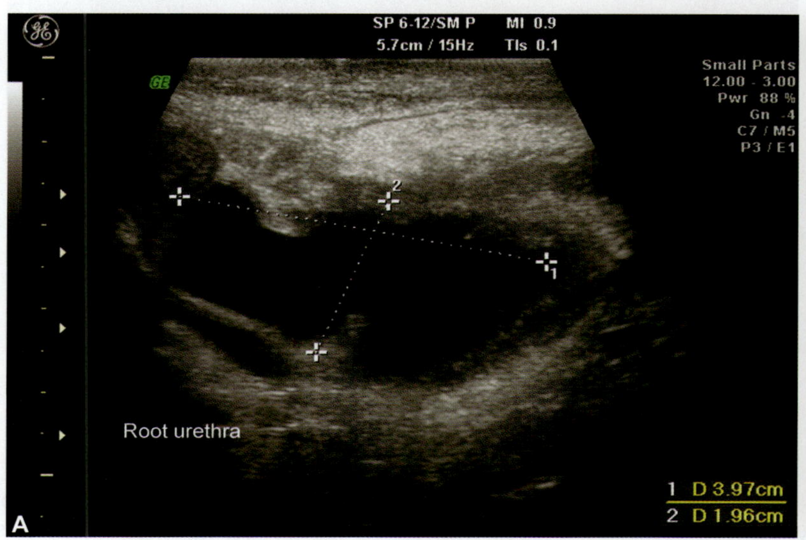

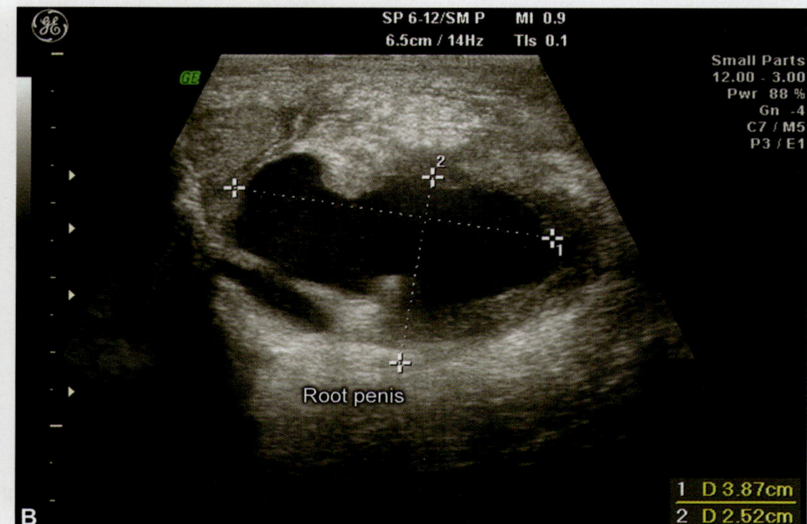

FIGURES 14.11A and B

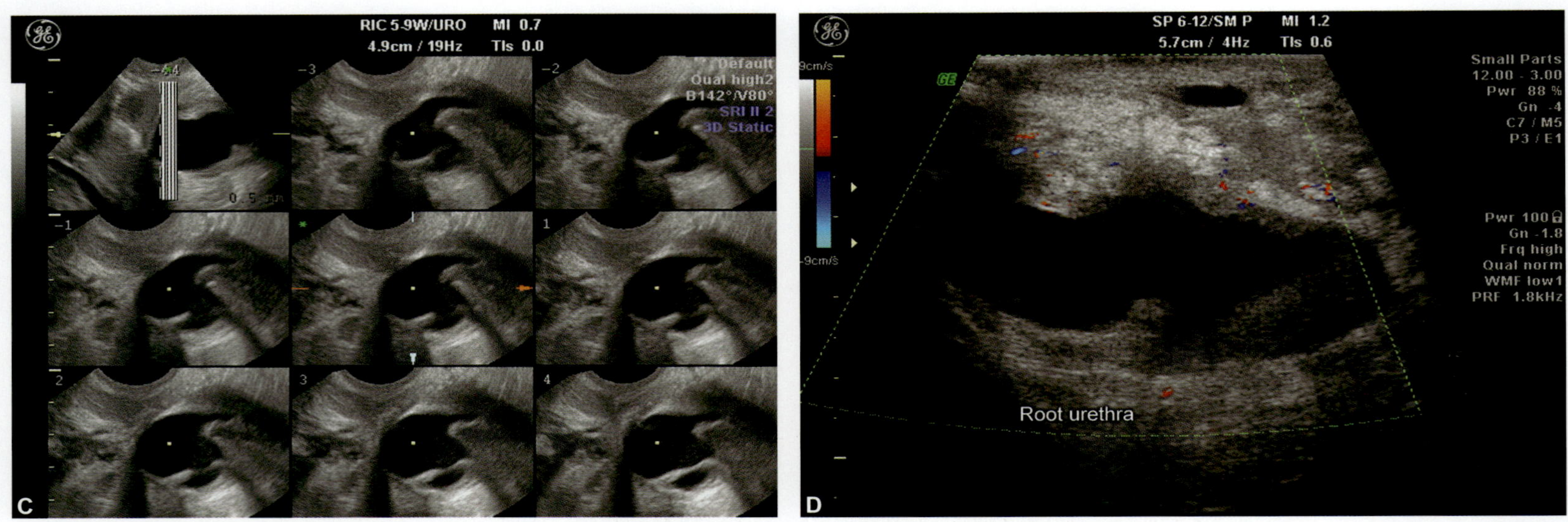

FIGURES 14.11C and D

FIGURES 14.11A to D: A patient presented with injury to the penis in a trauma. HRSG shows pocket of low level echo collection at the proximal urethra, which gets distended on urination suggestive of urethral injury with extravasations of urine. Associated hematoma formation is also seen at the site of injury. 3D tomography ultrasound imaging shows communication of urethra with urinoma.

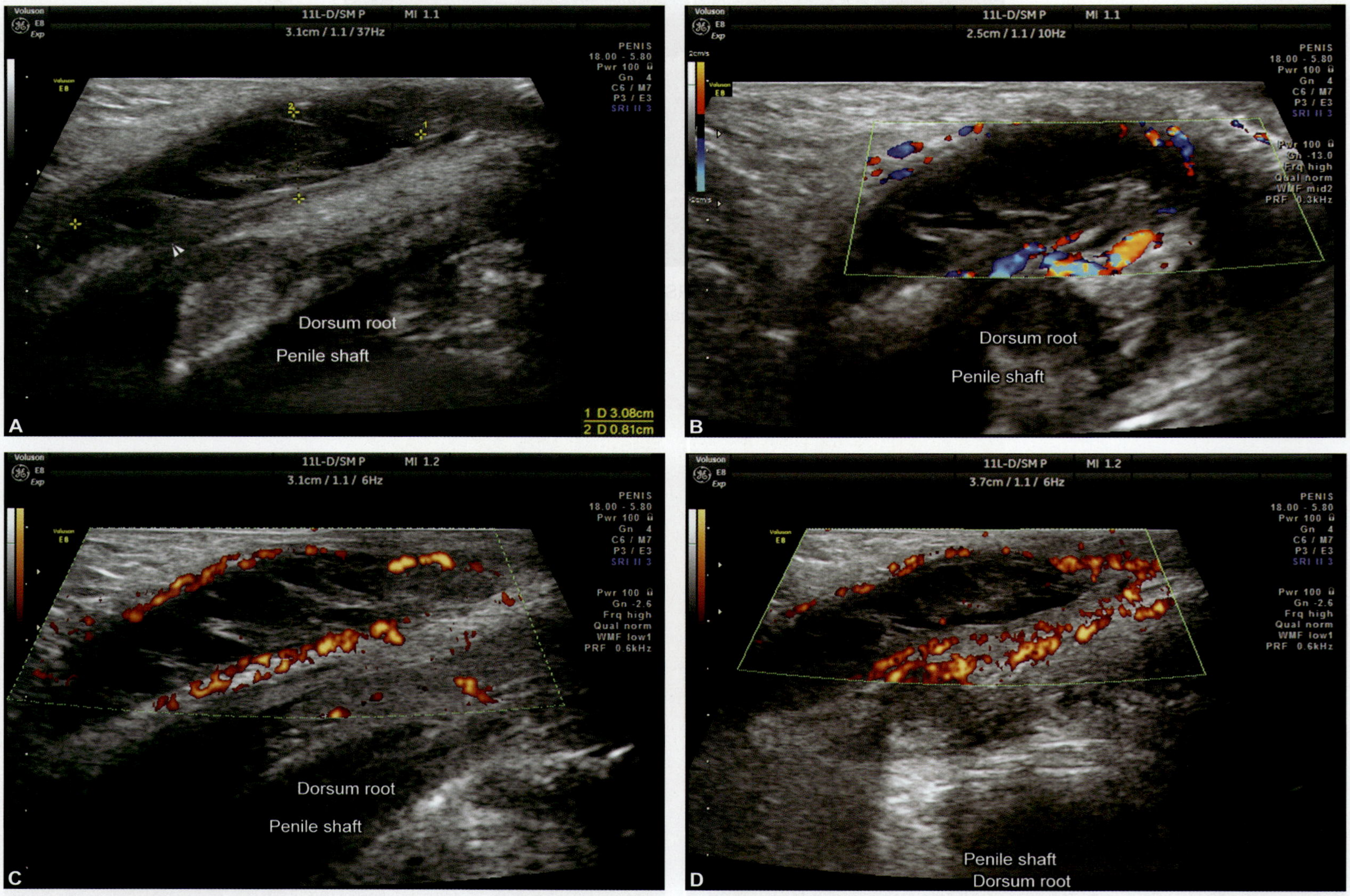

FIGURES 14.12A to D: Penile abscess. A patient presented with painful swelling at the root of penis on dorsal aspect. HRSG shows a pocket of thick collection at the root of penis. Associated soft tissue edema is also seen. Thick collection is seen in it. On color flow imaging, increased flow is seen in the penile tissue. But no flow is seen in the abscess cavity. Findings are suggestive of acute pyogenic abscess.

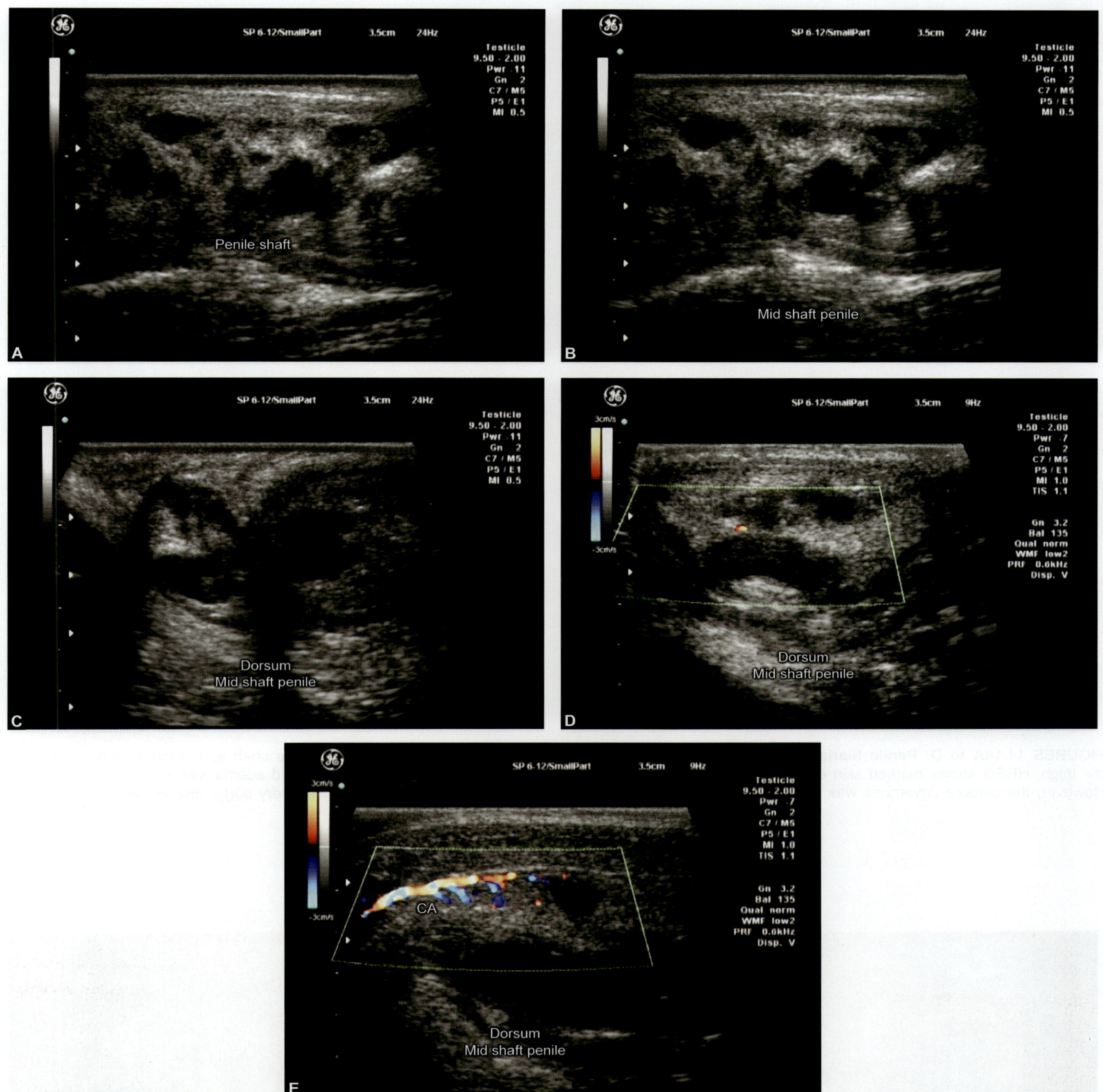

FIGURES 14.13A to E: Penile tuberculosis. A young patient presented with multiple nodular masses in the shaft of the penis. HRSG shows multiple hypoechoic areas in the proximal and mid part of the shaft. They are discrete in distribution with cystic degeneration. Low level echoes are seen in them. No calcification is seen. Normal texture is lost and the penile shaft gives moth eaten appearance. On color flow imaging, no flow was seen in the abscesses. However, normal flow was seen in the cavernosal arteries. Biopsy of the masses confirmed tuberculosis.

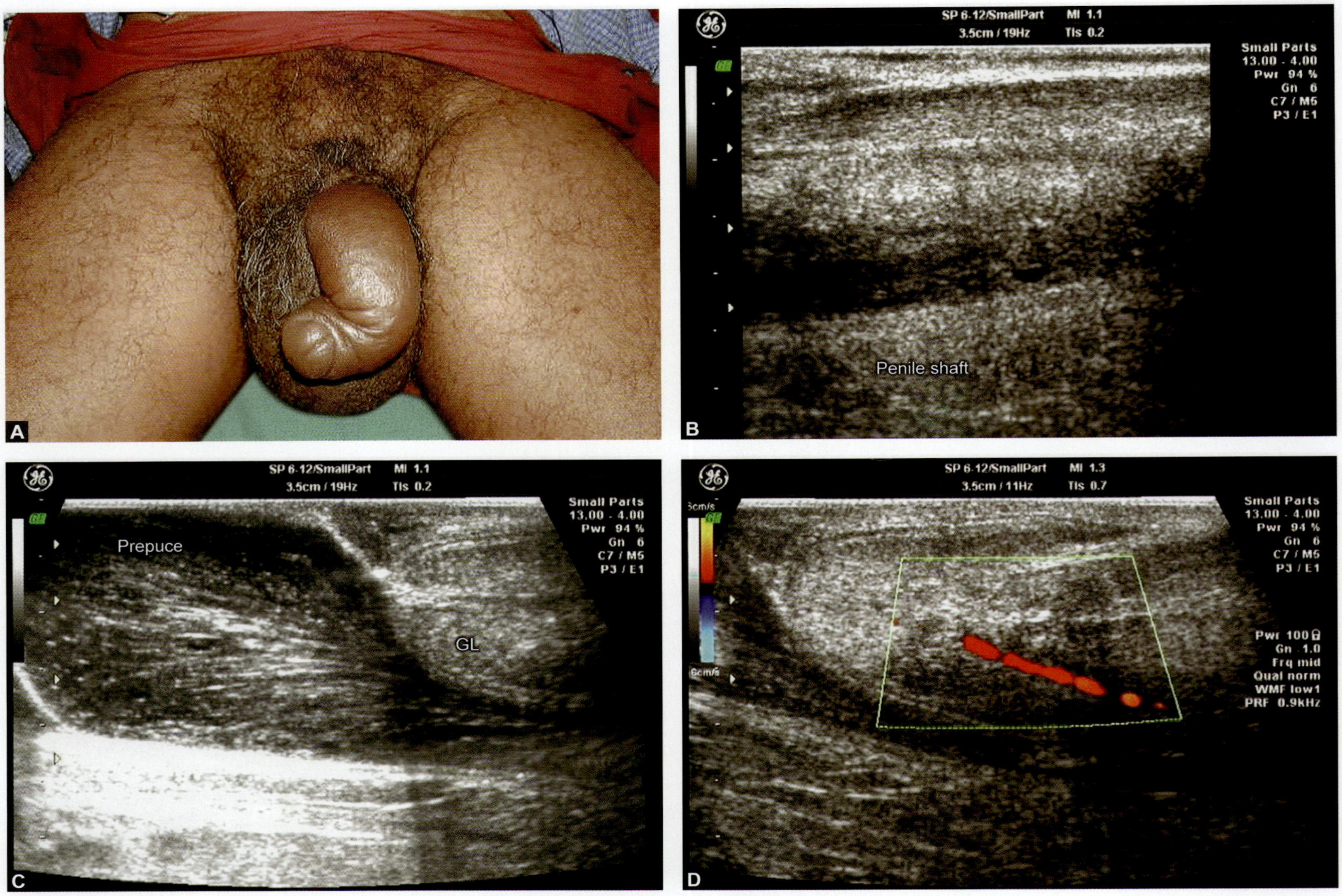

FIGURES 14.14A to D: Penile filariasis. A patient presented with marked soft tissue edema over the penile shaft and scrotum with edema over the thigh. HRSG shows marked skin edema over the penile skin. Subcutaneous edema was presented. Marked edema was seen over the prepuce. However, the corpora cavernosa was normal. On color flow imaging normal flow was seen in dorsal penile artery suggestive of filariasis.

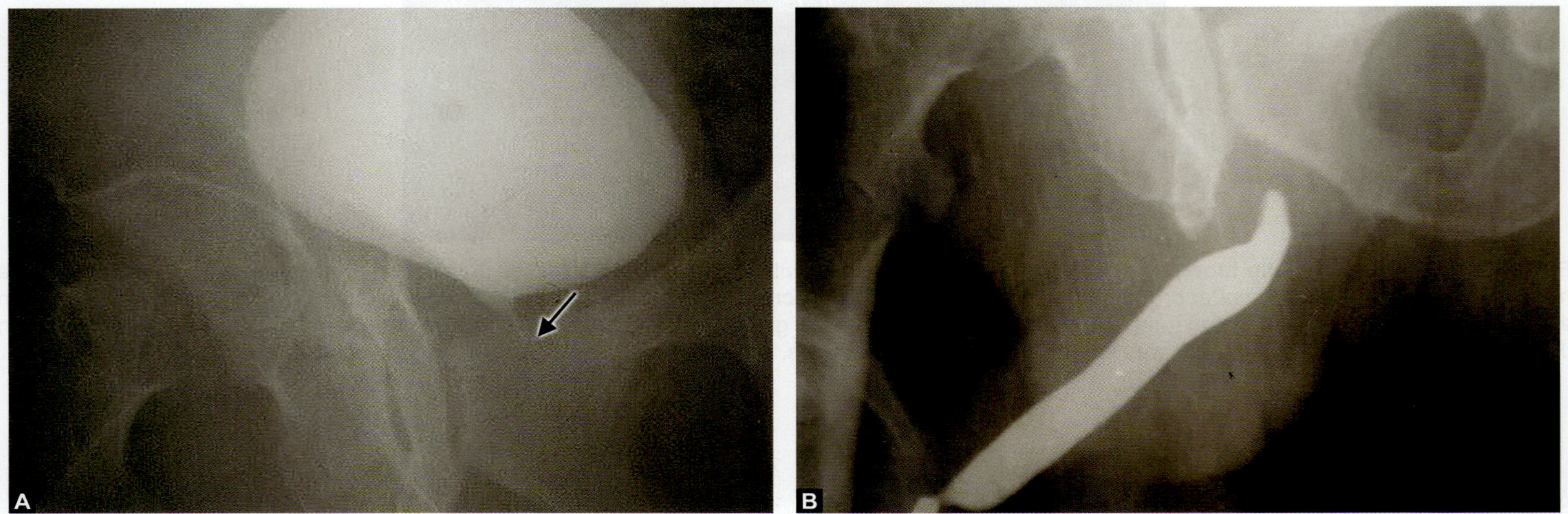

FIGURES 14.15A and B

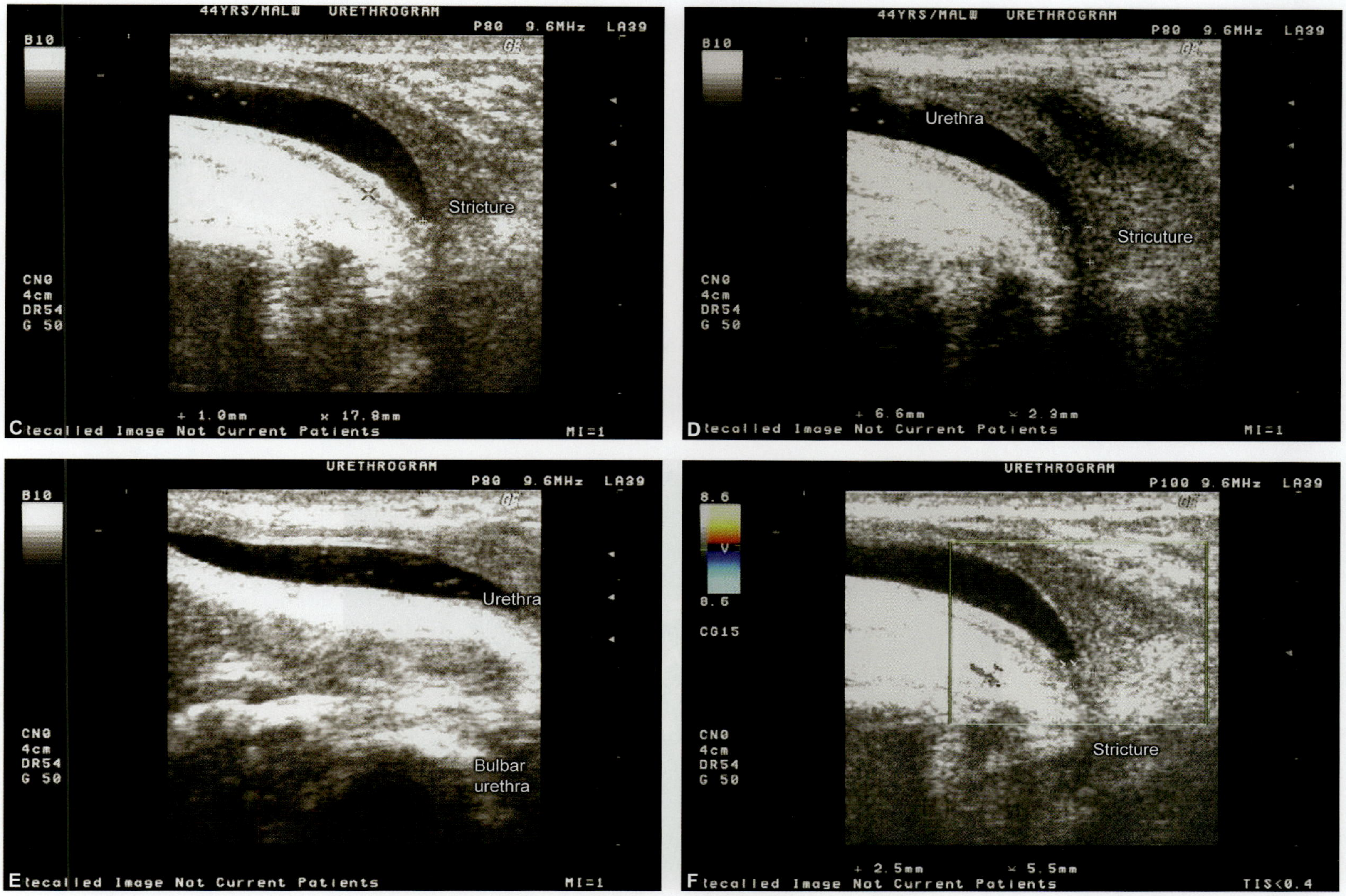

FIGURES 14.15C to F

FIGURES 14.15A to F: Bulbar urethral stricture. Micturating urethrogram shows complete stricture of urethra. Beaking of urethral stricture is seen. Retrograde urethrogram shows sudden cut-off of the urethral lumen and non-visualization of bulbar urethra in a case of post-traumatic urethral rupture. Sono-urethrogram shows completely obliterated lumen of bulbar urethra. A hypoechoic soft tissue shadow is seen obliterating the lumen of urethra suggestive of marked peri-urethral fibrosis. The length of urethral structure is around 15 mm. The distal urethra is seen distended. The middle and the distal urethra are seen normally with smooth mucosal lining. Color flow imaging through the obliterated urethral structure does not show any flow of the water jet suggestive of completely obliterated lumen by the periurethral fibrosis.

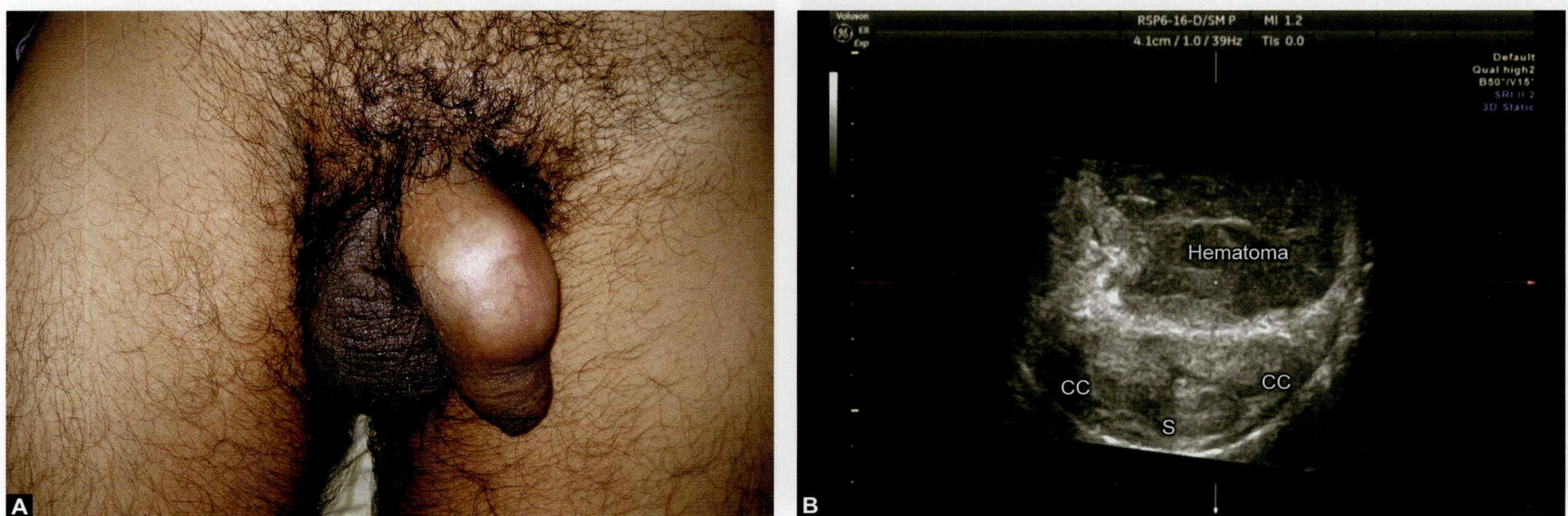

FIGURES 14.16A and B

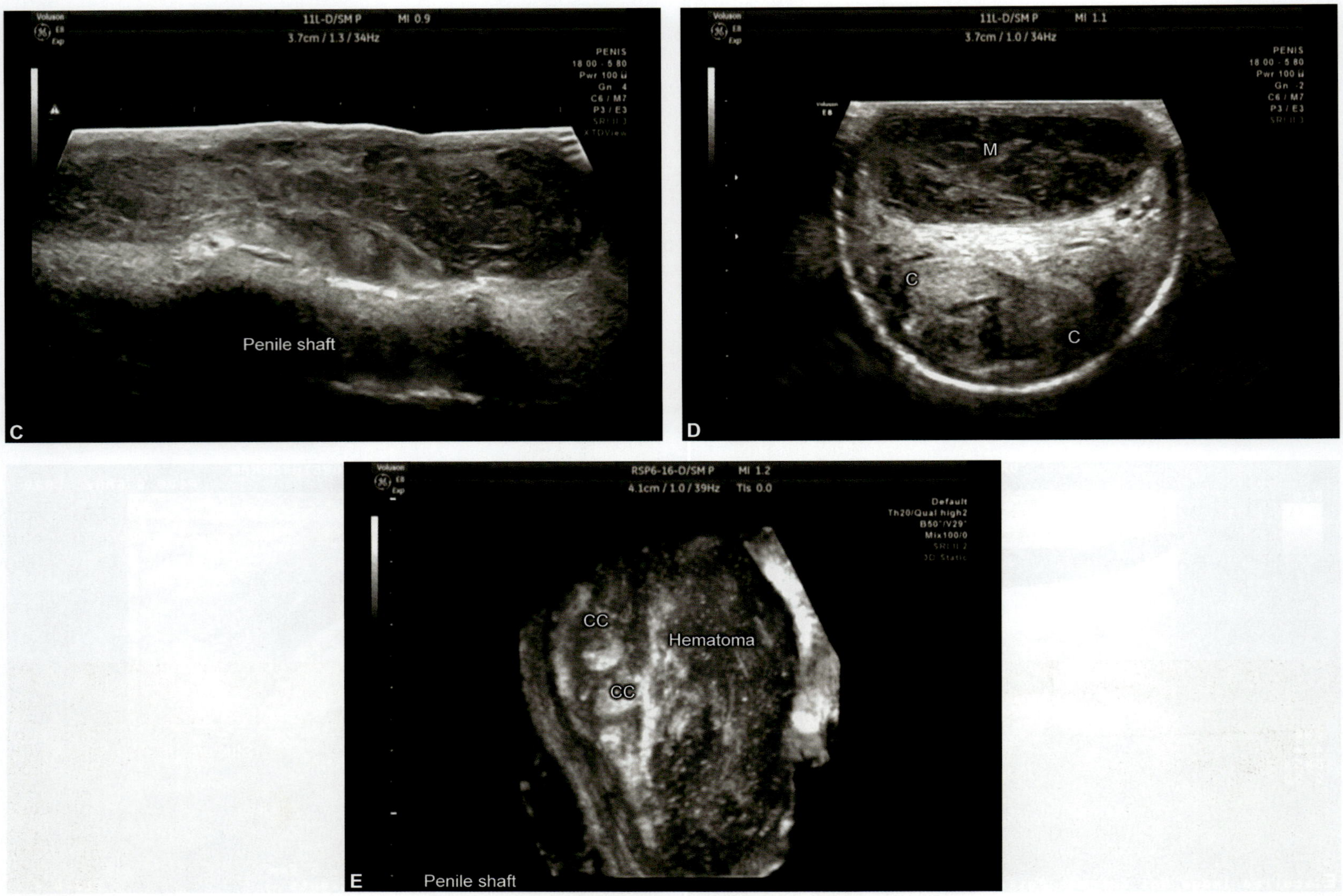

FIGURES 14.16C to E

FIGURES 14.16A to E: Penis trauma with rupture of tunica albuginea. A patient sustained penile trauma. HRSG shows a pocket of low level echo collection in mid shaft part of the penis. There is evidence of rupture of tunica albuginea seen on right side. Hematoma formation is seen. Pressure is seen on corpora cavernosa. 3D imaging shows big hematoma formation with rupture of tunica albuginea. The hematoma is seen pressing and compressing the corpora cavernosa.

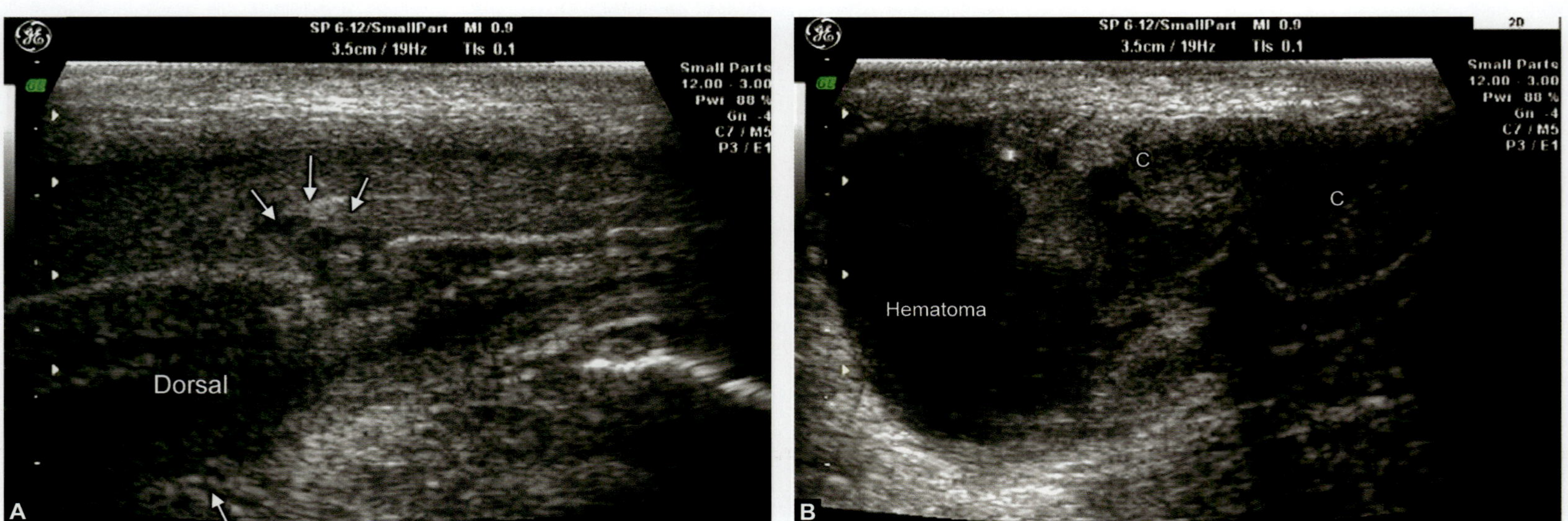

FIGURES 14.17A and B

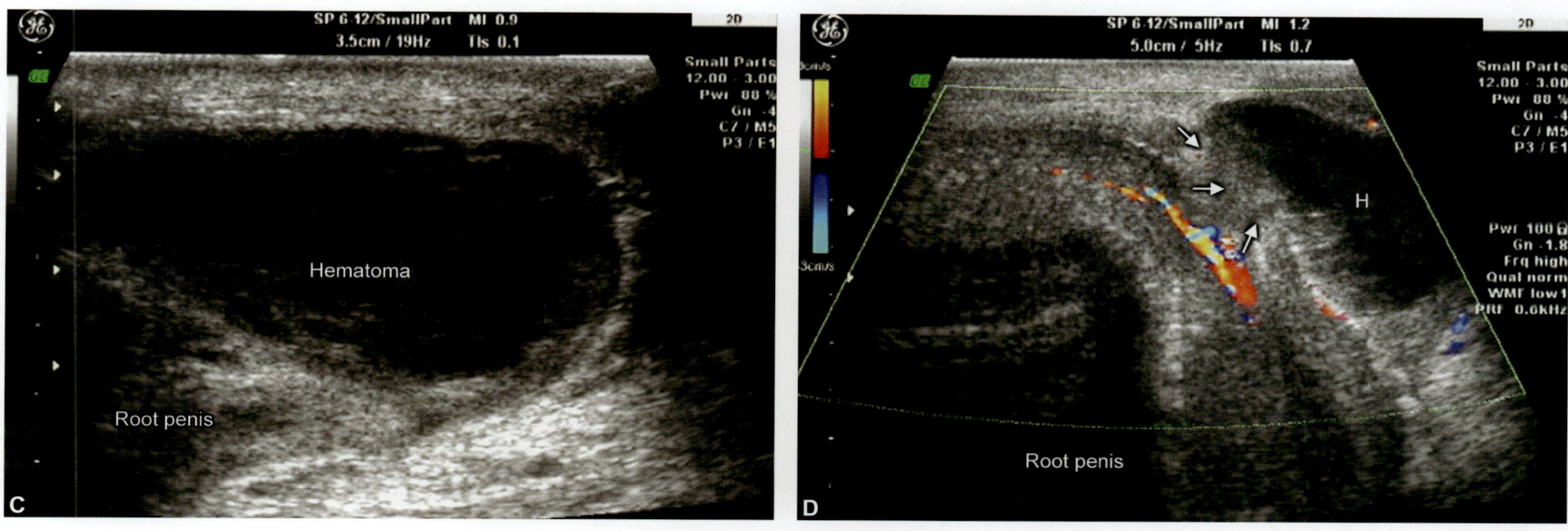

FIGURES 14.17C and D

FIGURES 14.17A to D: Fracture penis with hematoma formation. A patient presented with trauma to the penis during erection. HRSG shows a hypoechoic cleft in corpora cavernosa at the root of penis suggestive of rupture. A big low level echo complex pocket is seen at the site of rupture suggestive of hematoma formation. It is seen collecting on the right side of penile shaft and compressing the left corpora cavernosa. On color flow imaging, blood flow is seen in cavernosal artery.

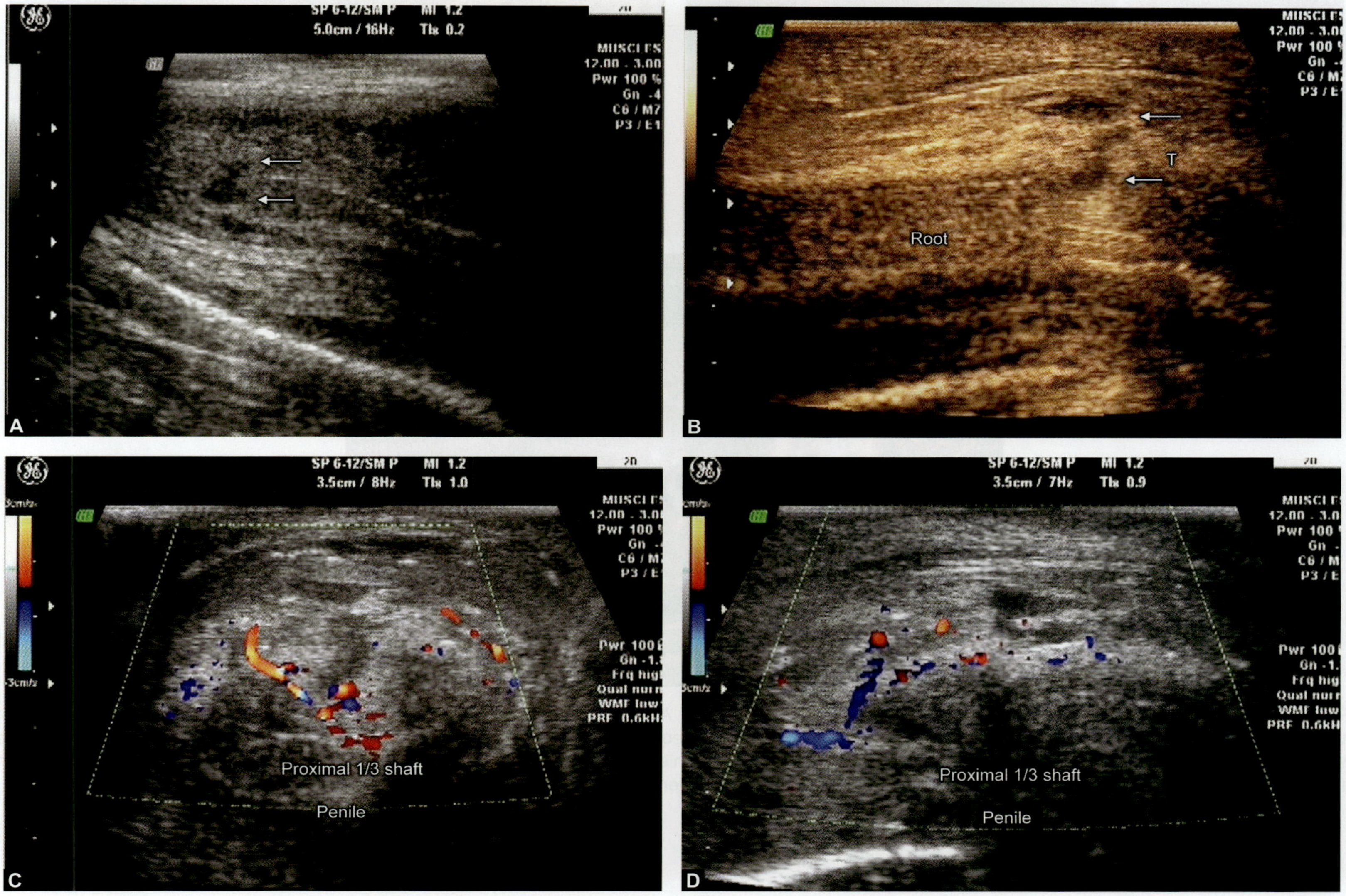

FIGURES 14.18A to D: Rupture of corpora cavernosa with hematoma formation. A patient sustained trauma to penis during intercourse. HRSG shows rupture of corpora cavernosa in its proximal part. Both corpora cavernosa show rupture. Hypoechoic cleft is seen at the site of rupture. There is also evidence of tear seen in the tunica albuginea at the root of penis. Associated hematoma formation is also seen.

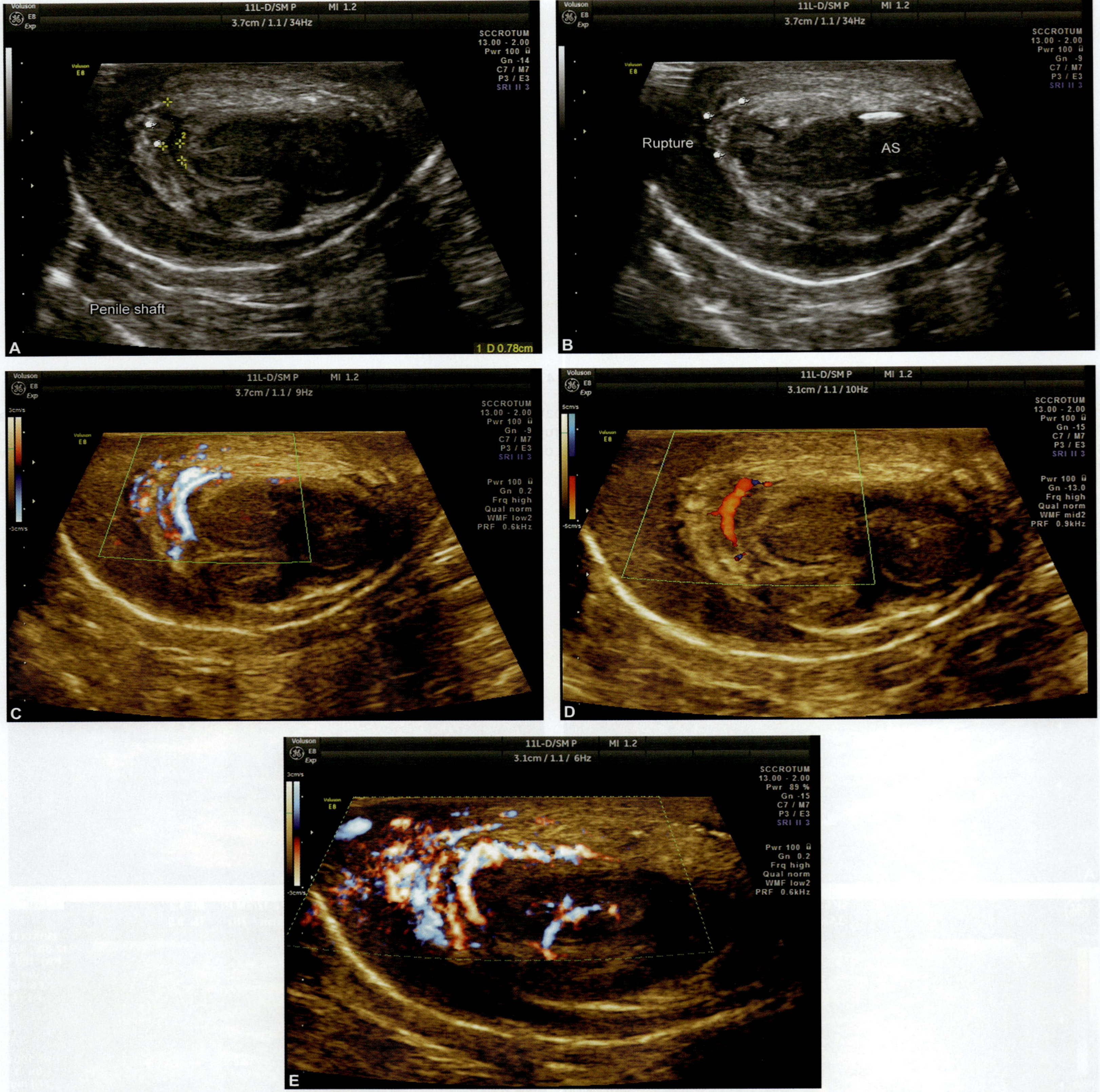

FIGURES 14.19A to E: Rupture of tunica albuginea with calcification. A patient presented with history of penile trauma. HRSG shows rupture of tunica albuginea at the proximal part of penile shaft on right side. A hypoechoic cleft is seen at the site of rupture. Dense echogenic calcified plaque is also seen on the anterior aspect of tunica albuginea, which is accompanied with acoustic shadowing. On color flow imaging, increased flow is seen at the site of rupture suggestive of acute injury. Associated soft tissue edema is also present.

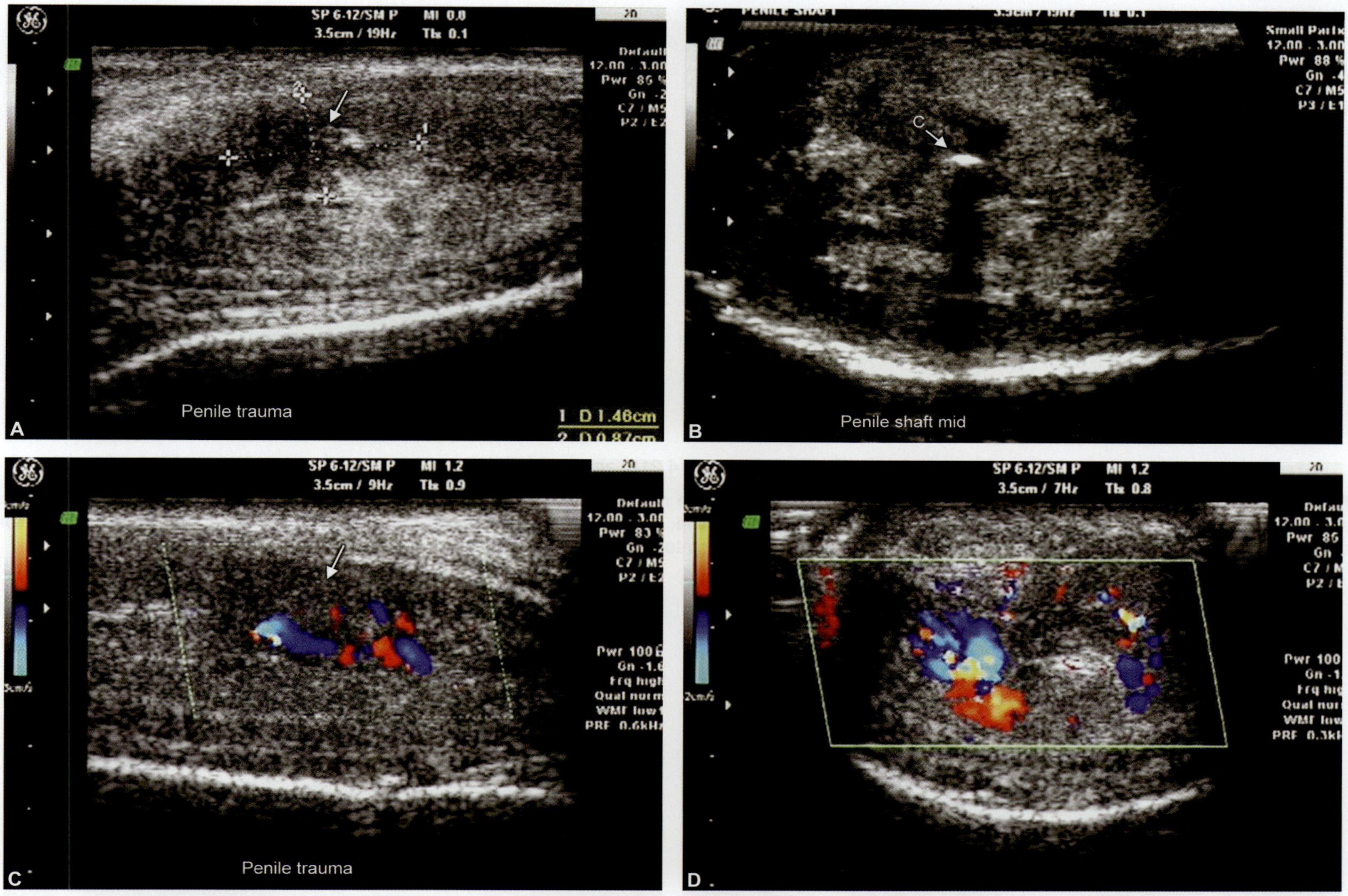

FIGURES 14.20A to D: Penile trauma with rupture of corpora cavernosa. A patient presented with trauma to the penis with failure to erection. HRSG shows a big hypoechoic cleft in the corpora cavernosa in the mid part of penile shaft. Irregular hypoechoic areas are seen in the penile shaft. Echogenic calcified plaques are also seen at the site of rupture. On color flow imaging, multiple vessels are seen at the site of rupture. Few vessels are seen communicating each-other suggestive of traumatic arteriovenous malformation (AVM). Patient was not having optimum arterial flow because of AVM and failed to achieve tumescence.

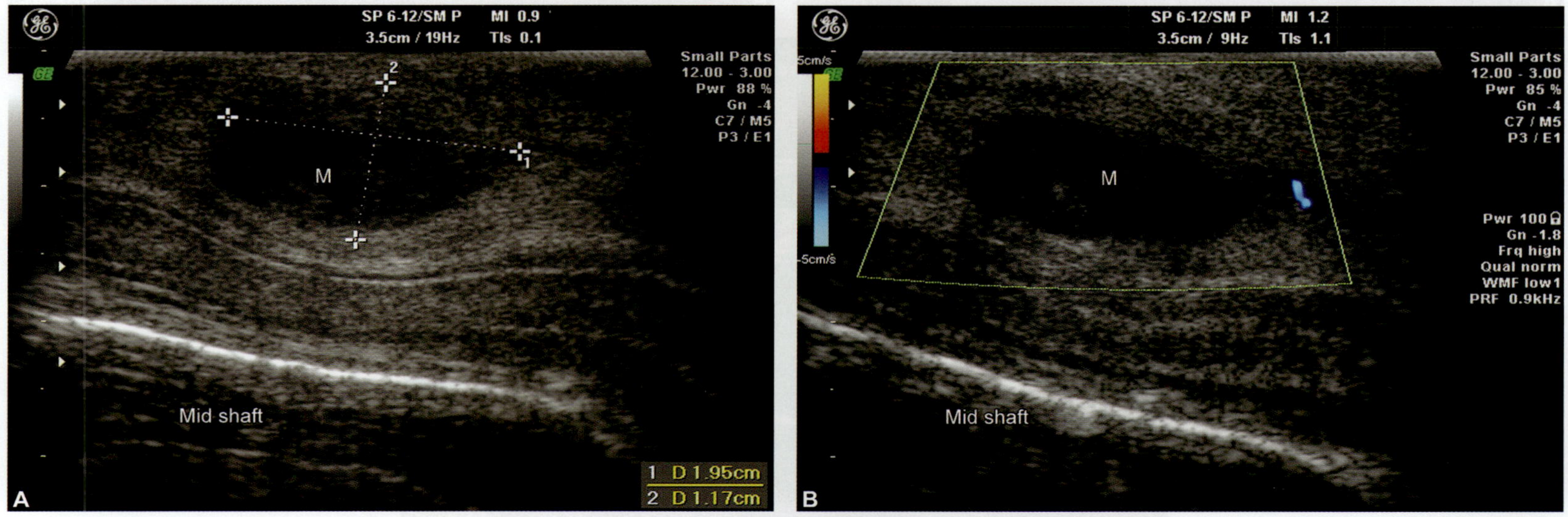

FIGURES 14.21A and B

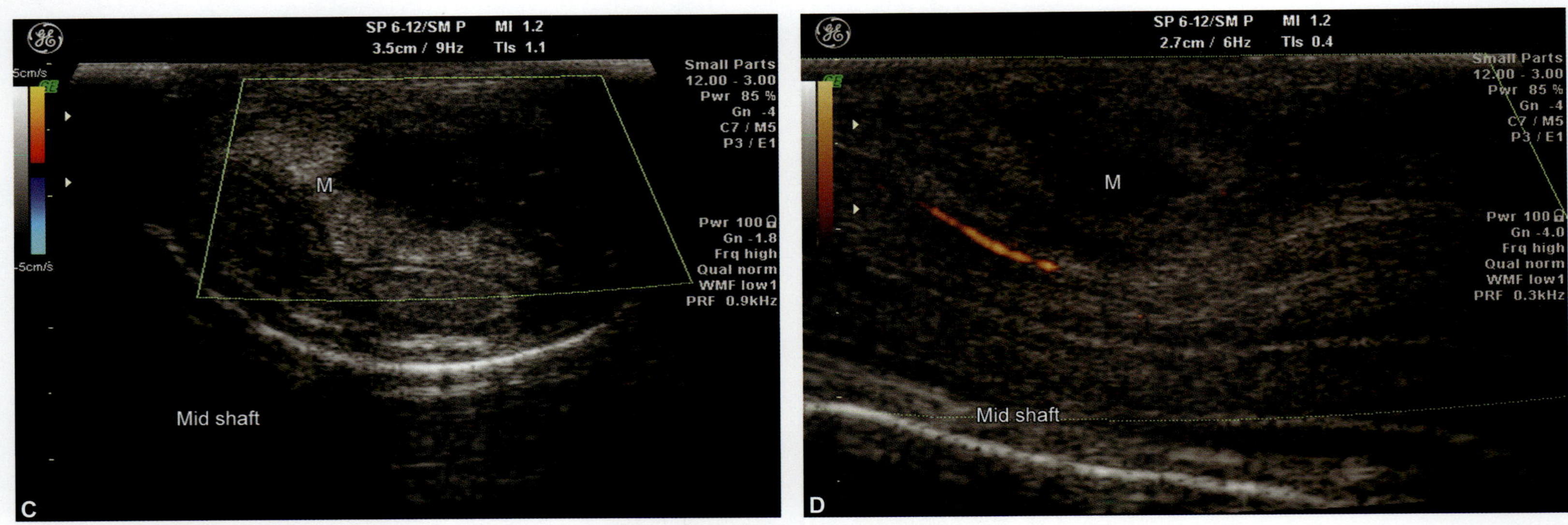

FIGURES 14.21C and D

FIGURES 14.21A to D: Penile mass. A patient presented with soft tissue nodular mass on the ventral aspect in the mid part of penis. HRSG shows a complex echo mass in the mid part of penis. It shows irregular outline. Low level echoes are seen in it. But no perifocal edema is present. On color flow imaging, poor flow is seen in it suggestive of chronic inflammatory mass. Biopsy of the mass confirms tubercular mass.

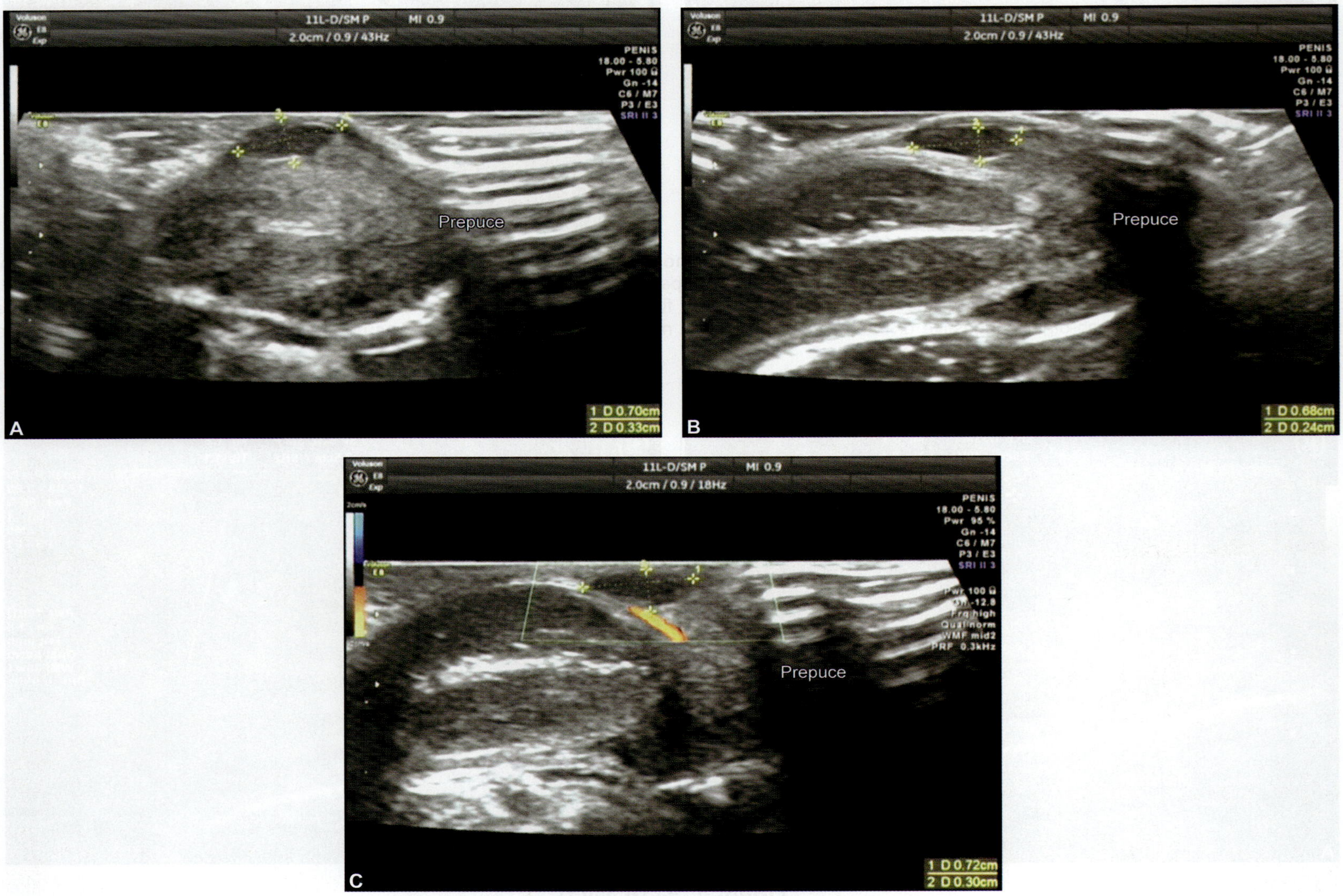

FIGURES 14.22A to C: A 4-year-child presented with small nodule at prepuce. HRSG shows a well-defined hypoechoic nodular shadow at the prepuce. It measures 7 × 3 mm in size. No calcification is seen in it. No cystic degeneration is seen. On color flow imaging, no flow is seen in it. Findings are consistent with neurofibroma.

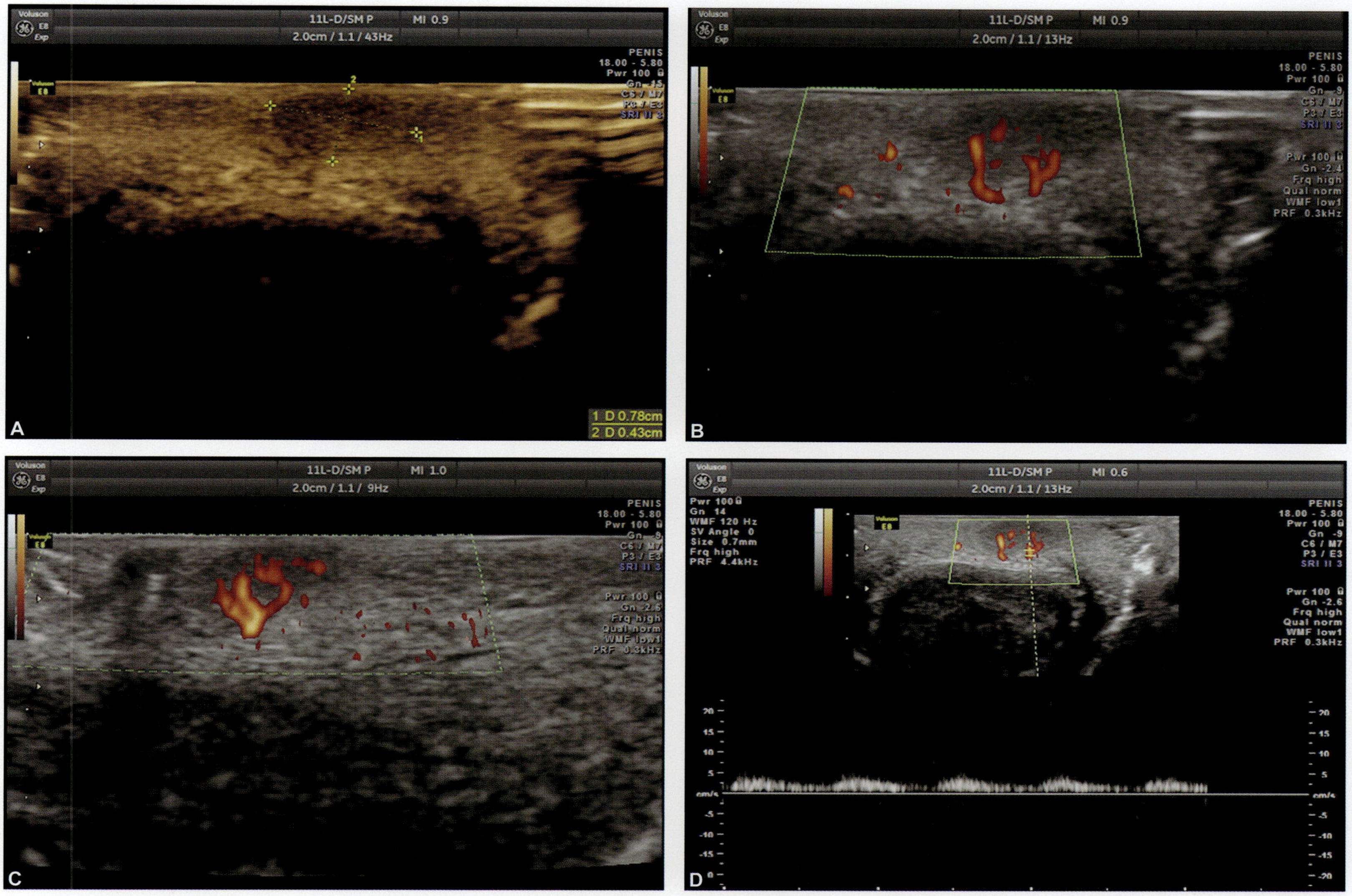

FIGURES 14.23A to D: A patient presented with soft tissue nodular shadow on the superior aspect of glans. HRSG shows a well-defined nodular shadow on the superior surface of glans in its proximal part. It is homogeneous and hypoechoic in texture. No calcification is seen in it. No cystic degeneration is seen. On color flow imaging, multiple small vessels are seen feeding it. On spectral Doppler tracing, low arterial flow is seen in it. It is seen confined to the superficial planes. The penile shaft is normal in appearance.

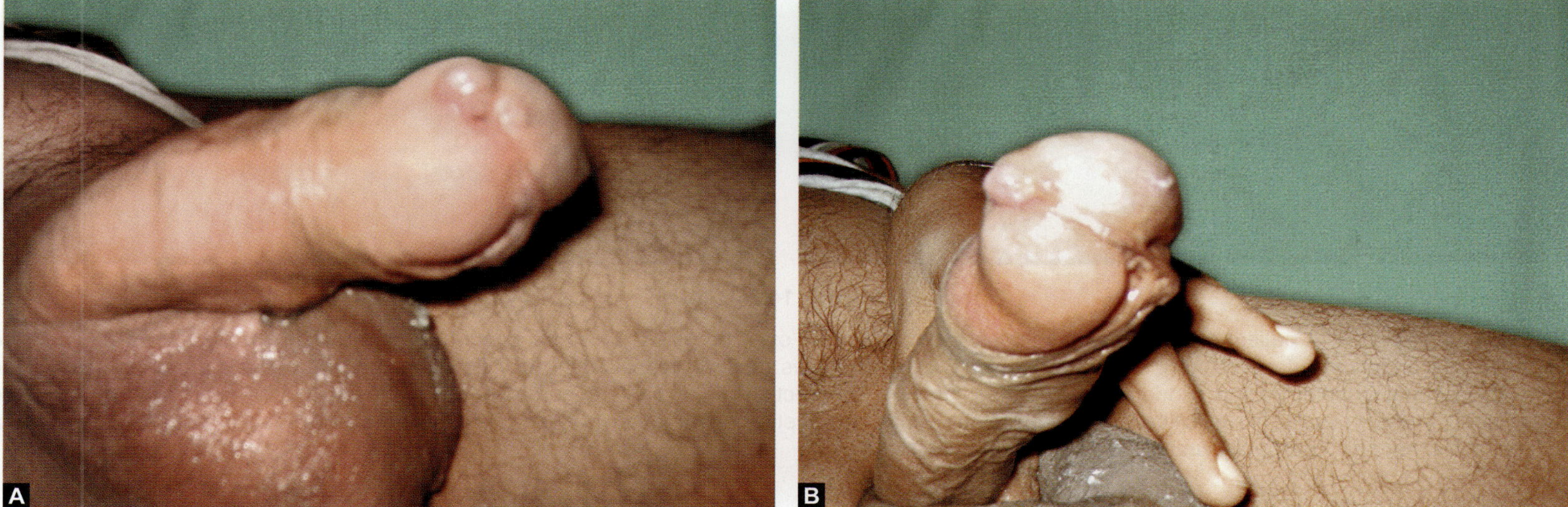

FIGURES 14.24A and B

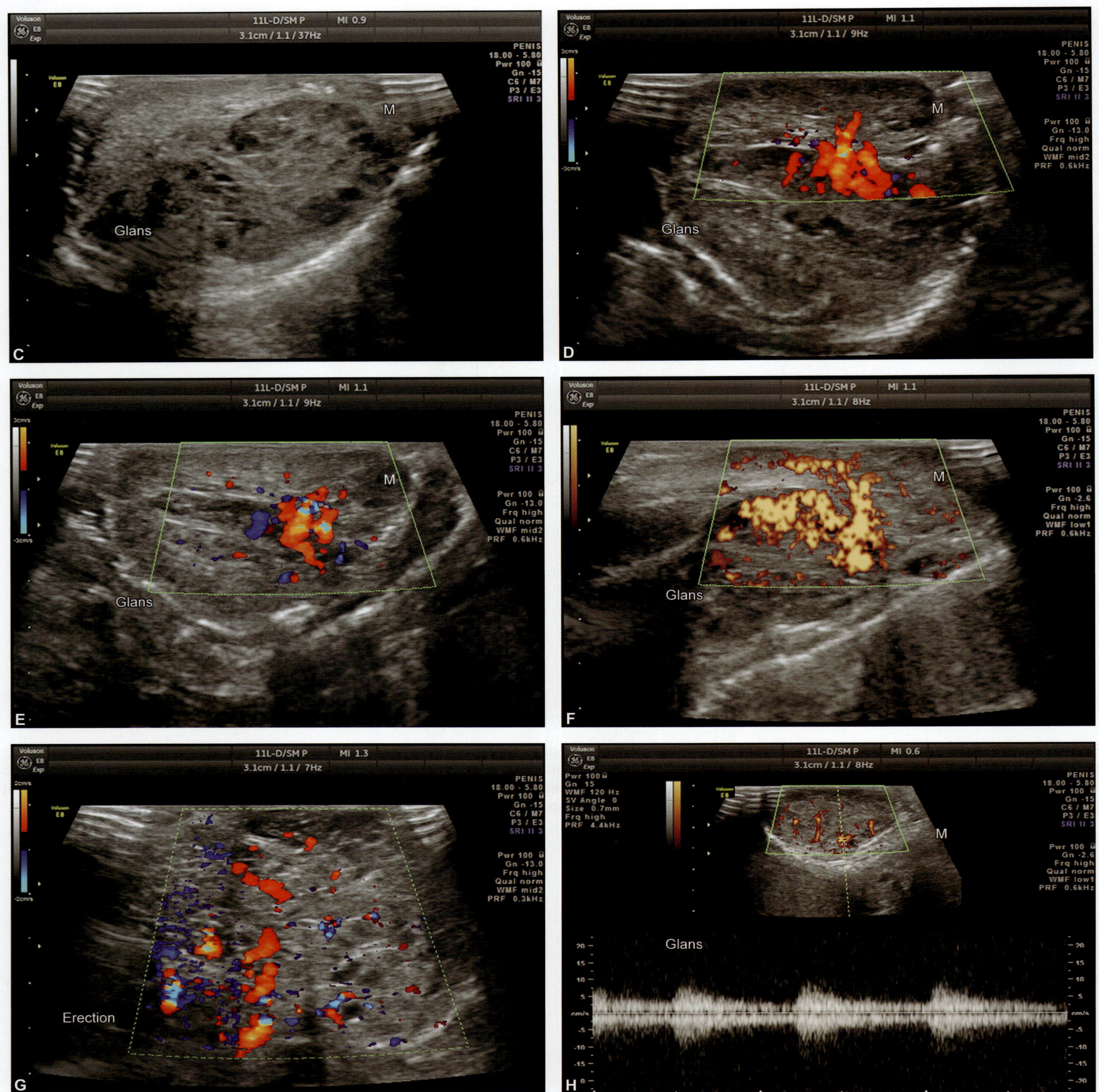

FIGURES 14.24C to H

FIGURES 14.24A to H: A patient presented with soft tissue nodular mass over the glans, which becomes hard on erection. HRSG shows a soft tissue mass over the superior surface of the glans of the penis. The mass shows multiple vessels. On color flow imaging, the vessels are seen feeding the mass. On spectral Doppler tracing, moderate arterial flow is seen. On erection of the penis engorgement of the vessels is seen. Pooling of the blood is also seen in the vessels. No calcification is seen in the mass. No cystic degeneration is seen. Rest of the penile shaft is normal. The corpora cavernosa are normal. The penile urethra is normal.

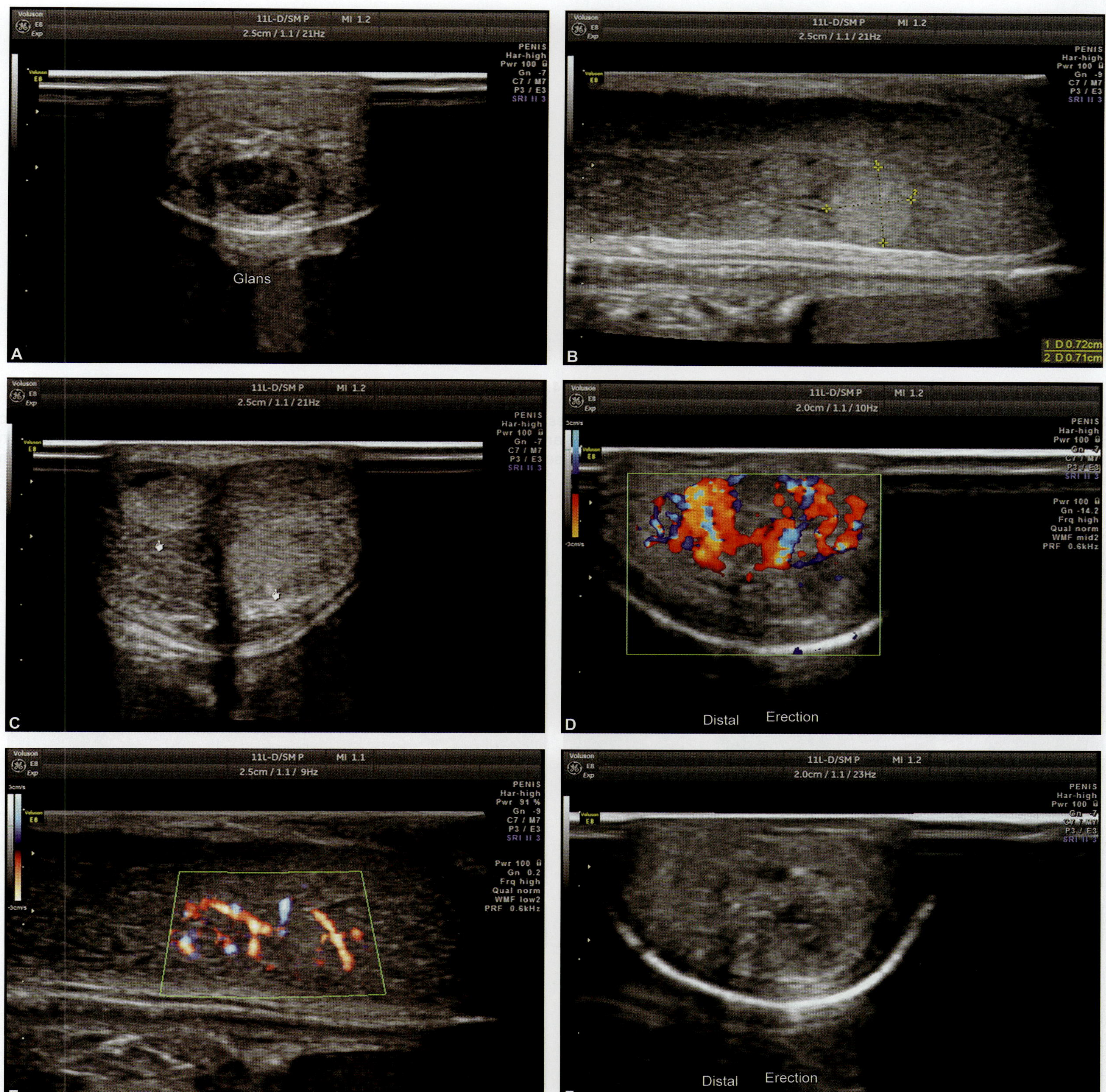

FIGURES 14.25A to F

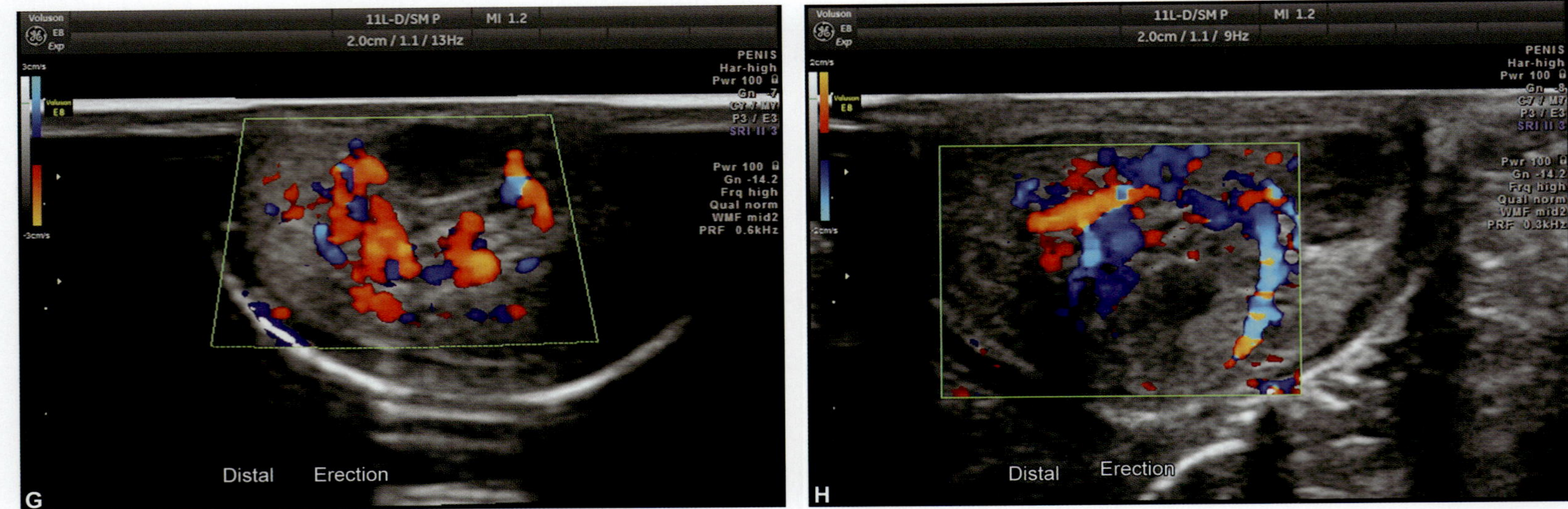

FIGURES 14.25G and H

FIGURES 14.25A to H: A 14-year-old boy presented with nodular masses in the distal part of penile shaft. HRSG shows homogeneous echogenic mass in the distal 1/3rd part of corpora cavernosa on both sides. They are echogenic in texture. No calcification or cystic degeneration is seen in them. On color flow imaging, multiple vessels are seen feeding the masses. On erection, the vessels got engorged and high flow is seen in them suggestive of arteriovenous malformation.

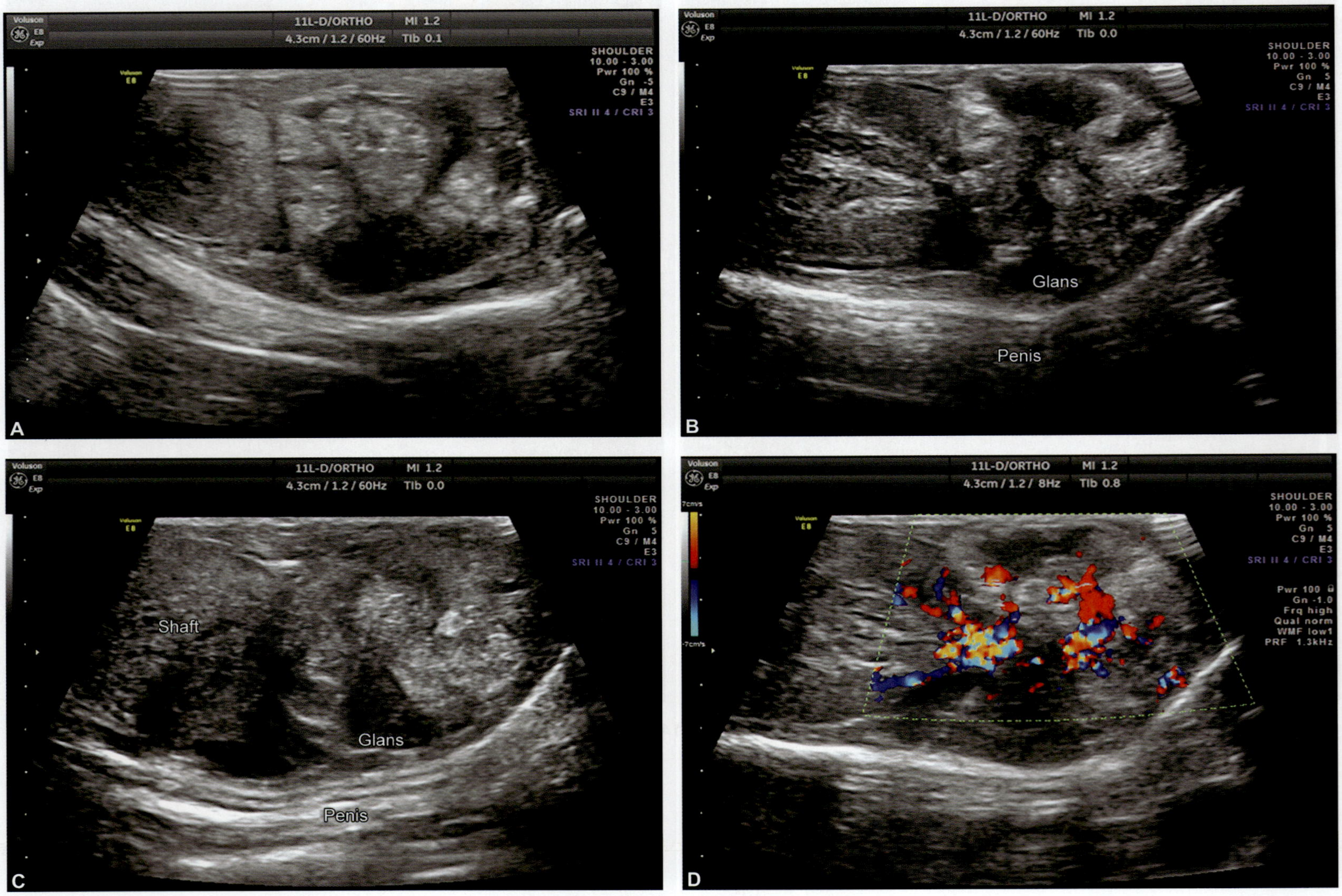

FIGURES 14.26A to D

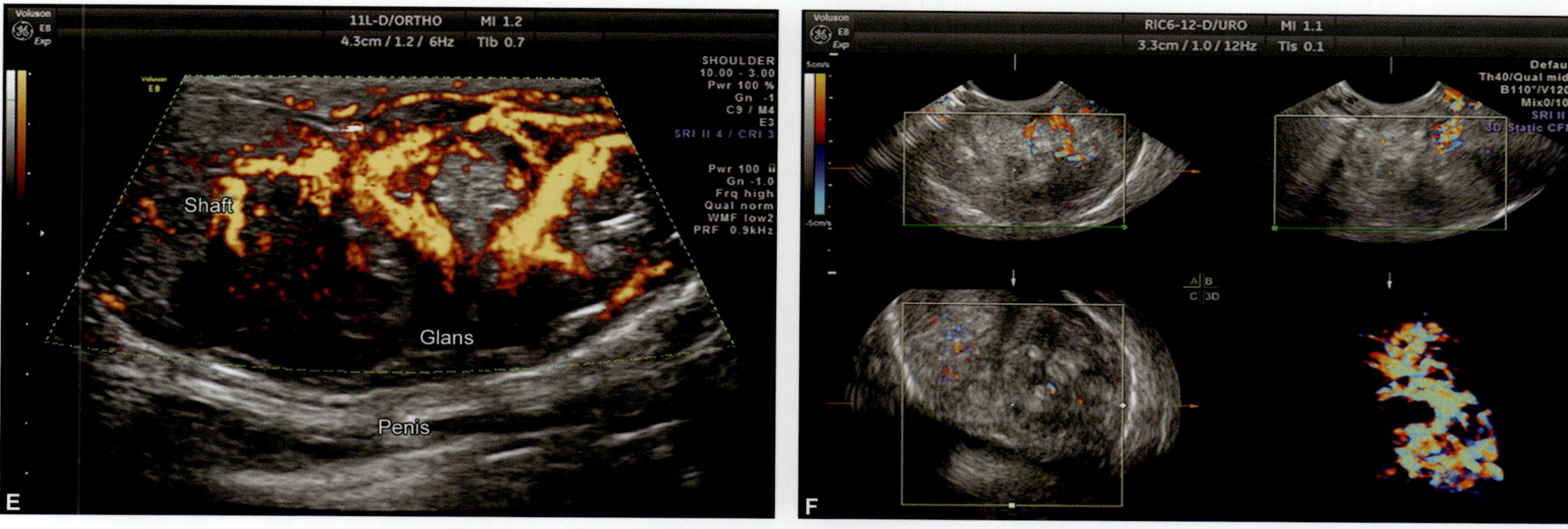

FIGURES 14.26E and F

FIGURES 14.26A to F: A patient presented with soft tissue mass over the glans of penis. HRSG shows a heterogeneous mass over the glans of penis. It is predominately solid. No calcification is seen in it. It is seen invading the distal part of penile shaft. On color flow imaging, multiple vessels are seen feeding the mass suggestive of carcinoma penis. Patient also had enlarged lymph nodes in inguinal region.

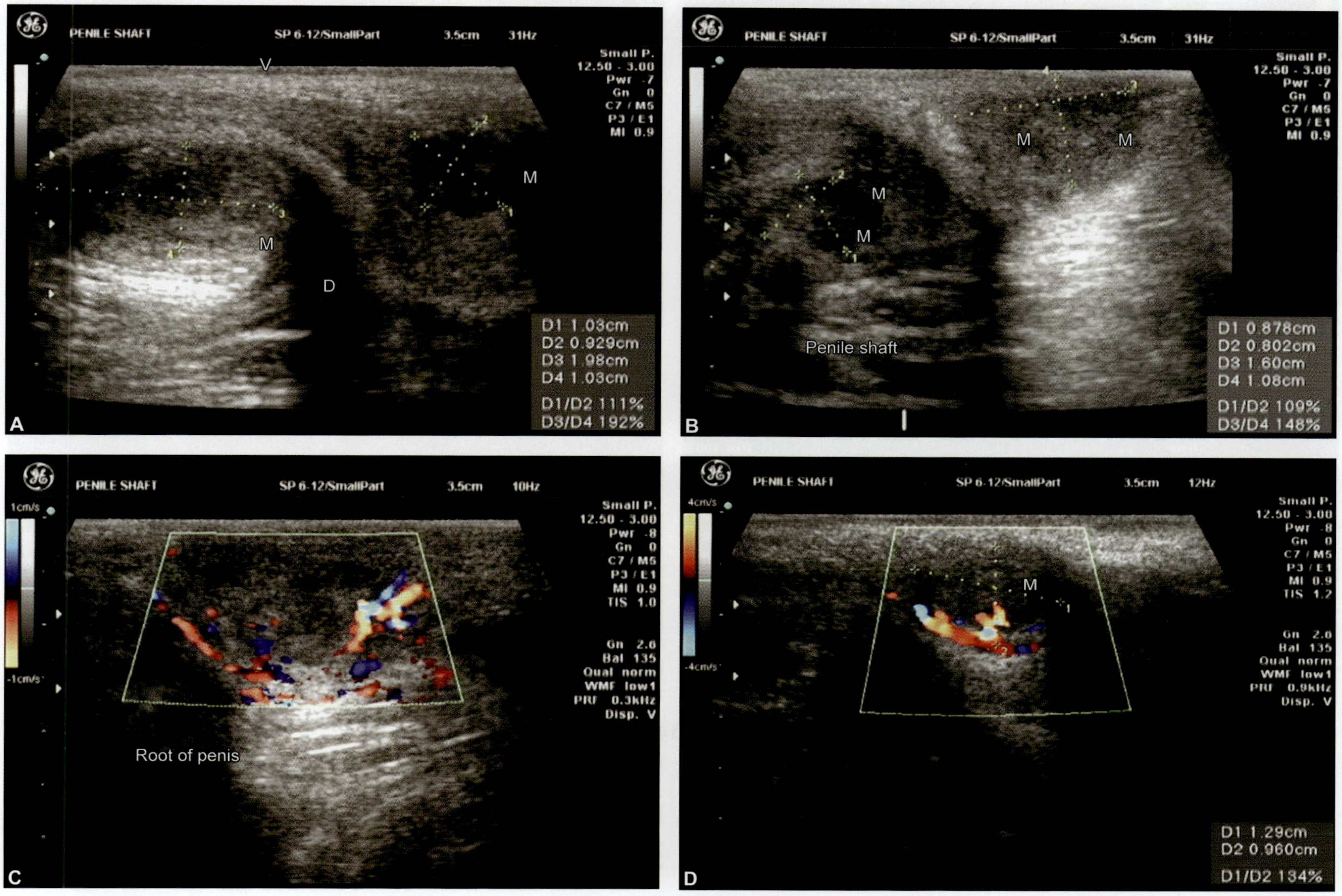

FIGURES 14.27A to D: Carcinoma penis. A patient presented with irregular mass at the root of the penis. HRSG showed and irregular heterogeneous mass at the root of the penis. Margins were irregular. It was seen invading the corpora. The mass was seen invading the root of the penis. There was also evidence of big heterogeneous mass seen invading the ventral side of the penile shaft. The capsule was broken. On color flow imaging, few vessels were seen feeding the mass. Biopsy of the mass confirms carcinoma penis.

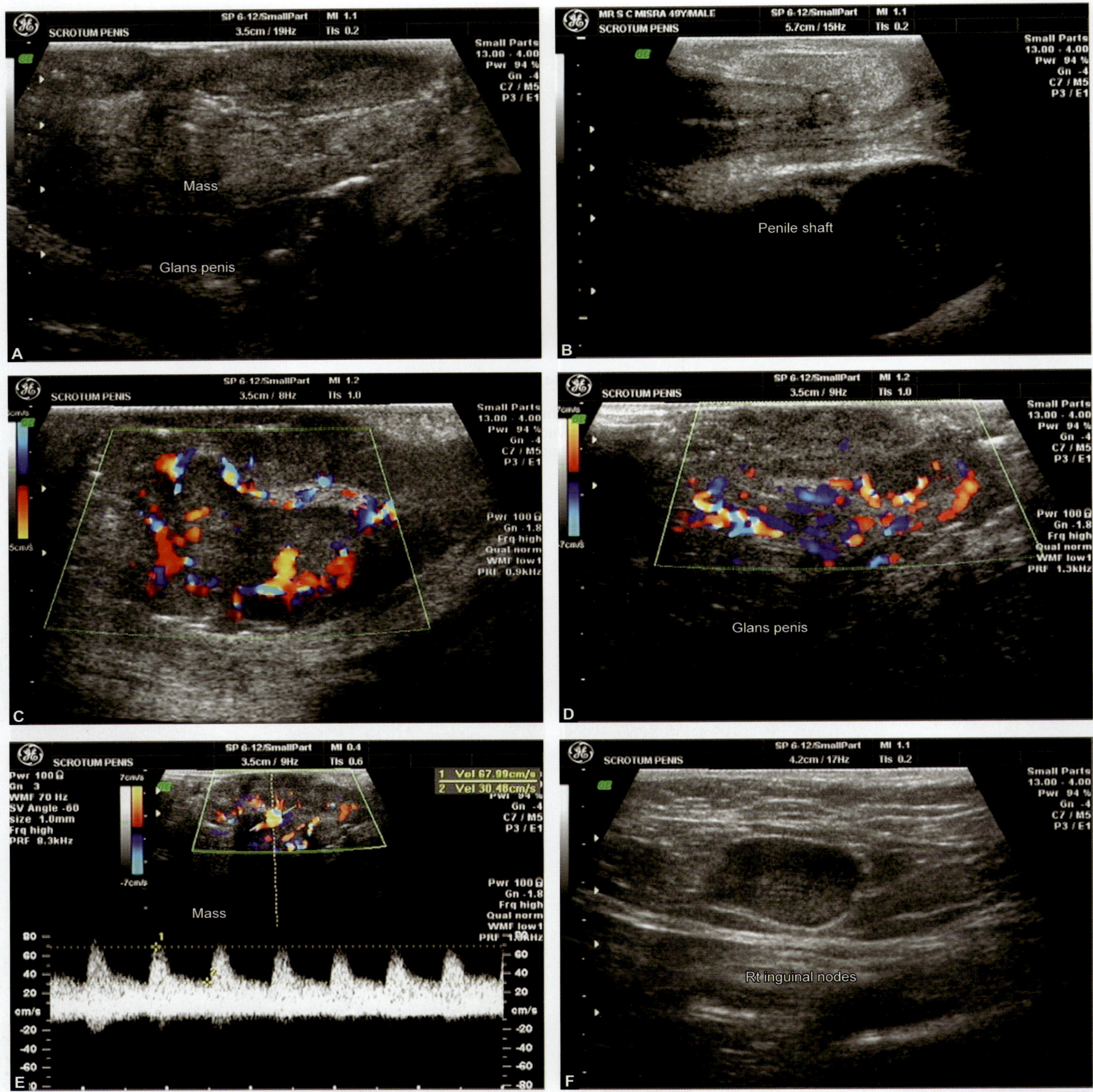

FIGURES 14.28A to F

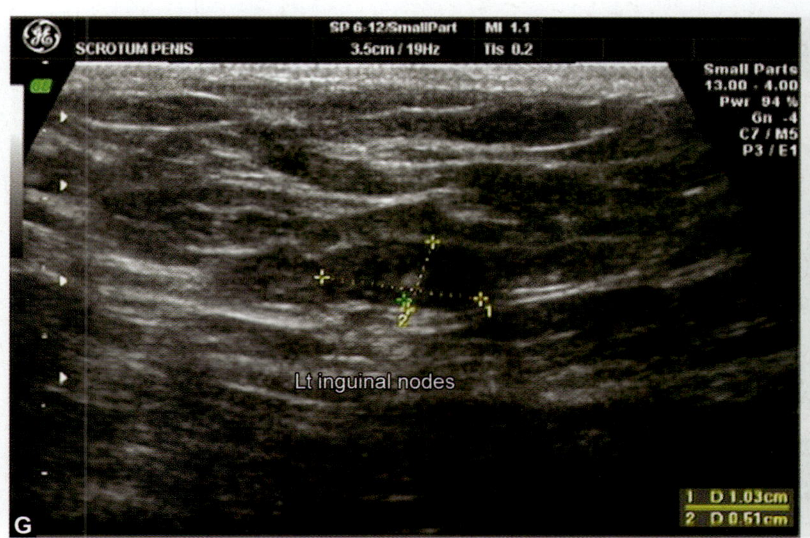

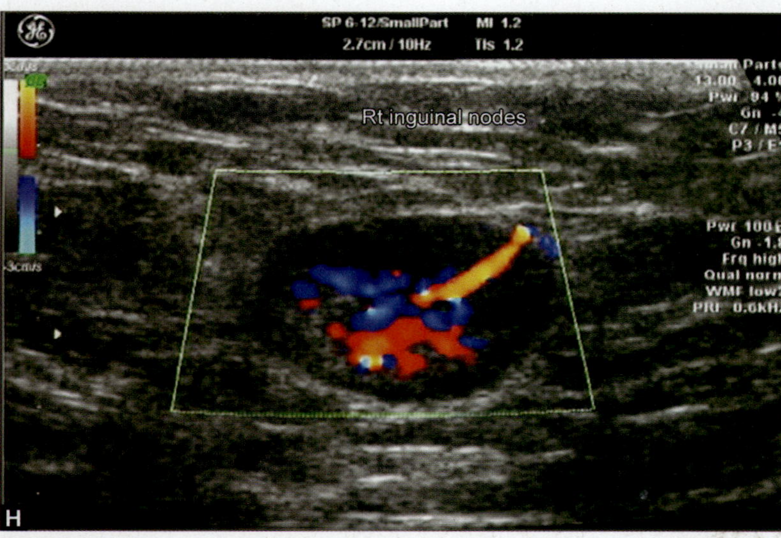

FIGURES 14.28G and H

FIGURES 14.28A to H: Carcinoma of the glans penis. A middle aged patient presented with heterogeneous soft tissue mass over the glans of the penis. Irregular masses were seen over the glans on HRSG. The mass was seen invading the distal penile shaft. On color flow imaging, multiple vessels were seen feeding the mass. On spectral Doppler tracing, high arterial flow was seen. Enlarged nodes were also seen in both inguinal regions. They were hypoechoic in texture. Lymph node hilum was lost. On color flow imaging high flow was seen in the lymph nodes. Biopsy of the mass confirms carcinoma penis.

ERECTILE DYSFUNCTION

High-resolution ultrasound with color flow imaging is an excellent modality for evaluation of erectile dysfunction. The various causes of erectile dysfunction are as follows:

1. Vasculogenic
2. Metabolic
3. Psychogenic
4. Hypogonadism
5. Trauma
6. Idiopathic

High-resolution ultrasound can tell with confidence about the penile shaft anatomy and any other pathology whereas color Doppler ultrasound tells about arterial and venous flow in dorsal penile artery, deep dorsal vein of penis and both cavernosal arteries. It is an important investigation to rule of vasculogenic causes of erectile dysfunction. Normal Doppler flow pattern shows gradual increase in the peak systolic value in cavernosal artery. It can be more than 30 cm/sec to achieve tumescence. There is high systolic flow and obliterated diastolic flow seen on tumescence of penis. Reversal of arterial flow is seen in cavernosal arteries because of distention of sinusitis and obliterated venous flow is seen because of obliteration of deep dorsal vein of penis due to tightening of tunica albuginea.

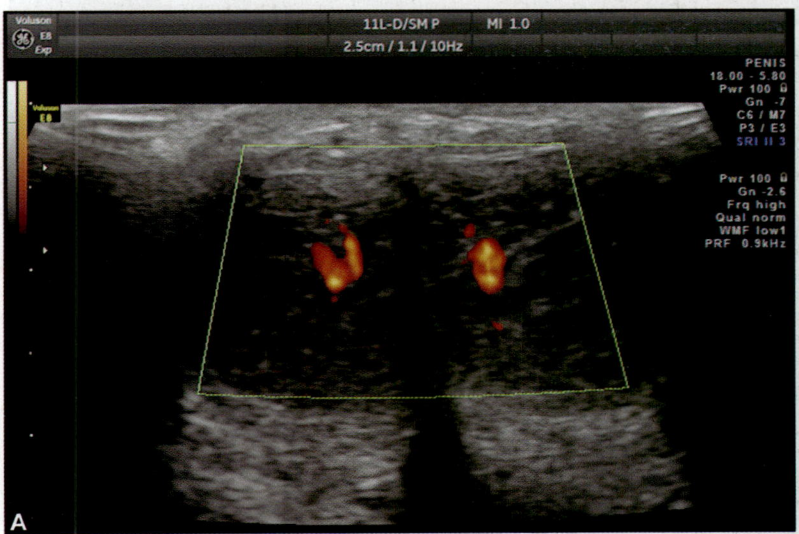

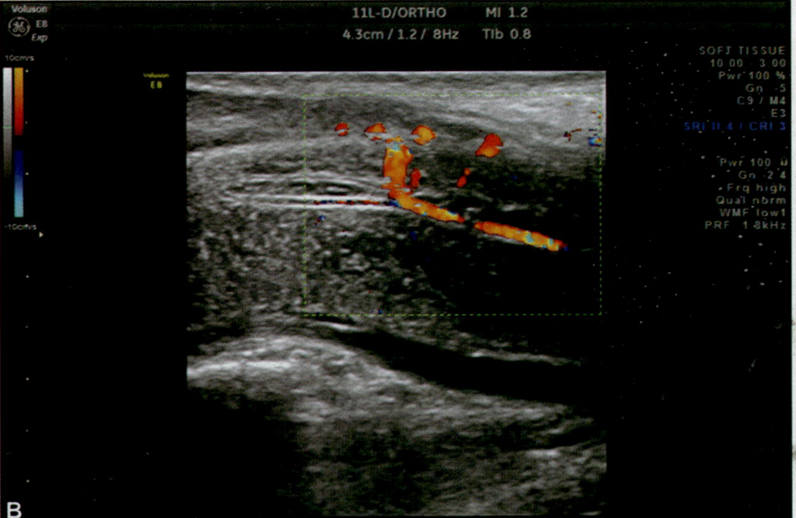

FIGURES 14.29A and B

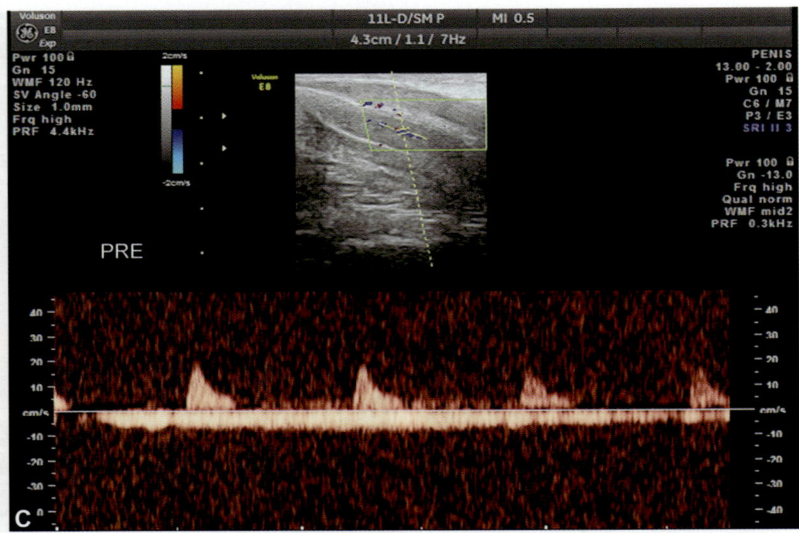

FIGURE 14.29C

FIGURES 14.29A to C: Normal cavernosal artery flow in neutral position. Color Doppler ultrasound shows normal flow in both cavernosal arteries in neutral position. Short systolic and early diastolic flow is seen in cavernosal arteries.

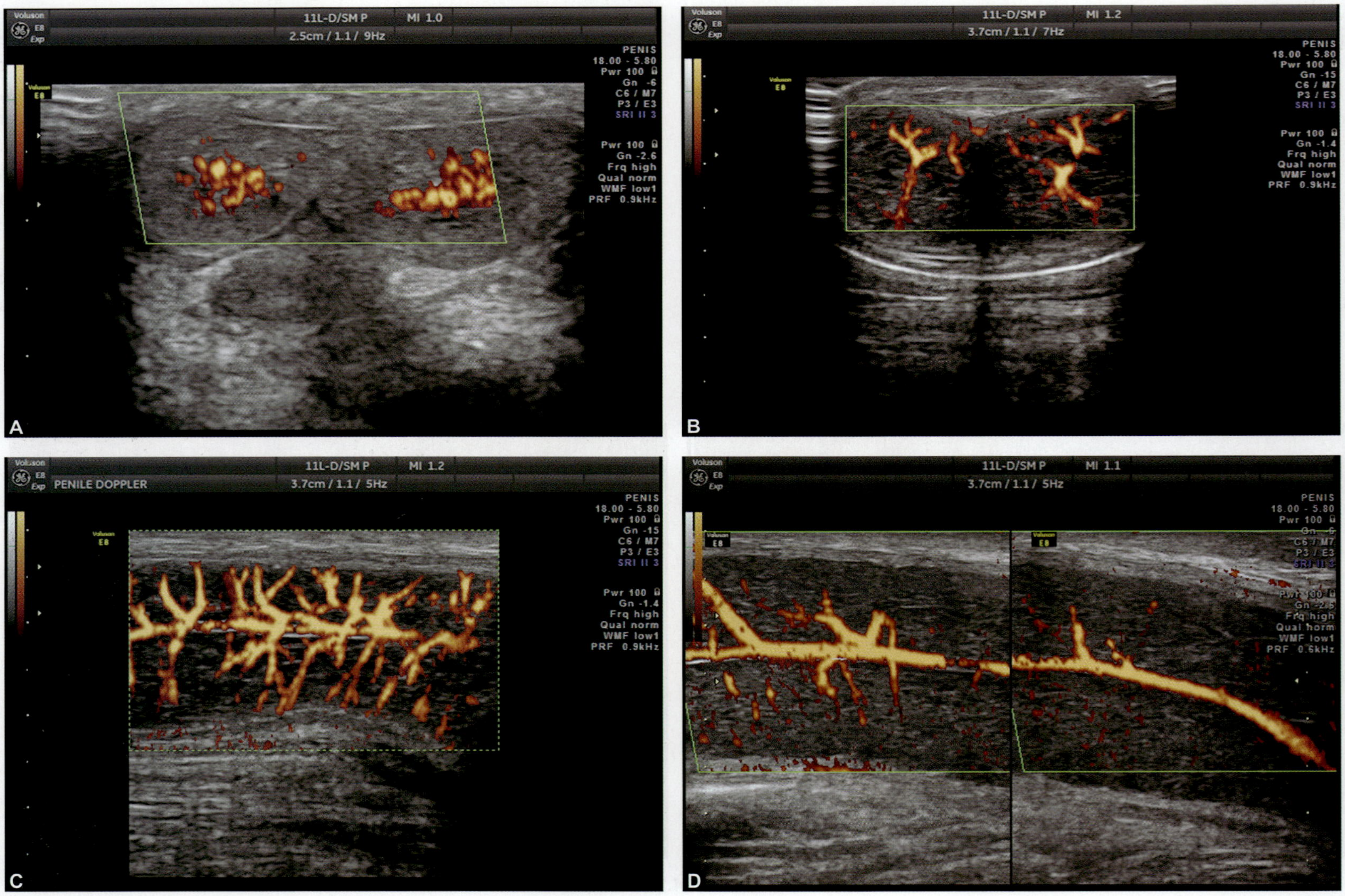

FIGURES 14.30A to D: Normal branching of cavernosal arteries. The power Doppler ultrasound shows multiple branches of cavernosal arteries supplying the corpora cavernosa on both sides.

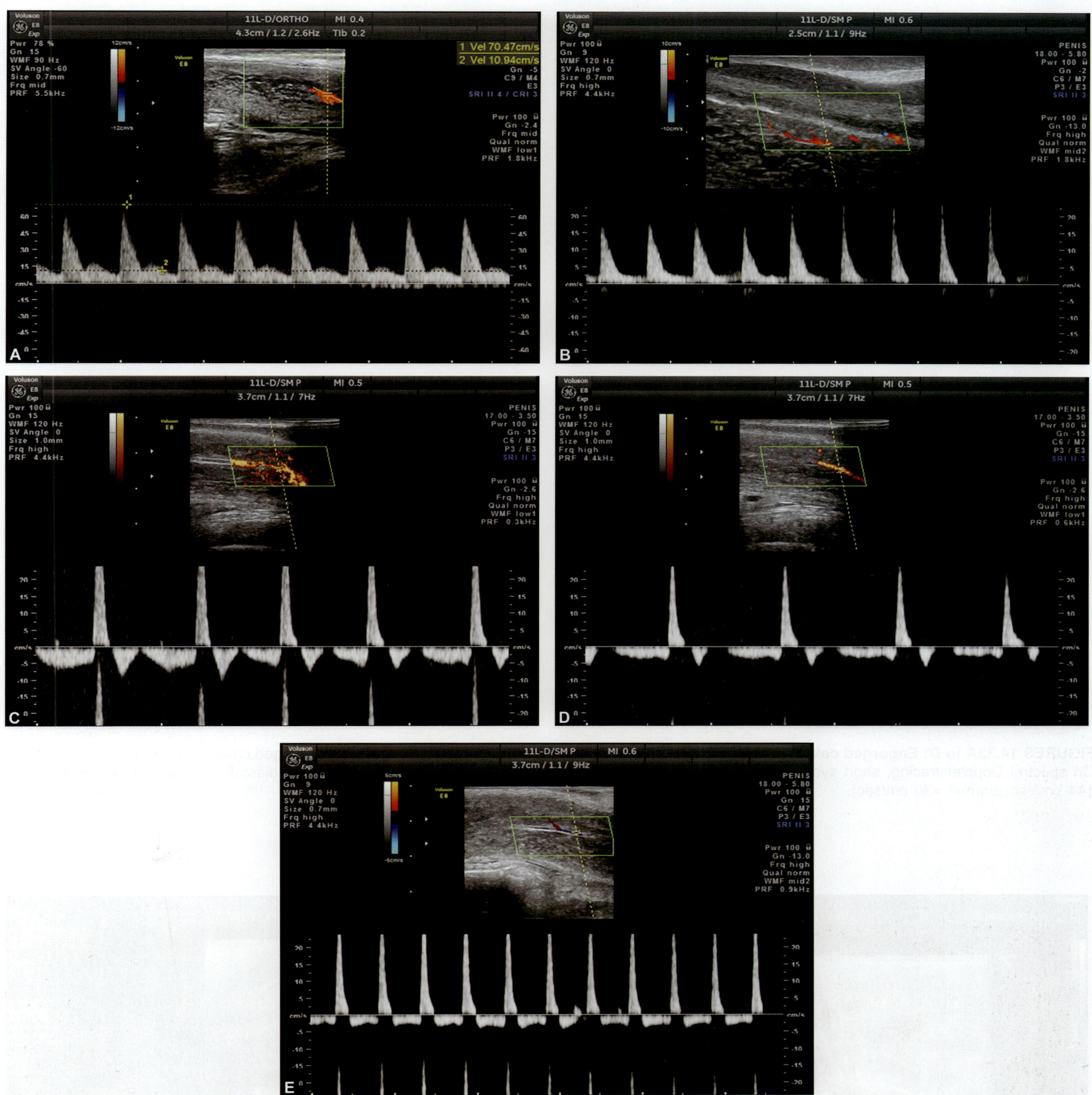

FIGURES 14.31A to E: Normal arterial flow pattern in cavernosal artery after giving 30 mg papaverine injection in cavernosa. In early phase of injection, high systolic and short diastolic flow is seen in cavernosal artery. As the patient starts achieving tumescence high systolic and obliterated diastolic flow is seen. On achieving complete tumescence, reversal of diastolic flow is seen and in tight erection, obliterated flow is seen in cavernosal artery.

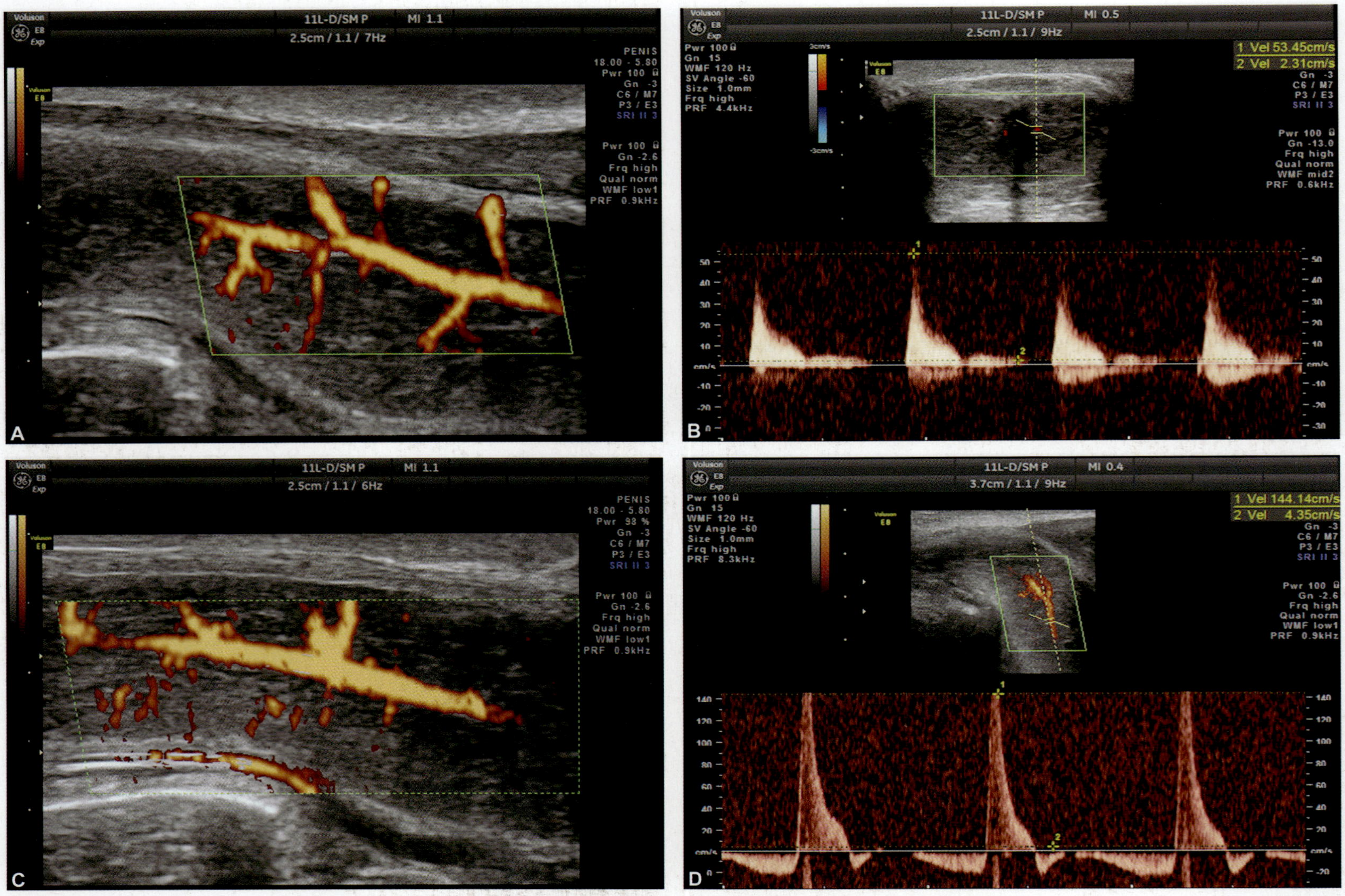

FIGURES 14.32A to D: Engorged cavernosal artery and its branches. Color Doppler ultrasound shows engorged cavernosal artery and its branches. On spectral Doppler tracing, short systolic and obliterated diastolic flow is seen. Figures C shows reversal of diastolic flow and high systolic flow of 144 cm/sec (normal >30 cm/sec).

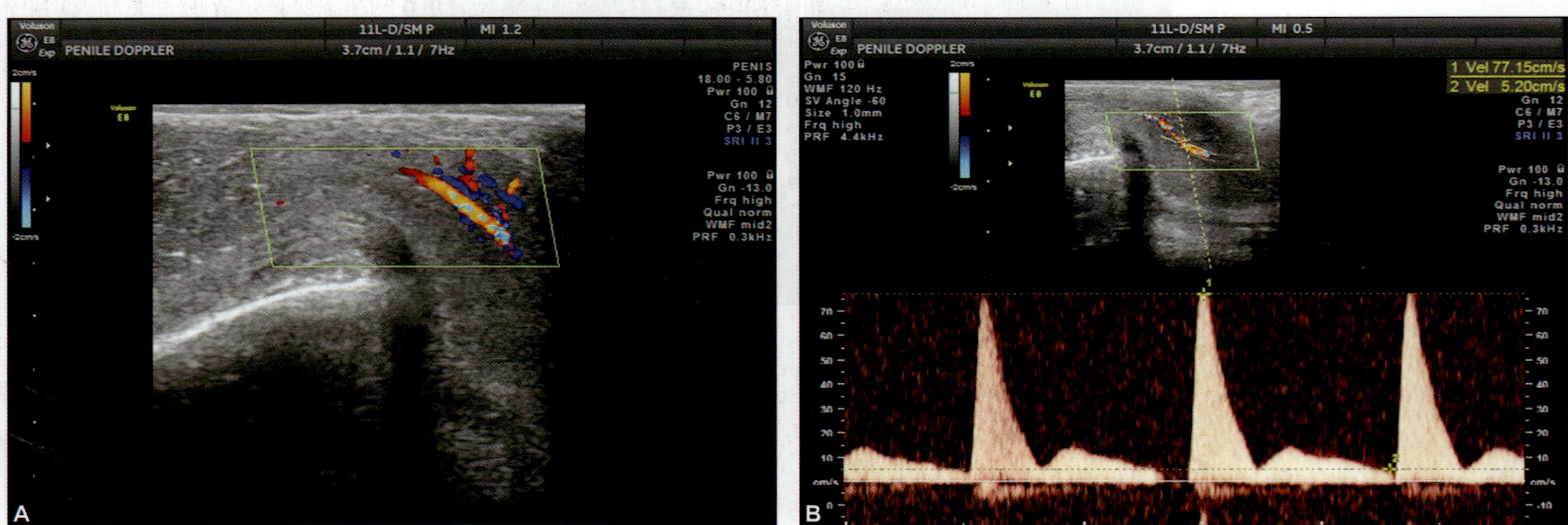

FIGURES 14.33A and B

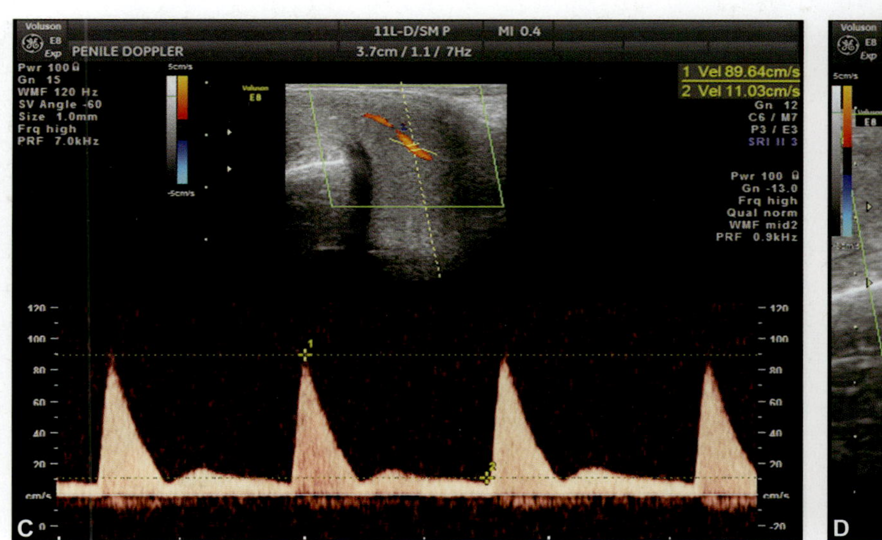

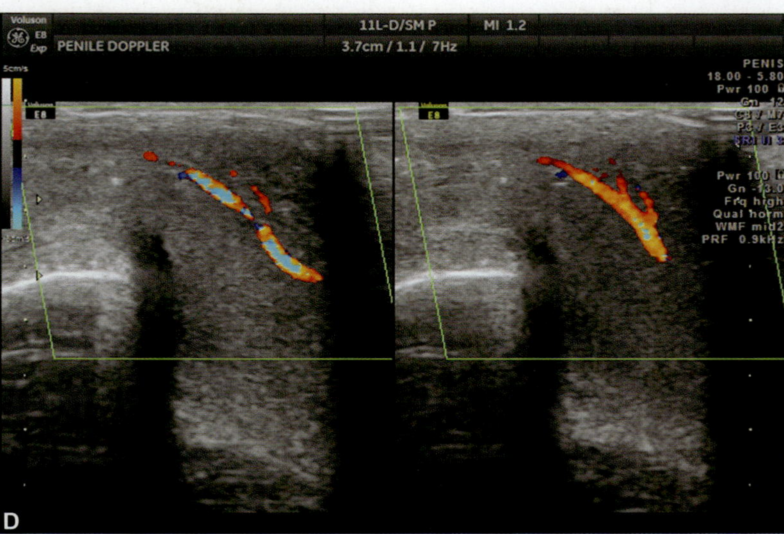

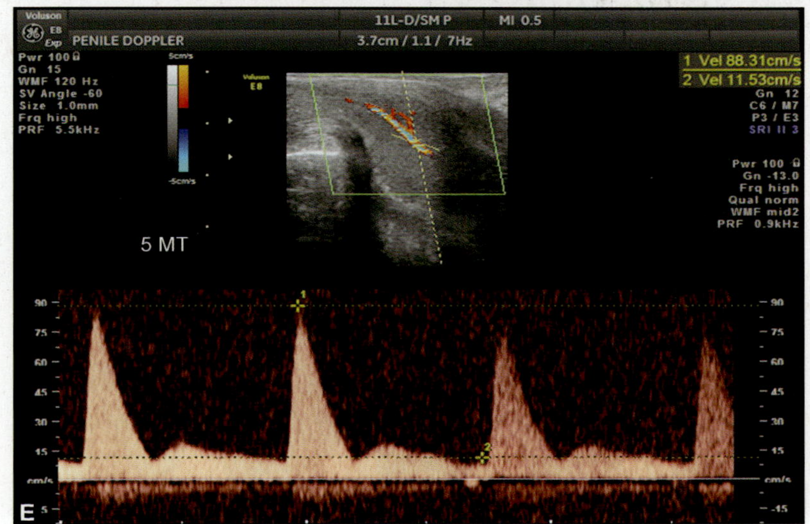

FIGURES 14.33C to E

FIGURES 14.33A to E: Persistent venous leak. A patient presented with history of erectile dysfunction. HRSG with color Doppler imaging shows persistent venous leak. Though, arterial flow is normal, it is 77.1 cm/sec, but no obliteration or reversal of diastolic flow is seen. Persistent prolonged high diastolic flow is seen in cavernosal artery. It is 11cm/sec suggestive of persistent venous leak (normal <3 cm/sec).

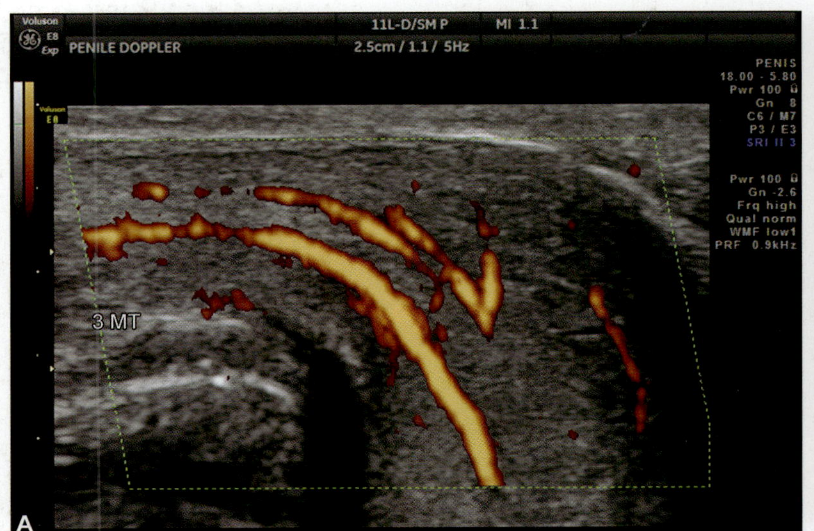

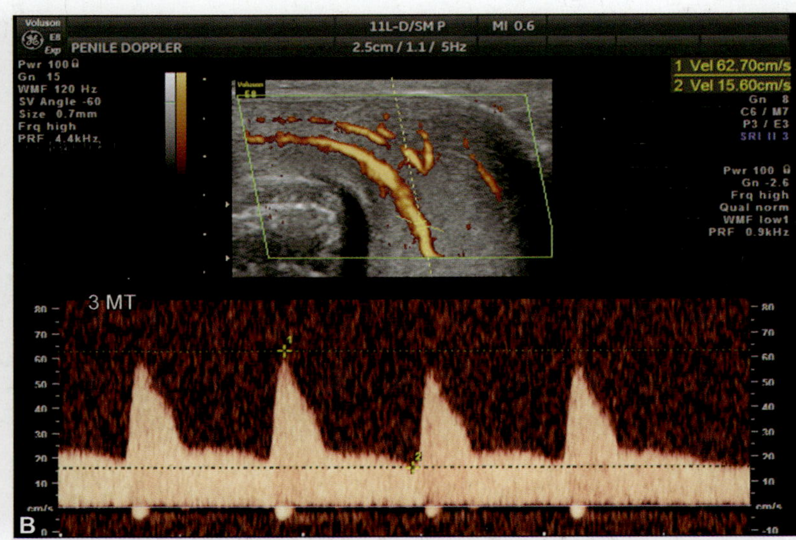

FIGURES 14.34A and B

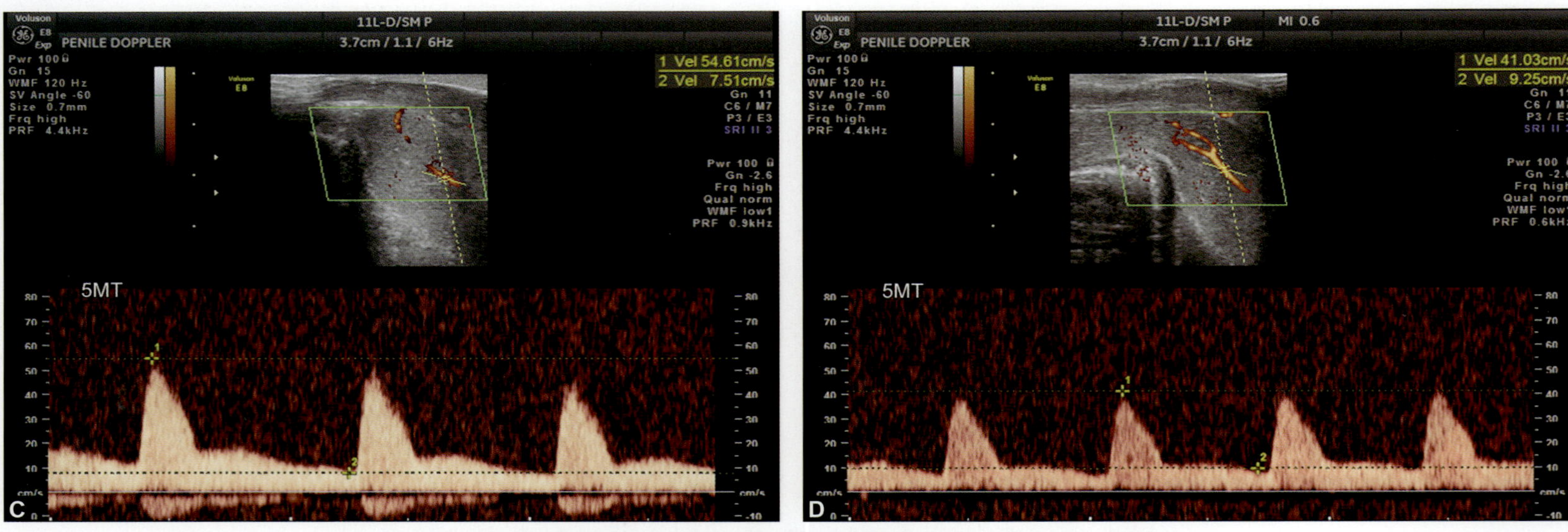

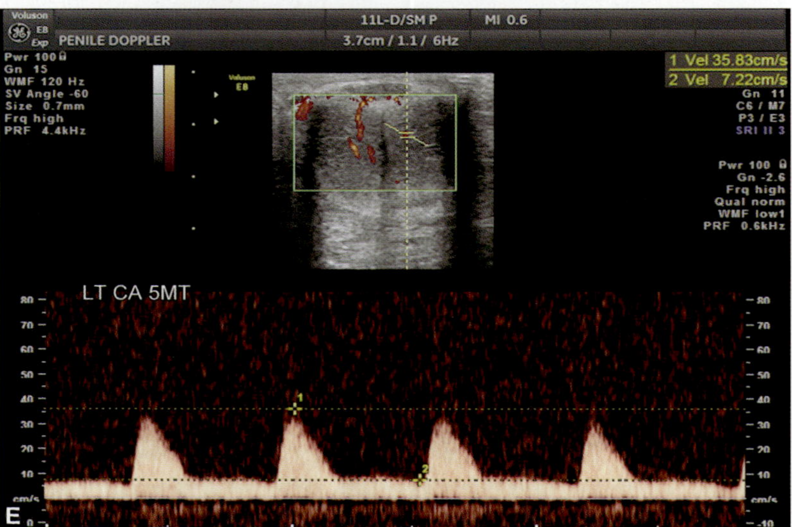

FIGURES 14.34C to E

FIGURES 14.34A to E: Persistent venous leak. A patient of erectile dysfunction shows persistent high diastolic flow suggestive of venous leak. The diastolic flow was not obliterated. No reversal of flow seen in the arterial cycle. The persistent diastolic flow was seen with velocity of 7.2 cm/sec.

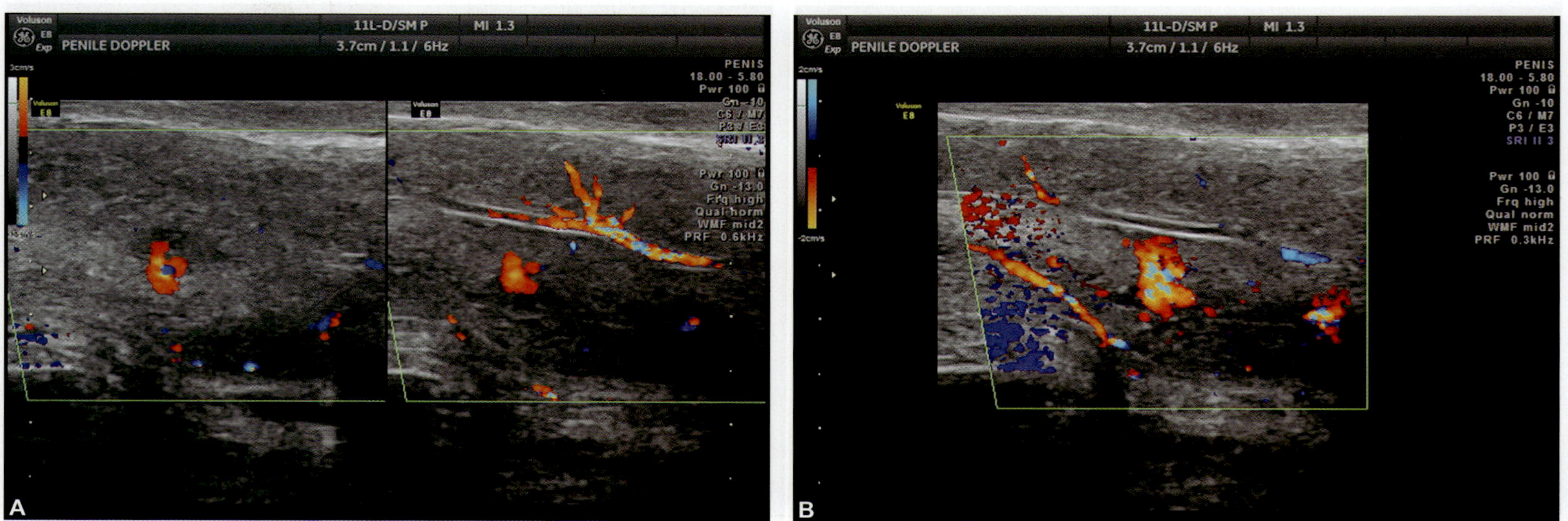

FIGURES 14.35A and B: Venous malformation. A patient presented with erectile dysfunction. HRSG shows an irregular hypoechoic low level echo mass in corpora cavernosa. On color flow imaging, pooling of blood is seen in it suggestive of venous malformation. Patient failed to achieve tumescence due to diverting of blood in venous malformation.

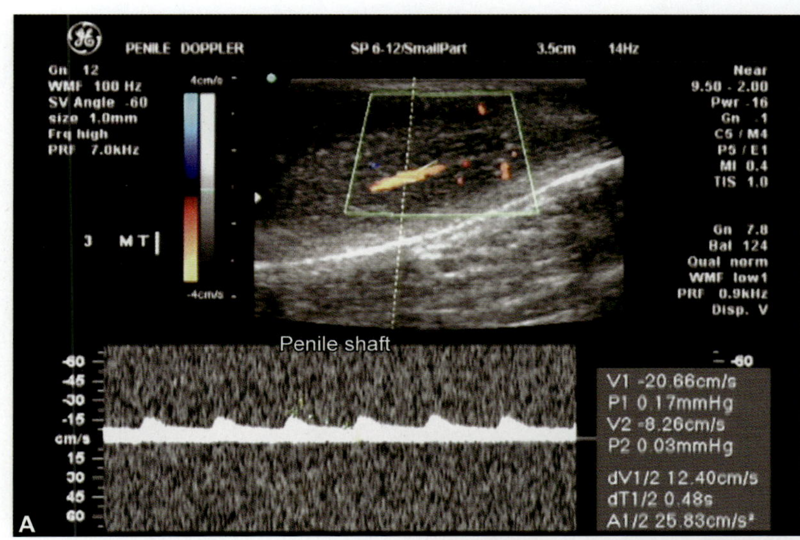

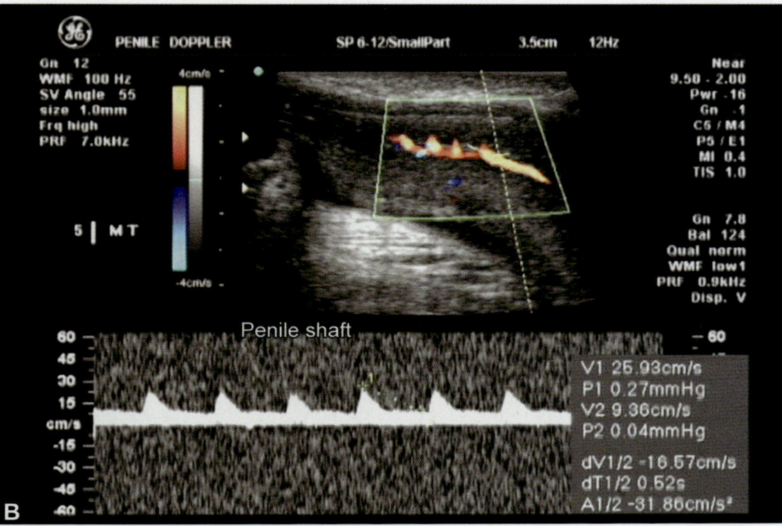

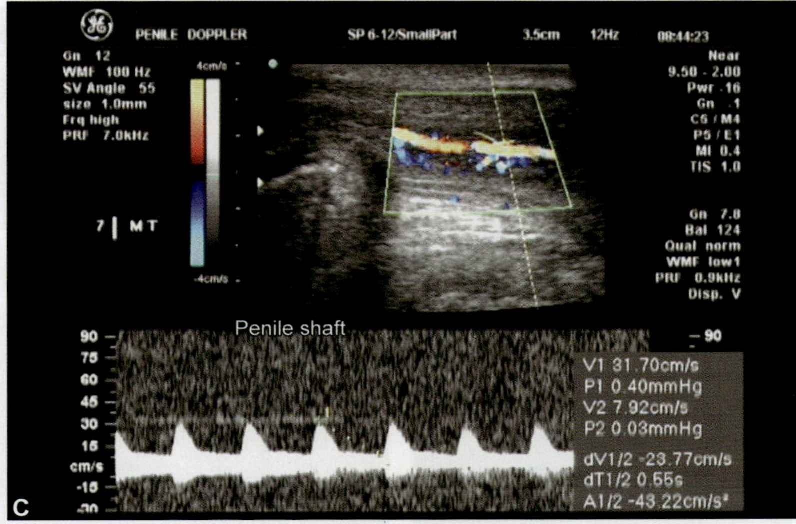

FIGURES 14.36A to C: Arterial insufficiency. The Doppler spectral waveform shows increased systolic pressure. However, the systolic peak is less than normal limits and it is 15 cm/sec in its peak state. Partial tumescence is achieved not lasting for long time. Since, optimum arterial systolic pressure is not achieved. It suggests of arterial insufficiency. Prolonged diastolic flow is also seen.

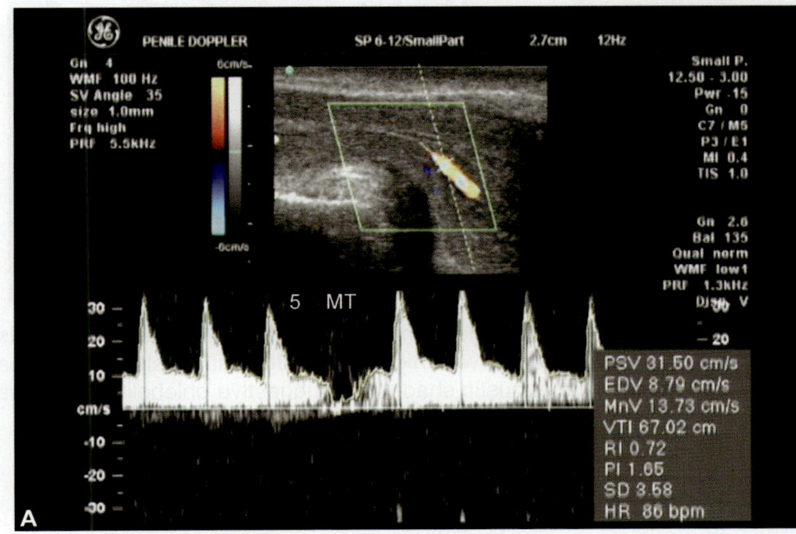

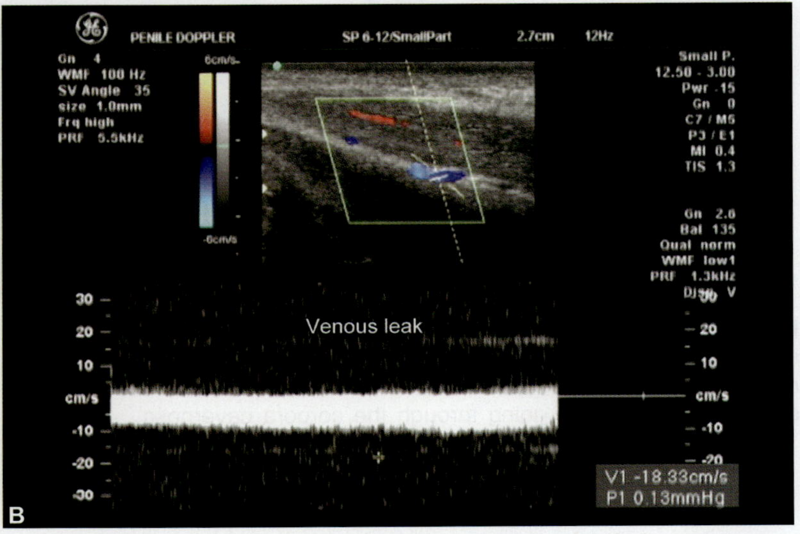

FIGURES 14.37A and B: Arterial insufficiency with venous leak. A patient of erectile dysfunction showed arterial insufficiency with venous leak. Doppler study shows suboptimal arterial flow after injecting vasodilating drug. The maximum peak arterial velocity was achieved 31.5 cm/sec. However, persistent high diastolic flow was also seen suggestive of venous leak. There is evidence of high flow seen in the veins of the penis. No obliteration of venous flow seen throughout the study.

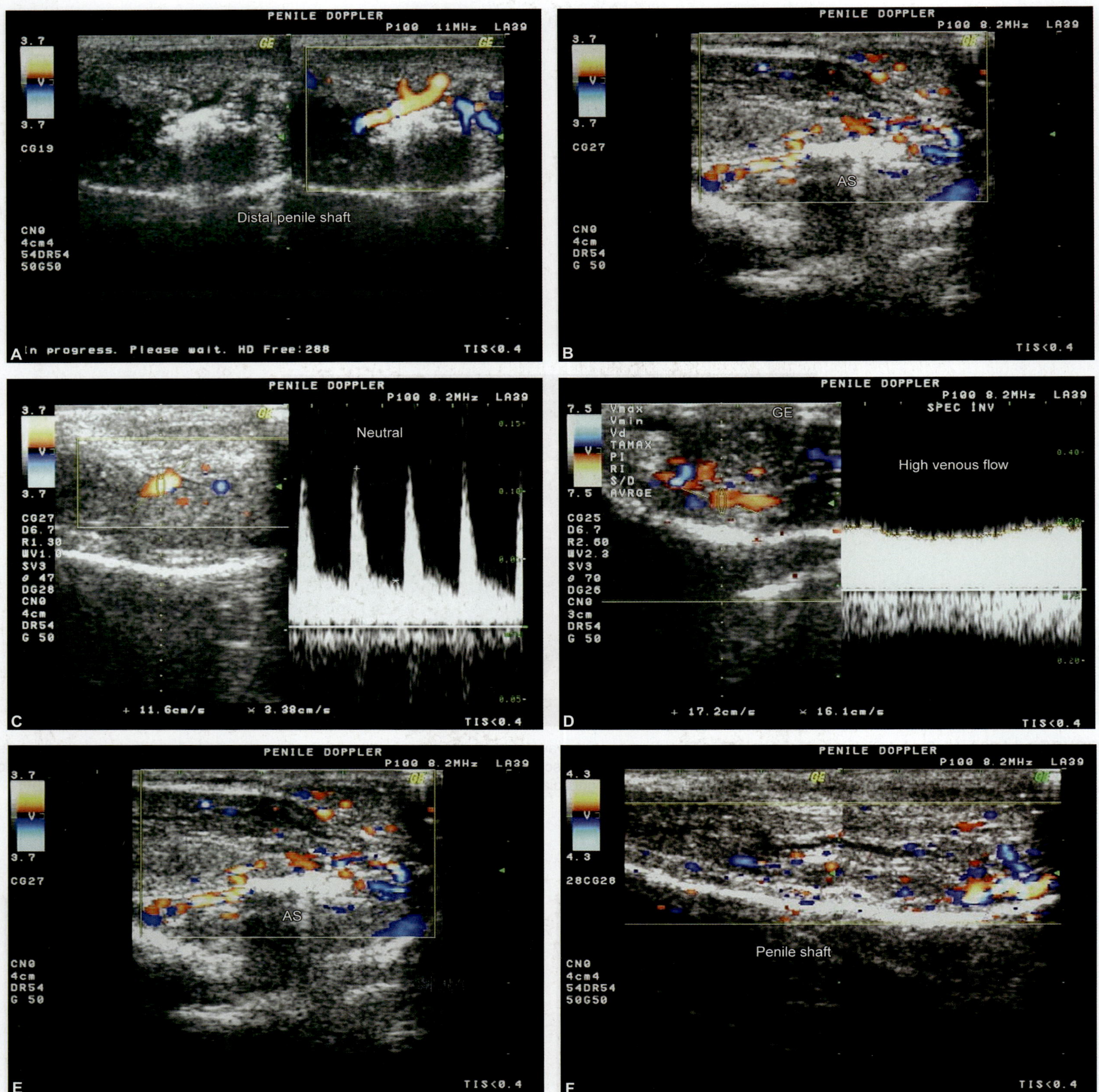

FIGURES 14.38A to F: Venous malformation. A patient presented with impotence. HRSG and color flow imaging shows multiple dilated vessels in the distal part of the corpora cavernosa. On color flow imaging pooling of the blood is seen in them with high venous flow suggestive of venous malformation. Echogenic calcified shadows are also seen in the veins, which are accompanied with acoustic shadowing suggestive phlebolith. Tortuous dilated veins are seen going through the corpora cavernosa.

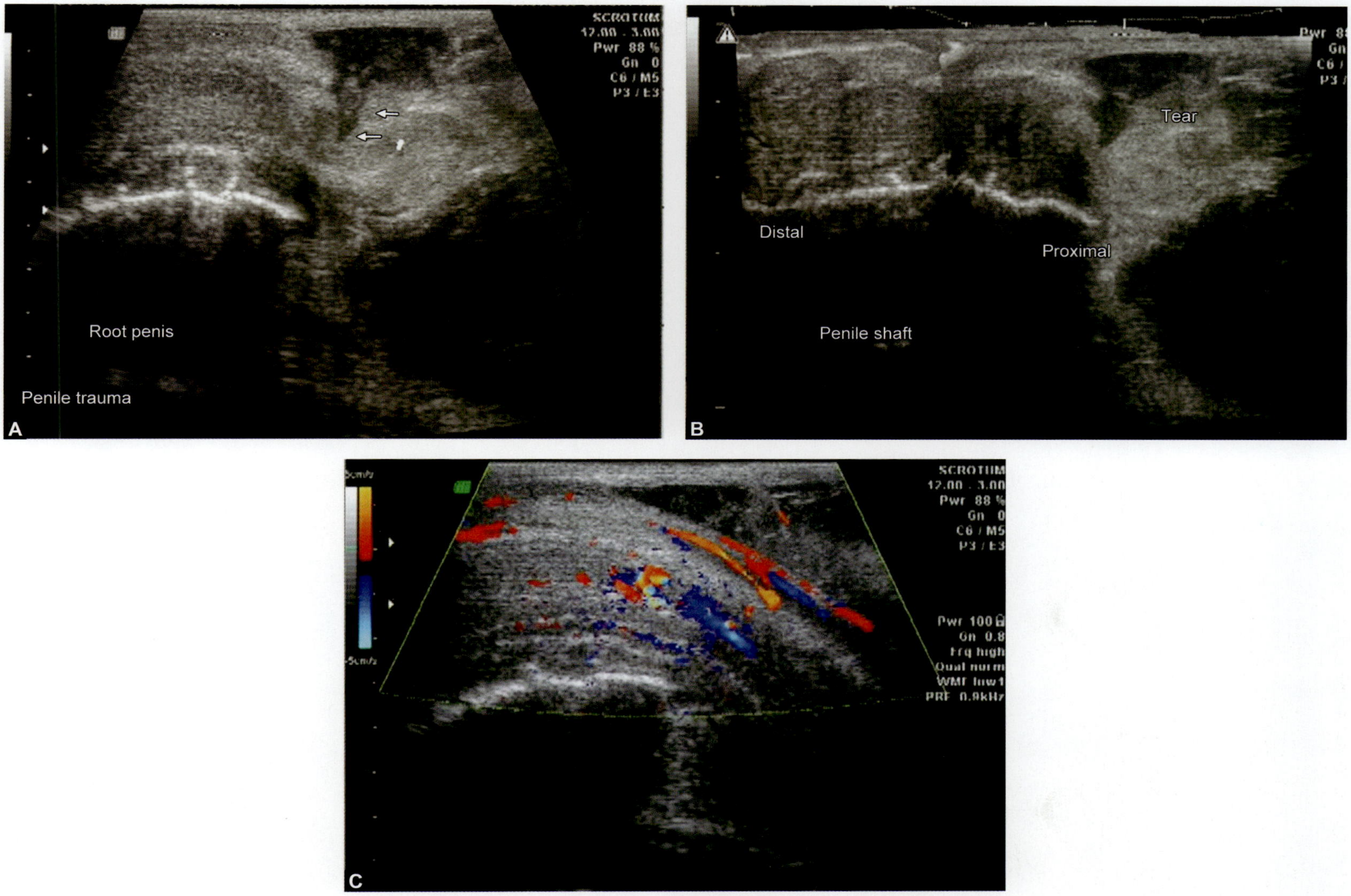

FIGURES 14.39A to C: Penile trauma with erectile dysfunction. A patient sustained penile trauma and developed erectile dysfunction. HRSG shows rupture of tunica albuginea at the root of penis. A big cleft is seen going into corpora cavernosa suggestive of fracture of penis. On color flow imaging, persistent venous leak is seen. The arterial flow is also suboptimal resulting into erectile dysfunction.

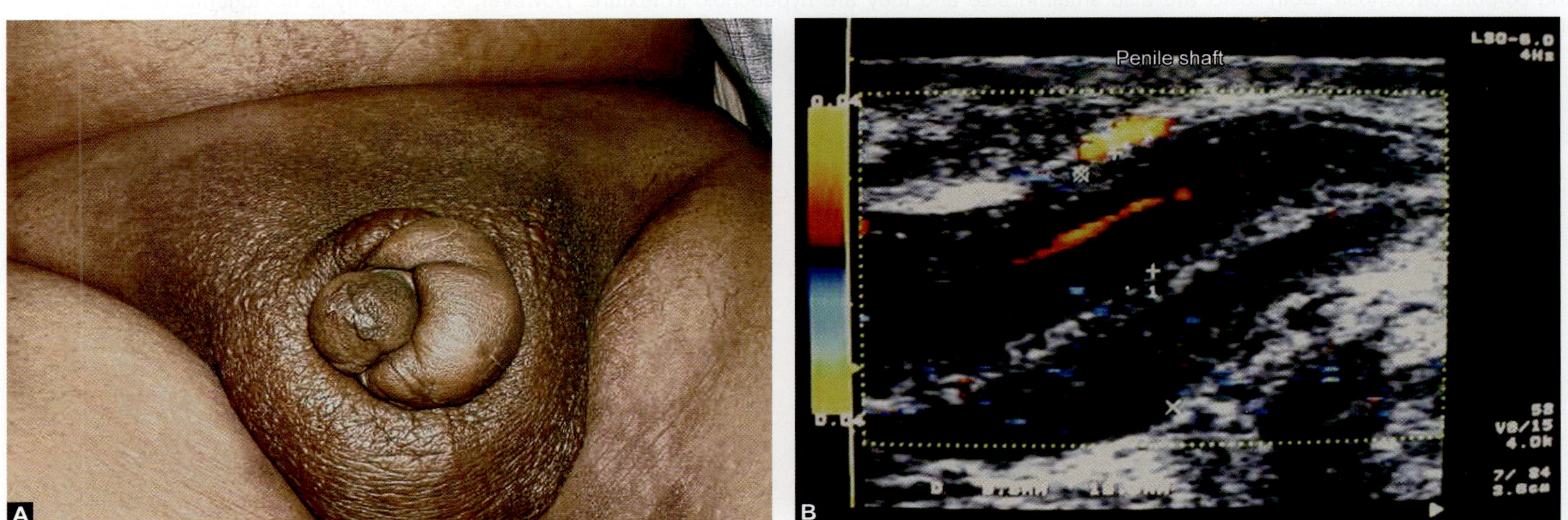

FIGURES 14.40A and B

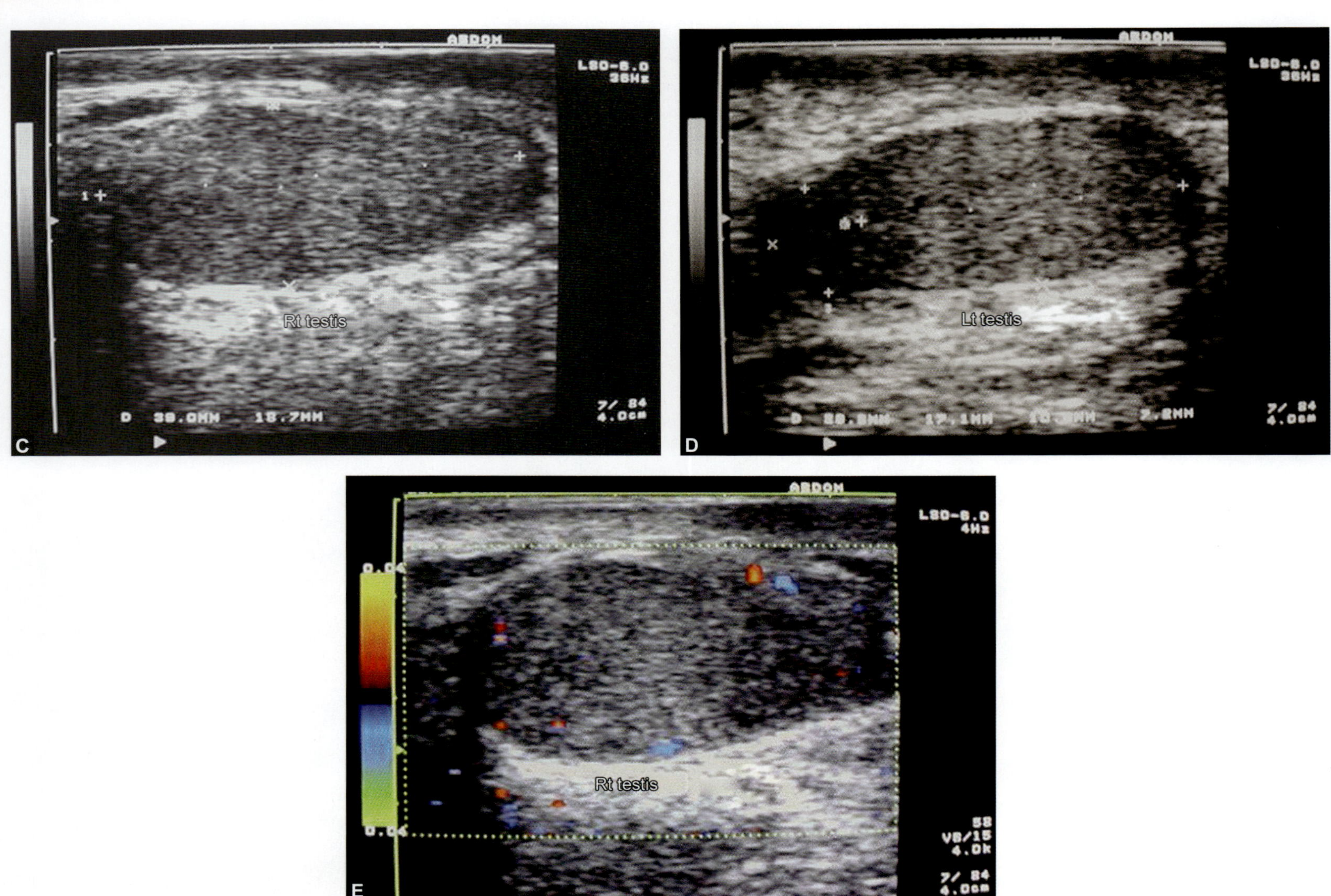

FIGURES 14.40C to E

FIGURES 14.40A to E: Filarial penis and scrotum. A young man presented with impotence. The penis is markedly edematous and flaccid in position. It is seen as a coiled collapsed organ. Marked skin edema is present. HRSG and color flow imaging shows hypoechoic corpora cavernosa. On color flow and Doppler ultrasound, low flow is seen in cavernosal artery after injecting vasodilating agent suggestive of arterial insufficiency and edema in the corpora cavernosa. Both testis are also small in size and they are hypoechoic in texture. However, echogenicity is homogeneous. On color flow imaging poor flow is seen in the testis suggestive of arterial insufficiency.

CHAPTER 15

Anterior Abdominal Wall

PK Srivastava

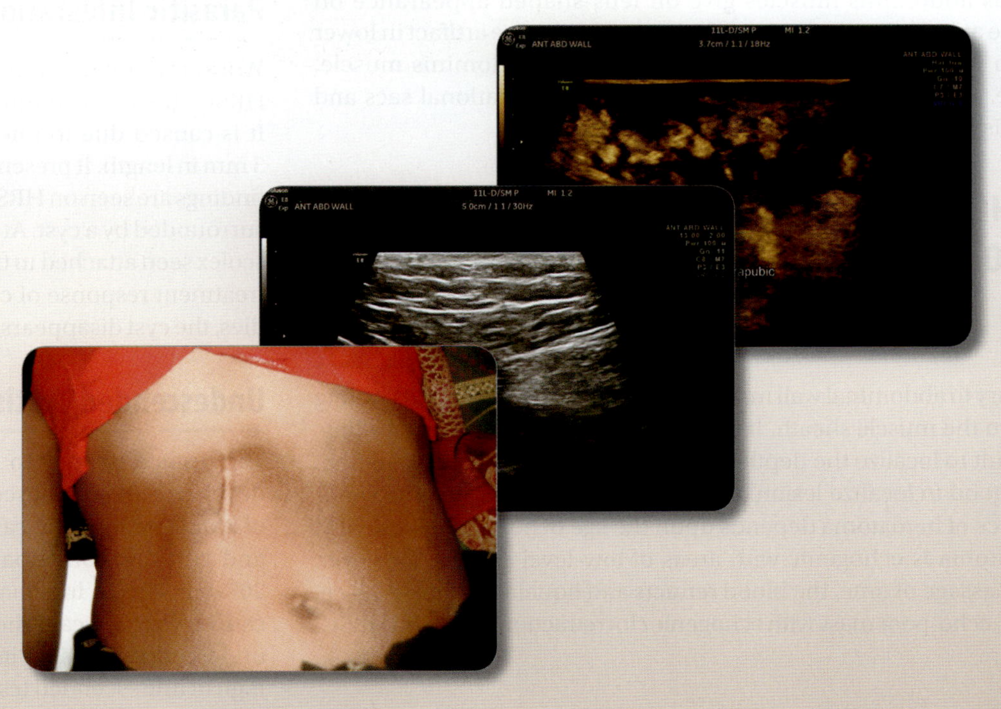

INTRODUCTION

Abdominal wall provides the access to ultrasonographic beam to examine internal abdominal organs. A common indication for anterior abdominal wall imaging is to examine a palpable mass in abdominal wall. High-resolution sonography (HRSG) can demonstrate about the nature of the mass whether it is solid or cystic. It also tells about the location of the mass whether it is intra-abdominal or in the abdominal wall.

Normal Anatomy

Anterior abdominal wall is a layered structure. The outermost layer is skin, the superficial fascia, subcutaneous fat, muscles, transversalis fascia and extraperitoneal fat. The muscle layer contains paired midline rectus muscles, anteriolateral external oblique, internal oblique and transversus abdominis arise from fifth, sixth and seventh ribs and extend inferiorly and insert in pubic crest. They are wrapped in rectus sheath. The rectus sheath is formed by aponeurosis of internal oblique, external oblique and transversus muscles. The transversalis fascia lies deep to muscle layers. It contains little fat and separates the muscle layers from peritoneum.

Sonographic Appearance of Abdominal Wall

High-resolution sonography can very well-demonstrate the normal layer of abdominal wall. A linear transducer of 10 MHz is choice of transducer to study abdominal wall. The skin stands out clearly as an echogenic line. Subcutaneous fat is seen beneath the skin as hypoechoic layer. Musculofascial layer is more echogenic than subcutaneous fat. High-resolution transducer can show individual muscle bundles. The extra-peritoneal fat is seen as an echo-poor fat line posterior to the muscle. The rectus abdominis muscles give on lens-shaped appearance on transverse axis. This may give a confusing double image artifact in lower abdomen when imaging is done through rectus abdominis muscle. Therefore, a single gestational sac is seen as two gestational sacs and can be misdiagnosed as twin pregnancy.

PATHOLOGICAL LESIONS OF ANTERIOR ABDOMINAL WALL

Trauma

Blunt injury to abdominal wall may lead to tearing of muscles and pooling of blood in the muscle sheath. It presents as a palpable tender swelling. It is difficult to localize the depth of hematoma on clinical examination. HRSG is good to localize lesion and also status of the lesion. The sono-appearance of hematoma depends upon the age of hematoma. Initially, the hematoma is echogenic with areas of low-level echoes. However, with the passage of time, the blood retracts and liquefaction takes place. Therefore, echo-poor mass with echogenic clot retraction is seen on HRSG.

Abscess

Anterior abdominal wall abscess may develop to any region. However, most common factor is post-surgical abscess formation in abdominal wound. HRSG can demonstrate the different states of abscess. Pus collection is seen in the subcutaneous tissue. The abscess cavity shows thick echo collection. Echogenic debris is also seen on HRSG. Ultrasonographic-guided drainage can be performed to speed-up the healing process. At times gas is also seen in the abscess cavity. Communication of abscess cavity to deep layers of abdominal wall can be easily picked up of HRSG. Only removal of stitch can release the pus and helps the wound to heal spontaneously.

Foreign Body

Foreign body entrapped in anterior abdominal wall is very rare and most commonly is seen due to post-surgical complication. Fever, persistent lump and tenderness in local area are most common features complained by the patient. HRSG can very well-demonstrate the nature of the mass, its consistency and location. Most common cause is a sponge, which is left in the abdomen after surgery. HRSG can show the layers of sponge. It may be seen as an echogenic mass with granuloma formation. The adherent blood gives a hyper-reflective appearance.

Muscle Tumors

Abdominal wall tumors are uncommon. The most common primary tumors are desmoid tumors of muscles. They take origin from fascia of aponeurosis. They are well-defined hypoechoic masses with homogenous texture. HRSG guided fine-needle aspiration cytology (FNAC) can be done to confirm the diagnosis.

Metastatic Lesions

Metastatic deposits can be found in the abdominal wall. The most common metastatic nodules are seen in metastatic melanoma. However, secondaries from lymphoma, carcinoma of lung, breast, ovary and colon can go the abdominal wall. HRSG shows multiple hypoechoic nodular masses in abdominal wall.

Parasitic Infestations

Worm infestation to muscles and cyst formation can be picked up on HRSG. The most common worm infestation to muscles is cysticercosis. It is caused due to infestation of ***Taenia solium***. The worm is about 3 mm in length. It presents as subcutaneous nodule. Typical sonographic findings are seen on HRSG. The scolex is highly reflective nodule, which is surrounded by a cyst. At times two or three cysts are seen with echogenic scolex seen attached to their walls. HRSG is also very good to monitor the treatment response of cysticercosis with medical treatment. The worm dies, the cyst disappears, and only localized thickening of muscle is seen.

Undescended Testis

The testis descends to its normal position in scrotum in the normal development. The descent of testis can arrest at any place from hilum of kidney to inguinal canal. In all undescended testis 80% are palpable and 20% are nonpalpable. But out of these 20% nonpalpable testis, 20% are seen in inguinal canal, and 20% are found in abdomen. HRSG can very well-locate the site of the nonpalpable testis. Localization of undescended testis is important, as incidence of neoplastic changes is high in undescended testis. The undescended testis can be easily located in the inguinal canal at root of scrotum in suprapubic area and medial side of thigh on HRSG. However, arrest of testis in abdominal cavity is difficult to find out on ultrasonography due to retroperitoneal fat.

Recanalization of Umbilical Vein

Recanalization of umbilical vein can be detectable on HRSG. The appearance is irregular and the vein can be traced downward in venous overload.

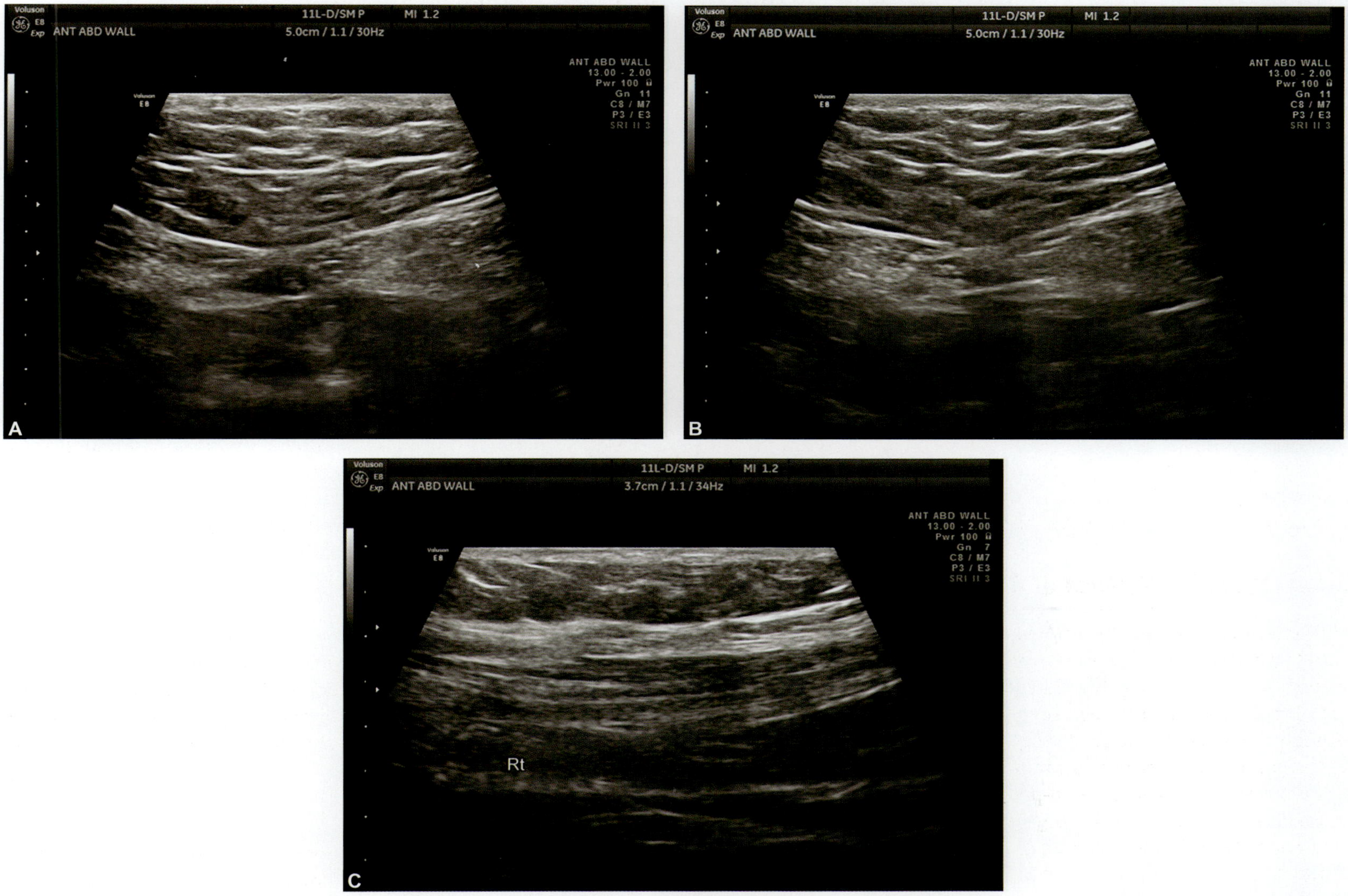

FIGURES 15.1A to C: Normal anatomy. High-resolution sonography (HRSG) shows normal anatomy of the anterior abdominal wall. Bright echogenic line is skin. The hypoechoic layer posterior to the skin is subcutaneous fat. The rectus muscle bundles are seen as a lens shaped structure. Extraperitoneal fat is seen as a hypoechoic layer posterior to the muscle bundle.

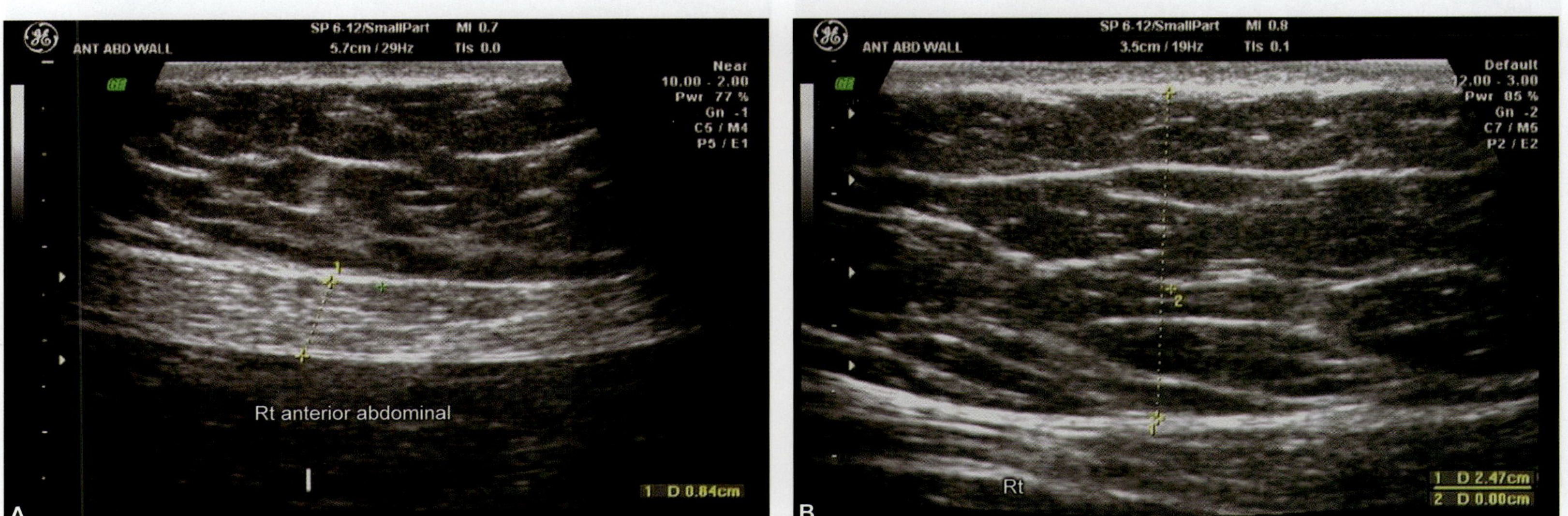

FIGURES 15.2A and B: Thickened subcutaneous fat. A patient presented with lump with epigastric lesion. HRSG shows increased amount of pad of fat in the epigastric lesion. No evidence of any mass lesion is seen.

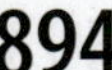

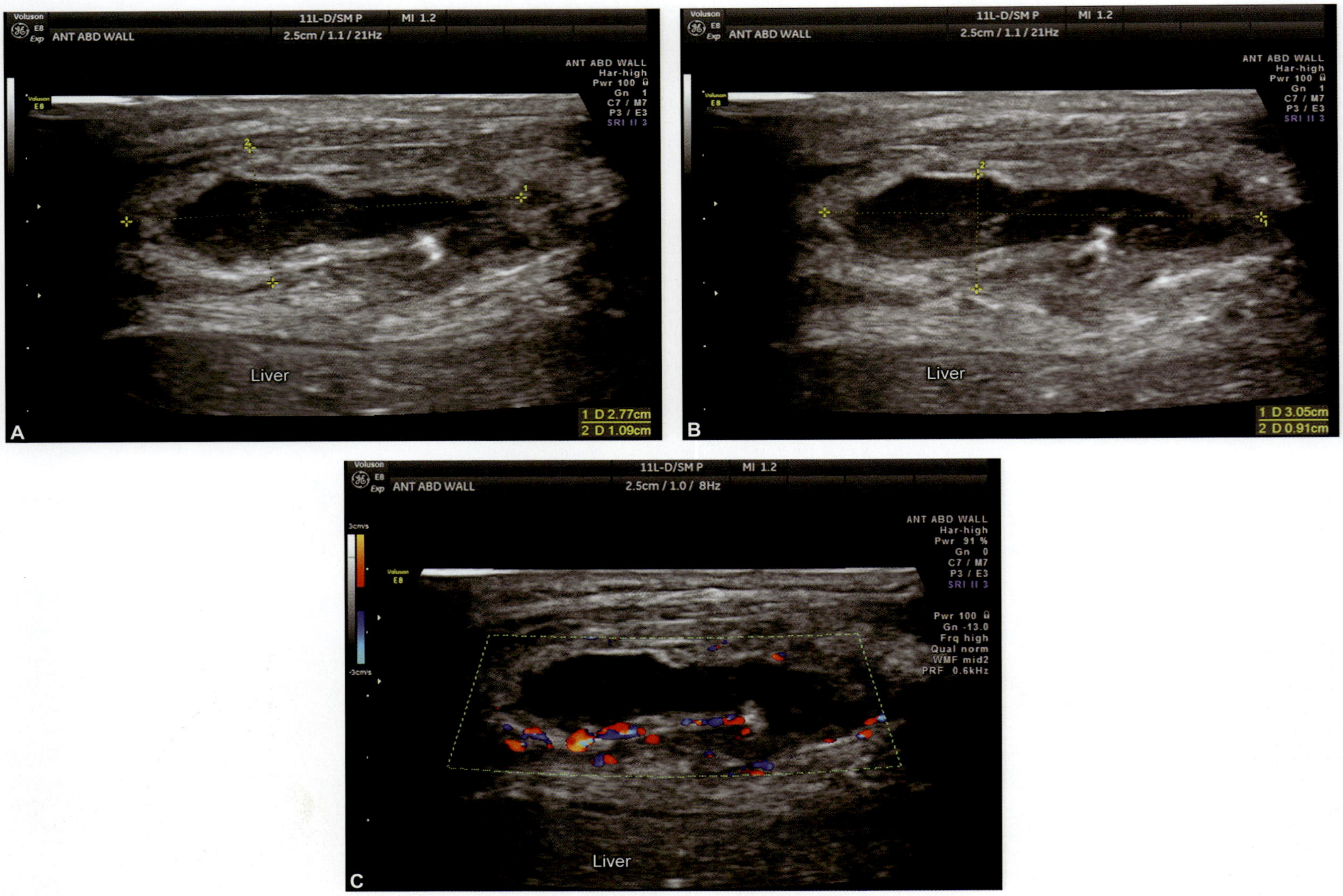

FIGURES 15.3A to C: Anterior abdominal wall abscess. A 5-year-old boy presented with painful soft tissue in the anterior abdominal wall in right subcostal region. HRSG shows a pocket of thick collection in the anterior abdominal wall. It is seen in the subcutaneous tissue plane. It measures 30 x 10 mm in size. Thick echoes are seen in it with central area of necrosis. Associated perifocal edema is also present suggestive of pyogenic abscess.

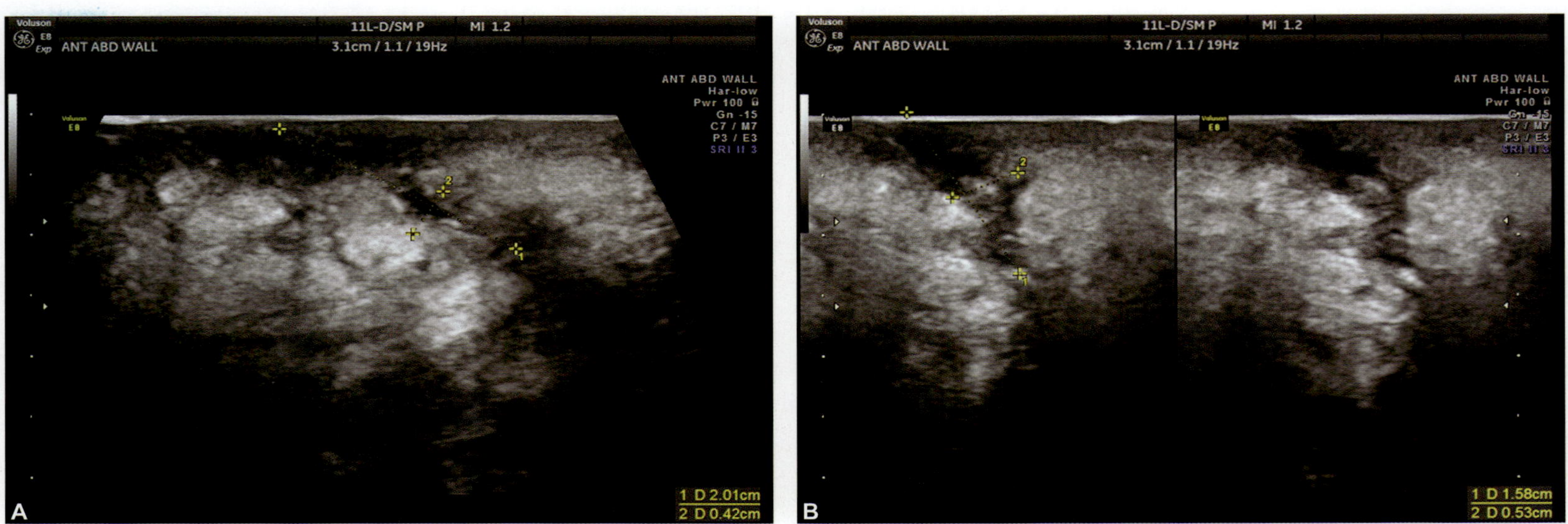

FIGURES 15.4A and B

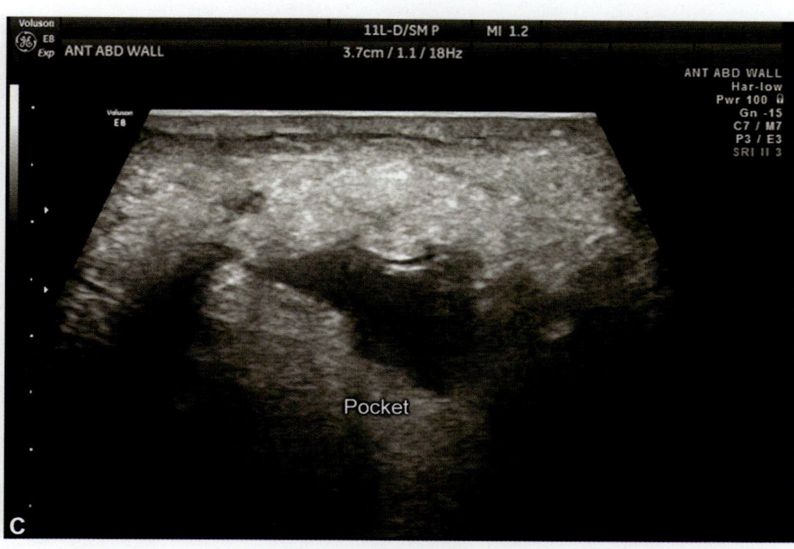

FIGURE 15.4C

FIGURES 15.4A to C: A patient presented with soft tissue swelling in the right subcostal region. HRSG shows irregular ill-defined low level echo complex mass in the subcutaneous tissue plane. Central area of necrosis is seen. Associated soft tissue edema is also present. Breaking down of the fat tissue is seen suggestive of fat necrosis. Findings are suggestive of acute cellulitis with abscess formation.

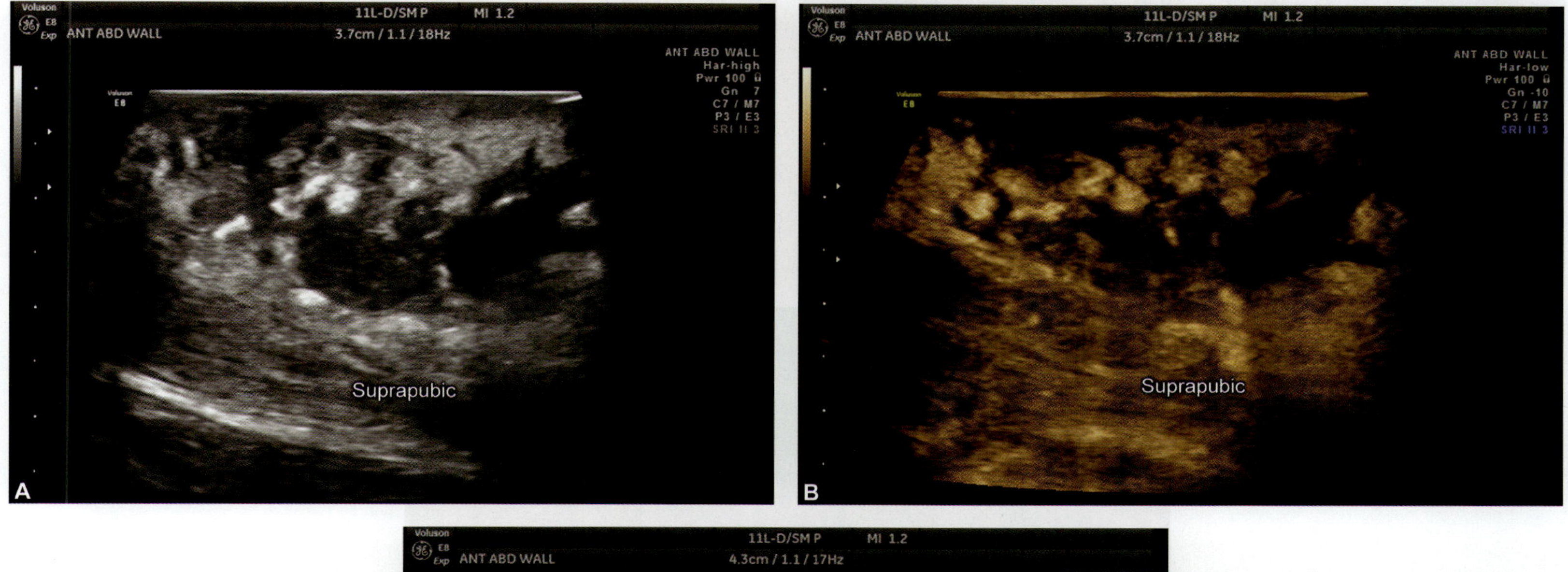

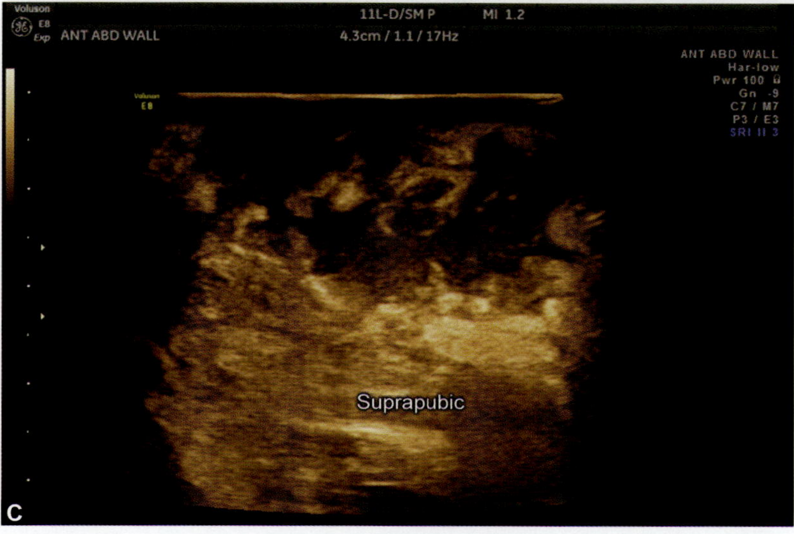

FIGURES 15.5A to C: Acute fluminating cellulitis with tissue necrosis. A patient presented with acute pain in the suprapubic region with soft tissue swelling after underwent cesarean operation. HRSG shows irregular ill-defined hypoechoic mass in the suprapubic region. Fat necrosis is also seen in it. Necrotizing fat lobules are seen floating in it. Small amount of fluid collection is seen in it suggestive of acute infection with fat necrosis.

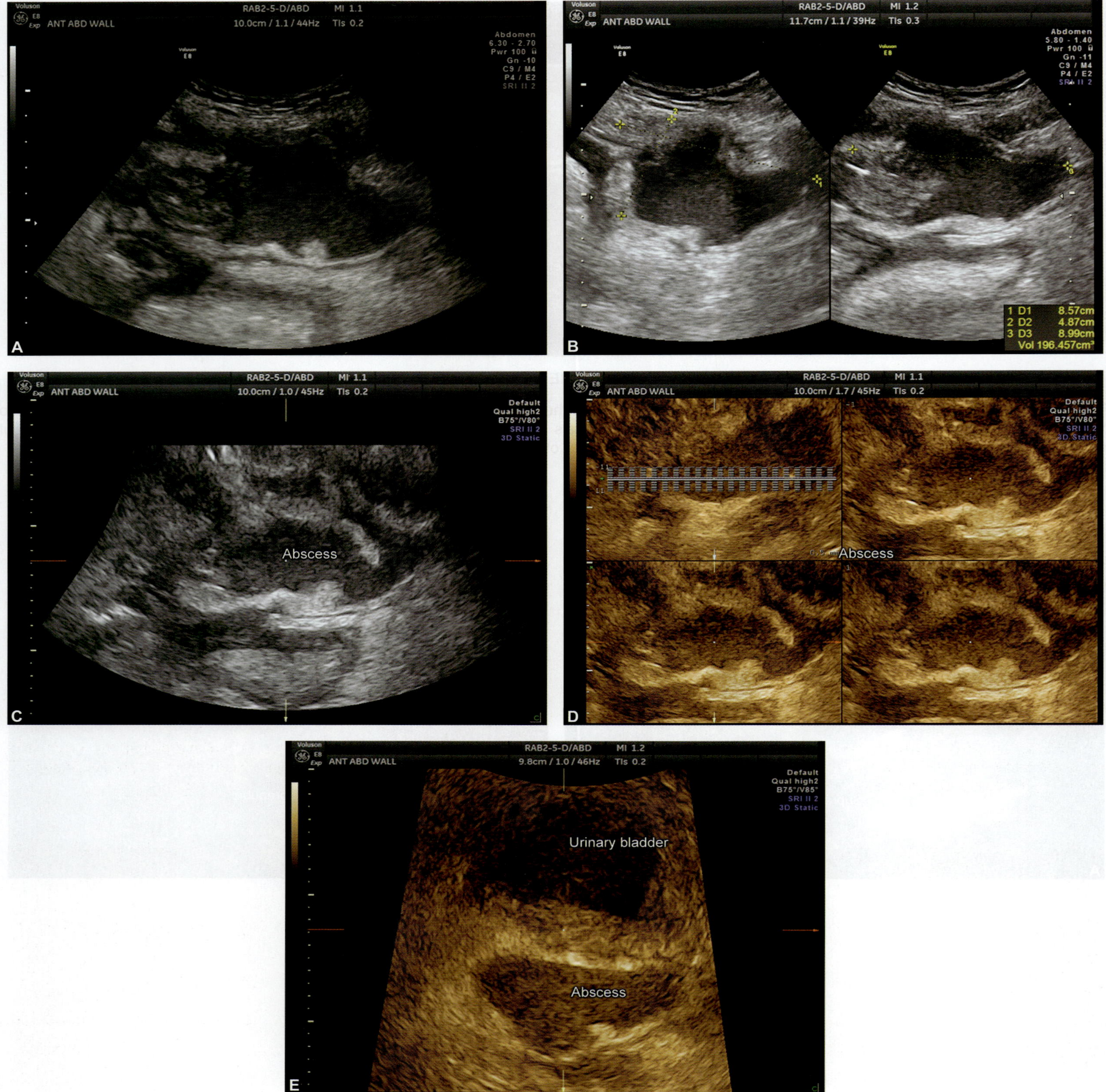

FIGURES 15.6A to E: HRSG shows a thick pocket of collection seen in the anterior abdominal wall in the suprapubic region. The collection shows low level echoes. However, capsule of the collection is ill-defined. It is seen anterior to the bladder. Volume of the collection is more than 200 cc. On color flow imaging, no flow is seen in it. Normal anatomic relations are distorted. Findings are suggestive of pocket of thick collection in the suprapubic region in the anterior abdominal wall with multiple internal echoes suggestive of pyogenic abscess.

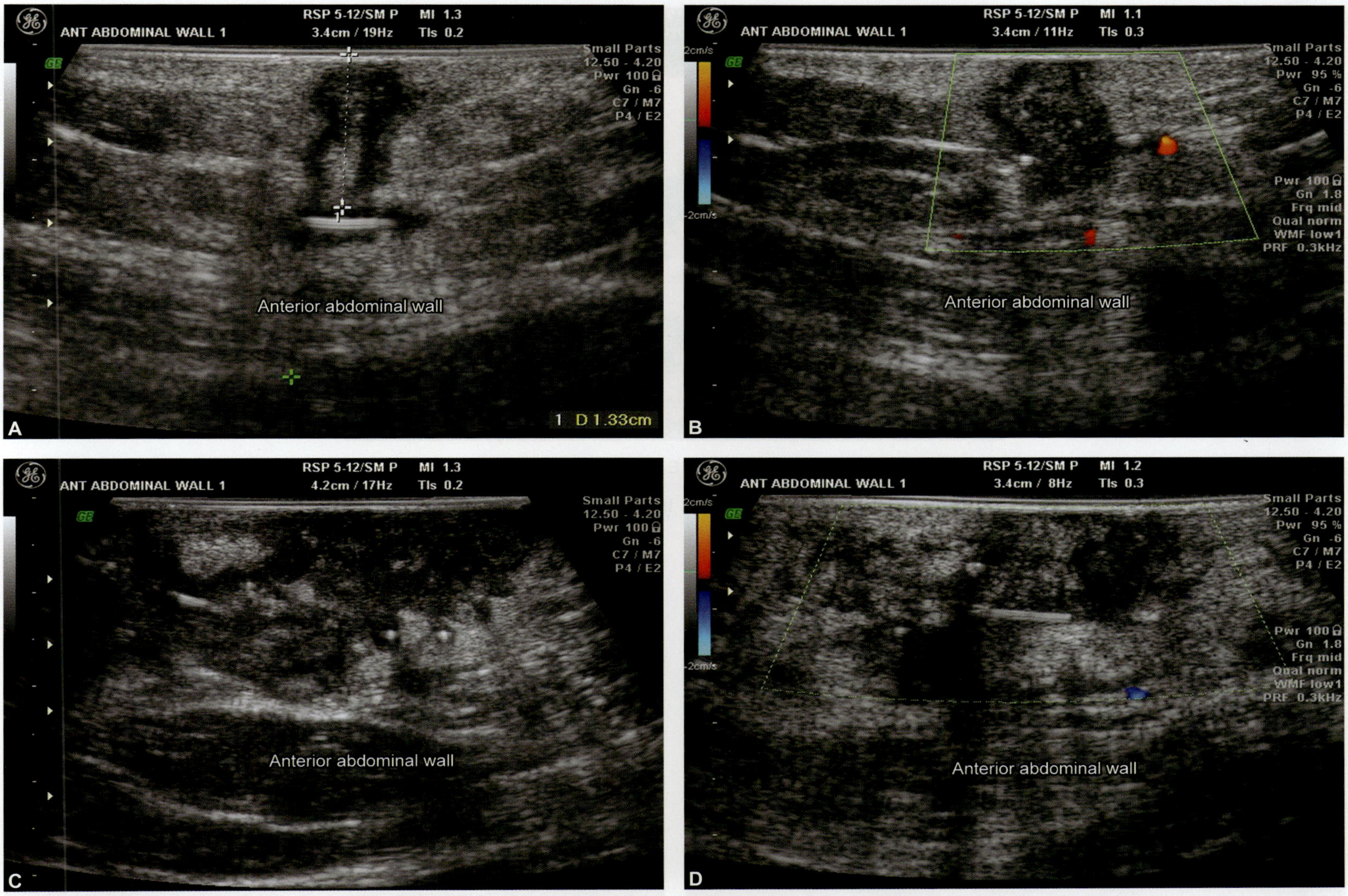

FIGURES 15.7A to D: Suture granuloma with abscess formation. A patient presented with discharging sinus in the supraumbilical region after underwent laprotomy. HRSG shows an irregular ill-defined low level echo complex collection along the suture line. Echogenic thread like shadow is seen in it suggestive of suture and obliquely running sinus is seen running to the skin. Associated fat necrosis is also seen in it.

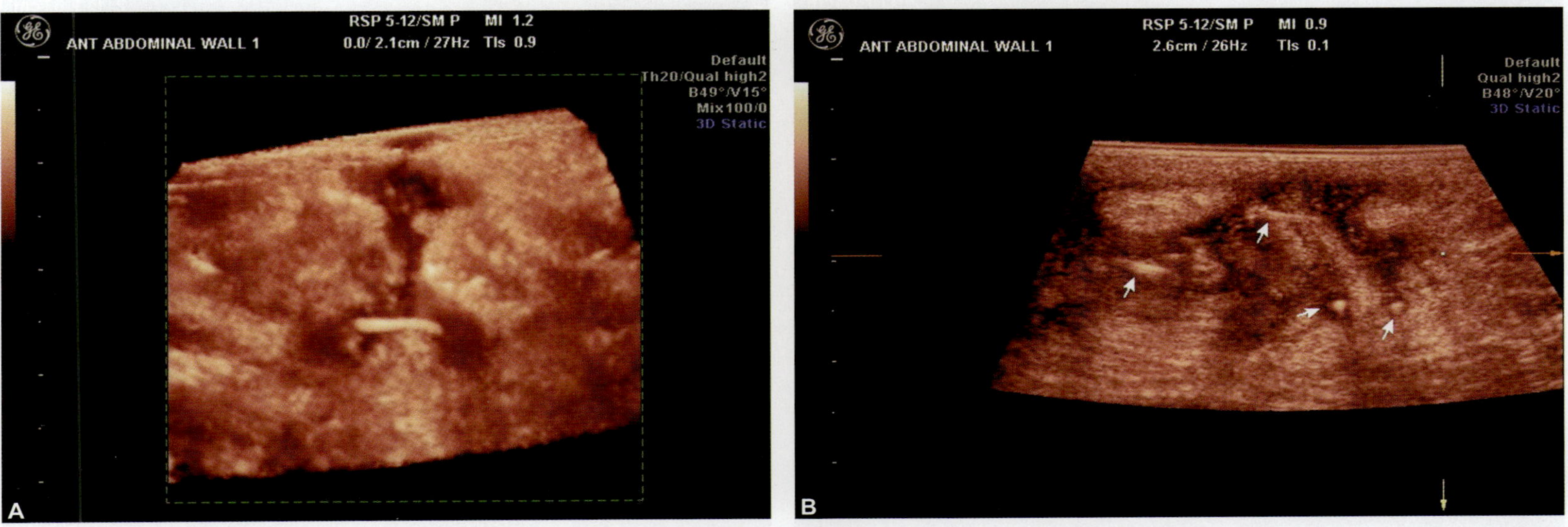

FIGURES 15.8A and B

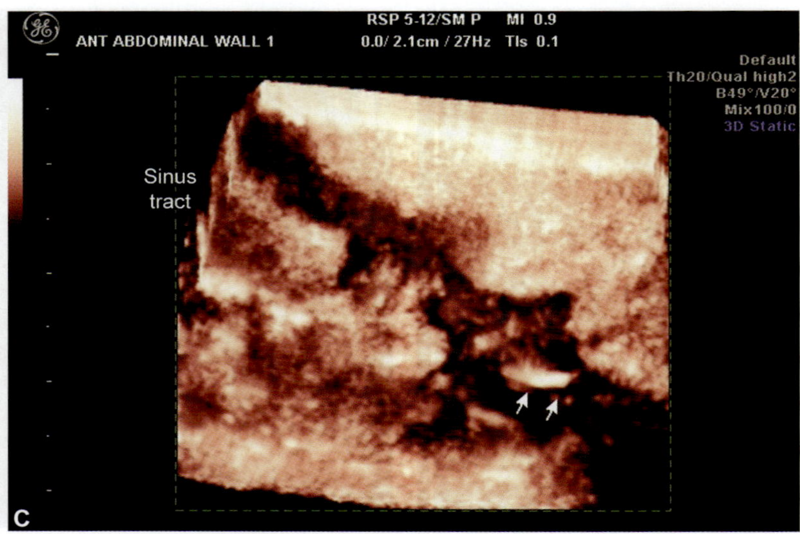

FIGURE 15.8C

FIGURES 15.8A to C: The 3D ultrasound shows the sinus tract and embedded suture very clearly.

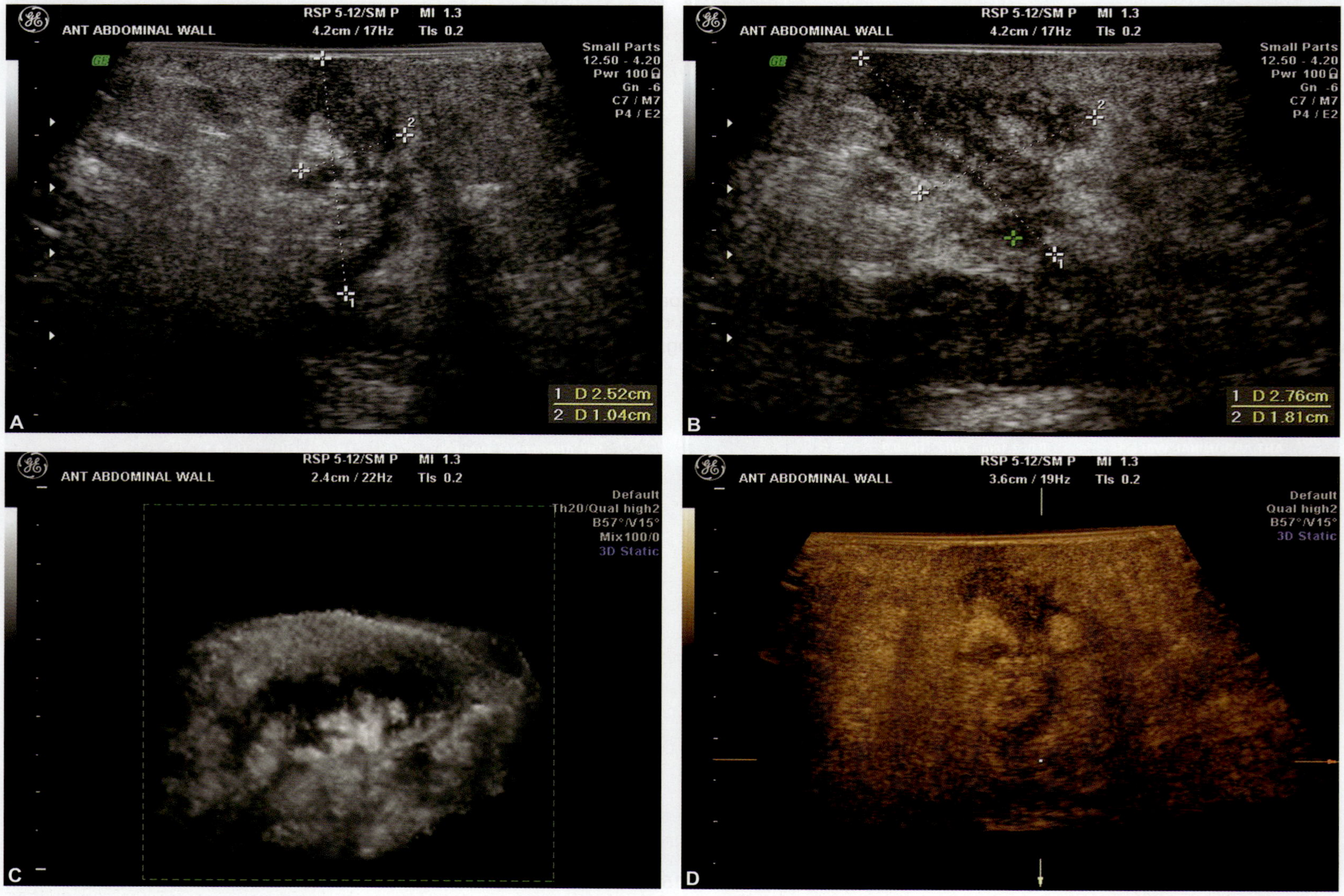

FIGURES 15.9A to D: Suture granuloma with sinus formation. There is evidence of low level echo complex mass in anterior abdominal wall. The mass measures 25 x 15 mm in size. It is irregular in outline. Multiple internal echoes are seen into it. But no cystic degeneration is seen. No necrosis is seen. Perifocal edema is present. A sinus is running from it. It is 3 cm deep from the skin. Associated edema is present. But no evidence of any foreign body is seen. The abdominal wall shows subcutaneous edema. Dermis and hypodermis edema is present. On color flow imaging, increased flow is seen around it. Biopsy confirmed chronic granulomatous mass suggestive of tuberculosis.

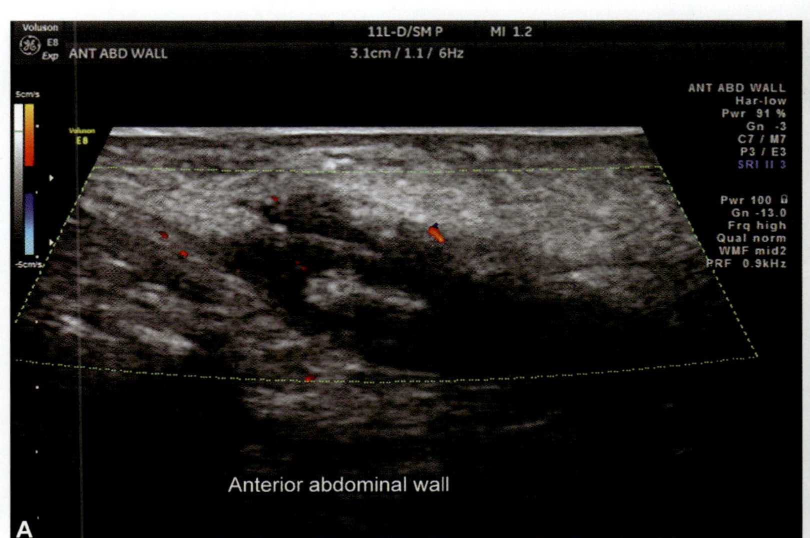

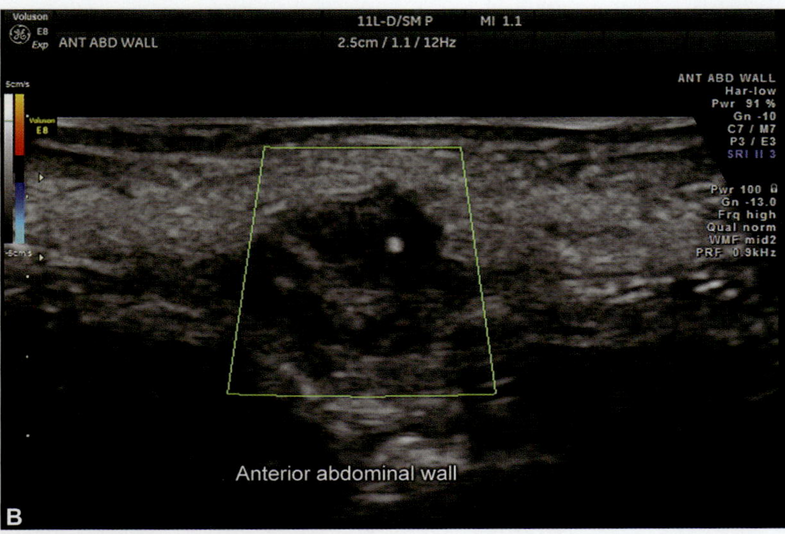

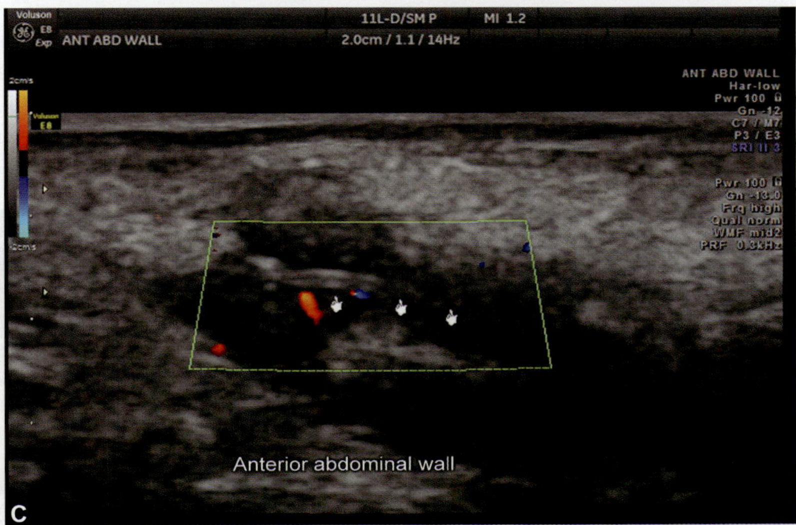

FIGURES 15.10A to C: Suture granuloma. A patient presented with discharging sinus and nodular mass along the suture line after having operation. HRSG shows an irregular ill-defined low level echo complex mass seen in the anterior abdominal wall in the subcutaneous tissue plane. It is seen extending from the suture line below to infraumbilical region. Entanglement of the thread is seen into it. Associated fat necrosis is also seen. An echogenic linear thread-like shadow is seen embedded in it. Associated subcutaneous tissue edema is seen around it. But no sinus formation is seen. No free fluid collection is seen. It is seen below the fat layer. On color flow imaging, few vessels are feeding it.

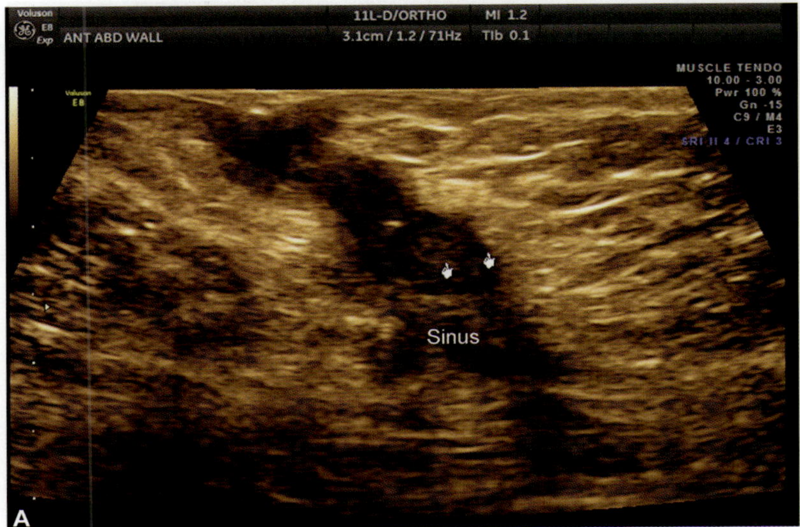

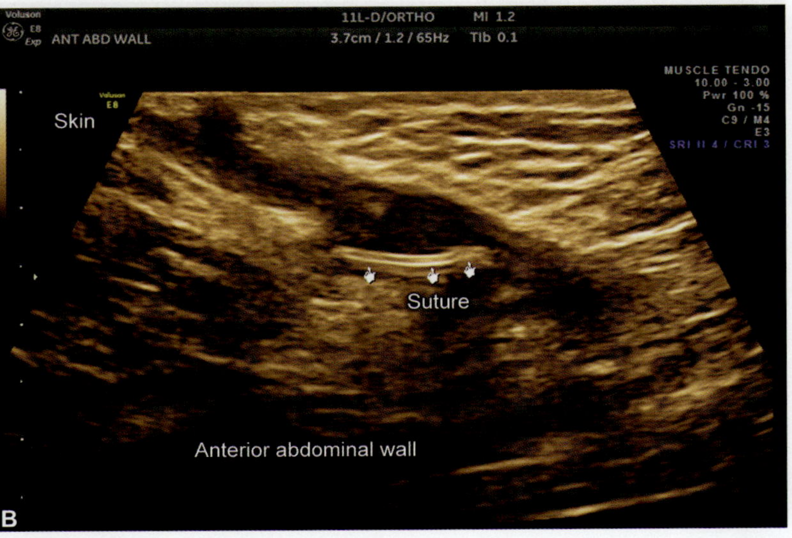

FIGURES 15.11A and B

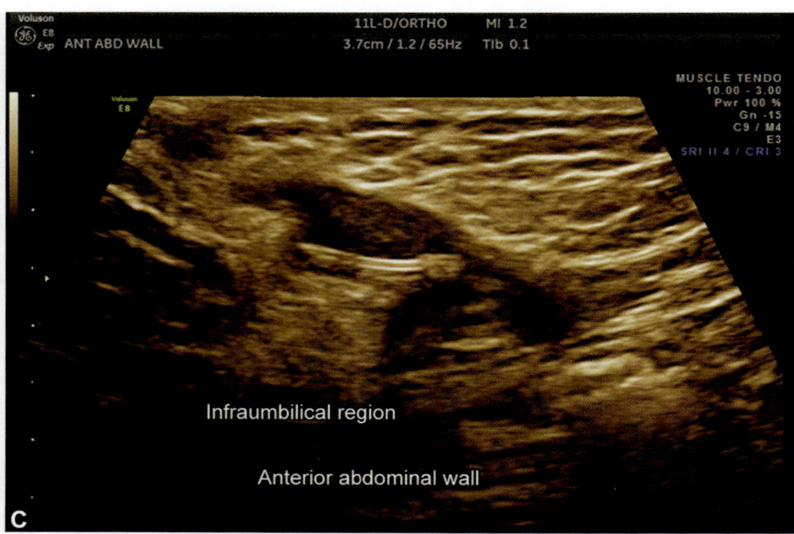

FIGURE 15.11C

FIGURES 15.11A to C: Suture granuloma with discharging sinus. HRSG shows a obliquely running sinus in anterior abdominal wall in infraumbilical region. Echogenic suture material is seen embedded in it. Thick echoes are seen around the suture with soft tissue formation suggestive of suture granuloma formation. Low level echoes are also seen in the sinus.

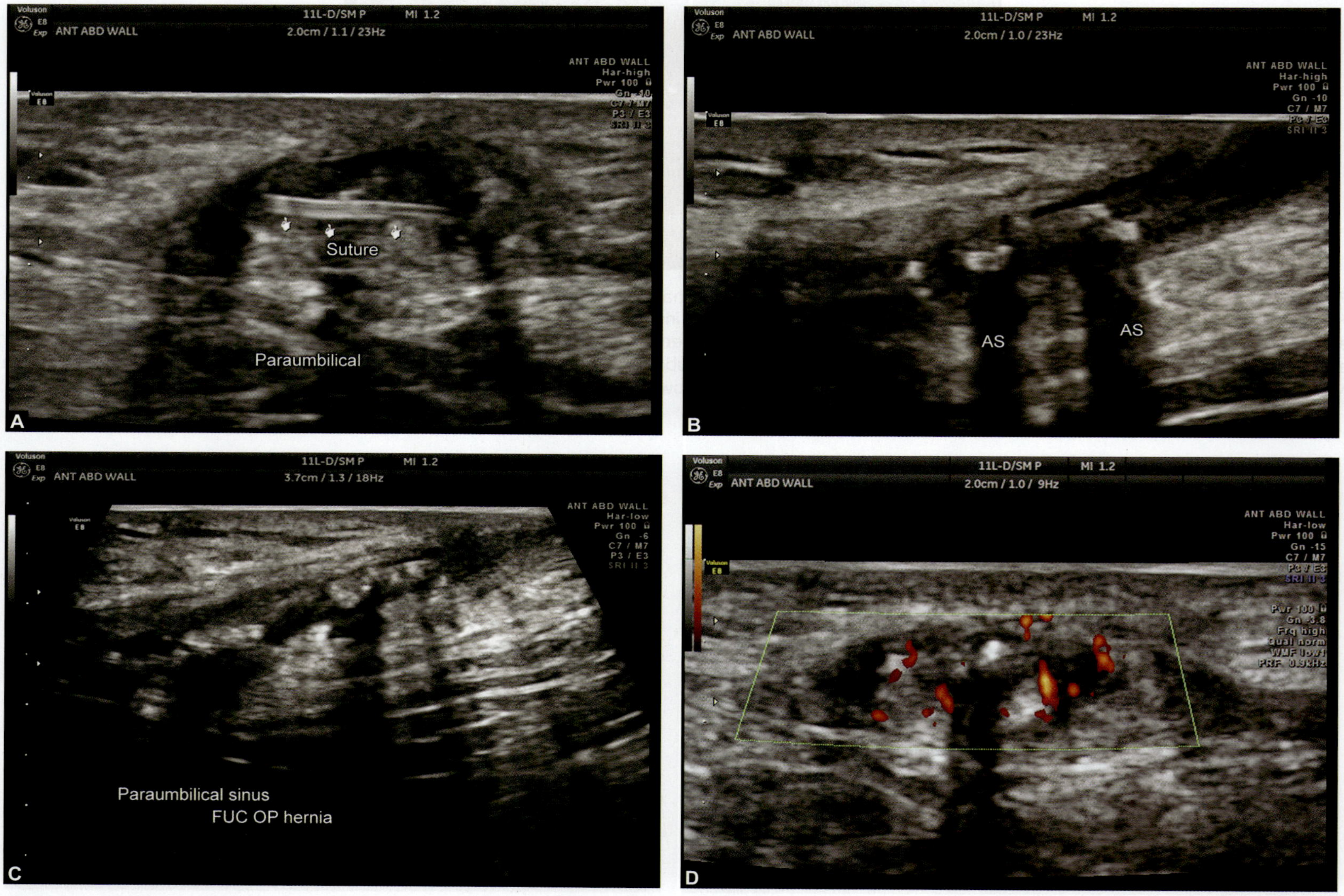

FIGURES 15.12A to D: Suture granuloma with mass formation with discharging sinus. A patient presented with soft tissue mass in the paraumbilical region after underwent surgery for hernia. HRSG shows irregular ill-defined mass in the paraumbilical region. Echogenic suture material is seen embedded in it, which shows acoustic shadowing. Thick echoes are seen around it. An obliquely running sinus is also seen from the mass to the skin. Thick echoes are seen in it. On color flow imaging, increased flow is seen in the granulomatous mass.

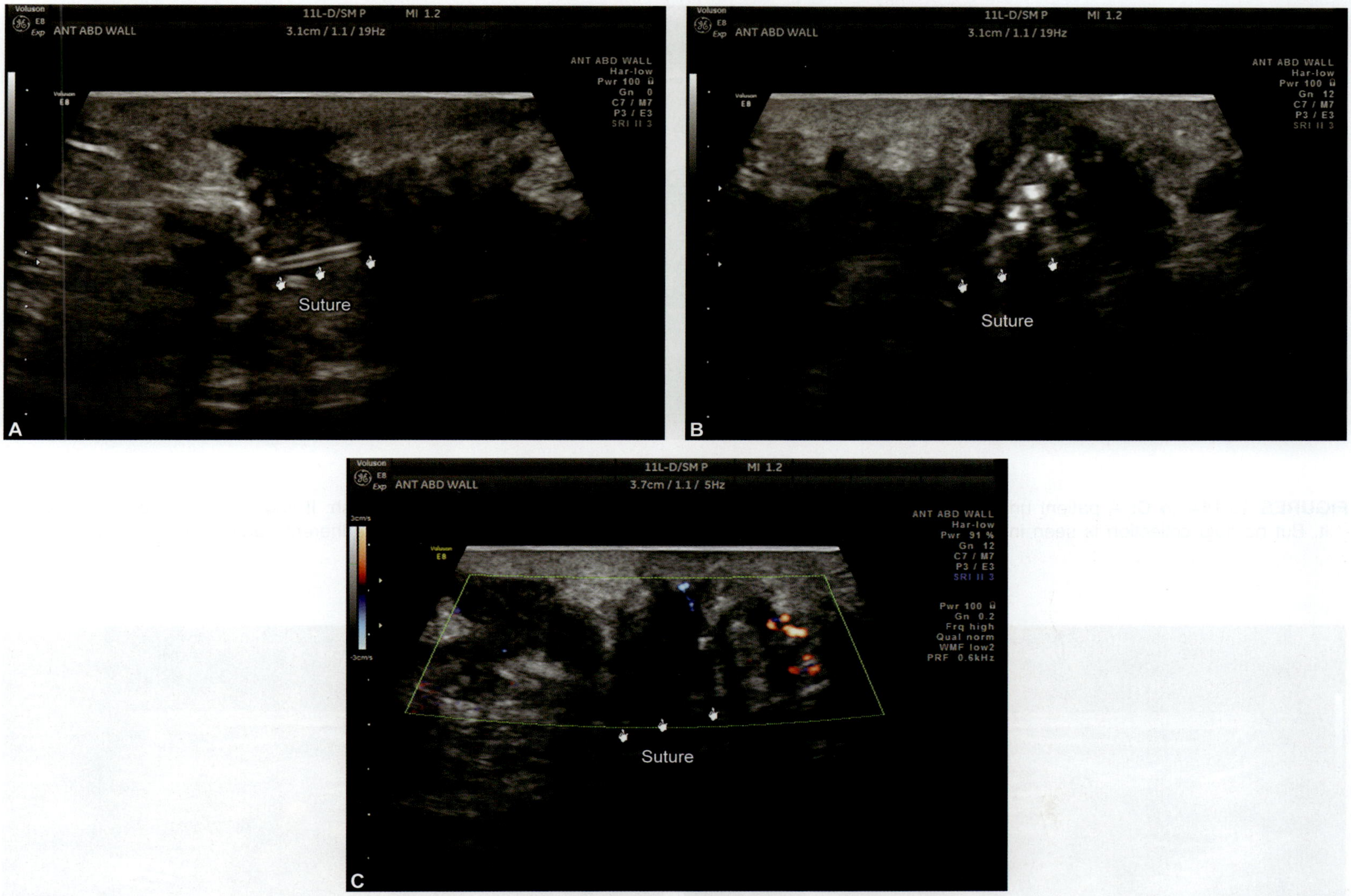

FIGURES 15.13A to C: Suture granuloma formation. A patient presented with painful nodular mass in the anterior abdominal wall. HRSG shows irregular ill-defined inhomogeneous mass in supraumbilical region. Multiple echogenic thread-like shadows are seen embedded in it suggestive of suture material. Associated perifocal edema is also present suggestive of suture granuloma formation.

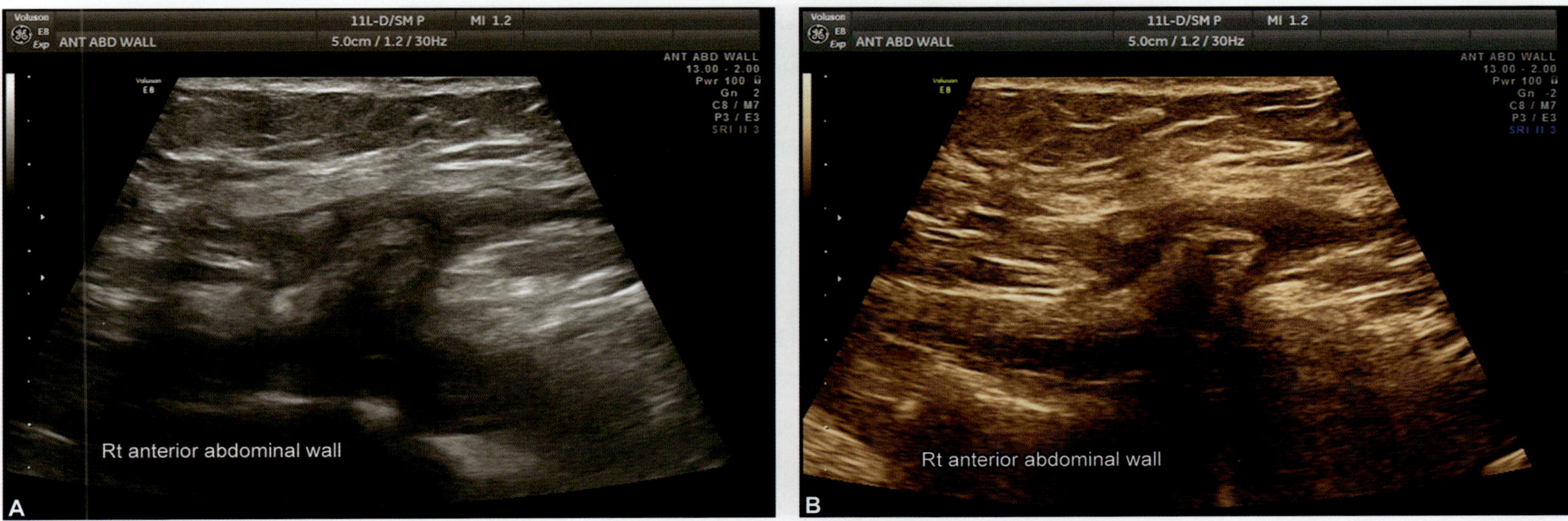

FIGURES 15.14A and B

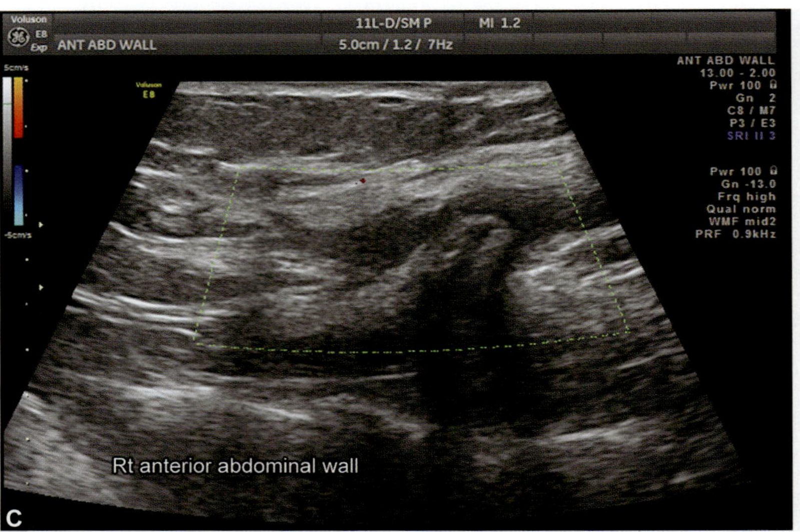

FIGURE 15.14C

FIGURES 15.14A to C: A patient underwent hernioplasty. HRSG shows a bowel loop bulging below the mesh. It shows soft tissue edema around it. But no fluid collection is seen in the bowel loop. The mesh is seen intact. Findings are suggestive of adherent bowel loop below the mesh.

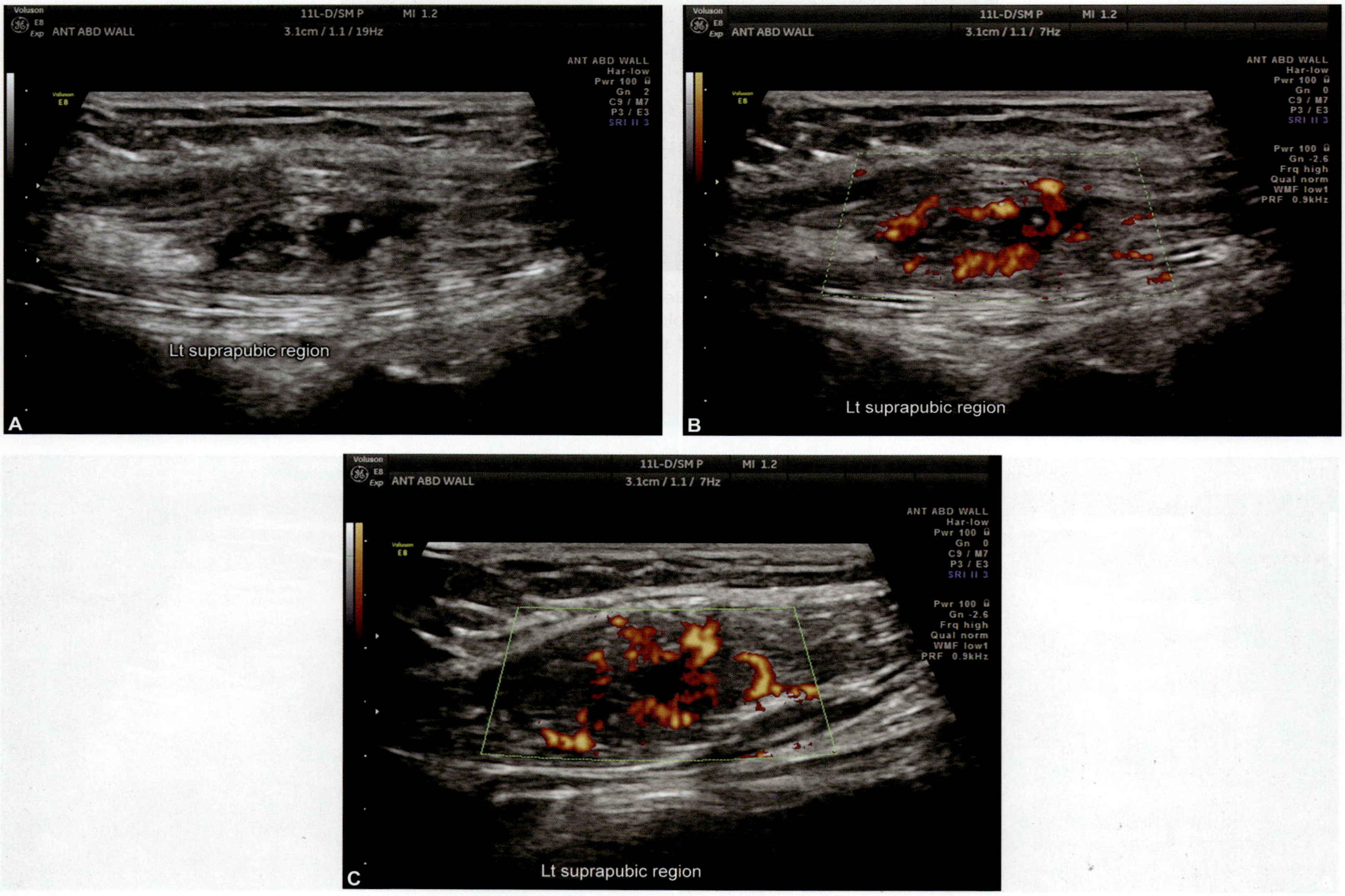

FIGURES 15.15A to C: Cysticercus cyst with inflammation. A patient presented with painful nodular swelling in the left suprapubic region. HRSG shows a thick walled cystic mass seen in the muscle belly of anterior abdominal wall in suprapubic region measuring 15 x 7mm in size. Thick echoes are seen into it. Echogenic nidus is also seen into it. The nidus measures 3 x 2 mm in size. Associated perifocal edema is present. Multiple internal echoes are seen in it. On color flow imaging, multiple vessels are seen feeding the capsule suggestive of inflamed cysticercus cyst with myositis.

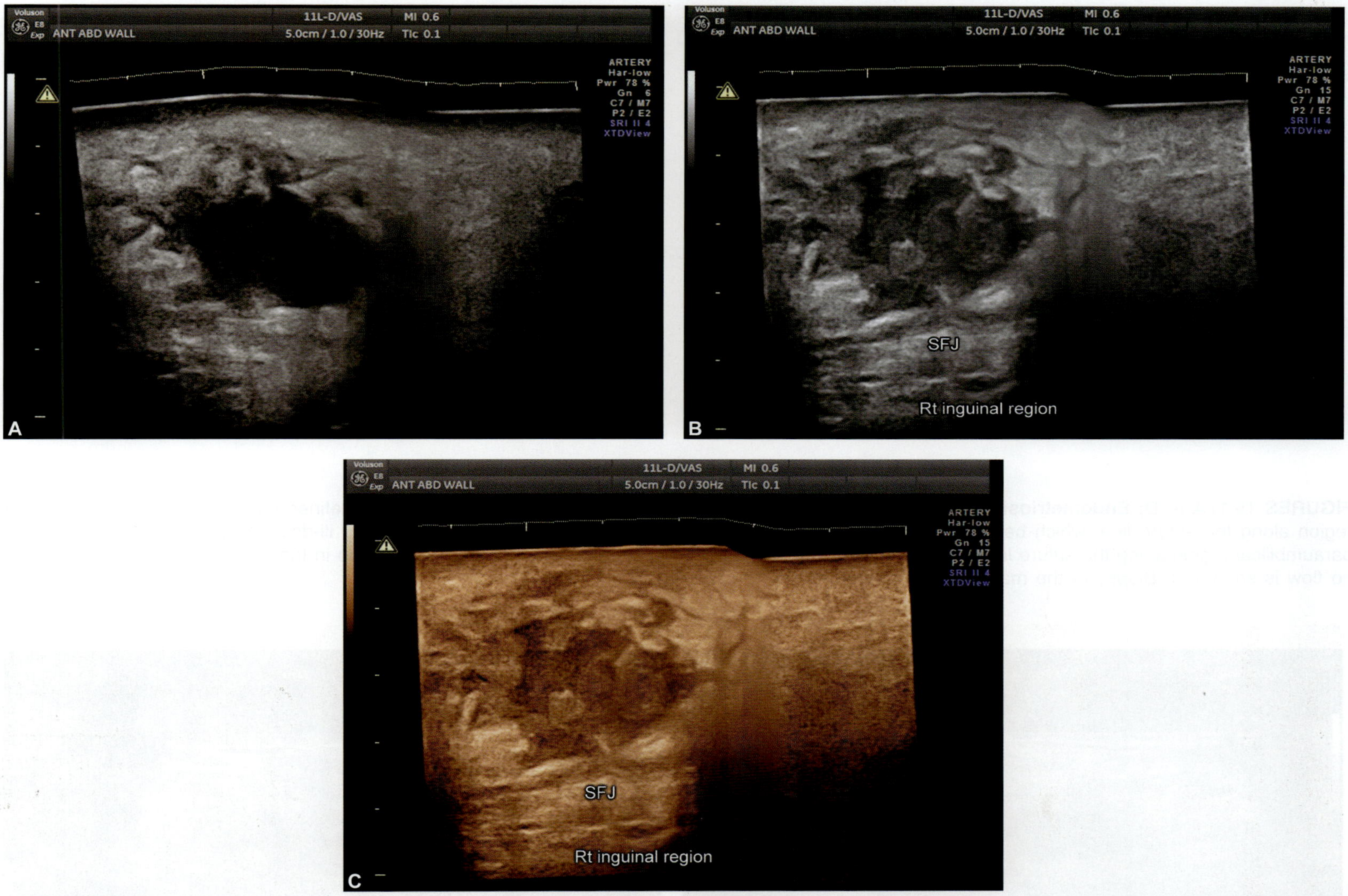

FIGURES 15.16A to C: A patient presented with painful swelling in the right inguinal region. HRSG shows a low level echo complex mass seen in the right inguinal region. Central area of necrosis is seen into it. Marked soft tissue edema is also seen. Perifocal edema is present suggestive of an abscess. But no cystic degeneration is seen.

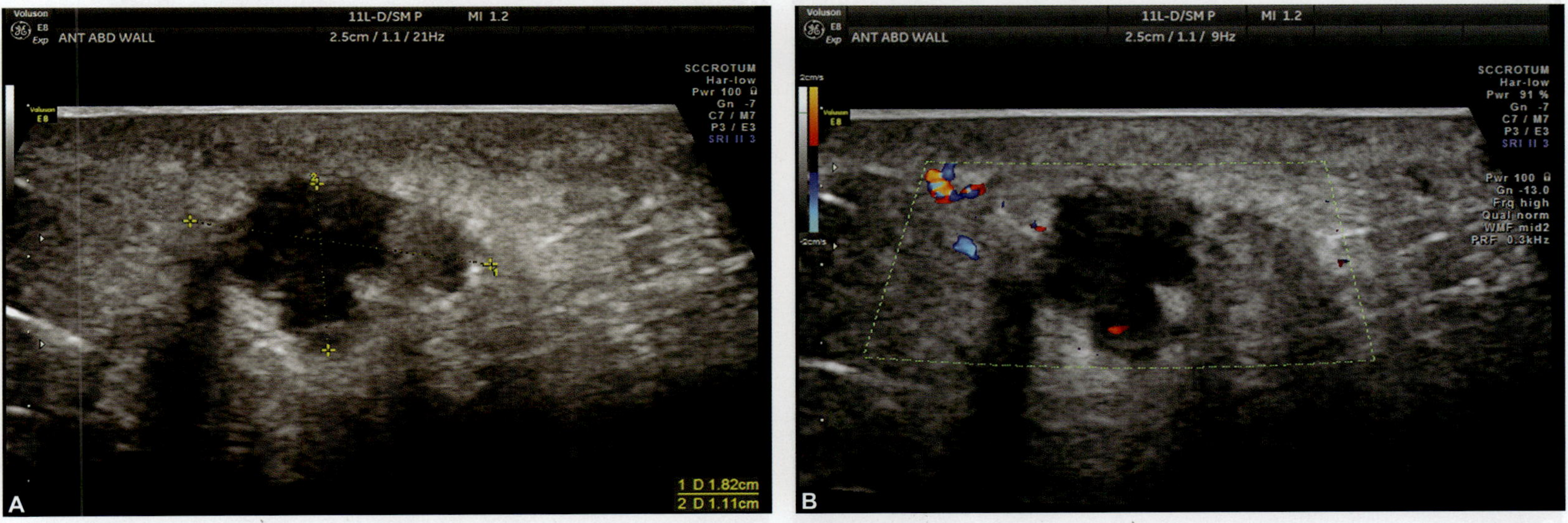

FIGURES 15.17A and B

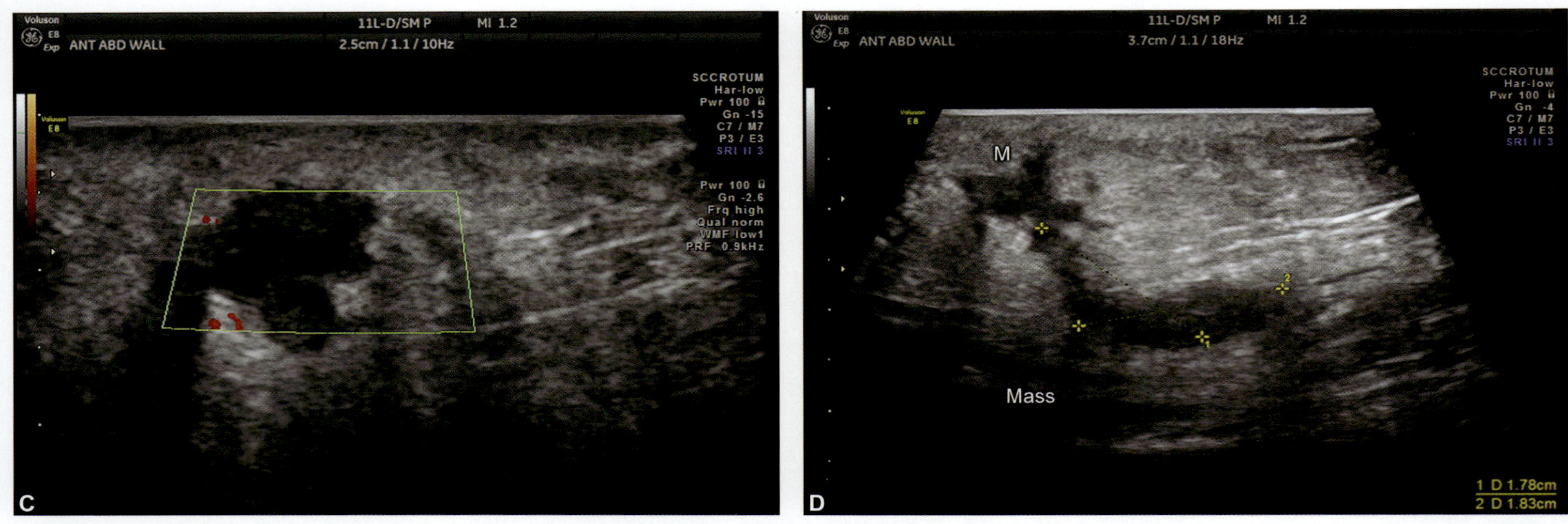

FIGURES 15.17C and D

FIGURES 15.17A to D: Endometriosis in the anterior abdominal wall. A patient presented with irregular ill-defined nodular mass in the suprapubic region along the suture line, which become painful when patient has menstrual period. HRSG shows irregular ill-defined soft tissue mass in the left paraumbilical region along the suture line. Margins are shaggy. An irregular sinus tract is seen going down deep in the muscle. On color flow imaging, no flow is seen in it. Biopsy of the mass confirmed endometrial tissue deposits.

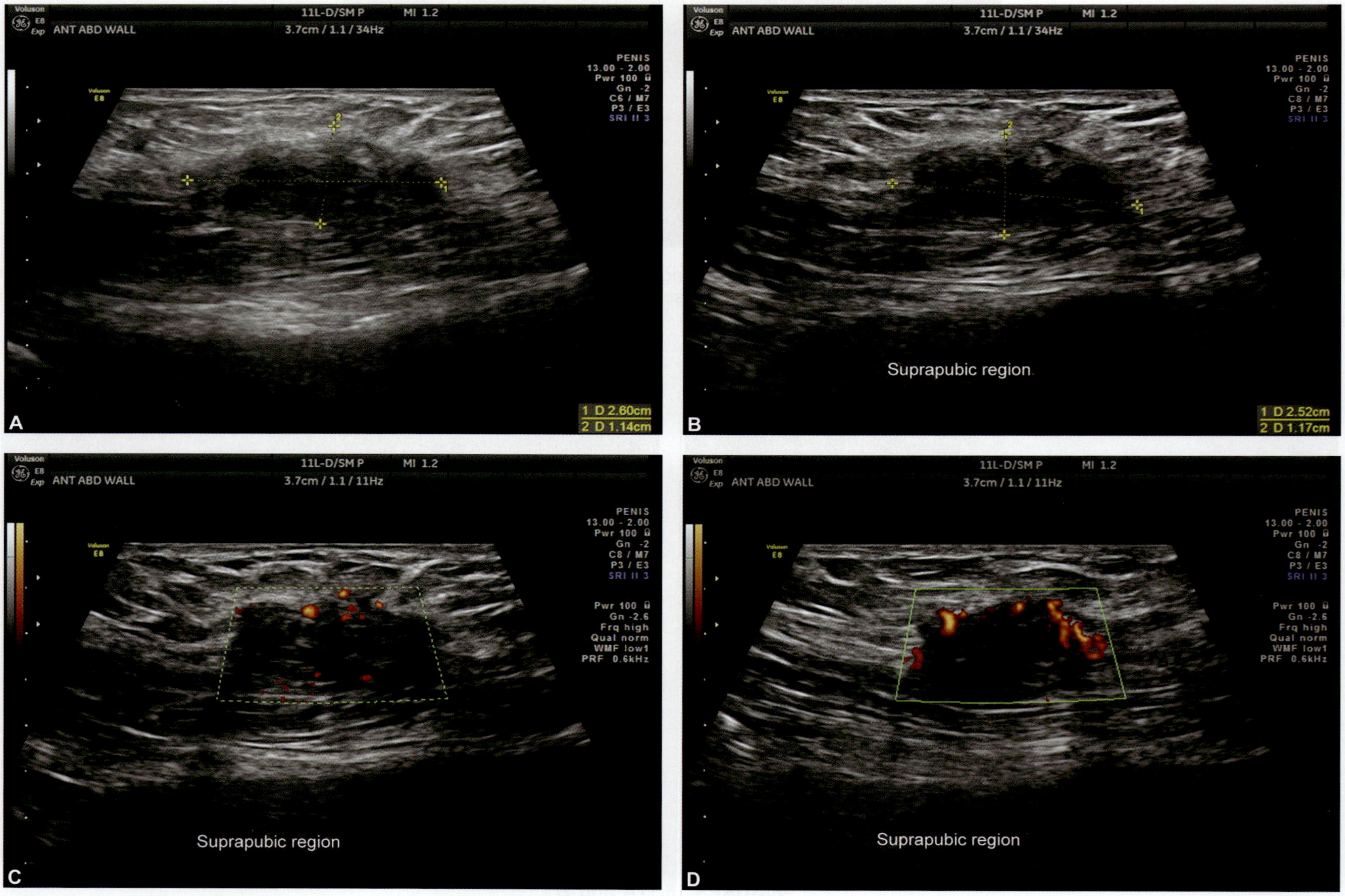

FIGURES 15.18A to D: Endometriosis. A patient presented with in painful swelling increased in size on menstrual period. HRSG shows an irregular ill-defined inhomogeneous low level echo complex mass in the anterior abdominal wall in the suprapubic region. It is seen above the parietal layer and 1cm deep from the skin. It measures 25 x 12 mm in size. No calcification is seen into it. No cystic degeneration is seen. On color flow imaging, low flow is seen into it. It is not seen invading the deep layer. No sinus formation is seen.

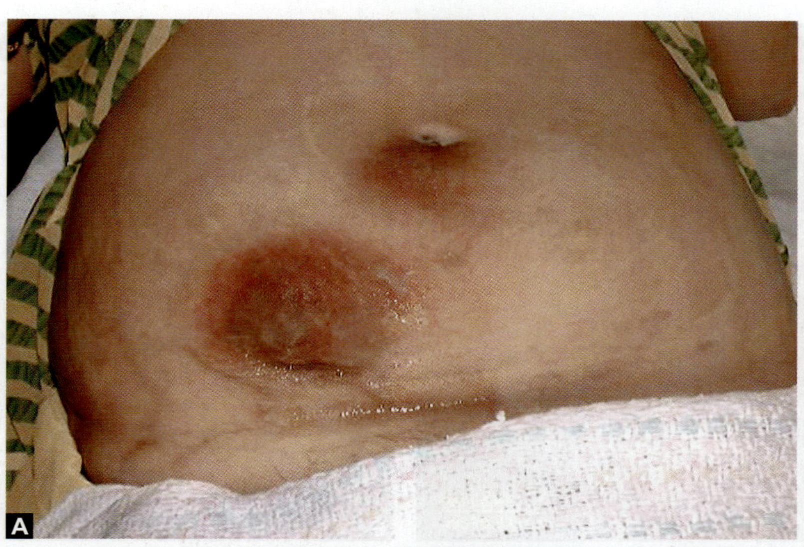

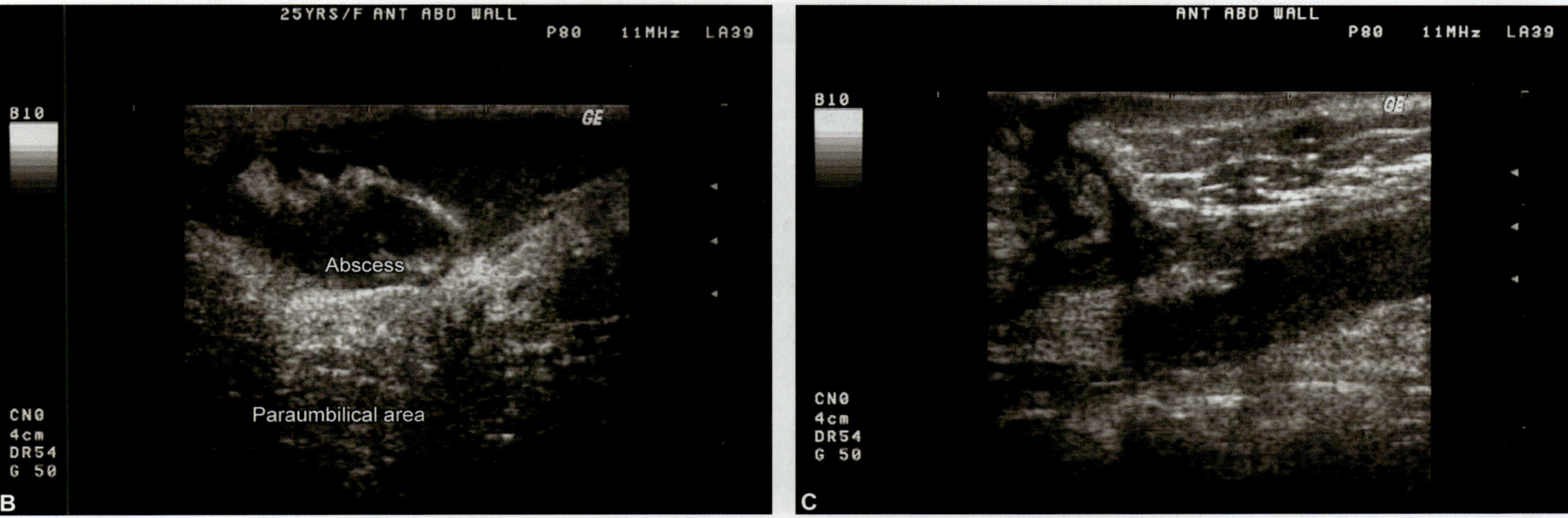

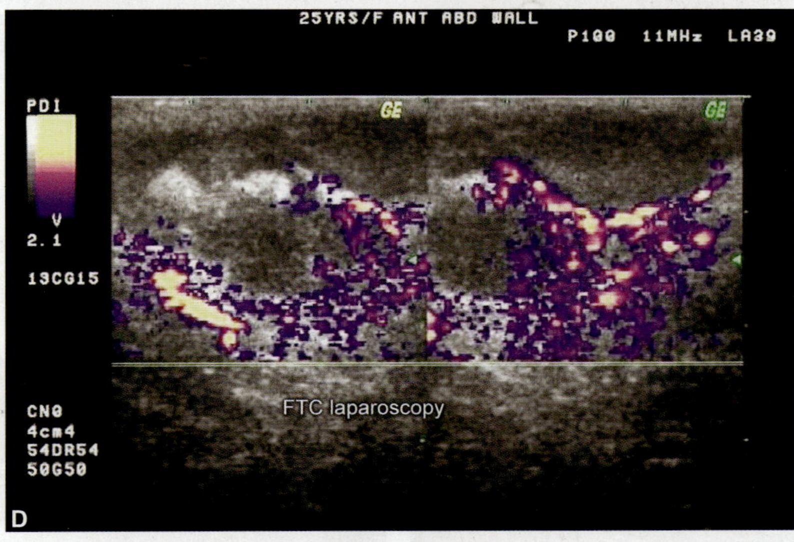

FIGURES 15.19A to D: Anterior abdominal wall abscess after laproscopic surgery. A patient presented with marked swelling on the anterior abdominal wall in right iliac fossa region. It was red and hot with fullness of the anterior abdominal wall. HRSG shows thick lowlevel echo collection in the parietal layers. The collection is seen crossing the midline and going to the left side. Perifocal edema is also presented suggestive of diffuse abscess. On color flow imaging, peripheral flow seen in the abscess.

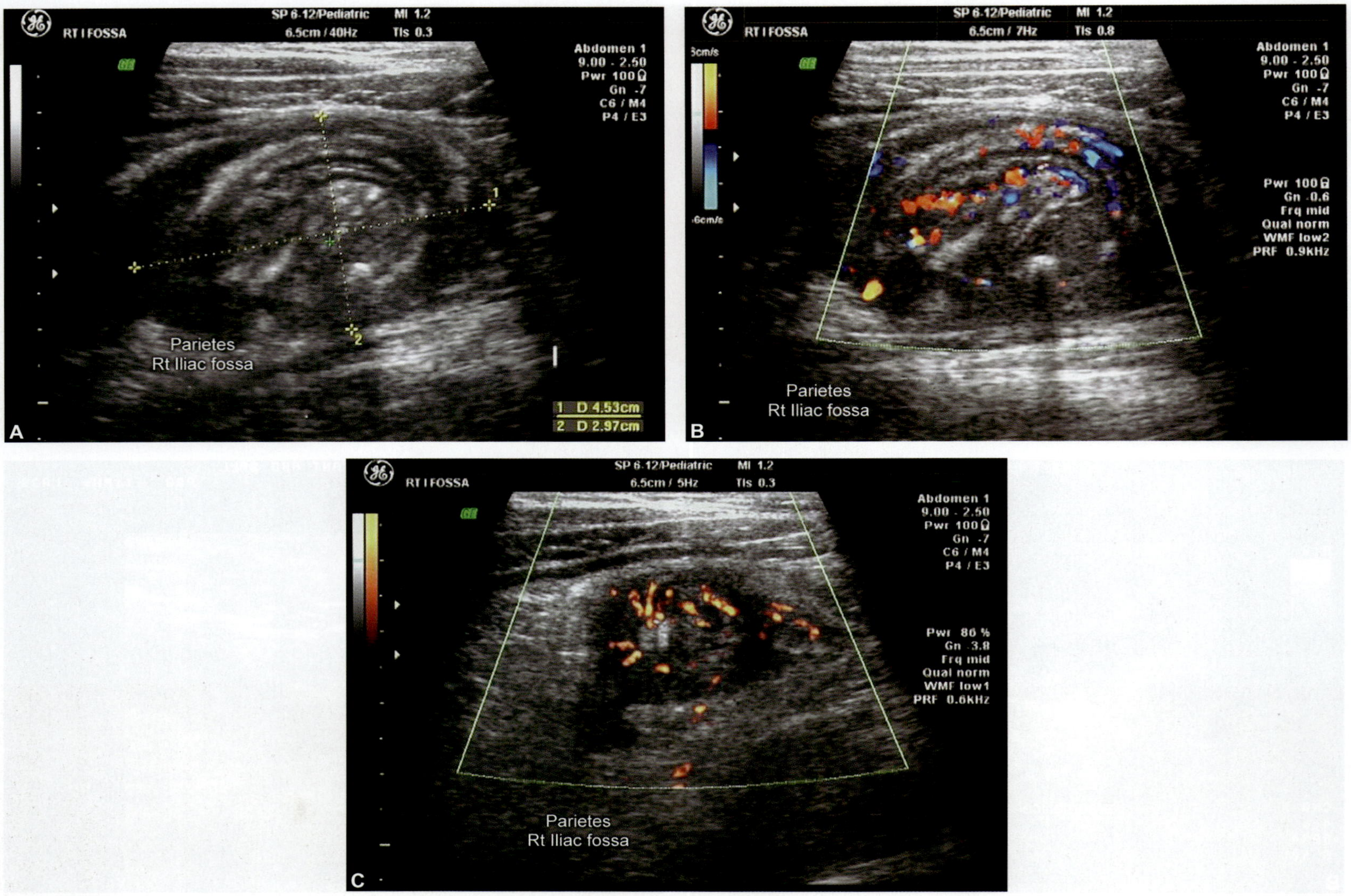

FIGURES 15.20A to C: Parietal abscess in right iliac fossa. HRSG shows well-defined parietal abscess in the right iliac fossa. The abscess is seen confined to the parietes. Layering sign is positive. Perifocal edema is present. It was mistaken as appendicitis on clinical examination. On color flow imaging wall hyperemia is seen in the abscess. Multiple vessels are seen feeding the abscess.

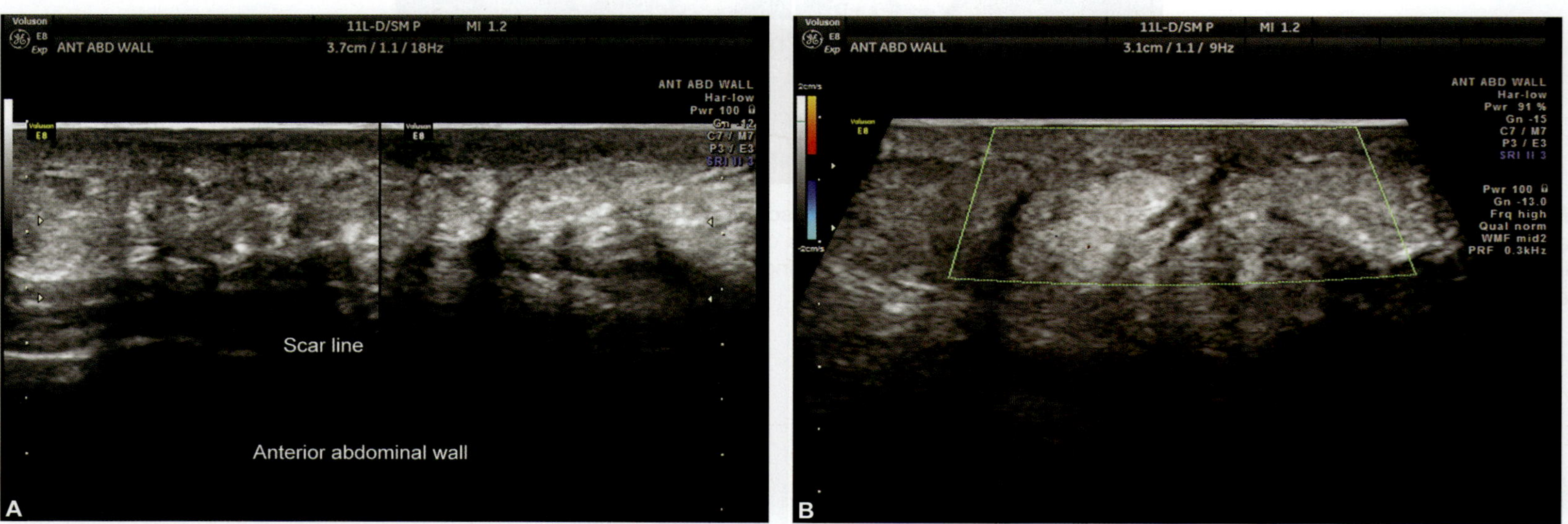

FIGURES 15.21A and B

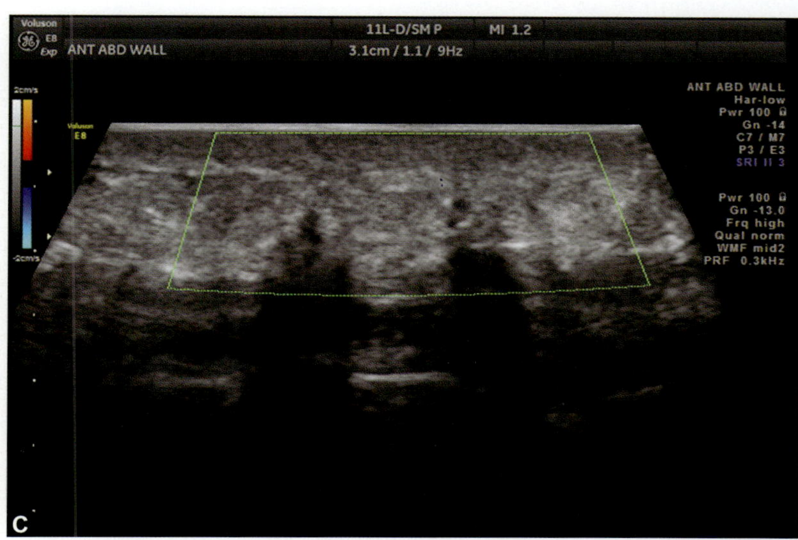

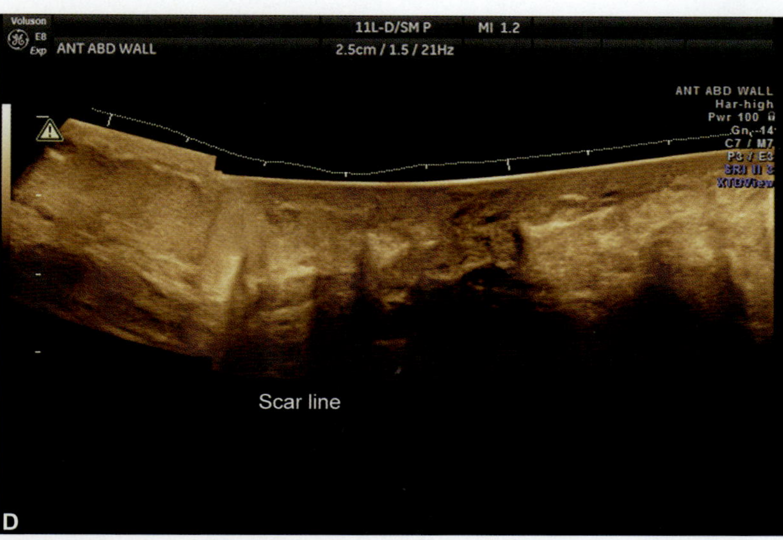

FIGURES 15.21C and D

FIGURES 15.21A to D: Radiation dermatitis. A patient underwent radiotherapy for carcinoma gallbladder. HRSG shows diffuse irregular ill-defined thickening of anterior abdominal wall tissue along the suture line. Multiple echogenic shadows are seen along it. Calcified specks are also seen in it. The dermis and hypodermis show inhomogeneous texture. The fascia is also inflamed. No mass is seen. No calcification is seen. On color flow imaging, poor flow is seen in it suggestive of chronic radiation dermatitis.

ANTERIOR ABDOMINAL WALL TRAUMA

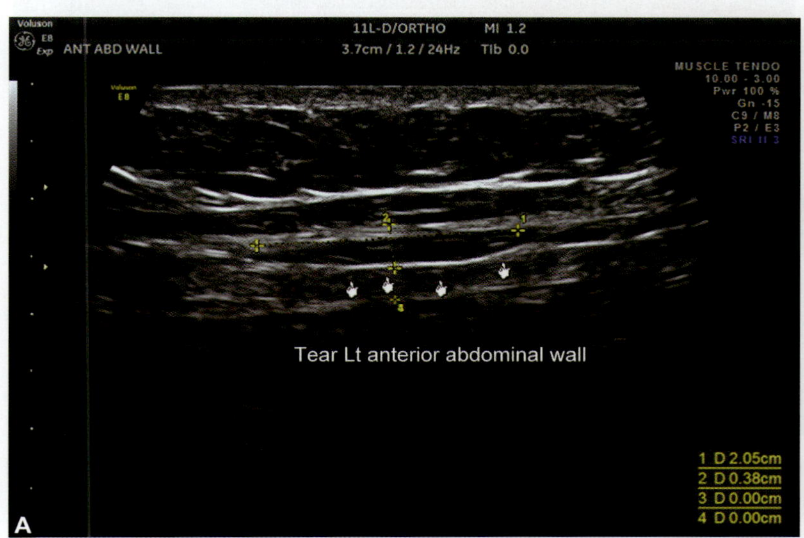

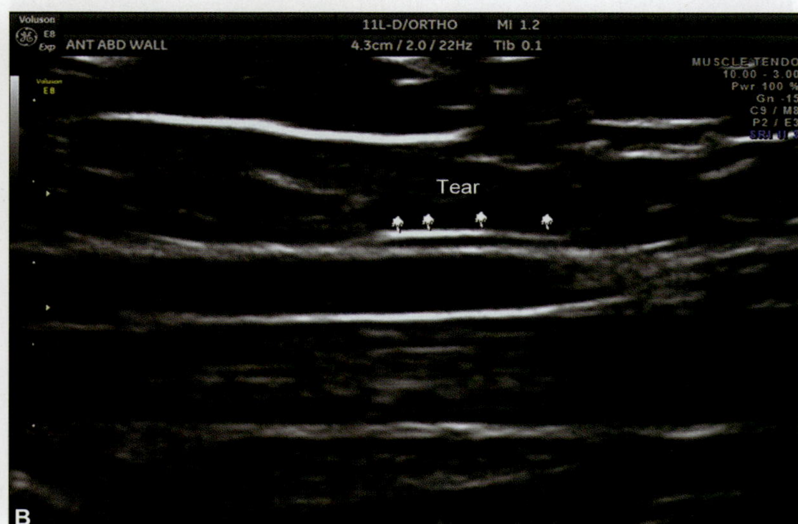

FIGURES 15.22A and B: Anterior abdominal wall tear. A patient presented with pain in left anterior abdominal wall. HRSG shows a hypoechoic cleft in the rectus abdominis muscle on the left side. It is linear and shows low level collection in it.

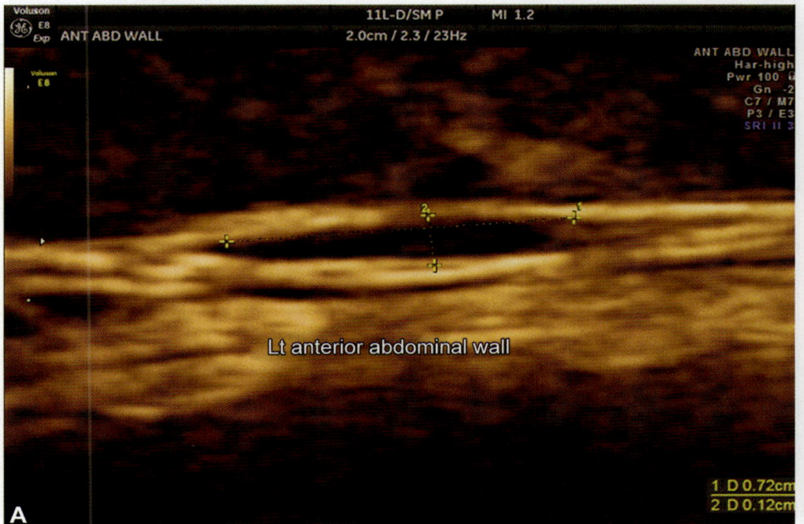

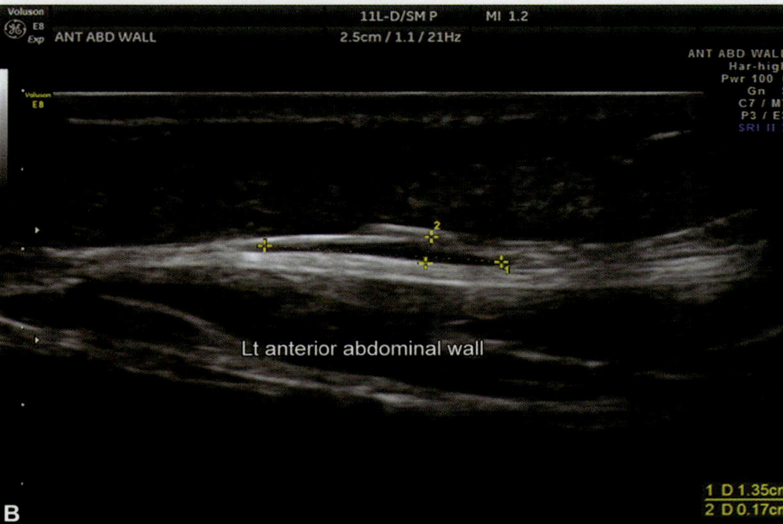

FIGURES 15.23A and B

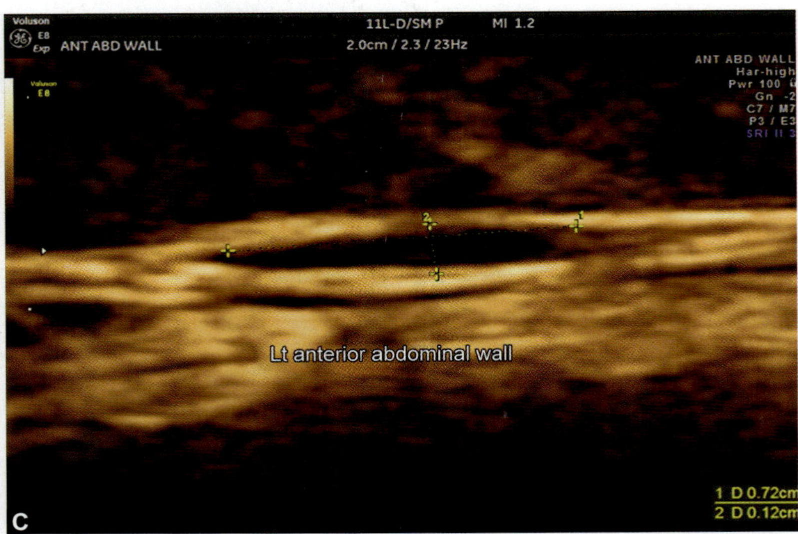

FIGURE 15.23C

FIGURES 15.23A to C: A young man presented with pain in left anterior abdominal wall while moving and bending. HRSG shows a hypoechoic cleft in the transverse oblique muscle in its mid part. A hypoechoic cleft is seen in the muscle. Low level echoes are seen in the tear.

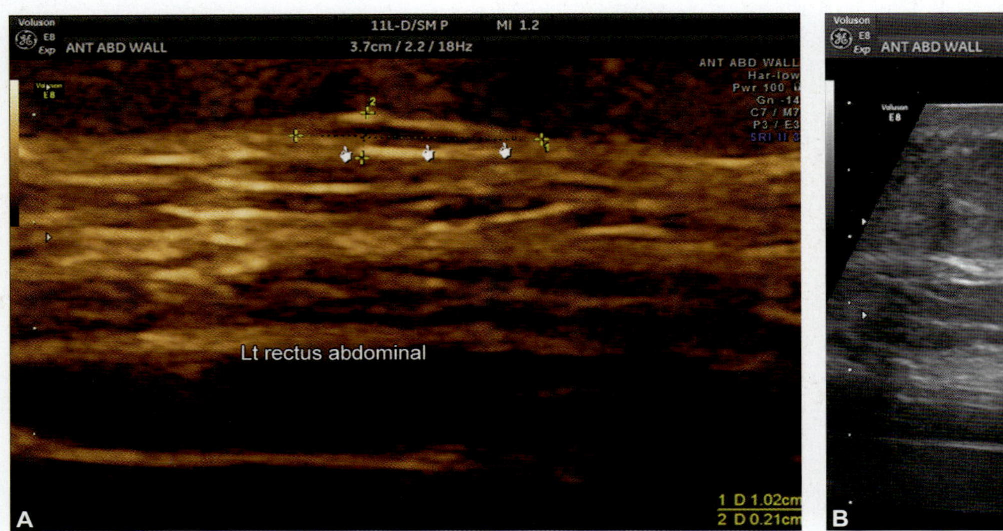

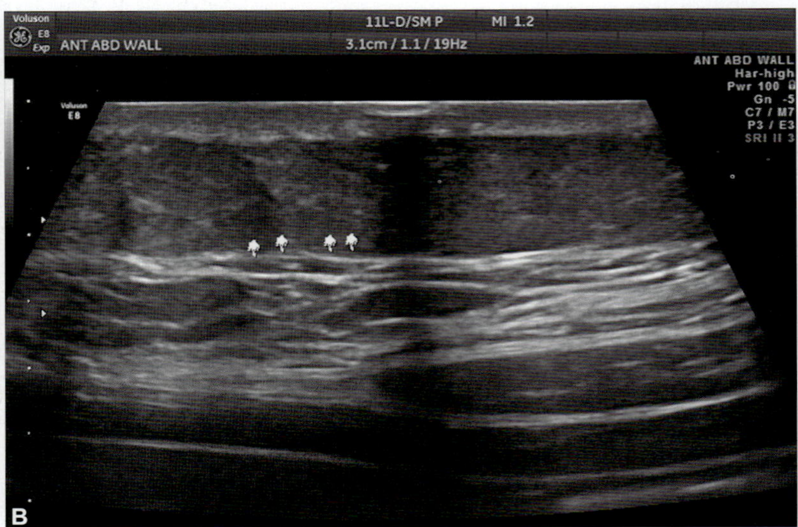

FIGURES 15.24A and B: Tear in rectus abdominis muscle. A patient presented with pain while bending and stretching abdomen. HRSG shows a hypoechoic cleft in left rectus abdominis muscle. The muscles fibers are seen torned.

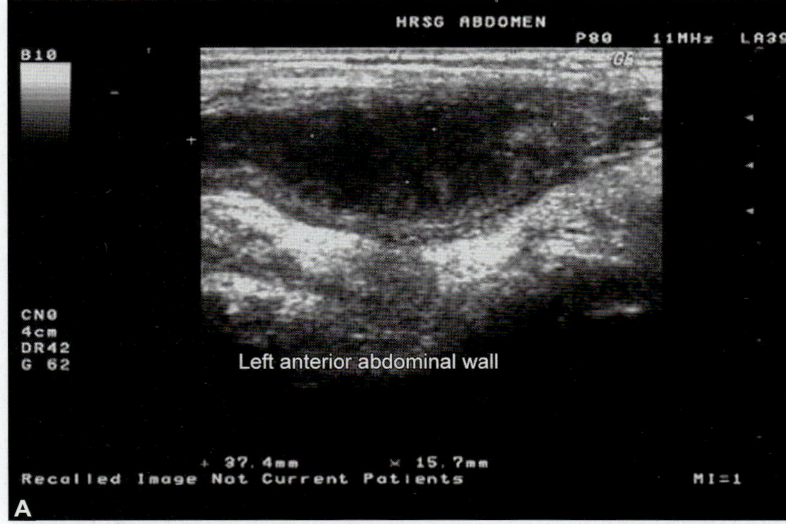

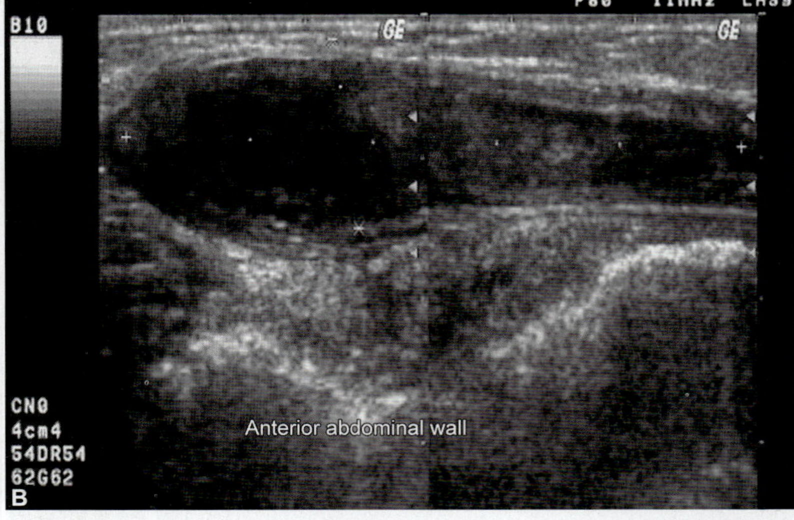

FIGURES 15.25A and B: Rectus sheath hematoma. A young child sustained blunt injury abdomen by a fall. HRSG shows thick low level collection in the rectus sheath. Echogenic shadows are seen floating into it suggestive of rectus sheath hematoma.

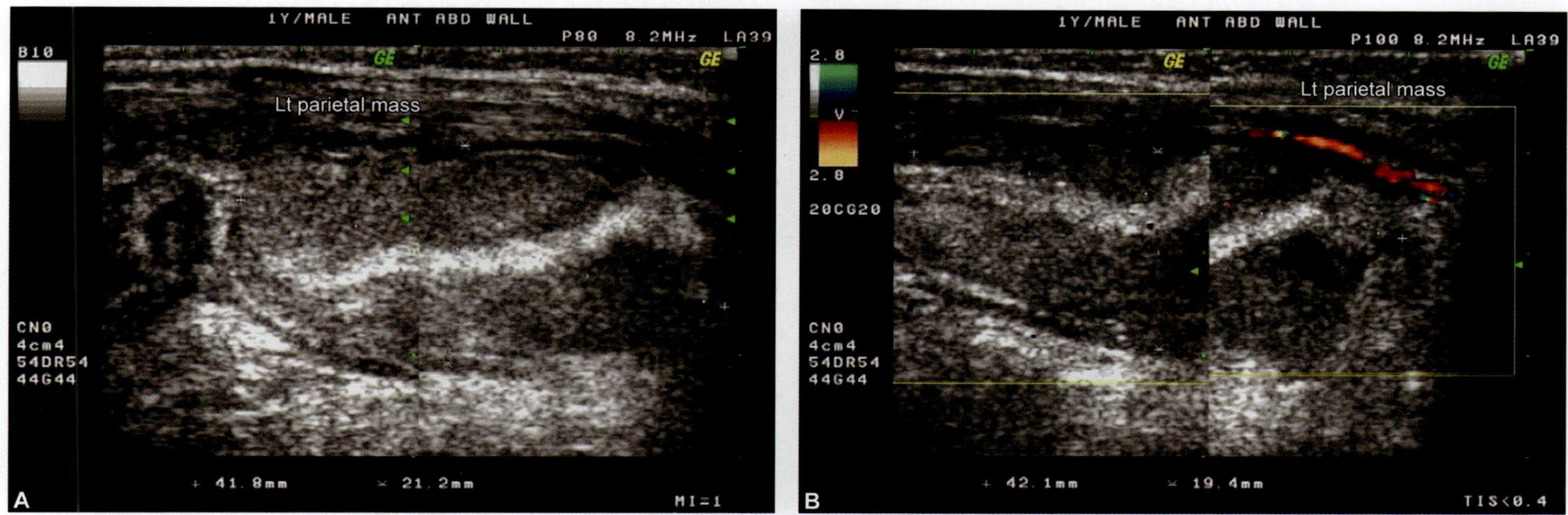

FIGURES 15.26A and B: Parietal hematoma. A young child sustained blunt injury to the anterior abdominal wall by a fall. HRSG shows a big echogenic collection in the parietal layers. Thick echoes are seen in it. No evidence of any necrosis or cystic degeneration is seen. On color flow imaging, no flow is seen in it. Blood came out on aspiration suggestive of fresh hematoma.

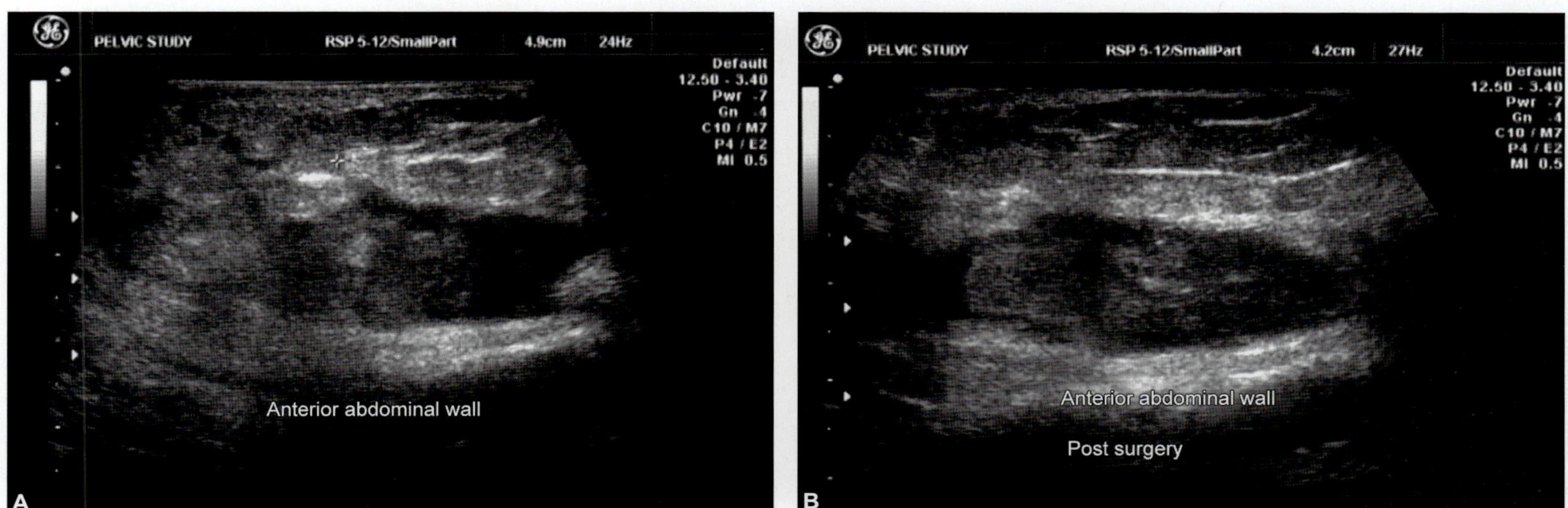

FIGURES 15.27A and B: Postsurgical hematoma. HRSG shows thick collection in the anterior abdominal wall after the surgery. The collection is seen confined in the anterior abdominal wall. Echogenic shadows are seen in them. They are irregular in outline. Aspiration suggests hemorrhagic collection suggestive of hematoma.

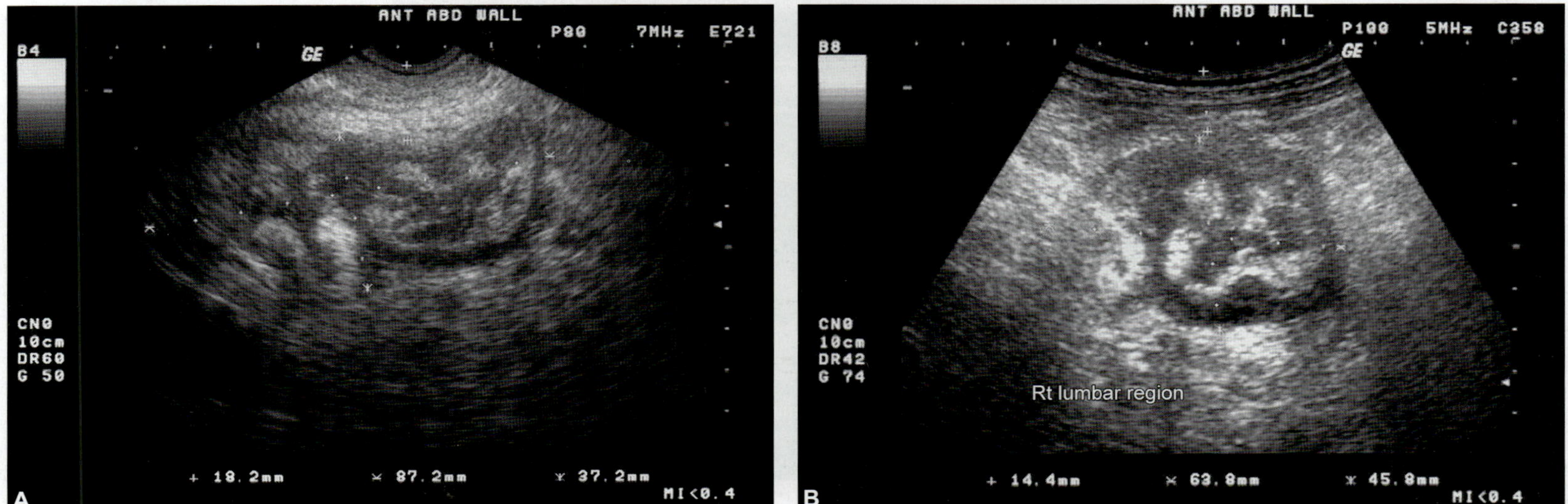

FIGURES 15.28A and B

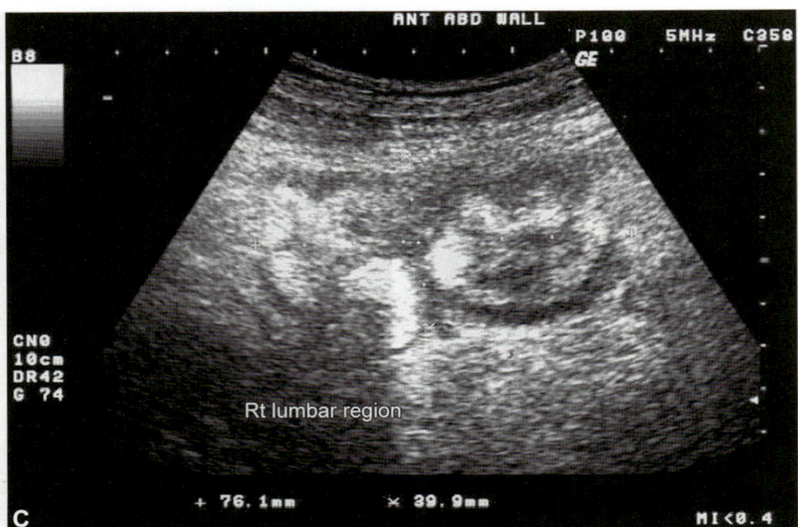

FIGURE 15.28C

FIGURES 15.28A to C: Organized hematoma in the right anterior abdominal wall. A patient presented a painful swelling in the right paralumbar region. HRSG shows a big irregular heterogeneous mass, which was confined into the anterior abdominal wall muscles. Margins are shaggy. Echogenic debris is seen in it. But no evidence of any cystic degeneration is seen. Biopsy of the mass confirmed organised hematoma.

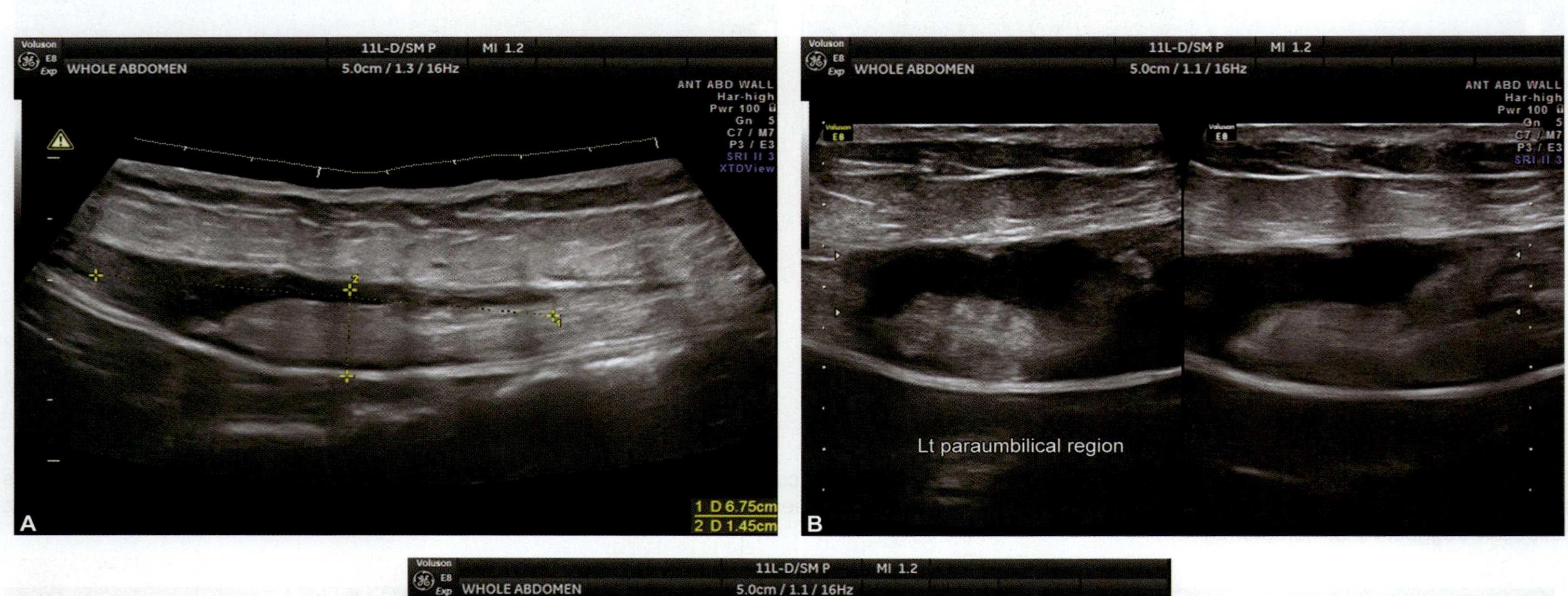

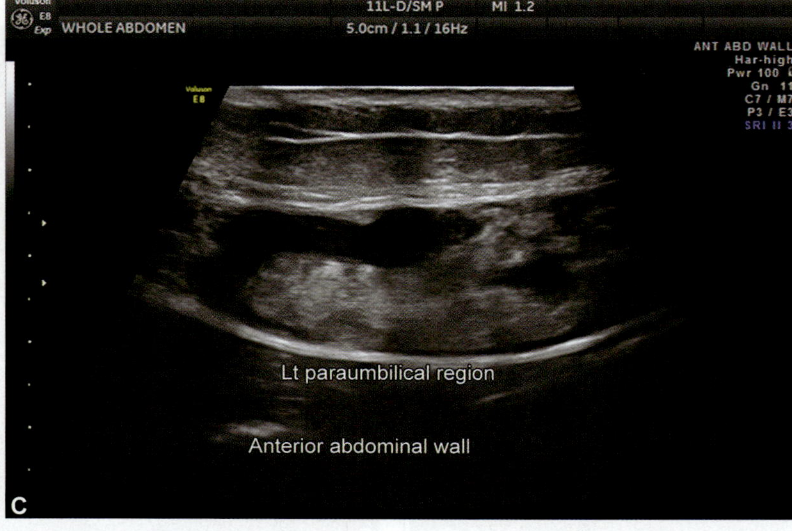

FIGURES 15.29A to C: A patient presented with painful soft tissue swelling after sustaining direct trauma to anterior abdominal wall. HRSG shows a big pocket of echogenic collection in anterior abdominal muscle in left paraumbilical region. Echogenic shadows are seen in it. Low level echoes are also seen in it. On aspiration biopsy, blood was aspirated. Findings left are suggestive of old hematoma formation.

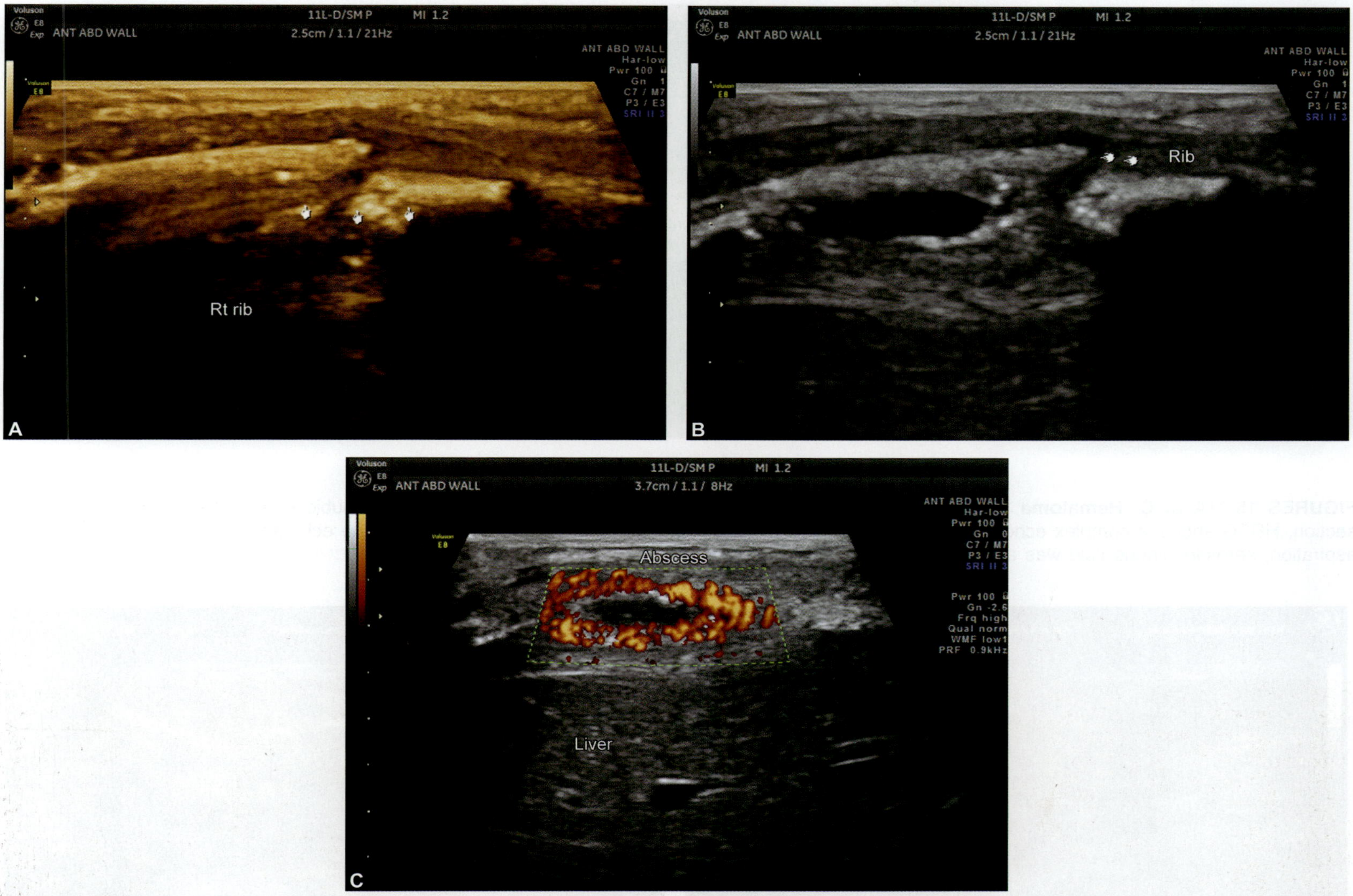

FIGURES 15.30A to C: Rib fracture with hematoma formation with muscle tear. A 9-year-old young child sustained anterior abdominal wall trauma and presented with painful swelling in the right subcostal region. HRSG shows fracture of 11th rib. The fractured segments are seen close to each other. There is also intercostal muscle tear seen. A pocket of low level echo collection is seen at the site of fracture suggestive of hemorrhagic collection. On color flow imaging, increased flow is seen around it suggestive of secondary infection.

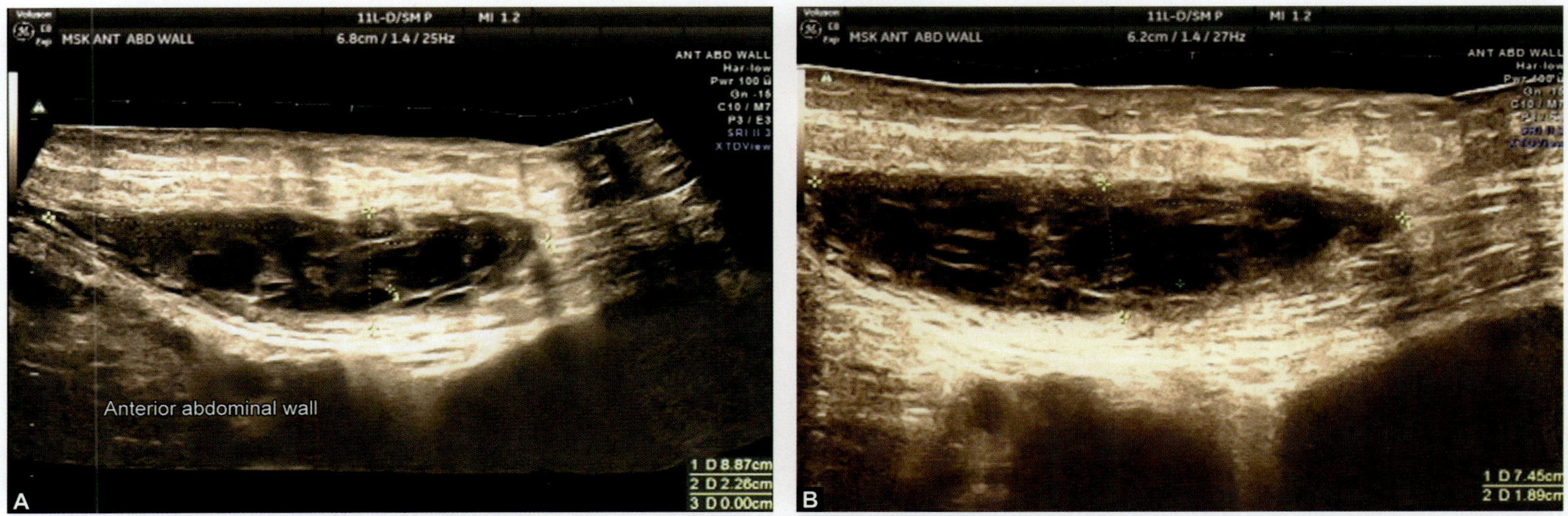

FIGURES 15.31A and B

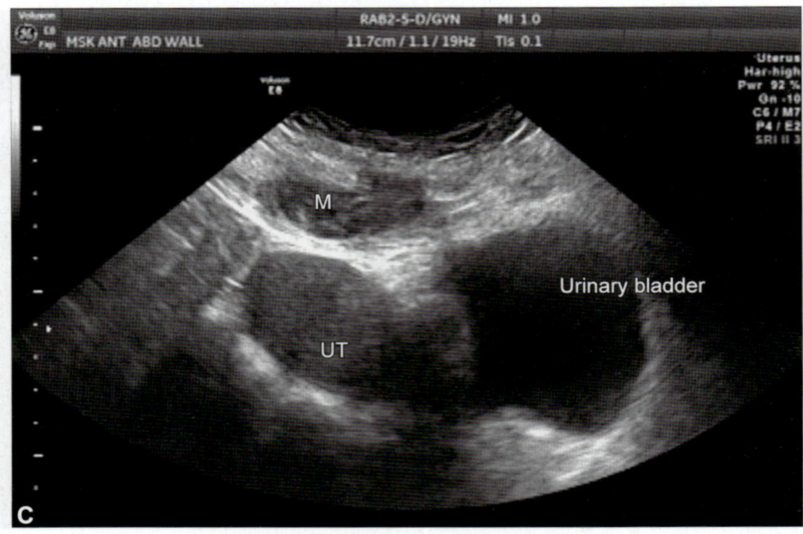

FIGURE 15.31C

FIGURES 15.31A to C: Hematoma under resorption. A patient presented with soft tissue mass in suprapubic region after underwent cesarean section. HRSG shows a complex echo mass in suprapubic region. Multiple internal echoes are seen in it. Fine echogenic strands are also seen. On aspiration, serosanguinous fluid was aspirated. Findings are suggestive of old hematoma under resorption.

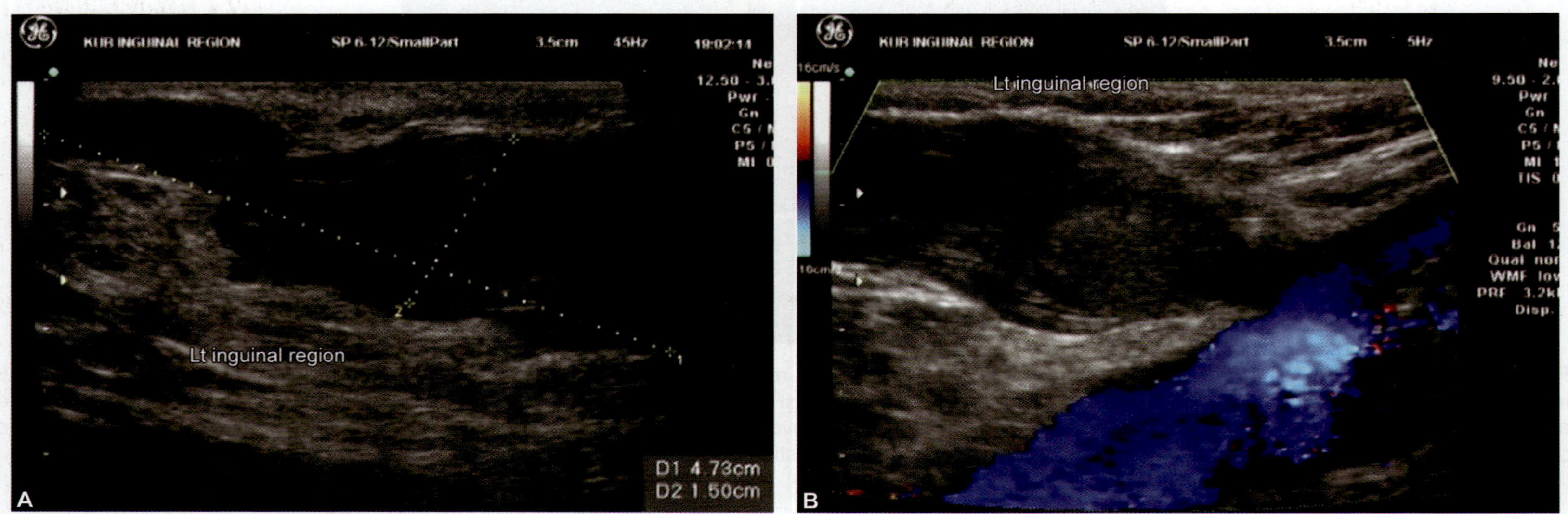

FIGURES 15.32A and B: Inguinal hematoma. A patient presented with hard lump in right inguinal region after femoral angiography. HRSG shows a big low level echo complex mass in the left inguinal region. Multiple internal echoes are seen in it suggestive of hematoma formation. Mild pressure is seen on common femoral vein.

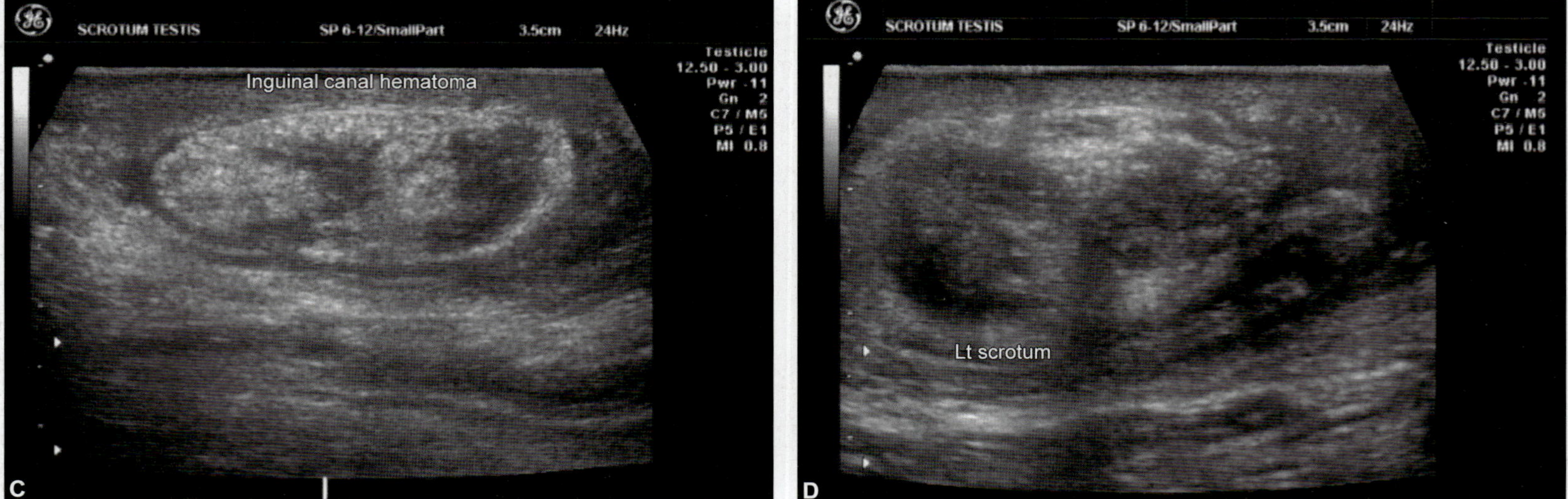

FIGURES 15.32C and D: Inguinal canal hematoma. A young boy presented with inguinoscrotal swelling after sustaining trauma. HRSG shows echogenic collection in inguinal canal suggestive of hematoma formation. Left testis is also enlarged, edematous and hypoechoic in texture. Echogenic shadows are seen in epididymis suggestive of post-traumatic epididymoorchitis.

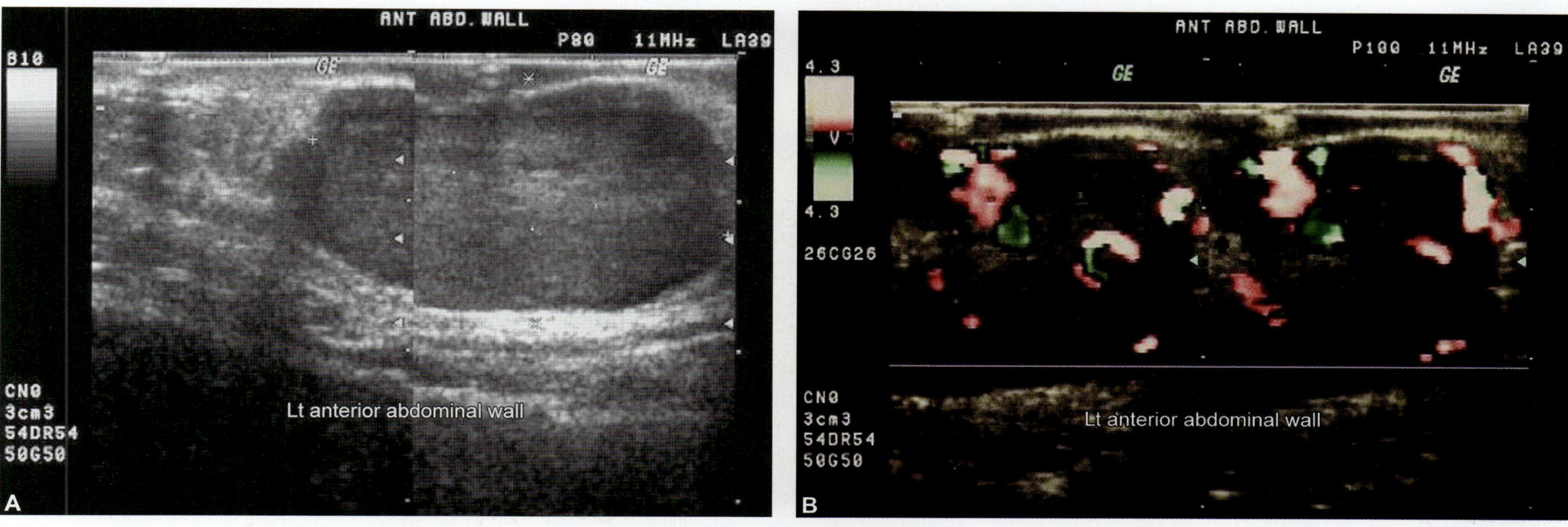

FIGURES 15.33A and B: Bleeding hematoma in the anterior abdominal wall. A patient presented progressively increasing mass in the anterior abdominal wall after sustaining blunt trauma. HRSG shows a big low level echo collection in the anterior abdominal wall. Homogeneous echoes are seen in it with floating debris. On color flow imaging, multiple vessels are seen in the collection. Aspiration of the collection came out to be fresh blood.

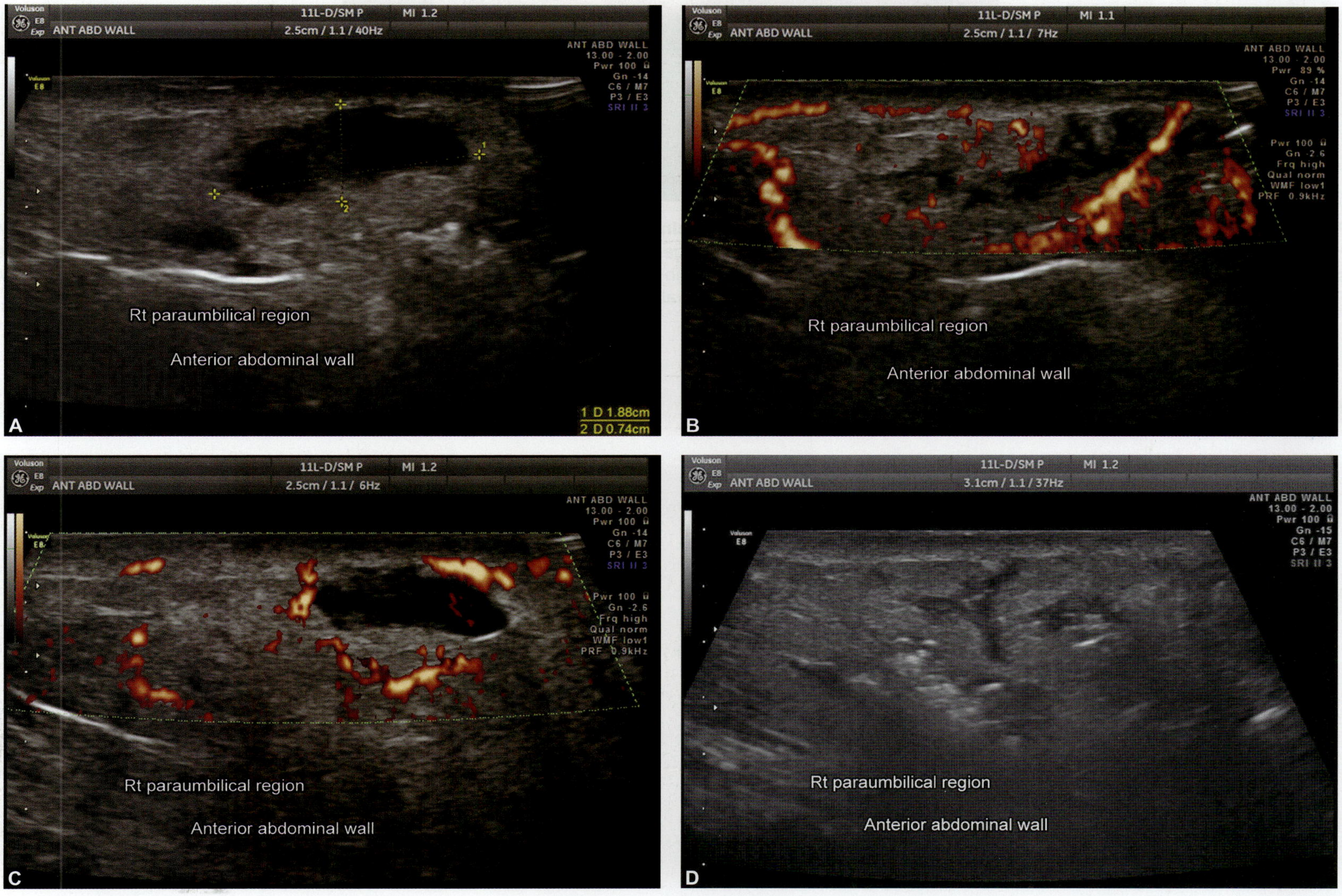

FIGURES 15.34A to D: A patient presented with soft tissue mass after sustaining trauma in anterior abdominal wall. HRSG shows an irregular ill-defined inhomogeneous mass in the right paraumbilical region. The mass measures 25 x 10 mm in size. It is hypoechoic in texture. Low level echo are seen in it. Associated perifocal edema is also present. On color flow imaging, increased flow is seen around it. Findings are suggestive of post-traumatic hematoma with super added infection.

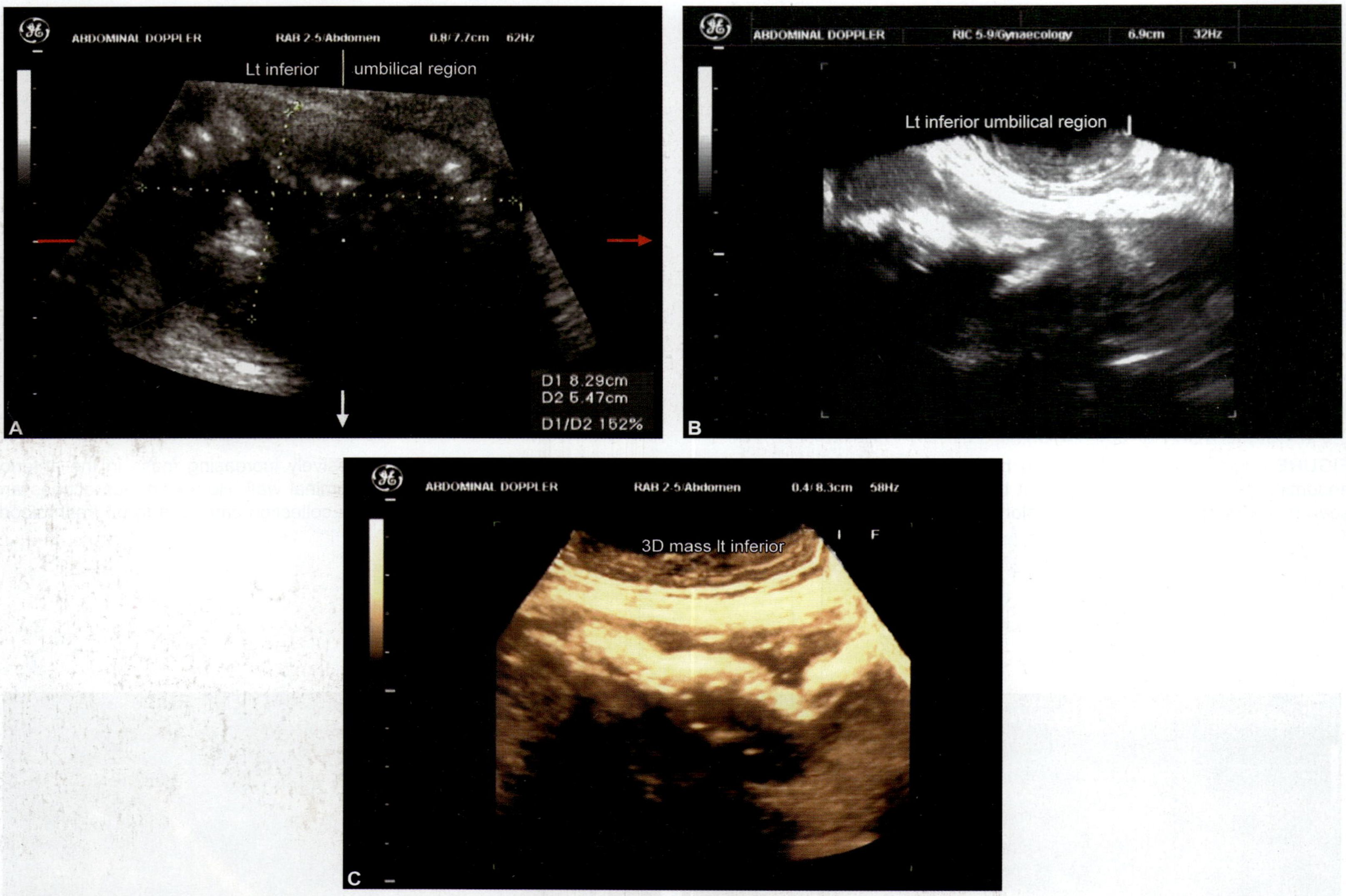

FIGURES 15.35A to C: Foreign body (Sponge) in the anterior abdominal wall. A patient presented with soft tissue mass after the post surgery. HRSG shows a complex echo mass in the left infraumbilical region. Echogenic calcification is also seen in it. It casts acoustic shadowing masking the scanning field. 3D imaging of the mass shows a complex echo shadow in the anterior abdominal wall. On color Doppler imaging it shows no flow. Postoperative finding confirmed a sponge in the left anterior abdominal wall.

ANTERIOR ABDOMINAL WALL HERNIA

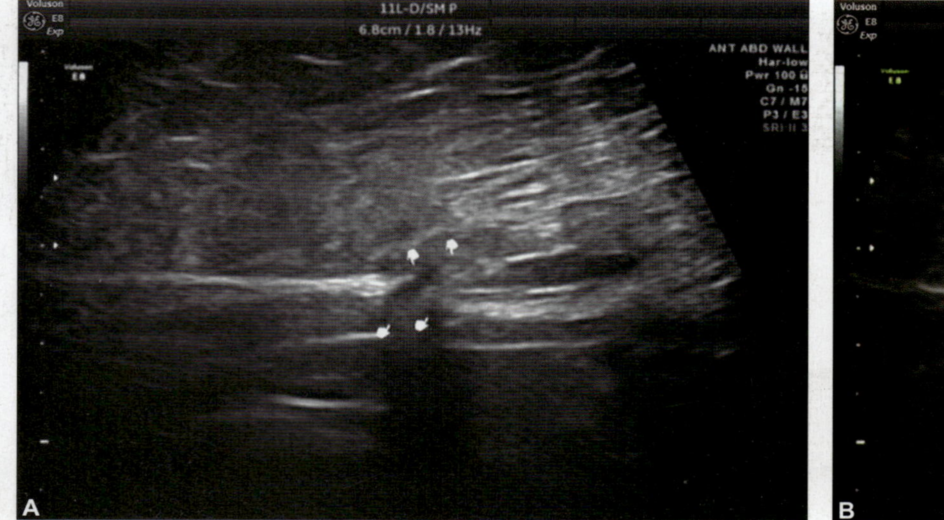

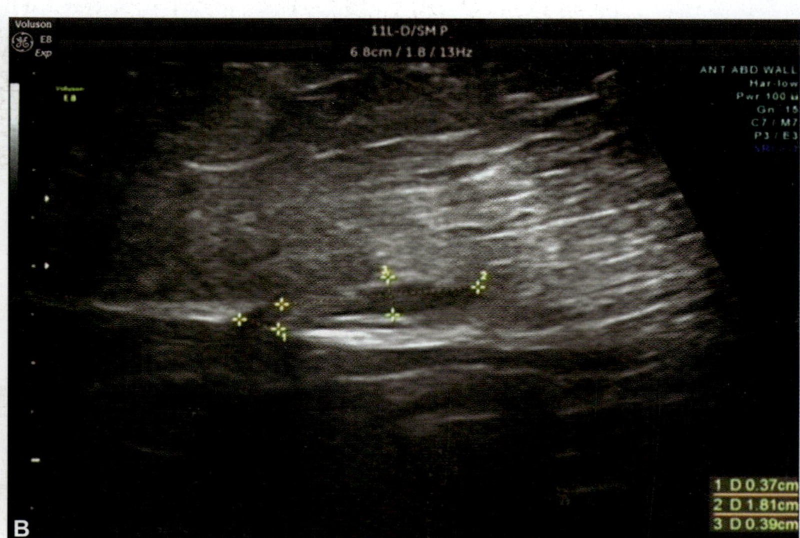

FIGURES 15.36A and B

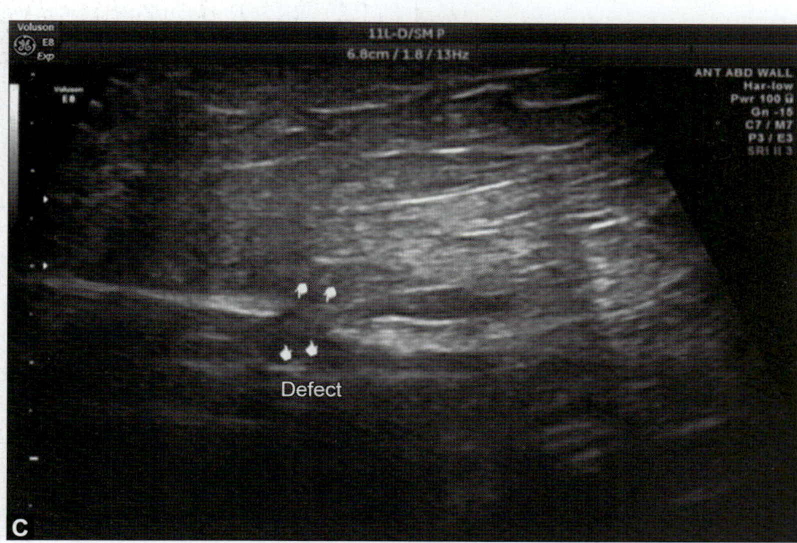

FIGURE 15.36C

FIGURES 15.36A to C: Spigelian hernia. A patient presented with recurrent vomiting after having food. HRSG shows a defect in the spigelian aponeurosis of transverse abdominis muscle lateral to the umbilicus. On dynamic scanning, a bowel loop is seen herniating through the defect suggestive of spigelian hernia.

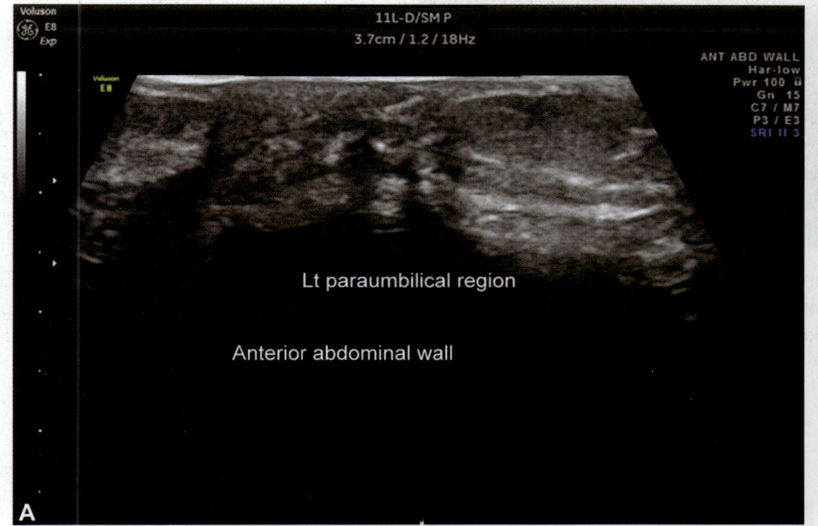

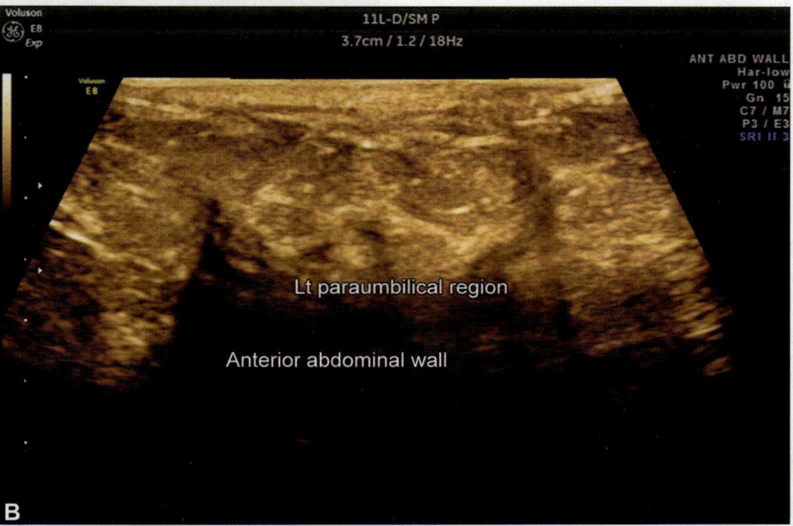

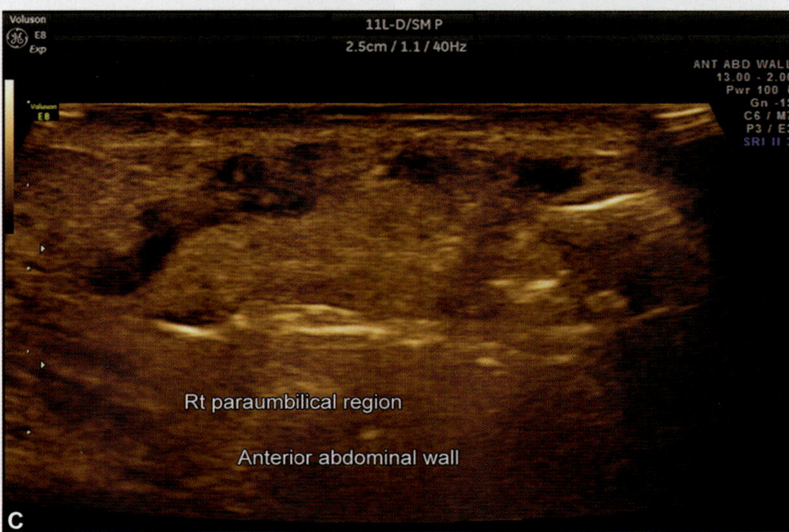

FIGURES 15.37A to C: Left paraumbilical hernia. HRSG shows big defect in left transverse abdominal muscle. A membrane is seen herniating through it suggestive of omental hernia. But no bowel loop herniation is seen.

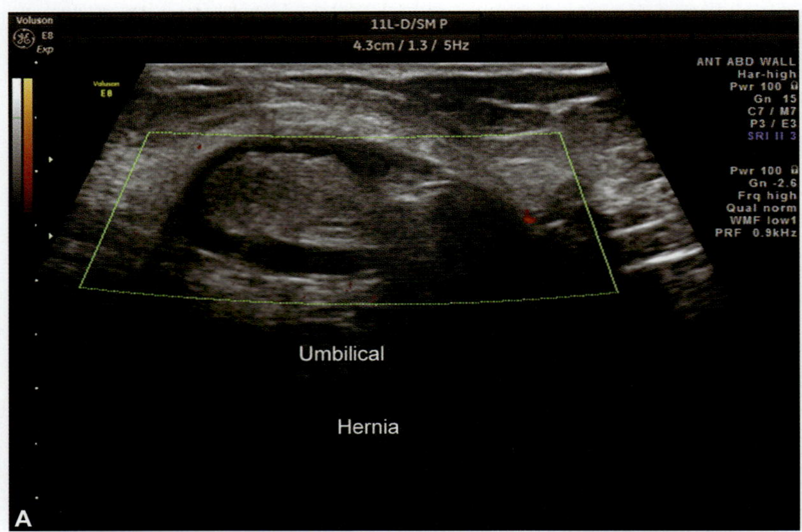

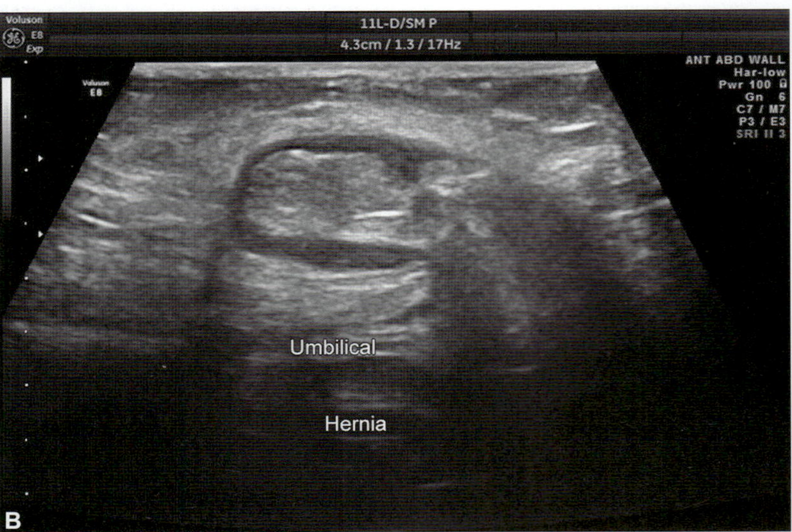

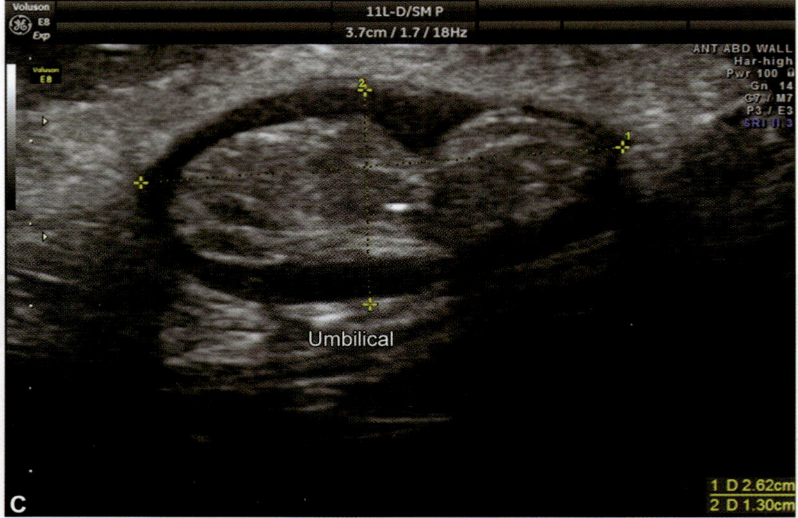

FIGURES 15.38A to C: Anterior abdominal wall hernia. A patient presented with anterior abdominal wall hernia in supraumbilical region. HRSG shows a big defect in anterior abdominal wall muscle. A bowel loop is seen herniating through defect. Air and fluid movement is seen in herniating bowel loop. On transverse axis imaging, the herniated bowel loop looks like a mass. However, on dynamic scanning and pressure, it is seen.

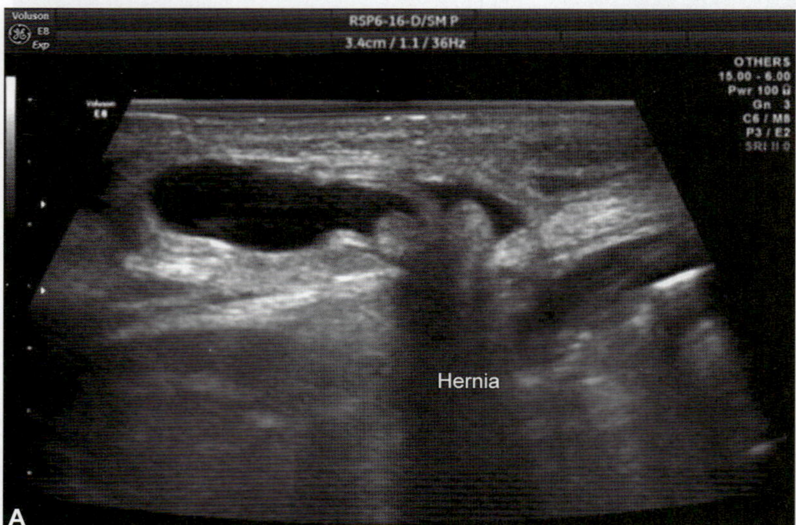

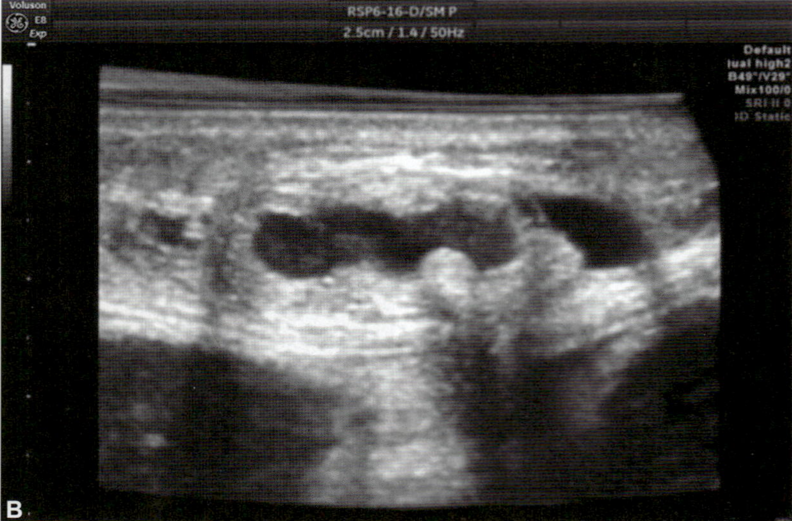

FIGURES 15.39A and B

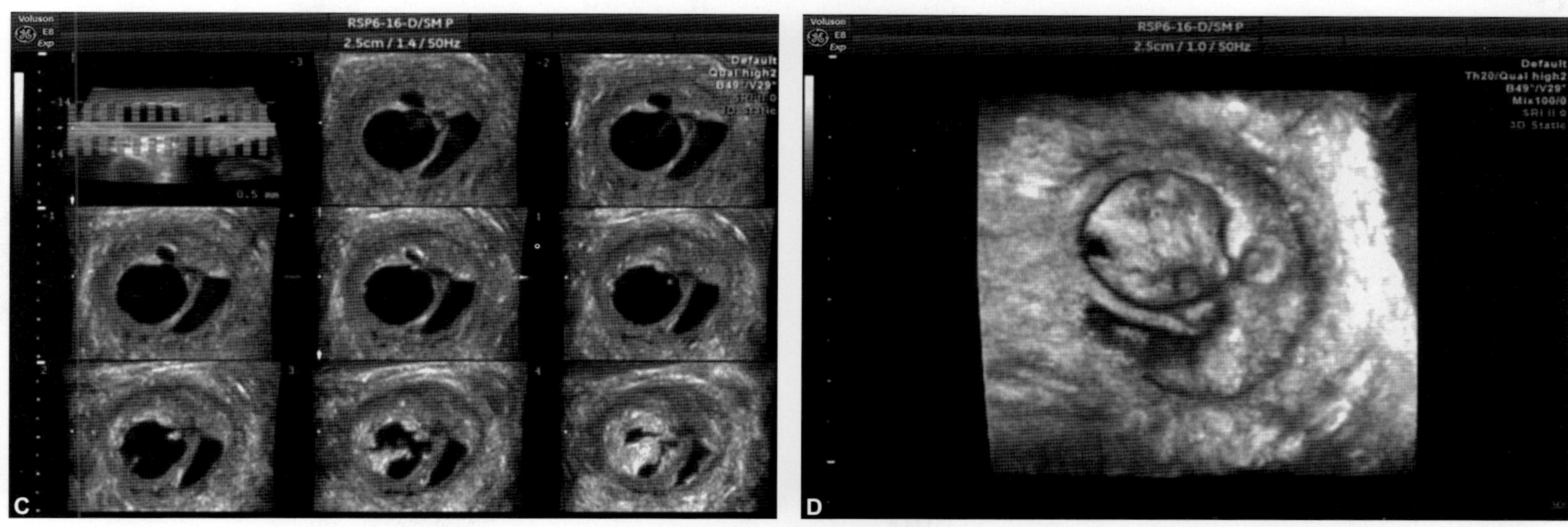

FIGURES 15.39C and D

FIGURES 15.39A to D: Obstructed hernia. A lady presented with painful swelling in supraumbilical region. HRSG shows a defect in anterior abdominal wall muscle. A bowel loop is seen herniating through defect. The bowel loop is seen stuck in hernial sac. An echogenic band is seen in the sac, which is seen obstructing the reduction of bowel loop. On 3D ultrasound, the band is clearly seen and bowel loop got stuck in the sac because of the band.

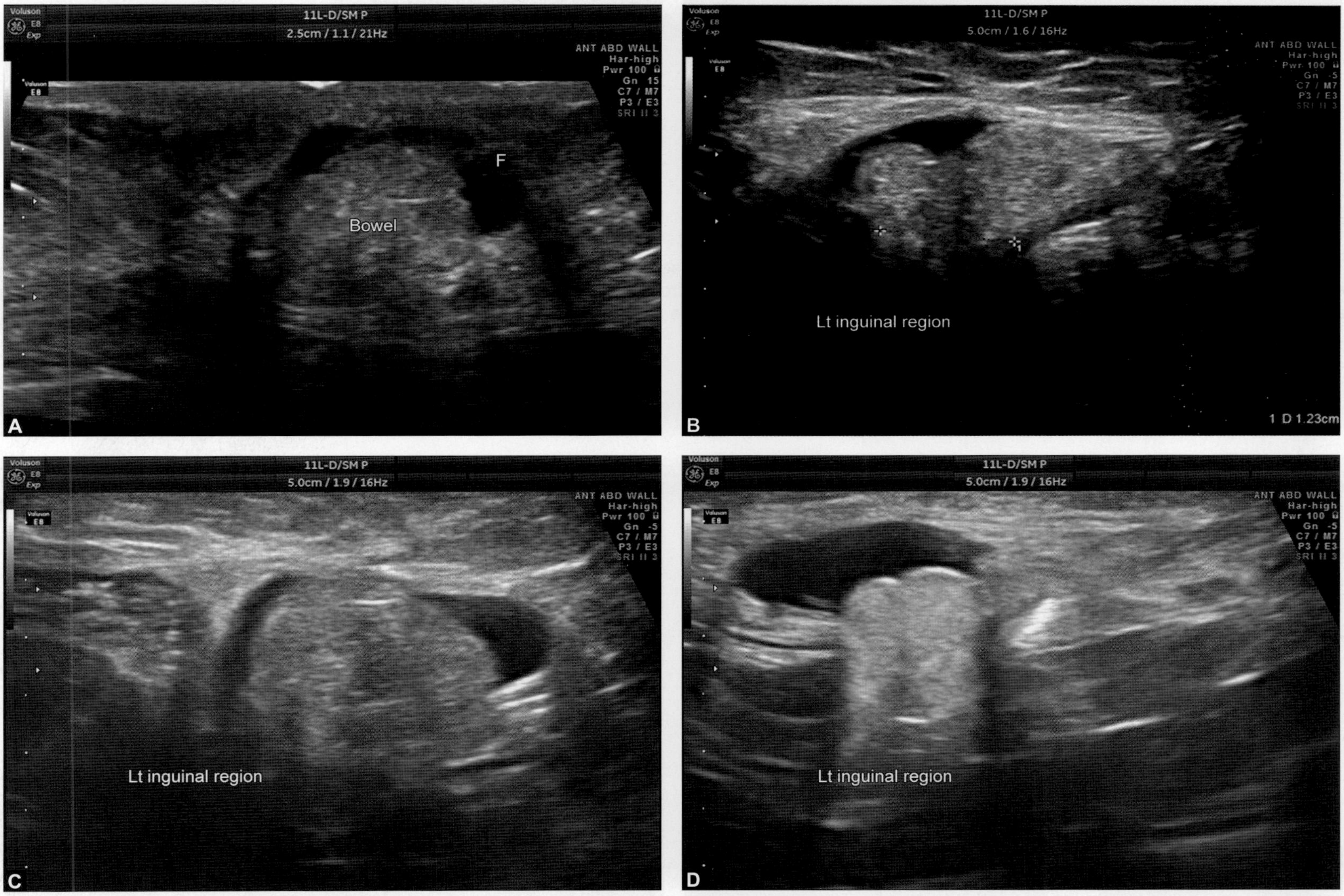

FIGURES 15.40A to D: Big left inguinal hernia. A patient presented with soft tissue swelling in the left inguinal region. HRSG shows a defect in the left inguinal canal. A bowel loop is seen herniating through defect. Fluid movement is seen in the bowel loop. No evidence of any bowel loop obstruction is seen.

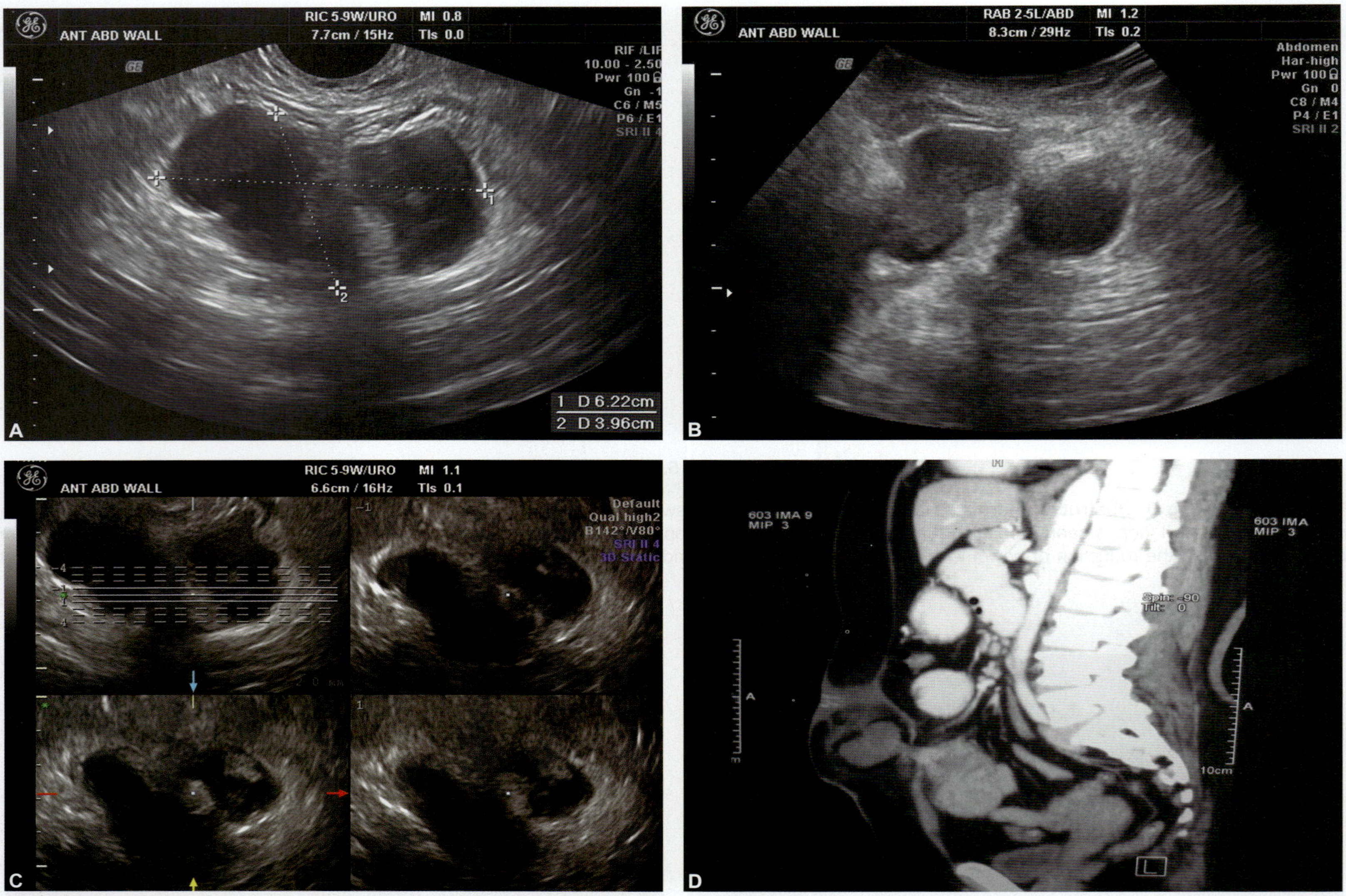

FIGURES 15.41A to D: Obstructed infraumbilical hernia. A patient presented with acute pain with vomiting. HRSG shows a defect in the anterior abdominal wall in infraumbilical region. A bowel loop is seen coming out from the defect. An echogenic band is seen in the bowel loop, which is not allowing loop to be reduced suggestive of obstructed hernia. CT scan of the same patient also shows infraumbilical hernia with obstructed bowel loops.

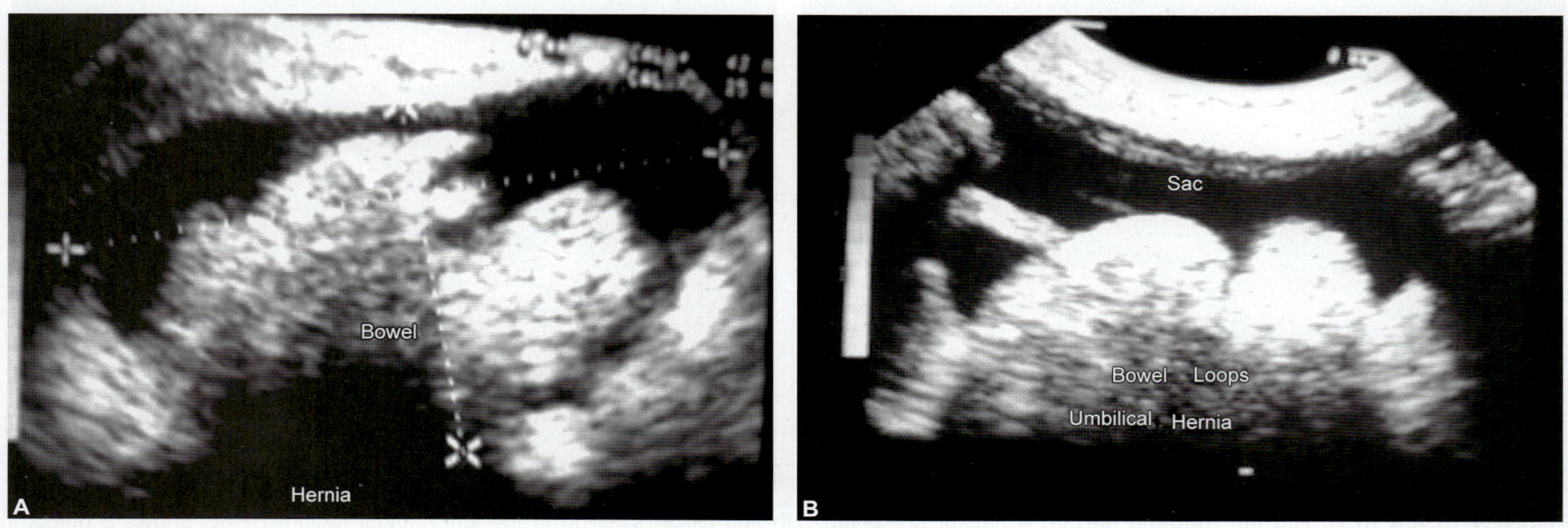

FIGURES 15.42A and B: Paraumbilical hernia. HRSG shows floating bowel loops in the soft tissue mass in paraumbilical region. Fluid collection is also seen in it suggestive of paraumbilical hernia. Echogenic band is seen in the umbilical hernia obstructing the reduction of the bowel loops.

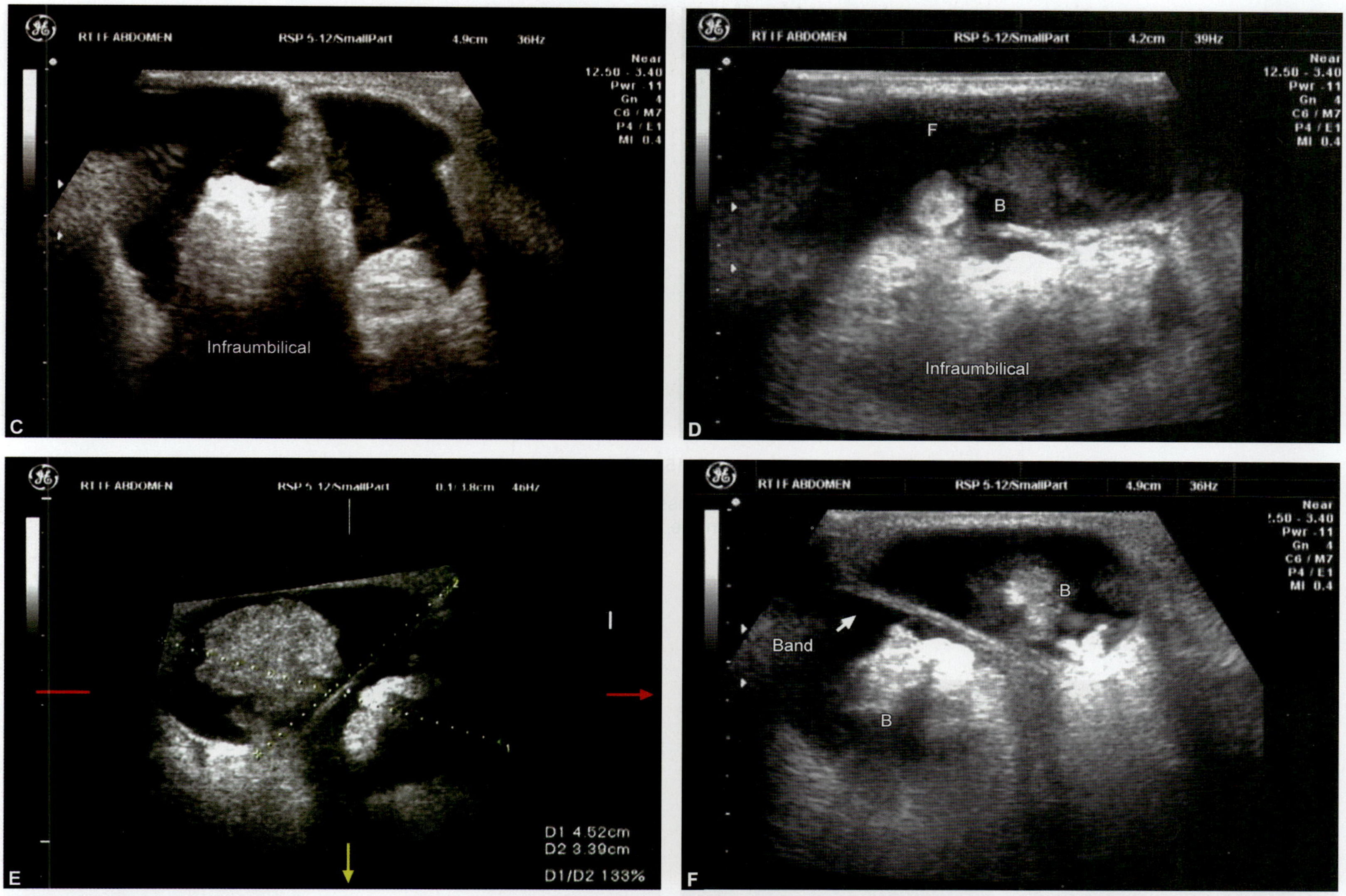

FIGURES 15.42C to F: Umbilical hernia. HRSG shows herniating bowel loops in infraumbilical region. The bowel loops are seen echogenic floating gas-containing shadows floating in the hernial sac. 3D imaging with surface rendering shows the details of the hernial sac. An echogenic band is seen dividing the sac into two. The bowel loops are floating in both the sacs. However, no evidence of any knotting is seen. The band results in strangulation and entanglement of bowel loops. Therefore, color Doppler imaging is important to rule out strangulation.

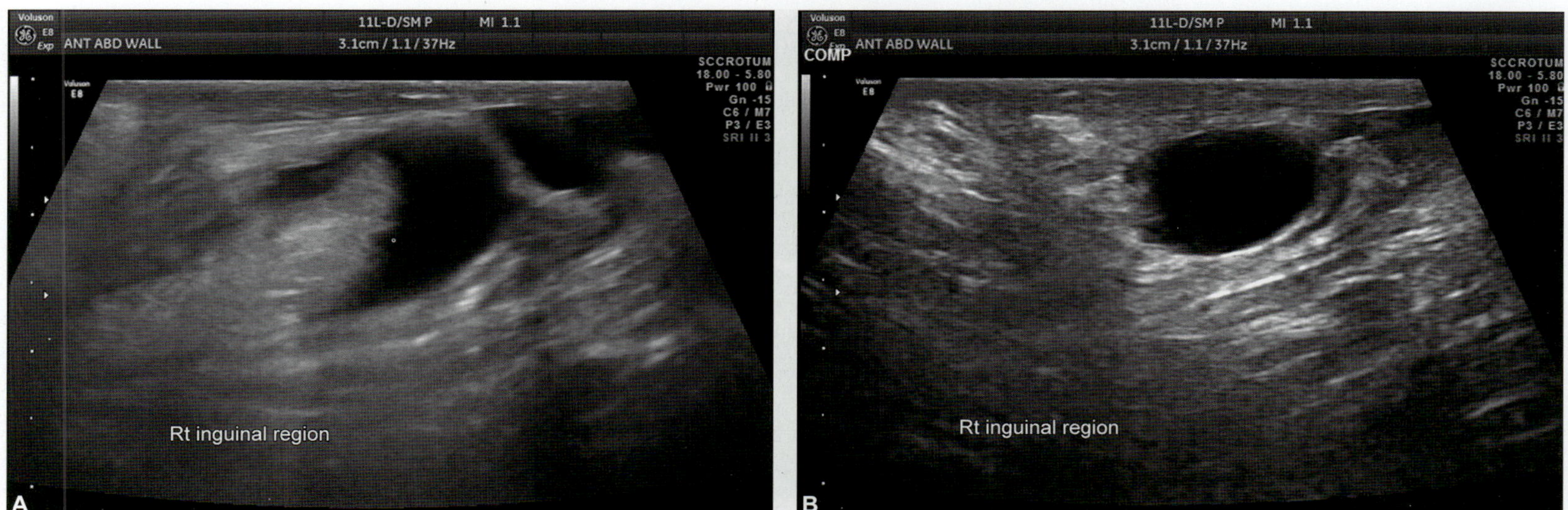

FIGURES 15.43A and B

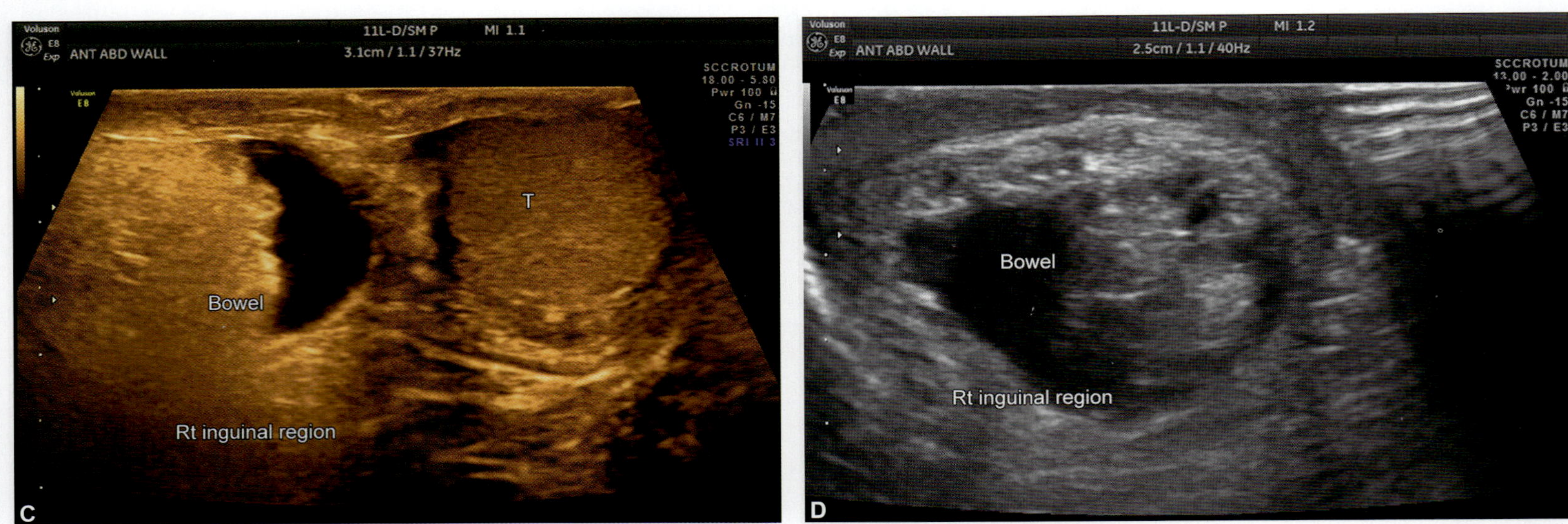

FIGURES 15.43C and D

FIGURES 15.43A to D: Inguinal hernia. A patient presented with soft tissue swelling in right inguinal canal. HRSG shows a bowel loop herniating in right inguinal canal. Fluid movement is also seen in the bowel loop. But no evidence of scrotal herniation is seen.

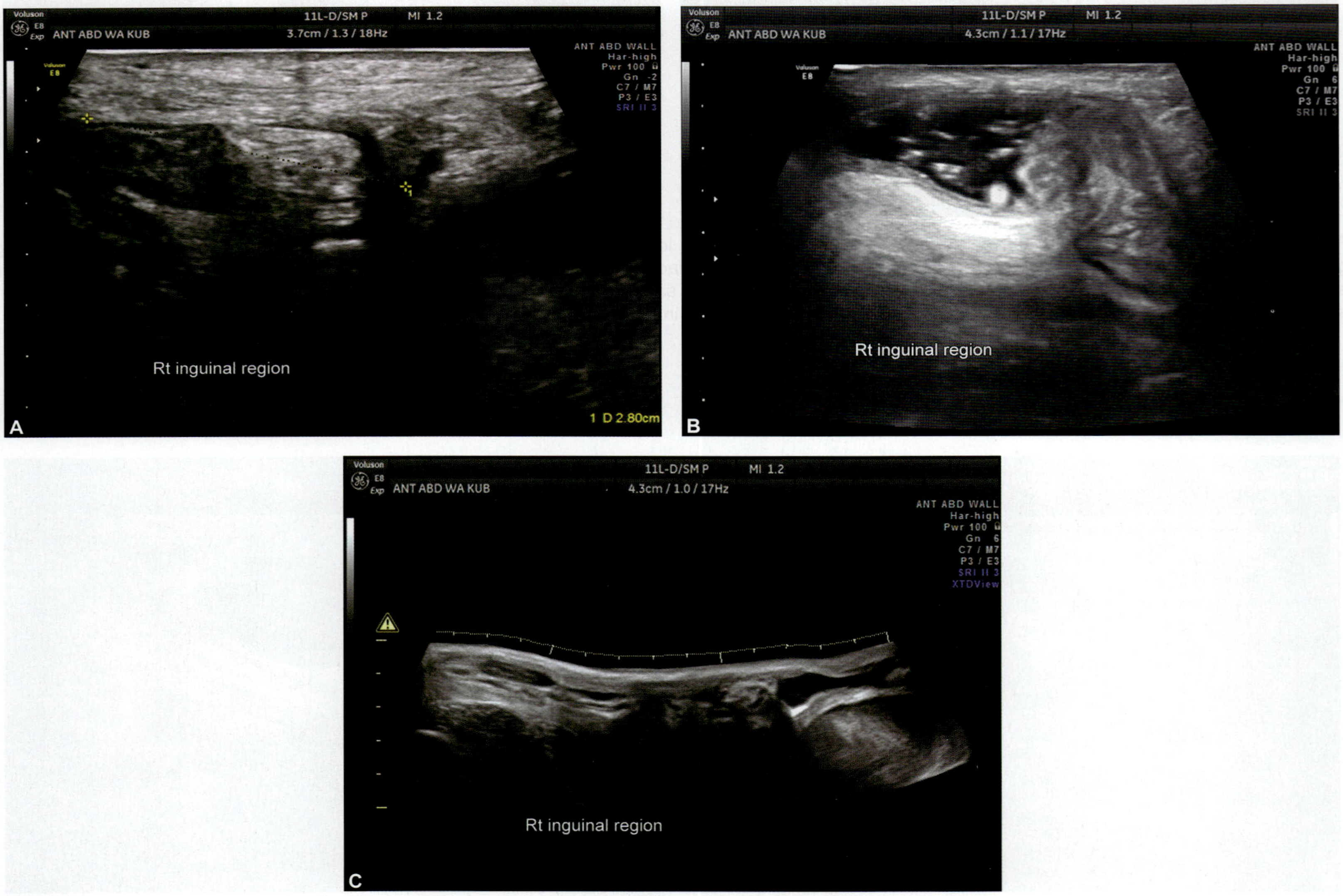

FIGURES 15.44A to C: Inguinal hernia. A young girl presented with soft tissue swelling in right inguinal region. HRSG shows a bowel loop herniation in the right inguinal region. Fluid movement is seen in the bowel loop. No evidence of any obstruction of bowel loop is seen. The suprapubic region and both labia are normal.

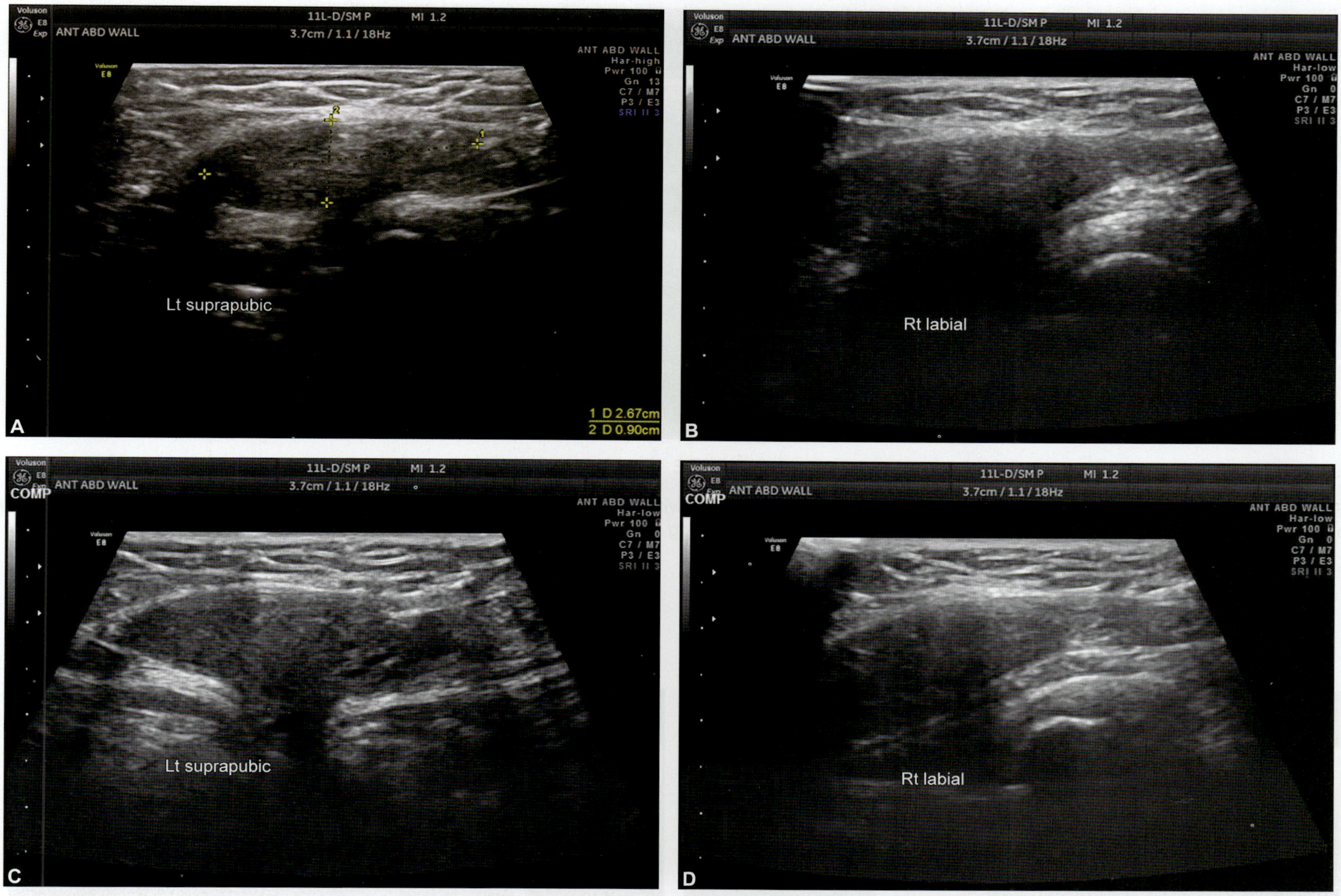

FIGURES 15.45A to D: A patient presented with bilateral inguinal swelling. HRSG shows membranous shadows herniating in both inguinal regions. However, no bowel loop herniation is seen suggestive of omental hernia.

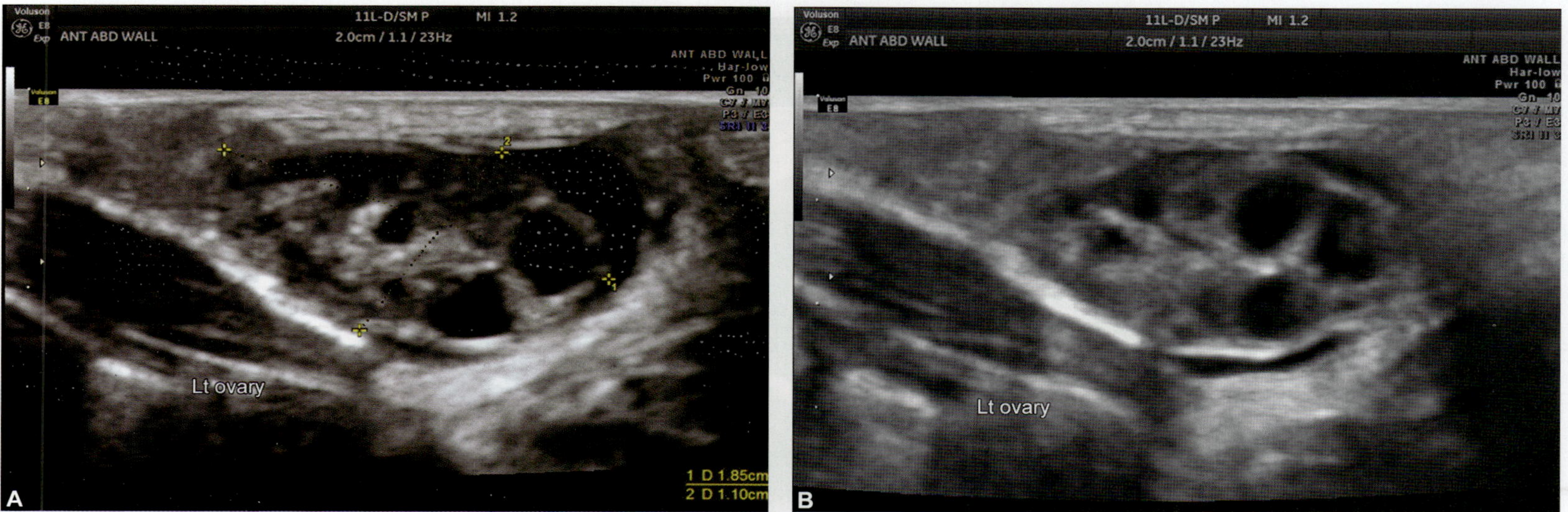

FIGURES 15.46A and B

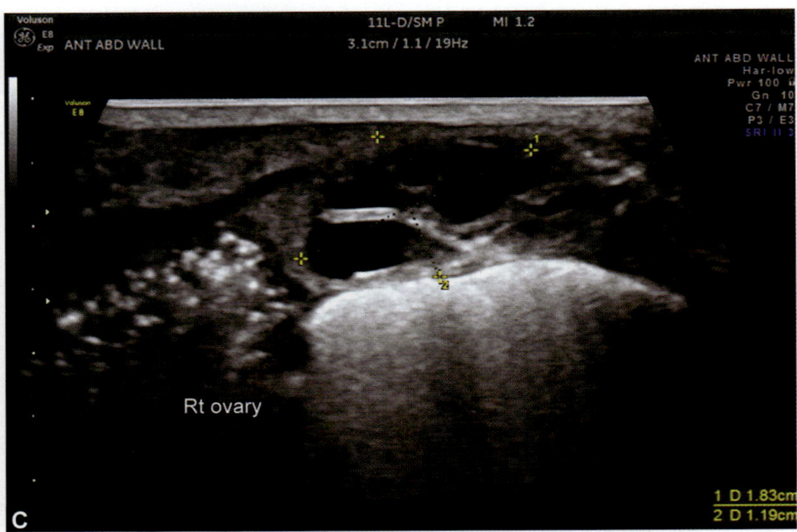

FIGURE 15.46C

FIGURES 15.46A to C: Ovarian hernia. A 1.5 month old baby presented with left inguinal canal swelling. HRSG shows enlarged edematous left ovary herniating in the left inguinal canal. The right ovary is also seen herniating on the right side. The ovaries are edematous and hypoechoic in texture.

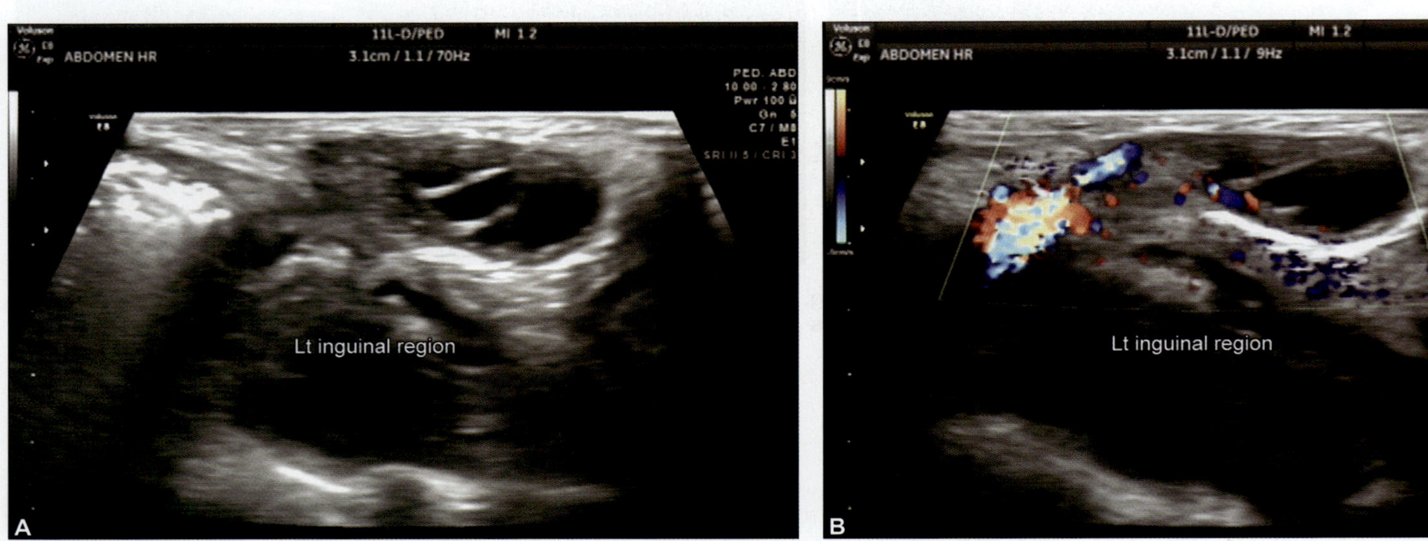

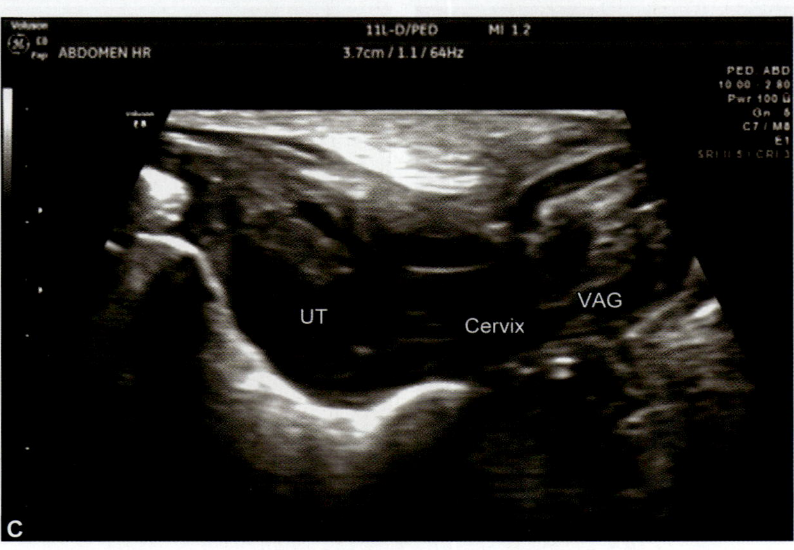

FIGURES 15.47A to C: Ovarian hernia in the left inguinal region. A 2 months old baby presented with painful swelling in the left inguinal region. HRSG shows edematous, enlarged left ovary herniating in left inguinal region. Few vessels are also seen in the herniating sac.

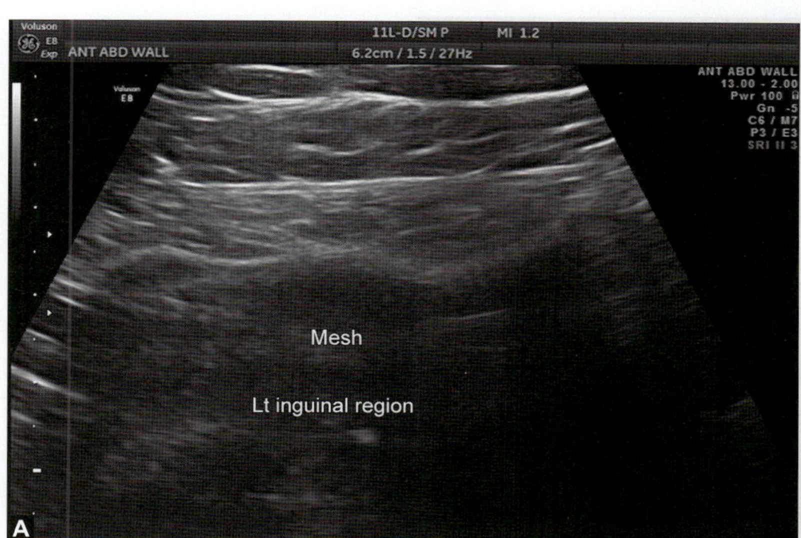

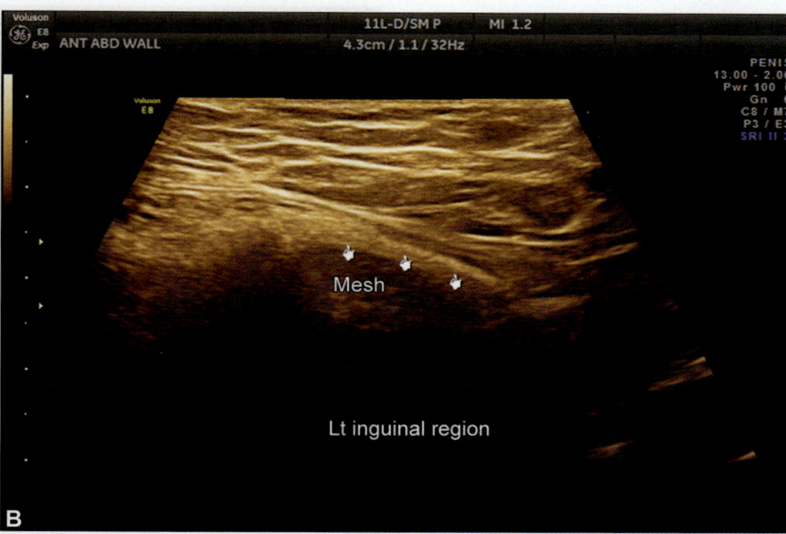

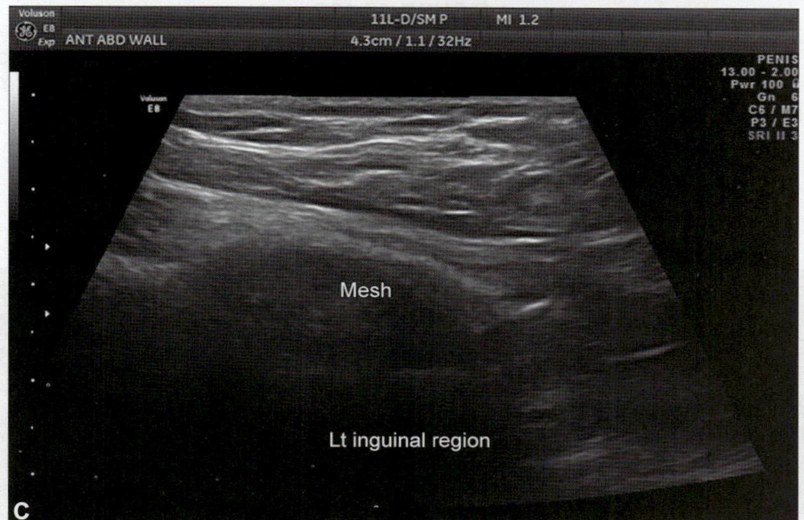

FIGURES 15.48A to C: Intact mesh. A patient underwent hernioplasty with mesh in position. HRSG shows echogenic linear shadow in left inguinal region suggestive of mesh in position. The bowel loops are seen below the mesh. No defect is seen in the mesh.

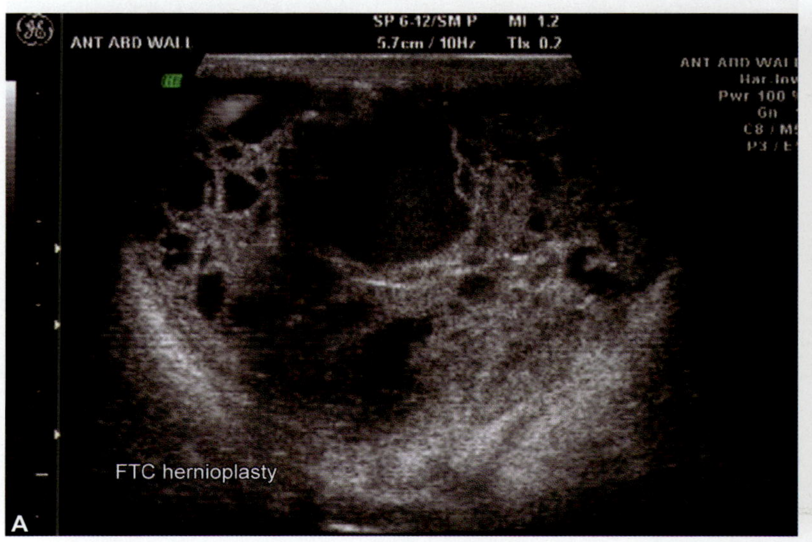

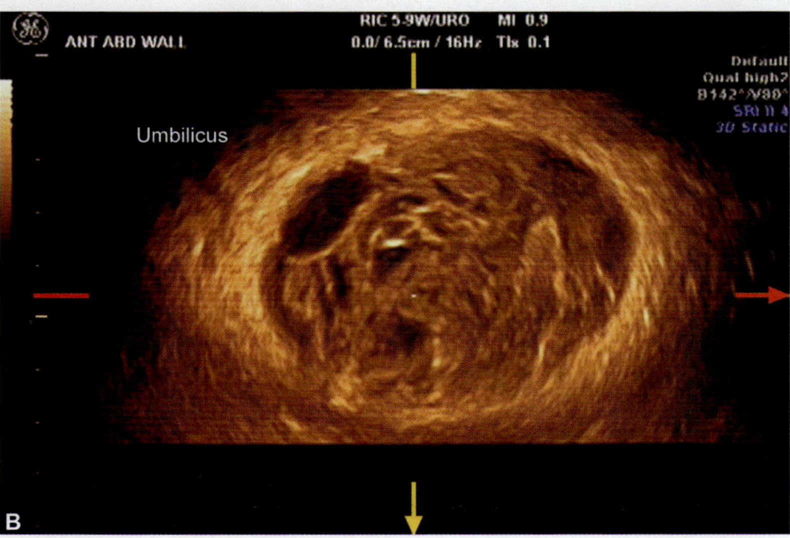

FIGURES 15.49A and B

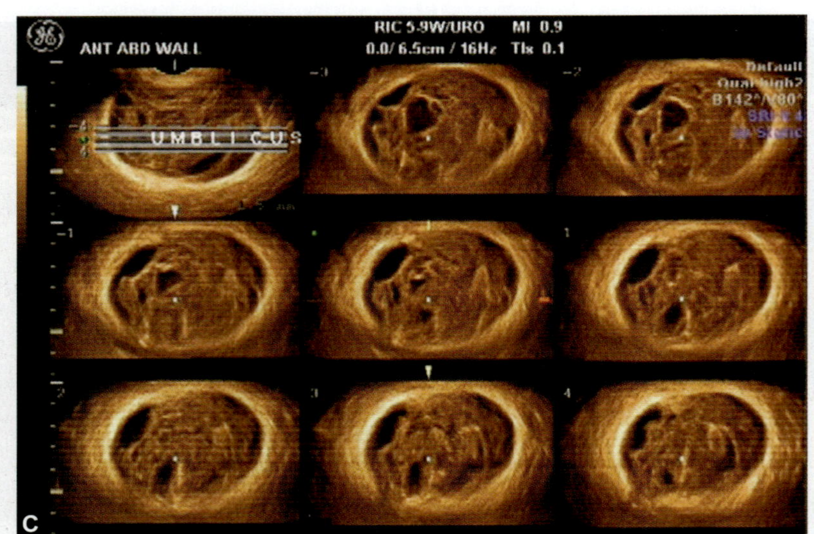

FIGURE 15.49C

FIGURES 15.49A to C: Rupture of the mesh with herniating bowel loop. A patient presented with lump in right paraumbilical region. HRSG shows rupture of the mesh with entanglement of bowel loops. The bowel loops are edematous and looks like a clumped mass. 3D ultrasound with tomographic ultrasound imaging beautifully shows the clumping of bowel loops.

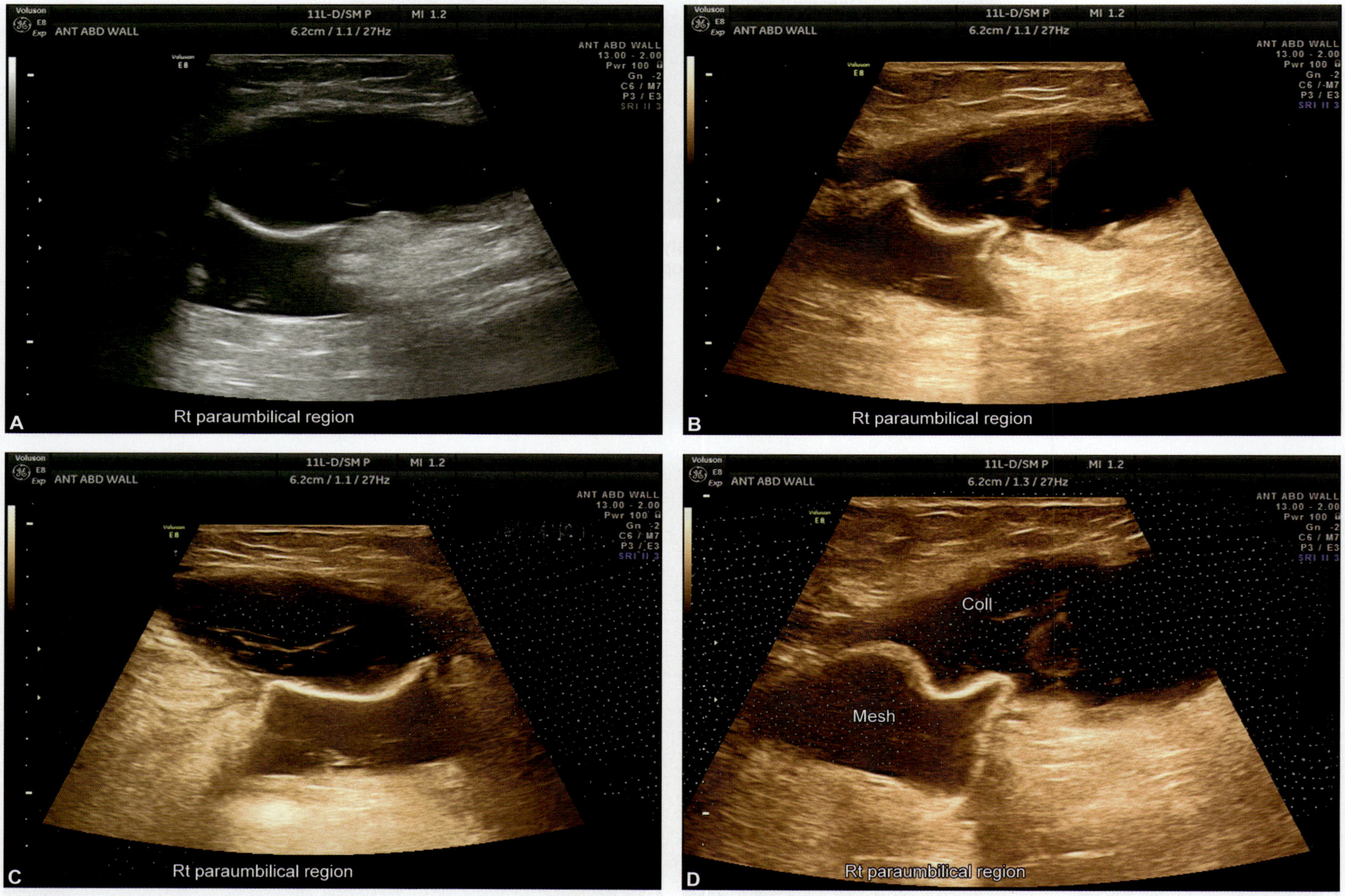

FIGURES 15.50A to D

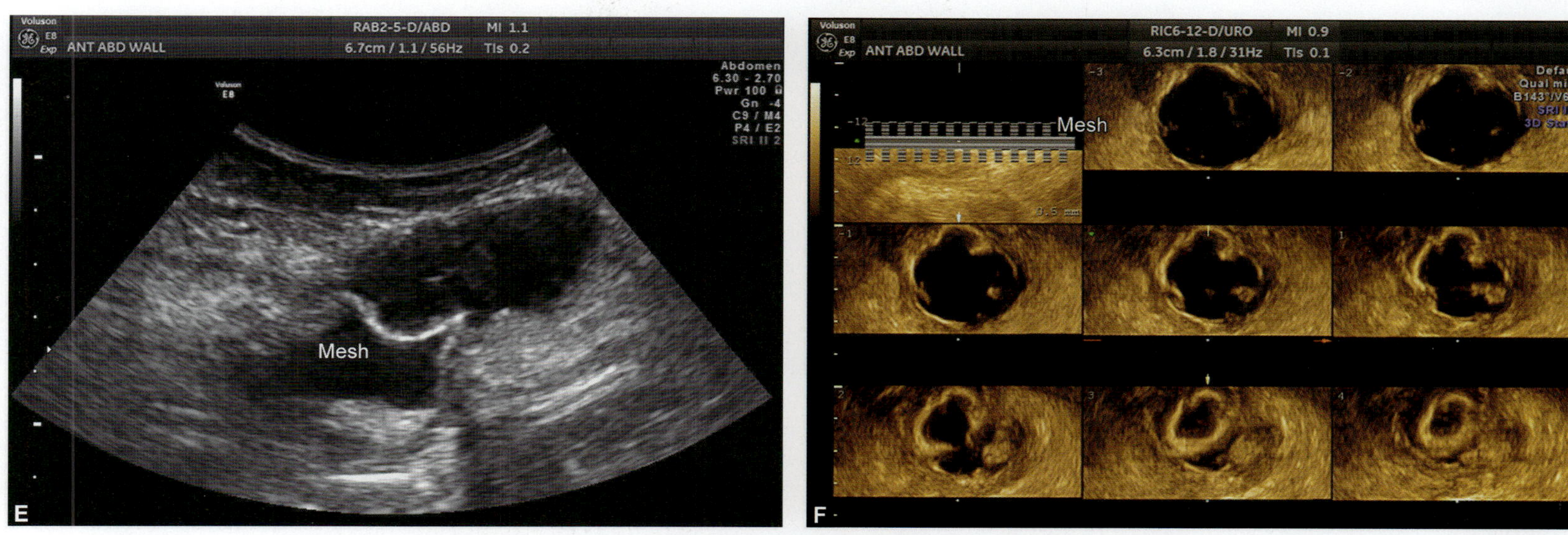

FIGURES 15.50E and F

FIGURES 15.50A to F: Ruptured mesh with collection in paraumbilical region. A patient underwent hernioplasty and he presented with pain and lump in paraumbilical region. HRSG shows an echogenic shadow floating in the paraumbilical region suggestive of rupture of the mesh and floating bowel loops. Moderate amount of collection is also seen in the ruptured mesh.

ANTERIOR ABDOMINAL WALL MASSES

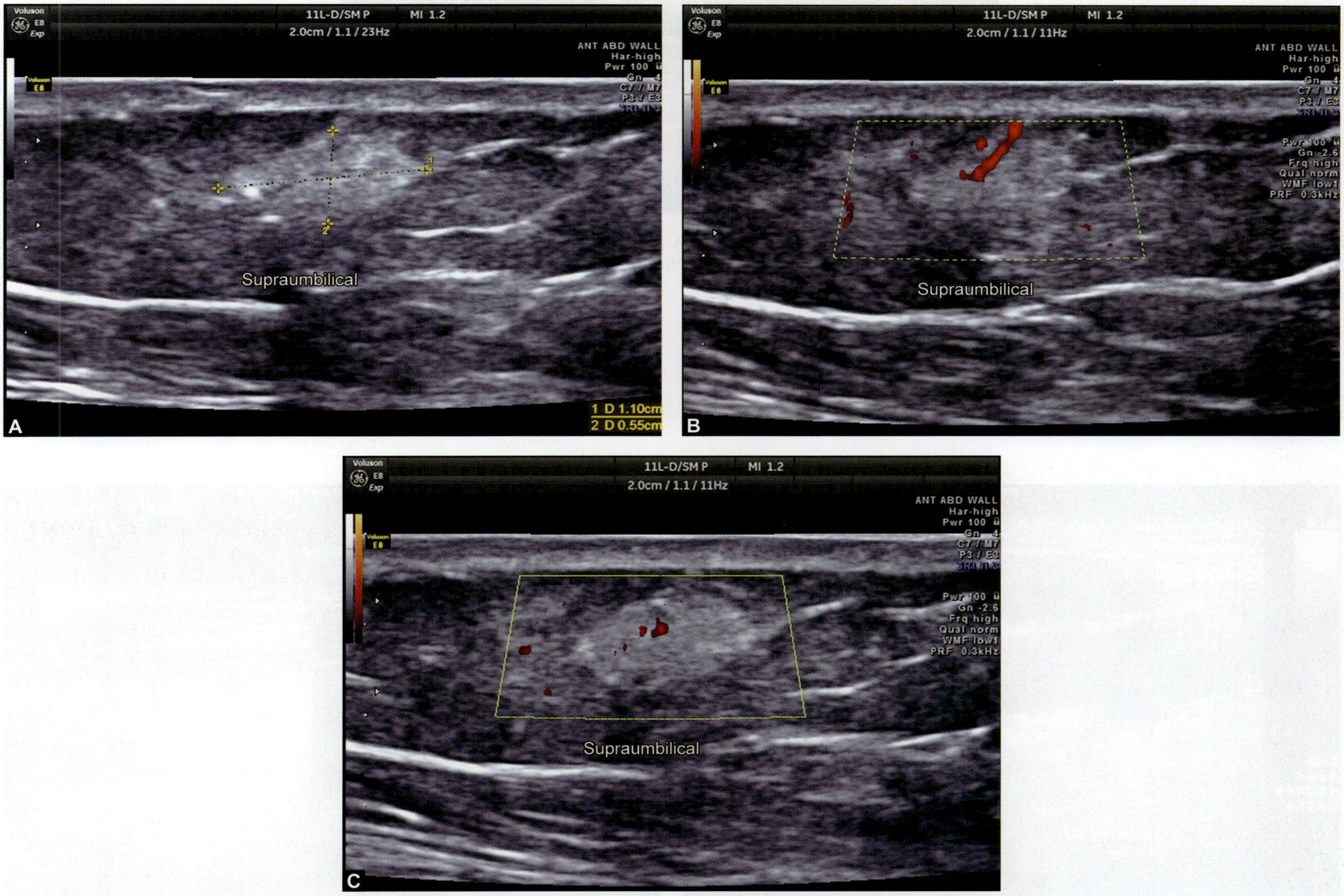

FIGURES 15.51A to C: Anterior abdominal wall lipoma. A patient presented with small nodular shadow in the anterior abdominal wall supraumbilical region. HRSG shows a well-defined echogenic soft tissue mass in supraumbilical region. It measures 10 x 6 mm in size. It is homogeneous in texture. Echo-texture is similar to the fat. No evidence of any calcification is seen it. No cystic degeneration is seen. Findings are suggestive of lipoma.

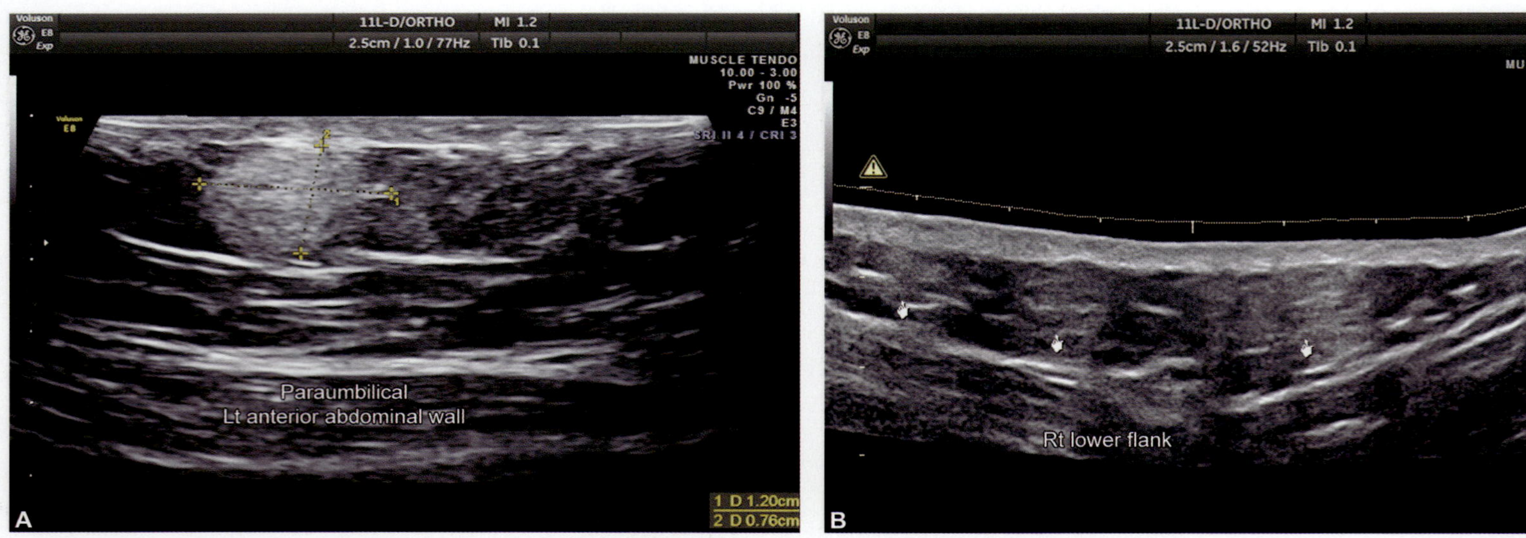

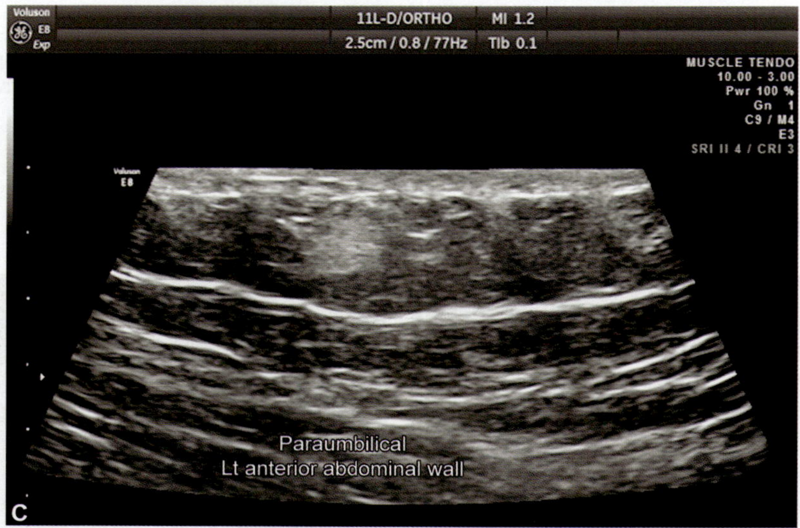

FIGURES 15.52A to C: Multiple lipomas in anterior abdominal wall. A patient presented with multiple nodular shadows in left anterior abdominal wall paraumbilical region right lower flank. HRSG shows well-defined echogenic masses in anterior abdominal wall. The echo-texture is similar to the fat suggestive of multiple lipomas.

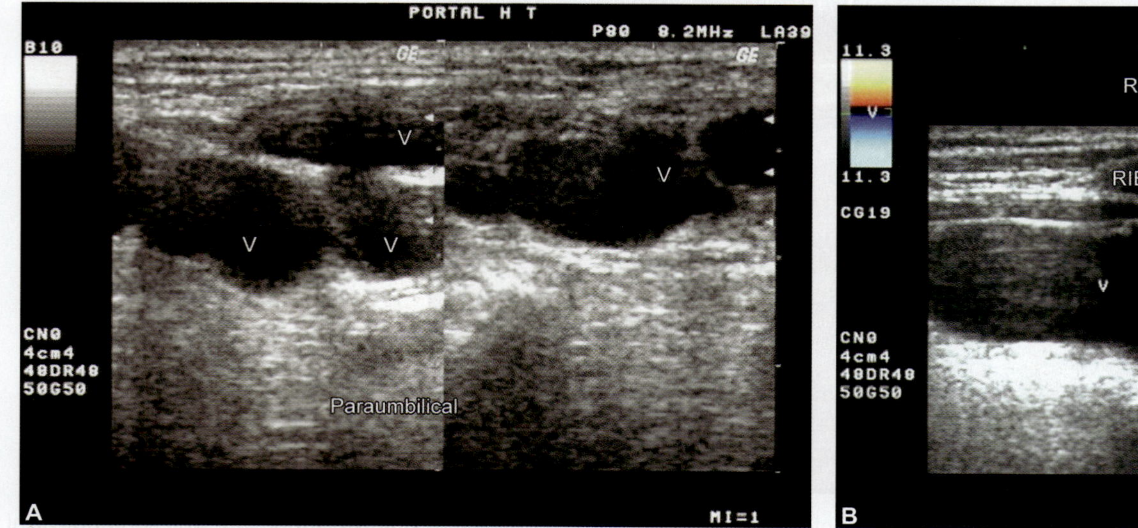

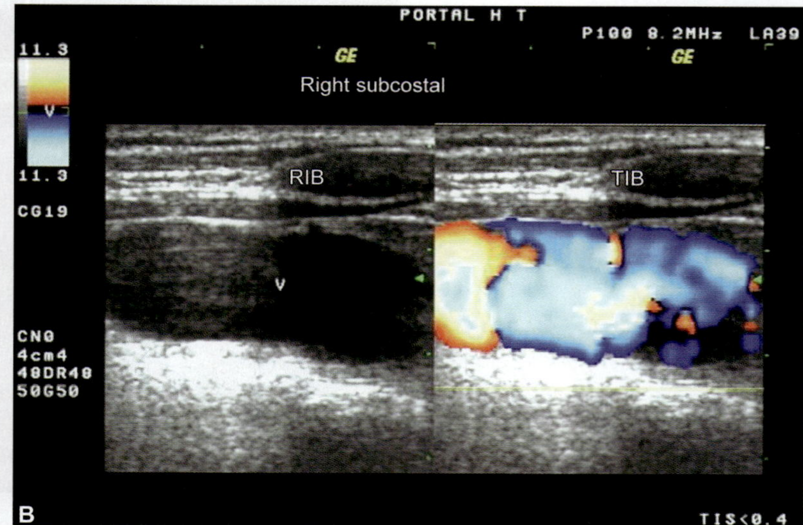

FIGURES 15.53A and B

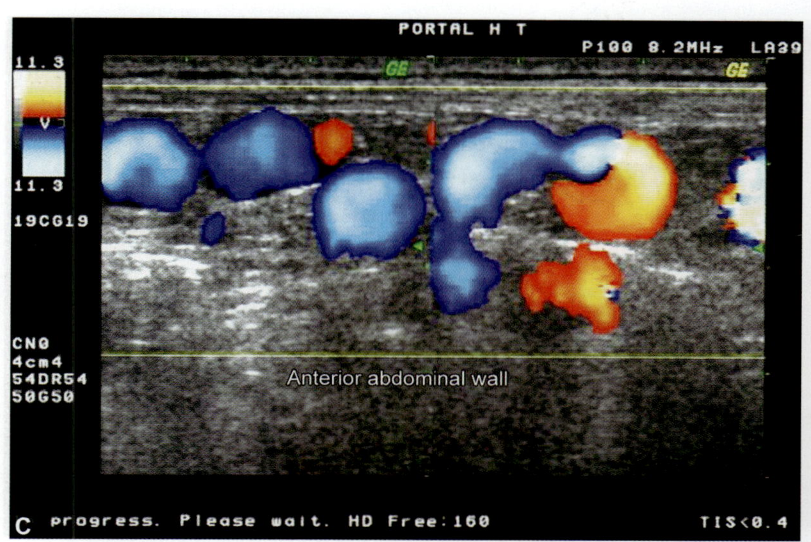

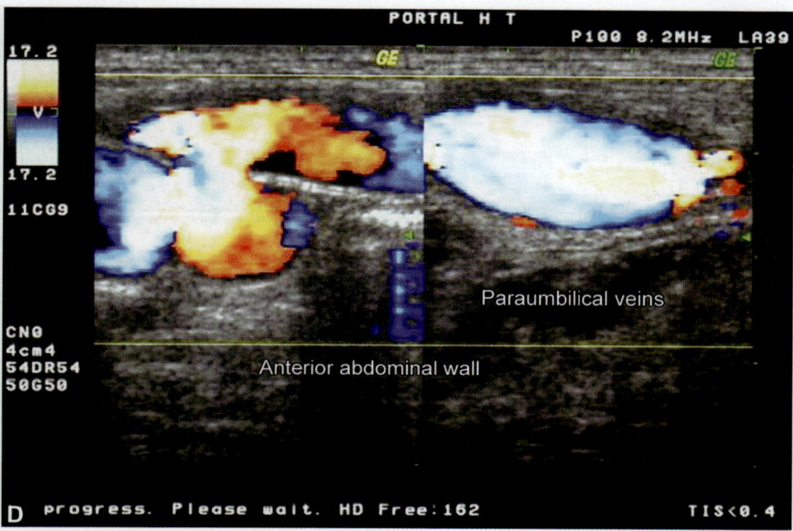

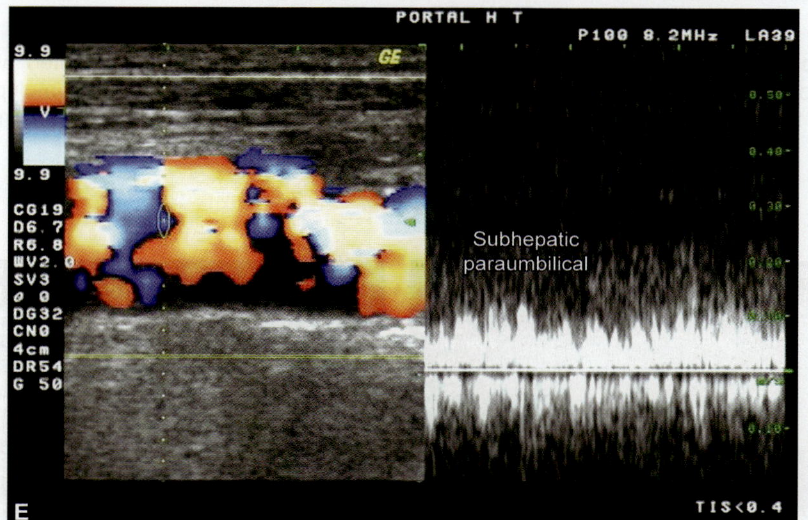

FIGURES 15.53C to E

FIGURES 15.53A to E: Umbilical vein canalization. HRSG shows multiple dilated vessels in the anterior abdominal wall along the paraumbilical region in a known case of portal hypertension. On color Doppler imaging blood flow is seen in it. Multiple dilated varices are also seen along the vein. On color flow imaging, multiple dilated varices are seen along the vein, which are confirmed on color flow imaging. Figure 11.95 Spectral Doppler tracing shows high venous flow in it.

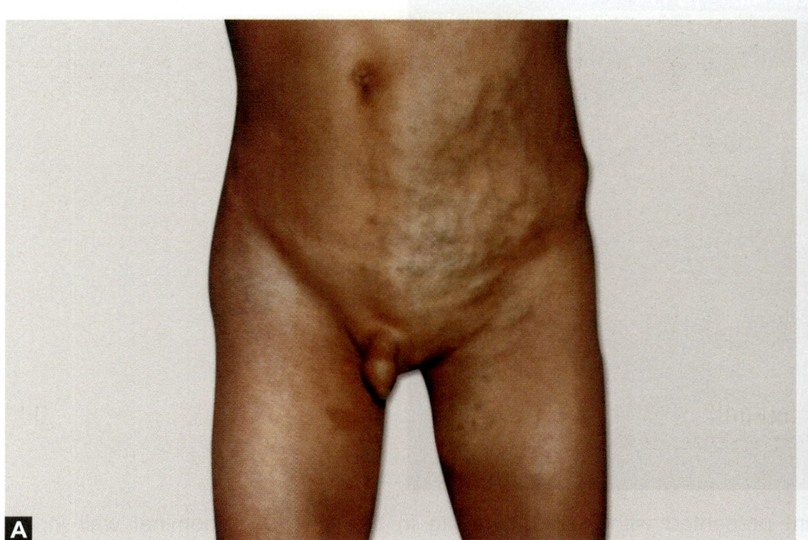

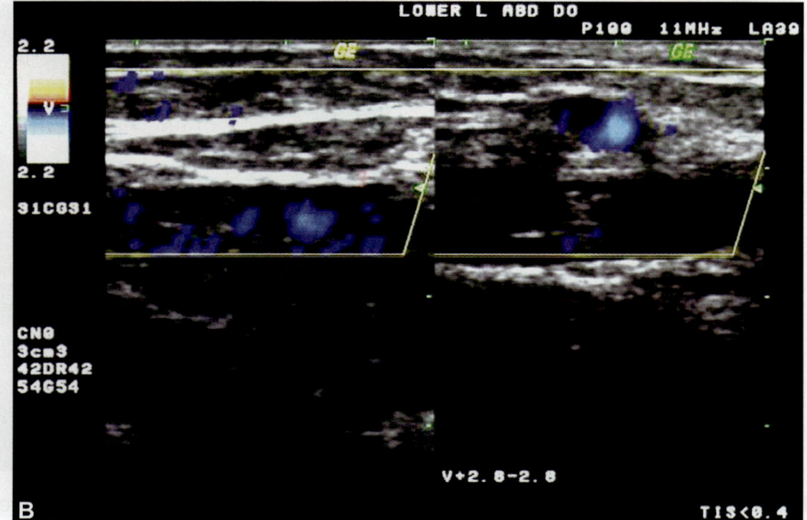

FIGURES 15.54A and B

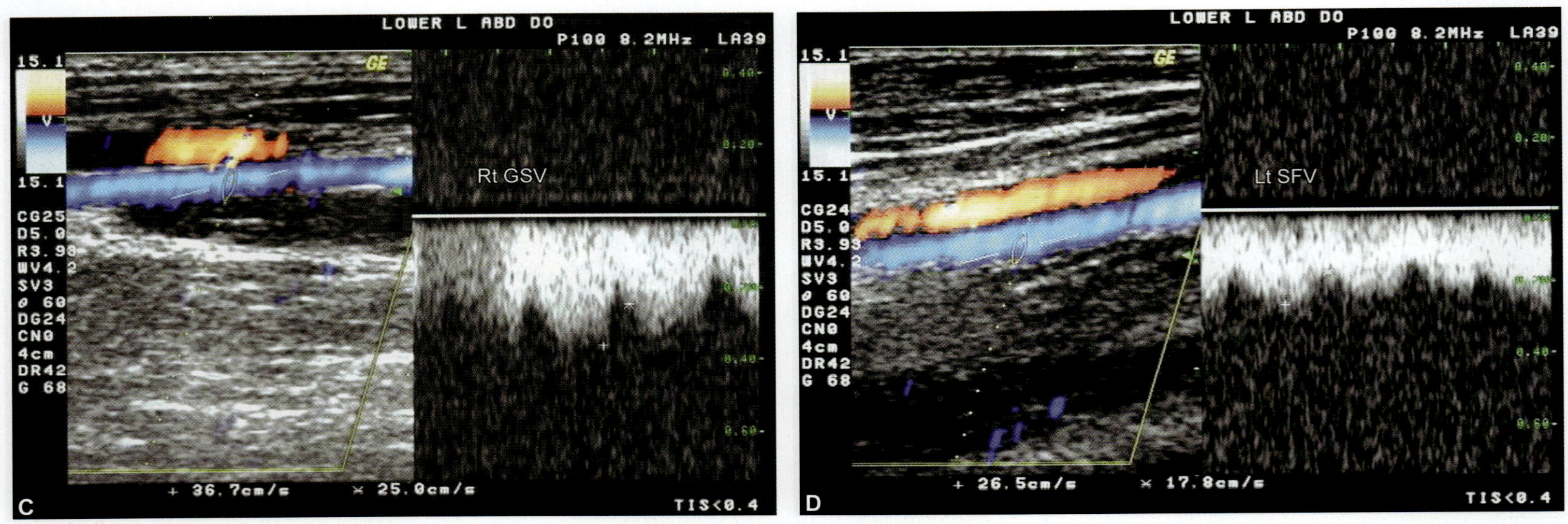

FIGURES 15.54C and D

FIGURES 15.54A to D: Local venous malformation anterior abdominal wall. A young child presented with multiple dilated vessels in the left anterior abdominal wall, inguinal region and the medial part of upper thigh. Color Doppler imaging shows multiple venous dilatations over the anterior abdominal wall. On spectral Doppler tracing, high pulsatile flow is seen in the superficial femoral and common femoral arteries on both sides.

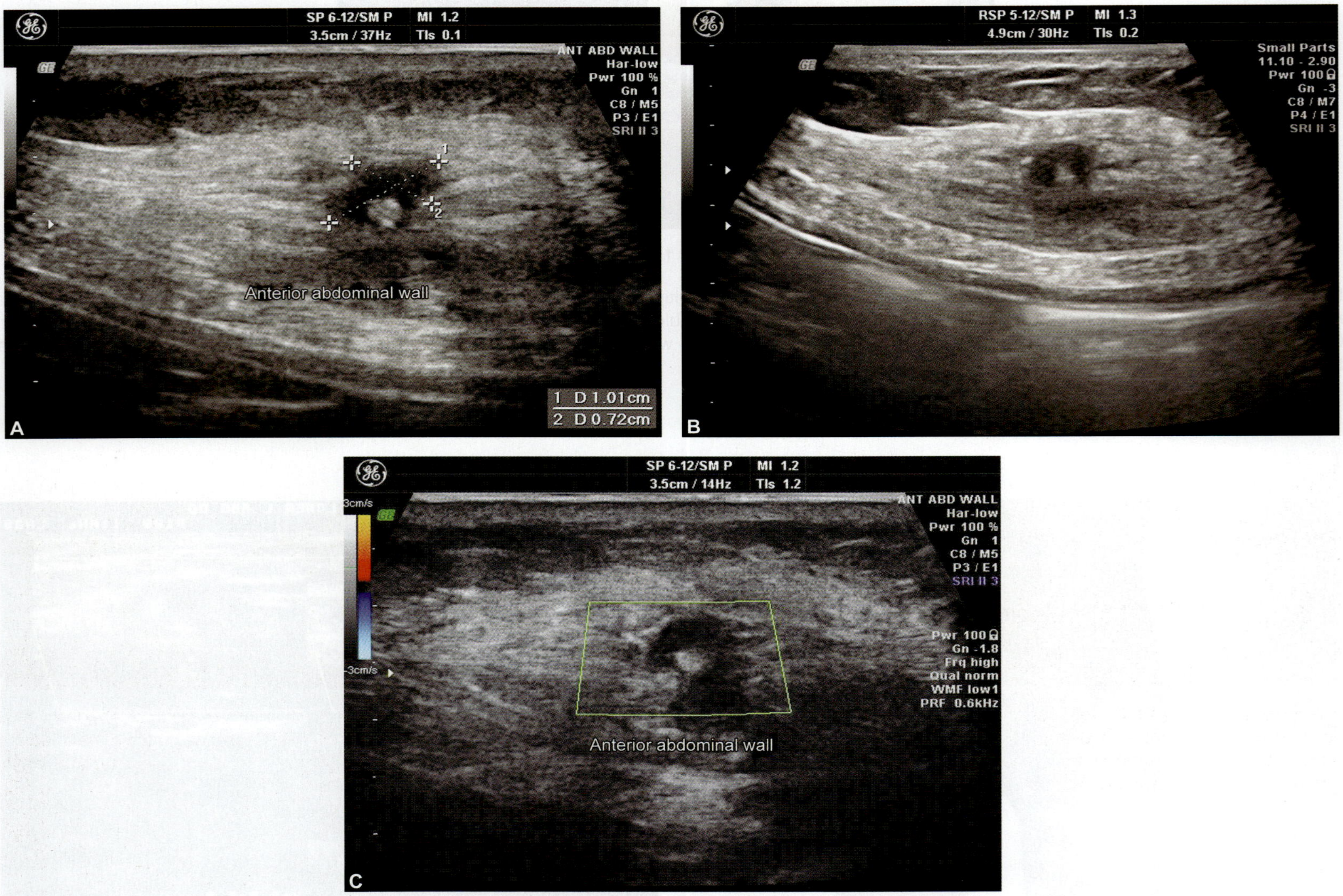

FIGURES 15.55A to C: Anterior abdominal wall cysticercus. A patient presented with painful swelling in the anterior abdominal wall in right hypochondrium. HRSG shows a thick walled cyst in the anterior abdominal wall muscle. An echogenic nidus is seen fixed with the cyst wall. Associated perifocal edema is present. Findings are suggestive of cysticercus cyst.

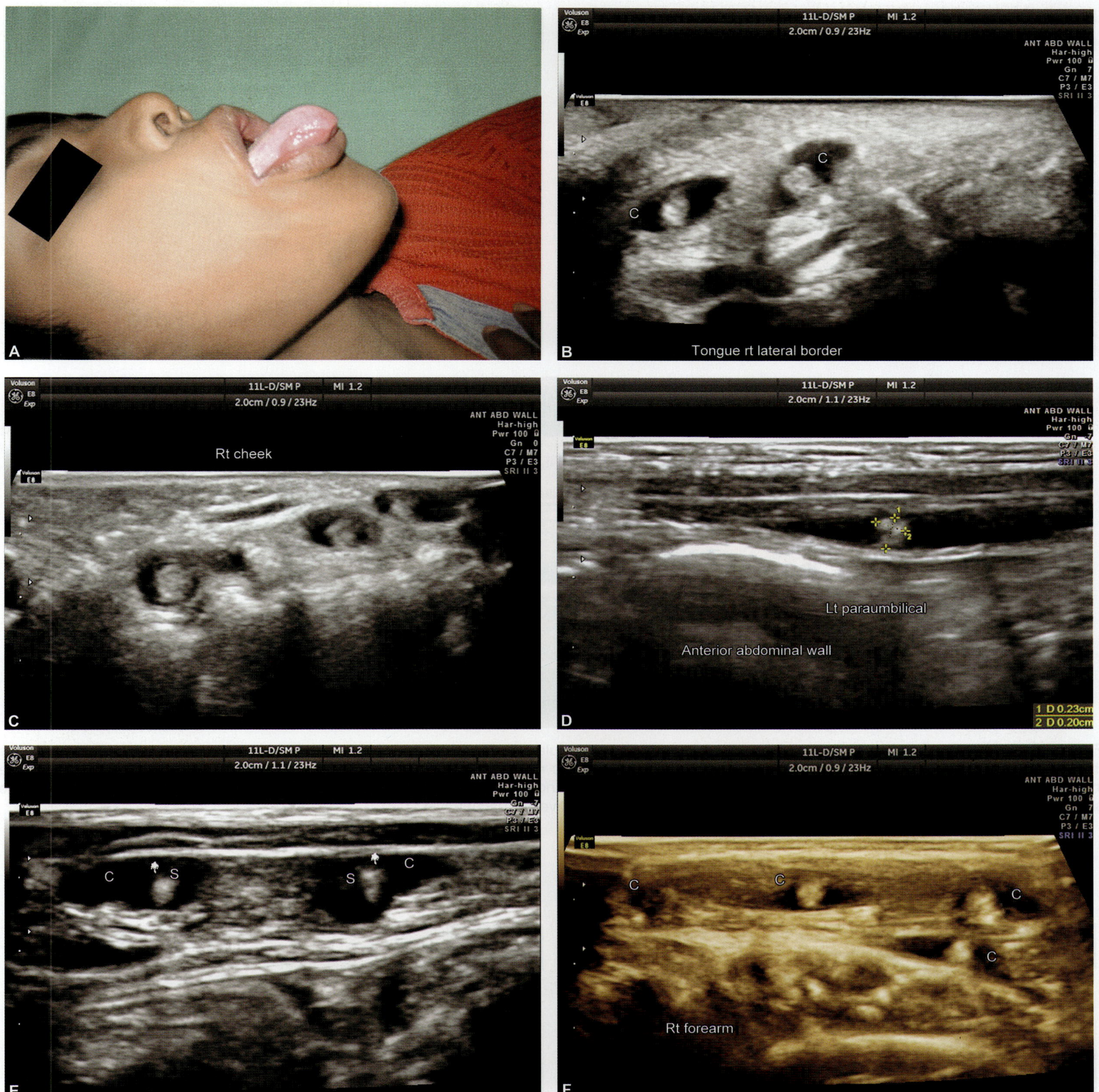

FIGURES 15.56A to F: Cheek, tongue and anterior abdominal wall cysticercus cyst. A young boy presented with multiple nodular shadows over the right cheek, lateral side of right tongue and anterior abdominal wall right paraumbilical region and right arm. HRSG shows multiple well-defined cystic masses. Echogenic nidus are seen in the cyst, which are eccentric in position suggestive of typical cysticercus cyst at different parts of body. This patient is a case of disseminated cysticercus cyst.

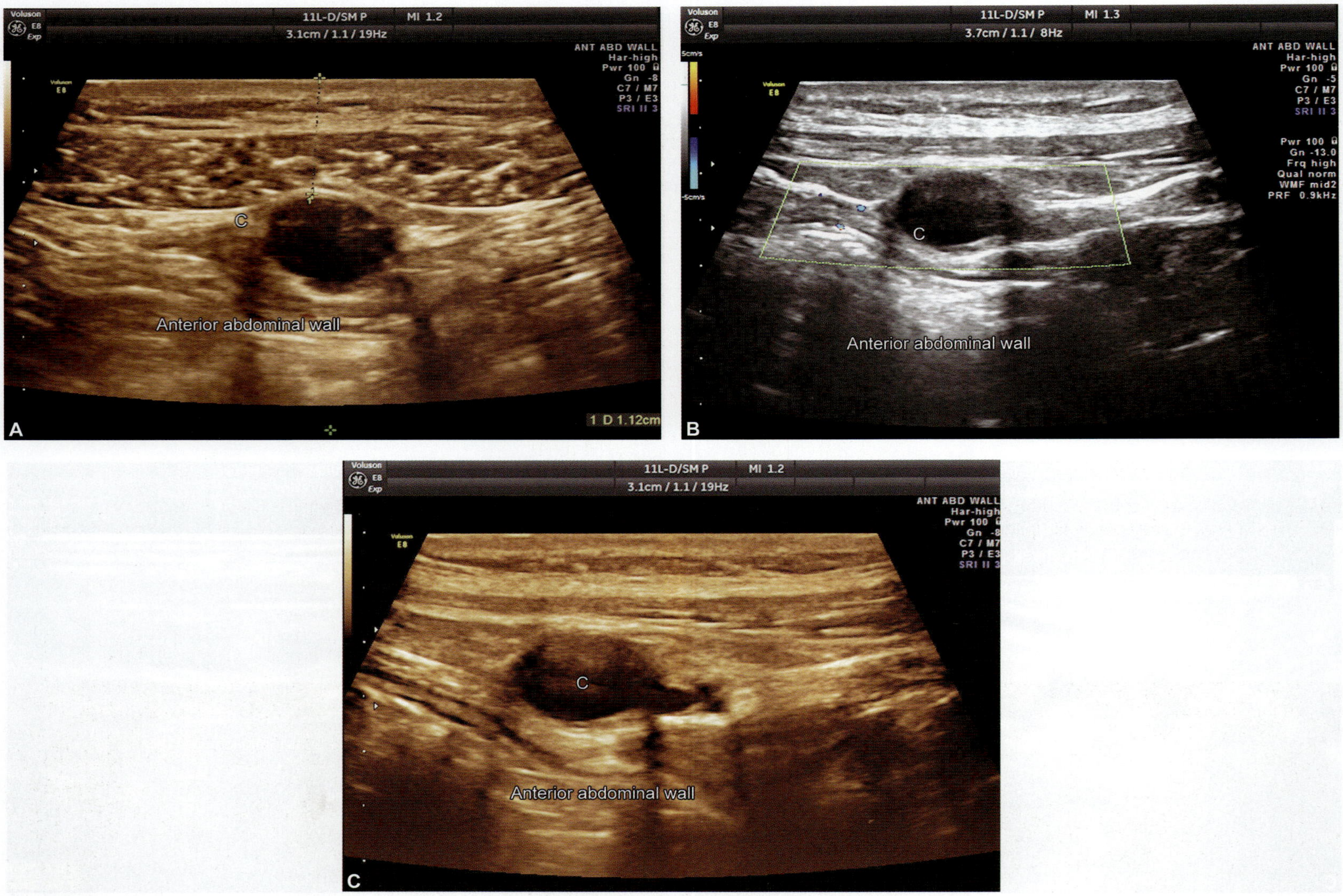

FIGURES 15.57A to C: Urachal cyst. A patient presented with a small nodular shadow in suprapubic region. HRSG shows a well-defined homogeneous thin walled cystic shadow in the anterior abdominal wall in the suprapubic region. It is seen in the mid-line. It shows a tounge like projection on the inferior site of the cyst. No septation seen. No calcification seen. The tounge-like projection measures 7 x 2 mm in size. It is 1.2mm deep from the skin. On color flow imaging, no flow is seen into it. Findings are suggestive of urachal cyst.

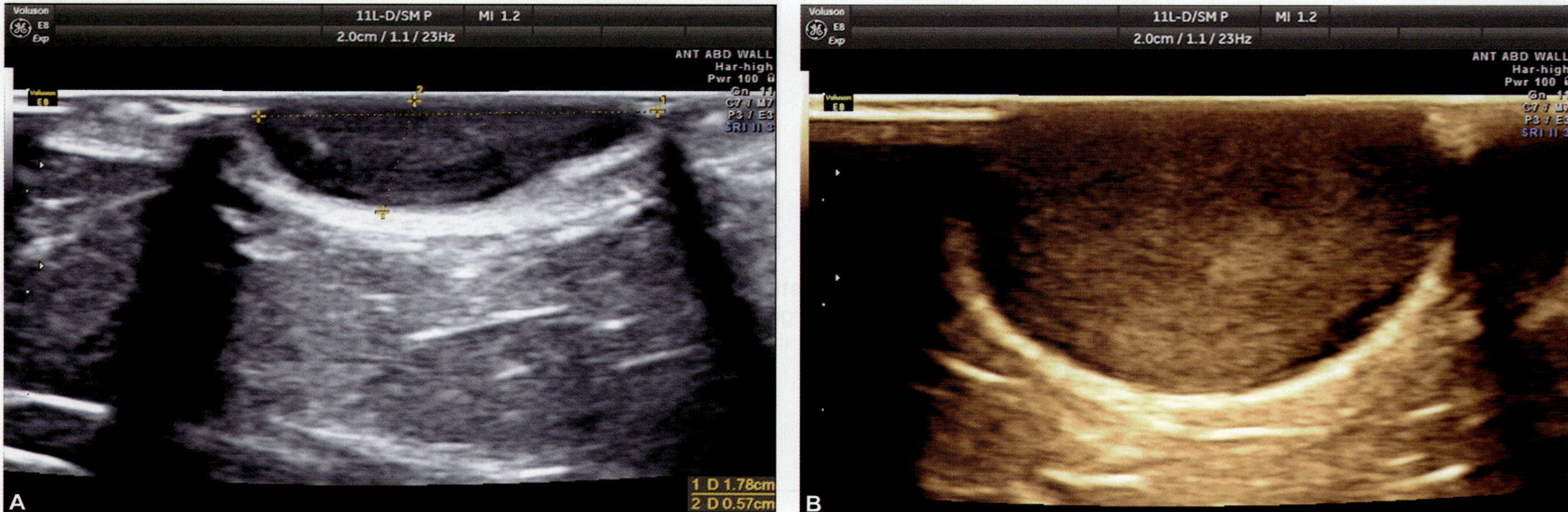

FIGURES 15.58A and B

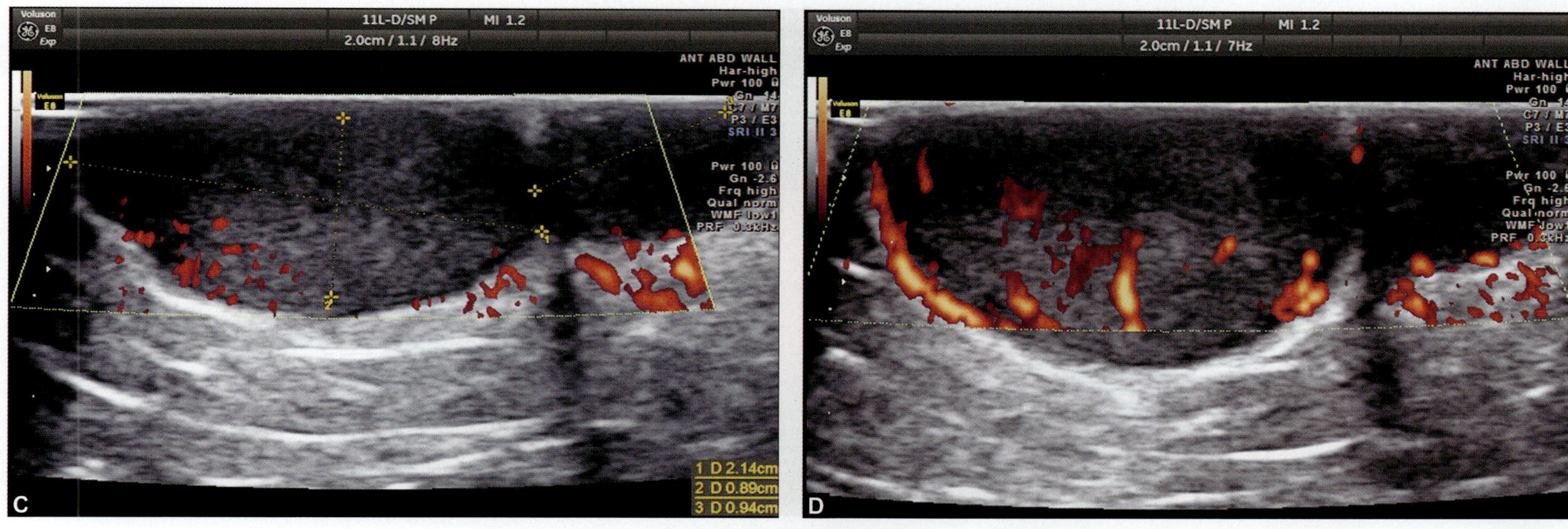

FIGURES 15.58C and D

FIGURES 15.58A to D: Multiple neurofibromas in anterior abdominal wall. A patient presented with multiple nodular shadows on anterior abdominal wall. HRSG shows multiple well-defined hypoechoic nodular masses in anterior abdominal wall. They are seen in subcutaneous tissue plane and discrete in distribution. They are hypoechoic in texture with homogeneous in texture. Few masses show lobulation. On color flow imaging, few vessels are seen feeding the masses. Findings are suggestive of multiple discrete neurofibromas.

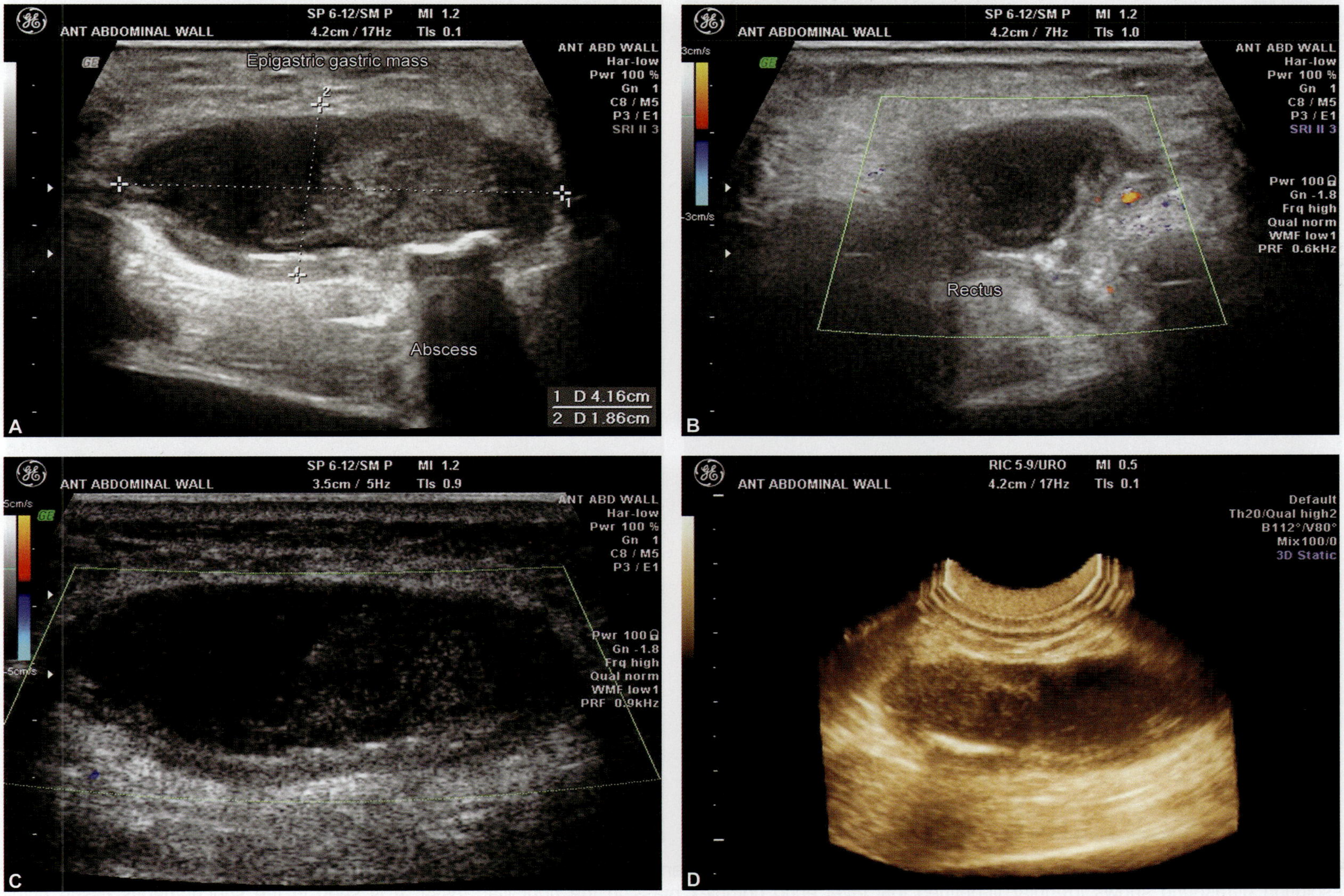

FIGURES 15.59A to D

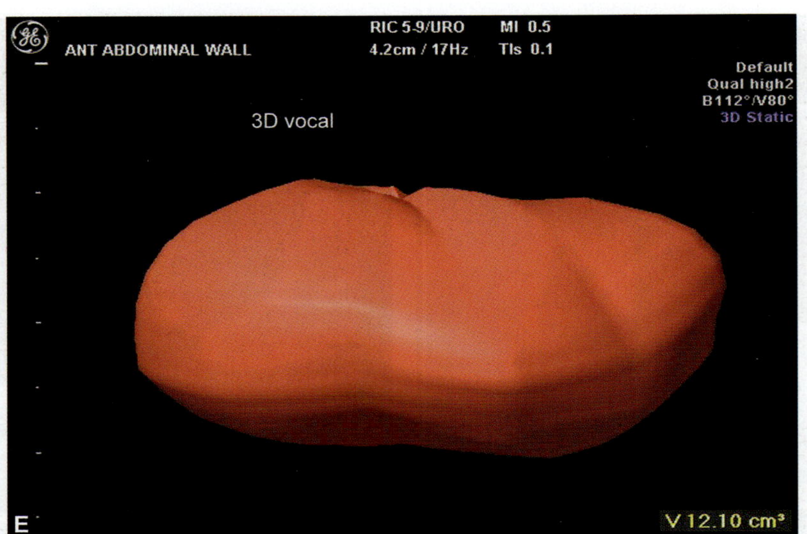

FIGURE 15.59E

FIGURES 15.59A to E: Organized abscess. A patient presented with loculated semi-hard mass in epigastric region in anterior abdominal wall. HRSG show a thick walled low level echo complex mass in the epigastric region. It is seen in the subcutaneous plane. Thick echoes are seen into it. Echogenic debris is also seen. There is also evidence of peripheral calcification seen in the mass. On color flow imaging, no flow is seen into it. No septation is seen. The rectus abdominal muscle is normal. 3D vocal imaging shows semi-solid nature of the mass. Aspiration biopsy confirms organized abscess.

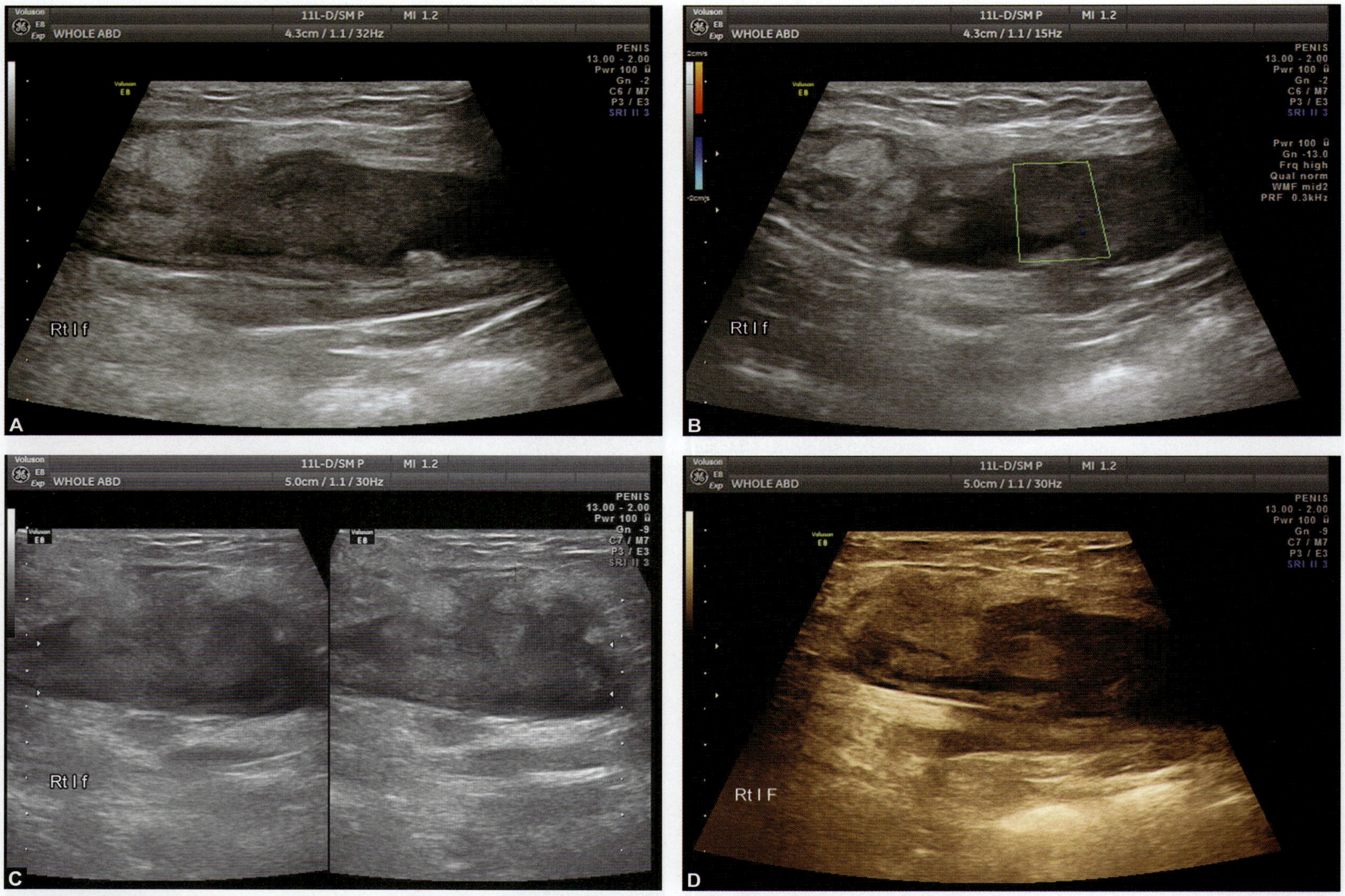

FIGURES 15.60A to D: Caseating necrotic nodal mass. A patient presented with painful soft tissue mass in right iliac fossa in its lower part. High resolution ultrasound shows irregular ill-defined low level echo complex mass in the right iliac fossa. It is seen in the subcutaneous tissue plane. Thick echoes are seen in it. It is 60 x 20 mm in size and volume is 20 cc. Associated perifocal edema is present. But no cystic degeneration is seen. No other focal mass lesion is seen. No free fluid is seen in the peritoneal cavity. No retroperitoneal lymph node enlargement is seen. Findings are suggestive of caseating necrotic nodal mass. The patient was known case of abdominal tuberculosis.

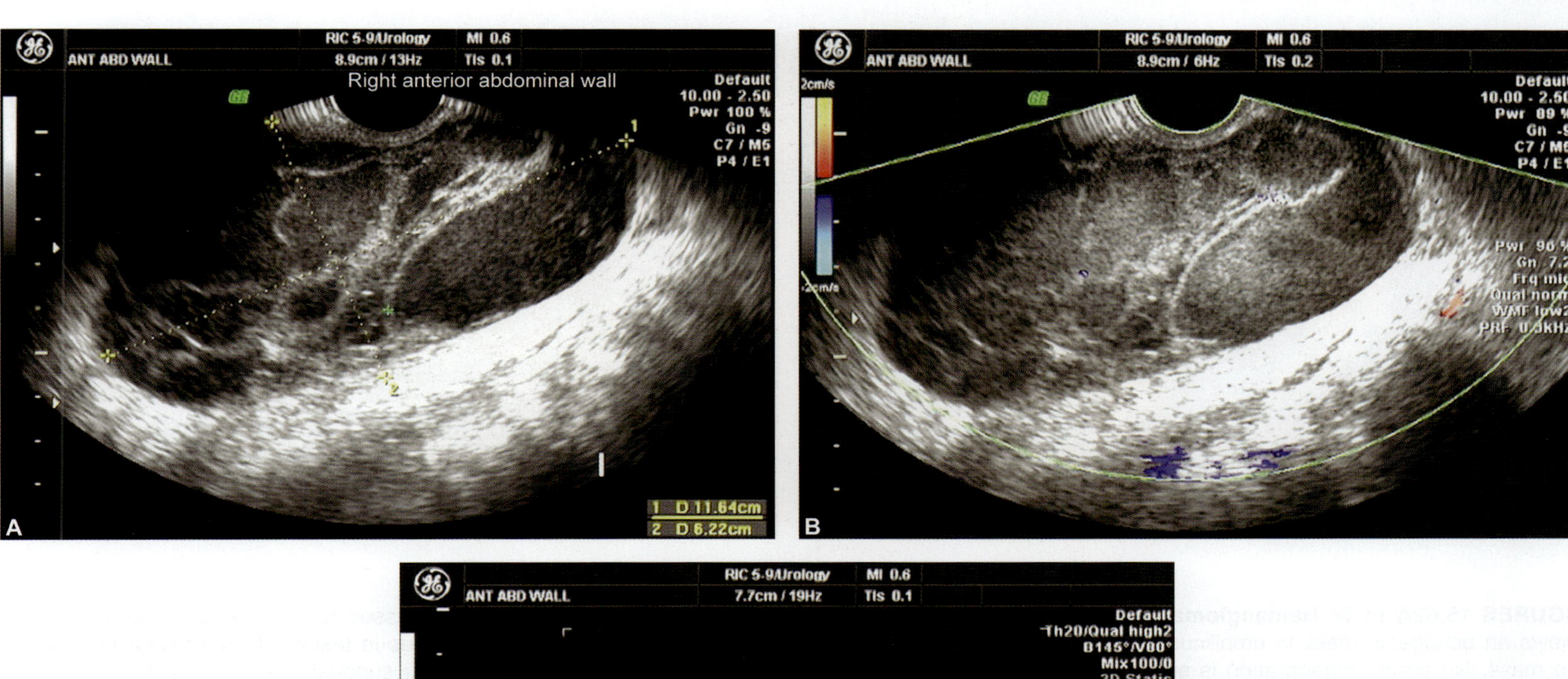

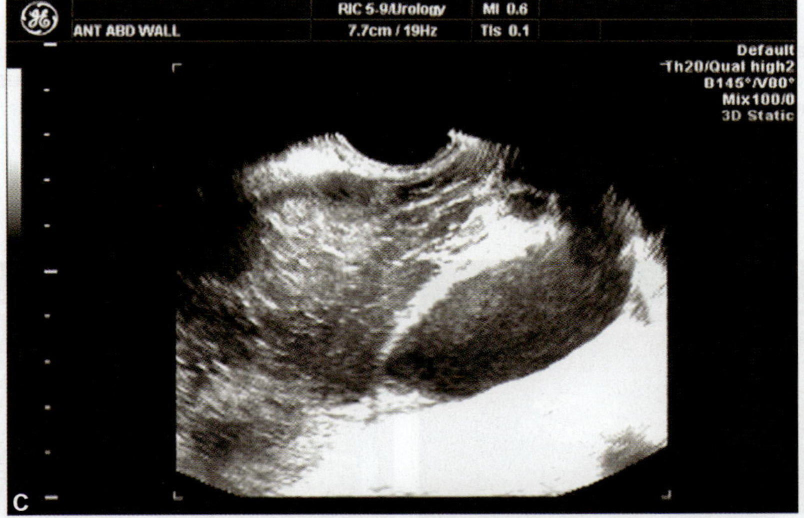

FIGURES 15.61A to C: FTC operated liposarcoma anterior abdominal wall collection. An operated patient of liposarcoma presented with cystic mass confined to the anterior abdominal wall on the right side. HRSG shows a big loculated collection in the anterior abdominal wall. Thick echoes are seen floating into it. On color flow imaging no flow is seen in the collection. Echogenic septa are also seen in it. 3D imaging of the same patient shows the collection confined to the anterior abdominal wall.

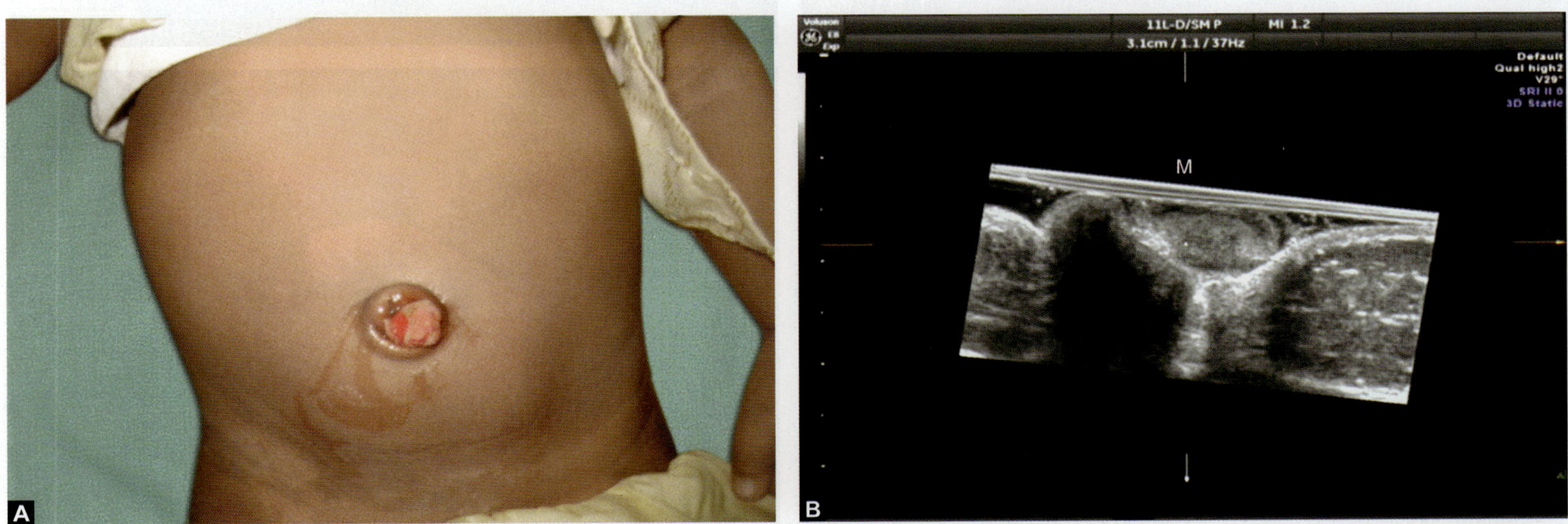

FIGURES 15.62A and B

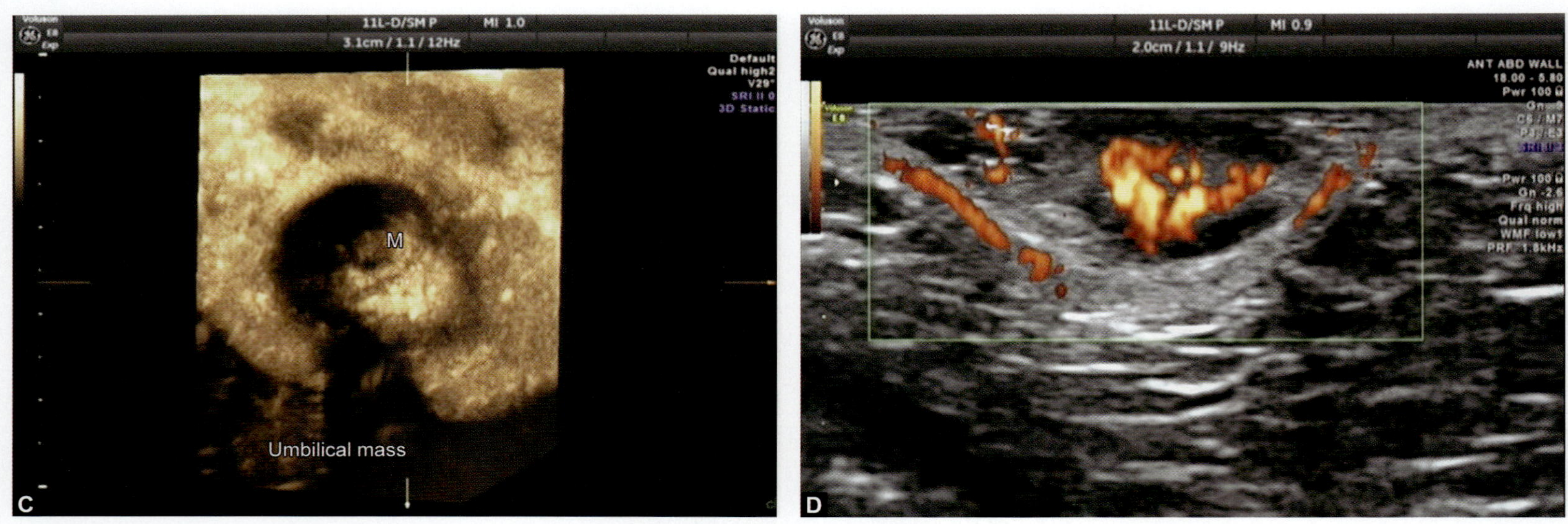

FIGURES 15.62C and D

FIGURES 15.62A to D: Hemangioma in anterior abdominal wall. A 8-month-old baby presented with soft tissue mass over the umbilicus. HRSG shows an echogenic mass in umbilicus. 3D ultrasound shows mass is confined to umbilicus. It is homogeneous in texture. No calcification is seen in the mass. No cystic degeneration is seen. On color flow imaging, multiple vessels are seen feeding the mass suggestive of hemangiomatous mass.

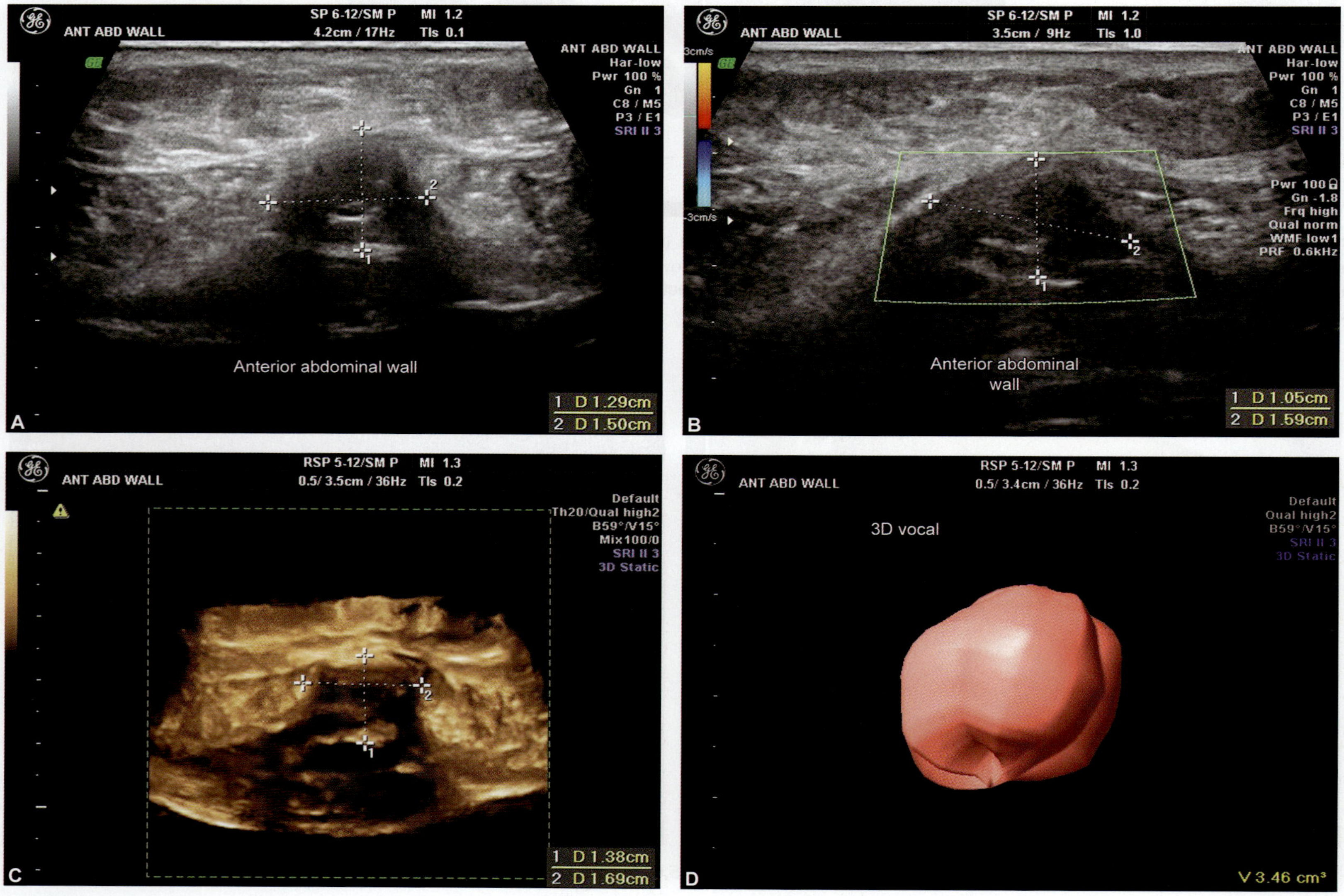

FIGURES 15.63A to D: Desmoid tumor of anterior abdominal wall. A patient presented with hard nodular mass in the anterior abdominal wall. HRSG shows a well-defined hypoechoic mass in anterior abdominal wall below the epigastric region. It is seen in the rectus muscle. Peripheral calcification is seen in it. But no cystic degeneration is seen. 3D ultrasound shows the mass very clearly. Biopsy of the mass confirms desmoid tumor.

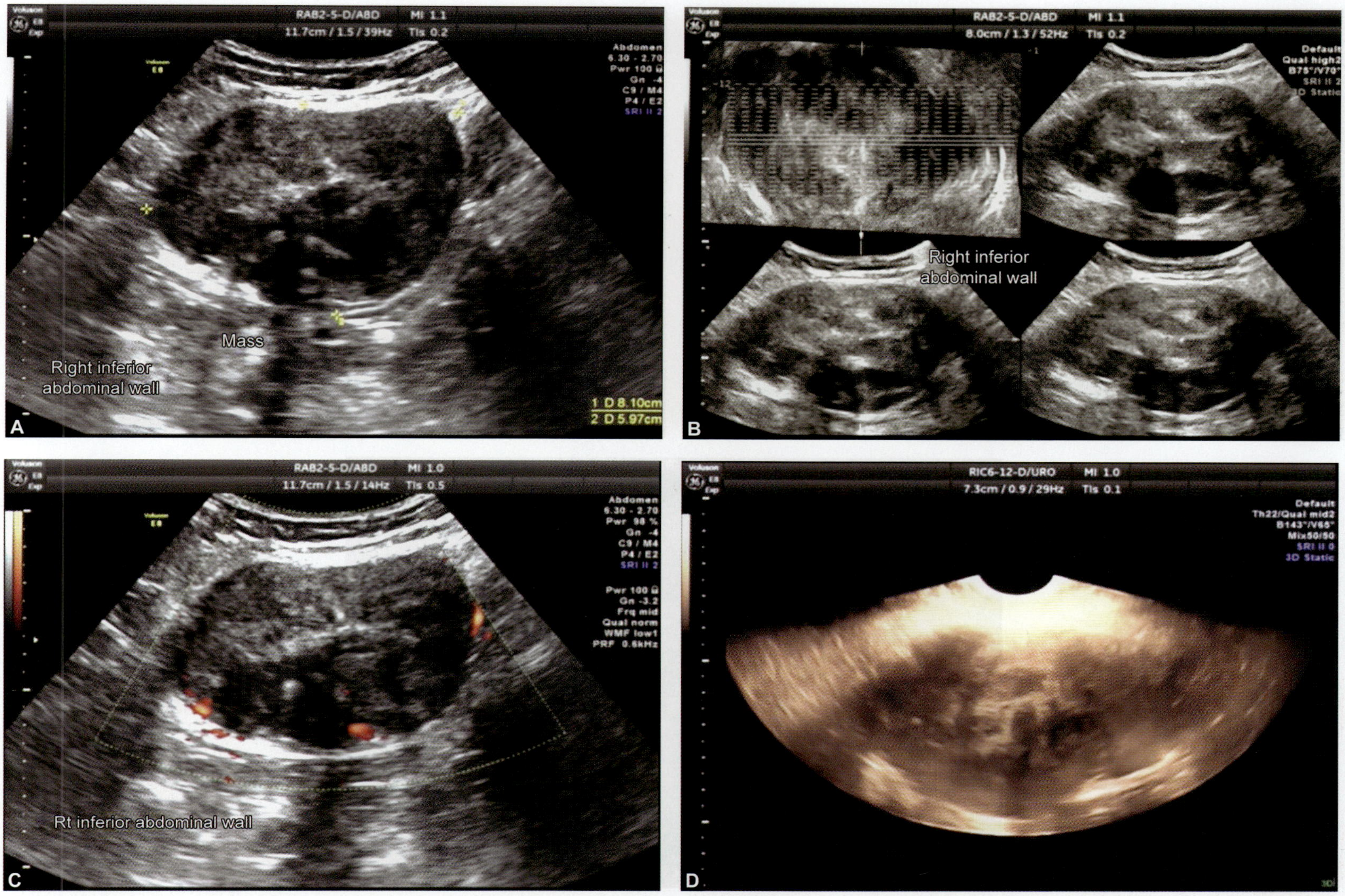

FIGURES 15.64A to D: Desmoid tumor in anterior abdominal wall. A patient presented with well-defined well-encapsulated mass in anterior abdominal wall. HRSG shows a big well-encapsulated soft tissue mass in the anterior abdominal wall in right iliac fossa. The mass is predominantly solid. Echogenic foci are also seen in it. No calcification is seen in the mass. On color flow imaging, poor flow is seen in the mass. 3D ultrasound shows the mass clearly. Biopsy of the mass confirms big desmoid tumor.

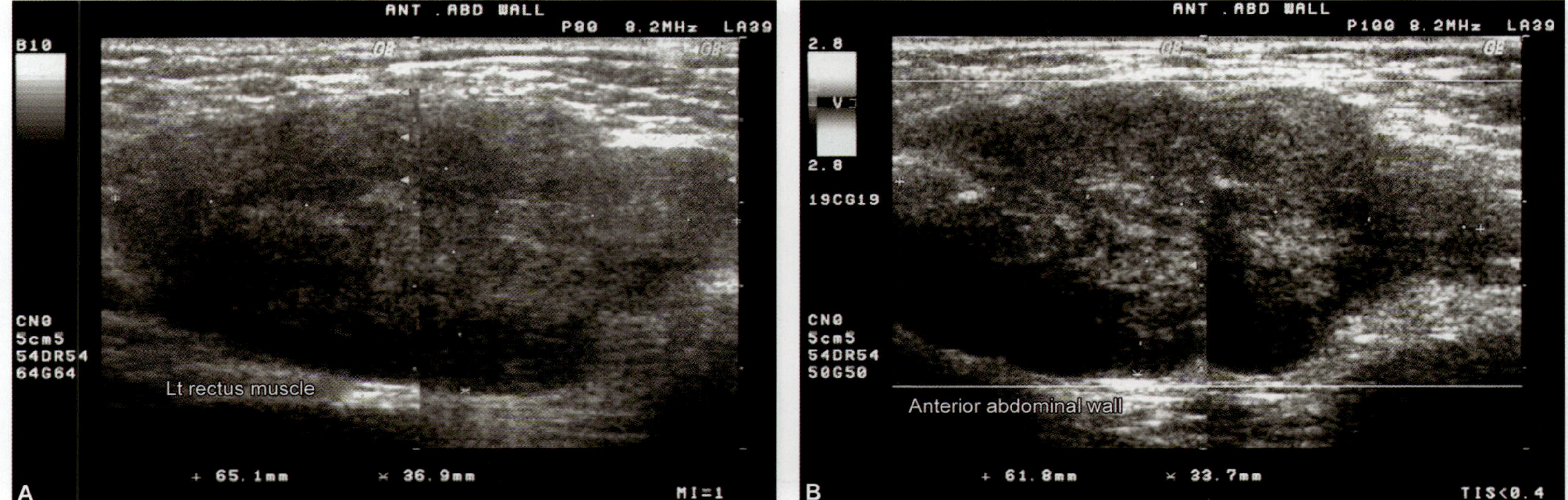

FIGURES 15.65A and B

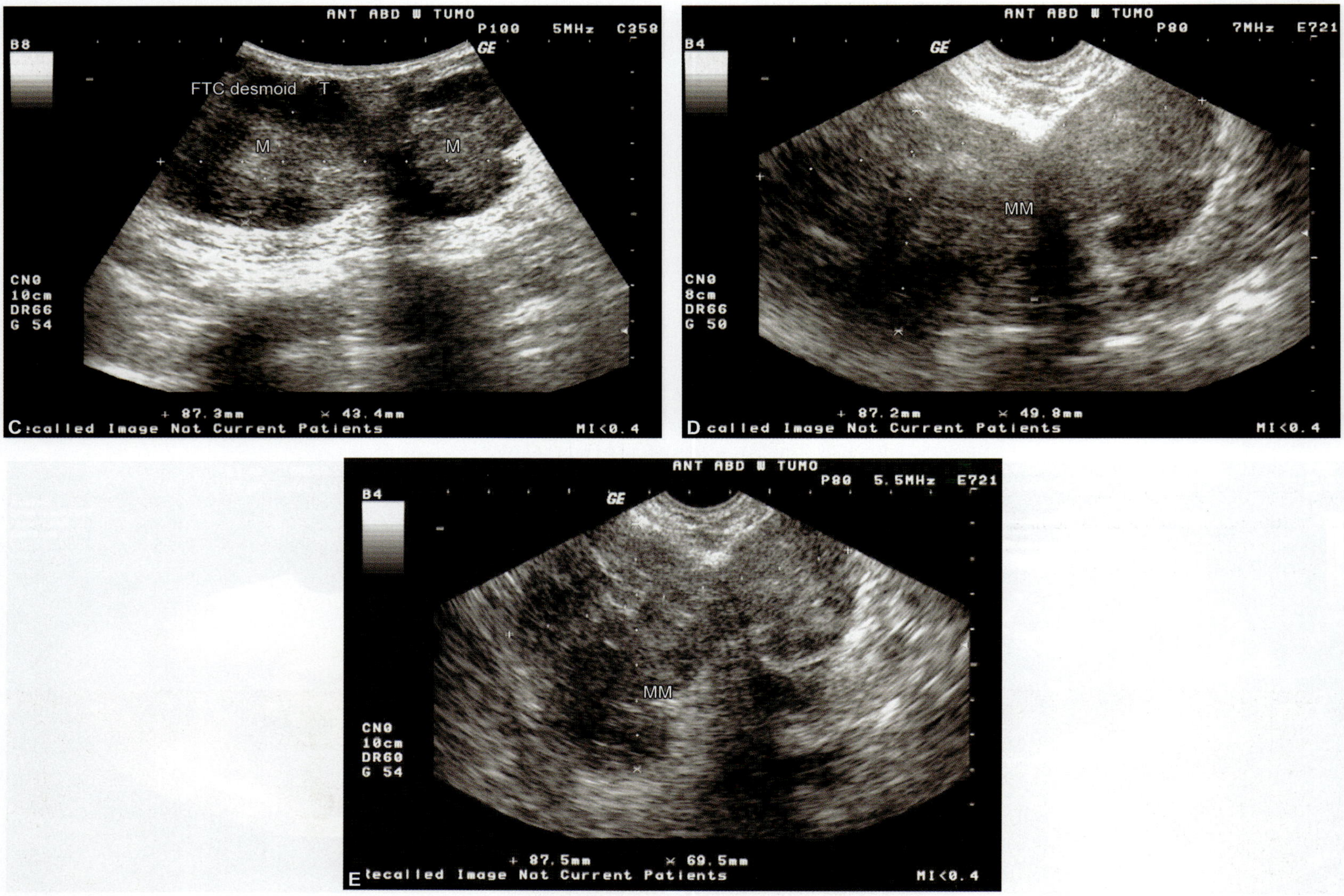

FIGURES 15.65C to E

FIGURES 15.65A to E: Big desmoid tumor in the anterior abdominal wall. A patient presented with big mass in the anterior abdominal wall. HRSG shows a well-defined lobulated mass in the anterior abdominal wall. The mass is homogeneous in texture. No calcification or necrosis is seen. On color flow imaging, no flow was seen in the mass. Biopsy of the mass confirms desmoid tumor.

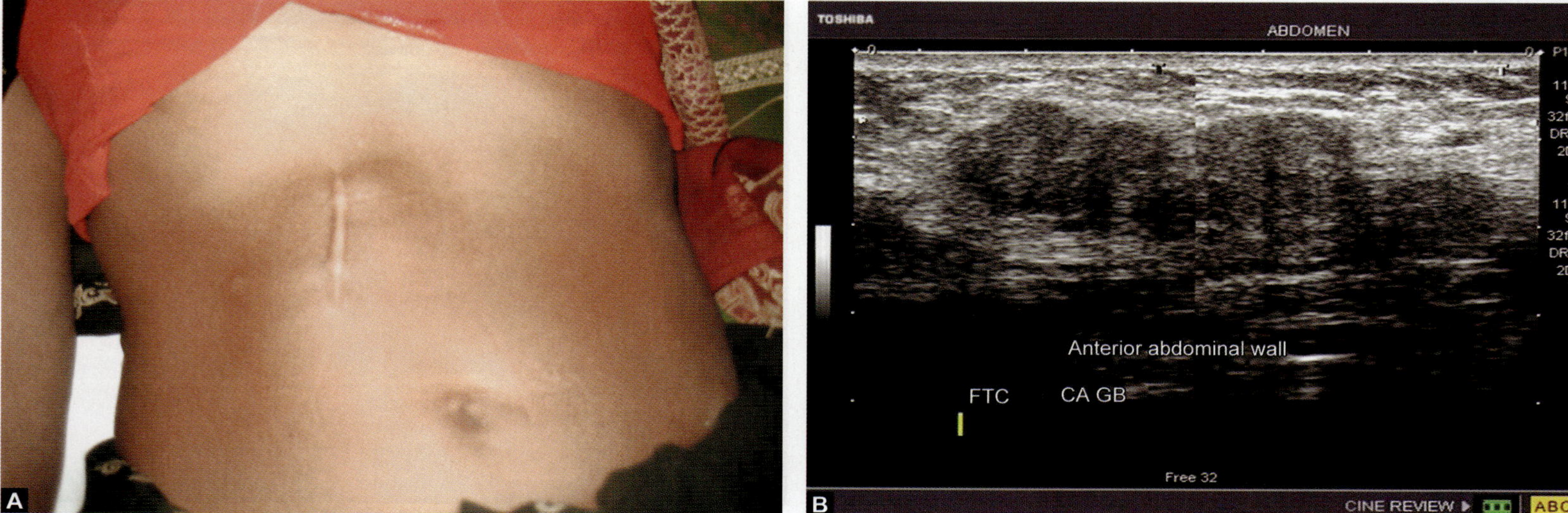

FIGURES 15.66A and B

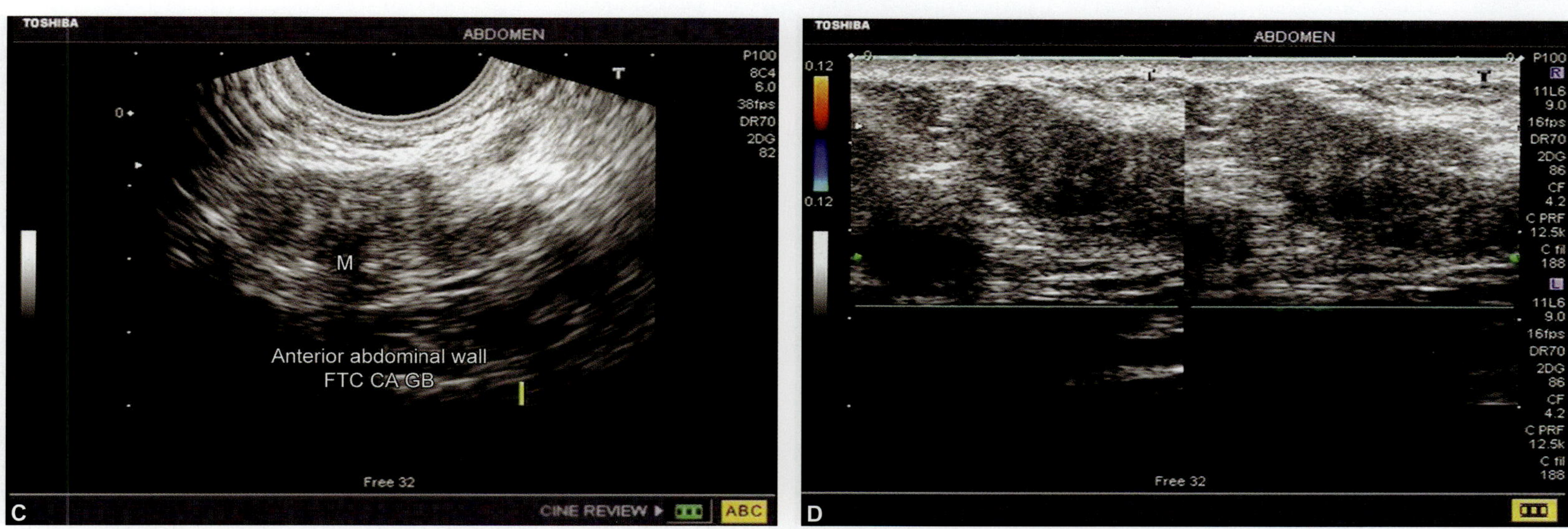

FIGURES 15.66C and D

FIGURES 15.66A to D: Carcinoma gallbladder metastasis in anterior abdominal wall. An operated case of carcinoma gallbladder presented with soft tissue mass in anterior abdominal wall along the suture line. HRSG shows a big irregular ill-defined lobulated mass in anterior abdominal wall. It is hypoechoic in texture. No calcification or cystic degeneration is seen in the mass. On color flow imaging, poor flow is seen in the mass. The mass is seen invading the anterior abdominal wall muscles. Biopsy confirms metastatic deposits of CA GB.

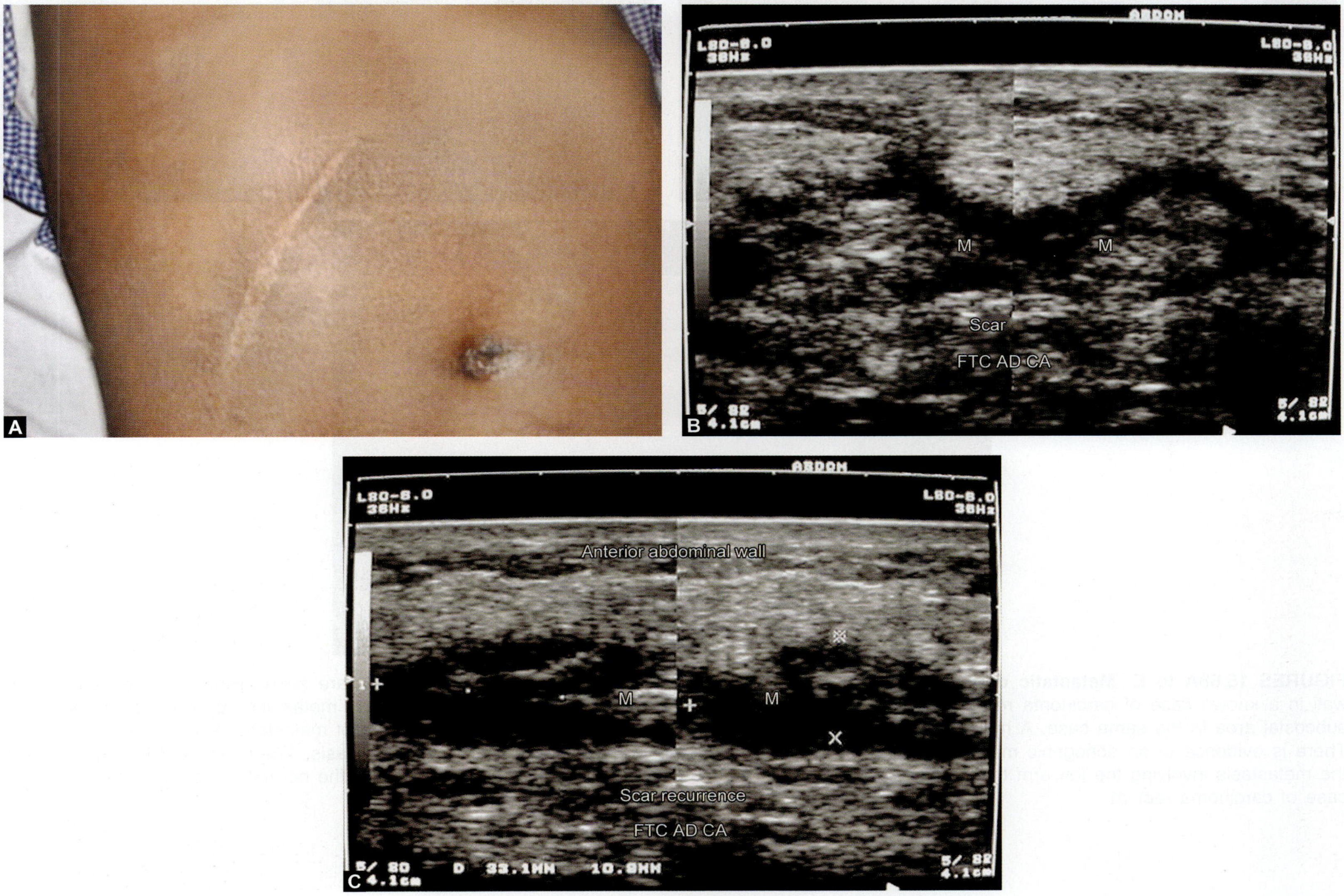

FIGURES 15.67A to C: Scar recurrence of operated carcinoma gallbladder. A young man operated for carcinoma gallbladder presented with soft tissue bulge along the suture line. HRSG shows infiltrating metastatic deposits in the anterior abdominal wall and along the suture line suggestive of scar recurrence. The mass is also seen infiltrating the parietal layer of the abdominal wall and going posteriorly.

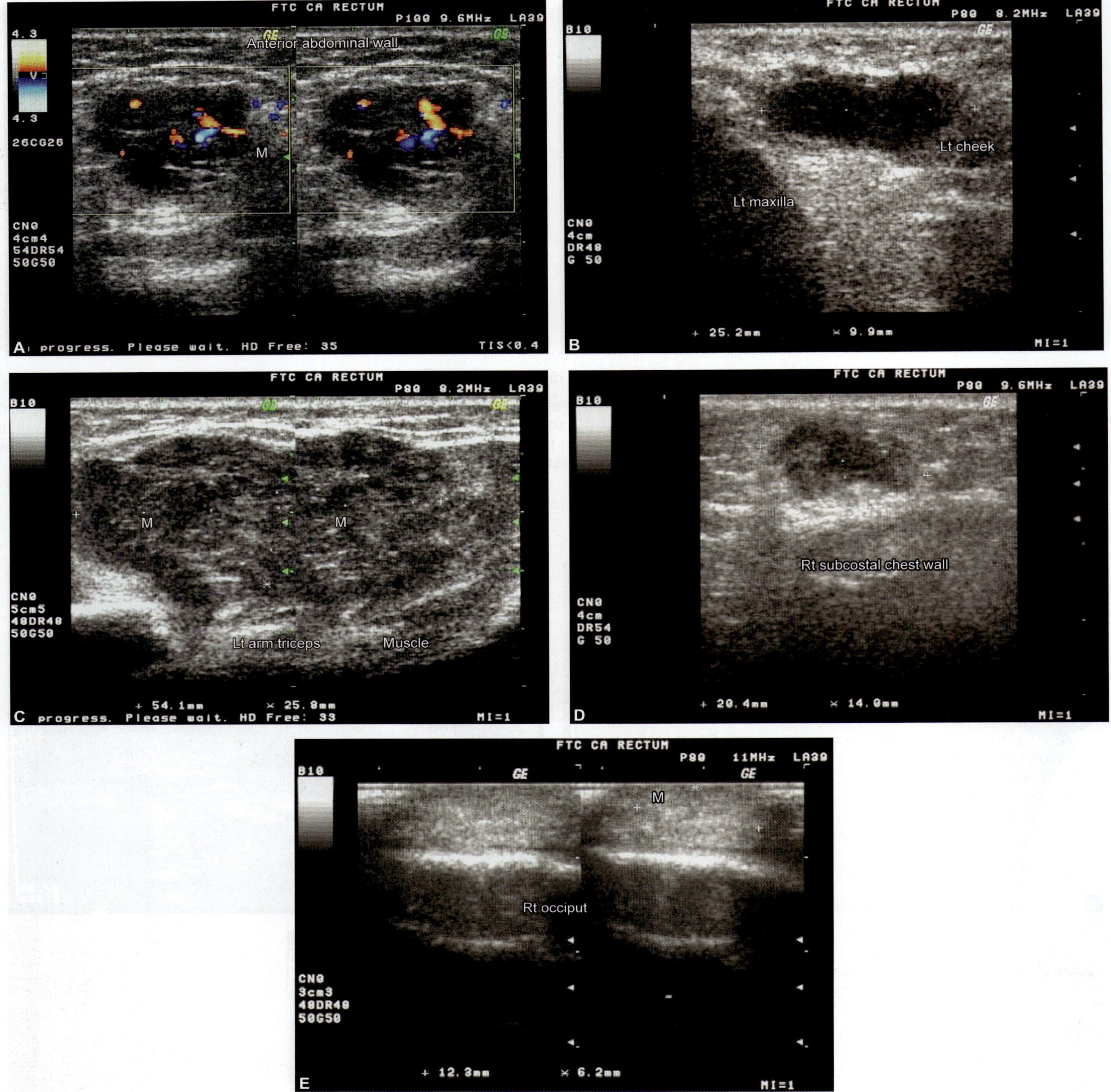

FIGURES 15.68A to E: Metastatic deposits in carcinoma rectum. Irregular hypoechoic nodular masses are seen infiltrating anterior abdominal wall in a known case of carcinoma rectum. On color flow imaging, moderate flow is seen in the mass. The metastatic deposit is also seen in left subcostal area in the same case. A hypoechoic irregular mass is also seen over the left maxilla suggestive of metastatic deposit in the same case. There is evidence of an echogenic mass seen over the right occiput in the same case suggestive of metastasis. The muscle infiltration is seen by the metastasis involving the left arm triceps muscle. Big irregular mass is seen in the muscle belly distorting the normal muscle texture in the same case of carcinoma rectum.

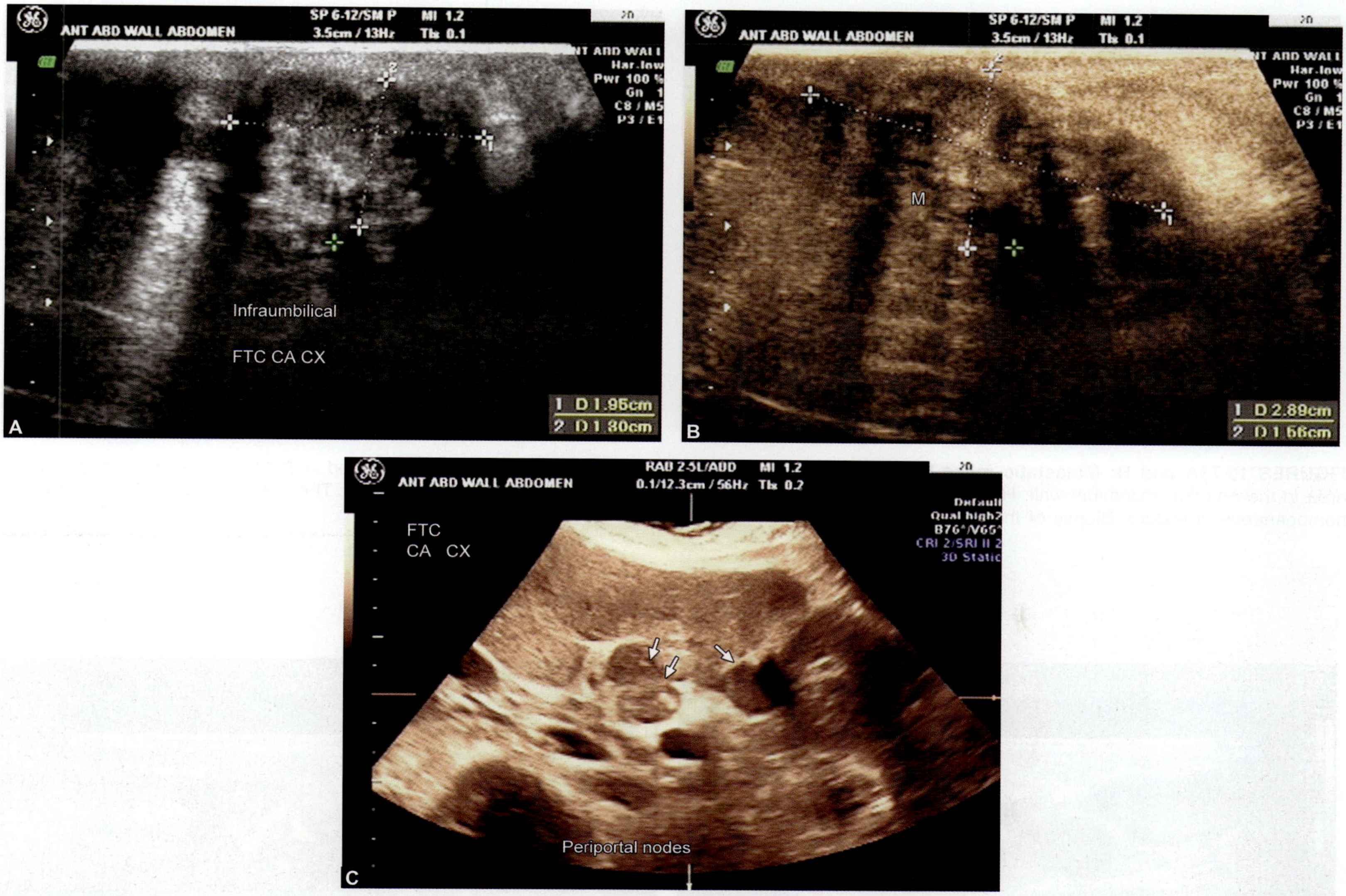

FIGURES 15.69A to C: Carcinoma cervix metastasis. A patient known case of operated carcinoma cervix presented with mass in suprapubic region in anterior abdominal wall. HRSG shows a big irregular ill-defined heterogeneous mass in anterior abdominal wall suprapubic region. The mass is predominantly solid. No calcification or cystic degeneration is seen in the mass. Multiple enlarged nodal shadows are also seen in retroperitoneum and periportal regions suggestive of metastatic nodes. Biopsy of the mass confirms metastatic mass of CA cervix.

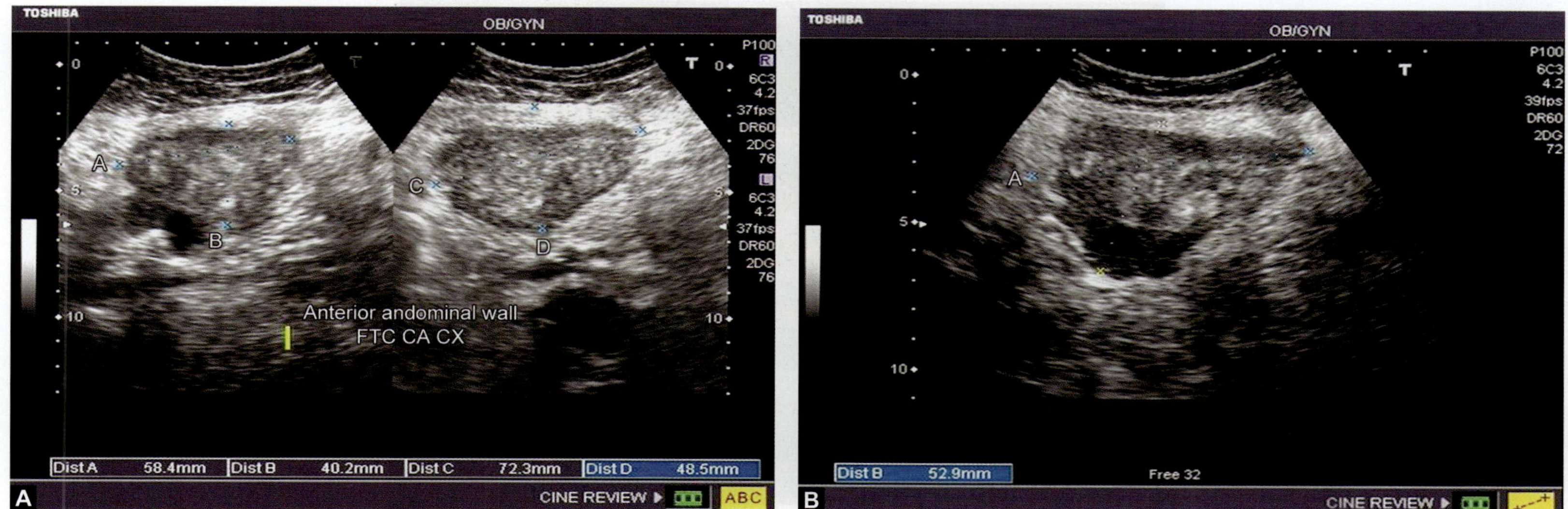

FIGURES 15.70A and B: Metastatic mass of carcinoma cervix. A known case of operated carcinoma cervix presented with hard lump in anterior abdominal wall in suprapubic region. HRSG shows a big heterogeneous solid mass in suprapubic region suggestive of metastatic mass of CA cervix. Biopsy of the mass confirms ultrasound findings.

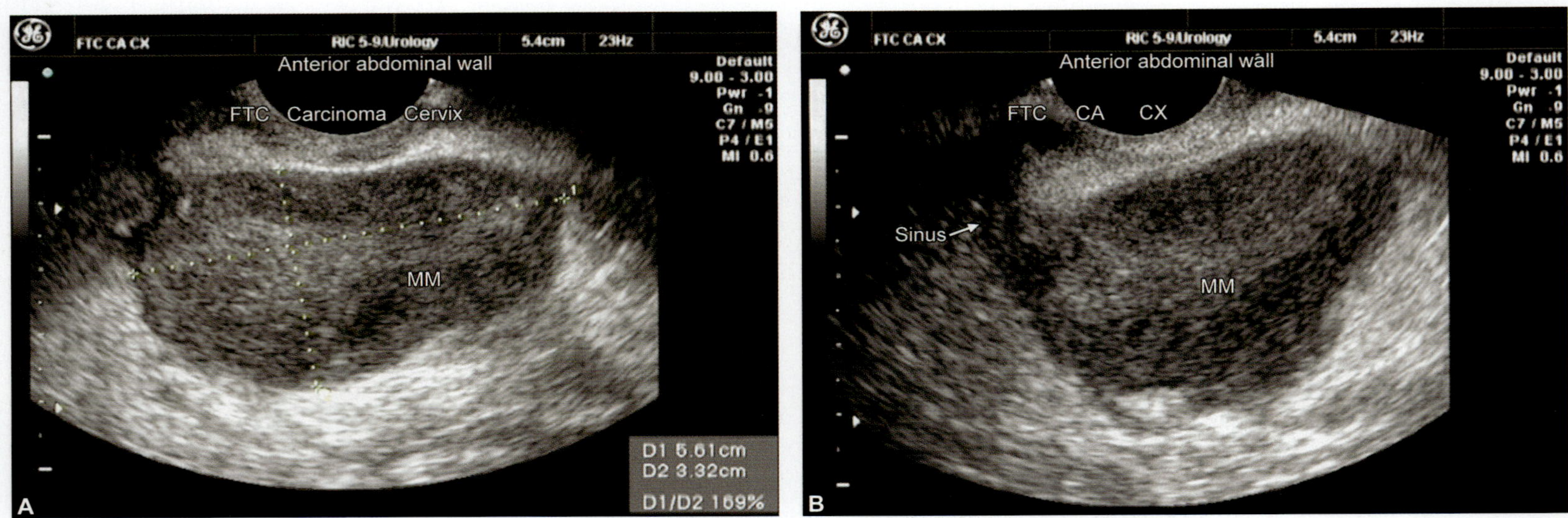

FIGURES 15.71A and B: Metastatic mass from carcinoma cervix. A known patient of CA cervix presented with soft tissue mass in suprapubic area in the anterior abdominal wall. HRSG shows a well-defined irregular mass in the anterior abdominal wall. The mass was irregular in outline but homogeneous in texture. Biopsy of the mass confirms metastatic deposits.

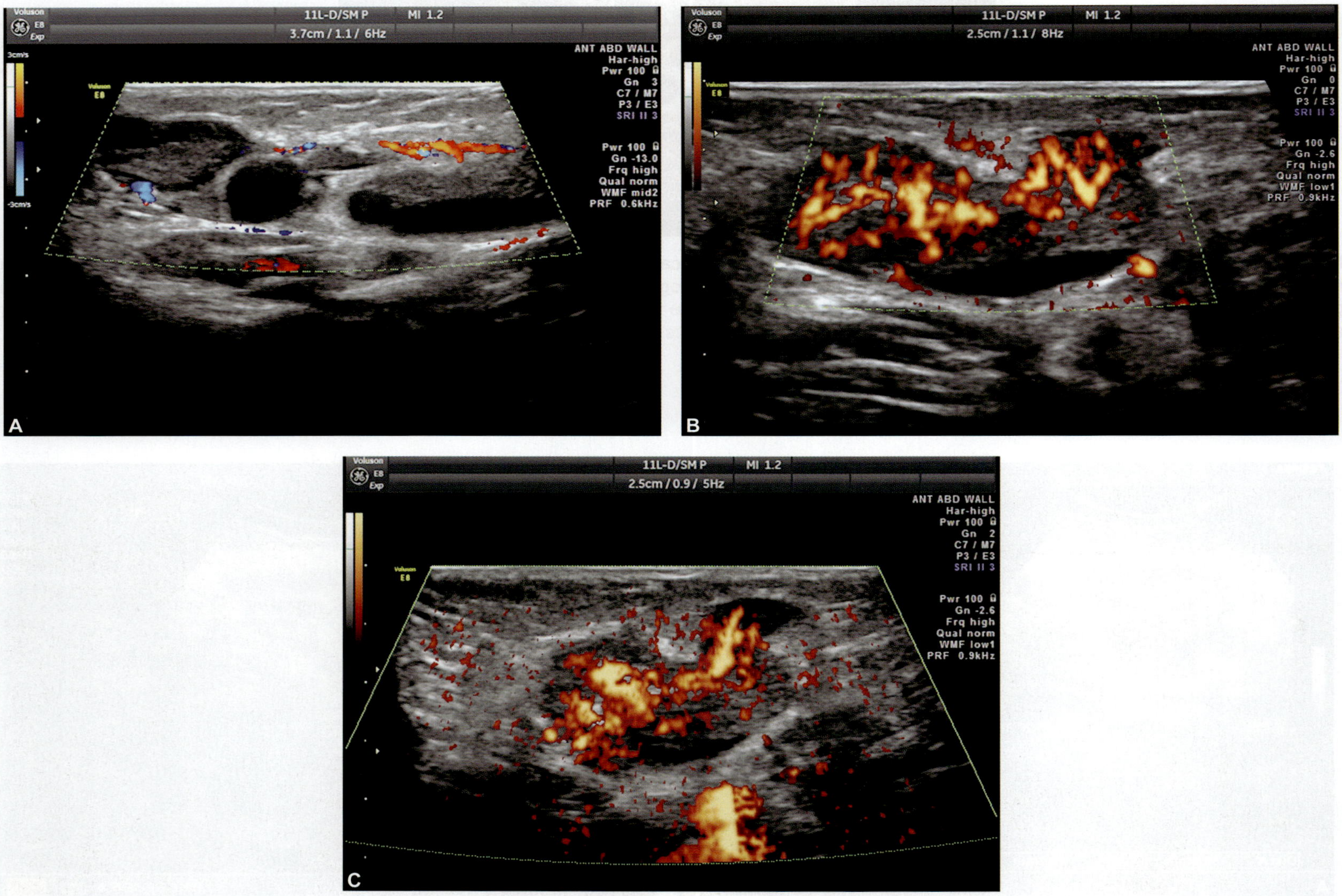

FIGURES 15.72A to C: A 9-year-old girl presented with heterogeneous mass in anterior abdominal wall. The mass is predominantly solid. On color flow imaging, multiple vessels are seen feeding the mass. Multiple enlarged nodes are also seen in retroperitoneum and right paraumbilical region. Biopsy of the mass confirms lymphoma.

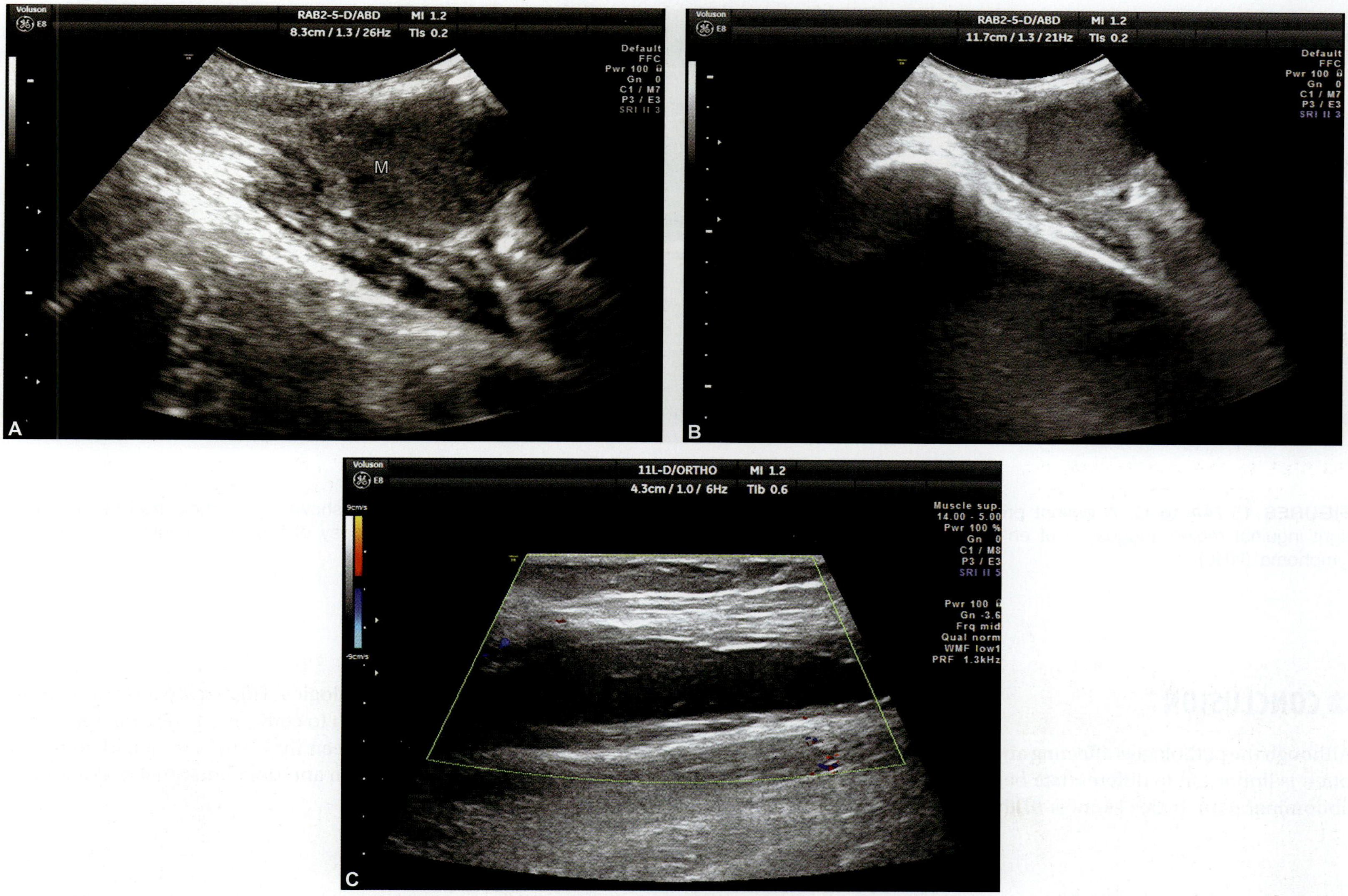

FIGURES 15.73A to C: A known case of sarcoma chest wall muscle presented with soft tissue masses over the left subcostal region. HRSG shows irregular hypoechoic mass in the left subcostal region. There is also evidence of small amount of fluid collection seen in the left subcostal region. Low level echoes are seen in the collection. Biopsy of the mass confirms metastatic deposits.

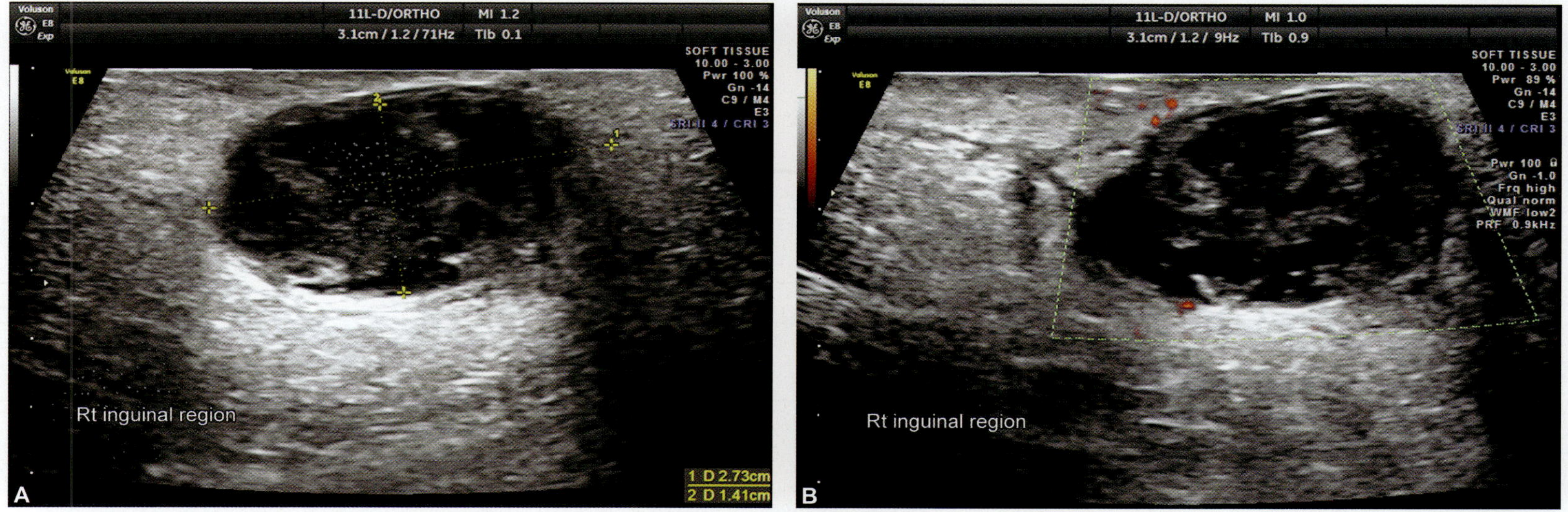

FIGURES 15.74A and B

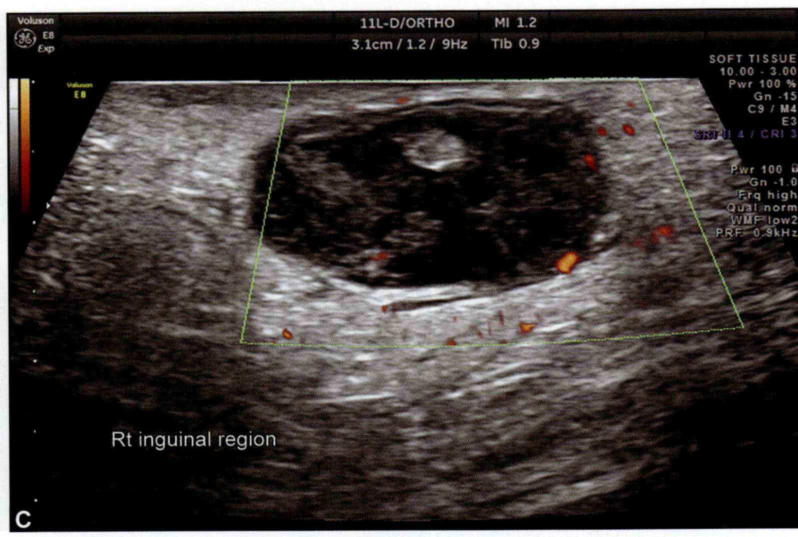

FIGURE 15.74C

FIGURES 15.74A to C: A patient presented with multiple nodular shadows in right inguinal region. HRSG shows hypoechoic nodular masses in right inguinal region suggestive of enlarged lymph nodes. Area of necrosis is seen in the lymph nodes. Biopsy of the mass confirms non-Hodgkin lymphoma (NHL).

CONCLUSION

Although the pathologies affecting anterior abdominal wall are limited, but it is important to differentiate between abdominal wall and intra-abdominal pathologies as most of the time, intra-abdominal masses mimic as abdominal wall pathologies. High-resolution sonography (HRSG) is very good investigation to confirm the localization of mass, its nature and differentiate between intra-abdominal and abdominal mass. It is first line investigation in anterior abdominal wall trauma.

Index

Page numbers followed by *f* refer to figure.

A

Abdomen
- blunt injury 908*f*
- causes of acute 606
- pain in lower 682*f*

Abdominal cavity 508*f*
Abdominal mass, unexplained 742
Abdominal muscle
- anterior 910*f*
- left transverse 915*f*

Abdominal pain, lower 676*f*
Abdominal wall 892
- abscess, anterior 894*f*, 905*f*
- anterior 606, 891, 892, 907, 909*f*, 910*f*, 913*f*, 914, 914*f*, 916*f*, 925, 925*f*, 929*f*, 934*f*-937*f*, 940*f*
- cysticercus, anterior 213*f*, 928*f*
- deep layers of 892
- endometriosis in anterior 904*f*
- hemangioma in anterior 934*f*
- layer of 892
- left anterior 908*f*
- liposarcoma anterior 933*f*
- local venous malformation anterior 928*f*
- multiple
  - lipomas in anterior 926*f*
  - neurofibromas in anterior 931*f*
- right anterior 910*f*
- tissue, anterior 907*f*

Abscess 288, 444, 753*f*, 892
- acute 311*f*
  - pyogenic 267*f*
- anaerobic scrotal 769*f*, 770*f*
- cavity, communication of 892
- cold 303*f*
- collar stud 294*f*, 296*f*, 297*f*, 299*f*, 302*f*
- formation 618*f*
  - suture granuloma with 897*f*
- in prostate, pyogenic 679*f*
- intratesticular 768*f*
- lachrymal sac 170*f*
- localized pyogenic 311*f*
- organized 147*f*, 932*f*
- penile 866*f*
- periorbital 161
- prostatic 661, 678*f*
- pyogenic 371*f*, 472*f*
  - suprasternal 310*f*
- rectal 652*f*
- retrobulbar 146*f*
- scrotal 770*f*
- states of 892
- subdiaphragmatic 512*f*
- supraclavicular 306*f*
- testicular 771*f*

Acoustic shadowing, posterior 563
Adenocarcinoma 159*f*, 599
- follicular 281*f*, 283*f*
- parotid, malignant 402*f*

Adenoma
- anatomical site of 661
- benign 279*f*
- follicular 257, 268*f*, 269*f*
- long axis of 550
- parotid 384*f*
  - benign 384*f*
- pleomorphic 381

Adenomata 550
Adenomatoid tumor 800, 805*f*
Adrenal rest tumors 800
Adrenocorticotrophic hormone 800
Air bronchogram 495
Ambiguous genitalia 839, 840, 849*f*-853*f*
American College of Radiology 564
Anaplastic carcinoma 274
Anechoic cystic mass 777
Anechoic fluid collection 777
Aneurysm brachiocephalic trunk 335*f*
Aneurysmal dilatation 332
Angiolymphoma 359*f*, 360*f*
Anophthalmia 5
- bilateral 8*f*

Anteriovenous malformation 339*f*
Antibioma 311*f*, 599
Appendicitis, acute 606, 610*f*, 611*f*-613*f*
Appendix
- long 612*f*
- perforation of 606
- torsion of 749

Arachnoiditis, basal 428*f*
Arterial flow 749
- assessment of 858

Arterial insufficiency 887*f*
Arteriogenic impotence 859
Arteriovenous fistulae 120
Arteriovenous malformation 187*f*, 462
Artery
- cavernosal 858, 859
- centrifugal 743
- centripetal 743
- cremasteric 742
- dorsal penile 858
- engorged cavernosal 884*f*

Asteroid hylosis 36, 45*f*
Atomach, majority of carcinoma 598
Atresia, duodenal 598
Atrophic thyroiditis 234

B

Basedow's disease 234, 245*f*
Biconvex reflective body 69
Biopsy 686
- gonadal 840
- guidance 655
- of tumor 344
- open 159*f*
- prostatic 686
- rhabdomyosarcoma 155
- ultrasound-guided 564

Bladder infections 750
Bladder neck 655
Bleeding aneurysm 482*f*
Bleeding hematoma 913*f*
Blood
- flow 332
  - in cancers 686
- in muscle sheath 892
- supply 742
  - to scrotum 742
- vessel 742

Body of epididymis 742
Bone 186
Bowel diverticuli 630*f*
Bowel loop 599, 606
- ascaris in 631*f*
- dilated 633*f*
- drain in adjacent 606
- herniation 792*f*

Bowel lymphoma with metastasis 648*f*
Bowel mass, exophytic 647*f*
Bowel pathology 598
Bowel tuberculosis 628*f*, 629*f*
Bowel wall 598
- structure of 598

Bowel, fecaliths in large 641*f*
Brachytherapy 655
Brain
- abscess 445*f*-447*f*, 455*f*, 457
  - multiple 454*f*, 455*f*
- development of 415
- edema 449*f*, 452*f*, 457
- neonatal 410
- neurosonography of neonatal 409
- parenchyma 137*f*, 419*f*, 427*f*, 444, 449*f*
  - thinning of 455*f*
- parenchymal flow, normal 413*f*

Branchial cleft 288
- cyst 314*f*

Branchial cyst, infected 315*f*
Breast 515, 516
- abscess 533*f*, 534*f*
  - diagnosis of 530
  - formation 532*f*
  - lactating 535*f*
  - loculated 549*f*
- accessory 521*f*
- bilateral
  - accessory 520*f*
  - filarial 544*f*
- calcification in 560*f*
- cancer, confirmation of 563
- carcinoma 110*f*, 285*f*, 563, 580*f*, 582*f*

bronchus 514*f*
male 593*f*
nonpalpable 581*f*
chemoreduction of carcinoma 590*f*
comparison of both 516
cyst 550
cystic mass in left 545*f*
cysticercus cyst in 545*f*
detection of carcinoma 563
diffuse
enlargement of glandular tissue in both 528*f*
glandular tissue enlargement of left 525*f*
enlargement
increased left 524*f*
unilateral 522*f*, 525*f*
fibroadenoma in 551*f*, 554*f*
left 551*f*
filarial 543*f*
mass in right 544*f*
galactocele right 536*f*
heterogeneous mass in
left 570*f*
right 576*f*
hypertrophy 522*f*
imaging, reporting and data system 564
implant 594
inflammatory carcinoma 585*f*
irregular
ill-defined nodule in left 566*f*
nodular mass in left 567*f*
nodularity in upper part of right 565*f*
lesion
malignant 563
mammographic suspicion of 564
lipoma 562*f*
lump
for biopsy 564
malignant 550
malignancy 564
malignant mass in 581*f*
mass
benign 550
in left 575*f*
inflammatory 530
mouse 550
normal 517*f*
right 577*f*, 578*f*
ruptured 547*f*
sarcoma 587*f*
sonoappearance of 516
surgery, augmentation 594, 595*f*
tissue 516
tuberculosis 538*f*
tumor, multifocal malignant 574*f*
ultrasonographic appearance of 516
ultrasonography, advantage of 516
unilateral hypertrophy of 523*f*
upper part of 534*f*
varies, normal 516
with fibroadenoma 546*f*

C

Canal hematoma, inguinal 912*f*
Cancer, pathognomonic of 686
Canthus cysticercosis 115*f*
Canthus dermoid, lateral 118*f*
Carotid artery 234
bifurcation 313
Carotid body tumor 323*f*, 324*f*
chemodectomas 313
Cartilage 186
of nose, hypertrophy of 218*f*
Cataract 24
mature 27*f*
post-traumatic 30*f*, 39*f*, 70*f*, 71*f*
surgery 35*f*, 43, 56*f*, 62*f*, 64*f*, 65*f*, 68*f*, 72*f*, 113*f*
traumatic 32*f*
Cataractous lens 71*f*
dislocated 109*f*
Caudothalamic groove, region of 424, 444
Cavernosal artery 883*f*
normal 882*f*
branching of 882*f*
Cavernous hemangioma 86*f*, 124*f*
Cavernous venous malformation 332, 398*f*, 462
Cavum septum pellucidum 415
Cell carcinoma
small 178*f*
transitional 706*f*
Cellulitis 294*f*
Central artery retina thrombosis 123*f*
Central corneal opacity 24*f*
Cerebellar tonsils 415
Cerebellum 410
Cerebral
arteries 414*ff*
cortex 455*f*
hemorrhage 435*f*
Cervical masses 288
Cervical tumors, malignant 344
Cervix metastasis, carcinoma 939*f*
Cervix, carcinoma of 655
Cheek cyst 211*f*
Chest wall 462, 495
abscess 467*f*
anterior 469*f*
anterior 472*f*
cystic hygroma 475*f*
muscle tear 468*f*
Chiari malformation 415
Chilaiditi syndrome 509*f*
Cholesterol crystals 777
Choriocarcinoma 800
Choroid 60, 68, 112*f*, 162
detachment 46*f*
invasion 110*f*
osteoma 112*f*
plexus 416*f*
cyst 416*f*
cyst, small 417*f*, 427*f*
plexus papilloma 424
Choroidal angioma 112*f*
Choroidal calcification 66*f*, 67*f*
Choroidal detachment 60, 61*f*-65*f*
postsurgical 63*f*, 64*f*
post-traumatic 68*f*
Choroidal excavation 107*f*
Choroidal flow 5*f*
Choroidal melanoma 108*f*
Choroidal metastasis 110*f*, 111*f*
carcinoma prostate 114*f*
Choroidal osteoma 112*f*
Choroidal swelling, causes of 60
Chromosome, development of abnormal 840
Chymosis 70*f*, 169*f*
Ciliary artery, posterior 5*f*
Cilliary body 36
melanoma 104*f*, 105*f*
Cingulate gyrus 415
Clitoris, hypertrophy of 853*f*
Coat's disease 20*f*, 21*f*, 47, 56*f*, 89, 93, 97*f*
Cocoon formation 628*f*
Coloboma 16*f*, 17*f*, 98*f*
Colon pseudotumor pattern 598
Colon, acute inflammation of 621*f*
Congenital
adrenal
hyperplasia 800
hypertrophy 852*f*
anomalies 5, 415
benign mass 313
buphthalmos 18*f*
cataract 5, 26*f*-28*f*
bilateral 18*f*
mature 28*f*
cystic eye 8*f*, 12*f*
exophthalmos 5, 13*f*
glaucoma 17*f*
masses 288
ocular tumors 5
orbital cyst 5
retinoblastoma 18*f*, 90*f*
rhabdomyosarcoma 155*f*
Conjunctiva 88*f*, 173*f*
carcinoma 173*f*
Conjunctival cyst 88*f*, 89*f*
Cord cysts, multiple 739*f*, 829*f*, 830*f*
Cord hematocele formation 785*f*
Cord hematoma, fresh 786*f*
Cord varices, left 834*f*, 835*f*
Cornea 84*f*, 88*f*
thickened opaque 26*f*
thickness of 162
Corneal opacification 24
Corneal ulcer 34*f*
Coronal scans 410
Corpora amylacea 658*f*
cause bright reflections 654
Corpora cavernosa 862*f*
dorsal columns of 858
rupture of 873*f*
Corporal tissue 858
Corpus amylacea 671*f*
Corpus callosum, agenesis of 415, 415*f*, 416*f*
Corpus spongiosum, column of 858
Corticosteroid therapy 143
Craniostenosis 13*f*
Cremasteric vein drains 742
Crohn's disease 599
Crouzon's disease 13*f*
Cushing's syndrome 800
Cyst 175*f*, 800
collapsed flattened 117*f*
colloid 258*f*, 260*f*-262*f*
cord 738*f*
daughter 140*f*
enteric duplication 635*f*
epidermoid 804*f*
epididymal 801*f*-803*f*
hydatid 546*f*
intraocular 113*f*
lacrimal ductal 161, 176*f*
lymphatic 319*f*
malignant 403*f*
multiple 11*f*
small 176*f*
of rete testes 746*f*

ovarian 606
porencephalic 430*f*, 449*f*
pseudo pancreatic 598
retention 374*f*, 383*f*
Cystic adenomatoid malformation 504*f*, 506*f*
Cystic degeneration 222*f*, 696*f*
of thalamus 457
Cystic fibrosis 599
Cystic glioma of optic nerve 152*f*
Cystic hygroma 288, 289*f*, 291*f*, 318*f*, 474*f*, 842*f*
anterior chest wall 476*f*
Cystic mass 115*f*, 131*f*, 175*f*, 398*f*, 457, 504*f*, 803*f*
irregular 8*f*
malignant 282*f*
multiloculated 131*f*
Cystic necrosis 550
Cystic swelling 257, 368*f*, 382*f*
Cystic tumors 444
Cystic wall 797*f*
Cysticercosis 119
lateral rectus muscle 136*f*
orbital 134
response of 892
Cysticercus cyst 53*f*, 97*f*, 113*f*, 115*f*-117*f*, 137*f*, 138*f*, 468*f*, 483*f*, 929*f*
ruptured 54*f*
with inflammation 902*f*
Cysticercus infestation 134
Cytomegalovirus 444

D

Dacryops 161
Dandy-Walker cyst 429*f*
Dandy-Walker malformation 415
Dandy-Walker variant 415
Dementia 116*f*
Dense calcified cataract 31*f*
Dense intragel hemorrhage 37*f*, 38*f*, 41*f*-44*f*
Dense peripheral calcification 31*f*
Dermoid cyst 161, 174*f*, 178*f*
of face 216*f*
Desmoid tumor 892, 934*f*-936*f*
Diabetic retinopathy 36
Diaphragm, normal 509*f*
Diktyoma 79, 86*f*, 87*f*
Diplopia 126*f*, 128*f*, 139*f*, 143*f*, 174*f*
Diverticulosis 599
Dorsal vein, deep 881
Drusen body 98*f*
Duct extension 563
Ductal carcinoma 582*f*
Ductal papilloma, small 560*f*
Duodenal mass 646*f*
Duodenal obstruction, causes of 598
Duodenum
inflammatory 607*f*
wall of 598
Dysembryogenetic components 800

E

Echoes, homogeneous 655
Echogenic bands, multiple 498*f*
Ectopic thyroid 237*f*, 238*f*
Edema 60, 444, 563, 749
perifocal 168*f*
Edematous parenchyma 452*f*, 457
Edematous uvea 59*f*
Ejaculatory duct 712, 730*f*
calculus 732*f*-734*f*
normal 661*f*, 713*f*, 732*f*
pathologies 729
small calculi in 735*f*
Embryonal carcinoma 800
Embryonal cell carcinoma 800
Empyema 495
appendix 624*f*
case of 495
pleural effusion of 495
thorax 500*f*
Encephalocele, occipital 419*f*
Endocrine neoplasia, part of multiple 274
Endocrinological syndromes 800
Endometriosis 904*f*
Endophthalmitis 60, 69, 93, 99*f*, 100*f*
Epididymal cyst, big 738*f*
Epididymis 738*f*, 767*f*, 805*f*
abscess 753*f*
in form of enlargement 777
largest portion of 742
lesions of 800
tail of 753*f*
Epididymitis 750
acute 750*f*-752*f*, 755*f*, 759*f*
with funiculitis, chronic 758*f*, 832*f*
Epididymo-orchitis
acute 750, 755*f*, 759*f*-762*f*, 766*f*, 768*f*, 771*f*
bilateral 777*f*
Epithelioma 85*f*
Erectile dysfunction 881, 889*f*
causes of 881
Erectile function of penis
pathological 859
physiological 859
Esophagus, carcinoma 642*f*
Ethmoid, blowout fracture of 68
Ewing's sarcoma 160*f*
of maxilla 228*f*
sternum 489*f*
Ewing's tumor 160*f*
Exophthalmos, bilateral 13*f*, 144*f*
Expulsive choroidal detachment 112*f*, 113*f*
Extraglandular mass 381
Extralobar sequestration 505*f*
Extranodal tumor extension 344
Extraocular muscle 5*f*
Extratesticular
abnormalities 838
collection, chronic 796*f*
Eye 1
agenesis of 5
appearance of 2
bilateral small 12*f*, 95*f*
coloboma of 16*f*, 17*f*, 93, 98*f*
conditions of 93
cross section of 2*f*
kinetic movements of 36
length of 2
posterior segment of 4*f*, 38*f*, 40*f*, 41*f*, 51*f*, 76*f*, 78*f*, 93*f*, 96*f*, 103*f*, 107*f*, 109*f*, 131*f*
quadrant of 69
reflex, white 16*f*, 17*f*, 20*f*, 26*f*, 29*f*, 42*f*, 56*f*, 87*f*, 91*f*, 92*f*, 94*f*, 96*f*-99*f*, 100*f*
segment of 2
small shrunken 100*f*
suspensary ligament tear 69*f*
trauma 68, 71
Eyeball 2*f*
anterior displacement of 119
bilateral agenesis of 6*f*
displacement of 130*f*, 135*f*, 148*f*, 170*f*

F

Face 185
disfigurement of 186
Facial nerve 354*f*
branches of 354*f*
intraglandular portion of 352
pressure of 365*f*
Fascia of aponeurosis 892
Fasciaeo nerve tumor 215*f*
Fascial defects 186
Fascial nerve tumor 326*f*
Fat
extraperitoneal 892
graft 220*f*
necrosis 530, 547*f*, 548*f*
with abscess formation 549*f*
pad graft 222*f*, 224*f*
degeneration 223*f*
Female pseudohermaphroditism 840, 852*f*
Fetal
cataract 3*f*
eyes, normal lens of 3*f*
lung 496*f*
thorax 504*f*, 508*f*
Fetus, large bowel loop obstruction in 633*f*
Fibroadenoma 550, 557*f*
big 552*f*
capsular calcification in 559*f*
dense capsular calcification in 559*f*
dense peripheral calcification in small 558*f*
macrocalcification in 558*f*
multiple 552*f*
Fibroadipose tissue, amount of 516
Fibroblast 840
Fibromuscular stroma, anterior 654
Fibrosis 858
Fibrotic bands 234
Fibrous tissue
consists of dense 654
linear bands of 234
Fine needle aspiration cytology 274, 285*f*, 286*f*, 313, 516, 800, 892
Fluid and inflammatory cells 495
Fluid collection
amount of 606
case of 151
Fluid, pressure of 499*f*
Focal masses 661
Focal retinal detachment 57*f*
Foley's catheter 858, 673*f*
deflation of 655
Follicular adenoma, big 271*f*
Follicular carcinoma 274, 281*f*
Forehead vascular mass 196*f*
Foreign body 892
trauma 74*f*
Fossa cyst, small posterior 415
Fossa, large posterior 415
Fracture 777
of bone, formation of 441*f*
Funiculitis 756*f*, 831*f*
with small hydrocele 757*f*, 831*f*

G

Gallbladder
carcinoma 937f
metastasis, carcinoma 937f
Gas pattern 598
Gastric
atresia, types of 598
band 604f
bezoars 598
diaphragm 598, 603f
tumors, benign 598
Gastrointestinal masses, malignant 642
Gastrointestinal neoplasms 800
Gastrointestinal tract 597, 598
moving roundworm in 631f
obstruction 632
roundworm in 630f
Genital skin, culture of 840
Germ cell
origin 800
tumor 806f, 807f
small 808f
Giant fibroadenoma 556f
with necrosis 542f
Giant lobulated fibroadenoma 556f
Giant retinal tear 55f
Gland
abscess, lachrymal 171f
acute inflammation of 370f
capsule of 661
cysts, lacrimal 175f
diffuse enlargement of 379f
external 655
internal 655
lacrimal 175f
lateral dimensions of 661
parenchyma of 234
remains hypoechoic, inner 661
small shrunken 234
swelling of 370f
tumor 655
lacrimal 161
zonal anatomy of 661
Glandular tissue 654
breaking down of 360
Glans penis, carcinoma of 881f
Glioma 119
Gliosis 454f, 455f
Gliotic cysts 455f
Goiter, multinodular 250f
Gonadal agenesis, pure 853f
Gonadal dysgenesis, mixed 852f
Gonadostromal tumors 800
Granuloma formation, suture 901f
Granuloma, suture 286f, 899f, 900f
Granulomatous disease, chronic 599
Granulomatous wart, chronic 826f
Graves' disease 144f
Gunshot injury 76f
Gut wall 598
Gynecomastia
bilateral 528f
unilateral 526f

H

Haemophilus influenzae 444
Hair follicles 161
Hamartoma 598, 800
Hashimoto's thyroiditis 234, 252f
Head
bending of 120
epididymal 742
Head and neck cancer 343, 349
mass 343
Hemangioma 119, 125, 332, 462
Hemangiomatous mass 342f, 477f
Hematocele 777
chronic 799f
formation, acute torsion with 780f
Hematogeneous metastasis 800
Hematogeneous spread of infection 661
Hematoma 550
age of 892
depth of 892
formation 871f, 911f
in scrotal wall, calcified 821f
inguinal 785f, 912f
intratesticular 777
postsurgical 909f
under resorption 912f
Hematuria, painless 707f, 709f
Hemorrhage 25f, 41f, 43f, 69, 72f, 113f, 332, 425, 777, 800
acute 296f
cause of 36
grades of 425
intragel 31f, 36f-42f, 43, 49f, 102f, 106f, 117f
intraventricular 425, 433, 433f-435f
location of 36
posterior segment 42f
postsurgery 44f
secondary 425
sequelae of 424
severity of 36
subchoroidal 68f, 161f
subependymal 425
subhyloid 40f
subretinal 48f, 50f, 93f
subvitreal 36, 40f, 41f
suggestive of 381
vitreal 41f
vitreous 42f
Hemorrhagic cyst 264f
Hemorrhagic cystic eye 39f
Hemorrhagic degeneration 234
Hemorrhagic epididymitis, traumatic 788f
Hemorrhagic nodule 257
Hemospermia 719f
Hemothorax 495
Hernia 914, 916f
diaphragmatic 504f, 509f, 511f
inguinal 791f, 920f
inguinoscrotal 789f
obstructed 917f
infraumbilical 641f, 918f
omental 793f
ovarian 922f
strangulated 749
umbilical 919f
Heterogeneous
cystic mass 152f
enlarged prostate 695f
mass 160f, 275f, 571f
irregular 692f, 910f
multinodular 513f
nonvascular cystic mass 161
soft tissue mass 108f
texture 313
Hormone therapy 698f
Human face 186
Hydatid cyst 134, 119, 140f, 263f, 313, 331f, 513f
of lung 503f
orbit 139f
peripheral chest 479f
retrobulbar 140f
thyroid 263f
Hydrocele 742, 749, 750, 795f
bilateral 797f
diagnosis of 777
inflammation, causes of 777
inguinal 790f, 792f, 794f
Hydrocephalus 410, 424, 431f, 447f, 448f, 450f, 451f, 455f
associated 415
gross 427f, 428f, 431f
mild 415
production of 424
Hyloid artery 10f
Hyperemia, reactive 749
Hypermature cataract 29f, 31f, 96f
Hyperplasia
multinodular 251f
of transition zones 655
Hyperplastic polyps 598
Hyperplastic primary vitreous, persistent 5, 89, 93
Hypertrophic
primary vitreous, bilateral proliferate 10f
pyloric stenosis 598, 599f
Hypertrophy, diffuse 200f, 662f
Hyphema 24
anterior chamber 25f, 70f
posterior 36
Hypodermis edema 774f
Hypoechoic edematous optic nerve 123f
Hypoechoic fluid collection 777
Hypoechoic mass, irregular 688f, 690f-692f, 696f
ill-defined 693f, 761
Hypoechoic nodular mass 278f, 514f, 576f, 689f, 815f
Hypoechoic nodule 662f, 687f
Hypoechoic solid mass 800
Hypoechoic texture of mass 563
Hypogonadism 881
Hypoplastic cerebellar hemispheres 415
Hypopyon 24

I

Ileocecal tuberculosis 627f
Iliac fossa
left 851f
right 845f
Immunochemotherapy for diseases 801
Impotence
pathological causes of 858
vengeance 859
Infarction 444
periventricular 425
Infection 777
antenatal 444
postnatal 444
Infertility 655
evaluation of 742
patients with 709

Inflammation 563, 742
acute 360, 361*f*
chronic 661
Inflammatory cells 161
Inflammatory disease 599
Inflammatory disorders, acute 750
Inflammatory masses 141, 288
Infraorbital cysticercus 175*f*
Inguinal canal
left 792*f*
right 794*f*
Inguinal collection, right 794*f*
Inguinal hernia
left 917*f*
right side 794*f*
Inguinal region
left 922*f*
right 903*f*
Inguinal swelling
bilateral 921*f*
right 794*f*
Inguinal testes, atrophic 824*f*
Inguinoscrotal hernia, right 792*f*
Injury, penetrating 75*f*
Intercostal muscle 468*f*
tear 464*f*
Intersex disorder 840
Intestinal obstruction, cause of 599
Intestine volvulus, small 640*f*
Intracerebral circulation 444
Intracerebral vessels 444
Intraconal fat 144*f*
Intracranial
hemorrhage 424
infections 444
masses 444
pressure 444
tumor glioma 459*f*
Intraductal carcinoma 578*f*, 583*f*, 584*f*
Intraluminal crystalloid, small 655
Intraocular
cysticercus cyst 93, 113*f*
damage 71
lens 69
tumors 2, 79
Intraparenchymal hemorrhage 425
Intrascrotal masses 838
Intrascrotal vas deferens, normal 746*f*
Intravaginal torsion 749
Intraventricular septa poses, development of 444
Iris cyst 81*f*
Iris mass 82*f*, 85*f*
Ischemia, consequence of 425
Isoechoic mass 800
Isthmus adenoma 168*f*

J

Jejunum with valvulae 598
Jugular vein 234
ectasia, internal 337*f*, 338*f*

K

Keratitis 13*f*, 152*f*
Keratomalcia 16*f*
Kidney 599
Klinefelter syndrome 840*f*

L

Lacrimal duct 161
ductal ectasia of 161, 176*f*
palpebral part of 176*f*
Langerhans cell histiocystosis 154*f*
Larynx
and laryngopharynx, carcinoma of 344
tumor of 344
Leiomyosarcoma 599
Lens
dislocation of 33*f*
hard calcified 30*f*
normal 4*f*
post-trauma dislocated 71*f*
status of 68
subluxation of 71*f*
thickening of 51*f*
traumatic 32*f*
Lesion
nature of 516
orbital 119
status of 892
Leukemia 750
metastatic deposits of 814*f*
Leukemic deposits 155*f*
Leukomalacia, periventricular 424, 425
Leukoria 86*f*
Leydig cell 800
tumor 742
Lid abscess 167*f*, 168*f*
Lid
abscess, upper 169*f*
bilateral swelling of 172*f*
carcinoma of 161
lower 181*f*
squamous carcinoma of 179*f*
swelling, painful 169*f*
tumors 161
Limbal mass 83*f*, 84*f*
Lip 186
Lipoma 313, 925*f*
of corpus callosum 415
scrotum 826*f*
Liver 495
reflection of 462
Lobar holoprosencephaly 424*f*
Longus colli muscle posteriorly 274
Lows Ley's classification 654
Ludwig angina 305*f*
Lumbosacral meningocele 420*f*
Lumbosacral meningomyelocele 423*f*
Lung 599
collapse of 495
collapsed portion of 495
mass, peripheral 503*f*
parenchyma 495
Lymph edema, causes of 800
Lymph node 313, 343, 344, 858
chains of 343
disease, primary 313
enlargement 344
malignant enlarged 347*f*
mass 288, 313, 343
metastasis 274
of neck 343
reflectivity of 343
shape 344
sinus 344
size 344
Lymphadenitis, nonspecific 313
Lymphangioma 119, 120, 131*f*, 205*f*, 207*f*, 320*f*, 341*f*
neck 290*f*
Lymphatic
dilated 837*f*
leukemia, acute 111*f*, 155*f*, 161*f*
vessel 742
Lymphoid tumor 156*f*
Lymphoma 119, 345, 495, 599, 742, 750
bilateral orbital 183*f*
orbital 156*f*
testes 816*f*, 817*f*
Lymphoproliferative masses 119

M

Macrophthalmos 5
Macular degeneration 36
Male breast carcinoma 591*f*, 592*f*
Male infertility
cause of 827
evaluation of 712, 742
with azoospermia 718*f*
with oligospermia 714*f*
Male pseudohermaphroditism 840, 845*f*, 848*f*-851
Mass 183
appendiceal 606
heterogeneous 777
nodular 699*f*
intermedia 415
large size of 313
lesions, extratesticular 742
malignant 403*f*
nature of 344
mobile 332
mobility of 550
nature of 161, 332, 892
palpable 516
penile 874*f*
periorbital 161
Masseter muscle
cysticercus cyst 214*f*
hypertrophy 217*f*
tumors of 227*f*
Mastitis, acute 531*f*
Mebobian cell tumor 172*f*
Meckel's diverticulum, obstructed 619*f*
Mediastinum testes, normal 744*f*
Medullary carcinoma 274
thyroid 348*f*
Medulloepithelioma 79
Meibomian cells 161
Melanoma 2, 102*f*, 107*f*, 109, 109*f*, 111*f*, 112*f*, 800
collar button 102*f*, 104*f*
discoid 100*f*, 101*f*
Meningioma 119, 150
Meningitis 444, 449*f*
hydrocephalus 450*f*
pyogenic 450*f*
Meningocele 420*f*
anterior 418*f*
occipital 417*f*
sacral 420*f*, 421*f*
Mesenchymal origin 800
Metastatic deposits in testes 815*f*
Metastatic disease 800
evaluation of 742, 838

Metastatic lesions 892
Metastatic lymph node disease, detection of 344
Metastatic tumors 495
Microabscess 360
Microphthalmos 5, 13*f*
Micturating urethrogram 869*f*
Milk during pregnancy, secretion of 516
Miosis 24
Mucocele 161
    appendix 616*f*
Mucoepidermoid carcinoma 161
Mucoid degeneration 368*f*
Mucoproteins, globules of 98*f*
Mucoviscidosis 634*f*
Multiple cystic encephalomalacia 444
Muscle 892, 910*f*
    atrophy of 313
    bundles 892
    fibers 908*f*
    of face 186
    of proximal urethra 654
    smooth 654
    tear 911*f*
    tumors 892
Myositis 141*f*

N

Natural human reproduction 858
Neck 287
    abscess 293*f*, 294*f*
    anterior
        part of 234, 257
        triangle of 288
    malignant masses 343
    masses 288, 349
        benign 313
    posterior triangle of 288
    spindle cell carcinoma of 407*f*
    trauma 342
    tuberculosis 303*f*
    vessels 288, 313
Necrotic nodal mass, caseating 932*f*
Necrotizing colitis, acute 623*f*
Neoplasm
    follicular 274
    malignant 274
Nerve
    calcification 150*f*
    tumors of 288, 313
Neural tube
    closure, disorders of 415
    disorders of 415
Neurilemmoma 151
Neuritis 149*f*
Neuroblastoma 157*f*
    metastasis, primary 158*f*
Neurocysticercosis 137*f*
Neurofibroma 172*f*, 800
    lid 162*f*
    occiput 330*f*
Nipple
    papilloma at 550*f*
    retracted 518*f*
Node, central part of 344
Nodular hyperplasia 234
Nodular mass
    complex 265*f*
    multiple 700*f*
Non-follicular adenomas 257
Non-germ cell tumor 800
Non-Hodgkin lymphoma 300*f*, 301*f*
    metastasis of 159*f*
Nonrhegmatogeneous retinal detachment 47
Nonseminomatous germ cell tumors 800
Nucleus, calcification of 27*f*

O

Occult testicular neoplasm 742
Ocular
    cysticercosis 115*f*
    melanoma 100, 106*f*, 113*f*
    muscles 2
        hypotoni of 60
    tumors 79
Oligospermia 722*f*, 729*f*
Opaque corneal membrane 14*f*
Opaque hemithorax, case of 495
Opaque lens, thickened 28*f*
Opaque ocular media 24
Opaque, cause of 36
Ophthalmic vein 121*f*
    dilated superior 119
    superior 121*f*, 122*f*
    thrombosis, superior 122*f*
Ophthalmoscopy 98*f*
Optic nerve 2*f*, 4*f*, 5*f*, 59*f*, 93*f*, 126*f*, 149*f*, 150*f*, 152*f*, 153*f*, 183*f*
    cyst 119
    diffuse edema of 149*f*
    edema 149*f*
    glioma 119, 150
    head 50*f*, 100*f*, 116*f*
        calcification of 98*f*
    meningioma 152*f*
    tumors of 151, 153*f*
Optic neuritis 151
Orbit 1, 119
    intraconal part of 121*f*, 126*f*
Orchitis 750
Organogenesis, disorders of 415
Osteomyelitis 462
Osteosarcoma 160*f*
    of tibia 160*f*
    tibia, metastatic deposits 160*f*

P

Paget's disease 565*f*
Pain in left scrotum, acute 759*f*
Pain, acute 113*f*, 116*f*, 749
Palpable tender swelling 892
Palpebral fissure, small 6*f*, 8*f*
Pancreas, annular 598
Papaverine injection 858
Papillary adenocarcinoma 278*f*
    thyroid 278*f*
Papillary carcinoma 274, 278*f*, 279*f*
    invasive 276*f*
    occult 277*f*
    thyroid, invasive non-palpable 278*f*
Papilloma
    ductal 561*f*, 562*f*
    multiple 708*f*
Papillomata 550
Parapharyngeal malignant mass 346*f*
Parasitic cyst 462
Parasitic infestation 119, 186, 331, 892
    of orbit 134
    retrobulbar 134
Parathyroid
    adenoma 272*f*, 273*f*, 322*f*
    gland 288
Paraumbilical hernia 915*f*, 918*f*
Parietal abscess 453*f*
    in right iliac fossa 620*f*, 906*f*
Parietal bone
    fracture 438*f*
    hematoma 437*f*
Parietal cyst 446*f*
Parietal hematoma 909*f*
Parotid abscess 215*f*, 365*f*, 367*f*
    subacute 364*f*
Parotid chain 343
Parotid cyst, simple 382*f*
Parotid duct 366*f*
Parotid gland 353*f*-355*f*, 361*f*, 367*f*-369*f*, 374*f*, 375*f*, 382*f*, 383*f*, 386*f*, 387*f*, 393*f*, 398*f*, 405*f*
    acute inflammation of 360, 362*f*
    normal 355*f*
    tumors of 381
Parotid mass 405*f*
    detection of 381
Parotitis, acute 363*f*
    narcotizing 364*f*
Pelvis 827
Penile carcinoma 858
Penile edema 772*f*
Penile erectile dysfunction, assessment of 858
Penile filariasis 868*f*
Penile shaft, distal part of 878*f*, 879*f*
Penile urethra, assessment of 858
Penis
    carcinoma of 858, 879*f*
    distal part of 858
    dorsal vein of 861*f*
    filarial 80*f*
    fracture 871*f*
    glans of 879*f*
    root of 865*f*
    small 855*f*
        rudimentary 854*f*
    trauma 870*f*
Peptic ulcer, perforated 606
Perineal pain 674*f*
    acute 678*f*
    and fever 678*f*
Periprostatic
    fluid collection 702*f*
    vessels, multiple 658*f*
Peristalsis 598
Periurethral glands 656*f*
Periurethral glandular tissue 661
Peyronie's disease 858, 861*f*, 865*f*
Photophobia 96*f*
Phyllodes tumor 589*f*
Plaque
    calcified 858, 862*f*
    dense calcified 865*f*
    number of 858
    surgical removal of 858
Porencephalic cyst
    formation of 425
    post meningitis 451*f*
Postmenopausal breast 530*f*

Post-surgery scrotal abscess 767*f*
Potato tumor 323*f*
Pregnancy, ectopic tubal 606
Proliferative gynecomastia 529*f*
Proliferative vitreoretinopathy 44*f*, 47, 68
Proptosis 119, 121*f*, 122*f*, 124*f*, 125*f*, 139*f*, 143*f*, 145*f*, 152*f*-154*f*
  bilateral 148*f*, 183*f*
    orbital 145*f*
  causes of 119
Prostate
  abnormal 655
  abscess in left lobe of 679*f*
  adenocarcinoma 696*f*
  apex of 654
  base of 655
  cancer of 655, 686
  cancer
    resembling 661
    staging of 655
  carcinoma of 114*f*, 685, 698*f*
  color Doppler of 686
  enlarged 692*f*
  gland
    biopsies of 686
    diffuse enlargement of 662*f*, 664*f*, 665*f*, 670*f*
    edematous hypoechoic 676*f*
    heterogeneous 696*f*
    normal 655, 656*f*
  heterogeneous mass in 695*f*
  hyperplasia 685
  internal texture of 655
  invasive adenocarcinoma of 698*f*, 699*f*
  lobes of 662*f*
  peripheral zone of 685
  sarcoidosis 668*f*
  soft enlargement of 661
  specific antigen 685, 686
    age-related 686
    density 686
    velocity 686
  transrectal ultrasound 731*f*
  zonal anatomy of 654
Prostatic abscess
  big 680*f*, 684*f*
  multiple 681*f*, 682*f*
Prostatic calcifications 654
Prostatic cancer
  diagnosis of 654, 685
  evaluation of 686
Prostatic carcinoma 800
Prostatic disease, diagnosis of 654
Prostatic disorders 654
Prostatic ellipse 685
Prostatic enlargement, benign 673*f*
Prostatic hypertrophy, benign 661, 663*f*, 686
Prostatic infarct 686
Prostatic inflammation 655, 686
Prostatic malignancy, diagnosis of 686
Prostatic sphincter, internal 654
Prostatic tunnel after turp 671*f*
Prostatic varices 675*f*, 739*f*
Prostatitis 661, 750
  acute 674*f*, 676*f*, 677*f*
  chronic 661, 662
Pseudokidney sign 598, 648*f*
Pseudoproptosis 119, 148*f*
Pseudotumor 143*f*, 161
  inflammatory orbital disease 119
  orbit 143*f*
Pubic crest 892
  insert in 892
Pubis bone 654
Pupil, lesions of 36
Pus collection 613*f*
Pyloric canal
  length of 598
  normal 604*f*
Pyloric muscle 598, 601*f*
  hypertrophy, gross 600*f*
Pyloric spasm 602*f*, 632*f*
Pyloric stenosis 601*f*
Pyoceles 777
Pyogenic ventriculitis 448*f*, 449*f*
Pyoophthalmos 46*f*, 68
Pyospermia 723*f*
Pyothorax 497*f*

R

Rectal examination
  digital 654
  post digital 686
Recti muscles, normal 142*f*
Rectus abdominis muscle
  left 908*f*
  tear in 908*f*
Rectus cysticercosis, lateral 137*f*
Rectus cysticercus
  cyst, superior 135*f*
  superior 136*f*
Rectus muscle
  enlargement, bilateral 158*f*
  lateral 143*f*
  medial 141*f*
  myositis of superior 142*f*, 143*f*
  superior 136*f*, 142*f*, 143*f*
Rectus sheath hematoma 908*f*
Refractive media 2
Renal
  carcinoma 800
  vein thrombosis, left 827
  vein, left 827
Reticuloendotheliosis 158*f*
Retina 36, 47, 96*f*, 105*f*, 162
  artery of 2
  central artery of 5*f*
  detachment of surrounding 68
  pathology of 47
  posterior surface of 89
  surface of 89
Retinal artery 21*f*
Retinal buckle 58*f*
  applications 57*f*
Retinal cyst 54*f*
  formation 12*f*, 55*f*
  multiple 54*f*
Retinal detachment 29*f*, 33*f*, 42*f*, 47, 50*f*, 53*f*, 57*f*, 58*f*, 79*f*, 97*f*, 102*f*, 106*f*, 108f 116*f*
  exudative 21*f*, 47, 89
  partial 48*f*
  postsurgical 56*f*
  tabletop 49*f*
  total 51*f*, 52*f*
  tractional 48*f*, 49*f*
Retinal membranes 117*f*
Retinal tear, chronic 54
Retinoblastoma 2, 89, 90*f*-92*f*, 93, 94*f*, 98*f*
  bilateral 92*f*
  circumference 89
  hallmark of 89
  multifocal 91*f*-93*f*
  retrobulbar extension of 93*f*
Retinochoroid layer 100*f*
Retinoschisis 47*f*
Retrobulbar
  cystic dermoid 140*f*
  cysticercus 135*f*
  fat 2*f*, 12*f*, 145*f*
  hemangioma 131*f*, 134*f*
  hematoma 148*f*
Retrolental fibroplasia 12*f*
Retrolental hyperplasia 5
Retrolental membrane 24
Retromammary layer 516
Retroperitoneal nodes 812*f*
Rhabdomyosarcoma 119
  muscle 155*f*
  of urinary bladder 705*f*
Rhegmatogeneous retinal detachment 47
Rib
  bony tumors of 462
  fracture 911*f*

S

Salivary gland 288, 349, 351, 397
  masses 381
    malignant 399
Sarcoma breast 588*f*
Sarcoma chest wall muscle 941*f*
Scalp
  hematoma 437*f*, 439*f*
  infection 445*f*
  injury 441*f*
  mass 443*f*
  metastasis 443*f*
Schwann cell
  neuromas 326*f*
  proliferation of 151
Sclera 78*f*, 88*f*, 162
Scleral rupture 68
Scolex of parasite 134
Scrotal abscess, left 766*f*
Scrotal collection, chronic 821*f*
Scrotal disorders, acute 742, 838
Scrotal fluid, evaluation of 742
Scrotal infections 750
Scrotal lymph edema 800
Scrotal mass 742, 800
  common 800
  right 819*f*
Scrotal mouse 748*f*
Scrotal pain, acute 750
Scrotal pathology
  acute 749
  diagnosis of 742
  evaluation of 838
Scrotal pearls 822*f*
Scrotal sac 749
Scrotal skin 777, 800
Scrotal sonography 742
Scrotal swelling
  left 817*f*
  right 795*f*
Scrotal wall 749, 750
  cellulitis 774*f*

edema 773*f*
Scrotum 890*f*
cause of
acute 749
enlarged 777
diffuse cellulitis of 772*f*
examination of 742
hyperemia of 749
inner wall of 742
painful swelling in left 754*f*, 765*f*
Sebaceous cyst 470, 825*f*
Seminal vesicle 712, 724*f*, 725*f*, 730*f*
abscess 721*f*
absent 715*f*
right 715*f*
ampulla of 714*f*
calculus
left 727*f*
multiple 727*f*
right 726*f*
congenital anomalies of 712
cyst 717*f*, 719*f*
abnormal 716*f*
right 729*f*
dilated engorged 717*f*
distended 725*f*
engorged 713*f*
evaluation of 709
fossa, right 715*f*
left 715*f*
males consists of 712
mouth of 727*f*
normal 660*f*, 712*f*, 713*f*
ampulla of 714*f*
right 729*f*, 731*f*
small left 715*f*
Seminal vesicular tissue 686
Seminal vesiculitis
bilateral 720*f*
chronic 721*f*
Seminoma testes 811*f*, 812*f*
with distant metastasis 810*f*
with metastasis 810*f*, 812*f*
with multiple metastasis 813*f*
Seminomatous germ cell tumors 800
Sentinel node 355*f*
Septicemia 454*f*
Septo-optic dysplasia 415, 423*f*
Septum pellucidum 423*f*
Sertoli cell 800
Sex development
disorder of 840, 855
types of 840
Sialectasis, chronic 371*f*
Sinus
formation, suture granuloma with 898*f*
tract 898*f*
Sinusitis, distention of 881
Skin
and skin edema 563
thickening 563
Skull, inner table of 424
Soft tissue
edema 774*f*, 868*f*, 895*f*
intraconal mass 183*f*
mass 88*f*, 102*f*, 106*f*, 107*f*, 118*f*, 129*f*, 154*f*, 162*f*, 172*f*-173*f*, 387*f*, 389*f*, 879*f*, 913*f*
in left breast 555*f*
in rectal canal 652*f*
multilobulated 393*f*
of lower lid 173*f*
nodular mass 876*f*
planes 332
swelling 22, 23*f*, 118*f*, 163*f*, 165*f*, 175*f*, 358*f*, 374*f*, 379*f*, 380*f*, 382*f*, 383*f*, 388*f*, 389*f*, 394*f*, 395*f*, 408*f*, 468*f*, 483*f*, 785*f*, 846*f*, 895*f*
painful 910*f*
Solid pleural tumor 462
Sonomammography, advantages of 564
Sperm transport system 711
evaluation of 712, 739
Spermatic cord, axis of 749
Spermatic vein valves 827
Spermatozoa 800
Spigelian hernia 915*f*
Spinal accessory chain 343
Spleen 495
Sponge, layers of 892
Squamous cell carcinoma 181*f*
Staphyloma 148*f*
anterior 5, 14*f*, 80*f*, 81*f*
posterior 148*f*
Sternocleidomastoid muscle
anterior margins of 288
border 288
Sternocleidomastoid tumor 290*f*, 291*f*
Stomach 598
thickening of 598
tumors of 598
wall 598
Subcutaneous fat 892
Subcutaneous layer 516
Subcutaneous soft tissue edema 481*f*
Subdiaphragmatic collection 511*f*
Subdural hematoma, chronic 439*f*
Sublingual
dermoid 288, 320*f*
gland adenoma 392*f*
ranula 304*f*, 395*f*, 396*f*
Submandibular chain 343
Submandibular fossa 394*f*
Submandibular gland 355*f*, 369*f*, 372*f*, 374*f*, 376*f*, 379*f*, 380*f*, 383*f*, 388*f*, 389*f*, 395*f*, 403*f*, 406*f*
abscess 371*f*
calculus 376*f*, 378*f*, 379*f*
cyst 383*f*
fossa 355*f*, 369*f*, 381*f*, 393*f*, 395*f*
inflammation 369*f*
pleomorphic adenoma 391*f*
ranula 393*f*-395*f*
tuberculosis 373*f*
Subvitreal space 36
Swelling, chronic non-tender 369*f*
Symphysis pubis 654

T

Taenia solium 892
Tenon's capsule separates 2
Teratocarcinoma 800
Teratoma 800
disorders 415
Testes 741, 742, 749
absence of palpable 840
acute torsion of left 779*f*
adrenal rest tumors of 800
and cord, mobility of 749
atrophic 827*f*
bilateral
atrophic 822*f*
ectopic 849*f*
chronic torsion of 783*f*
crossed 853*f*
cysts, bilateral rete 747*f*
descent of 892
echogenicity of 742
edematous right 771*f*, 783*f*, 784*f*, 787*f*
enlarged
edematous left 778*f*, 779*f*
heterogeneous right 807*f*
enlargement of 750
evaluation of undescended 742
fracture of 787*f*
hemorrhage in 749
heterogeneous mass in 811*f*
hypoechoic 750
compared to 742
implants, bilateral scrotal 824*f*
infarction of 749
left 761*f*
microlithiasis of 820*f*
neoplasms of 800
normal 743*f*, 744*f*
partial torsion of 779*f*, 782*f*
pole of 742
right 812*f*, 815*f*
rotation of 749
small seminoma 808*f*
supernumerary 749*f*
swollen left 764*f*
teratoma 819*f*
tunica of 800
undescended 742, 892
upper pole of 742
Testicular artery 742
Testicular collection, loculated 796*f*
Testicular contusion 777
Testicular echo texture 800
Testicular flow, normal 745*f*
Testicular hematoma, huge 819*f*
Testicular infarcts 763*f*, 764*f*
Testicular inflammation 749, 750
Testicular involvement 742
Testicular nodules, extra 801
Testicular rupture 777
Testicular swelling, left 817*f*
Testicular torsion 749
neonatal 773*f*
with necrosis 783*f*
Testicular trauma 749, 777
causes of 777
with hematoma formation 788*f*
Testicular tuberculosis, primary 801
Testicular tumors 800
encountered with 777
Testicular vasculitis 749
Thalamic cyst 430*f*
Thalamic gliosis 457
Thoracic cavity 496*f*
Thoracic meningomyelocele 422*f*
Thyroglossal cyst 238*f*, 292*f*
Thyroglossal duct cyst 288, 293*f*
infected 313*f*
Thyroid 233, 278*f*, 288
aberrant 239*f*
adenomas, manifestation of 257

cancer 274
cyst 257, 261*f*
simple 257*f*, 259*f*
diffuse hyperplasia of 234
disease, diffuse 234
dysfunction, chronic 252*f*
enlargement
acute 248*f*
diffuse 247*f*, 249*f*
gland 234
anterior surface of 234
malignant tumors of 274
pathology of 234
imaging 234
invasive adenocarcinoma 284*f*
malignancy, total 274
malignant tumor 274
neoplasms, total 274
nodule
benign 257
solitary 234, 257
normal 236*f*
occult primary carcinoma of 277*f*
true cysts of 257
Thyroiditis 234
acute 240*f*, 241*f*, 242*f*
chronic 234, 253*f*, 256*f*
calcific 256*f*
Thyrotoxicosis 145*f*, 243*f*
acute 244*f*
Tissue
cystic mass, soft 8*f*
necrosis 895*f*
solid 508
Tongue
cysticercus 213*f*
papilloma 198*f*
Tonsil infections 344
Torsion with necrosis, chronic 781*f*
Torsion, chronic 784*f*
Tortuous tubular structure 742
Toxocara 93
infection 96*f*
Transrectal ultrasound plug 655
Transversalis fascia 892
Transversus muscles 892
Trauma 186, 742, 881, 892, 907
blunt 37*f*
penetrating 75*f*, 78*f*
penile 873*f*, 889*f*
posterior segment 68
post-surgical 33, 186
Triorchidism 749*f*
Tubercular abscess 266*f*, 298, 308*f*, 369*f*, 372*f*, 471*f*, 472*f*, 483*f*, 538*f*, 540*f*, 693*f*, 775*f*
chronic 374*f*, 404*f*
left breast 540*f*
with sinus formation 776*f*
Tubercular epididymitis 805*f*, 806*f*
Tubercular paravertebral abscess 312*f*
Tubercular prostatitis 683*f*
Tubercular seminal vesiculitis 728*f*, 729*f*
Tuberculosis 801
of bowel 599
of breast 530
of scrotum 801
penile 867*f*
Tumor 79, 186, 599, 800
benign 288, 313, 495
calcified focus in 567*f*
carcinoid 599
echogenic
pattern of 274
well-defined 313
echogenicity 685
foci, contralateral 685
growth
assess regression of 89
retrobulbar extension of 89
homogeneous echo texture of 800
malignant 288, 344
mass
invasion of 274
multiple 93*f*
neovascularization of 2
neurogenic 325
of anterior chamber 79
oval shape of 800
primary 495
volume, estimation of 685
Tunic albuginea cysts, multiple 799*f*
Tunica albuginea 777, 800
bright 777
calcification in 861*f*, 862*f*, 864*f*
cyst 797*f*
rupture of 870*f*, 872*f*
stretches 859
superior part of 797*f*
tightening of 881
upper part of 797*f*
with calcification, rupture of 872*f*
Tunica vaginalis
layer of 742, 777
thickening of 801
visceral layer of 742
Turner's syndrome 842*f*

U

Urachal cyst 930*f*
Urethra 655, 858
complete stricture of 869*f*
distal part of 858
longest part of 858
part of 858
prostatic 737*f*
part of 713*f*, 858
rupture of 858
spongy 858
structure of 858
traverses, prostatic 654
Urethral meatus 840
distally blocked 858
Urethral sphincter, level of external 858
Urethral stricture, bulbar 869*f*
Urethrography, antegrade 858
Urinary bladder
carcinoma 701*f*, 706*f*
displaces 606
huge mass in 702*f*
mass 703*f*-705*f*
posterior wall of 664*f*
wall
carcinoma 708*f*
invasion 705*f*
Urinary tract, rest of 712
Urine
excretion of 858
retention of 664*f*, 669*f*, 674*f*, 678*f*, 694*f*, 701*f*
Urogenital
diaphragm 654
sinus 840
Utricle cyst 730*f*, 731*f*, 735*f*
calcified 733*f*
in prostate, calcified 731*f*
Uveitis 59*f*, 60*f*

V

Valsalva's maneuver 120, 827
Varicocele 742
causes of 827
evaluation of 742
Varicosed vessels, ligation of 827
Vas deference 712
in transverse plane 660*f*
normal 737*f*, 829*f*
Vascular mass 167*f*, 288, 332, 397, 462
of sclera 79
over anterior chest wall 478*f*
retrobulbar 130*f*
Vascular tumors 119
of orbit 119
Vasculogenic 881
impotence
assessment of 859
types of 858
Vein
canalization, umbilical 927*f*
drainage 749
emissary 859
of Galen 414*f*
aneurysm 444
umbilical 892
Vena cava, inferior 742
Venous
drain, blocked 749
drainage 742
flow 858
leak 887*f*
malformation 886*f*
obliterated 881
stasis 827
Ventricular system 410
Ventriculitis 444, 447*f*-450*f*, 451, 452*f*, 457
Vessels, multiple 110*f*, 164*f*
Viral infection 750
Vision
blurring of 25*f*, 124*f*, 149*f*
gradual loss of 150*f*
loss of 37*f*, 39*f*, 40*f*, 43*f*, 44*f*, 50*f*-52*f*, 55*f*, 56*f*, 62*f*, 64*f*, 66*f*, 68*f*, 75*f*, 76*f*, 78*f*, 86*f*, 102*f*, 106*f*, 108*f*, 112*f*, 113*f*, 153*f*, 155*f*, 159*f*
partial loss of 48*f*, 49*f*
sudden lose of 50*f*, 51*f*, 53*f*, 54*f*, 97*f*, 107*f*, 123*f*, 116*f*, 117*f*, 161*f*
Vitreal band formation 41*f*
Vitreoretinal bands 41*f*, 42*f*, 49*f*
multiple 49*f*
Vitreous body, assessment of 36
Vitreous cavity 87*f*
Vitreous detachment, posterior 36, 38*f*, 39*f*, 41*f*
Vitreous, retraction of 40*f*, 44*f*

W

Worms, bag of 827